# Oxford Textbook of
# Old Age
# Psychiatry

Edited by

## Robin Jacoby
The University of Oxford,
The Warneford Hospital, Oxford, UK

## Catherine Oppenheimer
The Warneford Hospital, Oxford, UK

## Tom Dening
Fulbourn Hospital, Cambridge, UK

## Alan Thomas
The University of Newcastle, Newcastle General Hospital,
Newcastle upon Tyne, UK

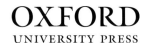
OXFORD
UNIVERSITY PRESS

# OXFORD
### UNIVERSITY PRESS

100538886

Great Clarendon Street, Oxford OX2 6DP

Oxford University Press is a department of the University of Oxford.
It furthers the University's objective of excellence in research, scholarship,
and education by publishing worldwide in

Oxford  New York

Athens  Auckland  Bangkok  Bogotá  Buenos Aires  Calcutta
Cape-Town  Chennai  Dar-es-Salaam  Delhi  Florence  Hong-Kong  Istanbul
Karachi  Kuala-Lumpur  Madrid  Melbourne  Mexico-City  Mumbai
Nairobi  Paris  São-Paulo  Singapore  Taipei  Tokyo  Toronto  Warsaw

with associated companies in  Berlin  Ibadan

Oxford is a registered trade mark of Oxford University Press
in the UK and in certain other countries

Published in the United States
by Oxford University Press Inc., New York

Psychiatry in the Elderly 1e published 1991
Psychiatry in the Elderly 2e published 1997
Psychiatry in the Elderly 3e published 2002

British Library Cataloguing in Publication Data

Data available

Library of Congress Cataloguing in Publication Data

Data available

ISBN 978-0-19-929810-5 (Pbk.)
ISBN 978-0-19-929809-9 (Hbk.)

10 9 8 7 6 5 4 3 2 1

Typeset in Minion
by Cepha Imaging Private Ltd, Bangalore, India
Printed in Great Britain
on acid-free paper by
Ashford Colour Press, Gosport, Hampshire

For our families
with love and gratitude
RJ, CO, TD, AT

# Preface

Although this book is now called *The Oxford Textbook of Old Age Psychiatry* it is in reality the fourth edition of *Psychiatry in the Elderly*. In the second edition we stated that each preface was part of a history of the book, and so we make no excuse for publishing here the prefaces to the first three editions.

When Alison Langton, then commissioning editor for Oxford Medical Books, approached one of us (RJ) in 1987 it was to write a single-author textbook of old age psychiatry to replace the classic one by the late Felix Post. Our response was that, because the speciality was by then well established, the time was ripe for a much larger multi-author book, to which Alison Langton and Oxford University Press (OUP) readily agreed. Clearly, the first edition was enough of a success to cause OUP to request a second, and so it has continued. That the first edition now looks very outdated is witness to the fact that old age psychiatry has continued to develop strongly in many countries.

The International Psychogeriatric Association has become an important forum for old age psychiatrists from all over the world to present their research both at conferences and in their journal, *International Psychogeriatrics*. Other journals, such as *The International Journal of Geriatric Psychiatry*, devoted to old age psychiatry have also developed over the last decade and have acquired respectable impact factors. The profile of Alzheimer's disease both in the scientific community and the world at large has become very strong, thanks to national Alzheimer's disease societies and Alzheimer's International. The personal stories of prominent persons, such as Ronald Reagan and Iris Murdoch, have also brought public attention to the problem of dementia, and have probably helped to attract money and scientific talent into research. The first generation of specific treatments for Alzheimer's disease (AD), the central cholinesterase inhibitors (ChEIs), are well established and university laboratories and pharmaceutical companies are already testing compounds that are designed to attack the pathogenesis rather than just increasing the bioavailability of a neurotransmitter,

as do the ChEIs. The search for modifiable risk factors is also intense, since, if one could delay the onset of AD for say only 5 years by modifying a particular risk factor, the total number of cases would significantly diminish. Dementia is, of course, not the whole of old age psychiatry but it is a large component and one for which there are grounds for considerable scientific optimism.

Where services are concerned, there are fewer reasons to be confident. There is no doubt that services for mentally ill old persons are developing and that research into how to make them better is also advancing. The problem is that resources are scarce in poorer countries, and in the richer ones cuts are being made under the cloak of cost-effectiveness, the result of which seems in the eyes of practitioners and patients alike to result in lower standards of care. Old age psychiatrists and those representing patients have to expend much time and energy in resolving tensions between their desire to improve services and a drive by holders of the purse-strings to restrict expenditure. One of our aims in presenting this book is to ensure that evidence is available to show healthcare managers and governments what is being achieved in our field, and what levels of service need to be provided.

As to the book itself, the basic plan remains unchanged from previous editions. Many new authors have been recruited, but those who have written for us before have all substantially revised their chapters. Most noticeably, we have two new editors, Tom Dening and Alan Thomas, since this is the last edition with which Robin Jacoby and Catherine Oppenheimer will be involved. We are as hopeful that our book will continue to thrive as we are confident that old age psychiatry will develop strongly.

Robin Jacoby, Oxford
Catherine Oppenheimer, Oxford
Tom Dening, Cambridge
Alan Thomas, Newcastle upon Tyne
March 2007

# Preface to the third edition

In the Preface to the second edition of this book we observed that in other books which have run into several editions, reproduction of preceding prefaces constitutes a kind of brief history of their development and the field they portray. With this one our own history continues.

The micro-development level we chronicle is the development of the book itself. We have been keen to introduce new elements and new authors, and to bear the changing needs of our readers in mind, while still preserving the sectional structure (Basic science, Clinical practice, Psychiatric services, and Specific disorders) which lends coherence, we hope, to the range of topics covered in the book. We have dispensed with certain chapters, such as those on nursing and occupational therapy, because these disciplines have developed to such an extent that they now merit their own specialized textbooks. For those subjects that have been retained from edition to edition we have engaged many new authors. This was a policy decision on our part; it is no reflection on our previous authors whose expertise and knowledge were crucial in establishing the book for what it is. Our intention, rather, is to maintain a fresh slant on the various topics, and always to afford opportunities to younger workers in the field. For this reason, we have also curtailed our own roles as contributors. All the chapters by authors who contributed to the second edition have been extensively revised and updated.

The macro-developmental level is the progress of old age psychiatry itself. We hope that this book reflects the development of the specialty over the last 5 years (1997–2001). As the number of old age psychiatrists increases in many countries, including the United Kingdom, the intellectual curiosity of its practitioners and their desire to seek a better deal for their patients also grows; so also does the range of professions involved in the field. This is manifest in the improvement in services and advances in research. Nothing is perfect, but opportunities for patients to be assessed, treated, and supported at home have increased, and more modern and home-like acute units and long-stay facilities have been opened. Better ways of monitoring and teaching improved standards of care of people in such facilities are emerging, and low standards of accommodation and care for sufferers are decreasingly acceptable to professionals, relatives, or the public in general. It is clear that the demand for better care is now louder in the halls of Western governments who, mindful that the increasing numbers of older people are also electors, have begun to pay attention to their voices, to assess unmet need, and to respond with more resources. Since resources go with power, the specialty is gradually finding its legitimate place among other branches of medicine. Old age psychiatry is being permitted to come in from the cold.

On the research front the exciting advances in molecular biology have continued, and much more is known now about the pathogenesis of the dementias, especially, but by no means exclusively, Alzheimer's disease (AD). This area of research has become one in which young scientists are eager to work, for the ultimate prizes are great. Over the past 5 years or so the search for a cure for AD has become passionate, comparable to the search for a cure for cancer. We have also seen the introduction of the central cholinesterase inhibitors, the first specific treatments for AD. As we write, we might have just learnt of one of the greatest advances in treatment for this condition ever made: immunization against Aβ protein. If this proves to be effective, the shadow of AD may really begin to lift. It may of course be a false dawn. What is sure, however, is that neuroscientists will be trying hard to prove wrong those who asserted that the cure for AD will come by serendipity rather than from systematic research. Whoever turns out to be correct, we remain optimistic that something approaching a cure will come within the foreseeable future, and what could be more exciting for our field than that?

*Oxford*　　　　　　　　　　　　　　　　　　　　　　R.J.
November 2001　　　　　　　　　　　　　　　　　　C.O.

# Preface to the second edition

As good a reason as any for updating this book is to document the many advances in the scientific basis of old age psychiatry since the first edition was published. The most striking must surely be those in the molecular biology of dementia, especially Alzheimer's disease. Research in this area is moving at such a pace, it is likely that the time taken to prepare, print and publish this book will see developments too recent to be included. Nevertheless, it is important for *Psychiatry in the elderly* to give the practising old age psychiatrist a review of scientific progress which is as current as publishing technology allows.

One of our first steps in planning this second edition was to conduct a modest readership survey by asking for comments from consultants and senior trainees working in the UK. While it was not possible to implement all their suggestions, we hope that the respondents will recognize their contribution to the finished work. As to specific changes, these fall into four main categories. First, there are the chapters by the same authors on the same subjects as in the first edition. Each of these has been revised and updated; none remains unchanged.

Second, there are reviews of new topics by new authors. Our editorial choice here reflects the advances in the field, such as the molecular biology and molecular genetics of dementia (Chapter 7), or the changed context in which old age psychiatry is practised, for example the economics of long-term care provision (Chapter 23) and the links between medical and social services (Chapter 12). In 1988 when *Psychiatry in the elderly* was first mooted it was still possible for old age psychiatrists in this country to devote most of their energies to clinical work and to ignore the economic and managerial context in which they practised. In the mid- to late-1990s changes in the structure of the National Health Service, competition for resources, budgetary limitations, and legislation such as the Community Care Act 1992, have made it essential for old age psychiatrists to understand and participate in the economic as well as clinical management of services. Clearly, a textbook of old age psychiatry needs to reflect this change.

Third, there are new authors writing on subjects that were covered by others in the first edition. Old age psychiatry has been proud from the outset to encompass clinicians who practise in a wide variety of personal styles, while all are rooted firmly in the same philosophy and basic science. The second edition gave us the opportunity to ask new authors to write on 'old' topics, and so to introduce changes of perspective which reflect this diversity in clinical practice.

The fourth and final category of change is the exclusion of some themes which were dealt with in the first edition. These were descriptions of specific services, teaching, and research. Our first instinct was to have much more on services than in the first edition, in order to include accounts from the many developed and developing countries in which this book has been read. In the end, it became too difficult to draw the line between what should and should not be included. We have therefore narrowed the choice down to a description of the general principles of service provision which can be applied across local and national boundaries. Teaching and research are similarly large areas which are now comprehensively covered in specialist texts. Old age psychiatry has come of age, and research and teaching are part of the culture, as in other branches of medicine or psychiatry, so they need no special mention here.

We have chosen to reprint the preface to the first edition. In other books (on any subject), which have run into several editions, reproduction of preceding prefaces constitutes a kind of brief history of their development and of the field they portray. Without making immodest assumptions about the future we hope that the two prefaces will help our readers to see how *Psychiatry in the elderly* and psychiatry in old age are developing, whilst the underlying aims and design of the book remain the same. To choose a minor example, in the earlier preface (in the heyday of political correctness) we mentioned that our editorial ruling on gender references was non-restrictive to reflect the 'variety that corresponds to life'. We have applied a similar ruling to the second edition, but now, where authors are describing personal interactions (the heart of old age psychiatry), we have sought to avoid the awkward 'they/their' in favour of a *non-exclusive* he, or she, or him, or her.

The final paragraph of the first preface would serve just as well for this one. We hope to remain true to the spirit that informs, stimulates debate, and encourages enquiry. Old age psychiatry has indeed matured since the first edition, but science and practice continue to make such great advances that much remains to be learnt in what is still one of the most rewarding and enjoyable activities which medicine has to offer.

*Oxford*                                                                    R.J.
February 1996                                                          C.O.

# Preface to the first edition

Old age psychiatry has become established as a specialty within its own right. Although many countries now recognize and practise it, Britain was one of the first. Here, the evolution and development were determined by demographic changes, academic advances, and service innovations. Academically there were the landmark studies of Roth, Post, and others. Service provision came in different forms, such as hospital joint assessment units, or domiciliary based services. The particular type of service was often dictated by the geographical nature of the district (urban or rural), and by the resources available, but above all by the drive and enthusiasm of individual practitioners. In 1973 the Royal College of Psychiatrists set up a special interest group, which in 1978 became the Section for the Psychiatry of Old Age. This has acted as a forum for debate and the exchange of ideas, as a channel of communication to the Government and to colleagues in other specialties and disciplines, and as a means of influencing opinion and setting standards. It was the Section of the College which in 1988 facilitated and organized recognition in Britain of old age psychiatry as a specialty, although unofficial recognition had come several years before. It was also prominent members of the Section who helped to ensure the representation of old age psychiatry at international conferences and in the World Psychiatric Association. The formative influence of consumer interests such as the Alzheimer's Disease Association and Age Concern, and of those interested in ethics, health economics, and gerontology should also be acknowledged in the drive to improve standards and focus attention on resource and research priorities.

In the USA interest in old age psychiatry followed that in Britain. The same demographic changes -'the greying of America' - were a powerful motivating force but scientifically the origins were different and emerged more from the basic sciences of gerontology. In the United States, too, old age psychiatry has now become a specialty in its own right. Wherever it is practised, old age psychiatry has overlapping frontiers and works in the closest partnership with other medical specialties and other disciplines, such as social work.

*Pari passu* with the emergence of specialty status and increased service provision there came interesting and important findings from basic scientific research, clinical psychiatry, and therapeutics. The care of the elderly mentally ill ceased to focus exclusively on custodial management, and began to concentrate much more on active intervention in all types of cases, with consequent improvement in prognosis and quality of life. Such has been the importance of discoveries in neuropathology and neurochemistry that there is an increasing need for a good clinical base from which further advances can be made; a need which has been translated into a demand for more resources and more well trained specialists. Clinical training in old age psychiatry is now an integral part of basic postgraduate psychiatric education, and also forms part of the undergraduate curriculum. General practitioners are expected to acquire knowledge and experience in this field. There are also schemes and courses in many countries for higher professional training and for updating practising specialists. It is in the context of a relatively new, but now firmly established, specialty with increasing academic, service, and training needs that this book should find a useful place.

The book can be seen as a two-storey building on prepared foundations. Section I - Basic science, the first of the three main sections, provides the foundations: a broad underpinning from neurochemistry through to sociology. The ground floor, Section II - Clinical practice, deals with the three principal clinical activities: assessment, treatment, and the provision of services. These are covered in detail, and from the different professional viewpoints which make up psychiatry for elderly people. The top floor, Section III - Specific disorders and medico-legal issues, describes the specific disorders with which psychogeriatricians and their colleagues deal every working day: dementia, the functional psychoses, and other less common but no less important conditions.

The book has been written by 43 authors drawn from all the relevant specialties and disciplines. The choice of a large number of contributors was deliberate: reviewers often praise single-author books for their unity of style, but we believe that there is much to be gained from a rich variety of style and perspective. The conjunction of disparate viewpoints is a great strength of old age psychiatry rather than a weakness. One small way in which this is reflected is the editorial ruling on the use of pronouns to refer to women and men (he/she, him/her), or ways of avoiding gender reference (their, person, and so on). We chose not to impose an editorial rule for the simple reason that variety corresponds to life, where staff and patients are of either sex.

We should mention here that there are some points of this book which overlap with each other. This is not a matter of editorial oversight, but a considered decision to permit the reader to view topics from more than one side. Where such overlap occurs, however, we hope the reader will find it complementary rather than repetitive.

An example of this would be the quotation of two different definitions of dementia in Chapter 17. In Section A (Epidemiology of dementia) Cooper quotes the WHO definition, whilst in Section B (Alzheimer's disease) Wilcock and Jacoby cite a Royal College of Physicians' report, each definition serving the points the authors wish to make and neither excluding the other.

Another reason for allowing this sort of overlap is to ensure that each contribution not only fits into the overall plan, but is also self-contained, We have no wish to force the reader into frequent cross-referencing moves a hundred pages forwards or backwards. Of course, appropriate cross-references are still made in the text, but we hope readers will be able to use the book in different ways. Some will follow it systematically from start to finish, whilst others should he able to dip into it to refresh themselves on a particular topic, or to turn to it by way of reference to a specific subject.

Where there are contradictory views, it is for the reader to decide which speaks with greater force. Our view of the reader is of a participant whose needs we have kept in mind at every stage in the composition of the book. We encouraged some contributors to write from personal experience because the body of knowledge in their field is still sparse. Moreover, there are some relatively uncharted areas that are mentioned only in passing and not given the prominence their clinical importance deserves, such as the quality of life in extended care or bereavement in old age. We hope that younger colleagues will feel stimulated in future to explore these areas and extend knowledge for all. Old age psychiatry is a young subject, many aspects of which are not established; some are well defined, but others are much less clear. We want the reader to be critical about what is known and inventive about what remains to be discovered.

We hope that this book will appeal to trainees in psychiatry. Because, however, the field is in its essence multidisciplinary, it should also be of value to a much wider readership. For instance, it may be useful to specialist teams in local area offices of social services departments, to nurses, general practitioners, general psychiatrists, managers, and care staff. We hope that these colleagues will be able to refer to the appropriate section of this book to supplement or refresh their knowledge.

Our authors have been chosen mostly but not exclusively from Britain. Because mental health legislation and the provision of services are essentially determined by national, social and political factors, we have been unable, nor have we wished, to avoid the British context. It simply has to be said that where required, for example with services, we have spelt out the principles on which specific provisions are based; principles which are generally and internationally recognized.

Much work has gone into the preparation of this book. Those who have contributed to it will be rewarded if it succeeds in its purpose of informing all those who read it, stimulating disagreement and enquiry, and enlightening and attracting many to what is a fascinating, worthwhile, and above all enjoyable field of endeavour.

*London and Oxford*  R.J.
December 1990  C.O.

# Brief contents

# Contents

# List of contributors

**Elizabeth Anderson**, University Teacher, Bradford Dementia Group, University of Bradford, Bradford BD5 OBB, UK.

**Eia Asen**, Consultant Psychotherapist, Marlborough Family Service, 38 Marlborough Place, London NW8 0PJ, UK

**Peter J. S. Ashley**, Alzheimer's Society and NHS Electronic Social Care Records Board, London, UK.

**Kathleen Bailey**, Senior Social Work Practitioner, Specialist Team for Older People, Shotover Centre, Oxford OX4 2RA, UK.

**Clive Baldwin**, Senior Lecturer, Bradford Dementia Group, University of Bradford, Bradford BD5 0BB, UK.

**Robert Baldwin**, Consultant Old Age Psychiatrist, Edale House, Manchester Royal Infirmary, Manchester M13 9WL, UK.

**Alan H. Bittles**, Professor of Community Genetics, Centre for Comparative Genomics, Murdoch University, Perth, WA 6150, Australia.

**Bradley F. Boeve**, Associate Professor of Neurology, Department of Neurology, Mayo Clinic, Rochester, Minnesota, USA.

**Walter Pierre Bouman**, Consultant Psychiatrist-Sexologist, University Hospital, Nottingham NG7 2UH, UK.

**Dawn Brooker**, Professor of Dementia Care Practice and Research, Bradford Dementia Group, University of Bradford, Bradford BD5 0BB, UK.

**Fay Brown**, Senior Social Work Practitioner, Specialist Team for Older People, Mount House, Church Green. Witney OX28 6AZ, UK.

**Jennifer Court**, Research Associate in Neurochemistry, Institute for Ageing and Health, Newcastle University, Newcastle upon Tyne NE4 6BE, UK.

**Tom Dening**, Consultant Psychiatrist, Fulbourn Hospital, Cambridge CB1 5EF, UK.

**Vincent Deramecourt**, Neurologist, Centre Hospitalier et Universitaire, EA 2691, Lille, France.

**Seena Fazel**, Clinical Senior Lecturer in Forensic Psychiatry, The Warneford Hospital, Oxford OX3 7JX, UK.

**Hans Förstl**, Professor of Psychiatry and Psychotherapy, Technical University Munich, Klinikum rechts der Isar, D-81675 Munich, Germany.

**Duncan Forsyth**, Consultant Geriatrician, Addenbrooke's Hospital, Cambridge University Hospitals Foundation Trust, Cambridge CB2 2QQ, UK.

**Jane Fossey**, Consultant Clinical Psychologist, The Fulbrook Centre, Churchill Hospital, Oxford OX3 7JU, UK.

**Laura Fratiglioni**, Professor of Neuroepidemiology, Aging Research Center, Karolinska Institutet and the Stockholm Gerontology Research Center, SE-11330 Stockholm, Sweden.

**Jane Garner**, Consultant Psychotherapist, Mental Health Unit, Chase Farm Hospital, Enfield EN2 8JL, UK.

**Andrew Graham**, Consultant Neurologist, Addenbrooke's Hospital, Cambridge CB2 2QQ, UK.

**Helen J. Graham**, Senior Lecturer in General Practice and Primary Care, Kings College London School of Medicine, Sherman Education Centre, Guys Hospital, London SE1 9RT, UK.

**Sarah Harper**, Professor of Gerontology, Director, Oxford Institute of Ageing, University of Oxford, Oxford OX1 3UQ, UK.

**Daniel Harwood**, Honorary Senior Clinical Lecturer, University of Southampton, St Mary's Hospital, Newport PO30 5TG, UK.

**Frank Hentschel**, Professor and Head of the Division of Neuroradiology, Central Institute for Mental Health, Faculty of Clinical Medicine Mannheim, University of Heidelberg, Germany.

**Nathan Herrmann**, Professor of Psychiatry, University of Toronto, Sunnybrook Health Sciences Centre, Toronto, Ontario M4N 3M5, Canada.

**Rolf D. Hirsch**, Professor of Psychogerontology, University of Erlangen-Nürnberg, Rheinische Kliniken Bonn, D-5311 Bonn, Kaiser-Karl-Ring 20, Germany.

**John R. Hodges**, MRC Professor of Behavioural Neurology, University of Cambridge, Addenbrooke's Hospital, Cambridge CB2 2QQ, UK.

**Anna Hoerder-Suabedissen**, Postdoctoral Fellow, The Department of Physiology, Anatomy and Genetics, University of Oxford, South Parks Road, Oxford OX1 3QX, UK.

**Jenny Hogg**, Consultant Geriatrician, Queen Elizabeth Hospital, Gateshead NE9 6SX, UK.

**Tony Holland**, Professor of Learning Disability, University of Cambridge, Douglas House, Cambridge CB2 2AH, UK.

**Clive Holmes**, Professor of Biological Psychiatry, University of Southampton, Memory Assessment and Research Centre, Southampton SO30 3JB, UK.

**John Holmes**, Senior Lecturer in Liaison Psychiatry of Old Age, University of Leeds, Academic Unit of Psychiatry and Behavioural Sciences, 15 Hyde Terrace, Leeds LS2 9LT, UK.

**Gareth Hoskins**, Principal, Gareth Hoskins Architects, Atlantic Chambers, 45 Hope Street, Glasgow G2 6AE, UK.

**Robert Howard**, Professor of Old Age Psychiatry and Psychopathology, King's College London, Institute of Psychiatry, London SE5 8AF, UK.

**Paul Hubbard**, Post-Doctoral Research Fellow, Neuroscience Division, Medical School, University of Birmingham, Birmingham B15 2TT, UK.

**Julian Hughes**, Consultant in Old Age Psychiatry, North Tyneside General Hospital, North Shields NE29 8NH, UK.

**Robin Jacoby**, Professor Emeritus of Old Age Psychiatry, University of Oxford, The Warneford Hospital, Oxford OX3 7JX, UK.

**Ian A. James**, Consultant Clinical Psychologist, Newcastle Challenging Behaviour Service, Newcastle General Hospital, Newcastle upon Tyne NE4 6BE, UK.

**Christoper M. Kipps**, Honorary Consultant Neurologist & Research Associate, University of Cambridge, Addenbrooke's Hospital, Cambridge CB2 2QQ, UK.

**Brian Lawlor**, Professor of Old Age Psychiatry, Trinity College Dublin, St. Patrick's Hospital, James's Street, Dublin 8, Ireland.

**Florence Lebert**, Psychogeriatrician, Centre Hospitalier et Universitaire, EA 2691, Lille, France.

**James Lindesay**, Professor of Psychiatry for the Elderly, University of Leicester, Leicester General Hospital, Leicester LE5 4PW, UK.

**Denzil Lush**, Senior Judge of the Court of Protection, London N19 5SZ, UK.

**Jenny McCleery**, Consultant Psychiatrist, The Fiennes' Centre, Horton Hospital, Banbury, Oxfordshire OX16 9BF, UK.

**Rupert McShane**, Honorary Senior Clinical Lecturer in Psychiatry, University of Oxford, The Warneford Hospital, Oxford OX3 7JX, UK.

**Mary Marshall**, Emeritus Professor, University of Stirling, Department of Applied Social Science, Colin Bell Building, University of Stirling, Stirling FK9 4LA, UK.

**Alisoun Milne**, Senior Lecturer in Social Gerontology, University of Kent, Canterbury CT2 7LZ, UK.

**Zoltán Molnár**, Professor of Developmental Neuroscience, The Department of Physiology, Anatomy and Genetics, University of Oxford, South Parks Road, Oxford OX1 3QX, UK.

**Urs P. Mosimann**, Senior Lecturer in Old Age Psychiatry, Institute for Ageing and Health, Newcastle University, Newcastle upon Tyne NE4 6BE, UK.

**Zsuzsanna Nagy**, University Lecturer, Neuroscience Division, Medical School, University of Birmingham, Birmingham B15 2TT, UK.

**John T. O'Brien**, Professor of Old Age Psychiatry, Institute for Ageing and Health, Newcastle University, Newcastle upon Tyne NE4 6BE, UK.

**Henry O'Connell**, Senior Registrar in Old Age Psychiatry, Department of Old Age Psychiatry, St Camillus' Hospital, Shelbourne Road, Limerick, Ireland.

**Daniel W. O'Connor**, Professor of Old Age Psychiatry, Monash University, Kingston Centre, Cheltenham 3191, Victoria, Australia.

**Desmond O'Neill**, Associate Professor of Medical Gerontology, Trinity College Dublin, Adelaide and Meath Hospital, Dublin 24, Ireland.

**Catherine Oppenheimer**, Consultant Psychiatrist, The Fulbrook Centre, The Churchill Hospital, Oxford OX3 7JU, UK.

**Florence Pasquier**, Professor of Neurology, Centre Hospitalier et Universitaire, EA 2691, Lille, France.

**Jane Pearce**, Consultant Psychiatrist, The Fulbrook Centre, The Churchill Hospital, Oxford OX3 7JU, UK.

**Margaret Ann Piggott**, Research Associate in Neurochemistry, Institute for Ageing and Health, Newcastle University, Newcastle upon Tyne NE4 6BE, UK.

**Harvey D. Posener**, Solicitor, 31/32 Ely Place, London EC1 6TD, UK.

**Martin Prince**, Professor of Epidemiological Psychiatry, King's College London, Institute of Psychiatry, London SE5 8AF, UK.

**Chengxuan Qiu**, Research Scientist in Epidemiology, Aging Research Center, Karolinska Institutet and the Stockholm Gerontology Research Center, SE-11330 Stockholm, Sweden.

**Craig Ritchie**, Senior Clinical Research Fellow, Department of Psychological Medicine, Imperial College London, Charing Cross Campus, London W6 8LN.

**Karen Ritchie**, Director Epidemiology of Pathologies of the Nervous System Research Group, French National Institute of Health and Medical Research (INSERM), Hôpital Val d'Aurelle, Montpellier 34298, France.

**Louise Robinson**, Senior Lecturer in Primary Care, Newcastle University, Newcastle upon Tyne, NE2 4AA, UK.

**Kenneth I. Shulman**, Professor of Psychiatry, University of Toronto, Sunnybrook Health Sciences Centre, Toronto, Ontario M4N 3M5, Canada.

**Robert Stewart**, Clinical Senior Lecturer, King's College London, Institute of Psychiatry, London SE5 8AF, UK.

**Eva von Strauss**, Associate Professor of Caring Sciences, Aging Research Center, Karolinska Institutet and the Stockholm Gerontology Research Center, SE-11330 Stockholm, Sweden.

**Alan Thomas**, Senior Lecturer in Old Age Psychiatry, Institute for Ageing and Health, Newcastle University, Newcastle upon Tyne NE4 6BE, UK.

**Bodo R. Vollhardt**, Senior Psychiatrist, Department of Gerontopsychiatry, Rheinische Kliniken Bonn, D-5311 Bonn, Kaiser-Karl-Ring 20, Germany.

**Gordon Wilcock**, Professor of Clinical Gerontology, University of Oxford, The John Radcliffe Hospital, Oxford OX3 9DU, UK.

**Philip Wilkinson**, Honorary Senior Clinical Lecturer in Psychiatry, University of Oxford, The Warneford Hospital, Oxford OX3 7JX, UK.

**Lorna Wilson**, Senior Social Work Practitioner, Specialist Team for Older People, Calthorpe House, Banbury OX16 8EX, UK.

**Gill Windle**, Centre for Social Policy, Research & Development, University of Wales Bangor LL57 2PX, UK.

**Robert Woods**, Professor of Clinical Psychology of Older People, University of Wales Bangor LL57 2PX, UK.

# SECTION I

# Basic science

# Biological aspects of human ageing

## Alan H. Bittles

## Introduction

The overall goal of this chapter is to review present knowledge of the biological processes that govern human ageing. Almost inevitably, during the last decade the Human Genome Project has had a strong impact on research into the biological aspects of ageing, with DNA analysis now offering major insights into changes in gene expression with advancing age. Nonetheless, a key consideration that still needs to be addressed is the nature of the relationship between ageing and evolution, and whether ageing should be considered as an adaptive or a non-adaptive trait. In other words, did senescence evolve as a direct result of natural selection in order to limit lifespan, or did increases in longevity follow random events which ordinarily would be expected to restrict that lifespan? Although adaptive theories have their attractions, it is non-adaptive hypotheses which primarily regard senescence as an evolutionary by-product that are now favoured (Kirkwood, 2002).

A second basic issue concerns the onset of ageing and, more specifically, its timing. Is ageing in mammals and other genera part of an overall developmental process commencing at conception or birth, or can a specific switch be observed later in life? To a large extent this question echoes the adaptive/non-adaptive conundrum, and although convincing evidence is available for significant changes in gene expression with advancing age, the concept of specific ageing genes and their activation in adulthood appears improbable (Partridge and Gems, 2002).

## Ageing and the human lifespan

The nature of the relationship between ageing and lifespan is of potential importance in biological, clinical, and demographic terms. Although ageing cannot be adequately described merely by lifespan, actuarial study of a population provides valuable insights into the process of ageing, and it is widely accepted that lifespan is a constitutional feature of the phenotype of a species. The plasticity of the human lifespan has been amply demonstrated by the major increases experienced by the populations of virtually all countries during the 20th century, with the Japanese currently the longest-lived national population, with mean life expectancies of 79 and 86 years for males and females, respectively (PRB, 2006).

A formula to describe the exponential rise in death rate between sexual maturity and old age was derived by Gompertz in 1825 and, with the effective decline of extrinsic causes of mortality during the 20th century, evidence in support of an intrinsic mortality schedule has gradually become more obvious. Contrary to Gompertzian prediction, laboratory-based studies on *Drosophila* have shown a flattening in age-specific mortality rates at advanced ages (Carey *et al.*, 1992), which has been interpreted as evidence that the lifespan of this species may not be rigidly defined (Curtsinger *et al.*, 1992). However, further *Drosophila* research showed that reproduction influenced both death rates and mortality in females, suggesting that ageing may have evolved primarily because of the damaging effects of reproduction earlier in life, as opposed to the action of late-acting detrimental mutations (Sgrò and Partridge, 1999). This means that the deceleration in death rates reported in *Drosophila* at greater ages might at least in part reflect waning of the wave of mortality induced by reproduction (Reznick and Ghalambor, 1999).

The maximum reported lifespan of humans is approximately 120 years, and there are conflicting opinions as to whether or not this apparent upper limit is likely to be extended within the foreseeable future (Wilmoth *et al.*, 2000; Olshansky *et al.*, 2001; Oeppen and Vaupel, 2002). Twin studies have indicated that 25–33% of the variance in human longevity is attributable to genetic factors (Herskind *et al.*, 1996; Ljungquist *et al.*, 1998), and a study of centenarians showed that their siblings also had significantly increased life expectancies (Perls *et al.*, 1998). A further example of this phenomenon is the family of Jeanne Calment who died in France in 1997 aged 122 years. Among her 55 immediate relatives whose life histories were studied, 24% lived to over 80 years of age compared with just 2% of a matched control group (Robine and Allard 1998).

Comparable surveys have since been conducted at the population level in Okinawa, an island prefecture of southern Japan that has the largest prevalence of very long-lived individuals in the world, and in The Netherlands which displays a similar mean life expectancy to other high-income European countries. In Okinawa, both the male and female siblings of centenarians experienced approximately half the mortality of birth cohort-matched, non-centenarian siblings (Willcox *et al.*, 2006). The cumulative survival advantages of the Okinawan centenarian sibling cohort increased across the lifespan. By comparison with their matched birth cohorts, female centenarian siblings had a 2.58-fold likelihood, and males siblings a 5.43-fold likelihood, of attaining 90 years. In the Dutch study, the survival of families with at least two long-lived siblings, defined as males aged 89 years or above and females aged 91 years or above, was compared with data from the general Dutch population. The results were calculated in terms of standardized mortality ratios (SMRs) and showed that the siblings of long-lived persons had a mean SMR of 0.66. Similar survival benefits were observed in the parents (SMR = 0.76) and offspring (SMR = 0.65) of the long-lived individuals, whereas the spouses of the long-lived subjects had a mean SMR of 0.95 (Schoenmaker *et al.*, 2006). On the basis of these data the authors concluded that their study sample was 'genetically enriched for extreme longevity'.

Of course the enhanced lifespan of individuals who exhibit above average longevity may be primarily associated with resistance to major life-threatening pathologies. This possibility was demonstrated in a large-scale Japanese survey which found that the risk of mortality from stroke, cardiovascular disease, and all causes was 20–30% lower in men and women whose fathers died at ≥80 years compared with those whose fathers' age at death was <60 years, with a similar picture when their mothers' age at death was ≥85 years, compared with <65 years (Ikeda *et al.*, 2006). However, a conflicting picture often is obtained in such surveys, as in a Finnish study of the relationship between apolipoprotein E (ApoE) genotype and plasma C-reactive protein (CRP) levels in nonagenarians. People with the *APOE* ε4/ε4 genotype had the highest total cholesterol and low-density lipoprotein (LDL) levels and there was a highly significant inverse relationship between ε4 frequency and age. At the same time, ε4ε4 individuals also had the lowest CRP levels, which may explain why some ε4 allele carriers can attain old age despite their increased risk of hypercholesterolaemia (Rontu *et al.*, 2006).

The relationship between ageing and the human lifespan has important practical connotations. For example, in considering future geriatric medical and social support needs, Fries (1980) assumed a maximum human lifespan of approximately 85 years, and on this basis he predicted a future compression of mortality and morbidity in human populations, with most people enjoying robust good health until shortly before their death. If this assumption was correct, no appreciable future increase in the numbers of very old individuals would be expected. In addition, the average period of reduced vigour in the elderly would decrease, a smaller proportion of the total lifespan would be occupied by chronic disease, and there would be an overall reduction in the requirement for health care by older persons. Although the assumption of a maximum lifespan of 85 years is unrealistic, subsequent longitudinal studies have indicated that optimum postponement of disability and compression of morbidity can be achieved by individuals following a healthier lifestyle (Vita *et al.*, 1998; Fries, 2005).

The rapid increases in mean life expectancy enjoyed by the populations of economically developed countries during the 19th and 20th centuries may have peaked (Olshansky *et al.*, 1990; Wilmoth and Horiuchi, 1999), and may even reverse in the near future (Olshansky *et al.*, 2005). But there seems little doubt that in both developed and developing countries the numbers of the oldest old, i.e. persons who are aged 80 years or more, will continue to increase to a significant degree. Indeed, changes of this nature have already been documented for a wide range of countries (Kannisto *et al.*, 1994). Further, while an autopsy study on persons aged 85 years and above reported no diagnosable, fatal pathology in at least 30% of

cases (Kohn, 1982a), with advancing age there is an increasing probability of cumulative physiological dysregulation.

The concept of an 'allostatic load' has been advanced to describe the price paid during the course of one's lifespan in adapting to physical and psychological stresses, with the neuroendocrine, sympathetic nervous, immune and cardiovascular systems, and metabolic pathways all potentially involved (McEwen, 1998, 2002). In health, the actions of biological mediators of stress are beneficial, but their chronic stimulation can result in regulatory imbalance and subsequent pathophysiological changes (McEwen and Wingfield, 2003). Empirical studies utilizing a range of biomarkers based on physical measurements and blood and urine assays have indicated increased physiological dysregulation and functional decline over 70 years of age (Seeman *et al.*, 2001; Seplaki *et al.*, 2006). Therefore, as previously proposed, any increase in the numbers of very old persons can be expected to be accompanied by a disproportionately higher prevalence of individuals with major age-related pathologies (Schneider and Brody, 1983; Brody, 1985).

# Theories of ageing

Theories of ageing usually reflect the scientific background and research interests of their proponents and are best interpreted with this fact in mind. Although the idea of a single 'magic bullet' cause of ageing was initially popular, it quickly became apparent that this was fallacious in complex biological species, and with this recognition earlier organ- and system-based theories (reviewed in Bittles, 1997) were gradually discounted. Just as the ageing phenotype shows marked variation in different members of a species, so there are many influences, both genetic and non-genetic, which interact to produce that phenotype. Through time, observational studies conducted by different groups of researchers coalesced into discrete theories of ageing. The various basic theories advanced have been summarized in two main categories, genome-based and stochastic theories, each subdivided under a number of discrete topic headings (Table 1.1).

## Genome-based theories

As the name indicates, genome-based theories are founded on the postulate that ageing is primarily associated with changes in the

**Table 1.1** Theories of ageing

| Theory | Source |
| --- | --- |
| **Genome-based theories:** | |
| Information transfer | Orgel (1963, 1973), Ly *et al.* (2000) |
| Somatic mutation | Szilard (1959), Curtis and Miller (1971) |
| Epigenetic mechanisms | Holliday (1987), Wojdacz and Hansen (2006) |
| Mitochondrial decline | Linnane *et al.* (1989), Bua *et al.* (2006) |
| Telomere loss | Harley *et al.* (1990), Harley (2005) |
| **Stochastic theories:** | |
| Rate-of-living | Sacher (1976) |
| Waste product accumulation | Fleming *et al.* (1985) |
| Macromolecule cross-linkage | Bjorksten (1968), Kohn (1982b) |
| Post-synthetic modification | Martin *et al.* (1993) |
| Free radical damage | Harman (1956), Gutteridge *et al.* (1986) |

genetic constitution of the organism. The major general theories which were advanced in the past differed in emphasis as to whether ageing was encoded genetically, represented an intrinsic failure in information flow, or was the result of extrinsic damage to the genome. To a large extent, support for genome-based theories was derived from the remarkable constancy in the life expectancy of various species, both mammalian and non-mammalian, and theories proposing a primarily genetic basis for ageing were greatly strengthened by the demonstration that human diploid cells exhibited a finite lifespan when cultured in the laboratory (Hayflick and Moorhead, 1961; Hayflick, 1965). While there are strong evolutionary advantages to species for genetic control of developmental changes from conception to reproductive adulthood, the case for ageing genes is much less convincing, since in the wild few if any species succeed in surviving to reach their maximum lifespan. Studies on *Drosophila* have confirmed that ageing is associated solely with the accumulation of deleterious mutations late in life, with no evidence to support the action of pleiotropic genes exerting beneficial effects early in life but detrimental outcomes in late adulthood (Hughes *et al.*, 2002).

## Information transfer

The ability of an organism to produce functional proteins is dependent on the fidelity of genetic information encoded in the DNA, on unimpaired transcription of this information from DNA to RNA, and on its subsequent translation into peptides and proteins. Each of these processes is subject to error, and during the life-course of an organism the sequence of information transfer steps is continuously operational. Therefore the potential for mistakes is large and would be expected to grow exponentially with increasing chronological age. Since a number of the proteins produced may be involved as surveillance enzymes to maintain the accuracy of the entire system, feedback mechanisms could lead to its collapse, resulting in a phenomenon initially termed error catastrophe (Orgel, 1963, 1973). DNA microarray analysis has shown an age-related down-regulation of genes specifically involved in the $G_2$–M phase of the cell cycle (Ly *et al.*, 2000), interpreted as evidence of increasing mitotic errors in dividing cells during the post-reproductive stage of life. If this is correct, these errors could ultimately result in chromosomal abnormalities and the misregulation of genes centrally involved in the ageing process. More specifically, mutations in the nuclear structural protein lamin A, known to cause the premature ageing syndrome Hutchinson–Gilford progeria, may also be implicated in normal ageing (Scaffidi and Misteli, 2006).

## Somatic mutation

Since DNA specifies the production of peptides and proteins essential for the maintenance of life, it was reasoned that the characteristic physiological decrements associated with ageing could have arisen from accumulated mutations in the nuclear DNA (nDNA) of somatic cells (Szilard, 1959). An inverse correlation was reported between the lifespan of a number of mammalian species and the incidence of chromosome abnormalities with increasing age (Curtis and Miller, 1971). However, rather than being indicative of a causal relationship, these findings could be as readily explicable by the ability of an animal to tolerate DNA damage via the repair of damaged molecules (Hart and Setlow, 1974). As more than 130 human DNA repair genes have been identified, the capacity of cellular DNA to resist attack by endogenous reactive species and environmental agents is considerable (Wood *et al.*, 2001).

## Epigenetic mechanisms

Rather than senescence involving defects in DNA or protein, it has been proposed that epigenetic errors, i.e. errors in the control of gene expression, may be major primary causal factors (Holliday, 1987). Epigenetic modification of promoter regions of genes has been implicated as an important regulatory mechanism of gene expression, with hypermethylation silencing a gene whereas the hypomethylation of previously methylated sequences permits their expression (Wojdacz and Hansen, 2006). The pattern of methylation is established during development and is cell type-specific, and changes in methylation occur both during ageing and in cancer cells. The advantage of this model of ageing over other genetic theories is its lack of requirement for an evolutionary preservation of genes which, in former generations, would seldom have been expressed.

## Mitochondrial decline

A more feasible connection between nDNA and ageing may be via the critical role of the nucleus in the maintenance of mitochondrial structure and function. Mitochondria are the subcellular organelles primarily responsible for aerobic energy production in humans, and throughout animal and insect phyla. The mammalian mitochondrial genome is characterized by its extremely compact organization, with a virtual absence of introns. The 16,569 nucleotides that comprise the human mitochondrial genome encode 13 polypeptides, all of which are constituents of the respiratory chain: subunits I, II, and III of cytochrome *c* oxidase, subunits 6 and 8 of ATPase, cytochrome *b*, and seven subunits of NAD dehydrogenase, along with 2 rRNAs and 22 tRNAs required for synthesis of the polypeptides (Anderson *et al.*, 1981; Chomyn *et al.*, 1986; Tzagoloff and Myers, 1986). Despite the obvious importance of mitochondrial DNA (mtDNA) in mitochondrial propagation and the maintenance of cellular respiration, the majority of proteins involved in the regulation of transcription, translation, and replication of mtDNA are encoded in the nuclear genome, which also encodes 70 subunits of the mitochondrial respiratory chain. The nuclear-encoded precursors of mitochondrial proteins carry specific targeting sequences and are imported into the organelle via a specific, energy-dependent system located in the outer mitochondrial membrane (Voos *et al.*, 1994). This implies the operation of a highly coordinated mechanism for the expression of the nuclear and mitochondrial genomes, with greatest vulnerability in those mitochondrial enzymes which include subunit polypeptides transcribed and translated from both nuclear and mitochondrial loci.

Across species, the mitochondria of old organisms show a decrease in number, an increase in size, and the occurrence of structural abnormalities. These changes are of considerable metabolic significance, given the central role occupied by mitochondria in energy production. Therefore, it is significant that recent studies have demonstrated increased levels of mtDNA deletions in aged human neurons (Bender *et al.*, 2006), heart (Mohamed *et al.*, 2006), and skeletal muscle (Bua *et al.*, 2006).

## Telomere loss

Telomeres are specialized structures critical to the maintenance of DNA stability and replication, located at the terminus of the DNA helix. Telomere synthesis occurs via the action of the enzyme telomerase during early embryonic and fetal development. Thereafter, telomerase activity declines and telomere synthesis is down-regulated in all human somatic cells before birth, but telomerase continues to be expressed in tumour tissue and transformed cells. Following the observation that human diploid fibroblasts in culture exhibit progressive loss of telomeres, it was proposed that telomere length could predict the potential number of divisions achievable by a cell strain in culture (Harley *et al.*, 1990; Harley, 1991). Experiments using vectors encoding the catalytic subunit of human telomerase to induce activity of the enzyme in previously telomerase-negative normal human cell strains showed that the resultant cell clones continued to divide vigorously long after cessation of mitosis in the cells from which they were derived (Bodnar *et al.*, 1998). On the basis of these results, telomere shortening fulfilled the essential criteria for a candidate marker of cellular senescence.

In addition to their apparent role as a biomarker of senescence, telomeres have also been implicated in various chronic disease states. Thus, people with shortened telomeres are at increased risk of dying from disorders such as heart disease, stroke, or infection (Harley, 2005), and shortened telomeres have been reported in women with long-term chronic stress (Epel *et al.*, 2004). Obesity and cigarette smoking, which are associated with oxidative stress and are important risk factors for many age-related diseases, result in increased loss of telomeres (Valdes *et al.*, 2005). Although humans have a common telomere profile found on lymphocytes, amniocytes, and fibroblasts that seems to be preserved throughout life (Graakjaer *et al.*, 2006), the rate of telomere loss with ageing varies between chromosomes (Britt-Compton *et al.*, 2006). There is also evidence that in addition to the common human profile, each person exhibits an individual telomere profile (Graakjaer *et al.*, 2006).

Given the relationship between telomere loss and both ageing and age-related pathologies, pharmacological activation of telomerase has been identified as a possible treatment for chronic or degenerative diseases (Harley, 2005). The reconstitution of telomerase activity in normal human cells by the expression of telomerase reverse transcriptase (hTERT) results in an immortal phenotype. However, DNA microarray analysis showed that the gene expression profiles of these immortalized cells and normal human cells differed significantly (Lindvall *et al.*, 2003), and other workers have demonstrated that, after prolonged laboratory cultivation, cells with abnormal cell-cycle control parameters can gradually take over the population (van Waarde-Verhagen *et al.*, 2006). If these findings are confirmed, attempts to restore telomere length therapeutically as a means of promoting longevity could prove counter-productive.

## Non-genetic/stochastic theories

Theories in this category are based on the assumption that cumulative minor, adverse random changes occur through time which ultimately overwhelm the capacity of an organism to survive, with ageing representing the preceding period of functional decline. The mechanisms which have been advanced can be categorized under five headings.

### Rate of living

Initial evidence for the rate of living theory came from the observation that in a variety of species, including *Drosophila* and rotifers, optimum lifespan was achieved when the organisms were maintained at suboptimal temperatures. As there is a general correlation between temperature and reaction rates, it was reasoned that the abbreviated lifespan observed at higher temperatures reflected the adverse effects of faster rates of living, presumably associated with energy expenditure.

A clear inverse relationship between basal metabolic rate and longevity was demonstrated in mammals (Sacher, 1976), and taken as corroborative evidence of lifespan being governed by the rate of living of the particular species. Unfortunately, theories of this type tend to be imprecise in defining the nature of the salient factor(s) controlling ageing and lifespan, although it has been proposed that the rate of living theory could be re-formulated as a stress theory of ageing (Parsons, 1995). According to this modified theory, resistance to external stress is the primary inherited trait that determines lifespan, and organisms which have evolved to a more stress-resistant genotype exhibit the greatest longevity.

### Waste product accumulation

Ageing has been ascribed to the accumulation of waste products within cells, on the assumption that these products interfere with normal cellular metabolism and function in a mainly non-specific manner. Ultimately, this results in dysfunction and death at cellular and organ levels. The molecule that has been principally implicated in accumulation theories is lipofuscin, a highly insoluble, pigmented compound present with advancing age in the cells of many mammalian tissues, including neurons, cardiac muscle fibres, and the adrenal cortex. Lipofuscin is believed to be derived by auto-oxidation from incompletely degraded cellular materials, in particular the lipid component of cell mitochondrial membranes (Fleming *et al.*, 1985). As such it appears probable that the build-up of lipofuscin, which has not been demonstrated to critically affect cell function, may be secondary to an age-related decline in the function of cellular catabolic processes.

### Macromolecule cross-linkage

With increasing chronological age many macromolecules of biological importance gradually develop cross-links, either covalent in nature or via hydrogen bonding. The establishment of cross-linkage changes the chemical and physical properties of molecules and, for example, cross-linkage of the extracellular protein collagen has been held to be responsible for the loss of elasticity in mammalian blood vessels and skin with advancing age (Bjorksten, 1968; Kohn, 1982b). Since DNA and RNA are believed to be potential intracellular targets for cross-linking agents, alterations in their structure could have serious functional implications for cellular information flow.

### Post-synthetic modification

The existence of cross-linkage in older organisms is indisputable, and the resultant molecular aggregation and immobilization predictably could compromise cellular metabolism and function. Similar end-effects could follow the post-synthetic modification of proteins, with non-enzymic glycosylation (glycation) being a potentially important example that has been associated with ageing. Glycation results from the initial reaction of glucose with the amino group of lysine residues, which then proceed to form a Schiff base and progressively more complex compounds termed advanced glycosylation end (AGE) products (Martin *et al.*, 1993).

In effect, cross-linkage or any modification of proteins that leads to decreased proteolysis could be considered a specific form of accumulation but, as with general accumulation theories, the extent to which abnormal proteins accumulate is uncertain. Progressive age-related increases in cross-linkage have been observed in collagen, which is subject to turnover throughout life (Schnider and Kohn, 1981). By contrast, little change was reported in the level of glycation in lens crystallin proteins obtained from subjects aged between 10 and 80 years (Patrick *et al.*, 1990). Thus, in common with the majority of ageing theories, cross-linkage and post-synthetic mechanisms primarily appear to represent examples of a cause versus effect debate.

### Free radical damage

Oxidative damage initiated by the action of highly reactive free radicals was first proposed as a significant factor in ageing by Harman (1956). A number of reactive species are derived from molecular oxygen, including the superoxide and hydroperoxyl radicals, hydrogen peroxide, hydroxyl radical, and singlet oxygen. Polyunsaturated fatty acid side chains of cell and organelle membranes serve as highly susceptible targets for the action of oxygen radicals, with the lipids undergoing a chain reaction, known as lipid peroxidation, that may result in severe damage and the eventual death of the cell (Gutteridge *et al.*, 1986). It also has been proposed that DNA may be the critical target molecule for free radical damage, with mtDNA especially susceptible (Hudson *et al.* 1998) because of its proximity to the site of free radical production in the inner mitochondrial membrane (Frisard and Ravussin, 2006).

Lesser concentrations of free radicals also are formed during phagocytosis, in prostaglandin synthesis, and in the cytochrome P-450 system, and non-enzymatic reactions of oxygen with organic compounds provide a further minor source (Harman, 1986). It has, however, been suggested that only terminally differentiated cells, such as those of the brain, heart, and muscle are severely affected, since in fast-replicating cells frequent turnover of macromolecules can take place during mitochondrial division at mitosis. Support for this idea is provided by marked age-dependent increases in oxidative damage to mtDNA, and to a lesser extent nDNA, in human brain (Mecocci *et al.*, 1993), and there also is an age-associated decline in respiratory chain function in skeletal muscle (Trounce *et al.*, 1989; Boffoli *et al.*, 1994; Hsieh *et al.*, 1994).

An inverse correlation has been demonstrated between the longevity of mammalian species and rates of peroxidation, at least partially determined by the antioxidant defences utilized by each species (Cutler, 1985, Ku *et al.*, 1993). In humans a wide variety of antioxidants have been identified including ascorbate, α-tocopherol, β-carotene, glutathione, and the enzymes superoxide dismutase, peroxidase, and catalase. There has been little evidence that these antioxidants produce a significant extension of maximum lifespan, but a series of experiments in the nematode *Caenorhabditis elegans* (*C. elegans*) using small, synthetic superoxide dismutase/catalase mimetics to augment their natural antioxidant systems succeeded in significantly extending both mean and maximum lifespan (Melov *et al.*, 2000). Further work on the same model system has indicated that oxidative damage to neurons may act as a primary determinant of lifespan (Wolkow *et al.*, 2000). Using transgenic mice, over-expression of the enzyme catalase targeted to mitochondria resulted in an approximately 20% extension to both mean and maximum lifespan, with concomitant delays in cardiac pathology and cataract development (Schriner *et al.*, 2005).

Considerable overlap is apparent between many of the theories which have been advanced to explain ageing. Earlier, non-genome theories such as wear and tear, rate of living, accumulation, and cross-linkage are to a large extent phenomenological, and

the observations on which they were based can probably be more convincingly discussed in terms of oxidative damage, which in turn results in the accumulation of modified proteins (Stadtman, 1992).

## The genetics of ageing

### Genetic models of life expectancy

The main rationale behind the genetic study of ageing is species-specific variation in maximum lifespan potential, which suggests that there are underlying differences in the genetic constitution of species controlling the rate of ageing. Although, as noted earlier, the nature of the relationship between ageing and lifespan requires qualification.

Initial attempts to specify the number of genes involved in the increase in maximum lifespan potential that accompanied the evolution of *Homo sapiens* were based on rates of amino acid substitution in proteins, an approach which yielded estimates of between 70 and 240 genes (Sacher, 1975; Cutler, 1975). Subsequent studies on evolutionary changes in lifespan assumed the involvement of chromosomal rearrangements at a large number of gene loci, rather than the point mutations on which the first estimates were based. By enumeration of the genetic variants associated with development of the senescent phenotype, it has been calculated that while approximately 1000 genes are implicated in regulating features of ageing, up to 6900 genes might be involved peripherally in the overall ageing phenotype (Martin, 1989). As the human genome has been shown to comprise some 30,000 genes, if these estimates are realistic they would imply that over 20% of the genome was involved in some aspect of ageing or lifespan control.

Much of the more recent work on the genetic control of lifespan has been based on species such as *C. elegans*, *Drosophila*, and *Saccharomyces* which have a short natural lifespan, with the aim of isolating strains that exhibit an extended lifespan and identifying the specific mutations associated with this lifespan expansion. In *C. elegans* it was shown that mutation of the *age-1* gene resulted in significant lifespan extension, in combination with thermotolerance (Lithgow *et al.*, 1994) and resistance to oxidative damage (Larsen, 1993). A doubling of lifespan was achieved in *C. elegans* with a low-activity mutation of the *daf-2* gene, a homologue of insulin and insulin-like growth factor receptors (Lin *et al.*, 1997). The same research group has suggested that lifespan is regulated by germ-line stem cells, through the control of a longevity-promoting steroid hormone (Arantes-Oliviera *et al.*, 2002), while in some cases an increase in the lifespan of *C. elegans* is accompanied by resistance to the growth of lethal germ-line tumours (Pinkston *et al.*, 2006). By comparison, the microRNA *lin-4* gene involved in nematode larval development regulates lifespan in the adult, and over-expression of *lin-4* results in *C. elegans* with an extended lifespan (Boehm and Slack, 2005).

Parallel studies on the appropriately named *methuselah* mutant of the fruit fly *Drosophila melanogaster* exhibited both a 35% increase in mean lifespan and enhanced resistance to various forms of stress, including starvation, high temperature, and free radical damage (Lin *et al.*, 1998). Stress resistance has been reported in other long-lived *Drosophila* mutants, such as *chico* and *InR*, with the implication that homologues of genes active in the insulin/insulin-like growth factor signalling pathway controlling lifespan may be responsible (Clancy *et al.*, 2001; Tatar *et al.*, 2001). The experimental evidence therefore suggests the evolutionary conservation of homologous mechanisms that extend lifespan in *C. elegans* and *Drosophila* (Giannakou *et al.*, 2004). However, it has been emphasized that insulin-like receptor mutants demonstrate dramatically reduced fitness, even in species maintained under favourable laboratory conditions (Jenkins *et al.*, 2004).

### Genetic models of ageing

During the last decade extensive studies based on DNA microarrays have been employed to investigate changes in gene expression that accompany ageing. Initial experiments conducted on over 6000 genes in mouse skeletal muscle showed differential gene expression patterns with ageing, indicative of a marked stress response and lower expression of metabolic and biosynthetic genes (Lee *et al.*, 1999). Subsequent investigations on mouse oocytes (Hamatani *et al.*, 2004) and rat digestive tract tissue (Englander, 2005) showed similar general age-related patterns of gene expression. However, in mouse oocytes the expression of genes involved in chromatin structure, DNA methylation, genome stability, and RNA helicases also altered with ageing, while in the rat digestive tract the magnitude and trend of age-associated changes differed in tissue sampled from the colon and duodenum.

Microarray analysis has now been applied to a wide variety of human tissues, and to cells from various tissues cultured *in vitro*, with arrays of more than 15,000 genes examined. Not surprisingly, increased and decreased gene expression was found in multiple genes in studies of the retina (Yoshida *et al.*, 2002), lens epithelia (Hawse *et al.*, 2004), kidney (Melk *et al.*, 2005), oral keratinocytes (Kang *et al.*, 2003), dermal fibroblasts (Yoon *et al.*, 2004), and sebocytes (Makrantonaki *et al.*, 2006). With such a variety of tissues and different test protocols it is difficult to summarize the results obtained. However, a bioinformatics analysis identified an 'ageing transcriptome', which appeared to be conserved across all mammalian cell types (Wennmalm *et al.*, 2005), comprising deregulation of mitosis, cell adhesion, transport, signal transduction, mitochondrial function, and inflammatory response, and with a reduction in processes dependent on energy metabolism and mitochondrial function. A study based on muscle samples from 81 volunteers aged 16 to 89 years has confirmed the existence of a common ageing signature. Of the 31,948 individual human genes analysed, i.e. representing almost the entire human genome, 250 age-regulated genes and three genetic pathways displayed altered levels of expression in the elderly that correlated both with chronological and physiological age (Zahn *et al.* 2006).

## Methods for the modification of ageing

Inherited factors clearly play a major role in ageing, and in determination of the human lifespan. However, adopting a different stance, if ageing also is stochastic in nature then it should be possible to retard development of the ageing phenotype by altering the relative influence of contributory environmental variables. Although many theories have been proposed and experimentally tested, the only method so far proven to increase maximum lifespan in mammals is dietary restriction, the provision of a diet reduced in total amount but otherwise nutritionally adequate, which to date has been demonstrated in species ranging from yeasts to mammals.

### Ageing and dietary restriction in rodents

The phenomenon of dietary food restriction, also commonly referred to as calorie restriction, was first reported in albino rats (McCay *et al.*, 1935). In these experiments, animals which were chronically underfed from birth remained pre-pubertal as a result of their retarded growth and development (McCay *et al.*, 1939). In more recent food restriction experiments, rodents typically were fed a diet corresponding to approximately 60% of that ingested by *ad libitum* fed controls, commencing either soon after weaning or in young adulthood, with both regimens equally efficacious in increasing maximum lifespan (Yu *et al.*, 1985). Dietary restriction in rodents also retarded the development of tumours and other chronic diseases of late adulthood (Weindruch and Walford, 1982; Holehan and Merry, 1986; Masoro, 1988), and has been shown to offer protection against radiation-induced myeloid leukaemia (Yoshida *et al.*, 1997).

Dietary restriction has been associated with immune theories of ageing, since delayed maturation of the immune system is predicted to result from the general retardation in growth and development of treated animals. Although this may be beneficial to old animals in terms of reduced autoimmunity, it is difficult to comprehend how a delay in the development of full immune competence could be other than detrimental to young animals, especially when reared under natural conditions.

A correlation between food restriction and diminished free radical damage has been claimed, secondary to lower metabolic activity and hence reduced oxygen consumption (Harman, 1986), and dietary restriction has been shown to attenuate age-related increases in rodent skeletal muscle enzyme activities (Luhtala *et al.*, 1994). But long-term food restriction did not result in a sustained reduction in metabolic rate (McCarter *et al.*, 1985), and the addition of antioxidants to the diet of rodents failed to increase maximum lifespan (Harman, 1986). Nevertheless, it has been claimed that adoption of an appropriately nutritious diet supplemented by one or more free radical reaction inhibitors would increase mean life expectancy at birth by 5 or more years (Harman, 1992).

More direct DNA microarray studies on the effects of caloric restriction in retarding mammalian ageing showed that by comparison with control mice, the transcriptional patterns of calorie-restricted animals indicated a metabolic shift towards increased protein turnover and decreased macromolecular damage (Lee *et al.*, 1999). Later skeletal muscle studies on rats maintained on a restricted diet (representing 60% of the control diet) for 36 weeks indicated increased transcription of genes involved in reactive free oxygen scavenging, tissue development, and energy metabolism, with decreased expression of genes involved in signal transduction, stress response, and structural and contractile proteins (Sreekumar *et al.*, 2002). Subsequently it was reported that dietary restriction can both reduce oxidative stress and attenuate age-dependent endogenous oxidative damage while maintaining ATP production (Lopez-Lluch *et al.*, 2006).

### Non-human primates

While experiments based on rodents can provide meaningful insights into the underlying mechanisms associated with dietary restriction, long-term confirmatory studies on non-human primates are necessary to provide results that can more readily be applied to humans (Roth *et al.*, 2004). Preliminary studies conducted on rhesus macaque monkeys aged approximately 20 years, and which had been maintained on a reduced caloric intake for between 9 and 10 years, suggested that long-term calorie restriction caused beneficial alterations in glycogen metabolism (Ortmeyer et al., 1994) and mitigated against the development of insulin resistance in older animals (Bodkin et al., 1995).

To standardize the conduct of subsequent investigations, and thus facilitate inter-study comparisons, two basic experimental criteria were proposed by Pugh et al. (1999): (1) the test and control animals should be individually housed, and (2) all animals in the control group should consume the same number of calories per day. These criteria were voluntarily adopted for most of the studies listed in Table 1.2, which illustrates the major findings obtained with dietary restriction experiments. Two points should be made: (1) while a number of the calorie restriction experiments have been conducted for 10 years or more, most animals still have not attained a very advanced age since rhesus macaques may live to approximately 40 years, and (2) quite small numbers of monkeys have been involved, averaging approximately 20 dietary-restricted animals per study with a comparable number of untreated controls.

A wide range of potentially beneficial outcomes have been reported, in particular an improvement in glucose tolerance (Lane et al., 1995), a lower core body temperature (Lane et al., 1996), attenuated decline in dehydroepiandrosterone sulphate (DHEAS) levels (Lane et al., 1997), decreased triglycerides and increased HDL2b (Verdery et al., 1997), with lower weight, lean body mass, and fat, and lower energy expenditure (DeLany et al., 1999). Since these promising early results a number of the reported outcomes have been more equivocal, and it will be interesting to see how the picture of dietary restriction develops as the animals reach ages equivalent to the oldest old in human terms—in particular whether, as in the rodent studies, they exhibit reduced rates of tumour formation and significant increases in maximum lifespan.

## Dietary restriction in humans

Given the quite limited information so far available from non-human primate experiments, dietary restriction in humans raises potential ethical concerns and may affect the quality of life of subjects (Dirks and Leeuwenburgh, 2006). A potential disadvantage of food restriction that may extend into adulthood was indicated in human studies which showed that poor early growth resulted in lower adult levels of the hormone thymosin $\alpha$1, produced by the thymus and essential both for T-cell function and in the overall regulation of the immune system (Clark et al., 1989). Nonetheless, a number of human experimental studies have been reported, including a 6-day investigation on eight adults and eight pubertal children involving a 50% caloric reduction (Smith et al., 1995). There was a significant reduction in the nitrogen balance of both adults and children and their insulin-like growth factor-1 (IGF-1) levels also decreased, but mixed results were obtained in the assays of insulin-growth factor-binding proteins. A study based on 18 individuals, who for 6 years had adopted a restricted food intake with the aim of slowing ageing, reported reduced body mass index and percentage body fat, lower levels of systolic and diastolic blood pressure, fasting glucose and insulin, serum total cholesterol, low-density lipoprotein, ratio of total cholesterol to high-density lipoprotein cholesterol, triglycerides, C-reactive protein, and platelet-derived growth factor, all of which would be consistent with protection against atherosclerosis (Fontana et al., 2004).

In a recent randomized control trial, a group of 48 overweight, non-obese males and females were recruited to one of four groups for a 6-month period: (1) controls (on a weight maintenance diet), (2) 25% calorie restriction of baseline energy requirements, (3) 12.5% calorie restriction plus 12.5% increase in energy expenditure by structured exercise, (4) a very low calorie diet of 890 kcal/day until 15% weight loss, followed by a weight maintenance diet (Heilbronn et al., 2006). The tests undertaken included body composition measures, 24-h energy expenditure, core body temperature, glucose, insulin and DHEAS levels, protein carbonyls, and DNA damage markers. The main findings were that fasting insulin levels and core body temperature were lowered by prolonged calorie restriction; however, given the study design no conclusions could be drawn as to the effects of dietary restriction on the attenuation of ageing in humans.

**Table 1.2** Dietary restriction in non-human primates

| Test protocol | Measures and results | Source |
|---|---|---|
| 30% reduction in calories for 7 years | Improved glucose tolerance and lower insulin response | Lane et al. (1995) |
| 30% reduction in calories for 6 years | 0.5°C reduction in core body temperature | Lane et al. (1996) |
| 30% reduction in calories for 6 years | Enhanced behavioural activity measures | Weed et al. (1997) |
| 30% reduction in calories for 2–3 years | Prolonged decrease in resting energy expenditure in males | Ramsey et al. (1997) |
| 30% reduction in calories for 3–6 years | Attenuation of post-maturational decline in dehydroepiandrosterone sulphate (DHEAS) levels in males | Lane et al. (1997) |
| 30% reduction in calories for 6–7 years | Decreased triglyceride levels, and increased levels of HDL2b | Verdery et al. (1997) |
| 30% reduction in calories for 6–7 years | No effect on a battery of haematological and blood biochemistry tests | Nakamura et al. (1998) |
| Unspecified level of calorie restriction for 10 years | Lower weight, lean body mass, and fat; lower total daily energy expenditure; lower thyroxine (T4) but not triiodothyronine (T3) | DeLany et al. (1999) |
| 30% reduction in calories for 5 years | Reduced locomotor activity in females aged 6–26 years | Moscrip et al. (2000) |
| 30% reduction in calories for > 2 years | Reduced circulating lipoprotein (a) levels in males but not females | Edwards et al. (2001) |
| 30% reduction in calories for 6–11 years | Reduced total T3 levels but not free or total T4; increased thyroid-stimulating hormone (TSH) levels | Roth et al. (2002a) |
| 30% reduction in calories for 11–13 years | No effect on striatal volume | Matochik et al. (2004) |

# Ageing as an energy crisis

The literature on ageing often appears vast and confusing, and with many apparently contradictory findings reported, which is not especially surprising given the complex issues to be examined, the length of the human lifespan, and the varied endogenous and environmental insults potentially involved. There has been an ongoing tendency to concentrate on theories that postulate a single cause of ageing. Given the widely variant nature of the ageing phenotype, it is difficult to perceive how such an extreme degree of pleiotropy could have been encoded or otherwise resulted from a unimodal origin. Much of the confusion inherent in theories of ageing also results from ambitious claims made on behalf of processes and systems that have been only marginally testable and so cannot readily be proved or disproved.

In evolutionary terms, senescence was suggested to be the end result of an energy conservation strategy operating in somatic cells (Kirkwood, 1977). During the course of an organism's lifespan, total available energy has to be differentially allocated to a variety of functions, including macromolecular synthesis and degradation, cell and organ maintenance, and reproduction of the species. Since the energy supply is finite, and to ensure propagation of the species by the successful transmission of genes to future generations, a compromise has to be reached between the energy made available for each function. According to the disposable soma theory, the proposed accommodation in energy saving is achieved by maintenance of absolute or near-absolute accuracy in germ cell replication but less rigorous error correction in somatic cells (Kirkwood and Holliday, 1986).

Minimally, this would provide an explanation for the puzzling inability of organisms to maintain existing structure and function despite having completed morphogenesis (Williams, 1957), and support for the theory is provided by the observation of a negative relationship between longevity and fecundity in mammals (Holliday, 1996). Likewise, in a study of the British aristocracy, female longevity was negatively correlated with a woman's number of progeny and positively correlated with age at first childbirth (Westendorp and Kirkwood, 1998). Extending this line of reasoning, if maintenance of the energy supply is a critical factor in ageing, then in the event of a reduction in energy production or supply all energy-dependent processes in somatic cells would suffer in proportion to their energy requirements. A simple check on the implications of this prediction can be made by reference to experimentally derived correlates of mammalian longevity, associated either with energy production or processes which appear to be energy dependent.

For that reason, and given the integral role that appears to be played by the mitochondria in apoptosis (Kujoth *et al.*, 2005), investigators have sought to link functional decline in mitochondria to somatic mutation, and to free radical-induced damage, particularly to the inner mitochondrial membrane. As the inner membrane is the site of the electron transport chain, and enzymes of the tricarboxylic acid cycle (TCA) are located within the mitochondrial matrix, oxidative damage by free radicals generated as by-products of cell respiration could severely compromise the ability of an organism to produce ATP and so meet its energy requirements. Cross-sectional experimental studies on invertebrates and rodents have indicated major morphological and functional changes in mitochondria with ageing, and similar observations

were reported in the mitochondria of individuals aged from 60 to 80 years (Tauchi and Sato, 1985; Beregi, 1986), and cultured human cells close to termination of their *in vitro* lifespan (Johnson, 1979).

In humans, analysis of mtDNA after amplification revealed the age-dependent presence of a 4977 base pair (bp) deletion in mtDNA from a wide variety of tissues, including heart, brain, liver, kidney, spleen, and skeletal muscle (Cortopassi and Arnheim, 1990; Ikebe *et al.*, 1990; Linnane *et al.*, 1990; Yen *et al.* 1991). This deletion also was detected in ovarian tissue, but only after onset of the menopause (Kitagawa *et al.*, 1993). The mtDNA region deleted occurs between base pairs 8470 and 13,459 of the mitochondrial genome; genes encoded in this region include subunits 6 and 8 of ATP synthase, subunit CO3 of the cytochrome oxidase complex, and subunits ND3, -4L, -4 and -5 of the NADH–coenzyme Q reductase complex (Linnane *et al.* 1990). Further age-dependent deletions have since been described, ranging in size from 6063 bp to 10,422 bp (Corral-Debrinski *et al.*, 1992; Hsieh *et al.*, 1994; Pang *et al.*, 1994), and specific age-related point mutations in human mtDNA also have been detected (Münscher *et al.*, 1993; Zhang *et al.*, 1993).

This evidence provides valuable support for the hypothesis that the accumulation of somatic mtDNA deletions and other forms of mutation may be an important determinant of ageing (Linnane *et al.*, 1989; Hudson *et al.*, 1998), and cytoplasmic segregation of the mutant genomes could lead to cells with variable bioenergetic capacities. Whether the appearance of mtDNA mutations is spontaneous and/or provoked by free radical damage, it seems probable that once initiated the problem would be exacerbated by the organization of mtDNA, with its virtual absence of introns (Anderson *et al.*, 1981), lack of histone protection (Richter *et al.*, 1988), and no excision or recombinational repair (Clayton, 1982). The subsequent segregation patterns of mutant mtDNA per cell via the process of heteroplasmy, and the effects on cellular bioenergetic capacities, would be largely dependent on the essentially stochastic process of mitochondrial replication in diluting out defective genomes (Hart and Turturro, 1987). It was claimed that non-availability of this option is a critical component in the age-dependent functional decline of fixed, post-mitotic cells (Miquel, 1991), and specific missense mutations in the *CO1* and *CO2* genes of cytochrome c oxidase, each of which is exclusively encoded in the mitochondria, have been shown to segregate at higher frequency with late onset Alzheimer's disease (Davis *et al.*, 1997). In other cell types, mitochondrial turnover may be a significant factor in reducing adverse age-related responses.

The number of mtDNA genomes per cell equally could be a critical factor in determining the extent to which respiration of the organism will be adversely affected. Human cells typically contain hundreds of mitochondria, all of which appear to be polyploid. Mitochondria and mitochondrial genome numbers are tissue-dependent and their concentration is proportional to respiratory demand, being highest in tissues such as muscle (Holt and Jacobs, 1994). In persons over 80 years of age, randomly deleted mtDNA affected up to 70% of mtDNA molecules (Chabi *et al.*, 2005), and abnormalities of the mitochondrial electron transport system in skeletal muscle fibres increased from 6% at the age of 49 to 31% by 92 years of age (Bua *et al.*, 2006).

From the results of microarray studies conducted on different species there seems to be unanimous agreement that mitochondrial function is compromised with increasing age, which suggests that the main driving force behind ageing is a gradual deficiency in available energy. As an organism ages, the demands placed upon the free energy pool alter and increase from a primarily anabolic role to meeting the requirements of ever-increasing repair and catabolic functions, including those imposed by specific disease-related insults. With damage to the mitochondrial inner membrane and/or mtDNA an organism must increasingly rely on alternative, less efficient pathways for its energy needs and, ultimately, these pathways may no longer be capable of meeting the energy requirements necessary to sustain life.

## Ageing and the concept of healthy life expectancy

Given the projected global numbers of persons over 60 years of age, and more especially those aged 80 years or more, progress in understanding the nature of the disorders that frequently accompany ageing is timely. Rather than concentrate only on life expectancy, there has been a major push by health planners to develop ancillary measures which would be of greater practical value in assessing the adverse effects of ageing, and hence the potential capabilities or disabilities of older people. Active Life Expectancy (ALE) is defined as the period of life that is free of disabilities with respect to the basic Activities of Daily Living (ADL), e.g. eating, getting in and out of bed, bathing and toiletry needs, dressing, and indoor mobility (Manton and Land, 2000). This approach has been extended by weighting specific physical and cognitive dysfunctions to produce measures of Disability-Adjusted Life Years (DALY) and Quality-Adjusted Life Years (QALY).

Based on a comparable indicator, Disability Adjusted Life Expectancy (DALE) which estimates the number of years that might be expected to be spent in 'full health', tables of healthy life expectancy were compiled for babies born in 1999 (WHO, 2000). Under this system the number of years of healthy life expectancy can be calculated after weighting the period of predicted ill-health according to the perceived severity of the disorder(s). A common finding in developed countries was that although females enjoyed higher DALE scores they also could expect more years of disability than males, thus emphasizing the greater probability of disability at more advanced ages.

Measures such as DALE, DALY, and QALY have been criticized because of their dependence on subjective judgements regarding the level of health care required to maintain an individual in a given state of health, and this criticism can become even more significant in international, cross-cultural comparisons. Despite these limitations, the concept of healthy life expectancy should be useful in practical terms when applied to the general ageing population, and given access to better quality data the initial estimates can be adjusted and regularly updated. However, application of the approach to specific population subgroups could prove difficult without major modifications in rationale, for example people with intellectual disability whose life expectancy has increased to a remarkable extent during the last 50 years (Bittles et al., 2002; Bittles and Glasson, 2004).

## Future prospects

There has been major progress in elucidating the nature of the genomic changes which cause and/or accompany ageing, extending even to topics such as the greying of hair (Nishimura et al., 2005). While the claim that 'ageing is no longer an unsolved problem in biology' (Holliday, 2006) can probably be sustained in general terms, much significant detail remains to be identified and incorporated into what is clearly a multicausal process. However, modification of the ageing phenotype at the cellular level no longer seems unrealistic, and for the first time in human history the majority of those living in economically developed countries and entering old age can look forward with confidence to an extended state of healthy life expectancy.

Dietary restriction experiments on non-human primates are rapidly approaching the stage where data that are meaningful in terms of human ageing should be produced. It has already been claimed that mortality rates are reduced in dietary-restricted monkeys and, as in other species, healthy men who have lower core body temperatures, lower insulin levels, and higher DHEAS levels show greater survival times (Roth et al., 2002b). If dietary restriction is confirmed as advantageous to survival and health in non-human primates, considerable effort may be necessary to establish the age at which the procedure can safely be instituted without compromising normal development, the length of time over which it can be used, and the levels of food restriction that are optimal—especially since intermittent fasting without a reduction in overall food intake was shown to have similar effects to dietary restriction in reducing serum glucose and insulin levels, and increasing stress resistance in rodents (Anson et al., 2003).

Another alternative approach to food restriction could be to employ pharmaceutical mimetics of dietary restriction, such as 2-deoxyglucose to inhibit glycolysis and metformin to enhance the action of insulin (Ingram et al., 2004; Spindler, 2006). While a large potential market can be predicted for such products, the entire topic of anti-ageing medicine is controversial and cogent guidelines for its application and control have yet to be developed (Olshansky et al., 2002; Juengst et al., 2003).

At a more basic level, research on adult stem cells may reveal further insights into ageing. According to cell type, adult stem cells mainly undergo chronological ageing, as in skeletal muscle, or exhibit a combination of chronological and replicative ageing, typified by haematopoietic stem cells (Rando, 2006). It is still unclear whether the overall decline in tissue regenerative capacity with advancing age is caused by the intrinsic ageing of stem cells or by increasing impairment of stem cell function in an aged tissue environment. An answer to this fundamental question is needed if the application of stem cell therapy to counteract the functional declines and degenerative diseases typical of human ageing is to become a reality.

## References

Anderson, S., Bankier, A.T., Barrell, B.G. et al. (1981). Sequence and organisation of the human mitochondrial genome. Nature, 290, 457–65.

Anson, R.M., Guo, Z., de Cabo, R. et al. (2003). Intermittent fasting dissociates beneficial effects of dietary restriction on glucose metabolism and neuronal resistance to injury from calorie intake. Proceedings of the National Academy of Sciences USA, 100, 6216–20.

Arantes-Oliviera, N., Apfeld, J, Dillin, A., and Kenyon, C. (2002). Regulation of life-span by germ-line stem cells in Caenorhabditis elegans. Science, 295, 502–5.

Bender, A., Krishnan, K.J., Morris, C.M. et al. (2006). High levels of mitochondrial DNA deletions in substantia nigra neurons in aging and Parkinson disease. Nature Genetics, 38, 515–17.

Beregi, E. (1986). Relationship between ageing of the immune system and ageing of the whole organism. In *Dimensions in ageing* (ed. M. Bergener, M. Ermini, and H.B. Stahelin), pp. 35–50. Academic Press, London.

Bittles, A.H. (1997). Biological aspects of human ageing. In *Psychiatry in the elderly*, 2nd edn (ed. R. Jacoby and C. Oppenheimer), pp. 3–23. Oxford University Press, Oxford.

Bittles, A.H. and Glasson, E.J. (2004). Clinical, social and ethical aspects of the changing life expectancy of people with Down syndrome. *Developmental Medicine and Child Neurology*, **46**, 282–6.

Bittles, A.H., Petterson, B.A., Sullivan, S.G., Hussain, R., Glasson, E.J., and Montgomery, P.D. (2002). The influence of intellectual disability on life expectancy. *Journal of Gerontology Series A, Biological Sciences and Medical Sciences*, **57A**, M470–M472.

Bjorksten, J. (1968). The crosslinkage theory of aging. *Journal of the American Geriatrics Society*, **16**, 408–27.

Bodkin, N.L., Ortmeyer, H.K., and Hansen, B.C. (1995). Long-term dietary restriction in older-age rhesus monkeys: effects on insulin resistance. *Journal of Gerontology Series A, Biological Sciences and Medical Sciences*, **50**, B142–B147.

Bodnar, A.G., Ouellette, M., Frolkis, M. *et al.* (1998). Extension of life-span by introduction of telomerase into normal human cells. *Science*, **279**, 349–52.

Boehm, M. and Slack, F. (2005). A developmental timing microRNA and its target regulate life span in *C. elegans*. *Science*, **310**, 1954–7.

Boffoli, D., Scacco, S.C., Vergari, R., Solarino, G., Santacroce, G., and Papa, S. (1994). Decline with age of the respiratory chain activity in human skeletal muscle. *Biochimica et Biophysica Acta*, **1226**, 73–82.

Britt-Compton, B., Rowson, J., Locke, M., Mackenzie, I., Kipling, D., and Baird, D.M. (2006). Structural stability and chromosome-specific telomere length is governed by cis-acting determinants in humans. *Human Molecular Genetics*, **15**, 725–33.

Brody, J.A. (1985). Prospects for an ageing population. *Nature*, **315**, 463–6.

Bua, E., Johnson, J., Herbst, A. *et al.* (2006). Mitochondrial DNA-deletion mutations accumulate intracellularly to detrimental levels in aged human skeletal muscle fibers. *American Journal of Human Genetics*, **79**, 469–80.

Carey, J.R., Liedo, P., Orozco, D., and Vaupel, J.W. (1992). Slowing of mortality rates at older ages in large Medfly cohorts. *Science*, **258**, 457–61.

Chabi, B., de Camaret, B.M., Chevrollier, A., Boisgard. S., and Stepien, G. (2005). Random mtDNA deletions and functional consequence in aged human skeletal muscle. *Biochemical and Biophysical Research Communications*, **332**, 542–9.

Chomyn, A., Cleeter, M.W.J., Ragan, C.I., Riley, M., Doolittle, R.F., and Attardi, G. (1986). URF6, last unidentified reading frame of human mtDNA, codes for an NADH dehydrogenase subunit. *Science*, **234**, 614–18.

Clancy, D.J., Gems, D., Harshman, L.G. *et al.* (2001). Extension of life-span by loss of *chico*, a *Drosophila* insulin receptor substrate protein. *Science*, **292**, 104–6.

Clark, G.A., Aldwin, C.M., Hall, N.R., Spiro, A., and Goldstein, A. (1989). Is poor early growth related to adult immune aging? *American Journal of Human Biology*, **1**, 331–7.

Clayton, D.A. (1982). Replication of animal mitochondrial DNA. *Cell*, **28**, 693–705.

Corral-Debrinski, M., Shoffner, J.M., Lott, M.T., and Wallace, D.C. (1992). Association of mitochondrial DNA damage with aging and coronary atherosclerotic heart disease. *Mutation Research*, **275**, 169–80.

Cortopassi, G.A. and Arnheim, N. (1990). Detection of a specific mitochondrial DNA deletion in tissues of older humans. *Nucleic Acids Research*, **18**, 6927–33.

Curtis, J.H. and Miller, K. (1971). Chromosome aberrations in liver cells of guinea pigs. *Journal of Gerontology*, **26**, 292–4.

Curtsinger, J.W., Fukui, H.H., Townsend, D.R., and Vaupel, J.W. (1992). Demography of genotypes: failure of the limited life-span paradigm in *Drosophila melanogaster*. *Science*, **258**, 461–3.

Cutler, R.G. (1975). Evolution of human longevity and the genetic complexity governing aging rate. *Proceedings of the National Academy of Sciences USA*, **72**, 4664–8.

Cutler, R.G. (1985). Peroxide-producing potential of tissues: inverse correlation with longevity of mammalian species. *Proceedings of the National Academy of Sciences USA*, **82**, 4798–802.

Davis, R.E., Miller, S., Herrnstadt, C. *et al.* (1997). Mutations in mitochondrial cytochrome *c* oxidase genes segregate with late-onset Alzheimer disease. *Proceedings of the National Academy of Sciences, USA*, **94**, 4526–31.

DeLany, J.P., Hansen, B.C., Bodkin, N.L., Hannah, J., and Bray, G.A. (1999). Long-term calorie restriction reduces energy expenditure in aging monkeys. *Journal of Gerontology Series A, Biological Sciences and Medical Sciences*, **54**, B5–B11.

Dirks, A.J. and Leeuwenburgh, C. (2006). Caloric restriction in humans: potential pitfalls and health concerns. *Mechanisms of Development and Ageing*, **127**, 1–7.

Edwards, I.J., Rudel, L.L., Terry, J.G. *et al.* (2001). Caloric restriction lowers plasma lipoprotein (a) in male but not female rhesus monkeys. *Experimental Gerontology*, **36**, 1413–18.

Englander, E.W. (2005). Gene expression changes reveal patterns of aging in the rat digestive tract. *Ageing Research Reviews*, **4**, 564–78.

Epel, E., Blackburn, E.H., Lin, J. *et al.* (2004) Stress and ageing. *Proceedings of the National Academy of Sciences USA*, **101**, 17312–15.

Fleming, J.E., Miquel, J., and Bensch, K.G. (1985). Age dependent changes in mitochondria. In *Molecular biology of aging* (ed. A.D. Woodhead, A.D. Blackett, and A. Hollaender), pp. 143–56. Plenum, New York.

Fontana, L., Meyer, T.E., Klein, S., and Holloszy, J.O. (2004). Long-term calorie restriction is highly effective in reducing the risk for atherosclerosis in humans. *Proceedings of the National Academy of Sciences USA*, **101**, 6659–63.

Fries, J.F. (1980). Aging, natural death and the compression of morbidity. *New England Journal of Medicine*, **303**, 130–5.

Fries, J.F. (2005). Frailty, heart disease, and stroke: the compression of morbidity paradigm. *American Journal of Preventive Medicine*, **29**, 164–8.

Frisard, M. and Ravussin, E. (2006). Energy metabolism and oxidative stress: impact on the metabolic syndrome and the aging process. *Endocrine*, **29**, 27–32.

Giannakou, M.E., Goss, M., Jünger, M.A., Hafen, E., Leevers, S.J., and Partridge, L. (2004). Long-lived *Drosophila* with over-expressed dFOXO in adult fat body. *Science*, **305**, 361.

Graakjaer, J., Londono-Vallejo, J.A., Christensen, K., and Kolvraa, S. (2006). The pattern of chromosome-specific variations in telomere length in humans shows signs of heritability and is maintained through life. *Annals of the New York Academy of Sciences*, **1067**, 311–16.

Gutteridge, J.M.C., Westermarck, T., and Halliwell, B. (1986). Oxygen radical damage in biological systems. In *Free radicals, aging and degenerative diseases*, Modern Aging Research Vol. 8 (ed. J.E. Johnson, R. Walford, D. Harman, and J. Miquel) pp. 99–139. Alan R. Liss, New York.

Hamatani, T., Falco, G., Carter, M.G. *et al.* (2004). Age-associated alteration of gene expression patterns in mouse oocytes. *Human Molecular Genetics*, **13**, 2263–78.

Harley, C.B. (1991). Telomere loss: mitotic clock or genetic time bomb? *Mutation Research*, **256**, 271–82.

Harley, C.B. (2005). Telomerase therapeutics for degenerative diseases. *Current Molecular Medicine*, **5**, 205–11.

Harley, C.B., Futcher, A.B., and Greider, C.W. (1990). Telomeres shorten during ageing of human fibroblasts. *Nature*, **345**, 458–60.

Harman, D. (1956). Aging: a theory based on free radical and radiation chemistry. *Journal of Gerontology*, **11**, 298–300.

Harman, D. (1986). Free radical theory of aging: role of free radicals in the origination and evolution of life, aging, and disease processes. In *Free radicals, aging and degenerative diseases*, Modern Aging Research Vol. 8 (ed. J.E. Johnston, R. Walford, D. Harman, and J. Miquel), pp. 3–49. Alan R. Liss, New York.

Harman, D. (1992). Free radical theory of aging. *Mutation Research*, **275**, 257–66.

Hart, R.W. and Setlow, R.B. (1974). Correlation between deoxyribonucleic acid excision repair and lifespan in a number of mammalian species. *Proceedings of the National Academy of Sciences USA*, **71**, 2169–73.

Hart, R.W. and Turturro, A. (1987). Review of recent biological research in the theories of aging. In *Review of biological research in aging*, Vol. 3 (ed. M. Rothstein), pp. 15–21. Alan R. Liss, New York.

Hawse, J.R., Hejtmancik, J.F., Horwitz, J., and Kantarow, M. (2004). Identification and functional clustering of global gene expression differences between age-related cataract and clear human lenses and aged human lenses. *Experimental Eye Research*, **79**, 935–40.

Hayflick, L. (1965). The limited *in vitro* lifetime of human diploid cell strains. *Experimental Cell Research*, **37**, 614–36.

Hayflick, L. and Moorhead, P.S. (1961). The serial cultivation of human diploid cell strains. *Experimental Cell Research*, **25**, 585–621.

Heilbronn, L.K., de Jonge, L. Frisard, M.I. *et al.* (2006). Effect of 6-month calorie restriction on biomarkers of longevity, metabolic adaptation, and oxidative stress in overweight individuals: a randomized controlled trial. *Journal of the American Medical Association*, **295**, 1539–48.

Herskind, A.M., McGue, M., Holm, N.V., Sørensen, T.I.A., Harvald, B., and Vaupel, J.W. (1996). The heritability of human longevity: a population-based study of 2872 Danish twin pairs born 1870–1900. *Human Genetics*, **97**, 319–23.

Holehan, A.M. and Merry, B.J. (1986) The experimental manipulation of ageing by diet. *Biological Reviews*, **61**, 329–68.

Holliday, R. (1987). The inheritance of epigenetic defects. *Science*, **238**, 163–70.

Holliday, R. (1996). The evolution of human longevity. *Perspectives in Biology and Medicine*, **40**, 100–7.

Holliday, R. (2006). Aging is no longer an unsolved problem in biology. *Annals of the New York Academy of Sciences*, **1067**, 1–9.

Holt, I.J. and Jacobs, H.T. (1994). The structure and expression of normal and mutant mitochondrial genomes. In *Mitochondria: DNA, proteins and disease* (ed. V. Darley-Usmar and A.H.V. Schapira), pp. 27–54. Portland, London.

Hsieh, R.-H., Hou, J.-H., Hsu, H.-S., and Wei, Y.-H. (1994). Age-dependent respiratory function decline and DNA deletions in human muscle mitochondria. *Biochemistry and Molecular Biology International*, **32**, 1009–22.

Hudson, E.K., Hogue, B.A., Souza-Pinti, N.C. *et al.* (1998). Age-associated change in mitochondrial DNA damage. *Free Radical Research*, **29**, 573–9.

Hughes, K.A., Alipaz, J.A., Drnevich, J.M., and Reynolds, R.M. (2002). A test of evolutionary theories of aging. *Proceedings of the National Academy of Sciences USA*, **99**, 14286–91.

Ikebe, S., Tanaka, M., Ohno, K. *et al.* (1990). Increase of deleted mitochondrial DNA in the striatum in Parkinson's disease and senescence. *Biochemistry and Biophysics Research Communications*, **170**, 1044–8.

Ikeda, A., Iso, H., Toyoshima, H. *et al.* (2006). Parental longevity and mortality amongst Japanese men and women: the JACC Study. *Journal of Internal Medicine*, **259**, 285–95.

Ingram, D.K., Anson, R.M., de Cabo, R. *et al.* (2004). Development of calorie restriction mimetics as a prolongevity strategy. *Annals of the New York Academy of Sciences*, **1019**, 412–23.

Jenkins, N.L., McColl, G., and Lithgow, G.J. (2004). Fitness costs of extended lifespan in *Caenorhabditis elegans*. *Proceedings of the Royal Society B: Biological Sciences*, **271**, 2523–6.

Johnson, J.E. (1979). Fine structure of IMR-90 cells in culture as examined by scanning and transmission electron microscopy. *Mechanisms of Ageing and Development*, **10**, 405–43.

Juengst, E.T., Binstock, R.H., Meglman, M.J., and Post, S.G. (2003). Antiaging research and the need for public dialogue. *Science*, **299**, 1323.

Kang, M.K., Kameta, A., Shin, K.H., Baluda, M.A., Kim, H.R., and Park, N.H. (2003). Senescence-associated genes in normal human oral keratinocytes. *Experimental Cell Research*, **287**, 272–81.

Kannisto, V., Lauritsen, J., Thatcher, A.R., and Vaupel, J.W. (1994). Reductions in mortality at advanced ages. *Population and Development Review*, **20**, 793–810.

Kirkwood, T.B.L. (1977). Evolution of ageing. *Nature*, **270**, 301–4.

Kirkwood, T.B. (2002). Evolution of ageing. *Mechanisms of Ageing and Development*, **123**, 737–45.

Kirkwood, T.B.L. and Holliday, R. (1986). Ageing as a consequence of natural selection. In *The biology of human ageing* (ed. A.H. Bittles and K.J. Collins), pp. 1–16. Cambridge University Press, Cambridge.

Kitagawa, T., Suganuma, N., Nawa, A. *et al.* (1993). Rapid accumulation of deleted mitochondrial deoxyribonucleic acid in postmenopausal ovaries. *Biology of Reproduction*, **49**, 730–6.

Kohn, R.R. (1982a). Causes of death in very old people. *Journal of the American Medical Association*, **247**, 2793–7.

Kohn, R.R. (1982b). *Principles of mammalian aging*, 2nd edn. Prentice-Hall, Englewood Cliffs, NJ.

Ku, H-K., Brunk, U.T., and Sohal, R.S. (1993). Relationship between mitochondrial superoxide and hydrogen peroxide production and longevity of mammalian species. *Free Radicals in Biology and Medicine*, **15**, 621–7.

Kujoth, G.C., Hiona, A., Pugh, T.D. *et al.* (2005). Mitochondrial DNA mutations, oxidative stress, and apoptosis in mammalian aging. *Science*, **309**, 481–4.

Lane, M.A., Ball, S.S., Ingram, D.K. *et al.* (1995). Diet restriction in rhesus monkeys lowers fasting and glucose-stimulated glucoregulatory end points. *American Journal of Physiology*, **268**, E941–E948.

Lane, M.A., Baer, D.J., Rumpler, W.V. *et al.* (1996). Calorie restriction lowers body temperature in rhesus monkeys, consistent with a postulated anti-aging mechanism in rodents. *Proceedings of the National Academy of Sciences USA*, **93**, 4159–64.

Lane, M.A., Ingram, D.K., Ball, S.S., and Roth, G.S. (1997). Dehydroepiandrosterone sulfate: a biomarker of primate aging slowed by calorie restriction. *Journal of Clinical Endocrinology and Metabolism*, **82**, 2093–6.

Larsen, P.L. (1993). Ageing and resistance to oxidative damage in *Caenorhabditis elegans*. *Proceedings of the National Academy of Sciences USA*, **90**, 8905–9.

Lee, C.-K., Klopp, Weindruch, R., and Prolla, T.A. (1999). Gene expression profile of aging and its retardation by caloric restriction. *Science*, **285**, 1390–3.

Lin, K., Dorman, J.B., Rodan, A., and Kenyon, C. (1997). *daf-16*: an HNF-3/ forkhead family member that can function to double the life-span of *Caenorhabditis elegans*. *Science*, **278**, 1319–22.

Lin, Y.-J., Seroude, L., and Benzer, S. (1998). Extended life-span and stress resistance in the *Drosophila* mutant *methuselah*. *Science*, **282**, 943–6.

Lindvall, C., Hou, N.M., Komurasaki, T. *et al.* (2003). Molecular characterization of human telomerase reverse transcriptase-immortalized human fibroblasts by gene expression profiling: activation of the epiregulin gene. *Cancer Research*, **63**, 1743–7.

Linnane, A.W., Marzuki, S., Ozawa, T., and Tanaka, M. (1989). Mitochondrial DNA mutations as an important contributor to ageing and degenerative diseases. *Lancet*, **1**, 642–5.

Linnane, A.W., Baumer, A., Maxwell, R.J., Preston, H., Zhang, C., and Marzuki, S. (1990). Mitochondrial gene mutation: the ageing process and degenerative diseases. *Biochemistry International*, **22**, 1067–76.

Lithgow, G.J., White, T.M., Hinerfeld, D.A., and Johnson, T.E. (1994). Thermotolerance of a long-lived mutant of *Caenorhabditis elegans*. *Journal of Gerontology*, **49**, B270–B276.

Ljungquist, B., Berg, S., Lanke, J., McClearn, G.E., and Pedersen, N.L. (1998). The effect of genetic factors for longevity: a comparison of identical and fraternal twins in the Swedish Twin Registry. *Journal of Gerontology Series A, Biological Sciences and Medical Sciences*, **53**, M441–M446.

Lopez-Lluch, G., Hunt, N., Jones, B. *et al.* (2006). Calorie restriction induces mitochondrial biogenesis and bioenergetic efficiency. *Proceedings of the National Academy of Sciences USA*, **103**, 1768–73.

Luhtala, T.A., Roecker, E.B., Pugh, T., Feuers, R.J., and Weindruch, R. (1994). Dietary restriction attenuates age-related increases in rat skeletal muscle antioxidant enzyme activities. *Journal of Gerontology*, **49**, B231–B238.

Ly, D.H., Lockhart, D.J., Lerner, R.A., and Schultz, P.G. (2000). Mitotic misregulation and human aging. *Science*, **287**, 2486–92.

McCarter, R., Masoro, E.J., and Yu, B.P. (1985). Does food restriction retard aging by reducing the metabolic rate? *American Journal of Physiology*, **248**, E488–E490.

McCay, C.M., Crowell, M.F., and Maynard, L.A. (1935). The effect of retarded growth upon the length of lifespan and upon the ultimate body size. *Journal of Nutrition*, **10**, 63–79.

McCay, C.M., Ellis, G.H., Barnes, L.L., Smith, C.A.H., and Sperling, G. (1939). Clinical and pathological changes in aging and after retarded growth. *Journal of Nutrition*, **18**, 15–25.

McEwen, B.S. (1998). Stress, adaptation, and disease. Allostasis and the allostatic load. *Annals of the New York Academy of Sciences*, **840**, 33–44.

McEwen, B.S. (2002). Sex, stress and the hippocampus: allostasis, allostatic load and the aging process. *Neurobiology and Aging*, **23**, 921–39.

McEwen, B.S. and Wingfield, J.C. (2003). The concept of allostasis in biology and biomedicine. *Hormones and Behavior*, **43**, 2–15.

Makrantonaki, E., Adjaye, J., Herwig, R. *et al.* (2006). Age-specific hormonal decline is accompanied by transcriptional changes in human sebocytes *in vitro*. *Ageing Cell*, **5**, 331–44.

Manton, K.G. and Land, K.C. (2000) Active life expectancy estimates for the U.S. elderly population: a multidimensional continuous-mixture model of functional change applied to completed cohorts, 1982–1986. *Demography*, **37**, 253–65.

Martin, G.M. (1989). Genetic modulation of the senescent phenotype in *Homo sapiens. Genome*, **31**, 390–7.

Martin, G.R., Danner, D.B., and Holbrook, N.J. (1993). Aging – causes and defenses. *Annual Review of Medicine*, **44**, 419–29.

Masoro, E.J. (1988). Food restriction in rodents: an evaluation of its role in the study of aging. *Journal of Gerontology*, **43**, B59–B64.

Matochik, J.A., Chefer, S.I., Lane, M.A. *et al.* (2004). Age-related decline in striatal volume in rhesus monkeys: assessment of long-term calorie restriction. *Neurobiology of Aging*, **25**, 193–200.

Mecocci, P., MacGarvey, U., Kaufman, A.E. *et al.* (1993). Oxidative damage to mitochondrial DNA shows marked age-dependent increases in human brain. *Annals of Neurology*, **34**, 609–16.

Melk, A., Mansfield, E.S., Hsieh, S.C. *et al.* (2005). Transcriptional analysis of the molecular basis of human kidney using cDNA microarray profiling. *Kidney International*, **68**, 2667–79.

Melov, S., Ravenscroft, J., Malik, S. *et al.* (2000). Extension of life-span with superoxide dismutase/catalase mimetics. *Science*, **289**, 1567–9.

Miquel, J. (1991). An integrated theory of aging as the result of mitochondrial-DNA mutation in differentiated cells. *Archives of Gerontology and Geriatrics*, **12**, 99–117.

Mohamed, S.A., Hanke, T., Erasmi, A.W. *et al.* (2006). Mitochondrial DNA deletions and the aging heart. *Experimental Gerontology*, **41**, 508–17.

Moscrip, T.D., Ingram, D.K., Lane, M.A., Roth, G.S., and Weed, J.L. (2000). Locomotor activity in female rhesus monkeys: assessment of age and calorie restriction effects. *Journal of Gerontology Series A, Biological Sciences and Medical Sciences*, **55**, B373–B380.

Münscher, C., Müller-Höcker, J., and Kadenbach, B. (1993). Human ageing is associated with various point mutations in tRNA genes of mitochondrial DNA. *Biological Chemistry Hoppe-Seyler*, **374**, 1099–104.

Nakamura, E., Lane, M.A., Roth, G.S., and Ingram, D.K. (1998). A strategy for identifying biomarkers of aging: further evaluation of haematology and blood chemistry data from a calorie restriction study in rhesus monkeys. *Experimental Gerontology*, **33**, 421–43.

Nishimura, E.K., Granter, S.R., and Fisher, D.E. (2005). Mechanisms of hair graying: incomplete melanocyte stem cell maintenance in the niche. *Science*, **307**, 720–4.

Oeppen, J. and Vaupel, J.W. (2002). Broken limits to life expectancy. *Science*, **296**, 1029–30.

Olshansky, S.J., Carnes, B.A., and Cassel, C. (1990). In search of Methusaleh: estimating the upper limits to human longevity. *Science*, **250**, 634–40.

Olshansky, S.J., Carnes, B.A., and Desesquelles, A. (2001). Prospects for human longevity. *Science*, **291**, 1491–2.

Olshansky, S.J., Hayflick, L., and Carnes, B.A. (2002). Position statement on human aging. *Journal of Gerontology Series A, Biological Sciences*, **57A**, B292–B297.

Olshansky, S.J., Passaro, D.J., Hershow, R.C. *et al.* (2005). A potential decline in life expectancy in the United States in the 21st century. *New England Journal of Medicine*, **352**, 1138–45.

Orgel, L.E. (1963). The maintenance of the accuracy of protein synthesis and its relevance to aging. *Proceedings of the National Academy of Sciences USA*, **49**, 517–21.

Orgel, L.E. (1973). Ageing of clones of mammalian cells. *Nature*, **243**, 441–5.

Ortmeyer, H.K., Bodkin, N.L., and Hansen, B.C. (1994). Chronic calorie restriction alters glycogen metabolism in rhesus monkeys. *Obesity Research*, **2**, 549–55.

Pang, C.-Y., Lee, H.-C., Yang, J.-H., and Wei, Y.-H. (1994). Human skin mitochondrial DNA deletions associated with light exposure. *Archives of Biochemistry and Biophysics*, **312**, 534–8.

Parsons, P.A. (1995). Inherited stress resistance and longevity: a stress theory of ageing. *Heredity*, **74**, 216–21.

Partridge, L. and Gems, D. (2002). Mechanisms of ageing: public or private? *Nature Reviews Genetics*, **3**, 165–75.

Patrick, J.S., Thorpe, S.R., and Baynes, J.W. (1990). Nonenzymatic glycosylation of protein does not increase with age in normal lenses. *Journal of Gerontology*, **45**, B18–B23.

Perls, T.T., Bubrick, E., Wager, C.G., Vijg, J., and Kruglyak, L. (1998). Siblings of centenarians live longer. *Lancet*, **351**, 1560.

Pinkston, J.M., Garigan, D., Hansen, M., and Kenyon, C. (2006). Mutations that increase the life span of *C. elegans* inhibit tumor growth. *Science*, **313**, 971–5.

PRB (2006). *World population data sheet, 2006*. Population Reference Bureau, Washington, DC.

Pugh, T.D., Klopp, R.G., and Weindruch, R. (1999). Controlling caloric consumption: protocols for rodents and rhesus monkeys. *Neurobiology of Aging*, **20**, 157–65.

Ramsey, J.J., Roecker, E.B., Weindruch, R., and Kemnitz, J.W. (1997). Energy expenditure of adult male rhesus during the first 30 mo of dietary restriction. *American Journal of Physiology*, **272**, E910–E917.

Rando, T.A. (2006) Stem cells, ageing and the quest for immortality. *Nature Genetics*, **441**, 1080–1086.

Reznick, D.N. and Ghalambor, C. (1999). Sex and death. *Science*, **286**, 2458–9.

Richter, C., Park, J.W., and Ames, B.N. (1988). Normal oxidative damage to mitochondrial and nuclear DNA is extensive. *Proceedings of the National Academy of Sciences USA*, **85**, 6465–7.

Robine, J.M. and Allard, M. (1998). The oldest old. *Science*, **279**, 1834–5.

Rontu, R., Ojala, P, Hervonen, A. *et al.* (2006). Apolipoprotein E genotype is related to plasma levels of C-reactive protein and lipids and to longevity in nonagenarians. *Clinical Endocrinology*, **64**, 265–70.

Roth, G.S., Handy, A.M., Mattison, J.A., Tilmont, E.M., Ingram, D.K., and Lane, M.A. (2002a). Effects of caloric restriction and aging on thyroid hormones of rhesus monkeys. *Hormone and Metabolic Research*, **34**, 378–82.

Roth, G.S., Lane, M.A., Ingram, D.K. *et al.* (2002b). Biomarkers of caloric restriction may predict longevity in humans. *Science*, **297**, 811.

Roth, G.S., Mattison, J.A., Ottinger, M.A., Chachich, M.E., Lane, M.A., and Ingram, D.K. (2004). Ageing in rhesus monkeys: relevance to human health interventions. *Science*, **305**, 1423–5.

Sacher, G.A. (1975). Maturation and longevity in relation to cranial capacity in hominid evolution. In *Antecedents of man and after, Vol. 1 Primates: functional morphology and evolution* (ed. R. Tuttle), pp. 417–41. Mouton, The Hague.

Sacher, G.A. (1976). Evaluation of the entropy and information terms governing mammalian longevity. In *Cellular ageing: concepts and mechanisms*, Interdisciplinary Topics in Gerontology Vol. 9 (ed. R.G. Cutler), pp. 69–82. Karger, Basel.

Scaffidi, P. and Misteli, T. (2006). Lamin A-dependent nuclear defects in human aging. *Science*, **312**, 1059–63.

Schneider, E.L. and Brody, J.A. (1983). Aging, natural death, and the compression of morbidity: another view. *New England Journal of Medicine*, **309**, 854–5.

Schnider, S.L. and Kohn, R.R. (1981). Effects of age and diabetes mellitus on the solubility of collagen and nonenzymatic glycolysation of human skin collagen. *Journal of Clinical Investigation*, **67**, 1630–5.

Schoenmaker, M. de Craen, A.J., de Meijer, P.H. *et al.* (2006). Evidence of genetic enrichment for exceptional survival using a family approach: the Leiden Longevity Study. *European Journal of Human Genetics*, **14**, 79–84.

Schriner, S.E., Linford, N.J., Martin, G.M. *et al.* (2005) Extension of murine life span by overexpression of catalyse targeted to mitochondria. *Science*, **308**, 1909–11.

Seeman, T.E., McEwen, B.S., Rowe, J.W., and Singer, B.H. (2001). Allostatic load as marker of cumulative biological risk: MacArthur studies of successful aging. *Proceedings of the National Academy of Sciences USA*, **98**, 4770–5.

Seplaki, C.L., Goldman, N, Weinstein, M., and Lin, Y.-H. (2006). Measurement of cumulative physiological dysregulation in an older population. *Demography*, **43**, 165–83.

Sgrò, C.M. and Partridge, L. (1999). A delayed wave of death from reproduction in *Drosophila*. *Science*, **286**, 2521–4.

Smith, W.J., Underwood, L.E., and Clemmons, D.R. (1995). Effects of caloric or protein restriction on insulin-like growth factor-1 (IGF-1), and IGF-binding proteins in children and adults. *Journal of Clinical Endocrinology and Metabolism*, **80**, 443–9.

Spindler, S.R. (2006). Use of microarray biomarkers to identify longevity therapeutics. *Aging Cell*, **5**, 39–50.

Sreekumar, R., Unnikrishnan, J., Fu, A. *et al.* (2002). Effects of caloric restriction on mitochondrial function and gene transcripts in rat muscle. *American Journal of Physiology, Endocrinology and Metabolism*, **283**, E38–E43.

Stadtman, E.R. (1992). Protein oxidation and aging. *Science*, **257**, 1220–4.

Szilard, L. (1959). On the nature of the ageing process. *Proceedings of the National Academy of Sciences USA*, **45**, 30–45.

Tatar, M., Kopelman, A., Epstein, D., Tu, M.-P., Yin, C.-M., and Garofolo, R.S. (2001). A mutant *Drosophila* insulin receptor homolog that extends life-span and impairs neuroendocrine function. *Science*, **292**, 107–10.

Tauchi, H. and Sato, T. (1985). Cellular changes in senescence: possible factors influencing the process of cellular ageing. In *Thresholds in ageing* (ed. M. Bergener, M. Ermini, and H.B. Stahelin), pp. 91–113. Academic, London.

Trounce, I., Bryne, E., and Marzuki, S. (1989). Decline in human skeletal muscle mitochondrial respiratory chain function: possible factor in ageing. *Lancet*, **1**, 637–9.

Tzagoloff, A. and Myers, A.M. (1986). Genetics of mitochondrial biogenesis. *Annual Review of Biochemistry*, **55**, 249–85.

Valdes, A.M., Andrew, T., Gardner, J.P. *et al.* (2005). Obesity, cigarette smoking, and telomere length in women. *Lancet*, **366**, 662–4.

van Waarde-Verhagen, M.A., Kampinga, H.H., and Linskens, M.H. (2006). Continuous growth of telomerase-immortalised fibroblasts: how long do cells remain normal? *Mechanisms of Ageing and Development*, **127**, 85–7.

Verdery, R.B., Ingram, D.K., Roth, G.S., and Lane, M.A. (1997). Caloric restriction increases HDL2 levels in rhesus monkeys (*Macaca mulatta*). *American Journal of Physiology*, **273**, E714–E719.

Vita, A.J., Terry, R.B., Hubert, H.B., and Fries, J.F. (1998). Aging, health risks, and cumulative disability. *New England Journal of Medicine*, **338**,1035–41.

Voos, W., Moczko, M., and Pfanner, N. (1994). Targeting, translocation and folding of mitochondrial preproteins. In *Mitochondria: DNA, proteins and disease* (ed. V. Darley-Usmar and A.H.V. Schapira), pp. 55–80. Portland, London.

Weed, J.L., Lane, M.A., Roth, G.S., Speer, D.L., and Ingram, D.K. (1997). Activity measures in rhesus monkeys on long-term calorie restriction. *Physiology and Behavior*, **62**, 97–103.

Weindruch, R. and Walford, R.L. (1982). Life span and spontaneous cancer incidence in mice dietarily restricted beginning at one year of age. *Science*, **215**, 1415–18.

Wennmalm, K., Wahlestedt, C., and Larsson, O. (2005). The expression signature of *in vitro* senescence resembles mouse but not human aging. *Genome Biology*, **6**, R109.

Westendorp, R.G.J. and Kirkwood, T.B.L. (1998). Human longevity at the cost of reproductive success. *Nature*, **396**, 743–6.

WHO (2000). *The World Health Report 2000. Health systems: improving performance*. World Health Organization, Geneva.

Willcox, B.J., Willcox, D.C., He, Q., Curb, J.D., and Suzuki, M. (2006). Siblings of Okinawan centenarians share lifelong mortality advantages. *Journal of Gerontology Series A, Biological Sciences and Medical Sciences*, **61**, 345–54.

Williams, G.C. (1957). Pleiotropy, natural selection and the evolution of senescence. *Evolution*, **11**, 398–411.

Wilmoth, J.R. and Horiuchi, S. (1999). Rectangularization revisited: variability of age at death within human populations. *Demography*, **36**, 475–95.

Wilmoth, J.R., Deegan, L.J., Lundström, H., and Horiuchi, S. (2000). Increase of maximum life-span in Sweden, 1861–1999. *Science*, **289**, 2366–9.

Wojdacz, T.K. and Hansen, L.L. (2006). Techniques used in studies of age-related DNA methylation changes. *Annals of the New York Academy of Science*, **1067**, 479–87.

Wolkow, C.A., Kimura, K.D., Lee, M.-S., and Ruvkun, G. (2000). Regulation of *C. elegans* life-span by insulin-like signaling in the nervous system. *Science*, **290**, 147–50.

Wood, R.D., Mitchell, M., Sgouros, J., and Lindahl, T. (2001). Human DNA repair genes. *Science*, **291**, 1284–9.

Yen, T.C., Su, J.H., King, K.L., and Wei, Y.H. (1991). Ageing-associated 5 kb deletion in human liver mitochondrial DNA. *Biochemistry and Biophysics Research Communications*, **178**, 124–31.

Yoon, I.K., Kim, H.K., Kim, Y.K. *et al.* (2004). Exploration of replicative senescence-associated genes in human dermal fibroblasts by cDNA microarray technology. *Experimental Gerontology*, **39**, 1369–78.

Yoshida, K. Inoue, T., Nojima, K., Hribayashi, Y., and Sado, T. (1997). Calorie restriction reduces the incidence of myeloid leukemia induced by a single whole-body radiation in C3H/He mice. *Proceedings of the National Academy of Sciences USA*, **94**, 2615–19.

Yoshida, S., Yashar, B.M., Hiriyanna, S., and Swaroop, A. (2002). Microarray analysis of gene expression in the aging human retina. *Investigative Ophthalmology and Visual Science*, **43**, 2554–60.

Yu, B.P., Masoro, E.J., and McMahan, C.A. (1985). Nutritional influences on aging of Fischer 344 rats: I. Physical, metabolic, and longevity characteristics. *Journal of Gerontology*, **40**, 657–70.

Zahn, J.M., Sonu, R., Vogel, H. *et al.* (2006). Transcriptional profiling of aging in human muscle reveals a common aging signature. *PLoS Genetics*, **2**, e115.

Zhang, C., Linnane, A.W., and Nagley, P. (1993). Occurrence of a particular base substitution (3243 A to G) in mitochondrial DNA of tissues of ageing humans. *Biochemical and Biophysical Research Communications*, **195**, 1104–10.

# 2

# Sociological approaches to age and ageing

## Sarah Harper

## Introduction

Current sociological approaches to understanding ageing can be seen to address the theoretical constructs of *continuity and discontinuity* of the life course, and the *configuration and reconfiguration* of public and private personal networks. Changes which occur in later life, such as retirement and widowhood, lead to discontinuities in roles and relationships and require the reconfiguration of social networks. However, there are many roles and relationships which remain the same as we age, allowing continuity and the maintenance of stable personal networks.

Sociological approaches have, however, tended to neglect the actual concept of *age* itself. While concepts of *class*, *race* and *gender* have been explored fully, the variable *age* is less well understood. Yet the concepts of *age* and *ageing* need to be explored at various dichotomous levels: historically and contemporarily; individually and societally; biologically and socially.

## Understanding concepts in age and ageing

### Old age in history

There have been several analyses of the experiences and representations of age and ageing over time (Finley, 1984; Minois, 1989; Pelling and Smith, 1991; Parkin, 1992; Achenbaum, 1995; Shahar, 1997). As Kertzer (1995) points out, our notion of the historical reality of later life sits somewhere between images of a time in which the old were treated with respect, when they occupied positions of power by virtue of their control over family holdings, and when they were surrounded and supported by married children and grandchildren; and a time when old people crowded meagre public charitable facilities to allow them to survive in a society that gave little support to those lacking the ability or the health to earn their daily living. In the first scenario modernization is heralded as the tragic perpetrator/executor of doom, with older people as the victims of progress. In the second, modernization brings with it welfare reforms and older people are the beneficiaries of social programmes and intergenerational transfers. In fact, historically the social and political arrangements for older adults have varied considerably between and within societies, and over time, and were moderated by factors such as class and gender.

Pictures which emerge from these suggest that there was always a clear understanding of the heterogeneity of later life, and that the experience of ageing and old age was acutely different for men and for women. There was a recognition that old age could be broadly divided into a more active span and a more frail one, but also that capacity varied in later life, and was not necessarily in line with chronological age. Old age has thus been long divided into what in early modern England was called the 'green old age', a time of fitness and activity, albeit with some failing powers, and a final phase of decrepitude and frailty (Thane, 2000). This division is still recognized today in the notions of the Third and Fourth Ages. The Third Age is now associated with healthy active retirement, and as such is even conceived as commencing at age 50 (Harper and Leeson, 2004), and the period of increasing disability that may occur sometime between 80 and 100 is noted as the Fourth Age.

### Age as a concept

While there is an extensive literature on the meaning of *old age*, analysis of the notion of age *per se* has been less well rehearsed (Kertzer and Keith, 1984; Kertzer and Schaie, 1989). Yet, within Western societies, the naturalness of the use of *chronological age* in the marking of our lives is instilled within us from our early socialization. So culturally immersed are we, that the view is almost taken for granted that there is no satisfactory alternative to chronology as an indicator of age. This is reflected in a spectrum of ways: from the social recognition of the importance of annual ageing, with the emphasis on anniversaries such as birthdays, to the legal entrenchment of chronological age as a marker for a series of life transitions—age of consent, age of majority, age of retirement, etc.

One standpoint (Hazelrigg, 1997), however, is that age *per se* explains very little, perhaps nothing of abiding interest. Age itself is not a cause of anything. It is part of the trait description of persons, a classification variable, the title of a set of categories in a particular classification system. Even its use as a social marker tells us very little about any contemporary individual of that age. The fact that individuals are enfranchised in many European countries at 18 tells us little about the maturity of a particular 18-year-old, other than that they live in a society which regards 18 to be the norm for the population of attaining some level of political maturity. Similarly the fact that the pensionable age for many individuals throughout the West is 65 again does not inform us about any particular 65-year-old, other than that they live in a society which regards 65 to be the age at which the majority of the working population require some kind of supplementary assistance to maintain an income. Indeed, as we shall discuss later, this is based on an historical model which, in most cases, is now bereft of any relevance to contemporary health or capability status. One could thus argue that the labels 'aged 18' and '65' simply tell us that the particular individuals have survived for 18 and 65 years, respectively.

Mate selection appears to be age sensitive to some degree. Firstly, it is age sensitive in that the sexual intercourse component of mating behaviour is proscribed in most Western societies until an age-eligibility threshold has been reached, though this age varies between societies. It also appears to be age sensitive in that the ages of most couples fall within a short chronological range, on average within a 5-year band. This may be an outcome of selection on age, or it may be a proxy for other traits such as fecundity or congruent life expectancy. Alternatively, it may be a factor of proximity and availability, for at the time of initial mate selection younger people are legally inaccessible and those who are older fall outside the range of normal social interaction as delimited by education, or have already been selected. Analysis of age variation among couples in second and subsequent marital and cohabiting unions reveals greater variance than in first union, on average up to 15 years for example.

## Age as a variable

A key question is whether age is able to have the same analytical coherency as race, class, or gender. Riley, for example, regards age as a classification variable of social status (Riley, 1987), while Minkler and Estes (1999) deny that age *per se* has any salience as an analytical variable, arguing instead that it is only through its association with gender and class that we can understand its relationship to power structures and access to resources. Hazelrigg (1997) argues that beyond its use by individuals and groups to date events, a simple marker in the regulation of the process of living, age itself is of little importance. There are hierarchies of power where gender is the determining factor, others where class is dominant, and yet others, as we shall see, where age is key. On the whole, sex, race, and ethnicity are fixed characteristics of individuals, class and religion have the potential to be mobile, while mobility across age strata is universal.

## Age and the individual

From the perspective of the individual, age classification introduces signposts *linking memory and anticipation, an iteratively remembered past and an iteratively expected future* (Hazelrigg, 1997). Age classification is thus integral to the normal organization of consciousness. As Mead's extensive work on life history, reminiscence, and autobiography informs us, one interacts retrospectively with one's younger selves, recalling earlier states of self-hood; and prospectively with one's older selves, anticipating later states of self-hood (Mead, 1934). What is of interest is that we as individuals are able both to conceptualize age as an internal process, a marker, a lived experience, and a regulator of consciousness and memory, and at the same time accept the reality of age as an institutionalized series of sequences and an externally articulated attribute.

Modern life is lived in two separate registers. On the one hand, most of a life experience is formed directly and indirectly in a highly standardized sequence of institutionalized events—schooling, work, parenting, retirement. On the other hand, there are those aspects of life experiences that are not institutionalized and structurally stabilized in recognized life course sequences—self-image, personal satisfaction, existential aesthetics, etc. (Hazelrigg,1997)

Tensions arise when the two registers fail to coincide—that is the internal register falls out of synchrony with that regulated by society. This may be referred to as 'off time' (Hochschild, 1973). Examples include middle-aged couples falling in love and publicly exhibiting displays of physical affection and romance, or older people adopting student-style lives (Hagestad, 1986). Off time may also include the experience of being forced, through illness or external factors, to fall outside the normal behaviour range as defined for one's age.

## Age and society

For both the individual and society, age conveniently dissects the life course into more manageable components. With the arrival of capitalism and industrialization, chronological age was a useful tool to divide and regulate the population (Thomas, 1979; Marshall, 1985; Kohli, 1986; Keith *et al.*, 1994) and for coping with the need for rationalization, succession, social control, and integration. Age defined the responsibilities of citizenship, including adulthood and labour-force participation, regulating the entry and exit to economic activity (Hazelrigg, 1997). Others argue that that the task of the individual is to build and maintain a stable identity. An institutionalized life course is one way to regulate this individual change over time. It arrays ages of self-hood into a predictable sequence of states and transitions that satisfies many of the demands of population management on a societal scale (Fortes, 1984).

## Age stratification

*Age stratification theory* was proposed by Riley and colleagues (Riley *et al.*, 1972) in the 1970s. Age is defined as both a process and a structure, with individual ageing comprising psychological and biological development alongside the experience of entering and exiting social roles (Riley and Riley, 1994) Using the dual concepts of *allocation*, the process whereby individuals are assigned and reassigned to roles, and *socialization*, the instructing of individuals as to how to perform new life course roles, they suggested that these two concepts moderate between social structures relating to individuals of given ages and social structures relating to roles open to individuals of given ages (with their age-related expectations and sanctions). Age stratification theory thus promotes the idea that societies organize the distributions of rewards and opportunities, and develop sets of behavioural expectations based on the stratifying characteristics of its members, with chronological age as a central element in the system (McMullin, 2000). Societies are structured and individuals stratified on the basis of age. Over time two separate processes occur as the age structures change and individuals themselves age. These processes are both independent and separate and also, at some level, interdependent.

As Harper (2006) concludes, age is an *indicator*, as opposed to a determinant, of biological and psychological changes; it can be a *determinant* of individuals' allocated roles, independent of their biological or psychological capacity; it has *analytical value* as a descriptive variable; and it identifies at any given time point *birth-cohort membership*, and thus potentially shared cohort life experiences.

## Age and the life course

The life course in complex societies is thus based on a combination of generational and chronological age (Elder, 1985; Hagestad and Neugarten, 1985; Fry, 1999). It is necessary to combine age with other social characteristics (gender, race, and class, for example) to understand specific life experiences for men and women across the life course.

Two life-course themes—*timing* and *process*—have been identified. *Timing* relates to the incidence, duration, and sequence of roles throughout the life course (Moen, 1996). Thus, understanding an individual's life-course employment history is more useful than understanding their employment position at any one point. *Process* focuses on ageing as a series of life transitions (Elder, 1985). Each phase of life is understood in relation to prior phases, and is mediated by other variables of gender, class, and race. The transition to parenthood, for example, is experienced very differently by men and women, and the transition to parent of a non-dependent child, the so-called *empty nest syndrome*, is mediated both by gender and by the experience of active parenting itself.

A starting point for life-course analysis is the acknowledgement of the historical *context* within which different cohorts experience different aspects of the life course. It is clearly important to recognize the cohort and period influences here (Elder and O'Rand, 1995). As Harper (2006) explores, while most older men experienced a long period of economic activity followed by abrupt retirement, many older Western women experienced their younger lives within a framework of primary domestic duties, supplemented by intermittent economic activity. As a result, most older women replaced low earning capacity or economic dependence in younger life, with low incomes in old age. Cohorts in mid life, however, have had very different social and economic frameworks within which to live out their lives. Half the labour force in many countries is now female, and full-time economic employment (with or without domestic responsibilities, childcare in particular) is becoming a widespread experience for many women. Despite this, there are still considerable disparities in the earning capacity of mid-life men and women. However, it is likely that future cohorts of older women will have higher incomes relative to the older women of today, and the gender disparity in incomes will be lower.

## Age in cultural contexts

The intersection of age with gender, race, and class, or status groups, thus produces specific life experiences for men and women across the life course. The connection of the life course with age is far weaker in traditional societies. Various anthropological studies (Makoni and Stroeken, 2002) have highlighted alternative ways in which the life course might be structured, though by the late 20th century the influence of the state and penetration of chronological age as an ordering variable was evident in most of the research sites. In Stroeken's study of the Sukama of north-west Tanzania, for example, rather than individuals being marked by a physical body, they were defined by a zone, incorporating the large network of their life-course events. The social status of elderhood was thus measured by the accumulated wealth of alliances, offspring, and livestock, which could not be diminished through ill-health or loss of mental capacity. The Gussui of south-western Kenya (Okemwa, 2002) have a similar notion of elderhood. However, they have adapted this traditional seniority gradation, based on networks and affiliations, to modern demands, and have incorporated such aspects as the role of entrepreneur into the criteria for achieving successful seniority status. As a consequence, elders no longer have a precise measure by which to gauge their successful attainment of elderhood.

Neither the !Kung nor Herero, hunter-gatherer and Bantu pastoralist peoples, respectively, of Botswana, have a concept of chronological age. They were unable to perceive similarities between members of different age groups, nor conceive that there should be any. Their concept of ageing is of a slow inexorable process of physical decline, but with a tempo of this process which varies widely among individuals, so that a person who retains health at age 70 does much the same thing every day as does a 50-year-old (Okemwa, 2002). While the Herero or !Kung mark changes in age by physical transitions, the Tuareg, semi-nomadic people in northern Niger, use social transitions. Courtship, marriage, childbirth, and grandchildren mark the steps in ageing, not number of years survived (Rasmussen, 1997).

# Understanding old age as post-reproductive life

The percentage of people surviving to old age, and extreme old age, within each cohort has increased significantly over the past 100 years. A key question thus concerns the role of this extensive post-reproductive portion of the lifespan found in humans. Indeed, modern female humans within economically advanced societies can expect to live nearly one-third of their adult lives in a post-reproductive state.

The existence of an extensive post-reproductive life in humans has inspired an at times heated debate between biologists and anthropologists. The discussion can be simply put as follows. Some believe that the female menopause is an adaptive consequence of natural selection, probably as a solution to the trade-off between investing in additional offspring, or in existing offspring and their children (Hill and Hurtado, 1991; Kaplan, 1997). If this long post-reproductive period of the lifespan was formed through evolution, what is its role? And, given the very rapid changes in modern environments, what kinds of responses and variability might occur. Others argue that this post-reproductive life of human females is a modern effect due to environmentally induced increases in longevity (Austad, 1997). In other words, the protection offered by our current environment has enabled us to live much longer than the period within which natural selection has moulded our reproductive capacity.

## The evolution of the menopause

Most arguments have accepted the longevity of humans as given, and then asked what type of selective forces would result in the menopause. Selection for the cessation of reproduction has generally been seen as a solution to trade-offs between two broad types of investment. Firstly, a trade-off between early and late reproduction, secondly between the reproductive value of existing kin and the production of additional descendants. Both cases rely on the assumption that the children of older women will be of a lower reproductive value. This is due to the increased chance of less viable children following from genetic abnormalities, or due to the higher probability of the parents dying while the children are still young and vulnerable.

Kaplan (1997) suggests that perhaps the cost of increasing the length of the reproductive period is a decrease in energy available for reproduction early in life. Thus selection might favour allocating more resources to the early reproductive period, at the expense of ending reproduction in mid-life. Two assumptions operate. Firstly, given that the children of older women are assumed to be of a lower reproductive value, the cost of the menopause would therefore be low. Secondly, by ceasing to reproduce, older people can bring benefits, by investing in the reproduction of their offspring and other kin. This has been called the *grandmother hypothesis*. Thus if the cost of the menopause is low, and the benefits are high, the existence of the menopause could maximize the biological fitness of the species (Kaplan, 1997).

Carey and Gruenfelder (1997), for example, point out that there is clearly some association between extended longevity of a species and complex social structures, and that older group members appear to play an important role in sustaining the latter. Older members of a variety of non-human species play important roles in the cohesion and dynamics of their populations, serving as guardians, leaders, teachers, caregivers, and midwives, sometimes in an apparently altruistic role (Altmann, 1980; Hrdy, 1981; L.L. Rogers, 1987; Hill and Hurtado, 1991; A.R. Rogers, 1993). Post-reproductive female life appears common among most primate species, particularly chimpanzees and gorillas (Caro et al., 1995). In Hrdy's and Altman's work we find examples of both leadership and caregiving roles. Thus both male and female older primates take on leadership of their troops, with the specific gender varying between primate species. Older females also play an important role in caregiving, with evidence from vervets that the presence of grandmothers can more than halve infant mortality (Fairbanks and McGuire, 1986). In addition, as Hrdy points out, in some species, the rank of the older females is passed on to their daughters, thus carrying on into subsequent generations all the advantages or disadvantages that the rank may hold. Finally, Hrdy also highlights the altruistic role some older female primates play in risking their own lives to defend the troop. A similar, apparently altruistic, role, is also found in female black bears (Rogers 1987), who frequently shift their territories away from areas overlapping with their daughters, thereby reducing their own foraging area in favour of their offspring.

Let us now move to explore two frameworks within which ageing and later life are constructed. The first adopts the perspective of the individual: their position and experience of work and retirement. The second focuses on family, intergenerational relationships, and the changing roles of individuals within them.

## Understanding retirement

The acceptance of mass retirement for all at broadly fixed chronological but increasingly younger ages, in order to carry out a fulfilled leisure- and consumption-based healthy period of late life is historically very new. It is a post-war phenomenon. It arose in the second half of the 20th century to cope with specific health and socio-economic needs of the then older population, and in response to the changing demands of the labour market. Mass withdrawal by workers at state pension age has been extended to ever younger ages over the last 30 years through the spread of early retirement practices (Harper and Laslett, 2005).

To put this in a historical perspective, there has been a steady withdrawal in most OECD countries from employment at earlier ages throughout the 20th century (Costa, 1998). In the UK in 1881, when male life expectancy at birth was less than 42 years, three-quarters of men aged over 65 were economically active (Riddle, 1984). By 1931 male life expectancy at birth had risen to 58; 70% of those aged 65–69 were still economically active, and 37% of those over 70. Thirty years later, male life expectancy at birth had reached 67 years of age, and economic activity had fallen to 40% for those aged 65–69 and 10% for those over age 70 (Harper and Laslett, 2005).

The figures in the immediate post-war period are confused. Firstly there was a male labour shortage due to the impact of the Second World War. It is likely that this in part was compensated for by older male workers remaining longer in employment. In 1948 there was the introduction of public pensions conditional on retirement from full-time employment, and it is likely that this began to encourage retirement at 65, though the effects would have been staggered over the next 20 years. Older workers found the increase in pace required by the increasing mechanization of many production processes more difficult than younger workers and this too may have encouraged retirement (Le Gros Clark, 1968). Similarly, employers, coping with increasing bureaucratized organizations with a heavy administrative structure, used a retirement age to regulate the workforce (Harper and Thane, 1986; Harper 1989).

This period saw a steady move towards fixed retirement ages. While around one quarter of firms had fixed retirement ages in the 1940s and 1950s (Ministry of Labour 1945–55; Shenfield 1997), these had increased to two-thirds by the early 1960s (Acton Society Trust, 1960; Heron and Chown, 1961), particularly in large, technological industries with complex administrative structures (Green, 1963). By the mid-1960s, major industries such as such as chemicals, iron and steel, and the nationalized coal mines and railways, all operated with rigid retirement ages. Alongside this ran growing ageism towards older workers. Already by 1957, there was a recognition that discrimination by employers against men over 50 was becoming widespread (Shenfield, 1957; Industrial Welfare Society, 1951).

The medical profession supported the *retirement impact hypothesis* (McMahon and Ford, 1995) leading to widespread public acceptance that retirement led to ill-health, deterioration, and death:

> The literature is overwhelming in its indications that retirement is detrimental to the health of older men.
>
> Anderson and Cowan (1954, p. 1346)

> …the weight of medical opinion is that sudden demise of mental and bodily functions, previously regularly exercised, such as may happen through retirement is likely to cause atrophy and degeneration which are harmful to the health of older persons.
>
> Shenfield (1997, p. 59)

Indeed the literature, far from being overwhelming, was negligible in the UK (Harper, 1989), and under debate in the USA (Granick, 1952). Yet, it was clearly useful for the government in its campaign to retain older workers to promote such views:

> After six weeks of this existence, life began to pall. He became unsettled, restless and irritable. He really had nothing to do and longed to be back at work. He was repeatedly asked to take up some hobby, which he readily promised to do but his restlessness prevented him from seriously attempting it and a laissez-faire attitude resulted.

Eventually getting up in the morning became an effort, and in a short time all his interest in everything flagged. The peace of death came to him soon.

Ministry of Health Circular (1954)

There was a dramatic shift in attitudes over the second half of the 20th century, so that a period of funded leisure after leaving employment is now generally regarded as everyone's right. However, as Harper and Thane (1986) point out, current retirement expectations are a post-1960s phenomenon, which arose during the second half of the 20th century in order to cope with the specific socio-economic needs of the growing older population, and in response to the changing administrative and personnel management demands of growing corporations (Harper, 1989; Harper and Thane, 1989).

The introduction of widespread state and increasing employer-based pensions allowed retirement to occur by choice among a healthy active population. No longer was retirement confined to old frail workers, who were either pushed out of the labour market by employers or forced to exit due to ill-health. Retirement was now a choice (Carter and Sutch, 1996). The increase in late life health, and the spread of private pensions and occupational pensions, encouraged the growth of late life consumption and leisure activities. Retirement based on leisure has replaced retirement out of physical necessity. By the 1980s, the internalization of the period of funded leisure at the end of one's working life had become firmly established. The notion of retirement has thus been redefined from one of *Rest* in the 1940s and 1950s, to *Reward* in the 1970s to a *Right* by the 1980s (Harper, 2000).

It is, however, the rapid increase in early retirement which has caused most concern. Economic analysis suggests that retirement incentives exist within many national pension systems. As an influential study by Gruber and Wise (1999) reports, part of the diffusion of early retirement practices is motivated by retirement incentives in current pension schemes. State social security provision in some countries offers considerable incentives to early retirement, and may account for a significant part of the long-term decline in rates of economic activity for older men. Disability and unemployment programmes have provided early retirement benefits well before the official retirement age. Similarly, accumulated wealth, savings behaviour, and the availability of other sources of income in later life, including state as well as private benefits, are also influential.

Changes within the work environment and labour market still both force and encourage workers to withdraw. These include structural, sectoral, and technological changes, as well as evidence that employers retain ageist attitudes towards older workers. There is some evidence that age discrimination by employers encourages early withdrawal from the labour market and that push factors, such as redundancy or fixed retirement ages, are responsible for a large percentage of early retirements (McKay and Middleton, 1998; Scales and Scase, 2000). There is evidence of a lack of practices aimed at including older workers, lack of training, and lack of flexible working arrangements (David and Pilon, 1990; Gibson, 1993; Lussier and Wister, 1995; Bellemarre et al., 1998); and evidence that employers are also reluctant to employ older workers (Harper et al, 2006). There are perceived factors which might discourage employers from recruiting older workers: the perception that they lack appropriate skills, lack qualifications, and offer a low return on training investment (Leeson and Harper, 2006).

Health attitudes and behaviours towards disability and frailty have also been important factors, with evidence that retirees are more likely to be in poor health or to have more functional limitations (Quinn et al., 1998; Uccello and Mix, 1998; Humphrey et al., 2003). While ill-health may be given as a socially acceptable reason for retirement (Casey, 1998), there does seem to be consistent evidence that between one-fifth and one-quarter of retirements prior to age 65 can genuinely be assigned to the category of being promoted by 'ill-health' (Maule et al., 1996; Tanner, 1997).

Finally, as Harper (2006) discusses, there is evidence that the current older cohorts have internalized the notion of retirement, including early retirement, as an extended period of funded leisure and consumption after leaving work, and expectations of this are considerably entrenched (Scales and Scase, 2000). Such expectations are now strongly held not only by the employee, but also by his or her partner and wider family (Mutran et al., 1997; Harper, 1999). In particular, both high job satisfaction and having a working spouse decreased the likelihood of retirement, this latter finding being supported elsewhere (Henretta et al., 1993; Uccello and Mix, 1998) including findings that male retirement was nearly twice as likely if the spouse had retired (Henretta et al., 1993). This suggests that social factors are also significant at the individual level of choice. While it might appear counter-intuitive, given that on economic grounds one spouse might be more able to retire if the other was still working, here clearly couples were perceiving retirement as a time of leisure, in which they could carry out jointly shared activities. This is compounded by the growing responsibilities that many of these cohorts have for kin care and support, especially for their parents (Kodz et al., 1999; Anderson, 2001). The interaction of all of these factors with health status and disability in these ages may account for more than a third of early retirements.

Finally, those taking early retirement thus include two distinct groups (Day, 1995; Mutran et al., 1997; Quinn et al., 1998; Uccello and Mix, 1998; Humphrey et al., 2003):

Professional and managerial workers, with high levels of education, and secure well funded pension plans have a higher than average likelihood of withdrawing from economic activity, especially if their pension plan includes a defined benefit component. This may be tempered however by a restraining factor of high enjoyment of work, but also encouraged by increasing levels of stress in these high level occupations. A second group of early retirees comprise those with low levels of education and manual or semi-skilled occupations, who may be being encouraged or forced to take early retirement through employer instigated redundancy schemes. These may be involuntary or nominally voluntary but set in a context of discriminatory and uncomfortable working conditions.

Harper (2006)

## The impact of changing family structures on old age

The second half of the 20th century saw the emergence of a variety of new family structures. Reconstituted stepfamilies, single-parent families, and cohabiting couples now comprise around 25% of Western European families, living alongside European-style nuclear family households, and the various ethnic minority households with their own distinctive family forms. Three main trends can be identified: the ageing of individuals, life transitions, and demographic and social changes, which have impacted upon family structures, roles, relationships, and responsibilities. There has been a general ageing of life transitions, in particular that of the birth of the first child and of leaving the parental home. These have delayed the transition to grandparenthood and the *empty nest syndrome*, and in some cases resulted in childlessness. The demographic factors of falling fertility and mortality have resulted in vertically shaped families, and both the lengthening of adult unions and increases in divorce. Social changes have contributed to the increase in divorce, cohabitation, and reconstituted families. These have all affected the experience of kinship roles, relationships, and responsibilities in old age.

## Impact of ageing life transitions

While public and legal institutions may be lowering the age threshold into full legal adulthood (age of thresholds for inheritance, suffrage, jury service, alcohol and cigarette purchase, licensed driving having all fallen in many societies over the last half century), individuals themselves are choosing to delay many of those transitions which demonstrate a commitment to full adulthood—full economic independence from parents, formal adult union through marriage or committed long-term cohabitation, and parenting (Harper, 2004a,b). As Harper (2006) argues, the *ageing of life transitions* occurs as individuals recognize the general lengthening of their own lifespan and those of their peers. For women in particular, an ever-lengthening lifespan allow them the liberty to delay childbirth. Because infant mortality has fallen, and because early death through disease, war, famine, and (for women) reproduction is no longer the common experience, individuals feel more comfortable about establishing marital unions later in life, bearing children later, and having fewer children.

### Delayed childbirth

There has been in many OECD countries, and indeed also now in some parts of Asia and Latin America, a consistent delaying in birth of first child, with the mean age of first birth in the EU, for example, rising from 24 to 28 in the last four decades of the 20th century (Table 2.1).

Delaying the birth of the first child may lead to long intergenerational spacings, and a transition to both parenthood and grandparenthood at a later age than has been the recent historical norm. It delays the age at which the parent experiences the child leaving the family home, which is also being delayed by a general increase in the age at which the child '*flies the nest*'.

### Delayed independent living

Within most countries of the EU and the USA, young people are *leaving home* at a later age. Within Europe, every EU15 member state, with the exception of Denmark and The Netherlands, saw an increase between 1987 and 1996 in those aged 20–29 years continuing to live with their parents. In 1996, more than 80% of Spanish, Portuguese, and Italian men and women aged 20–24 years lived in the parental home, and over 50% of 25–29 year olds. The proportion of young adults who live with their parents has also increased in the USA. In 1997, 15% of men and 8% of women aged 25–34 years lived at home with their parents, an increase since 1970 of 10% and 7%, respectively (Goldscheider and Goldscheider, 1994). Furthermore, even those children who choose to spend a protracted period of time outside the parental home before setting up their own home increasingly remain economically dependent on their parents through, for example, subsidized boarding and rental

**Table 2.1** Mean age of women at birth of first child in the European Union, 1960–2000. Source: Council of Europe (2001), European Demographic Data Sheet (2006).

|                  | 1960 | 1970 | 1980 | 1990 | 1995 | 2000 | 2004       |
|------------------|------|------|------|------|------|------|------------|
| Austria          |      |      | 24.3 | 25.0 | 25.6 | 26.3 | 27.0       |
| Belgium          | 24.8 | 24.3 | 24.7 | 26.4 |      |      | 27.6       |
| Denmark          | 23.1 | 23.8 | 24.6 | 26.4 | 27.4 |      | 28.4       |
| Finland          | 24.7 | 24.4 | 25.6 | 26.5 | 27.2 | 27.4 | 27.8 (2003) |
| France           | 24.8 | 24.4 | 25.0 | 27.0 | 28.1 | 28.7 | 28.4       |
| Germany          | 25.0 | 24.0 | 25.0 | 26.6 | 27.5 | 28.0 | 29.0       |
| Greece           |      | 24.5 | 24.1 | 25.5 | 26.6 | 27.3 | 28.0 (2003) |
| Ireland          |      | 25.5 | 25.5 | 26.6 | 27.3 | 27.8 | 28.5       |
| Italy            | 25.7 | 25.0 | 25.0 | 26.9 | 28.0 |      | 28.7 (2001) |
| Luxembourg       |      |      |      |      | 27.4 | 28.4 | 28.6       |
| Netherlands      | 25.7 | 24.8 | 25.7 | 27.6 | 28.4 | 28.6 | 28.9       |
| Portugal         |      |      | 24.0 | 24.9 | 25.8 | 26.4 | 27.1       |
| Spain            |      | 25.1 | 25.0 | 26.8 | 28.4 | 29.0 | 29.2 (2003) |
| Sweden           | 25.5 | 25.9 | 25.3 | 26.3 | 27.2 | 27.9 | 28.6       |
| United Kingdom   |      |      |      | 27.3 | 28.3 | 29.1 | 27.5       |

expenses, assistance with home buying, and prolonged and expensive investment in education.

This extended economic dependence on parents not only delays the individual's full transition to independent adulthood, but also the experience for the parents of losing the last child from the family home—the *empty-nest syndrome*—the extended post-parental period following the departure from the family home of the child or children. In some societies, this is associated with a period of apparent grieving, especially for mothers.

These two phenomena, delayed first birth and delayed independence from parents, are clearly linked, and in addition they are influencing a third phenomenon, increasing childlessness.

### Childlessness

The later an individual has a child, the fewer children that individual has, with significant implications for their care and support in later life. As Uhlenberg has pointed out, in terms of support for older people the critical distinction is between one and none. Significantly, though, increasing childlessness in cohorts born after 1960 means that fewer adult children will have simultaneous commitments to an older parent and to children. So childlessness in today's younger cohorts paradoxically leads to more time being available for caregiving to older relatives. Furthermore, in both the USA and the UK, the highest percentage within the last century of very old women without children or with just one child occurred in the 1990s, among cohorts born at the around the beginning of the 20th century. One-quarter of these women had no children, and a further quarter had just one child. The proportion of women over 85 years of age with two or more surviving children will actually increase over the next decades, from less than 50% in 1995 to almost 75% by 2015. However, even though this will be followed by an increasing proportion of women with just one or no children, it will not return to the levels of the 1990s—according to current predictions, which run to 2050.

## Demographic ageing

As Harper (2006) points out:

> [T]he shift from a high-mortality/high-fertility society to a low-mortality/low-fertility society, results in an increase in the number of living generations, and a decrease in the number of living relatives within these generations. Increased longevity may increase the duration spent in certain kinship roles, such as spouse, parent of non-dependent child, sibling. A decrease in fertility may reduce the duration of others, such as parent of dependent child, or even the opportunity for some roles, such as sibling.

## Verticalization of family structures

The lengthening of lives combined with a fall in fertility has lead to *intragenerational contraction* and *intergenerational extension*. This is a decrease in the number of members within each generation, and an increase in vertical ties, or in other words an increase in the number of living generations with typically longer gaps between them (Shanas, 1980; Hagestad, 1986, 1988; Bengtson *et al.*, 1990; Lowenstein, 2003; Harper, 2004a; Katz *et al.*, 2005). Individuals will thus grow older having more vertical than horizontal linkages in the family. For example, vertically, a four-generation family structure has three tiers of parent–child relationships, two sets of grandparent–grandchild ties, and one great-grandparent–grandchild linkage. Within generations of this same family, horizontally, ageing individuals will have fewer brothers and sisters. In addition, at the level of extended kin, family members will have fewer cousins, aunts, uncles, nieces, and nephews. However, while the number of living generations will increase, the absolute number of living relatives will decrease (Harper, 2003).

Family members are spending more time in intergenerational family roles than before: more time as parents and children, more time as grandchildren, and more time as great-grandchildren/ great-grandparents. Both the Health and Retirement Survey (HRS, 2004) and the AARP Intergenerational Linkages Survey report more than half of the respondents being members of four-generation families (Bengtson and Harootyan, 1994; Bengtson, 1995; Soldo and Hill, 1995), while Hagestad (1988) reports that a fifth of all women surviving to beyond age 80 years will spend some time in a five-generation family as great-great-grandmothers.

## Lengthening adult unions and parent–child relationships

The common experience of length of marriage at the beginning of the 20th century in the USA was under 25 years for a White couple, and as low as 10 years for an African-American couple (Morgan and Kunkel, 1998). However, as life expectancy has increased, so the potential length of marriage has also lengthened. So that by the end of the 20th century, the majority of those marriages not terminated by divorce were exceeding 40 years (Myers, 1990). Marital satisfaction within these long marriages tends to rise in later life to levels expressed by younger married people, after a typical dip in mid-life (Bengtson *et al.*, 1990). The dimensions which make early and late life marriage happy and successful differ, however, with elements such as physical attraction and passion being replaced by familiarity and loyalty (Reiss, 1960; Brehm, 1992).

Increasing longevity also means that most parent–child relationships will be lived out as predominantly non-dependent adult dyads, this despite the delaying of childbirth. The common experience for many parents and children is around 60 years of joint life, of which under one-third is spent in the traditional parent/dependent-child

relationship. Around one-quarter of UK women and nearly 40% of US women aged 55–63 still have a surviving parent. These women have thus spent around 60 years as a child, some 40 of these years in an adult relationship with a living parent (Grundy, 1999). This relies on *re-bonding* in adulthood, sometimes also referred to as 'reverse bonding' (Harper, 2006). Under such experiences we see a loosening of the association between marital and parental roles As the common experience of parenthood moves to more than 50 years of shared life, parents and children are adjusting to spending most of their relationship as independent adults. Similarly husbands and wives are spending fewer years of their joint lives as parents of young children

> …Relationships which have historically been based on a hierarchy which existed in part to support successful reproduction must move to greater equality, both child-parent, and husband-wife, as traditional roles based on parenthood give way to companionate relationships.

Harper (2006)

However, not only will parents and children spend longer in non-dependent relationships, but the time spent as a child with a dependent parent is also increasing. Within the USA, for example, the time spent as the daughter of a parent over 65 now exceeds the time spent as the mother of a child under 18. This must, however, include the caveat that, while for much of the last two centuries a high proportion of those over 65 would be in varying degrees of dependency on others for some aspect of their daily living, this is now no longer the case. Indeed given that it is now not until after the age 80 of that the crucial stage for relying on children for assistance is reached (Uhlenberg, 1995), we should perhaps be comparing age over 80 with under 18. What is then apparent is that adult US women now spend more time *without* a dependent—albeit a dependent child or potentially dependent parent—than with one.

This has important implications for our understanding of the *sandwich generation*, or *women in the middle phenomenon* (Rossi, 1987) whereby women in particular are faced with coping with simultaneous demands from dependent parents and children. It is thus not that unusual for a mid-life woman to be an active grandmother with childcare responsibilities, mother of a new parent, and daughter of an increasingly frail elderly mother (Harper, 2005).

## Impact of divorce on old age

Owing to the reduction in early widowhood, the rate of marital dissolution has remained remarkably constant, with divorce replacing death as the primary cause of marital break-up. In the 18th century, for example, the average length of an American marriage was 12 years, and well over half of all children spent a part of their childhood in a single-parent or step-family. It has been argued that the potential length of marital unions has placed strains on such relationships, and is a contributory factor in divorce levels. The decline in death rates has made divorce more likely, or even more essential. This, combined with the relaxation of religious and social control, has made divorce more possible. The picture has the additional complexity that widowhood is predominantly a late-life experience, while divorce has been a young and mid-life phenomenon, but it is becoming increasingly common in older age groups.

Most of the research has been on divorce in younger life, but there is now a small but growing literature on the impact of divorce in old age—both early life divorce which does not lead to remarriage or repartnering, and late life divorce itself. Dissolution in younger life often leads to remarriage or cohabitation by one or both partners, introducing a variety of complex reconstituted family structures, which impact upon both reciprocal family care and intergenerational transmission. Dissolution in later life can lead to loneliness, lack of support and care, and loss of roles.

In comparison with non-married people, married people have an advantage which may be measured across both health and socioeconomic variables (Waite, 1995; Waite and Bachrach, 2000). As Waite has pointed out, intact husband–wife families provide a multiple support system for a spouse in terms of emotional, financial, and social exchanges, and married people tend to enjoy higher levels of health and survival, social participation, and life satisfaction than persons who are not married (Waite and Bachrach, 2000). Not only do married people appear to have an advantage in terms of both health and longevity, but this mortality differential between the married and non-married population appears to have increased over the past decades. Among the non-married category at all ages, most studies find the divorced have the highest mortality rate, followed by the widowed, and then the never-married. Divorced men are at an extra disadvantage in relation to widowed men, however, in that they frequently also lose social support networks, which appear more likely to be retained by both widowed men, and widowed and divorced women. Given that women generally have stronger and more multifaceted networks than men, they are able to retain stronger social support following divorce.

Each successive US cohort entering old age in the 20th century experienced lower mortality rates, increasing widowhood, and higher divorce rates over its lifetime. There are indications that this trend is likely to continue, resulting in larger proportions of non-married older persons in the second quarter of this century (Uhlenberg, 1994). The differential implications of widowhood versus death is clearly at their most acute in late life.

Between 1980 and 1996 the percentage of divorced people over 65 in the USA almost doubled from 3.5 to 6.4% (US Bureau of the Census, 1997). These figures emerge from a complex interaction of an increased divorce rate in mid and late life, with a fall, in all age groups, in the rates of remarriage following divorce. At the beginning of the last century, the number of widowed US men aged 55–64 outnumbered those divorced by 20 to 1. By the end of the century divorced men and women outnumbered those widowed, with three times as many male divorcees as widowers. Given the declining mortality for men, and lack of remarriage generally and particularly among older ages, this trend will continue into old age for the next few decades at least. Trends suggest that those currently in mid-life will also be experiencing high rates of divorce in later life.

Research looking at the differing impact of divorce and widowhood on family and intergenerational relationships has suggested that there are significant gender differences in the experience of these. Women face economic decline through both widowhood and divorce, but are able to maintain strong family and other relationships, while men are cut off from personal relationships through divorce to a far greater degree than through widowhood (Hughes and Waite, 2004).

In addition, as Harper (2006) points out, the recombination of new kin relationships following divorce is far more complex than it is following death. In the latter, while new combinations are formed, and have been historically so, there is but one family line to follow.

Marriages cut short by death have only to integrate biographies from the past on remarriage, while those ended by divorce have also to include the new kin narratives, which develop in parallel with their own new family lines.

Older divorced women are as likely as widowed women to co-reside with a child, and supportive intergenerational relationships are likely to continue for widowed, divorced, and married older women. Eighty to ninety per cent of all children live with their mothers after divorce. Mother–child relations for older divorced women remain quite similar to those of women who do not divorce, with, if anything, an intensification of mother–child relationships among divorced women. There is some evidence that maternal attachment by children increases after divorce, and that women intensify their kin relationships generally after divorce (Hagestad, 1986).

Divorced older men appear to do far worse than their younger counterparts. Among older age groups, for example, mortality among divorced men is particular high in relation to married men (Uhlenberg, 1995). In addition, interaction between fathers and their children tends to decline significantly following divorce. Among nationally representative divorced men aged 50–79 years, only half of the fathers saw or communicated with at least one child weekly, only 11% maintained contact with more than one child, and one-third had no contact at all with their children (US National Survey of Families and Households). One US study went so far as to suggest that half of adolescents living with their mothers after divorce had no contact with their fathers (Cherlin, 1992; Bornat *et al.*, 1998). This thus suggests that these men are less likely to have adult children available for them in time of need.

Most studies exploring the impact of divorce on well-being and standard of living have indicated that immediately after divorce younger cohorts appear to experience a general improvement in their economic situation for men, and a significant decline for women (Waite and Bachrach, 2000). However, the interruption of savings and destruction of assets associated with divorce are likely to depress the economic well-being of both men and women divorced in later life. Indeed, the rather limited empirical evidence we have suggests that divorce is associated with lower economic well-being among all older people. Thus, US data on both income and wealth indicate that older persons who are married enjoy much higher standards of living than non-married older persons, with the highest rates of poverty being experienced by those who are divorced—as much as three or four times the married rate (Waite and Bachrach, 2000). Uhlenberg's work on older divorced women, for example, which controlled for both race and educational attainment, found that these women were more likely to continue to work in later life and to reduce living expenses by sharing their homes. In addition, compared with those who were married, never-married, or widowed, divorced men and women both reported higher levels of dissatisfaction with their economic condition (Uhlenberg, 1995). In summary, while older divorced men and women both experience the highest poverty rates of any unmarried group, divorced men experience the highest mortality rates, have weaker social support networks, and have less contact with their children (Fox and Kelly, 1995, Waite, 1995).

Divorce, especially divorce which is not followed by remarriage, is an increasingly common experience, particularly among this age group, and has negative consequences for both men and women, especially in their old age. However, as divorce becomes the common experience of many more older people, the effects of being divorced in later life may be very different in the future. Even so, the prevalence of living alone in old age will increase, especially for men, who formerly escaped being alone in old age due to their greater likelihood of dying before their spouse. In addition, under a regime of low fertility both men and women will have fewer children, and in all Western industrialized countries geographical mobility results in separation from children. Given that, as we discussed earlier, children currently have a higher propensity to remain with the mother after a marital divorce or cohabitation split, an increasing number of men may find themselves without support from a child in later life.

# Social change

## Impact of increasing cohabitation on old age

The second concern is over the increase in *cohabitation*. It is now recognized that there are different types of cohabitation: a series of short-term, frequently dissolved temporary relationships; single pre-marriage cohabitation; and long-term stable marital-type unions. Thus, many of the existing and future consensual unions may well support the long-term vertical and lateral kin relationships developed through marriage. However, most studies do not distinguish between the different forms of cohabitation (Lesthaege, 1992; Lewin, 1992). While demographically most people still end up in a marital union at some time in their lives, and most cohabitations will end up as marriages, we still know little about the impact of a period of cohabitation on later life or on wider family relationships (Haskey, 1992; McRae, 1993). Indeed our general understanding of cohabitation, particularly outside the Scandinavian countries, is limited. The debate as to the processes behind its growth continues to be polarized between those who see it is a protest against conventional living and those who regard it as a practical living arrangement for turn-of-the-century industrialized society (Lesthaege, 1992).

There is discussion, for example, as to whether marital union between existing cohabitating partners is in some sense different from other marriages, since in the former case the existing union is transformed without any actual change in living arrangements (thus they are termed transformations). It is unclear as to whether such transition to marriage necessitates an alteration in the norms and expectations of the relationship, or whether marriage following cohabitation is primarily a confirmation of the relationship which has been already established (Lewin, 1992). Most of the consensual unions which are not dissolved evolve into marriages with high levels of dissolution risks. Indeed, if couple formation and dissolution rates remain constant, only 10% of all consensual unions compared with 70% of all marriages would last until death.

Perhaps the potentially biggest impact is from the growth of cohabitations in later life, particularly following divorce, as these are less likely to end in marriage. By 1998 around 15% of all cohabitations in Australia, for example, were among the 40–59 year age group (Australian Bureau of Statistics, 1998). It may be that such late life alliances do not provide the stability for the extensive cross-kin interactions and relationships which are supported within marriage-based families or step families. This may be particularly important in terms of reciprocal care in late life. However, the assertion that these relationships are less stable is based primarily on evidence from younger cohabiting couples. As older adults move to this form of mid- and late-life union, the picture may be very different.

## Reconstituted families and old age

The new family forms emerging this century include the linking of multi-'bean pole' families, thereby creating the horizontal or extended step family. Second marriages and subsequent birth of children often have to be assimilated into the on-going relationship between a former husband and wife, in addition to the assimilation of a former spouse's latest offspring, and the inclusion of step siblings and half-siblings from current and previous marriages. The process by which family members set about rewriting their new roles and relationships, becoming in essence new kin to each other, is unclear. Indeed, while the downward generations are often considered, few have explored this question in relation to antecedent generations—how modern families incorporate grandparents, step-grandparents, and grandparents-in-law into the complex network of modern Western kinship. Following the dissolution of a marriage with children, new relationships pivoting around those children must be sustained and re-created, including maintaining extended family relationships, which though cast off by the parents are blood-linked to the children. Among the most viable of these are grandparents. One family today may well have several lateral tiers of grandparents, each with a biological link to one or more children of a reconstituted family.

## Grandparenting

As was indicated earlier, demographic and life-course changes have changed the experience of grandparenting. The opportunity for greater interaction across generations has increased because of the increase in the number of living grandparents (Uhlenberg, 1980).

As Kornhaber (1996) argues, conceptualizing grandparenthood as a developmental process is helpful in understanding its many complexities and variations, the factors which promote successful grandparenting, and the conflicts which lead to dysfunctional grandparenting. In particular, how an individual proceeds from parenthood to grandparenthood, and even great-grandparenthood, determines both their self-identity and their roles and functions as a grandparent. In addition, interaction between family members is an important determinant of family life in later years: the experience of the relationship that grandchildren have with their grandparents earlier will partially determine the way they take on the role and relate to their own grandchildren later on in life (King and Elder,1997)

Our understanding of grandparent relationships has drawn on concepts from family sociology. The work of Bengtson on solidarity within multigenerational families is of importance here; he also emphasizes a life-course perspective and the inclusion of cohort and period effects into our understanding (Bengtson *et al.*, 1996). This perspective is also clearly described by Szinovacz (1998), who argues that grandparents whose cohort values an active and companionate relationship with grandchildren, and whose life stage and that of their grandchildren is unencumbered with other commitments, will have higher role involvement than others in the role. Other sociological theories which have been applied to the study of grandparenthood include *role theory*, which has been adopted to suggest that a successful transition to grandparenthood requires some socialization to the role, and appropriate life-course timing (Szinovacz, 1998); and *social stress theory*, which is used to argue that stress associated with transition to grandparenthood is related to the number, type, and context of the transitions, and moderated by gender, education, income, and race (Szinovacz, 1998).

Various roles of grandparenthood have been identified. Bengtson (1985), for example, identifies what he refers to as five separate symbolic functions of grandparents: being there; grandparents as national guard; family watchdog; arbiters who perform negotiations between (family) members; and participants in the social construction of family history. Harper *et al.*'s (2004) study of grandmothers identifies grandmother as carer, replacement partner (confidante, guide, and facilitator), replacement parent (listener, teacher, and disciplinarian), and as family anchor (transferring values, attitudes, and history).

Currently, women can expect to become grandmothers in their 50s and 60s due to the early first age of births in the 1960s and 1970s. In addition, grandparental roles are lasting far longer due to increased longevity (Watkins *et al.*, 1987) and with that the grandparent is more likely to be able to build a relationship with their grandchild into their adulthood (Hagestad, 1988). As a result many grandmothers in particular now face simultaneous demands as children of possibly frail and dependent parents, mothers, and grandmothers, as well as possibly still being in full or part-time economic employment (Harper, 2005). Grandmothers have more influence in almost every value domain over their grandchildren than do grandfathers (Roberto and Stroes, 1995). Cunningham-Burley (1986) notes that grandparenthood is an especially desirable status for grandmothers, and Thompson *et al.* (1990) and Dench *et al.* (1999) both identify grandmothers as the 'central' grandparent. Thompson *et al.* (1990) in their study found that grandchildren only ever mentioned grandmothers, implying that they are regarded as the single real grandparent. One obvious reason for this is that child rearing has been a culturally encouraged area of competence for women throughout their life course, thus grandmothers are most often drawn into caring for their grandchildren (Hagestad and Neugarten, 1985; Hagestad, 1986).

Maternal grandmothers are consistently noted as having the most contact and closest relationship with their grandchildren. Findings show that maternal grandparents are more likely to have frequent contact with grandchildren, and that grandchildren tend to have a stronger bond with maternal grandparents (Henretta *et al.*, 1993; Harper *et al.*, 2004). However, paternal grandparents play an important role, and this is evident especially where grandsons are concerned (Barranti, 1985). Emphasis on maternal grandmothers has perpetuated the matrifocal tilt in grandparent research, supporting the notion that familial continuity is most likely to persist through women, and that women of all ages are likely to retain the closest links with their child and grandchild (Matthews and Sprey, 1984; Hagestad and Neugarten, 1985). Maternal grandmothers are also considered more influential than paternal grandparents in terms of promoting 'closeness' and a 'sense of security' (Hyde and Gibbs, 1993). Harper *et al.* (2004) also found that grandmothers through the maternal line generally held the strongest involvement with grandchildren, though this is mediated by the grandmother's age, health, and proximity to her grandchildren.

Research into the role of grandfathers has been limited (Kivett, 1991; Radin *et al.*, 1991; Mann, 2007). However, it has been proposed that men become more nurturing as they get older and it could be hypothesized that these qualities might be expressed in relationships with their grandchildren (Dench *et al.*, 1999). Similarly, the need to consider grandfathers as important resources for teenage mothers who are rearing their children has been stressed (Radin *et al.*, 1991). Harper *et al.* (2004) also found that grandfathers could act as replacement partners and replacement fathers in female single-parent households.

## Family care in old age

Increasing life expectancy at later ages implies that more members of successive cohorts reach the age at which help with activities of daily living may be required, and family members are a likely source of at least some of this help. Given the rapidly changing demography of the family, and the impact this is having on kin roles and relationships, there are concerns that families will be unable to sustain the increasing care of the elderly which will be required. Declining fertility implies a reduction in the number of kin available to provide care, changing family structures and age transitions influence the availability and willingness of younger generations to care, and changing female activity across the life course, in particular, reduces the availability and willingness of women to care (Wolf and Soldo, 1994). In addition, the increase in the number of step and reconstituted—so-called 'blended'—families suggests that kin networks will increasingly comprise family members with highly diverse levels of connectedness and commitment to each other (Finch and Wallis, 1994; Wachter, 1997; Bornat *et al.*, 1998, 1999; Haskey, 1998; Dimmock *et al.*, 2004).

Intergenerational transfers of care and services generally flow from older to younger generations, declining during the life course. However, in later life the flow from younger to older generations increases and comes to dominate the intergenerational exchange (HRS, 2004). From a peak of parent to child transfers when the parents are in their early 60s, and/or the children are young adults, this declines rapidly, so that as the parent reaches their mid-70s the child to parent transfers begin to dominate (Kohli and Kunemund, 2003; Litwin, 2004).

However, despite the growth in individual household living and individualistic values, in complex recombinant families, and in dispersed living arrangements (Grundy, 1987; Grundy and Harrop, 1992; McGlone, 1996; Mason, 1999; Scott *et al.*, 1999) families still play an important role in late life, remaining committed, both in terms of expressed attitudes and behaviour, to caring for and supporting their kin.

Around two-thirds of the care provided to older people within the EU comes from within the family (Anderson, 2004). In the UK, in particular, spouses and children supplement formal care for elderly people by up to 80% of required community based care (Green, 1988; Arber and Gilbert, 1989; Arber and Ginn, 1992; Twigg, 1992; Askham, 1998). Family structure, including number and proximity of children, cultural values, which determine the kin relationship, gender, or numerical positioning of the child, followed by family history and personal characteristics, are key in the decision as to who should provide primary care and support to a frail older relative. This is likely to be a spouse or child, and most likely a daughter. Although men, particularly husbands, are increasingly providing care, the majority of carers are still female (Finch, 1989; Harper and Lund, 1989; Dwyer and Coward, 1991; Marks 1996; McGarry, 1998; Ikels, 2004).

Given the high reliance on family caregivers, current concerns include the lack of children, increasing levels of female employment, and unstable adult relationships.

### Lack of children

The availability of children to provide care depends on the number of offspring and their individual characteristics. The child's employment, geographical distance from the parent, and presence of their own children affects the caregiving network, by raising or lowering that child's availability (Anderson, 2001). For example, Henretta reports for the USA that having one's own children or having more education reduce the probability of providing elder care (Wolf *et al.*, 1997). Alternatively, children who have received earlier financial help from the parent are more likely to provide care for a parent later (Henretta *et al.*, 1997).

### Cohabitation

The concern that consensual unions will not provide stable extensive cross-kin relationships is based on evidence from younger cohabiting couples. Many of the existing and future consensual unions will be formed in mid and later life by older adults, and may well support the long-term vertical and lateral kin relationships developed through marriage. In addition, while divorce may be replacing death in long marriages, those marriages which do survive appear to provide a strong base for elder care, particularly by the spouse. There is some valid concern, however, over the rise in divorce and the impact this has on men. Interaction between fathers and their children tends to decline significantly following divorce, indicating that these men are less likely to have adult children available for them in time of need (Harper, 2004a).

### Female employment

There is concern that increasing levels of mid-life female employment reduce the time available to provide care for a dependent parent. The percentage of women aged between 45 and 65 in the US labour market has risen since 1960 from one-third to two-thirds (US Bureau of the Census, 1998; Johnson and Lo Sasso, 2004). However, the relationship between female caring and labour market responsibilities is complex, and one cannot make direct predictions (Wolf and Soldo, 1994). There does appear, however, to be a negative, but rather small effect, on both hours worked and amount of care given (University of Wisconsin, 2003; National Institute on Aging/Duke University, 2006; US Census Bureau, 2006; United States Bureau of Labor Statistics, 2007). This suggests that as more women assume important roles in the labour market, providing time-intensive personal care assistance will become increasingly difficult for them. In particular Johnson and Lo Sasso (2004) suggest that devoting time to the informal care of elderly parents may be incompatible with full-time paid employment at mid-life. It is clear that special work arrangements, including flexible work schedules and part-time work, may be necessary if persons with frail family members are to balance successfully their work and caregiving responsibilities.

It is also important to recognize that increasingly it is spouses who care for each other in later life. For example, over a quarter of men in a German study were giving care to a spouse, and 10% of men in their 80s in England are primary caregivers for their wives. Furthermore, of those men who were caring, 60% were caring full time. Data from the Berlin Ageing Study (BASE) also highlights the importance of extended kin in providing support for older generations. In particular, extended relatives may take over specific functions when central family relationships drop out from the older adult's personal network (Litwak, 1985).

## Attitudes towards providing care

The prevailing view is that modern nuclear-based families are not as willing or as able to provide care for older frail dependents as in the past (Cowgill and Holmes, 1972). It is argued that the extended family encouraged respect and prestige for elders. This sense of obligation towards kin was a manifestation of family culture, and took priority over individual needs and personal happiness (Hareven, 1982, 1996). The conjugal or nuclear family, on the other hand, is seen as lacking the resources to provide care and support for elderly dependents. Furthermore, it encourages independent adult living, which places older dependent adults in an ambiguous position because the concept of full personhood is closely tied to the ability to live alone. Thus the ideal of the nuclear family household makes living in an independent household an indicator of full adult status, something which young people strive for and older people resist giving up. This results in problematic re-entry into an extended family household when widowhood or increasing frailty occur (Goode, 1964; Keith *et al.*, 1994).

This view has been questioned on two levels. Macfarlane (1978) points out that from at least medieval times the English family has operated primarily on individual rather than collective principles, while Finch (1989) argues that there is actually little normative agreement in Britain on the obligations and responsibilities of adults towards other adult kin; and that furthermore, these obligations vary between cohorts. In addition there are considerable cultural differences, in some cases defined by law and policy.

Within the EU15 for example, there appears to be a spectrum of responsibility defined at the national level. At one end of this spectrum stand the Scandinavians, whose intergenerational contract has allowed the development of policy focused on individual entitlements and citizenship rights for all, with those in need expecting to receive state rather than family support. At the other end are the southern Europeans, who expect to rely almost exclusively upon the extended family. The expected obligations of those in the UK and Ireland are nuclear family-based, and mixed. Clearly, however, there are subtle difference in family responsibilities (Reher, 1998; Segalen, 1997; Murphy, 2001).

In terms of attitudes towards families, it is clear that the family still acts in a supportive manner towards its kin in times of need. Thus Scandinavian research has highlighted the importance of kinship within a modern welfare state, and indicated both increased contact with family members and a significant move towards a more positive view on the family as a supportive institution (Leeson, 2004). Data from northern Europe suggest that the vast majority of mid-life adult children would provide for their parents in a variety of practical ways. Southern European societies still support strong imperatives to care for needy relatives, and even US families continue to reveal a strong sense of obligation between the generations (Bengtson *et al.*, 2002). A recent global survey has also indicated that family obligations, and in particular the role of the family in self identification, still rank high in Western society (Leeson and Harper, 2007).

Households and family networks are becoming smaller, adult unions are changing, and life-course changes, particularly for women, are reducing opportunities for caregiving. However, family ties are remaining strong both in contact and attitude, and older adults are providing and will continue to provide major sources of elder care as their healthy life expectancy increases. This care will probably increasingly come from spouses rather than children, as the life trajectory and demands across the life course change, particularly for women. In addition, increasing healthy life expectancy not only means delaying morbidity, but also increasing the number of healthy late-life carers. Families are also providing support through reciprocal financial transfers. The indications are that families will continue to care, but that older people themselves will also become increasingly independent in their care and support needs.

## Conclusion

As this chapter has explored, though age is often understood as a determinant of biological and psychological changes, it is but an *indicator* of these changes. However, it can be a *determinant* of individuals' allocated roles, independent of their biological or psychological capacity. Age also has *analytical value* as a descriptive variable; and it identifies at any given time point *birth-cohort membership*, and thus potential shared cohort life experiences.

Exploration of the changing roles and relationships which occur in old age have also highlighted the tension between the continuity and discontinuity of the late age life course, and the potential for configuration and reconfiguration of public and private personal networks. Retirement, ill-health, widowhood, divorce, and grandparenthood, for example, result in the renegotiation of roles within the family and wider community, and the reconfiguration of social networks. Alternatively, many older people maintain continuity in their relationships with partners and children throughout their lives, and the introduction of early retirement has meant that some of the transitions previously arising in old age now occur in mid-life, allowing time for adjustment and reconfiguration of personal networks.

## Acknowledgements

I would like to acknowledge the assistance of Sue Marcus in the preparation and development of this chapter.

## References

Achenbaum, W.A. (1995). *Crossing frontiers: gerontology emerges as a science*. Cambridge University Press, Cambridge.

Acton Society Trust (1960). *Retirement: a study of current attitudes and practices*. Acton Society Trust, London.

Altmann, J. (1980). *Baboon mothers and infants*. Harvard University Press, Cambridge, MA.

Amato, P.R. (1994). Life-span adjustment of children to their parents' divorce. *Future Child*, **4**, 143–64.

Anderson, J.M. (2001). *Models for retirement policy analysis*. Society of Actuaries, Schaumburg, IL.

Anderson, M. (1985). The emergence of the modern life cycle in Britain. *Social History*, **10**, 69–87.

Anderson, R. (2004). Working carers in the European Union. In *Families in ageing societies: a multi-disciplinary approach* (ed. S. Harper), pp. 95–113. Oxford University Press, Oxford.

Anderson, W. and Cowan, N. (1956). Work and retirement: influences on the health of older men. *Lancet*, **271**, 1344–8.

Arber, S.L. and Gilbert, G.N. (1989). Men: the forgotten carers. *Sociology*, **23**, 111–18.

Arber, S. and Ginn, J. (1992). Class and caring: a forgotten dimension. *Sociology*, **26**, 619–34.

Askham, J. (1998). Supporting caregivers of older people: an overview of problems and priorities. *World Congress of Gerontology, Adelaide, Australia: 'Ageing beyond 2000: one world one future'*. International Association of Gerontology, Adelaide.

Austad, S. (1997). Postreproductive survival in nature. In *Between Zeus and the salmon: the biodemography of longevity* (ed. K.W. Wachter and C.E. Finch), pp. 161–74. National Academy Press, Washington, DC.

Australian Bureau of Statistics (1998). *Australian social trends*. Australian Bureau of Statistics, Canberra.

Barranti, C.C.R. (1985). The grandparent/grandchild relationship: family resource in an era of voluntary bonds. *Family Relations*, **34**, 343–52.

Bellemare, D. *et al.* (1998). *Le paradoxe de l'âgisme dans une société vieillissante; enjeux et défis de gestion*. Ed. St-Martin, Montreal.

Bengtson, V.L. (1985). Diversity and symbolism in grandparental roles. In *Grandparenthood* (ed. V.L. Bengtson and J.F. Robertson), pp. 11–24. Sage Publications, Beverly Hills, CA.

Bengtson, V.L. (1995). Hidden connections: intergenerational linkages in American society. In *Adult intergenerational relations: effects of societal change* (ed. V.L. Bengtson, K.W. Schaie and L. Burton). Springer, New York.

Bengtson, V.L. and Dannefer, D. (1987). Families, work and aging: implications of disordered cohort flow for the twenty-first century. In *Health in aging: sociological issues and policy directions* (ed. R.A. Ward and S.S. Tobin). Springer, New York.

Bengtson, V.L. and Harootyan, R.A. (eds) (1994). *Intergenerational linkages: hidden connections in American society*. Springer, New York.

Bengtson, V.L. *et al.* (1990). Families and aging: diversity and heterogeneity. In *Handbook of aging and the social sciences*, 3rd edn (ed. R.H. Binstock and L.K. George), pp. 263–87. Academic Press, San Diego.

Bengtson, V.L. *et al.* (1996). Paradoxes of families and aging. In *Handbook of aging and the social sciences*, 5th edn (ed. R.H. Binstock and L.K. George), pp. 254–82. Academic Press, New York.

Bengtson, V.L. *et al.* (2002). Solidarity, conflict, and ambivalence: complementary or competing perspectives on intergenerational relationships? *Journal of Marriage and the Family*, **64**, 568–76.

Bornat, J. *et al.* (1998). Generational ties in the 'new' family: changing contexts for traditional obligations. In *The 'new' family?* (ed. E.B. Silva and C. Smart). Sage, London.

Bornat, J. *et al.* (1999). Stepfamilies and older people: evaluating the implications of family change for an ageing population. *Ageing and Society*, **19**, 239–61.

Brehm, S.S. (1992). *Intimate relationships*. McGraw-Hill, New York.

Bumpass, L.L. *et al.* (1991). The impact of family background and early marital factors on marital disruption. *Journal of Family Issues*, **12**, 22–42.

Carey, J.R. and Gruenfelder, C. (1997). Population biology of the elderly in human aging. In *Between Zeus and the salmon: the biodemography of longevity* (ed. K.W. Wachter and C.E. Finch) pp. 127–60. National Academy Press, Washington, DC.

Caro, T.M. *et al.* (1995). Termination of reproduction in nonhuman and human female primates. *International Journal of Primatology*, **16**, 205–20.

Carter, S.B. and Sutch, R. (1996). Myth of the industrial scrap heap: a revisionist view of turn-of-the-century American retirement. *Journal of Economic History*, **56**, 5–38.

Casey, B. (1998). *Incentives and disincentives to early and late retirement*. Organisation for Economic Co-operation and Development, Paris.

Cherlin, A.J. (1992). *Marriage, divorce, remarriage*. Harvard University Press, Cambridge, MA.

Cherlin, A.J. and Furstenberg, F.F. (1985). Styles and strategies of grandparenting. In *Grandparenthood* (ed. V.L. Bengston and J.F. Robertson), pp. 97–116. Sage, Beverly Hills, CA.

Costa, D.L. (1998). *The evolution of retirement: an American economic history, 1880–1990.* University of Chicago Press, Chicago.

Cowgill, D.O. and Holmes, L.D. (1972). *Aging and modernization.* Appleton-Century-Crofts, New York.

Cunningham-Burley, S. (1986). Becoming a grandparent. *Ageing & Society*, **6**, 453–71.

David, H. and Pilon, A. (1990). Les pratiques d'entreprises manufacturières à l'égard de leur main-d'oeuvre vieillissante. In *Le vieillissement au travail: une question de jugement. Actes du colloque de l'IRAT* (ed. H. David), pp. 88–91. IRAT, Montreal.

Day, L. (1995). Recent fertility trends in industrialized countries: toward a fluctuating or a stable pattern? *European Journal of Population*, **11**, 275–88.

Dench, D. *et al.* (1999). The role of grandparents. In *British social attitudes: the 16th report* (ed. R. Jowell, J. Curtice, A. Park, and K. Thomson). Ashgate (in association with National Centre for Social Research), Aldershot.

Dimmock, B. *et al.* (2004). Intergenerational relationships among stepfamilies in the UK. In *Families in ageing societies: a multi-disciplinary approach* (ed. S. Harper), pp. 95–113. Oxford University Press, Oxford.

Disney, R. *et al.* (1997). *The dynamics of retirement: analysis of the ONS Retirement Survey.* Department of Social Security, Washington, DC.

Dwyer, J.W. and Coward, R.T. (1991). A multivariate comparison of the involvement of adult sons versus adult daughters in the care of impaired adults. *Journal of Gerontology Series B, Psychological Sciences and Social Sciences*, **46B**, S259–S269.

Elder, G.H. (1985). Perspectives on the life course. In *Life course dynamics: trajectories and transitions, 1968–1980* (ed. G.H. Elder), pp. 23–49. Cornell University Press, Ithaca.

Elder, G.H. and O'Rand, A.M. (1995). Adult lives in a changing society. In *Sociological perspectives on social psychology* (ed. K.S. Cook, G.A. Fine, and J.S. House), pp. 452–75. Allyn and Bacon, Boston.

Emerson, A. (1959). The first years of retirement. *Occupational Physiology*, **34**, 197–208.

Esping-Andersen, G. (1990). *The three worlds of welfare capitalism.* Polity, Cambridge.

ESRC, EPSRC BBSRC, MRC, and AHRC (2006). *New dynamics of ageing; a cross-council research programme* (available at: http://newdynamics. group.shef.ac.uk/downloads/nda-full_programme_specification.pdf).

Fairbanks, L.A. and McGuire, M.T. (1986). Age, reproductive value, and dominance-related in vervet monkey females: cross-generational influences on social relationships and reproduction. *Animal Behavior*, **34**, 1710–21.

Finch, J. (1989). *Family obligations and social change.* Polity, Cambridge.

Finch, J. and Wallis, L. (1994). Inheritance, care bargain and elderly people's relationships with their children. In *Community care: new agendas and challenges from the UK and overseas* (ed. D. Challis, B. Davies, and K. Stewart). Arena, in association with the British Society of Gerontology, Aldershot.

Finley, M.I. (1984). *The legacy of Greece: a new appraisal.* Oxford University Press, Oxford.

Fogerty, J.R. (1992). *Growing old in England, 1878–1949.* Australian National University, Canberra.

Fortes, M. (1984). Age, generation and social structure. In *Age and anthropological theory* (ed. D.I. Kertzer and J. Keith), pp. 99–122. Cornell University Press, Ithaca, NY.

Fox, G.L. and Kelly, R.F. (1995). Determinants of child custody arrangements at divorce. *Journal of Marriage and the Family*, **57**, 693–708.

Fry, C.L. (1999). Anthropological theories of age and aging. In *Handbook of theories of aging* (ed. V.L. Bengtson and K.W. Schaie), pp. 271–86. Springer, New York.

Gibson, C. (1993). The four baby booms. *American Demographics*, **15**, pp. 36–40.

Goldman, N. (1986). Effects of mortality levels on kinship. In *Consequences of mortality trends and differentials* (ed. UN Department of International Economic and Social Affairs). United Nations, New York.

Goldscheider, F.K. and Goldscheider, C. (1994). Leaving and returning home in twentieth century America. *Population Bulletin*, **48**, 1–34.

Goode, W.J. (1964). *The family.* Prentice-Hall, Englewood Cliffs, NJ.

Granick, S. (1952). Adjustment of older people in two Florida communities. *Journal of Gerontology*, **7**, 419–25.

Green, G. (1963). *The trade unions. Preparation for Retirement First National Conference.*

Green, H. (1988). *Informal carers: a study carried out on behalf of the Department of Health and Social Security as part of the 1985 General Household Survey.* UK Government Social Survey Department, HMSO, London.

Gruber, J. and Wise, D.A. (1999). *Social security and retirement around the world.* University of Chicago Press, Chicago.

Grundy, E. (1987). Household change and migration among the elderly in England and Wales. *Espace, Population, Sociétés*, **1**, 109–23.

Grundy, E. (1999). Household and family change in mid and later life in England and Wales. In *Changing Britain: families and households in the 1990s* (ed. S. McRae), pp. 201–28. Oxford University Press, Oxford.

Grundy, E. and Harrop, A. (1992). Co-residence between adult children and their elderly parents in England and Wales. *Journal of Social Policy*, **21**, 325–48.

Hagestad, G.O. (1986). Dimension of time and the family. *American Behavioral Scientist*, **29**, 679–94.

Hagestad, G.O. (1988). Demographic change and the life course: some emerging trends in the family realm. *Family Relations*, **37**, 405–10.

Hagestad, G. and Neugarten, B. (1985). Age and the life course. In *Handbook of aging and the social sciences*, 2nd edn (ed. R.H. Binstock and E. Shanas), pp. 35–61. van Nostrand Reinhold, New York.

Hareven, T.K. (1982). *Family time and industrial time: the relationship between the family and work in a New England industrial community.* Cambridge University Press, Cambridge.

Hareven, T.K. (ed.) (1996). *Aging and generational relations: life-course and cross-cultural perspectives.* Aldine de Gruyter, New York.

Harper, S. (1989). The impact of the retirement debate on post-war retirement trends. In *Post-war Britain, 1945–64: themes and perspectives* (ed. A. Gorst, L. Johnman, and W.S. Lucas), pp. 95–108. Pinter, in association with the Institute of Contemporary British History, London.

Harper, S. (1999). *A review of British social gerontology.* Nuffield Foundation, London.

Harper, S. (2000). Ageing 2000—questions for the 21st century. *Ageing & Society*, **20**, 111–22.

Harper, S. (2003). Changing European families as population ages. *European Journal of Sociology*, **44**, 155–84.

Harper, S. (2004a). The challenge for families of demographic ageing. In *Families in ageing societies: a multi-disciplinary approach* (ed. S. Harper), pp. 6–30. Oxford University Press, Oxford.

Harper, S. (ed.) (2004b). *Families in ageing societies: a multi-disciplinary approach*, p. 212. Oxford University Press, Oxford.

Harper, S. (2005) Understanding grandparenthood. In *The Cambridge handbook of age and ageing* (ed. M.L. Johnson). Cambridge University Press, Cambridge

Harper, S. (2006). *Ageing societies.* Hodder Arnold, London.

Harper, S. and Laslett, P. (2005). The puzzle of retirement and early retirement. In *Understanding social change* (ed. A.F. Heath, J. Ermisch, and D. Gallie). Oxford University Press (for British Academy), Oxford.

Harper, S. and Leeson, G.W. (2004) Time to reclaim old age [editorial]. *Generations Review*, **14**, 2–3.

Harper, S. and Lund, D.A. (1990). Wives, husbands, and daughters caring for institutionalized and noninstitutionalized dementia patients: toward a model of caregiver burden. *International Journal of Ageing and Human Development*, **30**, 241–62.

Harper, S. and Thane, P. (1986). *The social construction of old age in post-war Britain – 1945–1965*. Goldsmith College, University of London, London.

Harper, S. and Thane, P. (1989). The consolidation of 'old age' as a phase of life, 1945–65. In *Growing old in the twentieth century* (ed. M. Jefferys), pp. 43–61. Routledge, London.

Harper, S. *et al.* (2004) *Grandmother care in lone parent families*, Research Report. Oxford Institute of Ageing, Oxford.

Harper, S. *et al.* (2006). Attitudes and practices of employers towards ageing workers: evidence from a global survey on the future of retirement. *Ageing Horizons*, **5**, 31–42.

Haskey, J. (1992). *Pre-marital cohabitation and the probability of subsequent divorce*. Office for National Statistics, London.

Haskey, J. (1998). Families: their historical context, and recent trends in the factors influencing their formation and dissolution. In *The fragmenting family: does it matter?* (ed. K. Kiernan, P.M. Morgan, and M.E. David). Institute of Economic Affairs, Health and Welfare Unit, London.

Hazelrigg, L. (1997). On the importance of age. In *Studying aging and social change: conceptual and methodological issues* (ed. M.A. Hardy), pp. 93–128. Sage Publications, Thousand Oaks, CA.

Henretta, J.C. *et al.* (1993). Joint role investments and synchronization of retirement: a sequential approach to couples' retirement timing. *Social Forces*, **71**, 981–1000.

Henretta, J.C. *et al.* (1997). Selection of children to provide care: the effect of earlier parental transfers. *Journals of Gerontology Series B, Psychological Science and Social Science*, **52**, 110–19.

Heron, A. and Chown, S.M. (1961). Ageing and the semi-skilled: a survey in manufacturing industry on Merseyside. *Medical Research Council Annual Report*, **40**, pp. 1–59.

Hill, K. and Hurtado, A.M. (1991). The evolution of premature reproductive senescence and menopause in human females: an evaluation of the 'grandmother hypothesis'. *Human Nature*, **2**, 313–50.

Hochschild, A.R. (1973). *The unexpected community*. Prentice-Hall, Englewood Cliffs, NJ.

Hrdy, S. (1981). 'Nepotists' and 'altruists': the behaviour of old females among macaques and langur monkeys. In *Other ways of growing old: anthropological perspectives* (ed. P. Amoss and S. Harrell). Stanford University Press, Stanford, CA.

HRS (2004). *A longitudinal study of health, retirement, and aging*. Health and Retirement Study, National Institute on Aging and Michigan University.

Hughes, M.E. and Waite, L.J. (2004). The American family as a context for healthy aging. In *The family in an aging society: a multi-disciplinary approach* (ed. S. Harper), pp. 176–89. Oxford University Press, Oxford.

Humphrey, A. *et al.* (2003). *Factors affecting the labour market participation of older workers*. Corporate Document Services, Leeds.

Hutchens, R.M. (1986). Delayed payment contracts and a firm's propensity to hire older workers. *Journal of Labor Economics*, **4**, 439–57.

Hyde, V. and Gibbs, I. (1993). A very special relationship: granddaughters' perceptions of grandmothers. *Ageing and Society*, **13**, 83–96.

Ikels, C. (2004). *Filial piety: practice and discourse in contemporary East Asia*. Stanford University Press, Stanford, CA.

Industrial Welfare Society (1951). *The employment of elderly workers*. IWS, London.

Jensen, P.H. (1999). *Activation of the unemployed in Denmark since the early 1990s. Welfare or Workfare?* Aalborg University, Aalborg.

Johnson, R.W. and Lo Sasso, A.T. (2004). Family support of the elderly and female labour supply: trade-offs among caregiving, financial transfers, and work—evidence from the US Health and Retirement Survey. In *Families in ageing societies: a multi-disciplinary approach* (ed. S. Harper) pp. 114–42. Oxford University Press, Oxford.

Kaplan, H. (1997). The evolution of the human life course. In *Between Zeus and the salmon: the biodemography of longevity* (ed. K.W. Wachter and C.E. Finch), pp. 175–211. National Academy Press, Washington, DC.

Katz, R. *et al.* (2005). Theorizing intergenerational family relations: solidarity, conflict and ambivalence in cross-national contexts. In *Sourcebook of family theory and research* (ed. V. Bengtson *et al.*), pp. 393–420. Sage, Thousand Oaks, CA.

Keith, J. *et al.* (1994). *The aging experience: diversity and commonality across cultures*. Sage, Thousand Oaks, CA.

Kertzer, D.I. (1995). Toward a historical demography of aging. In *Aging in the past: demography, society, and old age* (ed. D.I. Kertzer and P. Laslett), pp. 363–83. University of California Press, Berkeley.

Kertzer, D.I. and Keith, J. (eds) (1984). *Age and anthropological theory*. Cornell University Press, Ithaca, NY.

Kertzer, D.I. and Schaie, K.W. (eds) (1989). *Age structuring in comparative perspective*. L. Erlbaum Associates, Hillsdale, NJ.

Kilbom, A. (1999). Evidence-based programs for the prevention of early exit from work. *Experimental Aging Research*, **25**, 291–9.

King, V. and Elder, G.H.J. (1997). The legacy of grandparenting: childhood experiences with grandparents and current involvement with grandchildren. *Journal of Marriage and the Family*, **59**, 848–59.

Kivett, V.R. (1991). Centrality of the grandfather role among older rural black and white men. *Journal of Gerontology: Social Sciences*, **46**, S250–S258.

Kivnick, H.Q. (1983). Dimensions of grandparenthood meaning: deductive conceptualization and empirical derivation. *Journal of Personality and Social Psychology*, **44**, 1056–68.

Kodz, J. *et al.* (1999). *The fiftieth revival*. Institute of Employment Studies, Brighton.

Kohli, M.(1986). The world we forgot: an historical review of the life-course. In *Later life: the social psychology of aging* (ed. V.W. Marshall), pp. 271–303. Sage, Beverly Hills, CA.

Kohli, M. and Kunemund, H.(2003) Intergenerational transfers in the family: what motivates giving?. In *Global aging and challenges to families* (ed. V.L. Bengtson and A. Lowenstein). Aldine de Gruyter, New York.

Kornhaber, A. (1996). *Contemporary grandparenting*. Sage Publications, Thousand Oaks, CA.

Le Gros Clark, F. (1968). *Pensioners in search of a job*. Nuffield Foundation, London.

Leeson, G.W. (2004). *Sociale netwaerk*. Aelder Sagen, Copenhagen.

Leeson, G.W. and Harper, S. (2006) *Future of Retirement II. Report to HSBC*. HSBC, London.

Leeson, G.W. and Harper, S. (2007) *Future of Retirement III. Report to HSBC*. HSBC, London.

Lesthaege, R. (1992). Beyond economic reductionism: the transformation of the reproductive regimes in France and Belgium in the 18th and 19th centuries. In *Fertility transitions, family structure, and population policy* (ed. C. Goldscheider). Westview Press, Boulder, CO.

Lewin, B. (1992). Unmarried cohabitation: a marriage form in a changing society. *Journal of Marriage and the Family*, **44**, 763–73.

Lindley, R.M. (1999). Population ageing and the labour market in Europe. *Rivista Italiana di Economia, Demografia e Statistica*, **LIII**, 167–92.

Litwak, E. (1985). *Helping the elderly: the complementary roles of informal networks and formal systems*. Guilford Press, New York.

Litwin, H. (2004). Intergenerational exchange patterns and their correlates in an aging Israeli cohort. *Research on Aging*, **26**, 202–23.

Lowenstien, A. (2003). Contemporary later-life family transitions: revisiting theoretical perspectives on aging and the family—toward a family identity framework. In *The need for theory: critical approaches to social gerontology* (ed. S. Biggs *et al.*). Baywood Publishing Co., Amityville, NY.

Lussier, G. and Wister, A.V. (1995). A study of workforce aging of the British Columbia public service 1983–1991. *Canadian Journal on Aging*, **14**, 480–97.

Lyng, K. (1998). Working life, aging and life course – work environment and personnel policy. *Productive ageing*. Institute of Occupational Health Promotion, Vienna.

Macfarlane, A. (1978). *The origins of English individualism: the family, property and social transition*. Blackwell, Oxford.

McGarry, K. (1998). Caring for the elderly: the role of adult children. In *Inquiries in the economics of aging* (ed. D. Wise). Chicago: University of Chicago Press, Chicago.

McGlone, F. *et al.* (1999). Kinship and friendship: attitudes and behaviour in Britain 1986–1995. In *Changing Britain: Families and Households in the 1990s* (ed. S. McRae), pp. 144–55. Oxford University Press, Oxford.

McKay, S. and Middleton, S. (1998). *Characteristics of older workers: secondary analysis of the Family and Working Lives Survey.* Department for Education and Skills, Suffolk.

McMahon, C. and Ford, T. (1955). Surviving the first five years of retirement. *Journal of Gerontology*, **10**, 212–15.

McMullin, B. (2000). John von Neumann and the evolutionary growth of complexity: looking backward, looking forward—. *Artificial Life*, **6**, 347–61.

McNicol, J. (1998). *The politics of retirement in Britain, 1878–1948.* Cambridge University Press, Cambridge.

McRae, S. (1993). Returning to work after childbirth: opportunities and inequalities. *European Sociological Review*, **9**, 125–38.

Makoni, S. and Stroeken, K. (eds) (2002). *Ageing in Africa: sociolinguistic and anthropological approaches.* Ashgate, Aldershot.

Mann, R. (2007). Out of the shadows: grandfatherhood and old age masculinities. *Journal of Aging Studies*, doi: 10.1016/j.jaging.2007.05.008.

Marks, N.F. (1996). Caregiving across the lifespan: national prevalence and predictors. *Family Relations*, **45**, 27–36.

Marmot, M. *et al.* (eds) (2003). *Health, wealth and lifestyles of the older population in England: the 2002 English Longitudinal Study of Ageing.* Institute for Fiscal Studies, London.

Marshall, V.W. (1985). Aging and dying in pacific societies. In *Aging and its transformations: moving toward death in pacific societies* (ed. D.A. Counts and D.R. Counts). University Press of America, Lanham, MD.

Mason, J. (1999). Living away from relatives: kinship and geographical reason. In *Changing Britain, families and households in the 1990s* (ed. S. McRae), pp. 156–75. Oxford University Press, Oxford.

Matthews, S.H. and Sprey, J. (1984). The impact of divorce on grandparenthood: an exploratory study. *The Gerontologist*, **24**, 41–7.

Maule, A.J. *et al.* (1996). Early retirement decisions and how they affect later quality of life. *Ageing and Society*, **16**, 177–204.

Mead, G.H. (1934). *Mind, self & society: from the standpoint of a social behaviorist.* University of Chicago Press, Chicago.

Millar, J. (1998). *Kinship obligations in Western Europe. Ageing and the family.* Conference, University of Oxford.

Ministry of Labour (1945–55). Unpublished memos. UK Ministry of Labour, London.

Minkler, M. and Estes, C.L. (eds) (1999). *Critical gerontology: perspectives from political and moral economy.* Baywood, Amityville, NY.

Minois, G. (1989). *History of old age: from antiquity to the Renaissance.* University of Chicago Press, Chicago.

Moen, P. (1996). Gender, age and the life course. In *Handbook of aging and the social sciences*, 4th edn (ed. R.H. Binstock and L.K. George), pp. 171–87. Academic Press, San Diego.

Morgan, L.A. and Kunkel, S. (1998). *Aging: the social context.* Pine Forge Press, Thousand Oaks, CA.

Murphy, M. (2001). Family and kinship networks in the context of ageing societies. *Conference on Population Ageing in the Industrialized Countries: Challenges and Responses.* Nihon University Population Research Institute, Tokyo.

Mutran, E.J. *et al.* (1997). Factors that influence attitudes toward retirement. *Research on Aging*, **19**, 251–73.

Myers, D. (ed.) (1990). *Housing demography: linking demographic structure and housing markets.* University of Wisconsin Press, Madison, WI.

National Institute on Aging/Duke University (2006). *National long term care survey.* Duke University, Durham, NC.

Neugarten, B.L. (1982). *Age or need?: public policies for older people.* Sage Publications, Beverly Hills, CA.

Neugarten, B. and Weinstein, K. (1964). The changing American grandparent. *Journal of Marriage and the Family*, **26**, 199–204.

Okemwa, S.N. (2002). Privileged authority of elders and the contested graduations of seniority. In *Ageing in Africa: sociolinguistic and anthropological approaches* (ed. S. Makoni and K. Stroeken). Ashgate, Aldershot.

Parkin, T.G. (1992). *Demography and Roman society.* Johns Hopkins University Press, Baltimore, MD.

Pelling, M. and Smith, R.M. (1991). *Life, death, and the elderly: historical perspectives.* Routledge, London.

Quinn, J.F. *et al.* (1998). *Microeconometric analysis of the retirement decision: United States.* Organisation for Economic Co-operation and Development, Paris.

Radin, N. *et al.* (1991). Grandfathers, teen mothers and children under 2. In *The influence of grandfathers on the young children of teen mothers: an international perspective* (ed. P.K. Smith), pp. 85–99. Routledge & Kegan Paul, London.

Ransom, R.L. and Sutch, R. (1986). The labor of older Americans: retirement of men on and off the job, 1870–1937. *Journal of Economic History*, **46**, 1–30.

Rasmussen, S.J. (1997). *The poetics and politics of Tuareg aging: life course and personal destiny in Niger.* Northern Illinois University Press, DeKalb.

Reher, D.S. (1998). Family ties in Western Europe: persistent contrasts. *Population and Development Review*, **24**, 203–34.

Reiss, I.L. (1960). Toward a sociology of the heterosexual love relationships. *Marriage and Family Living*, **22**, 139–45.

Riddle, S. (1984). Age, obsolescence and unemployment: old men in the British industrial system. *Ageing and Society*, **4**, 517–24.

Riley, M.W. (1987). On the significance of age in sociology. *American Sociological Review*, **52**, 1–14.

Riley, M. and Riley Jr, J. (1994). Age integration and the lives of older people. *Gerontologist*, **34**, 110–15.

Riley, M.W. *et al.* (eds) (1972). *Aging and society: a sociology of age stratification.* Russell Sage Foundation, New York.

Roberto, K. and Stroes, J. (1995). Grandchildren and grandparents: roles, influences and relationships. In *The ties of later life* (ed. J. Hendricks), pp. 141–53. Baywood, New York.

Rogers, A.R. (1993). Why menopause? *Evolutionary Ecology*, **7**, 406–20.

Rogers, L.L. (1987). Factors influencing dispersal in the black bear. In *Mammalian dispersal patterns: the effects of social structure on population genetics* (ed. B.D. Chepko-Sade and Z.T. Halpin). University of Chicago Press, Chicago.

Rossi, A. (1987). Parenthood in transition: from lineage to child to self-orientation. In *Parenting across the life span: biosocial dimensions* (ed. J.B. Lancaster, J. Altmann, A. Rossi, and L. Sherrod). A. de Gruyter, New York.

Salais, R. (2003). Work and welfare: towards a capability approach. In *Governing work and welfare in a new economy: European and American experiments* (ed. J. Zeitlin and D.M. Trubek). Oxford University Press, Oxford.

Saller, R. (1991). European family history and Roman law. *Continuity and Change*, **36**, 335–46.

Scales, J. and Scase, R. (2000). *Fit and fifty.* ESRC, Swindon.

Scott, E. *et al.* (1999). *My children come first: welfare-reliant women's post-TANF views of work-family tradeoffs, and marriage.* Northwestern University/University of Chicago Joint Center for Poverty Research, Chicago.

Segalen, M. (1997). Introduction. In *Family and kinship in Europe* (ed. M. Gullestad and M. Segalen). Pinter, London.

Shahar, S. (1997). *Growing old in the Middle Ages: 'winter clothes us in shadow and pain'.* Routledge, London New York.

Shanas, E. (1980). Older people and their families: the new pioneers. *Journal of Marriage and the Family*, **42**, 9–15.

Shenfield, B.E. (1957). *Social policies for old age.* Routledge & Kegan Paul, London.

Soldo, B.J. and Hill, M. (1995). Family structure and transfer measures in the health and retirement study: background and overview. *Journal of Human Resources*, **30**, S108–S137.

Szinovacz, M. (1998). Grandparents today: a demographic profile. *Gerontologist*, **38**, 37–52.

Tanner, S. (1997). The dynamics of retirement behaviour. In *The dynamics of retirement: analyses of the retirement surveys* (ed. R. Disney, E.M.D. Grundy and P. Johnson). The Stationary Office, London.

Taylor, P. and Walker, A. (1994). The ageing workforce: employers' attitudes towards older workers. *Work, Employment and Society*, **8**, 569–91.

Thane, P. (2000). *Old age in English history: past experiences, present issues.* Oxford University Press, Oxford.

Thomas, K. (1979). Age and authority in early modern England. *Proceedings of the British Academy*, **42**, 206–48.

Thompson, P. *et al.* (1990). Grandparenthood. In *I don't feel old, the experiences of later life* (ed. P. Thompson, C. Itzin, and M. Abendstern), pp. 174–213. Oxford University Press, Oxford.

Twigg, J. (ed.) (1992). *Carers: research and practice.* HMSO, London.

Uccello, C.E. and Mix, S.E. (1998). *Factors influencing retirement: their implications for raising retirement age.* AARP, Washington, DC.

Uhlenberg, P. (1980). Death and the family. *Journal of Family History*, **5**, 313–20.

Uhlenberg, P. (1994). Implications of being divorced in later life. *United Nations International Conference on Ageing Population in the Context of the Family (Ageing and the Family).* UN Department for Economic and Social Information and Policy Analysis, New York, Kitakyushu, Japan.

Uhlenberg, P. (1995). Demographic influences on intergenerational relationships. In *Adult intergenerational relations: effects of societal change* (ed. V.L. Bengtson, K.W. Schaie, and L. Burton). Springer, New York.

United States Bureau of Labor Statistics (2007). *National Longitudinal Survey of Mature Women.* United States Bureau of Labor Statistics, Washington, DC.

University of Wisconsin (2003). *National Survey of Families and Households.* University of Wisconsin, Madison.

US Bureau of the Census (1997). *Current population report.* US Government Printing Office, Washington, DC.

US Bureau of the Census (1998). *Current population report.* US Government Printing Office, Washington, DC.

US Census Bureau (2006). *Survey of Income and Program Participation.* US Census Bureau, Washington, DC.

Wachter, K.W. (1997). Kinship resources for the elderly. *Philosophical Transactions of the Royal Society of London, Series B: Biological Sciences*, **352**, 1811–17.

Waite, L.J. (1995). Does marriage matter? *Demography*, **32**, 483–507.

Waite, L.J. and Bachrach, C. (eds) (2000). *The ties that bind: perspectives on marriage and cohabitation.* Aldine de Gruyter, New York.

Watkins, S.C. *et al.* (1987). Demographic foundations of family change. *American Sociological Review*, **52**, 346–58.

Wolf, D.A. and Soldo, B.J. (1994). Married women's allocation of time to employment and care of elderly parents. *Journal of Human Resources*, **29**, 1259–76.

Wolf, D.A. *et al.* (1997). The division of family labor: care for elderly parents. *Journal of Gerontology Series B, Psychological Sciences and Social Sciences*, **52B**, 102–09.

Zeilig, H. and Harper, S. (2000). *Locating grandparents.* Oxford Centre on Population Ageing, University of Oxford, Oxford.

# 3

# Cognitive change in old age

## Elizabeth Anderson

Cognitive change in old age happens. The cells of the brain, just like those of all other bodily organs, are vulnerable to the processes of cellular senescence (for reviews see Kemper, 1994; Raz, 2000; Whalley, 2001; Hedden and Gabrieli, 2004). It was once thought that there is a significant loss of neurons during old age, but modern techniques suggest that the shrinkage of grey matter in old age is primarily due to fluid loss and loss of synaptic density rather than cell death. However, within the neural networks of the brain there is a loss of synaptic connectivity in old age and a reduction in the efficiency of dendritic remodelling. Old age is also associated with white matter change, particularly the deterioration of the myelin sheath. There are changes to the neurochemistry of the brain, particularly within the dopamine system (Backman and Farde, 2005). Thus, although cells do not die in large numbers as part of the normal ageing process there are functional alterations that would be expected to affect the processing power of the brain.

However, whilst it is clear that the brain undergoes change in old age, the relationship between the brain and the cognitive functions it produces is complex, to say the least. The brain is unique amongst bodily organs in that the relationship between the physical substrate of the brain and the mental functions it supports remains a deeply contested philosophical issue. It is difficult, therefore, to understand the true significance of the brain alterations reviewed above for cognition. The shrinkage of the cerebral cortex and the loss of synaptic density appear to begin in early adulthood and both follow a linear trajectory of decline across the lifespan into old age (Hedden and Gabrieli, 2004; Raz, 2005) and yet it is clear that cognition is not affected at this early age. Within the brain the passage of time is not only associated with the downward trajectory of biological ageing, but also the upward trajectory of learning from experience. In general, it appears that the elderly brain does become slower to learn but it never loses the capacity to learn (Nyberg, 2005) and information and skills learnt throughout the lifespan appear resilient to old age (Horn and Cattell, 1967).

There is, however, a loss of intellectual speed and flexibility which is observed even amongst the 'super-elderly', that is, very intelligent elderly people in very good health (Nielson et al., 2002; Morcom et al., 2003; Hedden and Gabrieli, 2004). This suggests that everyone experiences some loss of cognitive power in old age but that usually the cognitive decline is mild and the impact of such decline on everyday life is minimal. The experience of some loss in the speed, flexibility, and learning capacity of the mind in old age is likely to cause some frustration, and perhaps a little loss of pride, but to the extent that most elderly people have found a way of life well-suited to their character and skill, the need for active cognitive skills is much reduced in old age. This reflects the ancient view of old age as a time of reflection and wisdom rather than active intelligence. Whalley (2001) describes the difference between intelligence and wisdom as being that, 'intelligence is used to answer the question concerning how something should be done, whilst wisdom asks whether it should be done at all' (p. 67). By the latter decades of life most of the important questions of life have usually been answered and concepts related to wisdom (Baltes, 1993) or 'ego-integrity' (Erikson, 1982) appear to be central in determining whether people cope successfully with the negative changes of old age or not.

However, whilst the recent evidence suggests that cognitive change happens to everyone, there is marked variation in the rate of change from one individual to the next (reviewed by Hedden and Gabrieli, 2004). Many lifespan studies suggest considerable stability of intellectual ability from youth to old age (McClearn et al., 1997; Deary et al., 2000) but the increased variability in cognitive ability in elderly relative to young samples reveals that cognition is influenced by a greater range of factors in old age than in youth. This may reflect differences in factors that affect the rate of biological ageing itself, and also factors that affect the chances of developing the neurodegenerative conditions which can lead to dementia, particularly Alzheimer's disease and cerebrovascular disease. The extent to which biological ageing and these age-related diseases are truly separable remains controversial. The progressive nature of dementing conditions makes it extremely difficult to distinguish between the earliest signs of a neurodegenerative process and the normal effects of brain ageing. When cognitive ability in both demented and non-demented people is measured using the Mini Mental State Examination (Folstein et al., 1975), or an equivalent instrument, there is no sign of bimodality in the distribution of scores to suggest that elderly people divide into two separate populations of the demented and non-demented (Brayne and Calloway, 1988). Neither do longitudinal studies tracking cognitive change within individuals reveal a critical cut-off point which marks the onset of dementia (Whalley, 2002). There appears to be no pathological or physiological marker that clearly distinguishes between elderly people with and without dementia (see Huppert *et al.*, 1994). A large epidemiological study in a community-based population examining the prevalence of the pathologies associated with dementia found that the majority of elderly people who were not demented at death had some features of either Alzheimer's disease or cerebrovascular disease in their brains (Esiri *et al.*, 2001).

Such findings provide strong support for the continuum hypothesis in which 'normal ageing' and 'dementia' are seen as lying along a continuum of cognitive decline in old age, ranging from the very mild declines experienced by the 'super-elderly' through to the catastrophic declines associated with severe dementia. The continuum of change at the cognitive level, however, should not be seen as implying that there is a common process of 'brain ageing' that accounts for all cognitive decline in old age. With Alzheimer's disease being the dominant cause of dementia, and with age being the dominant risk factor for this condition, the continuum model of dementia is often viewed as being interchangeable with the question, 'Is Alzheimer's disease a true disease or accelerated ageing?'. It is easy to demonstrate that this is an over-simplistic and misleading question. Other dementias which are not caused by Alzheimer's disease are not considered to be the same disease. If not all dementias are caused by Alzheimer's disease then it is most unlikely that all 'normal ageing' is caused by Alzheimer's disease. Furthermore, epidemiological studies of nonagenarians and centenarians argue against the view that everyone would get Alzheimer's disease were they to live long enough. This view was based on an extrapolation of the rapid rise in risk for this condition observed during the eighth and ninth decades of life, but it seems that there is little increase in risk beyond the age of 90, and that the risk may even drop (Crystal *et al.*, 1993; Ritchie and Kildea, 1995; Lautenschlager *et al.*, 1996). The underlying causes of the dementia syndrome become increasingly multifactorial as age advances and vascular factors may become more dominant relative to Alzheimer's pathology in accounting for dementia amongst the oldest old (Crystal *et al.*, 1993; Skoog *et al.*, 1993). This suggests that the decline of cognition in extreme old age is associated with the accumulation of a mild level of separate (distinct) challenges to the brain, rather than the intensification of a single process.

Nonetheless, the overlap between normal ageing and Alzheimer's disease remains a problem. At the level of molecular biology most theories of Alzheimer's disease and theories of biological ageing overlap and merge into each other (for reviews see Whalley, 2001, 2002). This situation, whereby the mechanisms of biological ageing and age-related brain pathologies are hard to differentiate, sits alongside the view of many epidemiologists and ageing experts that ageing is nonetheless a multifactorial phenomenon. They would say that when it comes to understanding age-related disease it is best to focus on the specifics relating to the particular disease process, rather than to hope for the discovery of a common mechanism of ageing that will explain all age-related diseases ranging from cancer to dementia (Peto and Doll, 1997; Buckner, 2005). With respect to cognition it is quite clear that there are many challenges to the brain in old age, and that each individual almost certainly experiences a unique cocktail of these factors. In the next section the characteristics of the pattern of cognitive change observed in non-demented elderly subjects will be reviewed. In the succeeding section this pattern will be contrasted with the cognitive profile of early Alzheimer's disease, so as to demonstrate that, even though subclinical signs of this disease are often found in the brains of the normal elderly, it is unlikely that these small accumulations are the cause of the normal pattern of cognitive change in old age. On balance it is best, therefore, to conceive of Alzheimer's disease as an age-related disease that needs to be distinguished from the normal patterns of cognitive change in old age. Reconciliation of the two lines of evidence reviewed above may be achieved if biological ageing is shown to create the conditions in which the operation of other genetic and environmental factors can trigger the cascade that leads to Alzheimer's disease.

## Patterns of cognitive change in old age

Before beginning a brief review of the now considerable body of literature concerning changes to cognition in old age, a few words about the organization of cognition within the brain will be helpful. Prior to the latter decades of the last century, neuroscience was dominated by a debate as to whether the brain acted as an undifferentiated whole to produce intellectual functions or whether the brain was divided, with different parts being specialized to perform specific cognitive functions (see introductory chapter in Kandel *et al.*, 1995 for discussion). Advances during the 20th century have led to agreement that intelligent behaviour is a combination of specialized functions interacting with some general factor, captured by the layperson's notion of intelligence or, more formally, by either Spearman's concept of 'g' (Spearman, 1927) or the cognitive psychologists' notion of 'general processing capacity' (see the next section for further discussion). The general picture to emerge from the cognitive study of ageing is that there is little evidence for age-related decline in the specialized cognitive functions, but that when a test is made difficult by requiring active manipulation of information, age-related deficits occur in all the cognitive domains, suggesting that old age has a deleterious effect on the general factor that determines efficiency throughout the system. The idea that the primary effect of old age is to leave the fundamental architecture of cognition unchanged but to reduce overall 'processing capacity' is an old one (Welford, 1958) that is well-expressed by this quotation from Craik and Rabinowitz (1984, p.472):

> …many age-related decrements appear to reflect inefficiencies of processing, or to be strategic in nature, rather than to be reflections of broken or lost components.

The major challenge is to provide a theoretical definition of 'processing capacity' and to determine the extent to which a particular cognitive activity demands 'processing capacity'. The issue remains controversial and will be followed up in the next section.

### Changes in intelligence and problem-solving

Much of the early work on cognition and ageing used psychometric tests of intelligence (for reviews see Schaie, 1996; Woodruff-Pak, 1997; Stuart-Hamilton, 2000). It soon became apparent that the effect of old age upon intelligence was not uniform. Doppelt and Wallace (1955), for example, reported that the Performance IQ subtests from the WAIS (Wechsler Adult Intelligence Scale; Wechsler, 1981) were more sensitive to age than the Verbal IQ subtests. The finding of Doppelt and Wallace has been replicated so frequently that it has become known as the 'classic ageing pattern' (Botwinick, 1977).

Early explanations for the classic ageing pattern focused on the idea that the right cerebral hemisphere may be more vulnerable to the effects of age than the left. However, today the most widely accepted explanation derives from Horn and Cattell's (1967) theory that there are two sources of intelligent behaviour. The first, which Horn and Cattell refer to as 'fluid intelligence', is that typically associated with the concept of intelligence, whereby a person relies on his/her own reasoning powers to identify structure in the problem and apply appropriate strategies to reach a solution. 'Crystallized intelligence', by contrast, is developed through education and experience, and represents the well-learnt information, skills, methods, and habits that can be brought to bear on problems and activities. Horn and Cattell argue that fluid intelligence deteriorates in old age, but that crystallized intelligence is robust. The insensitivity of Verbal IQ subtests to old age is attributed to the fact that performance in these tests is determined by the size of a person's general knowledge and vocabulary, paradigm examples of crystallized intelligence. In the Performance IQ subtests, on the other hand, the materials presented are novel and must be actively manipulated, usually within a stringent time limit. In these tests prior knowledge is of little value and fluid intelligence becomes dominant in determining success.

The notion that fluid intelligence is vulnerable to old age is supported by studies of problem-solving. These studies have shown the elderly to be less strategic and flexible in their thought processes relative to the young (see Denney and Denney, 1973, 1974 for reviews). The elderly have been found to be poorer at abstracting structure from problems and at using feedback to abstract concepts and rules (for reviews see Arenberg, 1982; Reese and Rodeheaver, 1985; Woodruff-Pak, 1997).

Whilst these studies show that the elderly are challenged more than the young by novel problems, it should be noted that, in accordance with Horn and Cattell's (1967) distinction, problem-solving skills relating to well-practised activities are maintained in old age. Charness (1981a,b), for example, has studied chess-playing skills in young and old experts. Charness's experiments revealed that whilst the elderly chess players were impaired in the immediate recall of board positions, they matched the performance of young players in problem-solving tasks which required selection of the best next move. Indeed, the results showed that the elderly were able to select the best move more quickly than the young. Charness suggests that this is because their knowledge base is better organized through practice and experience, meaning that moves the young may evaluate and reject are not even considered by elderly players. Salthouse (1984) reached a similar conclusion in a study of typing experts. In this series of studies the elderly typists showed equivalent speed and accuracy in their typing, even though their basic perceptuomotor skills, measured by tapping speed and reaction time, were slower. The elderly maintained their typing speed because they were able to look further ahead in order to prepare for the coming text. As argued in the introduction, it seems probable that the preservation of 'crystallized' skills and techniques mitigates declining neural efficiency, allowing most elderly people to maintain active, independent, and fulfilling lives (Baltes, 1993).

## Changes in memory

Declining memory function is one of the most common complaints of elderly people. The word 'memory' covers a huge range of different learning and knowledge functions. In old age memory problems are particularly related to the ability to learn new information that can be consciously recalled at some later time. Within the cognitive

literature this form of memory has been referred to as 'declarative memory', 'explicit memory', or 'episodic memory' (see Schacter, 1994 for a full review of the cognitive theory of memory). Evidence from neuroscience suggests that this particular memory function is highly distributed, depending upon interactions between many brain structures, in particular the cerebral cortex and the circuits that run through the hippocampus (and associated medial temporal lobe structures) and the diencephalon. The highly distributed nature of this memory function no doubt explains why this kind of memory is so vulnerable to a variety of challenges to the brain (Lezak, 1995). There is certainly no doubt that this form of memory is very sensitive to the effects of age (Burke and Light, 1981; Poon 1985; Craik and Jennings, 1992). Figure 3.1 shows that performance in the paired associate learning tests of the Wechsler Memory Scale shows a slow decline from the age of 50 onwards. Other forms of memory, however, are less vulnerable. For example, there is little change in the amount of information that can be held within the mind for a few seconds (Babcock and Salthouse, 1990) or to the established knowledge base, as reviewed above.

Memory for contextual detail is particularly vulnerable in old age (Craik and Rabinowitz, 1984; Byrd, 1985; Holland and Rabbitt, 1990). In experiments where the ability of the old and young to recognize items from a learning list is equated, the elderly are less likely to detect subtle perceptual changes, such as a change in right/ left orientation (Bartlett et al., 1983), additions or deletions (Pezdek, 1987), or a change in colour (Park and Puglisi, 1985). Deficits in remembering the format in which information was presented, such as whether words were presented in spoken or written format (Lehmann and Mellinger, 1984), in upper or lower case (Kausler and Puckett, 1981a), or in a male or female voice (Kausler and Puckett, 1981b), have also been found. Cohen and Faulkener (1989), Guttentag and Hunt (1988), and Hashtroudi et al. (1990) conducted studies in which subjects were asked to learn a list of actions.

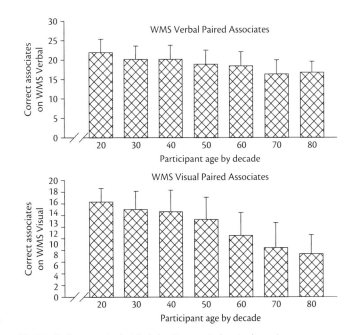

**Fig. 3.1** Performance in the Wechsler Memory Scale paired associates test declines in old age. Reprinted from Woodruff-Pak (1997, p. 38). Copyright (1997), with permission from Blackwell Publishing Ltd.

Subjects performed half of these actions and imagined the other half. All three studies found that the elderly were impaired relative to the young at remembering whether they performed the action or merely imagined it.

This suggests that the memory traces created by elderly subjects are lacking in detail, which may in turn affect the ability to retrieve key information successfully at later times (Mitchell and Johnson, 2000). However, there have been numerous demonstrations that if the elderly are given appropriate guidance during learning then this difficulty can be ameliorated. In most memory tests the subject is given no guidance as to how the learning task should be approached. Under such conditions the elderly are less likely to engage in strategies which promote elaborative encoding (for reviews see Craik, 1977; Burke and Light, 1981). In 1972, Craik and Lockhart performed experiments with young subjects which suggested that the key to a successful mnemonic strategy is to attend to the meaning of material to be learnt (technically termed as engaging in semantic processing). Semantic processing can be enforced by asking subjects appropriate questions about each item in the learning set (such as to categorize it, to rate its pleasantness, or to think of an associate). When elderly subjects are asked such orienting questions at the time of learning, the age difference in later memory performance is usually found to diminish (for reviews see Light, 1991; Craik and Jennings, 1992). Age differences in memory for spatial materials can also be reduced by presenting the material in an integrated and meaningful framework (Waddell and Rogoff, 1981; Park et al., 1990; Sharps, 1991).

Just as procedures which compensate for the strategic imbalance between the old and the young reduce age deficits, procedures which exacerbate the strategic difference increase the size of the age deficit. For example, Rabinowitz (1989) provided subjects with unlimited time during the learning phase and allowed them to make notes in order to boost their memory performance. Rabinowitz found greater age differences in an unstructured learning condition than in a structured condition where the experimenter controlled the pace of learning and note-making was not allowed. Erber et al. (1980) found that when subjects were asked to make judgements at encoding which hinder memory, the young were better able to compensate against the inappropriate strategy.

There is little doubt that unless considerable support is provided during learning, the elderly do not encode information into long-term memory as efficiently as the young. Effects relating to the need for internally driven, as opposed to externally supported, processing are also apparent at the retrieval stage. Age deficits in memory performance systematically decline in passing from free recall memory tests, to cued recall tests, to recognition tests (Schonfield and Robertson, 1966; Perlmutter, 1979; Craik and McDowd, 1987; Whiting and Smith, 1997). Indeed, many studies have found no age deficits in recognition tests, but age differences in recognition are found when the difficulty of the test is increased, either by providing inadequate guidance during learning (Craik and Simon, 1980) or by using lures that are very similar to the presented items (Till et al., 1982; Bartlett and Leslie, 1986). There is also evidence that the elderly rely more on feelings of familiarity in making recognition judgements than on true retrieval of the material (Fell, 1992; Perfect et al., 1995). The elderly are better at recognizing typical rather than atypical incidents from a scenario (Hess et al., 1989) and are more likely to be misled by plausibility in making recognition judgements (Reder et al., 1986; Cohen and Faulkner, 1989).

In the free recall of texts or incidents the elderly sometimes 'remember' plausible but absent information (Spilich, 1983; Cohen et al., 1994).

With respect to old learning and the store of information built up throughout the lifespan, evidence suggests that there is no significant loss of knowledge during old age. In the discussion on intelligence it has already been noted that the elderly are not impaired in tests of vocabulary and general knowledge (Botwinick, 1977; Perlmutter, 1979; Salthouse, 1988). Furthermore, there appears to be no change to the organization of information within long-term memory (see Light, 1992 for a detailed review). A technique which has been used extensively to examine the organization of established information in long-term memory is priming, whereby the presentation of priming information facilitates the processing of any subsequent information related to the priming material. For example, subjects are quicker to decide that 'doctor' is a word if they have recently encountered the word 'nurse'. A number of experiments have shown that although the elderly are always slower to make lexical decisions, they nonetheless benefit to the same degree as the young from the presentation of related words (Howard et al., 1981; Howard, 1983; Burke and Yee, 1984).

However, although a variety of paradigms point towards no loss of established information in old age, the retrieval difficulties which apply to newly learnt information appear to apply equally to well-established information (Reder et al., 1986; Holland and Rabbitt, 1990). Although the elderly are accurate when making semantic judgements they are slower to make those judgements (Meuller et al., 1980, Petros et al., 1983; Byrd, 1984). When asked to generate members of a category, the elderly typically generate fewer category members in a given time than do the young (Howard, 1980; Obler and Albert, 1985; Brown and Mitchell, 1991). Furthermore, access is not only slower but also less reliable. The elderly also show deficits in picture naming tests, particularly for items which are encountered only infrequently, such as 'trellis' or 'sextant' (Albert et al., 1988; Bowles, 1989; La Rue, 1992). Analysis of picture naming errors reveals that the elderly are prone to circumlocutions ('an artistic thing for flowers' for 'trellis'), nominalizations ('ringer' for 'bell'), and comments which indicate knowledge of the concept but not the name ('I have one of these on my porch but I cannot think of its name'). These error types suggest that the conceptual information remains in long-term memory but that the transmission of information from long-term memory to the lexicon is unreliable (Bowles, 1989; Kempler and Zelinski, 1994). This interpretation of the naming problem is supported by several studies reporting an increase in the number of 'tip of the tongue' (TOT) experiences in old age, particularly with respect to rare words and proper nouns (Cohen and Faulkener, 1986; Maylor, 1990a; Burke et al., 1991). When the elderly find themselves in a TOT state they are less able than the young to provide partial information, such as the first letter or number of syllables (Cohen and Faulkener, 1986; Maylor, 1990b), but the rate with which TOT states spontaneously resolve is equivalent (Burke et al., 1991). This again suggests a temporary access problem rather than loss of the concept.

Access to established information also appears to be less flexible in old age. For example, in a standard vocabulary test where the subject is given the word and must indicate its definition the elderly do not show impairments. However, the elderly are impaired in the less familiar task of providing the name in response to the definition (Bowles, 1989; Maylor, 1990b). This reduced flexibility is reflected in Holland and Rabbitt's (1990) finding that the recent and remote reminiscences of the old are impoverished in detail relative to those of the young (for further discussion of remote memories in old age see Cohen and Faulkener, 1987; Fitzgerald, 1988; Craik and Jennings, 1992). Rabbitt (1989) found that elderly people who had lived in Oxford for at least 30 years reported fewer landmarks on a mental walk down the high street than middle-aged people who had lived in Oxford for the same amount of time. When the subjects were cued for missing landmarks the size of the age deficit was significantly reduced, although not eliminated. This finding again reveals impaired access to well-established information in old age, particularly when retrieval is unsupported.

In conclusion, old age is a time when it is harder to learn new information. The memory traces generated by the elderly are lacking in contextual detail, and under unstructured learning conditions age-related deficits with encoding new information have been extensively documented. However, it seems probable that these deficits can be reduced by structuring the learning episode and supporting retrieval. There appears to be no loss of well-established information from long-term memory in old age and also no disruption to the organization of this knowledge. However, as with newly learnt information, access to well-established information is impaired when the difficulty of retrieval is increased, either because self-initiated search strategies must be used, the information or the mode of access is less familiar, or the potential for interference is increased (Reder et al., 1986).

## Changes in language

In general it is not difficult to communicate with elderly people, and formal studies demonstrate the essential preservation of the semantic and syntactic processes which associate meaning with the symbols and structures of language (Burke and Harrold, 1988; Light, 1992). The preservation of vocabulary has already been noted, whilst the previous subsection reviewed evidence that the organization of knowledge remains unchanged in old age. In free speech and writing there is no evidence for a restriction in the range of vocabulary used in old age and discourse is meaningful and grammatical in structure (Kempler and Zelinski, 1994). The processes that parse and interpret sentential structures remain intact during old age (Stine et al., 1989). Indeed, it seems that the elderly can use their powers of comprehension to overcome some perceptual difficulties associated with their declining sensory powers (Cohen and Faulkener, 1983; Wingfield et al., 1985; Stine et al. 1989; Tun and Wingfield, 1993).

However, the elderly do encounter some problems with the use and comprehension of language. 'Tip of the tongue' experiences and naming difficulties increase in old age, as discussed in the last subsection, and the elderly can also experience difficulty in following conversations when many participants are involved and the topic of the conversation is unfamiliar. Although the speech of the elderly remains free of syntactic error, several studies have noted a decrease in the range and complexity of syntactic constructions used by elderly subjects both in spoken (Kynette and Kemper, 1986) and written (Kemper 1987, quoted in Stuart-Hamilton, 2000) discourse. The effect of syntactic complexity is also apparent in the comprehension performance of the elderly, as indexed by disproportionately poor performance relating to sentences with a complex syntactic structure relative those with a simple structure (Davis and Ball, 1989; Norman et al., 1991; Obler et al., 1991).

The elderly are impaired when required to reason or to make logical deductions on the basis of verbal information (Cohen, 1981; Light et al., 1982). For example, Riegel (1959) found impairment in a verbal analogies test whilst Light and Albertson (1988) found that the elderly have particular trouble answering questions presented in a double negative format. The problem persists even when the question remains present during inferential processing, showing that this is a problem with the reasoning required, and not a problem with memory (Cohen, 1981).

Memory demands can, however, affect comprehension. Comprehension studies which present the text as a whole and then test comprehension at the end by either asking questions or requiring recall have generally found impairments (Cohen, 1979; Spilich, 1983; Till, 1985). It seems probable that these impairments reflect the problems with memory and new learning which were reviewed in the previous section, rather than problems with comprehension processes themselves. Light and Albertson (1988) investigated the capacity of the elderly to detect anomalies in written material (using a paradigm first used by Cohen, 1979). They compared short stories in which the material intervening between the two bits of conflicting information involved a shift of topic (example 1), with stories in which the intervening material maintained attention to the key facts (example 2):

1 Next door to us there's an old man who's completely blind. He lives with his unmarried sister who works as housekeeper for a banker. She works long hours and rarely seems to get any time off to be with her brother. We often see him sitting on his porch reading his newspaper.

2 Next door to us there's an old man who's completely blind. He lives quite alone and nobody ever goes to visit him, but he seems to manage quite well. He has a guide dog and goes out every day to do his shopping. We often see him sitting on his porch reading his newspaper.

Light and Albertson replicated Cohen's finding that the elderly are impaired in detecting the anomaly in examples of the first kind, but they found no differences between the young and old in examples of the second kind. Further results suggest that the problem with maintaining comprehension over more than one topic relates to the need to retrieve information relating to the earlier topic. When the elderly fail to detect the anomaly in the examples above, they also fail to answer the more straightforward question 'What handicap did the old man have?'. Thus, it seems that the elderly can use their knowledge of language and the world to make appropriate inferences, but that problems with memory can lead to difficulties with remembering what is what and who is who when reading or listening to long passages of material.

In conclusion, the processes underlying language are essentially unchanged by old age. However, comprehension can be impaired under two situations. The first is when earlier information is required from memory, and the second is when comprehension demands problem-solving. The phenomenon observed with respect to intelligence and memory appears again with respect to language skills: there is preservation of the fundamental abilities, but these abilities become compromised under demanding situations.

## Changes in spatial cognition

The study of spatial skills in old age has been neglected relative to memory and language but studies of everyday usages of spatial information suggest minimal change to the fundamentals of spatial cognition (see Kirasic, 1989 for a review). This supports the informal opinion one would form based on the fact that elderly people do not get lost in their homes or neighbourhood and are able to manipulate clothes, household objects, appliances, and tools appropriately (assuming their are no motoric difficulties). A small-scale diary study by Kirasic (1989) documenting a week in the lives of three elderly women confirms that problems with orientation within the home and travel within the locality do not occur. All difficulties reported by these women related to problems with memory rather than spatial cognition, such as losing things in the home, entering rooms to discover that the purpose of the visit was forgotten, and remembering where the car was parked in large car parks.

Most evidence on spatial performance has been generated indirectly through studies of intelligence. It was noted in the subsection on changes in intelligence and problem-solving that intelligence subtests which involve a component of spatial manipulation have been found to be very sensitive to age (Meudell and Greenhalgh, 1987; Koss *et al.*, 1991; Schaie, 1996). People over the age of 60 perform more than one standard deviation below the average performance of the young in the Performance IQ subtests from the WAIS (Doppelt and Wallace, 1955). Salthouse (1982) also reports a decline of 5–10% per decade in the WAIS subtests which involve spatial manipulations (object assembly, block design, picture completion, and picture arrangement). Both these studies are cross-sectional, and thus are likely to over-estimate age effects due to cohort effects (for discussion of the methodological issues associated with cross-sectional research see Schaie, 1996; Woodruff-Pak, 1997), but Schaie's extensive longitudinal study of different generational cohorts confirms that individuals begin to show decline in spatial intelligence tests after the age of 50.

The particular sensitivity of psychometric tests with a spatial component has been interpreted as indicating the greater vulnerability of the right hemisphere of the brain relative to the left (Schaie and Schaie, 1977; Goldstein and Shelly, 1981), but there is no evidence to suggest that the right hemisphere ages more rapidly than the left. It seems more likely that the sensitivity of spatial psychometric tests is due to dependence upon 'fluid intelligence' (Horn and Cattell, 1967; Ardila and Rosselli, 1989), as explained earlier.

As within the other cognitive domains examined, age deficits in spatial cognition can be ameliorated by increasing the familiarity of the task or the material. Kirasic (1980, quoted in Kirasic, 1989) demonstrated that the elderly are poor at generating internal perspectives relating to a mock town (which they were required to learn in an earlier phase of the experiment), but are less impaired with reference to their home town. In a subsequent study, Kirasic (1981, quoted in Kirasic, 1989) found the elderly to be impaired when completing shopping tasks in an unfamiliar supermarket, but not when shopping in their own supermarket. Scheidt and Schaie (1978) found that the everyday spatial tasks which created most concern for the elderly were those which involved unfamiliar environments in which little help was available. Driving in heavy traffic and moving into a new home were paradigm examples of the types of activity which caused low confidence and anxiety in the elderly, whilst shopping in a familiar supermarket was not approached with fear or apprehension. The studies of Charness (1981a,b) and Salthouse (1984) examining chess and typing performance (respectively) also show that when people have expertise relating to particular forms of spatial cognition, old age does not

affect their competence (see subsection 'Changes in intelligence and problem-solving').

In summary, although most psychometric tests of spatial cognition reveal dramatic age impairments, it seems likely that this is because these tests demand the high-level manipulation of unfamiliar and abstract information, rather than because spatial cognition *per se* is especially vulnerable to the ageing process. As in the other cognitive domains reviewed, when the familiarity of the material or the task is increased, the observed age deficits in spatial cognition are reduced. The findings from laboratory studies are supported by investigations into the everyday activities of the elderly which suggest that problems with spatial cognition are only prominent if there is a memory demand or if the situation is unfamiliar and complex.

# Explaining cognitive change in old age

The evidence reviewed in the previous section suggests that age deficits appear in all cognitive domains, but only when the demands made upon cognition are high. These changes can cause some frustration or inefficiency during everyday life, but on the whole the impact of these changes is minimal and certainly not disabling. This is consistent with the view expressed by Craik and Rabinowitz (1984) that old age does not affect the structure of specific cognitive components but rather affects processing efficiency throughout the cognitive system. It was noted earlier that the problem of defining 'processing capacity' has so far proven intractable, but at a descriptive level it can be said that the elderly show impairments in tests when one or more of the following apply:

1 the material and the task are unfamiliar;

2 internal (mental) manipulation of the material is required;

3 optimal performance depends upon the generation of strategies.

The main debate within cognitive psychology concerns whether the effects of age upon the system are specific or general. Theories for specific change focus on the vulnerability of the frontal lobes and the 'executive' functions that control the high-level conscious processing that occurs within the 'attentional spotlight'. General theories propose that there is a general loss of processing speed throughout the cognitive system. Support for each position will be outlined, before concluding with the suggestion that there may less distinction between these two positions than the long-standing debate implies.

## Specific theories of cognitive change in old age

Specific theories of cognitive change in old age focus on attentional functions that derive from the information-processing models of the mind developed by cognitive psychologists during the late 1950s to early 1970s (Broadbent, 1958; Kahneman, 1973). Within such models it is assumed that perceptual processes can simultaneously extract large amounts of information from the environment and process it to a low level. However, the amount of information that can be processed to a high level (for example, to determine identity, consider implications, perform transformations, or memorize information) is strictly limited. It is further assumed that the cognitive system contains a central attentional component which selects the information that will be processed and filters out irrelevant information. The central attentional component is thought to possess a limited quantity of processing resources which can be deployed to undertake the high-level processing of the selected information. Any deterioration either in the efficiency of this component, or in the amount of processing resources it has at its disposal, would appear to predict the patterns of cognitive change observed in old age.

The notion of the central attentional component is also associated with the concept of working memory, the idea of a mental space in which a limited amount of information can be consciously attended to and processed. Baddeley (1986) postulated that the working memory system is divided into the three components and comprises a 'central executive' which controls and allocates resources across two specialized 'slave systems', the phonological loop (dedicated to verbal processing), and the visuospatial sketchpad (dedicated to visual processing). Tests that purport to measure the processing capacity of working memory correlate with performance in the 'difficult' cognitive tests of memory, language and visuospatial function that are vulnerable to age effects (Engle, 1996; Park *et al.*, 1996), leading further support to the idea that it is an alteration in working memory function which is at the heart of cognitive change in old age.

Today it might be fair to say that the concept of the 'working memory system' largely covers conscious processing throughout the whole cognitive system. The functions of the central executive have been mapped onto the association areas of the frontal lobe (particularly the dorsolateral regions (BA 9, 46 and 47) and anterior cingulate), whilst the 'slave systems' can be mapped onto the specialized perceptual and knowledge functions supported by the different regions of cerebral cortex behind the central fissure—that is, the cortex of the occipital lobe (visual perception), the temporal lobe (language and knowledge), and the parietal lobe (spatial cognition). Many of the long-standing problems associated with defining working memory may arise because the concept derives from hierarchical models of the mind, in which it is assumed that information passes through an ordered set of stages from perception to selection to apprehension to thought to decision, with the underlying representations becoming increasingly advanced at each stage. Findings from neuroscience and neuroimaging suggest that this one-way hierarchy is too simplistic. More recent theories see high-level control as operating not upon advanced forms of representation, but rather upon original perceptions, as illustrated by these quotations from Posner and Raichle (1994, p. 147):

> Attention can amplify computations within particular areas, but often appears to do so by reentering the same area that initially performed the computations, not by activating new higher-level association areas. [p. 147]

> Computer models of neural networks whose computations require closely coordinated cooperative activity among many areas also suggest the importance of information being fed back to sensory-specific areas for additional computation. [p. 144]

> In general one thinks of brain circuitry as formed of fixed anatomical connections between brain areas or between neurons within an area. However, it is well known that any brain area can be anatomically connected to any other area by either direct or indirect routes. In higher cognition, the act of attending organizes the circuitry between brain areas. [p. 147]

This hypothesis suggests that, in complex situations, the appropriate use of function-specific brain regions behind the central fissure

depends upon the efficiency of a network located in the frontal lobe. The conclusions concerning cognition in old age, namely, that although there is no direct damage to cognitive modules there is impairment in the ability to use them flexibly, could be explained by a disruption to the anterior cingulate/dorsolateral prefrontal network. The similarity between the cognitive profile of normal ageing and that associated with damage to the frontal lobes has long been noted, and there are many theories that propose a specific decline in the integrity and efficiency of the frontal lobe to account for cognitive ageing (Albert and Kaplan, 1980; Dempster, 1992; West, 1996; Woodruff-Pak, 1997).

An example of such a theory which has captured considerable interest is Hasher and Zacks' (1988) proposal that the apparent limitations in working memory capacity are caused by interference or 'cross-talk' between the various bits of information present in working memory at any one time. It has already been noted above that memory becomes increasingly prone to interference effects in old age. Efficient performance of a task requires that only information relevant to the task in hand be present within working memory. The most effective way in which relevant information can be sifted from irrelevant information is through a combination of facilitatory processes and inhibitory processes (Houghton and Tipper, 1994). Hasher and Zacks propose that ageing has a specific impact upon the efficiency of inhibitory processes. This proposal is supported by recent neuroimaging evidence provided by Milham *et al.* (2002), who compared brain activation in young and old subjects during the performance of the Stroop task, in which a prepotent response to read colour words must be inhibited in order to name the contrasting colour of the ink. Old age was associated with poorer performance together with under-activation of the dorsolateral prefrontal cortex and over-activation of areas in temporal cortex and inferior frontal cortex known to be important for word recognition and speech. This pattern suggests that inefficiency in the frontal regions can lead to activity lower down the cortical hierarchy that is not relevant to the task. Hasher and Zacks' theory has stimulated a wealth of experiments examining the inhibitory powers of the elderly which have shown that the elderly are more susceptible to a wide variety of distractions than the young (for a review see Zacks and Hasher, 1997).

Frontal lobe theories of cognitive ageing are supported not only by the cognitive profile of old age, but also by neuroanatomical evidence for greater change in the frontal lobe than in the posterior regions of the brain. MRI investigations show greater volume loss in the frontal lobe (see Fig. 3.2), corresponding with the results of post-mortem studies that indicate a greater loss of synaptic density (Gibson, 1983; Adams, 1987). During development the frontal lobe is a late myelinating region. The demyelination that occurs during old age appears to follow a 'last in, first out' pattern with the white matter of the prefrontal lobe being particularly vulnerable (Bartzokis *et al.*, 2003). At a functional level, there is corresponding evidence for pronounced hypometabolism within the frontal regions (Coffey *et al.*, 1992; Baron and Godeau, 2000). There is, therefore, plenty of neuroanatomical evidence to support frontal lobe theories of cognitive ageing.

In recent times, these theories have stimulated a large number of functional imaging studies examining the patterns of brain activation that underpin cognitive activities in the old and young. The nascent body of evidence emerging from these studies is hard to interpret. Findings are not merely random and diverse but often

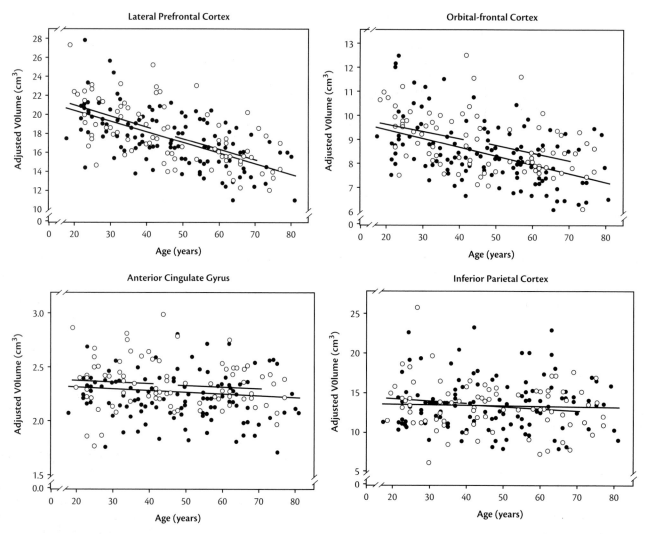

**Fig. 3.2** Rate of grey matter volume loss is greater in the frontal lobe than other lobes. Reprinted from N. Raz *et al.* (2004). Aging, sexual dimorphism, and hemispheric asymmetry of the cerebral cortex: replicability of regional differences. Neurobiology of Aging, 25, 377–96. Copyright (2004), with permission from Elsevier.

contradictory (see the reviews in Cabeza *et al.*, 2005). Studies vary widely in terms of the particular type of neuroimaging technology used, study design, cognitive task, subject selection, and theoretical focus so it is difficult to correlate discrepancies in results with methodological differences. However, the trends that do seem to be emerging point again towards the frontal lobe.

The characteristic pattern of particularly poor memory for context (see pp. 35–36) points towards deficiencies in frontal lobe involvement rather than deficiencies in medial temporal lobe involvement (Schacter *et al.*, 1997). This is supported by neuroimaging findings showing that during encoding, older adults underactivate the left prefrontal cortex (Grady *et al.*, 1995, 2002; Cabeza *et al.*, 1997; Stebbins *et al.*, 2002), an area known from the study of young subjects to be central to the encoding processes of episodic memory (Tulving *et al.*, 1994). Similarly, Jonides *et al.* (2000) have linked the greater interference in age-sensitive working memory tests to the under-activation of left prefrontal regions.

However, standing alongside these observations of reduced activity in the prefrontal regions in old age are observations of increased activity in other situations. Whilst the encoding processes of episodic memory are associated with the left prefrontal lobe, homologous areas in the right prefrontal lobe are important for retrieval (Tulving *et al.*, 1994). On the basis that left prefrontal activity is reduced during encoding in old age, it might be expected that right prefrontal activity would be reduced during retrieval. The evidence, however, shows no reduction in right prefrontal activity but an increase in left prefrontal activity during this phase of a memory test (Cabeza *et al.*, 1997). Cabeza *et al.* (2002) interpret these increased activations as representing compensatory functions within the prefrontal cortex in old age, the left and right sides starting to work together to compensate for biological change. Grady (2005), however, notes that the over-activation could indicate functional breakdown within the ageing brain. This would support a 'de-differentiation hypothesis' of ageing—a breakdown in the functional specificities of the cortical regions in old age, meaning that the prefrontal areas come to be involved in an increasingly diverse range of tasks.

There is evidence for both these aspects of the de-differentiation hypothesis. Beginning with the first point, there is evidence for the breakdown of other functional divisions in addition to the reduced lateralization between encoding and retrieval processes in episodic memory tests that has already been noted. In working memory tasks activation in young subjects is strongly lateralized according to the nature of the material to be processed; verbal materials activate the left prefrontal lobe whilst visual materials activate the right. This asymmetry also appears to lose definition in old age (Jonides *et al.*, 2000; Rympa and d'Eposito, 2000; Reuter-Lorenz *et al.*, 2000). Grady and colleagues have focused on the functional division between the dorsal (spatial processing) and ventral (object and face processing) streams of visual processing (Ungerleider and Mishkin, 1982). Old subjects show more activation in the dorsal stream when processing faces and more activation in the ventral stream when processing locations (Grady *et al.*, 1994; Grady, 2005).

With regard to the second point, the involvement of the prefrontal cortex in an increasingly diverse range of tasks, this area does appear to be activated in elderly subjects by simple tasks which do not activate the prefrontal lobe in youth. Reuter-Lorenz and Sylvester (2005) argue that study of ageing at the cognitive level alone may have been misleading concerning the nature of cognitive change in old age. Typically, the rote maintenance of information in mind is not associated with age effects. However, as soon as a demand to process or manipulate that information is introduced, age effects reliably appear (Babcock and Salthouse, 1990). Reuter-Lorenz and Sylvester argue that this does not show that rote maintenance processing is invulnerable to old age whilst active processing is, but that declines in rote maintenance 'merely escape detection with the use of behavioural measures alone' (p. 191). Their neuroimaging studies show an involvement of the prefrontal lobe in rote maintenance in old age that is absent in youth. Reuter-Lorenz and Sylvester conclude that ageing effects are system-wide and that age effects are only seen in 'difficult' tasks because it is only in these tasks that the compensatory reserve is exceeded.

DiGirolamo *et al.* (2001) have also found that old subjects activate the prefrontal cortex in tasks with low attentional demands that do not active the prefrontal cortex in the young. Grady (2002) found a similar pattern in a meta-analysis of face processing tasks. The face tasks were made harder either by introducing a memory demand or by degrading the quality of the photographs. Elderly subjects activated prefrontal cortex in response to both difficulty manipulations, whilst young subjects called upon prefrontal cortex only in response to the memory demand. Maylor and Wing (1996) found that postural stability was more seriously affected by concurrent cognitive demands in elderly people than the young, further suggesting that activities that in youth make little demand on executive control may increasingly rely on this control in old age.

## General theories of cognitive change

The greater involvement of the prefrontal lobe in a wide range of 'simple' activities could indicate that there are changes spread throughout the system that must be compensated for. Or it could indicate that the attentional system in the frontal lobe, as conceptualized by Posner and Raichle (1994) has lost strength, leading to a loss of focus and control throughout the cerebral cortex. The idea that change may be widespread throughout the system is supported by further findings from neuroimaging of alterations in the pattern of brain activation in conditions with minimal cognitive involvement, for example in response to photic stimulation (Ross *et al.*, 1997) or in performing a simple button-pressing task (Mattay *et al.*, 2002). It seems probable that the cognitive profile of old age is due to a combination of 'top-down' effects, mediated primarily by a loss of power in the central executive systems of the brain, and 'bottom-up' effects that affect the efficiency of the whole system.

'Bottom-up' effects may be due in part to the loss of sensory sensitivity, particular with respect to vision and hearing, that is another inevitable feature of old age. It has long been suggested that sensory decline is related to mild cognitive decline (Baltes and Lindenberger, 1997). Like most factors implicated in cognitive ageing, it is likely that sensory loss plays a role (see Stuart-Hamilton, 2000 for a more detailed review) but it is unlikely to provide the sole explanation (Lindenberger *et al.*, 2001). A far more influential general theory has been the 'generalized slowing hypothesis' which claims that the cognitive effects of old age can be accounted for by a basic loss in the speed of processing that operates throughout the entire system. It is certainly the case that the reaction times of the elderly are slower than those of the young, regardless of the task performed (Cerella, 1985), and thus, there is evidence for a general slowing of processing in old age. The generalized slowing hypothesis is most strongly supported by partial correlation analyses which show that measures of speed can account for most of the age-related variance in a wide variety of higher cognitive tests, regardless of whether those tests have a time limit or not (Salthouse, 1993). Calculations show that around 90 to 99% of the variance shared between age and higher cognition is also shared with speed measures (Salthouse, 1993).

Traditionally, these speeded measures have been pitted against working memory measures to determine which concept is the most effective at explaining age-related cognitive change. Speeded measures tend to out-perform working memory measures in statistical models of cognitive ageing, lending support to the generalized slowing hypothesis (Salthouse and Babcock, 1991). However, the Salthouse effect depends critically upon the type of speeded tests chosen to measure the purported basic element of 'processing speed'. Salthouse emphasizes the simplicity of his speeded measures, but if the speeded task becomes too simple then the power is lost. A paradigm example of an effective task, widely used by Salthouse and colleagues, is the Digit Symbol subtest from the WAIS (Wechsler, 1981). In this test the subject must decode numbers into symbols as fast as he/she can with reference to the key provided. Simpler speed tests, such as simple reaction time or copying rather than decoding symbols, are much less effective in explaining age-related variance in cognitive performance (Milwain, 1999). Although simple on the surface, Digit Symbol in fact involves coordination of a large number of component processes. Speed in this task requires the maintenance of a strong mental focus and resistance to interference or distraction. This brings the issue, once more, back to the specific functions of the frontal lobe. When searching for a theory of cognitive ageing it seems that any particular line of evidence appearing to support one explanation tends to go full circle, coming back to the explanation that was initially excluded.

These circles may suggest that the differences between the generalized slowing hypothesis and executive theories of cognitive ageing are more apparent than real. Indeed, although 'the central executive' has been defined to be a specific component of the cognitive system, its functions have always been general, in that they relate to the control of processing throughout the rest of the cognitive system. So there is some blurring between what is meant by 'specific' and 'general' from the outset. At the neuroanatomical level, whilst the frontal lobe remains central, the focus is being expanded to recognize that other structures, such as the thalamus (van der Werf *et al.*, 2001) and basal ganglia are also likely be important in explaining cognitive ageing. These frontostriatal circuits are implicated in both cognitive speed and executive functions (Hedden and Gabrieli, 2004), as is white matter change (Ylikoski *et al.*, 1993), another factor increasingly implicated in explaining cognitive decline in old age (Gunning-Dixon and Raz, 2000). Gunning-Dixon and Raz note that the association between global measures of white matter integrity and cognitive function is consistent with a generalized detrimental effect on neural transmission speed and interneuronal connectivity but also note that within their analysis it was impossible to say whether regional measures of white matter damage (i.e. which lobe) would yield more specific information. To the extent that white matter damage is also more severe in the frontal lobe (Bartzokis *et al.*, 2003) there is again blurring between 'specific' and 'general' with respect to this factor. There is also evidence that frontal lobe functions are highly dependent upon dopamine function throughout the frontostriatal loops and the whole cerebral cortex. The dopamine system has been singled out as being especially affected during normal ageing (Hedden and Gabrieli, 2004; Backman and Farde, 2005). Computerized simulations of the down-regulation of dopaminergic function in old age suggest a decrease in the signal-to-noise ratio throughout the neural networks, which affects the stability and distinctness of representations within memory. The performance characteristics of the 'elderly neural networks' mirror many of the phenomena (e.g. the reduced flexibility of access and loss of contextual detail) reviewed earlier (Li, 2005). These performance characteristics may also be related to the loss of functional definition within the cerebral cortex observed in the neuroimaging studies reviewed above.

Before moving onto the next section, we should consider a final issue which may be relevant. This concerns the availability and management of energy in old age. In the considerable theoretical discussions of the cognitive psychologists not much is made of the choice of the word 'effortful' to describe the type of processing which is particularly vulnerable to old age (Hasher and Zacks, 1979). Use of the word 'effortful' implies that the vulnerable processes are those that are quite literally experienced as being hard work. Alterations in energy availability and the management of energy could, therefore, be important in understanding the nature of cognitive ageing, particularly the move away from strategic forms of cognitive processing in old age.

Verhaeghen and Marcoen (1996) ran a study investigating the effects of mnemonic training upon memory ability in old age. The elderly did benefit from the mnemonic training, but to a lower degree than the young. An interesting feature of this study is that a significant number of elderly people decided not use the mnemonic in memory tests, especially when study time was short. This suggests that the move away from strategic cognitive processing in old age reflects not only a deficit in the ability to undertake strategic processing (a 'processing deficit') but also a conscious decision not to use such forms of processing (a 'production deficit'). Cognitive psychologists tend to refer to non-use of strategic forms of processing as a 'deficit' or 'non-compliance' but the decision not to use these forms of processing may be a reflection of wisdom

rather than failure. It seems probable that elderly subjects are aware both of their falling energy levels and of reductions in their processing abilities. They may, therefore, make a decision not to bother to use cognitive strategies because the costs outweigh the benefits. When it comes to coping with mild declines in memory ability it makes more sense, from the perspective of both regulating energy expenditure and improving the chances of success, to write a list than to engage in mnemonic training. If the central nervous system does have less energy available to it in old age, there may be readjustments at both a conscious (decisional) and non-conscious (automatic) level gearing the system away from high-demand executive or strategic processing.

At a broad level the evidence from EEG studies (as reviewed by Whalley, 2001) and blood-flow studies (as reviewed by Baron and Godeau, 2000) supports the idea that the elderly brain is less energetic than the young brain. There is also no doubt that elderly people are more likely to experience fatigue than the young. Changes in sleep patterns, which are extremely common if not universal during old age (Whalley, 2001), may also be significant, given that disturbed sleep is associated with alterations in the neurochemistry of the cerebral cortex and the disruption of the 'executive abilities' that are characteristically sensitive to old age (Salzarulo *et al.*, 1997; Beebe and Gozal, 2002; Jelicic *et al.*, 2002). However, the specifics of how energy availability changes in old age and how this impacts upon the brain and cognitive function remain unknown.

## Comparison of cognitive change in old age and in early Alzheimer's disease

The previous section has reviewed the changes associated with old age at some length. It was noted at the outset that the main reason for understanding the mild cognitive changes which appear to be a universal of old age is to answer the question of whether the dementias represent distinct disease states or whether they are extreme variants of the normal ageing process. From the last section it is apparent that there are a number of changes within the brain that could be associated with cognitive decline in old age, but amongst these many changes mild degrees of Alzheimer's pathology have not featured. It is plausible, however, that the mild degree of Alzheimer's pathology commonly observed in the brains of elderly people without dementia (Esiri *et al.*, 2001) could be responsible for some of the changes currently associated with normal ageing. Both Alzheimer's disease and normal ageing are strongly associated with memory problems, in particular the ability to learn new information and consciously recall it after a significant lapse of time. And, furthermore, neither old age nor Alzheimer's disease is a purely amnesic syndrome, in that deficits are also seen in other cognitive domains such as language and visuospatial functions. There is no doubt that whatever the resource is that underlies 'the central executive', 'effortful processing', and 'processing speed', it is very sensitive to Alzheimer's disease as well as to normal ageing (Jorm, 1986; Baddeley *et al.*, 1991; Bayles *et al.*, 1991; Nebes and Brady, 1992). Variables that affect performance in cognitive tests often affect performance in a qualitatively similar manner in old age and Alzheimer's disease even though the Alzheimer's patients perform at a significantly lower level overall (Martin *et al.*, 1985; Nebes, 1992). Free recall tests, for example, which demand internally driven search strategies and place heavy demands on effortful processing, show the strongest age effects, but are also the most effective at discriminating between the non-demented and the mildly demented. It has been argued that the degree of deficit seen in a memory test, for both the normal elderly and Alzheimer's patients, is determined by the degree to which the test demands effortful processing (Huppert, 1994).

However, qualitative similarities relating to the need for effortful processing need to be viewed with caution. Tests demanding effortful processing are known to be exquisitely sensitive to any form of challenge to the brain (Grafman *et al.*, 1990; Lezak, 1995). In other words, the tests that are most sensitive to normal ageing are those that are highly sensitive to any form of brain damage, but also highly unspecific with regard to the type of brain damage. Thus, it is dangerous to read too much into the similarity between normal ageing and Alzheimer's disease on the basis that 'difficult' tasks are those that are most sensitive to both challenges.

More detailed investigations into the nature of the memory deficit in dementia of the Alzheimer's type (DAT) reveal that whilst there are many similarities to normal old age there are also important differences, which suggest a particular problem in the consolidation of memories over time in DAT that is absent in normal ageing (Grober and Buschke, 1987; Hart *et al.* 1988; Dannenbaum *et al.*, 1988; Pepin and Eslinger, 1989; Christensen *et al.*, 1998). Furthermore, it appears that various forms of automatic processing relating to memory, that are not vulnerable to normal ageing, are vulnerable to Alzheimer's disease (Weingartner *et al.*, 1981; Grafman *et al.*, 1990). Overall, this evidence points towards medial temporal lobe damage as being central to the memory deficit of DAT (Corkin, 1982). Later neuropathological research showing that the medial temporal lobe is at the epicentre of the Alzheimer's disease process (Braak and Braak, 1991) has supported Corkin's conclusion based on the neuropsychological profile of DAT.

The conclusion that the memory symptoms of Alzheimer's disease are a reflection of a primary breakdown of memory functions, rather than secondary to a loss of processing resources, is further underscored by the fact that the memory deficit in Alzheimer's disease is disproportionate relative to measures of overall cognitive ability. Partial correlation techniques show that whilst measures of cognitive speed can account for the vast majority of age-related variance in memory performance (see p. 41), such measures cannot account for memory loss in Alzheimer's disease (Sliwinski and Buschke, 1997). Petersen *et al.* (1994) equated non-demented and demented patients on a test of overall cognitive ability (the Mini Mental State, Folstein *et al.*, 1975) but found that even when overall cognitive function was matched in this way, the memory function of the demented patients was still significantly worse than that of the non-demented subjects. A more detailed consideration of these relationships can be found in Milwain (1999).

Furthermore, whilst access to established information in long-term memory follows qualitatively similar patterns in old age and Alzheimer's disease (Nebes 1989; Bayles *et al.*, 1991), there is evidence for a substantial deterioration in the substrate of the knowledge base in Alzheimer's disease that is lacking in normal ageing (Chertkow and Bub, 1990; Hodges *et al.*, 1992; Hodges *et al.*, 1996). Priming procedures that are automatic, and do not demand effortful processing, reveal abnormalities in Alzheimer's patients (Shimamura *et al.*, 1987; Salmon *et al.*, 1988) but not in the normal elderly (see above; reviewed by Light, 1992). We saw above that age has minimal impact upon the forms of visuospatial processing associated with everyday life. This again contrasts with the symptoms of Alzheimer's disease where problems with copying and drawing, navigating the familiar local environment, and praxic skills, such as dressing or using household objects, are common. Overall, Alzheimer's disease seems seriously to undermine familiar and well-practised skills and knowledge in addition to the more active types of processing that are particularly vulnerable to normal ageing. Loss of some kind of central resource seems to provide a good account of the cognitive profile of normal ageing, but is not a sufficient explanation for the symptoms of Alzheimer's disease. It is this loss of understanding relating to the familiar and well-practised that makes Alzheimer's disease, unlike normal ageing, such a devastating condition. With reference to the quotation from Craik and Rabinowitz (1984) cited earlier, the evidence suggests that the cognitive symptoms of Alzheimer's disease represent both a loss of processing power and broken components. The idea of 'broken components' is congruent with the particular vulnerability to Alzheimer's disease of the association areas of the cortex in the temporal and parietal lobes that support language, knowledge, and praxic functions.

This does not, however, rule out early stage Alzheimer's pathology as being the prime cause of the mild processing deficit associated with normal ageing. The loss of processing ability associated with normal ageing could be accounted for by a low level of pathology with a limited spatial extent, while the more fundamental breakdown of the cognitive architecture seen in Alzheimer's disease reflects a dense pathology with a diffuse spatial extent. However, were normal ageing primarily due to Alzheimer's disease taking hold within the medial temporal lobe, then the cognitive profile would be one of disproportionate memory loss, and it has already been seen that the memory loss associated with normal ageing is proportionate. Disproportionate memory loss in old age is associated with a high risk of developing diagnosable Alzheimer's disease over the following few years (Morris *et al.*, 1991; Bondi *et al.*, 1994; Linn *et al.*, 1995; Bowen *et al.*, 1997). It is now recognized that Alzheimer's disease has an amnesic prodrome (Hodges, 1998) that precedes the diagnosis of dementia by as much as 5 years. There is, therefore, overlap within the non-demented population between those with normal ageing and those with incipient Alzheimer's disease, and the evidence points not towards a continuum but to the need to distinguish between these two processes. Whilst the medial temporal lobe has been observed to decline with increasing age (Geinisman *et al.*, 1995; Small, 2001), and lower medial temporal lobe volumes are associated with poorer memory amongst the non-demented elderly (Golomb *et al.*, 1994; de Toledo-Morrell *et al.*, 2000; Rosen *et al.*, 2003), there is increasing belief that these observations reflect undetected Alzheimer's disease rather than normal ageing. Small entorhinal cortex volumes predict precipitous cognitive decline towards Alzheimer's disease (de Toledo-Morrell *et al.*, 2000; Killiany *et al.*, 2002). Small *et al.* (2002) concluded that there is evidence for normal change within the medial temporal lobe, but that such changes are confined to the dentate gyrus and subiculum. Volume loss in the entorhinal cortex, on the other hand, is a sign of pathological change. Longitudinal measures of change in the medial temporal lobe also suggest that whilst there is a mild reduction in medial temporal lobe volume with advancing age, Alzheimer's disease is associated with some kind of catastrophic trigger that markedly accelerates the trajectory of change (see Fig. 3.3).

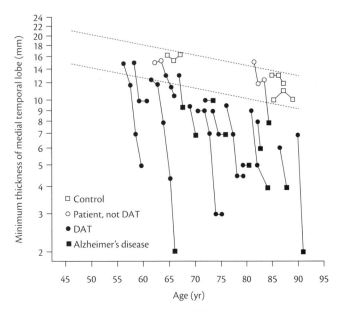

**Fig. 3.3** Rapid atrophy of the medial temporal lobe in Alzheimer's disease. Reprinted from Jobst *et al.* (1994). Copyright (1994), with permission from Elsevier.

The markers of Alzheimer's disease found in the non-demented elderly tend to be limited to the occasional neurofibrillary tangle within the entorhinal cortex or hippocampus (Mann *et al.* 1987; Bouras *et al.*, 1994) and diffuse (not neuritic) amyloid deposits in the cerebral cortex (Mann *et al.*, 1990; Delaere *et al.*, 1993). Although amyloid deposition may be involved in triggering the cascade that leads to dense Alzheimer's pathology and cell death, diffuse amyloid deposition itself correlates weakly with cognitive ability in Alzheimer's disease (Arriagada *et al.*, 1992; Delaere *et al.*, 1993; Nagy *et al.*, 1996) and is not associated with poor performance in neuropsychological tests in non-demented samples (Dickson *et al.*, 1991). Thus, whilst development of these mild markers of Alzheimer's disease in old age may be almost inevitable, it is unlikely the changes have any noticeable cognitive effect. Neuropathological investigations have also led to the conclusion that some other event is required to catalyse the process from these mild signs to full blown Alzheimer's disease (Ulrich, 1985). Overall the evidence leads to this positive conclusion: it is not the case that all old people are harbouring incipient Alzheimer's disease, and the changes of normal cognitive ageing are more likely to be due to the changes reviewed earlier.

## Preventing cognitive decline in old age

The continuum hypothesis of normal ageing and dementia is built upon the claim that the categories of 'normal ageing', 'mild cognitive impairment', and 'dementia' are highly heterogeneous conditions lying along a continuum of cognitive change in old age. This claim is true, but it does not imply a single continuum of underlying change. It leaves room for the belief that within the brains of the elderly, both pathological and non-pathological influences are operating to varying degrees. Naturally, the further one moves along the spectrum towards dementia the more likely it is that pathological influences are involved and dominant.

A recent analysis of a cohort of 150 people attending the Dundee Memory Clinic (Selwyn *et al.*, 2006) reported that 44% of

these people with concerns about their cognition were diagnosed with Alzheimer's disease (AD), 11% with vascular dementia (VD), 7% with mixed AD and VD, 5% with alcohol-related cognitive impairment, 17% with mood disorder, and 9% with a non-progressive impairment following a cerebrovascular event. One person had hypothyroidism and another complications following meningitis. However, despite the heterogeneous nature of the sample, 83% had some form of vascular risk, and control of vascular risk is emerging as the most important modifiable factor for preventing cognitive decline and dementia in old age (Whalley, 2001; Purandare *et al.*, 2005).

It is increasingly apparent that the preparation for old age is a life-long endeavour. As noted above, the control of vascular risk is becoming a central issue in the prevention of dementia, with growing evidence suggesting that what is good for the heart is also good for the head (Whalley, 2001). Anyone seeking to protect their cognition in old age is well advised to eat a healthy diet, low in fat and cholesterol and high in fish (Reqeujo *et al.*, 2003; Jorm, 2005) and vegetables (Kang *et al.*, 2005). The association between elevated homocysteine levels and risk for Alzheimer's disease (Clarke *et al.*, 1998; Morris, 2003) means that it may be particularly important to ensure that the diet includes adequate levels of folic acid and vitamin $B_{12}$—although, on the basis of existing evidence, dietary supplements are not associated with any clear benefit (Whalley, 2001; Malouf *et al.*, 2003). Physical exercise and an active lifestyle are associated with more constant blood flow to the brain in old age (as reviewed by Whalley, 2001). A study by Colcombe *et al.* (2003) found that aerobic fitness was associated with higher brain tissue density in the grey matter of the cerebral cortex and white matter of the frontal lobe, further suggesting associations between physical fitness and the health of the brain. However, cognitive measures were not included in the study design and (as with many associations in dementia research), the direction between cause and effect remains unknown. Stress management during life may be another modifiable factor. Parallels between the effects of stress and the consequences of ageing have long been noted (Selye, 1970) and there is growing evidence that glucocorticoids and other stress-related hormones may damage the hippocampus (Lupien *et al.*, 1998; Porter and Landfield, 1998). People who learn how to manage their stress effectively may be at lower risk for cognitive impairment or dementia during their old age (Pruessner *et al.*, 2004).

There is growing interest in the idea that mental exercise may protect cognition in old age, often marketed under the rubric of 'use it or lose it'. Recent television adverts suggest that practice with specialist puzzles for the Nintendo will produce observable improvements in cognition. Practice effects mean that this is probably true, but such claims need to be treated with caution. Studies from cognitive psychology show that training on a specific cognitive task will cause improvement in that task but that the benefits do not generalize to other forms of cognitive activity (Nyberg, 2005). Extensive training with the Nintendo is not guaranteed to have any impact on the everyday frustrations of getting old, such as forgetting names or struggling to understand the instruction manual for a new gadget. In a study of extensive mnemonic training for the elderly Baltes and Kliegl (1992) concluded that 'there is a robust, if not irreversible, negative age difference in some basic components of the mind' (p. 124). However, interventions targeted at frontal lobe, rather than mnemonic, functions have been found to be effective in a recent study (Levine *et al.* 2007).

If a person enjoys doing crosswords or sudoku puzzles, then all to the good, but if the activity is not enjoyable and is being undertaken specifically for the purposes of protecting cognition, then they would be better advised to focus on maintaining a healthy lifestyle including a good diet, plenty of physical exercise and keeping up the social contacts and activities they do enjoy. Indeed, if a person is very anxious about losing cognition then engagement with such puzzles could increase stress and possibly accelerate the ageing of his or her brain (Porter and Landfield, 1998).

To the extent that there is a valid difference between normal cognitive decline in old age and the accumulative forms of damage that lead to dementia, preventive medicine would seem to be more appropriately directed at the latter than the former. The effects of normal ageing upon cognition, although detectable in psychological studies, are so mild that it is unnecessary to seek to eliminate cognitive decline in old age altogether. Nonetheless, just as a considerable market has grown up for products promising to stave off the normal effects of age upon beauty, so such a market for products promising to stave off these effects upon the intellect is likely to grow, even in the absence of any evidence to suggest that such a change is pathological, or even meaningful, in terms of its impact on everyday life and well-being. For example, there have been suggestions that *Gingko biloba* may be effective in augmenting cognitive function in the elderly. The data remain inconclusive, and there has not been adequate research into the potential side-effects of this herbal remedy, but the US market for this product is already estimated to be US$ 240 billion per annum (Lee and Birks, 2004). There has also been interest in the use of the anticholinesterases to reverse the cognitive effects of normal ageing, but here it is relatively clear that the likelihood of unpleasant side-effects out-weighs the possibilities of any benefits (Rose, 2005). More recently attention has turned to procaine products as a potential anti-ageing treatment for cognition. The efficacy and safety of these products has also not been fully investigated and yet it is estimated that more than 50 million people around the world are already using them in the hope of boosting cognition (Szatmari and Bereczki, 2006).

Although there is no good evidence to support the use of any of the products above, scientific advancement does seem to be providing the means by which old age can be fought more successfully than in the past. The quest for immortality, of course, is very ancient so it is not surprising that products promising to maintain youthful appearance and zeal are in high demand. The question as to whether this quest is right, in moral terms, or whether people should accept the inevitability of old age and death with good grace, is very difficult. Marketing material for drugs promising to protect cognition in old age often blurs this moral issue by raising the prospect of incipient dementia as one of the reasons for using these products. The evidence reviewed in this chapter suggests that for the majority of elderly people mild cognitive decline is not indicative of incipient dementia. It may be unwelcome but it is not cause for fear. It is important that the fear of dementia is kept to its proper proportions and it should not be misused for cynical purposes.

Furthermore, recent evidence already suggests that the predicted dementia crisis will hit the disadvantaged sectors of society harder than the advantaged sectors, with repeated findings that a low intellect, poor education, and low socio-economic status are all factors associated with a greater risk of dementia (reviewed by Whalley, 2001). The possibility, or perhaps probability, of efficacious 'smart drugs' becoming available on the private market will only widen the gulf between the late life prospects for those who get off to a good start in life and those who do not. As knowledge of the processes of normal ageing within the brain grows many of the persistently difficult questions left unanswered in this chapter will be answered, but difficult ethical questions will take their place (Rose, 2005).

## References

Adams, I. (1987). Plasticity of the synaptic contact zone following loss of synapses in the cerebral cortex of aging humans. *Brain Research*, **424**, 343–51.

Albert, M.S. and Kaplan, E. (1980) Organic implications of neuropsychological deficits in the elderly. In *New directions in memory and aging: Proceedings of the George A. Talland Memorial Conference* (ed. L.W. Poon). Lawrence Erlbaum Associates, Hillsdale, NJ.

Albert, M.S., Heller, H.S., and Milberg, W. (1988). Changes in naming ability with age. *Psychology and Aging*, **3**, 173–8.

Ardila, A. and Rosselli, M. (1989). Neuropsychological characteristics of normal aging. *Developmental Neuropsychology*, **5**, 307–20.

Arenberg, D. (1982). Changes with age in problem-solving. In *Aging and Cognitive Processes* (ed. F.I.M. Craik and A.S. Trehub). Plenum, New York.

Arriagada, P.V., Growdon, J.H., Hedley-Whyte, E.T., and Hyman, B.T. (1992) Neurofibrillary tangles but not senile plaques parallel duration and severity of Alzheimer's disease. *Neurology*, **42**, 631–9.

Babcock, R.L. and Salthouse, T.A. (1990). Effects of increased processing demands on age differences in working memory. *Psychology and Aging*, **5**, 421–8.

Backman, L. and Farde, L. (2005). The role of dopamine systems in cognitive aging. In *Cognitive Neuroscience of Aging* (ed. R. Cabeza, L. Nyberg, and D. Park). Oxford University Press, New York.

Baddeley, A.D. (1986). *Working memory.* Oxford University Press, Oxford.

Baddeley, A.D., Bressi, S., Della Sala, S., Logie, R.H., and Spinnler, H. (1991). The decline of working memory in Alzheimer's disease. *Brain*, **114**, 2521–42.

Baltes, P.B. (1993). The aging mind: potential and limits. *The Gerontologist*, **33**, 580–94.

Baltes, P.B. and Kliegl, R. (1992). Further testing of limits of cognitive plasticity: negative age differences in a mnemonic skill are robust. *Developmental Psychology*, **28**, 121–5.

Baltes, P.B. and Lindenberger, U. (1997). Emergence of a powerful connection between sensory and cognitive functions across the adult life span: a new window to the study of cognitive aging? *Psychology and Aging*, **12**, 12–21.

Baron, J.C. and Godeau, C. (2000). Human aging. In *Brain mapping: the systems* (ed. A.W. Toga and J.C. Mazziotta). Academic Press, San Diego.

Bartlett, J.C. and Leslie, J.E. (1986). Aging and memory for faces versus single views of faces. *Memory and Cognition*, **14**, 371–81.

Bartlett, J.C., Till, R.E., Gernsbacher, M., and Gorman, W. (1983). Age-related differences in memory for lateral orientation of pictures. *Journal of Gerontology*, **38**, 439–46.

Bartzokis, G., Cummings, J.L., Sultzer, D., Henderson, V.W., Nuechterlein, K.H., and Mintz, J. (2003). White matter structural integrity in healthy aging adults and patients with Alzheimer disease. *Archives of Neurology*, **2003**, 393–8.

Bayles, K.A., Tomoeda, C.K., Kasniak, A.W., and Trosset, M.W. (1991). Alzheimer's disease effects on semantic memory: loss of structure or impaired processing? *Journal of Cognitive Neuroscience*, **3**, 166–82.

Beebe, D.W. and Gozal, D. (2002). Obstructive sleep apnea and the prefrontal cortex: towards a comprehensive model linking nocturnal upper airway obstruction to daytime cognitive and behavioral deficits. *Journal of Sleep Research*, **11**, 1–16.

Bondi, M.W., Monsch, A.U., Galasko, D., Butters, N., Salmon, D.P., and Delis, D.C. (1994). Preclinical cognitive markers of dementia of the Alzheimer type. *Neuropsychology*, **8**, 374–84.

Botwinick, J. (1977). Intellectual abilities. In *The handbook of the psychology of aging* (ed. J.E. Birren and K.W. Schaie). Van Nostrand Reinhold, New York.

Bouras, C., Hof, P.R., Giannakopoulos, P., Michel, J.-P., and Morrison, J.H. (1994). Regional distribution of neurofibrillary tangles and senile plaques in the cerebral cortex of elderly patients: A quantitative evaluation of a one-year autopsy population from a geriatric hospital. *Cerebral Cortex*, **4**, 138–50.

Bowen, J., Teri, L., Kukull, W., McCormick, W., McCurry, S., and Larson, E.B. (1997). Progression to dementia in patients with isolated memory loss. *The Lancet*, **349**, 763–5.

Bowles, N.L. (1989). Age and semantic inhibition in word retrieval. *Journal of Gerontology: Psychological Sciences*, **44**, P88–P90.

Braak, H. and Braak, E. (1991). Neuropathological staging of Alzheimer-related changes. *Acta Neuropathologica*, **82**, 238–59.

Brayne, C. and Calloway, P. (1988). Normal ageing, impaired cognitive function and senile dementia of the Alzheimer's type: a continuum? *Lancet*, **ii**, 1265–7.

Broadbent, D.E. (1958). *Perception and communication*. Pergamon, Oxford.

Brown, A.S. and Mitchell, D.B. (1991). Age differences in retrieval consistency and response dominance. *Journal of Gerontology: Psychological Sciences*, **46**, P332–P339.

Buckner, R. (2005). Three principles for cognitive aging research. In *Cognitive neuroscience of aging* (ed. R. Cabeza, L. Nyberg, and D. Park). Oxford University Press, New York.

Burke, D.M. and Harrold, R.M. (1988). Automatic and effortful semantic processes in old age: experimental and naturalistic approaches. In *Language, memory and aging* (ed. L.L. Light and D.M. Burke). Cambridge University Press, Cambridge.

Burke, D.M. and Light, L.L. (1981). Memory and aging: the role of retrieval processes. *Psychological Review*, **90**, 513–46.

Burke, D.M. and Yee, P.L. (1984). Semantic priming during sentence processing by young and older adults. *Developmental Psychology*, **20**, 903–10.

Burke, D.M., Mackay, D.G., Worthley, J.S., and Wade, E. (1991). On the tip of the tongue: what causes word finding failures in young and older adults? *Journal of Memory and Language*, **30**, 542–79.

Byrd, M. (1984). Age differences in the retrieval of information from semantic memory. *Experimental Aging Research*, **10**, 29–33.

Byrd, M. (1985). Age differences in the ability to recall and summarise text information. *Experimental Aging Research*, **11**, 87–91.

Cabeza, R., Grady, C., Nyberg, L., McIntosh, A., Tulving, E., and Kapur, S. (1997). Age-related differences in neural activity during memory encoding and retrieval: a positron emission tomography study. *Journal of Neuroscience*, **17**, 391–400.

Cabeza, R., Anderson, N.D., Locantore, J.K., and McIntosh, A.R. (2002). Aging gracefully: compensatory brain activity in high-performing older adults. *Neuroimage*, **17**, 1394–402.

Cabeza, R., Nyberg, L., and Park, D. (2005). *Cognitive neuroscience of aging*. Oxford University Press, New York.

Cerella, J. (1985). Information processing rates in the elderly. *Psychological Bulletin*, **98**, 67–83.

Charness, N. (1981a). Aging and skilled problem solving. *Journal of Experimental Psychology: General*, **110**, 21–38.

Charness, N. (1981b). Search in chess: aging and skill differences. *Journal of Experimental Psychology: Human Perception and Performance*, **7**, 467–76.

Chertkow, H. and Bub, D. (1990). Semantic memory loss in dementia of the Alzheimer's type. *Brain*, **113**, 397–417.

Christensen, H., Kopelman, M.D., Stanhope, N., Lorentz, L., and Owen, P. (1998). Rates of forgetting in Alzheimer's dementia. *Neuropsychologia*, **36**, 547–57.

Clarke, R., Smith, A.D., Jobst, K.A., Refsum, H., Sutton, L., and Ueland, P. (1998). Folate, vitamin B12 and serum total homocysteine levels in confirmed Alzheimer's disease. *Archives of Neurology*, **55**, 1449–55.

Coffey, C.E., Wilkinson, W.E., Parashos, L.A. *et al.* (1992). Quantitative cerebral anatomy of the aging human brain: a cross-sectional study using magnetic resonance imaging. *Neurology*, **42**, 527–36.

Cohen, G. (1979). Language comprehension in old age. *Cognitive Psychology*, **11**, 412–29.

Cohen, G. (1981). Inferential reasoning in old age. *Cognition*, **9**, 59–72.

Cohen, G. and Faulkener, D. (1983). Word recognition: age differences in contextual facilitation effects. *British Journal of Psychology*, **74**, 239–51.

Cohen, G. and Faulkener, D. (1986). Memory for proper names: age differences in retrieval. *British Journal of Developmental Psychology*, **4**, 187–97.

Cohen, G. and Faulkener, D. (1987). Life span changes in autobiographical memory. In *Practical aspects of memory: current research and issues* (ed. M.M. Gruneberg, P.E. Morris, and R.N. Sykes). John Wiley and Sons, Chichester.

Cohen, G. and Faulkener, D. (1989). Age differences in source forgetting: effects on reality monitoring and on eyewitness testimony. *Psychology and Aging*, **4**, 10–17.

Cohen, G., Conway, M.A., and Maylor, E.A. (1994). Flashbulb memory in young and older adults. *Psychology and Aging*, **9**, 454–63.

Colcombe, S., Erickson, K.I., Raz, N. *et al.* (2003). Aerobic fitness reduces brain tissue loss in aging humans. *Journal of Gerontology A, Biological Sciences and Medical Sciences*, **58A**, 176–80.

Corkin, S. (1982). Some relationships between global amnesias and the memory impairments in Alzheimer's disease. In *Alzheimer's disease: a report of progress* (ed. S. Corkin, K.L. Davis, J.H. Growdon, E. Usdin, and M.J. Wutrman). Raven, New York.

Craik, F.I.M. (1977). Age differences in human memory. In *Handbook of the psychology of aging* (ed. J.E. Birren and K.W. Schaie). Van Nostrand Reinhold, New York.

Craik, F.I.M. and Jennings, J.M. (1992). Human memory. In *Handbook of aging and cognition* (ed. F.I.M. Craik and T.A. Salthouse). Erlbaum, Hillsdale, NJ.

Craik, F.I.M. and Lockhart, R.S. (1972). Levels of processing: a framework for memory research. *Journal of Verbal Learning and Verbal Behavior*, **11**, 671–84.

Craik, F.I.M. and McDowd, J.M. (1987). Age differences in recall and recognition. *Journal of Experimental Psychology: Learning, Memory and Cognition*, **13**, 474–9.

Craik, F.I.M. and Rabinowitz, J.C. (1984). Age differences in the acquisition and use of verbal information: a tutorial review. In *Attention and performance X: control of language processes* (ed. H. Bouma and D. Bouwhuis), pp. 471–99. Lawrence Erlbaum Associates, Hillsdale, NJ.

Craik, F.I.M. and Rabinowitz, J.C. (1985). The effects of presentation rate and encoding task on age-related memory deficits. *Journal of Gerontology*, **40**, 309–15.

Craik, F.I.M. and Simon, E. (1980). Age differences in memory: the roles of attention and depth of processing. In *New directions in memory and aging* (ed. L.W. Poon, J.L. Fozard, L.S. Cermak, D. Arenberg, and L.W. Thompson). Lawrence Erlbaum Associates, Hillsdale, NJ.

Crystal, H.A., Dickson, D.W., Sliwinski, M.J. *et al.* (1993). Pathological markers associated with normal aging and dementia in the elderly. *Annals of Neurology*, **34**, 566–73.

Dannenbaum, S.E., Parkinson, S.R., and Inman, V.W. (1988). Short-term forgetting: comparison between patients with dementia of the Alzheimer type, depressed and normal elderly. *Cognitive Neuropsychology*, **5**, 213–33.

Davis, G.A. and Ball, H.E. (1989). Effects of age on comprehension of complex sentences in adulthood. *Journal of Speech and Hearing Research*, **32**, 143–50.

de Toledo-Morrell, L., Goncharova, I., Dickerson, B., Wilson, R.S., and Bennett, D.A. (2000). From healthy aging to early Alzheimer's disease: *in vivo* detection of entorhinal cortex atrophy. *Annals of the New York Academy of Sciences*, **911**, 240–53.

Deary, I.J., Whalley, L.J., Lemmon, H., Crawford, J.R., and Starr, J.M. (2000). The stability of individual differences in mental ability from childhood to old age: follow up of the 1932 Scottish mental survey. *Intelligence*, **27**, 1–7.

Delaere, P., He, Y., Fayet, G., Duyckaerts, C., and Hauw, J.-J. (1993). Beta-amyloid deposits are constant in the brain of the oldest old: An immunocytochemical study of 20 French centanarians. *Neurobiology of Aging*, **14**, 191–4.

Dempster, F.N. (1992). The rise and fall of the inhibitory mechanism: toward a unified theory of cognitive development and aging. *Developmental Review*, **12**, 45–75.

Denney, D.R. and Denney, N.W. (1973). The use of classification for problem solving: a comparison of middle and old age. *Developmental Psychology*, **9**, 275–8.

Denney, N.W. and Denney, D.R. (1974). Modelling effects on the questioning strategies of the elderly. *Developmental Psychology*, **10**, 458.

Dickson, D.W., Crystal, H.A., Mattiace, L.A. *et al.* (1991). Identification of normal and pathological aging in prospectively studied non-demented elderly humans. *Neurobiology of Aging*, **13**, 179–89.

Digirolamo, G.J., Kramer, A.F., Barad, V. *et al.* (2001). General and task-specific frontal lobe recruitment in older adults during executive processes: a fMRI investigation of task-switching. *Neuroreport*, **12**, 2065–71.

Doppelt, J.W. and Wallace, W.L. (1955). Standardization of the Wechsler Adult Intelligence Scale for older persons. *Journal of Abnormal and Social Psychology*, **51**, 312–30.

Engle, R.W. (1996). Working memory and retrieval: an inhibition-resource approach. In *Working memory and human cognition* (ed. J.T. Richardson, R.W. Engle, L. Hasher, R.H. Logie, E.R. Stoltzfus, and R.T. Zacks). Oxford University Press, Oxford.

Erber, J.T., Herman, T.G. and Botwinick, J. (1980). Age differences in memory as a function of depth of processing. *Experimental Aging Research*, **6**, 341–8.

Erikson, E.H. (1982). *The life cycle completed: a review.* Norton, New York.

Esiri, M.M., Matthews, F., Brayne, C., and Ince, P.G. (2001). Pathological correlates of late-onset dementia in a multicentre, community-based population in England and Wales. *Lancet*, **357**, 169–75.

Fell, M. (1992). Encoding, retrieval and age effects on recollective experience. *The Irish Journal of Psychology*, **13**, 62–78.

Fitzgerald, J.M. (1988). Vivid memories and the reminiscence phenomenon: the role of a self narrative. *Human Development*, **31**, 261–73.

Folstein, M.F., Folstein, S.E. and McHugh, P.R. (1975). Mini-mental state: a practical method for grading the cognitive state of patients for the clinician. *Journal of Psychiatric Research*, **12**, 189–98.

Geinisman, Y., de Toledo-Morrell, L., Morrell, F., and Heller, R.E. (1995). Hippocampal markers of age-related memory dysfunction: behavioral, electrophysiological and morphological perspectives. *Progress in Neurobiology*, **45**, 223–52.

Gibson, P.H. (1983). EM study of the numbers of cortical synapses in the brains of aging people and people with Alzheimer-type dementia. *Acta Neuropathologica*, **62**, 127–33.

Goldstein, G. and Shelly, C.H. (1981). Does the right hemisphere age more rapidly than the left? *Journal of Clinical Neuropsychology*, **3**, 65–78.

Golomb, J., Kluger, A., de Leon, M.J. *et al.* (1994). Hippocampal formation size in normal human aging: A correlate of delayed secondary memory performance. *Learning and Memory*, **1**, 45–54.

Grady, C.L. (2002). Age-related differences in face processing: a meta-analysis of three functional neuroimaging experiments. *Canadian Journal of Psychology*, **56**, 208–20.

Grady, C.L. (2005). Functional connectivity during memory tasks in healthy aging and dementia. In *Cognitive neuroscience of aging* (ed. R. Cabeza, L. Nyberg, and D. Park), pp. 286–308. Oxford University Press, New York,

Grady, C.L., Maisog, F.M., Horwitz, B., Ungerleider, L.G., Mentis, M.J., and Salerno, J.A. (1994). Age-related changes in cortical blood flow activation during visual processing of faces and location. *Journal of Neuroscience*, **14**, 1450–62.

Grady, C.L., McIntosh, A.R., Horwitz, B. *et al.* (1995). Age-related reductions in human recognition memory due to impaired encoding. *Science*, **269**, 218–21.

Grady, C.L., Bernstein, L.J., Beig, S., and Sigenthaler, A.L. (2002). The effects of encoding task on age-related differences in the functional neuroanatomy of face memory. *Psychology and Aging*, **17**, 7–23.

Grafman, J., Weingartner, H., Lawlor, B., Mellow, A.M., Thompson-Putman, K., and Sunderland, T. (1990). Automatic memory processes in patients with dementia-Alzheimer's type (DAT). *Cortex*, **26**, 361–71.

Grober, E. and Buschke, H. (1987). Genuine memory deficits in dementia. *Developmental Neuropsychology*, **3**, 13–36.

Gunning-Dixon, F.M. and Raz, N. (2000). The cognitive correlates of white matter abnormalities in normal ageing: a quantitative review. *Neuropsychology*, **14**, 224–32.

Guttentag, R.E. and Hunt, R.R. (1988). Adult age differences in memory for imagined and performed actions. *Journal of Gerontology: Psychological Sciences*, **43**, P107–P108.

Hart, R.P., Kwentus, J.A., Harkins, S.W., and Taylor, J.R. (1988). Rate of forgetting in mild Alzheimer's-type dementia. *Brain and Cognition*, **7**, 31–8.

Hasher, L. and Zacks, R.T. (1979). Automatic and effortful processes in memory. *Journal of Experimental Psychology: General*, **108**, 356–88.

Hasher, L. and Zacks, R.T. (1988). Working memory, comprehension and aging: a review and a new view. In *The psychology of learning and motivation* (ed. G.H. Bower). Academic Press, San Diego, CA.

Hashtroudi, S., Johnson, M.K., and Chrosniak, L.D. (1990). Aging and qualitative characteristics of memories for perceived and imagined complex events. *Psychology and Aging*, **5**, 119–26.

Hedden, T. and Gabrieli, J.D.E. (2004). Insights into the ageing mind: a view from cognitive neuroscience. *Nature Neuroscience*, **5**, 87–97.

Hess, T.M., Donley, J., and Vandermaas, M.O. (1989). Aging-related changes in the processing and retention of script information. *Experimental Aging Research*, **15**, 89–96.

Hodges, J.R. (1998). The amnestic prodrome of Alzheimer's disease. *Brain*, **121**, 1601–2.

Hodges, J.R., Salmon, D.P., and Butters, N. (1992). Semantic memory impairment in Alzheimer's disease: failure of access or degraded knowledge? *Neuropsychologia*, **1992**, 301–14.

Hodges, J.R., Patterson, K., Graham, N., and Dawson, K. (1996). Naming and knowing in dementia of the Alzheimer's type. *Brain and Language*, **54**, 302–25.

Holland, C.A. and Rabbitt, P. (1990). Autobiographical and text recall in the elderly: an investigation of a processing resource deficits. *The Quarterly Journal of Experimental Psychology*, **42A**, 441–70.

Horn, J.L. and Cattell, R.B. (1967). Age differences in fluid and crystallized intelligence. *Acta Psychologica*, **26**, 107–29.

Houghton, G. and Tipper, S.P. (1994). A model of inhibitory mechanisms in selective attention. In *Inhibitory processes in attention, memory and language* (ed. D. Dagenbach and T.H. Carr). Academic Press, San Diego, CA.

Howard, D.V. (1980). Category norms: a comparison of the Battig and Montague (1969) norms with the responses of adults between the ages of 20 and 80. *Journal of Gerontology*, **35**, 225–31.

Howard, D.V. (1983). The effects of aging and degree of association on the semantic priming of lexical decisions. *Experimental Aging Research*, **9**, 145–51.

Howard, D.V., McAndrews, M.P., and Lasaga, M.I. (1981). Semantic priming of lexical decisions in young and old adults. *Journal of Gerontology*, **36**, 707–14.

Huppert, F.A. (1994). Memory function in dementia and normal aging – dimension or dichotomy? In *Dementia and normal aging* (ed. F.A. Huppert, C. Brayne, and D.W. O'Connor). Cambridge University Press, Cambridge.

Huppert, F.A., Brayne, C., and O'Connor, D.W. (eds) (1994). *Dementia and normal aging.* Cambridge University Press, Cambridge.

Jelicic, M., Bosma, H., Rudolf, W.H.M. *et al.* (2002). Subjective sleep problems in later life as predictors of cognitive decline. Report from the Maastricht Ageing Study (MAAS). *International Journal of Geriatric Psychiatry*, **17**, 73–7.

Jobst, K.A., Smith, A.D., Szatmari, M. *et al.* (1994). Rapidly progressing atrophy of medial temporal lobe in Alzheimer's disease. *Lancet*, **343**, 829–30.

Jonides, J., Marshuetz, C., Smith, E.E., Reuter-Lorenz, P.A., Koeppe, R.A., and Hartley, A. (2000). Age differences in behavior and PET activation reveal differences in interference resolution in verbal working memory. *Journal of Cognitive Neuroscience*, **12**, 188–96.

Jorm, A.F. (1986). Controlled and automatic processing in senile dementia: a review. *Psychological Medicine*, **16**, 77–88.

Jorm, A.F. (2005). Risk factors for Alzheimer's disease. In *Dementia* 3rd edn. (ed. A. Burns, J. O'Brien, and D. Ames). Hodder Arnold, London.

Kahneman, D. (1973). *Attention and effort*, pp. 1–12. Prentice-Hall, Englewood Cliffs, NJ.

Kandel, E.R., Schwartz, J.H., and Jessell, T.M. (1995). *Essentials of neural science and behavior.* Prentice-Hall, Englewood Cliffs, NJ.

Kang, J.H., Ascherio, A., and Grodstein, F. (2005). Fruit and vegetable consumption and cognitive decline in aging women. *Annals of Neurology*, **57**, 713–20.

Kausler, D.H. and Puckett, J.M. (1981a). Adult age differences in memory for modality attributes. *Experimental Aging Research*, **7**, 117–25.

Kausler, D.H. and Puckett, J.M. (1981b). Adult age differences in memory for sex of voice. *Journal of Gerontology*, **36**, 44–50.

Kemper, T.L. (1994). Neuroanatomical and neuropathological changes during aging and dementia. In *Clinical neurology of aging*, 2nd edn (ed. M.L. Albert and E. Knoefel). Oxford University Press, New York.

Kempler, D. and Zelinski, E.M. (1994). Language in dementia and normal aging. In *Dementia and normal aging* (ed. F.A. Huppert, C. Brayne, and D.W. O'Connor). Cambridge University Press, Cambridge.

Killiany, R.J., Hyman, B.T., Gomez-Isla, T. *et al.* (2002). MRI measures of entorhinal cortex versus hippocampus in preclinical Alzheimer's disease. *Neurology*, **58**, 1188–96.

Kirasic, K.C. (1989). Acquisition and utilization of spatial information by elderly adults: implications for day-to-day situations. In *Everyday cognition in adulthood and late life* (ed. L.W. Poon, D.C. Rubin, and B.A. Wilson). Cambridge University Press, Cambridge.

Koss, E., Haxby, J.V., Decarli, C., Schapiro, M.B., Friedland, R.P., and Rapaport, S.I. (1991). Patterns of performance preservation and loss in healthy aging. *Developmental Neuropsychology*, **7**, 99–113.

Kynette, D. and Kemper, S. (1986). Aging and the loss of grammatical forms: a cross-sectional study of language performances. *Language and Communication*, **6**, 65–72.

la Rue, A. (1992). *Aging and neuropsychological assessment.* Plenum Press, New York.

Lautenschlager, N.T., Cupples, L.A., Rao, V.S. *et al.* (1996). Risk of dementia among relatives of Alzheimer's disease patients in the MIRAGE study: what is in store for the oldest old? *Neurology*, **46**, 641–50.

Lee, H. and Birks, J. (2004). Gingko biloba for cognitive improvement in healthy individuals (protocol). *Cochrane Database of Systematic Reviews*, 1, CD004671.

Lehmann, E.B. and Mellinger, J.C. (1984). Effects of aging on memory for presentation modality. *Developmental Psychology*, **20**, 1210–17.

Levine, B., Stuss D.T., Winocur G., Binns M.A., Fahy L., Mandic M., Bridges K., Robertson I.H. (2007). Cognitive rehabilitation in the elderly: effects on strategic behavior in relation to goal management. *Journal of the International Neuropsychological Society*, **13**, 143–152.

Lezak, M. (1995). *Neuropsychological assessment.* Oxford University Press, New York.

Li, S.-C. (2005). Neurocomputational perspectives linking neuromodulation, processing noise, representational distinctiveness and cognitive aging. In *Cognitive neuroscience of aging* (ed. R. Cabeza, L. Nyberg, and D. Park). Oxford University Press, New York.

Light, L.L. (1991). Memory and aging: four hypotheses in search of data. *Annual Review of Psychology*, **42**, 333–76.

Light, L.L. (1992). The organization of memory in old age. In *Handbook of aging and cognition* (ed. F.I.M. Craik and T.A. Salthouse). Lawrence Erlbaum Associates, Hillsdale, NJ.

Light, L.L. and Albertson, S.A. (1988). Comprehension of pragmatic implications in young and older adults. In *Language, memory and aging* (ed. L.L. Light and D.M. Burke). Cambridge University Press, Cambridge.

Light, L.L., Zelinski, E.M., and Moore, M. (1982). Adult age differences in reasoning from new information. *Journal of Experimental Psychology: Learning, Memory and Cognition*, **8**, 435–47.

Lindenberger, U. and Baltes, P.B. (1994). Sensory functioning and intelligence in old age: a strong connection. *Psychology and Aging*, **9**, 339–55.

Lindenberger, U., Scherer, H., and Baltes, P.B. (2001). The strong connection between sensory and cognitive performance in old age: not due to sensory acuity reductions operating during cognitive assessment. *Psychology and Aging*, **16**, 196–205.

Linn, R.T., Wolf, P.A., Bachman, D.L. *et al.* (1995). The 'preclinical phase' of probable Alzheimer's disease. *Archives of Neurology*, **52**, 485–90.

Lupien, S., de Leon, M.J., de Santi, S. *et al.* (1998). Cortisol levels during human aging predict hippocampal atrophy and memory deficits. *Nature Neuroscience*, **1**, 69–73.

McClearn, G.E., Johansson, B., Berg, S. *et al.* (1997). Substantial genetic influence on cognitive ability in twins 80 or more years old. *Science*, **276**, 1560–3.

Malouf, R., Grimley Evans, J., and Areosa Sastre, A. (2003). Folic acid with or without vitamin B12 for cognition and dementia. *Cochrane Database of Systematic Reviews*, 4, CD004514.

Mann, D.M.A., Tucker, C.M., and Yates, P.A. (1987). The topographic distribution of senile plaques and neurofibrillary tangles in the brains of non-demented persons of different ages. *Neuropathology and Applied Neurobiology*, **13**, 123–9.

Mann, D.M.A., Brown, A.M.T., Prinja, D., Jones, D., and Davies, C.A. (1990). A morphological analysis of senile plaques in the brains of non-demented persons of different ages using silver, immunocytochemical and lectin histochemical staining techniques. *Neuropathology and Applied Neurobiology*, **16**, 17–25.

Martin, A., Brouwers, P., Cox, C., and Fedio, P. (1985). On the nature of the verbal memory deficit in Alzheimer's disease. *Brain and Language*, **25**, 323–41.

Mattay, V.S., Fera, F., Tessitore, A. *et al.* (2002). Neurophysiological correlates of age-related changes in human motor function. *Neurology*, **58**, 630–5.

Maylor, E.A. (1990a). Age, blocking and the tip of the tongue state. *British Journal of Psychology*, **81**, 123–34.

Maylor, E.A. (1990b). Recognizing and naming faces: aging, memory retrieval and the tip of the tongue state. *Journal of Gerontology: Psychological Sciences*, **45**, P215–P226.

Maylor, E.A. and Wing, A.M. (1996). Age differences in postural stability are increased by additional cognitive demands. *Journal of Gerontology: Psychological Sciences*, **51B**, 143–54.

Meudell, P.R. and Greenhalgh, M. (1987). Age related differences in left and right hand skill and in visuo-spatial performance: their possible relationships to the hypothesis that the right hemisphere ages more rapidly than the left. *Cortex*, **23**, 431–45.

Meuller, J.H., Kausler, D.H. and Faherty, A. (1980). Age and access time for different memory codes. *Experimental Aging Research*, **6**, 445–9.

Milham, M.P., Erickson, K.I., Banich, M.T., and Kramer, A.F. (2002). Attentional control in the aging brain: insights from an fMRI study of the Stroop task. *Brain and Cognition*, **49**, 277–96.

Milwain, E.J. (1999). *An evaluation of memory loss in old age and Alzheimer's disease.* Department of Experimental Psychology, University of Oxford.

Mitchell, K.J. and Johnson, M.K. (2000). Source monitoring: attributing mental experiences. In *The Oxford handbook of memory* (ed. E. Tulving and F.I.M. Craik). Oxford University Press, New York.

Morcom, A.M., Good, C.D., Frackowiak, R.J., and Rugg, M.D. (2003). Age effects on neural correlates of successful memory encoding. *Brain*, **126**, 213–29.

Morris, J.C., McKeel, D., Storandt, M. *et al.* (1991). Very mild Alzheimer's disease: informant-based clinical, psychometric and pathologic distinction from normal ageing. *Neurology*, **41**, 469–78.

Morris, M.S. (2003). Homocysteine and Alzheimer's disease. *Lancet Neurology*, **2**, 425–8.

Nagy, Z., Esiri, M.M., Jobst, K.A. *et al.* (1996). Clustering of pathological features in Alzheimer's disease: Clinical and neuroanatomical aspects. *Dementia and Geriatric Cognitive Disorders*, **7**, 121–7.

Nebes, R. (1989). Semantic memory in Alzheimer's disease. *Psychological Bulletin*, **106**, 377–94.

Nebes, R. (1992). Cognitive dysfunction in Alzheimer's disease. In *The handbook of aging and cognition* (ed. F.I.M. Craik and T.A. Salthouse). Erlbaum, Hillsdale, NJ.

Nebes, R. and Brady, C. B. (1992). Generalized cognitive slowing and severity of dementia in Alzheimer's disease: implications for the interpretation of response-time date. *Journal of Clinical and Experimental Neuropsychology*, **14**, 317–30.

Nielson, K.A., Langenecker, S.A., and Garavan, H. (2002). Differences in the functional neuroanatomy of inhibitory control across the adult life span. *Psychology and Aging*, **17**, 56–71.

Norman, S., Kemper, S., Kynette, D., Chenug, H., and Anagnopoulos, C. (1991). Syntactic complexity and adult's running memory span. *Journal of Gerontology: Psychological Sciences*, **46**, P346–P351.

Nyberg, L. (2005). Cognitive training in healthy aging. In *Cognitive neuroscience of aging* (ed. R. Cabeza, L. Nyberg, and D. Park). Oxford University Press, New York.

Obler, L.K. and Albert, M.L. (1985). Language skills across adulthood. In *Handbook of the psychology of aging*, 2nd edn (ed. J.E. Birren and K.W. Schaie). Van Nostrand Reinhold, New York.

Obler, L.K., Fein, D., Nicholas, M., and Albert, M.L. (1991). Auditory comprehension and aging: decline in syntactic processing. *Applied Psycholinguistics*, **12**, 433–52.

Park, D.C. and Puglisi, J.T. (1985). Older adults' memory for the color of pictures and words. *Journal of Gerontology*, **40**, 198–204.

Park, D.C., Smith, A.D., Morrell, R.W., Puglisi, J.T., and Dudley, W.N. (1990). Effects of contextual integration on recall of pictures by older adults. *Journal of Gerontology: Psychological Sciences*, **45**, P52–P57.

Park, D.C., Smith, A.D., Lautenschlager, G. *et al.* (1996). Mediators of long-term memory performance across the life-span. *Psychology and Aging*, **11**, 621–37.

Pepin, E.P. and Eslinger, P.J. (1989). Verbal memory decline in Alzheimer's disease: a multiple-process deficit. *Neurology*, **39**, 1477–82.

Perfect, T.J., Williams, R.B., and Anderton-Brown, C. (1995). Age differences in reported recollective experience are due to encoding effects, not response bias. *Memory*, **3**, 169–86.

Perlmutter, M. (1979). Age differences in adults' free recall, cued recall and recognition. *Journal of Gerontology*, **34**, 533–9.

Petersen, R.C., Smith, G.E., Ivnik, R.J., Kokmen, E., and Tangalos, E.G. (1994). Memory function in very early Alzheimer's disease. *Neurology*, **44**, 867–72.

Peto, R. and Doll, R. (1997). There is no such thing as ageing: old age is associated with disease but does not cause it. *British Medical Journal*, **315**, 1030–2.

Petros, T.V., Zehr, H.D., and Chabot, R.J. (1983). Adult age differences in accessing and retrieving information from long-term memory. *Journal of Gerontology*, **38**, 589–92.

Pezdek, K. (1987). Memory for pictures: a lifespan study of memory for visual detail. *Child Development*, **58**, 807–15.

Poon, L.W. (1985). Differences in human memory with aging: nature, causes and clinical implications. In *Handbook of the psychology of aging*, 2nd edn (ed. J.E. Birren and K.W. Schaie). Van Nostrand Reinhold, New York.

Porter, N.M. and Landfield, P. (1998). Stress hormones and brain aging: adding injury to insult? *Nature Neuroscience*, **1**, 3–4.

Posner, M.I. and Raichle, M.E. (1994). *Images of mind*, pp. 153–80. Scientific American Library, New York.

Pruessner, J.C., Lord, C., Meaney, M., and Lupien, S. (2004). Effects of self-esteem on age-related changes in cognition and the regulation of the hypothalamic-pituitary-adrenal axis. *Annals of the New York Academy of Sciences*, **1032**, 186–90.

Purandare, N., Ballard, C., and Burns, A. (2005). Prevention of Alzheimer's disease. In *Dementia*, 3rd edn (ed. A. Burns, J. O'Brien, and D. Ames). Hodder Arnold, London.

Rabbitt, P.M.A. (1989). Inner-city decay? Age changes in structure and process in recall of familiar topographical information. In *Everyday cognition in adulthood and late life* (ed. L.W. Poon, D.C. Rubin, and B.A. Wilson). Cambridge University Press, Cambridge.

Rabinowitz, J.C. (1989). Age deficits in recall under optimal study conditions. *Psychology and Aging*, **4**, 378–80.

Raz, N. (2000). Aging of the brain and its impact on cognitive performance: integration of structural and functional findings. In *Handbook of aging and cognition*, 2nd edn (ed. F.I.M. Craik and T.A. Salthouse). Erlbaum, Mahwah, NJ.

Raz, N. (2005). The aging brain observed *in vivo*: differential changes and their modifiers. In *Cognitive neuroscience of aging* (ed. R. Cabeza, L. Nyberg, and D. Park). Oxford University Press, New York.

Reder, L.M., Wible, C., and Martin, J. (1986). Differential memory changes with age: exact retrieval versus plausible inference. *Journal of Experimental Psychology: Learning, Memory and Cognition*, **12**, 72–81.

Reese, H.M. and Rodeheaver, D. (1985). Problem solving and complex decision making. In *Handbook of the psychology of aging*, 2nd edn (ed. J.E. Birren and K.W. Schaie). Van Nostrand Reinhold, New York.

Requejo, A.M., Ortega, R.M., Robles, F., Navia, B., Faci, M., and Aparicio, A. (2003). Influence of nutrition on cognitive function in a group of elderly, independently living people. *European Journal of Clinical Nutrition*, **57**(Suppl. 1), S54–S57.

Reuter-Lorenz, P.A. and Sylvester, C.-Y. C. (2005). The cognitive neuroscience of working memory and aging. In *Cognitive neuroscience of aging* (ed. R. Cabeza, L. Nyberg, and D. Park). Oxford University Press, New York.

Reuter-Lorenz, P.A., Jonides, J., Smith, E.E. *et al.* (2000). Age differences in the frontal lateralization of verbal and spatial memory revealed by PET. *Journal of Cognitive Neuroscience*, **12**, 174–87.

Riegel, K.F. (1959). A study of verbal achievements of older persons. *Journal of Gerontology*, **14**, 453–6.

Ritchie, K. and Kildea, D. (1995). Is senile dementia 'age-related' or 'ageing-related'? Evidence from meta-analysis of dementia prevalence in the oldest old. *Lancet*, **346**, 931–4.

Rose, S. (2005). *The 21st century brain*. Jonathan Cape, London.

Rosen, A.C., Prull, M.W., Gabrieli, J.D.E. *et al.* (2003). Differential associations between entorhinal and hippocampal volumes and memory performance in older adults. *Behavioral Neuroscience*, **117**, 1150–60.

Ross, M.H., Yurgelen-Todd, D.A., Renshaw, P.F. *et al.* (1997). Age-related reduction in functional MRI response to photic stimulation. *Neurology*, **48**, 173–6.

Rympa, B. and d'Esposito, M. (2000). Isolating the neural mechanisms of age-related changes in human working memory. *Nature Neuroscience*, **3**, 509–15.

Salmon, D.P., Shimamura, A.P., Butters, N., and Smith, S. (1988). Lexical and semantic priming deficits in patients with Alzheimer's disease. *Journal of Clinical and Experimental Neuropsychology*, **10**, 477–94.

Salthouse, T.A. (1982). *Adult cognition*, pp. 51–82. Springer, New York.

Salthouse, T.A. (1984). Effects of age and skill in typing. *Journal of Experimental Psychology: General*, **113**, 345–71.

Salthouse, T.A. (1988). Effects of aging on verbal abilities: examination of the psychometric literature. In *Language, memory and aging* (ed. L.L. Light and D.M. Burke). Cambridge University Press, Cambridge.

Salthouse, T.A. (1993). Speed mediation of adult age differences in cognition. *Developmental Psychology*, **29**, 722–38.

Salthouse, T.A. and Babcock, R.L. (1991). Decomposing adult age differences in working memory. *Developmental Psychology*, **27**, 763–76.

Salzarulo, P., Formicola, G., Lombardo, P. *et al.*(1997). Functional uncertainty, aging, and memory processing during sleep. *Acta Neurologica Belgica*, **97**, 118–22.

Schacter, D.L. (1994). Priming and multiple memory systems: perceptual mechanisms of implicit memory. In *Memory systems 1994* (ed. D.L. Schacter and E. Tulving). MIT Press, Cambridge, MA.

Schacter, D.L., Koutsaal, W., and Norman, K.A. (1997). False memories and aging. *Trends in Cognitive Sciences*, **1**, 229–36.

Schaie, K.W. (1996). Intellectual development in adulthood. In *Handbook of the psychology of aging*, 4th edn (ed. J.E. Birren and K.W. Schaie). Academic Press, San Diego, CA.

Schaie, K.W. and Schaie, J.P. (1977). Clinical assessment and aging. In *Handbook of the psychology of aging*, 1st edn (ed. J.E. Birren and K.W. Schaie). Van Nostrand Reinhold, New York.

Scheidt, R.J. and Schaie, K.W. (1978). A taxonomy of situations for an elderly population: generating situational criteria. *Journal of Gerontology*, **33**, 848–57.

Schonfield, D. and Robertson, B.A. (1966). Memory storage and aging. *Canadian Journal of Psychology*, **20**, 228–36.

Selwyn, J., Findlay, D.J. and McMurdo, M.E.T. (2006). Diagnoses and vascular risk factors in a cohort of 150 attendees at a memory clinic. *International Journal of Geriatric Psychiatry*, **21**, 1001–2.

Selye, H. (1970). Stress and aging. *Journal of the American Geriatrics Society*, **18**, 669–80.

Sharps, M.J. (1991). Spatial memory in young and elderly adults: the category structure of stimulus sets. *Psychology and Aging*, **6**, 309–12.

Shimamura, A.P., Salmon, D.P., Squire, L., and Butters, N. (1987). Memory dysfunction and word priming in dementia and amnesia. *Behavioral Neuroscience*, **101**, 347–51.

Skoog, I., Nilsson, L., Palmertz, B., Andreasson, L.-A., and Svanborg, A. (1993). A population based study of dementia in 85-year olds. *New England Journal of Medicine*, **328**, 153–8.

Sliwinski, M. and Buschke, H. (1997). Processing speed and memory in aging and dementia. *Journal of Gerontology: Psychological Sciences*, **52B**, P308–P318.

Small, S.A. (2001). Age-related memory decline: current concepts and future directions. *Archives of Neurology*, **58**, 360–4.

Small, S.A., Tsai, W.Y., Delapaz, R., Mayeux, R., and Stern, Y. (2002). Imaging hippocampal function across the human life span: Is memory decline normal or not? *Annals of Neurology*, **51**, 290–5.

Spearman, C. (1927). *The abilities of man*. Macmillan, New York.

Spilich, G.J. (1983). Life-span components of text processing: structural and procedural differences. *Journal of Verbal Learning and Verbal Behavior*, **22**, 231–44.

Stebbins, G.T., Carrillo, M.C., Dorfman, J. *et al.* (2002). Aging effects on memory encoding in the frontal lobes. *Psychology and Aging*, **17**, 44–55.

Stine, E.L., Wingfield, A., and Poon, L.W. (1989). Speech comprehension and memory through adulthood: the roles of time and strategy. In *Everyday cognition in adulthood and late life* (ed. L.W. Poon, D.C. Rubin, and B.A. Wilson). Cambridge University Press, Cambridge.

Stuart-Hamilton, I. (2000). *The psychology of ageing*, 2nd edn. Jessica Kingsley, London.

Szatmari, M. and Bereczki, D. (2006). Procaine treatments for cognition and dementia (protocol). *Cochrane Database of Systematic Reviews*, 2, CD005993.

Till, R.E. (1985). Verbatim and inferential memory in young and elderly adults. *Journal of Gerontology*, **40**, 316–23.

Till, R.E., Bartlett, J.C., and Doyle, A.H. (1982). Age differences in picture memory with resemblance and discrimination tasks. *Experimental Aging Research*, **8**, 179–84.

Tulving, E., Kapur, S., Craik, F.I.M., Moscovitch, M., and Houle, S. (1994). Hemispheric encoding/retrieval asymmetry in episodic memory: positron emission tomography findings. *Proceedings of the National Academy of Sciences USA*, **91**, 2016–20.

Tun, P.A. and Wingfield, A. (1993). Is speech special? Perception and recall of spoken language in complex environments. In *Adult information processing: limits on loss* (ed. J. Cerella, J. Rybash, W. Hoyer, and M.L. Commons). Academic Press, San Diego, CA.

Ulrich, J. (1985). Alzheimer changes in nondemented patients younger than sixty-five: possible early stages of Alzheimer's disease and senile dementia of the Alzheimer type. *Annals of Neurology*, **17**, 273–7.

Ungerleider, L.G. and Mishkin, M. (1982). Two cortical visual systems. In *Analysis of visual behavior* (ed. D.J. Ingle, M. Goodale, and R.J.W. Mansfield). MIT Press, Cambridge, MA.

van der Werf, Y., Tisserand, D.J., Visser, P.J. *et al.* (2001). Thalamic volume predicts performance on tests of cognitive speed and decreases in healthy aging: a magnetic resonance imaging-based volumetric analysis. *Cognitive Brain Research*, **11**, 377–85.

Verhaeghen, P. and Marcoen, A. (1996). On the mechanisms of plasticity in young and older adults after instruction in the method of loci: evidence for an amplification model. *Psychology and Aging*, **11**, 164–78.

Waddell, K.J. and Rogoff, B. (1981). Effect of contextual organization on spatial memory of middle-aged and older women. *Developmental Psychology*, **17**, 878–85.

Wechsler, D. (1981). *WAIS-R Manual*. The Psychological Corporation, New York.

Weingartner, H., Kaye, W., Smallberg, S.A., Ebert, M.H., Gillin, J.C., and Sitaram, N. (1981). Memory failures in progressive idiopathic dementia. *Journal of Abnormal Psychology*, **90**, 187–96.

Welford, A.T. (1958). *Aging and human skill*, pp. 1–16. Oxford University Press, Oxford.

West, R.L. (1996). An application of prefrontal cortex function theory to cognitive aging. *Psychological Bulletin*, **120**, 272–92.

Whalley, L.J. (2001). *The ageing brain*. Phoenix, London.

Whalley, L.J. (2002). Brain aging and dementia: what makes the difference? *British Journal of Psychiatry*, **181**, 369–71.

Whiting, W.L. and Smith, A.D. (1997). Differential age-related processing limitations in recall and recognition tasks. *Psychology and Aging*, **12**, 216–24.

Wingfield, A., Poon, L.W., Lombardi, L., and Lowe, D. (1985). Speed of processing in normal aging: effects of speech rate, linguistic structure and processing time. *Journal of Gerontology*, **40**, 579–85.

Woodruff-Pak, D. (1997). *The neuropsychology of aging*, p. 38. Blackwell, Oxford.

Ylikoski, R., Ylikoski, A., Erkinjuntti, T., Sulkava, R., Raininko, R., and Tilvis, R. (1993). White matter changes in healthy elderly persons correlate with attention and speed of mental processes. *Archives of Neurology*, **50**, 818–24.

Zacks, R.T. and Hasher, L. (1997). Cognitive gerontology and attentional inhibition: a reply to Burke and McDowd. *Journal of Gerontology: Psychological Sciences*, **52B**, P274–P283.

# 4

# Epidemiology

## Martin Prince

## What is epidemiology?

Last's *Dictionary of Epidemiology* (Last, 1995) defines epidemiology as

> The study of the distribution and determinants of health-related states or events in specified populations, and the application of this study to the control of health problems.

Epidemiology is concerned with the health states of populations, communities, and groups. The health state of individuals is the concern of clinical medicine. Epidemiology may simply describe the distribution of health states (extent, type, severity) within a population. This is *descriptive epidemiology*.

Alternatively it may try to explain the distribution of health states. This is *analytical epidemiology* (Fig. 4.1). The basic strategy is to compare the distribution of disease between groups or between populations, looking for *associations* between hypothesized *risk factors* (genes, behaviours, lifestyles, environmental exposures) and *health states*. These associations may or may not indicate that the hypothesized risk factor has caused the disease.

## What do epidemiologists do?

Epidemiological studies are generally not controlled experiments. Observations are made on individuals living freely in the 'real world'; these non-experimental studies are referred to as 'observational'. There is much background noise, so it is difficult to make clear-cut inferences from the resulting data. Observed associations between risk factors and diseases may represent the effects of chance (random error), or bias or confounding (non-random error). Occasionally the apparent risk factor may be a consequence rather than a cause of the disease. This is called 'reverse causality' (Box 4.1).

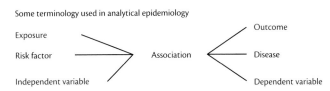

Some terminology used in analytical epidemiology

**Fig. 4.1** Some terminology used in analytical epidemiology.

---

> **Box 4.1** Possible explanations for an observed association
>
> - Chance
> - Bias
> - Confounding
> - Reverse causality
> - Valid association (may or may not be causal)

Two key functions for epidemiologists are therefore to design and analyse their studies in such a way as to maximize the *precision* and *validity* of their findings:

- *Maximizing precision* reduces random error. The two main sources of random error are sampling error and measurement error. Precision may be increased by ensuring an adequate sample size and by maximizing the accuracy of the measures.

- *Maximizing validity* implies the avoidance of non-random error. Non-random error arises from bias and confounding. These concepts will be dealt with in more detail later in this chapter. The error is non-random, because its effects are unequal (differential) between the two or more groups which are being compared.

If the precision and validity of epidemiological studies are adequate, and the effects of chance, bias, confounding, and reverse causality can be confidently excluded, then and only then can tentative causal inferences be made from observed associations. Identification of causal factors may lead to strategies for prevention.

For ethical reasons, it is generally not possible in human populations to study under experimental conditions the effects of factors thought likely to increase the risk of disease. However, causal inferences made from observational (non-experimental) studies can be assessed further by testing the disease-preventing effects of reducing or eliminating exposure to potential risk factors under experimental conditions. Thus epidemiologists have tested the effects of:

- laying babies on their backs on sudden infant death syndrome (cot death)

- reducing dietary fat on coronary heart disease
- iodine supplementation on cretinism.

The optimal experimental design is the randomized controlled trial, in which the allocation to either the active intervention arm or the control or placebo arm is randomly determined.

Epidemiology has been described as the basic science of public-health medicine; in reality these are complementary disciplines. Without epidemiology there can be no evidence-based direction to public health policy. Without public-health medicine, epidemiological findings cannot be prioritized and converted into practical policies.

## Context

### Mental health in an ageing world

Six per cent of the world's population is accounted for by those aged 65 years or over. However, this proportion varies according to region—17% in the UK (one of the world's 'oldest' countries), 14% in Europe, 13% in the USA, but only 3% in African countries and 5% in Latin America and Southeast Asia. In many developing countries, children account for around half of the total population. Given these indices, it is perhaps surprising to learn that two-thirds of the world's older citizens live in the developing world. This proportion is set to increase to three-quarters by 2020. The apparent paradox is explained by the vast size of some of the populations of developing countries; India alone has a population of 1 billion, of whom 4%, or 40 million, are aged 65 or over. The rapid increase in the absolute and relative numbers of older persons in the developing world is explained by the phenomenon of demographic ageing. The proportion of older persons in the population increases partly as a result of increasing life expectancy, but more particularly because of falling fertility rates in response to declining child mortality, education, and economic development; in classical demographic theory this is the third and final 'demographic transition' before the achievement of population stability. The rates of demographic ageing currently seen in China, India, and parts of Latin America are completely unprecedented in world history, and will have far-reaching consequences for the health and welfare needs of their populations. The hope is that economic growth will match the growing needs for care of dependent older persons, but there is as yet little evidence of policy development or service planning.

Demographic ageing will lead to large increases in the numbers of people with dementia. In 2005 Alzheimer's Disease International commissioned a panel of experts to review all available epidemiological data and reach a consensus estimate of prevalence in each world region, and the numbers of people affected. Evidence from well-conducted, representative epidemiological surveys was lacking in many regions. The 2005 panel estimated that 24.3 million people have dementia, with 4.6 million new cases of dementia annually (one new case every 7 seconds). The numbers of people affected will double every 20 years to 81.1 million by 2040. Most people with dementia live in developing countries, 60% in 2001 rising to 71% by 2040. Rates of increase are not uniform; numbers in developed countries are forecast to increase by 100% between 2001 and 2040, but by more than 300% in India, China, and their south Asian and western Pacific neighbours (Fig. 4.2).

The final demographic transition is now under way in most developing countries (other than sub-Saharan Africa) but is largely complete in Great Britain and in Western Europe. Warnes (1989) points out that the ageing of these populations has been neither very recent nor particularly rapid. What is new is the public awareness of these changes. Over the last 100 years, annual mortality rates have declined from 3% to 1%, and expectation of life has nearly doubled. The increase over the last 100 years in the proportion of the British population aged over 65 from approximately 5% to approximately 16% has been gradual and relatively painless in economic terms. There may, however, be a 'sting in the tail' of demographic ageing. By 2040 in the UK, the proportion of those aged 60 and over will have increased from 21% to 26% (Table 4.1). However, over the same time the proportion of the oldest old will have nearly doubled from 6% to 11% (OPCS, 1991). It is this increase in the numbers and relative proportions of the oldest old which accounts for the continuing projected increase in the numbers of persons with dementia in the world's developed regions (see Fig. 4.2).

## Epidemiological methods

### Measurement in psychiatric epidemiology

The science of the measurement of mental phenomena, psychometrics, is central to quantitative research in psychiatry. Without appropriate, accurate, stable, and unbiased measures, research is doomed to fail. Most measurement strategies are based on eliciting symptoms, either by asking the subject to complete a self-report questionnaire or by using an interviewer to question the subject. Some of these questionnaires or interviews are long, detailed,

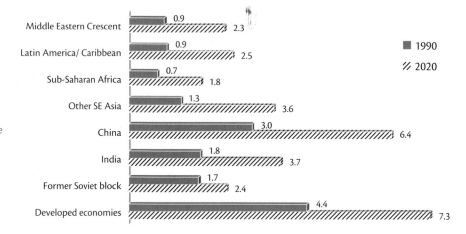

**Fig. 4.2** Projected changes in absolute numbers of those with dementia, by world region. Assumptions: (1) World Bank medium range population growth projections; (2) constant prevalence of dementia (3% of all those aged 60 and over) across time and region.

**Table 4.1** UK Population trends (standard projection assumptions)

|  |  | 2001 | 2011 | 2021 | 2041 |
|---|---|---|---|---|---|
| 60–64 | Male | 1.4 | 1.8 | 1.8 | 1.5 |
|  | Female | 1.4 | 1.9 | 1.9 | 1.5 |
| 65–74 | Male | 2.2 | 2.4 | 2.8 | 2.9 |
|  | Female | 2.6 | 2.7 | 3.2 | 3.2 |
| 75–84 | Male | 1.3 | 1.3 | 1.5 | 1.9 |
|  | Female | 2.0 | 1.9 | 2.0 | 2.7 |
| 85+ | Male | 0.3 | 0.4 | 0.4 | 0.6 |
|  | Female | 0.8 | 0.9 | 0.9 | 1.1 |
| All 60+ | Male | 5.2 | 5.9 | 6.5 | 6.9 |
|  | Female | 6.8 | 7.4 | 8.0 | 8.5 |
| Whole population | Male | 29.0 | 29.3 | 29.6 | 29.2 |
|  | Female | 30.0 | 30.1 | 30.3 | 29.9 |

Figures in millions of population.

Source: OPCS (1987).

comprehensive clinical diagnostic assessments. Others are much briefer, designed either to screen for probable cases or as scalable measures in their own right—of a trait or dimension such as depression, neuroticism, or cognitive function. Researchers in other medical disciplines sometimes criticize psychiatric measures for being vague or woolly, because they are not based on biological markers of pathology. For this very reason, psychiatry was among the first medical disciplines to develop internationally recognized operationalized diagnostic criteria. At the same time the research interview has become progressively refined, such that the processes of eliciting, recording, and distilling symptoms into diagnoses or scalable traits are now also highly standardized. These criticisms are therefore mainly misplaced.

Our confidence in our measures is based on our understanding of their psychometric properties, principally their validity and reliability. Validity refers to the extent to which a measure really does measure what it sets out to measure. Reliability refers to the consistency of a measure when applied repeatedly under similar circumstances. Put simply, a measure is reliable if you use it twice to measure the same thing and arrive at the same answer. A measure is valid if you measure the same thing twice using two different measures, one known to be valid, and come to the same answer. The reliability and validity of all measures need to be cited in research grant proposals and research publications. If they have not been adequately established, particularly if the measure is new, then the investigators need to do this themselves in a pilot investigation. A resource guide to commonly used; and well-validated measures, with an emphasis upon those validated upon older populations, is given in the appendix at the end of this chapter.

## Domains of measurement

Measures in common use in psychiatric epidemiology can be thought of as covering six main domains:

1 Demographic status: age, gender, marital status, household circumstances, occupation.

2 Socio-economic status: social class, income, wealth, debt.

3 Social circumstances: social network, social support.

4 Activities, lifestyles, behaviours: a very broad area, whose contents are dictated by the focus of the research. Examples would include tobacco and alcohol consumption, substance use, diet, and exercise. Some measures such as recent exposure to positive and negative life events may be particularly relevant to psychiatric research.

5 Opinions and attitudes: an area of measurement initially restricted to market research organizations, but increasingly being adopted by social science and biomedical researchers.

6 Health status: measures can be further grouped into

(a) specific measures of 'caseness' (i.e. dichotomous diagnoses such as schizophrenia) or dimensions, (i.e. continuously distributed traits such as mood, anxiety, neuroticism, and cognitive function);

(b) global measures, e.g. subjective or objective global health assessment, disablement (impairment, activity and participation) and health-related quality of life; and

(c) measures reflecting the need for, or use of health services.

## Caseness and dimensions
### Measures of 'caseness'

At first sight, the concept of psychiatric caseness can seem arbitrary, confusing, and possibly even unhelpful. For example, a recent review of 40 community-based studies of the prevalence of late-life depression concluded that there was wide variation in reported prevalence, but that the most important source of variation seemed to be the diagnostic criteria that were used to identify the cases (Beekman *et al.*, 1999). Thus the 15 studies that identified cases of major depression meeting DSM criteria had a weighted average prevalence of 2% (range 0–3%). Twenty-five studies using other criteria gave a weighted average prevalence of 13% (range 9–18%). Is the correct prevalence of late-life depression 2% or 13%? Surely both these contrasting estimates cannot be 'right'. In our confusion, we are led to ask the question 'What is a case of depression?'. The answer will depend always on the purpose for which the measurement is being made. The question should therefore not be 'what is a case?' so much as 'a case for what?'.

Diagnostic criteria for a disease can be classified as broad or narrow, and as more or less operationalized. Broader criteria include diffuse and less severe forms of the disorder, narrow criteria exclude all but the most clear-cut and severe cases. Operationalized criteria make explicit a series of unambiguous rules according to which people either qualify or do not qualify as cases. DSM-IV major depression criteria (American Psychiatric Association, 1994) are both narrow and strictly operationalized. In the other studies included in the review late-life depression was both more broadly and more loosely defined. Operationalized criteria were not used; for these studies the threshold was defined in terms of the concept of 'clinical significance', a level of depression that a competent clinician would consider to merit some kind of active therapeutic intervention. The narrow criteria for major depression define a small proportion of persons with an unarguably severe form of depressive disorder, implying strong construct validity. Since the criteria are strictly operationalized they can also be applied reliably. This might then be a good case definition for the first studies investigating the efficacy of a new treatment for depressive disorder. Major depression might also be a good 'pure' case definition for a genetic linkage study, aiming to identify gene loci predisposing to depression in a multiply affected family pedigree. However, these criteria will not suit all purposes. One cannot presume, for instance, that the findings from the drug efficacy studies will generalize to the broader group of depressed patients whom clinicians typically diagnose and treat, but who do not meet criteria for major depression. Also, major depression criteria arguably miss much of the impact of depressive disorder within a community population. Depressed persons are known to be heavy users of health and social services. However, the very small number of cases of major depression account for a tiny proportion of this excess, which is mainly made up of cases of 'common mental disorder' a term used to describe collectively the 'neuroses'—depressive, anxiety, and somatization disorders, with mixed forms being especially frequent.

### Measures of dimensions

The idea of a psychiatric disorder as a dimension can be difficult for psychiatrists to grasp. They are used to making a series of dichotomous judgements in their clinical practice. Is this patient depressed? Does he/she need treatment? Should she/he be admitted? Does he/she have insight? Is she/he a danger to her/himself? As Pickering commented (when arguing that hypertension was better understood as a dimensional rather than a dichotomous disorder) 'doctors can count to one but not beyond'. It is important to recognize that a dimensional concept need not contradict a categorical view of a disorder. As with the relativity of the concept of 'a case', it may be useful under some circumstances to think categorically and in others dimensionally. There is for instance a positive correlation between the number of symptoms of depression experienced by a person and

- the impairment of their quality of life
- the frequency with which they use GP services and
- the number of days they take off work in a month.

Thus a dimensional perspective, even more so than broadly-based diagnostic criteria, can offer useful insights into the way in which the consequences of mental disorder are very widely distributed in the community.

From a technical point of view, continuous measures of dimensional traits such as depression, anxiety, neuroticism, and cognitive function offer some advantages over their dichotomous equivalents, major depression, generalized anxiety disorder, personality disorder, and dementia. These diagnoses tend to be rather rare—collapsing a continuous trait into a dichotomous diagnosis may mean that the investigators are in effect throwing away informative data; the net effect may be loss of statistical power to demonstrate an important association with a risk factor, or a real benefit of a treatment.

### Validity

*Construct validity* refers to the extent to which the construct that the measure seeks to address is real and coherent, and then also to the relevance of the measure to that construct. Construct validity cannot be demonstrated empirically, but evidence can be sought to support it. For example, the scope and content of the construct can be identified in open-ended interviews and focus group discussions with experts or key informants. These same informants can review the proposed measure and comment on the appropriateness of the items (face validity).

*Concurrent validity* is tested by the extent to which the new measure relates, as hypothesized, to other measures taken at the same time (hence concurrent). There are four main variants: criterion, convergent, divergent, and known group validity.

*Criterion validity* is tested by comparing measures obtained with the new instrument to those obtained with an existing *criterion* measure. The criterion is the current 'gold standard' measure and is usually more complex, lengthier, or more expensive to administer, otherwise there would be little point in developing the new measure! In psychiatry there are generally no biologically based criterion measures as, for example, bronchoscopy and biopsy for carcinoma of the bronchus. The first measures developed for psychiatric research were compared with the criterion or 'gold standard' of a competent psychiatrist's clinical diagnosis. More recently, detailed standardized clinical interviews such as SCAN have taken the place of the psychiatrist's opinion.

*Convergent and divergent validity* should be tested in relation to each other. A measure will be more closely related to an alternative measure of the same construct than it will be to measures of different constructs. Thus the general health questionnaire (GHQ, a measure of psychiatric morbidity) should correlate more strongly with the Beck Depression Scale than with a physical functioning scale, or with a measure of income.

*Known group validity* can be assessed where no established gold standard external criterion exists. Thus a new questionnaire measuring the amount of time parents spend in positive joint activities with their children could be applied to two groups of parents, identified by their health visitors or teachers as having contrasting levels of involvement with their children: if the measure successfully distinguished members of the two groups, it would possess known group validity.

*Predictive validity* assesses the extent to which a new measure can predict future variables. Thus depression may predict time off work, or use of health services; cognitive impairment may predict dementia.

### Reliability

*Test–retest reliability (intra-measurement reliability)* tests the stability of a measure over time. The measure is administered, and then after an interval of time is administered again to the same person, under the same conditions (e.g. by the same interviewer). The selection of the time interval is a matter of judgement. Too short and the respondent may simply recall and repeat their response from the first testing. Too long, and the trait that the measure was measuring may have changed, e.g. they may have recovered from their depression.

Inter-observer reliability tests the stability of the measure when administered or rated by different investigators. Administering the measure to the same person under the same conditions by first one and then the other interviewer tests inter-interviewer reliability. Having the same interview rated by two or more investigators tests inter-rater reliability.

### Measuring reliability

Intra-measurement and inter-observer reliability are assessed using measures of agreement. For a continuous scale measure the appropriate statistic would be the intra-class correlation. For a categorical measure the appropriate statistic is Cohen's kappa; this takes into account the agreement expected by chance, and is independent of the prevalence of the condition in the test population.

The internal consistency of a measure indicates the extent to which its component parts (in the case of a scale, the individual items) address a common underlying construct. This is conventionally considered a component of reliability. For a scale it is usually measured using Cronbach's coefficient alpha, which varies between 0 and 1. A coefficient alpha of 0.6 to 0.8 is moderate but satisfactory, above 0.8 indicates a highly internally consistent scale. Another measure of internal consistency is the split-half reliability, a measure of agreement between subscales derived from two randomly selected halves of the scale.

## Study designs

As with the plots of Hollywood movies, there have only ever been a limited number of epidemiological designs in general use. However, the details of the study designs, and the conduct and analysis of these studies has become increasingly refined and sophisticated. Studies may be experimental or non-experimental (observational). Observational studies may use observations made on individuals, or aggregated data from groups or populations. They may be descriptive or analytical in purpose and design. Figure 4.3 summarizes the main types of study design.

On the following pages, the essentials of these basic types of study design are illustrated with reference to the epidemiology of mental health conditions in later life.

## Descriptive studies

Prevalence is defined as the proportion of persons in a defined population that have the disease under study at a defined time period. This may be point prevalence (prevalence at the instant of the survey), 1-month prevalence (prevalence at any time over the month before the study), and so on. The prevalence of dementia (and of the common subtype, Alzheimer's disease) increases exponentially with increasing age, and is therefore generally quoted in the form of age-specific rates in 5-year age bands. Thus the EURODEM consortium meta-analysis (Hofman et al., 1991) for European population-based studies applying DSM-III dementia criteria reported the following prevalences: 1% (65–69 years), 4% (70–74), 6% (75–79), 13% (80–84), 22% (85–89), 32% (90–94). The overall prevalence for those aged 65 years and over is in the region of 6%.

Incidence risk is defined as the probability of occurrence of disease in a disease-free population (population at risk) during a specified time period. The annual incidence risk for dementia again typically increases exponentially with increasing age. The overall incidence risk for those aged 65 years and over has been reported to lie between 1% and 2%. Note that the *prevalence* of dementia is approximately three to six times greater than the annual *incidence*

risk. Prevalence ($P$) is approximately equal to the product of incidence ($I$) and disease duration ($T$): $P = I \leftrightarrow T$. Disease is terminated either by death or recovery. For conditions with high short-term mortality rates (lung cancer) or short-term recovery rates (common cold) prevalence and incidence rates are similar. Dementia is a more chronic condition.

Most functional mental illnesses, including depression, do not fit the classical incidence model in that they are typically relapsing and remitting disorders. Some authors prefer therefore to talk of onset rates rather than incidence. Typically around 12% of those not suffering from depression will have experienced an onset at follow-up 1 year later (Prince et al., 1998). However, much may have occurred in the intervening year. Few population-based studies have assessed the natural course of the disorder in the community with frequent repeated assessments. In a small Dutch community-based sample (Beekman et al., 1995) older participants were assessed with a postal questionnaire on five occasions over 1 year. Forty-eight per cent of the older population met CES-D criteria for 'depression of clinical significance' at one time or another over the course of the year. Most followed a variable, or relapsing and remitting, course. While half of all incident episodes were brief and self-limiting, 43% of prevalent cases at baseline remained depressed at each assessment throughout the subsequent year.

### The cross-sectional survey

The cross-sectional survey is the basic descriptive study. All members of a population, or a representative sample of the population are surveyed simultaneously for evidence of the disease under study (the outcome) and for exposure to potential risk factors.

Cross-sectional surveys can be used to measure the prevalence of a disorder within a population. This may be useful for:

- planning services—identifying need, both met and unmet;
- drawing public and political attention to the extent of a problem within a community;
- making comparisons with other populations or regions (in a series of comparable surveys conducted in different populations);
- charting trends over time (in a series of comparable surveys of the same population repeated over time).

They can also be used to compare the characteristics of those in the population with and without the disorder, thus:

- identifying cross-sectional associations with potential risk factors for the disorder;
- identifying suitable (representative) cases and controls for population-based case–control studies.

| Non-experimental | | | | | Experimental |
|---|---|---|---|---|---|
| Descriptive | | Analytic | | | |
| 1. Population prevalence/ incidence a. Geographic variation b. Temporal ('secular') variation | 2. Ecological correlation | 3. Cross-sectional survey | 4. Case-control study | 5. Cohort study | 6. Randomised controlled trial |

**Fig. 4.3** The main types of study design.

Findings from population-based cross-sectional surveys can be generalized to the base population for that survey, and to some extent to other populations with similar characteristics. The main drawback of cross-sectional surveys for analytical as opposed to descriptive epidemiology, is that they can only give clues about aetiology. Because exposure (potential risk factor) and outcome (disease or health condition) are measured simultaneously one can never be sure, in the presence of an association, which led to which. The technical term is 'direction of causality'.

Cross-sectional surveys are generally inefficient designs for the study of rare disorders, such as, for example, late-onset schizophrenia. With a population prevalence of less than 1%, non-cases will out-number cases by more than 100 to 1. However, all participants in the survey will need to be screened for the presence of the disorder. If all the true cases are to be identified, many false positives will also have to be processed. Cases will be over-represented in inpatient facilities and in residential and nursing home settings. These populations may be difficult to access by standard community survey techniques. In the community sufferers often live alone and may be unlikely to open their doors to researchers or consent to interview. Unless special attempts are made to sample these sub-populations there is a clear risk that an unrepresentative sample of cases will be identified, leading to bias.

The base population in cross-sectional surveys must be defined. This could be, for instance,

- all inpatients in a hospital
- all hospital inpatients in a given country
- all residents of a city borough aged 65 and over
- all residents of a country (aged 18–60).

Firstly it is necessary to identify a sampling frame of all eligible persons. Criteria for eligibility need to be thought through carefully, but usually a place of residence criterion and a period criterion are included; thus all residents of a defined area, resident on a particular day or month. Participants may (rarely) need to be excluded from the survey because of health or other circumstances that render their participation difficult or impossible. These exclusion criteria should ideally be specified in advance. Every effort should be made to be as inclusive as possible, in order to maximize the potential for generalization of the survey findings. Sampling frames for population-based surveys require an accurate register of all eligible participants in the base population. In most countries, such registers are drawn up and updated regularly for general population censuses, for taxation and other administrative purposes, and for establishing voting entitlement in local and national elections. However, there are problems associated with using such registers. Some may not contain all of the information (e.g. age, sex, and address) that is needed to identify and contact a sample of older adults. Many governments will either not allow researchers to have access to these registers, or will set limits on the information that can be gleaned from them or limit the way in which the data are used. Also many administrative registers are surprisingly inaccurate. This is particularly the case for older people who may have moved address without informing the relevant agency, or have moved or died in the interval between regular updates of the register. Because of these deficiencies, some population-based surveys draw up their own register by carrying out a door-knock census of the area to be surveyed. While this is practical for a small

catchment area survey, a survey of a larger base population such as the population of a whole country would need a different strategy. Often investigators draw a random sample of households, which are then visited by researchers who interview either all eligible residents, or individuals selected at random from among the eligible residents in the household.

Descriptive studies of disease frequency can be used to generate hypotheses about disease aetiology, particularly where the prevalence and incidence of a disease varies by geographical region (geographical variation) or over time (secular variation).

Geographical variation. The EURODEP consortium estimated the prevalence of late-life depression in a series of European population-based studies of those aged 65 years and over (Copeland *et al.*, 1999a). They reported considerable (over two-fold) variation in the prevalence of the disorder (see Fig. 4.4). The studies had all used the same semistructured clinical assessment interview, the Geriatric Mental State, and had used similar sampling strategies. Regional clusters of low or high prevalence for a disorder are of great interest to epidemiologists, as they may give important clues about its aetiology. The relationship between sun exposure and melanoma was established in this way. The prevalence of the disease in light-skinned persons increased as one approached the equator. The high prevalence of motor neuron type diseases in Guam, and the rarity of multiple sclerosis in southern Africa are other examples of regional differences that have led to theories about the aetiology of those diseases. In the EURODEP consortium study, there was no clear pattern discernible to explain the origins of the differences in prevalence, and this remains an important area for further study. Identification of large differences in social or environmental characteristics of the low- and high-prevalence populations could lead to further hypothesis-driven research, or to attempts at community-level intervention.

The consensus, until recently, has been that there are no important regional differences in the frequency of dementia or Alzheimer's disease (AD). Jorm *et al.* (1987) reviewed 47 studies of the prevalence of dementia published between 1945 and 1985. Much of the variability in prevalence between studies was explained by the different methods used by the investigators, involving principally

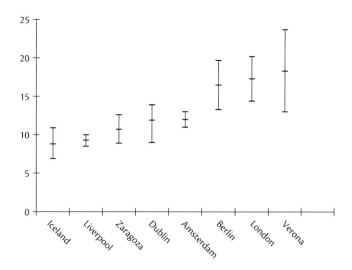

**Fig. 4.4** The EURODEP consortium: the prevalence (%) of late life depression in Europe (from Copeland *et al.* 1999a).

sampling, inclusion and exclusion criteria, research instruments, and diagnostic criteria. Corrada (1995) reviewed AD prevalence surveys published between 1984 and 1993, with a very similar pattern of findings. Since then the research methods for these investigations have been increasingly refined and standardized. The EURODEM consortium found that among European studies using similar methodologies and diagnostic criteria, there were only trivial differences in the age-specific prevalence of dementia (12 studies) (Hofman *et al.*, 1991) and AD (six centres) (Rocca *et al.*, 1991), concluding that 'ecological comparisons were unlikely to be informative about aetiology'. However, the large majority of these studies have been carried out in urban, developed-country settings. Other evidence suggests that AD may be less common in rural than urban areas, and in developing compared with developed regions

A recent review of population-based dementia prevalence studies in the developing world (10/66 Dementia Research Group, 2000) identified a large variation in the age-adjusted prevalence of dementia, from 1.3% to 5.3% for all those aged 60 or over, and from 1.7% to 5.2% for all those aged 65 and over. This may represent genuine differences in the prevalence of dementia, or may simply be an artefact of the methodological differences between the studies. Two of the developing-country studies (Hendrie *et al.*, 1995a; Chandra *et al.*, 1998) reported a strikingly low prevalence of dementia (Fig. 4.5). These are also the two developing-country studies with the most rigorously developed culture- and education-fair dementia diagnostic procedures, which had furthermore been harmonized for use in US–Nigeria and US–India transnational studies. The Nigerian study supported earlier observations on the rarity of AD in Ibadan, and on the absence of amyloid

plaques and neurofibrillary tangles in an unselected brain autopsy series (Osuntokun *et al.*, 1992). There seems to be a general trend, supported by the panel of experts reviewing the global literature on prevalence (Ferri *et al.*, 2005), towards a lower prevalence of dementia, at least in south Asia and in sub-Saharan Africa, compared with that seen in Europe and North America.

It is important, however, to understand that even striking differences in disease frequency between studies and populations may have mundane explanations:

1 Diagnostic procedures for psychiatric disorders that have been standardized in one setting must not be applied indiscriminately to another. They may turn out to be culturally biased, giving a misleadingly high or low estimate of the prevalence of the disease. It may be that mild dementia is underdetected in developing countries because of difficulties in establishing the criterion of social and occupational impairment.

2 Other methodological differences between studies, for example in sampling procedures and in inclusion and exclusion criteria, may have important effects on prevalence estimates.

3 Low prevalence may be accounted for either by selective out-migration of susceptible persons, or by in-migration of those unlikely to develop the disorder, and vice versa for high prevalence.

4 As prevalence is the product of incidence and duration, low prevalence rates may indicate a high recovery rate or a low survival rate for those with the disorder, rather than a true difference in incidence. One obvious explanation for the low prevalence of dementia and AD seen in Nigeria and in India is that it simply reflects a particularly high mortality rate among people with dementia in developing countries. Thus the incidence rate for dementia may be similar between the two settings, but survival with the disease may be longer in developed countries allowing cases to accumulate, and resulting in higher point prevalence estimates. Several factors may be implicated; intercurrent illnesses are more likely to be treated, diagnoses are more likely to lead to access to the full range of specialist dementia services available in most developed countries, including formal support for caregivers, and provision for residential and nursing home care. Thus, only longitudinal studies, with their capacity for disaggregating the frequency of new cases and their duration, will suffice to understand and explore geographical variation in dementia. Incidence rates from Nigeria and India are also much lower than those from the developed West (Hendrie *et al.* 2001; Chandra *et al.* 2001).

*Temporal (secular) variation.* Secular trends (changes over time in disease frequency) may help to generate or support aetiological hypotheses. Doll and Hill's studies into the association between smoking and lung cancer were preceded by the observation that by the middle years of the 20th century the UK faced a rapidly growing epidemic of the disease among males. This was temporally related, with a time lag for the cancer to develop, to the rise in cigarette smoking during and after the First World War. In the field of mental health, it is rare for data on disease frequency to have been collected and collated in a reliable way over long periods of time, such as to allow valid secular comparisons to be made. One example is that of schizophrenia, where, it has been suggested, falling first admission rates may reflect an underlying progressive fall in disease incidence (Der *et al.*, 1990).

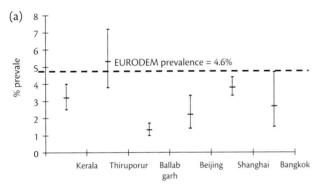

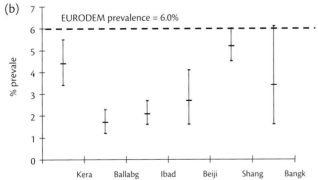

**Fig. 4.5** The prevalence of dementia in six developing country studies: (a) for those aged 60 and over and (b) for those aged 65 and over. Prevalence is adjusted for age and sex (Ballabgarh and Beijing) or for age (Thiruporur, Ibadan, Shanghai, Bangkok, and EURODEM), using the Kerala population as standard.

**Table 4.2** Lifetime prevalence of major depression by age and gender

| Age | Men | Women |
|---|---|---|
| 18–29 | 6.4% | 10.6% |
| 30–44 | 6.6% | 15.3% |
| 45–64 | 3.6% | 9.3% |
| 65+ | 1.6% | 3.3% |

Source: United States Epidemiological Catchment Area (ECA) survey (Weissman *et al.*, 1988).

The USA Epidemiological Catchment Area (ECA) survey (Weissman *et al.*, 1988) reported a decline in the prevalence of major depression with increasing age, not only for prevalence over the past year, but also for lifetime diagnoses (see Table 4.2).

These data could be interpreted as evidence of a cohort effect, with successive birth cohorts (presumably as a consequence of their life experiences) carrying an increasing propensity for major depression. However, these cross-sectional findings need not imply that the lifetime prevalence of depression is increasing. Alternative explanations include a selective tendency for older people not to recall earlier undiagnosed episodes (Giuffra and Risch, 1994), and a selective mortality of those most vulnerable to repeated severe episodes of depression (Ernst and Angst, 1995; van Ojen *et al.*, 1995). A broad review of this area reported similar findings for most psychiatric diagnoses, including schizophrenia, and concluded that cohort trends cannot be safely extrapolated from cross-sectional data (Simon and VonKorff, 1992).

Two epidemiological programmes have continued to survey the residents of the same area over long periods of time, and are therefore in the unusual position of being able to comment on the trends in the prevalence of dementia over time. The Lundby study in Sweden (Rorsman *et al.*, 1986) reported no significant change in the prevalence or incidence of either multi-infarct dementia or what was described at the time as 'senile dementia' over the period from 1947 to 1972. In Rochester in the USA (Beard *et al.*, 1991) the meticulously maintained health-care register suggested no change in the prevalence of either AD or dementia between 1975 and 1980. However, despite the recent stability of prevalence rates we cannot exclude the possibility that dementia is a more common disease nowadays than say 100 or even 50 years ago, at a time when developed countries were still developing. Accounts of typical cases of AD are to be found in historical sources, centuries before Alois Alzheimer's description of early onset cases. However, up to the last 20 to 30 years, we lack any kind of hard data on prevalence that would allow valid comparison with modern studies. Recent research suggests that vascular disease predisposes to AD as well as to vascular dementia (Hofman *et al.*, 1997). Smoking seems to increase the risk for AD as well as vascular dementia (Ott *et al.*, 1998). Long-term follow-up studies show that high blood pressure (Skoog *et al.*, 1996; Kivipelto *et al.*, 2001) and high cholesterol levels (Kivipelto *et al.*, 2001) in middle age each increase the risk of going on to develop AD in later life.

Changes in vascular risk exposures, particularly reduction in smoking, together with improvements in treatment of hypertension and established vascular disease, have led to a reduction in cardiovascular and cerebrovascular morbidity and mortality in many populations in the developed world. It will be both interesting and important in the future to monitor whether these changes have a discernible effect on the age-specific incidence of dementia and AD. Recent standardization of research methods and the establishment of precise baseline estimates in large population-based samples will assist such future secular comparisons. Any reductions in age-specific incidence rates are likely still to be accompanied by an increase in the absolute numbers of those with dementia, because of the continuing ageing of the population in developed and, particularly, developing-country populations.

## Analytical studies

Analytical studies differ from descriptive studies in that they are designed to address one or more specific hypotheses regarding the aetiology of a health condition. The basic strategy involves a comparison of the distribution of disease between groups or between populations, looking for associations between hypothesized risk factors and health experiences. There are two common types of study, the case–control study and the cohort study.

### Case–control studies

Case–control studies are relatively quick and cheap, and are useful for the initial investigation of the aetiology of rare conditions. As such, they would be particularly appropriate for the study of a condition such as late-onset schizophrenia. Surprisingly, there are few examples in the literature, and these are in effect clinical case series with small and potentially biased control comparison groups (Prager and Jeste, 1993; Phillips *et al.*, 1997; Brodaty *et al.*, 1999;). In the field of old age psychiatry the case–control study has been used primarily for the study of the aetiology of dementia.

Case–control studies aim to recruit, from a notional base population, a random sample of all persons with the disease under study (cases) and a random sample of persons without the disease (controls). The odds of being exposed to the presumed causal agent for cases is compared with the odds of being exposed for controls. The resulting measure of effect, an odds ratio (OR), will approximate to the relative risk (RR) if the disease is rare. The OR begins to depart significantly from the RR when the prevalence of the disease in the population reaches 10% (Box 4.2).

*Bias* can be a particular problem in case–control studies unless great care is taken with the study design. Selection of subjects is crucial. The chances of being selected as a case or as a control must not depend on exposure, as this would lead to *selection bias*. An example of this problem occurred in an Australian case–control study reporting on the association between arthritis and AD (Broe *et al.*, 1990). Cases were referred from primary care to a secondary-care dementia service. Controls were selected from among *attendees* at the same primary-care practice. Of course, the controls would have required a reason to attend the practice, and arthritis is a common pathology in older people. Hence, the selection procedures

---

**Box 4.2** Case–control studies

|  | Cases | Controls |
|---|---|---|
| Exposure$^+$ | $a$ | $b$ |
| Exposure$^-$ | $c$ | $d$ |

Odds of being exposed if a case = $a/c$

Odds of being exposed if a control = $b/d$

Odds ratio = $\dfrac{a/c}{b/c} = ad/bc$

would have been likely to produce a spurious, biased inverse association between arthritis and risk of AD. The authors themselves highlighted this difficulty. In case–control studies, since cases have already developed the disease, inquiry into exposure to risk factors is generally retrospective. The methods used to ascertain exposure must be applied symmetrically to both cases and controls in order to reduce *information bias* (observer bias or recall bias). It has been suggested that recall bias might have accounted for the often reported association between head injury with loss of consciousness and AD (Mortimer *et al.*, 1991). Histories are taken from an informant for both case and control. However, the informant for the case may be more likely to recall and report the head injury that occurred many years before, than the informant for the control, because they had been seeking a plausible explanation for their relative's decline into dementia; this phenomenon is sometimes referred to as making an 'effort after meaning'. Thus, the fact that the outcome has already occurred at the time when the exposure (risk factor) is ascertained can lead to bias. This facet of the case–control design also limits the inferences to be drawn from positive findings, in that it is usually impossible to determine the direction of causality for the association. Thus for an association between depression and AD, has the depression caused the AD or the AD caused the depression (Jorm *et al.*, 1991) ?

Given the inherent limitations of the case–control design, research into the aetiology of dementia has now largely progressed to the use of the cohort study design. However, the efficiency of the case–control study means that examples continue to appear in the literature. A useful variant of the case–control study is the nested case–control study in which recently incident cases recruited from an ongoing cohort study are compared with suitable controls from the same cohort for exposures that would be prohibitively expensive or impractical to have measured on all participants at the outset of the study. Thus Bots *et al.* (1998) have reported an association between thrombin–antithrombin complex (TAT) and dementia, having compared 277 cases with 298 controls recruited from within the larger Rotterdam longitudinal survey, suggesting that increased thrombin generation may have a role to play in the aetiology of dementia. Case–control studies may also in the future have a role in the elucidation of gene–environment interactions. The detection of such interactions requires very large numbers of cases, the logistics of which might be managed more effectively in a case–control design.

### Cohort studies

Cohort studies compare the incidence of new cases of the disease under study in groups of persons free of the disease at outset but who are a) exposed and b) not exposed to a hypothesized risk factor. The ratio of incidence risk between the two groups gives a risk ratio (RR) which is the measure of effect for a cohort study (Box 4.3).

Cohort studies have two principal advantages over case–control studies. Firstly, the longitudinal perspective allows the direction of causality to be established. Since exposed and unexposed are both free of the disease at the outset of the study, the onset of disease among the exposed implies that the exposure has led to the disease rather than vice versa. Secondly, information bias is limited, for at the time when the exposure is ascertained neither the participant nor the investigator should be influenced by the disease outcome, which has not yet occurred. However, cohort studies can be lengthy and costly, as the sample size needs to be large enough and the period of follow-up long enough to accumulate sufficient numbers of incident cases of the disease to make a statistically meaningful comparison between the two groups. For these reasons they are not the first choice of study design for rare conditions.

The defining characteristics, the advantages and disadvantages of case-control and cohort studies are described and compared in Table 4.3.

There is little doubt that the longitudinal perspective of the cohort study can clarify and sometimes change findings from cross-sectional or retrospective (e.g. case–control study) research. In the first instance, factors associated cross-sectionally with prevalent cases may be differentially associated with the incidence and the chronicity of disease episodes. Thus in one community-based study, disablement arising from health conditions was associated with the *onset* of episodes of depression but not with their *duration*, which was predicted rather by social support and social engagement at baseline (Prince *et al.*, 1998). Secondly, in case–control studies, selection effects or prevalence bias can give misleading results. In aetiological research into AD, the consensus from the earlier case–control studies was that smoking appeared to be a protective factor reducing the risk for AD, and with a negative dose–response effect; the more one smoked, the lower the risk of AD (Graves *et al.*, 1991). The first findings from a major cohort study suggest that the opposite may be true, that smoking increases the risk for AD, particularly in men (Ott *et al.*, 1998). Factors found to be associated with case outcomes in case–control studies may be factors predicting survival with the disease, rather than the onset of the disease itself. Doubt has also now been cast upon the consistent finding from case–control studies of an association between head injury with loss of consciousness and AD (Mortimer *et al.*, 1991).

**Table 4.3** Case–control and cohort studies. Characteristics, advantages, and disadvantages

| | Case–control | Cohort |
|---|---|---|
| Subjects selected according to: | Caseness | Exposure |
| Perspective: | Retrospective (subjects recall exposure) | Prospective (usually) (observers attend outcome) |
| Sources of bias: | Selection Information (recall and observer) | Information (observer only) Non-response |
| Resources: | Quick Relatively cheap | Lengthy Relatively expensive |
| Useful for: | Rare outcomes Single outcomes Multiple exposures | Rare exposures Single exposures Multiple outcomes |
| Measure of effect | Odds ratio | Relative risk |

---

**Box 4.3** The cohort study

| | Cases | Non-cases | Total |
|---|---|---|---|
| Exposed$^+$ | $a$ | $b$ | $a + b$ |
| Exposed$^-$ | $c$ | $d$ | $c + d$ |

Incidence risk in exposed $= a/(a + b)$

Incidence risk in non-exposed $= c/(c + d)$

Risk ratio $= \dfrac{a/(a+b)}{c/(c+d)}$

This has not been borne out in a large cohort study (Mehta *et al.*, 1999). Recall bias, or selective mortality, may have explained the positive association from case–control studies.

Many of the obstacles associated with cohort studies are eliminated where the outcome may be cheaply and conveniently ascertained in an existing cohort, in which appropriate baseline exposure measures have already been made for another purpose. Thus Jones *et al.* (1994) used data on child development gathered during the UK National Survey of Health and Development, based on a representative sample of all babies born in one week in 1946, and related it to their future risk of developing schizophrenia. The continuing regular surveillance of the birth cohort helped to identify those who had developed the disorder. In the UK there is no national register of schizophrenia cases but the 1946 cohort could also be cross-linked with the Mental Health Enquiry, a central register of all admissions to psychiatric hospitals, with ICD diagnoses on discharge. There is growing interest in the notion that mental health conditions of later life, particularly dementia, may have their antecedents in early life. Such associations across the entire lifespan can only feasibly be studied using historical cohort designs. One fascinating example of such a study is the Nun Study (Snowdon *et al.*, 1996). This study assessed verbal ability by analysing for density of ideas and grammatical complexity the autobiographies the nuns had written as young adults. Their cognitive function was assessed approximately 58 years later and those nuns who subsequently died had a neuropathological examination. Low idea density and grammatical complexity in young adulthood were associated with poorer cognitive functioning in old age. More surprising was the finding, among the nuns who had died and consented to post mortem, that low idea density at age 18 was strongly correlated with AD pathology.

## Randomized controlled trials

Randomized controlled trials (RCTs) are often seen as the prerogative of health services and clinical researchers, rather than epidemiologists. However, epidemiologists are commonly involved in this area of research.

Randomized controlled trials are in a sense a special variant of the cohort study, in which the exposure has been allocated at random, instead of recruiting participants who happen, for whatever reasons, to be exposed or not exposed. The design is particularly attractive to epidemiologists, in that it effectively eliminates the problem of confounding. This is because, when randomization has been effective, all potential confounding variables can be assumed to be evenly distributed between the intervention and control conditions, and therefore any observed difference in outcome can be safely assumed to be causally associated with the randomized variable. Thus, where the condition of equipoise is met—when there is genuine uncertainty as to the balance of risks and benefits associated with the randomized condition—the randomized controlled trial is the best design for assessing the effect of a protective factor identified in observational epidemiology.

These conditions apply particularly to the testing of apparent protective effects of medications identified in case–control and cohort studies. Thus, there is a body of evidence from observational epidemiology suggesting around a 40% risk reduction for AD in those older people using non steroidal anti-inflammatory drugs (Stewart *et al.*, 1997), and in post-menopausal women prescribed hormone replacement therapy (HRT) (Tang *et al.*, 1996). The consistency and strength of these protective associations argues for a causal association. However, there is a substantial and insuperable problem with all of these observational studies. The dementia syndrome is known to have a long pre-clinical prodrome, therefore even in cohort studies there is the possibility that older people who are developing AD may be less likely to present to doctors in such a way as would elicit a prescription. Alternatively, their general health status may be sufficiently impaired that their doctor would perceive a contraindication to prescription of these medications. This methodological problem has been neatly termed 'confounding by indication and contraindication' (Andersen *et al.*, 1995). The question can only be settled in a large, well-designed RCT in which the prescription is allocated at random, rather than on the presentation of the patient and the clinical decision-making of the doctor. Reports from epidemiological studies that certain prescribed medications, non-steroidal anti-inflammatory drugs, HRT, and cholesterol-lowering therapies, were associated with reduced risk for dementia are now being investigated in randomized controlled trials. The Women's Health Initiative HRT Preventive Trial was designed primarily to test the effects of HRT on cardiovascular disease and stroke. It was stopped early when it became apparent that randomization of post-menopausal women to HRT was associated with an increase, rather than an anticipated (based on earlier findings from observational epidemiological studies) reduction, in cardiovascular disease endpoints. Although underpowered, subsequent analyses of data on dementia outcomes showed that women randomized to HRT had nearly double the risk of going on to develop dementia in the short follow-up period (Shumaker *et al.*, 2004).

Certain risk exposures identified in observational studies may be amenable to clinical intervention. It would, of course, be unethical to *increase* blood pressure levels in a RCT, as a definitive test of the hypothesis that hypertension is associated with increased risk for AD or cognitive decline, but it is possible to piggy-back the question onto an RCT which is designed primarily to test the hypothesis that lowering blood pressure levels may reduce the incidence of these outcomes. Two RCTs of this kind have suggested no effect of antihypertensive treatment on cognitive decline (SHEP Cooperative Research Group, 1991; Prince *et al.*, 1996), while one RCT has suggested a protective effect of such treatment for dementia (Forette *et al.*, 1998). Another trial, involving older participants with mild to moderate hypertension, showed no benefits of antihypertensive therapy (using candesartan) on either cognitive decline or dementia (Lithell *et al.*, 2003).

Older persons are commonly excluded from RCTs, often for no good reason. Thus, the evidence base for the efficacy and effectiveness of commonly available therapies can often not be extended to older people, in whom the balance of risks and benefits may be somewhat different. Gerson, reviewing double-blind, placebo-controlled antidepressant drug trials, focusing on older people and reported between 1964 and 1986, located 25 studies, many of which were 'plagued with methodological difficulties' (Gerson *et al.*, 1988). The studies were small, and in total only 746 participants aged 60 and over were involved.

The evidence base has now developed significantly; the recent large-scale IMPACT trial randomized 1801 primary care patients aged 60 and older with major depression, dysthymia, or both to a 12-month collaborative care intervention or 'treatment as usual' (Hunkeler *et al.*, 2006). The intervention involved education, behavioural activation, antidepressants, problem-solving, and relapse prevention. Those given the intervention had better outcomes than the 'treatment as usual' group for continuation of antidepressant treatment, depressive symptoms, remission of depression, physical functioning, quality of life, and satisfaction with care at 18 and 24 months.

Most RCTs are conducted in secondary care settings, thus in the case of depression those that are recruited generally have more severe forms of the disorder. The evidence base for non-major depression, accounting for around 90% of cases of depression of clinical significance in population-based studies, scarcely exists. This restriction of the evidence base is compounded when RCTs in clinical settings address the efficacy of treatments under ideal conditions (recruiting unusually fit older people lacking co-morbidity), rather than their effectiveness under more routine clinical conditions. This process is particularly evident in the evidence base for the effectiveness of pro-cholinergic therapies for dementia, where the exclusion criteria clearly do not reflect the profile of the patients for whom the drug may be prescribed in routine clinical practice (Table 4.4). The AD2000 trial of long-term donepezil therapy in the UK aimed to recruit patients that more accurately reflected the target population for the medication (Courtney *et al.*, 2004). It found much smaller effect sizes on cognitive function than the drug-company sponsored efficacy trials, with no differences between donepezil and placebo on risks of entering institutional care, progression of disability, or death, or upon behavioural and psychological symptoms, carer psychopathology, costs of formal care, or unpaid caregiver time. Epidemiologists, with their focus upon the representativeness of the populations that they recruit, and the consequent generalizability of findings, can make a contribution to the design of trials that seek to assess the effectiveness rather than efficacy of new interventions.

### Genetic epidemiology studies
#### Association studies
Dementia epidemiologists are currently in a unique position. The discovery in 1992 of the association between the *APOE* gene and risk for both the dementia syndrome and AD (Saunders *et al.*, 1993)

**Table 4.4** Exclusion criteria for a procholinergic drug trial in Alzheimer's disease

| |
|---|
| Over 85 |
| Unable to walk freely with help |
| Visual/hearing impairment |
| Psychiatric or neurological disorder |
| Past or present active disease (GI, CV, renal, hepatic, endocrine) |
| Any diabetes |
| Obstructive lung disease |
| Oncology, haematology onset in last 2 years |
| $B_{12}$ or folate deficiency |
| Alcohol or drug abuse |
| Anticonvulsant medication |
| Anticholinergic medication |
| Antidepressant medication |
| Antipsychotic medication |
| Other drugs with CNS activity |

has ushered in a new phase in epidemiological research that will undoubtedly serve as a model for research into other chronic conditions. However, as yet, despite extensive research, the *APOE*/dementia association remains the only locus that has been reliably identified as having a major effect on risk for a common chronic disorder. The finding of the association with the *APOE* gene is now among the most replicated findings in biomedicine, with over 1000 positive reports in the literature. Research has now moved on to second-order considerations:

1 The association appears to be modified by age (decreasing effect size with increasing age) and by race (lower effect sizes in Africans and Asians, compared with Caucasians) (Farrer *et al.*, 1997). The age effect is most likely to be explained by differential mortality; those who survive to a great age despite the *APOE* ε4 allele may have other genetic or constitutional characteristics that protect against neurodegeneration.

2 The apparent effect of race is more interesting. One striking finding is the apparent lack of an association in Nigeria and Kenya (Kalaria *et al.*, 1997; Gureje *et al.* 2006), despite a higher than usual prevalence of the ε4 allele in Africa, and typically robust associations in an African-American sample (Hendrie *et al.*, 1995b). As we have seen, the prevalence of AD in the Nigerian sample was only about a quarter of that in Europe and the USA. These findings are strongly suggestive of a gene–environment interaction, in which the *APOE* gene is not a direct risk factor for AD but modifies the effect of one or more environmental factors that are common exposures in the developed world but very rare exposures in sub-Saharan Africa. The US/Nigerian researchers are currently investigating the role of vascular disease and its risk factors that are common in African-Americans and rare in Nigeria. Other researchers, employing a similar model, have suggested that widely differing levels of exposure to cholesterol (Chandra and Pandav, 1998) or toxic effects on the developing brain (Prince, 1998) may have been responsible both for the difference in disease frequency and the differences in level of association with *APOE*.

3 Observational epidemiology has already suggested that *APOE* may interact with a variety of environmental exposures that have the capacity to insult the brain at different stages over the life course. Thus apolipoprotein E (ApoE) seems to modify mortality after stroke (Corder *et al.*, 2000), the association between atherosclerosis and both cognitive decline (Slooter, 1998) and dementia (Hofman *et al.*, 1997), the association between white matter lesions and dementia (Skoog *et al.*, 1998), and the association between head injury (Mayeux *et al.*, 1995) and boxing (Jordan *et al.*, 1997) and AD. These findings suggest a mechanism for the operation of ApoE as a neuroprotective factor influencing the growth and regeneration of peripheral and central nervous system tissues in normal development and in response to injury (Prince, 1998).

## Conclusion

There is a continuing need for further epidemiological research into the mental health problems of ageing populations. Priorities will include:

1 Descriptive studies of the extent and distribution of both functional illness and dementia in the developing world. Very few

reliable studies have been conducted, and awareness of the extent of the problem posed by demographic ageing in these regions is very limited.

2 Comparative epidemiological studies validating and then further exploring possible differences in the prevalence and incidence of late-life mental disorders between different geographical regions and populations.

3 Monitoring of age-specific incidence rates for dementia in the developed world for evidence of possible reductions in incidence, in response to striking improvements in population health (e.g. nutrition, education, and vascular health).

4 More epidemiological studies are needed in all world regions to monitor continuously the response of health systems and health services to the needs of older people with functional mental illness and dementia. For example, the most recent epidemiological studies in the UK are already 15 years out of date, over which interval of time there have been profound changes in patterns of awareness and help-seeking, and of service provision and delivery.

5 Further large-scale population-based cohort and case–control studies focusing on interactions between genetic and environmental risk factors. At present the focus is upon *APOE* and dementia, but it is likely in the next few years that further genes for dementia, and also perhaps genes for functional disorders will be identified, revolutionizing and energizing the study of these disorders too.

6 Pragmatic trials of the effectiveness of common therapies for dementia and late-life depression in the settings where, and among the patient groups to whom, they are typically administered.

# Appendix: a resource guide to measures in common use in psychiatric epidemiology

This is a selection of the more rigorously constructed, best-validated, and most widely used measures. The choice reflects to some extent the author's bias towards briefer measures.

## Scalable measures with validated screening properties

### Measuring psychiatric disorder

◆ GHQ (General Health Questionnaire): self-administered (5 minutes).
Goldberg, G. and Williams, P. (1988). *A user's guide to the General Health Questionnaire*. NFER-Nelson, Windsor.
Goldberg, D.P., Gater, R., Sartorius, N., *et al.* (1997). The validity of two versions of the GHQ in the WHO study of mental illness in general health care. *Psychological Medicine*, **27**, 191–7.

◆ CIS-R (Clinical Interview Schedule – Revised): interviewer or self-(computer) administered (20–30 minutes) NB: not specifically validated in older persons.
Lewis, G., Pelosi, A.J., Araya, R., and Dunn, G. (1992). Measuring psychiatric disorder in the community: a standardized assessment for use by lay interviewers. *Psychological Medicine*, **22**, 465–86.

### Measuring depression

◆ CES-D (Centre for Epidemiological Studies – Depression): self-administered (5–10 minutes).

Radloff, L.S. (1977). The CES-D scale: a self report depression scale for research in the general population. *Applied Psychological Measurement*, **1**, 385–401.

◆ ZDS (Zung Depression Scale): self-administered (5–10 minutes).
Zung, W.W.K. (1965). A self-rating depression scale. *Archives of General Psychiatry*, **12**, 62–70.

◆ GDS (Geriatric Depression Scale) (over 65s): self-administered (5–10 minutes).
Yesavage, J., Rose, T., and Lum, O. (1983) Development and validation of a Geriatric Depression Screening Scale: a preliminary report. *Journal of Psychiatric Research*, **17**, 43–9.

### Measuring cognitive function (and screening for dementia)

◆ MMSE (Mini-Mental State Examination): interviewer administered (10–15 minutes).
Folstein, M.F., Folstein, S.E., and McHugh, P.R. (1975). 'Mini-mental State': a practical method for grading the cognitive state of patients for the clinician. *Journal of Psychiatric Research*, **12**, 189–98.

◆ TICS-m (Telephone Interview for Cognitive Status): interviewer administered (over the telephone, 10–15 minutes).
Brandt, J., Spencer, M. and Folstein, M. (1988). The Telephone Interview for Cognitive Status. *Neuropsychiatry, Neuropsychology and Behavioral Neurology*, **1**, 111–17.

◆ CSI-D (Cognitive Screening Instrument for Dementia): interviewer administered to subject (5–10 minutes) and informant (10 minutes).
Hall, K.S., Hendrie, H.H., Brittain, H.M. *et al.* (1993). The development of a dementia screening interview in two distinct languages. *International Journal of Methods in Psychiatric Research*, **3**, 1–28.

◆ IQ-CODE (Informant Questionnaire on Cognitive Decline in the Elderly): interviewer administered to informant (10 minutes).
Jorm, A.F. (1994). A short form of the Informant Questionnaire on Cognitive Decline in the Elderly (IQCODE): development and cross-validation. *Psychological Medicine*, **24**, 145–53.

## Instruments generating diagnoses according to established algorithms

### Assessing a comprehensive range of clinical diagnoses

◆ CIDI (Composite International Diagnostic Interview): interviewer administered (2 hours in its full form, although shorter versions, CIDI-PC and UM-CIDI, have also been developed). NB: not specifically validated in older persons.
Wittchen, H.U. (1994). Reliability and validity studies of the WHO Composite International Diagnostic Interview (CIDI): a critical review. *Journal of Psychiatric Research*, **28**, 57–84.
World Health Organization (1990). *Composite International Diagnostic Interview (CIDI, Version 1.0)*. World Health Organization, Geneva.

◆ SCAN and PSE: clinician administered (1½ to 2 hours).
Wing, J.K. (1983). Use and misuse of the PSE. *British Journal of Psychiatry*, **143**, 111–17.
Wing, J.K. (1996). SCAN and the PSE tradition. *Social Psychiatry and Psychiatric Epidemiology*, **31**, 50–4.

◆ GMS (Geriatric Mental State) (over 65s): interviewer administered (25–40 minutes).

Copeland, J.R.M., Dewey, M.E., and Griffith-Jones, H.M. (1986). A computerised psychiatric diagnostic system and case nomenclature for elderly subjects: GMS and AGECAT. *Psychological Medicine*, **16**, 89–99.

◆ CAMDEX (over 65s): interviewer administered to subject and informant (1 hour).

Roth, M., Tym, E., Mountjoy, C.Q. *et al.* (1986) CAMDEX. A standardised instrument for the diagnosis of mental disorder in the elderly with special reference to the early detection of dementia. *British Journal of Psychiatry*, **149**, 698–709.

### Assessing personality disorder

◆ SAP (Standardized Assessment of Personality): interviewer administered to informant (20–30 minutes).

Pilgrim, J.A. and Mann, A.H. (1990). Use of the ICD-10 version of the Standardized Assessment of Personality to determine the prevalence of personality disorder in psychiatric in-patients. *Psychological. Medicine*, **20**, 985–92.

Pilgrim, J.A., Mellers, J.D., Boothby, H.A., and Mann, A.H. (1993). Inter-rater and temporal reliability of the Standardized Assessment of Personality and the influence of informant characteristics. *Psychological. Medicine*, **23**, 779–86.

## Measures of other variables, relevant to mental disorder

### Measuring stable traits

◆ EPQ (Eysenck Personality Questionnaire): neuroticism/extroversion/introversion.

Eysenck, H. (1959). The differentiation between normal and various neurotic groups on the Maudsley Personality Inventory. *British Journal of Psychology*, **50**, 176–7.

### Measuring life events

◆ LTE (the List of Threatening Events): self-report or interviewer administered (5–10 minutes).

Brugha, T.S., Bebbington, P., Tennant, C., and Hurry, J. (1985). The list of threatening experiences: a subset of 12 life event categories with considerable long-term contextual threat. *Psychological Medicine*, **15**(1), 189–94.

### Measuring social support

◆ SPQ (the Social Problems Questionnaire): self-report or interviewer administered (10 minutes).

Corney, R.H. and Clare, A.W. (1985). The construction, development and testing of a self-report questionnaire to identify social problems. *Psychological Medicine*, **15**, 637–49.

◆ CPQ (the Close Persons Questionnaire): interviewer administered (10–20 minutes).

Stansfeld, S. and Marmot, M. (1992) Deriving a survey measure of social support: the reliability and validity of the Close Persons Questionnaire. *Social Science and Medicine*, **35**, 1027–35.

### Describing social network

◆ Social Network Assessment Instrument: self-report or interviewer administered (5–10 minutes).

Wenger, G.C. (1989). Support networks in old age: constructing a typology. In *Growing old in the twentieth century* (ed. M. Jeffreys). Routledge, London.Quality of Life

◆ WHOQOL-BREF: self-report or interviewer administered (10–15 minutes).

World Health Organization (1997). *Measuring quality of life. The World Health Organization quality of life instruments. The WHOQOL – 100 and the WHOQOL-BREF*. WHO/MNH/PSF/97.4. World Health Organization, Geneva. (e-mail: whoqol@who.ch)

### Global health/disablement

◆ LHS (the London Handicap Scale): self-report or interviewer administered (5–10 minutes).

Harwood, R.H., Gompertz, P., and Ebrahim, S. (1994). Handicap one year after a stroke: validity of a new scale. *Journal of Neurology, Neurosurgery and Psychiatry*, **57**, 825–9.

◆ SF-12 (Short Form – 12; reduced version of MOS SF-36): self-report or interviewer administered (5–10 minutes).

Jenkinson, C. and Layte, R. (1998) Development and testing of the UK SF-12. *Journal of Health Services Research and Policy*, **2**(1), 14–18.

A fuller account of validated health measures, with particular reference to older subjects, is contained in:

Prince, M.J., Harwood, R., Thomas, A. and Mann, A.H. (1997). Gospel Oak V. Impairment, disability and handicap as risk factors for depression in old age. *Psychological Medicine*, **27**, 311–21.

## References

10/66 Dementia Research Group (2000). Dementia in developing countries. a consensus statement from the 10/66 Dementia Research Group. *International Journal of Geriatric Psychiatry*, **15**, 14–20.

American Psychiatric Association (1994). *Diagnostic and statistical manual of mental disorders*, 4th edn. American Medical Association, Washington, DC.

Andersen, K., Launer, L.J., Ott, A., Hoes, A.W., Breteler, M.M., and Hofman, A. (1995). Do nonsteroidal anti-inflammatory drugs decrease the risk for Alzheimer's disease? The Rotterdam Study. *Neurology*, **45**, 1441–5.

Beard, C.M., Kokmen, E., Offord, K., and Kurland, L.T. (1991). Is the prevalence of dementia changing? *Neurology*, **41**, 1911–14.

Beekman, A.T.F., Deeg, D.J.H., Smit, J.H. and van Tilburg, W. (1995). Predicting the course of depression in the older population: results from a community-based study in the Netherlands. *Journal of Affective Disorders*, **34**, 41–9.

Beekman, A.T.F., Copeland, J.R.M., and Prince, M.J. (1999). Review of community prevalence of depression in later life. *British Journal of Psychiatry*, **174**, 307–11.

Bots, M.L., Breteler, M.M., van Kooten, F. *et al.* (1998). Coagulation and fibrinolysis markers and risk of dementia. The Dutch Vascular Factors in Dementia Study. *Haemostasis*, **28**, 216–22.

Brodaty, H., Sachdev, P., Rose, N., Rylands, K., and Prenter, L. (1999). Schizophrenia with onset after age 50 years. I: Phenomenology and risk factors. *British Journal of Psychiatry*, **175**, 410–15.

Broe, G.A., Henderson, A.S., Creasey, H., *et al.* (1990). A case-control study of Alzheimer's disease in Australia. *Neurology*, **40**, 1698–707.

Chandra, V. and Pandav, R. (1998). Gene–environment interaction in Alzheimer's disease: a potential role for cholesterol. *Neuroepidemiology*, **17**, 225–32.

Chandra, V., Ganguli, M., Pandav, R., Johnston, J., Belle, S., and DeKosky, S.T. (1998). Prevalence of Alzheimer's disease and other dementias in rural India. The Indo-US study. *Neurology*, **51**, 1000–8.

Chandra, V., Pandav, R., Dodge, H.H. *et al.* (2001). Incidence of Alzheimer's disease in a rural community in India: the Indo-US study. *Neurology*, **57**, 985–9.

Copeland, J.R.M., Hooijer, C., Jordan, A. (1999a). Depression in Europe: geographical distribution among older people. *British Journal of Psychiatry*, **174**, 312–21.

Copeland, J.R., McCracken, C.F., Dewey, M.E. *et al.* (1999b). Undifferentiated dementia, Alzheimer's disease and vascular dementia: age- and gender-related incidence in Liverpool. The MRC-ALPHA Study. *British Journal of Psychiatry*, **175**, 433–8.

Corder, E.H., Basun, H., Fratiglioni, L. *et al.* (2000). Inherited frailty. ApoE alleles determine survival after a diagnosis of heart disease or stroke at ages 85+. *Annals of the New York Academy of Sciences*, **908**, 295–8.

Corrada, M., Brookmeyer, R., and Kawas, C. (1995). Sources of variability in prevalence rates of Alzheimer's disease. *International Journal of Epidemiology*, **24**, 1000–5.

Courtney, C., Farrell, D., Gray, R. *et al.* (2004). Long-term donepezil treatment in 565 patients with Alzheimer's disease (AD2000): randomised double-blind trial. *Lancet*, **363**, 2105–15.

Der, G., Gupta, S., and Murray, R.M. (1990). Is schizophrenia disappearing? *Lancet*, **335**, 513–16.

Ernst, C. and Angst, J. (1995). Depression in old age. Is there a real decrease in prevalence? A review. *European Archives of Psychiatry and Clinical Neuroscience*, **245**, 272–87.

Farrer, L.A., Cupples, L.A., Haines, J.L. *et al.* (1997). Effects of age, sex, and ethnicity on the association between apolipoprotein E genotype and Alzheimer disease. A meta-analysis. APOE and Alzheimer Disease Meta Analysis Consortium. *Journal of the American Medical Association*, **278**, 1349–56.

Ferri, C.P., Prince, M., Brayne, C. *et al.* (2005). Global prevalence of dementia: a Delphi consensus study. *Lancet*, **366**, 2112–17.

Forette, F., Seux, M.L., Staessen, J.A. *et al.* (1998). Prevention of dementia in randomised double-blind placebo-controlled Systolic Hypertension in Europe (Syst-Eur) trial. *Lancet*, **352**, 1347–51.

Gerson, S.C., Plotkin, D.A., and Jarvik, L.F. (1988). Antidepressant drug studies, 1964-1986: empirical evidence for aging patients. *Journal of Clinical Psychopharmacology*, **8**(5), 311–21.

Giuffra, L.A. and Risch, N. (1994). Diminished recall and the cohort effect of major depression: a simulation study. *Psychological Medicine*, **24**, 375–83.

Graves, A.B., van Duijn, C.M., Chandra, V. *et al.* (1991). Alcohol and tobacco consumption as risk factors for Alzheimer's disease: a collaborative re-analysis of case-control studies. EURODEM Risk Factors Research Group. *International Journal of Epidemiology*, **20**(Suppl. 2), S48–S57.

Gureje, O., Ogunniyi, A., Baiyewu, O. *et al.* (2006). APOE epsilon4 is not associated with Alzheimer's disease in elderly Nigerians. *Annals of Neurology*, **59**, 182–5.

Hendrie, H.C., Osuntokun, B.O., Hall, K.S. *et al.* (1995a). Prevalence of Alzheimer's disease and dementia in two communities: Nigerian Africans and African Americans. *American Journal of Psychiatry*, **152**, 1485–92.

Hendrie, H.C., Hall, K.S., Hui, S. *et al.* (1995b). Apolipoprotein E genotypes and Alzheimer's disease in a community study of elderly African Americans. *Annals of Neurology*, **37**, 118–20.

Hendrie, H.C., Ogunniyi, A., Hall, K.S. *et al.* (2001). Incidence of dementia and Alzheimer disease in 2 communities: Yoruba residing in Ibadan, Nigeria, and African Americans residing in Indianapolis, Indiana [see comment]. *Journal of the American Medical Association*, **285**, 739–47.

Hofman, A., Rocca, W.A., Brayne, C. *et al.* (1991). The prevalence of dementia in Europe: a collaborative study of 1980–1990 findings. Eurodem Prevalence Research Group. *International Journal of Epidemiology*, **20**, 736–48.

Hofman, A., Ott, A., Breteler, M.M.B. *et al.* (1997). Atherosclerosis, apolipoprotein E, and prevalence of dementia and Alzheimer's disease in the Rotterdam Study. *Lancet*, **349**, 151–4.

Hunkeler, E.M., Katon, W., Tang, L. *et al.* (2006). Long term outcomes from the IMPACT randomised trial for depressed elderly patients in primary care. *British Medical Journal*, **332**, 259–63.

Jones, P., Rodgers, B., Murray, R., and Marmot, M. (1994). Child development risk factors for adult schizophrenia in the British 1946 birth cohort. *Lancet*, **344**(8934), 1398–402.

Jordan, B.D., Relkin, N.R., Ravdin, L.D., Jacobs, A.R., Bennett, A., and Gandy, S. (1997). Apolipoprotein E epsilon4 associated with chronic traumatic brain injury in boxing. *Journal of the American Medical Association*, **278**, 136–40.

Jorm, A.F., Korten, A.E., and Henderson, A.S. (1987). The prevalence of dementia: a quantitative integration of the literature. *Acta Psychiatrica Scandinavica*, **76**, 465–79.

Jorm, A.F., van Duijn, C.M., Chandra, V. *et al.* (1991). Psychiatric history and related exposures as risk factors for Alzheimer's disease: a collaborative re-analysis of case-control studies. EURODEM Risk Factors Research Group. *International Journal of Epidemiology*, **20**(Suppl. 2), S43–S47.

Kalaria, R.N., Ogeng'o, J.A., Patel, N.B. *et al.* (1997). Evaluation of risk factors for Alzheimer's disease in elderly east Africans. *Brain Research Bulletin*, **44**, 573–7.

Kivipelto, M., Helkala, E.L., Laakso, M.P. *et al.* (2001). Midlife vascular risk factors and Alzheimer's disease in later life: longitudinal, population based study. *British Medical Journal*, **322**, 1447–51.

Last, J.M. (1995). *A dictionary of epidemiology*, 3rd edn. Oxford University Press, New York.

Lithell, H., Hansson, L., Skoog, I. *et al.* (2003). The Study on Cognition and Prognosis in the Elderly (SCOPE): principal results of a randomized double-blind intervention trial. *Journal of Hypertension*, **21**, 875–86.

Mayeux, R., Ottman, R., Maestre, G. *et al.* (1995). Synergistic effects of traumatic head injury and apolipoprotein-e4 in patients with Alzheimer's disease. *Neurology*, **45**, 555–7.

Mehta, K.M., Ott, A., Kalmijn, S. *et al.* (1999). Head trauma and risk of dementia and Alzheimer's disease: The Rotterdam Study. *Neurology*, **53**, 1959–62.

Mortimer, J.A., van Duijn, C.M., Chandra, V. *et al.* (1991). Head trauma as a risk factor for Alzheimer's disease: a collaborative re-analysis of case-control studies. EURODEM Risk Factors Research Group. *International Journal of Epidemiology*, **20**(Suppl. 2), S28–S35.

OPCS (Office of Population Censuses and Surveys) (1991). *National population projections: mid 1989 based*. OPCS Monitor PP 2 91.1. HMSO, London.

Osuntokun, B.O., Ogunniyi, A.O., and Lekwauwa, U.G. (1992). Alzheimer's disease in Nigeria. *African Journal of Medicine and Medical Sciences*, **21**, 71–7.

Osuntokun, B.O., Sahota, A., Ogunniyi, A.O. *et al.* (1995). Lack of an association between apolipoprotein E epsilon 4 and Alzheimer's disease in elderly Nigerians. *Annals of Neurology*, **38**(3), 463–5.

Ott, A., Slooter, A.J.C., Hofman, A. *et al.* (1998). Smoking and risk of dementia and Alzheimer's disease in a population-based cohort study: the Rotterdam Study. *Lancet*, **351**, 1841–3.

Phillips, M.L., Howard, R., and David, A.S. (1997). A cognitive neuropsychological approach to the study of delusions in late-onset schizophrenia. *International Journal of Geriatric Psychiatry*, **12**, 892–901.

Prager, S. and Jeste, D.V. (1993). Sensory impairment in late-life schizophrenia. *Schizophrenia Bulletin*, **19**, 755–72.

Prince, M. (1998). Is chronic low-level lead exposure in early life an aetiological factor in Alzheimer's disease ? *Epidemiology*, **9**, 618–21.

Prince, M.J., Bird, A.S., Blizard, R.A., and Mann, A.H. (1996). Is the cognitive function of older patients affected by antihypertensive treatment? Results from 54 months of the Medical Research Council's treatment trial of hypertension in older adults. *British Medical Journal*, **312**, 801–5.

Prince, M.J., Harwood, R., Thomas, A., and Mann, A.H. (1998). A prospective population-based cohort study of the effects of disablement and social milieu on the onset and maintenance of late-life depression. Gospel Oak VII. *Psychological Medicine*, **28**, 337–50.

Rocca, W.A., Hofman, A., Brayne, C. *et al.* (1991). Frequency and distribution of Alzheimer's disease in Europe: a collaborative study of 1980–1990 prevalence findings. The EURODEM-Prevalence Research Group. *Annals of Neurology*, **30**, 381–90.

Rorsman, B., Hagnell, O., and Lanke, J. (1986). Prevalence and incidence of senile and multi-infarct dementia in the Lundby Study: a comparison between the time periods 1947–1957 and 1957–1972. *Neuropsychobiology*, **15**, 122–9.

Saunders, A.M., Strittmatter, W.J., Schmechel, D. *et al.* (1993). Association of apolipoprotein E allele e4 with late-onset familial and sporadic Alzheimer's disease. *Neurology*, **43**, 1467–72.

SHEP Cooperative Research Group (1991). Prevention of stroke by antihypertensive drug treatment in older persons with isolated systolic hypertension. Final results of the systolic hypertension in the elderly program (SHEP). *Journal of the American Medical Association*, **265**, 3255–64.

Shumaker, S.A., Legault, C., Kuller, L. *et al.* (2004). Conjugated equine estrogens and incidence of probable dementia and mild cognitive impairment in postmenopausal women: Women's Health Initiative Memory Study. *Journal of the American Medical Association*, **291**, 2947–58.

Simon, G.E. and VonKorff, M. (1992). Reevaluation of secular trends in depression rates. *American Journal of Epidemiology*, **135**, 1411–22.

Skoog, I., Lernfelt, B., Landahl, S. *et al.* (1996). 15-year longitudinal study of blood pressure and dementia [see comments]. *Lancet*, **347**, 1141–5.

Skoog, I., Hesse, C., Aevarsson, O. *et al.* (1998). A population study of apoE genotype at the age of 85: relation to dementia, cerebrovascular disease, and mortality. *Journal of Neurology, Neurosurgery and Psychiatry*, **64**, 37–43.

Slooter, A.J., van Duijn, C.M., Bots, M.L. *et al.* (1998). Apolipoprotein E genotype, atherosclerosis, and cognitive decline: the Rotterdam Study. *Journal of Neural Transmission. Supplementum*, **53**, 17–29.

Snowdon, D.A., Kemper, S.J., Mortimer, J.A. *et al.* (1996). Linguistic ability in early life and cognitive function and Alzheimer's disease in late life: findings from the Nun Study. *Journal of the American Medical Association*, **275**, 528–32.

Stewart, W.F., Kawas, C., Corrada, M., and Metter, E.J. (1997). Risk of Alzheimer's disease and duration of NSAID use. *Neurology*, **48**, 626–32.

Tang, M.X., Jacobs, D., Stern, Y. *et al.* (1996). Effect of oestrogen during menopause on risk and age at onset of Alzheimer's disease. *Lancet*, **348**, 429–32.

van Ojen, R., Hooijer, C., Jonker, C. *et al.* (1995). Late-life depressive disorder in the community, early onset and the decrease of vulnerability with increasing age. *Journal of Affective Disorders*, **33**, 159–66.

Warnes, A.M. (1989). Elderly people in Great Britain: variable projections and characteristics. *Care of the Elderly*, **1**, 7–10.

Weissman, M.M., Leaf, P.J., Tischler, G.L. *et al.* (1988). Affective disorders in five United States communities. *Psychological Medicine*, **18**, 141–53.

# 5

# Neuropathology

Zsuzsanna Nagy and Paul Hubbard

## Introduction

The aim of this chapter is to review the changes that occur in the human brain during normal ageing and in the processes of neurodegenerative diseases, such as Alzheimer's disease (AD), vascular dementia (VD), Parkinson's disease (PD), and dementia with Lewy bodies (DLB), as well as some less common causes of dementia in old age. Anatomical diagrams of the brain regions referred to in this chapter are provided in Figs 5.1–5.3. These diagrams are designed to illustrate the major areas of the brain affected by age-related diseases and include the *nucleus basalis* (Figs 5.1, 5.3), *globus pallidus* and *amygdala* (Fig. 5.1), the *hippocampus* (Fig. 5.2), the *raphe nuclei* and the *locus coeruleus* (Fig. 5.3).

## Normal ageing and the brain

### Changes in neurons

The human brain consists of two main cellular components, neurons and glia. Neurons exhibit enormous variety in terms of their size and shape, the length and number of processes they possess, and the distribution and number of synaptic contacts that they make. Neuronal cell division is limited in the post-natal brain, though neurons continue to grow as the body develops and the restructuring of synaptic connections (synaptic plasticity) continues throughout life. Neurons are therefore a dynamic cell type that undergo constant changes during life. However, within the scope of this chapter it is more appropriate to discuss the differences between mature young and ageing brains. The reasons for these age-related changes are poorly understood. However, two recent hypotheses dominate the field of ageing research. One theory postulates that the presence of reactive oxygen species and other free radicals generated as a by-product of the highly active metabolism of neurons is responsible for the age-related degenerative changes (Berr, 2002; Mariani *et al.*, 2005). The other theory attributes the age-related changes to the toxic effects of the excitatory neurotransmitter, glutamate (Beal, 2000; Perry *et al.*, 2000). To a certain extent both phenomena probably contribute to the neuronal cell loss and functional decline seen in the elderly. While the causes of neuronal damage in ageing are disputed, the mechanisms by which neurons die seem to be better understood. The realization that neuronal death, both in ageing and neurodegenerative diseases, occurs via a mechanism which is very similar to programmed cell death

(apoptosis), an active process that plays an important part in normal brain development was an exciting step forward in understanding the ageing process (Glasgow and Perez-Polo, 2000; Krantic *et al.*, 2005).

There are four aspects of neuronal changes which occur during ageing: changes in neuronal numbers, changes in size, changes in the constitution of the cytoplasm, and changes in neuronal processes and connections. Changes in glial cells, consisting mainly of an increase in astrocytes and microglia, accompany these neuronal changes.

### Changes in neuronal numbers

There are several populations of neurons known to become depleted in ageing brains. These include many regions of the cerebral cortex, the hippocampus (subiculum and dentate hilus), the substantia nigra, and Purkinje cells of the cerebellum. The extent of

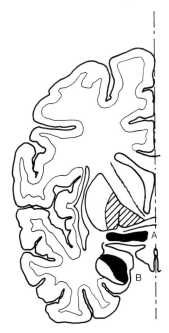

A Nucleus basalis (contains tangles; lies ventral to globus pallidus)

B Corticomedial amygdala (contains plaques and tangles)

**Fig. 5.1** Low-power view of a coronal section through the left cerebral hemisphere to show the position of the nucleus basalis (A), lying ventral to the globus pallidus and close to the amygdala (B).

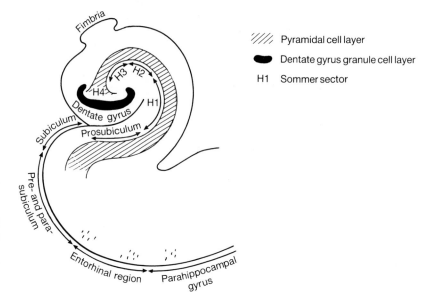

//// Pyramidal cell layer

● Dentate gyrus granule cell layer

H1    Sommer sector

**Fig. 5.2** Diagram of a coronal section of the right hippocampus showing the main anatomical features of the region and the subdivision of the pyramidal cell layer into regions CA1–4. Indicated as dots in the entorhinal region are the positions of large stellate neurons that are highly susceptible to neurofibrillary tangle formation in old age and Alzheimer's disease.

this cell loss is variable (Finch, 2003), depending on the brain region examined, and can range from comparatively low-level losses, such as in the inferior frontal gyrus (1% cell loss per year over the age of 70; Anderson *et al.*, 1983) and in Purkinje cells of the cerebellum (2.5% per decade of adult life), to somewhat higher values in the hilus and subiculum of the hippocampus (37% and 43%, respectively, between the ages of 13 and 101 years; Davies *et al.*, 1992; West *et al.*, 1994; Simic *et al.*, 1997). However, this depletion does not necessarily result in impaired function, a phenomenon which may be due to compensation where many brain regions have an overprovision of neurons in the first place. In addition, neuronal loss in the specific areas mentioned above is not necessarily indicative of a global decline in numbers of neurons. Many other regions of the brain, such as cranial nerve nuclei and the dentate nucleus of the cerebellum, are spared from significant loss during ageing. The reasons for this differential vulnerability between different regions of the brain are not clear but may be due to differences in neuronal plasticity (Arendt, 2003, 2004).

## Changes in neuronal size

In many of the regions of the aged brain affected by neuronal cell loss there is also a reduction in the size of neuronal cell bodies (or soma) (Meier-Ruge, 1988). Examples of regions where neuronal soma size has been shown to be reduced include areas of the cortex and the putamen, a nucleus of the basal ganglia. This change can complicate attempts to estimate cell numbers, since larger neurons, such as Purkinje and pyramidal neurons, come to resemble small neurons, while small neurons, such as the granule cells, may end up with soma similar in size to that of glia, and as a result may be unintentionally discounted from studies.

The loss and shrinkage of neurons is accompanied by a slow but steady reduction in the volume and weight of the brain, occurring from approximately 50 years of age. The normal weight of an adult human brain varies from 1240–1680 g in men, and 1130–1510 g in women, but this can decrease as the brain ages. As the brain shrinks, the ventricles and subarachnoid space enlarge to fill the intracranial space, and the ratio of brain volume to cranial cavity

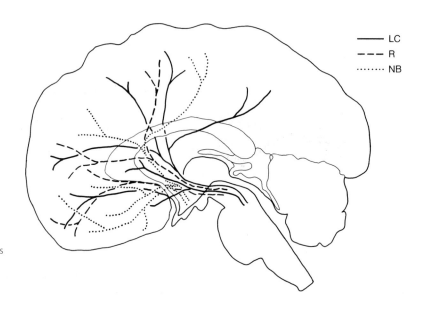

—— LC

--- R

······ NB

**Fig. 5.3** Diagram of a sagittal section through the brain to show the origins and widespread cortical distribution of axonal processes of neurons situated in the nucleus basalis (NB) (cholinergic), raphe nuclei (R) (serotonergic), and locus coeruleus (LC) (noradrenergic).

volume is reduced from 92% earlier in adult life to 83% by the ninth decade. The meninges surrounding the brain show slight thickening from collagen deposition.

## Changes to the constitution of the cytoplasm

A most obvious change to the cytoplasmic constituents of neurons in the aged brain is the accumulation of a granular pigment in the cytoplasm, called lipofuscin. This process begins early in life and progresses as the brain ages. Lipofuscin is a complex of substances which includes lysosomal enzymes, lipids, and partially degraded and obsolete cellular components. The extent of lipofuscin accumulation varies between brain nuclei, with the inferior olive (brainstem), thalamic nuclei, including lateral geniculate nuclei (LGN), and anterior horn motor neurons particularly affected. Another substance that accumulates in the aged brain is neuromelanin. Neuromelanin is chemically related to lipofuscin.

Changes also occur to the neuronal cytoskeleton as the brain ages. The cytoskeleton forms the internal framework of neurons and is responsible for maintaining their shape and connections. The cytoskeleton also performs important transport functions in neurons: it assists in the transfer of substances produced in the soma, such as enzymes and other proteins, moving them along dendrites and axons, and it provides the return transport of synaptic substances to the soma. There are three main components of the cytoskeleton: microfilaments, intermediate filaments (or neurofilaments in neurons), and microtubules. Microfilaments are principally composed of the protein actin, neurofilaments contain at least three neurofilamentary proteins, and microtubules are composed of tubulin. Links between the cytoskeleton, the cell membrane, and extracellular matrix (ECM) are maintained by many proteins. One such protein that has important implications in the ageing brain is *tau*. Tau is a microtubule-associated protein (MAP) that accumulates in neurons in the ageing brain. Accumulations of tau form ultrastructurally detectable abnormal, helically wound, paired filaments which form neurofibrillary tangles (NFT) in some neurons. Pyramidal neurons in the hippocampus and large stellate cells in superficial layers of the entorhinal cortex are particularly susceptible to these type of changes, though usually only a small proportion of cells are affected (Fig. 5.4).

Accompanying this alteration is the formation of argyrophilic or *senile plaques* (SP), abnormal extracellular deposits of -amyloid protein in a roughly spherical formation, in some cases with a core at the centre. SP lacking a core are sometimes referred to as 'primitive' or 'diffuse' and those with one as 'mature' (Fig. 5.5a, b). SP have a wider distribution than NFT in normal brains, occurring in the neocortex (cortex outside the hippocampus and entorhinal cortex) and amygdala as well as in the hippocampus and entorhinal cortex. There is no clearly defined and widely agreed cut-off between the numbers and distribution of SP in normal ageing and those in AD. Of particular importance for higher mental function is the accumulation of plaques with abnormal, tau-positive neuritic components to them. These may be present, but only in small numbers, in normal ageing. Criteria have been put forward for making a distinction between normal ageing and AD based on a requirement for more numerous neuritic SP to be found in the neocortex in AD (Mirra *et al.*, 1991) (see also AD below).

A further cytoskeletal abnormality that occurs to a mild degree in the normal aged brain is the development of Hirano bodies. Hirano bodies are eosinophilic rod- or carrot-shaped structures that occur either in or close to pyramidal neurons in the hippocampus. These bodies contain large amounts of the microfilament protein actin. Like the SP and NFT mentioned earlier, these are

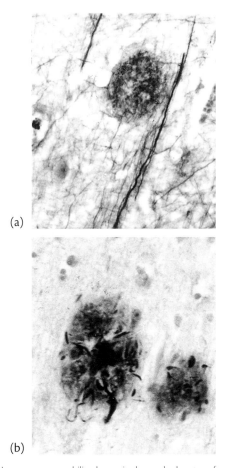

(a)

(b)

**Fig. 5.5** (a) Immature argyrophilic plaques in the cerebral cortex of a case of Alzheimer's disease (×400). Methenamine silver stain. (b) Example of a mature plaque in the cerebral cortex of an undemented elderly subject (×200). There is a well-defined core and condensation of surrounding neuritic processes to form a corona. Von Braunmühl silver stain.

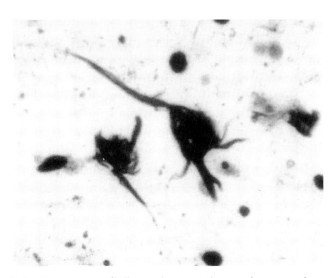

**Fig. 5.4** Numerous neurofibrillary tangles in cortical neurons from a case of severe Alzheimer's disease (×400). Gallyas silver impregnation.

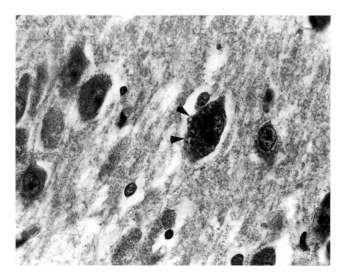

**Fig. 5.6** Granulovacuolar degeneration in the cytoplasm of a hippocampal pyramidal cell from a case of Alzheimer's disease (×1000). Note granules of differing size occupying pale vacuoles. Haematoxylin and eosin stain.

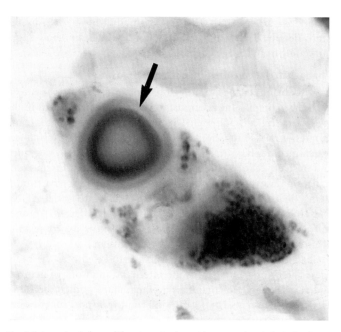

**Fig. 5.7** Lewy body (arrow) forming a laminated intracytoplasmic inclusion in a melanin-containing neuron in the substantia nigra from a case of Parkinson's disease (×800).

more numerous in AD than in the healthy aged brain. Their presence is also often accompanied by granulovacuolar degeneration—the appearance in pyramidal neurons of a cluster of vacuoles containing dense granules (Fig. 5.6). Granulovacuolar degeneration also occurs in normal ageing but it is much more common in AD.

In addition to the cytoplasmic abnormalities mentioned above a fourth pathological marker may also be present in aged brains. Lewy bodies (LB) are named after Friederich Lewy, an early 20th century neuropathologist who originally described LBs in 1912, as eosinophilic intra-cellular inclusions in parkinsonian patients. They are found in the substantia nigra and locus coeruleus in a small number of brains of healthy aged patients. LBs are particularly associated with neuronal loss and damage in both PD and DLB (discussed below). They take the form of a single spherical body, or small cluster of bodies, and have a 'laminated' appearance under the microscope with a dense core of mainly granular material at the centre, and radiating fibrillary material in the outer corona (Fig. 5.7). A major component of LB is the protein -synuclein. The gene on chromosome 4 coding for this protein has recently been recognized as the site of mutation in rare, dominantly inherited, early onset Parkinson's disease (Polymeropoulos *et al.*, 1997).

A further biochemical alteration in ageing brains, which can be shown by immunolabelling, is the occurrence of deposits of *ubiquitin*, particularly in the hippocampus. These take the form of small granules or threads in white and grey matter. Ubiquitin, as its name implies, is a protein that is widespread in animal cells. It becomes complexed to proteins which are destined for degradation, though that is not its only role. In addition to forming granular deposits of unknown significance in normal aged brains, ubiquitin is also found as a constituent of senile plaques, neurofibrillary tangles, Lewy bodies, Pick bodies, Hirano bodies, fibrillary inclusions in motor neurons in motor neuron disease, and the granules of granulovacuolar degeneration.

In about 30% of aged brains some foci of -amyloid deposition are present in the walls of leptomeningeal and cortical blood vessels. When such deposits are present in normal aged brains they

are usually small and very frequently widespread, usually in superficial cortical areas and in the leptomeninges overlying all the cerebral lobes. Occasionally they occur in leptomeninges over the cerebellum, but the hippocampus tends to be spared. The nature of the amyloid deposited in blood vessels is the same as that found in SP and is described in more detail below.

### Changes in neuronal processes and connections

Much less is known about the changes that occur to neuronal cell processes and connections in the central nervous system (CNS) as the brain ages (Masliah *et al.*, 2006). However, there are indications from Golgi impregnation studies that cortical neurons in the aged brain have a reduced number of dendritic spines. Other dendrites show excessive, branched extensions as if in compensation for the loss of others. It is also likely that neuronal cell processes are reduced in either calibre or length during ageing. Using an antibody to synaptophysin as a marker for synaptic terminals, immunocytochemical studies indicate a reduction in synapses in the frontal cortex of 15–25% between the ages of 16 and 98 years (Masliah *et al.*, 1993).

### Changes in glia

In addition to neuronal changes it is also important to mention glial changes during ageing. There are three main glial cell types in the brain (see the textbook by Kettenmann and Ransom in Further reading for a review). These are: the oligodendrocytes, which ensheath neurons in insulating myelin; the astrocytes, which provide structural, nutritional, and environmental support for neurons; and the microglia, the immune cells of the CNS.

The majority of studies of the aged brain focus on astrocytes. Astrocytes are highly reactive cells which respond to any type of damage to the nervous system. Following neuronal injury astrocytes become hypertrophic, enlarging their cell bodies and processes, and they move towards the site of injury to form a protective scar. Thus, dense focal collections of astrocytic processes accompany any local damage to the CNS. In normal ageing a more diffuse and less conspicuous glial scarring occurs, particularly in the subpial and ependymal layers. Another familiar change that occurs with ageing is the accumulation of *corpora amylacea*, most commonly in subpial and perivascular and subependymal regions. These are spherical bodies 20–50 mm across, sometimes laminated, and stained strongly by periodic acid Schiff stain. Ultrastructural examination has shown that they are mostly situated in astrocyte processes, though similar bodies can also be found in axons.

## Pathological changes in dementia

In large published autopsy series there is a general consensus that the most common cause of dementia in old age is Alzheimer's disease (Jellinger *et al.*, 1990; Esiri *et al.*, 1997a; Barker *et al.*, 2002; Attems *et al.*, 2005; Bennett *et al.*, 2006). However, there is considerable variation in the proportion of cases attributed to AD. In most series this proportion lies between one-half and three-quarters. Differences in the referral pattern of cases included in these studies may partly account for this variation. For example, of cases of dementia diagnosed in Oxford and referred to autopsy during the 1990s, 50% of those coming from geriatric psychiatrists were diagnosed neuropathologically as suffering from AD. Causes of dementia that give rise to physical disability, particularly Parkinson's disease and cerebrovascular disease, were more frequently present in the physicians' series. To obtain a true indication of the relative importance of different causes of dementia, community-based, prospectively assessed subjects need to be studied and followed to autopsy (Attems *et al.*, 2005; Bennett *et al.*, 2006). The cause of death in most cases of dementia, regardless of the type of dementia, is bronchopneumonia or pulmonary embolism. In the terminal stages of dementia subjects may become severely wasted.

### Alzheimer's disease

It is difficult to define the pathology of AD precisely at present. The reason for this is that the individual pathological components typical of AD brains all occur to some extent in normal ageing. The main difference between AD and the pathology attributable to normal ageing is the extent and distribution of the pathological components. Therefore the criteria for classifying the characteristic pathological features of AD are as follows:

1 The presence of numerous senile plaques, particularly neuritic SP, in the cerebral cortex, hippocampus, and certain subcortical nuclei—particularly the amygdala, nucleus basalis, locus coeruleus, and hypothalamus. Suggestions have been made about how many SP need to be found in cerebral cortex in order for a neuropathological diagnosis to be made (CERAD; Mirra *et al.*, 1991). The CERAD diagnosis is based on a semiquantitative estimate of SPs in the most severely affected foci of the neocortex. The frequencies of SP required to make a diagnosis of AD depend on age and on whether or not the patient was clinically diagnosed with dementia. The protocol allows the neuropathologist to make a diagnosis of definite, probable, or possible AD. The CERAD protocol has a wider acceptance than earlier criteria suggested by Khachaturian (1985), or Tierney *et al.* (1988) (Fig. 5.8).

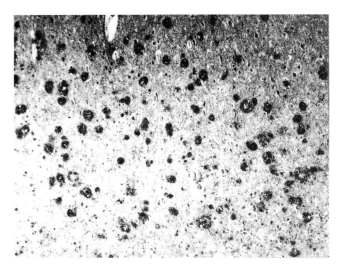

**Fig. 5.8** Low-power views of methenamine silver-stained area of association cortex in a case of Alzheimer's disease showing the abundance of plaques that is characteristic of this disease.

2 The presence of neurofibrillary tangles. Some NFT, particularly those in the hippocampus and transentorhinal cortex, appear as extracellular structures. This is because the neurons that contained them have degenerated. NFT are also commonly present in AD in the amygdala, nucleus basalis, some hypothalamic nuclei, raphe nuclei of the brainstem, and locus coeruleus of the pons (see Figs 5.1–5.3 for the positions of these nuclei). Brains from elderly subjects with only mild AD-related pathology have NFT but these are confined to the transentorhinal cortex. Those with slightly more pathology also show NFT in the hippocampus, and those with the most severe pathology and clinical AD show extension of NFT to neocortical and subcortical sites (Braak *et al.*, 1991). Recognition of this progression has led to the development of Braak staging of Alzheimer-type pathology, which recognizes entorhinal (stages 1 and 2), limbic (stages 3 and 4), and neocortical (stages 5 and 6) stages. Symptoms of dementia tend to develop in the limbic stages (Nagy *et al.*, 1999).

3 β-Amyloid protein deposits other than in SP. Amyloid deposits also occur in small leptomeningeal and cortical blood vessel walls in almost all cases of AD. Their extent is variable, from very slight to extensive. If extensive, the vessels may show secondary changes such as occlusion and recanalization of the lumen or slight haemorrhage around them (Fig. 5.9).

4 Frequent granulovacuolar degeneration and abundant Hirano bodies in the hippocampus.

Accompanying these changes substantial loss of neurons (30% or more) has been demonstrated among populations that are susceptible to NFT formation. This neuronal cell loss is particularly marked in pyramidal cell populations of the neocortex and hippocampus (Mountjoy 1988), though this has been debated (Regeur *et al.*, 1994; Korbo *et al.*, 2004). Cell loss is accompanied by an increase in astrocytic and microglial reaction in the cortex and white matter. In prospective studies correlations with severity of dementia have been shown between NFT counts and neuronal cell loss in the cerebral cortex and hippocampus (Wilcock and Esiri, 1982; Arriagada *et al.*, 1992; Nagy *et al.*, 1995). More recent studies indicate that the

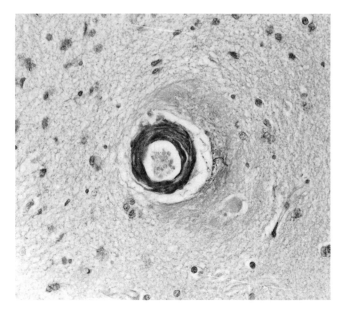

**Fig. 5.9** Example of a cortical arteriole containing amyloid in its wall from a case of Alzheimer's disease (×400). β-Amyloid immunohistochemistry.

main determinants of cognitive deficit are the accumulation of hyperphosphorylated tau protein and neuritic plaques (Smith *et al.*, 2000) while other studies indicate that synaptic loss is the main correlate of disease severity (Scheff and Price, 2003; Scheff *et al.*, 2006).

Behavioural abnormalities, in contrast to cognitive decline, correlate best with changes associated with subcortical pathology (Esiri, 1996). Excessive wandering and over-activity correlate with reduction in the level of cortical choline acetyltransferase activity, reflecting damage to basal forebrain cholinergic nuclei (Minger *et al.*, 2000). Depression in AD correlates with reductions in the density of 5-HT (serotonin) endings in the cortex, reflecting raphe pathology (Chen *et al.*, 1996) or with an a noradrenergic/cholinergic imbalance in the locus coeruleus (Forstl *et al.*, 1992, 1994). In another study aggressive behaviour in AD has been found to correlate with loss of cells in the rostral locus coeruleus (Matthews *et al.*, 2002) and with preservation of nigral neurons (Victoroff *et al.*, 1996).

The weight and volume of the brain, particularly in the cerebral hemispheres, is reduced in AD, though there is much overlap in the range of weight and volume loss between normal individuals and patients with AD (Fig. 5.10). Figures of about 7–8% reduction in brain weight in series of AD patients compared with normal have been described. Occasionally there is severe generalized cortical atrophy in AD, usually in the relatively young patients. The volumes of white matter and of deep grey matter are also reduced in AD, and the amygdala, hippocampus, and parahippocampal gyrus may be selectively affected, causing a compensatory dilatation of the inferior horns of the ventricles (Fig. 5.11). The volume reduction in the hippocampus and amygdala can be detected during life on temporal lobe oriented CT scans or MRI (Jobst *et al.*, 1994; Smith and Jobst, 1996). The cortical ribbon in coronal slices of the brain may appear marginally narrowed in some cases.

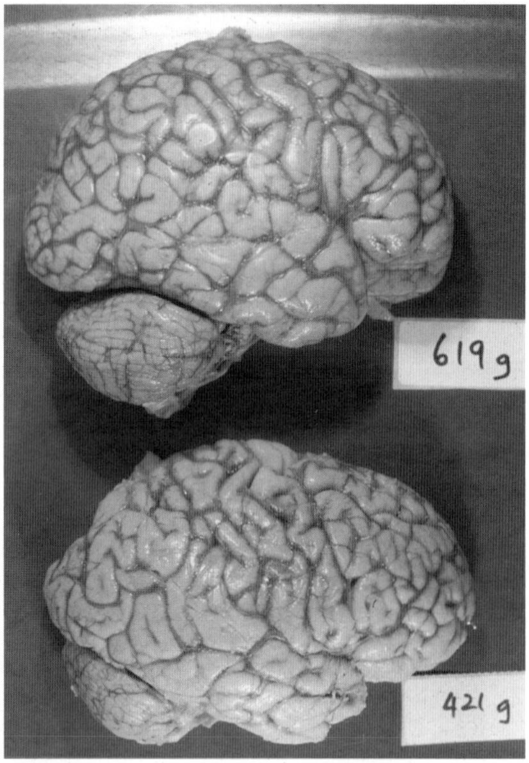

**Fig. 5.10** Right lateral views of the brain from an elderly non-demented subject (above) and a case of Alzheimer's disease (below). The cerebrum is slightly smaller and the cortical sulci are slightly wider in the case of Alzheimer's disease. The weights given to the right are for the respective cerebral hemispheres.

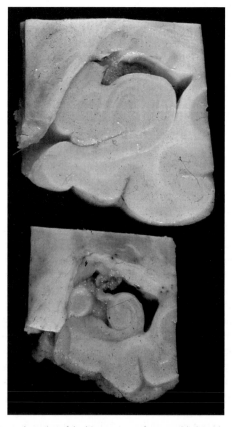

**Fig. 5.11** Coronal section of the hippocampus from an elderly undemented subject (above) and a case of Alzheimer's disease (below). Note atrophy of the hippocampus and adjacent temporal lobe cortex in Alzheimer's disease.

## Anatomical considerations

As indicated above, SP and NFT are much more numerous and widely distributed in AD than in normal ageing. However, they are not randomly scattered throughout the cortex and subcortical nuclei, but show a distribution that is closely linked to neuroanatomical connections (Braak and Braak, 1991; Arendt, 2004). This is particularly true of NFT. In general, areas of association cortex without, or with only one, intervening synapse to the entorhinal cortex are severely affected, while association cortical regions separated by two or more synapses are affected to a lesser degree. The primary motor and somatosensory cortices, far removed from entorhinal cortex, are relatively spared. The primary olfactory cortex, unlike other sensory cortices, is also affected, in keeping with its relatively close anatomical links to the entorhinal cortex. It is of interest that more peripheral parts of the olfactory system are also affected in AD (Harrison *et al.*, 1989; McShane *et al.*, 2001). It is therefore not surprising that considerable olfactory deficits, exceeding those found in normal ageing, have been recorded in patients with early AD.

Regarding the involvement of subcortical nuclei in the pathological changes of AD, it is generally the case that nuclei receiving a heavy input of afferent fibres *from* the cortex develop SP while those that have many fibres projecting *to* the cortex develop NFT (Pearson and Powell, 1989). Basal forebrain and brainstem nuclei that diffusely innervate the cortex and hippocampus are among the nuclei that lose neurons and develop tangles in AD: these are the nucleus basalis (cholinergic), raphe nuclei (serotonergic), and locus coeruleus (noradrenergic). Loss of pigmented cells in the locus coeruleus is usually sufficiently severe to impart abnormal pallor to this nucleus, visible to the naked eye. Loss of transmitters released in the cortex by these nuclei are among the most prominent neurochemical effects of AD.

## Relationship of senile plaques to neurofibrillary tangles in Alzheimer's disease

The paired helical filaments that compose NFT are also detectable ultrastructurally in the abnormal neuritic processes found in SPs. The most prominent protein antigen detectable in NFT, hyperphosphorylated tau, is also detectable in the neuritic corona of SP in cases of AD that have plentiful NFT. This suggests that the axons of neurons with NFT in their soma might be the neuritic components of senile plaques. This relationship between SP and NFT is supported by studies of the hippocampus (Hyman *et al.*, 1986). When there are NFT-bearing neurons in the entorhinal cortex then SP are also found where the axons of these neurons terminate in the dentate fascia of the hippocampus. Evidence from Down's syndrome subjects in whom AD pathology almost invariably develops by late middle age, suggests that diffuse SP develop first, followed by neuritic SP and NFT (Mann and Esiri, 1989).

The presence of diffuse amyloid deposits, unaccompanied by neurofibrillary pathology, in the brain of healthy elderly individuals indicates that amyloid deposition on its own is not sufficient to trigger the development of AD and related dementia. Although several hypotheses have been put forward, the link between the development of the different features of AD (i.e. amyloid deposition, neurofibrillary degeneration, and neuronal death) remained elusive. However, recent evidence from sporadic AD and Down's syndrome patients raised the possibility that these features may be the end result of a common mechanism triggered in the brain by age- or damage-related loss of synapses (Arendt, 2001). It has been suggested that synaptic loss and/or the loss of synaptic remodelling ability in the brain may result in the loss of the differentiated phenotype of neurons (Nagy, 2000; Arendt, 2003). These neurons, although unable to complete cell division, attempt to re-enter the cell cycle. As a consequence of this aberrant cell cycle re-entry, and a subsequent regulatory failure, neurons may either develop Alzheimer-type pathology or die via an apoptosis-like mechanism (Nagy *et al.*, 1998). The factors responsible for this aborted attempt of neurons to divide are to yet be elucidated.

## Alzheimer's disease and other pathology

The pathological changes of AD may be found in conjunction with signs of other CNS disease, most commonly Parkinson's disease or cerebrovascular disease. The relationship of Parkinson's disease to AD is discussed below. The relationship to vascular disease was thought to be partly due to chance—both conditions being common in old age. However, recent evidence indicates that the two diseases may share common risk factors, such as elevated plasma homocysteine levels (Clarke *et al.*, 1998; Hogervorst *et al.*, 2002) and the apolipoprotein E (ApoE) genotype 4 (Strittmatter *et al.*, 1993) suggesting common pathogenic pathways (Skoog *et al.*, 1999) (see Chapter 7).

Amyloid deposition in blood vessel walls in AD is usually mild and not associated with local ischaemic or haemorrhagic lesions. However, occasionally it is severe and widespread and then it may be associated with thrombotic occlusion of small leptomeningeal and cortical blood vessels, leading to the formation of multiple small cortical infarcts, or ischaemic damage to subcortical white matter. Occasionally, leakage of blood from amyloid-infiltrated superficial vessels results in small or massive intra-cerebral and subarachnoid haemorrhage. Small haemorrhages may be asymptomatic, but evidenced at autopsy by the presence of focal areas of rusty discoloration of the leptomeninges, where haemoglobin has been processed to the brown pigment haemosiderin. The massive haemorrhages may be fatal. Their position, relatively peripherally situated in one cerebral lobe (lobar haemorrhage), distinguishes them from the common major haemorrhages due to hypertension and rupture of short, penetrating arterioles, which are generally centred on the basal ganglia. Cerebral amyloid angiopathy accounts for about 10% of major intra-cerebral haemorrhages in the elderly. They usually occur in subjects who are not known to have been demented previously, but whose brains nevertheless show at least some of the pathology of AD at autopsy. Possession of the ApoE 2 genotype increases risk of haemorrhage from amyloid angiopathy (Nicoll *et al.*, 1997).

## Cerebrovascular dementia

Ischaemic dementia is the next most common cause of adult dementia after AD. Ischaemic brain lesions often coexist with those of AD. Even when the severity of AD-type pathology is insufficient to diagnose AD, the pathological changes may summate with multiple small vascular lesions to give rise to symptoms of dementia (Nagy *et al.*, 1997). Recent evidence indicates that the presence of even minimal cerebrovascular pathology lowers the threshold for cognitive deficit and results in clinical dementia in patients with pre-clinical Alzheimer-related pathology (Esiri *et al.*, 1999).

### Lesions in grey matter

One of the important underlying processes leading to ischaemic dementia is atheromatous arterial degeneration, causing narrowing of the arteries or ulceration of their surface. This arterial degeneration predisposes to thrombus formation and embolization. The internal carotid, vertebral, basilar, and other large cerebral arteries can be affected, leading to embolic or thrombotic occlusion of small arterial branches. Less commonly, thrombosis may occur in the small vessels themselves. This gives rise to multiple small cortical infarcts which may be widely distributed but are particularly common in territories supplied by the middle and posterior cerebral arteries. (Occlusion of larger vessels is likely to lead to larger infarcts, which give a stroke-like illness rather than dementia.) In studies of dementia associated with stroke, multiple infarcts (including bilateral infarcts and recurrent infarcts) distinguished demented from non-demented subjects at autopsy (del Ser *et al.*, 1990; Pohjasvaara *et al.*, 1998; Schmidt *et al.*, 2000). Since mural thrombus in the vertebrobasilar vasculature can give rise to emboli distributed in both right and left posterior cerebral artery territories (including the hippocampus), infarction or hypoxia may develop in both hippocampi and give rise to a severe memory deficit (Fig. 5.12). Bilateral infarction in boundary zone territories in both cerebral hemispheres is liable to develop following a precipitate fall in blood pressure, for example during cardiac arrest. Infarcts (lacunae) may be found in deep grey matter as well as cortex.

Other causes of multiple small infarcts in grey and white matter, resulting in dementia in old age, include various forms of vasculitis

such as polyarteritis nodosa, systemic lupus erythematosus, and granulomatous arteritis. These are all conditions that are only rarely encountered. A common condition that may exacerbate the damage produced when circulation is compromised is iron-deficiency anaemia.

### Lesions in white matter

Well-defined infarcts are less common in white matter than in grey matter, but white matter frequently suffers from more diffuse ischaemic hypoxic damage. Frequently, the basis of this type of damage is long-standing hypertension, which leads to hyalinization of the arteriolar walls and increased tortuosity of vessels in the white matter and deep grey matter. Rarefaction of white matter around these arterioles follows, possibly from the high pulse pressure inside the vessels. The resulting condition of the brain, sometimes referred to as 'cribriform state' (*état cribré*), resembles a fine sponge to naked eye examination, with each tiny vessel being surrounded by a widened perivascular space in which there are likely to be a few pigment-containing macrophages, and beyond that a zone of poorly myelinated, loosened white matter (Fig. 5.13). These changes may be maximal in temporal lobe white matter or basal ganglia and thalamus, or may be widespread in cerebral white matter. The white matter volume is then correspondingly reduced and the lateral ventricles enlarged. The vessels themselves show reduplication of the intimal lining and collagenous deposition in the media. The internal elastic lamina may also show reduplication and there may be two or three small vascular channels replacing a normal single

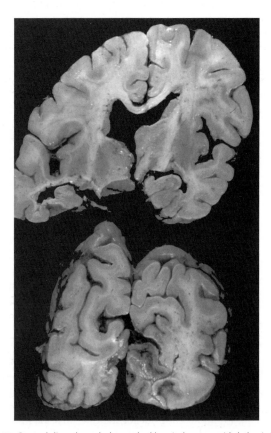

**Fig. 5.12** Coronal slices through the cerebral hemispheres at mid-thalamic level (above) and in the parieto-occipital region (below). Infarcts in posterior cerebral artery territory are present on both sides, in the hippocampus on the left in the top slice and in the right calcarine cortex on the right in the lower slice. The right hippocampus was included in the damage in an intermediate slice. The patient was an 84-year-old female with a 5-year history of confusion and memory loss with some episodes of aggression.

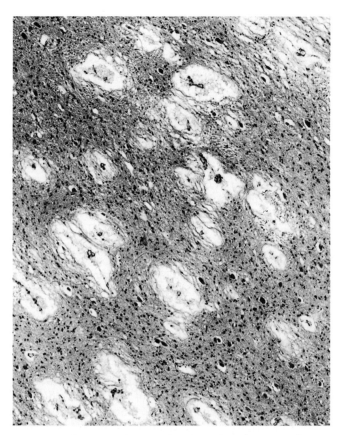

**Fig. 5.13** Low-power view of a section from the cerebrum from a case of *état cribré* in which there is dilatation of the perivascular spaces and rarefaction of adjacent tissue (×80).

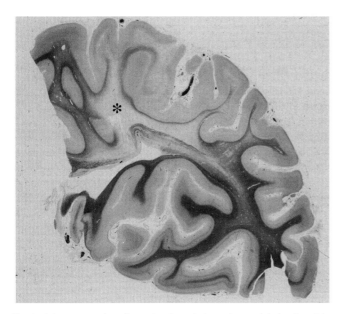

**Fig. 5.14** Low-power view of a section through the parieto-occipital region of the left cerebral hemisphere from a case of progressive dementia complicating long-standing hypertension in a woman of 71 years (×1). The section has been stained for myelin and shows loss of myelin in inferior parietal and occipital white matter (*) with sparing only of the immediately subcortical myelin. The damage to white matter was attributable to occlusion and narrowing by intimal proliferation of many small arterioles in the white matter.

one, indicating thrombosis with recanalization or tortuosity. Although these changes are classically seen in elderly subjects with long-standing hypertension, they may also occur in the sixth to tenth decades in the absence of a strong history of hypertension. There is reason to believe that this type of vascular disease is the commonest form of vascular dementia (Esiri *et al.*, 1997a; Esiri, 2000; Rossi *et al.*, 2004). Such lesions may be the only ones demonstrable in the brains of subjects with a history of progressive dementia, or they may be combined with grey matter infarcts and/or AD pathology. In some cases, the white matter rarefaction may be unusually diffuse and widespread. This pathological picture is known as Binswanger's disease (Fig. 5.14). Many cases of this sort will be shown at autopsy to have an enlarged heart with a hypertrophied left ventricle.

## Parkinson's disease and dementia with Lewy bodies

Parkinson's disease (PD) was first described by James Parkinson in 1817 as the 'shaking palsy'. Within the spectrum of neurodegenerative diseases there is considerable overlap between Alzheimer's and Parkinson's diseases. A substantial minority of patients with idiopathic PD have dementia (termed Parkinson's disease with dementia, PDD) and a similar minority of patients with AD have symptoms of parkinsonism (Leverenz and Sumi, 1986) (see Chapter 27iv). There has therefore been considerable interest in discovering a possible relationship between these two diseases and in clarifying the reasons for the development of dementia in PD and of symptoms of parkinsonism in AD. Indeed, there are similarities in the areas affected in PD and AD. For example, it is worth noting that both PD and AD patients have pathological changes in the nucleus basalis, a major source of cholinergic input to the cerebral cortex.

As mentioned previously, the major pathological feature of PD is the Lewy body (LB). LBs may be found beyond the nuclei conventionally recognized to be regularly affected in PD, and may occur in large numbers in cerebral cortex, particularly in demented subjects (Braak *et al.*, 2003). When dementia develops in patients previously diagnosed with PD a further diagnosis of PDD may be made. PDD resembles a condition known as diffuse or cortical Lewy body disease, or dementia with Lewy bodies (DLB), in which Lewy bodies occur throughout the limbic and cortical regions. DLB is generally distinguished clinically from PD by the time of onset of dementia. That is, using the consensus guidelines for DLB, PD patients developing dementia 12 months or more after the diagnosis of parkinsonian symptoms should be regarded as having PDD rather than DLB (McKeith and Mosimann, 2004).

The detection of widespread LBs has been made easier by using immunolabelling with antibodies to ubiquitin or -synuclein, with which LBs react. It has been suggested that in the past cases of diffuse LB disease may have gone undetected, and that diffuse LB disease is not rare, as was believed a few years ago, but is as common, or nearly as common, as vascular disease among the causes of dementia (Lennox *et al.*, 1989). Indeed, recent studies have shown that the prevalence of DLB in the over 65s is 0.7%, suggesting that DLB could account for up to 10% of all dementias (Stevens *et al.*, 2002). Furthermore a study of patients over 85 found that 5.0% met consensus criteria for DLB (3.3% probable, 1.7% possible) representing 22% of all dementia cases (Rahkonen *et al.*, 2003).

Most patients with PD do not suffer from the full clinical picture of dementia, despite having poorer cognitive function than age- and education-matched controls. In such cases the pathology, consisting of LB formation, neuron loss, and gliosis, occurs predominantly in subcortical and brainstem nuclei, particularly in nuclei containing melanized neurons. Thus, the naked-eye lesion characteristic of PD is pallor of the (normally pigmented) brainstem nuclei, the substantia nigra, and locus coeruleus. Studies of PD subjects with the full picture of dementia have found a variety of pathologies that might explain the dementia:

1 More cell loss seen in the nucleus basalis than in non-demented PD subjects.

2 Cortical LBs: these are often combined with the presence of diffuse SP (but not always neuritic SP, so CERAD criteria for AD may not be met) (Hurtig *et al.*, 2000). Patients suffering from DLB, with many cortical Lewy bodies, frequently develop severe dementia and may show a fluctuating course in the early stages of their illness. Patients with DLB are also likely to suffer from persistent (usually visual) hallucinations (Byrne *et al.*, 1990; McKeith *et al.*, 1994; Papapetropoulos *et al.*, 2006), and are usually sensitive to the effect of neuroleptic drugs (McKeith *et al.*, 1992; McShane *et al.*, 1997). Cortical Lewy bodies are particularly numerous in cingulate, insular, and parahippocampal cortices (Braak *et al.*, 2003). They have a less distinctive appearance than Lewy bodies in the substantia nigra, showing less clear lamination (Fig. 5.15). A constant accompaniment of cortical Lewy bodies is the presence of many abnormal α-synuclein immunoreactive neurites, termed Lewy neurites. These are particularly numerous in the hippocampus in the CA2–3 region where they have been correlated with dementia severity in some reports (Churchyard and Lees, 1997).

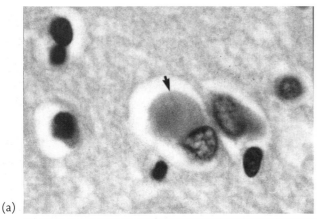

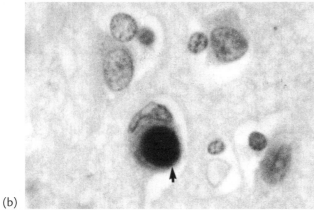

**Fig. 5.15** Cerebral cortex from a case of diffuse Lewy body disease: (a) stained with haematoxylin and eosin (×400) and (b) stained an antibody to α-synuclein (×200). The intracytoplasmic Lewy body inclusions are strongly reactive for α-synuclein. Lewy neurites are also evident with immunolabelling.

3 Classical AD pathology with classical subcortical PD pathology. There are usually a few cortical Lewy bodies present in such cases.

However, some cases show only the expected subcortical PD pathology, with or without a few cortical Lewy bodies and with or without some ischaemic vascular pathology. Many subjects with numerous cortical LBs have clinical features of parkinsonism, even though dementia may be the presenting complaint. When the density of cortical LBs has been quantified, a positive correlation with the severity of dementia has been demonstrated, suggesting a relationship between the presence of LBs and neuronal dysfunction (Lennox *et al.*, 1989; Hurtig *et al.*, 2000).

In DLB the LBs are found to be most numerous in entorhinal, temporal, insular, olfactory, and cingulate cortices, where they occur mainly in small- and medium-sized pyramidal cells in the deeper cortical layers (layers V and VI). Additionally, cases with cortical LBs almost invariably also show cell loss and LBs in the substantia nigra. Interestingly, LBs are relatively rare in the hippocampus, especially when compared with the amygdala in which LBs are more common. The reason for these regional differences in LB pathology in such anatomically closely related regions is unknown. It is also important to note that some cases of DLB present with large numbers of diffuse SP. Because Lewy bodies can be difficult to detect in the cerebral cortex unless they are specifically looked for, it is possible that some of these patients were previously regarded as cases of AD with SP predominating, when actually they were cases of DLB (Hansen *et al.*, 1993).

## Brain damage due to alcohol

There is a wide spectrum of neuropathological change that may be found in the brains of subjects with a prolonged high intake of alcohol. Features of Wernicke's encephalopathy are common, as is cerebellar cortical degeneration (Fadda and Rossetti, 1998). Those who have developed cirrhosis of the liver and terminal liver failure may have features of acute hepatic encephalopathy. Since alcoholics are prone to repeated falls, they commonly develop brain damage due to head injury, such as cortical contusions and subdural haematomas. Cerebrovascular disease is also common in alcoholics. Exceptionally, the pathological features of Marchiafava–Bignami disease or central pontine myelinolysis may be found. Recent studies indicate that the brain shrinkage due to uncomplicated alcoholism is mainly due to white matter loss that, to some extent, appears to be reversible (Harper, 1998). While alcohol-related neuronal loss has been well documented in the superior frontal cortex (Harper *et al.*, 1987) hypothalamus (Harper, 1998), and cerebellum (Fadda and Rossetti, 1998), findings on hippocampus and amygdala are more controversial (Harper, 1998).

## Wernicke's encephalopathy and cerebellar degeneration in alcoholics

The lesions of Wernicke's encephalopathy have been found in 1.7–2.7% of unselected autopsies and are probably frequently undetected unless they are specifically sought. They are due to a deficiency of vitamin $B_1$ (thiamine). The lesions chiefly affect the grey matter around the third ventricle and aqueduct and in the floor of the fourth ventricle. The mamillary bodies are particularly liable to be affected. The appearance of the lesions depends on how acute they are. In the initial stages there are petechial haemorrhages, but more commonly the pathology is seen at a chronic stage when there is brown discoloration and atrophy of the areas affected. The lesions cannot be reliably detected by naked-eye examination alone. Microscopy shows, in the acute stage, prominent enlargement of the endothelial cells of capillaries and some red blood cells and macrophages in perivascular tissue. Surrounding astrocytes are enlarged but neurons are usually relatively well preserved. In the chronic stage, there is an increased content of reticulin in perivascular spaces and some prominence of endothelium with a few scattered haemosiderin-containing macrophages. The dorsal medial thalamic nuclei, as well as the mamillary bodies, are at risk for developing these lesions and their involvement may explain the prominence of memory disturbances in such patients. Although alcoholic patients with Wernicke's syndrome develop neurofibrillary pathology in the nucleus basalis, the loss of cholinergic cells in this region is minor and it is not related to the profound memory disorder (Cullen *et al.*, 1997).

The cerebellar degeneration seen in alcoholics is distinctive for its relatively selective involvement of the superior vermis. To the naked eye, the affected cerebellar folia appear shrunken; microscopically they show severe loss of Purkinje cells, patchy loss of granule cells, and gliosis of the Bergmann glia (astrocytes) extending into the molecular layer of the cortex. Cerebellar cortical degeneration in alcoholics may occur in conjunction with Wernicke's encephalopathy, but it is not clearly due to thiamine deficiency. Similarly, the cortical degeneration and cognitive deficits seen in Korsakov's syndrome cannot be explained by thiamine deficiency alone (Homewood *et al.*, 1999). It has been found recently that the ApoE genotype has a significant role in determining whether patients suffering from Korsakov's syndrome will develop a global cognitive deficit or not (Muramatsu *et al* 1997).

## Hydrocephalus

A small number of demented patients are found at autopsy to have marked dilation of the lateral ventricles without significant cerebral atrophy (Fig. 5.16). The third ventricle may also be dilated. The appearances suggest an obstructive hydrocephalus and this impression may be borne out by the presence of defects in the septum. Rarely, there is an obvious tumour mass obstructing the flow of cerebrospinal fluid, for example a non-functioning pituitary adenoma, but this is exceptional. In some cases, there may be thickening of the leptomeninges, providing an explanation for obstruction to circulation of the cerebrospinal fluid in the subarachnoid space, but most cases show no clear evidence of such obstruction to flow. Alternatively, there may be signs of old intracerebral or subarachnoid haemorrhage, or head injury, perhaps sufficient to have impaired uptake of cerebrospinal fluid at the arachnoid villi. These cases usually lack classical clinical features of raised intracranial pressure but show the triad of dementia, incontinence, and ataxia that characterize 'normal pressure (or more correctly, intermittently raised pressure) hydrocephalus' (see Chapter 27vi). It may be significant that a high percentage of such cases display small foci of deep cerebral vascular damage which may result in transient obstruction to flow of cerebrospinal fluid by haemorrhage into the ventricles (Esiri, 1997).

## Pick's disease

Pick's disease is a rare, autosomal dominant disease, though occasional apparently sporadic cases can also be encountered. It is sometimes called *lobar atrophy* because of the distinctive naked-eye atrophy of the cortex that characterizes the brain in most cases of

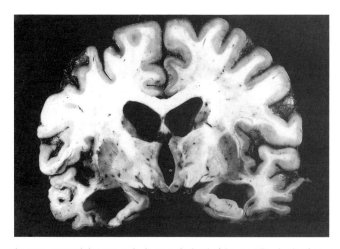

**Fig. 5.17** Coronal slice across the brain at the level of the mamillary bodies from a case of Pick's disease. In this case the atrophy is confined to the temporal lobes, in which the cortex is narrowed and the sulci are widened. The inferior horns of the ventricles are correspondingly grossly dilated while the main body of the lateral ventricles and third ventricle are only mildly dilated. The corpus callosum and frontal cortex are relatively well preserved.

this disease. The atrophy usually affects most prominently the frontal and/or temporal poles of the cerebral hemispheres. In the temporal lobes, the posterior two-thirds of the superior temporal gyrus are relatively spared. There may be asymmetry, with one cerebral hemisphere more affected than the other. The degree of atrophy present in the most severely affected parts of the cortex is usually more marked than that seen in AD. The overlying leptomeninges are usually considerably thickened. The deep grey matter, particularly the caudate nuclei, and the white matter are atrophic. The lateral ventricles, particularly the frontal and inferior horns, are grossly dilated to compensate for this atrophy and the corpus callosum is thin (Fig. 5.17).

On microscopy, neuronal loss in affected parts of the cortex is usually obvious, or even extreme, with few surviving large pyramidal neurons. This cell loss is accompanied by marked astrocytosis in both grey and white matter. Myelin staining in atrophic white matter is poor, reflecting diffuse loss of myelinated fibres. Some remaining cortical neurons show expansion and enlargement by argyrophilic bundles of neurofilaments that immunolabel for tau (Fig. 5.18). Expanded cells of this sort are called Pick cells; rounded, perinuclear condensations of such filaments are called Pick bodies. These cells can frequently be detected in the dentate fascia of the hippocampus as well as scattered in the cortex, though here their numbers may be low if most cells have disappeared. Pick bodies give immunocytochemical reactions for neurofilaments and ubiquitin. Some microscopic features of AD, particularly granulovacuolar degeneration, may be found in Pick's disease.

*Dementia of frontal lobe type* (Chapter 27v) is primarily a clinical diagnosis. These patients typically present with alteration in personality, disinhibited behaviour, neglect of personal appearance, loss of social awareness, and impulsive or ill-considered action. The condition encompasses several different pathological conditions. Some cases are diagnosed post-mortem as typical or atypical Pick's disease (Brun *et al.*, 1994). Atypical Pick's disease has the macroscopic appearance in the brain of Pick's disease but lacks Pick cells or Pick bodies. Other cases are categorized as '*non-specific frontal lobe dementia*', and have less marked frontal and/or temporal lobe

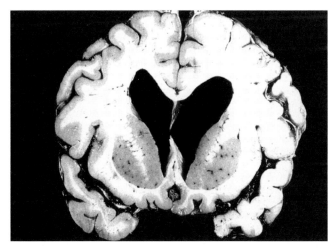

**Fig. 5.16** Coronal slice across the frontal lobes of a case of dementia due to hydrocephalus in a male of 76 years. The frontal horns of the ventricles are markedly dilated. This is not due to compensatory dilatation following atrophy, because the cortical gyri are well preserved and the sulci are narrow, while the corpus callosum is of good width. The appearance is typical of that seen in 'normal pressure' hydrocephalus.

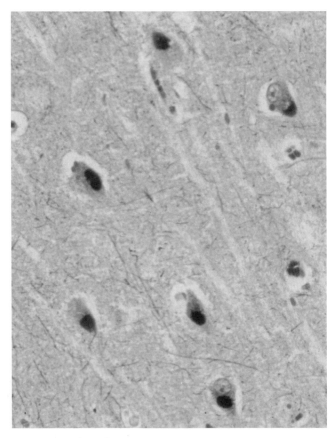

**Fig. 5.18** Neurons containing condensed, rounded Pick bodies (dark) immunolabelled with an antibody to tau protein (×200).

atrophy than in Pick's disease. Microscopically, such cases usually have a characteristic microvacuolation of layer 2 of the cortex of the frontal and temporal lobes, together with some shrinkage and loss of cortical pyramidal neurons in these lobes, and astrocytosis of deep cortex and subcortical white matter. They do not show Pick cells or Pick bodies. Subcortical nuclei including the substantia nigra, striatum, and medial thalamus may show neuron loss and gliosis. Non-specific frontal lobe dementia shows neuropathological similarities in the cerebral cortex to the rare cases of *dementia associated with motor neuron disease* (Kew and Leigh, 1992), but in these cases there are, in addition, neuropathological features of motor neuron disease, with degeneration of upper and lower motor neurons.

## Frontal lobe dementia associated with mutations in the tau gene located on chromosome 17

Recent reports have documented 20 or so different mutations in the gene encoding microtubule-associated protein tau on chromosome 17, which are linked to frontotemporal dementia and parkinsonism (Poorkaj *et al.*, 1998; Spillantini *et al.*, 1998). Many of these mutations are associated with a reduced ability of tau to interact with microtubules (Arawaka *et al.*, 1999; Sahara *et al.*, 2000), an abundance of tau pathology in the form of neurofibrillary tangles in both neuronal and glial cells, and neuropil threads in the brains of these affected. The ultrastructure of the filaments that accumulate differs somewhat from that of classical Alzheimer tangles in that (in isolated material) there is an abundance of straight

filaments and wide twisted ribbons (Heutink, 2000). Although most reported cases have presented primarily with dementia, some have had a clinical and pathological phenotype more akin to progressive supranuclear palsy or corticobasal degeneration. The reasons for the widely variable phenotypic expression remain unexplained at present, but the recognition of these tau gene mutations represents an important new development in the understanding of neurodegeneration.

## Huntington's disease (HD)

Huntington's disease is an autosomal dominant disease determined by a gene on chromosome 4. The molecular biology of the disease is relatively well understood (Ho *et al.*, 2001; MacDonald *et al.*, 2003). Although symptoms of fidgetiness progressing to chorea, and alterations in mood or behaviour progressing to dementia, characteristically occur in the middle decades of adult life, some cases present later and come under the care of geriatric psychiatrists.

By the time of death, the brain is usually small, although external evidence of cortical atrophy is rarely severe. The characteristic pathology is seen when the brain is sliced: selective atrophy of the caudate nucleus and putamen (Fig. 5.19). The subcortical degeneration is paralleled by the degeneration of pyramidal cells in the primary motor cortex (Macdonald and Halliday, 2002). The globus pallidus may also be atrophic, particularly in its external segment. Microscopy shows severe loss of small neurons together with gliosis in the caudate nucleus and putamen, with relative sparing of large- and medium-sized neurons. The neurons most at risk contain gamma aminobutyric acid (GABA). Neuron loss in the basal ganglia is most severe in cases showing advanced chorea (Vonsattel *et al.*, 1985). The motor dysfunction is the best correlate of neuronal loss (Rosenblatt *et al.*, 2003). The dementia, which has been described as subcortical in its pattern of deficits, may be related to cell loss in the frontal cortex: this can be documented using quantitative methods though it may not be evident on inspection. Some cases show more widespread neuron loss, for example in certain thalamic and hypothalamic nuclei, substantia nigra (*zona reticularis*), and dentate nuclei of the cerebellum.

In a mouse model of Huntington's disease the pathological features and symptoms can be reversed by switching off activation of the mutant gene (Yamamoto *et al.*, 2000). Although the report

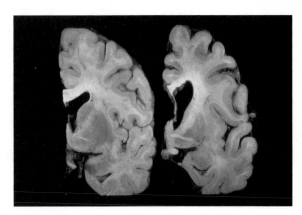

**Fig. 5.19** Coronal slices through the frontal and temporal lobes from a case of Huntington's disease (right) and control (left). Note dilated ventricle and the reduced volume of caudate nucleus in Huntington's disease.

generated optimism, and the search for therapeutic targets continues (Berman and Greenamyre, 2006), the treatment options remain very limited (Bonelli and Wenning, 2006).

## Progressive supranuclear palsy and corticobasal degeneration

Progressive supranuclear palsy is a rare, sporadic disease occurring in the fifth to seventh decades. It is characterized clinically by ataxia, dysarthria, nuchal rigidity, and slowly progressive loss of upward gaze. Some patients have impaired cognitive abilities, though these are different from those in AD and suggestive of a subcortical dementia (Snowden *et al.*, 1987). The most obvious pathological changes are found in the globus pallidus, subthalamic nucleus, substantia nigra, red nucleus, and dentate nucleus of the cerebellum. In these areas there is atrophy, loss of neurons, and gliosis. Some remaining neurons contain NFT in their cell bodies, as do some glial cells in a similar distribution. At the ultrastructural level these tangles differ from those in AD in being composed predominantly of straight, 15-nm diameter filaments but, like NFT, they contain tau and ubiquitin.

Corticobasal degeneration has emerged as a distinct disease entity only recently. Clinically it represents a heterogeneous group of 'Parkinson's plus' syndromes with features of cortical and basal ganglionic dysfunction. However, it has emerged that some patients present with a dementia syndrome alone. Pathologically, corticobasal degeneration is characterized by neuronal loss and gliosis in the frontal and parietal cortices and in the basal ganglia (Gras *et al.*, 1994). The same areas are affected by abundant cytoplasmic inclusions of the hyperphosphorylated form of the microtubule-associated protein tau, similar to that found in AD (Li *et al* 1998).

## Paraneoplastic syndrome

Rapidly progressive dementia may form the presenting clinical picture in some forms of paraneoplastic syndrome. In this syndrome, various neurological deficits result from a probable autoimmune attack against neural antigens, this response being triggered by the presence of a carcinoma, often occult. The commonest form of carcinoma to be associated with this syndrome is small cell (or oat cell) carcinoma of the lung, and the neurological involvement can occur at any level of the neuraxis, from the cerebral cortex to peripheral nerves. In cases with dementia, the pathological changes are those of an encephalitis involving the temporal lobe and hippocampus, though other areas may also be affected such as the basal ganglia, thalamus, and brainstem. In these areas there are perivascular lymphocytic infiltrates, microglial proliferation, astrocytosis, and variable, but usually patchy, loss of neurons. Some cases have a circulating antibody that reacts with the nuclei of a variety of neurons, but it remains to be shown that this has an aetiological role in the syndrome (Darnell, 1996; Musunuru and Darnell, 2001).

## Creutzfeldt–Jakob disease

Sporadic Creutzfeldt–Jakob disease (CJD) is a very rare cause of rapidly progressive dementia, occasionally presenting in an elderly person but more characteristically in the fifth or sixth decade. A few cases are familial (probably fewer than 10%). In most cases death occurs within 6–12 months of the onset of symptoms. Neurological deficits, particularly ataxia, are likely to be present in addition to dementia.

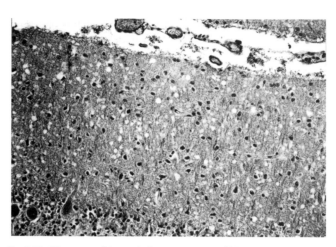

**Fig. 5.20** Microscopy of the cerebellar cortex in Creutzfeldt–Jakob disease. There is loosening of the neuropil and a spongy appearance in the molecular layer. (Haematoxylin and eosin stain, ×100).

At autopsy, the brain usually appears normal to naked-eye inspection. With microscopy, the characteristic feature is a spongy or vacuolar change in the neuropil of grey matter, particularly in cerebral and cerebellar cortex (Fig. 5.20). The vacuoles measure 50–200 mm across, and occur within the processes of neurons. Accompanying this change there is loss of neurons and reactive astrocytosis in similar distribution. These pathological changes resemble those of similar spongiform encephalopathies in animals, such as scrapie in sheep and bovine spongiform encephalopathy (BSE). All these diseases are experimentally transmissible to laboratory animals, with similar symptoms developing months or years after intra-cerebral inoculation of affected brain homogenates. The infective agent of scrapie, the most extensively studied of the spongiform encephalopathies, has several unusual properties such as resistance to normal agents that inactivate bacteria and viruses, failure to provoke an immune response, and no well-characterized ultrastructure. No nucleic acid has been unequivocally demonstrated in the agent and the high-infectivity fraction of the brain homogenates has been found to consist largely of a protein. This observation has led to the suggestion that the agent may itself be a protein, termed prion protein, the amino acid sequence of which is identical to a normal cellular membrane-associated protein of unknown function (DeArmond and Prusiner, 1995; Prusiner, 1995). An important difference between the two proteins derives from the fact that only the disease version is resistant to degradation by certain cellular proteases and it tends to polymerize to form minute amyloid fibrils. Much active research is engaged in defining more of the properties of prions and their normal cellular counterparts. There are other human diseases related to CJD: kuru, a now almost extinct cerebellar degeneration occurring in a remote tribe in Papua New Guinea, and Gerstmann–Sträussler syndrome, which is inherited and in which cerebellar ataxia forms a prominent clinical feature. In this disease, amyloid plaques containing prion protein antigen are found in the brain, and the gene coding for the cellular, prion-like protein is abnormal, resulting in a protein with an abnormal sequence. A different prion gene mutation is associated with a condition known as fatal familial insomnia. Recently a new form of human prion disease has emerged in the UK, known as variant (v or nv) CJD. This is closely linked to the recent epidemic there of BSE (Will 2004, 2005). This condition, in which prominent protease-resistant prion protein-containing plaques as well as spongiform change and gliosis occur in the brain has not been described in anyone beyond the sixth decade.

## Human immunodeficiency virus (HIV type I), AIDS, and dementia

HIV-1 causes neurological symptoms in a significant proportion of cases of AIDS (Neuenburg *et al.*, 2002). Dementia is one of the most prominent features of AIDS encephalopathy, a degenerative condition of the brain which appears to be related to HIV-1 infection itself rather than to other CNS complications of immunodeficiency such as other infections or lymphoma (Everall *et al.*, 2005). In Western countries most cases of HIV-1 encephalopathy occur in young or middle aged male homosexuals or intravenous drug abusers, but some cases occur in elderly males. In developing countries millions of cases have occurred in heterosexuals. Blood transfusions as well as sexual contact can transmit the disease.

The pathology of HIV-1 encephalopathy is found mainly in the white matter of the cerebral and cerebellar hemispheres and in deep grey matter (Gray *et al.*, 1996; Esiri *et al.*, 1997b). These areas show diffuse lack of normal staining quality of myelin (Fig. 5.21) sometimes with patchy axonal, as well as myelin, damage. These changes are associated with an infiltrate of macrophages and increased microglial cells as well as reactive astrocytosis. In the most severely affected cases, multinucleated giant cells of macrophage origin are found in affected white matter and basal ganglia. These cells and other macrophages and microglia contain productive infection with HIV-1. Exactly how this infection causes the white matter damage is still uncertain, but there are two

mechanisms thought likely to play a part. Firstly, some protein products coded for by the virus and shed from infected cells, particularly the envelope protein gp120, are known to have toxic effects on cultured neurons *in vitro*. When expressed in transgenic mice in astrocytes, gp120 produced neuropathological changes similar to those seen in human HIV encephalopathy (Toggas *et al.*, 1994). Secondly, HIV-infected macrophages, microglia, and multinucleated cells secrete cytokines, such as tumour necrosis factor alpha, that are capable of damaging neurons and myelin. In addition to white matter damage due to HIV infection, there is also loss of cortical neurons and reduction in dendritic spines and synapses in those that remain (Everall, 2000), but the extent of the contribution of this damage to the clinical state is still unclear.

## The problem of dementia of uncertain aetiology

In most large autopsy series of dementia there is a small percentage of cases in which no definite cause for the dementia can be ascertained, despite careful examination of the brain. It is likely that some other causes for dementia will be identified if post-mortem studies are extended. Examples of relatively recently described diseases which can present with dementia are progressive supranuclear palsy, non-specific frontal lobe dementia, diffuse Lewy body disease, the chromosome 17 tau mutations, and AIDS. It is therefore important that clinicopathological studies should continue to be carried out on cases of dementia. This calls for frank discussion with relatives about the importance of autopsy examination of the brain in unusual cases of dementia so that their informed consent can be gained.

## Other neuropathological conditions associated with dementia in the elderly

There are a number of other conditions that may occasionally give rise to dementia in the elderly, such as metachromatic leucodystrophy, damage due to head injuries or herpes simplex encephalitis, tumours (particularly gliomas and meningiomas), and cerebral metastases. Consideration of the pathology of these varied conditions is beyond the scope of this chapter but can be found in Graham and Lantos (1997) and other similar textbooks.

## Further reading

Graham, D.I. and Lantos, P.L. (2002). *Greenfield's neuropathology*, 7th edn. Arnold, London.

Esiri, M.M., Lee, V.M.-Y., and Trojanowski, J.Q. (2004). *The neuropathology of dementia*, 2nd edn. Cambridge University Press, Cambridge.

Kettenmann, H. and Ransom, B. (2004). *Neuroglia*, 2nd edn. Oxford University Press, Oxford.

Markesbery, W.R. (ed.) (1998). *Neuropathology of dementing disorders*. Arnold, London.

## References

Anderson, J.M. *et al.* (1983). The effect of advanced old age on the neurone content of the cerebral cortex. Observations with an automatic image analyser point counting method. *Journal of the Neurological Sciences*, **58**(2), 235–46.

Arawaka, S. *et al.* (1999). The tau mutation (val337met) disrupts cytoskeletal networks of microtubules. *Neuroreport*, **10**(5), 993–7.

Arendt, T. (2001). Alzheimer's disease as a disorder of mechanisms underlying structural brain self-organization. *Neuroscience*, **102**(4), 723–65.

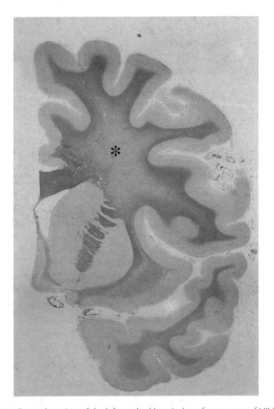

**Fig. 5.21** Coronal section of the left cerebral hemisphere from a case of HIV encephalopathy. The section has been stained to show myelin and there is a diffuse deficiency of myelin in the deep white matter (*).

Arendt, T. (2003). Synaptic plasticity and cell cycle activation in neurons are alternative effector pathways: the 'Dr. Jekyll and Mr. Hyde concept' of Alzheimer's disease or the yin and yang of neuroplasticity. *Progress in Neurobiology*, **71**(2–3), 83–248.

Arendt, T. (2004). Neurodegeneration and plasticity. *International Journal of Developmental Neuroscience* **22**(7): 507–14.

Arriagada, P.V. et al. (1992). Neurofibrillary tangles but not senile plaques parallel duration and severity of Alzheimer's disease. *Neurology*, **42**, 631–9.

Attems, J. et al. (2005). Cause of death in demented and non-demented elderly inpatients; an autopsy study of 308 cases. *Journal of Alzheimers Disease*, **8**(1): 57–62.

Barker, W.W. et al. (2002). Relative frequencies of Alzheimer disease, Lewy body, vascular and frontotemporal dementia, and hippocampal sclerosis in the State of Florida Brain Bank. *Alzheimer Disease and Associated Disorders*, **16**(4), 203–12.

Beal, M.F. (2000). Energetics in the pathogenesis of neurodegenerative diseases. *Trends in Neuroscience*, **23**(7), 298–304.

Bennett, D.A. et al. (2006). Neuropathology of older persons without cognitive impairment from two community-based studies. *Neurology*, **66**(12), 1837–44.

Berman, S.B. and Greenamyre, J.T. (2006). Update on Huntington's disease. *Current Neurology and Neuroscience Reports*, **6**(4), 281–6.

Berr, C. (2002). Oxidative stress and cognitive impairment in the elderly. *Journal of Nutrition, Health & Aging*, **6**(4), 261–6.

Bonelli, R.M. and Wenning, G.K. (2006). Pharmacological management of Huntington's disease: an evidence-based review. *Current Pharmaceutical Design*, **12**(21), 2701–20.

Braak, H. and Braak, E. (1991). Neuropathological stageing of Alzheimer-related changes. *Acta Neuropathologica*, **82**(4), 239–59.

Braak, H. et al. (2003). Staging of brain pathology related to sporadic Parkinson's disease. *Neurobiology of Aging*, **24**(2), 197–211.

Brun, A. et al. (1994). Clinical and neuropathological criteria for frontotemporal dementia. *Journal of Neurology, Neurosurgery and Psychiatry*, **57**, 416–18.

Byrne, E. J. et al. (1990). Diffuse Lewy body disease: the clinical features. *Advances in Neurology*, **53**, 283–6.

Chen, C.P. et al. (1996). Presynaptic serotonergic markers in community-acquired cases of Alzheimer's disease: correlations with depression and neuroleptic medication. *Journal of Neurochemistry* **66**, 1592–8.

Churchyard, A. and Lees, A.J. (1997). The relationship between dementia and direct involvement of the hippocampus and amygdala in Parkinson's disease. *Neurology*, **49**(6), 1570–6.

Clarke, R. et al. (1998). Folate, vitamin B12, and serum total homocysteine levels in confirmed Alzheimer disease. *Archives of Neurology*, **55**(11), 1449–55.

Cullen, K.M. et al. (1997). The nucleus basalis (Ch4) in the alcoholic Wernicke–Korsakoff syndrome: reduced cell number in both amnesic and non-amnesic patients. *Journal of Neurology, Neurosurgery and Psychiatry*, **63**(3), 315–20.

Darnell, R.B. (1996). Onconeural antigens and the paraneoplastic neurologic disorders: at the intersection of cancer, immunity, and the brain. *Proceedings of the National Academy of Sciences USA* **93**(10), 4529–36.

Davies, D.C. et al. (1992). The effect of age and Alzheimer's disease on pyramidal neuron density in the individual fields of the hippocampal formation. *Acta Neuropathologica*, **83**(5), 510–17.

DeArmond, S.J. and Prusiner, S.B. (1995). Etiology and pathogenesis of prion diseases. *American Journal of Pathology*, **146**(4), 785–811.

del Ser, T. et al. (1990). Vascular dementia. A clinicopathological study. *Journal of the Neurological Sciences*, **96**(1), 1–17.

Esiri, M. (1996). The basis of behavioural disturbances in dementia. *Journal of Neurology, Neurosurgery & Psychiatry*, **61**, 127–30.

Esiri, M. (1997). Hydrocephalus. In *Neuropathology of dementia* (ed. M. Esiri and J. Morris), pp. 332–43. Cambridge University Press, Cambridge.

Esiri, M.M. (2000). Which vascular lesions are of importance in vascular dementia? *Annals of the New York Academy of Sciences*, **903**, 239–43.

Esiri, M. and Kennedy, P. (1997). Viral diseases. *Greenfield's neuropathology*, 6th edn, Vol 2 (ed. D. Graham and P. Lantos), pp. 3–63. Arnold, London.

Esiri, M. et al. (1997a). Ageing and the dementias. *Greenfield's neuropathology*, 6th edn, Vol 2 (ed. D. Graham and P. Lantos). pp. 153–233. Arnold, London.

Esiri, M.M. et al. (1997b). Neuropathological assessment of the lesions of significance in vascular dementia. *Journal of Neurology, Neurosurgery & Psychiatry*, **63**(6), 749–53.

Esiri, M.M. et al. (1999) Cerebrovascular disease and threshold for dementia in the early stages of Alzheimer's disease. *Lancet*, **354**(9182), 919–20.

Everall, I.P. (2000). Neuronal damage – recent issues and implications for therapy. *Journal of Neurovirology*, **6**(Suppl. 1), S103–S105.

Everall, I.P. et al. (2005). The shifting patterns of HIV encephalitis neuropathology. *Neurotoxicity Research*, **8**(1–2), 51–61.

Fadda, F. and Rossetti, Z.L. (1998). Chronic ethanol consumption: from neuroadaptation to neurodegeneration. *Progress in Neurobiology*, **56**(4), 385–431.

Finch, C.E. (2003). Neurons, glia, and plasticity in normal brain aging. *Neurobiology of Aging*, **24**(Suppl. 1): S123–S127 (discussion S131).

Forstl, H. et al. (1992). Clinical and neuropathological correlates of depression in Alzheimer's disease. *Psychological Medicine*, **22**(4), 877–84.

Forstl, H. et al. (1994). Disproportionate loss of noradrenergic and cholinergic neurons as cause of depression in Alzheimer's disease – a hypothesis. *Pharmacopsychiatry*, **27**(1), 11–15.

Glasgow, J. and Perez-Polo, R. (2000). One path to cell death in the nervous system. *Neurochemical Research*, **25**(9–10), 1373–83.

Graham, D.I. and Lantos, P.L. (eds) (2002). *Greenfield's neuropathology*, 7th edn. Arnold, London.

Gras, P. et al. (1994). Cortico-basal degeneration: a new entity. *Presse Medicale*, **23**(38), 1772–4.

Gray, F. et al. (1996). Neuropathology of early HIV-1 infection. *Brain Pathology*, **6**(1), 1–15.

Hansen, L.A. et al. (1993). Plaque-only Alzheimer disease is usually the Lewy body variant, and vice versa. *Journal of Neuropathology & Experimental Neurology* **52**(6): 648–54.

Harper, C. (1998). The neuropathology of alcohol-specific brain damage, or does alcohol damage the brain? *Journal of Neuropathology & Experimental Neurology*, **57**(2), 101–10.

Harper, C. et al. (1987). Are we drinking our neurones away? *British Medical Journal (Clinical Research ed.)*, **294**(6571), 534–6.

Harrison, P.J. and Pearson, R.C. (1989). Olfaction and psychiatry. *British Journal of Psychiatry*, **155**, 822–8.

Heutink, P. (2000). Untangling tau-related dementia. *Human Molecular Genetics*, **9**(6), 979–86.

Ho, L.W. et al. (2001). The molecular biology of Huntington's disease. *Psychological Medicine*, **31**(1), 3–14.

Hogervorst, E. et al. (2002). Plasma homocysteine levels, cerebrovascular risk factors, and cerebral white matter changes (leukoaraiosis) in patients with Alzheimer disease. *Archives of Neurology*, **59**(5), 787–93.

Homewood, J. and Bond, N.W. (1999). Thiamin deficiency and Korsakoff's syndrome: failure to find memory impairments following nonalcoholic Wernicke's encephalopathy. *Alcohol*, **19**(1), 75–84.

Hurtig, H.I. et al. (2000). Alpha-synuclein cortical Lewy bodies correlate with dementia in Parkinson's disease. *Neurology*, **54**(10), 1916–21.

Hyman, B. T., G. W. Van Hoesen, et al. (1986). Perforant pathway changes and the memory impairment of Alzheimer's disease. *Annals of Neurology*, **20**(4), 472–81.

Jellinger, K. et al. (1990). Clinicopathological analysis of dementia disorders in the elderly. *Journal of the Neurological Sciences*, **95**(3), 239–58.

Jobst, K.A. et al. (1994). Rapidly progressing atrophy of medial temporal lobe in Alzheimer's disease. *Lancet* **343**(8901), 829–30.

Kew, J. and Leigh, N. (1992). Dementia with motor neurone disease. *Baillieres Clinical Neurology*, **1**(3), 611–26.

Khachaturian, Z.S. (1985). Diagnosis of Alzheimer's disease. *Archives of Neurology*, **42**(11), 1097–105.

Korbo, L. *et al.* (2004). No evidence for loss of hippocampal neurons in non-Alzheimer dementia patients. *Acta Neurologica Scandinavica*, **109**(2), 132–9.

Krantic, S. *et al.* (2005). Molecular basis of programmed cell death involved in neurodegeneration. *Trends in Neuroscience*, **28**(12), 670–6.

Lennox, G. *et al.* (1989). Diffuse Lewy body disease: correlative neuropathology using anti-ubiquitin immunocytochemistry. *Journal of Neurology, Neurosurgery & Psychiatry*, **52**(11), 1236–47.

Leverenz, J. and Sumi, S.M. (1986). Parkinson's disease in patients with Alzheimer's disease. *Archives of Neurology*, **43**(7), 662–4.

Li, F. *et al.* (1998). Regional quantitative analysis of tau-positive neurons in progressive supranuclear palsy: comparison with Alzheimer's disease. *Journal of the Neurological Sciences*, **159**(1), 73-81

MacDonald, M.E. *et al.* (2003). Huntington's disease. *Neuromolecular Medicine*, **4**(1–2), 7–20.

Macdonald, V. and Halliday, G. (2002). Pyramidal cell loss in motor cortices in Huntington's disease. *Neurobiology of Disease*, **10**(3), 378–86.

McKeith, I. *et al.* (1992). Neuroleptic sensitivity in patients with senile dementia of Lewy body type. *British Medical Journal*, **305**(6855), 673–8.

McKeith, I.G. *et al.* (1994). An evaluation of the predictive validity and inter-rater reliability of clinical diagnostic criteria for senile dementia of Lewy body type. *Neurology*, **44**(5), 872–7.

McKeith, I.G. and Mosimann, U.P. (2004). Dementia with Lewy bodies and Parkinson's disease. *Parkinsonism and Related Disorders*, **10**(Suppl. 1): S15–S18.

McShane, R. *et al.* (1997). Do neuroleptic drugs hasten cognitive decline in dementia? Prospective study with necropsy follow up. *British Medical Journal*, **314**(7076), 266–70.

McShane, R.H. *et al.* (2001). Anosmia in dementia is associated with Lewy bodies rather than Alzheimer's pathology. *Journal of Neurology, Neurosurgery & Psychiatry*, **70**(6), 739–43.

Mann, D.M. and Esiri, M.M. (1989). The pattern of acquisition of plaques and tangles in the brains of patients under 50 years of age with Down's syndrome. *Journal of the Neurological Sciences*, **89**(2–3), 169–79.

Mariani, E. *et al.* (2005). Oxidative stress in brain aging, neurodegenerative and vascular diseases: an overview. *Journal of Chromatography. B, Analytical Technologies in the Biomedical and Life Sciences*, **827**(1), 65–75.

Masliah, E. *et al.* (1993). Quantitative synaptic alterations in the human neocortex during normal aging. *Neurology*, **43**(1), 192–7.

Masliah, E. *et al.* (2006). Synaptic remodeling during aging and in Alzheimer's disease. *Journal of Alzheimers Disease*, **9**(3, Suppl.): 91–9.

Matthews, K.L. *et al.* (2002). Noradrenergic changes, aggressive behavior, and cognition in patients with dementia. *Biological Psychiatry*, **51**(5), 407–16.

Meier-Ruge, W. (1988). Morphometric methods and their potential value for gerontological brain research. In *Histology and histopathology of the ageing brain*, Interdisciplinary Topics in Gerontology Vol. 25 (ed. J. Ulrich), pp. 90–100. Karger, Basel.

Minger, S.L. *et al.* (2000). Cholinergic deficits contribute to behavioral disturbance in patients with dementia. *Neurology*, **55**(10), 1460–7.

Mirra, S.S. *et al.* (1991). The Consortium to Establish a Registry for Alzheimer's Disease (CERAD). Part II. Standardization of the neuropathologic assessment of Alzheimer's disease. *Neurology*, **41**(4), 479–86.

Mountjoy, C. (1988). Number of plaques and tangles, loss of neurons: their correlation with deficient neurotransmitter synthesis and the degree of dementia. In *Histology and histopathology of the ageing brain*, Interdisciplinary, Topics in Gerontology Vol 25 (ed. J. Ulrich), pp. 74–89. Karger, Basel.

Muramatsu, T. *et al.* (1997). Apolipoprotein E epsilon 4 allele distribution in Wernicke-Korsakoff syndrome with or without global intellectual deficits. *Journal of Neural Transmission*, **104**(8–9), 913–20.

Musunuru, K. and Darnell, R.B. (2001). Paraneoplastic neurologic disease antigens: RNA-binding proteins and signaling proteins in neuronal degeneration. *Annual Review of Neuroscience*, **24**, 239–62.

Nagy, Z. (2000). Cell cycle regulatory failure in neurones: causes and consequences. *Neurobiology of Aging*, **21**(6), 761–9.

Nagy, Z. *et al.* (1995). Relative roles of plaques and tangles in the dementia of Alzheimer's disease: correlations using three sets of neuropathological criteria. *Dementia*, **6**(1), 21–31.

Nagy, Z. *et al.* (1997). The effects of additional pathology on the cognitive deficit in Alzheimer disease. *Journal of Neuropathology & Experimental Neurology*, **56**(2), 165–70.

Nagy, Z. *et al.* (1998). The cell division cycle and the pathophysiology of Alzheimer's disease. *Neuroscience*, **87**(4), 731–9.

Nagy, Z. *et al.* (1999). The progression of Alzheimer's disease from limbic regions to the neocortex: clinical, radiological and pathological relationships. *Dementia and Geriatric Cognitive Disorders*, **10**(2), 115–20.

Neuenburg, J.K. *et al.* (2002). HIV-related neuropathology, 1985 to 1999: rising prevalence of HIV encephalopathy in the era of highly active antiretroviral therapy. *Journal of Acquired Immune Deficiency Syndromes*, **31**(2), 171–7.

Nicoll, J.A. *et al.* (1997). High frequency of apolipoprotein E epsilon 2 allele in hemorrhage due to cerebral amyloid angiopathy. *Annals of Neurology*, **41**(6), 716–21.

Papapetropoulos, S. *et al.* (2006). Cortical and amygdalar Lewy body burden in Parkinson's disease patients with visual hallucinations. *Parkinsonism and Related Disorders*, **12**(4), 253–6.

Pearson, R. and Powell, T. (1989). The neuroanatomy of Alzheimer's disease. *Reviews in Neuroscience*, **1**, 101–21.

Perry, G. *et al.* (2000). Oxidative damage in Alzheimer's disease: the metabolic dimension. *International Journal of Developmental Neuroscience*, **18**(4–5), 417–21.

Pohjasvaara, T. *et al.* (1998). Clinical determinants of poststroke dementia. *Stroke*, **29**(1), 75–81.

Polymeropoulos, M.H. *et al.* (1997). Mutation in the alpha-synuclein gene identified in families with Parkinson's disease. *Science*, **276**(5321), 2045–7.

Poorkaj, P. *et al.* (1998). Tau is a candidate gene for chromosome 17 frontotemporal dementia. *Annals of Neurology*, **43**(6), 815–25.

Prusiner, S.B. (1995). Molecular genetics and biophysics of prions. *Uirusu*, **45**(1), 5–42.

Rahkonen, T. *et al.* (2003). Dementia with Lewy bodies according to the consensus criteria in a general population aged 75 years or older. *Journal of Neurology, Neurosurgery & Psychiatry*, **74**(6), 720–4.

Regeur, L. *et al.* (1994). No global neocortical nerve cell loss in brains from patients with senile dementia of Alzheimer's type. *Neurobiology of Aging*, **15**(3), 347–52.

Rosenblatt, A. *et al.* (2003). Predictors of neuropathological severity in 100 patients with Huntington's disease. *Annals of Neurology*, **54**(4), 488–93.

Rossi, R. *et al.* (2004). Association between subcortical vascular disease on CT and neuropathological findings. *International Journal of Geriatric Psychiatry*, **19**(7), 690–5.

Sahara, N. *et al.* (2000). Missense point mutations of tau to segregate with FTDP-17 exhibit site-specific effects on microtubule structure in COS cells: a novel action of R406W mutation. *Journal of Neuroscience Research*, **60**(3), 380–7.

Scheff, S.W. and Price, D.A. (2003). Synaptic pathology in Alzheimer's disease: a review of ultrastructural studies. *Neurobiology of Aging*, **24**(8), 1029–46.

Scheff, S.W. *et al.* (2006). Hippocampal synaptic loss in early Alzheimer's disease and mild cognitive impairment. *Neurobiology of Aging*, **27**(10), 1372–84.

Schmidt, R. *et al.* (2000). Vascular risk factors in dementia. *Journal of Neurology*, **247**(2), 81–7.

Simic, G. *et al.* (1997). Volume and number of neurons of the human hippocampal formation in normal aging and Alzheimer's disease. *Journal of Comparative Neurology*, **379**(4), 482–94.

Skoog, I. *et al.* (1999). Vascular factors and Alzheimer disease. *Alzheimer Disease and Associated Disorders*, **13**(Suppl. 3), S106–S114.

Smith, A.D. and Jobst, K.A. (1996). Use of structural imaging to study the progression of Alzheimer's disease. *British Medical Bulletin*, **52**(3), 575–86.

Smith, M.Z. *et al.* (2000). Coexisting pathologies in the brain: influence of vascular disease and Parkinson's disease on Alzheimer's pathology in the hippocampus. *Acta Neuropathologica*, **100**(1), 87–94.

Snowden, J. *et al.* (1987). The subcortical dementias. In *Degenerative neurological disease in the elderly* (ed. R. Griffiths and S. McCarthy), pp. 157–68. Wright, Bristol.

Spillantini, M.G. *et al.* (1998). Frontotemporal dementia and parkinsonism linked to chromosome 17: a new group of tauopathies. *Brain Pathology*, **8**(2), 387–402.

Stevens, T. *et al.* (2002). Islington study of dementia subtypes in the community. *British Journal of Psychiatry*, **180**, 270–6.

Strittmatter, W.J. *et al.* (1993). Apolipoprotein E: high-avidity binding to beta-amyloid and increased frequency of type 4 allele in late-onset familial Alzheimer disease. *Proceedings of the National Academy of Sciences USA*, **90**(5), 1977–81.

Tierney, M.C. *et al.* (1988). The NINCDS-ADRDA Work Group criteria for the clinical diagnosis of probable Alzheimer's disease: a clinicopathologic study of 57 cases. *Neurology*, **38**(3), 359–64.

Toggas, S.M. *et al.* (1994). Central nervous system damage produced by expression of the HIV-1 coat protein gp120 in transgenic mice. *Nature*, **367**(6459), 188–93.

Victoroff, J. *et al.* (1996). Physical aggression is associated with preservation of substantia nigra pars compacta in Alzheimer disease. *Archives of Neurology*, **53**(5), 428–34.

Vonsattel, J.P. *et al.* (1985). Neuropathological classification of Huntington's disease. *Journal of Neuropathology & Experimental Neurology*, **44**(6), 559–77.

West, M.J. *et al.* (1994). Differences in the pattern of hippocampal neuronal loss in normal ageing and Alzheimer's disease. *Lancet*, **344**(8925), 769–72.

Wilcock, G.K. and Esiri, M.M. (1982). Plaques, tangles and dementia. A quantitative study. *Journal of the Neurological Sciences*, **56**(2–3), 343–56.

Will, R. (2004). Variant Creutzfeldt–Jakob disease. *Folia Neuropathologica*, **42**(Suppl. A): 77–83.

Will, R.G. (2005). Commentary: The risk of variant Creutzfeldt–Jakob disease: reassurance and uncertainty. *International Journal of Epidemiology*, **34**(1), 52–3.

Yamamoto, A. *et al.* (2000). Reversal of neuropathology and motor dysfunction in a conditional model of Huntington's disease. *Cell*, **101**(1), 57–66.

# 6

# Neurochemical pathology of neurodegenerative disorders of old age

Margaret Ann Piggott and Jennifer Court

## Introduction

Increased age is the consistent risk factor associated with several discrete dementing illnesses, amongst which this chapter will focus on the neurodegenerative disorders Alzheimer's disease (AD), Lewy body dementia, which incorporates dementia with Lewy bodies (DLB) and Parkinson's disease dementia (PDD), and frontotemporal dementia; and vascular dementia which results from cerebrovascular disease. These different conditions, which give rise to dementia syndromes, each have a distinct neurochemical pathology, with important implications for treatment. A detailed understanding of the neurotransmitter function in each condition can lead to rational drug design and treatment strategies appropriate for each group of patients. Neurochemical pathology in transmitter systems subserving principal features of these disorders will be reviewed, noting where these are amenable to pharmacotherapy, and the major documented transmitter changes for these illnesses are summarized in tabular form.

## Alzheimer's disease

Alzheimer's disease is the most common age-associated dementia, with incidence rising from 4% at 65 to 20% after the age of 80 (Evans *et al.*, 2004). Several neurotransmitter systems are affected in AD, potentially having combined effects resulting in a range of clinical symptoms.

### Acetylcholine

The cholinergic system, arising from the basal forebrain (including septal, diagonal band, and Meynert nuclei which constitute the cholinergic projections to the neocortex), innervates all areas of the cerebral cortex including hippocampus, and also the reticular nucleus of the thalamus. Cholinergic brainstem neurons (from the pedunculopontine and laterodorsal tegmental nuclei) innervate the thalamus and cerebellum. In contrast, the highly cholinergic putamen and caudate nucleus do not receive such inputs, but have intrinsic cholinergic neurons (large striatal interneurons). Activation of cholinergic receptors is pro-cognitive, especially by improving attention (Voytko, 1996; Perry *et al.*, 1999). The importance of acetylcholine (ACh) to cognitive impairment in AD was recognized over 25 years ago, with several early reports highlighting the significant reduction in both cholinergic basal forebrain

neurons (Whitehouse *et al.*, 1982) and cortical choline acetyltransferase (ChAT) (the enzyme that synthesizes acetylcholine) and acetylcholinesterase (AChE) activities (Perry *et al.*, 1978; Francis *et al.*, 1999; Wilcock *et al.*, 1982) (see Table 6.1). These studies predominantly involved autopsy tissue, which of necessity reflect endstage processes; however, limited biopsy investigations were also undertaken (reviewed in Francis *et al.*, 1999). These latter studies of AD patients on average 3.5 years after diagnosis indicated that cholinergic neurotransmitter pathology is likely to occur relatively early in the course of the disease, with cortical cholinergic presynaptic markers (not only ChAT activity, but also high-affinity choline uptake and ACh synthesis) being reduced to about 50% of control values. *In vivo* mapping of cholinergic terminals in AD (single photon emission tomography, using [$^{123}$I]iodobenzovesamicol (IBVM), binding to the vesicular ACh transporter) also demonstrated reduced cholinergic innervation of the neocortex and hippocampus (Kuhl *et al.*, 1996). Cerebrospinal fluid (CSF) ACh content has recently been noted to be a third that of non-demented controls (Jia *et al.*, 2004). Significantly, *in vivo* (Kuhl *et al.*, 1996; Jia *et al.*, 2004) and biopsy studies (Francis *et al.*, 1999) have corroborated the association between cholinergic marker loss and the degree of cognitive impairment seen in autopsy investigations (Perry *et al.*, 1978; Wilcock *et al.*, 1982). In contrast, others have argued that there is an initial stabilization or possibly up-regulation of cortical ChAT activity during the early stages of AD (Davis *et al.*, 1999; DeKosky *et al.*, 2002), but since ChAT activity is not the rate-limiting step of ACh synthesis, such data do not preclude the likelihood of cortical cholinergic synaptic dysfunction occurring at an early stage of the disease (Terry and Buccafusco, 2003; Gauthier *et al.*, 2006; Ginsberg *et al.*, 2006).

Reduced thalamic and striatal ChAT activity in AD has also been observed in some, but not all, autopsy studies (Danielsson *et al.*, 1988; Reinikainen *et al.*, 1988; Xuereb *et al.*, 1990), including reduced ChAT immunoreactivity (34–46%) in the mediodorsal thalamic nucleus (Brandel *et al.*, 1991). Attenuated thalamic binding to the vesicular cholinergic transporter using IBVM has been reported in AD with early onset (Kuhl *et al.*, 1996). A marked reduction in the expression of ChAT mRNA has also been noted in the dorsal striatum in AD (Boissiere *et al.*, 1997). These studies indicate cholinergic dysfunction in AD extending beyond basal forebrain projections.

**Table 6.1** Alzheimer's disease

| | Cortex/hippocampus | Basal forebrain | Brainstem | Receptor/transporter polymorphisms | CSF |
|---|---|---|---|---|---|
| **Acetylcholine (ACh)** | | | | | |
| Acetylcholine | | | | | ↓ |
| Synthesis | ↓ | | | | |
| ChAT activity | ↓ | | | | |
| Vesicular ACh transporter | ↓ | | | | |
| AChE activity | ↓ | | | | |
| nAChRs | ↓↓ (particularly α4β2-containing) | | | | |
| mAChRs | ↔ (↓)M1[a], ↓(↔) M2[a] | | | | |
| Neuron loss | | ✓ | | | |
| **Serotonin (5-HT)** | | | | | |
| Serotonin | ↓ (in some areas) | | | | |
| Uptake | ↓ | | | | |
| 5-HIAA | ↓ | | | | ↓ (modest) |
| 5-HT$_2$Rs | ↓ (associated with aggression) | | | Assoc. psychosis | |
| 5-HT$_6$Rs | | | | Assoc. depression | |
| 5-HT transporter | | | | Assoc. aggression | |
| Neuron loss | | | ✓ Dorsal raphe (in some patients) | | |
| **Noradrenaline (NA)** | | | | | |
| Noradrenaline | ↓ (hippocampus) | | | | |
| MHPG | ↑ | | | | |
| Neuron loss | | | ✓ Locus coeruleus | | |
| **Glutamate (Glu)** | | | | | |
| Glutamate | ↓↔ | | | | ↓↑↔ |
| Uptake (Na$^+$-dependent D-Asp uptake) | ↓ | | | | |
| NMDARs by binding | ↓↔ | | | | |
| NMDAR1 protein mRNA | ↓ | | | | |
| AMPAR binding | ↓↑↔ | | | | |
| Kainate binding | ↓↑↔ | | | | |
| mGluRs and signalling | ↓ | | | | |
| Neuron loss | ✓ Correlated with dementia | | | | |
| Spermidine | ≠ | | | | |

Other post-mortem studies have demonstrated select changes in cholinergic receptors in AD. Multiple muscarinic, G-protein-linked acetylcholine receptors (mAChRs) are expressed in human brain (M1–5), the most prevalent being M1 (in cortical regions) and M2 (widely distributed). For M1 mAChRs (predominantly post-synaptic), ligand-binding studies tend to indicate no loss from neocortical areas (Lai *et al.*, 2001; Mulugeta *et al.*, 2003; Piggott *et al.*, 2003), although reductions in M1 binding in the hippocampus have been reported (Nordberg, 1992), especially late in the disease process (Rodriguez-Puertas *et al.*, 1997). However, declines in M1 immunoreactivity have been noted in neo- as well as archicortical regions (Flynn *et al.*, 1995; Shiozaki *et al.*, 2001). In addition, disruption of M1 signalling is indicated in AD with evidence of impaired coupling of M1 receptors to G-proteins and second messenger systems in several cortical regions (Ladner *et al.*, 1995; Jope, 1996; Perry *et al.*, 1998; Warren *et al.*, submitted), with coupling apparently being more impaired with increasing severity of dementia (Tsang *et al.*, 2006).

Reductions in cortical M2 mAChRs (considered predominantly pre-synaptic on cholinergic terminals) have been more consistently reported, but deficits have not been evident in all studies in neo- and archicortex (Flynn *et al.*, 1995; Lai *et al.*, 2001; Mulugeta *et al.*, 2003;

Piggott *et al.*, 2003). Although the density of these receptors appears unchanged in the thalamus in AD (Warren *et al.*, 2007), elevations have been observed in the striatum (Piggott *et al.*, 2003), and relative sparing of cortical M2 receptors in AD is apparently associated with psychosis (Lai *et al.*, 2001). There are also indications that M2–G-protein coupling is impaired in AD, notably in areas most affected by pathology (Cowburn *et al.*, 1996). Protocols to assess M4 mAChRs have offered little consistency. Whilst an immunoprecipitation study indicated increases in frontal, temporal, and parietal cortices, in parallel with selective receptor binding data (Flynn *et al.*, 1995), others noted no change in receptor binding in frontal cortex and striatum, and reduced levels of M4 mAChRs in the mediodorsal nucleus of the thalamus (Warren *et al.*, 2007) and hippocampus in AD (Mulugeta *et al.*, 2003).

Deficits in ionotropic nicotinic acetylcholine receptors (nAChRs) are widely reported in the hippocampus and neocortex in AD (reviewed in Court *et al.*, 2001a) (Table 6.1). There are two major subtypes of these receptors, homomeric receptors that are composed of α7 subunits, and heteromeric receptors. The latter have recently been demonstrated to contain α4 and β2 subunits, by immunoprecipitation in human brain tissue (Gotti *et al.*, 2006). There are also populations of α2 subunits in the neocortex and

**Table 6.1**  (*cont.*)

| | Cortex/hippocampus | Basal forebrain | Brainstem | Receptor/ transporter polymorphisms | CSF |
|---|---|---|---|---|---|
| **GABA** | | | | | |
| GABA | ↓ (associated with depression) | | | | |
| GABA$_A$R/BZs | ↑ (associated with depression) | | | | |
| GABA$_A$ α1 and α5 subunit mRNA and α5 protein | ↓ | | | | |
| Benzodiazepine binding | ↓ (inverse correlation with tangles) | | | | |
| GABA$_B$R1 | ↓ (at latter stages) | | | | |
| **Peptides** | | | | | |
| Somatostatin | ↓ | | | | ↓ |
| NPY | ↔ (cortex)[b] | ↑ | | | ↓ |
| CRF/H | | | | | ↓↔ |
| β-END | | | | | ↓ |
| DSIP | | | | | ↓↑ |
| Galanin | | ↑ | | | |

[a] Receptors may not be coupled to G-proteins/second messenger systems.

[b] Cortical NPY-IR axons dystrophic.

Sources:

ACh: Jia *et al.* (2004), Francis *et al.* (1999), Whitehouse *et al.* (1982), Wilcock *et al.* (1982), Perry *et al.* (1978), Court *et al.* (2001), Flynn *et al.* (1995), Jope (1996), Cowburn *et al.* (1996).

5-HT: Procter *et al.* (1992), Halliday *et al.* (1992), Soininen *et al.* (1981), Bowen *et al.* (1983), Cross *et al.* (1983), Zarros *et al.* (2005), Sweet *et al.* (2001), Sukonick *et al.* (2001), Nacmias *et al.* (2001a,b), Mossner *et al.* (2000), Holmes *et al.* (1998).

NA: Arai *et al.* (1984), Mann *et al.* (1980), Herrmann *et al.* (2004).

Peptides: Allen *et al.* (1984), Dawbarn *et al.* (1986), Chan-Palay (1987), Edvinsson *et al.* (1993), Heilig *et al.* (1995), Koide *et al.* (1995), Martel *et al.* (1990), Chan-Palay (1988), Silva *et al.* (2005).

GABA: Iwakiri *et al.* (2005), Garcia-Alloza *et al.* (2006), Rissman *et al.* (2003, 2004).

Glu: Esiri (1991), Francis (2003), Penney *et al.* (1990), Amada *et al.* (2005), D'Aniello *et al.* (2005), Garcia-Alloza *et al.* (2006), Albasanz *et al.* (2005), Smith *et al.* (1985), Morrison and Kish (1995), Hynd *et al.* (2004), Armstrong *et al.* (2003).

Abbreviations: CSF, cerebrospinal fluid; ACh, acetylcholine; ChAT, choline acetyltransferase; AChE, acetylcholinesterase; nAChR, nicotinic acetylcholine receptor; mAChR, muscarinic acetylcholine receptor; 5-HT, serotonin (5-hydroxytryptamine); 5-HIAA, 5-hydroxy-indole acetic acid (metabolite of serotonin); 5-HTRs, 5-HT (serotonin) receptors; NA, noradrenaline; MHPG, 3-methoxy-4-hydrophenylglycol (metabolite of noradrenaline); D-Asp, D-aspartate; NMDA, *N*-methyl-D-aspartic acid; NMDARs, *N*-methyl-D-aspartic acid receptor (ionotropic glutamate receptor subtype); AMPAR, alpha-amino-3-hydroxy-5-methyl-4-isoxazolepropionic acid receptor (ionotropic glutamate receptor subtype); Kainate R, kainic acid receptor (ionotropic glutamate receptor subtype); mGluR, metabotropic glutamate receptor; GABAR, gamma-aminobutyric acid receptor; BZ, benzodiazepine; NPY, neuropeptide Y; NPY-IR, NPY immunoreactivity; CRF (CRH), corticotropin releasing factor (hormone); β-END, beta-endorphin; DSIP, delta sleep-inducing peptide; DA, dopamine; HVA, homovanillic acid; D2R, dopamine D2 receptor; α$_{1D}$R, α$_2$R; α-adrenergic receptor.

α6 and β3 in the striatum (Gotti *et al.*, 2006). Reductions in cortical heteromeric nAChRs have been observed universally in AD and this has been confirmed to be due to α4 and β2 loss (Gotti *et al.*, 2006). Cortical and hippocampal α7 receptor deficits have also been reported by some but not by all investigators (Court *et al.*, 2001a), possibly depending on disease severity. In addition, since α7 receptors are present on astrocytes and this population is up-regulated by gliosis in AD (Teaktong *et al.*, 2003), loss of this receptor subtype from neurons may be masked, when gross/bulk methodology is employed. A decline in the α4β2 subtype in the striatum has also been reported (Court *et al.*, 2001a) and such a deficit is likely to be due to nAChRs being lost from cortical inputs rather than nigrostriatal afferents (Court *et al.*, 2000; Pimlott *et al.*, 2004). Despite the high levels of nAChRs in the thalamus, significant deficits have not been observed in specific thalamic nuclei in AD, with the exception of a 25% reduction in α7 receptor binding in the reticular nucleus (Court *et al.*, 2001a), possibly reflecting the presence of this receptor on basal forebrain cholinergic inputs.

Cholinergic support via administration of cholinesterase inhibitors has been shown to have efficacy both in terms of attenuated cognitive deficits and improved activities of daily living (Birks, 2006). Perhaps it is not surprising that the effects, although significant, are small given the relative inefficiency of coupling and/or loss of acetylcholine receptors in AD. Possible cholinergic dysfunction in the thalamus in concert with that in other brain regions may have effects on the expression of behavioural and psychological symptoms of dementia (BPSD), since therapy with cholinesterase inhibitors (ChEI) also leads to some improvement in anxiety, depression, and apathy in AD (Feldman *et al.*, 2001). There may also be a relationship between reduced cholinergic transmission and the accumulation of AD-type pathology (Nordberg, 2006), with chronic cholinergic antagonism (in Parkinson's disease, PD) being associated with an increased density of plaques and tangles (Perry *et al.*, 2003). It has also been demonstrated that long-term exposure to nicotine (tobacco use) is associated with reduced AD pathology (Aβ deposition) (Hellstrom-Lindahl *et al.*, 2004; Court *et al.*, 2005). In addition, treatment with an M1 agonist can reduce CSF amyloid β 1–42 peptide in patients with AD (Hock *et al.*, 2003), and in model systems both amyloid and tau pathology (Caccamo *et al.*, 2006).

## Glutamate

The possible involvement of glutamatergic mechanisms in AD is a difficult and complex issue to investigate because of the participation of multiple receptor subtypes [*N*-methyl-D-aspartate (NMDA), amino-3-hydroxy-5-methyl-4-isoxazolepropionic acid (AMPA), kainate, and metabotropic glutamate receptor (mGluR)], subunits and subunit splice variants, and receptor modulation by many common endogenous molecules (e.g. $Mg^{2+}$, $Zn^{2+}$, and polyamines) (Francis, 2003; Hynd *et al.*, 2004). Furthermore, there is intimate involvement of both neurons and glia in glutamate transmission and possible glutamate neurotoxicity in AD (Boksha, 2004). Added to this, many of the reported changes in glutamatergic parameters in AD are inconsistent (see Table 6.1; Francis, 2003; Hynd *et al.*, 2004).

The measurement of glutamate itself as a marker of pre-synaptic glutamatergic transmission has been utilized, although this amino acid is not only synthesized in nerve terminals but is integral to protein, ammonia, and energy metabolism (Francis, 2003). Although some studies indicate reductions in brain and CSF glutamate content in AD, an almost equal number of reports demonstrate no change or even an increase in glutamate (notably in the CSF) (Smith *et al.*, 1985, Jimenez-Jimenez *et al.*, 1998; Francis, 2003; D'Aniello *et al.*, 2005; Garcia-Alloza *et al.*, 2006). The attrition of glutamatergic synapses and neurons in AD is supported by shrinkage of the cortical ribbon in AD, demonstrated both at autopsy and *in vivo*, at least in part as a consequence of the loss of a proportion of glutamatergic pyramidal neurons (Esiri, 1991). An estimate of glutamate uptake capacity ($Na^+$-dependent D-$[^3H]$ aspartate uptake *in vitro*) also demonstrated a potential decline in glutamatergic transmission (Francis, 2003) in the frontal and temporal cortex in AD. Conversely, an increase in the protein expression of some of the enzymes involved in glutamate metabolism (including glutamine synthetase and Glu dehydrogenase) has been observed in the pre-frontal cortex in AD (Burbaeva *et al.*, 2005), consistent with, and possibly a result of, increased local concentration of extracellular glutamate.

Reports of possible changes in the density of glutamate receptors in AD also tend to be inconsistent (Table 6.1). Investigating multiple receptors in the hippocampal formation Dewar *et al.* (1991) observed reductions of AMPA and kainate receptors in the subiculum and parahippocampal gyrus in AD, but not in the CA1 region. Penney *et al.* (1990) also observed no decline in quisqualate binding (to AMPA receptors) in the CA1 in AD, but reductions in non-quisqualate (putatively kainate receptors) in this region. In contrast, Geddes *et al.* (1992) noted an increase in AMPA receptors in the infragranular layer of the hippocampus and an increase in kainate binding in the outer half of the dentate gyrus molecular layer in AD. Hynd *et al.* (2004) concluded that published studies predominantly report a decline in NMDA receptor density in the hippocampus in AD. An increase in kainate binding, no change in quisqualate binding, but a reduction in NMDA receptors was observed in the frontal cortex (Chalmers *et al.*, 1990), whereas Cowburn *et al.* (1989) demonstrated a decline in kainate binding in the parietal cortex. Perhaps whether ionotropic glutamate receptors are affected in any brain region in AD is dependent on the degree of pathology. A reduction in mGluRs in the frontal cortex has been observed in AD and shown to be correlated with pathological staging and to be associated with reduced mGluR/phospholipase C (PLC) signalling and PLCβ1 isoform expression (Albasanz *et al.*, 2005). Further Aβ peptide has been shown *in vitro* to disrupt mGluR functions which are mediated via protein kinase C (PKC) (Tyszkiewicz and Yan, 2005).

Some recent studies have also investigated glutamate receptor subunit expression in AD. A reduction in the NR1 (NMDA receptor) subunit protein has been reported in the frontal cortex and hippocampus in AD (Amada *et al.*, 2005), whereas lower NR1 mRNA levels were observed in entorhinal and perirhinal cortices, but not in the hippocampal CA1, hilus, or subiculum (Ulas and Cotman, 1997). Studies investigating the isoform variants of NMDA receptors ($NR1_{1XX}$ with and $NR1_{0XX}$ lacking, respectively, the alternatively spiced exon 4) demonstrated that these were lower in AD cases in disease-susceptible areas, with the $NR1_{1XX}:NR1_{0XX}$ ratio being a possible index of disease severity (Hynd *et al.*, 2004). Armstrong *et al.* (2003) also investigated AMPA and NMDA receptor subunit protein expression in the hippocampus in mild to severe cases of AD and noted the relative preservation of subunits in severe cases (compared to mild) with the exception of reduced NR1 expression in the subiculum in the most severe cases (compared with the mild and moderate). In contrast, exposure to β-amyloid in Tg2576 APP mice and in cultured neurons has been shown to reduce post-synaptic densities of GluR1 and PSD-95 (a GluR recruiting and anchoring protein) (Almeida *et al.*, 2006).

In terms of the efficacy of glutamate NMDA receptor signals in AD it is worthy of note that the content of spermidine, a polyamine-positive modulator of these receptors, has been reported to be elevated in the temporal cortex (but not other brain regions) in this disorder (Morrison and Kish, 1995). The activity of ornithine decarboxylase, a key enzyme involved in polyamine synthesis, has also been reported to be increased in temporal cortex (but not in the hippocampus or occipital cortex) in AD (Morrison *et al.*, 1998). But since polyamine (spermine) enhancement of MK801 binding (a measure of NMDA channel opening) in areas susceptible to pathology has been shown to be attenuated in AD (Ragnarsson *et al.*, 2002), it may be doubtful whether an increase in polyamine content will result in increased NMDA receptor activity.

Given the likelihood of decreased glutamatergic transmission in AD, it is at first glance surprising that a glutamatergic (NMDA receptor) antagonist such as memantine has been used for therapy. But glutamate, via NMDA receptors, is also implicated in neurotoxic cascades that are likely to play a role in neurodegenerative disease (Francis, 2003; Hynd *et al.*, 2004). In states of reduced membrane potential (reduced oxygenation and energy metabolism) the voltage-dependent $Mg^{2+}$ blockage of NMDA receptors can be released leading to excessive and neurotoxic entry of $Ca^{2+}$ into neurons. So perhaps it is not surprising that memantine has been demonstrated to have efficacy in patients with a heavier burden of neuronal disruption and pathology, those with moderate or severe, but not mild, AD (Muir, 2006). Also, since memantine is an uncompetitive, low-affinity, open-channel blocker it is suggested that it may be of benefit in AD by limiting excessive glutamate transmission, as it were reducing signal to noise (Lipton, 2005). Further, glutamate may have a potentially adverse role in AD by increasing the production and secretion of Aβ via inhibition of an enzyme which may function as an α-secretase (tumour necrosis factor-alpha converting enzyme; see Chapter 7), as has been demonstrated in primary neuronal cultures (Lesne *et al.*, 2005). Stimulation of glutamate receptors on microglia (potentially via both mGluRs and NMDARs GluRs) may lead to neuronal cell death, via generation of tumour necrosis factor-alpha (Floden *et al.*, 2005; Taylor *et al.*, 2005); such a mechanism may act in concert with β-amyloid stimulation of microglia (Floden *et al.*, 2005). Other suggestions for memantine's mode of action in AD include the possibility that via NMDA inhibition it may offset the disinhibition of forebrain neuronal circuits resulting from reduced ACh, noradrenaline (NA), 5-hydroxytryptamine (5-HT), and histamine neurotransmission in AD (Schmitt, 2005).

## Gamma-aminobutyric acid (GABA)

There are also reports of changes in the major brain inhibitory system, which uses GABA as a transmitter, in AD; although alterations are generally only reported to occur at later stages of the disorder as pathology and clinical severity mount and to be associated with only selective receptors and subunits (Table 6.1). Reductions in cortical (frontal and temporal) levels of GABA have been recently observed at autopsy in association with depression (Garcia-Alloza *et al.*, 2006). An early study noted that the reduction in hippocampal benzodiazepine binding [to sites on $GABA_A$ receptors ($GABA_A$Rs)] was correlated to neurofibrillary tangle numbers (Penney *et al.*, 1990). In contrast, relatively increased $GABA_A$/ benzodiazepine binding sites have been associated with severe depression in AD (Garcia-Alloza *et al.*, 2006). Investigation of $GABA_A$ subunit expression indicates relative sparing in AD. Small reductions in $GABA_A$ α1 and α5 mRNA (20–35%) expression were observed in the hippocampus in moderate cognitive impairment and probable AD in comparison with a non-impaired group, and protein expression of α1, β1 and β2 $GABA_A$Rs was not changed, although α5 protein was reduced by 40% in the CA1/2 region in the most severe cases (Braak stages V–VI; see Chapter 5) (Rissman *et al.*, 2003). This was corroborated by a further study indicating that $GABA_A$R subunits were relatively preserved in a group of severe compared with mild AD patients, with the exception of α5 in regions CA1/2 and CA3 (Armstrong *et al.*, 2003). At early stages of AD no change or increased hippocampal $GABA_B$R1 immunoreactivity (on pyramidal neurons) has been reported, whereas advanced stages of the disease are associated with reduced expression in region CA1 as pyramidal neurons decline (Iwakiri *et al.*, 2005).

## Serotonin

Reductions in serotonin function in AD were noted as part of early investigations of neurochemical pathology in AD (Table 6.1), but deficits were not consistently observed or were restricted to, for example, the temporal lobe only (Perry *et al.*, 1993). Cell loss and tangle pathology in the raphe nuclei results in reduced cortical serotonin in AD, and several polymorphisms of serotonergic system genes have been reported to be linked to neuropsychiatric symptoms in AD, such as aggression (Mossner *et al.*, 2000; Sukonick *et al.*, 2001; Zarros *et al.*, 2005) and psychosis (Holmes *et al.*, 1998; Nacmias *et al.*, 2001).

Relatively retained serotonergic function may be related to increased expression of behavioural and neuropsychiatric features in dementia, such as aggression, anxiety, depressed mood, and agitation, while greater reduction of markers of serotonin innervation is related to cognitive impairment (Halliday *et al.*, 1992). It is the balance between transmitter systems which is probably important (Lanari *et al.*, 2006), as in the reported relative preservation of 5-HT markers in dementia with Lewy bodies, where in an environment of a much reduced cholinergic system there is increased likelihood of visual hallucinations (Perry *et al.*, 1990b).

Serotonin function has been linked to aggression in AD (reviewed Mintzer, 2001; Zarros *et al.*, 2005), with 5-HT2-type receptors relatively preserved (interpreted as relatively preserved cortical interneurons) in patients without aggressive behaviour (Procter *et al.*, 1992). Subsequently $5-HT_{2A}$ receptors were found to be reduced in the cortex in AD, more so in severely compared with mildly demented patients, and the reduction correlated with decline in the Mini-Mental State Examination (MMSE) independently of cholinergic loss, or the presence or absence of BPSD (Lai *et al.*, 2005), suggesting that AD patients with greater serotonergic loss may have faster disease progression. Cortical $5-HT_{1A}$ receptors are also lost, correlating with aggression (Lai *et al.*, 2003b), as are $5-HT_{(1B/1D)}$ and $5-HT_6$, correlated with MMSE score decline and overactivity with aggression, respectively (Garcia-Alloza *et al.*, 2004). However, $5-HT_4$ receptors, which are positively coupled to adenylyl cyclase and modulate the release of other transmitters, were unaltered in frontal and temporal cortex in AD (Lai *et al.*, 2003a). The status of $5-HT_4$ coupling has not been investigated.

As with muscarinic receptors, there may be a relationship between serotonin receptors and amyloid pathology, with activation of the $5-HT_4$ receptor stimulating the secretion of non-amyloidogenic soluble form of the amyloid precursor protein in model systems (Robert *et al.*, 2001; Lezoualc'h and Robert, 2003).

## Noradrenaline (NA)

Early studies revealed deficits in the NA system in the brains of AD patients, with reductions in NA being noted in the cingulate gyrus, substantia innominata, putamen, hypothalamus, medial nucleus of the thalamus, and globus pallidus (Arai *et al.*, 1984) (Table 6.1). Reduced numbers of neurons in the noradrenergic locus coeruleus were also observed in the majority of AD cases (Mann *et al.*, 1980). More recent evidence indicates that the surviving neurons may attempt to compensate by up-regulation of tyrosine hydroxylase mRNA and dendritic sprouting (Szot *et al.*, 2006), consistent with the majority of studies observing increased levels of the NA metabolite 3-methoxy-4-hydroxyphenylglycol (MHPG) in AD brain (Herrmann *et al.*, 2004) indicative of increased brain NA turnover. Indeed, it has been suggested that many of the behavioural and psychological symptoms of dementia, for example aggression and agitation, may be linked to increased NA activity or adrenoreceptor hypersensitivity in AD, and initial trials of β-adrenergic receptor blockers indicate some efficacy (Herrmann *et al.*, 2004).

## Dopamine

Although dopamine receptors decline continuously across the lifespan and may play a role in the gradual decline of cognitive ability, there is no particular loss of dopamine associated with features of AD. There is no significant loss of substantia nigra neurons, and no loss of striatal dopamine concentration or of receptors (R.H. Perry *et al.*, 1990; Piggott *et al.*, 1999), although there is some decline in dopamine transporter binding in the nucleus accumbens with increased age of onset in AD (Piggott *et al.*, 1999). No satisfactory neurochemical substrate for the movement disorder which emerges in many patients with AD progression has been established. However, rather than being dopamine-based it is likely to be due to Alzheimer pathology and atrophy in basal ganglia and brainstem nuclei, and/or extensive cholinergic derangement.

## Peptides

Reductions in a number of neuropeptides have been noted in the CSF and brain in AD, although initial studies have not always been replicated (see Table 6.1). Deficits in neuropeptide Y (NPY) and somatostatin have been reported most consistently. Reductions in CSF NPY were reported to correlate with disease duration (Edvinsson *et al.*, 1993) and appear to parallel the noted NPY deficits in plasma (Koide *et al.*, 1995) and hippocampus (Martel *et al.*, 1990), although no deficits in neocortex were observed (Allen *et al.*, 1984). In addition no change in hippocampal NPY binding was observed (Martel *et al.*, 1990). NPY may be neuroprotective as it inhibits evoked glutamate release, and thus NPY and NPY receptors may be therapeutic targets in neurodegenerative conditions (Silva *et al.*, 2005). Reduced cortical/hippocampal somatostatin levels and immunoreactivity have also been shown to correlate with disease severity (Allen *et al.*, 1984; Dawbarn *et al.*, 1986; Chan-Palay, 1987). The nucleus basalis of Meynert and substantia innominata are notable because of observed elevations in NPY and galanin, presumably the result of relative neuronal sparing and/or compensation mechanisms (Allen *et al.*, 1984; Chan-Palay, 1988).

## Vascular dementia

The term vascular dementia (VaD) is used to describe a heterogeneous group of neuropathologies resulting from vascular disease or injury. The pathological hallmarks can range from large focal lesions to a number of small-vessel diseases, and VaD frequently coexists with AD-type pathology. The site, extent, and combination of lesions inevitably affect any resulting neurochemical deficit(s). Hence it is not easy to assess the generality of the relatively small-scale studies of neurochemical changes in VaD that have been published to date. None the less, the occurrence of brain neurotransmitter deficits in VaD has been indicated by autopsy, CSF, and *in vivo* positron emission tomography (PET) investigations (see Table 6.2) (reviewed in Court *et al.*, 2003; Court and Perry, 2003).

## Acetylcholine

Deficits in cortical and hippocampal cholinergic innervation in VaD (predominantly multi-infarct dementia, MID), assessed by ChAT activity and high-affinity choline uptake have been observed in a number of studies (reviewed in Court *et al.*, 2003; Court and Perry, 2003; Roman and Kalaria, 2006). However, one early investigation of the number of neurons in the nucleus basalis of Meynert did not observe any reduction in MID (Mann *et al.*, 1986), indicating that declines in cortical innervation in this condition are likely to be because of ischaemic disruption of cholinergic projections or neuronal function rather than extensive loss of cholinergic neurons, as is the case in AD. A more recent autopsy study suggests that reduced cortical ChAT only occurs in VaD when in combination with AD-type pathology, and not in 'pure VaD' (Perry *et al.*, 2005). This contrasts with rodent model studies indicating that cholinergic deficits can be the result of cerebral ischaemia

**Table 6.2** Vascular dementia

| | Cortex/hippocampus | Basal forebrain | Brainstem | Basal ganglia | CSF |
|---|---|---|---|---|---|
| **Acetylcholine (Ach)** | | | | | ↓ |
| ChAT activity | ↔↓ | | | ↓ (striatum) | |
| High-affinity choline uptake | ↓ | | | | |
| nAChRs | | | | | |
| Neuron loss | ↔↓ (α4β2-containing) | ↔ | | | |
| **Serotonin (5-HT)** | | | | ↓ (striatum) | ↓ |
| Uptake | ↔ | | | ↔ | |
| 5-HIAA | ↓ | | | ↓ | |
| 5-HT1ARs | ↔ | | | | |
| 5-HT$_2$Rs | ↔ | | | | |
| Neuron loss | | | No (dorsal raphe) | | |
| **Dopamine** | | | | | |
| Dopamine | | | | | ↑ |
| HVA | | | | | ↓ |
| DA uptake sites | | | | ↓ (caudate) | |
| $^{18}$F-fluorodopa influx rate | | | | ↓ (striatum) | |
| **Noradrenaline (NA)** | | | | | |
| Neuron loss | | | No (locus coeruleus) | | |
| **Peptides** | | | | | |
| Somatostatin | | | | | ↓ |
| CRF/H | | | | | ↔↓ |
| β-END | | | | | ↓ |
| DSIP | | | | | ↔ |
| ACTH | | | | | ↔ |

Based on reviews (Court *et al.*, 2003; Court and Perry, 2003; Roman and Kalaria, 2006) and references cited for Table 6.1, with the addition of Perry *et al.* (2005), Heilig *et al.* (1995), Mann *et al.* (1986), Gottfries *et al.* (1994), and Keverne *et al.* (in press).

See Table 6.1 for abbreviations.

(reviewed in Court *et al.*, 2003), and with a recent observation in human post-mortem tissue of reduced cortical ChAT in CADASIL, a genetic condition with severe vascular pathology (Keverne *et al.*, 2007).

There is limited and conflicting evidence to date in relation to changes in muscarinic receptors in VaD (increases, no change, and decreases have all been reported) with little exploration of selected subtype changes (M1–5) and none of functional coupling. Evidence from M5-deficient mice indicates that this muscarinic subtype particularly mediates acetylcholine dilation of cerebral blood vessels (Araya *et al.*, 2006). The most recent and extensive study of nAChRs indicated no loss of cortical heteromeric receptor binding or of α4 (and α7) subunit immunoreactivity (when smoking status, which affects receptor binding, was taken into account) (Martin-Ruiz *et al.*, 2000). This is in striking contrast to AD, DLB, and PD. The apparent intactness of at least nicotinic cholinergic receptors in combination with reduced cholinergic innervation indicates that cholinergic medication may be efficacious in VaD, and this has some support from recent trials (Erkinjuntti *et al.*, 2004; Roman *et al.*, 2005) (see Chapter 27iv for details).

### Biogenic amines

Disruption of dopaminergic function is also suggested by alterations in dopaminergic parameters in the CSF and striatum in VaD (Table 6.2). The apparently elevated dopamine/homovanillic acid ratio in the CSF, possibly suggestive of reduced brain dopamine metabolism, together with reduced striatal dopamine uptake markers, indicate impaired striatal function (reviewed Court *et al.*, 2003). This, in common with reduced ChAT observed in the caudate and putamen (the large interneurons of the striatum are cholinergic) (see Table 6.2), is possibly due to the particular susceptibility of the lenticulostriate vessels to embolic obstruction. Further indication of non-specific disruption of the striatum in VaD is indicated by reduced levels of serotonin (5-HT) and its metabolite 5-hydroxy indole acetic acid (5-HIAA), although no decline in 5-HT uptake sites was observed in this region (Gottfries *et al.*, 1994).

Reduced 5-HT and/or 5-HIAA have also been noted in the CSF, hippocampus, and hypothalamus. In contrast, no reduction in neocortical 5-HT uptake sites or receptors was observed in addition to no diminution in the number of dorsal raphe serotonergic neurons (reviewed Court *et al.*, 2003). This is again suggestive of local attrition of neuronal fields rather than primary neuronal loss. No reduction in the number of noradrenergic neurons in the locus coeruleus was noted.

### Neuropeptides

Neuropeptide profiles in VaD have some overlap with AD. Reductions in a number of neuropeptides in the CSF in VaD have been reported, including somatostatin and β-endorphin, and in some studies, corticotrophin-releasing hormone/factor (Heilig *et al.*, 1995) (Table 6.2). In contrast, some neuropeptides including somatostatin and neurotensin have been found to be increased in a number of brain regions, particularly the hypothalamus, possibly the result of reduced inhibitory serotonergic tone (Gottfries *et al.*, 1994).

Since neurotransmitters modulate cerebral blood flow (reviewed Court *et al.*, 2002) it is possible that neurotransmitter changes in VaD not only contribute to behavioural and cognitive symptoms

via direct effects on neuronal circuits, but also further compromise cerebral perfusion and blood–brain barrier control. Hence rational transmitter based therapies may be of particular significance in VaD.

## Dementia with Lewy bodies and Parkinson's disease dementia

Dementia with Lewy bodies (DLB) and Parkinson's disease dementia (PDD) have clinicopathological features in common with AD, as well as distinguishing features. These differences include fluctuations in attention, alertness, and cognitive performance varying over minutes as well as days and weeks; persistent visual hallucinations; spontaneous parkinsonism; repeated falls; and sensitivity to neuroleptics. DLB and PDD are virtually indistinguishable pathologically, but differ by clinical history in that PDD starts with levodopa-responsive PD at least 1 year before the onset of dementia; while in DLB, parkinsonism (extrapyramidal symptoms, EPS) starts later, and a proportion (about 20%) have no EPS. These clinical differences between AD and DLB/PDD reflect distinct neurochemical profiles, which have treatment implications such as response to cholinesterase inhibitors and levodopa, and the importance of avoiding neuroleptic exposure in DLB/PDD. The neurotransmitter changes in DLB and PDD are summarized in Table 6.3.

### Dopamine

#### Pre-synaptic dopaminergic measures

Reduced substantia nigra (SN) neuron density and low dopamine concentration in the caudate nucleus were first reported in DLB in the early 1990s (R.H. Perry., 1990; Perry *et al.*, 1990c; Marshall *et al.*, 1994). Subsequently, dopamine concentration and dopamine transporters were shown to be reduced in posterior striatum even in DLB cases with little movement disorder (Piggott *et al.*, 1999; Piggott, unpublished) (see Fig. 6.1). The pattern of dopamine loss in DLB is less selectively focused on the posterior putamen than in PD, and the caudate is more affected (Piggott *et al.*, 1999). This is a reflection of the pattern of SN neuron loss with relative sparing of the medial SN in PD. SN and dopamine transporter loss in DLB are also more symmetric between hemispheres than in PD (Ransmayr *et al.*, 2001; O'Brien *et al.*, 2004; Walker *et al.*, 2004).

Loss of dopamine transporter affecting both caudate and putamen rostrocaudally in DLB has been confirmed *in vivo* (Walker *et al.*, 2004; Colloby *et al.*, 2005). Imaging dopamine transporters by single photon emission computed tomography (SPECT) and PET is now an established investigation for assisting differentiation of DLB from AD (Hu *et al.*, 2000; O'Brien *et al.*, 2004). Reduced nigrostriatal dopamine is the most likely substrate for the parkinsonism of DLB, as in PD, but it may be that a moderate reduction in dopaminergic input results in more severe movement disorder in DLB than it would in PD. This is because of the lack of other compensatory changes such as increased turnover of dopamine which occurs in PD to a much greater extent than in DLB, and lack of up-regulation of dopamine D2 receptors in DLB, which occurs in PD (Piggott *et al.*, 1999), as well as the likelihood of other changes in the neurotransmitter system contributing to the movement disorder of DLB as evidenced by the axial predominance and relative levodopa resistance (Bonelli *et al.*, 2004).

**Table 6.3** Dementia with Lewy bodies and Parkinson's disease dementia

| | Cortex/hippocampus | Basal forebrain | Brainstem | Basal ganglia |
|---|---|---|---|---|
| **Acetylcholine (ACh)** | | | | |
| ChAT activity | ↓↓ | | | |
| Vesicular ACh transporter | ↓ | | | |
| nAChRs | ↓ (α4,β2-containing) | | | ↓ (α4,6,β2,3 subunit*) |
| M1 mAChRs | ↑ (with hallucinations) | | | ↓ (striatum) |
| M2/M4 mAChRs | ↑ | | | ↔ |
| Neuron loss | | ✓✓ | ✓ (probably) PPN/LDTg | |
| **Serotonin (5-HT)** | | | | |
| Uptake | ↓↓ | | | |
| 5-HT1ARs | ↑ (with depression) | | | |
| 5-HT$_2$Rs | ↓ | | | ↓ |
| Neuron loss | | | ✓ Raphe | |
| **Dopamine** | | | | |
| Dopamine | | | | ↓ |
| HVA | | | | ↓ |
| DA uptake sites | | | | ↓ (striatum) |
| ¹⁸F-fluorodopa influx rate | | | | ↓ (striatum) |
| Neuron loss (substantia nigra pars compacta) | | | | ↔✓ (DLB), ✓✓✓ (PDD) |
| D2Rs | ↓↓ | | | ↓ (striatum and thalamus) |
| D1 and D3 Rs | | | | ↔ (striatum) |
| **Noradrenaline (NA)** | | | | |
| Noradrenaline | | | | ↓ (striatum) |
| Neuron loss | | | ✓ Locus coeruleus | |
| α$_{1D}$ Rs | ↓ | | | |
| α$_2$ Rs | ↑ | | | |

Sources:

ACh: Gotti *et al.* (2006), Perry *et al.* (1990a,b, 1995), Reid *et al.* (2000), Ballard *et al.* (2000), Tiraboschi *et al.* (2000, 2002), Piggott *et al.* (2003), Kuhl *et al.* (1996).

DA: Hu *et al.* (2000), Perry *et al.* (1990a,c), Piggott *et al.* (1999), Marshall *et al.* (1994).

5-HT: Langlais *et al.* (1993), Ohara *et al.* (1998), Perry *et al.* (1993), Cheng *et al.* (1991), Chen *et al.* (1998), Sharp *et al.* (submitted).

NA: Cash *et al.* (1987), Zweig *et al.* (1993), Leverenz *et al.* (2001), Szot *et al.* (2006), Langlais *et al.* (1993).

See Table 6.1 for abbreviations and PPN/LDTg, pedunculopontine tegmental nucleus and laterodorsal tegmental nucleus.

Nigrothalamic dopamine is also likely to be reduced in DLB and PDD. The thalamus receives dopamine via nigrostriatal collaterals, which have been shown to have depleted dopamine transporter immunoreactivity in the 1-methyl-4-phenyl-1,2,3,6-tetrahydropyridine (MPTP)-treated monkey model of PD (Freeman *et al.*, 2001).

### Post-synaptic dopaminergic measures

In post-mortem analysis, dopamine D2 receptor density is up-regulated in PD without dementia, in the striatum by >70%

(Piggott *et al.*, 1999) and in all examined regions of the thalamus (~100%) (Piggott *et al.*, 2007). In DLB there is a slight reduction (17%) in D2 receptor density in the striatum (Piggott *et al.*, 1999). D2 receptor density was lowest in cases which had severe neuroleptic sensitivity and was slightly higher in cases which were tolerant of neuroleptic treatment (Piggott *et al.*, 1998); it may be that cases with lower D2 density are more at risk of sudden catastrophic blockade due to the D2 antagonist action of neuroleptics. Failure to up-regulate D2 receptors in DLB could be due to intrinsic striatal

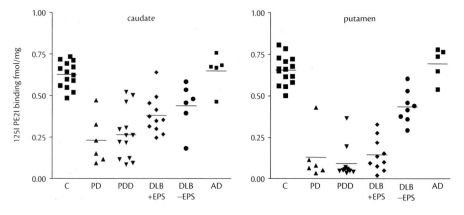

**Fig. 6.1** Dopamine concentration and dopamine transporters in caudate and putamen. C = Control; PD = Parkinson's Disease; PDD = Parkinson's Disease Dementia; DLB = Dementia with Lewy Bodies; +EPS, −EPS = with or without extrapyramidal symptoms; AD = Alzheimer's Disease.

pathology, with β-amyloid and synuclein pathology reported, (A.J. Harding, unpublished; Duda *et al.*, 2002), or perhaps to deficits in other systems, for example in thalamo-striatal afferents or the cholinergic system.

In the thalamus there is a tendency for lower D2 binding in all regions in DLB without EPS (DLB – EPS), slight but significant up-regulation only in ventrointermedius (motor function) and laterodorsal (association) nuclei in DLB with EPS (DLB + EPS), and moderate, significant up-regulation in PDD cases in the ventrointermedius nucleus alone (Piggott *et al.*, 2007). D2 receptor binding in the thalamus in DLB and PDD binding did not vary with cognitive decline or visual hallucinations, but was significantly higher with increased EPS (Piggott *et al.*, 2007). Although somewhat confounded by neuroleptic use, in DLB and PDD there was higher thalamic D2 binding in cases with disturbances of consciousness, particularly in the reticular nucleus (Piggott *et al.*, 2007). D2 receptors located on reticular nucleus GABA-ergic neurons, being inhibitory, will probably help maintain thalamic and cortical activity, thus enabling fluctuations. In an environment of reduced transmitter concentration, relatively higher D2 receptor concentration may amplify small transmitter changes leading to variations in consciousness and attention. Similarly, there were more nicotinic receptors in some thalamic nuclei in cases with variations in consciousness (Pimlott *et al.*, 2004) (see below), possibly suggesting that combined cholinergic and dopaminergic therapy is required to treat disturbed consciousness in DLB.

In temporal cortex (Brodmann area 21) in DLB and PDD, D2 receptors are significantly reduced (>40%), and are also reduced in cases with concomitant Alzheimer pathology, but are not reduced in pure AD (Piggott, in press). The reduced temporal cortical D2 density correlated with cognitive decline, but not with hallucinations or delusions, suggesting that neuroleptics may have a deleterious effect on cognition in DLB.

Dopamine D1 and D3 receptors in the striatum were not altered in DLB in a post-mortem study mainly involving cases with little or no parkinsonism (Piggott *et al.*, 1999).

## Acetylcholine

### Pre-synaptic changes

Cholinergic system changes in DLB are summarized in Table 6.3. Cholinergic losses are generally greater than in AD, both in terms of pre-synaptic cortical activities and additionally in the striatum and in the projection from the pedunculopontine nucleus to the thalamus. As in AD, there is consistent involvement of the nucleus basalis of Meynert, but with Lewy body pathology and more extensive cell loss (Tiraboschi *et al.*, 2000). Within the cerebral cortex, ChAT and acetyl cholinesterase (AChE) losses determined postmortem exceed those in AD (in which they are particularly pronounced in the hippocampus) and are apparent early in the disease course (Perry *et al.*, 1990a,b, Tiraboschi *et al.*, 2002). In PD with dementia, *in vivo* imaging of the vesicular ACh transporter showed extensive losses (Kuhl *et al.*, 1996). As in AD, cholinergic loss and ChAT reductions are correlated with cognitive decline in DLB (Perry *et al.*, 1990c; Samuel *et al.*, 1997; Tiraboschi *et al.*, 2002), and in PD (Perry *et al.*, 1985; Kuhl *et al.*, 1996; Mattila *et al.*, 2001; Bohnen *et al.*, 2006). ChAT deficits are greater in some visual cortical areas in DLB cases with visual hallucinations compared with those without, for example in Brodmann area 36 of the temporal

cortex (Perry *et al.*, 1990a; Ballard *et al.*, 2000). It may be that a propensity to visual hallucinations is increased with much reduced acetylcholine combined with a relatively active serotonergic system (Perry *et al.*, 1990b).

### Nicotinic receptor changes

Neocortical binding to nAChRs containing α4 and β2 subunits is reduced in DLB in common with AD (Perry *et al.*, 1990d; Gotti *et al.*, 2006), but unlike in AD, in DLB there is an apparent correlation between this nAChR deficit and cortical ChAT reduction (Reid *et al.*, 2000). Somewhat surprisingly, heteromeric nAChR binding was relatively preserved in the temporal cortex in cases of DLB with disturbed consciousness (Ballard *et al.*, 2002b). Since patients with disturbances of consciousness are able, some of the time, to be more alert than at other times, the neurotransmitter systems must be capable of reaching the higher level of awareness. When the cholinergic system is very low, a higher density of nicotinic receptors may enable small transmitter fluctuations to lead to variations in consciousness and attention. Whether cortical α7-containing receptors are reduced generally in DLB is equivocal (Reid *et al.*, 2000; Gotti *et al.*, 2006), but it is perhaps most likely to occur in DLB cases with hallucinations (Court *et al.*, 2001b).

In the striatum nAChRs are more reduced in DLB and PD than is the case in AD, notably of the α6-, α4-, β2-, and β3-containing subtypes (Gotti *et al.*, 2006). Reduced nAChR binding in this region, which is at least in part on dopaminergic terminals, is as severe in DLB as PD (Perry *et al.*, 1995; Gotti *et al.*, 2006), perhaps indicating that loss of these receptors occur at a relatively early stage of nigrostriatal degeneration (Perry *et al.*, 1995). In contrast, α4β2-containing nAChRs visualized with [125I]-5-IA85380 were not generally reduced in the thalamus in DLB (although there were reductions in PD), significant deficits being only observed in cases without variations in consciousness (Pimlott *et al.*, 2004). Reduced α7 receptor binding has also been noted in the reticular nucleus of the thalamus in DLB (in common with AD), a region innervated by cholinergic neurons from the basal forebrain (Court *et al.*, 1999).

Loss of nAChRs in DLB is likely to reflect reduced cholinergic innervation (cortex and thalamus), dopaminergic innervation (striatum), and also attenuation of pre- and post-synaptic receptors including those on glutamatergic, GABA-ergic, and serotonergic neurons (cortex, thalamus, and basal ganglia).

### Muscarinic receptor changes

Although pre-synaptic losses are extensive in DLB, post-synaptically there is less neuronal damage than in AD (Tiraboschi *et al.*, 2000; O'Brien *et al.*, 2001). Muscarinic M1 receptor modulation differs between DLB and AD. While unchanged or slightly reduced in the cortex in severe AD, with defective coupling, in DLB M1 receptors have been reported to be up-regulated in temporal and parietal cortex (Perry *et al.*, 1990d; Ballard *et al.*, 2000), and higher in frontal cortex in PDD and DLB compared to AD (Warren *et al.*, submitted). Such up-regulation in the temporal cortex in DLB was associated with delusions (Ballard *et al.*, 2000). Additionally, coupling to G-protein second messenger systems is found to be preserved in DLB compared with AD, in temporal cortex (Perry *et al.*, 1998) and in frontal cortex (Warren *et al.*, submitted). Despite these findings based on receptor-binding assays, immunohistochemistry indicates reduced M1 expression in selected subfields of the hippocampus (Shiozaki *et al.*, 2001). In contrast to the neocortex, striatal M1 receptor binding is reduced, in parallel with D2 receptors, in DLB (M1 and D2 are distributed together mainly on the same population of striatum to external globus pallidus projection neurons) (Piggott et al., 2003). This is possibly why cholinesterase inhibitor therapy tends not to provoke worsening of parkinsonism in DLB patients.

In DLB and PDD, M4 receptors are raised in cingulate cortex with impaired consciousness (Teaktong et al., 2005), and in the insula cortex with the symptom of delusions, while M2 receptors tend to be higher in relation to the severity and duration of extra-pyramidal symptoms in putamen and insula cortex (Piggott, unpublished). M2 binding was higher in cingulate cortex compared to controls, and higher M2 and M4 cingulate binding was associated with visual hallucinations (Teaktong et al., 2005). In contrast, in thalamus M4 receptors are reduced in DLB while M2 are unchanged (Warren et al., 2007). M4 receptors have also been reported to be reduced in DLB in temporal cortex (Shiozaki et al., 1999).

### Serotonin

Lewy body pathology and neuron loss have been reported in the raphe nucleus in DLB (Langlais et al., 1993), although no significant neuron loss was found in one recent study (Benarroch et al., 2005). Reduced serotonin has been reported in striatum and cortex in DLB (Langlais et al., 1993; Perry et al., 1993; Ohara et al., 1998), but not in another study of the putamen (Piggott and Marshall, 1996). Serotonin transporter binding is reduced by about 70% in temporal and parietal cortex in DLB, and $5\text{-HT}2_{2A}$ receptors are reduced by 50% in putamen in PD (Piggott, unpublished), with $5\text{-HT}2_{2A}$ receptors also reduced in temporal cortex in DLB and PDD (Cheng et al., 1991). Depression is a frequent symptom in PD and DLB but a link between serotonin loss and depression remains to be clarified. There is no evidence that selective serotonin reuptake inhibitors are effective in depression in PD (Ghazi-Noori et al., 2003), and untreated PD patients with depression showed no differences in CSF serotonin metabolites compared with patients without depression (Kuhn et al., 1996). DLB patients with a history of major depression actually had relatively higher serotonin transporter binding in parietal cortex than cases without (Ballard et al., 2002a). There is, however, an increase in the numbers of $5\text{-HT}_{1A}$ receptors in temporal cortex in DLB and PDD with depression (S.I. Sharp et al., unpublished), and in PD $5\text{-HT}_{1A}$ receptors are increased in frontal and temporal cortex compared with controls (although any relationship to depression was not assessed in this study) (Chen et al., 1998). Treatment of depression in DLB and PDD may be more efficacious with a $5\text{-HT}_{1A}$ antagonist.

Greater preservation of serotonergic function may be related to more behavioural and psychological symptoms in DLB than in AD. Patients with visual hallucinations show a relative preservation of 5-HT markers and also have markedly reduced cholinergic parameters (Perry et al., 1990b, 1993; Cheng et al., 1991).

### Glutamate

Excitatory amino acid transmission occurs between several components of the basal ganglia circuit, which are likely to be affected in PDD and DLB, and excitotoxic mechanisms have been implicated in the progress of neurodegenerative diseases. In PD increased output from the subthalamic nucleus is part of the neurochemical pathology of the disorder, and glutamate antagonists have been used therapeutically. However, there have been few investigations of glutamate markers. No change was shown in glutamate transporter protein in cortex in two DLB cases (Scott et al., 2002), no change in NMDA receptor immunoreactivity in entorhinal cortex and hippocampus (Thorns et al., 1997), and no reduction in glutamate in CSF (Molina et al., 2005). GluR2/3 AMPA receptor immunoreactivity was, however, decreased in entorhinal cortex and hippocampus (Thorns et al., 1997), and group I metabotropic mGluRs were reduced in DLB (Albasanz et al., 2005), but these reductions were in cases with Alzheimer pathology. Further studies are needed to determine the extent of glutamate receptor changes in DLB/PDD.

### GABA

While anxiety and insomnia are common complaints in DLB which may respond to treatment with benzodiazepines, and GABA-ergic systems are probably affected in DLB, there are few published reports of GABA-ergic changes in DLB. Selective dendritic derangement of GABA-ergic medium spiny neurons in the caudate have been reported, and suggested to be linked to disrupted executive function (Zaja-Milatovic et al., 2006), and similar disruption in the motor putamen in late-stage PD has been found (Zaja-Milatovic et al., 2005). However, there was no change in benzodiazepine binding ($GABA_A$ receptor) in the striatum in DLB, with a slight increase in the globus pallidus (Suzuki et al., 2002). No difference in GABA CSF concentration between controls and DLB has been found (Molina et al., 2005).

### Noradrenaline

Degeneration of the locus coeruleus has been reported in PD, and suggested to be linked to symptoms of mood disorder and subtle cognitive change (Scatton et al., 1983; Cash et al., 1987), and this loss is more extensive in PDD than PD (Cash et al., 1987; Zweig et al., 1993) and DLB (where it is equivalent to AD; Leverenz et al., 2001; Szot et al., 2006). Locus coeruleus neuron loss correlates with cognitive decline (Szot et al., 2006). Szot et al. (2006) found evidence of compensation for the neuron loss in the remaining locus coeruleus neurons in AD and DLB, but in both disorders there was reduced $\alpha_{1D}$ and $\alpha_{2C}$ adrenergic receptor mRNA in hippocampus. $\alpha_2$-Adrenergic receptor density was increased slightly in DLB in frontal cortex (Leverenz et al., 2001).

Noradrenaline system changes in limbic areas may contribute to depression and to behavioural symptoms such as aggression and pacing, to cognitive decline in cortical areas, and to movement disorder in basal ganglia; but in the main these relationships are still to be investigated. In DLB, noradrenaline is much reduced in putamen (Langlais et al., 1993), which could mitigate symptoms of parkinsonism.

## Frontotemporal dementia

The current designation of frontotemporal dementia (FTD) groups together Pick's disease, primary progressive aphasia, and semantic dementia. FTD involves atrophy and neuron loss in the frontal and temporal lobes to greater or lesser extents, without amyloid plaques but with tau pathology. There is also variable degeneration, often asymmetric, in the substantia nigra, hippocampus, thalamus, striatum, and amygdala (Barnes et al., 2006). Studies of neurotransmitter changes in FTD are relatively few, and involve a small number of cases, often single case studies. Study findings are summarized in Table 6.4.

**Table 6.4** Frontotemporal dementia

| | Cortex/hippocampus | Basal forebrain | Brainstem | Basal ganglia |
|---|---|---|---|---|
| **Acetylcholine (ACh)** | | | | |
| ChAT activity | ↔ | | | ↓ (thalamus) |
| mAChRs | ~↓ | | | |
| Neuron loss | | ↔ | ↓ (?) | |
| **Serotonin (5-HT)** | | | | |
| Serotonin | ↓↓ | ↓↓ | | ↓↓ |
| Uptake | ↔↓ | | | ↓ |
| 5-HT1ARs | ↓ | | | |
| 5-HT₂Rs | ↓ | | | ↓ |
| Neuron loss | | | ✓✓ Raphe | |
| **Dopamine** | | | | |
| Dopamine | ↓ | | ↓ (substantia nigra) | ↓↓ (striatum) |
| DA uptake sites | | | | ↓↓ (striatum) |
| **Noradrenaline (NA)** | | | | |
| Noradrenaline | | | | ↓ (thalamus) |
| Neuron loss | | | ↔ or ✓ Locus coeruleus | |

Sources:

ACh: Di Lazzaro *et al.* (2006), Foster *et al.* (1998), Huey *et al.* (2006), Hansen *et al.* (1988), Weinberger *et al.* (1991), Odawara *et al.* (2003).

5-HT: Nagaoka *et al.* (1995), Gilbert *et al.* (1988), Francis *et al.* (1993), Sparks and Markesbery (1991), Franceschi *et al.* (2005), Procter *et al.* (1999).

DA: Rinne *et al.* (2002), Knopman *et al.* (1990), Nagaoka *et al.* (1995).

NA: Yang and Schmitt (2001), Arima and Akashi (1990), Nagaoka *et al.* (1995).

See Table 6.1 for abbreviations.

## Acetylcholine

Cholinergic systems have generally been reported as normal in FTD (Di Lazzaro *et al.*, 2006), with sparing of the nucleus basalis of Meynert (Foster *et al.*, 1998; reviewed in Huey *et al.*, 2006). Some studies have found deficits, however; for example in muscarinic receptors in temporal cortex in Pick's disease (Hansen *et al.*, 1988; Weinberger *et al.*, 1991) or in atypical Pick's disease (Odawara *et al.*, 2003). In the thalamus, ChAT levels were reduced (by 40%) in anterior and ventral posteriolateral nuclei in two cases (Piggott, unpublished), perhaps similar to progressive supranuclear palsy where cortical cholinergic receptors are unchanged but there are thalamic losses in regions innervated by the cholinergic pedunculopontine and laterodorsal tegmental nuclei of the brainstem (Warren *et al.*, 2007). Acetylcholinesterase inhibitor treatment in FTD is generally not helpful (Huey *et al.*, 2006), although there is one report of benefit to behavioural symptoms but not to cognition (Lampl *et al.*, 2004).

## Dopamine

Basal ganglia involvement with substantia nigra cell loss occurs in many patients and is the likely cause of parkinsonian symptoms. A PET study in 12 FTD patients found dopamine transporter loss correlated with severity of motor items from the Unified Parkinson's Disease Rating Scale (Rinne *et al.*, 2002). In this study the average reduction in putamen was 82% of control, while in caudate it was down by 86%. This is similar to the reduction found in a post-mortem study, with severe loss of caudate and putamen dopamine concentration and transporter binding in three sporadic FTD cases of older onset (52, 67, and 80 years) (Piggott, unpublished). This group also had lowered dopamine content in hippocampus and frontal cortex. The temporal and frontal predilection cortical sites for atrophy in FTD normally receive strong dopaminergic inputs, and mesocortical dopamine insufficiency is likely to contribute to the non-motor features of depression and dementia in FTD (Knopman *et al.*, 1990). In one young FTD case (28 years) with behavioural changes, striatal dopamine loss was profound in the caudate and putamen, but deficits were also seen in the substantia nigra, nucleus basalis, locus coeruleus, raphe nucleus, lateral thalamus, and occipital cortex (Nagaoka *et al.*, 1995).

## Serotonin

Serotonergic deficits are the most consistent neurochemical finding in FTD, revealed in both autopsy and imaging studies. In the young case of FTD reported by Nagaoka *et al.* (1995) there was a 50% reduction in serotonin in striatum, lateral thalamus, nucleus basalis of Meynert, and hippocampus, and in another case there was a 30–50% reduction in substantia nigra, striatum, and hypothalamus (Gilbert *et al.*, 1988). In 12 FTD cases there was a 40% reduction in neuron number in the raphe (Yang and Schmitt, 2001). Serotonin reuptake site density has been found in some studies to be unchanged or increased (Sparks and Markesbery 1991; Francis *et al.*, 1993), but in three post-mortem cases, using cyanoimipramine to visualize 5-HT transporter (5-HTT), densities were reduced by >40% in putamen and by 30–50% in cingulate and insula cortex (Piggott, unpublished). The HVA:5-HIAA ratio in CSF correlated significantly with aggressiveness and agitation in 13 FTD patients (but did not in AD) (Engelborghs *et al.*, 2004).

Post-synaptic serotonin receptor binding is reduced in FTD; a PET study in eight patients found 5-HT₂ₐ receptor density reduced in orbitofrontal, frontal medial, and cingulate cortex (Franceschi *et al.*, 2005). In post-mortem studies, serotonin binding was reduced by 50% in hypothalamus, temporal, and frontal cortex (Sparks and Markesbery, 1991), while post-synaptic 5-HT₁ₐ receptors were low in frontal cortex (Francis *et al.*, 1993; Procter *et al.*, 1999).

5-HT2 binding was reduced by 30% in caudate, putamen, and cingulate cortex in three cases (Piggott, unpublished).

FTD patients often have symptoms of stereotyped compulsive behaviour, impulsivity, and of food cravings, which could be caused by serotonin deficiency (Miller *et al.*, 1995). Although large studies of effective treatments have yet to be published, the behavioural symptoms of FTD can improve with serotonin reuptake inhibitors according to some (Swartz *et al.*, 1997; Ikeda *et al.*, 2004; Moretti *et al.*, 2003; Mendez *et al.*, 2005), but not all reports (Deakin *et al.*, 2004).

## Glutamate

AMPA receptors are reduced in both temporal and frontal lobes in FTD with no reduction of kainate receptors, while in a group with Pick's disease, NMDA receptors were additionally lost, suggesting selective loss of different populations of cortical pyramidal neurons (Procter *et al.*, 1999).

## Noradrenaline

The locus coeruleus is spared in FTD (Yang and Schmitt, 2001), or may have decreased neuron number in Pick's disease (Arima and Akashi, 1990). In the single young case of FTD (Nagaoka *et al.*, 1995), noradrenaline concentration was less than 20% of normal in the lateral thalamus and the nucleus basalis of Meynert, and slightly reduced in the locus coeruleus, amygdala, and medial thalamus, although pathology in the locus coeruleus appeared slight. Idazoxan, an $\alpha_2$ noradrenergic receptor antagonist, may improve attention, verbal fluency, and planning (Coull *et al.*, 1996).

## Neuropeptides

Neuropeptides may be reduced in FTD, with low CSF levels of somatostatin, neuropeptide Y, antidiuretic hormone, and corticotrophin-releasing factor reported (Minthon *et al.*, 1990; Edvinsson *et al.*, 1993), with concentrations of somatostatin and neuropeptide Y related to agitation, irritability, and restlessness (Minthon *et al.*, 1997).

## References

Albasanz, J.L., Dalfo, E., Ferrer, I., and Martin, M. (2005). Impaired metabotropic glutamate receptor/phospholipase C signaling pathway in the cerebral cortex in Alzheimer's disease and dementia with Lewy bodies correlates with stage of Alzheimer's-disease-related changes. *Neurobiology of Disease*, **20**, 685–693.

Allen, J.M., Ferrier, I.N., Roberts, G.W. *et al.* (1984). Elevation of neuropeptide Y (NPY) in substantia innominata in Alzheimer's type dementia. *Journal of the Neurological Sciences*, **64**, 325–331.

Almeida, C.G., Takahashi, R.H., and Gouras, G.K. (2006). Beta-amyloid accumulation impairs multivesicular body sorting by inhibiting the ubiquitin-proteasome system. *Journal of Neuroscience*, **26**, 4277–4288.

Amada, N., Aihara, K., Ravid, R., and Horie, M. (2005). Reduction of NR1 and phosphorylated Ca2+/calmodulin-dependent protein kinase II levels in Alzheimer's disease. *Neuroreport*, **16**, 1809–1813.

Arai, H., Kosaka, K., and Iizuka, R. (1984). Changes of biogenic amines and their metabolites in postmortem brains from patients with Alzheimer-type dementia. *Journal of Neurochemistry*, **43**, 388–393.

Araya, R., Noguchi, T., Yuhki, M. *et al.* (2006). Loss of M5 muscarinic acetylcholine receptors leads to cerebrovascular and neuronal abnormalities and cognitive deficits in mice. *Neurobiology of Disease*, **24**, 334–344.

Arima, K. and Akashi, T. (1990). Involvement of the locus coeruleus in Pick's disease with or without Pick body formation. *Acta Neuropathologica*, **79**, 629–633.

Armstrong, D.M., Sheffield, R., Mishizen-Eberz, A.J. *et al.* (2003). Plasticity of glutamate and GABAA receptors in the hippocampus of patients with Alzheimer's disease. *Cellular and Molecular Neurobiology*, **23**, 491–505.

Ballard, C., Piggott, M., Johnson, M. *et al.* (2000). Delusions associated with elevated muscarinic M1 receptor binding in dementia with Lewy bodies. *Annals of Neurology*, **48**, 868–876.

Ballard, C., Johnson, M., Piggott, M. *et al.* (2002a) A positive association between 5HT re-uptake binding sites and depression in dementia with Lewy bodies. *Journal of Affective Disorders*, **69**, 219–223.

Ballard, C.G., Court, J.A., Piggott, M. *et al.* (2002b). Disturbances of consciousness in dementia with Lewy bodies associated with alteration in nicotinic receptor binding in the temporal cortex. *Consciousness and Cognition*, **11**, 461–474.

Barnes, J., Whitwell, J.L., Frost, C., Josephs, K.A., Rossor, M., and Fox, N.C. (2006). Measurements of the amygdala and hippocampus in pathologically confirmed Alzheimer disease and frontotemporal lobar degeneration. *Archives of Neurology*, **63**, 1434–1439.

Benarroch, E.E., Schmeichel, A.M., Low, P.A., Boeve, B.F., Sandroni, P., and Parisi, J.E. (2005). Involvement of medullary regions controlling sympathetic output in Lewy body disease. *Brain*, **128**, 338–344.

Birks, J. (2006). Cholinesterase inhibitors for Alzheimer's disease. *Cochrane Database of Systematic Reviews*, CD005593.

Bohnen, N.I., Kaufer, D.I., Hendrickson, R. *et al.* (2006). Cognitive correlates of cortical cholinergic denervation in Parkinson's disease and parkinsonian dementia. *Journal of Neurology*, **253**, 242–247.

Boissiere, F., Faucheux, B., Agid, Y., and Hirsch, E.C. (1997). Choline acetyltransferase mRNA expression in the striatal neurons of patients with Alzheimer's disease. *Neuroscience Letters*, **225**, 169–172.

Boksha, I.S. (2004). Coupling between neuronal and glial cells via glutamate metabolism in brain of healthy persons and patients with mental disorders. *Biochemistry (Moscow)*, **69**, 705–719.

Bonelli, S.B., Ransmayr, G., Steffelbauer, M., Lukas, T., Lampl, C., and Deibl, M. (2004). L-dopa responsiveness in dementia with Lewy bodies, Parkinson disease with and without dementia. *Neurology*, **63**, 376–378.

Bowen, D.M., Allen, S.J., Benton, J.S. *et al.* (1983). Biochemical assessment of serotonergic and cholinergic dysfunction and cerebral atrophy in Alzheimer's disease. *Journal of Neurochemistry*, **41**, 266–272.

Brandel, J.P., Hirsch, E.C., Malessa, S., Duyckaerts, C., Cervera, P., and Agid, Y. (1991). Differential vulnerability of cholinergic projections to the mediodorsal nucleus of the thalamus in senile dementia of Alzheimer type and progressive supranuclear palsy. *Neuroscience*, **41**, 25–31.

Burbaeva, G., Boksha, I.S., Tereshkina, E.B., Savushkina, O.K., Starodubtseva, L.I., and Turishcheva, M.S. (2005). Glutamate metabolizing enzymes in prefrontal cortex of Alzheimer's disease patients. *Neurochemistry Research*, **30**, 1443–1451.

Caccamo, A., Oddo, S., Billings, L.M. *et al.* (2006). M1 receptors play a central role in modulating AD-like pathology in transgenic mice. *Neuron*, **49**, 671–682.

Cash, R., Dennis, T., L'Heureux, R., Raisman, R., Javoy-Agid, F., and Scatton, B. (1987). Parkinson's disease and dementia: norepinephrine and dopamine in locus ceruleus. *Neurology*, **37**, 42–46.

Chalmers, D.T., Dewar, D., Graham, D.I., Brooks, D.N., and McCulloch, J. (1990). Differential alterations of cortical glutamatergic binding sites in senile dementia of the Alzheimer type. *Proceedings of the National Academy of Sciences USA*, **87**, 1352–1356.

Chan-Palay, V. (1987). Somatostatin immunoreactive neurons in the human hippocampus and cortex shown by immunogold/silver intensification on vibratome sections: coexistence with neuropeptide Y neurons, and effects in Alzheimer-type dementia. *Journal of Comparative Neurology*, **260**, 201–223.

Chan-Palay, V. (1988). Galanin hyperinnervates surviving neurons of the human basal nucleus of Meynert in dementias of Alzheimer's and Parkinson's disease: a hypothesis for the role of galanin in accentuating cholinergic dysfunction in dementia. *Journal of Comparative Neurology*, **273**, 543–557.

Chen, C.P., Alder, J.T., Bray, L., Kingsbury, A.E., Francis, P.T., and Foster, O.J. (1998). Post-synaptic 5-HT1A and 5-HT2A receptors are increased in Parkinson's disease neocortex. *Annals of the New York Academy of Science*, **861**, 288–289.

Cheng, A.V., Ferrier, I.N., Morris, C.M. *et al.* (1991). Cortical serotonin-S2 receptor binding in Lewy body dementia, Alzheimer's and Parkinson's diseases. *Journal of the Neurological Sciences*, **106**, 50–55.

Colloby, S.J., Williams, E.D., Burn, D.J., Lloyd, J.J., McKeith, I.G., and O'Brien, J.T. (2005). Progression of dopaminergic degeneration in dementia with Lewy bodies and Parkinson's disease with and without dementia assessed using [123]I-FP-CIT SPECT. *European Journal of Nuclear Medicine and Molecular Imaging*, **32**, 1176–1185.

Coull, J.T., Sahakian, B.J., and Hodges, J.R. (1996). The alpha(2) antagonist idazoxan remediates certain attentional and executive dysfunction in patients with dementia of frontal type. *Psychopharmacology (Berlin)*, **123**, 239–249.

Court, J.A. and Perry, E.K. (2003). Neurotransmitter abnormalities in vascular dementia. *International Psychogeriatrics*, **15**(Suppl. 1), 81–87.

Court, J., Spurden, D., Lloyd, S. *et al.* (1999). Neuronal nicotinic receptors in dementia with Lewy bodies and schizophrenia: α-bungarotoxin and nicotine binding in the thalamus. *Journal of Neurochemistry*, **73**, 1590–1597.

Court, J.A., Piggott, M.A., Lloyd, S. *et al.* (2000). Nicotine binding in human striatum: elevation in schizophrenia and reductions in dementia with Lewy bodies, Parkinson's disease and Alzheimer's disease and in relation to neuroleptic medication. *Neuroscience*, **98**, 79–87.

Court, J., Martin-Ruiz, C., Piggott, M., Spurden, D., Griffiths, M., and Perry, E. (2001a). Nicotinic receptor abnormalities in Alzheimer's disease. *Biological Psychiatry*, **49**, 175–184.

Court, J.A., Ballard, C.G., Piggott, M.A. *et al.* (2001b). Visual hallucinations are associated with lower alpha bungarotoxin binding in dementia with Lewy bodies. *Pharmacology Biochemistry and Behavior*, **70**, 571–579.

Court, J., Perry, E., and Kalaria, R. (2002). Neurotransmitter control of the cerebral vasculature and abnormalities in vascular dementia. In *Vascular cognitive impairment* (ed. T. Erkinjuntti and S. Gauthier), pp. 167–185. Martin Dunitz, London.

Court, J., Perry, E., and Kalaria, R. (2003). Neurochemical changes in vascular dementia. In *Cerebrovascular disease, cognitive impairment and dementia* (ed. D. Ames, E. Chui, L. Gustafson, and J. O'Brien), pp. 133–151. Martin Dunitz, London.

Court, J.A., Johnson, M., Religa, D. *et al.* (2005). Attenuation of Abeta deposition in the entorhinal cortex of normal elderly individuals associated with tobacco smoking. *Neuropathology and Applied Neurobiology*, **31**, 522–535.

Cowburn, R.F., Hardy, J.A., Briggs, R.S., and Roberts, P.J. (1989). Characterisation, density, and distribution of kainate receptors in normal and Alzheimer's diseased human brain. *Journal of Neurochemistry*, **52**, 140–147.

Cowburn, R.F., Wiehager, B., Ravid, R., and Winblad, B. (1996). Acetylcholine muscarinic M2 receptor stimulated [35S]GTP gamma S binding shows regional selective changes in Alzheimer's disease postmortem brain. *Neurodegeneration*, **5**, 19–26.

Cross, A.J., Crow, T.J., Johnson, J.A. *et al.* (1983). Monoamine metabolism in senile dementia of Alzheimer type. *Journal of Neurological Science*, **60**, 383–392.

D'Aniello, A., Fisher, G., Migliaccio, N., Cammisa, G., D'Aniello, E., and Spinelli, P. (2005). Amino acids and transaminases activity in ventricular CSF and in brain of normal and Alzheimer patients. *Neuroscience Letters*, **388**, 49–53.

Danielsson, E., Eckernas, S.A., Westlind-Danielsson, A. *et al.* (1988). VIP-sensitive adenylate cyclase, guanylate cyclase, muscarinic receptors, choline acetyltransferase and acetylcholinesterase, in brain tissue afflicted by Alzheimer's disease/senile dementia of the Alzheimer type. *Neurobiology of Aging*, **9**, 153–162.

Davis, K.L., Mohs, R.C., Marin, D. *et al.* (1999). Cholinergic markers in elderly patients with early signs of Alzheimer disease. *Journal of the American Medical Association*, **281**, 1401–1406.

Dawbarn, D., Rossor, M.N., Mountjoy, C.Q., Roth, M., and Emson, P.C. (1986). Decreased somatostatin immunoreactivity but not neuropeptide Y immunoreactivity in cerebral cortex in senile dementia of Alzheimer type. *Neuroscience Letters*, **70**, 154–159.

Deakin, J.B., Rahman, S., Nestor, P.J., Hodges, J.R., and Sahakian, B.J. (2004). Paroxetine does not improve symptoms and impairs cognition in frontotemporal dementia: a double-blind randomized controlled trial. *Psychopharmacology*, **172**, 400–408.

DeKosky, S.T., Ikonomovic, M.D., Styren, S.D. *et al.* (2002). Upregulation of choline acetyltransferase activity in hippocampus and frontal cortex of elderly subjects with mild cognitive impairment. *Annals of Neurology*, **51**, 145–155.

Dewar, D., Chalmers, D.T., Graham, D.I., and McCulloch, J. (1991). Glutamate metabotropic and AMPA binding sites are reduced in Alzheimer's disease: an autoradiographic study of the hippocampus. *Brain Research*, **553**, 58–64.

Di Lazzaro, V., Pilato, F., Dileone, M. *et al.* (2006). In vivo cholinergic circuit evaluation in frontotemporal and Alzheimer dementias. *Neurology*, **66**, 1111–1113.

Duda, J.E., Giasson, B.I., Mabon, M.E., Lee, V.M., and Trojanowski, J.Q. (2002). Novel antibodies to synuclein show abundant striatal pathology in Lewy body diseases. *Annals of Neurology*, **52**, 205–210.

Edvinsson, L., Minthon, L., Ekman, R., and Gustafson, L. (1993). Neuropeptides in cerebrospinal fluid of patients with Alzheimer's disease and dementia with frontotemporal lobe degeneration. *Dementia*, **4**, 167–171.

Engelborghs, S., Vloeberghs, E., Maertens, K., Marescau, B., and De Deyn, P.P. (2004). Evidence for an association between the CSF HVA:5-HIAA ratio and aggressiveness in frontotemporal dementia but not in Alzheimer's disease. *Journal of Neurology, Neurosurgery and Psychiatry*, **75**, 1080.

Erkinjuntti, T., Roman, G., Gauthier, S., Feldman, H., and Rockwood, K. (2004). Emerging therapies for vascular dementia and vascular cognitive impairment. *Stroke*, **35**, 1010–1017.

Esiri, M. (1991). Neuropathology. In *Psychiatry in the elderly* (ed. R. Jacoby and C. Oppenheimer), pp. 113–147. Oxford University Press, Oxford.

Evans, J.G., Wilcock, G., and Birks, J. (2004). Evidence-based pharmacotherapy of Alzheimer's disease. *International Journal of Neuropsychopharmacology*, **7**, 351–369.

Feldman, H., Gauthier, S., Hecker, J., Vellas, B., Subbiah, P., and Whalen, E. (2001). A 24-week, randomized, double-blind study of donepezil in moderate to severe Alzheimer's disease. *Neurology*, **57**, 613–620.

Floden, A.M., Li, S., and Combs, C.K. (2005). Beta-amyloid-stimulated microglia induce neuron death via synergistic stimulation of tumor necrosis factor alpha and NMDA receptors. *Journal of Neuroscience*, **25**, 2566–2575.

Flynn, D.D., Ferrari-DiLeo, G., Mash, D.C., and Levey, A.I. (1995). Differential regulation of molecular subtypes of muscarinic receptors in Alzheimer's disease. *Journal of Neurochemistry*, **64**, 1888–1891.

Foster, N.L., Sima, A.A.F., Minoshima, S., and Kuhl, D.E. (1998). Clinical and neuropathological correlations with PET in FTDP-17 and sporadic frontal dementia. *Neurobiology of Aging*, **19**, S296.

Franceschi, M., Anchisi, D., Pelati, O. *et al.* (2005). Glucose metabolism and serotonin receptors in the frontotemporal lobe degeneration. *Annals of Neurology*, **57**, 216–225.

Francis, P.T. (2003). Glutamatergic systems in Alzheimer's disease. *International Journal of Geriatric Psychiatry*, **18**, S15–S21.

Francis, P.T., Holmes, C., Webster, M.T., Stratmann, G.C., Procter, A.W., and Bowen, D.M. (1993). Preliminary neurochemical findings in non-Alzheimer dementia due to lobar atrophy. *Dementia*, **4**, 172–177.

Francis, P.T., Palmer, A.M., Snape, M., and Wilcock, G.K. (1999). The cholinergic hypothesis of Alzheimer's disease: a review of progress. *Journal of Neurology, Neurosurgery and Psychiatry*, **66**, 137–147.

Freeman, A., Ciliax, B., Bakay, R. *et al.* (2001). Nigrostriatal collaterals to thalamus degenerate in parkinsonian animal models. *Annals of Neurology*, **50**, 321–329.

Garcia-Alloza, M., Hirst, W.D., Chen, C.-H., Lasheras, B., Francis, P.T., and Ramirez, M.J. (2004). Differential involvement of 5-HT1B/1D and 5-HT6 receptors in cognitive and non-cognitive symptoms in Alzheimer's disease. *Neuropsychopharmacology*, **29**, 410–416.

Garcia-Alloza, M., Tsang, S.W., Gil-Bea, F.J. *et al.* (2006). Involvement of the GABAergic system in depressive symptoms of Alzheimer's disease. *Neurobiology of Aging*, **27**, 1110–1117.

Gauthier, S., Reisberg, B., Zaudig, M. *et al.* (2006). Mild cognitive impairment. *Lancet*, **367**, 1262–1270.

Geddes, J.W., Ulas, J., Brunner, L.C., Choe, W., and Cotman, C.W. (1992). Hippocampal excitatory amino acid receptors in elderly, normal individuals and those with Alzheimer's disease: non-N-methyl-D-aspartate receptors. *Neuroscience*, **50**, 23–34.

Ghazi-Noori, S., Chung, T.H., Deane, K., Rickards, H., and Clarke, C.E. (2003). Therapies for depression in Parkinson's disease. *Cochrane Database of Systematic Reviews*, CD003465.

Gilbert, J.J., Kish, S.J., Chang, L.J., Morito, C., Shannak, K., and Hornykiewicz, O. (1988). Dementia, parkinsonism, and motor neuron disease: neurochemical and neuropathological correlates. *Annals of Neurology*, **24**, 688–691.

Ginsberg, S.D., Che, S., Wuu, J., Counts, S.E., and Mufson, E.J. (2006). Down regulation of trk but not p75NTR gene expression in single cholinergic basal forebrain neurons mark the progression of Alzheimer's disease. *Journal of Neurochemistry*, **97**, 475–487.

Gottfries, C.G., Blennow, K., Karlsson, I., and Wallin, A. (1994). The neurochemistry of vascular dementia. *Dementia*, **5**, 163–167.

Gotti, C., Moretti, M., Bohr, I. *et al.* (2006). Selective nicotinic acetylcholine receptor subunit deficits identified in Alzheimer's disease, Parkinson's disease and dementia with Lewy bodies by immunoprecipitation. *Neurobiology of Disease*, **23**, 481–489.

Halliday, G.M., McCann, H.L., Pamphlett, R. *et al.* (1992). Brain stem serotonin-synthesizing neurons in Alzheimer's disease: a clinicopathological correlation. *Acta Neuropathologica*, **84**, 638–650.

Hansen, L.A., Deteresa, R., Tobias, H., Alford, M., and Terry, R.D. (1988). Neocortical morphometry and cholinergic neurochemistry in Pick's disease. *American Journal of Pathology*, **131**, 507–518.

Heilig, M., Sjogren, M., Blennow, K., Ekman, R., and Wallin, A. (1995). Cerebrospinal fluid neuropeptides in Alzheimer's disease and vascular dementia. *Biological Psychiatry*, **38**, 210–216.

Hellstrom-Lindahl, E., Mousavi, M., Ravid, R., and Nordberg, A. (2004). Reduced levels of Abeta 40 and Abeta 42 in brains of smoking controls and Alzheimer's patients. *Neurobiology of Disease*, **15**, 351–360.

Herrmann, N., Lanctot, K.L., and Khan, L.R. (2004). The role of norepinephrine in the behavioral and psychological symptoms of dementia. *Journal of Neuropsychiatry and Clinical Neurosciences*, **16**, 261–276.

Hock, C., Maddalena, A., Raschig, A. *et al.* (2003). Treatment with the selective muscarinic m1 agonist talsaclidine decreases cerebrospinal fluid levels of A beta 42 in patients with Alzheimer's disease. *Amyloid*, **10**, 1–6.

Holmes, C., Arranz, M.J., Powell, J.F., Collier, D.A., and Lovestone, S. (1998). 5-HT2A and 5-HT2C receptor polymorphisms and psychopathology in late onset Alzheimer's disease. *Human Molecular Genetics*, **7**, 1507–1509.

Hu, X.S., Okamura, N., Arai, H. *et al.* (2000). 18F-fluorodopa PET study of striatal dopamine uptake in the diagnosis of dementia with Lewy bodies. *Neurology*, **55**, 1575–1577.

Huey, E.D., Putnam, K.T., and Grafman, J. (2006). A systematic review of neurotransmitter deficits and treatments in frontotemporal dementia. *Neurology*, **66**, 17–22.

Hynd, M.R., Scott, H.L., and Dodd, P.R. (2004). Glutamate-mediated excitotoxicity and neurodegeneration in Alzheimer's disease. *Neurochemistry International*, **45**, 583–595.

Ikeda, M., Shigenobu, K., Fukuhara, R. *et al.* (2004). Efficacy of fluvoxamine as a treatment for behavioral symptoms in frontotemporal lobar degeneration patients. *Dementia and Geriatric Cognitive Disorders*, **17**, 117–121.

Iwakiri, M., Mizukami, K., Ikonomovic, M.D. *et al.* (2005). Changes in hippocampal GABABR1 subunit expression in Alzheimer's patients: association with Braak staging. *Acta Neuropathologica*, **109**, 467–474.

Jia, J.P., Jia, J.M., Zhou, W.D. *et al.* (2004). Differential acetylcholine and choline concentrations in the cerebrospinal fluid of patients with Alzheimer's disease and vascular dementia. *Chinese Medical Journal (English Edition)*, **117**, 1161–1164.

Jimenez-Jimenez, F.J., Molina, J.A., Gomez, P. *et al.* (1998). Neurotransmitter amino acids in cerebrospinal fluid of patients with Alzheimer's disease. *Journal of Neural Transmission*, **105**, 269–277.

Jope, R. (1996). Cholinergic muscarinic receptor signaling by the phosphoinositide signal transduction system in Alzheimer's disease. *Alzheimer's Disease Review*, **1**, 2–14.

Keverne, J.S., Low, W.C., Ziabreva, I., Court, J.A., Oakley, A.E., and Kalaria, R.N. (2007). Cholinergic neuronal deficits in CADASIL. *Stroke*, **38**, 188-191.

Knopman, D.S., Mastri, A.R., Frey, W.H.d, Sung, J.H., and Rustan, T. (1990). Dementia lacking distinctive histologic features: a common non-Alzheimer degenerative dementia. *Neurology*, **40**, 251–256.

Koide, S., Onishi, H., Hashimoto, H., Kai, T., and Yamagami, S. (1995). Plasma neuropeptide Y is reduced in patients with Alzheimer's disease. *Neuroscience Letters*, **198**, 149–151.

Kuhl, D.E., Minoshima, S., Fessler, J.A. *et al.* (1996). *In vivo* mapping of cholinergic terminals in normal aging, Alzheimer's disease, and Parkinson's disease. *Annals of Neurology*, **40**, 399–410.

Kuhn, W., Muller, T., Gerlach, M. *et al.* (1996). Depression in Parkinson's disease: biogenic amines in CSF of 'de novo' patients. *Journal of Neural Transmission*, **103**, 1441–1445.

Ladner, C.J., Celesia, G.G., Magnuson, D.J., and Lee, J.M. (1995). Regional alterations in M1 muscarinic receptor-G protein coupling in Alzheimer's disease. *Journal of Neuropathology and Experimental Neurology*, **54**, 783–789.

Lai, M.K., Lai, O.F., Keene, J. *et al.* (2001). Psychosis of Alzheimer's disease is associated with elevated muscarinic M2 binding in the cortex. *Neurology*, **57**, 805–811.

Lai, M.K., Tsang, S.W., Francis, P.T. *et al.* (2003a). [3H]GR113808 binding to serotonin 5-HT(4) receptors in the postmortem neocortex of Alzheimer disease: a clinicopathological study. *Journal of Neural Transmission*, **110**, 779–788.

Lai, M.K., Tsang, S.W., Francis, P.T. *et al.* (2003b). Reduced serotonin 5-HT1A receptor binding in the temporal cortex correlates with aggressive behavior in Alzheimer disease. *Brain Research*, **974**, 82–87.

Lai, M.K., Tsang, S.W., Alder, J.T. *et al.* (2005). Loss of serotonin 5-HT2A receptors in the postmortem temporal cortex correlates with rate of cognitive decline in Alzheimer's disease. *Psychopharmacology*, **179**, 673–677.

Lampl, Y., Sadeh, M., and Lorberboym, M. (2004). Efficacy of acetylcholinesterase inhibitors in frontotemporal dementia. *Annals of Pharmacotherapy*, **38**, 1967–1968.

Lanari, A., Amenta, F., Silvestrelli, G., Tomassoni, D., and Parnetti, L. (2006). Neurotransmitter deficits in behavioural and psychological symptoms of Alzheimer's disease. *Mechanisms of Ageing and Development*, **127**, 158–165.

Langlais, P.J., Thal, L., Hansen, L., Galasko, D., Alford, M., and Masliah, E. (1993). Neurotransmitters in basal ganglia and cortex of Alzheimer's disease with and without Lewy bodies. *Neurology*, **43**, 1927–1934.

Lesne, S., Ali, C., Gabriel, C. *et al.* (2005). NMDA receptor activation inhibits alpha-secretase and promotes neuronal amyloid-beta production. *Journal of Neuroscience*, **25**, 9367–9377.

Leverenz, J.B., Miller, M.A., Dobie, D.J., Peskind, E.R., and Raskind, M.A. (2001). Increased alpha 2-adrenergic receptor binding in locus coeruleus projection areas in dementia with Lewy bodies. *Neurobiology of Aging*, **22**, 555–561.

Lezoualc'h, F. and Robert, S.J. (2003). The serotonin 5-HT$_4$ receptor and the amyloid precursor protein processing. *Experimental Gerontology*, **38**, 159–166.

Lipton, S.A. (2005). The molecular basis of memantine action in Alzheimer's disease and other neurologic disorders: low-affinity, uncompetitive antagonism. *Current Alzheimer Research*, **2**, 155–165.

Mann, D.M., Lincoln, J., Yates, P.O., Stamp, J.E., and Toper, S. (1980). Changes in the monoamine containing neurones of the human CNS in senile dementia. *British Journal of Psychiatry*, **136**, 533–541.

Mann, D.M., Yates, P.O., and Marcyniuk, B. (1986). The nucleus basalis of Meynert in multi-infarct (vascular) dementia. *Acta Neuropathologica*, **71**, 332–337.

Marshall, E.F., Perry, E.K., Perry, R.H., McKeith, I.G., Fairbairn, A.F., and Thompson, P. (1994). Dopamine metabolism in post-mortem caudate nucleus in neurodegenerative disorders. *Neuroscience Research Communications*, **14**, 17–25.

Martel, J.C., Alagar, R., Robitaille, Y., and Quirion, R. (1990). Neuropeptide Y receptor binding sites in human brain. Possible alteration in Alzheimer's disease. *Brain Research*, **519**, 228–235.

Martin-Ruiz, C., Court, J., Lee, M. *et al.* (2000). Nicotinic receptors in dementia of Alzheimer, Lewy body and vascular types. *Acta Neurologica Scandinavica Supplement*, **176**, 34–41.

Mattila, P.M., Roytta, M., Lonnberg, P., Marjamaki, P., Helenius, H., and Rinne, J.O. (2001). Choline acetyltransferase activity and striatal dopamine receptors in Parkinson's disease in relation to cognitive impairment. *Acta Neuropathologica*, **102**, 160–166.

Mendez, M.F., Shapira, J.S., and Miller, B.L. (2005). Stereotypical movements and frontotemporal dementia. *Movement Disorders*, **20**, 742–745.

Miller, B.L., Darby, A.L., Swartz, J.R., Yener, G.G., and Mena, I. (1995). Dietary changes, compulsions and sexual behavior in frontotemporal degeneration. *Dementia*, **6**, 195–199.

Minthon, L., Edvinsson, L., Ekman, R., and Gustafson, L. (1990). Neuropeptide levels in Alzheimer's disease and dementia with frontotemporal degeneration. *Journal of Neural Transmission Supplement*, **30**, 57–67.

Minthon, L., Edvinsson, L., and Gustafson, L. (1997). Somatostatin and neuropeptide Y in cerebrospinal fluid: correlations with severity of disease and clinical signs in Alzheimer's disease and frontotemporal dementia. *Dementia and Geriatric Cognitive Disorders*, **8**, 232–239.

Mintzer, J.E. (2001). Underlying mechanisms of psychosis and aggression in patients with Alzheimer's disease. *Journal of Clinical Psychiatry*, **62**(Suppl. 21), 23–25.

Molina, J.A., Gomez, P., Vargas, C. *et al.* (2005). Neurotransmitter amino acid in cerebrospinal fluid of patients with dementia with Lewy bodies. *Journal of Neural Transmission*, **112**, 557–563.

Moretti, R., Torre, P., Antonello, R.M., Cazzato, G., and Bava, A. (2003). Frontotemporal dementia: paroxetine as a possible treatment of behavior symptoms. A randomized, controlled, open 14-month study. *European Neurology*, **49**, 13–19.

Morrison, L.D. and Kish, S.J. (1995). Brain polyamine levels are altered in Alzheimer's disease. *Neuroscience Letters*, **197**, 5–8.

Morrison, L.D., Cao, X.C., and Kish, S.J. (1998). Ornithine decarboxylase in human brain: influence of aging, regional distribution, and Alzheimer's disease. *Journal of Neurochemistry*, **71**, 288–294.

Mossner, R., Schmitt, A., Syagailo, Y., Gerlach, M., Riederer, P., and Lesch, K.P. (2000). The serotonin transporter in Alzheimer's and Parkinson's disease. *Journal of Neural Transmission Supplement*, **60**, 345–350.

Muir, K.W. (2006). Glutamate-based therapeutic approaches: clinical trials with NMDA antagonists. *Current Opinion in Pharmacology*, **6**, 53–60.

Mulugeta, E., Karlsson, E., Islam, A. *et al.* (2003). Loss of muscarinic M4 receptors in hippocampus of Alzheimer patients. *Brain Research*, **960**, 259–262.

Nacmias, B., Tedde, A., Forleo, P. *et al.* (2001a). Association between 5-HT2A receptor polymorphism and psychotic symptoms in Alzheimer's disease. *Biological Psychiatry*, **50**, 472–475.

Nacmias, B., Tedde, A., Forleo, P. *et al.* (2001b). Psychosis, serotonin receptor polymorphism and Alzheimer's disease. *Archives of Gerontology & Geriatrics*, **33**(Suppl.), 279–283.

Nagaoka, S., Arai, H., Iwamoto, N. *et al.* (1995). A juvenile case of frontotemporal dementia: neurochemical and neuropathological investigations. *Progress in Neuro-Psychopharmacology and Biological Psychiatry*, **19**, 1251–1261.

Nordberg, A. (1992). Neuroreceptor changes in Alzheimer disease. *Cerebrovascular and Brain Metabolism Reviews*, **4**, 303–328.

Nordberg, A. (2006). Mechanisms behind the neuroprotective actions of cholinesterase inhibitors in Alzheimer disease. *Alzheimer Disease and Associated Disorders*, **20**, S12–18.

O'Brien, J.T., Paling, S., Barber, R. *et al.* (2001). Progressive brain atrophy on serial MRI in dementia with Lewy bodies, AD, and vascular dementia. *Neurology*, **56**, 1386–1388.

O'Brien, J.T.D.M.M., Colloby, S.M., Fenwick, J.P. *et al.* (2004). Dopamine transporter loss visualized with FP-CIT SPECT in the differential diagnosis of dementia with Lewy bodies. *Archives of Neurology*, **61**, 919–925.

Odawara, T., Shiozaki, K., Iseki, E., Hino, H., and Kosaka, K. (2003). Alterations of muscarinic acetylcholine receptors in atypical Pick's disease without Pick bodies. *Journal of Neurology, Neurosurgery and Psychiatry*, **74**, 965–967.

Ohara, K., Kondo, N., and Ohara, K. (1998). Changes of monoamines in post-mortem brains from patients with diffuse Lewy body disease. *Progress in Neuro-Psychopharmacology and Biological Psychiatry*, **22**, 311–317.

Penney, J.B., Maragos, W.F., Greenamyre, J.T., Debowey, D.L., Hollingsworth, Z., and Young, A.B. (1990). Excitatory amino acid binding sites in the hippocampal region of Alzheimer's disease and other dementias. *Journal of Neurology, Neurosurgery and Psychiatry*, **53**, 314–320.

Perry, E.K., Tomlinson, B.E., Blessed, G., Bergmann, K., Gibson, P.H., and Perry, R.H. (1978). Correlation of cholinergic abnormalities with senile plaques and mental test scores in senile dementia. *British Medical Journal*, **2**, 1457–1459.

Perry, E.K., Curtis, M., Dick, D.J. *et al.* (1985). Cholinergic correlates of cognitive impairment in Parkinson's disease: comparisons with Alzheimer's disease. *Journal of Neurology, Neurosurgery and Psychiatry*, **48**, 413–421.

Perry, E.K., Kerwin, J., Perry, R.H., Irving, D., Blessed, G., and Fairbairn, A. (1990a). Cerebral cholinergic activity is related to the incidence of visual hallucinations in senile dementia of Lewy body type. *Dementia*, **1**, 2–4.

Perry, E.K., Marshall, E., Kerwin, J. *et al.* (1990b). Evidence of a monoaminergic-cholinergic imbalance related to visual hallucinations in Lewy body dementia. *Journal of Neurochemistry*, **55**, 1454–1456.

Perry, E.K., Marshall, E., Perry, R.H. *et al.* (1990c). Cholinergic and dopaminergic activities in senile dementia of Lewy body type. *Alzheimer Disease and Associated Disorders*, **4**, 87–95.

Perry, E.K., Smith, C.J., Court, J.A., and Perry, R.H. (1990d). Cholinergic nicotinic and muscarinic receptors in dementia of Alzheimer, Parkinson and Lewy body types. *Journal of Neural Transmission – Parkinson's Disease and Dementia Section*, **2**, 149–158.

Perry, E.K., Marshall, E., Thompson, P. *et al.* (1993). Monoaminergic activities in Lewy body dementia: relation to hallucinosis and extrapyramidal features. *Journal of Neural Transmission – Parkinson's Disease and Dementia Section*, **6**, 167–177.

Perry, E.K., Morris, C.M., Court, J.A. *et al.* (1995). Alteration in nicotine binding sites in Parkinson's disease, Lewy body dementia and Alzheimer's disease: possible index of early neuropathology. *Neuroscience*, **64**, 385–395.

Perry, E., Court, J., Goodchild, R. *et al.* (1998). Clinical neurochemistry: developments in dementia research based on brain bank material. *Journal of Neural Transmission*, **105**, 915–933.

Perry, E., Walker, M., Grace, J., and Perry, R. (1999). Acetylcholine in mind: a neurotransmitter correlate of consciousness? *Trends in Neurosciences*, **22**, 273–280.

Perry, E.K., Kilford, L., Lees, A.J., Burn, D.J., and Perry, R.H. (2003). Increased Alzheimer pathology in Parkinson's disease related to antimuscarinic drugs. *Annals of Neurology*, **54**, 235–238.

Perry, E., Ziabreva, I., Perry, R., Aarsland, D., and Ballard, C. (2005). Absence of cholinergic deficits in 'pure' vascular dementia. *Neurology*, **64**, 132–133.

Perry, R.H., Irving, D., Blessed, G., Fairbairn, A., and Perry, E.K. (1990). Senile dementia of Lewy body type. A clinically and neuropathologically distinct form of Lewy body dementia in the elderly. *Journal of the Neurological Sciences*, **95**, 119–139.

Piggott, M.A. and Marshall, E.F. (1996). Neurochemical correlates of pathological and iatrogenic extrapyramidal symptoms. In *Dementia with Lewy bodies: clinical, pathological, and treatment issues* (ed. R.H. Perry, I.G. McKeith, and E.K. Perry), pp. 449–467. Cambridge University Press, Cambridge.

Piggott, M.A., Perry, E.K., Marshall, E.F. *et al.* (1998). Nigrostriatal dopaminergic activities in dementia with Lewy bodies in relation to neuroleptic sensitivity: comparisons with Parkinson's disease. *Biological Psychiatry*, **44**, 765–774.

Piggott, M.A., Marshall, E.F., Thomas, N. *et al.* (1999). Striatal dopaminergic markers in dementia with Lewy bodies, Alzheimer's and Parkinson's diseases: rostrocaudal distribution. *Brain*, **122**, 1449–1468.

Piggott, M.A., Owens, J., O'Brien, J. *et al.* (2003). Muscarinic receptors in basal ganglia in dementia with Lewy bodies, Parkinson's disease and Alzheimer's disease. *Journal of Chemical Neuroanatomy*, **25**, 161–173.

Piggott, M.A., Ballard, C.G., Dickinson, H.O., McKeith, I.G., Perry, R.H., and Perry, E.K. (2007). Thalamic D2 receptors in dementia with Lewy bodies, Parkinson's disease, and Parkinson's disease dementia. *International Journal of Neuropsychopharmacology*, **10**(2), 231–244.

Piggott, M.A., Ballard, C.G., Rowan, E., Holmes, C., McKeith, I.G., Jaros, E., Perry, R.H., and Perry, E.K. Selective loss of dopamine D2 receptors in temporal cortex in dementia with Lewy bodies, association with cognitive decline. *Synapse* (in press).

Pimlott, S.L., Piggott, M., Owens, J. *et al.* (2004). Nicotinic acetylcholine receptor distribution in Alzheimer's disease, dementia with Lewy bodies, Parkinson's disease, and vascular dementia: *in vitro* binding study using 5-[(125)I]-a-85380. *Neuropsychopharmacology*, **29**, 108–116.

Procter, A.W., Francis, P.T., Stratmann, G.C., and Bowen, D.M. (1992). Serotonergic pathology is not widespread in Alzheimer patients without prominent aggressive symptoms. *Neurochemical Research*, **17**, 917–922.

Procter, A.W., Qurne, M., and Francis, P.T. (1999). Neurochemical features of frontotemporal dementia. *Dementia and Geriatric Cognitive Disorders*, **10**(Suppl. 1), 80–84.

Ragnarsson, L., Mortensen, M., Dodd, P.R., and Lewis, R.J. (2002). Spermine modulation of the glutamate(NMDA) receptor is differentially responsive to conantokins in normal and Alzheimer's disease human cerebral cortex. *Journal of Neurochemistry*, **81**, 765–779.

Ransmayr, G., Seppi, K., Donnemiller, E. *et al.* (2001). Striatal dopamine transporter function in dementia with Lewy bodies and Parkinson's disease. *European Journal of Nuclear Medicine*, **28**, 1523–1528.

Reid, R.T., Sabbagh, M.N., Corey-Bloom, J., Tiraboschi, P., and Thal, L.J. (2000). Nicotinic receptor losses in dementia with Lewy bodies: comparisons with Alzheimer's disease. *Neurobiology of Aging*, **21**, 741–746.

Reinikainen, K.J., Riekkinen, P.J., Paljarvi, L. *et al.* (1988). Cholinergic deficit in Alzheimer's disease: a study based on CSF and autopsy data. *Neurochemistry Research*, **13**, 135–146.

Rinne, J.O., Laine, M., Kaasinen, V., Norvasuo-Heila, M.K., Nagren, K., and Helenius, H. (2002). Striatal dopamine transporter and extrapyramidal symptoms in frontotemporal dementia. *Neurology*, **58**, 1489–1493.

Rissman, R.A., Mishizen-Eberz, A.J., Carter, T.L. *et al.* (2003). Biochemical analysis of GABA(A) receptor subunits alpha 1, alpha 5, beta 1, beta 2 in the hippocampus of patients with Alzheimer's disease neuropathology. *Neuroscience*, **120**, 695–704.

Rissman, R.A., Bennett, D.A., and Armstrong, D.M. (2004). Subregional analysis of GABA(A) receptor subunit mRNAs in the hippocampus of older persons with and without cognitive impairment. *Journal of Chemical Neuroanatomy*, **28**, 17–25.

Robert, S.J., Zugaza, J.L., Fischmeister, R., Gardier, A.M., and Lezoualc'h, F. (2001). The human serotonin 5-HT4 receptor regulates secretion of non-amyloidogenic precursor protein. *Journal of Biological Chemistry*, **276**, 44881–44888.

Rodriguez-Puertas, R., Pascual, J., Vilaro, T., and Pazos, A. (1997). Autoradiographic distribution of M1, M2, M3, and M4 muscarinic receptor subtypes in Alzheimer's disease. *Synapse*, **26**, 341–350.

Roman, G.C. and Kalaria, R.N. (2006). Vascular determinants of cholinergic deficits in Alzheimer disease and vascular dementia. *Neurobiology of Aging*, **27**, 1769–1785.

Roman, G.C., Wilkinson, D.G., Doody, R.S., Black, S.E., Salloway, S.P., and Schindler, R.J. (2005). Donepezil in vascular dementia: combined analysis of two large-scale clinical trials. *Dementia and Geriatric Cognitive Disorders*, **20**, 338–344.

Samuel, W., Alford, M., Hofstetter, C.R., and Hansen, L. (1997). Dementia with Lewy bodies versus pure Alzheimer disease: differences in cognition, neuropathology, cholinergic dysfunction, and synapse density. *Journal of Neuropathology and Experimental Neurology*, **56**, 499–508.

Scatton, B., Javoy-Agid, F., Rouquier, L., Dubois, B., and Agid, Y. (1983). Reduction of cortical dopamine, noradrenaline, serotonin and their metabolites in Parkinson's disease. *Brain Research*, **275**, 321–328.

Schmitt, H.P. (2005). On the paradox of ion channel blockade and its benefits in the treatment of Alzheimer disease. *Medical Hypotheses*, **65**, 259–265.

Scott, H.L., Pow, D.V., Tannenberg, A.E., and Dodd, P.R. (2002). Aberrant expression of the glutamate transporter excitatory amino acid transporter 1 (EAAT1) in Alzheimer's disease. *Journal of Neuroscience*, **22**, RC206.

Sharp, S.I., Ballard, C.G., Ziabreva, I. et al. Serotonin 1A receptor levels associated with depression in patients with Dementia with Lewy bodies and Parkinson's disease dementia. *American Journal of Geriatric Psychiatry* (submitted).

Shiozaki, K., Iseki, E., Uchiyama, H. *et al.* (1999). Alterations of muscarinic acetylcholine receptor subtypes in diffuse Lewy body disease: relation to Alzheimer's disease. *Journal of Neurology, Neurosurgery and Psychiatry*, **67**, 209–213.

Shiozaki, K., Iseki, E., Hino, H., and Kosaka, K. (2001). Distribution of M1 muscarinic acetylcholine receptors in the hippocampus of patients with Alzheimer's disease and dementia with Lewy bodies-an immunohistochemical study. *Journal of the Neurological Sciences*, **193**, 23–28.

Silva, A.P., Xapelli, S., Grouzmann, E., and Cavadas, C. (2005). The putative neuroprotective role of neuropeptide Y in the central nervous system. *Current Drug Targets CNS Neurological Disorders*, **4**, 331–347.

Smith, C.C., Bowen, D.M., Francis, P.T., Snowden, J.S., and Neary, D. (1985). Putative amino acid transmitters in lumbar cerebrospinal fluid of patients with histologically verified Alzheimer's dementia. *Journal of Neurology, Neurosurgery and Psychiatry*, **48**, 469–471.

Soininen, H., MacDonald, E., Rekonen, M., and Riekkinen, P.J. (1981). Homovanillic acid and 5-hydroxyindoleacetic acid levels in cerebrospinal fluid of patients with senile dementia of Alzheimer type. *Acta Neurologica Scandinavica*, **64**, 101–107.

Sparks, D.L. and Markesbery, W.R. (1991). Altered serotonergic and cholinergic synaptic markers in Pick's disease. *Archives of Neurology*, **48**, 796–799.

Sukonick, D.L., Pollock, B.G., Sweet, R.A. *et al.* (2001). The 5-HTTPR*S/*L polymorphism and aggressive behavior in Alzheimer disease. *Archives of Neurology*, **58**, 1425–1428.

Suzuki, M., Desmond, T.J., Albin, R.L., and Frey, K.A. (2002). Striatal monoaminergic terminals in Lewy body and Alzheimer's dementias. *Annals of Neurology*, **51**, 767–771.

Swartz, J.R., Miller, B.L., Lesser, I.M., and Darby, A.L. (1997). Frontotemporal dementia: treatment response to serotonin selective reuptake inhibitors. *Journal of Clinical Psychiatry*, **58**, 212–216.

Sweet, R.A., Pollock, B.G., Sukonick, D.L. *et al.* (2001). The 5-HTTPR polymorphism confers liability to a combined phenotype of psychotic and aggressive behavior in Alzheimer disease. *International Psychogeriatrics*, **13**, 401–409.

Szot, P., White, S.S., Greenup, J.L., Leverenz, J.B., Peskind, E.R., and Raskind, M.A. (2006). Compensatory changes in the noradrenergic nervous system in the locus ceruleus and hippocampus of postmortem subjects with Alzheimer's disease and dementia with Lewy bodies. *Journal of Neuroscience*, **26**, 467–478.

Taylor, D.L., Jones, F., Kubota, E.S., and Pocock, J.M. (2005). Stimulation of microglial metabotropic glutamate receptor mGlu2 triggers tumor necrosis factor alpha-induced neurotoxicity in concert with microglial-derived Fas ligand. *Journal of Neuroscience*, **25**, 2952–2964.

Teaktong, T., Graham, A., Court, J. *et al.* (2003). Alzheimer's disease is associated with a selective increase in alpha7 nicotinic acetylcholine receptor immunoreactivity in astrocytes. *Glia*, **41**, 207–211.

Teaktong, T., Piggott, M.A., McKeith, I.G., Perry, R.H., Ballard, C., and Perry, E. (2005). Muscarinic M2 and M4 receptors in anterior cingulate cortex: relation to neuropsychiatric symptoms in dementia with Lewy bodies. *Behavioural Brain Research*, **161**, 299–305.

Terry, A.V., Jr and Buccafusco, J.J. (2003). The cholinergic hypothesis of age and Alzheimer's disease-related cognitive deficits: recent challenges and their implications for novel drug development. *Journal of Pharmacology and Experimental Therapeutics*, **306**, 821–827.

Thorns, V., Mallory, M., Hansen, L., and Masliah, E. (1997). Alterations in glutamate receptor 2/3 subunits and amyloid precursor protein expression during the course of Alzheimer's disease and Lewy body variant. *Acta Neuropathologica*, **94**, 539–548.

Tiraboschi, P., Hansen, L.A., Alford, M. *et al.* (2000). Cholinergic dysfunction in diseases with Lewy bodies. *Neurology*, **54**, 407–411.

Tiraboschi, P., Hansen, L.A., Alford, M. *et al.* (2002). Early and widespread cholinergic losses differentiate dementia with Lewy bodies from Alzheimer disease. *Archives of General Psychiatry*, **59**, 946–951.

Tsang, S.W.Y., Lai, M.K.P., Kirvell, S. *et al.* (2006). Impaired coupling of muscarinic M1 receptors to G-proteins in the neocortex is associated with severity of dementia in Alzheimer's disease. *Neurobiology of Aging*, **27**, 1216–1223.

Tyszkiewicz, J.P. and Yan, Z. (2005). beta-Amyloid peptides impair PKC-dependent functions of metabotropic glutamate receptors in prefrontal cortical neurons. *Journal of Neurophysiology*, **93**, 3102–3111.

Ulas, J. and Cotman, C.W. (1997). Decreased expression of N-methyl-D-aspartate receptor 1 messenger RNA in select regions of Alzheimer brain. *Neuroscience*, **79**, 973–982.

Voytko, M.L. (1996). Cognitive functions of the basal forebrain cholinergic system in monkeys: memory or attention? *Behavioural Brain Research*, **75**, 13–25.

Walker, Z., Costa, D.C., Walker, R.W. *et al.* (2004). Striatal dopamine transporter in dementia with Lewy bodies and Parkinson disease: a comparison. *Neurology*, **62**, 1568–1572.

Warren, N.M., Piggott, M.A., Lees, A.J., Perry, E.K., and Burn, D.J. Cortical muscarinic receptors in progressive supranuclear palsy and other dementias. *Journal of Neural Transmission* (submitted).

Warren, N.M., Piggott, M.A., Lees, A.J., and Burn, D.J. (2007). Muscarinic receptors in the thalamus in progressive supranuclear palsy and other neurodegenerative disorders. *Journal of Neuropathology and Experimental Neurology*, **66**, 399–404.

Weinberger, D.R., Gibson, R., Coppola, R. *et al.* (1991). The distribution of cerebral muscarinic acetylcholine receptors in vivo in patients with dementia. A controlled study with 123IQNB and single photon emission computed tomography. *Archives of Neurology*, **48**, 169–176.

Whitehouse, P.J., Price, D.L., Struble, R.G., Clark, A.W., Coyle, J.T., and Delon, M.R. (1982). Alzheimer's disease and senile dementia: loss of neurons in the basal forebrain. *Science*, **215**, 1237–1239.

Wilcock, G.K., Esiri, M.M., Bowen, D.M., and Smith, C.C. (1982). Alzheimer's disease. Correlation of cortical choline acetyltransferase activity with the severity of dementia and histological abnormalities. *Journal of the Neurological Sciences*, **57**, 407–417.

Xuereb, J.H., Perry, E.K., Candy, J.M., Bonham, J.R., Perry, R.H., and Marshall, E. (1990). Parameters of cholinergic neurotransmission in the thalamus in Parkinson's disease and Alzheimer's disease. *Journal of the Neurological Sciences*, **99**, 185–197.

Yang, Y. and Schmitt, H.P. (2001). Frontotemporal dementia: evidence for impairment of ascending serotoninergic but not noradrenergic innervation. Immunocytochemical and quantitative study using a graph method. *Acta Neuropathologica*, **101**, 256–270.

Zaja-Milatovic, S., Keene, C.D., Montine, K.S., Leverenz, J.B., Tsuang, D., and Montine, T.J. (2006). Selective dendritic degeneration of medium spiny neurons in dementia with Lewy bodies *Neurology*, **66**, 1591–1593.

Zaja-Milatovic, S., Milatovic, D., Schantz, A.M. *et al.* (2005). Dendritic degeneration in neostriatal medium spiny neurons in Parkinson disease. *Neurology*, **64**, 545–547.

Zarros, A., Kalopita, K.S., and Tsakiris, S.T. (2005). Serotoninergic impairment and aggressive behavior in Alzheimer's disease. *Acta Neurobiologiae Experimentalis*, **65**, 277–286.

Zweig, R.M., Cardillo, J.E., Cohen, M., Giere, S., and Hedreen, J.C. (1993). The locus ceruleus and dementia in Parkinson's disease. *Neurology*, **43**, 986–991.

# 7

# The genetics and molecular biology of dementia

## Clive Holmes

Over the past 5 years it has become increasingly clear that neurodegenerative diseases that lead to dementia are often characterized by processes that result in the aberrant polymerization of proteins. A proportion of subjects with these diseases develop dementia as a direct result of the presence of mutations or polymorphisms in genes that influence these processes. An understanding of the biological effects of genetic variation is helping to elucidate the mechanisms that exist not only in subjects in whom a genetic aetiology has been determined but also in subjects with no clear familial basis. It is also increasingly clear that the spectrum of diseases that cause dementia, whilst often considered as separate disease entities clinically, have a great deal of overlap in their underlying pathogenesis. This brings hope that successful treatment strategies in one disease area may have beneficial effects in a wide range of neurodegenerative diseases.

## Alzheimer's disease

### Molecular biology

At post mortem Alzheimer's disease (AD) is characterized at the microscopic level by the presence of large numbers of classic (neuritic) senile plaques and neurofibrillary tangles. These pathological changes are associated with neuroinflammation and widespread neuronal cell loss.

### Senile plaques

In AD, senile plaques (SPs) can be broadly classified into two main categories, diffuse and classic (neuritic) plaques:

◆ *Diffuse plaques* are large (10–100 mm) areas of poorly defined beta amyloid (Aβ) deposition, detected using antibodies against Aβ. Diffuse plaques are found in the neocortex of non-demented elderly individuals without any neurofibrillary changes, suggesting that they precede neurofibrillary formation. The hypothesis that Aβ deposition in the form of diffuse plaques is an early event in the pathogenesis of AD has been given support by the lack of association of diffuse plaques with any neuritic change, increased astrocytic activity, and only minimal microglial involvement (Yamaguchi *et al.*, 1988).

◆ *Classical neuritic plaques* are larger (50–200 mm) and most clearly present in more severe AD. They consist of an amyloid core with radiating amyloid fibrils and are associated with a corona of degenerative neuronal cell processes (neurites), glial cell processes, astrocytes, and microglial cells. Neuritic processes are often dystrophic and contain paired helical filaments. Like diffuse plaques, the frequency of classic neuritic plaques does not correlate well with the severity of dementia. This has been interpreted as being because plaque frequency increases with severity up to a maximum point, regardless of plaque type, but then reaches a steady state or even decreases (Thal *et al.*,1997). However, it may be that plaques have a more benign role than has previously been assumed and that soluble Aβ is the more toxic species. Indeed, in support of this hypothesis, soluble Aβ correlates more strongly with dementia severity than plaque counts (McLean *et al.*, 1999).

### Amyloid and amyloid precursor protein

Both diffuse and classical plaques are principally composed of Aβ deposits. Aβ comprises aggregated straight, unbranching 4 kDa protein fibrils of 6–10 nm in length (Glenner *et al.*, 1984). Aβ is heterogeneous in size, between 37 and 43 amino acids in length, but the predominant species found in amyloid plaques is 42 amino acids long (Aβ42) (Iwatsubo *et al.* 1994). *In vitro* structural studies of Aβ using synthetic peptides have demonstrated the spontaneous assembly of Aβ into amyloid-like fibres. Fibrillogenesis is a two-step process involving an initial slow, lag period that reflects the thermodynamic barrier to the formation of a nucleation 'seed' followed by rapid fibril aggregation. Fibril aggregation is modulated by several factors. Thus, the longer forms of Aβ, i.e. Aβ42 or Aβ43 moieties, are considered to be more fibrillogenic and are deposited early in disease compared with the shorter Aβ40. In addition, the interaction with other elements including small metal ions (copper, iron and zinc) and other proteins including proteoglycans (McLaurin *et al.*, 2003) are known to facilitate aggregation.

Aβ peptides are derived from a larger protein called amyloid precursor protein (APP). The precise role of APP is unknown. However, it has been shown that secreted APP exerts neurotrophic and neuroprotective effects, indicating a possible role in learning and memory. In addition, C-terminal fragments of APP are also involved in interactions with a number of proteins including Fe65 (Cao and Sudhof, 2001) that may be involved in the activation of kinesin light chain (Kamal *et al.*, 2000) that may regulate axonal transport (Stokin *et al.*, 2005).

Several APP mRNA isoforms of different amino acid length arise through the alternative splicing of the *APP* gene including APP695, APP751, and APP770. These isoforms differ mainly by the absence (APP695) or presence (APP751 and APP770) of a Kunitz protease inhibitor (KPI) domain. APP695 is expressed almost exclusively in neurons but the longer isoforms are expressed in both neuronal and non-neuronal cells. These various isoforms of APP are modified by various mechanisms including glycosylation, sulphation, and phosphorylation in the endoplasmic reticulum before incorporation as a type-1 integral membrane protein (Caporaso *et al.*, 1992).

APP has a large amino (N)-terminal ectodomain, a single membrane-spanning domain, and a short carboxy (C)-terminal cytoplasmic domain. APP undergoes proteolytic cleavage by α-, β-, and γ-secretase activity to produce Aβ protein of varying lengths (Fig. 7.1). Access to APP by secretases is regulated by the binding of other proteins to APP including apolipoprotein E (ApoE) (Irizarry *et al.*, 2004).

Cleavage of α-secretase is the non-amyloidogenic secretory pathway, cutting the Aβ peptide in half between amino acids 16 and 17 resulting in a soluble fragment (sAPPα) and a membrane-bound C-terminal APP (C83) fragment. Under normal circumstances the α-secretase pathway is the predominant pathway accounting for 95% of APP processing. Cleavage by β-secretase at the N-terminus of Aβ between amino acids 671 and 672 leads to the production of a soluble APP fragment (sAPPβ) and a different membrane-bound C-terminal APP (C99) fragment. Both the C83 and the C99 fragments are targets for γ-secretase. C83 is processed to produce the APP intracellular domain and a 3 kDa protein called P3, whilst processing of C99 produces the APP intracellular domain and Aβ. γ-Secretase cleavage of C99 is not site specific and produces a variety of Aβ fragments between 37 and 43 amino-acids in length, although the major species are the shorter Aβ40 and the longer Aβ42 form (Wang *et al.*, 1996). Finally, the APP intracellular domain is released by a second γ-secretase cleavage at the S3-like recognition site within the transmembrane domain. This secondary γ-secretase cleavage is also non-specific and APP intracellular domains of varying lengths between 48 and 51 amino acids long are produced, although the major species is 50 amino acids long (Gu *et al.*, 2001).

The secretases that process APP come in a variety of different forms. Thus, three proteins have α-secretase activity: ADAM9

(a disintegrin and metalloprotease domain 9), ADAM10 and ADAM17 (also known as tumour necrosis factor-α converting enzyme; TACE) (Asai *et al.*, 2003). α-secretase activity, particularly ADAM17, can be stimulated by phorbol esters and diacyl glycerol via protein kinase C signalling pathways (Gillespie *et al.*, 1992) whilst ADAM10 is stimulated by low cholesterol levels (Kojro *et al.*, 2001) and may be influenced by a low-carbohydrate diet (Wang *et al.*, 2005). Two proteins have β-secretase activity: BACE1 (beta site APP cleaving enzyme 1) and BACE2 (beta site APP cleaving enzyme 2) (Vassar, 2004). High cholesterol levels stimulate β-secretase, increasing the production of Aβ (Refolo *et al.*, 2000).

γ-Secretase belongs to a family of intramembrane-cleaving proteases which carry out intramembrane proteolysis. γ-secretase is composed of at least four components, including the presenilin proteins, nicastrin (NCT) (Yu *et al.*, 2000), anterior-pharynx defective-1 (APH1), and presenilin enhancer-2 (PEN2) (Francis *et al.*, 2002; Goutte *et al.*, 2002). All four of these components are essential for γ-secretase activity. Presenilin appears to represent the catalytic component of γ-secretase (Wolfe, 2002). Two presenilin proteins have been identified, presenilin 1 (PS1) and presenilin 2 (PS2), both having a similar structure with eight transmembrane domains, with PS1 thought to be the major presenilin in γ-secretase (Herreman *et al.*, 1999). The catalytic activity of presenilin is dependent on two conserved aspartyl residues, one found in transmembrane domain six and the other in transmembrane domain seven. These aspartyl residues are required for the pairing (dimerization) of presenilin proteins that is required for γ-secretase activity (Cervantes *et al.*, 2004). A further five presenilin homologues are predicted to exist (Ponting *et al.*, 2002) and, in addition, three APH1 homologues have been identified, designated APH1a, APH1b and APH1c. These data suggests that a number of γ-secretase complexes can be generated incorporating different subunits of APH1 and presenilin (Shirotani *et al.*, 2004). A homocysteine-responsive endoplasmic reticulum protein (Herp) has been identified and found to enhance the γ-secretase activity (Sai *et al.*, 2002) and more recently it has been shown that homocysteic acid results in the accumulation of intracellular and extracellular Aβ42 in neuronal cells (Hasegawa *et al.*, 2005).

In addition to APP, it is important to recognize that γ-secretase processes a number of other targets including Notch proteins (Kopan and Ilagan, 2004). Notch proteins are a family of transmembrane receptors that determine cell fate with the phenotype of Notch knock-out mice being perinatally lethal (Donoviel *et al.*, 1999). Notch and APP compete with each other for processing by γ-secretase (Lleo *et al.*, 2003).

In normal metabolism, Aβ levels are regulated by amyloid-degrading enzymes including insulin-degrading enzyme and neprilysin. Insulin-degrading enzyme (IDE) and neprilysin degrade Aβ monomers, while other proteases cleave fibrillogenic and oligomeric forms. Interestingly, clinical and epidemiological studies have found that type 2 diabetes and hyperinsulinaemia increase the risk of developing AD. IDE degrades both insulin and amylin, peptides related to the pathology of type 2 diabetes, along with Aβ (Biessels and Kappelle, 2005). Thus hyperinsulinaemia found in type 2 diabetes may elevate Aβ through competition of insulin with Aβ for IDE. In addition, extracellular Aβ can be cleared and exported, via lipoprotein-related protein-mediated endocytosis (Kounnas *et al.*, 1995).

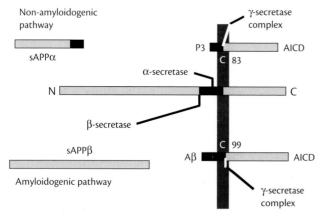

**Fig. 7.1** Amyloid precursor protein processing.

## Neurofibrillary tangles

Neurofibrillary tangles (NFTs) are also a major histological hallmark of AD. Like SPs, they are not specific to AD and occur in normal ageing, as well as in other neurodegenerative diseases including Down's syndrome, post-encephalitic parkinsonism, and frontotemporal lobe dementia with parkinsonism. NFTs are neuronal inclusions, and are composed mainly (95%) of paired helical filaments and a small proportion (5%) of straight filaments. Paired helical filaments have a diameter of 8–20 nm and are formed by two filaments wound round each other with a periodic twist every 18 nm resulting in a typical double helix. Straight filaments lack periodicity and have a diameter of 15 nm (Spillantini and Goedert, 1998). Paired helical filaments are chiefly composed of the microtubule-associated protein tau, which is involved in microtubule assembly and stabilization, and is in a hyperphosphorylated state in NFTs. NFTs also contain other proteins including actin and ubiquitin.

It is increasingly clear that whilst the overall correlation between NFT pathology and ante-mortem cognitive score is good (Riley et al., 2002) there is a degree of individual variability. Thus, some patients in the earliest transentorhinal stage of AD do, in fact, have identifiable memory impairment and some patients with more severe disease (Braak stages IV or higher) may have only mild cognitive impairment ante-mortem. Such variations between individuals may be explained by a number of other factors including age, the presence of cerebral atherosclerosis, and the degree of cerebral atrophy. Alternatively, in an analogous fashion to soluble Aβ and plaque formation, it may be that soluble tau, rather than NFTs, may be responsible for loss of neurons and impaired memory function in AD (Ramsden et al., 2005; SantaCruz et al., 2005; Spires et al., 2006).

## Tau

Tau, the major constituent of NFTs, is extensively spliced to form six isoforms that differ by the presence or absence of a 29 and/or 58 amino acid insert in the N-terminal domain, encoded by exons 2 and 3 on chromosome 17 and by the presence or absence of a 31 amino acid repeat, encoded by exon 10, in the C-terminal domain (Van et al., 2000). The inclusion of the 31 amino acid repeat generates a protein with four microtubule-binding domains, whereas its exclusion produces a protein with three microtubule-binding domains (Fig. 7.2).

Tau is normally located in axons, where it promotes assembly and stabilization of microtubules, and has roles in membrane interactions, enzyme anchoring, and cell transport. Tau is modified post-translationally, and these events affect both its structure and function. Abnormal phosphorylation of tau appears to inhibit the binding of tau to microtubules, leading to aggregation of tau and the formation of NFTs. In AD NFTs are reported to contain all six different isoforms of tau at similar concentrations (Goedert et al., 1992) although PHFs and SFs are formed from different species with PHFs being formed from three repeat tau and SFs from four repeat tau (Spillantini and Goedert, 1998). Tau in PHFs and SFs is abnormally phosphorylated in approximately 20 different sites (Grundke-Iqbal et al., 1986). Most of the phosphorylation sites flank microtubule-binding repeats and half of these have serine/threonine–proline motifs. A number of kinases have been shown to target these motifs, classified as proline-directed kinases, including CamK (Steiner et al., 1990); MAPK (Drewes et al., 1995); GSK3α/β (Hanger et al. 1992), and Cdk5 (Baumann et al., 1993). Of these kinases the two most important for the development of NFTs appear to be GSK3β and Cdk5 (Maccioni et al., 2001). These kinases are themselves regulated by various pathways such as Wnt and insulin signalling.

Whilst most studies support the role of NFTs as being the more toxic species other studies suggest that soluble forms of tau may also have a role. Thus, one study of transgenic mice over-expressing mutant tau has shown that if tau production is turned off then the mice show improvements in cognitive function despite a continued accumulation of NFTs (SantaCruz et al., 2005).

## Inflammation

Inflammation is a well-recognized phenomenon in AD (Mrak and Griffin, 2005). Central to this inflammation are cells of the mononuclear phagocyte lineage, the macrophages and microglia. Microglia are the most numerous of the macrophage populations of the central nervous system (CNS), characterized by their highly branched morphology and down-regulated phenotype. Microglia in the normal, healthy brain are characterized by low or undetectable levels of expression of cell surface antigens such as CD45 and MHC Class I and Class II, thus making these a highly atypical population of mononuclear phagocytes. They are, however, exquisitely sensitive to almost any disturbance of brain homeostasis and rapidly change their morphology and up-regulate expression of a spectrum of cell antigens: they are then referred to as 'activated microglia'. In AD microglia adopt a morphologically activated phenotype with enhanced expression of cell surface antigens.

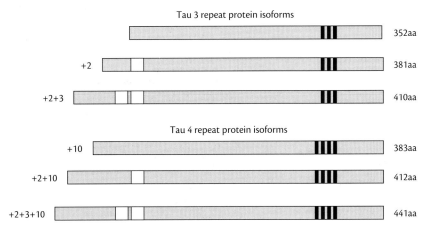

**Fig. 7.2** Tau isoforms (2 = exon 2; 3 = exon 3; 10 = exon 10).

In animal models of AD, microglia are described as morphologically activated and tend to be shown surrounding amyloid plaques, and in particular senile plaques (D'Andrea *et al.*, 2004). Microglia are involved in plaque clearance as shown by both *in vitro* (Frautschy *et al.*, 1998) and *in vivo* studies (Rivest, 2006), but their presence in AD suggests that they are not effectively removed from the brain parenchyma. One possible reason for this is that the microglia are not appropriately or robustly activated and it is therefore important to establish whether the stimulus for microglia activation is amyloid or some other product of neuronal damage, whether either one is an effective activator of microglia (Meda *et al.*, 2001), and whether the chronic exposure to the same stimulus over perhaps weeks or months, down-regulates the response. Though widely referred to as elevated (Mrak and Griffin, 2005), the cytokine profile in models of AD is, in fact, best described as muted. Thus, some investigators have failed to find increases in any pro-inflammatory cytokines (Quinn *et al.*, 2003; Sly *et al.*, 2001) and others reported very modest increases in some cytokines (Sly *et al.*, 2001). Minocycline, a drug widely believed to down-regulate microglial function, exacerbates amyloid deposition in an animal model of AD (Seabrook *et al.*, 2006). Together these data suggest that the pro-inflammatory response to neurodegeneration is kept under tight control, most likely by appropriate anti-inflammatory mediators such as IL-10 and TGF-β1. Indeed there is evidence that apoptotic cell death, such as that seen in a number of neurodegenerative diseases, actively suppresses the microglial synthesis of pro-inflammatory molecules, through display of moieties such as phosphatidylserine on their surface, engaging microglia receptors and inducing synthesis of the anti-inflammatory molecules PGE2 and TGF-β1 (Fadok *et al.*, 2001; De Simone *et al.*, 2003).

### Synaptic dysfunction and neuronal loss

The degree of cognitive impairment in patients with mild cognitive impairment (MCI) shows a significant correlation with degree of synaptic loss (Selkoe, 2002). In addition, subtle alterations of hippocampal synaptic efficacy occur prior to neuronal cell loss with the earliest symptoms of AD correlating with dysfunction of the cholinergic and glutamatergic synapses (Selkoe, 2002).

Neuronal loss in AD is predominantly of the large pyramidal neurons from layers three and five of the neocortex. Neocortical loss is most evident in the temporal and frontal lobes whilst the parietal and occipital lobes are less involved. There is also a substantial loss of large pyramidal neurons in the hippocampus, the nucleus basalis of Meynert, the locus coeruleus, and the raphe nuclei. Notably, whilst this pattern of neuronal loss correlates well with the distribution of tangle-bearing cells, neuronal cell loss exceeds the number of NFTs. This suggests that the tangle-bearing neurons are removed and/or some neurons die without forming tangles.

The death of populations of neurons in the brain regions affected in AD occurs over many years, which suggests that a relatively small number of neurons are dying at any one time. Such a spatiotemporal pattern of cell death is characteristic of a form of programmed cell death called apoptosis and contrasts with necrosis in which cells die *en masse*.

### Genetics

The potential importance of chromosome 21 in the development of AD was initially highlighted by the inevitable and early pathological changes of AD found in subjects with Down's syndrome, all of whom have three copies of chromosome 21 (Mann *et al.*, 1989). However, perhaps the clearest clinical evidence for a genetic contribution to the aetiology of AD is the existence of families in which the disease is transmitted in a clear autosomal dominant pattern and whose clinical features are largely present before the age of 65 years. Linkage studies of one of these large autosomal dominant pedigrees revealed the transmission, from generation to generation, of a single point mutation in the *APP* gene found on chromosome 21 in subjects developing early onset AD. Further studies of these families led to the discovery of other point mutations in the same gene and later to the presence of mutations in two other genes, Presenilin-1 (*PS-1*) and Presenilin-2 (*PS-2*) found on chromosomes 14 and 1, respectively. More recently, it has been shown that duplication of the *APP* gene on chromosome 21 is another determinant of AD (Rovelet-Lecrux *et al.*, 2006). The presence of other early onset AD families without linkage to these identified loci indicates the presence of other loci yet to be identified.

However, whilst familial early onset AD is important in our understanding of the biological mechanisms involved in the aetiology of AD it is important to realize that these loci account for less than 0.1% of the total of all AD cases and the vast majority occur after the age of 65 years with no clear autosomal pattern of inheritance. In these subjects a number of twin studies suggest an important role for genetic risk factors, with a higher pairwise concordance in monozygotic compared with dizygotic twins giving heritability estimates at around 0.6–0.7 (Bergem *et al.*, 1997). Obtaining a clear family history of dementia is often difficult because of the late onset of the condition, but a positive family history of dementia in first-degree relatives is considered to confer an increase in relative risk of between two- and six-fold compared with subjects without a positive family history. There is no consistent mode of inheritance, and both autosomal dominant and recessive inheritance has been proposed (Farrer *et al.*, 2003; Sleegers *et al.*, 2004). Identifying the genetic risk factors for late onset AD has proved to be a difficult task with the only accepted genetic risk factor being the ε4 allele of apolipoprotein E.

### APP mutations

The *APP* gene is located on chromosome 21q21 (Korenberg *et al.*, 1989). The first mutation to be identified was the 'London mutation' V717I which was shown to segregate within a single kindred of autopsy-confirmed AD (Goate *et al.*, 1991). To date, approximately 15 disease-causing mutations have been identified in APP accounting for 5% of autosomal dominant AD with an age of onset from 40 to 60 years of age. APP mutations are located in exons 16 and 17 where they cluster primarily around the major APP cleavage sites, suggesting that these mutations alter the processing of APP. Mutations like the Swedish mutation, close to the β-secretase site are thought to enhance the production of general Aβ levels, while mutations like the Flemish mutation, close to the α-secretase site cause impaired α-secretase activity with an increase in β- and γ-secretase activity, and a consequent increase in secreted Aβ. Mutations like the London mutation, next to the γ-secretase site, lead to a selective increase in the Aβ42 isoform. In addition to coding variants, *APP* promoter polymorphisms have also been identified as possible susceptibility factors for AD (Wavrant-De *et al.*, 1999) (Fig. 7.3).

More recently, it has been shown in French families that duplications of segments of chromosome 21, between 600 kb and 7 Mb in

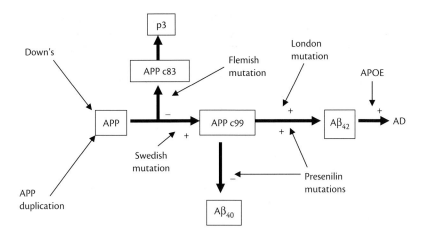

**Fig. 7.3** Genetic variation and pathways for Alzheimer's disease.

length, and all encompassing the *APP* gene, cause β-amyloidopathy (Rovelet-Lecrux *et al.*, 2006). The phenotype of individuals with *APP* duplications is variable, with some having a pure demented phenotype, others having a haemorrhagic phenotype, and others having a mixture of both. This phenotype is similar to that caused by the Flemish mutation in APP (A692G) and is intermediate between that of Dutch amyloid angiopathy (E693Q), in which amyloid deposition along blood vessels causes brain haemorrhage and AD.

### Presenilin mutations

Presenilin-1 protein is a transmembrane protein expressed in many tissues including the brain where it is enriched in neurons. In 1995 Sherrington and colleagues (Sherrington *et al.*, 1995) identified five missense mutations in this gene, later designated *PS1*, that segregate with individuals from families with autosomal dominant early onset AD. To date over 100 different mutations have been found in presenilin-1, which account for around 18–50% of all early onset (usually within the fourth decade) familial AD (Campion *et al.*, 1995; Cruts *et al.*, 1998). A third locus for familial AD was found by identifying a homologue to PS1 that was found to segregate with another well-established early onset AD kindred, formally known as the Volga-German kindred. This gene, with around 80% homology to PS1, was designated as presenilin-2 (Levy-Lahad *et al.*, 1995). PS2 mutations are relatively rare compared with PS1, with fewer than 10 being identified to date. Age of onset in these subjects is more variable with a number of subjects having onset after 65 years.

Mutations within presenilin are mainly found within the transmembrane region and in exon 8. To date, only missense mutations or inframe deletions in the presenilins have been associated with AD. Presenilin-1 mutations do not appear to alter the levels of Aβ40 but instead appear to increase the preferential γ-secretase cleavage at residue 42 increasing levels of Aβ42. PS2 mutations appear to decrease the levels of Aβ40, suggesting a partial loss of function.

### Apolipoprotein E

Linkage analysis of late onset families in 1991 suggested the existence of a susceptibility loci on chromosome 19q13.1–q13.3 (Pericak-Vance *et al.*, 1991). Subsequent association studies showed an increase in the presence of the *APOE* ε4 allele in familial cases compared to controls (Strittmatter *et al.*, 1993).

The *APOE* gene has three allele types, ε2, ε3, and ε4 and the protein isoforms differ in their amino-acids at positions 112 and/or 158: i.e. ε2 (Cys112, Cys158); ε3 (Cys112, Arg158); and ε4 (Arg112, Arg158). The ε4 allele exhibits a dose effect both in increasing risk (Roses *et al.*, 1995) and by decreasing the age of onset. Indeed, early studies indicated that the presence of the *APOE* ε4 allele is associated with an earlier age of onset of late onset AD of approximately 6 years in individuals who carried two copies of the *APOE* ε4 allele compared with non-carriers. This has led to the suggestion that the main reason that the *APOE* ε4 allele is a risk factor for AD is because of this age of onset effect since in old age AD and death are competing risks. Any factor which leads to an earlier age of onset of AD in the elderly (and hence the development of the disease prior to death!) will be associated with AD. Evidence confirming this hypothesis has come from a large study of approximately 5000 individuals (Meyer *et al.*, 1998). This study showed a clear decline in the relative risk of developing late onset AD in all subjects with increasing age but a clear plateau beyond which no further new cases of AD were reported. The age at which this plateau was reached was earlier in carriers of the *APOE* ε4 allele. Thus it appears clear that the *APOE* ε4 allele has its predominant effect by determining when, but not if, an individual develops late onset AD (Meyer *et al.*, 1998) with its greatest effects being between the ages of 60 and 80 years (Farrer *et al.*, 1997). In contrast to the ε4 allele, the *APOE* ε2 allele has a protective effect in late onset familial and sporadic AD (Beyer *et al.*, 2002).

Other studies (Bullido and Valdivieso, 2000) have also suggested an association between a number of polymorphisms within the transcriptional regulatory region of the *APOE* gene and late onset AD that is independent of *APOE* ε4 status. Based on these data it was suggested that there are two independent mechanisms by which the risk of late onset AD can be modified by the *APOE* gene. Firstly, by variations in the coding regions, which alter the functional properties of ApoE and secondly, by the presence of promoter variants which result in quantitative differences in ApoE expression (Artiga *et al.*, 1998). However, this hypothesis is controversial and other studies (Helisalmi *et al.*, 1999; Zurutuza *et al.*, 2000) have failed to lend support to the independence of *APOE* promoter variants in the development of AD.

The mechanism by which ApoE contributes to AD pathogenicity is still speculative. ApoE is synthesized by astrocytes and is the major lipoprotein and the major cholesterol transporter within the CNS. The different isoforms of ApoE have different efficiencies with regard to cholesterol efflux. Thus, ε4 is the least efficient

(Kojro *et al.*, 2001) and this may affect membrane fluidity that may in turn influence Aβ generation (Puglielli *et al.*, 2003). However, in addition to its role in cholesterol metabolism, the ε4 variant of ApoE has also been shown to be less efficient with regards to other pathways that may influence AD pathology, including neurite extension, binding and clearance of Aβ, antioxidant activity, and inhibition of tau phosphorylation by GSK3β (Strittmatter *et al.*, 1993; Yang *et al.*, 1997; Lauderback *et al.*, 2002; Cedazo-Minguez *et al.*, 2003; Dodart *et al.*, 2005). In addition ApoE also binds to a number of receptors including the low-density lipoprotein-related protein (Holtzman *et al.*, 1995) and ApoER2 (Weeber *et al.*, 2002) that have an important role in modulating hippocampal synaptic plasticity and learning.

### Novel genetic risk factors

A number of genetic simulations have indicated that there may be at least another four susceptibility loci for late onset AD, with a magnitude equal to or greater than the *APOE* ε4 allele (Daw *et al.*, 2000). Almost 1000 candidate association studies have been completed, and as a result around 300 candidate genes have been proposed to be risk factors for the development of AD. This includes positive associations with polymorphisms in β-secretase (Kirschling *et al.*, 2003), neprilysin (Clarimon *et al.*, 2003; Helisalmi *et al.*, 2004), insulin-degrading enzyme (Biessels and Kappelle, 2005), nicastrin (Dermaut *et al.*, 2002), angiotensin-converting enzyme (Kehoe *et al.*, 2003), lipoprotein receptor-related protein gene (Kang *et al.*, 1997), and various inflammatory cytokines, e.g. interleukin-1 (Nicoll *et al.*, 2000). Unfortunately, the only consistent finding remains that of *APOE* ε4, originally identified as a positional candidate. The high number of false positive findings found in candidate association studies has led many researchers to question this approach, and as such the focus of attention has switched to the identification of candidate genes through whole-genome scans as a way to identify susceptibility loci and then to focus on positional candidate genes. To date 13 genome scans have been carried out (Bertram and Tanzi, 2004; Lee *et al.*, 2004). The most consistent replications of findings have been on three chromosomes: 9p21, 10q21, and 12p11. These regions include a number of plausible biological candidates, such as *VLDL-r* (Chr9; Christie *et al.*, 1996), insulin-degrading enzyme (*IDE*), *PLAU* (Chr10; Bertram *et al.*, 2000; Finckh *et al.*, 2003), and *A2M*, *LRP* (Chr12; Lambert *et al.*, 1998a; Zappia *et al.*, 2002).

## Aetiological hypotheses of AD

The above description of the various biological processes and genetic changes found in AD stresses the need to establish an aetiological hypothesis that can explain the temporal and spatial relationship between the neuropathological and genetic features of the disease. A number of hypotheses have been put forward that stress a primary pathological event that initiates the rest of the neuropathological and clinical features of the disease. These include hypotheses based on disturbances of calcium homeostasis (LaFerla, 2002); the role of specific pathogens including *Chlamydia* and Herpes simplex (Robinson *et al.*, 2004). However, the current dominant hypothesis is the amyloid cascade hypothesis (Hardy and Higgins, 1992).

### The amyloid cascade hypothesis

This hypothesis initially stated that it was the excessive production of Aβ, and in particular the longer forms of Aβ, that was the key event in a chain of events that leads to the formation of amyloid plaques. The formation of plaques was then considered to initiate the development of the other neurodegenerative features of AD including NFTs; the disruption of synaptic connections; death of tangle-bearing neurons; and the loss of neurotransmitters. However, this hypothesis has undergone some revisions since it was first proposed, and increasing emphasis is now placed on the importance of the oligomers of Aβ rather than the plaques themselves.

Evidence that the accumulation of Aβ is the primary neuropathological insult is largely centred around the overwhelming genetic evidence already described that shows that subjects with mutations in APP or in other gene products (PSs) that process APP develop an early form of AD that is neuropathologically identical to late onset sporadic AD. Further support comes from the finding that Down's syndrome subjects with trisomy 21 and three copies of APP all develop the neuropathological features of AD by the fourth decade of life (Mann *et al.*, 1989) and that transgenic mice with pathogenic mutation of APP or PS have increased levels of amyloid plaques (Hsiao *et al.*, 1996). Furthermore, Aβ appears neurotoxic to cells (Goodman and Mattson, 1994). The mechanism of its neurotoxicity is unclear, but it is likely to have effects on multiple pathways including the activation of microglial cells leading to the production of pro-inflammatory cytokines (Mrak and Griffin, 2005), effects on insulin signalling (Xie *et al.*, 2002), inhibition of Wnt, a family of conserved signalling molecules involved in a plethora of fundamental developmental and cell biological processes (Caricasole *et al.*, 2003), disruption of mitochondrial function (Lustbader *et al.*, 2004), and the formation of ion channels (Kagan *et al.*, 2002). There is increasing evidence to suggest that soluble Aβ rather than its accumulation in plaques may be the more neurotoxic element. Thus, cognitive deficits in mice are caused by oligomeric Aβ assemblies (Westerman *et al.*, 2002; Billings *et al.*, 2005) before Aβ deposition (Arendash *et al.*, 2004) and the injection of isolated soluble Aβ from an amyloid mouse model into healthy rat brains triggers memory problems (Ashe, 2006).

The amyloid cascade hypothesis states that the formation of plaques precedes NFT formation. This is supported by the finding of multiple mutations in tau that lead to the development of frontotemporal dementia characterized by severe tangle pathology but with no amyloid plaque formation (Poorkaj *et al.*, 2001). However, the exact route by which aggregated Aβ results in the development of NFTs is unclear. A number of mechanisms have been proposed. Thus, Aβ inhibits insulin and Wnt pathways that negatively regulate GSK3β and other kinase activity (Caricasole *et al.*, 2003). Increased GSK3β activity is associated with increased phosphorylation of the critical residues of tau, resulting in tau being less able to bind to microtubules rendering the microtubules less stable and more likely to depolymerize. Alternatively, increased GSK3β activity may lead to the increased phosphorylation of kinesin light chains that results in a reduction in the levels of kinesin-1-mediated fast axonal transport (Pigino *et al.*, 2003). Either of these mechanisms lead to critical problems in sustaining axonal transport, and for cytoskeletal structure the loss of microtubule stability is thought to be a key factor in neuronal cell death. Alternatively, as previously stated, Aβ has also been shown to activate microglia leading to the generation of the pro-inflammatory cytokine interleukin-1 which has been hypothesized to have a pivotal role in perpetuating an inflammatory cascade by not only increasing the deposition of Aβ but also by contributing to tau phosphorylation (Griffin *et al.*, 1998). It should be noted that mouse models that over-express APP do not form tangles, and this has led to some question whether Aβ alone is sufficient to cause tangles (Ashe, 2006).

## Vascular dementia

The development of severe vascular dementia is usually the cumulative effect of multiple focal brain lesions with accumulating loss of neurons or axons. Less commonly a severe dementia may arise from a single focal strategic lesion, diffuse anoxic or ischaemic damage, or haemorrhage.

The main reason for cerebrovascular damage is substrate shortage, i.e. an inadequate supply of oxygen due either to failing heart or lung function or to an obstruction from stenosis or the occlusion of blood vessels. Occlusion occurs in the carotid artery, in the circle of Willis and its main vessels including the meningeal main arterial branches (large vessels) and in the intracerebral arteries (small vessels). In larger vessels, emboli and arteriosclerotic changes with thrombosis dominate, resulting in large infarcts, whereas fibrohyaline arteriosclerosis, collagen disease, and hypertensive angiopathy are more common when multiple smaller vessels are occluded, resulting in smaller infarcts.

Multi-infarct dementia is defined as resulting from occlusions of large vessels leading to large infarcts. It has been stated that an infarct size of 100 ml is required to produce dementia (Tomlinson, 1980) although the location and bilaterality are also important. An infarct may also be small and still cause a severe dementia if it is strategically placed. Thus, bilateral thalamic infarcts result in a sudden onset severe dementia with frontal traits. Although less common, the white matter may be most severely affected as in the subcortical sclerosis of Binswanger. In addition, vasculitides such as polyarteritis nodosum, granulomatous arteritis, sarcoidoisis, and rheumatoid arthritis may all be associated with multiple infracts and dementia. CADASIL (cerebral autosomal dominant arteriopathy with subcortical infarcts and leucoencephalopathy) was initially thought to be a rare disorder, but increasing numbers of families have now been identified. It appears to be due to the inheritance of mutations of the NOTCH3 gene located at the chromosome locus 19p13 (Kalaria et al., 2004) and is characterized by the accumulation of electron-dense granules in the media of arterioles. MRI reveals extensive cerebral white matter lesions and subcortical infarcts.

Haemorrhage as a cause of severe dementia is much less common that infarction. A major cause of haemorrhage is amyloid deposition in the walls of vessels affecting primarily the leptomeningeal and cortical vessels (cerebral amyloid angiopathy, CAA). Amyloid deposition increases with increasing age and is particularly prevalent in AD. Thus, severe CAA is associated with many of the genetic and other risk factors for AD. However, CAA can occur in the absence of plaques, as evidenced by hereditary cerebral haemorrhage with amyloidosis–Dutch type caused by a point mutation in APP (E693Q). Although the most common form of CAA is Aβ-CAA, hereditary cerebral haemorrhage with amyloidosis–-Icelandic type is caused by a point mutation in the cystatin C gene that leads to dementia and early onset haemorrhage (Levy et al., 1989).

## Mixed AD and vascular dementia

The proportion of patients with mixed pathology varies according to the strictness of the criteria utilized. Thus, the proportion of cases seen as having mixed dementia may be quoted to be as little as 3–5% (Jellinger, 2002) or up to 60–90% (Kalaria, 2000). Few and small vascular lesions may be of little consequence in themselves. However, there is increasing evidence to show that in combination with AD pathology the severity of the dementia is greater than anticipated from consideration of either pathology in isolation. For example, the Nun Study (Snowdon et al., 1997) found that less Alzheimer pathology was required to produce dementia if cerebrovascular disease is also present.

The biological relationship between vascular and AD pathology is an interesting one that has been highlighted both by the overlap between pathologies in subjects with APP mutations and duplications and by the finding of antibody-mediated damage to the microvasculature in AD in those receiving Aβ vaccination (Gandy and Walker, 2004). Indeed, recent data have confirmed an old view that amyloid plaques have at their centre an angiopathic blood vessel (Miyakawa et al., 1982; Kumar-Singh et al., 2005) and recent evidence shows that amyloid plaques represent the sites of microhaemorrhages (Cullen et al., 2005; Falangola et al., 2005). This has raised the possibility that Aβ may have a damage protection role in response to microhaemorrhages, possibly as an emergency sealant of the vasculature during haemorrhage or by reducing the brain's requirement for oxygen during an ischaemic event by acting as a neuronal depressant (Lambert et al., 1998b).

## Dementia with Lewy bodies

### Molecular biology

Dementia with Lewy bodies (DLB) has a variable burden of Alzheimer-type pathology, together with Lewy bodies in both the cortical and subcortical regions. Given that Alzheimer-type pathology is common in DLB it is not surprising to find CAA in many cases (Wu et al., 1992). However, even when plaque counts are high, DLB cases have mild or insignificant neocortical tau pathology. Lewy bodies are also present in other conditions including Down's syndrome and familial early Alzheimer's disease but are characteristically associated with idiopathic Parkinson's disease (PD).

Ultrastructurally, classical LBs are composed of filamentous and amorphous granular material. The central region contains dense material that lacks discernible detail, while the periphery has radially arranged filaments of 10 nm diameter. Most recently it has been demonstrated that a major component, possibly the core filamentous constituent of subcortical or cortical Lewy bodies is the protein α-synuclein. α-Synuclein is a pre-synaptic protein that exists in two alternatively spliced forms, with no recognizable secondary structures. The mechanism by which α-synuclein leads to DLB is unclear, although it may be due to abnormal interaction with neurofilaments or due to the self-aggregation of α-synuclein in an analogous fashion to tau and tangle formation. In addition to α-synuclein, ubiquitin is present in most classical and cortical LBs (Kuzuhara et al., 1988) and tau protein is also associated with a subset of LBs (Ishizawa et al., 2003).

In addition to Lewy bodies, DLB patients have neuronal degeneration in the substantia nigra that, in terms of severity, is between that seen in PD and normal control individuals of the same age and correlates well with parkinsonism. The mechanism of neuronal loss is unknown, but evidence, like in AD, supports apoptosis. Perhaps surprisingly, given the good correlation between synaptic loss and cognitive decline in AD, synaptic loss in pure DLB does not correlate with cognitive decline in DLB (Hansen et al., 1998) although a number of studies suggest that the density of LBs, particularly in the temporal cortex, does correlate with cognitive decline (Harding and Halliday, 2001).

## Genetics

No clear genetic risk factors have been identified in DLB although several genes have been implicated in familial PD. Mutations in the Iowa PD kindred overlap considerably with DLB (Gwinn-Hardy et al., 2000) and are due to a triplication of the α-synuclein gene. In addition, polymorphisms in the α-synuclein gene that appear to affect expression levels of α-synuclein may also be risk factors for the development of PD (Chiba-Falek et al., 2003). APOE ε4 is over represented in DLB with concurrent AD (Singleton et al., 2002). As shown in other studies (Snowdon, 1997) synergy may occur between the presence of amyloid plaques and LBs. Thus, transgenic mice expressing both α-synuclein and APP develop more LB-like inclusions than mice expressing α-synuclein alone (Masliah et al., 2001).

# Frontotemporal dementia

## Molecular biology

Frontotemporal dementia (FTD) is characterized by cerebral atrophy, principally in the cerebral hemispheres involving mostly the frontal, anterior parietal, cingulate, insular, and temporal regions. All of the variable clinical and pathological phenotypes share, to a greater or lesser degree, a non-Alzheimer-type histological profile. This is characterized by cerebral cortical neuronal loss, gliosis, and microvacuolar change due to shrinkage of nerve cell bodies and their processes. In addition, neuronal inclusions including Pick bodies and neurofibrillary tangles may or may not be present.

Antibodies to the heavy subtype of the neurofilament proteins but also to tau have been found to stain neuronal swellings in the neuropil in FTD (Zhou et al., 1998). Furthermore, ballooned cells (or Pick cells) which are found in FTD have been suggested to be a product of defective axoplasmic transport of neurofilaments (NFs) (Dickson et al., 1986). In one study, the ballooned cells contained phosphorylated epitopes that were immunoreactive to antibodies against the NFs but not against NFTs or Pick bodies (Dickson et al., 1986). Another study found that the ballooned cells also contained alpha B crystallin, a protein that, according to the investigators, was probably involved in the aggregation and remodelling of NFs (Lowe et al., 1992).

### Inflammation

The involvement of autoimmune mechanisms has been suggested for FTD (Marcinkowski, 1996) and increased serum levels of antibodies towards gangliosides have been found in FTD patients (Sjogren et al., 2001) as well as increased levels of TNF-α and TGF-β (Sjogren et al., 2004) suggesting that autoimmune and inflammatory mechanisms are involved in the pathophysiology of FTD. The main question is at what stage of the process these factors come into play; they may be primary events but could also be secondary to other initiating changes, for example mutations or acquired cytoskeleton changes.

### Genetics

Approximately 25–50% of FTD is familial, making the genetic contribution to these diseases substantial (Scarpini et al., 2006).

### Tau

In 1994, an autosomal dominant inherited form of FTD with parkinsonism was linked to chromosome 17q21.2 (Wilhelmsen et al., 1994). This was followed by the identification of other families with the same clinical features (Foster et al., 1997) which were designated as FTD and parkinsonism linked to chromosome 17 (FTDP-17). This hereditary tauopathy affects approximately 200 kindreds and about 600 individuals. The major neuropathological feature of FTDP-17 is a filamentous pathology made of hyperphosphorylated tau and the discovery of coding regions and intronic mutations in these families has confirmed the FTDP-17 locus to be the tau gene (Poorkaj et al., 1998).

Tau mutations in FTDP-17 are either missense, deletion, or silent mutations in the coding regions found in exons 1, 9, 10, 11, 12, or 13 or are mutations in the intron following exon 9 or 10. Most of the missense mutations appear to reduce the ability of tau protein to interact with microtubules, as shown by the reduced ability of mutant tau to promote microtubule assembly. There are some exceptions—thus two missense mutations in exon 10 deviate from this rule (N279K and S305N) in that they don't appear to reduce the ability of tau to promote microtubule assembly. Instead they act more like the intronic mutations and increase splicing of exon 10 (Hasegawa et al., 1999). In addition, two silent mutations in exon 10 (L284L (CTT to CTC) and N296N (AAT to AAC)) are believed to disrupt the exon splicing silencer sequence (D'Souza et al., 1999) and also increase splicing of exon 10. The intronic mutations in tau have their primary effects at the RNA level, resulting in the overproduction of tau isoforms with four microtubule-binding repeats. To date, there are around 40 known tau mutations. Although the frequency of tau mutations is low in sporadic FTD, the tau mutation frequency for affected individuals having a family history of a similar disorder is between 9.4% and 40.5% depending on the study and population examined (Houlden et al., 1999a; Rizzu et al., 1999; Poorkaj et al., 2001).

The morphologies of tau filaments and their isoform compositions appear to be determined by whether they are tau mutations affecting mRNA splicing of exon 10, or whether they are missense mutations located inside or outside exon 10 (Goedert, 1999). Mutations that affect splicing of exon 10 lead to the formation of wide twisted ribbon-like filaments that only contain four-repeat tau isoforms (Yasuda et al., 2000). Mutations within exon 10 that do not affect alternative mRNA splicing lead to the formation of narrow twisted ribbons that contain four-repeat tau isoforms, with a small amount of the most abundant three-repeat isoform (Mirra et al., 1999). Coding region mutations located outside exon 10 lead to tau pathology that is neuronal, without a significant glial component. Some of these mutations (exon 12 V337M and exon 13 R406W) lead to the formation of paired helical and straight filaments that contain all six tau isoforms, and are indistinguishable from those found in AD (Spillantini and Goedert, 1998). Others (exon 13 G389R; exon 9 G272V) produce tau filaments that resemble the characteristics of Pick's disease (Murrell et al., 1999). Thus, depending on the positions of the tau missense mutations, a filamentous tau pathology ensues that resembles either AD or Pick's disease.

The likely effect of the missense mutations is the reduced ability of mutant tau to bind to microtubules, resulting in microtubule destabilization and the consequent effects on axonal transport. Intronic mutations and those mutations in exon 10 that affect splicing of exon 10 lead to an increased ratio of four-repeat tau. Four-repeat tau has a greater ability to interact with microtubules than three-repeat tau (Goedert and Jakes, 1990) and it may be that the correct ratio of three- to four-repeat tau is essential for the normal function of tau.

### Progranulin

Whilst mutations in tau explain some of the inheritance of FTD linked with chromosome 17q21 it was also clear that some FTD families linked with chromosome 17q21 exist that had been extensively examined by genomic sequencing and fluorescent *in situ* hybridization but had no evidence of tau mutations. These patients consistently lacked tau-immunoreactive inclusion pathology and in contrast to the other families with tau mutations had ubiquitin-immunoreactive neuronal cytoplasmic inclusions with characteristic lentiform ubiquitin-immunoreactive intraneuronal inclusions. This research focused attention on other genes in a 19 cM region of chromosome 17q21 (Mackenzie *et al.*, 2006). Recent genetic work (Baker *et al.*, 2006; Cruts *et al.*, 2006) has now shown that null mutations (stop mutations; intronic mutations in splice donor sites and in the initiation codon) leading to a reduced transcription of a gene coding for a secreted growth factor called progranulin appear to be responsible. The progranulin gene is located 1.7 Mb distant from the tau gene and is involved in multiple processes including development, wound repair, and inflammation and has also been strongly linked to tumourigenesis. Interestingly, progranulin is increased in activated microglial cells in many neurodegenerative diseases including AD. The relative importance of this gene in the development of FTD is still being evaluated, but in a Belgian series of familial FTD patients, progranulin mutations were 3.5 times more frequent than mutations in tau, suggesting an important aetiological role (Cruts *et al.*, 2006).

### *PS1*

Whilst most work on PS1 mutations has focused on their role in Aβ processing, mutations in the *PS1* gene have also been found associated with FTD (Amtul *et al.*, 2002; Raux *et al.*, 2000b; Tang-Wai *et al.*, 2002; Dermaut *et al.*, 2005). Raux *et al.* (2000b) reported a PS1 mutation (L113P) in a family with six cases of clinically determined frontotemporal dementia. Two studies have shown that amino acid insertions in codon 352 of PS1 are associated with FTD (insR352 and insA352) (Raux *et al.*, 2000b; Tang-Wai *et al.*, 2002). More recently a G-to-T transversion in exon 6 of the *PS1* gene, resulting in a gly183-to-val substitution has also been implicated in frontotemporal dementia (Dermaut *et al.*, 2005). Four sibs of the proband had the mutation; one was clearly affected and three others showed evidence compatible with cognitive deterioration or early stage cognitive decline. Neuropathological examination of the proband showed tau-immunoreactive Pick bodies without Aβ plaques. It was suggested that the G183V mutation results in a partial loss of function of the presenilin-1 protein. In addition, mutant *PS1* knock-in mice exhibit an acceleration of tau pathology (Tanemura *et al.*, 2006). Thus, presenilin mutations might have a larger role to play in the aggregation of tau than was previously recognized.

### *APOE*

In FTD, the role of *APOE* ε4 has given conflicting results with some studies showing an increase in the ε4 allele frequency in Pick's disease (Farrer *et al.*, 1995), whereas others have found a normal frequency in FTD (Minthon *et al.*, 1997). Some have suggested that homozygosity of ε4 increases the risk for FTD (Stevens *et al.*, 1997) and that inheritance of ε4 lowers the age at onset of FTD in a dose-dependent manner (Farrer *et al.*, 1995). However, in FTDP-17, another investigation found no influence on age at onset for the *APOE* genotype (Houlden *et al.*, 1999b).

### Other genes

In addition to linkage to chromosome 17, linkage studies have also revealed the existence of two other genetically distinct groups of inherited FTD. FTD and motor neuron disease linked to chromosome 9 and FTD linked to chromosome 3 (Ashworth *et al.*, 1999; Hosler *et al.*, 2000; Kovach *et al.*, 2001). Ubiquitin inclusions have been found in FTD with motor neuron disease linked to chromosome 9 and tau inclusions have been found in neurons in families with chromosome 3 linkage, suggesting different genes; however, the genes on chromosome 9 and chromosome 3 remain to be identified. Genetic linkage studies are, however, closing in and more recently two independent linkage studies have narrowed down the linkage region for motor neuron disease to 9p13.2–21.3, a region with 103 known genes (Morita *et al.* 2006; Vance *et al.*, 2006).

## Huntington's disease

### Molecular biology

Huntington's disease (HD) is caused by an abnormal expansion of CAG-encoded polyglutamine repeats in a protein called huntingtin. In HD, expanded polyglutamine fragments, cleaved from their respective full-length proteins, form microscopically visible aggregates in affected individuals (Wellington *et al.*, 1998) and there is a correlation between the threshold for aggregation *in vitro* and the threshold for disease in humans, consistent with the idea that aggregation is related to pathogenesis (Scherzinger *et al.*, 1999; Ross and Poirier, 2004). In parallel to the molecular processes thought to occur in AD, huntingtin intermediates seem to have the major role in aggregate formation and toxicity. Globular and protofibrillar intermediates that form before mature huntingtin fibres appear to be crucial for toxicity. Protein aggregates or inclusions with huntingtin are present in regions of the brain that degenerate, but the neurons with inclusions do not correspond exactly to the neurons that degenerate. Inclusions are more enriched in populations of large interneurons than in medium spiny projection neurons, which are more susceptible to degeneration (Kuemmerle *et al.*, 1999). In addition, inclusion body formation improved survival and led to decreased levels of mutant huntingtin elsewhere in a neuron. Thus, it is possible that inclusion body formation, like amyloid plaques in AD, may function as a coping response to toxic mutant huntingtin (Arrasate *et al.*, 2004). One of the earliest events in the pre-symptomatic and early symptomatic stages of the disease is transcriptional up-regulation of the caspase 1 gene (Ona *et al.*, 1999). Nuclear translocation of N-terminal fragments of mutant huntingtin increases the expression of caspase-1, which may in turn activate caspase-3 and trigger apoptosis (Li *et al.*, 2000). Caspase-1 and -3 cleave huntingtin (Wellington *et al.*, 1998). As the disease progresses, caspase-mediated cleavage of huntingtin therefore increases the generation of huntingtin fragments and depletes wild-type huntingtin, suggesting both toxic effect of fragments and depletion of huntingtin might be responsible for the HD pathogenesis.

## Genetics

At the gene locus (4p16.3) implicated in HD, there are normally 10–29 (median, 18) consecutive repetitions of the CAG triplet that codes for glutamine. In contrast, HD patients have an expanded CAG repeat ranging from 36 to 121 repeats (median, 44). The length of the CAG repeat is inversely correlated with the age of disease onset (Kremer *et al.*, 1994). Therefore, earlier onset disease is associated with more CAG repeats, whereas fewer repeats lead to later onset disease.

## Conclusion

Recent years have seen further advances in our understanding of the genetic and molecular processes underlying a number of diseases that cause dementia. Indeed, research in genetic and molecular biology has already led to innovative treatment approaches based on the manipulation of these proposed aetiological mechanisms. In AD, for example, the next generation of drugs, passive and active immunization with Aβ, and disruption of plaque formation are aimed at the postulated starting points of this disease. These new therapeutic agents have been largely developed as a direct, or indirect, result of the intense study of a few individuals in whom the disease has been inherited in an autosomal dominant pattern. The assumption is that since these processes lead to the same end pathology, that the pathways to this pathology are the same. This assumption is now at the point at which these fundamental assumptions are about to be tested. The outcomes of these studies will need to be weighed carefully since they will have repercussions not only for the treatment of AD but for the adoption of similar strategies based on our knowledge of genetic and molecular biology in other neurodegenerative diseases.

## References

Amtul, Z., Lewis, P.A., Piper, S. *et al.* (2002). A presenilin 1 mutation associated with familial frontotemporal dementia inhibits gamma-secretase cleavage of APP and notch. *Neurobiology of Disease*, 9(2), 269–273.

Arendash, G.W., Garcia, M.F., Costa, D.A., Cracchiolo, J.R., Wefes, I.M., and Potter, H. (2004). Environmental enrichment improves cognition in aged Alzheimer's transgenic mice despite stable beta-amyloid deposition. *Neuroreport*, 15(11), 1751–1754.

Arrasate, M., Mitra, S., Schweitzer, E.S., Segal, M.R., and Finkbeiner, S. (2004). Inclusion body formation reduces levels of mutant huntingtin and the risk of neuronal death. *Nature*, 431(7010), 805–810.

Artiga, M.J., Bullido, M.J., Frank, A. *et al.* (1998). Risk for Alzheimer's disease correlates with transcriptional activity of the APOE gene. *Human Molecular Genetics*, 7(12), 1887–1892.

Asai, M., Hattori, C., Szabo, B. *et al.* (2003). Putative function of ADAM9, ADAM10, and ADAM17 as APP α-secretase. *Biochemical & Biophysical Research Communications*, 301(1), 231–235.

Ashe, K.H. (2006). Molecular basis of memory loss in the Tg2576 mouse model of Alzheimer's disease. *Journal of Alzheimer's Disease*, 9(3, Suppl.), 123–126.

Ashworth, A., Lloyd, S., Brown, J. *et al.* (1999). Molecular genetic characterisation of frontotemporal dementia on chromosome 3. *Dementia and Geriatric Cognitive Disorders*, 10(Suppl. 1), 93–101.

Baker, M., Mackenzie, I.R., Pickering-Brown, S.M. *et al.* (2006). Mutations in progranulin cause tau-negative frontotemporal dementia linked to chromosome 17. *Nature*, 442(7105), 916–919.

Baumann, K., Mandelkow, E.M., Biernat, J., Piwnica-Worms, H., and Mandelkow, E. (1993). Abnormal Alzheimer-like phosphorylation of tau-protein by cyclin-dependent kinases cdk2 and cdk5. *FEBS Letters*, 336(3), 417–424.

Bergem, A.L., Engedal, K., and Kringlen, E. (1997). The role of heredity in late onset Alzheimer disease and vascular dementia. A twin study. *Archives of General Psychiatry*, 54(3), 264–270.

Bertram, L. and Tanzi, R.E. (2004). Alzheimer's disease: one disorder, too many genes?. *Human Molecular Genetics*, 13(Special Issue 1), R135–R141.

Bertram, L., Blacker, D., Mullin, K. *et al.* (2000). Evidence for genetic linkage of Alzheimer's disease to chromosome 10q. *Science*, 290(5500), 2302–2303.

Beyer, K., Lao, J.I., Gomez, M. *et al.* (2002). Identification of a protective allele against Alzheimer disease in the APOE gene promoter. *Neuroreport*, 13(11), 1403–1405.

Biessels, G.J. and Kappelle, L.J. (2005). Increased risk of Alzheimer's disease in Type II diabetes: insulin resistance of the brain or insulin-induced amyloid pathology? *Biochemical Society Transactions*, 33(5), 1041–1044.

Billings, L.M., Oddo, S., Green, K.N., McGaugh, J.L., and LaFerla, F.M. (2005). Intraneuronal Abeta causes the onset of early Alzheimer's disease-related cognitive deficits in transgenic mice.[see comment]. *Neuron*, 45(5), 675–688.

Bullido, M.J. and Valdivieso, F. (2000). Apolipoprotein E gene promoter polymorphisms in Alzheimer's disease. *Microscopy Research and Technique*, 50(4), 261–267.

Campion, D., Flaman, J.M., Brice, A. *et al.* (1995). Mutations of the presenilin I gene in families with early-onset Alzheimer's disease. *Human Molecular Genetics*, 4(12), 2373–2377.

Cao, X. and Sudhof, T.C. (2001). A transcriptionally [correction of transcriptively] active complex of APP with Fe65 and histone acetyltransferase Tip60. *Science*, 293(5527), 115–120.

Caporaso, G.L., Gandy, S.E., Buxbaum, J.D., Ramabhadran, T.V., and Greengard, P. (1992). Protein phosphorylation regulates secretion of Alzheimer beta/A4 amyloid precursor protein. *Proceedings of the National Academy of Sciences USA*, 89(7), 3055–3059.

Caricasole, A., Copani, A., Caruso, A. *et al.* (2003). The Wnt pathway, cell-cycle activation and beta-amyloid: novel therapeutic strategies in Alzheimer's disease?. [Review]. *Trends in Pharmacological Sciences*, 24(5), 233–238.

Cedazo-Minguez, A., Popescu, B.O., Blanco-Millan, J.M. *et al.* (2003). Apolipoprotein E and beta-amyloid (1–42) regulation of glycogen synthase kinase-3beta. *Journal of Neurochemistry*, 87(5), 1152–1164.

Cervantes, S., Saura, C.A., Pomares, E., Gonzalez-Duarte, R., and Marfany, G. (2004). Functional implications of the presenilin dimerization: reconstitution of gamma-secretase activity by assembly of a catalytic site at the dimer interface of two catalytically inactive presenilins. *Journal of Biological Chemistry*, 279(35), 36519–36529.

Chiba-Falek, O., Touchman, J.W., and Nussbaum, R.L. (2003). Functional analysis of intra-allelic variation at NACP-Rep1 in the alpha-synuclein gene. *Human Genetics*, 113(5), 426–431.

Christie, R.H., Chung, H., Rebeck, G.W., Strickland, D., and Hyman, B.T. (1996). Expression of the very low-density lipoprotein receptor (VLDL-r), an apolipoprotein-E receptor, in the central nervous system and in Alzheimer's disease. *Journal of Neuropathology and Experimental Neurology*, 55(4), 491–498.

Clarimon, J., Munoz, F.J., Boada, M. *et al.* (2003). Possible increased risk for Alzheimer's disease associated with neprilysin gene. *Journal of Neural Transmission*, 110(6), 651–657.

Cruts, M., van Duijn, C.M., Backhovens, H. *et al.* (1998). Estimation of the genetic contribution of presenilin-1 and -2 mutations in a population-based study of presenile Alzheimer disease, *Human Molecular Genetics*, 7(1), 43–51.

Cruts, M., Gijselinck, I., van der Zee, J. *et al.* (2006). Null mutations in progranulin cause ubiquitin-positive frontotemporal dementia linked to chromosome 17q21. *Nature Cell Biology*, 442(7105), 920–924.

Cullen, K.M., Kocsi, Z., and Stone, J. (2005). Pericapillary haem-rich deposits: evidence for microhaemorrhages in aging human cerebral cortex. *Journal of Cerebral Blood Flow and Metabolism*, 25(12), 1656–1667.

D'Andrea, M.R., Cole, G.M., and Ard, M.D. (2004). The microglial phagocytic role with specific plaque types in the Alzheimer disease brain. [Review] *Neurobiology of Aging*, **25**(5), 675–683.

D'Souza, I., Poorkaj, P., Hong, M. *et al.* (1999). Missense and silent tau gene mutations cause frontotemporal dementia with parkinsonism-chromosome 17 type, by affecting multiple alternative RNA splicing regulatory elements. *Proceedings of the National Academy of Sciences USA*, **96**(10), 5598–5603.

Daw, E.W., Payami, H., Nemens, E.J. *et al.* (2000). The number of trait loci in late onset Alzheimer disease. *American Journal of Human Genetics*, **66**(1), 196–204.

De Simone, R., Ajmone-Cat, M.A., Tirassa, P., and Minghetti, L. (2003). Apoptotic PC12 cells exposing phosphatidylserine promote the production of anti-inflammatory and neuroprotective molecules by microglial cells, *Journal of Neuropathology and Experimental Neurology*, **62**(2), 208–216.

Dermaut, B., Theuns, J., Sleegers, K. *et al.* (2002). The gene encoding nicastrin, a major gamma-secretase component, modifies risk for familial early-onset Alzheimer disease in a Dutch population-based sample. *American Journal of Human Genetics*, **70**(6), 1568–1574.

Dermaut, B., Kumar-Singh, S., Rademakers, R., Theuns, J., Cruts, M., and van Broeckhoven, C. (2005). Tau is central in the genetic Alzheimer-frontotemporal dementia spectrum. *Trends in Genetics*, **21**(12), 664–672.

Dickson, D.W., Yen, S.H., Suzuki, K.I., Davies, P., Garcia, J.H., and Hirano, A. (1986). Ballooned neurons in select neurodegenerative diseases contain phosphorylated neurofilament epitopes. *Acta Neuropathologica*, **71**(3–4), 216–223.

Dodart, J.C., Marr, R.A., Koistinaho, M. *et al.* (2005). Gene delivery of human apolipoprotein E alters brain Abeta burden in a mouse model of Alzheimer's disease. *Proceedings of the National Academy of Sciences USA*, **102**(4), 1211–1216.

Donoviel, D.B., Hadjantonakis, A.K., Ikeda, M., Zheng, H., Hyslop, P.S., and Bernstein, A. (1999). Mice lacking both presenilin genes exhibit early embryonic patterning defects. *Genes and Development*, **13**(21), 2801–2810.

Drewes, G., Trinczek, B., Illenberger, S. *et al.* (1995). Microtubule-associated protein/microtubule affinity-regulating kinase (p110mark). A novel protein kinase that regulates tau-microtubule interactions and dynamic instability by phosphorylation at the Alzheimer-specific site serine 262. *Journal of Biological Chemistry*, **270**(13), 7679–7688.

Fadok, V.A., De Cathelineau, A., Daleke, D.L., Henson, P.M., and Bratton, D.L. (2001). Loss of phospholipid asymmetry and surface exposure of phosphatidylserine is required for phagocytosis of apoptotic cells by macrophages and fibroblasts. *Journal of Biological Chemistry*, **276**(2), 1071–1077.

Falangola, M.F., Lee, S.P., Nixon, R.A., Duff, K., and Helpern, J.A. (2005). Histological co-localization of iron in Abeta plaques of PS/APP transgenic mice. *Neurochemical Research*, **30**(2), 201–205.

Farrer, L.A., Abraham, C.R., Volicer, L. *et al.* (1995). Allele epsilon 4 of apolipoprotein E shows a dose effect on age at onset of Pick disease. *Experimental Neurology*, **136**(2), 162–170.

Farrer, L.A., Cupples, L.A., Haines, J.L. *et al.* (1997). Effects of age, sex, and ethnicity on the association between apolipoprotein E genotype and Alzheimer disease. A meta-analysis. APOE and Alzheimer Disease Meta Analysis Consortium. *Journal of the American Medical Association*, **278**(16), 1349–1356.

Farrer, L.A., Bowirrat, A., Friedland, R.P., Waraska, K., Korczyn, A.D., and Baldwin, C.T. (2003). Identification of multiple loci for Alzheimer disease in a consanguineous Israeli-Arab community. *Human Molecular Genetics*, **12**(4), 415–422.

Finckh, U., Van, H.K., Muller-Thomsen, T. *et al.* (2003). Association of late onset Alzheimer disease with a genotype of PLAU, the gene encoding urokinase-type plasminogen activator on chromosome 10q22.2. *Neurogenetics*, **4**(4), 213–217.

Foster, N.L., Wilhelmsen, K., Sima, A.A., Jones, M.Z., D'Amato, C.J., and Gilman, S. (1997). Frontotemporal dementia and parkinsonism linked to chromosome 17: a consensus conference. *Annals of Neurology*, **41**(6), 706–715.

Francis, R., McGrath, G., Zhang, J. *et al.* (2002). aph-1 and pen-2 are required for Notch pathway signaling, gamma-secretase cleavage of betaAPP, and presenilin protein accumulation. *Developmental Cell*, **3**(1), 85–97.

Frautschy, S.A., Yang, F., Irrizarry, M. *et al.* (1998). Microglial response to amyloid plaques in APPsw transgenic mice. *American Journal of Pathology*, **152**(1), 307–317.

Gandy, S. and Walker, L. (2004). Toward modeling hemorrhagic and encephalitic complications of Alzheimer amyloid-beta vaccination in nonhuman primates. *Current Opinion in Immunology*, **16**(5), 607–615.

Gillespie, S.L., Golde, T.E., and Younkin, S.G. (1992). Secretory processing of the Alzheimer amyloid beta/A4 protein precursor is increased by protein phosphorylation. *Biochemical and Biophysical Research Communications*, **187**(3), 1285–1290.

Glenner, G.G., Wong, C.W., Quaranta, V., and Eanes, E.D. (1984). The amyloid deposits in Alzheimer's disease: their nature and pathogenesis. *Applied Pathology*, **2**(6), 357–369.

Goate, A., Chartier-Harlin, M.C., Mullan, M. *et al.* (1991). Segregation of a missense mutation in the amyloid precursor protein gene with familial Alzheimer's disease. *Nature*, **349**(6311), 704–706.

Goedert, M. (1999). Filamentous nerve cell inclusions in neurodegenerative diseases: tauopathies and alpha-synucleinopathies. *Philosophical Transactions of the Royal Society B: Biological Sciences*, **354**(1386), 1101–1118.

Goedert, M. and Jakes, R. (1990). Expression of separate isoforms of human tau protein: correlation with the tau pattern in brain and effects on tubulin polymerization. *EMBO Journal*, **9**(13), 4225–4230.

Goedert, M., Spillantini, M.G., Cairns, N.J., and Crowther, R.A. (1992). Tau proteins of Alzheimer paired helical filaments: abnormal phosphorylation of all six brain isoforms. *Neuron*, **8**(1), 159–168.

Goodman, Y. and Mattson, M.P. (1994). Secreted forms of beta-amyloid precursor protein protect hippocampal neurons against amyloid beta-peptide-induced oxidative injury. *Experimental Neurology*, **128**(1), 1–12.

Goutte, C., Tsunozaki, M., Hale, V.A., and Priess, J.R. (2002). APH-1 is a multipass membrane protein essential for the Notch signaling pathway in *Caenorhabditis elegans* embryos. *Proceedings of the National Academy of Sciences USA*, **99**(2), 775–779.

Griffin, W.S., Sheng, J.G., Royston, M.C. *et al.* (1998). Glial-neuronal interactions in Alzheimer's disease: the potential role of a 'cytokine cycle' in disease progression. *Brain Pathology*, **8**(1), 65–72.

Grundke-Iqbal, I., Iqbal, K., Tung, Y.C., Quinlan, M., Wisniewski, H.M., and Binder, L.I. (1986). Abnormal phosphorylation of the microtubule-associated protein tau (tau) in Alzheimer cytoskeletal pathology. *Proceedings of the National Academy of Sciences USA*, **83**(13), 4913–4917.

Gu, Y., Misonou, H., Sato, T., Dohmae, N., Takio, K., and Ihara, Y. (2001). Distinct intramembrane cleavage of the beta-amyloid precursor protein family resembling gamma-secretase-like cleavage of Notch, *Journal of Biological Chemistry*, **276**(38), 35235–35238.

Gwinn-Hardy, K.A., Crook, R., Lincoln, S. *et al.* (2000). A kindred with Parkinson's disease not showing genetic linkage to established loci. *Neurology*, **54**(2), 504–507.

Hanger, D.P., Hughes, K., Woodgett, J.R., Brion, J.P., and Anderton, B.H. (1992). Glycogen synthase kinase-3 induces Alzheimer's disease-like phosphorylation of tau: generation of paired helical filament epitopes and neuronal localisation of the kinase. *Neuroscience Letters*, **147**(1), 58–62.

Hansen, L.A., Daniel, S.E., Wilcock, G.K., and Love, S. (1998). Frontal cortical synaptophysin in Lewy body diseases: relation to Alzheimer's disease and dementia. *Journal of Neurology, Neurosurgery and Psychiatry*, **64**(5), 653–656.

Harding, A.J. and Halliday, G.M. (2001). Cortical Lewy body pathology in the diagnosis of dementia. *Acta Neuropathologica*, **102**(4), 355–363.

Hardy, J. and Higgins, G.A. (1992). Amyloid deposition as the central event in the aetiology of Alzheimer's disease. *Trends in Pharmacological Sciences*, **12**, 383–388.

Hasegawa, M., Smith, M.J., Iijima, M., Tabira, T., and Goedert, M. (1999). FTDP-17 mutations N279K and S305N in tau produce increased splicing of exon 10. *FEBS Letters*, **443**(2), 93–96.

Hasegawa, T., Ukai, W., Jo, D.G. *et al.* (2005). Homocysteic acid induces intraneuronal accumulation of neurotoxic Abeta42: implications for the pathogenesis of Alzheimer's disease. *Journal of Neuroscience Research*, **80**(6), 869–876.

Helisalmi, S., Hiltunen, M., Valonen, P. *et al.* (1999). Promoter polymorphism (-491A/T) in the APOE gene of Finnish Alzheimer's disease patients and control individuals. *Journal of Neurology*, **246**(9), 821–824.

Helisalmi, S., Hiltunen, M., Vepsalainen, S. *et al.* (2004). Polymorphisms in neprilysin gene affect the risk of Alzheimer's disease in Finnish patients. *Journal of Neurology, Neurosurgery and Psychiatry*, **75**(12), 1746–1748.

Herreman, A., Hartmann, D., Annaert, W. *et al.* (1999). Presenilin 2 deficiency causes a mild pulmonary phenotype and no changes in amyloid precursor protein processing but enhances the embryonic lethal phenotype of presenilin 1 deficiency. *Proceedings of the National Academy of Sciences USA*, **96**(21), 11872–11877.

Holtzman, D.M., Pitas, R.E., Kilbridge, J. *et al.* (1995). Low density lipoprotein receptor-related protein mediates apolipoprotein E-dependent neurite outgrowth in a central nervous system-derived neuronal cell line. *Proceedings of the National Academy of Sciences USA*, **92**(21), 9480–9484.

Hosler, B.A., Siddique, T., Sapp, P.C. *et al.* (2000). Linkage of familial amyotrophic lateral sclerosis with frontotemporal dementia to chromosome 9q21-q22. *Journal of the American Medical Association*, **284**(13), 1664–1669.

Houlden, H., Baker, M., Adamson, J. *et al.* (1999a). Frequency of tau mutations in three series of non-Alzheimer's degenerative dementia. *Annals of Neurology*, **46**(2), 243–248.

Houlden, H., Rizzu, P., Stevens, M. *et al.* (1999b). Apolipoprotein E genotype does not affect the age of onset of dementia in families with defined tau mutations. *Neuroscience Letters*, **260**(3), 193–195.

Hsiao, K., Chapman, P., Nilsen, S. *et al.* (1996). Correlative memory deficits, Abeta elevation, and amyloid plaques in transgenic mice. *Science*, **274**(5284), 99–102.

Irizarry, M.C., Deng, A., Lleo, A. *et al.* (2004). Apolipoprotein E modulates gamma-secretase cleavage of the amyloid precursor protein. *Journal of Neurochemistry*, **90**(5), 1132–1143.

Ishizawa, T., Mattila, P., Davies, P., Wang, D., and Dickson, D.W. (2003). Colocalization of tau and alpha-synuclein epitopes in Lewy bodies. *Journal of Neuropathology and Experimental Neurology*, **62**(4), 389–397.

Iwatsubo, T., Odaka, A., Suzuki, N., Mizusawa, H., Nukina, N., and Ihara, Y. (1994). Visualization of A beta 42(43) and A beta 40 in senile plaques with end-specific A beta monoclonals: evidence that an initially deposited species is A beta 42(43). *Neuron*, **13**(1), 45–53.

Jellinger, K.A. (2002). The pathology of ischemic-vascular dementia: an update. *Journal of the Neurological Sciences*, **203–204**, 153–157.

Kagan, B.L., Hirakura, Y., Azimov, R., Azimova, R., and Lin, M.C. (2002). The channel hypothesis of Alzheimer's disease: current status. *Peptides*, **23**(7), 1311–1315.

Kalaria, R.N. (2000). The role of cerebral ischemia in Alzheimer's disease. *Neurobiology of Aging*, **21**(2), 321–330.

Kalaria, R.N., Viitanen, M., Kalimo, H., Dichgans, M., and Tabira, T. (2004). The pathogenesis of CADASIL: an update. *Journal of Neurological Science*, **226**(1–2), 35–39.

Kamal, A., Stokin, G.B., Yang, Z., Xia, C.H., and Goldstein, L.S. (2000). Axonal transport of amyloid precursor protein is mediated by direct binding to the kinesin light chain subunit of kinesin-I. *Neuron*, **28**(2), 449–459.

Kang, D.E., Saitoh, T., Chen, X. *et al.* (1997). Genetic association of the low-density lipoprotein receptor-related protein gene (LRP), an apolipoprotein E receptor, with late onset Alzheimer's disease. *Neurology*, **49**(1), 56–61.

Kehoe, P.G., Katzov, H., Feuk, L. *et al.* (2003). Haplotypes extending across ACE are associated with Alzheimer's disease. *Human Molecular Genetics*, **12**(8), 859–867.

Kirschling, C.M., Kolsch, H., Frahnert, C., Rao, M.L., Maier, W., and Heun, R. (2003). Polymorphism in the BACE gene influences the risk for Alzheimer's disease. *Neuroreport*, **14**(9), 1243–1246.

Kojro, E., Gimpl, G., Lammich, S., Marz, W., and Fahrenholz, F. (2001). Low cholesterol stimulates the nonamyloidogenic pathway by its effect on the alpha-secretase ADAM 10. *Proceedings of the National Academy of Sciences USA*, **98**(10), 5815–5820.

Kopan, R. and Ilagan, M.X. (2004). Gamma-secretase: proteasome of the membrane?, *Nature Reviews Molecular Cell Biology*, **5**(6), 499–504.

Korenberg, J.R., Pulst, S.M., Neve, R.L., and West, R. (1989). The Alzheimer amyloid precursor protein maps to human chromosome 21 bands q21.105-q21.05. *Genomics*, **5**(1), 124–127.

Kounnas, M.Z., Moir, R.D., Rebeck, G.W. *et al.* (1995). LDL receptor-related protein, a multifunctional ApoE receptor, binds secreted beta-amyloid precursor protein and mediates its degradation. *Cell*, **82**(2), 331–340.

Kovach, M.J., Waggoner, B., Leal, S.M. *et al.* (2001). Clinical delineation and localization to chromosome 9p13.3-p12 of a unique dominant disorder in four families: hereditary inclusion body myopathy, Paget disease of bone, and frontotemporal dementia. *Molecular Genetics and Metabolism*, **74**(4), 458–475.

Kremer, B., Goldberg, P., Andrew, S.E. *et al.* (1994). A worldwide study of the Huntington's disease mutation. The sensitivity and specificity of measuring CAG repeats. *New England Journal of Medicine*, **330**(20), 1401–1406.

Kuemmerle, S., Gutekunst, C.A., Klein, A.M. *et al.* (1999). Huntington aggregates may not predict neuronal death in Huntington's disease. *Annals of Neurology*, **46**(6), 842–849.

Kumar-Singh, S., Pirici, D., McGowan, E. *et al.* (2005). Dense-core plaques in Tg2576 and PSAPP mouse models of Alzheimer's disease are centered on vessel walls. *American Journal of Pathology*, **167**(2), 527–543.

Kuzuhara, S., Mori, H., Izumiyama, N., Yoshimura, M., and Ihara, Y. (1988). Lewy bodies are ubiquitinated. A light and electron microscopic immunocytochemical study. *Acta Neuropathologica*, **75**(4), 345–353.

LaFerla, F.M. (2002). Calcium dyshomeostasis and intracellular signalling in Alzheimer's disease, *Nature Reviews Neuroscience*, **3**(11), 862–872.

Lambert, J.C., Wavrant-De, V.F., Amouyel, P., and Chartier-Harlin, M.C. (1998a). Association at LRP gene locus with sporadic late onset Alzheimer's disease. *Lancet*, **351**(9118), 1787–1788.

Lambert, M.P., Barlow, A.K., Chromy, B.A. *et al.* (1998b). Diffusible, nonfibrillar ligands derived from Abeta1–42 are potent central nervous system neurotoxins. *Proceedings of the National Academy of Sciences USA*, **95**(11), 6448–6453.

Lauderback, C.M., Kanski, J., Hackett, J.M., Maeda, N., Kindy, M.S., and Butterfield, D.A. (2002). Apolipoprotein E modulates Alzheimer's Abeta(1–42)-induced oxidative damage to synaptosomes in an allele-specific manner. *Brain Research*, **924**(1), 90–97.

Lee, J.H., Mayeux, R., Mayo, D. *et al.* (2004). Fine mapping of 10q and 18q for familial Alzheimer's disease in Caribbean Hispanics. *Molecular Psychiatry*, **9**(11), 1042–1051.

Levy, E., Lopez-Otin, C., Ghiso, J., Geltner, D., and Frangione, B. (1989). Stroke in Icelandic patients with hereditary amyloid angiopathy is related to a mutation in the cystatin C gene, an inhibitor of cysteine proteases. *Journal of Experimental Medicine*, **169**(5), 1771–1778.

Levy-Lahad, E., Wijsman, E.M., Nemens, E. *et al.* (1995). A familial Alzheimer's disease locus on chromosome 1. *Science*, **269**(5226), 970–973.

Li, S.H., Lam, S., Cheng, A.L., and Li, X.J. (2000). Intranuclear huntingtin increases the expression of caspase-1 and induces apoptosis. *Human Molecular Genetics*, **9**(19), 2859–2867.

Lleo, A., Berezovska, O., Ramdya, P. *et al.* (2003). Notch1 competes with the amyloid precursor protein for gamma-secretase and down-regulates presenilin-1 gene expression. *Journal of Biological Chemistry*, **278**(48), 47370–47375.

Lowe, J., Errington, D.R., Lennox, G. *et al.* (1992). Ballooned neurons in several neurodegenerative diseases and stroke contain alpha B crystallin. *Neuropathology and Applied Neurobiology*, **18**(4), 341–350.

Lustbader, J.W., Cirilli, M., Lin, C. *et al.* (2004). ABAD directly links Abeta to mitochondrial toxicity in Alzheimer's disease. *Science*, **304**(5669), 448–452.

Maccioni, R.B., Munoz, J.P., and Barbeito, L. (2001). The molecular bases of Alzheimer's disease and other neurodegenerative disorders. *Archives of Medical Research*, **32**(5), 367–381.

Mackenzie, I.R., Baker, M., West, G. *et al.* (2006). A family with tau-negative frontotemporal dementia and neuronal intranuclear inclusions linked to chromosome 17, *Brain*, **129**(4), 853–867.

McLaurin, J., Go, M., and Kosaka, K. (2003). Factors regulating amyloid-b fibril formation and their potential for therapeutic intervention in plaque deposition. In *Alzheimer's disease and related disorders: recent advances*, pp. 541–547. 'Ana Aslan' International Academy of Aging, Bucharest.

McLean, C.A., Cherny, R.A., Fraser, F.W. *et al.* (1999). Soluble pool of Abeta amyloid as a determinant of severity of neurodegeneration in Alzheimer's disease. *Annals of Neurology*, **46**(6), 860–866.

Mann, D.M., Brown, A., Prinja, D. *et al.* (1989). An analysis of the morphology of senile plaques in Down's syndrome patients of different ages using immunocytochemical and lectin histochemical techniques. *Neuropathology and Applied Neurobiology*, **15**(4), 317–329.

Marcinkowski, T. (1996). The diseases of Alzheimer and Pick from the viewpoint of prevention, *Medical Hypotheses*, **46**(3), 180–182.

Masliah, E., Rockenstein, E., Veinbergs, I. *et al.* (2001). Beta-amyloid peptides enhance alpha-synuclein accumulation and neuronal deficits in a transgenic mouse model linking Alzheimer's disease and Parkinson's disease. *Proceedings of the National Academy of Sciences USA*, **98**(21), 12245–12250.

Meda, L., Baron, P., and Scarlato, G. (2001). Glial activation in Alzheimer's disease: the role of Abeta and its associated proteins. *Neurobiology of Aging*, **22**(6), 885–893.

Meyer, M.R., Tschanz, J.T., Norton, M.C. *et al.* (1998). APOE genotype predicts when–not whether–one is predisposed to develop Alzheimer disease. *Nature Genetics*, **19**(4), 321–322.

Minthon, L., Hesse, C., Sjogren, M., Englund, E., Gustafson, L., and Blennow, K. (1997). The apolipoprotein E epsilon4 allele frequency is normal in fronto-temporal dementia, but correlates with age at onset of disease. *Neuroscience Letters*, **226**(1), 65–67.

Mirra, S.S., Murrell, J.R., Gearing, M. *et al.* (1999). Tau pathology in a family with dementia and a P301L mutation in tau. *Journal of Neuropathology and Experimental Neurology*, **58**(4), 335–345.

Miyakawa, T., Shimoji, A., Kuramoto, R., and Higuchi, Y. (1982). The relationship between senile plaques and cerebral blood vessels in Alzheimer's disease and senile dementia. Morphological mechanism of senile plaque production. *Virchows Archiv B-Cell Pathology Including Molecular Pathology*, **40**(2), 121–129.

Morita, M., Al-Chalabi, A., Andersen, P.M. *et al.* (2006). A locus on chromosome 9p confers susceptibility to ALS and frontotemporal dementia. *Neurology*, **66**(6), 839–844.

Mrak, R.E. and Griffin, W.S. (2005). Glia and their cytokines in progression of neurodegeneration. [Review] *Neurobiology of Aging*, **26**(3), 349–354.

Murrell, J.R., Spillantini, M.G., Zolo, P. *et al.* (1999). Tau gene mutation G389R causes a tauopathy with abundant pick body-like inclusions and axonal deposits. *Journal of Neuropathology and Experimental Neurology*, **58**(12), 1207–1226.

Nicoll, J.A., Mrak, R.E., Graham, D.I. *et al.* (2000). Association of interleukin-1 gene polymorphisms with Alzheimer's disease. *Annals of Neurology*, **47**(3), 365–368.

Ona, V.O., Li, M., Vonsattel, J.P. *et al.* (1999). Inhibition of caspase-1 slows disease progression in a mouse model of Huntington's disease. *Nature*, **399**(6733), 263–267.

Pericak-Vance, M.A., Bebout, J.L., Gaskell, P.C., Jr *et al.* (1991). Linkage studies in familial Alzheimer disease: evidence for chromosome 19 linkage. *American Journal of Human Genetics*, **48**(6), 1034–1050.

Pigino, G., Morfini, G., Pelsman, A., Mattson, M.P., Brady, S.T., and Busciglio, J. (2003). Alzheimer's presenilin 1 mutations impair kinesin-based axonal transport. *Journal of Neuroscience*, **23**(11), 4499–4508.

Ponting, C.P., Hutton, M., Nyborg, A., Baker, M., Jansen, K., and Golde, T.E. (2002). Identification of a novel family of presenilin homologues. *Human Molecular Genetics*, **11**(9), 1037–1044.

Poorkaj, P., Sharma, V., Anderson, L. *et al.* (1998). Missense mutations in the chromosome 14 familial Alzheimer's disease presenilin 1 gene. *Human Mutation*, **11**(3), 216–221.

Poorkaj, P., Grossman, M., Steinbart, E. *et al.* (2001). Frequency of tau gene mutations in familial and sporadic cases of non-Alzheimer dementia. *Archives of Neurology*, **58**(3), 383–387.

Puglielli, L., Tanzi, R.E., and Kovacs, D.M. (2003). Alzheimer's disease: the cholesterol connection. *Nature Neuroscience*, **6**(4), 345–351.

Quinn, J., Montine, T., Morrow, J., Woodward, W.R., Kulhanek, D., and Eckenstein, F. (2003). Inflammation and cerebral amyloidosis are disconnected in an animal model of Alzheimer's disease. *Journal of Neuroimmunology*, **137**(1–2), 32–41.

Ramsden, M., Kotilinek, L., Forster, C. *et al.* (2005). Age-dependent neurofibrillary tangle formation, neuron loss, and memory impairment in a mouse model of human tauopathy (P301L). *Journal of Neuroscience*, **25**(46), 10637–10647.

Raux, G., Gantier, R., Martin, C. *et al.* (2000a). A novel presenilin 1 missense mutation (L153V) segregating with early-onset autosomal dominant Alzheimer's disease. *Human Mutation*, **16**(1), 95.

Raux, G., Gantier, R., Thomas-Anterion, C. *et al.* (2000b). Dementia with prominent frontotemporal features associated with L113P presenilin 1 mutation. *Neurology*, **55**(10), 1577–1578.

Refolo, L.M., Malester, B., LaFrancois, J. *et al.* (2000). Hypercholesterolemia accelerates the Alzheimer's amyloid pathology in a transgenic mouse model. *Neurobiology of Disease*, **7**(4), 321–331.

Riley, K.P., Snowdon, D.A., and Markesbery, W.R. (2002). Alzheimer's neurofibrillary pathology and the spectrum of cognitive function: findings from the Nun Study. *Annals of Neurology*, **51**(5), 567–577.

Rivest, S. (2006). Cannabinoids in microglia: a new trick for immune surveillance and neuroprotection. *Neuron*, **49**(1), 4–8.

Rizzu, P., van Swieten, J.C., Joosse, M. *et al.* (1999). High prevalence of mutations in the microtubule-associated protein tau in a population study of frontotemporal dementia in the Netherlands. *American Journal of Human Genetics*, **64**(2), 414–421.

Robinson, S.R., Dobson, C., and Lyons, J. (2004). Challenges and directions for the pathogen hypothesis of Alzheimer's disease. [Review] *Neurobiology of Aging*, **25**(5), 629–637.

Roses, A.D., Saunders, A.M., Alberts, M.A. *et al.* (1995). Apolipoprotein E E4 allele and risk of dementia. *Journal of the American Medical Association*, **273**(5), 374–375.

Ross, C.A. and Poirier, M.A. (2004). Protein aggregation and neurodegenerative disease. *Nature Medicine*, **10**(Suppl.), S10–S17.

Rovelet-Lecrux, A., Hannequin, D., Raux, G. *et al.* (2006). APP locus duplication causes autosomal dominant early-onset Alzheimer disease with cerebral amyloid angiopathy. *Nature Genetics*, **38**(1), 24–26.

Sai, X., Kawamura, Y., Kokame, K. *et al.* (2002). Endoplasmic reticulum stress-inducible protein, Herp, enhances presenilin-mediated generation of amyloid beta-protein. *Journal of Biological Chemistry*, **277**(15), 12915–12920.

SantaCruz, K., Lewis, J., Spires, T. *et al.* (2005). Tau suppression in a neurodegenerative mouse model improves memory function. *Science*, **309**(5733), 476–481.

Scarpini, E., Galimberti, D., and Bresolin, N. (2006). Genetics and neurobiology of frontotemporal lobar degeneration. *Neurological Science*, **27**(Suppl. 1), S32–S34.

Scherzinger, E., Sittler, A., Schweiger, K. *et al.* (1999). Self-assembly of polyglutamine-containing huntingtin fragments into amyloid-like fibrils: implications for Huntington's disease pathology. *Proceedings of the National Academy of Sciences USA*, **96**(8), 4604–4609.

Seabrook, T.J., Jiang, L., Maier, M., and Lemere, C.A. (2006). Minocycline affects microglia activation, Abeta deposition, and behavior in APP-tg mice. *GLIA*, **53**(7), 776–782.

Selkoe, D.J. (2002). Alzheimer's disease is a synaptic failure. *Science*, **298**(5594), 789–791.

Sherrington, R., Rogaev, E.I., Liang, Y. *et al.* (1995). Cloning of a gene bearing missense mutations in early-onset familial Alzheimer's disease. *Nature*, **375**(6534), 754–760.

Shirotani, K., Edbauer, D., Kostka, M., Steiner, H., and Haass, C. (2004). Immature nicastrin stabilizes APH-1 independent of PEN-2 and presenilin: identification of nicastrin mutants that selectively interact with APH-1. *Journal of Neurochemistry*, **89**(6), 1520–1527.

Singleton, A.B., Wharton, A., O'Brien, K.K. *et al.* (2002). Clinical and neuropathological correlates of apolipoprotein E genotype in dementia with Lewy bodies. *Dementia and Geriatric Cognitive Disorders*, **14**(3–4), 167–175.

Sjogren, M., Blomberg, M., Jonsson, M. *et al.* (2001). Neurofilament protein in cerebrospinal fluid: a marker of white matter changes, *Journal of Neuroscience Research*, **66**(3), 510–516.

Sjogren, M., Folkesson, S., Blennow, K., and Tarkowski, E. (2004). Increased intrathecal inflammatory activity in frontotemporal dementia: pathophysiological implications. *Journal of Neurology, Neurosurgery and Psychiatry*, **75**(8), 1107–1111.

Sleegers, K., Roks, G., Theuns, J. *et al.* (2004). Familial clustering and genetic risk for dementia in a genetically isolated Dutch population. *Brain*, **127**(7), 1641–1649.

Sly, L.M., Krzesicki, R.F., Brashler, J.R. *et al.* (2001). Endogenous brain cytokine mRNA and inflammatory responses to lipopolysaccharide are elevated in the Tg2576 transgenic mouse model of Alzheimer's disease. *Brain Research Bulletin*, **56**(6), 581–588.

Snowdon, D.A. (1997). Aging and Alzheimer's disease: lessons from the Nun Study. *Gerontologist*, **37**(2), 150–156.

Snowdon, D.A., Greiner, L.H., Mortimer, J.A., Riley, K.P., Greiner, P.A., and Markesbery, W.R. (1997). Brain infarction and the clinical expression of Alzheimer disease. The Nun Study. *Journal of the American Medical Association*, **277**(10), 813–817.

Spillantini, M.G. and Goedert, M. (1998). Tau protein pathology in neurodegenerative diseases. *Trends in Neuroscience*, **21**(10), 428–433.

Spires, T.L., Orne, J.D., SantaCruz, K. *et al.* (2006). Region-specific dissociation of neuronal loss and neurofibrillary pathology in a mouse model of tauopathy. *American Journal of Pathology*, **168**(5), 1598–1607.

Steiner, B., Mandelkow, E.M., Biernat, J. *et al.* (1990). Phosphorylation of microtubule-associated protein tau: identification of the site for Ca2(+)-calmodulin dependent kinase and relationship with tau phosphorylation in Alzheimer tangles. *EMBO Journal*, **9**(11), 3539–3544.

Stevens, M., van Duijn, C.M., De Knijff, P. *et al.* (1997). Apolipoprotein E gene and sporadic frontal lobe dementia. *Neurology*, **48**(6), 1526–1529.

Stokin, G.B., Lillo, C., Falzone, T.L. *et al.* (2005). Axonopathy and transport deficits early in the pathogenesis of Alzheimer's disease. *Science*, **307**(5713), 1282–1288.

Strittmatter, W.J., Saunders, A.M., Schmechel, D. *et al.* (1993). Apolipoprotein E: high-avidity binding to beta-amyloid and increased frequency of type 4 allele in late onset familial Alzheimer disease. *Proceedings of the National Academy of Sciences USA*, **90**(5), 1977–1981.

Tanemura, K., Chui, D.H., Fukuda, T. *et al.* (2006). Formation of tau inclusions in knock-in mice with familial Alzheimer disease (FAD) mutation of presenilin 1 (PS1). *Journal of Biological Chemistry*, **281**(8), 5037–5041.

Tang-Wai, D., Lewis, P., Boeve, B. *et al.* (2002). Familial frontotemporal dementia associated with a novel presenilin-1 mutation. *Dementia and Geriatric Cognitive Disorders*, **14**(1), 13–21.

Thal, D.R., Glas, A., and Schneider, W. (1997). Differential pattern of α amyloid, amyloid precursor protein and apolipoprotein E expression in cortical senile plaques. *Acta Neuropathologica*, **94**, 255–265.

Tomlinson, B.E. (1980). The structural and quantitative aspects of dementia. In *Biochemistry of dementia* (ed. P.J. Roberts), pp. 15–52. Wiley, New York.

Van, S.M., Lewis, J., and Hutton, M. (2000). The molecular genetics of the tauopathies. *Experimental Gerontology*, **35**(4), 461–471.

Vance, C., Al-Chalabi, A., Ruddy, D. *et al.* (2006). Familial amyotrophic lateral sclerosis with frontotemporal dementia is linked to a locus on chromosome 9p13.2–21.3. *Brain*, **129**(4), 868–876.

Vassar, R. (2004). BACE1: the beta-secretase enzyme in Alzheimer's disease. *Journal of Molecular Neuroscience*, **23**(1–2), 105–114.

Wang, J., Ho, L., Qin, W. *et al.* (2005). Caloric restriction attenuates beta-amyloid neuropathology in a mouse model of Alzheimer's disease. *FASEB Journal*, **19**(6), 659–661.

Wang, R., Sweeney, D., Gandy, S.E., and Sisodia, S.S. (1996). The profile of soluble amyloid beta protein in cultured cell media. Detection and quantification of amyloid beta protein and variants by immunoprecipitation-mass spectrometry. *Journal of Biological Chemistry*, **271**(50), 31894–31902.

Wavrant-De, V.F., Crook, R., Holmans, P. *et al.* (1999). Genetic variability at the amyloid-beta precursor protein locus may contribute to the risk of late onset Alzheimer's disease. *Neuroscience Letters*, **269**(2), 67–70.

Weeber, E.J., Beffert, U., Jones, C. *et al.* (2002). Reelin and ApoE receptors cooperate to enhance hippocampal synaptic plasticity and learning. *Journal of Biological Chemistry*, **277**(42), 39944–39952.

Wellington, C.L., Ellerby, L.M., Hackam, A.S. *et al.* (1998). Caspase cleavage of gene products associated with triplet expansion disorders generates truncated fragments containing the polyglutamine tract. *Journal of Biological Chemistry*, **273**(15), 9158–9167.

Westerman, M.A., Cooper-Blacketer, D., Mariash, A. *et al.* (2002). The relationship between Abeta and memory in the Tg2576 mouse model of Alzheimer's disease. *Journal of Neuroscience*, **22**(5), 1858–1867.

Wilhelmsen, K.C., Lynch, T., Pavlou, E., Higgins, M., and Nygaard, T.G. (1994). Localization of disinhibition-dementia-parkinsonism-amyotrophy complex to 17q21–22. *American Journal of Human Genetics*, **55**(6), 1159–1165.

Wolfe, M.S. (2002). APP, Notch, and presenilin: molecular pieces in the puzzle of Alzheimer's disease. *International Immunopharmacology*, **2**(13–14), 1919–1929.

Wu, E., Lipton, R.B., and Dickson, D.W. (1992). Amyloid angiopathy in diffuse Lewy body disease. *Neurology*, **42**(11), 2131–2135.

Xie, L., Helmerhorst, E., Taddei, K., Plewright, B., Van, B.W., and Martins, R. (2002). Alzheimer's beta-amyloid peptides compete for insulin binding to the insulin receptor. *Journal of Neuroscience*, **22**(10), RC221.

Yamaguchi, H., Hirai, S., Morimatsu, M., Shoji, M., and Harigaya, Y. (1988). Diffuse type of senile plaques in the brains of Alzheimer-type dementia. *Acta Neuropathologica*, **77**(2), 113–119.

Yang, D.S., Smith, J.D., Zhou, Z., Gandy, S.E., and Martins, R.N. (1997). Characterization of the binding of amyloid-beta peptide to cell culture-derived native apolipoprotein E2, E3, and E4 isoforms and to isoforms from human plasma. *Journal of Neurochemistry*, **68**(2), 721–725.

Yasuda, M., Maeda, S., Kawamata, T. *et al.* (2000). Novel presenilin-1 mutation with widespread cortical amyloid deposition but limited cerebral amyloid angiopathy. *Journal of Neurology, Neurosurgery and Psychiatry*, **68**(2), 220–223.

Yu, G., Nishimura, M., Arawaka, S. *et al.* (2000). Nicastrin modulates presenilin-mediated notch/glp-1 signal transduction and betaAPP processing. *Nature*, **407**(6800), 48–54.

Zappia, M., Cittadella, R., Manna, I. *et al.* (2002). Genetic association of alpha2-macroglobulin polymorphisms with AD in southern Italy. *Neurology*, **59**(5), 756–758.

Zhou, L., Miller, B.L., McDaniel, C.H., Kelly, L., Kim, O.J., and Miller, C.A. (1998). Frontotemporal dementia: neuropil spheroids and presynaptic terminal degeneration. *Annals of Neurology*, **44**(1), 99–109.

Zurutuza, L., Verpillat, P., Raux, G. *et al.* (2000). APOE promoter polymorphisms do not confer independent risk for Alzheimer's disease in a French population. *European Journal of Human Genetics*, **8**(9), 713–716.

# 8

# Psychometry in older persons

## Karen Ritchie

Psychometric assessment involves the quantification of observations of behaviour, cognition, and affect, and as such is an important adjunct to psychogeriatric assessment in both the clinical and research setting. The step from observation to measurement is also important in the contribution it frequently makes to furthering our understanding of a given health problem at a conceptual level. As Blalock (1970) has pointed out 'measurement considerations often enable us to clarify our theoretical thinking and to suggest new variables that should be considered....careful attention to measurement may force a clarification of one's basic concepts and theories'.

This chapter will first consider some of the theoretical issues specific to the psychometric evaluation of elderly populations, and secondly review the use which has been made of psychometric techniques in the evaluation of cognitive disorder in the elderly.

## Conceptual considerations

### Assessment models

Two principal models have governed our conceptualization of mental disorder. On the one hand the dichotomic medical model clearly distinguishes normal fluctuations in mental functioning (e.g. transient feelings of sadness or ageing-associated memory impairment) from psychopathology (e.g. a major depressive episode, dementia). This model construes psychiatric disorder as a disease process whose aetiology is separate from that of 'normal' ageing. Measures based on the medical model refer to pathological behaviours which are not seen in normal populations (for example, aphasia, apraxia, insomnia, hallucinations) and thus clearly differentiate healthy and unhealthy cohorts.

The psychological model, on the other hand, conceptualizes mental functioning in terms of a normal distribution. This model assumes that affective and cognitive problems are to some degree present in all elderly persons; poor mental health being defined in terms of degree of discomfort or a statistically significant deviation from an established norm. Measures based on this model are therefore dimensional rather than categorical and present the problem of determining a suitable cut-off point for 'abnormality'. The determination of an appropriate cut-off point for this type of measure is in part a statistical problem, but also depends on changing social conceptualizations of dysfunction. Increasing emphasis on the quality of life of the elderly and an increasingly optimistic view

of what should constitute the normal health status of the elderly person have undoubtedly led to a lowering of the threshold for what is considered 'acceptable' discomfort.

Given that the biological mechanisms underlying mental disorder are only partially understood (Michels and Marzuk, 1993), diagnosis commonly relies on observations of the non-specific behavioural consequences of mental disorder, which are dimensional rather than categorical variables. The situation thus frequently arises that mental disorders now commonly considered to be discontinuous with normal ageing (for example Alzheimer's disease, major depressive illness) are commonly diagnosed by reference to non-specific dimensional variables such as sadness, motor speed, or memory performance. As a result measures of mental health status in the elderly are often based on both the psychological and medical models. For example, neuropsychological measures of cognitive functioning commonly take the form of dimensional behavioural measures based on the psychological model such as word fluency and visual recall. Such tests also permit the investigator to observe the existence of dichotomous signs indicative of pathology according to the medical model, such as perseveration, dyskinesia, aphasia, and visual field neglect. More recently the development of functional neuroimaging techniques has served to draw together the two approaches by the visualization of the functional anatomical correlates of performance on laboratory tests of cognition in both normal and pathological states (Cabeza and Nyberg, 1997; Nyberg, 1998; Page, 2006).

When developing a measuring instrument for diagnosis or screening of mental disorder in the elderly, some consideration should be given to its underlying conceptual assumptions as these will play an important part in the scoring of items and in assessing validity. In the case of the medical model the power to discriminate may be improved by increasing the number of items relating to disease-specific symptoms and reducing those relating to non-specific symptoms. In the case of measures based on the psychological paradigm adjustment is more commonly required in the cut-off point according to symptom prevalence and severity in the target population. This point is discussed further below in relation to screening instruments.

### The definition of 'normality' in elderly populations

An important consideration in the development of measures of mental functioning in the elderly, irrespective of whether the medical or psychological model is adhered to, is the question of what is 'normal' at a given age. All too often 'normal' performance is taken to be the average performance of an age cohort in which elderly persons with mental disorder have been excluded. This practice has undoubtedly underestimated true normal performance due to the inclusion in the so-called normal group of persons with subclinical pathologies and other conditions likely to mask true ability (notably sensory impairments and coexisting physical illness). Advances in medical technology have also permitted the identification of previously unrecognized pathology in so-called 'normal' elderly brains, for example white matter lesions observed in normal elderly and persons with stable deficits (Breteler *et al.*, 1994; Skoog *et al.*, 1996).

Rapid changes over the last century in environmental factors likely to have an important influence on mental functioning (education, medical care, nutrition, protection from adverse environmental exposure) have given rise to important age-cohort effects. That is younger elderly are likely to have benefited from more favourable conditions than the oldest old—including greater familiarity with questionnaires and psychometric tests. As Schaie (1983) noted for example significant cross-sectional age-group differences in mean performance, but over a 20-year follow-up very little difference in longitudinal change before the 80s. Drawing on the example of cardiovascular disease, Manton and Stallard (1988) have also raised the point that disorders once thought to be an inevitable feature of the ageing process are now being redefined as pathologies '…age criteria are tending to disappear and what is considered to be the normal state for an elderly person is not very different from that of younger adults'. A recent study by Deary *et al.* (2006) associating cognitive tests in the elderly with density of white matter lesions found that this association was significantly modified by IQ at age 11, suggesting that cognitive dysfunction may be erroneously attributed to ageing-related changes rather than inherent ability.

## Measurement issues in geriatric assessment

In developing tests for elderly populations a number of specific problems arise. Perhaps the most important, and yet most neglected, is that of the heterogeneity observed within age cohorts. The performance of children is so highly predictable at a given age that it has been possible to constitute normative developmental scales which rapidly detect social and cognitive delays and abnormalities. With age, however, standard errors on almost all behavioural measures fan out to such an extent that the 'normal' performance of elderly age cohorts is extremely difficult to characterize. This is partly due to inter-individual differences in inherent ability and partly due to interaction with extrinsic factors such as varying general health profiles. This implies that with age normal levels of functioning should be established on increasingly large samples. In most cases the opposite has been the case so that normative data at high ages are usually unreliable.

A second issue, as touched on above, is the problem of the high prevalence of sensory impairment and multiple pathologies in elderly populations and the difficulties inherent in developing measures which are independent of these factors. It is known, for example, that respiratory disorders, which show increasing prevalence with age, may have an important impact on test performance (Grant *et al.*, 1982) as may also medications commonly taken by the elderly,

particularly those with anticholinergic effects (Ancelin *et al.*, 2006). Elderly populations have a high prevalence of sensory impairment. Very few tests have been developed specifically for elderly persons who have visual or auditory problems. The inventive clinician may consider, however, making use of the tactile tests included in child assessment batteries. Unfortunately many of the psychometric measures available for use with the elderly have been validated on 'selected' populations free of impairment and disease (and their validity on the majority of elderly persons who do not fall into this category remains unknown).

A further problem is the high level of illiteracy and low levels of education often found in elderly populations. Education differentials raise two major problems. The first has been the difficulties inherent in the development of 'education fair' measures which do not produce, for example, high false positive rates in the assessment of cognitive deficit in the poorly educated, or false negative rates in elderly persons with high levels of education. A number of statistical techniques have been developed which may assist in the evaluation of item bias such as the use of statistical weighting, using for example a non-parametric or stratified regression method (Kittner *et al.*, 1986), multicomponent latent trait models (MLTM), or item response theory (IRT) (Embretson and Yang, 2006). An example of the application of item response theory to a cognitive test battery is given by Lindeboom *et al.* (2004). The second problem is the question of whether in adjusting for education effects in psychometric tests the researcher is not in fact removing the effects of a true risk factor. This point has been discussed at length in relation to cognitive testing in the elderly by Berkman (1986).

High rates of institutionalization in elderly populations, particularly amongst the oldest old and the socially isolated, raises further difficulties in psychometric assessment. The imposition of institutional regimes makes, for example, the differentiation of aptitude (what the elderly person is actually able to do) from performance (that which he or she habitually does in everyday life) at times rather difficult. This factor is particularly likely to affect measures of the consequences of mental illness such as Activities of Daily Living scales and informant measures of performance. The stress associated with the move to long-term care and the isolated nature of institutional life together may have a significant effect on performance on both affective and cognitive measures. Performance on cognitive tests has been shown to drop significantly immediately after entry into an institution (Wells and Jorm, 1987; Ward *et al.*, 1990; Ritchie and Fuhrer, 1992) with only partial restitution after a 3-month period (Wells and Jorm, 1987). Ward *et al.* (1990) report a mean drop of four points on the Mini-Mental State Examination (Folstein *et al.*, 1975) and Ritchie and Fuhrer (1996) observed that elderly persons with mild senile dementia living in the community performed better on this test than normal elderly living in institutions. The principal difficulty lies in differentiating true changes in mental status which may be due to institutionalization (or to have been the cause of institutionalization) from transient adjustment effects.

A general problem has been that tests used with the elderly are commonly tests developed for use with younger adults. The problem is not only one of content (adapting test materials to older populations) but also lies at a more fundamental level—little thought has been given to the ways in which information processing might evolve at higher ages. Theories of cognitive development are primarily concerned with childhood changes, and it is assumed that cognitive processes once mature in early adolescence do not evolve further. Research in this area is clearly needed in order to determine whether differences between younger and older adults are due to deterioration or adaptive evolution of cognitive processes. For example, small children rely heavily on rote memory which requires no analysis of information content. With age there is an increasing ability to learn by association and condensation; new information is linked with existing information and retained in a summarized form. This permits the retention of larger amounts of information. Interestingly enough, assumptions that elderly people have poorer memories than younger persons is often based on performance on tests of rote recall (for example list learning) rather than précis recall (requesting the subject to retain a summary of a text) on which older persons perform better.

# Psychometric measures of cognitive functioning in the elderly

Interest in the assessment of cognitive functioning in the elderly has undoubtedly been further stimulated by concern on the part of both health planners and clinicians that ageing of the population may be giving rise to what Kramer (1980) has termed a 'rising pandemic of mental disorders and associated chronic diseases and 'disabilities'. For mental health service providers cognitive disorder is costly—not only does the elderly person with cognitive impairment require assistance with activities of daily living, but his or her judgement is also impaired so that assistance may also be required for decision-making. Additionally it has been demonstrated that the caregivers of elderly persons with cognitive disorders have a significantly increased risk of both physical and mental illness (Gilleard et al., 1984; Kiecolt-Glaser et al., 1987).

A large number of tests have appeared in the literature which aim not only to identify cognitive dysfunction in the elderly but also to assess its functional consequences for the purposes of planning care and evaluating the impact of therapeutic intervention. These instruments involve principally the direct examination of the elderly person through questions assessing memory, orientation, language, and visuospatial performance. Given the inherent difficulties involved in requesting autoevaluation from persons with cognitive difficulties, increasing interest has been given in recent years to informant measures which provide information on pre-morbid ability, degree of change over time, and ability to perform activities of daily living.

Within the field of geriatric psychiatry, psychometric evaluation of cognitive functioning has served three principal purposes; screening for cognitive impairment, differential diagnosis of disorders affecting intellectual performance, and evaluation of the consequences of cognitive impairment. Each of these shall be considered in turn. Table 8.1 provides summary information on most of the validated psychometric measures of cognitive performance which have been used with elderly subjects. The table indicates the name of the test, its more commonly known acronym, the country and the language in which it has been developed, and the purpose for which it has been developed. The three principal uses of cognitive measures (screening, diagnosis, and assessment of consequences) are discussed below.

## Screening tests

In medieval Britain the *Prerogativa Regis* (a Crown document later adopted as common law) established tribunals in 1392 for the screening of cognitive impairment in order to ensure protection of the afflicted individual and provide assistance in the management of his financial affairs (Tomlins, 1822). It is interesting to note that this examination consisted of questions to the individual relating to temporal and spatial orientation, memory, calculation, and reasoning. The content is in fact strikingly similar to the many screening tests for dementia in current use.

Screening tests for cognitive impairment in the elderly may generally be divided into three categories: (1) brief mental status examinations consisting of single-item assessments of orientation, memory and reasoning such as the Mini-Mental State Examination (Folstein et al., 1975), the Mental Status Questionnaire (Kahn et al., 1960), and the Abbreviated Mental Test (Qureshi and Hodkinson, 1974); (2) abbreviated neuropsychological batteries designed to target specific cognitive functions known to be affected by dementing disease such as the Iowa battery (Eslinger et al., 1985) and the Memory Impairment Screen (Buschke et al., 1999); and (3) informant tests designed to estimate the degree of cognitive decline from pre-morbid levels of functioning such as the proxy questionnaire from the Blessed Scale (Blessed et al., 1968), DECO (Ritchie and Fuhrer, 1992, 1996), the IQCODE (Jorm and Korten, 1988), and the CAMDEX family interview (Roth et al., 1988).

Preference has generally been given to the first type of test, undoubtedly because of its high face validity, although the other two methods have been found to be equally as discriminative. While formerly considered an adjunct to the clinical examination, informant report has now been demonstrated by a number of researchers to be as highly discriminant in screening for cognitive disorder as direct examination of the elderly person himself or herself, and less subject to education effects (Jorm and Korten, 1988; Ritchie and Fuhrer, 1992, 1996). Informant methods also appear unaffected by institutionalization (Ritchie and Fuhrer, 1992). A combination of informant and cognitive screening tests has been shown to have better discriminability than either method alone (Mackinnon and Mulligan, 1998).

Most screening tests show quite high levels of discriminability in case–control studies which are typically designed with an equal case to non-case ratio, using normal subjects free of likely confounding characteristics, and cases of cognitive impairment which are relatively clear-cut. However, performance on these same tests is seen to drop dramatically when used in the community setting. This is partly due to the fact that prevalence rates of cognitive disorder in the community are much lower than in case–control studies, and the level of cognitive impairment often much milder giving rise to poorer positive and negative predictive values. Brayne and Calloway (1991) have demonstrated for example that the positive predictive value of the Mini-Mental Status examination falls from 89% when the case:non-case ratio is 1:10, to only 59% when it is 1:50. Similarly Ritchie and Fuhrer (1996) observed that the discriminability of an informant questionnaire fell from 90% in a case–control study to 79% in a community study. Weinstein and Fineberg (1980) have pointed out that this problem can to a large extent be overcome by adjustment of the cut-off point of a screening test according to the predicted prevalence of the disease within the target population. A downward adjustment on an informant questionnaire was found by Ritchie and Fuhrer (1996) for example to improve discriminability in the community setting by 10%.

## Diagnostic instruments

Psychometric tests may also be used as an adjunct to differential diagnosis of disorders responsible for cognitive impairment in the elderly.

**Table 8.1** Psychometric tests developed for the assessment of cognitive performance in the elderly. The tests are classified according to function: screening of cognitive disorder (SC), assessment of a specific cognitive function (S), differential diagnosis (D), assessment of the impact of therapeutic intervention (T), estimation of pre-morbid intelligence level (P), or for the evaluation of the consequences of cognitive disorder (C)

| Test name | Author | Country | Function |
|---|---|---|---|
| AD8 Informant Interview | Galvin *et al.* (2005) | USA | SC |
| Alzheimer Disease Assessment Scale (ADAS) | Rosen *et al.* (1984) | USA | T |
| Amsterdam Dementia Screening Test (ADS) | De Jonghe *et al.* (1994) | Holland | SC |
| Alters Konzentrations Test (AKT) | Geiger-Kabisch *et al.* (1993) | Germany | SC |
| Behaviour Dyscontrol Scale (BDS) | Grigsby *et al.* (1992) | UK | S |
| Behavioral Pathology in AD (Behave-AD) | Harwood *et al.* (1998) | USA | C |
| Behavioral and Emotional Activities in Dementia | Sinha *et al.* (1992) | USA | T, C |
| Cognitive Abilities Screening Instrument (CASI) | Liu *et al.* (1994) | China | S |
| Canberra Interview for the Elderly (CIE) | Henderson *et al.* (1994) | Australia | D |
| Clock Drawing Test (CDT) | Ainslie and Murden (1993) | USA | SC |
| Cambridge Contextual Reading Test (CCRT) | Beardsall and Huppert (1994) | UK | P |
| Cognitive Performance Test (CPT) | Burns *et al.* (1994) | USA | C |
| CERAD Neuropsychological Battery | Welsh *et al.* (1994) | USA | D |
| Cognitive Screening Test (CST) | Ponds *et al.* (1992) | Holland | SC |
| Computerized Neuropsychological Test Battery (CNTB) | Veroff *et al.* (1991) | USA | C |
| Clifton Assessment Scale (CAPE) | Clarke *et al.* (1991) | UK | C |
| Cambridge Exam. for Mental Disorders (CAMDEX) | Roth *et al.* (1988) | UK | C, D |
| CAMDEX-N (Dutch version) | Neri *et al.* (1994) | UK | C, D |
| Dementia Rating Scale (DRS) | Rosser and Hodges (1994) | UK | C, D |
| Structural Interview for the Diagnosis of Alzheimer's Type and Multiinfarct Dementias (ENEDAM) | Morinigo *et al.* (1990) | Spain | D |
| Détérioration Cognitive Observée (DECO) | Ritchie and Fuhrer (1992) | France | SC |
| East Boston Memory (EBMT) | Albert *et al.* (1991) | USA | S, C |
| Extended Scale for Dementia (ESD) | Helmes *et al.* (1992) | Canada | C, D |
| Functional Assessment Staging (FAST) | Sclan and Reisberg (1992) | USA | S, C |
| Gedragsobservatieschool-geriatrie (GOS-G) | Gorissen (1994) | Holland | D |
| GPCOG Dementia in General Practice | Brodaty *et al.* (2002) | Australia | SC |
| Guy Advanced Dementia Schedule (Guy-ADS) | Ward *et al.* (1993) | UK | D, S |
| Global Deterioration Scale (GDS) | Eisdorfer *et al.* (1992) | USA | D, C |
| Hierarchic Dementia Scale (HDS) | Ronnberg and Ericsson (1994) | Sweden | D, C |
| Hasegawa Dementia Scale (HDS) | Gao (1991) | China | SC |
| Hierarchic Dementia Scale | Cole and Dastoor (1996) | Canada | SC |
| Hodkinson Test | Gomez de Caso (1994) | | D, C |
| Hodkinson Abbreviated Mental test | Rocca *et al.* (1992) | Italy | C, S |
| Informant Questionnaire on Cognitive Decline in the Elderly (IQCODE) | Jorm *et al.* (1991) | Australia | D, SC |
| Iowa Screening Test | Eslinger *et al.* (1985) | USA | S, SC |
| London Psychogeriatric Rating Scale (LPRS) | Reid *et al.* (1991) | UK | SC |
| Mattis Dementia Rating Scale | Coblentz (1973) | UK | SC |
| Mental Status Questionnaire (MSQ) | Kahn *et al.* (1960) | USA | SC |
| Mini-Mental State Examination (MMSE) | Folstein *et al.* (1975) | USA | SC |
| Mini-Object Test | Still *et al.* (1983) | USA | SC |
| Mémoire de Prose | Capitani *et al.* (1994) | Italy | C |
| Memory Impairment Screen (MIS) | Buschke *et al.* (1999) | USA | SC |
| Modified Ordinal Scales for Psychological Development (M-OSPD) | Auer and Reisberg (1996) | USA | C |
| N-ADL | Nishimura *et al.* (1993) | Japan | C |
| NM Scale | Nishimura *et al.* (1993) | Japan | C |
| National Adult Reading Test (NART) | Nelson (1982) | UK | P, C |
| Nurse's Observation Scale for Geriatric Patients (NOSGER) | Tremmel and Spiegel (1993) | UK | D, C |
| Nürnberg Alters Inventar (NAI) | Pek (1991) | Hungary | C, T |
| Neuropsychiatric Inventory (NPI) | Cummings *et al.* (1994) | USA | D |
| Observation Psycho Geriatrics (OPG) | Duine (1991) | Holland | C |
| Qualitative Evaluation of Dementia (QED) | Royall and Mahurin (1994) | USA | C |
| R148 Test of Cued Recall | Ivanoiu *et al.* (2005) | Belgium | S |
| Refined ADL Assessment Scale (R-ADL) | Tappen (1994) | USA | C, D |

**Table 8.1** (*cont.*)

| Test name | Author | Country | Function |
|---|---|---|---|
| Short Portable Mental Status Questionnaire (SPMSQ) | Albert *et al.* (1991) | USA | SC |
| Syndrom Kurztest (SKT) | Kim *et al.* (1993) | Germany | C, T |
| Structured Interview for the Diagnosis of Dementia of Alzheimer Type, Multi-Infarct Dementia and Dementias of Other Etiology (SIDAM) | Zaudig *et al.* (1992) | Germany | D |
| Structured Assessment of Independent Living Skills (SAILS) | Mahurin *et al.* (1991) | USA | C |
| Telephone Assessed Mental State (TAMS) | Lanska *et al.* (1993) | USA | D, SC |
| Troublesome Behaviour Scale (TBS) | Asada *et al.* (1994) | Japan | D |

These tests derive from experimental studies in cognitive psychology applied in clinical practice in the field of neuropsychology. Quantifiable tasks have thus been developed which are capable of isolating the specific cognitive subsystems affected by diseases and clinical syndromes such as working and semantic memory, attention, and visuospatial organization. Despite the proliferation of focalized testing methods now available in the field of cognitive processing research in normal adults, and their demonstrated utility in differential diagnosis, surprisingly few of these tests are being carried over into everyday clinical practice. A recent survey across developed countries suggests that reliance is still predominantly placed on older tests such as the Wechsler Memory and Intelligence scales (Sullivan and Bowden, 1997).

Neuropsychometric tests targeting specific cognitive processes have now been used in the differential diagnosis of senile dementia of the Alzheimer type (Almkvist *et al.*, 1993; Kertesz and Clydesdale, 1994; Rosser and Hodges, 1994), and subtypes of Alzheimer's disease (Mann *et al.*, 1992; Stern *et al.*, 1993; Richards *et al.*, 1993; Lundervold *et al.*, 1994), vascular dementia (Almkvist *et al.*, 1993; Kertesz and Clydesdale, 1994), fronto-temporal degeneration and Lewy body disease (Filley *et al.*, 1994; Grossman *et al.*, 1998), depression (Masserman *et al.*, 1992), Huntington's disease (Masserman *et al.*, 1992; Lundervold *et al.*, 1994; Rosser and Hodges, 1994; Rich *et al.*, 1997), progressive supranuclear palsy (Rosser and Hodges, 1994), and Parkinson's disease (Stern *et al.*, 1993; Lundervold *et al.*, 1994; Westwater *et al.*, 1997). Cognitive testing has also been used to monitor the effects of adverse environmental exposure, such as surgery and anaesthesia, in the elderly (Moller *et al.*, 1998; Ancelin *et al.*, 2001).

The psychometric tests used in the diagnosis of pathologies in elderly subjects have varied widely between studies, thus making comparisons between clinical centres very difficult. In response to this problem psychometric tests targeting specific cognitive functions have been incorporated into standardized comprehensive diagnostic batteries designed for the differential diagnosis of psychogeriatric illness, such as the CAMCOG which forms part of CAMDEX (Roth *et al.*, 1988), the mental status examination of the Canberra Interview for the Elderly (Henderson *et al.*, 1994), and the cognitive assessment component of the SIDAM (Zaudig *et al.*, 1991). The National Institute on Aging has also established a series of collaborative studies to standardize cognitive measurement in the elderly (Buckholtz and Radebaugh, 1994).

## Measurement of the consequences of psychiatric disorder

Increasing interest in the impact of psychiatric illness on the quality of life, on caregiving services, and on the caregivers themselves has led to the more recent development of psychometric tests designed to assess the *consequences* of cognitive disorder. In this context terms such as 'disability' and 'dependency' are often used, but with little precision. The International Classification of Functioning, Disability and Health (WHO, 2001) provides a useful conceptual framework for the consideration of the consequences of disease by differentiating three levels: functioning (the consequences of disease at the level of body organs and systems); disability (interference with the activities performed by the individual); participation (the social consequences of disease). At the impairment level psychometric tests measure changes in specific cognitive processes (memory, language, attention) as discussed above. Disability and handicap scales on the other hand describe the impact of cognitive dysfunction on behaviour and social adaptation. Examples of this type of scale are the Neuropsychiatric Inventory assessing behavioural and emotional changes in dementia (Cummings *et al.*, 1994), the Troublesome Behaviour Scale (Asada *et al.*, 1994), and the Refined ADL Assessment Scale (Tappen, 1994). Other scales assess deterioration in daily activities corresponding to specific changes in cognitive processing, for example the Functional Assessment Staging scale (Sclan and Reisberg, 1992), the BEHAVE-AD (Harwood *et al.*, 1998) and the Cognitive Performance Test (Burns *et al.*, 1994). Tests have also been developed to monitor residual functioning in severely impaired subjects based on the Piagetian model such as the M-OSPD (Auer and Reisberg, 1996) and the Hierarchic Dementia Scale (Cole and Dastoor, 1996).

## Computerized cognitive assessment

Although automated cognitive testing has been reported in the literature since the late 1960s, it has only become popular as a routine clinical procedure since the 1980s, principally due to three important developments: the ability to simulate complex imagery, the microcomputer, and the touch screen. The most important of these has undoubtedly been the development of the microprocessor, which has not only dramatically decreased the cost of automated testing, but also greatly increased its flexibility such that users can design their own testing programmes with little expense and transfer results to other software for analysis.

The most obvious advantage of computerized cognitive testing is the possibility of standardizing stimulus presentation; an advantage which has led to the computerization of popular manual tests such as the Progressive Matrices and Mill Hill Vocabulary Test (Watts *et al.*, 1982). By the end of the 1960s a review of cognitive tests which had been adapted for computer administration had already appeared in the literature (Gedye and Miller, 1969). A further advantage of computer administration is a significant reduction in administration time. Computerization also permits the use of extremely complex administration procedures which may be tailored to suit individual needs. This possibility has led to the development of 'adaptive' or 'tailored' testing in which the test content is determined for each individual as a function of each response that is made in the course of the testing period. In this way difficulty levels can be adjusted according to the ability of the subject.

Item selection algorithms generally follow one of three branching models; item to item via predetermined structures, subtest to subtest, or as a function of a complex rule specified by a mathematical testing model. Item to item branching strategies are the simplest form of adaptive testing with a triangular or pyramidal structure when drawn graphically. Inter-subtest branching strategies are similar except that each node in the diagram now consists of several items rather than one. This gives fewer nodes but allows for re-entrant nodes in which only a portion of the items in a subtest need to be administered before branching to another. Model-based branching is based on item response, or latent trait theory, assuming that item responses are probabilistically related by a specified function to a continuous underlying trait or ability. Theoretical models of branching systems and scoring methods for adaptive testing are described in greater detail by Vale (1981) and Dewitt and Weiss (1976). These articles also provide practical guidelines for the construction of branching strategies.

Reliable data recording has been a persistent problem in both research and clinical investigations, as it is at this point that both conscious and unconscious interviewer bias may exert a strong influence. This problem has been repeatedly reported in the literature relating to behavioural evaluation since the 1940s. Most of us are familiar with this type of problem, and no matter how well interviewers are trained the investigator can never be sure if the coded response is truly an accurate representation of the subject's behaviour. Computer testing has greatly alleviated this problem. Computerized testing provides an interactive environment in which the subject can respond directly to the stimulus via a keyboard or touch screen and the response is registered immediately by the programme without the intermediary of an interviewer or response coder. In this way investigators may incorporate into their programs a control system through which they may check at the end of a session that all items have been presented by the interviewer.

While earlier tests generally only recorded simple information such as 'right' or 'wrong', computer technology has permitted the development of complex automated decision-making. For example the program may automatically record persistent perseveration between tasks where subjects continue to attend to stimuli relevant to a previous task, or visual-field neglect where the subject responds only to items in one part of the screen. Direct interaction between the respondent and the testing apparatus permits the accurate recording of reaction times and response latencies. The latter is of particular interest in follow-up studies as increased response time in subsequent administrations of a test is often a more sensitive indicator of early cognitive deficit than error rate. In this way complex observations may be recorded even where the examination is carried out by lay interviewers. For example Fagot et al. (1993) describe a haptic recognition task in which the computer records the number and duration of hand contacts with each stimulus, and the ECO cognitive battery for the elderly (Ritchie et al., 1993) automatically records visual field neglect and rotation errors in a matching to sample task.

In the early years of the development of computerized tests investigators (and in particular clinicians) expressed doubts as to the feasibility of presenting elderly subjects with computer hardware, and thus frequently rejected computerized testing as being detrimental to the clinician–patient relationship. On the other hand, the growing number of reports of the use of computerized testing with the elderly suggest that there is in practice very little difficulty (Morris, 1985; Carr et al., 1986). In the first place many elderly persons now own their own personal computers and many others have had some experience with them. Additionally, elderly people generally find computer-generated tests far more interesting and less threatening than paper and pencil tests administered by an interviewer—the latter situation is often negatively associated with school experiences, and the elderly person often feels that he or she is being judged by the younger interviewer.

For readers interested in the use of computerized cognitive assessment some points are perhaps worth noting. Development of a computerized test or battery of tests involves firstly the selection of both hardware and software. The options available are currently so numerous that it is not possible to cover them all within the scope of this chapter. Researchers are generally guided by practical limitations. In computerized testing for laboratory research of a specific cognitive function the user generally seeks out the hardware and software which are best able to demonstrate and manipulate the cognitive function under investigation. On the other hand if the tests are designed for multicentre use, then standardization becomes an important consideration and preference may be given to widely used material such as PC or Macintosh which have user-friendly software packages such as Hypercard, Flash, or Java, which are well-suited to the development and rapid modification of adaptive cognitive tests. If the test is to be used in general population studies, light-weight portable hardware is now available which is highly shock-resistant.

If response latencies are to be recorded in different research sites, then care should be exercised to ensure standardization of hardware—furthermore, the accurate recording of reaction times remains a problematic area when standardized packages such as Flash and Java are used which may confound processing time with subject responses, with absolute timing only reaching one-tenth of a second, which while generally adequate for the estimation of response time in clinical studies may not be adequate for experimental examination of reaction time. Timing accuracy can be increased for PC through BIOS-modifying software (see Graves and Bradley, 1991 for a description of this procedure) and for Macintosh using special public domain software timing routines as described by Westall et al. (1986, 1989).

Display clarity depends upon the graphic standard used by the software. The relative advantages of different standards should be taken into consideration in the selection of test software. Earlier standards such as CGA (colour graphics adapter) give figures with relatively poor resolution so that stimuli requiring finer detail or portraying dimensionality are best programmed by more advanced graphics standards such as EGA (enhanced graphics adapter) or VGA (visual graphics array). On the other hand, with lower resolution graphics can be drawn more quickly on the screen and the display and response timing of the test is easier to coordinate.

When adapting existing paper and pencil cognitive tests for computer administration, reliability and validity should be established, even where this has previously been done for the manually administered form. Watts *et al.* (1982) have shown for example that the computerized version of the Ravens Progressive Matrices gave absolute levels which were approximately 5 points lower than obtained by the paper and pencil version of the test. Furthermore, normative data collected using one type of visual display unit may not apply if the display type and quality are altered—especially when changing from a cathode ray tube to the liquid crystal displays used in laptop machines. It may also be necessary to test alternative administration methods to reduce error due to test presentation method. Banderet *et al.* (1988) compared two versions of a computerized addition task with the original paper and pencil version. The first version required subjects to enter answers from a keyboard, and despite pre-test typing practice, subjects were 35% slower with the keyboard than with the paper and pencil version. Furthermore scores obtained from the computer version were less stable over time. An alternative computerized multiple-choice version was found to be not only more stable than either the paper and pencil or original computer task, but also more sensitive to the experimental conditions.

Finally, while as noted above subject acceptance is generally not a problem, Kane and Kay (1992) stress that previous experience with computers may constitute an important source of variance in test performance in the elderly, especially when the subject is required to manipulate a number of keys on a keyboard. Variation between subjects is likely to be even greater with cross-cultural data collection and in groups with a wide age range. It is thus important to standardize as far as possible subject familiarity. This should not be left to the interviewer, who may introduce significant error variance at this point. The test program should incorporate standardized practice trials which bring all subjects up to an equivalent pre-test level of competency in manipulating response devices, before commencing the testing procedures.

Table 8.2 provides examples of computerized cognitive tests developed since the 1980s which have been used with elderly persons, and the hardware required for their administration. The availability of software such as Java and Flash has now made test development so easy that research groups often develop testing for a specific project without publishing or copyrighting the battery itself. For this reason it is not possible to provide an exhaustive repertoire of currently used computerized tests.

## Conclusion

A large number of psychometric tests have been developed for the evaluation of the mental health status of elderly people. In this chapter we have considered developments specifically in the field of cognitive dysfunction and its behavioural consequences. Computerized testing methods have greatly expanded the functions which may be measured, and also increased efficiency and reliability. Perhaps the greatest shortcoming at the moment is the assumption that information processing in the normal elderly is the same as that for young adults. Little consideration has been given to the possibility that an upper extension to existing theories of cognitive and emotional development may be required (that is beyond childhood and adolescence to different phases of adult life) if psychometric testing is to be adequately adapted to elderly populations.

**Table 8.2** Computerized cognitive tests suitable for use with elderly populations

| Test | Author | Hardware |
| --- | --- | --- |
| Adaptive Rate Continuous Performance Test (ARCPT) | Buschbaum and Sosteck (1980) | Apple II/PC |
| Automated Portable Test System (APTS) | Bittner *et al.* (1986) | PC |
| Automated Psychological Screening (B-MAPS) | Acker and Acker (1982) | PC/Macintosh |
| Cambridge Neuropsychological Test (CANTAB) | Sahakian and Owen (1992) | PC |
| Cambridge Mental Disorders of the Elderly (CAMDEX) | Roth *et al.* (1988) | PC |
| Computergestützte Neuropsychologische Testanordnung (CNAT) | Unpublished[a] | Atari |
| Evaluation Cognitive par Ordinateur (ECO) | Ritchie *et al.* (1993) | Macintosh |
| Geriatric Mental State (GMS-AGECAT) | Copeland *et al.* (1986) | PDP 11/34 |
| Memory Assessment Clinics Battery (MAC) | Larrabee *et al.* (1991) | AT&T 6300 |
| NeuroTrax Mindstreams | Dwolatzky *et al.* (2004) | PC |
| Psychomotor and Visuospatial Tasks | Hofman *et al.* (2000) | PC |
| Automated Neuropsychological Assessment Metrics (ANAM) | Kane *et al.* (2007) | PC |
| Walter Reed Performance Assessment Battery (WRPAB) | Thorne *et al.* (1985) | PC |

[a] Reischies, F.M. and Wilms, H.U., Psychiatrische Klinik und Poliklinik der Freie Universität Berlin, 1987.

## References

Acker, W. and Acker, C. (1982). *Bexley Maudsley Automated Psychological Screening and Bexley Maudsley Category Sorting Test: Manual*. NFER-Nelson, Windsor.

Ainslie, N.K. and Murden, R.A. (1993). Effect of education on the clock-drawing dementia screen in non-demented elderly persons. *Journal of the American Geriatrics Society*, **41**, 249–252.

Albert, M., Smith, L.A., Scherr, P.A., Taylor, J.O., Evans, D.A., and Funkenstein, H.H. (1991). Use of brief cognitive tests to identify individuals in the community with clinically diagnosed Alzheimer's disease. *International Journal of Neuroscience*, **57**(3–4), 167–178.

Almkvist, O., Backman, L., Basun, H., and Wahlund, L.O. (1993). Patterns of neuropsychological performance in Alzheimer's disease and vascular dementia. *Cortex*, **29**, 661–673.

Ancelin, M.-L., Artero, S., Portet, F., Dupuy, A.-M., Touchon, J., and Ritchie, K. (2006). Non-degenerative mild cognitive impairment in elderly people and use of anticholinergic drugs: longitudinal cohort study. *British Medical Journal*, **332**, 455–459.

Ancelin, M.L., de Roquefeuil, G., Ledesert, B., Bonnel, F., Cheminal, J.C., and Ritchie, K. (2001). Exposure to anaesthetic agents, cognitive functioning and depressive symptomatology in the elderly. *British Journal of Psychiatry*, **178**, 360–366.

Asada, T., Yoshioka, M., Morikawa, S. *et al.* (1994). Development of a troublesome behaviour scale (TBS) for elderly patients with dementia. *Japanese Journal of Public Health*, **41**(6), 518–527.

Auer, S.R. and Reisberg, B. (1996). Reliability of the Modified Ordinal Scales of Psychological Development: a cognitive assessment battery for severe dementia. *International Psychogeriatrics/IPA*, **8**, 225–231.

Banderet, L.E., Shukitt, B.L., Walthers, M.A., Kennedy, R.S., Bittner, A.C., and Kay, G.G. (1988). Psychometric properties of three addition tasks with different response requirements. *30th Annual Conference of the Military Testing Association, Arlington, VA, 1988*. US Army Research Institute of Environmental Medicine, Natick, MA 01760-5007, USA (Louis.Banderet@us.army.mil).

Beardsall, L. and Huppert, F.A. (1994). Improvement in NART word reading in demented and normal older persons using the Cambridge Contextual Reading Test. *Journal of Clinical and Experimental Neuropsychology*, **16**(2), 232–242.

Berkman, L.F. (1986). The association between educational attainment and mental status examinations: of etiologic significance for senile dementias or not ? *Journal of Chronic Disease*, **39**, 171–174.

Bittner, A.C., Carter, R.C., Kennedy, R.S., Harbeson, M.M., and Krause, M. (1986). Performance evaluation tests for environmental research (PETER): evaluation of 114 measures. *Perceptual and Motor Skills*, **63**, 683–708.

Blalock, H.M. (1970). The measurement problem. In *Methodology in social research* (ed. H.M. Blalock and A. Blalock). McGraw-Hill, New York.

Blessed, G., Tomlinson, B.E., and Roth, M. (1968). The association between quantitative measures of dementia and of senile change in the cerebral gray matter of elderly subjects. *British Journal of Psychiatry*, **114**, 797–811.

Brayne, C. and Calloway, P. (1991). The case identification of dementia in the community: a comparison of methods. *International Journal of Geriatric Psychiatry*, **5**, 309–316.

Breteler, M.M.B., van Amerongen, N.M., van Swieten, J.C. *et al.* (1994). Cognitive correlates of ventricular enlargement and cerebral white matter lesions on magnetic resonance imaging. The Rotterdam Study. *Stroke*, **25**, 1109–1115.

Brodaty, H., Pond, D., Kemp, N.M. *et al.* (2002). The GPCOG: a new screening test for dementia designed for general practice. *Journal of the American Geriatric Society*, **50**, 530–534.

Buckholtz, N.S. and Radebaugh, T.S. (1994). National Institute on Aging collaborative studies in the standardization of cognitive measures. *Alzheimer Disease and Associated Disorders*, **8**(Suppl.), 214–216.

Burns, T., Mortimer, J.A., and Merchak, P. (1994). Cognitive Performance Test: a new approach to functional assessment in Alzheimer's disease. *Journal of Geriatric Assessment and Neurology*, **7**, 46–54.

Buschbaum, M.S. and Sostek, A.J. (1980). An adaptive rate continuous performance test: vigilance and reliability for 400 male students. *Perceptual and Motor Skills*, **51**, 707–713.

Buschke, H., Kusianski, G., Katz, M. *et al.* (1999). Screening for dementia with the memory impairment screen. *Neurology*, **15**, 231–238.

Cabeza, R. and Nyberg, L. (1997). Imaging cognition: an empirical view of PET studies with normal subjects *Journal of Cognitive Neuroscience*, **9**, 1–26.

Capitani, E., Della-Sala, S., Laiacona, M., and Marchetti, C. (1994). Standardization and use of a test of memory of prose. *Bollettino di Psicologia Applicata*, **209**, 47–63.

Carr, A.C., Woods, R.T., and Moore, B.J. (1986). Automated cognitive assessment of elderly patients: a comparison of two types of response device. *British Journal of Clinical Psychology*, **25**(4), 305–306.

Clarke, M., Jagger, C., Anderson, J., Battcock, T., Kelly, F., and Stern, M.C.(1991). The prevalence of Dementia in a total population: a comparison of two screening instruments. *Age and Ageing*, **20**(6), 396–403.

Coblentz, J.M., Mattis, S., Zingesser, L.H., Kasoff, S.S., Wisniewski, H.M., and Katzman, R. (1973). Presenile dementia: clinical aspects and evaluation of cerebrospinal fluid dynamics; 1973; *Archives of Neurology*, **29**, 299–308.

Cole, M.G. and Dastoor, D.P. (1996). The Hierarchic Dementia Scale: conceptualization. *International Psychogeriatrics/IPA*, **8**, 205–212.

Copeland, J.R.M., Dewey, M.E., and Griffiths-Jones, H.M. (1986). A computerized diagnostic system and case nomenclature for elderly subjects: GMS and AGECAT. *Psychological Medicine*, **16**, 89–99.

Cummings, J.L., Mega, M., Gray, K., Rosenberg-Thompson, S., Carusi, D.A., and Gornbein, J. (1994). The Neuropsychiatric Inventory: comprehensive assessment of psychopathology in dementia. *Neurology*, **44**(12), 2308–2314.

De Jonghe, J.F., Krijgsveld, S., Staverman, K., Lindeboom, J., and Kat, M.G. (1994). Differentiation between dementia and functional psychiatric disorders in a geriatric ward of a general psychiatric hospital using the Amsterdam dementia screening test. *Nederlands Tijdschrift voor Geneeskunde*, **138**, 1668–1673.

Deary, J.J., Bastin, M.E., Pattie, A. *et al.* (2006). White matter integrity and cognition in childhood and old age. *Neurology*, **28**, 505–512.

Dewitt, L.J. and Weiss, D.J. (1976). Hardware and software evolution of an adaptive ability measurement system. *Behavior Research Methods and Instrumentation*, **8**, 104–107.

Duine, T.J. (1991). Validity of a new psychogeriatric behavior observation scale for application in nursing homes and homes for the aged. *Tijdschrift voor Gerontologie en Geriatrie*, **22**(6), 228–233.

Dwolatzky, T., Whitehead, V., Doniger, G.M. *et al.* (2004). Validity of the Mindstreams computerized cognitive battery for mild cognitive impairment. *Journal of Molecular Neuroscience*, **1**, 33–44.

Eisdorfer, C., Cohen, D., Paveza, G.J. *et al.* (1992). An empirical evaluation of the Global Deterioration Scale for staging Alzheimer's disease. *American Journal of Psychiatry*, **149**(2), 190–194.

Embretson, S.E. and Yang, X. (2006). Multicomponent latent trait models for complex tasks. *Journal of Applied Measurement*, **7**, 335–350.

Eslinger, P.J., Damasio, A.R., Benton, A.L., and Van Allen M. Neuropsychologic detection of abnormal mental decline in older persons. *Journal of the American Geriatric Society*, **25**(3), 670–674.

Fagot, J., Lacreuse, A., and Vauclair, J. (1993). Haptic discrimination of nonsense shapes: hand exploratory strategies but not accuracy reveal laterality effects. *Brain and Cognition*, **21**(2), 212–225.

Filley, C.M., Kleinschmidt-DeMasters, B.K., and Gross, K.F. (1994). Non-Alzheimer fronto-temporal degenerative dementia. A neurobehavioural and pathologic study. *Clinical Neuropathology*, **13**, 109–116.

Folstein, M.F., Folstein, S.E., and McHugh, P.R. (1975). 'Mini Mental State'. A practical method for grading the cognitive state of patients for the clinician. *Journal of Psychiatric Research*, **12**, 189–198.

Galvin, J.E., Roe, C.M., Powlishta, K.K. *et al.* (2005). The AD8: a brief informant interview to detect dementia. *Neurology*, **65**, 559–564.

Gao, Z. (1991). Assessment of Hasegawa's Dementia Scale for screening and diagnosis of dementia in the elderly. *Chinese Journal of Neurology and Psychiatry*, **24**(5), 258–261, 316.

Gedye, J.L. and Miller, E. (1969). The automation of psychological assessment. *International Journal of Man–Machine Studies*, **2**, 237–262.

Geiger-Kabisch, C. and Weyerer, S. (1993). The Geriatric Concentration Test. Results of a study of patients over 65 years of age in Mannheim. *Zeitschrift für Gerontologie*, **26**, 81–85.

Gilleard, C.J., Belford, H., Gilleard, E., Whittick, J.E., and Gledhill, K. (1984). Emotional distress among the supporters of the elderly mentally infirm. *British Journal of Psychiatry*, **145**, 172–177.

Gomez de Caso, J.A., Rodriguez-Artalejo, F., Claveria, L.E., and Coria, F. (1994). Value of Hodkinson's test for detecting dementia and mild cognitive impairment in epidemiological surveys. *Neuroepidemiology*, **13**(1–2), 64–68.

Gorissen, J.P. (1994). Structure of the Behavior Observation Scale-Geriatrics. *Tijdschrift voor Gerontologie en Geriatrie*, **25**(2), 58–62.

Grant, I., Heaton, R., McSweeney, A., Adams, K., and Timms, R. (1982). Neuropsychological findings in chronic obstructive pulmonary disease. *Archives of Internal Medicine*, **142**, 1470–1476.

Graves, R.E. and Bradley, R. (1991). Millisecond timing on the IBM PC/XT and PS/2: a review of the options and corrections for the Graves and

Bradley algorithm. *Behavior Research Methods Instruments and Computers*, **23**, 377–379.

Grigsby, J., Kaye, K., and Robbins, L.J. (1992). Reliabilities, norms and factor structure of the Behavioral Dyscontrol Scale. *Perceptual and Motor Skills*, **74**, 883–892.

Grossman, M., Payer, F., and Onishi, K. (1998). Language comprehension and regional cerebral defects in frontotemporal degeneration and Alzheimer's disease. *Neurology*, **50**, 157–163.

Harwood, D.G., Ownby, R.L., Barker, W.W., and Duara, R. (1998). The behavioural pathology in Alzheimer's Disease Scale (BEHAVE-AD). *International Journal of Geriatric Psychiatry*, **11**, 793–800.

Helmes, E., Merskey, H., Hachinski, V.C., and Wands, K. (1992). An examination of psychometric properties of the extended scale for dementia in three different populations. *Alzheimer Disease and Associated Disorders*, **6**(4), 236–246.

Henderson, A.S., Jorm, A.F., Mackinnon, A. *et al.* (1994). Survey of dementia in the Canberra population: experience with ICD-10 and DSM-III criteria. *Psychological Medicine*, **24**, 473–482.

Hofman, M., Seifritz, E., Krauchi, K. *et al.* (2000). Alzheimer's disease, depression and normal ageing: merit of simple psychomotor and visuospatial tasks. *International Journal of Geriatric Psychiatry*, **15**, 31–39.

Ivanoiu, A., Adam, S., Van der Linden, M *et al.* (2005). Memory evaluation with a new cued recall test in patients with mild cognitive impairment and Alzheimer's disease. *Journal of Neurology*, **252**, 47–55.

Jorm, A.S. and Korten, A. (1988). Assessment of cognitive decline in the elderly by informant interview. *British Journal of Psychiatry*, **152**, 209–213.

Jorm, A.F., Scott, R., Cullen, J.S., and Mackinnon, A.J. (1991). Performance of the informant questionnaire on cognitive decline in the elderly (IQCODE) as a screening test for dementia. *Psychological Medicine*, **21**(3), 785–790.

Kahn, R.L., Godfarb, A.I., and Pellack, M. (1960). Brief objective measures for the determination of mental status in the aged. *British Journal of Psychiatry*, **117**, 326–328.

Kane, R.L. and Kay, G.G. (1992). Computerized assessment in neuropsychology: a review of tests and test batteries. *Neuropsychology Review*, **3**(1), 1–117.

Kane, R.L., Roebuck-Spencer, T., Short, P., Kabat, M., and Wilken, J. (2007). Identifying and monitoring cognitive deficits in clinical populations using Automated Neuropsychological Assessment Metrics (ANAM) tests. *Archives of Clinical Neuropsychology*, **22**(Suppl. 1), 115–126.

Kertesz, A. and Clydesdale, S. (1994). Neuropsychological deficits in vascular dementia vs Alzheimer's disease. *Archives of Neurology*, **51**, 1226–1231.

Kiecolt-Glaser, J.K., Glaser, R., Shuttleworth, E.C., Dyer, C.S., Ogrocki, P., and Speicher, C.E. (1987). Chronic stress and immunity in family care-givers of Alzheimer's disease victims. *Psychosomatic Medicine*, **49**, 523–535.

Kim, Y.S., Nibbelink, D.W., and Overall, J.E. (1993). Factor structure and scoring of the SKT test battery. *Journal of Clinical Psychology*, **49**(1), 61–71.

Kittner, S.J., White, L.R., Farmer, M.E. *et al.* (1986). Methodological issues in screening for dementia: the problem of education adjustment. *Journal of Chronic Diseases*, **39**, 163–170.

Kramer, M. (1980). The rising pandemic of mental disorders and associated chronic diseases and disabilities. *Acta Psychiatrica Scandinavica*, **62**, 282–297.

Lanska, D.J., Schmitt, F.A., Stewart, J.M., and Howe, J.N. (1993). Telephone-assessed mental state. *Dementia*, **4**(2), 117–119.

Larrabee, G.J., West, R.L., and Crook, T.H. (1991). The association of memory complaint with computer-simulated everyday memory performance. *Journal of Clinical and Experimental Neuropsychology*, **13**(4), 466–478.

Lindeboom, R., Schmand, B., Holman, R., de Haan, R.J., and Vermeulen, M. (2004). Improved brief assessment of cognition in aging and dementia. *Neurology*, **63**, 543–546.

Liu, H.C., Chou, P., Lin, K.N. *et al.* (1994). Assessing cognitive abilities and dementia in a predominantly illiterate population of older individuals in Kinmen. *Psychological Medicine*, **24**, 763–770.

Lundervold, A.J., Karlsen, N.R., and Reinvang, I. (1994). Assessment of sub-cortical dementia in patients with Huntington's disease, Parkinson's disease, multiple sclerosis and AIDS by a neuropsychological screening battery. *Scandinavian Journal of Psychology*, **35**, 48–55.

Mackinnon, A. and Mulligan, R. (1998). Combining cognitive testing and informant report to increase accuracy in screening for dementia. *American Journal of Psychiatry*, **155**, 1529–1535.

Mahurin, R.K., DeBettignies, B.H., and Pirozzolo, F.J. (1991). Structured Assessment of Independent Living Skills: preliminary report of a performance measure of functional abilities in dementia. *Journal of Gerontology*, **46**(2), 58–66.

Mann, U.M., Mohr, E., Gearing, M., and Chase, T.N. (1992). Heterogeneity in Alzheimer's disease: progression rate segregated by distinct neuropsychological and cerebral metabolic profiles. *Journal of Neurology, Neurosurgery and Psychiatry*, **55**, 956–959.

Manton, K.G. and Stallard, E. (1988). *Chronic disease modeling: measurement and evaluation of the risks of chronic disease processes.* Charles Griffin, London.

Masserman, P.J., Delis, D.C., Butters, N., Dupont, R.M., and Gillin, J.C. (1992). The subcortical dysfunction hypothesis of memory deficits in depression: neuropsychological validation in a sub-group of patients. *Journal of Clinical and Experimental Neuropsychology*, **14**, 687–706.

Michels, R. and Marzuk, P.M. (1993). Progress in psychiatry. *New England Journal of Medicine*, **329**, 552–560.

Moller, J.Y., Cluitmans, P., and Rasmussen, L.S. (1998). Long-term postoperative cognitive dysfunction in the elderly: ISPOCD1 Study. *Lancet*, **351**, 857–861.

Morinigo, A., Zaudig, M., Mittelhammer, J., and Hiller, W. (1990). Description y validez 'Test–Retest' de le ENEDAM. *Actas Luso Espanolas de Neurologia Psiquitria y Ciencias Afines*, **18**(6), 396–402.

Morris, R.G. (1985). Automated clinical assessment. In *New directions in clinical psychology* (ed. F. Watts). John Wiley, Chichester.

Nelson, H.E. (1982). *National Adult Reading Test*. NFER-Nelson, London.

Neri, M., Roth, M., Mountjoy, C.Q., and Andermacher, E. (1994). Validation of the full and short forms of the CAMDEX interview for diagnosing dementia. *Dementia*, **5**(5), 257–265.

Nishimura, T., Kobayashi, T., Hariguri, S. *et al.* (1993). Scales for mental state and daily living activities for the elderly: clinical behavioral scales for assessing demented patients. *International Psychogeriatrics*, **5**(2), 117–134.

Nyberg, L. (1998). Mapping episodic memory. *Behavioural Brain Research*, **90**, 107–114.

Page, M.P. (2006). What can't functional imaging tell the cognitive psychologist? *Cortex*, **42**, 428–443.

Pek, G. and Fulop, T. (1992). The Hungarian version of the Nuremberg Geronto-psychological Inventory. *Orvosi Hetilap*, **132**(42), 2319–2322.

Ponds, R.W., Verhey, F.R., Rozendaal, N., Jolles, J., and Deelman, B.G. (1992). Screening for dementia: validity of the cognitive screening test and the Mini-Mental State Examination. *Tijdschrift voor Gerontologie en Geriatrie*, **23**, 94–99.

Qureshi, K.N. and Hodkinson, H.M. (1974). Evaluation of a ten-question mental test in the institutionalized elderly. *Age and Ageing*, **3**, 152–157.

Reid, D.W., Tierney, M.C., Zorzitto, M.L., Snow, W.G., and Fisher, R.H. (1991). On the clinical value of the London Psychogeriatric rating Scale. *Journal of the American Geriatrics Society*, **39**(4), 368–371.

Rich, J.B., Campodonico, J.R., Rothlind, J., Bylema, F.W., and Brandt, J. (1997). Perseverations during paired associate learning in Huntington's disease. *Journal of Clinical and Experimental Neuropsychology*, **19**, 191-203.

Richards, M., Bell, K., Dooneief, G. *et al.* (1993). Patterns of neuropsychological performance in Alzheimer's disease patients with and without extrapyramidal signs. *Neurology*, **43**, 1708–1711.

Ritchie, K. and Fuhrer, R. (1992). A comparative study of the performance of screening tests for senile dementia using receiver operating characteristics analysis. *Journal of Clinical Epidemiology*, **45**, 627–637.

Ritchie, K. and Fuhrer, R. (1996). The validation of an informant screening test for irreversible cognitive decline in the elderly: performance characteristics within a general population sample. *International Journal of Geriatric Psychiatry*, **11**, 149–156.

Ritchie, K., Allard, M., Huppert, F.A., Nargeot, C., Pinek, B., and Ledésert, B. (91993). Computerized cognitive examination of the elderly (ECO): the development of a neuropsychological examination for clinic and population use. *International Journal of Geriatric Psychiatry*, **8**, 700.

Rocca, W.A., Bonaiuto, S., Lippi, A. *et al.* (1992). Validation of the Hodkinson abbreviated mental test as a screening instrument for dementia in an Italian population. *Neuroepidemiology*, **11**(4–6), 288–295.

Ronnberg, L. and Ericsson, K. (1994). Reliability and validity of the Hierarchic Dementia Scale. *International Psychogeriatrics*, **6**(1), 87–94.

Rosen, W.G., Mohs, R.C., and Davis, K.L. (1984). A new rating scale for Alzheimer's disease. *American Journal of Psychiatry*, **4**, 1356–1364.

Rosser, A.E. and Hodges, J.R. (1994). The Dementia Rating Scale in Alzheimer's disease, Huntington's disease and progressive supranuclear palsy. *Journal of Neurology*, **241**(9), 531–536.

Roth, M., Huppert, F.A., Tym, E., and Mountjoy, C.Q. (1988). *CAMDEX: the Cambridge Examination for Mental Disorders of the Elderly*. Cambridge University Press, Cambridge.

Royall, D.R. and Mahurin, R. (91994). EXIT, QED, and DSM-IV: regional syndromes. *Journal of Neuropsychiatry and Clinical Neurosciences*, **6**(1), 60–62.

Royall, D.R., Mahurin, R.K., Cornell, J., and Gray, K.F. (1993). Bedside assessment of dementia type using the qualitative evaluation of dementia. *Neuropsychiatry-Neuropsychology and Behavioral Neurology*, **6**(4), 235–244.

Sahakian, B.J. and Owen, A.M. (1992). Computerized assessment in neuropsychiatry using CANTAB: discussion paper. *Journal of the Royal Society of Medicine*, **85**(7), 399–402.

Schaie, K.W. (1983). The Seattle Longitudinal Study: a twenty-one year exploration of psychometric intelligence in adulthood. In *Longitudinal studies of adult psychological development* (ed. K.W. Schaie). Guilford Press, New York.

Schneider, W. (1988). Micro Experimental Laboratory: an integrated system for IBM PC compatibles. *Behavior Research Methods, Instruments & Computers*, **20**, 206–217.

Sclan, S.G. and Reisberg, B. (1992). Functional assessment staging in Alzheimer's disease: reliability, validity, and ordinality. *International Psychogeriatrics*, **4**(Suppl. 1), 55–69.

Sinha, D., Zemlan, F.P., Nelson, S. *et al.* (1992). A new scale for assessing behavioral agitation in dementia. *Psychiatry Research*, **41**, 73–78.

Skoog, I., Berg, S., Johansson, B., Palmertz, B., and Andreasson, L.A. (1996). The influence of white matter lesions on neuropsychological functioning in demented and non-demented 85-year olds. *Acta Neurologica Scandinavica*, **93**, 142–148.

Stern, Y., Richards, M., Sano, M., and Mayeux, R. (1993). Comparison of cognitive changes in patients with Alzheimer's and Parkinson's disease. *Archives of Neurology*, **50**, 1040–1045.

Still, C., Goldsmith, T., and Mallin, R. (1983). Mini-object test: a new brief clinical assessment for aphasia–apraxia–agnosia. *Southern Medical Journal*, **76**, 52–54.

Sullivan, K. and Bowden, S. (1997). Which tests do neuropsychologists use ? *Journal of Clinical Psychology*, **53**, 657–661.

Tappen, R.M. (1994). Development of the refined ADL Assessment Scale for patients with Alzheimer's and related disorders. *Journal of Gerontological Nursing*, **20**(6), 36–42.

Thorne, D., Genser, S., Sing, H., and Hegge, F. (1985). The Walter Reed Performance Assessment Battery. *Neurobehavioral Toxicology and Teratology*, **7**, 415–418.

Tomlins, T.E. (1822). *Statutes of the realm*. Eyre and Strahan, London.

Tremmel, L. and Spiegel, R. (1993). Clinical experience with the NOSGER: tentative normative data and sensitivity to change. *International Journal of Geriatric Psychiatry*, **8**(4), 311–317.

Vale, C.D. (1981). Design and implementation of a microcomputer-based adaptive testing system. *Behaviour Research and Instrumentation*, **13**, 399–406.

Veroff, A.E., Cutler, N.R., Sramek, J.J., Prior, P.L., Mickelson, W., and Hartman, J.K. (1991). A new assessment tool for neuropsychopharmacologic research: the computerized Neuropsychological Test Battery. *Journal of Geriatric Psychiatry and Neurology*, **4**, 211–217.

Walczyk, J. (1993). A computer program for constructing language comprehension tests. *Computers in Human Behavior*, **9**(1), 113–116.

Ward, H.W., Ramsdell, J.W., Jackson, J.E., Renvall, M., Swart, J.A., and Rockwell, E. (1990). Cognitive function testing in comprehensive geriatric assessment: a comparison of cognitive test performance in residential and clinical settings. *Journal of the American Geriatrics Society*, **38**, 1088–1092.

Watts, K., Baddeley, A.D., and Williams, M. (1982). Automated tailored testing using Raven's Matrices and Mill Hill Vocabulary Tests: a comparison with manual administration. *International Journal of Man–Machine Studies*, **17**, 331–344.

Weinstein, M.C. and Fineberg, H.V. (1980). *Clinical decision analysis*. WB Saunders, Philadelphia.

Wells, Y. and Jorm, A.F. (1987). Evaluation of a special nursing home unit for dementia sufferers: a randomized controlled comparison with community care. *Australian and New Zealand Journal of Psychiatry*, **21**, 524–531.

Welsh, K.A., Butters, N., Mohs, R.C. *et al.* (1994). The Consortium to Establish a Registry for Alzheimer's Disease (CERAD). Part V. A normative study of the neuropsychological battery. *Neurology*, **44**, 609–614.

Westall, R., Perkey, M.N., and Chute, D.L. (1986). Accurate millisecond timing on Apple's MacIntosh using Drexel's millitimer. *Behavior Research Methods Instruments and Computers*, **18**, 307–311.

Westall, R., Perkey, M.N., and Chute, D.L. (1989). Millisecond timing on the Apple MacIntosh: updating Drexel's millitimer. *Behavior Research Methods, Instruments and Computers*, **21**, 540–547.

Westwater, H., McDowall, J., Siegert, R., Mossman, S., and Abenethy, D. (1997). Implicit learning in Parkinson's disease: evidence from a verbal version of the serial reaction time task. *Journal of Clinical and Experimental Neuropsychology*, **20**, 413–418.

WHO (2001). *International classification of functioning disability and health*. World Health Organization, Geneva.

Zaudig, M. (1992). A new systematic method of measurement and diagnosis of 'mild cognitive impairment' and dementia according to ICD-10 and DSM-III-R criteria. *International Psychogeriatrics*, **4**(Suppl. 2), 203–219.

Zaudig, M., Mittelhammer, J., Hiller, W. *et al.* (1991). SIDAM: a structured interview for the diagnosis of dementia of the Alzheimer type, multi-infarct dementia and dementias of other aetiology according to ICD-10 and DSM III-R. *Psychological Medicine*, **21**, 225–236.

# 9

# Principles of cerebral cortical development

## Anna Hoerder-Suabedissen and Zoltán Molnár

## Introduction

The brain is the seat of typically human traits like language, consciousness, and logical thinking. The millions of cells and billions of connections of the human brain are generated from the complex interactions between our unfolding genetic program and our environment. It is awe-inspiring how the activation of subsets of our 30,000 genes in different combinations and sequences can produce the most complex object in our known universe.

But a highly structured organ like the brain can only function if it is set up correctly. Gross anatomical malformations and their associated mental deficits usually become evident in the first few years of life, if not before. But subtle changes, such as slight changes in the ratios of different cell types or the strength of connections between brain regions, are less easy to identify and they are likely to contribute to, if not cause, diverse forms of mental illness. Development is the ultimate readout of our genome; the combination of genetic susceptibility and environmental perturbations could lead to several devastating diseases. Comprehending how the brain develops and gets modified throughout our life is an essential step to understanding how the brain adapts to pathological conditions caused either by genetic or environmental accidents at any age.

The construction of the brain follows an integrated series of developmental steps. It begins with the decision of a few early embryonic cells to become neural progenitors, and then the neural plate will form the neural tube, which will differentiate further using signals from outside and within the neural tissue. As connections form between nerve cells, and their electrical properties emerge, the brain begins to process information and to mediate behaviours even during embryonic life. Some of the underlying circuitry is built into the nervous system during embryogenesis. However, interactions with the world continuously update and adapt the brain's functional architecture. The mechanisms for these later plastic changes are probably a continuation of the processes that sculpt the brain during development. To understand the brain and its devastating diseases, we need to reveal the mechanisms that produce it and the ways in which it can constantly change throughout life.

## Why study brain development?

It could be argued that our 'ageing' process starts with the fertilization of the egg. Our unfolding genetic program and the environmental interactions throughout our life determine our ultimate capacities in old age. As progress has been made with the understanding of the aetiopathogenesis of numerous psychiatric and neurological diseases it has been realized that many of them have developmental origins (Polleux and Lauder, 2004; Harrison and Weinberger, 2005). Schizophrenia, autism, attention deficit hyperactivity disorder, dyslexia, and numerous forms of epilepsy are now widely considered to be brain developmental diseases. They are relatively common (schizophrenia, 1:100; autism, 1:166; dyslexia, 1:10) and they follow patients for the rest of their lives. Even the late onset schizophrenia cases which manifest themselves relatively late in life (after 40 or even 60) may be based on similar aetiological mechanisms as they exhibit identical symptoms. Understanding the interactions between the susceptibility genes and the environmental influences in these diseases is the current challenge of developmental neurobiology (Moldin et al., 2006).

Environmental influences can accelerate or delay the onset of various hereditary neurological symptoms in animal models (e.g. Huntington's and Alzheimer's diseases; Nithianantharajah and Hannan, 2006). This research will have considerable influence on the care given to patients with these illnesses. It has been recently revealed that the same mechanisms that are active during neuronal development and plasticity, and the same set of genes, are involved in the progression of numerous neurological diseases (Levitt et al., 2006).

Future research may also reveal the factors (genetic and environmental) that lead us to age differently. Ageing might limit the repertoire of the compensatory mechanisms to maintain our phenotype; therefore the differences in the environmental influences we experience, and the variations of our genome, are more exposed. We believe that a basic knowledge of the principles of neurodevelopment will be important for future generations of psychiatrists, even if they primarily work with elderly patients.

## How to study brain development?

A large portion of our knowledge of the mechanisms of brain development originates from animal models. Until recently our knowledge of human brain development was restricted to what could be gleaned from anatomical analysis of (sometimes severely degraded) post-mortem tissue. Thus animal models, and in particular rodents, were a major source of information about mammalian brain development. Despite recent advances in live imaging of human fetal and baby brains, rodents remain the preferred source of information on cell–cell interactions, gene function, molecular determinants of connectivity and brain arealization, as well as a good model to investigate the functional abnormalities present in psychiatric or neurodegenerative diseases (Goffinet and Rakic, 2000). Basic neuroscience research may provide most of the clues to understanding the aetiology and pathophysiology of these mechanisms. However, these animal models are just the starting point, and their validation in human development is essential (Molnár *et al.*, 2006a).

## Development of the mammalian brain: the outline of this chapter

This chapter is divided into several sections that follow the chronological development of the mammalian brain. Initially, a region of the embryo must be specified as future neural tissue, followed by the generation of neurons which then need to migrate to their final destination. Throughout this it is essential that positional information is provided to the developing neurons, and the initially rough subdivisions of the central nervous system are continuously refined as it matures. Therefore the next two sections will focus on the specification of future neural tissue, and the early types of signalling that contribute to the regionalisation of the central nervous system (p. 130–131). Then, specifically focussing on the cerebral cortex, we will describe in detail how different cell types are generated and comment on some general principles underlying the layered structure of the mature neocortex (pp. 131–136). The mature cortex is divided into different areas that usually carry out different functions, and the following sections (pp. 136–138) will cover some of the mechanisms that contribute to this so-called arealization. Dividing the cortex into regions can occur at several levels of organization, i.e. definition of broad areas must occur earlier than the exact establishment of topographical maps representing the sensory receptor surface in the brain. As the underlying mechanisms are diverse, they will be dealt with in separate sections (pp. 139–140), although the finished product is the result of a continuous process. Lastly, a short section (pp. 140–141) will cover the modifications that are known to occur both in development as well as in the mature brain and which are thought to underlie learning and memory, before concluding with an overview of the clinical relevance of developmental abnormalities.

## Specification of neural versus non-neuronal tissue

### Neural tube and early brain vesicle development

An integrated series of developmental steps transforms a thin layer of unspecified tissue into our central nervous system, which is able to process information and organize actions. There are numerous general mechanisms that permit this transformation: neural induction, neurulation, proliferation, migration, axonal outgrowth, synaptogenesis, differentiation, and apoptosis (Kandel *et al.*, 2000).

All neural tissue is derived from one continuous sheet of cells in the ectodermal layer at the dorsal midline of the gastrula stage embryo. The neural fate is the default outcome for ectodermal cells, but in the whole embryo they are subject to inhibitory signals from the bone morphogenetic protein family type of molecules. Inhibition of this bone morphogenetic protein signalling cascade is mediated by the (non-neural) tissue of the underlying mesoderm, and this allows ectodermal cells to form the columnar cell layer of the neural plate. The process is called *neuronal induction*.

Secreted factors that can act as neural-inducing molecules have now been identified and these include noggin, chordin, and fibroblast growth factor (Stern, 2006).

Shortly after its induction, the neural plate begins to fold inwards along the midline, such that the edges of the neural plate rise up to form the neural folds, the peaks of which eventually touch and fuse at the midline. Fusion of the neural folds results in the formation of the neural tube—a hollow cylinder along the rostro-caudal (head–tail) axis of the developing embryo. Closure of the neural fold does not occur simultaneously along the length of the embryo but rather begins in several places along the rostro-caudal axis and progresses bidirectionally along the axis from these initiation points, in a zipper-like fashion. The caudal regions of the neural tube develop into the spinal cord, whereas the rostral regions become the brain. Failure to close the neural tube results in a variety of neural tube defects (spinal disraphisms; associated with a failure of closure of the posterior neural arch, defined by their position and severity). If the early steps of neural tube closure fail, the entire back of the embryo remains open leading to anencephaly and embryonic lethality. The mildest form is spina bifida occulta, which is thought to reach a prevalence of 5–10% in the general population.

## Ventro-dorsal and rostro-caudal patterning of the neural tube

The cells within the neural tube must be given *positional information* to allow the right type of cell to develop in the right location. For example, in the mature spinal cord the ventral half mostly contains the cell bodies of motor neurons, whereas sensory neurons are located in the dorsal half. Thus, at some point during development, in regions on the ventral (front) side of the neural tube future motor neurons of the spinal cord will be induced to differentiate, while cells in the dorsal (back) half will give rise to sensory neurons. The subdivisions of the mature nervous system are set up during very early embryogenesis. Interestingly, the dorso-ventral patterning is achieved by diffusible signalling molecules that are produced outside of the neural plate, whereas rostro-caudal (head-to-tail) patterning is mediated by signals intrinsic to the neural plate.

The *ventro-dorsal patterning* molecules are secreted by nearby tissues, especially by the axial mesoderm (called the notochord) beneath the ventral midline, and by the ectoderm flanking the dorsal neural tube. The notochord, lying below the medial neural plate, induces the floor plate and motor neurons of the ventral neural tube, by a diffusible molecule belonging to the sonic hedgehog family of proteins. The epidermis that lies lateral to the neural plate represses ventral fates through a bone morphogenic protein (BMP) signal. Therefore, the exact cell fate is specified by the relative concentration of the two types of signals to which a given cell is exposed (Jessell, 2000). This graded type of signalling is common in the early development of the nervous system whenever positional information is required, and the reader will encounter graded signals (partly by the same family of molecules) again in the sections on cortical arealization.

On the other hand, the *rostro-caudal patterning* is regulated by signals within the neural tube. The genes controlling the development of the forebrain are distinct from those responsible for the development of the trunk, and regional differences along the rostro-caudal axis are also manifest very early during development. The hindbrain is strikingly segmented into structures called rhombomeres, which contain specific cranial nerve nuclei. Rhombomeres are specified in part by the activation of the Hox genes (Lumsden, 2004). The Hox or homeotic genes are genes which, when mutated, cause conversion of one part of the body into another. They were first discovered in flies, but they are highly conserved throughout evolution from flies, to rodents and humans.

# Generation of neurons and glia in the central nervous system

## Neurulation

The vertebrate brain and spinal cord develop from the neural tube. Within the neural tube the cells of the neuroectoderm divide to generate the neurons and glia, in a process referred to as *neurulation*. Neural precursor cells divide in the ventricular layer (those cell layers on the inside of what used to be the hollow neural tube) and most divisions are completed before birth. Neurons of the central nervous system and glial cells—except microglia—are derived from the neuroepithelium, while neurons of the peripheral nervous system (e.g. future neurons of the dorsal ganglia) derive from scattered neural crest cells that are located laterally on both sides of the neural tube. Within the neuroepithelium of the neural tube, cells divide repeatedly in a characteristic pattern of cell division. The cell proliferation is more rapid in the rostral regions of the neural tube, which bulges outwards to form three brain vesicles: the forebrain, the midbrain, and the hindbrain. Given the nature of this book, the remainder of this chapter will focus on the development of the telencephalic region and how that gives rise to the cerebral neocortex.

The primary divisions of the brain occur as three brain vesicles or swellings of the neural tube, known as the forebrain (prosencephalon), midbrain (mesencephalon), and hindbrain (rhombencephalon) (Fig. 9.1). The forebrain vesicle becomes subdivided into the paired telencephalic vesicles and the diencephalon, and the rhombencephalon subdivides into the metencephalon and the myelencephalon. These basic brain divisions can be related to the overall anatomical organization of the mature brain. As development proceeds, the rostral end of the neural tube undergoes a series of complex folds or flexures. At the junction of the spinal cord and hindbrain is the cervical flexure, and a more dramatic flexure occurs at the midbrain, the cephalic flexure. The pontine flexure has the effect of buckling the hindbrain. The eyes develop from the lateral part of the diencephalon, and as the telencephalon undergoes its massive enlargement into the cerebral hemispheres, the transverse fissure forms as the cortex sweeps back over the brainstem (Fig. 9.2). The retina with its diencephalic origin is a window to the brain, since numerous neurological symptoms can be detected by examining the eye. Eye developmental abnormalities very frequently accompany other brain developmental abnormalities, as they share the basic developmental mechanisms and genes.

## Origin and migration of cortical neurons

The uniformly six-layered mammalian neocortex can be divided both anatomically and functionally into different regions. The multitude of neurons that comprise the cortex differ from layer to layer and region to region, but they can none the less be subdivided into two functional groups: excitatory cells that primarily use the amino acid glutamate as a neurotransmitter, and inhibitory cells that mostly use the modified amino acid GABA (gamma-aminobutyric acid)

as a neurotransmitter. Alternatively, these same cells can be classified by their cell shape: the pyramidal cells equate to excitatory cells, while the non-pyramidal cells or interneurons, which can be much more varied in shape, represent the inhibitory cells (although some non-pyramidal shaped excitatory cells also exist). Pyramidal cells form the majority of projections out of the cortex, and GABA-ergic interneurons mostly form local projections. These two cell types are born in different regions of the developing brain, but eventually each of the six cortical layers with the exception of the neuron-free marginal zone will consist of a mixture of both cell types. The ratio of pyramidal to non-pyramidal cells varies slightly from region to region, but on average there are four times more excitatory than inhibitory cells in the cortex (Fig. 9.3).

The six layers of the neocortex develop from the thin-walled telencephalic vesicles over the course of days in mice and months in humans. Cell division primarily takes place in the germinal zone surrounding the lateral ventricle—aptly named the ventricular zone—and cells have to migrate to their final position in the cortex. In primates and humans this eventually amounts to up a centimetre or more of cellular travel, and ample scope for disorders of cell migration (Levitt, 2005; Lambert de Rouvroit and Goffinet, 2001).

Pyramidal neurons and interneurons are generated in different parts of the ventricular zone (VZ). The former arise from the VZ directly underneath the telencephalic wall and migrate radially outwards to form the cortex, whereas interneurons arise from the lateral and medial ganglionic eminences (future striatum or basal ganglia) and migrate laterally into the cortex (Marin and Rubenstein, 2003). But irrespective of their site of origin, cortical neurons eventually settle in the cortex in an inside-out manner, such that late-born cells settle in progressively more outward layers. For pyramidal neurons this means that the later born cells must migrate past their older cousins to reach their final position in cortex (Fig. 9.4).[1] Although the processes of interneuron and pyramidal cell migration occur simultaneously and are likely to influence each other, the following section will deal with each cell type separately to avoid confusion, but the figures apply to both.

## Pyramidal cells and radial migration

Pyramidal neurons arise from cell divisions in the ventricular zone underneath the future cortex, i.e. the cortical primordium or pallium (see Fig. 9.1). At the early stages of development, the cerebral wall consists of the ventricular zone where extensive cell proliferation takes place. Cell proliferation in the ventricular zone occurs asymmetrically such that the two daughter cells have different cell properties. One cell retains its progenitor characteristics, whereas the other cell migrates radially outwards along radial glia processes and eventually differentiates into a mature neuron. Initially, the very first born and still immature neurons will form the pre-plate. The cortical layers 2–6 are formed later, and during the formation of these later layers, the earlier generated pre-plate is split into an upper and a lower half, as the cells of cortical layers 2–6 settle in

---

[1]   Current knowledge about the cellular mechanisms of proliferation and cell migration as well as the molecular cues that direct these processes were derived from cell culture and mutant mouse studies (Kriegstein, 2005). The routes of migration taken were analysed by dye tracing techniques and retroviral labelling of clonally related cells in both wild-type and mutant mouse lines as well as in other rodents, carnivores, and primates (Wonders and Anderson, 2006).

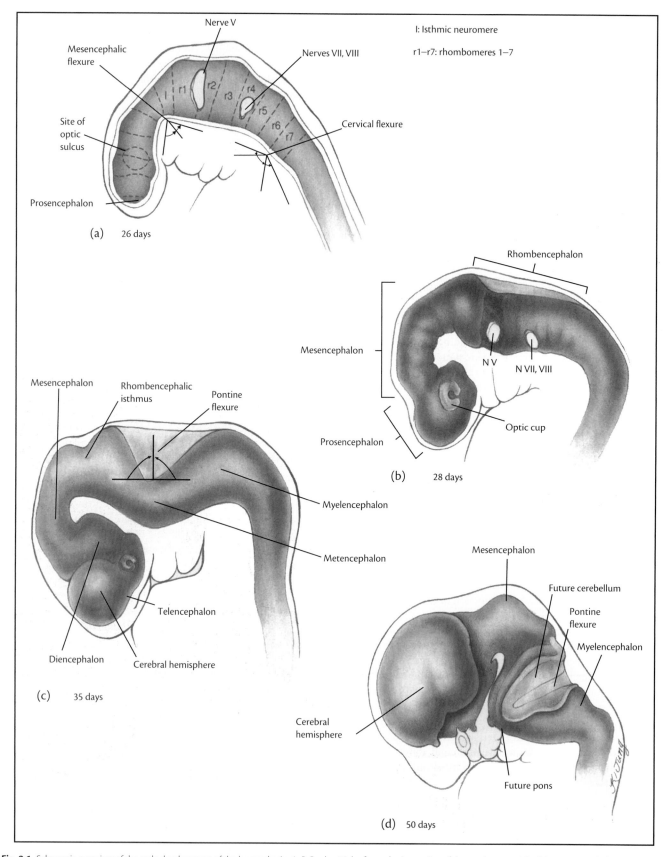

**Fig. 9.1** Schematic overview of the early development of the human brain. A, B: By day 26 the future brain consists of three primary vesicles (the prosencephalon, mesencephalon, and rhombencephalon) and is visibly segmented into neuromeres. Of these neuromeres, the seven rhombomeres and the isthmic segment are relatively distinct (dotted lines). Cephalic folding causes the neural tube to begin bending at the mesencephalic and cervical flexures. C, D: Further subdivision of the brain vesicles creates five secondary vesicles: the rhombencephalon divides into the diencephalon and telencephalon. The cerebral hemispheres appear and expand rapidly, covering the diencephalon. The pontine flexure folds the metencephalon back against the myelencephalon. (Figure adapted from Larsen, 1993, Fig. 13–1.)

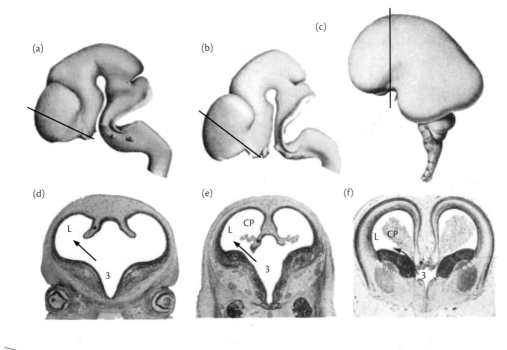

**Fig. 9.2** Figure illustrating the progressive enlargement of the human brain, disproportionate growth of the cerebral cortex, and development of the ventricular system. A–C: Brains at about 6, 7, and 15 weeks. D–F: Sections in the indicated planes. Note the gradual separation of the lateral ventricles (L) from the third ventricle (3) with the narrowing of the interventricular foramen (arrow). The thinned out roof of the neural tube begins to invaginate into the lateral ventricle at the choroid fissure. At 7 weeks (E) fronds of choroid plexus (CP) begin to form at the site of invagination. On the sections the progressive thickening of the cortex and the elaboration of the ganglionic eminence is apparent. (Adapted from Hochstetter, 1919; inspired by Nolte, 1999. A–C are reversed for consistency of orientation with Fig. 9.1.)

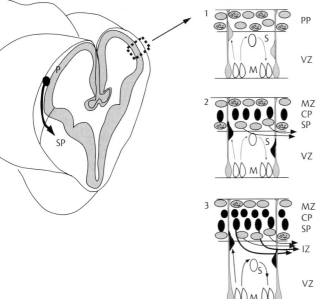

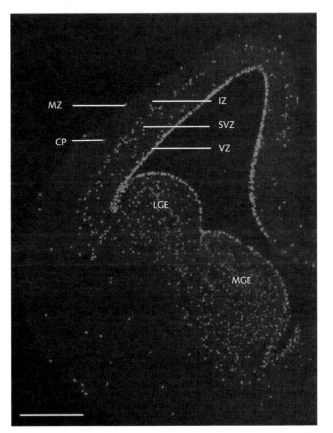

**Fig. 9.3** The early sequence of development in the mouse cortex (from Bellion and Métin, 2005). The diagram on the left shows the caudal half of an E13.5 mouse telencephalon after a coronal cut. The germinal zone (including ventricular zone, VZ) is indicated with grey shading. SP marks subplate projection leaving pallium(P). Radial line depicts the pallial subpallial boundary (PSPB). On the right panels (1–3) the sequence of pallial (P) development is shown schematically. There is a temporal delay of the dorsal regions compared to the lateral and a delay of the caudal regions compared to rostral according to the classical latero-medial and rostro-caudal gradient of proliferation and maturation in the cortex. The first post-mitotic cells accumulate at the pial surface in the pre-plate (1, PP). Cortical cells generated thereafter migrate within the PP and form the cortical plate (2, CP) that divides the PP in two layers, the marginal zone (MZ) and the subplate (SP). Soon after leaving the VZ, early post-mitotic cortical neurons extend efferent axons in the intermediate zone that is oriented toward the ventral subpallium (see arrow on the tip of the descending fibre on the scheme on the left). Neurons in the PP, SP, or layer VI could contribute to the early efferent projection extending in the intermediate zone (IZ). (Reproduced with permission from Bellion and Métin (2005).)

**Fig. 9.4** Coronal section through the right hemisphere of an E14 rat brain (similar level to the one shown in Fig. 9.3) stained with H3 (anti-phosphohistone) antibody to reveal the sites of cell divisions. Most of the divisions occur in the ventricular zone (VZ) lining the cortical neuroepithelium. There is a second major row of divisions in the subventricular zone (SVZ), but there are further scattered divisions in the marginal zone (MZ), cortical plate (CP), and intermediate zone (IZ). There are large number of divisions in the medial and lateral ganglionic eminences (LGE, MGE). Scale bar: 100 μm. (Figure adapted from Molnár *et al.*, 2006b.) See Plate 1 for a colour version of this figure.

between in an inside-first, outside-last pattern. This latter process of cortical development is directed by a signalling molecule called reelin, which is secreted by cells of the marginal zone (upper half of the former pre-plate). But equally important is the scaffold of radial glia.

At the beginning of corticogenesis, post-mitotic neurons migrate radially outwards to form the pre-plate (also referred to as primordial plexiform layer). The pre-plate is on the outside of the cerebral wall and is populated by neurons in an outside-in sequence, such that later born cells settle underneath the earlier born cells. The pre-plate and ventricular zone are separated by the intermediate zone (IZ), which consists of tangentially oriented fibres and will eventually develop into the white matter underneath the cortex (Fig. 9.3, third panel). Some cells in the pre-plate derive from the subpallium and arrive in the pre-plate by tangential migration, described later.

Throughout all stages of corticogenesis, the entire width of the cerebral wall is spanned by radial glia, with each cell having one process that touches the ventricular wall and one that reaches to the outer edge of the developing cortex. These cells are neural progenitors, but they also serve as scaffold and probably provide positional information for the radially migrating future pyramidal cells. Future pyramidal cells migrate into the pre-plate and split it into two parts, the subplate at the lower edge and the marginal zone at the outer edge of cortex.

Although initially derived from the same cell population, and indistinguishable from each other, the cells located in the marginal zone develop different neurochemical properties from those of the subplate. Most notably, the marginal zone contains the reelin-expressing Cajal–Retzius cells. Reelin is a secreted signalling molecule, and the reelin-mediated signalling pathway is essential to provide radially migrating cells with positional information. In the absence of reelin signalling (e.g. in the Reeler mouse or shaking rat Kawasaki) the cortex is formed in the opposite order, such that later born cells settle underneath their earlier born cousins (Rakic and Caviness, 1995; Higashi *et al.*, 2005). Humans homozygous for mutations in the reelin gene present with severe lissencephaly. The lissencephalic cortex is essentially four-layered and neurons of pallial origin settle in an outside-in manner such that the earlier born, large pyramidal cells of the normal layer 5 reside in the outermost layer of the cortex (Golden and Harding, 2004). Reduced levels of reelin have also been reported in post-mortem brain tissue from schizophrenic patients, but no obvious migration defect has been described, apart from reports of abnormally many cells in the subplate. Nonetheless, subtle migration deficits might well be present.

Towards the later stages of corticogenesis a further compartment of cell division—the subventricular zone (SVZ)—can be identified. The SVZ lies in between the VZ (ventricular zone) and the IZ (intermediate zone) and gives rise to the supragranular cell layers. The cells in the supragranular layers are still initially derived from the VZ, but as they migrate radially outwards, they arrest their migration in the SVZ and undergo one final, this time symmetric, cell division (Kriegstein and Noctor, 2004; Lukaszewicz *et al.*, 2005). The two resulting cells then continue to migrate along the radial glia until they get to their final destination in the supragranular layers. It has been suggested that this mode of division and the compartmentalization of the germinal zone is linked to the expansion of the mammalian cerebral cortex (Martinez-Cerdeno *et al.*, 2006; Molnár *et al.*, 2006a,b). Because the majority of pyramidal neurons migrate only radially, cells derived from the same progenitor cell settle in a single column above their site of origin. They also disperse slightly in a horizontal direction to allow for the increase in cortical surface area during corticogenesis.

The cellular and molecular mechanisms involved in radial migration have been extensively studied (Rakic, 2000). Radially migrating cells can move in either of two ways; translocation or locomotion (Nadarajah and Parnavelas, 2002). Translocating cells extend a long leading process all the way to the pia and the nucleus is moved along this process until it reaches the correct laminar position, and the leading process is subsequently retracted. Locomoting cells on the other hand are freely migrating—usually along radial glia—and have relatively short leading and longer trailing processes. During locomotion, pyramidal neurons have a simple bipolar shape and adhere closely to the radial glia. It has been suggested that translocation is the preferred mode of migration during early corticogenesis, when the pre-plate forms and the cortical wall is still relatively thin, whereas locomotion is predominantly used during later stages of corticogenesis.

Such a switch in the mode of migration is an attractive model for explaining abnormalities of lamination, where the pre-plate forms normally but the subsequent formation of the cortical laminae is disrupted. Time-lapse imaging in slice cultures revealed that neurons generated in the cortical proliferative zones at later stages of development pass through four different phases of migration, each characterized by changes in cell shape, direction of movement, and speed of migration (Kriegstein and Noctor, 2004). In phase one, newly generated neurons move radially away from the ventricle to the SVZ.

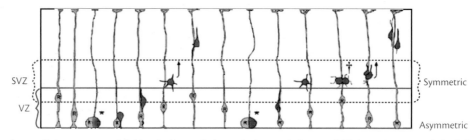

**Fig. 9.5** Figure demonstrating the two distinct programs of divisions in the germinal zone. In the ventricular zone (VZ) there are asymmetrical cell divisions (*) and immature neurons migrate out into the cortex (arrow). With this mode of division radial glia (R) directly give rise to neurons. With the second mode of division radial glia gives rise to neurons via intermediate progenitors, which produce neurons with symmetric cell division (see cross) in subventricular zone (SVZ). (Figure adapted from Noctor *et al.* (2004) with permission.) See Plate 2 for a colour version of this figure.

In phase two, they pause in the IZ–SVZ for up to a day in mice and adopt a multipolar morphology. Cells in this second phase are highly dynamic, extending and retracting processes. During this phase, neurons are capable of moving tangentially away from their guiding radial glia cell.

The third phase of migration is not undertaken by all cells, but those neurons that pass through the third phase extend a process towards the ventricle and often also translocate the cell body toward the ventricle. Once they reach the ventricle, they enter phase four of migration (or directly progress from stage two to stage four). The neurons extend a pia-directed leading process, take on the bipolar morphology of migrating neurons with a relatively short leading process, and begin radial migration to the cortical plate. Different phases of migration are probably regulated by different molecular signals. The protein product of the X-linked doublecortin (*DCX*) gene for example is necessary for the transition from the second phase of undirected movement to the final radially directed migration.[2] It was discovered in DCX-knockdown mice that the migrating pyramidal cells that succeeded in reaching the cortex did not always migrate to the correct layer. Electrophysiological recordings from neurons in the Dcx-knockdown mice demonstrate that the abnormally located neurons are active and integrated into the cortical circuitry (Bai et al., 2003), albeit at the wrong position (Fig. 9.6).

## Interneuron generation and tangential migration

For pyramidal cells, the normal mode of cell division and radial migration results in clonally related cells forming a single column in the cortex. By contrast, interneurons derived from the same progenitor cell are found across the entire expanse of the mature cortex (Marin and Rubenstein, 2003). This is the direct result of a different form of migration. The cells are generated in the ganglionic eminence, the primordium of the striatum (also referred to as subpallium, see Fig. 9.2) and migrate horizontally into the cortex, thereby crossing the striatocortical junction. This tangential form of migration came as a great surprise to many researchers, as there was a long-standing dogma that the neurons of the cortex and basal ganglia derive from different progenitor populations and do not intermix.

In mice, the time window in which inhibitory interneurons are born is similar to that of pyramidal cells, and there is evidence to suggest that early born interneurons settle in the lower cortical layers, and later born cells in the upper cortical layers, in a pattern similar to pyramidal neurons. Moreover, the route of migration chosen, and the final destination in the rostro-caudal dimension of the cortex, appear to be determined by both the time and place of birth of interneurons. Cells deriving from the medial ganglionic eminence spread throughout the cortex, while cells derived from the central ganglionic eminence were later found primarily in the caudal aspect of the telencephalic vesicle. The route taken, and the cytoskeletal mode of cell movement, differ between these two cell populations. There is mounting evidence that the wide diversity of interneurons (as characterized by different molecular markers) reflects their origin

from different regions of the subpallium (Nery et al., 2002; Butt et al., 2005; Métin et al., 2006; Wonders and Anderson, 2006) (Fig. 9.7).

Whether the different cell types use the same substrate for migration is unknown, but migrating cells of subpallial origin have repeatedly been observed in close contact with Tag-1-expressing corticofugal fibres in the internal capsule and intermediate zone (Denaxa et al., 2001). Therefore the Tag-1-expressing corticofugal fibres could be envisaged as playing a similar scaffold role in the striatum as the radial glia cells do in the telencephalic wall.

Migrating interneurons must cross the pallial–subpallial boundary to enter the telencephalon. Once inside the telencephalon, interneurons further migrate within the intermediate zone. From the IZ, they can either enter the cortex directly by migrating radially or obliquely into it, or they detour into the ventricular zone first. Cells choosing the latter route arrest their cell movement in the VZ for a short period before resuming their migration radially outwards, possibly along radial glia cells. Interneurons that migrate out of the ventricular zone settle in the same cortical layers as pyramidal cells born at the same time of gestation, and is has been suggested that they might receive positional information during their waiting period in the VZ. Whether the two types of migration reflect further underlying differences in the cells that follow them is currently unknown, but should be testable. Some interneurons also move all the way out to the marginal zone, from where they descend into the cortex; and also settle in the same layer as isochronical pyramidal neurons of pallial origin. Whether interneurons receive signals from glia and/or pallial neurons instructing them to settle in a particular layer, or whether interneurons instruct pyramidal neurons, is still open to debate, although the evidence for the former hypothesis is beginning to look stronger.

Given the differences in distance that laterally migrating interneurons and radially migrating pyramidal cells have to negotiate, it is amazing that cells of the same age still manage to settle in the same layers. It has been suggested (Kriegstein and Noctor, 2004) that the second phase of pyramidal cell migration serves to delay their outward movement sufficiently for isochronic interneurons to arrive in the intermediate zone, so that both cell types can conclude their migration together. Experimental evidence indicates that older interneurons derived from the subpallium can adopt the laminar position of younger pyramidal cells that they come into contact with. This suggests that extrinsic factors may be involved in determining which layer migrating interneurons will occupy. On the other hand, the laminar position of early born pyramidal neurons is determined even before the final cell division is complete.

Interneuron migration is influenced by a complex interplay of motogenic and repulsive factors (expressed mostly at their site of origin) and permissive or chemoattractive cues in the cortex. Interneurons appear capable of sensing cell surface or diffusible factors at their growth cones. Interneurons redirect their orientation of movement by extending new neurites in the new direction of movement and retracting processes in the previous direction. This frequently results in migrating cells with split neurites, allowing the cells to respond to small regional differences in the concentration of chemoattractive cues (Métin et al., 2006).

## Cell death during early cortical development

Several lines of evidence indicate that programmed cell death (apoptosis) is a major contributing factor to the formation of the vertebrate brain from very early stages (Buss et al., 2006). In the past, most

---

[2]  Manipulation of the levels of Dcx protein present in the mouse cortex resulted in heterotopias in the intermediate zone and white matter when Dcx levels were reduced, as expected from the comparison with *DCX* heterozygous women who present with double-cortex or subcortical band heterotopia (Bai et al., 2003).

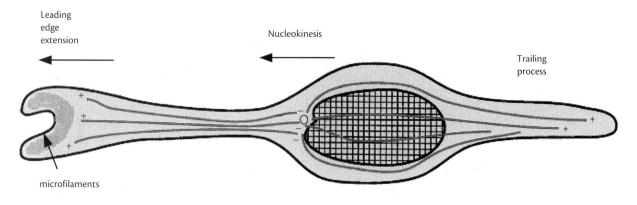

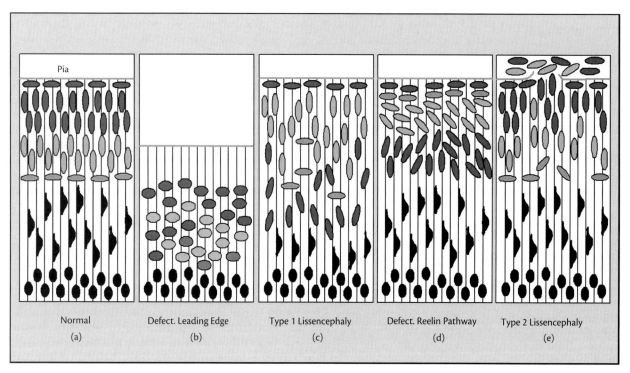

**Fig. 9.6** Schematic view of a migrating neuron and chart of the common migration disorders (from Lambert de Rouvroit and Goffinet, 2001). The leading edge extension of a migrating neuron occurs by polymerization of the actin meshwork (brown), while nucleokinesis is dependent on microtubules (red) organized with their minus end radiating from the microtubule organizing centre (yellow dot). The retraction of the trailing process is generally not considered important. (A) A graphical representation of the normal development of the cerebral cortex. The black, round cells at the bottom of the panel represent neural progenitors as well as radial glia along which immature neurons migrate (black bipolar cells). The former pre-plate cells are represented in pink (subplate) and red (marginal zone) with the cortical plate (future cortical layers 2–6) neurons indicated in blue and green. The lower, green cells are born at an earlier stage than the upper, blue cells. (B) In disorders where the molecular assembly of the leading edge of a migrating cell is defective, no or only very few migrating cells can be identified, and the cortex is thinner and more disorganized. Moreover, the marginal zone cells are not in the outermost cell layer and therefore cannot set up the signalling gradient of reelin. (C) In the type 1 lissencephalic brain, the pre-plate becomes split by the invading cortical plate cells as normal, but the cortical plate cells settle in the wrong order, with younger cells remaining underneath the older cells. Not all cortical plate cells arrive in the cortical plate, thereby also giving the appearance of a disrupted subplate (pink cells). (D) If any aspect of the reelin signalling pathway is defective, the pre-plate remains unsplit with the cortical plate cells settling underneath and in the wrong order. (E) In type 2 lissencephaly, some cortical plate neurons migrate beyond their target and even past the marginal zone cells, generating a disordered outermost cell layer composed of heterochronic neurons. See Plate 3 for a colour version of this figure.

research has been focused on histogenetic cell death occurring at late developmental stages, where it is primarily involved in eliminating 'incorrect' axonal connections after neurons have attained their final positions. But recently the use of methods that identify dying cells (by exposing their fragmented nuclear DNA) suggested that apoptosis in the ventricular zone is more significant than previously assumed (Blaschke *et al.*, 1998). This is supported by evidence from transgenic mice with disruption of the cell death pathway. Reducing cell death in the neuroepithelium (Casp-9 KO) increases the founder cell population and leads to a 'larger brain' (Rakic, 2000).

## Cortical organization

The mammalian neocortex is considered to be the most recently evolved part of the central nervous system, and responsible for the

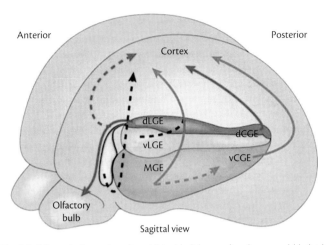

**Fig. 9.7** Schematic illustration of established (solid arrows) and proposed (dashed arrows) pathways of migration of cortical interneurons (from Wonders and Anderson, 2006). Blue arrows represent somatostatin (SST)- or parvalbumin (PV)-containing interneuron progenitors. Red arrows represent calretinin (CR)-containing interneuron progenitors. Black arrows represent the potential migration of cortical interneuron progenitors, the subtype of which has yet to be determined. SST and PV interneurons primarily migrate from the Nkx2.1-expressing domain of the medial ganglionic eminence (MGE) and might also arise from the ventral caudal ganglionic eminence (vCGE), which also expresses Nkx2.1 (blue shading). These interneurons have also been shown to migrate caudally from the MGE into the CGE (Butt *et al.*, 2005; Yozu *et al.*, 2005). CR interneurons primarily arise from the dorsal CGE (dCGE). The dorsal lateral ganglionic eminence (dLGE) expresses **ER81** (red shading) and also generates CR interneurons destined for the olfactory bulb, which might contribute to the cortical CR interneuron population. Progenitors from the ventral LGE (vLGE; green shading) also migrate to the cortex, and could represent an undetermined subgroup of cortical interneurons. Finally, Vax1-expressing progenitors of the septal region (yellow shading) might generate cortical interneurons of an unknown subgroup (Taglialatela *et al.*, 2004). (Figure reproduced with permission of *Nature Reviews Neuroscience*.) See Plate 4 for a colour version of this figure.

higher cognitive functions (sight, smell, and touch, as well as language, episodic memory, thought, and consciousness) in humans. The mature or adult cortex, in humans a highly convoluted and in most rodents and some carnivores an essentially agyric sheet of cells on the outside of the brain, can be divided into functional as well as anatomical domains, the boundaries of which are often (but not always) identical. This is a clear manifestation of the principle that specialized function requires specialized structures (Krubitzer and Kaas, 2005).

## Regionalization

The segregation in time and place of birth for pyramidal cells and interneurons might be necessary to produce cell variety. The type of nerve cell formed is influenced by environmental signals presented by the surrounding tissues, which regulate tissue-intrinsic gene expression, as mentioned above. These external signals change with time, so the ability to form specific cell types is gradually restricted as development proceeds. Cell determination (commitment of progenitor cells to a particular fate) is an essential early step in the development of cell lineages, and current evidence indicates that common mechanisms operate in different tissues to regulate this step (Hevner *et al.*, 2006).

Recently, several transcription factors have emerged as important players in cell fate specification in rodents (Molyneaux *et al.*, 2005; Guillemot *et al.*, 2006; Nelson *et al.*, 2006). They are believed to orchestrate the cell-type-specific expression of functional proteins,

such as the enzymes necessary for neurotransmitter generation. Many of these recently identified transcription factors are again expressed in gradients across the developing cortex or brain as a whole, and the combinatorial expression of these factors does not just determine the fates of different cortical cells, but also sets up the basic coordinates for cortical arealization and basic connectivity (see below).

Small variations in the level of expression of some of these factors can occur naturally. These variations may underlie fundamental individual differences in how the early brain develops. This could provide an attractive explanation of an early influence on what the (intellectual) strengths of the mature brain will be. Therefore there is current excitement around the composite analysis of gene expression patterns. Such analysis will allow us to identify molecularly distinct progenitor domains in the telencephalon, to elucidate genetic interactions underlying the generation of unique cellular phenotypes, and hence to understand the process of regionalization of the cerebral cortex.

Areas of the neocortex can be defined by their anatomical structure or by the function they serve, and accordingly two schools of thought exist on how this regionalization is initially set up during the development of the cerebral cortex.

The 'anatomical' or intrinsic school of thought proposed that a complex interplay of molecular signalling pathways determines the anatomical structure of the cortex, including the type of connections that exist between different areas (Rakic, 1988). In this view, the 'hardware' determines the function that a particular area can carry out. The alternative school of thought maintains that, within limits, the initial organization is not predetermined, but emerges as a result of the complex interplay of developing connections, such that an area that receives a lot of functional input of one kind, will subsequently adapt to specialize in processing this type of information (O'Leary, 1989).

Although these models were initially proposed as mutually exclusive hypotheses of arealization, it is now believed that a combination of both occurs. The gross structure is determined by molecular markers that guide (or repel), for example, long-range connections from the visual areas of the thalamus to future visual areas of the cortex. The fine structure at the cellular level is not predetermined, but is rather the result of initially widespread connectivity of which only highly active connections survive to form the final network (Innocenti and Price, 2005). Future development depends on the balance between intrinsic versus activity determined mechanisms (Rash and Grove, 2006).

## External and intrinsic signalling centres

The cortex, just like the neural tube, is patterned by a combination of extrinsic and intrinsic signals. The first regional differences are imposed onto the cortical neuroepithelium from adjacent signalling centres (Grove and Fukuchi-Shimogori, 2003). These centres set up gradients of various diffusible signalling molecules collectively referred to as morphogens [e.g. fibroblast growth factor 8 (FGF8), bone morphogenetic proteins (BMPs), etc.]. Each morphogen is capable of altering gene expression in responsive cells, and the exact concentrations of each morphogen to which an area is exposed lead to the first regional differences in the cortex. Experimental increase or decrease in the production of one of these morphogens can shift the boundaries of cortical areas, and presumably natural variation occurs as well.

Recent studies have started to define these extrinsic candidate molecules that control the patterns of expression of regulatory genes and transcription factors within the cortex (Rash and Grove, 2006). The factors intrinsic to the cortex in turn control the expression of membrane-bound or soluble guidance molecules, which modulate pathfinding and establishment of axonal connections. Some of the identified extrinsic signalling molecules include FGF8, Sonic hedgehog (Shh), BMP-2, -4, -6 and -7 and Wnt2b, -3a, -5a and -7a. Their interactions control the regional expression of specific transcription factors and regulatory genes. A graded or restricted expression of different genes that encode transcription factors, nuclear receptors, cell adhesion molecules, axon guidance receptors, and ligands has been described for many areas of the embryonic forebrain. Many of these region-specific and lamina-specific gene expression patterns are present before the first thalamic afferents invade the cerebral cortex. For example, mutant mice exist in which thalamocortical innervation of the cortex fails, but the initial region-specific and lamina-specific expression patterns develop none the less (Miyashita-Lin *et al.*, 1999; Nakagawa *et al.*, 1999).

Combinatorial expression of transcription factors is different between the pallium and subpallium, and modulates the molecular patterning of the striato-cortical junction as well as influencing axon pathfinding (López-Bendito and Molnár, 2003; Price *et al.*, 2006). But despite the numerous examples of intrinsic mechanisms of cortical map formation, cortical areas do not appear to be fully pre-programmed, and differences also arise from local interactions with afferent neurons. Thalamic axons, which later will carry most sensory information from the environment, reach the cortex at a very early stage, before the majority of cortical neurons have even been born. Recent work points to the crucial role of the early developing thalamocortical projections and their interactions with the developing cortical circuitry in establishing some aspects of the functional and structural organization of cortical maps, although other aspects of cortical arealization do not require thalamic input (Miyashita-Lin *et al.*, 1999) (Fig. 9.8).

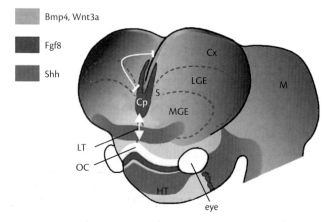

**Fig. 9.8** Summary of proposed interactions between patterning centres (from Storm *et al.*, 2006). Schema of a frontolateral view of the telencephalon showing the patterning centres as marked by expression of the genes indicated, the cross-regulation between the Fgf8 and Bmp4/Wnt3a-expressing centres, and the positive interactions between the Fgf8- and Shh-expressing domains. CP, commissural plate; Cx, cortex; HT, hypothalamus; LGE, lateral ganglionic eminence; LT, lamina terminalis; M, mesencephalon; MGE, medial ganglionic eminence; OC, optic chiasm; S, septum. See Plate 5 for a colour version of this figure.

## Formation of maps in the cortex

The development of innervation patterns and 'maps' in the brain depends on cascades of mechanisms. Topographic order is a very common feature of the brain. Information becomes distributed and represented spatially across structures of the central nervous system. This tendency of the brain to be organized in 'maps', as they are commonly known, is particularly clear in the major sensory and motor areas of the cerebral cortex. In visual, auditory, and somatosensory cortical areas, the representation of the receptor surface (retina, cochlea, skin) is arranged across the cortex in an isomorphic fashion. This is not to say that cortical maps are topologically simple, linear projections of receptor sheets: rather they are distorted and sometimes fragmented, in various interesting ways. In particular, a general feature of central sensory maps is that densely innervated regions of the receptor surface occupy a larger fraction of the map than regions that are more sparsely innervated. This anisotropy in central representation means that the local scale of the mapping is determined by the density and spatial arrangement of afferent fibres bringing information into the cortex from the periphery. In motor areas of the cerebral cortex, too, regions devoted to the richly innervated musculature of the hands and face (in humans) occupy larger regions than those concerned with the muscles of the trunk (Penfield and Rasmussen, 1950). This anisotropy obviously reflects the different volumes of neuronal machinery required for the control of richly, as opposed to sparsely, innervated muscle.

The development of these maps is gradual and based on a sequence of mechanisms. The representation can change throughout life due to plasticity of nerve connections (Krubitzer and Kaas, 2005). Several studies have shown that thalamocortical projections can influence the size and even the identity of specific cortical areas, in support of the view that activity in afferent fibres determines cortical areas. For example, reduction of thalamic input to the cortex following binocular enucleation alters cortical areal fate by creating a 'hybrid' visual cortex in place of area 17 (Rakic, 1988; Dehay *et al.*, 1996). Similarly, early ablation of thalamic nuclei leads to an alteration in the size and cell number in the corresponding area of the neocortex. These observations indicate that cortical regionalization is initially created by the graded expression of various genes, and that thalamic input controls the later stages of areal subdivision. The role of thalamic projections in determining cortical areas and architecture might not be limited to later stages, however. Recent *in vitro* studies indicate that thalamic afferents release a diffusible factor that promotes proliferation of neurons and glia in the proliferative zones of the cortex (Dehay *et al.*, 2001; Lukaszewicz *et al.*, 2005).

## Connectivity between regions

Thalamic axons arrive in the subplate (the first generated, largely transient cell population of the cerebral cortex), where they accumulate, before they develop transient side branches which enter the cerebral cortex (Kostovic and Rakic, 1980; Allendoerfer and Shatz, 1994). The thalamic axons then arborize and develop contacts with their ultimate target cells, mostly in layer 4. As the fibres grow directly to their correct target area, a detailed knowledge of the early regionalization of the telencephalon is required to explain the underlying guidance mechanisms

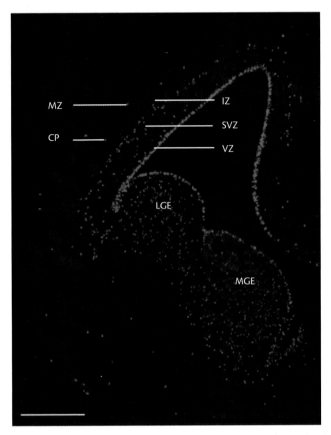

**Plate 1** Coronal section through the right hemisphere of an E14 rat brain(similar level to the one shown in Fig. 9.3) stained with H3 (anti-phosphohistone) antibody to reveal the sites of cell divisions. Most of the divisions occur in the ventricular zone (VZ) lining the cortical neuroepithelium. There is a second major row of divisions in the subventricular zone (SVZ), but there are further scattered divisions in the marginal zone (MZ), cortical plate (CP), and intermediate zone (IZ). There are large number of divisions in the medial and lateral ganglionic eminences (LGE, MGE). Scale bar: 100 μm. (Figure adapted from Molnár *et al.*, 2006b.) See also Figure 9.4 in the text.

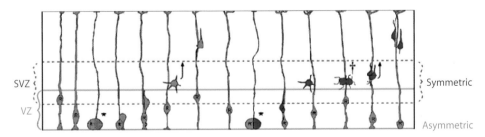

**Plate 2** Figure demonstrating the two distinct programs of divisions in the germinal zone. In the ventricular zone (VZ) there are asymmetrical cell divisions (*) and immature neurons migrate out into the cortex (arrow). With this mode of division radial glia (R) directly give rise to neurons. With the second mode of division radial glia gives rise to neurons via intermediate progenitors, which produce neurons with symmetric cell division (see cross) in subventricular zone (SVZ). (Figure adapted from Noctor *et al.* (2004) with permission.) See also Figure 9.5 in the text.

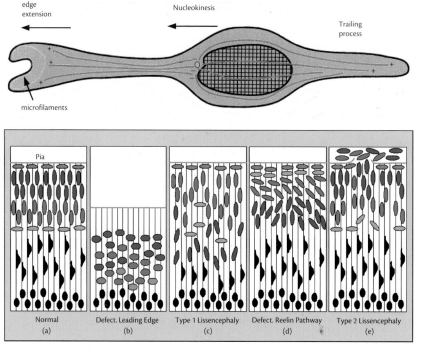

**Plate 3** Schematic view of a migrating neuron and chart of the common migration disorders (from Lambert de Rouvroit and Goffinet, 2001). The leading edge extension of a migrating neuron occurs by polymerization of the actin meshwork (brown), while nucleokinesis is dependent on microtubules (red) organized with their minus end radiating from the microtubule organizing centre (yellow dot). The retraction of the trailing process is generally not considered important. (A) A graphical representation of the normal development of the cerebral cortex. The black, round cells at the bottom of the panel represent neural progenitors as well as radial glia along which immature neurons migrate (black bipolar cells). The former pre-plate cells are represented in pink (subplate) and red (marginal zone) with the cortical plate (future cortical layers 2–6) neurons indicated in blue and green. The lower, green cells are born at an earlier stage than the upper, blue cells. (B) In disorders where the molecular assembly of the leading edge of a migrating cell is defective, no or only very few migrating cells can be identified, and the cortex is thinner and more disorganized. Moreover, the marginal zone cells are not in the outermost cell layer and therefore cannot set up the signalling gradient of reelin. (C) In the type 1 lissencephalic brain, the pre-plate becomes split by the invading cortical plate cells as normal, but the cortical plate cells settle in the wrong order, with younger cells remaining underneath the older cells. Not all cortical plate cells arrive in the cortical plate, thereby also giving the appearance of a disrupted subplate (pink cells). (D) If any aspect of the reelin signalling pathway is defective, the pre-plate remains unsplit with the cortical plate cells settling underneath and in the wrong order. (E) In type 2 lissencephaly, some cortical plate neurons migrate beyond their target and even past the marginal zone cells, generating a disordered outermost cell layer composed of heterochronic neurons. See also Figure 9.6 in the text.

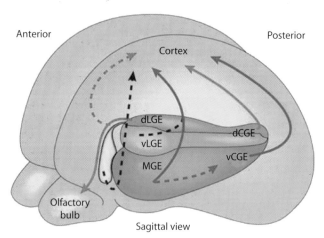

**Plate 4** Schematic illustration of established (solid arrows) and proposed (dashed arrows) pathways of migration of cortical interneurons (from Wonders and Anderson, 2006). Blue arrows represent somatostatin (SST)- or parvalbumin (PV)-containing interneuron progenitors. Red arrows represent calretinin (CR)-containing interneuron progenitors. Black arrows represent the potential migration of cortical interneuron progenitors, the subtype of which has yet to be determined. SST and PV interneurons primarily migrate from the Nkx2.1-expressing domain of the medial ganglionic eminence (MGE) and might also arise from the ventral caudal ganglionic eminence (vCGE), which also expresses Nkx2.1 (blue shading). These interneurons have also been shown to migrate caudally from the MGE into the CGE (Butt *et al.*, 2005; Yozu *et al.*, 2005). CR interneurons primarily arise from the dorsal CGE (dCGE). The dorsal lateral ganglionic eminence (dLGE) expresses **ER81** (red shading) and also generates CR interneurons destined for the olfactory bulb, which might contribute to the cortical CR interneuron population. Progenitors from the ventral LGE (vLGE; green shading) also migrate to the cortex, and could represent an undetermined subgroup of cortical interneurons. Finally, Vax1-expressing progenitors of the septal region (yellow shading) might generate cortical interneurons of an unknown subgroup (Taglialatela *et al.*, 2004). (Figure reproduced with permission of *Nature Reviews Neuroscience*.) See also Figure 9.7 in the text.

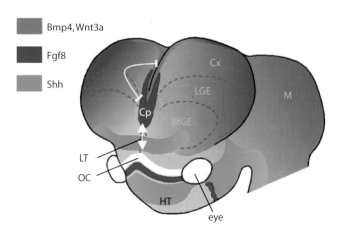

**Plate 5** Summary of proposed interactions between patterning centres (from Storm *et al.*, 2006). Schema of a frontolateral view of the telencephalon showing the patterning centres as marked by expression of the genes indicated, the cross-regulation between the Fgf8 and Bmp4/Wnt3a-expressing centres, and the positive interactions between the Fgf8- and Shh-expressing domains. CP, commissural plate; Cx, cortex; HT, hypothalamus; LGE, lateral ganglionic eminence; LT, lamina terminalis; M, mesencephalon; MGE, medial ganglionic eminence; OC, optic chiasm; S, septum. See also Figure 9.8 in the text.

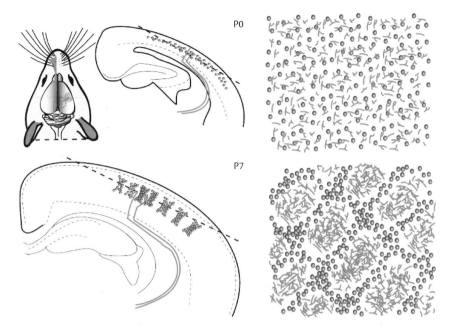

**Plate 6** Schematic overview of the development of the periphery-related thalamocortical patterning and the cytoarchitectural barrel pattern in the mouse from the initially uniform distribution of thalamocortical arbors (red) at birth ((P)ost-natal day 0) and layer 4 neurons (blue), to the ordered structure of the mature cortex which is achieved within a week (P7). Left column represents coronal, right column tangential sections. (From Molnár and Molnár, 2006.) See also Figure 9.9 in the text.

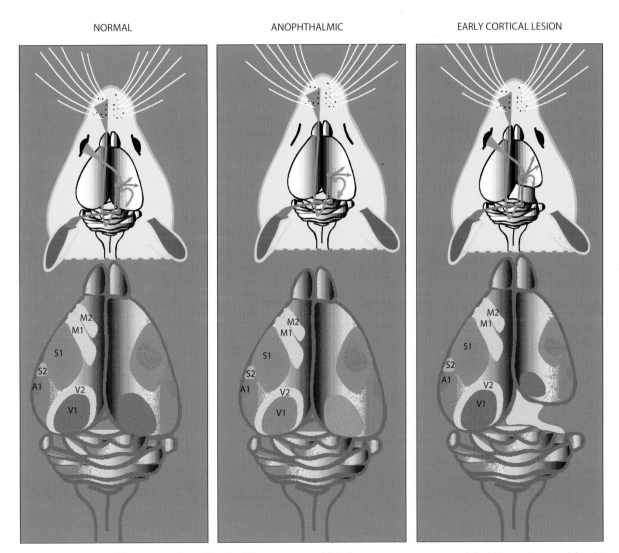

**Plate 7** Schematic representation of the sensory pathways from the different sensory modalities (upper row: somatosensory, red; visual, blue; auditory, purple) and the distribution of cortical areas (lower row: S1, primary somatosensory cortex red; V1, primary visual cortex blue; A1, primary auditory cortex, purple) in normal, anophthalmic, and early cortical lesioned animals. The normal thalamocortical relationship is maintained in anophthalmic mice, but the auditory and somatosensory modalities invade the visual thalamic nuclei (dLGN) and thus the cortex will be responsive to these modalities (Bronchti et al., 2000). The thalamocortical relations do not show major rearrangements. In contrast to this; after extremely early cortical lesions in the marsupial, cortical areas showed substantial rearrangements on the remaining cortical sheets, together with considerable rearrangements of the thalamic afferents (Huffmann et al., 1999). (From Molnár et al., 2006c.) See also Figure 9.10 in the text.

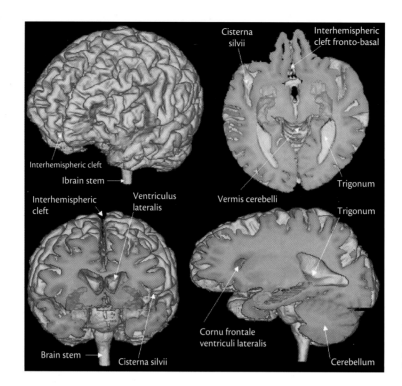

**Plate 8** Three-dimensional reconstruction of the amygdala (red)–hippocampus complex (blue) (MRI, $T_1$-weighted, 3D-MPRAGE, VOXIM). See also Figure 13.3 in the text.

(a)

(b)

(c)

(d)

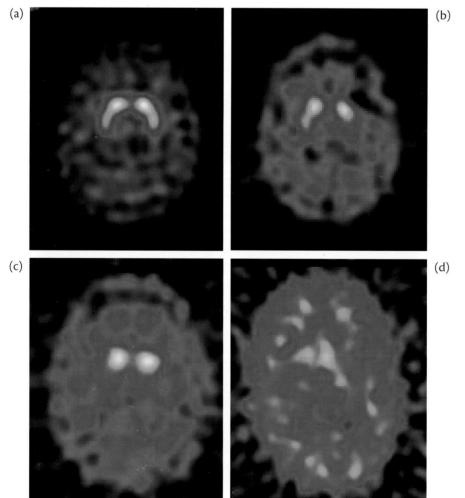

**Plate 9** Normal (a) and abnormal (b)–(d) FP-CIT SPECT images in subjects with dementia. (b) Asymmetric uptake in the putamen with near normal on one side (type 1). (c) Greatly reduced putamen uptake bilaterally (type 2). (d) Uptake is virtually absent (type 3). (Taken from McKeith *et al.* 2007, with permission.) See also Figure 27v.1 in the text.

(López-Bendito and Molnár, 2003). The mechanisms underlying thalamocortical and corticofugal axon pathfinding are likely to be similar, as there are numerous mouse mutants (such as *Pax6*, *Tbr1*, *Gbx2*, *Emx2*) in which both thalamocortical and corticofugal pathfinding is arrested or altered at the striatocortical junction (Molnár *et al.*, 2003). This zone, also called the pallial–subpallial boundary (PSPB; Fig 9.3), lies perpendicular to the trajectories of the thalamocortical projections, and their interactions with early corticofugal projections within this region are crucial for their deployment.

The release of attractive and repulsive factors and axon guidance molecules from the cortex is believed to play an important role in channelling the growing projections though the forebrain, and also in the homing in of specific sets of axons to particular cortical areas. All of the above-mentioned region-specific extracellular signalling molecules, ligands, and receptors could act to attract or repel specific sets of thalamocortical projections. Different classes of molecules are likely to serve different functions, which include broad growth-promoting properties, chemoattraction and chemorepulsion, specific substrates that indicate a route along which axons should grow, as well as those that prevent crossing of particular boundaries such as the midline or the hypothalamus. It is worth noting that a chemorepulsive cue for one group of axons may well be a chemoattractant to another group of axons growing in the opposite direction and expressing a different set of cell-surface receptors. Thus the role of a signalling molecule is defined by the cellular reaction to it, which in turn is dependent on its complement of cell surface receptors and intracellular signalling cascades.

The early deployment of thalamocortical connectivity is established in an autonomous fashion, before the afferents from the sensory periphery reach the dorsal thalamus, in accordance with the 'anatomical' or 'intrinsic properties' school of view. However, the sensory periphery can modify this juvenile topography after the initial targeting, during the process of thalamic fibre ingrowth and arborization (Price *et al.*, 2006), in accordance with the 'activity-dependent development' view. It has been proposed that while the thalamic axons accumulate in the subplate, they engage in activity-dependent interactions with these cells, and this in return might lead to their realignment before they enter the cortex.

When TTX (a sodium channel antagonist that blocks action potentials, and thereby nerve electrical activity) was delivered into the brain of cat fetuses at the time of arrival of thalamic projections to the subplate, abnormal connections were established by the axons from the lateral geniculate nucleus. Only a few thalamic fibres entered the visual cortex, and an aberrant topography was formed within the cortical plate. The exact nature of the required neural activity is not known.

Shortly before birth, most thalamic axons start to detach from the subplate and grow into the cortical plate, forming branches and synapses in the appropriate layer. It has been suggested that a 'stop' and/or a 'branch' signal in the cortex plays a role in the specific targeting of thalamic axons to their appropriate layer 4. Some of the layer-specific cell surface and extracellular matrix molecules might account for the molecular differences between the cortical layers that influence the termination of thalamocortical projections (Yamamoto *et al.*, 2000).

## Mouse model—barrel formation—as an example of map formation

The complexity of the interplay between invading axons and cortical cells is exemplified by the specialized cytoarchitectural formation of the mouse barrel cortex (Woolsey and Van der Loos, 1970; Van der Loos and Woolsey, 1973). The barrel cortex is a major part of the primary somatosensory cortex, in which the whiskers on the snout are represented topographically, such that one so-called 'barrel' in the cortical layer 4 corresponds to each whisker. Stimulation of a single whisker results in the activation of a well-defined cortical region—a barrel—corresponding to that particular whisker. The barrel-field is composed of 'barrel walls' made up of the cell bodies of the cortical layer 4 cells, each surrounding a 'barrel hollow' which contains the afferent thalamic axons as well as the dendrites of the cortical cells (Fig. 9.9). Several lines of evidence indicate that the morphological reorganization and differentiation of cortical neurons to form barrels depend, at least in part, on signals conveyed by invading thalamic axons (Erzurumlu and Kind, 2001; Molnár and Hannan, 2000).

Blocking or changing the flow of sensory input during the first post-natal week alters the pattern of cortical representation in accordance with the peripheral pattern. If the peripheral pattern is altered before the barrel cortex pattern is established, e.g. by removal of whiskers, the arrangement of barrels will develop differently to reflect the peripheral arrangement. Similar plastic changes in development are believed to occur in humans who lack one sensory modality (e.g. blindness for a variety of causes), in a more dramatic version such that the cortical areas usually reserved for that sensory modality are taken over by another one.

In mice with null mutations in either the monoamine oxidase A (*MAOA*) gene or the adenylyl cyclase 1 gene, ingrowing thalamic axons fail to segregate to form the primordial periphery-related pattern, and cortical cells do not rearrange as cytoarchitectural entities. A disruption of thalamocortical patterning is caused by elevated levels of 5-hydroxytryptamine (5-HT), but not other amines, in the *MAOA* knock-out mouse. Genetic removal of 5-HT1B receptors or pharmacological blockade of 5-HT synthesis in this mutant mouse restores normal patterning of thalamic axon terminals and near-normal segregation of cortical barrels.

Group I metabotropic glutamate receptors (mGluR1 and mGluR5) have been implicated in cortical and hippocampal plasticity. Post-synaptic molecules [such as the metabotropic glutamate receptor 5 (mGluR5), and the receptor-activated G-protein-coupled phosphodiesterase PLC1] also seem to be involved in cytoarchitectural differentiation imposed by thalamocortical axons within the cortex. Mice with a deletion of the *mGluR5* gene display normal segregation of large whisker thalamocortical axons, but only rows and not individual patches within rows form, and these mice lack barrels (Hannan *et al.*, 2001). The fact that deletion of *mGluR5* leads to the loss of barrels indicates that mGluR5 signalling is also crucial for transmitting the periphery-related pattern from thalamic axons to their post-synaptic target in the cortex.

Interestingly, in mice that lack the *PLC1* gene, defects in barrel formation have been described in the absence of defects in the patterning of thalamocortical axons. The expression of PLC1 in the developing cortex is mainly post-synaptic, and phosphoinositide hydrolysis following activation of the group I mGluRs is dependent on *PLC1* expression during the first post-natal week, indicating

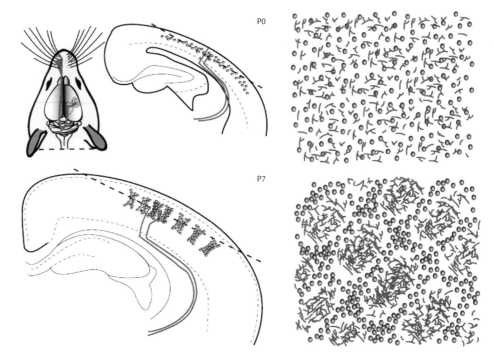

**Fig. 9.9** Schematic overview of the development of the periphery-related thalamocortical patterning and the cytoarchitectural barrel pattern in the mouse from the initially uniform distribution of thalamocortical arbors (red) at birth ((P)ost-natal day 0) and layer 4 neurons (blue), to the ordered structure of the mature cortex which is achieved within a week (P7). Left column represents coronal, right column tangential sections. (From Molnár and Molnár, 2006.) See Plate 6 for a colour version of this figure.

that mGluR5 activation of PLC1 is crucial for barrel formation. The mechanism responsible for the segregation of thalamic axons according to the peripheral pattern is not known. Activity mediated through *N*-methyl-ᴅ-aspartate receptors (NMDARs) does not seem to be involved, because deletion of the NMDAR1 (*NR1*) gene in excitatory cortical neurons did not completely prevent the formation of the periphery-related pattern of thalamo-cortical axons, but cytoarchitectural barrels failed to form (Erzurumlu and Kind, 2001).

### Plasticity during development

As described above, changes in the periphery result in changes in the anatomical structure of the brain at the cellular level—at least if the peripheral changes occur before or during the so-called 'critical period' (Fig 9.10)'. This is the period during which activity-dependent mechanisms determine the finer structure of the cerebral cortex, in which superfluous or wrong connections are reduced and the most active connections are strengthened, so influencing both long-range as well as local connectivity (Innocenti and Price, 2005).

### Plasticity during adulthood

Plastic changes need to continue throughout the life of an organism—how else would we learn? But whereas in development, the changes are at 'gross connectivity' level, i.e. whether particular regions are connected or not, in the adult brain, plasticity manifests itself mostly in the modification of existing circuits. Cells do not completely abandon a connection via synapses, or extend entire new axon collaterals. Instead, they modify the efficacy of the existing synaptic connections—either strengthening or weakening them. The cellular machinery needed to modify synaptic strengths is partly the same as that described above for the patterning of thalamic afferents and rearrangement of cortical layer 4 cells during barrel cortex development (Fig. 9.9).

Information processing in the brain is highly redundant, with multiple representations of information in different cell assemblies. Computational models of information encoding in the brain suggest that such representations, even within a cell assembly, are very robust, such that the necessary information can still be extracted even if the signal or encoding is severely degraded. The reason for saying so is partly theoretical: this is how we think information is encoded by neural assemblies. And partly it reflects a feature of the anatomy of the brain whereby (for example) sensory information is split into different aspects and processed by different areas in a redundant fashion. The effect of both these sources of redundancy in combination may help to explain why pathological changes in the brain can be demonstrated on post-mortem tissue without the patient having exhibited obvious signs of dementia prior to death.

Therefore the early pruning of 'wrong' connections in the brain probably does not extend to the wholesale removal of redundant connections, thereby providing scope for compensation as well as the basis for future modification in the form of learning. The existence of redundancy allows modification, without the need to modify all existing connections. This allows both memory retention (maintenance of previous connections) and acquisition of new memories (modification of redundant connections). As mentioned previously, in the mature brain much of this occurs not at the level of axon growth or removal, but rather as a change in the strength of existing connections, in the form of altered synaptic strengths.

### Implications for human disease

Specific causes of schizophrenia and other mental illnesses remain elusive. The most consistent hypothesis suggests that schizophrenia may result from a mutation in susceptibility genes that act on early stages of neurodevelopment, combined with environmental events occurring during pregnancy or the post-natal period (Lewis and Levitt, 2002). Recently, several susceptibility genes: neuregulin-1,

NORMAL                               ANOPTHALMIC                          EARLY CORTICAL LESION

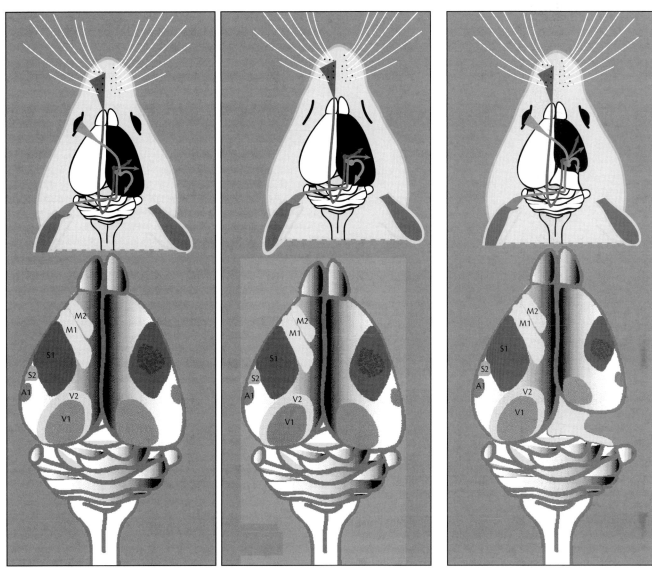

**Fig. 9.10** Schematic representation of the sensory pathways from the different sensory modalities (upper row: somatosensory, red; visual, blue; auditory, purple) and the distribution of cortical areas (lower row: S1, primary somatosensory cortex red; V1, primary visual cortex blue; A1, primary auditory cortex, purple) in normal, anophthalmic, and early cortical lesioned animals. The normal thalamocortical relationship is maintained in anophthalmic mice, but the auditory and somatosensory modalities invade the visual thalamic nuclei (dLGN) and thus the cortex will be responsive to these modalities (Bronchti *et al.*, 2000). The thalamocortical relations do not show major rearrangements. In contrast to this; after extremely early cortical lesions in the marsupial, cortical areas showed substantial rearrangements on the remaining cortical sheets, together with considerable rearrangements of the thalamic afferents (Huffmann *et al.*, 1999). (From Molnár *et al.*, 2006c.) See Plate 7 for a colour version of this figure.

dysbindin, *DAAO* (D-amino acid oxidase), *G72* (activator of DAAO), *RGS4* (regulator of G-protein signalling-4), and *COMT* (catecholamine-O-methyltransferase) have been identified. All of these have been implicated in early brain development and adult neuroplasticity (Harrison and Owen, 2003).

## Conclusion

The cerebral cortex provides the biological substrate for human cognitive capacity and is, arguably, the part of the brain that distinguishes us from other species. Therefore, understanding the evolution and development of this complex structure is central to our understanding of human intelligence and creativity, as well as of disorders of cognitive functions.

In recent years, the molecular and cellular processes underlying fundamental aspects of cortical development have begun to be elucidated in transgenic mouse models. Mouse genetics will continue to be at the centre stage of cortical research, but the insights into human development that we can gain from studying other species are limited. The enormous size of the human forebrain, the vast number of functionally specialized cortical areas, and the richness of human cognitive capacity, all demand explanations.

Evolutionary expansion in the size and complexity of the human cerebral cortex is probably a result of changes in the molecular mechanisms of cell proliferation and phenotypic differentiation.

Although the basic principles are similar in all mammalian species, the modulation of developmental mechanisms in human and non-human primates leads to the emergence of new neuronal subclasses and the addition of specialized cortical areas.

The sequence and combination of gene activation is carefully choreographed during brain development. Alterations in gene activation by environmental signals or by a disrupted genetic code can lead to several devastating diseases, some manifesting themselves relatively late in life, and only after further environmental and/or genetic influences. Developmental processes during embryonic and early post-natal life will have implications for the rest of our lives. In the light of the number of genes and their complex interactions during development, it is surprising that there are not more developmental abnormalities influencing our cognitive functions.

The nervous system evolved to be able to adapt to the environment exceptionally well, and this design allows it to cope with changes in the genotype with relatively few blips in the manifested phenotype. However, environmental influences can accelerate or delay the emergence of symptoms of a disease and disease progression (Nithiananatharajah and Hannan, 2006). Symptoms associated with ageing can show great individual variation, and understanding these variations will be an exciting area in old age psychiatry. Their origin may lie in the individual details of early development and plasticity, and in the infinite variability of interaction with the environment.

## References

Allendoerfer, K.L. and Shatz, C.J. (1994). The subplate, a transient neocortical structure: its role in the development of connections between thalamus and cortex. *Annual Review of Neuroscience*, **17**, 185–218.

Arlotta, P., Molyneaux, B.J., Chen, J., Inoue, J., Kominami, R., and Macklis, J.D. (2005). Neuronal subtype-specific genes that control corticospinal motor neuron development *in vivo*. *Neuron*, **45**(2), 207–21.

Bai, J., Ramos, R.L., Ackman, J.B., Thomas, A.M., Lee, R.V., and LoTurco, J.J. (2003). RNAi reveals doublecortin is required for radial migration in rat neocortex. *Nature Neuroscience*, **6**(12), 1277–83.

Bellion, A. and Métin, C. (2005) Early regionalisation of the neocortex and the medial ganglionic eminence. *Brain Research Bulletin*, **66**(4–6), 402–9.

Blaschke, A.J., Weiner, J.A., and Chun, J. (1998). Programmed cell death is a universal feature of neuroproliferative regions throughout the developing CNS. *Journal of Comparative Neurology*, **396**: 39–50.

Bronchti, G., Molnár, Z., Welker, E., Croquelois, A., and Krubitzer, L. (1999). Auditory and somatosensory activity in the 'visual cortex' of the anophthalmic mutant mouse. *Swiss Society for Neuroscience Meeting*, *Zürich*, Vol. 4, p. 22.

Buss, R.R., Sun, W., and Oppenheim, R.W. (2006). Adaptive roles of programmed cell death during nervous system development. *Annual Review of Neuroscience*, **29**, 1–35.

Butt, S.J., Fuccillo, M., Nery, S. *et al.* (2005). The temporal and spatial origins of cortical interneurons predict their physiological subtype. *Neuron*, **48**(4), 591–604.

Dasen, J.S., Liu, J.P., and Jessell, T.M. (2003). Motor neuron columnar fate imposed by sequential phases of Hox-c activity. *Nature*, **425**(6961), 926–33.

Dehay, C., Giroud, P., Berland, M., Killackey, H., and Kennedy, H. (1996). Contribution of thalamic input to the specification of cytoarchitectonic cortical fields in the primate effects of bilateral enucleation in the fetal monkey on the boundaries, dimensions, and gyrification of striate and extrastriate cortex. *Journal of Comparative Neurology*, **367**(1), 70–89.

Dehay, C., Savatier, P., Cortay, V., and Kennedy, H. (2001). Cell-cycle kinetics of neocortical precursors are influenced by embryonic thalamic axons. *Journal of Neuroscience*, **21**(1), 201–14.

Denaxa, M., Chan, C.H., Schachner, M., Parnavelas, J.G., and Karagogeos, D. (2001). The adhesion molecule TAG-1 mediates the migration of cortical interneurons from the ganglionic eminence along the corticofugal fiber system. *Development*, **128**(22), 4635–44.

Erzurumlu, R.S. and Kind, P.C. (2001). Neural activity: sculptor of 'barrels' in the neocortex. *Trends in Neuroscience*, **24**(10), 589–95.

Goffinet, A.M. and Rakic, P. (2000). *Mouse brain development*. Springer-Verlag, New York.

Golden, J.A. and Harding, B.N. (2004). Pathology and genetics. In *Developmental neuropathology*. ISN Neuropath Press, Basel.

Grove, E.A. and Fukuchi-Shimogori, T. (2003). Generating the cerebral cortical area map. *Annual Review of Neuroscience*, **26**, 355–80.

Guillemot, F., Molnár, Z., Tarabykin, V., and Stoykova, A. (2006). Molecular mechanisms of cortical differentiation. *European Journal of Neuroscience*, **23**(4), 857–68.

Hannan, A.J., Blakemore, C., Katsnelson, A. *et al.* (2001). PLC-beta1, activated via mGluRs, mediates activity-dependent differentiation in cerebral cortex. *Nature Neuroscience*, **4**(3), 282–8.

Harrison, P.J. and Owen, M.J. (2003). Genes for schizophrenia? Recent findings and their pathophysiological implications. *Lancet*, **361**(9355), 417–19.

Harrison, P.J. and Weinberger, D.R. (2005). Schizophrenia genes, gene expression, and neuropathology: on the matter of their convergence. *Molecular Psychiatry*, **10**(1), 40–68.

Hevner, R.F., Hodge, R.D., Daza, R.A., and Englund, C. (2006). Transcription factors in glutamatergic neurogenesis: conserved programs in neocortex, cerebellum, and adult hippocampus. *Neuroscience Research*, **55**(3), 223–33.

Higashi, S., Hioki, K., Kurotani, T., Kasim, N., and Molnár, Z. (2005). Functional thalamocortical synapse reorganization from subplate to layer IV during postnatal development in the reeler-like mutant rat (shaking rat Kawasaki). *Journal of Neuroscience*, **25**(6), 1395–406.

Hochstetter, F. (1919). *Beiträge zur Entwicklungsgeschichte des menschlichen Gehirns*, pt I. Franz Deuticke, Vienna.

Huffman, K.J., Molnár, Z., Van Dellen, A., Kahn, D.M., Blakemore, C., and Krubitzer, L. (1999). Formation of cortical fields on a reduced cortical sheet. *Journal of Neuroscience*, **19**(22), 9939–52.

Innocenti, G.M. and Price, D.J. (2005). Exuberance in the development of cortical networks. *Nature Reviews Neuroscience*, **6**(12), 955–65.

Jessell, T.M. (2000). Neuronal specification in the spinal cord: inductive signals and transcriptional codes. *Nature Reviews Genetics*, **1**(1), 20–9.

Kandel, E.R., Schwartz, J.H., and Jessel, T.M. (2000). Principles of neural science, 4th edn. Elsevier, Amsterdam.

Kostovic, I. and Rakic, P. (1980). Cytology and time of origin of interstitial neurons in the white matter in infant and adult human and monkey telencephalon. *Journal of Neurocytology*, **9**(2), 219–42.

Kostovic, I. and Rakic, P. (1990) Developmental history of the transient subplate zone in the visual and somatosensory cortex of the macaque monkey and human brain. *Journal of Comparative Neurology*, **297**(3), 441–70.

Kriegstein, A.R. (2005). Constructing circuits: neurogenesis and migration in the developing neocortex. *Epilepsia*, **46**(Suppl. 7), 15–21.

Kriegstein, A.R. and Noctor, S.C. (2004). Patterns of neuronal migration in the embryonic cortex. *Trends in Neuroscience*, **27**(7), 392–9.

Krubitzer, L. and Kaas, J. (2005). The evolution of the neocortex in mammals: how is phenotypic diversity generated? *Current Opinion in Neurobiology*, **15**(4), 444–53.

Lambert de Rouvroit, C. and Goffinet, A.M. (2001). Neuronal migration. *Mechanisms of Development*, **105**(1–2), 47–56.

Larsen, W.J. (1993). *Human embryology*. Churchill Livingstone, New York.

Levitt, P. (2005). Disruption of interneuron development. *Epilepsia*, **46**(Suppl. 7), 22–8.

Levitt, P., Ebert, P., Mirnics, K., Nimgaonkar, V.L., and Lewis, D.A. (2006). Making the case for a candidate vulnerability gene in schizophrenia: convergent evidence for Regulator of G-Protein Signaling 4 (RGS4). *Biological Psychiatry*, **60**(6), 534–7.

Lewis, D.A. and Levitt, P. (2002) Schizophrenia as a disorder of neurodevelopment. *Annual Review of Neuroscience*, **25**, 409–32.

López-Bendito, G. and Molnár, Z. (2003). Thalamocortical development: how are we going to get there? Nature Reviews Neuroscience, **4**(4), 276–89.

Lukaszewicz, A., Savatier, P., Cortay, V. et al. (2005). G1 phase regulation, area-specific cell cycle control, and cytoarchitectonics in the primate cortex. Neuron, **47**(3), 353–64.

Lumsden, A. (2004). Segmentation and compartition in the early avian hindbrain. Mechanisms of Development, **121**(9), 1081–8.

Marin, O. and Rubenstein, J.L. (2003). Cell migration in the forebrain. Annual Review of Neuroscience, **26**, 441–83.

Martinez-Cerdeno, V., Noctor, S.C., and Kriegstein, A.R. (2006). The role of intermediate progenitor cells in the evolutionary expansion of the cerebral cortex. Cerebral Cortex, **16**(Suppl. 1), i152–i161.

Métin, C., Baudoin, J.P., Rakic, S., and Parnavelas, J.G. (2006). Cell and molecular mechanisms involved in the migration of cortical interneurons. European Journal of Neuroscience, **23**(4), 894–900.

Miyashita-Lin, E.M., Hevner, R., Wassarman, K.M., Martinez, S., and Rubenstein, J.L. (1999). Early neocortical regionalization in the absence of thalamic innervation. Science, **285**(5429), 906–9.

Moldin, S.O., Rubenstein, J.L., and Hyman, S.E. (2006). Can autism speak to neuroscience? Journal of Neuroscience, **26**(26), 6893–6.

Molnár, Z. and Hannan, A. (2000). Development of thalamocortical projections in normal and mutant mice. In Results and problems in cell differentiation, Vol. 30 Mouse brain development (ed. A. Goffinet and P. Rakic), pp. 293–332. Springer-Verlag, Berlin.

Molnár, Z. and Molnár, E. (2006). Calcium and NeuroD2 control the development of thalamocortical communication. Neuron, **49**(5), 639–42.

Molnár, Z., Higashi, S., and Lopez-Bendito, G. (2003). Choreography of early thalamocortical development. Cerebral Cortex, **13**(6), 661–9.

Molnár, Z., Métin, C., Stoykova, A. et al. (2006a). Comparative aspects of cerebral cortical development. European Journal of Neuroscience, **23**(4), 921–34.

Molnár, Z., Tavare, A., and Cheung, A.F.P. (2006b). The origin of neocortex: lessons from comparative embryology. Evolution of nervous systems, Vol. 3: The evolution of nervous systems in mammals (ed. L.A. Krubitzer and J.H. Kaas), pp. 13–26. Elsevier, Oxford.

Molnár, Z., López-Bendito, G., Blakey, D., Thompson, A., and Higashi, S. (2006c). Earliest thalamocortical interactions. In Development and plasticity in sensory thalamus and cortex (ed. R. Erzurumlu, W. Guido, and Z. Molnár), pp. 54–78. Springer-Verlag, New York.

Molyneaux, B.J., Arlotta, P., Hirata, T., Hibi, M., and Macklis, J.D. (2005). Fezl is required for the birth and specification of corticospinal motor neurons. Neuron, **47**(6), 817–31.

Nadarajah, B. and Parnavelas, J.G. (2002). Modes of neuronal migration in the developing cerebral cortex. Nature Reviews Neuroscience, **3**(6), 423–32.

Nakagawa, Y., Johnson, J.E., O'Leary, D.D. (1999). Graded and areal expression patterns of regulatory genes and cadherins in embryonic neocortex independent of thalamocortical input. Journal of Neuroscience, **19**(24), 10877–85.

Nelson, S.B., Sugino, K., and Hempel, C.M. (2006). The problem of neuronal cell types: a physiological genomics approach. Trends in Neuroscience, **29**(6), 339–45.

Nery, S., Fishell, G., and Corbin, J.G. (2002). The caudal ganglionic eminence is a source of distinct cortical and subcortical cell populations. Nature Neuroscience, **5**(12), 1279–87.

Nithianantharajah, J. and Hannan, A.J. (2006). Enriched environments, experience-dependent plasticity and disorders of the nervous system. Nature Reviews Neuroscience, **7**(9), 697–709.

Noctor, S.C., Martinez-Cerdeno, V., Ivic, L., and Kriegstein, A.R. (2004). Cortical neurons arise in symmetric and asymmetric division zones and migrate through specific phases. Nature Neuroscience, **7**(2), 136–44.

Nolte, J. (1999). The human brain, 4th edn. Mosby, St Louis, MO.

O'Leary, D.D. (1989) Do cortical areas emerge from a protocortex? Trends in Neuroscience, **12**(10), 400–6.

Penfield, W. and Rasmussen, T. (1950). The cerebral cortex of man. Macmillan, New York.

Polleux, F. and Lauder, J.M. (2004). Toward a developmental neurobiology of autism. Mental Retardation and Developmental Disabilities Research Reviews, **10**(4), 303–17.

Price, D.J., Kennedy, H., Dehay, C. et al. (2006). The development of cortical connections. European Journal of Neuroscience, **23**, 910–20.

Rakic, P. (1988). Specification of cerebral cortical areas. Science, **241**(4862), 170–6.

Rakic, P. (2000). Molecular and cellular mechanisms of neuronal migration: relevance to cortical epilepsies. Advances in Neurology, **84**, 1–14.

Rakic, P. (2006). No more cortical neurons for you. Science, **313**(5789), 928–9.

Rakic, P. and Caviness, V.S., Jr (1995). Cortical development: view from neurological mutants two decades later. Neuron, **14**(6), 1101–4.

Rash, B.G. and Grove, E.A. (2006). Area and layer patterning in the developing cerebral cortex. Current Opinion in Neurobiology, **16**(1), 25–34.

Stern, C.D. (2006). Neural induction: 10 years on since the 'default model'. Current Opinion in Cell Biology, **18**(6), 692–7.

Storm, E.E., Garel, S., Borello, U. et al. (2006). Dose-dependent functions of Fgf8 in regulating telencephalic patterning centers. Development, **133**(9), 1831–44.

Taglialatela, P., Soria, J.M., Caironi, V., Moiana, A., and Bertuzzi, S. (2004). Compromised generation of GABAergic interneurons in the brains of Vax1–/– mice. Development, **131**, 4239–49.

Vanderhaeghen, P. and Polleux, F. (2004). Developmental mechanisms patterning thalamocortical projections: intrinsic, extrinsic and in between. Trends in Neuroscience, **27**(7), 384–91.

Van der Loos, H. and Woolsey, T.A. (1973). Somatosensory cortex: structural alterations following early injury to sense organs. Science, **179**(71), 395–8.

Walsh, C.A. and Goffinet, A.M. (2000). Potential mechanisms of mutations that affect neuronal migration in man and mouse. Current Opinion in Genetics and Development, **10**(3), 270–4.

Wonders, C.P. and Anderson, S.A. (2006). The origin and specification of cortical interneurons. Nature Reviews Neuroscience, **7**(9), 687–96.

Woolsey, T.A. and Van der Loos, H. (1970). The structural organization of layer IV in the somatosensory region (SI) of mouse cerebral cortex. The description of a cortical field composed of discrete cytoarchitectonic units. Brain Research, **17**(2), 205–42.

Yamamoto, N., Matsuyama, Y., Harada, A., Inui, K., Murakami, F., and Hanamura, K. (2000). Characterization of factors regulating lamina-specific growth of thalamocortical axons. Journal of Neurobiology, **42**, 56–68.

# SECTION II

# Clinical practice

# 10

# Psychiatric assessment of older people

Alan Thomas

The structure of the initial psychiatric assessment of older people is the same as in younger adults, comprising a thorough history, detailed mental state assessment, and a physical examination. However, the details and balance of each of these components vary considerably from the assessment in younger adults due to the high prevalence of physical morbidity and the crucial importance of proper cognitive assessment. In the same way, whilst the same kind of follow-up assessments, e.g. social work assessment and investigations such as neuroimaging, are needed, the assessments themselves are quite different.

## The venue for the initial assessment

Assessment of the older person with a possible mental illness may take place in a range of settings, as considered below, and whilst each has its strengths and weaknesses the evidence about the clinical and cost-effectiveness of these different approaches is poor (Parker et al., 2000). In practice the place where the initial assessment is conducted is constrained by the existing design of the local service, the manner of the referral, and the urgency of the clinical problem. The assessing clinician needs to show flexibility to adapt his or her assessment to the advantages and disadvantages of the different locations.

## Home-based assessment

Patients referred for old age psychiatric assessment should be seen initially at home. Such domiciliary assessment has several advantages over a hospital-based assessment for older people and is especially important for those with cognitive impairment. The patient is spared a time consuming, tiring, and perhaps expensive journey to clinic. Clinics, especially psychiatric ones, are too often unpleasant places to wait around and can be particularly distressing to frail, elderly, and cognitively impaired people. Unsurprisingly therefore when patients were asked they overwhelmingly opted for home-based assessment over clinic-based assessment or assessment at a primary care clinic (Jones et al., 1987). For the clinician, a home-based assessment provides a depth and quality of information that exposes the shallowness of what can be achieved in clinic, an aspect that frequently strikes medical students when visiting with consultants (Anderson and Aquilina, 2002). On arrival the doctor is already aware of the local environment, whether it is large houses with

spacious gardens or empty flats with boarded up windows, and the quality of the patient's own house before knocking on the door. On entering the doctor is rapidly able to determine the state of the entrance area and main room and can observe any hazards, such as loose carpets or objects strewn on the floor, as well as the general level of cleanliness. After politely seeking permission, a quick inspection of the kitchen, looking for out-of-date food, an empty fridge, or burned pans can be revealing. Interestingly, it was this aspect of home-based assessments, the ability to understand the home environment, which one study reported as the main reason general practitioners asked for such assessments (Hardy-Thompson et al., 1992). It is much easier for a key relative or carer to be present at the patient's home and often several are present. As well as providing corroboration for the history, this can assist the patient to remember and clarify important elements of the history and it may give an insight into family dynamics and the kind of relationships the patient enjoys. For those patients who have carers attending already there should be a written care plan available and daily notes from the carer(s) giving useful additional information. An informative practice is to ask the patient to produce their medication for checking, which, as well as confirming their current treatment, will often reveal evidence of erratic compliance. A domiciliary assessment also shows the patient at their best, giving a more realistic assessment of their mood, cognition, and general behaviour. Although most of these advantages will be familiar to clinicians practising in the field they are difficult to study, but one investigation reported a large reduction in non-attendance for home-based (1.7%) versus clinic-based (21.2%) assessments, leading to a more efficient use of valuable medical time (Anderson and Aquilina, 2002). This also results in patients being followed-up more effectively (Benbow, 1990) and non-attendance at clinics leads to important delays in assessment and on occasions assessment doesn't happen at all (Frankel et al., 1989).

## Assessment in residential homes

When a referred patient is living in a residential care facility this is usually because of the development of some form of behavioural disturbance in someone with a pre-existing illness, in most cases dementia. They have often therefore been previously assessed, and provided that their previous records are available this enables the psychiatrist to concentrate on the current issue(s). Where there has been no previous formal psychiatric assessment it can be very difficult to complete a full history because informants with a long-term knowledge of the patient are often not available. In some cases they may be available by telephone, but often a pragmatic approach is necessary, making the best use of available sources of information. As well as the referral letter, documents from social services recording the admission process to the home and care records can be consulted. This can furnish valuable information about the previous history. Care staff are usually able to provide a reasonable account about the current problems, although it is prudent to enquire how well the carer/informant knows the patient and for how long.

### Outpatient assessment

For most patients referred to old age psychiatric services an initial assessment in their own home remains the choice for the reasons outlined above. Whilst some people with functional illnesses, especially those who are physically fit, may be adequately assessed in an outpatient clinic, in practice it is usually difficult to identify with confidence such people from the referral letter alone. The main group where outpatient clinic assessment can be advantageous is in people with a possible early dementia, and over the last 10–15 years memory clinics, focusing on such patients, have become an increasingly prominent feature in old age psychiatry services (Lindesay *et al.*, 2002). Such clinics deal with younger, less cognitively impaired patients, and for those who have a dementia they are earlier in the course of their illness (Luce *et al.*, 2001). This development has been supported in England and Wales by the National Service Framework for Older People (standard 7 (7.49) (Health, 2001). The special elements of memory clinics are discussed in detail elsewhere (see Chapter 21).

### Inpatient assessment

A third to a quarter of new referrals to old age psychiatric services come from wards in general hospitals, and assessment here is a very different experience from home-based assessments and brings its own difficulties. The growing recognition that inpatient assessments require a different approach has led to the development in many places of specialist liaison old age psychiatric services. These services and the special approach and skills needed for inpatient old age psychiatry are discussed in Chapter 22.

## The psychiatric assessment

### Aims of the assessment

A psychiatric assessment aims to achieve much more than a diagnosis. A thorough assessment should enable the clinician to produce well-reasoned differential diagnoses and have some confidence in the most likely main diagnosis. But the initial assessment also aims to engage the patient and his or her family to facilitate further assessment as necessary and to foster cooperation in all aspects of future management. Thus the process of assessment should establish a good rapport with patients and their families and carers, and achieving such a positive relationship improves the quality of information obtained. There has been a marked trend recently towards disclosing the diagnosis of dementia, perhaps influenced by arrival of licensed treatments, and establishing a good rapport paves the way for dealing with this sensitive subject (Bamford *et al.*, 2004).

As well as eliciting information to determine a diagnosis it is important to identify other relevant problems which need dealing

with in their own right. The importance of non-cognitive symptoms in dementia (commonly referred to as behavioural and psychological symptoms in dementia, BPSD) is now well recognized (Finkel and Burns, 2000), yet these play no role in the diagnosis which is based on cognitive symptoms alone. And clarifying functional difficulties, such as with mobility or personal care, and the presence of other relevant medical illnesses is essential as well. Thus, for example, a summary of a patient's assessment should include, in addition to a diagnosis of dementia, reference to such issues as psychotic symptoms, mood disturbance, postural instability, and difficulties using stairs and bathing. The initial assessment should not, indeed cannot, aim to achieve a detailed understanding of all these matters, but should identify the range of issues which need further assessment. The initial assessment should therefore be holistic in aiming to achieve a clear overall understanding of the patient's complete set of needs.

### The initial assessment

Upon first meeting the patient a good handshake, polite smile, and clear explanation of who you are and why you have come begins the process of forming a working relationship. The referral letter should have identified the key issues but it is important at the outset to ensure they are correct and where the letter is unclear to ask what the main problems are. It is common for the patient to deny they have any problems, especially when they have cognitive impairment, and not infrequently the patient is found to have had no involvement in the referral process, which was initiated by concerned family members. Tact and sensitivity are needed to explain the concerns others have about the patient and to obtain patience and cooperation with the formal assessment itself. Seeking permission to speak with family or friends can be difficult in such circumstances but it is still important to try to do so. Explaining to the patient that understanding the whole picture is important and that it is standard practice to ask other people for information achieves consent in most cases.

### History

A careful and detailed history remains the most important element in the whole assessment; physical and mental state examinations and special investigations only serve to clarify and confirm the history. It is therefore vital to establish a good rapport and give adequate time to cover all the necessary aspects in the clinical history.

### Presenting complaint

One main problem may be given as the reason for referral but typically several interrelated issues are present. These need to be identified, clarified individually, and their relationship, temporal and otherwise, established. At the outset it is appropriate to check that patients understand why they are being assessed and that the presenting problems are all those that need to be discussed. This may reveal important issues, such as that the person resents having been referred and is angry with their husband or wife for having done so. The development of each key symptom can then be covered, asking about key aspects such as duration, pattern of onset, change through time, and any known precipitants. The timing of the onset of amnesia and cognitive decline is frequently difficult, but asking about this in relation to memorable dates can be useful, e.g. was the patient his or her usual self last birthday, or at Christmas, or on holiday last summer? In old age psychiatry people usually present with a history of insidious onset of amnesia, and whilst this is characteristic of Alzheimer's disease (AD), dementia with Lewy bodies (DLB) also presents this way and it is a common pattern in vascular dementia (VaD), especially of the subcortical type. The classic VaD presentation, a sudden onset of dementia and/or a stepwise deterioration, is unusual in old age psychiatry, probably because such patients usually present acutely to stroke services. A more rapid (but not sudden) onset of cognitive impairment, over a few days or weeks, is consistent with a delirium or a depression and should lead to questions to identify these syndromes, e.g. for delirium the presence of an infection or fluctuating consciousness and for depression of affective change and biological symptoms. In someone with an insidious onset of amnesia then questions to identify other cognitive symptoms may be appropriate, e.g. problems reading or writing, difficulties naming objects or recognizing objects or people, but such issues are usually identified more clearly during cognitive testing. Of more importance during history taking is covering the range of non-cognitive symptoms which occur in dementia. It is essential to ask about problems in everyday function, in order to identify needs for which further assessment and help can be given and to assess the severity of the dementia. These are usually divided into basic activities of daily living (ability to maintain personal care) and instrumental activities of daily living (more complex everyday tasks) and the use of a structured assessment tool, e.g. the Bristol Activities of Daily Living (Bucks et al., 1996), may help here. Behavioural and psychological disturbances are common in dementia, and questions about social interaction, mood, paranoia, hallucinations, wandering, aggression, sleep, and eating (both appetite and eating behaviour) are usually appropriate. Identifying such symptoms is important because they are frequently troublesome and when present usually cause more distress than cognitive symptoms. Specific symptoms are also important in the differential diagnosis of dementia. Thus changes in social interaction and eating behaviour are characteristic of frontotemporal dementia (FTD) (Neary et al., 1998) (Chapter 27vi) and visual hallucinations and sleep changes (especially REM sleep behaviour disorder, see Chapter 36) are diagnostic features of DLB (McKeith et al., 2005) (see Chapter 27v).

## Previous medical and psychiatric history

Often a referral from primary care will come with a computer printout of the patient's previous illnesses and medication. Whilst such records are helpful as a starting point they often contain errors and omissions and it is prudent to confirm these illnesses, especially where there is apparent contradiction, e.g. a history of hypothyroidism but no prescription for thyroxine. Questions about previous psychiatric history should always be asked, and any illnesses in the months before and since the onset of the presenting symptoms should be carefully assessed; cognitive decline and mood alterations after operations or major illnesses are not uncommon. If 'vascular factors', (stroke, transient ischaemic attacks, myocardial infarction, angina pectoris, peripheral vascular disease, diabetes, hypertension, and falls) were not covered in the presenting complaint they should be asked about here, as evidence in support of or against a diagnosis of VaD.

## Current medication

Whilst a good referral usually lists the currently prescribed treatments, it is prudent to check this information against the actual

medication the patient is taking by asking patients to produce their medication. As discussed earlier this helps identify problems with compliance but also enables one to check about non-prescribed, alternative treatments. The use of substances such as vitamins, ginseng, and gingko biloba is not uncommon in older people. Polite questioning about why these treatments, as well as the prescribed ones, are being taken can give useful insights into current concerns and may raise issues not identified elsewhere. Checking the treatment actually being taken may also reveal an important recent change of medication; it is not uncommon for medication to be altered in hospital and for the patient to be on different treatments from the referral letter. Treatments with adverse effects on cognition and behaviour may have been commenced, e.g. oxybutinin for urinary incontinence impairs cognition, and sometimes necessary treatments may have been stopped inadvertently, e.g. antihypertensives.

## Family history

Obtaining a family history of mental illness can be helpful because the major mental illnesses, including dementia, have a definite genetic contribution. In practice, however, it can be very difficult to determine the validity of the information given for at least two reasons. First younger informants may not be able to corroborate the information given by elderly patients and where cognitive impairment is present this may not be accurate. Second when informed that a parent had, for example, dementia it is not at all certain this term corresponds to the clinical diagnosis a psychiatrist would make. Thus the added diagnostic value of a family history of mental illness is unclear. Other family history about relationships with parents and siblings may be helpful in understanding certain behaviours or for 'functional illnesses' but again this information can be difficult to verify and is generally probably of less importance than in younger adults.

## Personal history

This naturally follows on from the family history and for early life often raises the same problems of corroborating information. For cognitively impaired patients it is usually helpful to move to the personal history near the beginning of the interview because patients can talk happily about their earlier life and are not distressed by difficulties in remembering recent events. Taking a detailed personal history serves two main functions in old age psychiatry. It enables the psychiatrist to assess the severity of amnesia without the use of cognitive testing, which can be upsetting for patients who are anxious or in denial. Thus names, dates, and anecdotes from early in life may be easily remembered but events later in working life and the names of children and especially grandchildren are forgotten; the approximate age at which memory fragments gives an indication of the severity of a dementia. The personal history is also important in old age psychiatry, as in general psychiatry, for understanding the patient as a person.

Obtaining a personal history in old age psychiatry follows the same chronological order as with younger adults but there is clearly more ground to cover. Generally events earlier in life will be less important, but care should be taken to sensitively ask about the quality of relationships and experiences at all stages of the patient's life. Unless issues emerge, questions about childhood can be restricted to those to do with happiness and friendships at school and contentedness with family life at home. Older people usually left full-time education at 14 or 15 and one should be careful about inferring intelligence levels from such information or from patients' own comments about their educational attainments. The subsequent history of further training and their occupational record gives a surer indication of their ability. When eliciting this information it is important to try and clarify the degree of autonomy and responsibility the patient enjoyed. Being told someone worked in a factory is of limited value: was this packing boxes, as a clerk, or a production manager? When, as is frequently the case, someone held many jobs over the decades of their working life it is necessary to focus on their longest employments and any jobs which had special importance. Comments made about a marriage or relationships may raise this as a natural topic for discussion, but if not then it is important to elicit a marital history, again focusing on the nature of the relationship enjoyed (or not) with the spouse and any children and grandchildren. Where there have been several marriages and sexual relationships then matters may be very sensitive and it may be appropriate to obtain only the broad outline about these. Another area requiring tactful enquiry is the current sexual activity and degree of satisfaction with this and in the marital relationship in general. Some couples may find such questions inappropriate but important information about the strength of the marriage may be revealed which impinge on the caregiving role. Bereavement and other loss events are obviously much more frequently experienced by older people. Most cope very well, recognizing this as an inescapable part of growing old, but the loss of children, even when they themselves may have become old, is a severe blow for many, and such losses often precipitate a search for help when other bereavements have been borne well. Again, most cope well with serious illnesses, probably again because they are regarded as inevitable, but some disabling illnesses do cause depressive reactions. Some people, especially men, find adapting to retirement difficult and this can create stress at home and consequent marital difficulty, and discreet questions about adapting to this major change are appropriate in those close to retirement. Another event which frequently causes problems, and one which is familiar to old age psychiatrists, is placement in residential care. Services and residential homes are aware of the difficulty a patient may have in adapting to this new situation but the spouse left behind has to adapt too and depression and alcohol abuse may result.

Clearly in taking a personal history in old age psychiatry there is an immense amount of information which could be obtained. Clinicians need to adapt their questions to the nature of the problem at hand, e.g. questions about relationships in earlier life are more important for people presenting with a depressive or anxiety disorder than for those with probable dementia.

## Personality

At the initial assessment the clinician can only begin to understand the personality of a new patient. There is limited value in asking either the patient or any informants directly about the patient's personality; such questions provoke stereotyped answers lacking in depth. If a detailed personal and social history has been obtained then the questions about relationships with family, at school, and at work along with achievements and activities at school, work, and elsewhere, will have shed light on enduring personality traits which may have changed with illness and are important in managing the patient. A few extra questions to clarify matters as this history is taken may be all that is needed at this stage. For older people with long-term functional illnesses then the effects of their chronic illness may now be indistinguishable from their personality, but developing an awareness of personality traits is still important in understanding their behaviour and relationships. For those with a more recent illness, especially a dementia, the pre-morbid personality moulds the presentation of the illness. Someone who has lived independently all their life, has strong opinions and has always had things their own way is unlikely to settle quietly into a nursing home! A referral from a ward or a residential home for 'aggressive behaviour' in such a person needs to be interpreted in this context of their personality, rather than lead to a prescription for antipsychotic medication.

## Social history

The social history follows smoothly from the personal history, bringing it up to date. The pattern of the patient's everyday life, their activities, relationships with family members and others, should be clarified and confirmed. The amount of care currently given to the patient, by family, friends, and formal carers needs to be elicited, and in addition to information from the patient and informant(s) a written care plan may be available which can provide evidence of day to day issues as well as of the programme of care. Other health professionals may be involved, e.g. a district nurse, and the patient may attend day care or have a respite care programme. Enquiring about the pattern of daily activity can bring out problems such as apathy or resistiveness, as well as providing further evidence about the extent of current difficulties. Having established an understanding of the pattern of living and current support the social history may conclude with more direct questions about the use of alcohol and other substances. The abuse of alcohol and benzodiazepines remain the major foci of concern, but increasingly old age psychiatrists will see people abusing other substances and should be alert to this possibility. In recent years the issue of driving motor vehicles has become a prominent issue as an increasing number of older people, including women, own and drive their own vehicles (Brown and Ott, 2004). If the patient is driving, the clinician may ask others about any concerns they may have or incidents which have occurred and will need to consider whether to ask the patient to stop driving if it appears he or she cannot safely drive any longer. Clinical assessment is difficult, because whilst several neuropsychological measures, especially visuospatial and attentional tests, correlate well with driving performance (Adler et al., 2005) such measures are not easily available and also do not provide definitive evidence. Hence this review recommended a driving assessment for all patients with Mini-Mental State Examination (MMSE) scores of less than 24 or where concern exists (Adler et al., 2005). These issues are discussed in detail in Chapter 44.

## Mental state examination

It is important to remember that the mental state examination is an assessment of the mental state of the patient at the time of the interview and so symptoms identified in the history, e.g. hallucinations, may not be manifest for recording as part of the patient's current mental state. The mental state assessment begins on arrival and continues throughout the interview and should be recorded in the standard way.

## Appearance and behaviour

Generally speaking older people have maintained more formal modes of dress and behaviour, with men frequently attired in suits and women in dresses. Although this is changing, it means the clinician may be informed that an apparently well-groomed man has slipped in his standards. It is a delicate matter to enquire directly about issues of dress and hygiene but it is appropriate to gently ask where there is an apparent discrepancy between the patient's state of grooming and that of the spouse or the surroundings in the home. Another important element to consider in assessing older people is the presence of sensory impairment. The severity of any deafness and blindness should also be noted both because of the influence it has on the assessment process, especially on cognitive testing, and of the importance in ensuring that handicaps related to these are addressed during the management of the patient's illness.

The clinician should be looking for the range of behavioural changes manifest in functional illnesses, e.g. poor eye contact in depression or suspiciousness in paranoid schizophrenia. In old age psychiatry, psychomotor changes can be especially prominent in the affective disorders, with agitation a common feature in depression. When a patient exhibits apparent psychomotor retardation it is important to consider whether this may be apathy or related to Parkinson's disease (bradykinesia) rather than a depressive illness. The high prevalence of parkinsonism in older people and the diagnostic importance of this in dementia, as a hallmark feature of DLB, means it is good practice to assess for parkinsonism in every new patient. This can be done briefly in most settings by carefully observing the patient at rest for tremor, examining the arms for rigidity, and asking the patient to take a short walk to watch for gait changes and postural instability. At the same time the examiner should look for focal neurological signs, especially those that may be due to stroke disease. Such an examination should not replace a more detailed physical examination (see Chapter 12) and is necessarily limited at an initial assessment in someone's home but it frequently adds important diagnostic information.

Apathy is highly prevalent even in early dementia (Mega et al., 1996) and is often mistaken for depression (Levy et al., 1998). The listless and disengaged presentation of someone with apathy can usually be distinguished from the withdrawn and retarded picture in depression, although it can be difficult especially in more severely impaired patients, and both may be present. At interview someone with apathy may appear uninterested and switched off when the clinician is discussing the situation with an informant but then warm up and engage well when directly addressed and show a reactive mood. On questioning why they have given up certain activities apathetic patients will intimate that they no longer have the drive to do them and in fact still enjoy visits from friends and family, whereas patients with depression will explain that they do not enjoy them any more, or at least not as they used to (anhedonia). Whilst 'frontal dementias' may be accompanied by an apathetic picture, a disinhibited presentation is also well recognized and much less likely to be due to a manic illness than in younger adults. Subtler aspects of disinhibited behaviour, such as overfamiliarity, may be difficult to distinguish from the normal range of social interaction, but more overt behaviours, such as coarse joking, sometimes occur, although even in such circumstances it is prudent to consider whether this may be an aspect of the patient's pre-morbid personality. In all cases it is prudent to observe the reaction of relatives and to gently enquire about whether such comments or interactions represent a change before regarding them as pathological.

## Speech

Occasionally when dealing with older people the clinician will encounter someone who is loud and garrulous, consistent with FTD or mania, but quiet and impoverished speech is much more common, being a feature of the major degenerative dementias and depression. Dysphasia is another key feature of early dementing illnesses and one which does not occur in depression. Thus whilst poverty of speech does not in itself help to distinguish depression from dementia, the presence or absence of dysphasia does. However, deafness is a frequent problem, and at interview it can be very difficult to distinguish whether an apparent failure to understand is because of receptive dysphasia or deafness. In milder dementia subtle difficulties occur in speech structure, especially in finding names, but these can be very difficult to detect at interview because patients can be adept at covering up these problems through the use of circumlocutions. Whilst instruments exist for formally assessing dysphasia (see Chapter 11 on cognitive assessment) these are not well suited to regular clinical practice.

## Mood

Abnormalities of mood follow the same pattern as in disorders of younger adults. Lowering of mood in a depressive illness is often accompanied by a more prominent anxiety than in earlier life, with other associated anxiety symptoms, and this can be misleading. The reluctance of many older people to express their feelings is better recognized and, although probably changing in the young-old compared with the old-old, the clinician still needs to be aware of this phenomenon. Elevation of mood in a manic illness tends to be attenuated, like the rest of the illness, in later life and also occurs in frontal dementias and where present in dementia it may be indicative of a more severe illness, especially when associated with agitation. A feature of mood disturbance more specific to old age psychiatry is the mood lability which occurs with cerebrovascular disease (Morris et al., 1993). Stroke disease, but also less obvious cerebrovascular disease, is frequently accompanied by mood abnormalities and whether the prevailing change is an elevation or a depression of mood it is often highly labile. Apparently spontaneous, but typically short-lived, episodes of weeping without any sustained lowering of mood should alert the clinician to the possibility this may be emotional lability related to stroke disease rather than a mood disorder as such (House et al., 1989) (see Chapter 29ii).

## Thought

Abnormalities in the form of thought occur in schizophrenia, depression, and bipolar disorder as in younger people but it is rare to encounter formal thought disorder in late onset schizophrenia. Incoherence of thought is, of course, common in dementing illnesses, and can occur early on but is more common in advanced disease.

Paranoid delusions, especially of theft, are extremely common in dementia and can be difficult to distinguish from the effects of amnesia and from related confabulation (Burns et al., 1990). Misidentification delusions are characteristic of dementia, and whilst the Capgras syndrome (more accurately a symptom) is the most well known, there are several variants (Harwood et al., 1999). All appear to be related to a failure to recognize or correctly identify an image. In the Capgras syndrome the patient believes a close relative has been substituted by an exact double. The 'mirror sign' occurs when the patient fails to recognize their image in the mirror, leading to them engaging this stranger in conversation or becoming angry at their presence. People seen on television are believed to be really present in the room with the patient in the 'TV sign' and in the phantom boarder syndrome the patient believes extra people are living in the house (perhaps after failing to recognize relatives). More sophisticated and complex delusions are unusual in dementia but remain typical of schizophrenia in either its early or late onset forms.

## Perception

Psychiatrists working with older people encounter patients with auditory hallucinations, and sometimes olfactory hallucinations, typical of schizophrenia but more frequently they encounter prominent and persistent hallucinations in other sensory modalities. This is a well-recognized consequence of the 'organic' nature of the illnesses which present to old age psychiatry. Visual and tactile hallucinations are frequently seen in patients with delirium in the general hospital but also in less overt delirium during home assessments. Complex and enduring visual hallucinations, characteristically of people and animals, are a core feature of DLB (McKeith *et al.*, 2005; Mosimann *et al.*, 2006) (see Chapter 27v) but it is always important to consider whether they may be due to a delirium. Often it can be difficult to be sure whether the visual hallucination is truly occurring in the absence of a real stimulus or whether it is a misperception resulting from poor eyesight or some other defect in visual processing. However, since such problems in visual processing commonly occur in DLB the presence of such phenomena suggests such a diagnosis even if frank hallucinations cannot be confirmed. Sometimes persistent, complex visual hallucinations are the only phenomenological feature confirmed during assessment; in particular, there may be no significant cognitive impairment or alteration in consciousness. Such patients are said to have Charles Bonnet syndrome and although many will proceed to decline cognitively, develop a dementia and other features of DLB, this does not appear to happen to everyone presenting in this way. Most old age psychiatrists are familiar with a similar phenomenon of persistent auditory hallucinations in clear consciousness and in the absence of cognitive decline (an auditory hallucinosis, sometimes called auditory Charles Bonnet syndrome). Typically such patients experience musical hallucinations for hours on end, hearing choirs singing hymns or bands playing old songs, and show good insight, often giving detailed descriptions of their hallucinations. Neither the visual or auditory variants of Charles Bonnet syndrome do well with antipsychotic treatment (Batra *et al.*, 1997).

## Cognition

Formal cognitive assessment is dealt with in detail in Chapter 11. However, the clinician should have been gleaning cognitive information throughout the assessment. A structured brief instrument for assessing cognition should be used as part of the cognitive assessment and although many are available the MMSE (Folstein *et al.*, 1975) appears to remain the favourite of most clinicians. Such instruments can provide an estimate of the extent of cognitive impairment and through repeated use over time enable the clinician to monitor illness progression or response to antidementia treatment; patients 'typically' decline at 2–3 points per year on the MMSE (Salmon *et al.*, 1990), but in clinical practice immense variability between patients is observed. Whilst dysphasia can be difficult to assess formally during a standard clinical assessment it can frequently be observed during the process of history and mental state assessment. More obviously, inconsistencies and gaps in the patient's account provide evidence of both the presence and the severity of amnesia. Other information on orientation, cognition, and perhaps spatial or executive dysfunction may also be detected. Whilst this information does not replace proper cognitive testing, it provides important additional evidence.

## Insight

Insight is a complex, variable, and multidimensional phenomenon (Howorth and Saper, 2003). In patients with 'functional' disorders the degree of insight varies in much the same way as in younger adults. It is good practice to record a brief description of the extent of insight rather than a summary phrase; to say 'she understands she has a depressive illness, of which her anxiety and tremor are manifestations, and is willing to take antidepressant medication for this' rather than simply 'full insight'. In people with moderate to severe dementia there is usually very little insight, just an awareness perhaps that one is not right and an acceptance that help is needed. However, patients may have more awareness of their illness than they are able to express verbally, perhaps due to better preservation of implicit memory (Howorth and Saper, 2003). Such insight appears to be greater for the amnesia than for the impact of the cognitive decline on their function and perhaps least for the impact of their illness on other people. In those with milder dementia there is typically more insight into the illness but the extent to which this is acknowledged varies considerably. Often the clinician suspects the patient and family are colluding in denying the severity of problems because they are aware of the implications. There has been a trend recently towards disclosure of the diagnosis of dementia, and whilst such openness is usually appropriate this may not always be the case, especially when the family appear to prefer denial. When prescription of antidementia treatment is indicated the issue of diagnosis is especially acute and difficult to avoid and sensitive handling of the issue is needed.

## Assessment of capacity

Capacity and decision-making have become increasingly prominent features of old age psychiatry practice and capacity assessment and the relevant legislation is dealt with in detail in Chapters 41–43. Key principles of the Mental Capacity Act 2005 (for England and Wales) are that capacity is specific to the time of the assessment and that it is functional in nature (capacity varies by the function being assessed). A formal assessment of capacity is not part of routine clinical assessment, and indeed for these reasons, strictly speaking, it cannot be made unless it is requested because the clinician needs to know what the patient is being assessed as being capable or incapable of deciding at any point in time. When making an assessment the clinician needs to determine whether the four aspects of capacity (sufficient information has been conveyed; this information can be retained for long enough to make a decision; an ability to weigh matters up is present; a decision can be communicated to others) are fulfilled for each particular decision-making issue (see Chapter 42).

## Physical examination

Even if assessing someone at home a brief physical assessment is appropriate. In those who are found to be physically unwell, perhaps delirious, this will need to include hydration status and cardiovascular, respiratory, and abdominal assessments prior to referral to colleagues at the general hospital. In routine practice the need is for a neurological examination, especially to look for features of stroke disease and parkinsonism. Power, tone, coordination, basic sensation, gait, and most cranial nerves can all be examined without the need for special equipment. Such an examination does not replace the need for a full assessment with related physical investigations later but does provide valuable evidence to clarify the potential causes of a dementia.

### The informant interview

Obtaining a history from a family member, friend, or carer who knows the patient helps fill out the history and ensure that all problems have been identified and understood. In those with cognitive impairment it is essential because the patient is unable to provide reliable information. A decision about how much useful information can be garnered from the patient can usually be made early in the interview. Those with early dementia or other cognitive impairment can typically give a reasonable account of their personal history until the recent past, and some information on major medical or psychiatric illnesses as well, but for the more impaired an informant is needed for this as well and the interview with the patient focuses on the mental state, especially the cognitive assessment.

Whilst most informants are reliable historians who desire appropriate treatment and help for the patient, this is not always the case and the assessing clinician should be alert to other possibilities. In some cases the informant is cognitively impaired themselves and on other occasions does not have sufficient knowledge of the patient. Occasionally conflict within the family is revealed by different opinions being offered and an informant may not be a disinterested party but one with his or her own views about what should be done, e.g. a patient kept inappropriately at home so benefits and allowances continue to be available.

### Further assessment

Following the initial assessment, the psychiatrist is usually in a position to make a differential diagnosis and plan further assessments to clarify or confirm this and to deal with other important issues which have arisen. Inpatient admission and assessment is only necessary in a small minority of cases, usually where there are severe behavioural disturbances or significant immediate risks. Such admission provides for a thorough assessment but one which is limited by it not taking place in the home environment. More frequent is further assessment through attendance at a day unit. This is a suitable setting for coordinating a full physical assessment and associated physical investigations and one which allows nursing staff to provide longer-term assessment of the patient's interaction with other people and to observe for significant psychopathology. In most cases further assessment can be satisfactorily carried out at home, with visits from other relevant professionals as required. For example, in patients with borderline or mild cognitive impairments, suggesting they may have an early dementia, a more detailed neuropsychological assessment by a psychologist is helpful to clarify the pattern and extent of any deficits. Where difficulties in everyday functioning have been identified or are likely to be present it is appropriate to refer to an occupational therapist for a detailed functional assessment. In such circumstances, and where financial issues arise and care plans may need adjustment, the

involvement of a social worker specializing in dealing with older people with mental illness is also necessary. Community psychiatric nurses are able to monitor changes in mental state in response to treatment and to deal with carer stress issues and related problems which may be present in their relationship with the patient.

## Principles of management

As explained earlier, the main elements of management for each patient should emerge as the assessment process unfolds. When the initial assessment leads to a diagnosis of a functional illness the appropriate pharmacological treatment can be initiated immediately and consideration given to the need for any additional psychosocial intervention. These treatments are broadly the same as for younger adults and their application to older people is discussed in later chapters (see Chapters 14 and 18). Involvement of other professionals, as outlined above under 'Further assessment', will usually lead to their involvement to deal with the particular needs identified and the psychiatrist has a coordinating and consultative role in managing the overall strategy. In more straightforward cases the different individuals involved gradually withdraw as problems are solved, symptoms improve, and the patient settles in to a stable existence again. In more complex cases this role leads to the calling of a case conference to facilitate the exchange of information and to ensure that everyone involved is 'singing from the same hymn sheet'. In people with dementia such a meeting is usually followed by a period in which the agreed management plan is enacted and, if successful, all settles down again. In those who have severe functional illnesses long-term follow-up by the psychiatrist and/or community nurse is usually the outcome, rather than discharge from the service. In the most resistant and severe illnesses closer long-term follow-up may be needed by regular attendance at a day unit, e.g. to monitor psychosis in people on clozapine or mood in those on combinations of antidepressants and mood stabilizers.

## References

Adler, G., Rottunda, S., and Dysken, M. (2005). The older driver with dementia: an updated literature review. *Journal of Safety Research*, **36**, 399–407.

Anderson, D.N. and Aquilina, C. (2002). Domiciliary clinics I: effects on non-attendance. *International Journal of Geriatric Psychiatry*, **17**, 941–4.

Bamford, C., Lamont, S., Eccles, M., Robinson, L., May, C., and Bond, J. (2004). Disclosing a diagnosis of dementia: a systematic review. *International Journal of Geriatric Psychiatry*, **19**, 151–69.

Batra, A., Bartels, M., and Wormstall, H. (1997). Therapeutic options in Charles Bonnet syndrome. *Acta Psychiatrica Scandinavica*, **96**, 129–33.

Benbow, S. (1990). The community clinic – its advantages and disadvantages. *International Journal of Geriatric Psychiatry*, **5**, 119–21.

Brown, L.B. and Ott, B.R. (2004). Driving and dementia: a review of the literature. *Journal of Geriatric Psychiatry and Neurology*, **17**, 232–40.

Bucks, R.S., Ashworth, D.L., Wilcock, G.K., and Siegfried, K. (1996). Assessment of activities of daily living in dementia: development of the Bristol Activities of Daily Living Scale. *Age and Ageing*, **25**, 113–20.

Burns, A., Jacoby, R., and Levy, R. (1990). Psychiatric phenomena in Alzheimer's disease. I: Disorders of thought content. *British Journal of Psychiatry*, **157**, 72–6, 92–4.

Finkel, S.I. and Burns, A. (2000). Behavioural and Psychological Symptoms of Dementia (BPSD): a clinical and research update: introduction. *International Psychogeriatrics*, **12**, 9–12.

Folstein, M.F., Folstein, S.E., and McHugh, P.R. (1975). 'Mini-mental state'. A practical method for grading the cognitive state of patients for the clinician. *Journal of Psychiatric Research*, **12**, 189–98.

Frankel, S., Farrow, A., and West, R. (1989). Non-admission or non-invitation? A case-control study of failed admissions. *British Medical Journal*, **299**, 598–600.

Hardy-Thompson, C., Orrell, M.W., and Bergmann, K. (1992). Evaluating a psychogeriatric domiciliary visit service: views of general practitioners. *British Medical Journal*, **304**, 421–2.

Harwood, D.G., Barker, W.W., Ownby, R.L., and Duara, R. (1999). Prevalence and correlates of Capgras syndrome in Alzheimer's disease. *International Journal of Geriatric Psychiatry*, **14**, 415–20.

Health, D.O. (2001). *National service framework – for older people*. Department of Health, London.

House, A., Dennis, M., Molyneux, A., Warlow, C., and Hawton, K. (1989). Emotionalism after stroke. *British Medical Journal*, **298**, 991–4.

Howorth, P. and Saper, J. (2003). The dimensions of insight in people with dementia. *Aging and Mental Health*, **7**, 113–22.

Jones, S.J., Turner, R.J., and Grant, J.E. (1987). Assessing patients in their homes. *Bulletin of the Royal College of Psychiatry*, **11**, 117–19.

Levy, M.L., Cummings, J.L., Fairbanks, L.A. *et al.* (1998). Apathy is not depression. *Journal of Neuropsychiatry and Clinical Neurosciences*, **10**, 314–19.

Lindesay, J., Marudkar, M., Van Diepen, E., and Wilcock, G. (2002). The second Leicester survey of memory clinics in the British Isles. *International Journal of Geriatric Psychiatry*, **17**, 41–7.

Luce, A., McKeith, I., Swann, A., Daniel, S., and O'Brien, J. (2001). How do memory clinics compare with traditional old age psychiatry services? *International Journal of Geriatric Psychiatry*, **16**, 837–45.

McKeith, I.G., Dickson, D.W., Lowe, J. *et al.* (2005). Diagnosis and management of dementia with Lewy bodies: third report of the DLB Consortium. *Neurology*, **65**, 1863–72.

Mega, M.S., Cummings, J.L., Fiorello, T., and Gornbein, J. (1996). The spectrum of behavioral changes in Alzheimer's disease. *Neurology*, **46**, 130–5.

Morris, P.L., Robinson, R.G., and Raphael, B. (1993). Emotional lability after stroke. *Australian and New Zealand Journal of Psychiatry*, **27**, 601–5.

Mosimann, U.P., Rowan, E.N., Partington, C.E. *et al.* (2006). Characteristics of visual hallucinations in Parkinson disease dementia and dementia with Lewy bodies. *American Journal of Geriatric Psychiatry*, **14**, 153–60.

Neary, D., Snowden, J.S., Gustafson, L. *et al.* (1998). Frontotemporal lobar degeneration: a consensus on clinical diagnostic criteria. *Neurology*, **51**, 1546–54.

Parker, G., Bhakta, P., Katbamna, S. *et al.* (2000). Best place of care for older people after acute and during subacute illness: a systematic review. *Journal of Health Services and Research Policy*, **5**, 176–89.

Salmon, D.P., Thal, L.J., Butters, N., and Heindel, W.C. (1990). Longitudinal evaluation of dementia of the Alzheimer type: a comparison of 3 standardized mental status examinations. *Neurology*, **40**, 1225–30.

# 11

# Clinical cognitive assessment

## Christopher M. Kipps and John R. Hodges

## Introduction

Cognitive symptoms arise from the location of brain dysfunction and are not linked directly to any particular pathology. In the early stages of disease, symptoms may be non-specific, and while certain symptom clusters are commonly seen in particular disorders, atypical presentations are not infrequent. For example, in Alzheimer's disease, patients may present with a focal language syndrome instead of the more commonly appreciated autobiographical memory disturbance despite identical pathology. In our approach to the cognitive assessment, we maintain a symptom-oriented approach. This facilitates the localization of pathology and subsequent clinical diagnosis, which may then be supplemented by associated neurological signs, imaging, or other investigations.

The purpose of the cognitive examination is to separate out those patients in whom a firm clinical diagnosis can be made from those in whom additional investigation is required. In this assessment, the history and clinical examination are completely intertwined, and the ability to respond to conversational clues or provide details of personal events is as much a consideration as any formal testing. Skilful examiners often weave their assessment into a relaxed conversation with a patient, making it more enjoyable for both. In neurodegenerative diseases in particular, poor memory and impaired insight make the perspective of an informant, who knows the patient well, essential.

A clear focus is needed from early in the consultation in order to direct the assessment to the areas of greatest relevance which need specific and more detailed examination. A list of particularly discriminating questions can be seen in Table 11.1. In the sections that follow, we divide the cognitive examination into a number of broad domains: attention and orientation, memory, language, executive function, apraxia, visuospatial ability, and behavioural.

## General assessment

We start by establishing a picture of pre-morbid functioning (e.g. education, employment, significant relationships). Learning a little about the patient's interests or hobbies allows one to tailor questions in the cognitive examination more precisely. The onset and time course of the deterioration is as important as the cluster of deficits, be they memory, language, visual function, behaviour, or indeed psychiatric, and often the first noted deficit has diagnostic relevance. It is frequently very helpful to ask the patient directly what they believe the reason is for their attendance in the clinic.

We try to interview both the patient and informant independently, even when the amount of information likely to be obtained from the patient is minimal. It allows a chance to assess both language and cooperation without assistance or interruption from the partner. Disparities between the two accounts are important as insight is often poor. A family history and risk factors, notably vascular, are particularly relevant, and should be specifically enquired about. Considerable, and sometimes repeated, probing may be needed as a history of suicide or alcohol dependency in close relatives may disguise an unrecognized early onset dementia. Concomitant illness and medication use frequently underlie, or complicate, cognitive complaints. We use a questionnaire filled out before the consultation, which saves time and helps draw attention to issues in the background history.

## Orientation and attention

Alertness and cooperation with the assessment should be noted, as these factors may impact on the subsequent findings. The level of alertness is an important clue to the presence of a delirium or the effects of medication. Delirium may be marked by both restlessness and distractibility, or the patient may be quiet, and drift off to sleep easily during the consultation. If there is any concern about the level of alertness of the patient, a review of the medication list is often helpful. It may be misleading, and is frequently hopeless, to perform a detailed cognitive assessment on a patient with diminished alertness. If that is the case, documentation of orientation and attention may be as much as can be achieved initially.

### Orientation

Orientation is usually assessed to time, place, and person; it is not particularly sensitive, and intact orientation does not exclude a significant memory disorder, particularly if there is concern about memory from an informant.

*Time* orientation is the most helpful, and should include the time of day. Many normal people do not know the exact date, and being out by 2 days or less is considered normal when scoring this formally. Time intervals are often poorly monitored by patients with delirium, moderate to severe dementia, and in the amnesic syndrome, and are easily tested by asking about the length of time spent in hospital.

**Table 11.1** Discriminating features in common neurodegenerative diseases

| Disease | Key questions to ask: Is there...? Do they...? | Clinical signs/ investigations |
|---|---|---|
| Alzheimer's disease | Repetition of the same question with rapid forgetting of the answer? Get lost on familiar routes? | MRI: Generalized atrophy, particularly medial temporal and hippocampal regions |
| Frontotemporal dementia (FTD)— behavioural variant | Loss of empathy Eating changes Stereotypic behaviours Social inappropriateness Disinhibition Lack of insight | MRI: Frontal and/or right predominant temporal lobe atrophy |
| FTD—semantic dementia | Difficulty with naming objects? An inability to understand words? | MRI: Anterior temporal lobe atrophy (usually left > right) |
| FTD—progressive non-fluent aphasia | Mispronunciation of words with insertion of repeated or incorrect syllables? | |
| FTD—motor neuron disease (MND) | Rapid progression of a behavioural syndrome and/or language deficits? Prominent delusions and/or hallucinations (transient) | Fasciculations (limb or tongue) Electromyography (EMG) |
| Progressive supranuclear palsy (PSP) | A history of falls Profound apathy Slowed movement and thinking? | Axial rigidity Vertical gaze palsy Loss postural reflexes |
| Lewy body disease | Visual hallucinations Fluctuating cognitive ability Falls REM sleep disorder | Mild parkinsonism Visuospatial dysfunction |
| Corticobasal degeneration | Difficulty using objects with one hand Limb having 'a mind of its own' Shock-like jerks | Limb apraxia Visuospatial dysfunction Parkinsonism May develop non-fluent language syndrome |
| Huntington's disease | Family history (autosomal dominant) | Generalized chorea Huntington's gene |
| Vascular dementia | Vascular risk factors May have step-wise decline, but frequently do not | Pyramidal signs Evidence of small and/or large vessel disease on brain imaging |
| Creutzfeldt– Jakob disease (CJD) | Rapid cognitive decline Movement disorder Neurosurgical procedure or graft | Ataxia, tremor, myoclonus MRI abnormalities on diffusion imaging |
| Variant CJD | Rapid cognitive decline Sensory disturbance Movement disorder | MRI—pulvinar sign |

*Place* should be confirmed, and asking what the name of the building is (e.g. outpatient clinic), rather than the name of the hospital, often produces a surprising lack of awareness of location. Since there are often visual and contextual cues present, this is less sensitive than orientation to time, and is particularly the case when assessing someone at home.

*Person orientation* includes name, age, and date of birth. Disorientation to name is usually only seen in psychogenic amnesia. In the aphasic patient, earlier conversation should have revealed the true deficit, but a mistaken label of 'confusion' is frequently applied because such patients either fail to comprehend the question, or, produce the wrong answer. Given a choice, they can usually pick out their own name.

### Attention

Attention can be tested in a number of ways including serial 7s, digit span, spelling WORLD backwards and recitation of the months of the year in reverse order. Although serial 7s is commonly used, it is frequently performed incorrectly by the elderly, as well as by patients with impaired attention. The order of the months of the year is a highly overlearned sequence, and so we prefer to test the ability to provide it in reverse order as a measure of sustained attention.

Digit span is a relatively pure test of attention, and is dependent on working memory, but it is not specific, and can be impaired in delirium, focal left frontal damage, aphasia, and moderate to severe dementia. It should, however, be normal in the amnesic syndrome (e.g. Korsakoff's syndrome or medial temporal lobe damage). Start with three digits, and ensure that they are spoken individually and not clumped together in the way that one might recite a telephone number (e.g. 3–7–2–5 and not 37–25 etc). Normal digit span is 6 ± 1, depending on age and general intellectual ability. In the elderly, or intellectually impaired, 5 can be considered normal. Reverse span is usually one less than forward span. In performing this test, it is helpful to write out the numbers to be used before starting.

## Memory

Complaints about poor memory are the most frequent reason for referral to a cognitive disorders clinic, and often provide a good starting point for the consultation despite not being very specific.

A useful framework for analysing memory complaints divides memory into several separate domains. *Episodic memory* (personally experienced events) comprises *anterograde* (newly encountered information) or *retrograde* (past events) components, and depends on the hippocampal–diencephalic system. A second important system involves memory for word meaning and general knowledge (*semantic memory*), the key neural substrate being the anterior temporal lobe. *Working memory* refers to the very limited capacity store which allows us to retain information for a few seconds, and uses the dorsolateral pre-frontal cortex. The term 'short-term' memory is applied, confusingly, to a number of different memory problems and is best avoided.

### Episodic memory

Anterograde memory loss is suggested by the following:

◆ forgetting recent personal and family events (appointments, social occasions)

- losing items around the home
- repetitive questioning
- inability to following and/or remember plots of movies, television programmes, details of current affairs
- deterioration of message-taking skills
- increasing reliance on lists.

Retrograde memory loss may involve:

- memory of past events (jobs, past homes, major news items)
- getting lost, with poor topographical sense (route-finding).

Specific questions about the route taken to the hospital or recent events on the ward can be tested directly during conversation. Recalling a name and address, or the names of three items, is also often used. If care is not taken to ensure proper registration of the items at the start of this test, the results may be confusing or misleading. Poor registration, usually a feature of poor attention or executive dysfunction, may invalidate the results of recall or recognition which test episodic memory. Free recall is harder than the recognition of an item from a list. Testing in the hearing impaired poses particular challenges, but verbal testing by the use of written instructions, in large print, can be used after handing the patient their spectacles.

Anterograde non-verbal memory can be assessed by asking a subject to copy and later recall geometric shapes. Alternatively, it is possible to hide several objects around the room at random, and ask the patient to search for them several minutes later. This is an easy task, and inability to perform well is a convincing sign of memory impairment.

Famous events, recent sporting results, or the names of recent prime ministers can all be used to test retrograde memory without an informant. More remote autobiographical memory assessment needs corroboration, and may be relatively preserved in early Alzheimer's disease. Autobiographical 'lacunes', where discrete periods of time or events are forgotten, are a characteristic feature of transient epileptic amnesia (TEA).

Memory loss and learning impairment out of proportion to other cognitive disturbance is known as the amnesic syndrome. Generally both anterograde and retrograde memory loss occur in parallel, such as in Alzheimer's disease or head injury, but dissociations occur. Disproportionately severe anterograde amnesia may be seen when there is hippocampal damage, particularly in herpes simplex encephalitis, focal temporal lobe tumours, or infarction. Confabulation, for example in Korsakoff's syndrome, might be grandiose or delusional, but more often involves the misordering and fusion of real memories which end up being retrieved out of context. A transient amnesic syndrome with marked anterograde, and variable retrograde, amnesia is seen in transient global amnesia (TGA), whilst 'memory lacunes', and repeated brief episodes of memory loss suggest transient epileptic amnesia (TEA).

Simply asking both patient and informant to give an overall memory rating (out of 10) is often helpful. It is seldom, if ever, that truly amnestic patients will give themselves scores such as 0 or 1, although their spouse might. The reverse is often true of those who forget primarily because of anxiety or depression.

## Working memory

Lapses in concentration and attention (losing your train of thought, wandering into a room and forgetting the reason, forgetting a phone number which has just been looked at) are common and increase with age, depression, and anxiety. Such symptoms are much more evident to patients than to family members and, in isolation, are usually not of great concern. It should be noted, however, that basal ganglia and white matter diseases may present with predominantly working memory deficits.

## Semantic memory

Patients with semantic breakdown typically complain of 'loss of memory for words'. Vocabulary diminishes and patients substitute words like 'thing'. There is a parallel impairment in appreciating the meaning of individual words which first involves infrequent or unusual words. Word-finding difficulty is common in both anxiety and ageing, but is variable and not associated with impaired comprehension. This is in stark contrast to the anomia (impaired naming) in semantic dementia which is relentlessly progressive and associated with both associative object agnosia (inability to recognize infrequently encountered objects) and atrophy of the anterior temporal lobe, usually on the left. Testing of language function is described in detail below.

# Language

The majority of language deficits are usually revealed within the first few minutes of listening to the patient speak, particularly where poor fluency, prosody, agrammatism, and articulation are involved. Evidence of word-finding impairments and paraphasic errors are also usually quickly apparent. Documenting several examples of these errors is often quite helpful to subsequent clinicians. Sometimes, however, a relatively fluent history may mask quite significant naming and single-word comprehension deficits, and it is important to assess this routinely with infrequently encountered words and with directed questioning.

## Naming

The degree of anomia is useful as an overall index of the severity of a language deficit, and is a prominent feature in virtually all post-stroke aphasic patients, in moderate stage Alzheimer's disease, as well as semantic dementia. Naming ability requires an integration of visual, semantic, and phonological aspects of item knowledge. There is a marked frequency effect, and rather than using very common items to test the patient, such as a *pen* or *watch*, it may be more informative to ask about a *winder*, *nib*, *cufflinks*, or a *stethoscope*. Line drawings in the Addenbrooke's Cognitive Examination (ACE-R; Fig. 11.1) are useful for assessing naming ability. *Phonemic paraphasias* (e.g. *'electrickery'* for *'electricity'*), and *semantic paraphasias* (*'clock'* for *'watch'*, or *'apple'* for *'orange'*) may also be seen, and reflect pathology in Broca's area and the posterior perisylvian region, respectively. Broad superordinate responses, such as *'animal'* may be given in response to pictures of, for example, a camel, with the progressive semantic memory impairment seen in semantic dementia. Posterior lesions, particularly of the angular gyrus, can produce quite pronounced anomia for visually recognized objects, and may be associated with alexia.

## Comprehension

Difficulty with comprehension is often (incorrectly) assumed to be a result of hearing impairment. However, conversely, always consider the possibility of deafness in a patient who fails to understand

ADDENBROOKE'S COGNITIVE EXAMINATION – ACE-R

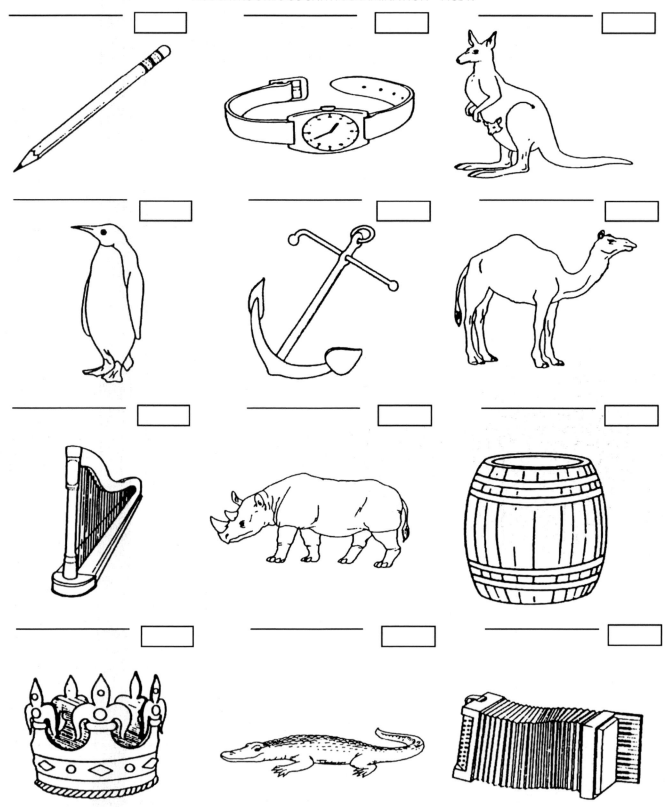

**Fig. 11.1** Line drawings used in Addenbrooke's Cognitive Examination (revised version) to assess naming and comprehension.

what is being asked. Complaints of difficulty using the telephone, or withdrawal from group conversations, may be more subtle clues to its presence. It is useful to assess comprehension in a graded manner, starting with simple and then more complex instructions.

Use several common items (coin, key, pen), and ask the patient to point to each one in turn in order to assess *single word comprehension*. There is a frequency effect, and if this test seems too easy, try harder items around the room. We also test comprehension by asking patients to define the meaning of words such as hippopotamus, caterpillar, encyclopaedia, emerald, and perimeter, which is done at the same time as assessing repetition (see below).

*Sentence comprehension* can be tested with several common items in order to devise syntactically complex commands. For example: *touch the pen, and then the watch*, followed by more difficult sentences such as *touch the watch, after touching the keys and the pen*. Alternatively, ask '*If the lion ate the tiger, who survived?*'. Syntactic ability is classically impaired with lesions of Broca's area or the anterior insular region, and is commonly accompanied by phonological errors and poor repetition.

### Repetition

Use a series of words and sentences of increasing complexity. Repetition of polysyllabic words such as '*hippopotamus*' or '*caterpillar*' followed by enquiry as to its meaning, assesses phonological, articulatory, and semantic processing simultaneously. Listen carefully for phonemic paraphasias during this task. *Sentence repetition* can be tested with the well-known phrase, '*No ifs, ands or buts*' which is somewhat surprisingly more difficult than repeating '*The orchestra played and the audience applauded*'.

### Reading

Failure to comprehend is usually accompanied by an inability to read aloud, but the reverse is not necessarily true. Test this either by writing a simple command '*Close your eyes*' or using a few phrases from a nearby newspaper. If a reading deficit is detected, this should be characterized further.

Patients with so-called *pure alexia* exhibit the phenomenon of letter-by-letter reading, with frequent errors in letter identification. *Neglect dyslexia*, seen in right hemisphere damage, is usually confined to the initial part of a word and can take the form of omissions or substitutions (e.g. *land* for *island*, and *fish* for *dish*). *Surface dyslexics* have difficulty in reading words with irregular spelling (e.g. *pint, soot, cellist, dough*), which indicates a breakdown in the linkage of words to their underlying semantic meanings and is one of the hallmarks of semantic dementia. *Deep dyslexics* are unable to read plausible non-words (e.g. *neg, glem, deak*), and make semantic errors (*canary* for *parrot*).

### Writing

Writing is more vulnerable to disruption than reading, and involves coordination of both central (spelling) and more peripheral (letter formation) components. Central dysgraphias affect both written and oral spelling. These syndromes are analogous to those seen in the acquired dyslexias, and can be tested similarly.

In general, intact oral spelling in the face of written spelling impairments suggests a writing dyspraxia or neglect dysgraphia. The former results in effortful, and often illegible, writing with frequent errors in the shape or orientation of letters. Copying is also abnormal. A mixed central and peripheral dysgraphia with spelling errors that tend to be phonologically plausible is commonly seen in corticobasal degeneration (CBD). Neglect dysgraphia results in misspelling of the initial part of words, and is frequently associated with other non-dominant parietal lobe deficits of visuospatial ability and perceptual function.

### Acalculia

Acalculia refers to the inability to read, write, and comprehend numbers, and is not exactly the same as an inability to perform arithmetical calculations (anarithmetria). Although simple calculation is sufficient for most purposes, a full assessment of this skill requires the patient to *write numbers to dictation, copy numbers* and *read them aloud*. The left angular gyrus appears to be important for these numeracy skills. The patient should also be asked to perform *oral arithmetic, written calculation*, and finally be tested in ability to reason arithmetically (e.g. *calculating change received when purchasing several items*). The integration of several skills is important here including the retrieval of stored arithmetic facts, and the ability to manipulate numerical quantities arithmetically.

## Executive and frontal lobe function

Impairments in this domain typically involve errors of goal setting, planning, judgement, initiation, flexibility, impulse control, and abstract reasoning. Although executive function is generally believed to a (dorsolateral) frontal lobe function, this set of skills is probably much more widely distributed in the brain. Head injury is a common cause of impaired executive function, which is also usually seen in Alzheimer's disease, even in the early stages. It is important not to forget that the majority of the frontal lobe is subcortical white matter, and consequently many of the leucodystrophies cause executive dysfunction, and discrete frontal lobe signs. Basal ganglia disorders also impair these skills, the prime example being progressive supranuclear palsy (PSP).

### Letter and category fluency

Letter and category verbal fluency are very useful tests, and poor performance on both is common in executive dysfunction. Patients are asked to produce as many words as possible starting with a particular letter of the alphabet (F, A, and S are the commonly used letters). Proper names, and the generation of exemplars from a single stem (e.g. pot, pots, potter) are not allowed. *Category fluency* is performed by, for example, asking for as many animals as possible in 1 minute. Young adults can produce 20 animals, 15 animals is low average, and fewer than 10 is definitely impaired. Letter fluency is usually more difficult (a score of 15 words per letter is normal), and subjects with subcortical or frontal pathology score poorly on both measures, but worse on letter fluency. In contrast, patients with semantic deficits, such as semantic dementia or Alzheimer's disease, have a more marked impairment for categories. Refinements, such as categories of dogs or type of fruit, can be introduced to detect more subtle deficits.

### Impulsivity, cognitive estimates, perseveration, and proverbs

Impulsivity, is thought to reflect failure of response inhibition, and is seen in inferior frontal pathology. It can be assessed using the Go–No-Go task. The examiner instructs the patient to tap once in response to a single tap, and to withhold a response for two taps.

**Fig. 11.2** Examples of meaningful and meaningless hand gestures that may be used in testing for limb apraxia. It is important to ensure that there is no physical limitation (e.g. severe arthritis, contractures, hemiplegic stroke) that prevents the patient from copying the gesture.

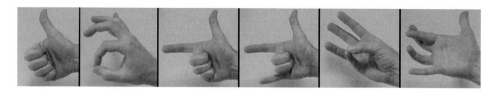

This test can be made more difficult by changing the initial rule after several trials (e.g. *tap once when I tap twice, and not at all when I tap once*). The ability to switch task, and the inhibition of inappropriate, or perseverative, responses can also be assessed by asking the patient to copy a short sequence of alternating squares and triangles, and then to continue across the page. Perseveration in drawing one or other of the shapes may be seen in frontal lobe deficits, but the test is relatively insensitive. A tendency to clap more than the same number of times as the examiner (usually three) also suggests perseveration. Further clinical examples include *palilalia or palalogia* which are characterized by the repetition of sounds or words, respectively, whilst the repetition of whatever is heard is known as *echolalia*.

The Cognitive Estimates Test may prompt bizarre or improbable responses in patients with frontal or executive dysfunction. Although it is a formal test, with defined scoring norms, it can be performed at the bedside by asking, for example, the population of a nearby city, of London, and of the UK, the height of the Post Office Tower, or the speed of a typical racehorse. Questions about the similarity between two conceptually similar objects can be used to assess inferential reasoning which may be impaired in the same way. Simple pairs such as 'apples and oranges' or 'desk and chair' are tested first, followed by more abstract pairs such as 'praise and punishment' or 'a poem and a statue'. Patients typically answer, quite concretely, that two objects are 'different' or that they are 'not similar' and are unable to form an abstract concept to link the pair. This often persists despite encouragement to consider other ways in which the items are alike. Testing of proverbs (too many cooks spoil the broth, etc.) probably measures a similar skill, but it is highly dependent on premorbid educational ability and cultural background.

The three-step Luria test, a motor sequencing task, is thought to be a left frontal lobe task, and is discussed more fully below.

### Behavioural assessment

Inappropriate behaviour is seldom, if ever, elicited from the history given by the patient, who may act quite normally during a clinical consultation. Direct questioning about conflict at work, with interpersonal relationships, or involvement with law enforcement agencies may be helpful in determining the degree of insight; however, the corroboration of the history from an informant, interviewed alone, is crucial. Spouses may mention embarrassing social behaviour, changes in food preference (in particular sweet foods), or inappropriate sexual behaviour. Ability to empathise, and judge the emotional state of others is particularly disrupted in the frontotemporal syndromes. The informant should also be questioned about irritability, anxiety, and poor judgement. Apathy or poor motivation is a common feature of Alzheimer's disease and frontotemporal and subcortical dementias, but does not

differentiate well between different aetiologies. Impulsiveness, which is sometimes demonstrated clinically by the Go–No-Go task described above, may be a marker of impaired inhibition, an inferior frontal lobe function.

To document behavioural impairment it is valuable to use one of the standardized inventories which list symptoms and their severity [e.g. Neuropsychiatric Inventory (NPI), Cambridge Behavioural Inventory (CBI), Frontal Behavioral Inventory (FBI)] which are either filled out by the carer prior to the consultation or are scored in a structured clinical interview.

The anatomical localization of many behavioural symptoms is poorly understood, but there is an increasing awareness of the role of the right hemisphere, particularly the medial (anterior cingulate) and inferior (orbital) frontal and anterior temporal regions.

## Apraxia

The inability to perform a movement with a body part despite intact sensory and motor function is termed apraxia. Theoretically, the concept can be divided into errors of action conception (knowledge of actions and of tool functions, e.g. the purpose of a screwdriver), and action production (generation and control of movement). Although a number of categories, such as limb-kinetic, ideomotor, and ideational apraxia, exist, these labels are seldom useful in clinical practice. It is more helpful to describe the apraxia by region (orobuccal or limb), and to provide a description of impaired performance, recording both spatial and temporal or sequencing errors on several different types of task.

A thorough assessment of apraxia should involve the following:

1 *Imitation of gestures*, both meaningful (e.g. wave, salute, hitch-hiking sign) and meaningless (body- and non-body-oriented hand positions). Meaningful gestures should also be tested to command (Fig. 11.2).

2 *Orobuccal movements* (blow out a candle, stick out your tongue, cough, lick your lips), and *the use of imagined objects* (comb your hair, brush your teeth, slice a loaf of bread) are assessed. A common error is to use a body part as a tool, such as a finger for a toothbrush; if repeated after being corrected, this can be considered pathological. Actual use of the object generally elicits better performance than when it is mimed, and is typical of so-called ideomotor apraxia.

3 *A sequencing task* such as the Luria three-step command (fist, edge, palm), or the Alternating Hand Movements test, completes the assessment. This latter task is performed, after demonstration, with arms outstretched, and alternate opening and closing of the fingers of one hand, while those of the other remain clenched in a fist.

**4** Lower limb apraxia may be demonstrated by an inability to trace patterns with the feet on the ground in response to command. Relative preservation of some movements (e.g. bicycling movements with the legs whilst lying down) in the presence of gait ataxia may also suggest an apraxic cause.

In general, apraxic signs are of limited localizing value, but the left parietal and frontal lobes appear to be of greatest importance. Orobuccal apraxia is closely associated with lesions of the left inferior frontal lobe and the insula, and commonly accompanies the aphasia caused by lesions of Broca's area. Progressive, isolated limb apraxia is virtually diagnostic of corticobasal degeneration.

## Visuospatial ability

Deficits in the visuospatial domain are quite commonly associated with neurodegenerative diseases, particularly Alzheimer's disease, but are often clinically silent and missed unless enquired about specifically. Getting lost in familiar surroundings (topographical disorientation), difficulties with dressing (dressing apraxia), misreaching for objects, or the failure to identify familiar faces are all markers of this type of impairment.

Visual neglect may produce a failure to groom one half of the body, or eat what is placed on one side of a plate. Visual hallucinations invariably suggest an organic cause, and are prominent in dementia with Lewy bodies and acute confusional states. Formed visual hallucinations may also be seen in the absence of cognitive impairment in the *Charles Bonnet syndrome*, and are often associated with poor eyesight; insight is generally retained.

Information from the visual cortex is directed towards the temporal or parietal cortex via one of two streams. The dorsal ('where') stream links visual information with spatial position and orientation in the parietal lobe, whereas the ventral ('what') stream links this information to the store of semantic knowledge in the temporal lobes. The frontal eye fields are important in directing attention towards targets in the visual field.

### Neglect

Neglect of personal and extrapersonal space is usually caused by lesions to the right hemisphere—usually the inferior parietal or pre-frontal regions. Deficits can be uncovered by simultaneous bilateral sensory or visual stimulation, or having the patient bisect lines of variable length. Letter and star cancellation tasks are similar, more formal tasks. Patients with object-centred neglect fail to copy one side of an object, and *neglect dyslexics* may not read the beginning of a line or word. Patients with *anosognosia* deny they are hemiplegic or even that the affected limb belongs to them.

### Dressing and constructional apraxia

Although deficits in dressing and constructional ability are termed apraxias, they are best considered as visuospatial, rather than motor impairments. Copying three-dimensional shapes such as a wire cube, interlocking pentagons or constructing a clock-face with numbers are good tests of constructional ability, and may also highlight neglect if it is present (Fig. 11.3). Left-sided lesions tend to cause over-simplification in copying, whereas right-sided lesions may result in abnormal spatial relationships between the constituent parts of the figure. Dressing apraxia is easily tested by having the patient put on clothing that has been turned inside-out.

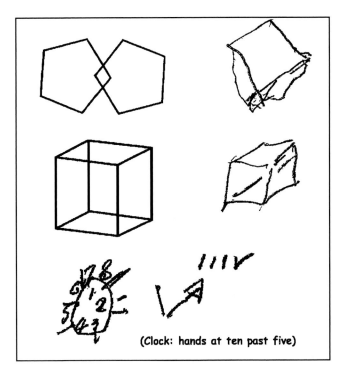

(Clock: hands at ten past five)

**Fig. 11.3** Examples of poor visuospatial performance when reproducing interlocking pentagons, the wire cube or drawing a clock face. This patient has dementia with Lewy bodies which frequently causes visuospatial impairment. Other common causes include Alzheimer's disease and corticobasal degeneration.

### Visual agnosias

Visual object agnosias cause a failure of object recognition despite adequate perception. Those with *aperceptive visual agnosia* have normal basic visual functions, but fail on more complex tasks involving object identification and naming. However, they are able to name objects to description, or by touch, indicating a preserved underlying semantic representation of the object. This phenomenon is described with bilateral occipito-temporal infarction. In cases of *associative visual agnosia*, the deficit reflects a disruption of stored semantic knowledge, and involves all modalities accessing this information. This is always secondary to anterior temporal lobe pathology, typically semantic dementia or herpes encephalitis. To test for these syndromes, it is necessary to assess object naming and description, along with naming unseen objects from their description, and the ability to provide semantic information about unnamed items.

### Prosopagnosia

*Prosopagnosics* cannot recognize familiar faces. Often other clues, such as gait, voice, or distinctive clothing, are used to aid identification. The deficit may not be entirely selective to faces, and often fine-grained identification within categories may also be impaired (e.g. makes of car, types of flowers). Patients are generally able to characterize individual facial features, and if the underlying (semantic) knowledge associated with a particular person is not disrupted, the ability to produce attributes of the face in question, if it is named, remains intact. An occipito-temporal lesion underlies this disability, and is often associated with a field defect, achromatopsia, or pure alexia. Whether it is necessary to have bilateral pathology remains controversial. Where there is anterior right temporal lobe involvement, as in the right temporal variant of semantic dementia, person-based social knowledge is often profoundly affected. These patients also find it difficult to judge facial affect. In delusional misidentification syndromes such as the *Capgras syndrome*, patients are convinced that an impostor, who looks identical, has replaced a close relative. It occurs in dementia and schizophrenia, and there is a suggestion that the linkage of affective attributes to a face may be disconnected from processing of its identification.

### Colour deficits

Colour processing deficits such as *achromatopsia* (loss of ability to discriminate colours) are often associated with pure alexia after medial occipito-temporal damage, following left posterior cerebral artery infarction. *Colour agnosia* impairs tasks requiring retrieval of colour information (e.g. 'What colour is a banana?') and *colour anomia* (e.g. 'What colour is this?') refers to a specific disorder of colour naming despite intact perception and colour knowledge, probably caused by a disconnection of the language structures in the temporal lobe from the visual cortex.

### Rare visual syndromes

A few rare syndromes are worthy of mention. *Balint's syndrome* consists of a triad of *simultanagnosia* (inability to attend to more than one item of a complex scene at a time), *optic ataxia* (inability to guide reaching or pointing despite adequate vision), and *oculomotor apraxia* (inability to voluntarily direct saccades to a visual target). Fields may be full when challenged with gross stimuli, and oculocephalic reflexes are intact. This syndrome results from bilateral damage including the superior parieto-occipital region, which disrupts the dorsal ('where') visual processing stream linking visual with parietal association areas. Possible causes include carbon monoxide poisoning, watershed infarction, leucodystrophy, and the posterior cortical variant of Alzheimer's disease. *Anton's syndrome* is a visual agnosia, in which the patient denies any deficit and may attempt to negotiate the environment, invariably without success. In the curious phenomenon known as *blindsight*, visual stimuli can induce a response despite cortical blindness. It is probably mediated by perceptual processing in subcortical structures and brainstem nuclei.

### Activities of Daily Living (ADL)

Recent research criteria for dementia include impaired ADLs in the definition of dementia. The ability to organize finances, use home appliances, drive safely, and organize medication regimens are higher-order (instrumental) ADLs which are usually impaired earlier in disease than more commonly assessed skills such as cooking, walking, personal hygiene, and continence (basic ADLs). This is an area in which a reliable informant, who knows the patients well, is essential.

### Driving

Driving is often a sensitive issue. Early cognitive impairment does not preclude driving, but should prompt discussion of driving ability. In general, spouses are fairly aware of changes in driving skill, and their concerns should not be dismissed lightly. Impairments in visuospatial ability (e.g. copying the wire cube, pentagons, drawing a clock face) are good markers of increased driving risk. Often, cessation of driving can be negotiated, but in extreme cases, where poor insight conflicts with a sensible approach, keys can be hidden, cars can be disabled, moved, or sold, and the licensing authority notified. An independent driving assessment may be very advisable.

## Cognitive assessment scales

Perhaps the most widely used cognitive rating scale is the Mini-Mental State Examination (MMSE), which although useful is weighted significantly towards aspects of memory and attention. However, it provides relatively little by way of language testing, minimal assessment of visuospatial ability, and no testing of executive performance. It is scored out of 30, with a score of 24 or less being regarded as abnormal. The patient's educational background, age, and first language should be considered. It has the benefit of being fast to administer, and well recognized as a screening instrument, but is quite insensitive, particularly in the context of frontal and subcortical pathology, as well as mild cognitive impairment.

The Addenbrooke's Cognitive Examination (ACE), has been developed in an attempt to address the deficiencies of the MMSE. It was designed to be sensitive to the early stages of frontotemporal dementia and Alzheimer's disease and has been shown to be sensitive to cognitive dysfunction in the Parkinson's-plus syndromes. The 100-point scale incorporates the items of the MMSE, but includes more tests of executive function, visuospatial skill, and more complex language assessment. The recently revised version (ACE-R) provides subscores for five domains: orientation and attention, memory, verbal fluency, language, visuospatial/perceptual functioning. A cut-off of 88 provides high sensitivity but lower specificity, while a cut-off of 82 has very high specificity for dementia at the cost of lower sensitivity.

The briefest of all of the screening examinations is the Mental Test Score (MTS), which is a 10-item scale assessing orientation, memory (anterograde and retrograde), and attention. A score of 6 or less is abnormal in the elderly, but as with the other cognitive rating scales, the profile of deficits is more instructive than the global score. It may help direct further, more detailed assessment, but offers no advantages over the other scales other than speed of administration.

## Formal neuropsychological assessment

Unfortunately, neuropsychological services are not always available. In general it is reasonable to reserve this facility for patients in whom we need more detailed assessment for diagnostic purposes, or those in whom we wish to better characterize deficits for the purposes of rehabilitation. Patients with clear-cut deficits of moderate severity are unlikely to need formal testing to reach a diagnosis. In contrast, neuropsychology has much to offer for patients in whom deficits are early and subtle, or who have marginal performance on cognitive screening scales.

## General neurological examination

A cognitive assessment is incomplete without a careful general neurological examination. There are a number of clinical features that have particular importance. Although in the early stages of many neurodegenerative diseases, clinical signs may be absent, this is not invariable. Table 11.2 highlights the important neurological findings associated with various cognitive disorders.

**Table 11.2** Associated neurological features in dementia

| Neurological feature | Common or early | Less common or late |
|---|---|---|
| Extrapyramidal: bradykinesia, rigidity, tremor | Parkinson's disease (PD), corticobasal degeneration (CBD), progressive supranuclear palsy (PSP), frontotemporal dementia (FTD), dementia with Lewy bodies (DLB), vascular dementia (VaD) | Alzheimer's disease (AD), dementia pugilistica, Wilson's disease (WD), neurodegeneration with brain iron accumulation (NBIA), leucodystrophies, dentato-rubro-pallido-luysian atrophy (DRPLA) |
| Chorea | Huntington's disease (HD), DRPLA | Autoimmune (systemic lupus erythematosus) |
| Eyes: impaired saccades and/or gaze palsy, visual hallucinations, Kayser–Fleischer rings | PSP, HD, Niemann–Pick type C (NPC), Wernicke–Korsakoff (WK), DLB, delirium, WD | |
| Frontal signs: utilization, grasp, palmo-mental, pout | Subcortical dementia, leucodystrophy, FTD, PSP, WD, frontal tumours, hydrocephalus | |
| Alien limb | CBD | Corpus callosum lesion |
| Dystonia | CBD, WD, HD | AD, Lesch–Nyhan |
| Myoclonus | Prion disease, CBD, familial AD, encephalopathy (asterixis) | Multisystem atrophy (MSA), DLB, post-anoxic, Whipple's (facial myorhythmia) |
| Ataxia | Prion diseases, multiple sclerosis, (MS), MSA, WK spino-cerebellar atrophy (SCA), NBIA, DRPLA, WD, leucodystrophy | |
| Orobuccal apraxia | CBD, progressive non-fluent aphasia (PNFA) | |
| Pyramidal signs | MND, MS, MSA, SCA, leucodystrophy, prion disease, hydrocephalus | FTD, familial AD |
| Peripheral neuropathy | Leucodystrophy (esp. metachromatic), deficiency states, NBIA, SCA syndromes | Neuroacanthocytosis |
| Muscle wasting, weakness and fasciculation | Motor neurone disease associated FTD (MND-FTD) | |
| Anosmia | Head injury, most neurodegenerative diseases (HD, PD, AD) | Anterior cranial fossa tumour |

# Conclusion

It is not possible to examine everything in the cognitive assessment, and as in most other areas of neurology, the history remains pre-eminent in guiding subsequent examination. The central role of a reliable informant, and the ability to immediately test hypotheses generated during the history-taking, distinguish this means of neurological assessment.

In some patients it is not possible to reach a firm diagnosis after a single cognitive assessment, even when in possession of a formal neuropsychological report. This is particularly true for the mild stages of neurodegenerative diseases where symptoms may be non-specific, and reflects the relative insensitivity of both clinical and imaging assessment to early pathology. The time-honoured method of longitudinal follow-up and repeated assessment in such cases is invaluable, and should not be forgotten.

## Selected further reading

Bak, T.H., Rogers, T.T., Crawford, L.M., Hearn, V.C., Mathuranath, P.S., and Hodges, J.R. (2005). Cognitive bedside assessment in a typical parkinsonian syndromes. *Journal of Neurology, Neurosurgery, and Psychiatry*, **76**(3), 420–422.

Dubois, B., Slachevsky, A., Litvan, I., and Pillon, B. (2000). The FAB: a Frontal Assessment Battery at bedside. *Neurology*, **55**(11), 1621–1626.

Heilman, K.M. and Valenstein, E. (2003). *Clinical neuropsychology*, 4th edn. Oxford University Press, Oxford.

Hodges, J.R. (2007). *Cognitive assessment for clinicians*, 2nd edn. Oxford University Press, Oxford.

Hodges, J.R. (2007). *Frontotemporal dementia syndromes*. Cambridge University Press, Cambridge.

Lezak, M.D. (2004). *Neuropsychological assessment*, 4th edn. Oxford University Press, Oxford.

Mathuranath, P.S., Nestor, P.J., Berrios, G.E., Rakowicz, W., and Hodges, J.R. (2000). A brief cognitive test battery to differentiate Alzheimer's disease and frontotemporal dementia. *Neurology*, **55**(11), 1613–1620.

Mioshi, E., Dawson, K., Mitchell, J., Arnold, R., and Hodges, J.R. (2006). The Addenbrooke's Cognitive Examination Revised (ACE-R): a brief cognitive test battery for dementia screening. *International Journal of Geriatric Psychiatry*, **21**(11), 1078–1085.

Sampson, E.L., Warren, J.D., and Rossor, M.N. (2004). Young onset dementia. *Postgraduate Medical Journal*, **80**(941), 125–139.

# 12

# Physical assessment of older patients

Duncan Forsyth

## Introduction

Mental health problems in older age may be the presenting feature of other medical illness, they may present with somatization, or they may exacerbate co-existent medical conditions. Thus the patient may first be referred to a geriatrician rather than an old age psychiatrist to exclude 'organic' pathology. Equally, colleagues in old age psychiatry may need to involve the geriatrician to assist in the management of co-existing medical problems and to advise regarding complex polypharmacy. All physicians should be aware of the potential psychological impact of ill-health and its treatments on patients and their carers.

As a broad general rule each individual tends to age at a relatively constant rate; in other words the ageing process is not a sudden occurrence, but its trajectory may be influenced by acute illness and chronic disease processes. Frail older people may deteriorate rapidly and are more likely to develop secondary complications due to their poor physiological reserve. The so-called non-specific presentation of disease typifies the geriatric giants with presentations of delirium, immobility (gone off feet), falls, incontinence, or increased dependency. This non-specific presentation of disease in older life can often mean that symptoms of disease are mistaken for the process of ageing or worse still assigned as not coping ('acopia') or 'social problems'. Although typical diagnostic features of particular disease processes may be obscured in older age, making the diagnostic process more difficult, diagnostic features are seldom completely absent and clues will be found if care and attention are taken with a good history (including corroborative history from relatives and carers) as well as a thorough physical examination and appropriate investigations. For example, whilst truly silent myocardial infarction may occur, and is commoner with increasing age (Muller *et al.*, 1990), most are not truly silent as they come to light as the result of a fall, evidence of left ventricular failure, or new onset atrial fibrillation. Atypical presentations of disease in older age have been overemphasized and, in the author's view, generally reflect inadequate assessment of the older person.

### Learning point

Patients admitted to the general hospital with a diagnosis of 'acopia' or as a 'social admission' generally have significant underlying pathology and are likely to benefit from comprehensive geriatric assessment.

Older people are more prone to multiple pathologies so that there may be several aetiologies for a given symptom, e.g. the combination of Parkinson's disease, osteoarthritis, poor visual acuity from senile macular degeneration, new-onset atrial fibrillation, and drug-induced orthostatic hypotension may combine to explain postural instability and falls. Thus, having found one possible cause for presenting symptoms the clinician should consider whether others may also be contributing (this is in contrast to Ockham's razor, which suggests one accepts the simplest explanation for an event unless there is reason to do otherwise); this will also require a judicious use of clinical acumen in apportioning clinical relevance to every possible diagnosis and determining to what extent each should be investigated and managed. Equally, the effects of several minor (individually unimpressive) interventions may combine to produce a major change, e.g. the combination of quadriceps exercises to help stabilize an osteoarthritic knee, analgesia for osteoarthritic pain, withdrawing diuretics to reduce postural hypotension, digoxin to slow atrial fibrillation, and treatment of mild Parkinson's may enable the physiotherapist to rehabilitate a previously immobile individual.

There is much contention in the literature regarding assessment scales, whether for disability, mobility, or cognition. It is not appropriate in the context of this chapter to discuss the pros and cons of all scales; suffice it to say that clinicians should use scales that they are familiar with and understand, and recognize their limitations and that it is the process of documenting change within these assessment scales which is most important in determining whether a particular treatment modality is working or whether a disease process is progressing. Any scales used need to be applicable to everyday clinical usage and may be different from those used in clinical trials, where more time is available to complete more complex assessment scales. A pragmatic approach is simply to be descriptive. For example, a person who can now walk using a Zimmer frame, with the assistance of one person and transfer with the help of one person is improving if one week earlier they needed two people to assist with transfers and could only stand with the help of two people. A smiling patient, who acknowledges your presence and initiates conversation, is responding to the antibiotics for their severe pneumonia, if several days earlier they could barely speak and showed no interest in their surroundings. On the other hand, the individual whose appetite and fluid intake is declining and who is becoming less engaged in their environment is developing some illness and needs further attention.

Wherever possible, and provided the patient is agreeable, it is useful to have a member of their family or carer in attendance when assessing the patient. The benefits are fourfold: additional information can be obtained from the third party; the family member/carer remains informed; carer strain may become evident; and a care plan is better developed.

### Learning point

Involving family or carers in the assessment process:

- assists with information gathering and communication
- provides an opportunity to educate the carer/family as well as the patient
- may help identify carer strain
- facilitates the care planning process

The impact of illness on any older person can be devastating both physically and psychologically (see later). It is important to warn family members that rarely will an individual with any background of a chronic progressive disease return to their prior level of function upon recovery from any acute illness. The extent of the difference in their level of functioning will be determined by the severity and duration of the acute illness. In those with cognitive impairment, it is a strong clinical impression that their cognitive abilities will not be the same after acute illness of any nature (shown schematically in Fig. 12.1).

It is beyond the scope of this chapter to cover the entire complexity of geriatric medicine, it will be more appropriate to address some broad principles and highlight specific areas that may commonly present as problems for the old age psychiatrist.

## Observation

General observation of the patient before and during the actual consultation can provide important clues, e.g. a resting tremor and shuffling gait suggests a parkinsonian syndrome; failure to make eye contact may alert to possible depression or a glass eye! Do not miss any opportunity to assess gait: watch the patient walk into the consultation room, lead you through their house, going to the toilet and so on. Do they require assistance with walking, transfers, and so on? The following may give vital clues to falls risk:

- ill-fitting footwear
- postural instability and tendency to lean backwards on standing or postural hypotension
- shuffling gait of extrapyramidal syndromes
- hemiplegic gait
- antalgic gait of osteoarthritic hips
- broad based gait of postural instability due to cerebellar or posterior spinocerebellar tract pathology, middle ear disease, or peripheral neuropathy
- inability to walk and talk at the same time
- taking more than four steps to turn through 180 degrees
- slow and careful gait of visual impairment.

Observing the face may reveal blunted facial expression of Parkinson's or depression; pallor of anaemia or lack of sun exposure

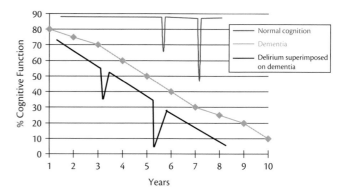

**Fig. 12.1** Impact of illness on cognitive trajectory.

(start to think about vitamin D deficiency and osteomalacia); vitiligo (which may mark other autoimmune conditions such as diabetes, pernicious anaemia, Addison's disease, or thyroid dysfunction); orofacial tardive dyskinesia; ptosis (if symmetrical this will be an ageing phenomenon, if unilateral this may be due to eye surgery or neurological disease); facial palsy of new or old stroke; or Bell's palsy.

Stooped posture may be the kyphosis of osteoporosis or due to Parkinson's. A tentative handshake may identify rotator cuff injury or painful inflammatory arthritis.

Evidence of self-neglect or inability to attend to oneself due to ill-health may be obvious with dirty clothes, hands, and face; unshaven and unkempt appearance; neglected nails.

Body habitus will separate the well nourished from the poorly nourished or cachexic due to underlying sinister pathology.

Initial conversation will identify whether speech is appropriate (delirium, psychosis), intelligible (e.g. dysarthria, dysphonia, or dysphasia suggesting neurological disease such as Parkinson's, stroke, tumour, encephalopathy, or motor neuron disease), plausible and accurate (delirium, dementia, delusional), hindered by shortness of breath (severe respiratory or cardiac disease); and whether mood is normal (depression, lability post-stroke).

### Learning point

The neuromuscular control of articulation is the same as for swallowing, so a dysarthric patient is highly likely to be dysphagic as well.

Being expert in the art of the 'non-touch' examination technique is a crucial part of the physical assessment of agitated, paranoid, or aggressive individuals. This will help reduce the chance of personal injury and also of unexpectedly coming in to contact with urine, blood, and faeces. For example, faecal soiling may alert to the possibility of constipation with overflow diarrhoea and the distended suprapubic region to agitation secondary to co-existent urinary retention. Asking a demented agitated patient why they keep hitting staff may also prove useful—'Because it hurts when they hold my arm' was the response from one old man with an undiagnosed fractured head of humerus. Whilst people with dementia are more prone to fall, their behaviour afterwards may be a consequence of the fall not of their pre-existing dementia. Check with their carers if there has been a change in behaviour, look carefully for fractures and consider the possibility of subdural haemorrhage. Also remember that the fall may have been precipitated by intercurrent illness or change in medication.

## Learning point

When faced with a behaviourally disturbed patient, check if this is usual for them. Where behaviour has changed consider the following common possibilities:

♦ pain, e.g. after a fall with or without fracture

♦ constipation

♦ urinary retention (more common in men than women)

♦ adverse drug reaction (has medication been changed recently?)

♦ infection

Blunted facial expression raises the possibility of a parkinsonian syndrome but in the absence of other extrapyramidal signs is more likely to be due to depression. However, the two do commonly coexist.

Inability to engage the patient in conversation requires a thorough assessment of hearing, e.g. look for wax, have they got a hearing aid that they should be wearing (is it in working order? see Table 12.1). The prevalence of hearing impairment increases with advancing age; over 80% of those aged over 80 years may benefit from a hearing aid. Whilst many older people with hearing impairment will have sensorineural deafness and benefit from a hearing aid, initial assessment must exclude blockage of the external auditory canal by wax. Early referral to the local audiology department is recommended for anyone with hearing impairment (not due to wax) for assessment (Sharaf *et al.*, 2006). Writing questions down or using a microphone and headset communicator may overcome any hearing impediment: if it does not, then, assuming that you are conversing in the patient's first language, consider the possibilities of aphasia (usually due to cerebrovascular disease), depression, and frontotemporal dementia.

## Learning point

Different tactics should be tried to facilitate listening for patients with hearing difficulties even if they have hearing aids. These include:

♦ attracting the person's attention before speaking

♦ face the person when speaking and make sure the light is on your face

♦ cutting down background noise whenever possible

♦ speak clearly and naturally, but not too quickly

♦ do not shout as this may cause distortion

♦ rephrasing the words where necessary—some words are more lip-readable than others

♦ checking that instructions have been understood correctly

♦ information could also be written down

Assessment of nutritional and hydrational status, including any records of food and fluid intake, supplemented by records of weight, will help assess the general impact of illness on the individual but does not necessarily give a clue as to the underlying diagnosis. However, absence of weight loss in someone complaining of weight loss and poor appetite, whether with or without other symptoms, suggests anxiety, depression, or attention-seeking behaviour. Failure to gain weight as expected with appropriate medical treatment should also raise the possibility of missed/inadequately treated co-morbidities, coexistent depression, or poor psychological adjustment to their illness. Similarly, lack of interest in personal care (dirty and dishevelled or simply just not wanting to get dressed or brush one's hair) may reflect apathetic delirium, subcortical or frontotemporal dementia, or depression.

In frail older individuals multiple pathology may complicate the assessment of gait, e.g. poor visual acuity may make the individual slow and cautious as will fear of further falls; diabetic peripheral neuropathy may cause a shuffling gait due to altered proprioception; and osteoarthritis of the lumbosacral spine and hips will cause the individual to move in a stiff and rigid manner. Care should also be taken to differentiate illusions in those with poor visual acuity from true hallucinations, thereby saving the individual from an unnecessary prescription of an antipsychotic.

Frail older people staying in hospital for a long time provide an opportunity to teach nursing and medical staff observational skills, so that they learn to recognize change in behaviour that alerts to underlying illness (Box 12.1).

## Immobility

This may be caused by pain or stiffness in joints (arthritis or infection), in muscles (trauma, polymyositis, polymyalgia rheumatica, Parkinson's disease), or bones (osteoporosis, osteomalacia,

**Table 12.1** Solving common problems with hearing aids

| Problem | Cause/solution |
|---|---|
| Hearing aid apparently not working | Check if aid is switched to the 'T' setting by accident |
| | Check volume at the correct level and not turned right down |
| | Check the battery is the right way round |
| | Try putting in a new battery |
| | For behind the ear (BTE) hearing aid, check that the tubing is not twisted, squashed, or split |
| | Check whether there are droplets of condensation in the tubing. If there are, gently pull the soft tubing off the hooked part of the aid and blow down the tubing to remove the droplets; and/or if it is a body-worn aid, the lead may need to be replaced |
| | Check that the ear mould (and ear) is not blocked with wax |
| Whistling, squealing, sizzling, or squeaking | This may be caused by 'feedback' when sound amplified by the hearing aid leaks out and is picked up by the hearing aid microphone. It may happen if: |
| | The ear mould is not put in properly—push it gently to check |
| | There is excess wax in the ear: patient's ears need to be checked |
| | The ear mould does not fit ear snugly enough (audiologist to review) |
| | The volume is set too high: check the volume control |
| | The ear mould has cracked or the plastic hook or tubing in a BTE aid has become loose or has split: hearing aid centre should be contacted for help |
| | The tubing in a BTE hearing aid has become hard causing the hearing aid not to work well. If it splits, the aid may start to whistle. It can be replaced by the patient or audiology staff |
| Buzzing noises | This might be due to switching the hearing aid to the 'T' setting by accident. Otherwise, buzzing generally means the hearing aid has developed a fault and needs to be repaired |

**Box 12.1**

An 82-year-old male was recovering from severe community acquired pneumonia with associated delirium. At week four his delirium had resolved and he was able to mobilize with the assistance of one person and a Zimmer frame. At week six on the day before transfer to a community rehabilitation unit the consultant noted that the patient was inattentive, drowsy, and engaged less in conversation than on his ward round 2 days earlier. Transfer to the rehabilitation unit was deferred and investigations revealed a urinary tract infection.

malignancy, Paget's disease). Immobility may also result from neurological weakness (stroke, peripheral neuropathy, motor neuron disease); muscle damage (myopathy, hypokalaemia, diabetic amyotrophy, disuse), or reduced exercise tolerance (cardiac or respiratory disease, anaemia). Immobility may be the psychological consequence of falling (fear of further falls). Other causes include painful bunions, foot ulceration, unsuccessful orthopaedic procedures, and sedation.

## Drug history

Any assessment is incomplete until all medications have been checked. Do not rely upon patient recollection but ask to see the drugs and then go through each concerning how they are taken (dose, frequency, and adherence) and ask about possible side-effects. Around 20–25% of older people are not taking drugs that their general practitioner (GP) expects them to be taking and about one-third will be taking drugs that their GP does not know about: this latter group will include complementary and alternative medicines (CAM) as well as over the counter (OTC) medications. Up to 50% may be taking their medicines incorrectly (Royal Pharmaceutical Society of Great Britain, 1997) and a similar percentage may be able to stop their drugs (Walma *et al.*, 1997).

### Learning point

- Do not assume that the patient is taking their medication as per the instructions on the bottle.

- Do not assume that the patient is taking the medication that their GP thinks they should be taking.

- Do not assume that the patient is only taking medication mentioned in any referral letter.

- Consider that any illness may be iatrogenic and assess medication accordingly.

The importance of medication risk in older age warranted a separate addendum to the National Service Framework for Older People (NSFOP), published in England in 2001 (Department of Health, 2001), and so this should be an integral part of the single assessment process (SAP), set out in Standard 2 of the NSFOP. Problems with medication are also often linked to stroke, falls, and mental health (Standards 5, 6, and 7 of the NSFOP). Risk factors for iatrogenic drug problems include:

- four or more drugs (remember OTCs),

- specific drugs, e.g. warfarin, non-steroidal anti-inflammatory drugs (NSAIDs), diuretics, digoxin,

- recent discharge from hospital,

- dementia,

- depression,

- poor vision/hearing/dexterity,

- living alone or low levels of support.

### Learning point

Reducing or omitting diuretics in hot weather can help reduce the incidence of postural hypotension and electrolyte imbalance in frail older people.

## Which drugs are really necessary and why?

Unfortunately, older people are largely excluded from clinical drug trials due to their high level of co-morbidities and so the evidence base for most pharmacological treatments is weak or non-existent in older age. Older people are at increased risk of adverse effects of drugs, due to altered pharmacokinetics and pharmacodynamics, but may also have more to gain (absolute risk reduction) from preventive therapies, as more events occur in older age, e.g. the absolute benefits of thrombolysis in acute myocardial infarction increase with age. The complex interaction of age and disease on drug metabolism, e.g. drug metabolism declines in delirium (White *et al.*, 2005), may enable the judicious manipulation of side-effects to advantage, e.g. in treating depression in Parkinson's disease the anticholinergic side-effects of tricyclic antidepressants (TCAs) may help reduce tremor.

In the later stages of dementia, or in an uncooperative patient, a decision may be needed as to which medications are really necessary. For example, in a bed-fast, severely demented individual with cardiovascular disease, is aspirin therapy still appropriate to reduce the possibility of a cardiovascular event? In an individual with severe dementia and inconsistent nutritional intake, for whom it has been agreed that artificial nutritional support is inappropriate, is continued bone prophylaxis with calcium and vitamin D supplements or a bisphosphonate appropriate? Would substitution of paracetamol for codeine-based analgesia reduce the necessity for regular laxatives? A medication review should be undertaken at every opportunity and advice sought from a consultant geriatrician if the old age psychiatrist is uncertain, e.g. is treatment with a statin still appropriate; would aspirin be safer than warfarin for stroke prevention?

## Examination

### General aspects

When examining a patient of the opposite sex it is essential to have a chaperone present. Examination technique will, by necessity, vary according to how cooperative the patient is and may not be completed in one go. Even the most expert clinician cannot get away entirely with the 'hands-off' approach outlined above. However, keen observation skills may focus the physical examination on to the essential and the not so essential aspects. Holding an agitated or paranoid patient down is more likely to lead to violent behaviour than to facilitate a successful examination. As a general rule, if the patient cannot comprehend the reason for the examination (whether this is cardiac auscultation or digital rectal examination) you will be unlikely to succeed. If at first you don't succeed try again later (Juss and Forsyth, 2005; Royal College of Physicians, 2006).

A calm reassuring manner, with appropriate introductions as to who you are, what you want to do, and why, will generally work (but not always). Gentle hand-holding is reassuring but can easily be turned in to a restraining hand if the patient becomes aggressive. Likewise, careful positioning of one's legs when facing the confused and agitated patient appears non-threatening but can also become a defensive block if the patient kicks out. Body language is important to maintain a non-threatening demeanour, on occasions even this can be misinterpreted, e.g. with a deaf patient, as one leans in to speak clearly in the proffered ear this can be mistaken for an affectionate greeting and you are greeted with an unexpected peck on the cheek!

Assessment of the confused individual must include assessment of cognition and a screen for delirium. Assessment scales commonly used by geriatricians include: Confusion Assessment Method (CAM) (Inouye *et al.*, 1990), Folstein Mini-Mental State Examination (MMSE) (Folstein *et al.*, 1975), CLOX or clock drawing test (Royall *et al.*, 1998), Informant Questionnaire on Cognitive Decline in the Elderly (IQCODE) (Jorm, 1994), and the Geriatric Depression Scale (GDS) (Yesavage and Brink, 1983) (see also Chapter 8).

## The mouth and its contents

Angular stomatitis is usually due to dribbling and may be seen in Parkinson's and in individuals with facial palsy or poorly fitting dentures; secondary infection may occur with candida. Herpes simplex and aphthous ulceration are often non-specific markers of ill-health. Oral candidiasis may reflect poor oral hygiene, diabetes, or recent treatment with antibiotics and can make swallowing very painful. Fasciculation of the tongue suggests motor neuron disease and requires further neurophysiological investigation, i.e. electromyography (EMG) and nerve conduction studies. Mouth ulceration is often due to ill-fitting dentures but the possibility of oral squamous cell carcinoma may need excluding.

Carious teeth may be the source of 'unexplained' fever and raised inflammatory markers and can make the clinician feel very foolish for not having looked in the mouth.

Dignity and nutrition are best maintained if dentures are well-fitting and worn. Labelling dentures should reduce the chances of them being lost by staff or confused patients.

## Skin

The dermis becomes thinner and more fragile with ageing due to changes in type-II collagen. Lack of elasticity with ageing renders skin turgor useless in the assessment of hydrational status.

Basal cell carcinoma is the most common skin malignancy and occurs most commonly on the face. It first appears as a pearly papule, which slowly and inexorably enlarges. Metastatic spread is rare. Squamous cell carcinoma presents as a reddened, indurated ulcer, nodule or plaque, which often arises in sun-exposed areas. It may metastasize. Malignant melanoma is an expanding pigmented lesion occurring anywhere on the body.

The risk of developing pressure sores is increased in those with poor mobility, oedematous skin, poor nutrition, poor circulation (peripheral vascular disease and cardiac failure), urinary and/or faecal incontinence, or with long-term steroid use. Every individual at risk should have their pressure points examined (occiput, ears, shoulders, elbows, sacrum, spine, ankles, feet, and heels).

Leg ulceration may be due to arterial or venous disease or often a mixture of both. A long history of recurrent ulceration, usually of the lower third of the shin above either malleolus, with surrounding eczema and hyperpigmentation and palpable (unless obscured by oedema) foot pulses is typical of venous ulceration. Arterial ulceration is distinguished by absent foot pulses and well circumscribed small punched-out ulcers often on the lateral leg or dorsum of the foot. Any ulceration will be painful; absence of pain usually implies coexistent peripheral neuropathy.

## Bruising and falls

The presence of bruising anywhere will usually be due to falls and should prompt a look for other injury, sprain, or fracture. Pain from this injury may explain altered behaviour or worsened cognition. Common sites for fragility fractures are the hip, wrist, head of humerus, and pelvis. Pelvic fracture should be suspected in anyone who fails to mobilize after a fall with no other obvious reason not to do so. Pain from pelvic fracture may radiate to the low lumbar spine and be misdiagnosed as osteoarthritis of the spine. Active flexion of the hip with extension of the knee (straight leg raising) contracts muscles attached to all surfaces of the pelvic ring. This simple test has a 95% positive predictive value and 90% negative predictive value for pelvic fracture and has greater diagnostic value than either downward pressure on the pubic bone or compression of the iliac rings (Ham *et al.*, 1996).

Bruising may result from elder abuse and should therefore always be accurately documented on body charts in the patient's records. Suspicious bruising includes: thumb marks (usually on limbs); bruising in the groins and inner thighs (most older people do not fall astride an object); multiple bruising of multiple ages (but this person may just be a frequent faller); bruising with other injuries suggestive of abuse, e.g. cigarette butt burns, scalds, friction burns. Bruising and a fearful or apprehensive patient should always make one consider the possibility of elder abuse (British Geriatrics Society, 2005a).

A focal neurological deficit or fluctuating cognition in the presence of bruising should raise the possibility of subdural haematoma. Fluctuating cognition without evidence of trauma or focal neurological deficit is almost always due to problems outside of the cranium causing delirium (Royal College of Physicians, 2006).

## Falls assessment and postural blood pressure

Measurement of resting (after 5 minutes, recumbent or semi-recumbent) and standing (after 2 minutes) blood pressure is mandatory in anyone who has fallen. Medication will need reviewing for drugs that might lower blood pressure either directly [vasodilators, volume depletors (diuretics)] or indirectly (centrally acting drugs affecting baroreceptor reflexes, e.g. antiparkinsonian medication, opiod analgesia, and antidepressants). Other causes of volume depletion should be excluded, e.g. diarrhoea, vomiting, blood loss, and dehydration.

Watching the patient walk will identify gait abnormalities, dangerous footwear, postural instability, and whether they can concentrate on other things whilst walking (walk and talk test). The shoulder-pull test may be required to identify postural instability. A pull on the individual's shoulders, whilst they stand with their feet slightly apart should not cause the individual to lose balance or retropulse; if either occur then they are posturally unstable. The author finds this to be a more useful test for postural instability than Romberg's test. Individuals who use a walking aid are (usually) by definition posturally unstable and so do not need this test!

A corroborative history will help determine whether there was any loss of consciousness; this is unlikely if the individual can recall the act of falling and coming to rest on the ground. However, many individuals, even those without cognitive impairment, do not remember falls that occurred within the last 3–12 months (Cummings *et al.*, 1988). If loss of consciousness is suspected then further tests are likely to be required to exclude a vascular (cardiac arrhythmia, acute coronary syndrome, pulmonary embolism, stroke, or acute severe blood loss) or cerebral (epilepsy) cause. Transient ischaemic attacks are focal neurological deficit resolving within 24 hours and do not cause loss of consciousness but may cause a fall.

Individuals with poor visual acuity are at increased risk of falling as are those who have not adjusted to wearing bi- or varifocal lenses (especially when going down steps) (British Geriatrics Society, 2003). Poorly fitting footwear and other environmental hazards should be sought and corrected.

The consequences of falls include: fracture (usually low-velocity osteoporotic), subdural haemorrhage; tissue and muscle necrosis from long periods of lying; acute tubular necrosis secondary to rhabdomyolysis; anaemia secondary to extensive bruising (beware the individual on anticoagulants); hypothermia; fear of further falls and resultant poor mobility. In the institutionalized elderly and those who are housebound, the risk of falls may reduce with vitamin D supplementation due to improvements in muscle strength and balance.

### Learning point

Falls assessment should include:

- check lying and standing blood pressure
- check temperature
- check for pain and document injuries (fractures and bruising)
- review medication for drugs that might cause postural hypotension
- review gait
- review footwear
- check balance, e.g. shoulder pull, walk and talk
- neurological examination
- musculoskeletal examination
- check vision and spectacles
- consider other investigations to look for a cause, e.g. ambulatory ECG recording, EEG, full blood count, vitamin D levels
- consider other investigations to look for complications, e.g. creatine kinase (CK), urea and electrolytes (U&Es), X-rays
- review home for environmental hazards
- assess cognition, e.g. dementia and/or delirium
- consider elder abuse—'Did they fall or were they pushed?'

### The neurological examination

The neurological examination can be an ordeal for all concerned, and is an excellent test of cognition on behalf of the examiner and the examinee. Talk the patient through what you are going to do in simple clear language—asking someone to relax all too frequently results in entirely the opposite response! Use observational skills as much as possible—muscle wasting is common with ageing and may lead to difficulties rising from a chair or opening the door to the examination room. Muscle wasting may be age related, secondary to disuse around arthritic joints, or reflect neurological disease (e.g. peripheral neuropathy, motor neuron disease, old polio). Reflexes may be difficult to elicit or interpret; and power and tone may be difficult to judge due to coexistent arthritis. Ankle jerks may be absent in around one in three normal older people. Pupils may be small and sluggish to react to light making fundoscopy difficult, even with mydriasis. Fundoscopy may also be hindered by cataracts. Position sense is generally retained in older age, whilst vibration sense may be lost or not understood. In general, testing sensation can be fraught with difficulty. Isolated upward gaze palsy is of dubious significance.

### Learning point

Progressive supranuclear palsy (PSP) may cause an isolated downward gaze palsy *not* isolated upward gaze palsy. In PSP upward gaze palsy occurs in the context of other gaze paresis. These individuals are at increased risk of falling going down stairs.

### Co-operative versus uncooperative patients

In individuals who demonstrate variable performance, physically and/or cognitively the differential diagnosis lies between:

- delirium
- personality disorder
- dementia, particularly dementia with Lewy bodies
- depression.

Differentiating these clinical conditions is generally easy, but can on occasions be difficult. For example, hypoactive delirium can be mistaken for subcortical dementia and depression, whilst agitated depression may be mistaken for symptoms of delirium. This may lead to inappropriate prescribing and/or lack of appropriate therapeutic interventions (e.g. rehabilitation).

Delirium is the most common complication of hospitalization among older adults, occurring in about one-third to two-fifths of elderly hospitalized patients. It is often not recognized in up to two-thirds of cases. Delirium may be precipitated by any drug or illness in susceptible individuals and often has more than one cause, usually outside of the brain. Delirium is associated with an excess mortality, increased lengths of stay, increased rates of institutionalization, and higher readmission rates. For a full account of the prevention, detection, and management of delirium the reader is referred to the Royal College of Physicians of London and British Geriatrics Society national guidelines (Royal College of Physicians, 2006). Serial recording of cognitive function will help differentiate delirium from dementia and can be useful in determining whether therapists should continue to try to engage the individual in rehabilitation. If delirium has been excluded then a trial of antidepressants may be warranted if depression cannot be excluded (in an effort to treat the treatable). Delirium symptoms may persist for several months after resolution of the precipitating cause(s) and may be a premonitory feature of dementia. Thus, individuals who have had delirium should be followed up after discharge.

The fluctuating course of delirium and its fluctuating recovery are often difficult for the patient's family to understand—they see someone recovering only to get worse and then recover and then deteriorate again. If medical and nursing staff do not recognize or understand delirium then their explanations to family members can seem confused and lead to hostility and complaints. A useful analogy is that of jet-lag: most people have experienced this form of delirium and can start to understand what is happening. The process of recovery is akin to setting your clock to local time, and so measures such as stopping delirium-inducing drugs or the resolution of infection do not immediately result in the body clock being reset or bring about an immediate resolution of confusion. As dementia is the commonest risk factor for developing delirium it is also worth advising relatives that the individual will rarely return to their prior level of function.

### Learning point

- Delirium is usually multifactorial with the cause(s) being outside of the brain.
- CT head scan is not necessary unless there is focal neurology or other reason to suspect intracranial pathology, e.g. falls and possible subdural haematoma.
- Delirium symptoms may persist for several months after resolution of the precipitating event.

### Investigations in an uncooperative patient

Even in cooperative patients one should always consider the utility of any investigation. Will the result influence this patient's management now or in the future? In uncooperative individuals one may need to practise empirical medicine and treat on the grounds of probabilities. Treatment may of course include masterly inactivity on the part of the doctor (so hard for many to practice!). Patients often do better when the doctor does nothing, as they are spared unnecessary and inappropriate interventions and their attendant complications.

### Learning point

Things that help win over even the most belligerent patients include:

- A calm and non distressing environment
- Friendly reassurance and consistent communication from staff
- Offering adequate fluids and nutrition
- Waiting for the individual to settle down before performing complex investigations.

Whilst waiting for a period of calm, attention to the basics of care (delirium prevention and management) will, for most individuals, be the most important aspects of their care. Time will also be well spent in reviewing which drugs are really necessary both now and for the future, if behavioural disturbance persists (see also later). For example, annoying already confused and agitated individuals by insisting that they take calcium and vitamin D supplements or aspirin is unnecessary, whilst coaxing them to take their antiparkinsonian medication may be time well spent. Parents quickly learn when coaxing their baby or toddler to take food or medicine what will or

will not work and how to prioritize what is really necessary: such skills are invaluable when dealing with a delirious frail older person (but you do not need to be a parent to have these skills)!

Faced with an uncooperative patient it will also be prudent to reduce nursing observations (measurements of blood pressure, pulse, temperature, etc.) to an absolute minimum. Indeed, such patients provide an ideal opportunity for staff to refine their people observation skills and to observe whether: the individual has started to accept or is taking less fluid and food; is more or less socially interactive; is wandering more or less; is starting to mobilize or has become less mobile; and so on. These simple observational skills help to determine whether the individual is improving or deteriorating. If the latter occurs a point will come at which they are no longer able to mount resistance to more detailed examination or investigation; hopefully this will not be beyond a point of salvation, but often is.

Sedating an uncooperative patient may be necessary to enable essential investigations to be performed, e.g. head CT scan when behavioural disturbance could be due to a subdural haemorrhage or intracranial tumour, and knowing would alter management plans. Sedation may also be necessary when the individual is a risk to themselves or others. However, in general, sedation is best avoided, as more often it makes things worse rather than better.

## Specific diseases

### Parkinson's disease

To diagnose a parkinsonian syndrome the individual *must* be bradykinetic and then have either rigidity and/or tremor. Tremor is common in older age, occurring in 10% of over 65-year-olds and is not always due to Parkinson's disease; equally not all Parkinson's patients have tremor. Tremor in Parkinson's is typically a rest tremor but may be present on action. Rigidity in older age is not always classical cogwheel in nature. Idiopathic Parkinson's disease can only be diagnosed if other parkinsonian syndromes have been excluded (Table 12.2). The diagnosis of idiopathic Parkinson's

**Table 12.2** Conditions to exclude before diagnosing idiopathic Parkinson's disease

| |
|---|
| Essential tremor |
| Drug induced parkinsonism: <br> phenothiazines <br> prochlorperazine <br> metoclopramide <br> tetrabenazine |
| Arteriosclerotic pseudo-parkinsonism (vascular parkinsonism) |
| Multisystem atrophy (MSA) |
| Progressive supranuclear palsy (PSP) |
| Dementia with Lewy bodies |
| Other causes of tremor: <br> drugs—lithium, amiodarone, SSRIs <br> anxiety <br> hyperthyroidism |
| MPTP (1-methyl-4-phenyl-1,2,3,6-tetrahydropyridine) exposure |
| Old age |

**Table 12.3** Diagnostic uncertainty in Parkinson's in older age

| | |
|---|---|
| Causes of diagnostic uncertainty in determining the presence of Parkinson's | The presence of co-morbidities (such as arthritis, depression, dementia, muscle weakness, involuntary movements) |
| | Non-specific presentation (falls, depression, slowing down, fatigue) |
| | Atypical presentation (dysphagia, pain, dysarthria) |
| | Tremor is common in older people and may be atypical and difficult to classify |
| | Tremor-dominant Parkinson's disease |
| | Minor signs of extrapyramidal disturbance in older people associated with cognitive impairment |
| Causes of diagnostic uncertainty in determining the cause | There are more causes of parkinsonism in older people |
| | Drug-induced parkinsonism increases in frequency with age |
| | Levodopa responsiveness is unreliable in older people as a marker for Parkinson's disease |
| | Vascular parkinsonism and parkinsonism associated with dementia become more prevalent with age and create diagnostic difficulty |

disease in older age can be extremely difficult due to the impact of other co-morbid conditions and the fact that there are more causes of parkinsonism in older age (Table 12.3).

Parkinson's patients with motor fluctuations can cause particular difficulties as they may be seen to undertake a task (e.g. walking or feeding themselves) for which they require assistance later the same day; this can lead to an incorrect assumption that they are manipulative or awkward. Assessment by a Parkinson's disease specialist should be undertaken to ensure optimal treatment for the Parkinson's (pharmacological and non-pharmacological) and to establish that the motor symptoms of Parkinson's are not being adversely affected by other extraneous events, e.g. physical illness, psychological stress, or other mental health problems. Sudden changes in the natural trajectory of the disease will always be due to the effect of extraneous factors on the patient's ability to compensate for their symptoms and the disability, i.e. the effect of physical (e.g. infection) or psychological stressors (e.g. anxiety).

**Learning point**

Parkinson's disease is a slowly progressive neurodegenerative disease which does not change suddenly. Sudden apparent change in Parkinson's symptomatology will always be due to the effects of some other event (physical or psychological), e.g. anxiety, infection, constipation, heat wave, or change in any medication.

For most patients with Parkinson's disease, it is crucial that they receive their medication at the appropriate time, whether or not this fits in with the timing of institutional drug round. It is imperative that the hospital ward does not 'run out' of the Parkinson's medication and that if a patient's medication is non-ward stock (which it usually will be) that the ward obtains a supply before the next dose of medication is due (whatever day of the week or time of day it is!). Failure to maintain normal dosing schedules runs the risk of:

- worsening Parkinson's symptoms
- decreased mobility

- increased rigidity and pain
- increased tremor
- slowed cognition with attendant increased anxiety and risk of complications
- dysphagia with inability to maintain hydration and nutritional intake
- aspiration or hypostatic pneumonia
- constipation
- urinary sepsis
- incontinence
- pressure sores
- falls
- delirium
- depression
- loss of faith in health professionals
- complaints and litigation.

If the Parkinson's patient has problems taking oral medication, e.g. due to dysphagia, acute illness, or severe psychomotor retardation, then urgent input from the Parkinson's specialist will be needed to consider alternatives to oral medication or advise whether the patient is in fact dying and medication is no longer appropriate.

A reasonable *aide-mémoire* for clinical pharmacology is that drugs that target a specific organ of the body will preferentially 'poison' that organ, i.e. drugs that act on the brain (e.g. Parkinson's drugs) will have cerebral side-effects, typically postural hypotension, delirium, agitation, and these will be more likely to occur in those who already have evidence of cognitive impairment.

The neuropsychiatry of Parkinson's disease is complex and fascinating. The cause of anxiety can often be very difficult to determine. This may be a response to motor fluctuations, particularly if they are unpredictable or a symptom of depression. Parkinson's symptoms may seem much worse than the disease actually is when the individual is depressed. Depression occurs in around two-thirds of community-dwelling Parkinson's patients (Meara *et al.*, 1999). Depressive symptoms of poor attention, poor initiation, poor construction, and increased perseveration all mimic Parkinson's dementia, so if in doubt a therapeutic trial of antidepressants may be warranted, whilst watching out for problems of postural hypotension.

Cognitive deficits in Parkinson's are commonly: executive function (most prominent and maybe earliest); higher-order attention; memory; and spatial skills (visuomotor processing and visual attention). Executive dysfunction underlies several impairments, including: memory dysfunction and problems with verbal fluency, reasoning, spatial skills, and complex attention. Executive dysfunction will limit the extent to which Parkinson's patients may be deemed competent to consent to medical treatments and/or clinical trials (Dymek *et al.*, 2001). Frontal executive dysfunction can be found in around one-third of newly diagnosed cases of Parkinson's disease (Foltynie *et al.*, 2004) and is a predictor for risk of developing subsequent Parkinson's dementia. The prevalence of dementia is 40% in all Parkinson's patients (Cummings, 1988) and correlates with age (0% < 50 years; 69% > 80 years) and duration of Parkinson's

(29% after 3 years and 78% after 8 years) (Lieberman *et al.*, 1979; Brown and Marsden, 1984; Aarsland *et al.*, 2003). Parkinson's dementia renders the individual more vulnerable to drug toxicity from their Parkinson's medications. Concomitant dementia represents a significant clinical problem in Parkinson's disease, and with it comes:

◆ increased carer strain (Aarsland *et al.*, 1999a)

◆ increased risk of institutionalization (Aarsland *et al.*, 2000)

◆ institutionalization, associated with increased mortality (Louis *et al.*, 1997).

Around 30% of Parkinson's patients develop hallucinations within the first 5 years after diagnosis (Fenelon *et al.*, 2000). These become permanent in over 80% (Graham *et al.*, 1997) and about 10% go on to develop psychosis with delusions (Jenkins and Groh, 1970; Aarsland *et al.*, 1999b). Psychosis is the single most important precipitant for long-term institutional care in Parkinson's (Aarsland *et al.*, 2000; Goetz *et al.*, 2001). Failing cognition or psychosis may make it necessary to sacrifice mobility in order to minimize psychotic symptoms and thereby preserve the sanity of carers and prevent the individual with Parkinson's disease being institutionalized. Close collaboration will be required with the local Parkinson's specialist in these circumstances as there is a complex interplay between symptoms and treatment effects when dealing with the neuropsychiatry of Parkinson's. There is now good evidence for potential benefit of rivastigmine in dementia associated with Lewy bodies (McKeith *et al.*, 2000) and dementia in Parkinson's disease (Emre *et al.*, 2004) (see Chapter 27v).

---

**Learning point**

Dementia in Parkinson's:

◆ has a frequency 6× that of age-matched controls.

Dementia in Parkinson's is more common:

◆ with age of onset of Parkinson's > 60 years

◆ in later stages of Parkinson's

◆ with more severe Parkinson's

◆ if psychosis and confusion develop with levodopa.

(Levy *et al.*, 2002)

---

## Stroke

New-onset stroke should be referred urgently to the local stroke physician for assessment of the type and size of stroke and for appropriate management to be instigated as well as for exclusion of possible brain tumour. The latter tends to have a more insidious onset of neurological deficit rather than the abrupt onset of cerebrovascular disease. Sudden severe headache with neurological deficit may represent subarachnoid haemorrhage and requires urgent assessment and investigation.

Transient neurological deficit (hemiplegia, dysphasia, hemianopia) resolving in under 24 hours is compatible with a diagnosis of transient ischaemic attack (TIA). The neurological deficit in TIAs is focal in nature and therefore does not result in loss of consciousness. The individual may fall due to their hemiparesis but there will not be any evidence of loss of consciousness. Transient neurological signs with loss of consciousness should raise the possibility of epilepsy or cardiac arrhythmia.

---

**Learning point**

◆ Once infarction has occurred, it is impossible to further damage that area of the brain, though lesser degrees of brain injury may be repeated.

◆ A person who has recurrent episodes of similar neurological deficit without cumulative long-term deficit may have: recurrent epileptic seizures with Todd's paresis or be failing to compensate for residual stroke deficit when stressed by additional illness.

---

Cerebrovascular disease is an important major cause of dementia, with atrial fibrillation perhaps being the single most important risk factor for multi-infarct dementia. Assessment of cognition is hindered in individuals who are dysphasic. The individual with hemianopia or visuospatial problems secondary to parietal lobe dysfunction may appear confused due to their dyspraxia or problems in negotiating their way through their environment due to hemianopia. For a comprehensive review of dyspraxias and dysphasias the reader is referred to Hodges (1994).

Routine administration of nutritional supplements to stroke patients does not improve overall outcome and should be reserved for those who are undernourished on admission or have deteriorating nutritional status after their stroke (FOOD Trial Collaboration, 2005). Early enteral feeding in those who are dysphagic after stroke reduces mortality but increases the number of severely disabled survivors. As dysphagia post-stroke recovers within 2 weeks in over 80% of cases, and most show signs of recovery within a few days, there is no need to rush into enteral feeding unless it is necessary for the management of diabetes or Parkinson's disease.

## Thyroid disease

Hypothyroidism should be considered in any depressed or apathetic individual. Symptoms of cold intolerance, constipation, tiredness, and slowing of mental and physical ability are indistinguishable from symptoms of depression. Alopecia, bradycardia, slow relaxing reflexes, hoarse or gruff voice, swelling of the face, ataxia, and, more rarely, pre-tibial myxoedema will help to confirm a clinical diagnosis of hypothyroidism. Anxiety and hyperactive, even paranoid, states may be due to thyrotoxicosis. Clinical signs of lid retraction, lid lag, and exophthalmos along with warm peripheries, fine tremor, and a tachycardia which persists during sleep all help confirm a clinical diagnosis of thyrotoxicosis. Less common is apathetic hyperthyroidism. Measurement of serum thyroid stimulating hormone (TSH) will help in the diagnosis of thyroid disorder. A normal TSH excludes hypo- and hyperthyroidism. However, an abnormal TSH, both high and low, may be due to non-thyroid disease, e.g. severity of illness (sick euthyroid) or the effects of drugs (amiodarone, steroids). In general a high TSH with a low serum thyroxine ($T_4$) indicates hypothyroidism; other combinations are likely to require specialist interpretation.

## Adrenal disease

General malaise, weight loss, hypotension, and falls may be due to hypoadrenalism, which may come on insidiously or may come to the fore more precipitously when an individual is stressed by infection. Hyperadrenalism, or Cushing's syndrome, is uncommon but may present with depression or psychosis, both of which may also occur with use of high-dose steroids in conditions such as asthma.

## Diabetes

Management of a psychiatric patient with diabetes should be a collaboration between the psychiatrist and the diabetologist. Particular attention needs to be given to the diabetic patient who by virtue of their psychiatric illness is either not eating or not taking their medication consistently. Under such circumstances the potential for either hypo- or hyperglycaemic complications is significant and may warrant inpatient treatment.

Careful assessment for complications of diabetes is required, with particular attention being paid to blood pressure, signs of cardiac failure, assessment of renal function including urinalysis for proteinuria and evidence of nephropathy, fundoscopy to assess for retinopathy, assessment for peripheral neuropathy, and evidence of neuropathic or arterial ulceration.

## Renal disease

Renal failure is rarely a cause of psychiatric symptoms except in a profoundly sick individual. Deterioration in renal function requires a review of medication that may adversely affect renal function, e.g. NSAIDs, angiotensin-converting enzyme inhibitors (ACEIs); a review of hydrational status and, in particular, a review of the need to continue diuretics and ACEIs in very hot weather or when the individual is suffering from a diarrhoeal illness; consideration of prostatic hypertrophy and obstructive uropathy in men (abdominal palpation will reveal the distended bladder and a rectal examination will reveal the enlarged prostate).

### Learning point

Urinary retention is uncommon in women and should lead to a search for pelvic or rectal tumour as well as a vaginal examination to exclude tumour and prolapse.

## Electrolyte imbalance

Hyponatraemia and hyper- and hypocalcaemia may all cause delirium or they may present with more subtle symptoms such as tiredness, constipation, reduced mobility. Hyponatraemia is most frequently secondary to diuretic drugs and selective serotonin reuptake inhibitor (SSRI) antidepressants. The syndrome of inappropriate antidiuretic secretion (SIADH) may occur with infection; renal, hepatic, cardiac, and pituitary dysfunction; or by inappropriate production of ADH in carcinoma of the bronchus. Hypercalcaemia is much more common than hypocalcaemia and should lead to a search for possible malignancy and measurement of parathormone to exclude hyperparathyroidism as well as a review of medications such as calcium and vitamin D supplements. Hypocalcaemia may be due to malabsorption, vitamin D deficiency, and hypoparathyroidism.

## Urinary tract infections

These are common and often present non-specifically with confusion, anorexia, or fatigue. Asymptomatic bacteriuria is frequent in older people and does not require treatment; if the individual is unwell and no other cause for their illness has been identified then this is not asymptomatic bacteriuria! Dipstick urinalysis that is positive for nitrites and leucocytes has a positive predictive value of over 90% for urinary tract infection. Negative dipstick testing of urine will obviate the need to send a urine sample to the laboratory unless there is unexplained fever, rising inflammatory markers, or delirium. All too frequently elderly people admitted to hospital will be treated for a presumed urinary tract infection when there is no evidence to support the presumption and the fact that they get better is mistakenly assigned to the treatment with antibiotics when in fact they were likely to get better anyway. Blind treatment with antibiotics runs the risk of antibiotic-associated diarrhoea (*Clostridium difficile* diarrhoea) and so should not be encouraged.

## Anaemia

This often presents with non-specific symptoms of malaise, poor mobility, apathy, possibly even self-neglect, falls, and confusion. Significant anaemia may occur due to extensive bruising after a fall, especially in those on antiplatelet agents or warfarin. Hypochromic microcytic anaemia is most likely to be due to blood loss from the bowel. This requires a review of medication (is the individual on aspirin, warfarin, steroids, or NSAIDs?) and a thorough abdominal examination, which must include a rectal examination. Other possible sources of bleeding may need to be considered, e.g. postmenopausal bleeding. Macrocytic anaemia may be due to alcohol excess, hypothyroidism, folate or $B_{12}$ deficiency, and it may contribute to dementia. Normochromic normocytic anaemia is often associated with chronic diseases such as rheumatoid arthritis and chronic renal failure.

Leuconychia and a smooth shiny tongue may be seen in chronic iron deficiency anaemia.

## Giant cell arteritis (temporal arteritis)

Giant cell arteritis (GCA) usually presents with headaches, visual disturbance, and tender scalp and sometimes causes pain around the shoulder girdle and pelvis (polymyalgia rheumatica). It may also present non-specifically with malaise, weight loss, fever, or stroke. There may be low-grade anaemia and mild abnormalities of liver function, and there will almost always be a raised erythrocyte sedimentation rate (ESR) or C-reactive protein (CRP). Temporal artery biopsy may be required to make the diagnosis. Urgent treatment with steroids is required to prevent blindness and, therefore, urgent referral should be made to a geriatrician.

# Specific problems
## Assessing pain in the cognitively impaired

Despite the high prevalence of pain amongst older people and its many consequences, pain is inadequately recognized and treated, especially in those with severe cognitive impairment. Barriers to assessment of pain include: the inability of some older people, especially those with severe dementia, to communicate their pain experience; and the misconception that pain is less severe in those with cognitive impairment. Use of surrogate reporters, direct observation of potential pain indicators, monitoring for changes in usual activity and behaviour, and ruling out pain as a possible cause of behaviours through non-drug and analgesic trials should improve the assessment and management of pain in those with cognitive impairment.

Unrelieved pain can have several adverse effects for the individual (Table 12.4) (Briggs, 2003), and these may lead to inappropriate management, e.g. disruptive behaviour may be inappropriately treated by sedation rather than by assessment of and alleviation of the pain. Poor pain management can also result in increased

**Table 12.4** Consequences of unrelieved pain

| Acute | Increased risk of complications: delirium, deep vein thrombosis, nausea and vomiting, respiratory infections<br>Increased mortality |
|---|---|
| Acute and chronic | Behavioural changes<br>Depression<br>Psychosocial effects: isolation, impaired mobility, disrupted sleep, changes in social roles and relationships<br>Increased length of hospital stay<br>Increased risk of institutionalization<br>Decrease in successful rehabilitation<br>Litigation |

complaints and litigation by patients' family members (advocates). Thus, it is important that we understand how those with dementia perceive pain, that we recognize their pain, and we treat it. A thorough systematic assessment is required in cognitively impaired older people to reveal covert pathology and to investigate and remedy symptoms such as pain. The given history may not be accurate or may be absent, which can mislead the clinician.

The experience of pain is inherently subjective and will be modulated by a variety of factors, which include: mood state; perception of control; expectations; social conditioning; cultural conditioning; and cognition. In cognitively impaired individuals both the experience and expression of pain may be altered. This poses difficulties in assessing pain, as all pain assessment scales require a reasonably high level of cognitive and language ability. Selecting accurate and useful assessment instruments for use in those with cognitive impairment is a major problem and becomes more problematic as cognition declines. Stolee *et al.* (2005) reviewed 30 instruments for assessing pain in cognitively impaired older people and found that for most reliability and validity data were basic or non-existent, and that none proved to be both valid and reliable.

Most of the available standardized pain assessment tools are primarily forms of self-report. The verbalization of pain can be difficult for patients who have cognitive impairment. Not only may they have problems localizing pain or describing its temporal relationship but they may even have problems saying whether or not they have pain. As dementia progresses and verbal skills decline, then carers and nursing and medical staff must increasingly rely on non-verbal cues of physical and emotional pain (Table 12.5). Common behaviours associated with pain are shown in Table 12.6,

**Table 12.5** Non-verbal cues in the expression of pain

| Agitation or irritability |
|---|
| Repetitive verbalization/shouting |
| Aggression |
| Fluctuating cognition |
| Falls/withdrawal |
| Decreasing functional ability |
| Sweating |
| Tachycardia/raised blood pressure |

**Table 12.6** Common pain behaviours in cognitively impaired elderly persons

| Facial expressions | Slight frown; sad, frightened face<br>Grimacing, wrinkled forehead, closed or tightened eyes<br>Any distorted expression<br>Rapid blinking |
|---|---|
| Verbalizations, vocalizations | Sighing, moaning, groaning<br>Grunting, chanting, calling out<br>Noisy breathing<br>Asking for help<br>Verbally abusive |
| Body movements | Rigid, tense body posture, guarding<br>Fidgeting<br>Repetitive rubbing of an area (perhaps indicating where pain is located)<br>Increased pacing, rocking<br>Restricted movement<br>Gait or mobility changes |
| Changes in interpersonal interactions | Aggressive, combative, resisting care<br>Decreased social interactions<br>Socially inappropriate, disruptive<br>Withdrawn |
| Changes in activity patterns or routines | Refusing food, appetite change<br>Increase in rest periods<br>Sleep, rest pattern changes<br>Sudden cessation of common routines<br>Increased wandering |
| Mental status changes | Crying or tears<br>Increased confusion<br>Irritability |
| Other restless or irritated behaviour | Pulling at tubes |

Adapted from: American Geriatrics Society Panel on Persistent Pain in Older Persons (2002).

but some patients demonstrate little or no specific behaviour associated with severe pain. Use of facial expressions or various behaviours may be difficult in patients with Parkinson's disease or facial palsy.

The altered affective response to pain, especially in people with Alzheimer's disease, may reflect pathology in the medial pain system, resulting in an inability to cognitively process the painful sensation in the context of prior pain experience, attitudes, knowledge, and beliefs (Scherder *et al.*, 2005). Reactions to painful sensations may therefore differ from the typical response expected from a cognitively intact older person. For example, constipation can cause great distress in the cognitively impaired older person and may lead to aggressive or agitated behaviours. As there is no evidence that those with dementia experience less pain, we should assume that any condition that is painful to a cognitively intact person would also be painful to those with advanced dementia who cannot express themselves. For example, pain should be considered as a possible explanation for a change in behaviour in an older person with advanced dementia. Although subtle changes in usual patterns of behaviour or activity do not always mean that the patient is in pain, they should raise the suspicion and lead to a thorough evaluation for possible pain-causing problems.

Simply observing an individual at rest may not identify pain behaviours which may only occur during activities such as transferring, walking, and repositioning.

Adequate pain assessment forms the basis for optimal pain control, and it has major implications for quality of life (QoL) and quality of care of older people. Unrelieved pain has been associated with altered immune function, impaired psychological function (e.g. depression, anxiety, and fear), impaired physical function (e.g. impaired mobility and gait, delayed rehabilitation, falls), sleep disturbance, compromised cognitive function, and decreased socialization (American Geriatrics Society, 2002). These may all result in increased dependency as well as increased use of health-care resources, with resultant increased costs. In those with severe cognitive impairment it is all too easy to attribute these effects to their dementia, rather than to unrecognized and untreated painful conditions. For instance, demented patients with persistent pain are more likely to be treated with benzodiazepines and antipsychotics than their non-demented counterparts (Balfour and O'Rourke, 2003).

An empirical trial of analgesia may be warranted if pain behaviours persist after other possible causes are ruled out or treated. The choice of an appropriate analgesic is challenging because it is difficult to determine the level of pain severity in persons with advanced dementia. Starting with paracetamol seems prudent, whilst titration to stronger analgesics may be necessary before ruling out pain as the aetiology for behaviour or activity changes. If analgesic use results in decreased pain-related behaviours, it seems reasonable to assume that pain was the likely cause and to continue pharmacological and/or non-pharmacological interventions. The increased susceptibility of cognitively impaired older people to adverse drug effects clearly necessitates very careful monitoring of any analgesic trial.

### Learning point

- Pain is under-reported and under-treated in cognitively impaired older people.

- Poorly treated pain is associated with increased disability, depression, behavioural problems (inappropriate prescription of neuroleptics), and worsening cognitive function.

- Most pain assessment scales rely upon verbal skills.

- Decline in verbal communication skills with worsening dementia makes assessment very difficult.

- A multifaceted approach using a combination of self-reported measures, family or carer input, measures of functional impairment/change, along with physiological or behavioural measures should improve the accuracy of pain assessment and improve the subsequent management of pain in this vulnerable group of older people.

### Learning point

In a communicative individual with cognitive impairment the following tips will assist in the assessment of pain:

- frame questions in the here and now

- use concrete questions with yes/no responses

- repeat the question

- use validating questions

- ensure communication aids (spectacles, hearing aids) are worn and functioning

- give adequate time for the individual to respond to questions

## Sleep disturbance

Sleep deprivation undermines daily performance and will hinder an individual's ability to both compensate for any disability and to give their optimum in rehabilitation. It is difficult to maintain sleep hygiene in hospital, especially in dormitory wards, so it is no wonder that an individual's performance upon returning home is often better than anticipated from their assessments in hospital. Poor sleep may be due to:

- noisy environment

- insomnia

- pain

- adverse effects of medication

- depression or anxiety

- prostatism

- detrusor instability

- delirium

- uncompensated cardiac failure

- chronic obstructive airways disease

- restless legs syndrome

- sleep apnoea

- REM behaviour sleep disorder

- caring role.

## Oedema

The commonest cause of swollen feet is venostasis oedema. This typically improves with foot elevation, e.g. lessens or disappears overnight only to return when the individual is upright. A previous history of varicose veins or veno-occlusive disease may be helpful clues. Clinical appearance of dry, scaly skin (varicose eczema), brown or purple pigmentation due to haemosiderin deposition in the subcutaneous tissues, venous ulceration, or the inverted champagne bottle appearance of lipodermatosclerosis all provide diagnostic pointers. Venous support stockings may help if the older person can put them on and tolerate wearing them. Before recommending support stockings care should be taken to exclude significant coexistent peripheral vascular disease by measuring the ankle–brachial pressure index (ABPI); an ABPI between 1.1 and 0.8 is normal. Leg elevation is generally all that is required, as well as reviewing the necessity for medication that might induce fluid retention, e.g. NSAIDs or steroids. As the problem is not one of fluid overload diuretics are rarely necessary and are highly likely to cause side-effects, e.g. electrolyte imbalance, dehydration, and postural hypotension.

Unilateral leg oedema may be due to deep vein thrombosis. If there is full-leg veno-occlusive disease (iliofemoral thrombosis) rectal and pelvic examinations are mandatory to look for possible pelvic tumours. Bilateral leg oedema with a raised jugular venous pressure would suggest right heart failure and in the context of acute shortness of breath should lead to the consideration of pulmonary embolism, especially if there is new-onset atrial fibrillation. An individual who is immobile may only have sacral oedema, especially if they have been bed-fast.

Other possible causes of oedema include hypoalbuminaemia, which may be due to malnutrition, malignancy, or nephrotic syndrome.

Assessment of the jugular venous pressure in old age can be very difficult, due to cervical flexion. Bilateral basal crepitations are common and do not in themselves constitute a diagnosis of heart failure. If heart failure is a possibility then the patient needs to be assessed by a geriatrician or a cardiologist.

## Weight loss

Weight loss in older age must always raise the possibility of underlying malignancy. Clues to a possible primary site may steer investigations, e.g. weight loss in an 80-year-old lifelong smoker should raise the possibility of lung cancer. Respiratory symptoms such as cough and haemoptysis may be further clues to a primary lung cancer; whilst altered bowel habit may suggest bowel cancer; and enlarged lymph nodes may reflect lymphoma or, if confined to a particular lymphatic drainage area, may point to the likely primary site, e.g. axillary lymph nodes suggesting breast cancer. Physical examination is not complete without a thorough examination of all lymphatic sites, breasts, thyroid, rectal, and pelvic examination. Other investigations will be guided by a process of probabilities, but a minimum would include chest X-ray, full blood count, erythrocyte sedimentation rate (ESR), serum immunoglobulins (to look for myeloma), serum calcium, liver and renal function tests.

Weight loss may be a manifestation of an individual's inability to care for themselves due to either physical or psychological disease. Weight loss may also be part of the later stages of a disease process, e.g. Parkinson's and Alzheimer's diseases.

Monitoring of current weights and review of previous weights will determine whether a complaint of weight loss is real or not. A slow decline in weight over many years may simply be part of the natural ageing process with loss of muscle and bone mass as well as natural shrinkage of internal organs.

## Dysphagia

Swallowing is a complex mechanism with no identified higher cortical control centre. Dysphagia may occur due to stroke of any size and at any site. There may be local problems such as ill-fitting or absent dentures; and oral pathology, such as a squamous cell carcinoma, needs to be excluded. Neuromuscular disorders, such as Parkinson's disease, motor neuron disease, and multiple sclerosis, may also cause dysphagia. Intrinsic obstructive disease of the oesophagus, such as oesophageal cancer, or extrinsic compression of the oesophagus from other cancers or from an enlarged left atrium must also be considered. There are obviously psychological causes of dysphagia, and one must also consider the possibility of oesophageal candidiasis, especially if the individual is malnourished or has recently been taking antibiotics. This list is by no means exhaustive.

Management of dysphagia should be considered a medical emergency—how many of us would care to go days (or even a day) without food? Urgent referral to a physician/geriatrician for investigation of non-psychological dysphagia is, therefore, important. Investigations are likely to include chest X-ray, barium swallow,

and upper gastrointestinal endoscopy. If the individual has complete dysphagia for fluids and solids, artificial nutritional support (parenteral or via nasogastric tube) may be required whilst a diagnosis is being sought. Dependent upon the cause of dysphagia, consideration will need to be given to the option of long-term artificial hydration and nutrition. Most commonly this would be by percutaneous endoscopic gastrostomy (PEG) feeding tube. Drug therapy of Parkinson's disease, sadly, provides limited improvement in dysphagic symptoms in Parkinson's.

**Learning point**

Dysphagia is a medical emergency—consider how long you would be prepared to go without food and do not allow your patients to be subjected to a longer period of starvation!

## Managing hydration and nutrition

Assessing hydrational status in older age can be very difficult due to reduced skin turgor, wasting of facial muscles, and difficulties in visualizing the jugular venous pressure. Postural hypotension or, for those who cannot stand, a fall in blood pressure on changing from lying to sitting in bed, may be the only reliable clinical sign of volume depletion.

Under-nutrition is a strong and independent predictor for morbidity and mortality. Older people may have difficulty maintaining adequate fluid and food intake due to the effects of ill-health, reduced mobility, delirium, dysphagia (remember oral and oesophageal thrush after a course of antibiotics), depression, and dementia. These all need to be differentiated from the reduction in oral intake that is part of the natural process of dying. If the individual is not dying then an appropriate management plan will depend upon the underlying cause for the inability to maintain adequate hydration and nutrition. Formal assessment of swallowing by a speech and language therapist with advice on how to enable swallowing, e.g. thickened fluids, and dietetic advice regarding nutritional support for those who are undernourished or at risk of becoming undernourished are essential and should be obtained as a matter of urgency. Without food and fluids, death will usually occur in less than 2 weeks. Without any food but with fluids the individual may survive many weeks, whilst with fluids and miniscule amounts of food they may survive for months.

Consideration needs to be given to the presentation of food (portion size, temperature, presentation), good oral hygiene, ensuring dentures are worn and well-fitting, and the use of subcutaneous fluids given overnight if daytime oral intake is inadequate. Overnight fluid supplementation has the advantage of allowing the individual to drink as much as they are able by day and does not restrict mobility or rehabilitation with intravenous lines. Nutrition assistants can also help encourage and increase oral intake. The management of diabetes and Parkinson's may cause particular problems if oral intake is poor or inconsistent and artificial hydration and nutritional support may be needed whilst a diagnosis is being sought and an appropriate treatment plan instigated; in such circumstances early resort to nasogastric feeding may be the most appropriate course of action.

The General Medical Council (2002) and British Medical Association (2001) guidance provide an explicit framework for making difficult decisions necessary to provide optimum care for individuals who are unable to maintain their own hydration and nutrition and are not competent to make decisions for themselves. Anorexia, weight loss, and dysphagia are common in advanced dementia and they may be precipitated or worsened by intercurrent infection, environmental change, depression, pain, poor oral hygiene, ill-fitting dentures, poor carer rapport, or lack of carer support. In the absence of a reversible cause for declining oral intake there is no evidence that artificial nutritional support using a PEG tube improves the prognosis in advanced dementia; there is no evidence that this intervention reduces aspiration risk, prolongs survival, improves quality of life, improves nutritional or functional status, or is well tolerated (Finucane *et al.*, 1999; Mitchell *et al.*, 2000, 2004). Where dietary intake is inadequate but death is not imminent, a second opinion should be sought from a senior clinician not involved in the individual's care before the decision to withhold artificial feeding is finalized (General Medical Council, 2002).

### Learning point

- Reduced oral intake is part of the natural dying process and needs to be differentiated from potentially treatable causes.

- PEG tube feeding in advanced dementia improves neither quality nor quantity of life.

- Before making a decision to withhold artificial hydration and nutrition, from an individual who lacks capacity, a second opinion should be obtained from an independent senior clinician.

## Palliative care

Most deaths occur in older age but sadly only one in four of us will die at home. Thus, a key part of the assessment of any older person should be the ability to recognize when death is imminent or when treatments are futile, in order that the individual, their family, and other carers (health and social) can be prepared for death and not strive officiously to try and prevent the inevitable (Finucane, 1999). Death does not always give warning of its proximity, but one should always be on the look out for it, especially in advanced or metastatic cancer; end-stage Parkinson's or dementia; as cardiac, respiratory, renal, or hepatic failure progresses. Death may be heralded by:

- failure to respond as anticipated to supportive therapy, e.g. lack of response to increasing doses of diuretics in cardiac failure;

- lack of response to potentially curative treatments, e.g. failure of infection to respond to antibiotics;

- increasing frequency of complications, e.g. rapid recurrence of aspiration pneumonia in dementia or Parkinson's;

- persistent coma after stroke;

- reducing fluid and nutritional intake in the absence of an obvious correctable cause.

The degree of warning that death is approaching may be very short, although in retrospect one can often appreciate that the warning signs were there for some time before they were recognized. There is an acknowledged need for palliative care in chronic progressive neurological diseases such as dementia (Hughes *et al.*, 2005; National Council for Palliative Care, 2006).

Once it has been recognized that the individual is dying, appropriate palliative care can be instigated with particular attention to pain control, anxiety and depression, nausea, breathlessness, delirium, constipation, insomnia, cough, hiccoughs, and any other symptoms that might occur (Ellershaw and Ward, 2003; Gold Standards Framework). The individual who is conscious and clear in mind may wish to say 'good-bye' to their loved ones and put their affairs in order. Likewise, their family and friends need to prepare themselves for the death and the grieving process, and may also need to say 'good-bye'. Health and social care staff also need to be prepared for the person's death and be confident of their role in the palliative care process.

## Psychological manifestations of disease

There are social and psychological aspects to all illnesses and it can be difficult to tell if psychological problems have taken over from the physical illness. Failure of an individual to achieve expected rehabilitation goals may be due to the development of depression or else that the patient does not share the same goals as the rehabilitation staff, e.g. lack of engagement with therapists after a fall may be because discharge from hospital means returning to a role of carer for their demented spouse. In this example, a discussion with the individual will reveal an unmet need for home care for their spouse and a need for a break from the caring role. Completing their rehabilitation as an inpatient rather than using an early supported discharge scheme may benefit the patient in the longer term, as the rehabilitation process offers a form of respite from their caring role.

Common medically unexplained symptoms that are due to psychological illness include fatigue, chest pain, dizziness, headache, back pain, and abdominal pain. A plethora of investigations will be normal but the individual, and often their family too, will not be satisfied and will seek consultations with multiple specialists. In older age there is often an underlying concern that the individual has cancer or other incurable disease; or this behaviour may emanate from social isolation or a fear of dependency. Recognizing the individual's concerns can allow the clinician to tackle the psychological problem and prevent unnecessary and repetitive investigations.

A stroll through my ward provides me with a good barometer as to how stressed the staff are. When staff are stressed this often turns out to be a transfer of anxieties from patients' relatives. Troublesome families, those that appear to demand inordinate amounts of time from health-care staff, are rarely the 'families from hell' that they are often portrayed to be. Of course, a small minority will never be satisfied no matter how good the care is. However, in general the family's anxieties stem from poor communication; concern regarding the nature, severity, and consequences of their loved one's illness; failure to grasp the information given to them (either it has not been made simple enough or was not detailed enough); lack of continuity in carers; or correctly identifying deficiencies in care (inadequate staffing levels or poor standards of care). Being aware of the ward 'barometric pressure' can allow timely input by a senior clinician at an early stage to deal with anxieties (family and staff) and defuse potential complaints (Table 12.7).

## Conclusions

In order that discharge planning may start on day one, frail older people must have access to early specialist comprehensive geriatric assessment (CGA) (British Geriatrics Society, 2005b), for it is

**Table 12.7** Common family concerns and likely explanation

| Concern | Explanation |
| --- | --- |
| Discharge will be too early | They feel home or residential care is needed<br>They were caring for their relative and have a holiday booked |
| Discharge home will be impossible | They do not understand what care is available<br>They do not appreciate to what extent recovery is possible<br>They are suffering from carer strain and need extra care |
| Nobody seems to know what is happening to my relative | Inconsistent staff<br>Over-reliance on agency and locum staff<br>Failure to appreciate that medical staff work shifts and not understanding that out-of-hours staff are not ward based<br>No firm diagnosis yet achieved (especially difficult for some to understand that medicine cannot always find the answers) |
| I get conflicting reports as to how my relative is doing | Lack of consistency in staff member liaising with the family<br>Inexperienced staff liaising with the family (nursing or medical)<br>Staff not adequately explaining delirium |

difficult to steer a course if you do not what the problems (diagnoses) are. A CGA is a multiprofessional endeavour and implies a team-based approach with clear understanding of community-based care and rehabilitation schemes. Admission assessment should include a structured description of the patient's pre-morbid function and mobility. This should be corroborated by discussion with relatives, or professionals who know the patient, as acute illness, pain, frailty, and cognitive impairment, as well as fears for the future, may compromise the accuracy of the patient's description.

The art within the science of physical assessment of older people is to engage eyes and ears with brain and only touch when necessary. Excellent observational skills are paramount and no clue must be missed or ignored. Fathoming the contribution of each and every pathological process in those with multiple pathologies can be complicated but immensely rewarding for the clinician and patient. Apparently minor changes to each of several pathological processes can easily multiply to have a major impact on an individual's physical well-being and quality of life. Complex decisions may be required as to the order of interventions most likely to provide the best results (akin to those puzzles that require you to determine the least number of moves needed to rearrange the puzzle into a certain order).

The concept of atypical presentation of disease in older age has been overstated (Isaacs, 1992). Falls, immobility, incontinence, delirium, and drug toxicity are typical presentations of pathology in frail older people. They result directly from physiological changes of ageing that can render an older person more vulnerable to stress and to changes in homeostatic processes, such as fluid balance (Rockwood *et al.*, 2004). Thus, functions that require integration of higher-order cortical process, such as staying upright, maintaining balance, or walking, are more likely to fail, resulting in falls, immobility, or delirium. These are not 'social' admissions or 'acopia'. These presentations of disease in older age demand rigorous assessment and interventions. If an individual cannot cope, it is either

because they have lost physical function, cognition, or confidence or because their social support network can no longer cope with their established care needs—either for physical or emotional/ psychological reasons. The latter would be a social presentation and would not require hospital admission but urgent social services input or respite care.

In patients with dementia, failure of language can provide particular problems in assessing pain, whilst failing cognition and language can hinder the neurological examination.

Psychological problems for the patient can slow recovery and hinder discharge planning. They need to be recognized, discussed, and appropriately managed. So-called 'problem families' are often not the problem and staff need to focus on the real issues, e.g. carer stress or poor communication, rather than becoming defensive or antagonistic.

## References

Aarsland, D., Larsen, J.P., Karlsen, K. *et al.* (1999a). Mental symptoms in Parkinson's disease are important contributors to caregiver distress. *International Journal of Geriatric Psychiatry*, **14**, 866–74.

Aarsland, D., Larsen, J.P., Cummins, J.L. *et al.* (1999b). Prevalence and clinical correlates of psychotic symptoms in Parkinson disease: a community-based study. *Archives of Neurology*, **56**, 595–601.

Aarsland, D., Larsen, J.P., Tandberg, E. *et al.* (2000), Predictors of nursing home placement in Parkinson's disease: a population-based, prospective study. *Journal of the American Geriatrics Society*, **48**, 938–42.

Aarsland, D., Andersen, K., Larsen, J.P. *et. al.* (2003). Prevalence and characteristics of dementia in Parkinson's disease: an 8 year prospective study. *Archives of Neurology*, **60**, 387–92.

American Geriatrics Society Panel on Persistent Pain in Older Persons (2002). Clinical practice guidelines: The management of persistent pain in older persons. *Journal of the American Geriatrics Society*, **50**, S205–S224.

Balfour, J.E. and O'Rourke, N. (2003). Older adults with Alzheimer disease, comorbid arthritis and prescription of psychotropic medications. *Pain Research and Management*, **8**, 198–204.

Briggs, E. (2003). The nursing management of pain in older people. *Nursing Standard*, **17**, 47–53.

British Geriatrics Society (2003). *Compendium document. The importance of vision in preventing falls*. http://www.bgs.org.uk/Publications/ Compendium/compend_4-7.htm (accessed 10 August 2006).

British Geriatrics Society (2005a). *Compendium document. Abuse of older people*. http://www.bgs.org.uk/Publications/Compendium/ compend_4-10.htm (accessed 10 August 2006).

British Geriatrics Society (2005b). *Compendium document. Comprehensive assessment for the older frail patient in hospital*. http://www.bgs.org.uk/ Publications/Compendium/compend_3-5.htm (accessed April 2007).

British Geriatrics Society (2005c). *Compendium document. The specialist health needs of older people outside an acute hospital setting*. http://www. bgs.org.uk/Publications/Compendium/compend_4-3.htm (accessed 10 August 2006).

British Medical Association (2001). *Withholding and withdrawing life-prolonging medical treatment: guidance for decision making*, 2nd edn. British Medical Association, London.

Brown, R.G. and Marsden, C.D. (1984). How common is dementia in Parkinson's disease? *Lancet*, **2**, 1262–5.

Cummings, J.L. (1988). The dementias of Parkinson's disease: prevalence, characteristics, neurobiology, and comparison with dementia of the Alzheimer type. *European Neurology*, **28**(Suppl. 1), 15–23.

Cummings, S.R., Nevitt, M.C., Kidd, S. (1988). Forgetting falls: the limited accuracy of recall of falls in the elderly. *Journal of the American Geriatrics Society*, **36**, 613–16.

Department of Health (2001). *National service framework for older people.* DoH, London.

Dymek, M.P., Atchison, P., Harrell, L., and Marson, D.C. (2001). Competency to consent to medical treatment in cognitively impaired patients with Parkinson's disease. *Neurology*, **56**, 17–24.

Ellershaw, J. and Ward, C. (2003). Care of the dying patient: the last hours or days of life. *British Medical Journal*, **326**, 30–4.

Emre, M., Aarsland, D., Albanese, A. *et al.* (2004). Rivastigmine for dementia associated with Parkinson's disease. *New England Journal of Medicine*, **351**, 2509–18.

Fenelon, G., Mahieux, F., Huon, R. *et al.* (2000). Hallucinations in Parkinson's disease: prevalence, phenomenology and risk factors. *Brain*, **123**, 733–45.

Finucane, T.E. (1999). How gravely ill becomes dying: a key to end-of-life care. *Journal of the American Medical Association*, **282**, 1638–45.

Finucane, T., Christmas, C., and Travis, K. (1999). Tube feeding inpatients with advanced dementia: a review. *Journal of the American Medical Association*, **47**, 1261–4.

Folstein, M.F., Folstein, S.E., and McHugh, P.R. (1975). 'Mini-mental state'. A practical method for grading the cognitive state of patients for the clinician. *Journal of Psychiatric Research*, **12**, 189–98.

Foltynie, T., Brayne, C.E., Robbins, T.W., and Barker, R.A. (2004). The cognitive ability of an incident cohort of Parkinson's patients in the UK. The CamPaIGN study. *Brain*, **127**, 550–60.

FOOD Trial Collaboration (2005). Effect of timing and method of enteral tube feeding for dysphagic stroke patients (FOOD): a multi-centred randomised controlled trial. *Lancet*, **365**, 764–72.

General Medical Council (2002). *Withholding and withdrawing life-prolonging treatments: good practice in decision making.* General Medical Council, London.

Goetz, C.G., Leurgans, S., Pappert, E.J. *et al.* (2001). Prospective longitudinal assessment of hallucinations in Parkinson's disease. *Neurology*, **57**, 2078–82.

Gold Standards Framework. www.goldstandardsframework.nhs.uk (accessed April 2007).

Graham, J.M., Grunewald, R.A., and Sagar, H.J. (1997). Hallucinosis in idiopathic Parkinson's disease. *Journal of Neurology, Neurosurgery and Psychiatry*, **63**, 434–40.

Ham, S.J., van Walsum, A.D., and Vierhout, P.A. (1996). Predictive value of the hip flexion test for fractures of the pelvis. *Injury*, **27**(8), 543–4.

Hodges, J.R. (1994). *Cognitive assessment for clinicians.* Oxford University Press, Oxford.

Hughes, J., Robinson, L., and Volicer, L. (2005). Specialist palliative care in dementia. *British Medical Journal*, **330**, 57–8.

Inouye, S.K., van Dyck, C.H., Alessi, C.A. *et al.* (1990). Clarifying confusion: the confusion assessment method. A new method for detection of delirium. *Annals of Internal Medicine*, **113**, 941–8.

Isaacs, B. (1992). *The challenge of geriatric medicine.* Oxford University Press, Oxford.

Jenkins, R.B. and Groh, R.H. (1970). Mental symptoms in Parkinsonian patients treated with L-dopa. *Lancet*, **2**, 177–9.

Jorm, A.F. (1994). A short form of the Informant Questionnaire on Cognitive Decline in the Elderly (IQCODE): development and cross-validation. *Psychological Medicine*, **24**, 145–53.

Juss, J. and Forsyth, D.R. (2005). *Delirium in the elderly. A case orientated CME module on delirium.* www.doctors.net.uk (go to education modules, Delirium in the Elderly; requires log-in) (accessed 30 July 2006).

Levy, G., Schupf, N., Tang, M.X. *et al. (2002)*. Combined effect of age and severity on the risk of dementia in Parkinson's disease. *Annals of Neurology*, **51**, 722–9.

Lieberman, A., Dziatolowski, M., Kupersmith, M. *et al.* (1979). Dementia in Parkinson disease. *Annals of Neurology*, **6**, 355–9.

Louis, E.D., Marder, K., Cote, L. *et al.* (1997). Mortality from Parkinson disease. *Archives of Neurology*, **54**, 260–4.

McKeith, I., Del Ser, T., Spano, P. *et al.* (2000). Efficacy of rivastigmine in dementia with Lewy bodies: a randomised, double-blind, placebo-controlled international study. *Lancet*, **356**, 2031–6.

Meara, R.J., Mitchelmore, E., and Hobson, J.P. (1999). Use of the GDS-15 as a screening instrument for depressive symptomatology in patients with Parkinson's disease and their carers in the community. *Age and Ageing*, **28**, 35–8.

Mitchell, S., Berkowitz, R., Lawson, F., and Lipsitz, L. (2000). A cross-sectional survey of tube-feeding decisions in cognitively impaired older persons. *Journal of the American Geriatrics Society*, **48**, 391–7.

Mitchell, S., Buchanan, J., Littlehale, S., and Hamel, M. (2004). Tube-feeding versus hand-feeding nursing home residents with advanced dementia: a cost comparison. *Journal of the American Dietetic Association*, **5**(2), S23–S29.

Muller, R.T., Gould, L.A., Betzu, R. *et al.* (1990). Painless myocardial infarction in the elderly. *American Heart Journal*, **119**, 202–4.

National Council for Palliative Care (2006). *Exploring palliative care for people with dementia: a discussion document.* National Council for Palliative Care, London.

Rockwood, K., Mtinski, A.B., and MacKnight, C. (2004). Some mathematical models of frailty and their clinical implications. *Age and Ageing*, **33**, 430–2.

Royal College of Physicians (2006). *The prevention, diagnosis and management of delirium in older people: national guidelines.* Royal College of Physicians, London. (Available at: http://www.rcplondon.ac.uk/pubs/books/pdmd/DeliriumConciseGuide.pdf, accessed 9 April 2007).

Royal Pharmaceutical Society of Great Britain (1997). *From compliance to concordance: achieving shared goals in medicine.* Royal Pharmaceutical Society of Great Britain, London.

Royall, D.R., Cordes, J.A., and Polk, M. (1998). CLOX: an executive clock drawing task. *Journal of Neurology, Neurosurgery and Psychiatry*, **64**, 588–94.

Scherder, E., Oosterman, J., Swaab, D. *et al.* (2005). Recent developments in pain in dementia. *British Medical Journal*, **330**, 461–4.

Sharaf, H., Fernihough, H., and Forsyth, D. (2006). Hearing aids: a clinician's guide. *CME Journal Geriatric Medicine*, **8**(2), 80–5.

Stolee, P., Hillier, I.M., Esbaugh, J. *et al.* (2005). Instruments for the assessment of pain in older persons with cognitive impairment. *Journal of the American Geriatrics Society*, **53**, 319–26.

Walma, E.P., Hoes, A.W., van Dooren, C. *et al.* (1997). Withdrawal of long-term diuretic medication in elderly patients: a double blind randomised trial. *British Medical Journal*, **315**, 464–8.

White, S., Calver, B.L., Newsway, V. *et al.* (2005). Enzymes of drug metabolism. *Age and Ageing*, **34**, 603–8.

Yesavage, J.A. and Brink, T.L. (1983). Development and validation of a geriatric depression screening scale: a preliminary report. *Journal of Psychiatric Research*, **17**, 37–49.

# 13

# Neuroimaging and neurophysiology in the elderly

## Frank Hentschel and Hans Förstl

## Introduction

Neuroimaging represents an essential part of the diagnostic work-up of dementing and other diseases in the elderly. The results offer important information on the nature of underlying brain changes and it can change the diagnosis in 30% of the patients attending a memory clinic (Hentschel *et al.*, 2005a). Findings may not usually represent characteristic 'qualitative' hallmarks of different nosological entities, but rather demonstrate the 'quantitative' severity and mixture of prevalent age-associated brain changes. Therefore a strict separation between a neurodegenerative or vascular aetiology of dementia is very often not possible and would not reflect the nature of the contributing pathophysiological factors.

Morphological neuroimaging in the elderly centres on the diagnosis and differential diagnosis of dementia:

- specific findings in patients with symptomatic dementia, e.g. brain tumours, subdural haematomas, hydrocephalus, herpes simplex encephalitis, Wernicke–Korsakoff encephalopathy, strategic infarcts etc.,

- admixtures of macro- or microangiopathy, and other brain changes

- patterns of atrophy in different forms of neurodegenerative disease, e.g. Alzheimer's disease, frontotemporal degeneration, etc.

One and a half per cent of 2013 consecutive patients admitted for the differential diagnosis of dementia showed specific findings, but only two needed specific interventions (Hentschel *et al.*, 2003a). A number of incidental observations are not related to clinical symptoms and do not necessarily imply therapeutic consequences, for example:

- limited white matter changes in microangiopathy and amyloidosis, 'leuco-araiosis';

- small, asymptomatic subdural haematomas (SDH);

- small meningiomas.

Other unexpected signs may be of pathognostic importance, for example (Ridha and Josephs, 2006):

- 'Mickey Mouse sign' in progressive supranuclear palsy;

- 'the face of the giant panda' in Wilson's disease;

- 'the eye of the tiger' in neurodegenerative iron accumulation (Fig. 13.1);

- 'pulvinar sign' in new variant Creutzfeldt–Jakob disease.

## Age-associated brain changes

Age is the fourth dimension of diagnostic neuroimaging. The mere prevalence of atrophy and other changes (Table 13.1) in the non-demented elderly prohibits the attribution of clinical significance to findings which would appear exceptional in the young.

Until the age of 65 most people only lose 0.24% of their brain volume per year and this hardly changes in the not (yet) dementing elderly (Mueller *et al.*, 1998). This atrophy is mostly cortical, primarily affecting the pre-frontal cortex, angular gyrus, superior parietal gyri, and hippocampus.

White matter changes in the elderly can only be regarded as clinically important if they are extensive and severe (Hentschel *et al.*, 2005b, 2007). Up to 18% of the healthy elderly show microbleeds leading to iron deposition and consequently to signals exceeding paradigm-related phenomena in functional neuroimaging (Roob *et al.*, 1999; Alemany *et al.*, 2006). The results of diffusion- and perfusion-weighted imaging (D-/PWI), diffusion tensor imaging (DTI), and spectroscopy are subject to remarkable age-related changes; only magnetization transfer rate (MTR) appears largely uninfluenced.

## EEG in normal ageing

Normal ageing is typically accompanied by a decrease in the posterior dominant power and frequency after the fifth decade, reduced alpha blocking after eye opening, and a mild and intermittent increase of theta activity which may be accentuated over the left temporal lobe. These changes may be less marked in strictly selected elderly normals. Until the 70s, beta-activity may increase, particularly during emotional stress; fast frontal beta power is correlated with cognitive performance. The photic driving response (the synchronization of the occipital EEG signal with rhythmical light stimuli) is impaired. After the age of 70, these alterations usually become more accentuated, but even then delta power is not increased in normals. There are complex gender differences in the pattern of age-related changes, and therefore gender-based norms are necessary for quantitative comparisons between normal and subtle pathology.

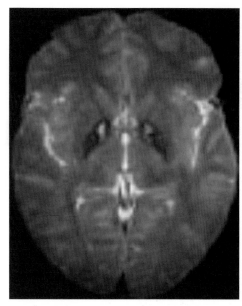

**Fig. 13.1** 'Eye of the tiger' sign due to the iron-accumulation in the basal ganglia during neurodegeneration [MRI, proton density-weighted (PD-w)]. The table shows sequences and notation for the figures in this chapter.

| Sequence | Characterized by |
|---|---|
| FLAIR transversal interleaved | TR 9000 ms, TI 2500 ms, TE 110 ms, 2 acqu.; 4 mm, gap 100%; FoV 220 mm |
| $T_1$-weighted SE transversal | TR 600 ms, TE 17 ms, 2 acqu.; 5 mm, gap 20%; FoV 220 mm |
| DE TSE transversal | TR 3400 ms, TE 105/15 ms; 2 acqu.; 5 mm, gap 20%; FoV 220 mm |
| $T_1$-weighted SE sagittal | TR 600 ms, TE 17 ms; 2 acqu.; 5 mm, gap 20%; FoV 220 mm |
| GE transversal | TR/TE 550/18 ms, 1 acqu.; 5 mm, gap 20%, FoV 220 mm |
| 3D-MP-RAGE | TR 11.4 ms, TE 4.4 ms, flip angle 12°, 1 acqu.; 1.0 mm, FoV 256 mm |

DE, double echo, instead of $T_2$-weighted and proton density weighted; GE, gradient echo; FLAIR, fluid attenuated inversion recovery; MP-RAGE, magnetization prepared rapid gradient echo; SE, spin echo; TSE, turbo spin echo; TR, repetition time; TE, spin echo time; TI, time of inversion pulse; $T_1$-weighted, longitudinal relaxation time, $T_2$-weighted, transversal relaxation time, FoV, field of view.

## Mild cognitive impairment

Structural studies reveal a continuous volume reduction of the hippocampus from health via mild cognitive impairment (MCI) towards Alzheimer's dementia (Xu *et al.*, 2000). The volumetric differentiation between 'normal ageing', MCI, and Alzheimer's has a low sensitivity and specificity, which is predetermined by the

**Table 13. 1** Morphological and functional age-associated brain changes

| |
|---|
| Brain atrophy with consequent ventricular and sulcal enlargement |
| White matter lesions, periventricular bands, 'leuco-araiosis' |
| Iron deposition in the basal ganglia and cortex/white matter margins after micro-infarction |
| Mild cerebral hypoperfusion |
| Mild cerebral hypometabolism |
| Altered cerebral metabolites |

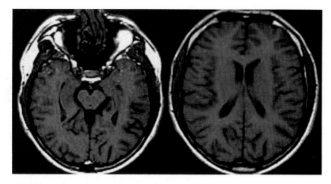

**Fig. 13.2** A 33-year-old patient with early onset Alzheimer's disease due to a presenilin-1 mutation at the stage of mild cognitive impairment [Mini-Mental State Examination (MMSE) 28/30]. Mediotemporal hypointensity; ventricular and perimesencephalic enlargement (MRI, $T_1$-weighted).

investigator's choice of comparison groups and statistics. It is completely irrelevant for practical diagnostic purposes. The subtle morphological changes affecting the entorhinal cortex, superior temporal gyrus, and the caudal part of the anterior cingulate gyrus are of scientific importance (Convit *et al.*, 1995; Albert, 2003; de Toledo-Morrell *et al.*, 2004). Total brain volume (hazard ratio, HR 1.4) and ventricular volume (HR 1.7) and the severity of white matter changes represent more robust harbingers of conversion from MCI to Alzheimer's disease (Jack *et al.*, 2005; van der Flier *et al.*, 2005; Fig. 13. 2).

The acetylcholine-deficit hypothesis of Alzheimer's disease has been the subject of investigations with functional (f)-MRI using various activation paradigms before and after the administration of acetylcholine-esterase inhibitors; these studies supported the pharmacological hypothesis and the clinical efficacy of cholinergic intervention (Grön *et al.*, 2006).

Hypoperfusion patterns are similar in many patients with MCI and Alzheimer's disease; hippocampus, entorhinal cortex, and subiculum are affected, while only the subiculum is functionally involved in 'normal ageing'.

**Table 13. 2** Typical patterns of atrophy in neurodegenerative forms of dementia

| | Neocortex and hemispheres | Hippocampus |
|---|---|---|
| Alzheimer's dementia (AD) | Frontal + temporal | Early, initially asymmetric, severe |
| Dementia with Lewy bodies | Temporal + parieto-occipital | Less than in AD |
| Frontotemporal degeneration | Frontal + temporal | Less + later |
| Corticobasal degeneration | Frontal + temporal, Rolando's region | Less + later |
| Semantic dementia | Anterior temporal lobe + left frontal lobe | Less + later |
| Progressive non-fluent aphasia | Posterior cingulate + praecuneus + left rostral temporal lobe | Less + later |
| + Macroangiopathy | + Focal infarct-related atrophy | (Less + later) |
| + Microangiopathy | + Diffuse white matter changes + global atrophy | (Less + later) |

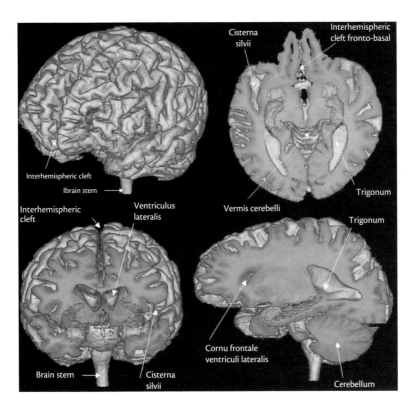

**Fig. 13.3** Three-dimensional reconstruction of the amygdala (red)–hippocampus complex (blue) (MRI, $T_1$-weighted, 3D-MPRAGE, VOXIM). See also Plate 8 for a colour version of this figure.

The prognostic value of diffusion tensor imaging (DTI; Fellgiebel *et al.*, 2005; Kantarci *et al.*, 2005; Ries *et al.*, 2006) and proton spectroscopy (H-MRS; Falini *et al.*, 2005; Modrego *et al.*, 2005) are currently under investigation. The prognostic shortcomings of morphological and functional neuroimaging are most of all a reflection of the heterogeneity of MCI.

## Structural and functional findings in neurodegenerative dementias

Clinically Alzheimer's disease (AD) is still diagnosed by excluding other causes of dementia. A combination of clinical examination with neuroimaging may improve diagnostic accuracy using neuropathology as the standard of comparison ('added value'). Some of the atrophic patterns in neurodegenerative dementias are typical, but they are in no way diagnostic (Table 13.2) (Fig. 13.3).

Temporal lobe atrophy progresses 10 times faster in AD than in 'normal ageing'. Indices of atrophy are statistically related to cognitive performance (Chetelat and Baron, 2003), and they are correlated with the severity of neuropathological change, for example the degree of cell loss in the subiculum and CA1 (Kril *et al.*, 2002).

Hippocampal imaging has proved a clinically useful and feasible method for identifying patients with early AD, and it has also gained some acceptance (Fig. 13.4). Subiculum and area CA1 are the most vulnerable structures which can be easily demonstrated with multishot, diffusion-weighted MR sequences. Atrophic changes are not only induced by Alzheimer neurodegeneration but also by ischaemic, toxicological, and traumatic lesions: therefore they are not diagnostically specific, but sensitive. Entorhinal and cingulate cortex are more difficult to visualize and their evaluation

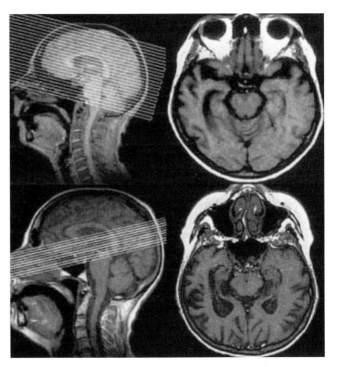

**Fig. 13.4** Alzheimer dementia. Standard slices yield inconspicuous views without obvious atrophy (scout view: above-left), while a different angulation (scout view: below-left) reveals medial temporal lobe atrophy with an enlarged hippocampal fissure (MRI, $T_1$-weighted; the studies were carried out on the same patient and on the same day).

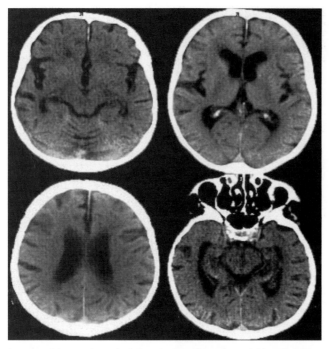

**Fig. 13.5** Alzheimer dementia. Enlarged Sylvian fissure (upper left), anterior horns (upper right), cella media (lower left), and micorangiopathic periventricular white matter changes (leuco-araiosis) (CT).

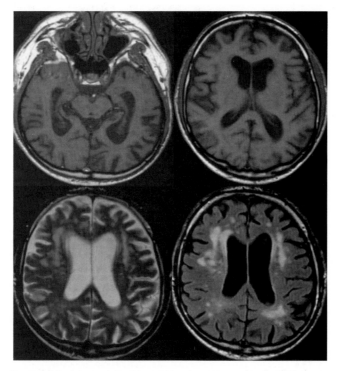

**Fig. 13.6** Mixed dementia in a 54-year-old patient with a positive family history. Hippocampal and pre-frontal atrophy with consequent enlargement of adjacent cerebrospinal fluid spaces (upper left and right). Confluent hyperintense periventricular white matter lesions (MRI, $T_2$-weighted lower left; FLAIR lower right).

has not entered diagnostic routines. The significance of corpus callosum measurements has not been reliably reproduced and cannot be considered clinically helpful.

White matter changes occur more frequently in patients with AD and their relatives. This may indicate a genetic and aetiological relationship to the neurodegeneration and not necessarily to a separate vascular pathology. Amyloid angiopathy, altered vascular permeability, autonomic dysregulation, and other mechanisms have been discussed (Gurol *et al.*, 2006; Lee and Markus, 2006; Figs. 13.5 and 13.6).

The frequent coincidence of atherosclerosis, e.g. of the circle of Willis, and increased cortical plaques and tangles underline molecular synergies between neurodegenerative and vascular pathology (Roher *et al.*, 2005). Both pathologies share several risk factors, for example age, hypertension, cardiac disease, diabetes mellitus, nicotine, and others.

Functional and quantitative neuroimaging changes in AD are summarized in Table 13.3.

## EEG in Alzheimer's disease

Conventional EEG in AD demonstrates an accentuation of age-related changes: a nearly symmetrical decrease of the occipital dominant rhythm and power, an increase of theta power and more specifically delta power in the later stages of illness. None of these findings are obligatory or diagnostic, and a normal conventional EEG recording can be considered compatible with a diagnosis of AD, whereas statistically a normal quantitative EEG has a high negative predictive power for AD. The usual findings in early AD are mild decreases of the mean EEG frequency, dominant occipital activity, decreased alpha/theta ratio, lower beta power, and increases of the relative and absolute theta power together with a disorganization of a EEG topography and impairment of the photic driving response. Significant decreases of normal alpha power (8–12 Hz) and increases of slow wave power in the delta and theta bands have been confirmed. The changes are particularly severe in early onset AD. The decreases of alpha and the increases of delta and theta power are correlated with the severity of cognitive deficits, e.g. memory, attention, and verbal tests. Both visually examined and

**Table 13.3** Miscellaneous functional and quantitative imaging changes in AD (Atiya *et al.*, 2003)

| | |
|---|---|
| fMRT, functional magnetic resonance tomography | Increased activation in order to compensate for deficits; decreased activation in later stages of illness (Rombouts *et al.*, 2005; Starr *et al.*, 2005) |
| ${}^1$H-MRS, proton magnetic resonance spectroscopy | Decreased *N*-acetylaspartate (NAA) indicating neuronal loss; increased myo-inositol indicating gliosis |
| P-MRS, phospho-MRS | Increased or decreased phospho-mono- or di-esters indicating altered membrane metabolism and phospholipid synthesis |
| MTR, magnetization transfer ratio | Different white matter texture indicating altered myelination |
| DTI, diffusion tensor imaging | Structural and functional alterations of subcortico-cortical and of cortico-cortical circuits (Rose *et al.*, 2000) |
| D-/PWI | Alterations of regional blood flow and volume |

quantitative EEG are widely underestimated in comparison to other much more expensive and fancy neuroimaging tools. A successful diagnostic discrimination between AD and normal aging can be achieved in more than 85% of cases if the synchronicity and complexity of the EEG signals are taken into consideration. Coherence or synchronicity may reflect neuronal coupling or connectivity, whereas complexity may reflect the subtlety of neuronal tuning. Relative theta power is a sensitive discriminator between ageing and dementia, whereas the occipital/frontal alpha ratio allows an efficient statistical distinction between groups of patients with AD and vascular dementia. Decreases of alpha and beta activity were found to be independent predictors of mortality.

## Frontotemporal degeneration

This is a heterogeneous group of prototypical diseases with a tendency to overlap and merge in the longer course of illness. The protean presentation facilitates a large number of misdiagnoses from schizophrenia to alcoholism, and various forms of dementia (Shi et al., 2005). One frequent morphological feature is an atrophy of the anterior temporal pole, while the mediotemporal lobe is less severely affected. A direct relationship between temporal lobe atrophy and semantic memory has been demonstrated. Posterior or progressive biparietal atrophies can be atypical early presentations of AD. Significant early hippocampal atrophy is an exclusion criterion for frontotemporal degeneration (FTD). A basic understanding of the principles of neuropsychology aids the localization of the disease process in individual patients (Table 13.4 and Fig. 13.7).

The EEG of patients with FTD often appears 'hyper-normal'.

## Dementia with Lewy bodies

Hippocampal atrophy and the enlargement of the surrounding cerebrospinal fluid spaces is less significant in patients with typical dementia with Lewy bodies (DLB) when compared with patients showing changes typical for AD. This corresponds to a lesser local neuronal loss in DLB. Parieto-occipital atrophy may represent another indicator of DLB, whereas vascular changes make this diagnosis less likely (McKeith et al., 2005). Functional neuroimaging studies demonstrate a decreased occipital perfusion with relatively well-preserved temporo-parietal perfusion in the Lewy body variant. Tracer studies reveal a more severe impairment of dopamine transport and function in the Lewy body variant compared with AD. A severe loss of choline acetyltransferase due to a double pathology from Lewy bodies combined with neurofibrillary tangles and Alzheimer plaques in the basal nucleus of Meynert may explain the greater slowing of the EEG in the Lewy body variant.

**Table 13. 4** Differential morphological brain changes in different prototypes of frontotemporal degenerations

| | Pattern of atrophy |
| --- | --- |
| Frontotemporal degeneration | Cortical pre-frontal + anterior cortical; little or no mediotemporal atrophy |
| Semantic dementia | Left temporal |
| Slowly progressive aphasia | Left frontal |
| Slowly progressive sociopathy | Right fronto-temporal |
| Corticobasal degeneration | Asymmetric Rolandic + substantia nigra atrophy + white matter changes |

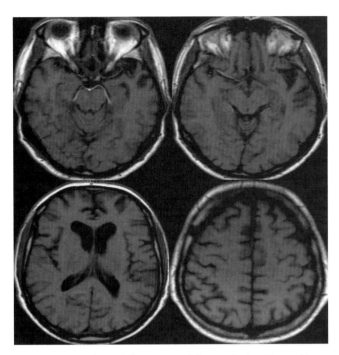

**Fig. 13.7** Semantic dementia/frontotemporal degeneration in a 73-year-old patient. Left superior temporal gyrus atrophy and mild left prefrontal atrophy with corresponding enlargement of cerebrospinal fluid spaces (MRI, $T_1$-weighted).

## Parkinson's disease dementia

Diagnostic criteria for Parkinson's disease mention a narrowing of the substantia nigra pars compacta which can be shown on heavily $T_2$-weighted ($T_2^\star$) MRI scans. Tracer studies, which show a decreased striatal uptake. Clear distinctions between pure AD on one extreme, pure Parkinson's disease at the other, and the Lewy body variant of AD in between cannot be drawn and it is better to think of these categories as part of a spectrum of neurodegenerative diseases, characterized by a mixture of plaques, neurofibrillary tangles, and Lewy bodies (and usually also superimposed vascular changes). Ten to 20% of all patients with Parkinson's disease develop severe dementia. Occasionally patients without significant Alzheimer-type changes can be observed, and in those dementia is correlated with the density of Lewy neurites in the area $CA_2$ hippocampal field. The disconnection between dentate gyrus, entorhinal cortex, septal nuclei, hypothalamus, and the $CA_1$ field may contribute to dementia in Parkinson's disease. Patients with Parkinson's disease dementia have more severe hippocampal atrophy than Parkinson's patients without dementia (Ramirez-Ruiz et al., 2005) and less severe cortical atrophy than in patients with AD (Tam et al., 2005).

Demented patients with Parkinson's disease cannot be distinguished reliably from patients with AD on the basis of functional neuroimaging studies, as both groups show changes in temporo-parietal and, occasionally frontal perfusion and metabolism. A decreased fluorodopa uptake in the caudate nucleus and frontal cortex is associated with impaired verbal fluency, working memory, and attentional functioning.

Striatal, cerebellar, and brainstem volumes are often normal in patients with pure idiopathic Parkinson's disease. Structural neuroimaging can help with the identification of patients with 'vascular parkinsonism', as patients with atypical parkinsonian syndromes demonstrate a number of morphological brain changes.

## Other dementias with motor deficits

Significant reductions in mean striatal and brainstem volumes can be seen in patients with *multiple system atrophy* and *progressive supranuclear palsy*. While patients with pure Parkinson's disease exhibit a loss of cholinergic innervation to the cerebral cortex, the PET study of acetylcholinesterase activity indicates a preferential loss of cholinergic innervation of the thalamus in progressive supranuclear palsy.

## Vascular dementias

Neuroimaging is obligatory for a diagnosis according to the NINDS-AIREN criteria and helps to distinguish between the following forms of vascular dementia:

- large-vessel infarcts localized in the anterior, medial, posterior cerebral arteries and watershed territories or association areas (so-called multi-infarct dementia, MID; Fig. 13.8);

- small-vessel disease affecting the basal ganglia and white matter with lesions that are multiple, diffuse, or extensive (extensive subcortical white matter lesions are frequently referred to as Binswanger's disease or subcortical vascular encephalopathy, SVE; Figs. 13. 9 and 13.10)

- bilateral paramedian thalamic or fornix infarcts, which lead to severe memory deficits (so-called strategic infarcts; Fig. 13.11).

There is not one form of vascular dementia, but a multitude of causes and vascular pathologies which can cause extensive cognitive impairment (Table 13.5). The identification of vascular factors in demented patients has been improved by advanced MRI techniques [e.g. fluid-attenuated inversion recovery (FLAIR) sequences].

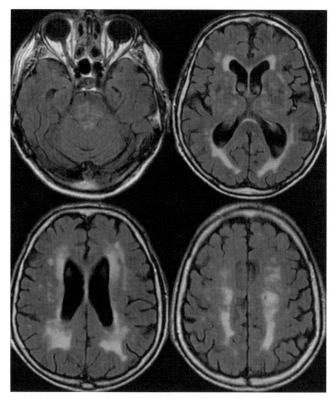

**Fig. 13.9** Moderate dementia in a 76-year-old patient with lacunar and diffuse subcortical brain changes including basal ganglia, thalamus and pons (MRI, FLAIR).

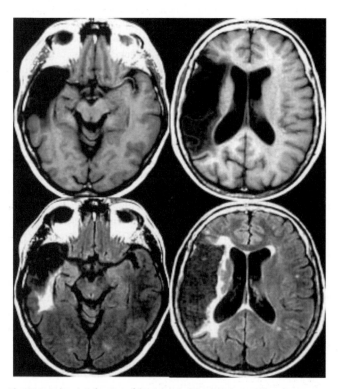

**Fig. 13.8** Ischemic infarction of the right medial cerebral artery. Sharply demarcated hypointense lesion with consequent ventricular enlargement (MRI, $T_1$-weighted; upper row). Bilateral subcortical microangiopathic white matter lesions ($T_2$-lower row).

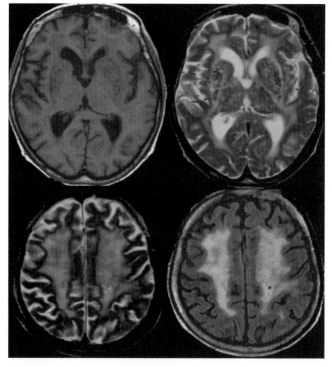

**Fig. 13.10** subcortical vascular encephalopathy (subcortical vascular encephalopathy, Binswanger's disease) in a 93-year-old patient with dementia. Enlarged Virchow–Robin spaces ('*état crible*'; MRI $T_1$- and $T_2$-weighted; upper row). Lacunes with hyperintense margins, hyperintense basal ganglia and thalamus lesions, Confluent microangiopathic white matter lesions ($T_2$-weighted; lower row).

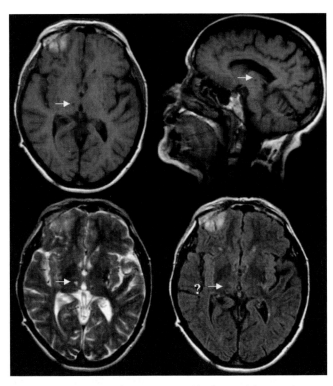

**Fig. 13.11** Right thalamic infarct in a 58-year-old patient with hypertension. Hypointensity in $T_1$-weighted images (upper row) and hyperintensity in $T_2$-weighted image (lower left). In this case $T_1$- and $T_2$-weighted appear diagnostically superior to the sensitive FLAIR sequence (lower right).

**Table 13. 5** Causes and forms of 'vascular dementia'

| Cause | Image |
|---|---|
| Macroangiopathy; thrombo-embolic infarction | Single territorial complete infarct or multiple complete infarcts ('multi-infarct dementia', MID); strategic infarcts (e.g. angular gyrus or thalamic infarcts); Waller's dying-back degeneration |
| Microangiopathy | Subacute incomplete white matter infarcts and complete lacunar infarcts ('subcortical vascular encephalopathy', SVE); the term 'Binswanger's disease' should be reserved for extensive and confluent lesions |
| Hypoxia or hypovolaemia | Hypoxic-ischaemic lesions in border zones |
| Amyloid angiopathy | Multiple or single ('atypic localized') haemorrhages and/or ischaemic infarcts |
| Intracranial bleeds; hypertonia, aneurysms | ('Typical localized') haemorrhage and tissue necrosis |
| Other causes (vasculitis, non-inflammatory angiopathies) | (Multiple) residual haemorrhagic or ischaemic lesions |
| Mixed | In elderly demented patients over the age of 50 vascular pathology is usually superimposed over neurodegenerative brain changes and mixed forms are therefore highly prevalent |

This is of great importance, as potential interventions go beyond simply symptomatic measures. Neurodegenerative changes of the Alzheimer type and also of other types can co-occur with vascular brain changes. Recent studies which document that one-sixth of the patients suffering ischaemic stroke suffered from pre-existing dementia, and that patients who show a pre-existing mediotemporally accentuated brain atrophy are preferentially liable to develop post-stroke dementia. Both the localization and the extent of brain damage determine the profile and severity of cognitive deterioration. The functional changes caused by vascular lesion are of decisive importance, and it appears that subcortical lacunar infarctions in the white matter, the basal ganglia, and the thalamus are the most critical. Diffusion-weighted MRI allows the identification of fresh infarcts and demonstrates, that vascular brain changes are on-going processes.

Cerebral autosomal dominant arteriopathy with subcortical infarcts and leucoencephalopathy (CADASIL) is a rare but important variant of vascular dementia. In this disease a significant inverse correlation between cognitive performance and lesion volume has been described.

### EEG in vascular dementias

Power spectra are linked to metabolic changes in vascular dementia and to clinical deficits. Event-related potentials (ERP) demonstrate a prolonged central processing time for novel stimuli. Focal EEG abnormalities—usually intermittent, lateralized slow waves, or spike and sharp waves—are found in 75% of patients with multi-infarct dementia. There are no significant differences between multi-infarct dementia, other forms of vascular dementia, and AD regarding the mean background parameters of qEEG, but the occipital/frontal power ratio is higher in any form of vascular dementia than in AD. Coherence is decreased between disconnected areas which are usually linked by short cortico-cortical and cortico-subcortical fibres. However, the differential diagnostic validity of EEG for vascular dementias appears clearly inferior to neuroradiological methods.

## Creutzfeldt–Jakob disease

Creutzfeldt–Jakob disease, a rapidly progressive form of dementia, is caused by proteinaceous infectious agents (prions). In the advanced stages of illness conspicuous sharp waves in the EEG which couple with myoclonic jerks can be observed.

Diffusion-weighted signal intensity can be increased early in the cortex and basal ganglia (Demaerel *et al.*, 2003; Parazzini *et al.*, 2003). Sometimes a rapidly progressive unspecific brain atrophy with occasional frontal accentuation and subcortical changes can be seen, but the absence of significant brain changes is much more characteristic in the early stage. The caudate nucleus and putamen show an increased signal in $T_2$-weighted imaging (Eschweiler *et al.*, 2003). The 'pulvinar sign', bilateral thalamic hyperintensity in $T_2$ proton-weighted images due to a thalamic gliosis is currently considered most distinctive (Fig. 13.12).

## AIDS–dementia complex

In global brain atrophy due to progressive white matter lesions the grey matter is almost unaffected. Focal perfusion changes are detected earlier than morphological changes and can be reversible.

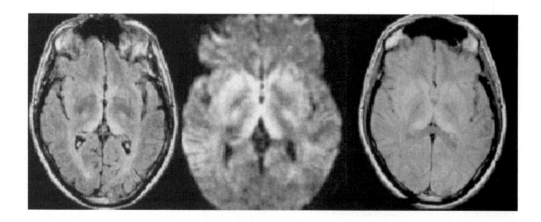

**Fig. 13.12** 'Pulvinar sign' in Creutzfeldt–Jakob-disease (MRI; left, FLAIR; middle, diffusion-weighted image, DWI; right, GE sequence).

The subacute encephalitis caused by HIV infection leads to periventricular circumscribed or confluent white matter lesions which need to be distinguished from a papova-viridae infection (progressive multifocal leucoencephalopathy, PML). Opportunistic infections of the central nervous system are frequent in patients with AIDS, and two of the most common cerebral complications—the *Toxoplasma gondii* abscess and lymphoma—are virtually indistinguishable by CT or MRI.

## Normal pressure hydrocephalus

Normal pressure hydrocephalus (NPH) is characterized clinically by a triad of fluctuating cognitive impairment, incontinence, and gait disturbance. Neuromorphologically large lateral ventricles and a small fourth ventricle, periventricular hypodensities, a small superior interhemispheric fissure, and small sulci are found. These morphological changes can be seen with cranial CT, whereas MRI

is necessary to observe the typical 'fluid void sign', a characteristic but non-specific phenomenon, which is also observed in 30% of the healthy elderly (Fig. 13.13). Hyperdynamic cerebrospinal fluid movement can cause a reversible signal extinction at the aqueduct but more often at the cerebrospinal junction. Volumetric measurements can distinguish NPH from AD in typical cases, but again the two diseases can coincide. If severe mediotemporal lobe atrophy is observed—an indication of AD—shunting will be of questionable benefit. No single morphological parameter can identify patients with NPH who will benefit from ventriculo-peritoneal shunting. Reductions of glucose metabolism and perfusion, frontally and periventricularly, are potentially reversible after an operation. A prevalent problem is not only the co-morbidity with AD, but also with other systemic and brain diseases. Tumours and inflammatory conditions have to be ruled out before the diagnosis of NPH is made.

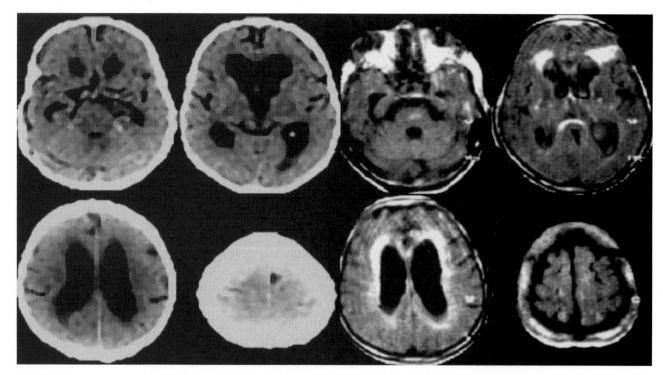

**Fig. 13.13** Normal pressure hydrocephalus (NPH). Enlarged lateral and third ventricles with leuco-araiosis (CT left) and frontal cerebrospinal fluid 'caps' and narrow subarachnoidal spaces (MRI, right; FLAIR, upper right).

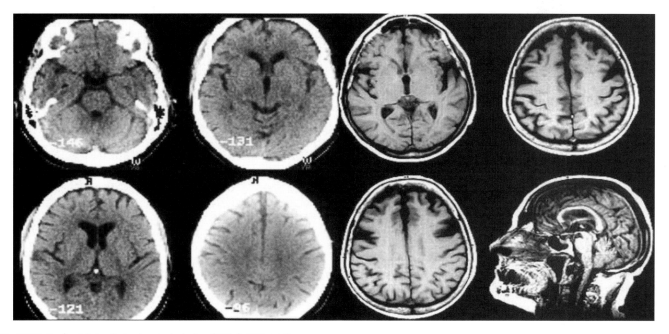

**Fig. 13.14** Pre-frontal atrophy in chronic alcoholism (CT, left; MRI, right).

## Alcohol-induced brain changes

A number of these changes can be visualized neuroradiologically, and they may occur in isolated or combined form:

♦ frontal cortical atrophy with widening of the rostral interhemispheric fissure and cerebellar atrophy, usually most pronounced around the vermis are common (Fig. 13.14);

♦ chronic subdural haematomata often after minor head injuries;

♦ Wernicke–Korsakoff encephalopathy sometimes with identifiable haemorrhagic changes in the mamillary bodies and tissue alterations in the dorso-medial thalamic nuclei;

♦ focal callosal atrophy and hemispheric white matter changes (Marchiafava–Bignami syndrome; Fig. 13.15); and

♦ central pontine or extrapontine myelinolysis, a frequent, but unspecific, outcome in chronic alcohol abuse following the

(rapid) normalization of hyponatraemia with intravenous fluids (Fig. 13.16).

MRI is clearly superior to CT in demonstrating the last three pathological changes. Other structural changes in the cortex or white matter are indicative of other pathology not directly related to alcohol (White *et al.*, 2005). Functional neuroimaging reveals a decrease of cerebral blood flow and metabolism which is most accentuated in the pre-frontal lobe and cerebellum. In alcohol-related dementia, infra- and supratentorial atrophy, enlargement of the third and lateral ventricles, an improvement in white matter volume and of hippocampal, hemispheric, and cerebellar volume were demonstrated in abstinent alcoholics.

The EEG shows increased slow-wave activity that persists during abstinence. The high prevalence of extensive cerebrovascular changes satisfying diagnostic criteria for vascular dementia in elderly male alcoholics represents an unexpected finding. Vascular changes can also play a major role in the mamillary pathology of the alcohol-related Wernicke–Korsakoff syndrome and in the white matter and corpus callosum lesions of the Marchiafava–Bignami disease

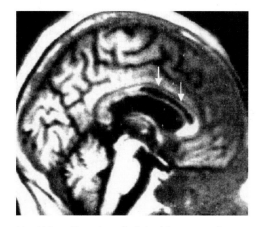

**Fig. 13.15** Marchiafava–Bignami myelinolysis of the corpus callosum (MRI, $T_1$-weighted).

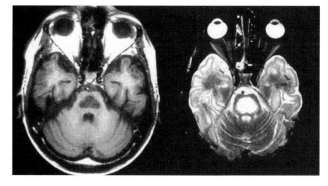

**Fig. 13.16** Pontine myelinolysis in chronic alcoholism (MRI, $T_1$-weighted left, $T_2$-weighted right).

and central pontine or extrapontine myelinolysis, demonstrated particularly well in MRI FLAIR sequences.

## Confusional states (delirium)

Little work has been done on the structural causes and functional changes in confusional states. Alcohol intoxication and alcohol withdrawal are well-known causes of confusional states. The Lewy body variant of AD is a form of dementia in which superimposed confusional states are of diagnostic significance. All forms of severe somatic or brain diseases leading to cerebral hypoperfusion, hypoxia, or a significant cholinergic/aminergic imbalance may cause confusional states. Therefore, the expected neuroimaging findings are highly variable and reflect the underlying illness.

A systematic investigation revealed that confusional states are more common in late onset (mixed) AD and in forms of vascular dementia with widespread cerebral damage, and much less frequent in the predominantly cortical forms of dementia.

Old studies, now almost forgotten, have repeatedly demonstrated the superior diagnostic validity of a simple EEG for the differential diagnosis of confusional states. Confusional states are associated with severe EEG alterations, whereas other more chronic and irreversible forms of cognitive impairment (for example AD) show much more subtle alterations which have often been detected only by quantitative EEG in the mild and moderate stages.

## Schizophrenia

Neuroimaging in elderly schizophrenic graduates confirms the importance of early brain changes for the development of illness, for example:

◆ widespread alterations of white matter integrity (decreased fractional anisotropy, FA; Hao et al., 2006);

◆ no correlation between duration of illness and hippocampal atrophy (i.e. no evidence of a 'neurotoxic' effect of psychosis; Ho et al., 2005).

The co-occurrence of late onset schizophrenia with neuroimaging evidence of organic brain changes exceeds expectation. White matter abnormalities indicating increased vascular risk, unsuspected vascular lesions, and ventricular enlargement have been described. Recent work has confirmed subcortical changes, e.g. increased periventricular and thalamic signal intensity in proton-weighted MRI sequences whereas the corpus callosum, cerebellum, and mediotemporal lobe structures appear largely intact.

## Depression

Somatic and brain diseases, often with a chronic course, and pain syndromes are frequently associated with depression in the elderly. Cerebrovascular abnormalities are often found in these conditions. A diagnosis of 'vascular depression' (Gaupp's disease) does not require a causal or temporal relationship between the development of psychopathology and a stroke. This is an important conceptual difference from post-stroke depression. An onset of depression after the age of 65 together with evidence of cerebrovascular disease or a vascular risk factor are sufficient. The diagnosis of 'vascular depression' is supported by cognitive deficits characterized by impaired planning and sequencing of 'purposeful' action;

psychomotor slowing, mildly depressive symptoms, e.g. feelings of guilt; impaired judgement; mildly impaired activities of daily living; and no family history of depression.

White matter hyperintensity is prevalent in patients with a late onset of depression and it is associated with increased plasma homocysteine levels with increased severity of depression (Cambell and MacQuenn, 2006). Vascular lesions in depressed patients generally carry an increased risk of drug-induced delirium (Firbank et al., 2005).

A mild volume reduction of grey matter of the pre-frontal, mediotemporal, caudate, hippocampal and amygdala volumes have been observed in vascular depression. The severity of the alterations may be correlated with cognitive impairment. It has been stressed in several studies that those morphological changes and the differences from elderly controls are not very large. Nevertheless, the observation of a poor treatment response in patients with subcortical and also with grey matter changes is of great clinical importance. SPECT and PET studies consistently demonstrate cerebral hypoperfusion in depressed elderly patients in the pre-frontal and paralimbic areas. The degree of hypoperfusion is correlated with age and with the severity of depression. An improvement of the affective state is accompanied by a normalization of cerebral perfusion. There is ample evidence for a relationship between vascular changes and depression in the elderly; the relationship is so comprehensive that it appears questionable to claim that vascular factors are relevant just in one subgroup of elderly depressed patients.

## Summary and recommendations

In elderly patients with psychiatric problems, morphological investigations by CT, MRI, and sometimes even functional neuroimaging with SPECT or PET, are strongly recommended if there is a suspicion of:

◆ degenerative dementia (for example AD, lobar atrophy, Huntington's disease, etc.);

◆ vascular changes (multiple cortical infarcts, subcortical vascular encephalopathy, thalamic infarction, etc.); or

◆ tumour, inflammation, post-traumatic brain lesions, hypoxia, and normal-pressure hydrocephalus as causes of secondary psychosis.

Little additional information can be gained by morphological or functional brain imaging and they should not be undertaken if:

◆ recent brain scans are available;

◆ no remarkable morphological and functional alterations can be expected (for example in long-lasting illnesses with pre-senile onset and no observable clinical change); or

◆ if the patient's condition does not allow a technically satisfactory examination.

EEG is a widely available, inexpensive, and non-invasive tool with excellent time-resolution, but limited spatial resolution. Its validity is probably underestimated in the UK and possibly overestimated elsewhere. Advanced and cheap methods of EEG analysis are widely available and their clinical importance is likely to increase in all parts of the world.

Paroxysmal discharges (spikes or sharp waves) and focal and generalized changes of the EEG background activity in organic brain disease can often be detected by the visual inspection of conventional analogue paper-and-ink recordings. New quantitative analysis of digitized EEG data (qEEG) offers an improved reliability and comparability between individuals or groups of patients and allows the investigation of subtle changes in the course of illness. A variety of statistical approaches and parameters has been employed in the investigation of elderly psychiatric patients, for example:

- spectral analysis or Fourier transformation of the EEG signal in a defined frequency band (delta, theta, alpha, beta power);

- correlations between different electrode locations yielding the coherence or synchronicity of the EEG signal;

- transformations derived from chaos theory yielding the dimensionality or complexity of the signals.

Conventional EEG will probably retain its importance for the diagnosis of acute and severe organic psychosis, even though it may be surpassed by qEEG in the early diagnosis of chronic degenerative brain disease. Our position is still critical regarding the clinical—not the scientific—importance of the impressive methodological advances in imaging that we have seen over the last 5 years.

# References

Albert, M.S. (2003). Detection of very early Alzheimer disease through neuroimaging. *Alzheimer Disease and Associated Disorders*, **17**(Suppl. 12), S63–S65.

Alemany, M., Stenborg, A., Terent, A. *et al.* (2006). Coexistence of microhemorrhages and acute spontaneous brain hemorrhage: correlation with sign of microangiopathy and clinical data. *Radiology*, **238**, 240–247.

Atiya, M., Hyman, B.T., Albert, M.S., and Killiany, R. (2003). Structural magnetic resonance imaging in established and prodromal Alzheimer disease: a review. *Alzheimer Disease and Associated Disorders*, **17**, 177–195.

Cambell, S. and MacQueen, G. (2006). An update on regional brain volume differences associated with mood disorder. *Current Opinion in Psychiatry*, **19**, 25–33.

Chetelat, G. and Baron, J.C. (2003). Early diagnosis of Alzheimer's disease: contribution of structural neuroimaging. *Neuroimage*, **18**, 525–541.

Convit, A., deLeon, M.J., Hoptman, M.J. *et al.* (1995). Age-related changes in the brain: I. Magnetic resonance imaging measures of temporal lobe volumes in normal subjects. *The Psychiatric Quarterly*, **66**, 343–355.

Demaerel, P., Sciot, R., Robbrecht, W. *et al.* (2003). Accuracy of diffusion-weighted MR imaging in the diagnosis of sporadic Creutzfeldt–Jakob disease. *Journal of Neurology*, **250**, 222–225.

Eschweiler, G.W., Wormstall, H., and Bartels, M. (2003). Was unterscheidet die Subtypen der Creutzfeldt- Jakob- Krankheit von anderen Demenzen mit initialen psychiatrischen Auffälligkeiten? *Nervenheilkunde*, **22**, 24–29.

Falini, A., Bozzali, M., Magnani, G. *et al.* (2005). A whole brain spectroscopy study from patients with Alzheimer's disease and mild cognitive impairment. *Neuroimage*, **26**, 1159–1163.

Fellgiebel, A., Müller, M.J., Wille, P. *et al.* (2005). Color-coded diffusion-tensor-imaging of posterior cingulate fiber tracts in mild cognitive impairment. *Neurobiology of Aging*, **26**, 1193–1198.

Firbank, M.J., O'Brien, J.T., Pakrasi, S. *et al.* (2005). White matter hyperintensities and depression – preliminary results from the LADIS study. *International Journal of Geriatric Psychiatry*, **20**, 674–679.

van der Flier, Wm., van der Vlies, A.E., Weverling-Rijnsburger, A.W.E. *et al.* (2005). MRI measures and progression of cognitive decline in nondemented elderly attending a memory clinic. *International Journal of Geriatric Psychiatry*, **20**, 1060–1066.

Grön, G., Brandenburg, I., Wunderlich, A.P., and Riepe, M.W. (2006). Inhibition of hippocampal function in mild cognitive impairment: targeting the cholinergic hypothesis. *Neurobiology of Aging*, **27**, 78–87.

Gurol, M.E., Irizarry, M.C., Smith, E.E. *et al.* (2006). Plasma beta-amyloid and white matter lesions in AD, MCI, and cerebral amyloid angiopathy. *Journal of Neurology*, **66**, 23–29.

Hao, Y., Liu, Z., Jiang, T. *et al.* (2006). White matter integrity of the whole brain is disrupted in first-episode schizophrenia. *NeuroReport*, **17**, 23–26.

Hentschel, F., Kreis, M., Damian, M. *et al.* (2003a). Evaluation of the contribution of the importance of neuroimaging for the diagnostics of dementias – comparison to the psychological diagnostics. *RöFo: Fortschritte auf dem Gebiete der Röntgenstrahlen und der Nuklearmedizin*, **175**, 1335–1343.

Hentschel, F., Kreis, M., Damian, M. *et al.* (2005a). The added clinical value of structural neuroimaging for the diagnosis and differential diagnosis of dementias: a memory clinic study. *International Journal of Geriatric Psychiatry*, **20**, 645–650.

Hentschel, F., Kreis, M., Damian, M. *et al.* (2005b). Quantification of microangiopathic lesions in brain parenchyma and age-adjusted mean scores for the diagnostic separation of normal from pathological values in senile dementia. *RöFo: Fortschritte auf dem Gebiete der Röntgenstrahlen und der Nuklearmedizin*, **177**, 864–871.

Hentschel,.F, Damian, M., Krumm, B., and Frölich, L. (2007). Age-correlated scores of microangiopathic brain lesions to differentiate cognitive normal subjects and patients with vascular dementia. *Acta Neurologica Scandinavica*, **115**, 174–180.

Ho, B.C., Alicata, D., Mola, C., and Andreasen, N.C. (2005). Hippocampus volume and treatment delays in first-episode schizophrenia. *American Journal of Psychiatry*, **162**, 1527–1529.

Jack, C.R., Shiung, M.M., Weigand, S.D. *et al.* (2005). Brain atrophy rates predict subsequent clinical conversion in normal elderly and amnestic MCI. *Journal of Neurology*, **65**, 1227–1231.

Kantarci, K., Petersen, R.C., Boeve, B.F. *et al.* (2005). DWI predicts future progression to Alzheimer disease in mild cognitive impairment. *Journal of Neurology*, **64**, 902–904.

Kril, J.J., Patel, S., Harding, A.J., and Halliday, G.M. (2002). Patients with vascular dementia due to microvascular pathology have significant hippocampal neuronal loss. *Journal of Neurology, Neurosurgery and Psychiatry*, **72**, 747–751.

Lee, J.M. and Markus, H.S. (2006). Does the white matter matter in Alzheimer disease and cerebral amyloid angiopathy? *Journal of Neurology*, **66**, 6–7.

McKeith, I.G., Dickson, D.W., Lowe, J. *et al.* (2005). Diagnosis and management of dementia with Lewy bodies. Third report of the LBD consortium. *Journal of Neurology*, **65**, 1863–1872.

Modrego, P.J., Fayed, N., and Pina, M.A. (2005). Conversion from mild cognitive impairment to probable Alzheimer´s disease predict by brain magnetic resonance spectroscopy. *American Journal of Psychiatry*, **162**, 667–675.

Mueller, E.A., Moore, M.M., Kerr, D.C.R. *et al.* (1998). Brain volume preserved in healthy elderly through the eleventh decade. *Journal of Neurology*, **51**, 1555–1562.

Parazzini, C., Mammi, S., Comola, M., and Scotti, G. (2003). Magnetic resonance diffusion- weighted images in Creutzfeldt–Jakob disease: a case report. *Neuroradiology*, **45**, 50–52.

Ramirez-Ruiz, B., Marti, M.J., Tolosa, E. *et al.* (2005). Longitudinal evaluation of cerebral morphological changes in Parkinson's disease with and without dementia. *Journal of Neurology*, **252**, 1345–1352.

Ridha, B. and Josephs, K.A. (2006). Young-onset dementia. a practical approach to diagnosis. *The Neurologist*, **12**, 2–13.

Ries, M.L., Schmitz, T.W., Kawahara, T.N. *et al.* (2006). Task-dependent posterior cingulate activation in mild cognitive impairment. *Neuroimage*, **29**, 485–492.

Roher, A.E., Esh, C., Kokjohn, T. *et al.* (2005). Atherosclerosis and AD: analysis of data from the US National Alzheimer's Coordinating Center. *Journal of Neurology*, **65**, 974.

Rombouts, S.A.R.B., Goekoop, R., Stam, C.J. *et al.* (2005). Delayed rather than decreased BOLD response as a marker for early Alzheimer's disease. *Neuroimage*, **26**, 1078–1085.

Rose, S., Chen, F., Chalk, J.B. *et al.* (2000). Loss of connectivity in Alzheimer's disease: an evaluation of white matter tract integrity with color coded MR diffusion tensor imaging. *Journal of Neurology, Neurosurgery and Psychiatry*, **69**, 528–530.

Roob, G., Schmidt, R., Kapeller, P. *et al.* (1999). MRI evidence of past cerebral microbleeds in a healthy elderly population. *Neurology*, **52**, 991–994.

Shi, J., Shaw, C.L., DuPlessis, D. *et al.* (2005). Histopathological changes underlying frontotemporal lobe degeneration with clinicopathological correlation. *Acta Neuropathologica*, **110**, 501–512.

Starr, J.M., Loeffler, B., Abousleiman, Y. *et al.* (2005). Episodic and semantic memory tasks activate different brain regions in Alzheimer disease. *Journal of Neurology*, **65**, 266–269.

Tam, C.W.C., Burton, E.J., McKeith, I.G. *et al.* (2005). Temporal lobe atrophy on MRI in Parkinson disease with dementia. A comparison with Alzheimer disease and dementia with Lewy bodies. *Journal of Neurology*, **64**, 861–865.

de Toledo-Morrell, L., Stoub, T.R., Bulgakova, M. *et al.* (2004). MRI-derived entorhinal volume is a good predictor of conversion from MCI to AD. *Neurobiology of Aging*, **25**, 1197–1203.

White, M.L., Zhang, Y., Andrew, L.G., and Hadley, W.L. (2005). MR imaging with diffusion-weighted imaging in acute and chronic Wernicke encephalopathy. *American Journal of Neuroradiology*, **26**, 2306–2310.

Xu, Y., Jack, C.R., O'Brien, P.C. *et al.* (2000). Usefulness of MRI measure of entorhinal cortex versus hippocampus in AD. *Neurology*, **54**, 1760–1767.

# 14

# Psychopharmacology in the elderly

Craig Ritchie

The use of drugs in older people presents the clinician with some unique challenges. The elderly are a distinct but heterogeneous population when considering the use of psychotropic medication. Gerontological factors such as altering pharmacokinetics and pharmacodynamics interact with clinical or geriatric factors such as concurrent medical illness, compliance, and polypharmacy to a greater or lesser degree to generate a different (and at times unpredictable) reaction to a drug in an older person compared with a younger person. This chapter will discuss psychopharmacology which is relevant specifically to older people; the pharmacodynamic effect of drugs (i.e. their mode of action) is the same as in younger populations and will not be dealt with here, an excellent review of this area being found elsewhere (Shiloh et al., 2002). Moreover, other chapters in this book discuss the treatments of specific mental illnesses and will discuss pharmacological interventions from a perspective of efficacy, effectiveness, and tolerability. Instead this chapter will focus on issues pertinent to prescribing psychotropics in older people and how age-related (gerontological) and geriatric issues affect this.

Despite the particular issues in prescribing psychotropics in older people (excepting dementia drugs), there are very few well-designed clinical trials of drugs commonly used in older people to educate clinicians with regard to their pharmacokinetics, efficacy, optimal dosing regimes, safety, and interactions (Ritchie, 2005; Marriot et al., 2006; Mottram et al., 2006; Rapoport et al., 2007). Instead, psychogeriatricians and other clinicians have to extrapolate findings from younger populations who have been subject to higher-quality research or prescribe from 'first principles' of physiology and pharmacology, supporting this with clinical experience.

## Clinical geriatrics and psychopharmacology

Clinical geriatrics (and psychogeriatrics) is concerned with the management of diseases or illness states in older people. The use of drugs in this context is informed by several relevant factors associated not with aging itself but with the presence of illness in older people.

### Polypharmacy

It is clear that older patients with increasingly greater physical co-morbidity are likely to be on a high number of concomitant medications, sometimes inappropriately. Highlighting this, a recent US study of 786 people over the age of 65 receiving home care showed that the average number of medications received was 8.0 (SD = 3.7), and the review noted that in almost one-third there was possible inappropriate use of at least one drug and in 10% there would have been dangerous drug interactions (Cannon et al., 2006). These data were entirely consistent with a pan-European study of 2707 people (again living at home) which showed that 20% of patients were being prescribed at least one drug inappropriately and this was more likely to occur in people receiving more drugs, those living in poorer socio-economic conditions, and those suffering from depression or being prescribed anxiolytics (Fialova et al., 2005). Polypharmacy increases the likelihood of drug–drug interactions, which will be discussed in more detail later.

### Compliance

Several terms are often now used to describe a patient's taking of medication: adherence, concordance, and compliance. Each has a slightly different meaning which articulates the relationship between prescriber and patient, though all are reasonably synonymous as a description of how much of a prescribed medication is taken. In the following, terms are used as they were by the authors cited. As well as the risks involved in polypharmacy, poor prescribing practice may also lead to uncertainty with regard to compliance or concordance between patient and the prescribing clinician (Bergman-Evans, 2006). From a large study in 11 European countries, Cooper et al. (2005) noted that 12.5% of 3881 older adults were not fully 'adherent' to their prescribed medication. Factors that raised the risk of non-adherence included problem drinking, cognitive impairment, and an absence of regular clinical review. However, interventions to improve compliance in older patients have been reported, with the most 'striking' improvement being noted with strategies incorporating telephone reminders to patients (van Eijken et al., 2003). Poor concordance or compliance is highly relevant clinically as makes it hard for a clinician to discern the tolerability or efficacy of a drug on the background of uncertainty regarding compliance.

### Patient co-morbidities

The compliance and polypharmacy issues discussed already could be considered non-biological or external factors which create challenges in using drugs in older patients. There are, however, very important biological or internal factors as well which are worth considering when using psychotropic medications in this population. Drug–patient interactions are relevant when the patient in question exhibits co-morbidities.

As a consequence of physical illness, older patients may be particularly vulnerable to the unwanted but well-recognized adverse effects of psychotropic medications. Examples of this include the increased risk of tardive dyskinesia with increasing age associated with conventional neuroleptics (Jeste, 2000), increased risk of delirium with drugs that have anticholinergic effects (Tune, 2001), or postural hypotension (Mukai and Lipsitz, 2002) with psychotropic drugs that inhibit α1-adrenergic and H1 histamine receptors. The elderly are more vulnerable to these effects because of, for example, an increased likelihood of substantia nigra or cholinergic pathway degeneration or autonomic instability, respectively. They are also less able to tolerate the consequences of such interactions. For example, an older person who suffers orthostatic hypotension may well fall and fracture a hip, whereas a younger person with a similar drop in blood pressure would simply feel a little light-headed.

There may be other characteristics of the individual who is receiving the drug that make them even more vulnerable to side-effects. By way of example there have been concerns raised regarding an increased risk of stroke with the use of atypical antipsychotics in the management of behavioural problems in dementia (Smith and Beier, 2004). If this risk is genuine, and this has recently been challenged (Schneider *et al.*, 2006), then it would appear to be restricted to only those with pre-existing cerebrovascular damage (Shah and Suh, 2005). This latter observation would explain why this putative safety concern has not been demonstrated in patients with schizophrenia (Ritchie, 2005). This example illustrates the point that medical morbidity can render the patient more vulnerable to side-effects which would not be observed in younger patients and in healthy older people.

In conclusion, because of the clinical or geriatric effects listed, i.e. polypharmacy, uncertainty about compliance, co-morbid physical illness, and an increased likelihood of developing symptomatic side-effects, much initial thought and ongoing vigilance needs to be exercised in prescribing psychotropics in older people.

# Gerontological changes and psychopharmacology

Gerontological changes are those, which are inherent to normal ageing (i.e. in the absence of any definable disease pathology) that may affect the use of psychotropic medication.

Ageing is associated with varying degrees of neuronal loss even without the development of a neurodegenerative disorder (Thal *et al.*, 2004) with some neurons, in particular cholinergic neurons, being more susceptible than others (McKinney and Jacksonville, 2005). In this context, a dose of drug given to an elderly person will lead to a greater proportion of receptors being occupied than would be observed if the same dose were given to a younger person. The effect of this would be to create both a greater efficacy of the drug as well as an increased likelihood of predictable side-effects, e.g. tardive dyskinesia (Jeste, 2000).

Even taken without the pharmacokinetic effects of ageing to be articulated below, these pharmacodynamic effects would argue for lower doses being required in older patients for similar efficacy and tolerability as is seen in younger populations.

## Unpredictable pharmacokinetics

This section will articulate gerontological changes that may take place which affect the pharmacokinetics of drugs in older people, i.e. what the body does to the drug. The manner in which the body interacts with drug can be summarized by the familiar acronym ADME [Absorption (of drug), Distribution (of drug), Metabolism (of drug), and Elimination (of drug)]. Polypharmacy, more prevalent in older people, may cause drug–drug interactions which take place usually through either effects on metabolism (e.g. cytochrome P-450 system) or the distribution of the drug (e.g. competition for plasma protein binding). This problem is particularly relevant in older people and it will be considered here in some detail.

### Absorption

Absorption of a drug is defined as the process by which the drug is moved from the site of administration into the plasma of the systemic circulation. By definition, then, drugs given intravenously are not absorbed.

The vast majority of psychotropic drugs are given orally with the exception of intramuscular long-acting depots of either traditional or atypical antipsychotics. Intramuscular injections of acute-acting psychotropics are also available for rapid tranquilization. There is little evidence to suggest that absorption of drugs following intramuscular injections is any different in older people than it is in younger people.

The only other means of administration used for psychotropic drugs are sublingual, and this applies to preparations of olanzapine (Zyprexa Velotabs) and risperidone (Quicklets), and intravenous (IV). Sublingual administration of drug is used to try and achieve more rapid absorption (Markowitz *et al.*, 2006) and decreased first-pass metabolism by the liver. There is little evidence to suggest that sublingual absorption of drugs is affected by ageing (Kharasch *et al.*, 2004). The IV preparations that are conceivably used in the elderly are of benzodiazepines, but as IV administration by definition avoids absorption, any age related differences with IV drugs are only related to distribution, metabolism, elimination, and pharmacodynamic changes.

Absorption of drugs given orally is through the gut wall, predominantly in the stomach or the small intestine. A drug's absorption is affected by its state of ionization and this is dependent upon pH. Psychotropic drugs are almost exclusively absorbed in the small intestine as at low gastric pH these drugs are highly ionized, which has the effect of inhibiting drug movement across lipid cell membranes. Occasionally drugs excreted in the bile are reabsorbed in the distal small bowel—so-called entero-hepatic circulation.

Therefore, there are three main factors that could influence the absorption of orally administered, psychotropic drugs into the systemic circulation and these are: bowel transit time, hepatic extraction from the portal circulation, and intraluminal gastrointestinal pH. Gastric emptying (Gainsborough *et al.*, 1993) and small bowel motility are not affected by normal ageing (Madsen and Graff, 2004); however, some drugs given in older people will affect gastric motility. Drugs with significant anticholinergic effects are commonly prescribed in older people and will tend to cause constipation or reduced gut motility through inhibition of the bowel's stimulation by the vagal nerve (Ness *et al.*, 2006); accordingly co-administered drugs will remain available for absorption for longer and hence may achieve higher plasma concentrations. However, as the steady state of a drug is determined predominantly by metabolism rather than absorption, delayed bowel transit time, in practice, has little effect on the steady state of drugs given chronically. More importantly, drugs which increase gastrointestinal motility may decrease the amount of drug absorbed leading to subtherapeutic levels of psychotropics; cholinergic, adrenergic, and serotonergic drugs may all lead to increased gastric motility and this should be borne in mind when prescribing drugs with these properties or, for similar reasons, in patients with diarrhoea with any other aetiology.

The other main factor which affects absorption of drug going into the systemic circulation is how much drug is extracted by the liver, also known as first-pass metabolism. There is ongoing debate about hepatic changes with ageing and their effect on drug absorption (Cusack, 2004). In normal ageing, liver weight decreases (Schmucker, 1998) and hepatocytes both decrease in number and metabolic function, not through a reduction in enzymic activity (Schmucker *et al*, 1990; Shimada *et al*, 1994) but possibly through a reduction in oxygen diffusion to hepatocytes following defenestration, thickening of the hepatic sinusoid endothelium, and infrequent development of the basal lamina (Le Couteur *et al*., 2001). This effect, known as pseudocapillarization, reduces the oxygen supply to hepatocytes which is necessary for energy-dependent phase 1 enzymic metabolism (Le Couteur *et al*.,1998, 1999, 2001; Cogger *et al*., 2003; McLean *et al*., 2003). Therefore decreased hepatic extraction (by reduced liver mass) is augmented by a reduction in metabolic enzyme function (by reduced hepatocyte oxygenation). Accordingly, more active drug is passed into the systemic circulation. The net effect of decreased liver mass and function with ageing is probably only relevant for drugs with a high extraction ratio, like clomethiazole, where there would be a reduction in the amount of drug removed from the portal circulation for metabolism—hence more parent drug passes into the systemic circulation. Beyond normal ageing in patients with impaired hepatic function through disease the use of most psychotropics is affected as first-pass metabolism decreases notably. In patients with hepatic disease a great deal of caution must be used in prescribing psychotropics (British National Formulary, 2006). However, for drugs (like diazepam) with a lower extraction ratio, the age-related reduction in liver size does not affect the drug's pharmacokinetics, though a reduction in enzymic metabolic degradation associated with ageing (Herrlinger and Klotz, 2001; Kinirons and O'Mahony, 2004) will reduce the amount of drug metabolized in the liver and hence increase the drug's bioavailability. The effects of ageing on hepatic drug metabolism will be revisited later in this chapter.

## Distribution

To achieve their effect, all psychotropic drugs must cross the blood–brain barrier; to do this these drugs must be highly lipophilic. This means that they will then be able to accumulate in body fat and have what is termed a high volume of distribution. The distribution of drugs is also affected by the amount of binding to plasma proteins that a drug exhibits.

Volume of distribution is the extent of distribution relative to the amount of drug in the plasma. It does not refer to any actual volume but rather defines the relationship between plasma drug concentrations and the amount of drug in the body. Accordingly, the volume of distribution (for drugs with very low plasma concentrations and high distribution to fat, for example), rather confusingly, can be greater than the 'total volume' of the body.

The formula below helps explain this:

volume of distribution (VD)
= amount of drug in body (mass)/plasma drug concentration.

A proportional increase in fat mass as people age (Kyle *et al*, 2001), due mainly to a reduction in muscle mass (Ruiz-Torres *et al*. 1995), may thus create a larger bioavailable store of parent drug in lipid than in younger, leaner patients. This may increase the drug's half-life, as has been observed with diazepam. The effect of this is to increase the length of time to reach steady state (if dosing intervals are reduced) but with little effect on its eventual steady-state plasma concentration, providing metabolic pathways are not compromised. If single doses are given, for example for tranquilization, then the higher volume of distribution in older people will prolong the duration of action of the drug. If dosing intervals are not adjusted, because most psychotropic drugs use metabolic pathways that (at therapeutic doses) are not saturated, there is unlikely to be accumulation of drug beyond the normally expected steady state. This is because the main influence on steady state is neither absorption nor distribution but metabolism. In conclusion, alterations to the volumes of distribution of drugs given chronically in older people will have little effect on steady state.

Distribution of a drug is also affected by binding to plasma proteins. Basic drugs bind mainly to albumin and acidic ones to $\alpha$1-glycoprotein. Most psychotropic drugs are basic. An alteration of plasma protein binding in drugs that are normally extensively protein bound (for example fluoxetine), may alter the free drug concentration. Protein binding can therefore be affected by a reduction in plasma albumin or competition between drugs for protein binding, as is the case with the co-administration of fluoxetine and warfarin. From this latter example, when prescribing SSRIs in patients on warfarin, the INR must be checked and adjustments of the dose of warfarin made accordingly.

Plasma albumin levels decrease slightly in normal ageing (Wallace and Verbeek, 1987) but more dramatically during acute illness, liver disease, post-operatively, and where malnutrition is present. In these circumstances to a greater or lesser degree, while total drug levels may remain constant the amount of free drug could increase.

## Metabolism

The metabolism of psychotropic drugs involves two types of process referred to as phase 1 and phase 2 metabolism. The aim of metabolism (or biotransformation) of drugs is to create molecules that are less lipid soluble (or more lipophobic). When in this state they do not easily diffuse from the distal tubule in the kidney back to the peritubular capillaries, after having passed there in the glomerular filtrate from plasma through Bowman's capsule into the renal tubule. The metabolism of drugs uses enzymes located on the endoplasmic reticulum of hepatic cells, though some metabolic enzymes are also located in luminal cells of the small intestine. Phase 1 metabolism involves oxidation, reduction, or hydrolysis and may result in molecules that retain some pharmacological activity, e.g. fluoxetine and its metabolite nor-fluoxetine. Sometimes products of phase 1 metabolism are sufficiently hydrophilic (or lipophobic) to be excreted in urine but often they require a further metabolic step to ensure excretion.

Phase 2 metabolism almost invariably leads to the creation of pharmacologically inactive compounds that are highly lipophobic. Phase 2 reactions involve the addition of a small, highly polar molecule to the parent compound or drug in a process known as conjugation. Conjugation may involve the addition of glucuronic acid, acetic acid, sulphuric acid, or an amino acid. These processes, like phase 1 reactions, take place predominantly in the liver's hepatocytes on smooth endoplasmic reticulum but other tissues may also be involved in phase 2 reactions, e.g. lung and kidney.

Phase 1 processes are energy dependent, requiring the presence of both nicotinamide adenine dinucleotide phosphate (NADPH) and the haem-containing protein cytochrome P-450. Various different types of cytochrome P-450 exist, known as isoenzymes, some of which are listed in Table 14.1. These enzymes are also sometimes referred to as microsomal enzymes, a microsome being a small vesicle that is derived from the endoplasmic reticulum; it is

these microsomes that actually contain the cell's cytochrome P-450 enzymes.

As noted previously, energy deficiency in ageing hepatocytes following pseudocapillarization and subsequent impairment in oxygen diffusion to the cell can lead to a reduction in the activity of microsomal enzymes. Reduced hepatic blood flow and reduced microsomal function could lead to a reduction in the metabolism of active drugs in older people. This, in theory, could lead to increases in steady-state concentrations of drugs in healthy elderly people. However, as stated previously this situation is much more likely to occur in the presence of hepatic failure or when drugs are competing for microsomal enzyme activity as described below.

**Table 14.1** Commonly used drugs in psychogeriatrics and their Cytochrome impact on the P450 system

| Drug | Is a substrate of... | Inhibitor of... | Stimulator of... |
|---|---|---|---|
| Venlafaxine | CYP2C; CYP2D6; CYP3A4 | CYP2C; CYP2D6; CYP3A4 | |
| Mirtazapine | CYP2D6; CYP1A2; CYP3A4 | None | |
| Duloxetine | CYP2D6, CYP1A2 | | |
| Fluoxetine | CYP1A2; CYP2C; CYP2D6; CYP3A4 | CYP2C; CYP2D6; CYP3A4 | |
| Paroxetine | CYP1A2; CYP2D6; CYP3A4 | CYP2D6 | |
| Citalopram | CYP2C; CYP3A4 | None | |
| Fluvoxamine | CYP1A2; CYP2C; CYP3A4 | CYP1A2; CYP2C; CYP3A4 | |
| St John's Wort | | CYP2D6, CYP3A4 | 'CYP450[a] |
| Nefazodone | CYP1A2; CYP2D6; CYP3A4 | CYP3A4 | |
| Haloperidol | CYP1A2; CYP2D6 | CYP2D6 | |
| Clozapine | CYP1A2; CYP2D6 | None | |
| Olanzapine | CYP1A2; CYP2D6 | None | |
| Risperidone | CYP2D6 | None | |
| Sulpiride | None | None | |
| Quetiapine | CYP3A4 | None | |
| Sertindole | CYP2D6; CYP3A4 | None | |
| Aripiprazole | CYP3A4; CYP2D6 | None | |
| Diazepam | CYP2C; CYP3A4 | None | |
| Clomethiazole | | CYP2E1 | |
| Temazepam | CYP2C19 | | |
| Lorazepam | Metabolized by glucuronation | | |
| Zopiclone | CYP2C8 | | |
| Zolpidem | CYP3A4 | | |
| Carbamazepine | CYP2D6; CYP3A4 | | CYP2D6 |
| Sodium valproate | CYP2D6 | | |
| Donepezil | CYP2D6; CYP3A4 | Not reported | Not known |
| Galantamine | CYP2D6; CYP3A4 | Not reported | Not reported |
| Rivastigmine | Very little CytoP450 metabolism | None | None |
| Memantine | Very little CytoP450 metabolism | None | None |
| Ginkgo biloba | Not reported | CYP3A4[b] | |

[a] Obach (2000).

[b] Yale and Glurich (2005).

This table can be supplemented with an excellent US website that details the pharmacokinetics and pharmacodynamics of most psychotropics (http://www.rxlist.com/drugs/alpha_a.htm) or, from Canada, http://redpoll.pharmacy.ualberta.ca/drugbank/index.html.

Drug–drug interactions often take place as a result of the drugs' impact on phase 1 reactions (Table 14.1).

Three scenarios can occur. Firstly, two (or more) drugs can compete to be a substrate for phase 1 enzymes. Secondly one (at least) drug may inhibit a specific or group of cytochrome P-450 isoenzymes. Thirdly, drugs may induce the activity and/or production of cytochrome P-450 isoenzymes. As the last process is an adaptive or physiological response, it has been questioned whether older people are able to induce cytochrome P-450 isoenzymes, though recent research has demonstrated that the ability of drugs to induce the activity of cytochrome P-450 isoenzymes does not diminish with healthy ageing (Cusack, 2004). Hence enzyme induction described in younger populations remains relevant in the elderly. Moreover, phase 2 conjugation reactions are little affected by age (Durnas et al., 1990).

It is also recognized that the activity of certain metabolic pathways can show variation at a population level, i.e. people can be grouped into effective (or fast) acetylators and ineffective (or slow) acetylators. Genetic polymorphisms that predict this grouping can be discerned through reasonably straightforward genomic analysis. This technology, if applied judiciously, may help clinicians predict who is more or less likely to have low (or higher) plasma levels of drug following the same dose based on their genotype. This observation comes within the broader and emerging field of pharmacogenetics.

Prediction through genetic analysis of a patient's ability to metabolize drug, prior to commencing treatment would help avoid tolerability issues that may aid compliance. This technology in theory offers a great deal (particularly in managing depression; Steimer et al., 2001) but its use has been very limited in practice (Nebert et al., 2003). However, the use of this technology in older people may be of particular benefit given the high levels of polypharmacy and greater susceptibility to the toxic effect of drugs.

Table 14.1 lists commonly used psychotropic medication and which isoenzyme is involved in its metabolic biotransformation. A drug's effect to either inhibit or induce the isoenzyme's activity is also presented.

### Excretion

Drugs are excreted either in faeces or in urine. Psychotropic drugs are mainly excreted (eliminated) through the kidneys. As all psychotropic drugs are lipid soluble (lipophilic), they need to be metabolized through phase 1 and phase 2 reactions (as above) to make them more water soluble, as it in this state that they less able to move passively across lipid cell membranes. Free drug (whether lipophilic or hydrophilic) in plasma is able to pass from the plasma into the renal tubules from Bowman's capsule in the glomerular filtrate. Large plasma proteins do not pass into the glomerular filtrate under physiological conditions, so protein-bound drug cannot pass into the renal tubule. As well as passive movement through glomerular filtration into the renal tubule (which usually accounts for about 20% of free drug), the remaining 80% of drug retained in the peritubular capillaries may be subject to active secretion into the renal tubule, though this does not happen to an appreciable extent with psychotropic drugs. Once in the renal tubule, lipid-soluble drugs will diffuse passively back into the peritubular capillaries and hence back into the systemic circulation. Through metabolic processes described above, lipid-soluble drugs are made more water soluble or hydrophilic and hence do not leave the renal tubule and are eliminated in the urine.

Gerontological effects on renal clearance of drugs have an important effect on prescribing in the elderly. Kidneys change with normal ageing; they shrink, the intra-renal vascular intima thickens, and glomeruli become sclerotic with both processes impairing diffusion. There is also infiltration of chronic inflammatory cells and fibrosis in the renal stroma (Muhlberg and Platt, 1999; Cusack, 2004). A reduction in the number of glomeruli is observed as well as an impairment in function of those surviving (Hoang et al., 2003). Some drugs which are hydrophilic (e.g. antibiotics) will be more affected by renal impairment than those that are hydrophobic (e.g. psychotropics) (Meyers and Wilkinson, 1989). The latter group are rendered inactive by biotransformation to their hydrophilic product that remains in the systemic circulation. Hence dose reduction of psychotropic medication in the context of normal ageing is not usually necessary for renal reasons, and even in mild renal failure little adjustment of these drugs are necessary (Table 14.2) (British National Formulary, 2006). This is not the case with more severe renal impairment.

In order to decide whether there is a need to adjust psychotropic drug dosage on the basis of renal impairment one requires a measure of the patient's renal function. This is usually described by the creatinine clearance which is a surrogate of the glomerular filtration rate (GFR). To measure this from serum creatinine levels the Cockcroft–Gault formulae is used:

$$\text{creatinine clearance (ml/min)} = \frac{(140 - \text{age}) \times \text{weight(kg)} \times 1.23}{\text{creatinine (μmol/l)}}$$

In women multiply this result by 0.85 instead of 1.23 (Cockcroft and Gault, 1976). A web-based calculator can be used to help with this calculation (see http://nephron.com/cgi-bin/CGSI.cgi).

However, this method to ascertain renal function has been criticized as underestimating renal function in healthy, elderly patients (Fliser et al., 1999). Despite these caveats, thresholds do exist which are used to quantify renal failure into mild (20–50 ml/min), moderate (10–20 ml/min), and severe (< 10 ml/min). These may be helpful in assisting with dose selection in older patients and should therefore be used routinely.

## Conclusions

Pharmacodynamics have not been discussed in detail in this chapter as the mode of action of each psychotropic drug is similar between young and old. Alterations to dosing and administration of drugs in older people is driven by pharmacokinetic differences and the increased frailty of older people. This frailty will lead to side-effects of drugs having a greater effect on the patient's well-being. Polypharmacy, mediated by multiple medical problems, is also a problem, and though not unique to the elderly is certainly more commonly observed in older people. Ironically this group is less likely to tolerate the polypharmacy that they are exposed to.

As a result of both the geriatric and gerontological changes articulated above, clinicians should obviously exercise caution in prescribing psychotropics in the elderly. On balance (Fig. 14.1) gerontological factors tend to increase the bioavailability of drugs in older people so we won't go far wrong if we simply adhere to the familiar adage 'start low and go slow'.

Finally, as can be seen from the review of this area, much work needs to be done to test whether what is considered from first principles actually translates into being clinically relevant. The only way

**Table 14.2** Commonly prescribed psychotropic drugs in older people and modification necessary in presence of renal impairment. Advice from British National Formulary, March 2006. Absence of advice does not necessarily equate to an absence of concern but rather indicates that no information is available. Also, adjustments listed are for adults and further adjustments may be necessary or advised in elderly *per se*

| Drug (degree of impairment) | Comment |
|---|---|
| Anxiolytics and hypnotics (severe) | Start with small doses due to increased cerebral sensitivity |
| Amisulpiride | Halve dose if GFR between 30–60 ml/min; take third of dose if GFR between 10–30 ml/min; intermittent treatment recommended at reduced dose if GFR < 10 ml/min |
| Antipsychotics (severe) | Start with small doses; increased cerebral sensitivity (see specific advice on amisulpiride, clozapine, olanzapine, quetiapine, risperidone and sulpiride) |
| Chloral hydrate (severe) | Avoid |
| Clozapine (severe) | Avoid |
| Duloxetine | Avoid if GFR < 30 ml/min |
| Fluvoxamine (moderate) | Start with smaller doses |
| Galantamine (severe) | Avoid |
| Lithium (mild) | Avoid if possible or reduce dose and monitor plasma concentrations carefully |
| Lithium (moderate) | Avoid |
| Lofepramine (severe) | Avoid |
| Memantine | Reduce dose to 10 mg a day if GFR 40–60 ml/min. Should be avoided if GFR < 10 ml/min |
| Mirtazapine | Manufacturers advise caution |
| Olanzapine | Consider starting dose of 5 mg |
| Paroxetine | Reduce dose if GFR < 30 ml/min |
| Quetiapine | Manufacturer advises initial dose of 25 mg daily increased in daily steps of 25–50 mg |
| Risperidone | Manufacturer advises initial oral dose of 0.5 mg b.d. increased in steps of 0.5 mg b.d. to 1–2 mg b.d.; if an oral dose of at least 2 mg daily is tolerated then can give 25 mg IM every 2 weeks of Risperdal Consta. |
| Sulpiride | Avoid if possible, or reduce dose |
| Valproate (mild to moderate) | Reduce dose |
| Venlafaxine | Use half normal dose if GFR 10–30 ml/min; avoid if GFR < 10 ml/min |

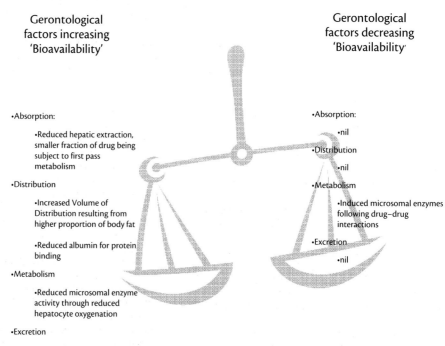

**Fig. 14.1** Gerontological factors and influence on bioavailability of drugs.

to achieve this is to undertake well-designed clinical trials; accordingly psychogeriatricians should be advocating to research funders, both public and commercial, on behalf of their patients that they should be subject to the benefits (enjoyed by younger populations) of a better evidence base. This will only come from better clinical trials research in this population.

## References

Bergman-Evans, B. (2006). Evidence-based guideline, improving medication management for older clients. *Journal of Gerontological Nursing*, **32**(7), 6–14.

British National Formulary (2006). BMJ Publishing Group, London.

Cannon, K.T., Choi, M.M., and Zuniga, M.A. (2006). Potentially inappropriate medication use in elderly patients receiving home health care: a retrospective data analysis. *American Journal of Geriatric Pharmacotherapy*, **4**(2), 134–143.

Cockcroft, D.W. and Gault, M.H. (1976). Prediction of creatinine clearance from serum creatinine. *Nephron*, **16**, 31–41.

Cogger, V.C., Warren, A., Fraser, R. *et al.* (2003). Hepatic sinusoidal pseudocapillarisation with aging in the non-human primate. *Experimental Gerontology*, **38**, 1101–1107.

Cooper, C., Carpenter, I., Katona, C. *et al.* (2005). The AdHOC Study of older adults' adherence to medication in 11 countries. *American Journal of Geriatric Psychiatry*, **13**(12), 1067–1076.

Cusack, B.J. (2004). Pharmacokinetics in Older Persons. *American Journal of Geriatric Pharmacotherapy*, **2**(4), 274–302.

Durnas, C., Loi, M., and Cusack, B.J. (1990). Hepatic drug metabolism and aging. *Pharmacokinetics*, **19**, 359–389.

Fialova, D., Topinkova, E., Gambassi, G. *et al.* (2005). Potentially inappropriate medication use among elderly home care patients in Europe. *Journal of the American Medical Association*, **293**(11), 1348–1358.

Fliser, D., Bischoff, I., Hanses, A. *et al.* (1999). Renal handling of drugs in the healthy elderly. Creatinine clearance underestimates renal function and pharmacokinetics remain virtually unchanged. *European Journal of Clinical Pharmacology*, **55**, 205–211.

Gainsborough, N., Maskrey, V.L., Nelson, M.L. *et al.* (1993). The association of age with gastric emptying. *Age and Ageing*, **22**, 37–40.

Herrlinger, C. and Klotz, U. (2001). Drug metabolism and drug interactions in the elderly. *Best Practice and Research in Clinical Gastroenterology*, **15**, 897–918.

Hoang, K., Tan, J.C., Derby, G. *et al.* (2003). Determinants of glomerular hypofiltration in aging humans. *Kidney International*, **64**, 1417–1424.

Jeste, D.V. (2000). Tardive dyskinesia in older patients. *Journal of Clinical Psychiatry*, **61**(Suppl. 4), 27–32.

Kharasch, E.D., Hoffer, C., and Whittington, D. (2004). Influence of age on the pharmacokinetics and pharmacodynamics of oral transmucosal fentanyl citrate. *Anesthesiology*, **101**, 738–743.

Kinirons, M.T. and O'Mahony, M.S. (2004). Drug metabolism and ageing. *British Journal of Clinical Pharmacology*, **57**, 540–544.

Kyle, U.G., Genton, L., Slosman, D.O., and Pichard, C. (2001). Fat-free mass percentiles in 5225 healthy subjects aged 15 to 98 years. *Nutrition*, **17**(7–8), 675.

Le Couteur, D.G. and McLean, A.J. (1998). The aging liver. Drug clearance and an oxygen diffusion barrier hypothesis. *Clinical Pharmacokinetics*, **34**, 359–373.

Le Couteur, D.G., Hickey, H.M., Harvey, P.J., and McLean, A.J. (1999). Oxidative injury reproduces age-related impairment of oxygen-dependent drug metabolism. *Pharmacology and Toxicology*, **85**, 230–232.

Le Couteur, D.G., Cogger, V.C., Markus, A.M. *et al.* (2001). Pseudocapillarization and associated energy limitation in the aged rat liver. *Hepatology*, **33**, 537–543.

McKinney, M. and Jacksonville, M.C. (2005). Brain cholinergic vulnerability: relevance to behaviour and disease. *Biochemical Pharmacology*, **70**(8), 1115–1124.

McLean, A.J., Cogger, V.C., Chong, G.C. *et al.* (2003). Age related pseudo-capillarization of the human liver. *Journal of Pathology*, **200**, 112–117.

Madsen, J.L. and Graff, J. (2004). Effects of ageing on gastrointestinal motor function. *Age and Ageing*, **33**, 154–159.

Markowitz, J.S., DeVane, C.L., Malcolm, R.J. *et al.* (2006). Pharmacokinetics of olanzapine after single-dose oral administration of standard tablet versus normal and sublingual administration of an orally disintegrating tablet in normal volunteers. *Journal of Clinical Pharmacology*, **46**(2), 164–171.

Marriott, R.G., Neil, W., and Waddingham, S. (2006). Antipsychotic medication for elderly people with schizophrenia. *Cochrane Database Systematic Review*, CD005580.

Meyers, B.R. and Wilkinson, P. (1989). Clinical pharmacokinetics of antibacterial drugs in the elderly. Implications for selection and dosage. *Clinical Pharmacokinetics*, **17**, 385–395.

Mottram, P., Wilson, K., and Strobl, J. (2006). Antidepressants for depressed elderly. *Cochrane Database Systematic Review*, CD003491.

Muhlberg, W. and Platt, D. (1999). Age-dependent changes of the kidneys: pharmacological implications. *Gerontology*, **45**, 243–253.

Mukai, S. and Lipsitz, L.A. (2002). Orthostatic hypotension. *Clinics in Geriatric Medicine*, **18**(2), 253–268.

Nebert, D.W., Jorge-Nebert, L., and Vessell, E.S. (2003). Pharmacogenomics and 'individualised drug therapy': high expectations and disappointing achievements. *American Journal of Pharmacogenomics*, **3**(6), 361–370.

Ness, J., Hoth, A., Barnett, M.J. *et al.* (2006). Anticholinergic medications in community-dwelling older veterans: prevalence of anticholinergic symptoms, symptom burden, and adverse drug events. *American Journal of Geriatric Pharmacotherapy*, **4**(1), 42–51.

Obach, R.S. (2000). Inhibition of human cytochrome P450 enzymes by constituents of St. John's Wort, an herbal preparation used in the treatment of depression. *Journal of Pharmacology and Experimental Therapeutics*, **294**(1), 88–95.

Rapoport, M., Polson, C., and Ritchie, C.W. (2007). Pharmacological treatment of psychosis and depression in neurological disease in older adults. In *Cambridge textbook of effective treatments in psychiatry* (ed. P. Tyrer and K. Silk). Cambridge University Press, Cambridge.

Ritchie, C.W. (2005). The use of antipsychotic medication for schizophrenia occurring in late life. In *Psychosis in the elderly* (ed. A. Hassett, D. Ames, and E. Chiu). Taylor and Francis, Abingdon.

Ruiz-Torres, A., Gimeno, A., Munoz, F.J., and Vicent, D. (1995). Are anthropometric changes in healthy adults caused by modifications in dietary habits or by aging? *Gerontology*, **41**, 243–251.

Schmucker, D.L. (1998). Aging and the liver: an update. *Journals of Gerontology. Series A, Biological Sciences and Medical Sciences*, **53**, B315–B320.

Schmucker, D.L., Woodhouse, K.W., Wang, R.K. *et al.* (1990). Effects of age and gender on in vitro properties of human liver monooxygenases. *Clinical Pharmacology and Therapeutics*, **48**, 365–374.

Schneider, L.S., Tariot, P.N., Dagerman, K.S. *et al.* (2006). Effectiveness of atypical antipsychotic drugs in patients with Alzheimer's disease. *New England Journal of Medicine*, **355**(15), 1525–1538.

Shah, A. and Suh, G.H. (2005). A case for judicious use of risperidone and olanzapine in behavioural and psychological symptoms of dementia (BPSD). *International Psychogeriatrics*, **17**(1), 12–22.

Shiloh, R., Nutt, D., and Weizman, A. (2002). *Atlas of psychiatric pharmacotherapy*. Martin Dunitz, London.

Shimada, T., Yamazaki, H., Mimura, M. *et al.* (1994). Interindividual variations in human liver cytochrome P-450 enzymes involved in the oxidation of drugs, carcinogens and toxic chemicals: Studies with liver microsomes of 30 Japanese and 30 Caucasians. *Journal of Pharmacology and Experimental Therapeutics*, **270**, 414–423.

Smith, D.A. and Beier, M.T. (2004). Association between risperidone treatment and cerebrovascular adverse events: examining the evidence and postulating hypotheses for an underlying mechanism. *Journal of the American Medical Directors Association*, **5**(2), 129–132.

Steimer, W., Muller, B., Leucht, S., and Kissling, W. (2001). Pharmacogenetics: a new diagnostic tool in the management of antidepressive drug therapy. *Clinica Chimica Acta*, **308**(1–2), 33–41.

Thal, D.R., Del Tredici, K., and Braak, H. (2004). Neurodegeneration in normal brain aging and disease. *Science of Aging Knowledge Environment*, **2004**(23), pe26 (2004).

Tune, L.E. (2001). Anticholinergic effects of medication in elderly patients. *Journal of Clinical Psychiatry*, **62**(Suppl. 21), 11–14.

van Eijken, M., Tsang, S., Wensing, M. *et al.* (2003). Interventions to improve medication compliance in older patients living in the community: a systematic review of the literature. *Drugs and Aging*, **20**(3), 229–240.

Wallace, S.M. and Verbeek, R.K. (1987). Plasma protein binding of drugs in the elderly. *Clinical Pharmacokinetics*, **12**, 41–72.

Yale, S.H. and Glurich, I. (2005). Analysis of the inhibitory potential of Ginkgo biloba, Echinacea purpurea, and Serenoa repens on the metabolic activity of cytochrome P450 3A4, 2D6, and 2C9. *Journal of Alternative and Complementary Medicine*, **11**(3), 433–439.

# 15

# Electroconvulsive therapy

Daniel W. O'Connor

## Introduction

Electroconvulsive therapy (ECT) is a demonstrably safe and effective treatment for severe depression, mania, catatonia, and some cases of schizophrenia. Its use is increasing in many countries, especially as a treatment of late life depression. It is important, therefore, that old age psychiatrists, most of whom prescribe it, have a good understanding of its uses, benefits, and risks. Most investigators have failed to distinguish between older and younger patients in their reports and so much of the evidence presented in this chapter is generic in nature and readers must apply the information as best they can to their own practice. The areas of greatest concern to old age psychiatrists, namely the medical and cognitive sequelae of ECT in frail aged patients, have been addressed in greater depth and are given suitable prominence here.

The mechanisms of action of ECT are poorly understood. ECT has clear anticonvulsant properties, as shown by a rise in seizure threshold as treatment progresses (Krystal *et al.*, 1998), inviting parallels with the mood-stabilizing effects of anti-epileptic medications like sodium valproate and carbamazepine. Cerebral blood flow and metabolism both fall with ECT (Nobler *et al.*, 1994; Michael *et al.*, 2003), and frontal EEG activity slows (Sackeim *et al.*, 1996), but links between these changes and clinical outcome are uncertain (Grover *et al.*, 2005). Contrary to expectation, ECT has no proven, consistent links with changes in the production, reuptake, and metabolism of the neurotransmitters serotonin and noradrenaline, which explains perhaps its benefits in patients resistant to pharmacotherapy (Grover *et al.*, 2005). Further research is required. ECT certainly works better than placebo and its effects cannot be ascribed solely to psychological mechanisms.

## Patterns of use

ECT declined in use from the 1970s onwards due to the advent of antidepressant and antipsychotic medications, and to its depiction in the popular and professional media as a tool to control aberrant behaviour, but the tide has now turned. Few countries publish figures but, in those that do, treatment rates have risen in Australia (Doessel *et al.*, 2006), the USA (Rosenbach *et al.*, 1997), and doubtless other countries too, based on the numbers of research publications.

Treatment rates still vary widely from 1.9 per 100,000 population in The Netherlands in 1999 (Van der Wurff *et al.*, 2004)

to 20 per 100,000 in Australia in 2002 (Doessel *et al.*, 2006). Within the USA, rates in 1989 ranged from 4 to 810 per 100,000 in different metropolitan areas. Predictors included the number of psychiatrists, their country of origin and treatment orientation, urban residency, and the stringency of State laws (Hermann *et al.*, 1995; Rosenbach *et al.*, 1997). Clinical application is shaped therefore by national, educational, legal, and practical parameters.

ECT is prescribed more to older people than younger ones in Australia (Wood and Burgess, 2003), Denmark (Munk-Olsen *et al.*, 2006), the United States (Olfson *et al.*, 1998), and probably most other countries. In Victoria, Australia, where rates are collated accurately in public and private hospitals, applications rose steeply with age until 85 years (Wood and Burgess, 2003), most probably because of an age-related intolerance of antidepressant and antipsychotic medications coupled with an increase in depressive psychomotor retardation and psychotic symptoms, both of which predict a good response to ECT (Fig. 15.1). It might also reflect a view by psychiatrists that severely depressed old people benefit more from medically oriented therapies. It is conceivable, therefore, that treatment patterns will change yet again now that medications are safer and the role of psychotherapy is expanding.

## Does ECT work?

### Depression

A series of randomized, controlled trials in the 1970s and 1980s established that real ECT was superior to simulated 'treatments' that entailed an anaesthetic but no electrical stimulation. In a meta-analysis of these studies, depressed patients given real ECT progressed faster and scored 9.7 fewer points on the 64-point Hamilton Depression Rating Scale (HDRS) 2–4 weeks later (UK ECT Review Group, 2003).

ECT also proved superior to a range of older and newer antidepressants and lithium, over periods of 3–12 weeks, in all but two of the 13 studies summarized by the UK ECT Review Group (2003). This difference in response translated to 5.2 fewer points on the HDRS. In one of the largest trials, 66% of patients given ECT had no or few symptoms after 4 weeks compared with 42% on those on imipramine 200 mg daily (Medical Research Council, 1965).

ECT can certainly work quickly and effectively when administered by skilled clinicians to carefully selected patients. In a large,

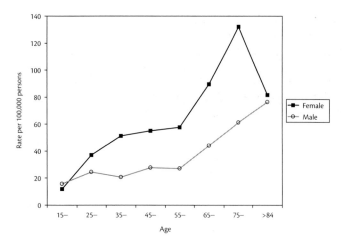

**Fig. 15.1** ECT application rates per 100,000 for age- and sex-specific populations in 1998–9, Victoria, Australia (Wood and Burgess, 2003).

prospective North American study in which 253 depressed patients were given supra-threshold, bilateral treatments, 13% improved after one treatment as shown by a drop of 50% or more in HDRS scores, and 75% remitted after seven sessions (Husain *et al.*, 2004). The same might not apply, though, when patients with complex, chronic conditions are treated in mainstream facilities using sub-optimal methods. As an example, in a survey of seven hospitals in New York where treatment practices varied widely, HDRS scores fell to normal in only 47% of cases; 40% of accrued improvement was lost within 10 days; and relapse rates ranged from 46% to 79% across sites (Prudic *et al.*, 2004).

There are remarkably few prospective, controlled studies of ECT in the elderly. When O'Leary *et al.* (1994) extracted data from a larger study regarding its 35 aged subjects, scores on the HDRS fell 31.7 points on average after six real ECTs versus 10.3 with simulated ones. Bilateral ECT worked a little better and faster than unilateral treatment. Similarly, Flint and Rifat (1998) found in an open, non-random trial that 88% of aged patients with depressive psychoses responded positively to ECT within 6 weeks compared with 25% of those treated with adequate doses of nortriptyline and perphenazine. HDRS scores fell to 10 or less 3 weeks sooner with ECT than medication.

Most other reports are of uncontrolled case series of markedly depressed old people with high rates of melancholia and psychosis. In the four largest series, outcomes were variously defined but mostly positive. Benbow (1987) discharged 52% of patients as 'well' and another 28% as 'improved', while Godber *et al.* (1987) found that 74% of patients made a 'full recovery' or were 'much improved'. In a report by Tew *et al.* (1999), 41% of their 'oldest-old' patients made a complete recovery, as did 39% of those described by Brodaty *et al.* (2000).

### Response predictors

Response to ECT is not well predicted by depression severity *per se* (Clinical Research Centre, 1984; Hickie *et al.*, 1996; Petrides *et al.*, 2001). Outcome correlates more specifically with depressive psychosis and melancholia (especially as reflected by *objective* signs of psychomotor agitation and retardation), either separately or together. Psychotic symptoms increase the likelihood of a positive response, though not to a major degree (Clinical Research Centre, 1984;

Mulsant *et al.*, 1991; O'Connor *et al.*, 2001; Petrides *et al.*, 2001). Depressed patients with psychotic symptoms scored 5.9 points less on average on the HDRS than non-psychotic patients after treatment by Mulsant *et al.* (1991) and 8% less in a report by Petrides *et al.* (2001). The *combination* of psychotic symptoms with observable psychomotor change has stronger predictive capacity. Deluded–retarded cases in one placebo-controlled trial lost 34.7 points on the HDRS in contrast to 16.2 in the retarded, non-deluded group and 10.7 in the non-retarded, non-deluded group (Buchan *et al.*, 1992).

Traditional teaching holds that ECT works best for aged patients, but the evidence is mixed. Older patients responded better to ECT than younger ones in three studies (Wilkinson *et al.*, 1993, Wesson *et al.*, 1997; O'Connor *et al.*, 2001) but not in two others (Hickie *et al.*, 1996; Petrides *et al.*, 2001). ECT's benefits might rise with age if older depressed people are more subject to delusions and hallucinations, but most studies suggest that they are not (Wilkinson *et al.*, 1993; Brodaty *et al.*, 2000; O'Connor *et al.*, 2001). It seems, therefore, that psychomotor changes and psychosis are more important than age *per se*.

Certain factors *reduce*, but do not preclude, the likelihood of responding to ECT. These include a failed response to adequate doses for an adequate period of appropriate medications (Prudic *et al.*, 1990); severe subcortical, grey matter hyperintensities on MRI brain scan (Steffens *et al.*, 2001), and personality disorder (Black *et al.*, 1988).

### Dementia and other organic mental disorders

Two thirds of the British old age psychiatrists surveyed by Benbow (1991) agreed that ECT was 'often or sometimes' appropriate when depression overlaid on dementia failed to respond to antidepressant medication. Published reports are favourable, with improvement rates, however defined, of up to 80% in cases of depression co-morbid with Alzheimer's disease, vascular dementia, Lewy body dementia, and frontotemporal dementia (Price and McAllister, 1989; Rao and Lyketsos, 2000; Rasmussen *et al.*, 2003). These reports take the form of small, retrospective case series that are subject to bias: positive reports are more likely to be published than negative ones. To counter this, Nelson and Rosenberg (1991) compared 21 consecutive patients with dementia and co-morbid major depression with 84 similarly aged, non-demented ones. The dementia group derived almost as much benefit from ECT. While confusion post-ECT was commoner and correlated with the degree of dementia, cognition improved in many instances as depression remitted and Mini-Mental State Examination (MMSE) scores improved on average by 1.6 points. Confusion complicated ECT in half the cases described by Rao and Lyketsos (2000) but it lasted only a few days and all treatments continued uneventfully. Few reports provide follow-up data, though in one relapse rates were high (Rasmussen *et al.*, 2003). With respect to mania in dementia, McDonald and Thompson (2001) described two patients who responded well to ECT in the short-term but required ongoing treatment to hold symptoms at bay.

ECT is not a standard treatment of the disturbed behaviours like screaming and aggression that arise in mid- to late-stage dementia, except where patients have co-morbid depression and fail to respond to antidepressant medication. Notwithstanding this, there are detailed reports of patients who were not obviously depressed but benefited greatly from ECT (Carlyle *et al.*, 1991;

Holmberg *et al.*, 1996; Grant and Mohan, 2001). Their disturbed behaviours, which posed serious risk to themselves and others, resolved quickly, but about half required occasional maintenance treatments.

ECT can also be delivered safely and effectively to patients with mental disorders secondary to stroke (Currier *et al.*, 1992); Huntington's disease (Ranen *et al.*, 1994), head injury (Kant *et al.*, 1999), and mental handicap (van Waarde *et al.*, 2001) though relapse rates tend to be high.

## Schizophrenia, mania, and catatonia

All major clinical guidelines accept acute schizophrenia, schizoaffective disorder, mania, and catatonia as possible indications for ECT (American Psychiatric Association, 2001; Royal College of Psychiatrists, 2005; Royal Australian and New Zealand College of Psychiatrists, 2005) and most old age psychiatrists agree with this position (Benbow, 1991).

The use of ECT in acute schizophrenia plummeted once antipsychotic medications became available in the 1950s. ECT works a little faster than antipsychotics, and is just as effective in reducing psychotic symptoms (Abraham and Kulhara, 1987), but medications are simpler to administer on a long-term basis and are preferred by most patients. Despite recent pharmacological advances, there remain patients who do not respond to medications or cannot tolerate them or require urgent intervention to prevent self-injury. Naturalistic and case report studies suggest, but do not prove, that half or more of those who fail to respond to standard medications improve substantially once ECT is added (Gujavarty *et al.*, 1987; Chanpattana and Chakrabhand, 2001). Responders are typically younger than non-responders, have more positive symptoms, and have been unwell for shorter periods (Chanpattana and Chakrabhand, 2001) but old age is not a barrier to recovery. Kramer (1999) described five women aged 58 to 74 years whose florid schizophrenia or schizoaffective disorders improved dramatically with ECT.

In earlier times, mania often respond favourably to ECT (Davies, 1983; Cawte, 1999) and, more recently, ECT performed as well or better than pharmacotherapy in two small randomized, controlled trials (Mukherjee *et al.*, 1988; Small *et al.*, 1988). Clinical experience suggests that manic patients who cannot tolerate antipsychotic or mood-stabilizing medications, or are so manic that they look to be delirious, respond best to ECT. 'Delirious mania' is life-threatening and ECT is possibly safer than pharmacotherapy (Friedman *et al.*, 2003). There is little information regarding older patients in particular.

The prevalence of catatonia has declined in recent decades but it arises occasionally in schizophrenia, depression, mania, and organic conditions like brain tumour, head trauma, stroke, encephalitis, and metabolic disturbance with any or all of the following signs: mutism, negativism, echolalia, echopraxia, muscle rigidity, posturing, and waxy flexibility. Its severest form, lethal catatonia, is associated with extreme agitation, stupor, fever, sweating, and autonomic instability and can lead to dehydration, exhaustion, and death if left untreated. It must be distinguished from neuroleptic malignant syndrome and malignant hyperthermia by means of a reliable medication history. ECT is recognized in clinical guidelines as an effective treatment of catatonia though, as with schizophrenia, core symptoms usually persist (American Psychiatric Association, 2001; Royal College of Psychiatrists, 2005; Royal Australian and New Zealand College of Psychiatrists, 2005).

## Other conditions

ECT can improve tremor, rigidity, bradykinesia, and gait in Parkinson's disease for periods of several weeks but is rarely used for this indication (Kennedy *et al.*, 2003). It is of greater benefit in neuroleptic malignant syndrome, a condition that overlaps in form with catatonia and is precipitated by antipsychotic medication (see above). Patients who fail to respond to supportive therapy, benzodiazepines, and dopamine agonists, or whose lives are in danger, may benefit from a brief course of ECT. Care is required, however, since patients are often medically unstable and require constant monitoring (Troller and Sachdev, 1999).

## Relapse and maintenance therapy

Relapse is common in the period following ECT. In a study by Sackeim *et al.* (2001), patients whose major depression remitted successfully with ECT were randomly assigned to receive placebo, nortriptyline, or a combination of nortriptyline and lithium carbonate. Over the ensuing 24 weeks, 84% of those on placebo relapsed compared with 60% in the nortriptyline group and 39% of those on combination therapy. Relapse was commoner in patients who had failed to respond to previous pharmacotherapy. In a naturalistic, prospective study of outcomes in patients treated in seven New York hospitals, relapse rates averaged 64% over a 24-week period and were higher in cases of psychotic depression (31% versus 22%), co-morbid psychiatric disorder (43% versus 27%), and personality disorder (23% versus 14%). Relapse occurred mostly within the first 12 weeks of follow-up (Prudic *et al.*, 2004).

It is now standard practice to introduce an antidepressant medication, either alone or together with an antipsychotic or mood stabilizer, once ECT stops. Where this is known to be ineffective or unsafe, continuing or maintenance ECT is an option. Continuation therapy (C-ECT) follows directly from an acute course of ECT with the object of preventing relapse. Treatment intervals are typically stretched from weekly to monthly depending on progress. Maintenance ECT (M-ECT) refers somewhat arbitrarily to treatments extending beyond 6 months, and occasionally for years, where the risk of relapse is known to be high (Fink *et al.*, 1996). Intervals between treatments are typically extended until breakthrough symptoms provide clues to the optimal schedule for each person.

M-ECT is clearly helpful in some instances. In a retrospective chart review by Russell *et al.* (2003) of 43 consecutive patients with unipolar depression, bipolar disorder, or schizoaffective disorder, days in hospital fell from an average of 18.9 per year before M-ECT to 3.2 afterwards. In a similar review of 10 depressed patients by Thornton *et al.* (1990), hospital admissions fell from 3.1 per person before M-ECT to 0.3 in the same period after it. Stronger evidence comes from a retrospective, case–control study by Gagné *et al.* (2000) in which 29 depressed ECT responders who received both C-ECT and antidepressant medication were compared with an equal number of controls who took medication only. Over a 2-year period, 93% of the C-ECT group remained well compared with 52% of controls. No significant differences emerged, however, in an earlier case–control study of depressed patients by Schwarz *et al.* (1995). M-ECT has also been used to limit relapse in bipolar disorder and schizophrenia (Vanelle *et al.*, 1994; Chanpattana *et al.*, 1999).

Many of the patients enrolled in M-ECT programmes are elderly, but few authors have focused just on this age group.

Duncan *et al.* (1990), Thienhaus *et al.* (1990), Loo *et al.* (1991), and Dubin *et al.* (1992) all describe positive responses to M-ECT in aged people who had relapsed on many other treatments. The National Institute for Clinical Excellence (2003), in a review of ECT, concluded that maintenance therapy could not be recommended on the grounds that its longer-term benefits and risks had yet to be established. While case reports are subject to publication bias, and lack the authority of controlled trials, painstaking clinical histories are still persuasive. M-ECT looks to be safe and there is no evidence of progressive cognitive impairment (Rami *et al.*, 2004), even in a patient who received 430 treatments over an 8-year period (Barnes *et al.*, 1997).

Since M-ECT is usually delivered on an outpatient basis, patients must be cooperative, medically stable, and fully acquainted with all requirements. Processes must also be in place to conduct physical and mental state checks at predetermined intervals; to gauge the intervals between treatments, and to decide when treatment comes to an end (Fink *et al.*, 1996).

## Treatment

### Anaesthesia

The ideal anaesthetic induction agent ensures rapid, painless unconsciousness, an adequate seizure, and speedy recovery with minimal post-ECT confusion (Folk *et al.*, 2000). Methohexital has a rapid onset, short duration of action, and no anticonvulsant properties. By contrast, propofol is more painful on injection and raises seizure thresholds, though not to a significant degree in usual doses. Its major advantage is that pulse rate and blood pressure are more stable (Fredman *et al.*, 1994). Ketamine is generally avoided because of slower induction, delayed recovery, nausea, and ataxia. (Folk *et al.*, 2000).

Muscle relaxants like succinylcholine virtually eliminate the risk of fractures during ECT, though two cases of vertebral compression fractures were reported by Mulsant *et al.* (1991) in patients known to be osteoporotic. Doses of relaxant can be increased if desired in these situations. There is no uniform view on the routine use of anticholinergics (usually atropine or glycopyrrolate) just prior to treatment to reduce salivation and bradycardia. Many centres now use them selectively given the risks of tachycardia due to unopposed sympathetic activity, myocardial ischaemia, and post-ECT confusion (Tiller and Lyndon, 2003).

### Seizure threshold

Tonic–clonic seizures are critical to ECT's success (Cronholm and Ottosson, 1960) and the electrical charge must therefore exceed seizure threshold to ensure that a convulsion ensues. Thresholds vary tenfold or more between patients but are mostly low at between 20 and 100 millicoulomb (mC) (Shapira *et al.*, 1996; Boylan *et al.*, 2000; Tiller and Ingram, 2006). Increasing age, male gender, and bilateral electrode placement all predict higher initial thresholds (Colenda and McCall, 1996; Sackeim *et al.*, 1987). Older men prescribed bilateral ECT will therefore have higher mean thresholds than younger women prescribed unilateral ECT.

Electrical charge is not critical in itself. What matters more is that energy levels exceed threshold by a defined amount. Bilateral ECT is effective at, or just above, seizure threshold. Unilateral ECT is not, as shown in a critical study by Sackeim *et al.* (2000) in which 'low-dose' unilateral treatment (50% above threshold) was much

less effective than 'high-dose' unilateral treatment (500% above threshold). 'Moderate-dose' ECT (150% above threshold) occupied an intermediate position. 'High-dose' unilateral ECT worked almost as well as bilateral ECT (50% above threshold) in lifting depressive symptoms (Fig. 15.2).

### Stimulus dosing

In former times, the same electrical dose was given to every patient. There is no place for this now: treatments are individualized to maximize efficacy and reduce side-effects. There is debate, however, about how best to achieve this. One approach, called stimulus dose titration, entails giving one or more stimulations in the first session to ascertain threshold. A commonly used protocol recommends that, for women receiving unilateral ECT, electrical charge is delivered at 32, 48, and then 80 mC until a convulsion is provoked. Once threshold is established, a therapeutic stimulus is delivered at between three and six times this level, depending on local practice. A 'multiplier' of three is recommended by the Royal Australian and New Zealand College of Psychiatrists (2005). Other authorities are less specific (Royal College of Psychiatrists, 1995; American Psychiatric Association, 2001). For bilateral ECT, the 'multiplier' is typically one and a half times threshold.

In experienced hands, stimulus titration takes just a few minutes to complete. Inexpert clinicians are less sure-handed, resulting in longer anaesthesia and slower recovery. There is also a risk that repeated subconvulsive stimulations will precipitate cardiac arrhythmias. This certainly happened in the 1940s and 1950s, prior to the routine use of muscle relaxation and oxygenation, but is rarely seen now (Beale *et al.*, 1994; McCall *et al.*, 1994).

Age-based dosing strategies are simpler, faster, and possibly safer for old, frail patients. In this approach, a 70-year-old having *unilateral* ECT is given 70% (about 400 mC) of the maximal charge delivered by modern machines. While this approach is not as individualized as stimulation titration, it seems to work well enough. According to Tiller and Ingram (2006), only 2% of their female patients and 7% of males would have received doses too low to prove therapeutic. Against this, doses would have been too high, in their view, at seven or more times threshold for 30% of women and 8% of men. Since their patients' ages covered a wide range, excessive dosing would doubtless be less of a problem in geriatric settings where thresholds are higher.

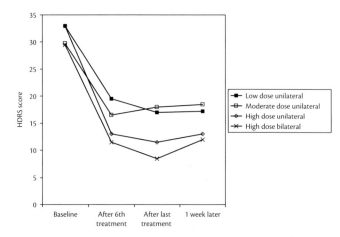

**Fig. 15.2** Hamilton Depression Rating Scale (HDRS) scores for patients treated with high- and low-energy, unilateral and bilateral ECT (Sackeim *et al.*, 2000).

'Full age' dosing is certainly excessive with *bilateral* ECT where stimuli should exceed threshold just by 50% (Enns and Karvelas, 1995). 'Half age' dosing, which entails giving a 60-year-old just 30% maximal energy (or about 190 mC), is preferable. Petrides and Fink (1996) found this method satisfactory in a small survey of 35 adult patients. There is an urgent need for large-scale studies of the pros and cons of these various approaches in genuinely old, frail patients. In the meantime, clinicians are divided in their approach: some prefer dose titration, others prefer age-based formulae, and a few use high, fixed doses for all patients (Colenda and McCall, 1996).

### Seizure monitoring

Threshold levels rise by 50% on average as treatment progresses, more for bilateral than unilateral ECT, and electrical charge must rise to keep pace if this happens (Sackeim *et al.*, 1987; Shapira *et al.*, 1996; Krystal *et al.*, 1998). It is not practicable to check and recheck patients' thresholds week after week. Instead, clinicians make judgements based on visual and EEG monitoring of seizure duration and morphology. This is an imprecise science. ECT machines now produce measures of seizure duration, amplitude, interhemispheric synchronicity, and post-seizure electrical suppression but none of this information can be interpreted exactly.

Short, powerful, well-suppressed convulsions, and a rise in threshold over time, correlate weakly with better outcomes (Krystal *et al.*, 1998; Perera *et al.*, 2004) but what is cause and what is effect is not clear. Studies by Nobler *et al.* (1993) and Perera *et al.* (2004) suggest that patients who respond well to ECT possess this sort of profile from the outset. A good 'electrical picture' might therefore predict recovery, not cause it. To complicate matters, older people typically have shorter, weaker, and less synchronous seizures, irrespective of clinical outcome, and their thresholds rise faster as treatment progresses (Nobler *et al.*, 1993). In the absence of clear evidence, it seems reasonable to increase electrical charge by 50% at a step if seizures become obviously shorter and weaker. Clinicians will naturally differ to some extent in how they interpret technical parameters (Little *et al.*, 2002).

### Electrode placement

Low-dose unilateral ECT is relatively ineffective and should not be administered. High-dose unilateral treatment, in which charge exceeds threshold three- to fivefold, works almost as quickly and effectively as bilateral (actually bi-temporal) ECT and causes less cognitive impairment. This will be discussed later (see Cognition). Efforts continue to find ways to boost efficacy while minimizing adverse effects. One alternative to the standard bi-temporal approach is bifrontal ECT in which the electrodes are placed 3 to 5 cm above the outer angle of both orbits. The technique dates from the 1970s (Abrams and Taylor, 1973) and resurfaced recently because of hopes of a better cognitive profile. It looks promising. In two randomized controlled trials, both with relatively young patients, bifrontal ECT proved just as potent an antidepressant as bi-temporal and high-dose right unilateral ECT, and caused less cognitive disruption than either (Bailine *et al.*, 2000; Ranjkesh *et al.*, 2005). It is not innocuous though. Among 14 genuinely aged patients who received bifrontal ECT, 12 recovered quickly but five had 'noticeable cognitive side effects' (Little *et al.*, 2004). The technique warrants more detailed investigation.

### Concomitant medications

Benzodiazepines raise seizure thresholds and should therefore be avoided, reduced, or stopped if possible (Pettinati *et al.*, 1990), but modest doses (e.g. lorazepam up to 3 mg daily) have little impact in reality (Boylan *et al.* 2000) and are permitted in most ECT trials to lessen anxiety and agitation. Mood stabilizers that are also anticonvulsants (e.g. valproate and carbamazepine) should be stopped if possible.

Medications with anticholinergic properties (e.g. tricyclic antidepressants, digoxin, prednisone, and warfarin) are possibly more hazardous, especially when taken in combination, given their link with worsened cognition post-ECT. Mondimore *et al.* (1983) found that eight of their 12 patients with high serum anticholinergic levels lost two or more points on the MMSE after a single ECT compared with only one of eight patients with lower anticholinergic levels.

Lithium might be hazardous too when combined with ECT given occasional reports of severe confusion, prolonged seizures, and catatonia, even with 'normal' blood levels (Sartorius *et al.*, 2005). By way of confirmation, rates of confusion were higher at 22% in 27 patients given lithium and ECT concurrently, compared with 12% in those whose lithium was stopped just prior to ECT, and 6% in those with no exposure (Penney *et al.*, 1990). Against this, Dolenc and Rasmussen (2005) cite case reports in which lithium and ECT were combined safely. Though the risk of serious mishap is slight, lithium should be stopped or replaced with another mood stabilizer before starting ECT.

### Treatment frequency

Once-weekly ECT works too slowly. When 15 elderly depressed patients were randomly assigned to either one or three bilateral treatments each week, all of them improved but the latter group recovered faster (Kellner *et al.*, 1992). Since better outcomes might result just from more treatments, Shapira *et al.* (1998) added simulated sessions in their comparison of twice versus three times weekly bilateral ECT in a randomized controlled trial involving 31 patients. The two schedules had similar antidepressant effects but thrice weekly ECT caused much more cognitive impairment. In a small, less sophisticated comparison of two and three times weekly unilateral ECT, psychiatric and cognitive outcomes were barely different a fortnight later (McAllister *et al.*, 1987). There is no compelling reason, therefore, to administer either unilateral or bilateral ECT more than twice weekly.

## Safety

ECT is generally very safe. Mortality rates in the USA are less than 2 per 100,000 applications (Shiwach *et al*, 2001; Nuttall *et al.*, 2004), and have fallen in recent decades, placing the risk of ECT at the bottom of the range for procedures entailing general anaesthesia (Abrams, 1997). This is not because treatment is reserved for physically fit patients. The reverse is often the case. ECT is given quite commonly to patients with serious medical co-morbidities compounded by dehydration, inanition, and exhaustion secondary to depression or psychosis. It might actually be safer than psychiatric medications in such circumstances. In a chart review by Zielinski *et al.* (1993), 11 of 21 patients with cardiac disease were forced to discontinue treatment with tricyclic antidepressants because of cardiovascular complications compared with only two of 40 similar patients given ECT. Similarly, rates of cardiovascular and gastro-intestinal adverse events were commoner in 39 very old medically treated depressives compared with 39 carefully matched patients treated with ECT. Their rates of hypertension, myocardial infarction, and heart failure were virtually identical (Manly *et al.*, 2000). There are risks, however, as the following sections make clear.

## Cardiovascular effects

ECT exerts its effect on the heart principally by direct neuronal transmission of impulses from the hypothalamus to the heart via parasympathetic and sympathetic tracts. During and immediately after electrical stimulation, an intense parasympathetic surge flows through the vagal nerve to the heart resulting in a transient sinus bradycardia with periods of asystole lasting for 2 s on average but occasionally for 5 s or more (Burd and Kettl, 1998). A sympathetic surge then follows, leading to an average rise in blood pressure of 55 mmHg, and in pulse rate of 37 beats per minute, together with clinically benign premature atrial and ventricular contractions. Rare complications at this time include acute myocardial infarction and ventricular fibrillation (Burd and Kettl, 1998). Pulse rates and blood pressure both rise more during bilateral than unilateral ECT, and more with higher than lower energy levels (Gangadhar *et al.*, 2000). Cardiac function usually returns to normal within 15 min but ST changes and bursts of bi- or trigeminy are a little commoner than usual in the following 24 h (Huuhka *et al.*, 2003).

## Frequency and severity of adverse events

Aged patients are at higher risk of adverse events. In a report by Burke *et al.* (1987), 15% of their patients aged 60 years and over experienced a cardiorespiratory complication (mostly changes in blood pressure) compared with 3% of younger patients, and 15% sustained a fall versus none in the younger group. Rates of post-ECT confusion were 18% and 13%, respectively. Altogether, 35% of older patients had a complication but most were transient and settled spontaneously. Side-effects also rose with age in a chart review by Alexopoulos *et al.* (1984). Cardiovascular complications arose in 19% of their patients aged 65 years and over versus 1% of younger patients, and 14% had neurological complications (mostly confusion) compared with 12%. Apart from an 87-year-old man who died of a myocardial infarction 48 h after his second treatment, most patients went on to complete their course.

Octogenarians were found by Cattan *et al.* (1990) to have adverse events roughly twice as often as 'younger old' patients. Cardiovascular complications and falls were both more frequent in very old patients than younger ones at 36% versus 12%, and 36% versus 14%, respectively. Confusion was the commonest problem, arising in 59% and 45% of the two groups. Outcomes were more benign in the patients aged 75 years and over described by Gormley *et al.* (1998), of whom 7% suffered prolonged confusion and 4% became manic. All problems resolved within 2 weeks. Similarly, 32% of the patients aged 85 years and over of Tomac *et al.* (1997) experienced prolonged confusion and 10% fell. One of the 34 patients sustained a fracture between treatments and six died of causes unrelated to ECT within 45 days after the last treatment, attesting to their very high rates of physical co-morbidity.

Other uncommon side-effects include dental injury, fractures secondary to falls (de Carle and Kohn, 2001), and vertebral compression fractures due to poorly modified seizures (Mulsant *et al.*, 1991). Very rare sequelae include stroke (Bruce *et al.*, 2006),

transient cortical blindness (Sonavane *et al.*, 2006), and status epilepticus (Srzich and Turbott, 2000). Neurological asymmetries are common after ECT but generally resolve within 20 min (Kriss *et al.*, 1978).

## Prevention and management

Contraindications to ECT include recent myocardial infarction and stroke, severe valvular heart disease, clinically significant arrhythmias, unstable angina, uncompensated cardiac failure, and cardiac and arterial aneurysms, but these rules are not absolute. Profoundly depressed patients who refuse to eat or drink or take essential medications might respond better to ECT than other treatments after a detailed evaluation of their mental and physical health (American Psychiatric Association, 2001; Royal College of Psychiatrists, 2005). ECT has certainly been applied safely and effectively in profoundly depressed patients with cerebral aneurysms and angiomas (Kang and Passmore, 2004); inoperable aortic aneurysms (Porquez *et al.*, 2003), and recent myocardial infarction (Magid *et al.*, 2005).

Examples of the strategies required to minimize risk in medically compromised patients are furnished by Hay (1989) and Regestein and Reich (1985). These include: pre-treatment with atropine or glycopyrrolate to prevent tachycardia (though atropine may worsen confusion); pre-treatment with beta-blockers to limit hypertension and bradycardia (though unopposed parasympathetic activity may worsen bradycardia); reductions in anticoagulant therapy in patients at risk of haemorrhage; and additional muscle relaxation in patients with fractures or marked osteoporosis. A careful physical examination, ECG, measures of renal function, and detailed discussions with medical and anaesthetic colleagues are vital. Other laboratory and imaging results add little extra information (Abramczuk and Rose, 1979; Lafferty *et al.*, 2001). Patients with implanted cardiac pacemakers can receive ECT safely. Cardioverter defibrillators should have their defibrillation and anti-tachycardia functions deactivated just prior to treatment (Bowley and Walker, 2005).

# Cognition
## Objective changes

No evidence has emerged from numerous anatomical and imaging studies that ECT causes altered brain structure, neuronal death, or cerebral atrophy (Devanand *et al.*, 1994; Ende *et al.*, 2000). There is no doubt, however, that ECT can result in objective cognitive disruption. Three time-frames have been identified. In the short-term, wakening from ECT is often followed by a brief period of confusion and disorientation. This typically lasts just for a few minutes but extends occasionally for hours or even days. Risk factors for emergent delirium include: bilateral electrode placement (Sackeim *et al.*, 1993); high electrical dose relative to threshold (Sackeim *et al.*, 1993); a sinusoidal waveform (Daniel and Crovitz, 1986); advanced age (Alexopoulos *et al.*, 1984; Tomac *et al.*, 1997); pre-existing dementia (Rao and Lyketsos, 2000); and concomitant anti-cholinergic medications (Mondimore *et al.*, 1983).

As ECT progresses, both new learning and recall of past events are compromised to varying degrees. In a study by McCall *et al.* (2002) of patients given high-dose (eight times threshold) unilateral ECT, scores on the Rey Auditory–Verbal Learning Test fell from 6.2 at baseline to 1.9 after the last treatment. By contrast, moderate-dose

(2.5 times threshold) unilateral ECT is relatively innocuous (Ng *et al.*, 2000). Recall of past events diminishes too, more for public events than personal ones, and more for recent events than long distant ones. As a result, knowledge of recent public incidents (e.g. a political news story) is roughly eight times more compromised than knowledge of remote personal episodes (e.g. a family anecdote) (Lisanby *et al.*, 2000). Risk factors for anterograde and retrograde amnesia include bilateral electrode placement (Lawson *et al.*, 1990; McElhiney *et al.*, 1995; Sackeim *et al.*, 2000); high electrical dose relative to threshold (Sackeim *et al.*, 2000; McCall *et al.*, 2002); advanced age (Zervas *et al.*, 1993), and limited education (Legendre *et al.*, 2003). Impaired cognition at baseline and prolonged disorientation after treatment also increase the risk of retrograde amnesia (Sobin *et al.*, 1995). Other possible factors include substance abuse, neurological disorders, and cardiac disease (Sackeim, 2000).

Memory typically improves quickly once ECT stops. It is not enough to return to baseline though. Depression inhibits cognitive speed, attention, recall, and executive function, and these elements should therefore improve in line with mood. If cognition after ECT is no better than before, it follows that treatment has failed or that ECT hinders cognition as much as depression (that is, one amnesic condition has been replaced with another). Typically, new learning improves steadily over a 1 to 6 month period (Lawson *et al.*, 1990; Sackeim *et al.*, 1993; McElhiney *et al.*, 1995; McCall *et al.*, 2002). In a trial by McCall *et al.* (2002) of high-dose unilateral (eight times threshold) versus standard bilateral treatment, verbal and visual memory both improved over the ensuing 4 weeks.

Recovery of past memories is less complete. At 2-month review, patients given ECT by Lisanby *et al.* (2000) recounted personal information, both recent and remote, as well as controls but forgot about a third of the recent impersonal events they had known just prior to treatment. Also, knowledge of events in the days or weeks prior to treatment may never be recovered. This happens more with bilateral than unilateral ECT (Lisanby *et al.*, 2000) and seems not to be influenced by current mood state (McElhiney *et al.*, 1995).

Remarkably few studies have focused on older people despite their higher rates of cognitive impairment, physical morbidity, and polypharmacy, and most studies that do so are small, naturalistic, and possibly unrepresentative of general clinical practice. Acute confusion is certainly commoner (see above). In other respects, ECT seems benign. In a group of patients aged 20 to 65 years, older age was associated with greater anterograde and retrograde amnesia immediately after a course of bilateral ECT and again 6 months later (Zervas *et al.* 1993). By contrast, Rubin *et al.* (1993) found that scores on the MMSE fell by three points on average during treatment (mostly bilateral) in 48 aged patients (mean age 76 years) but rose quickly and exceeded baseline scores prior to discharge from hospital. Similarly, 12 older patients (mean age 69 years) performed better on a range of neuropsychological tests 1 week after a course of unilateral or bilateral ECT (Russ *et al.*, 1990).

In the longer term, some cases of dementia must be expected in older age groups because of the established links between depression on the one hand and incipient cerebrovascular and Alzheimer's diseases on the other. While rates look high at 14% in the patients aged 65+ years followed for 3 years by Godber *et al.* (1987) and 36% in those aged 75+ years followed for 5 years by Brodaty *et al.* (2000), there is no reason to believe that ECT plays a causative role.

## Subjective reports

While complaints of poor memory subside as depression remits (Cronholm and Ottosson, 1963; Coleman *et al.*, 1996; Freeman and Kendall, 1980; McCall *et al.*, 1995), between 29% and 88% of patients describe persistent forgetfulness in the coming weeks and months (Squire and Slater, 1983; Brodaty *et al.*, 2001; Rose *et al.*, 2003; Philpot *et al.*, 2004). Gaps in memory of the 6 months before treatment and the 2 months after are common and well tolerated (Freeman *et al.*, 1980). Of more concern to patients are 'holes' in past memories and difficulties with remembering faces, names, and lists (Freeman *et al.*, 1980). Risk factors for subjective memory deficits include bilateral electrode placement and high electrical charge (Squire and Slater, 1983; Coleman et al., 1996) but rates seem not to be influenced by patients' ages (Brodaty *et al.*, 2001).

Subjective complaints correlate poorly with scores on cognitive tests though the tests employed by Sienaert *et al.* (2005) and Coleman *et al.* (1996) were rudimentary. More detailed serial assessments, with special attention to retrograde memory, might prove more revealing. There is no doubt, however, that complaints correlate strongly with current mood. Patients whose depressions persist despite treatment report more memory difficulties, perceive ECT more negatively, and are reluctant to have it again (Cronholm and Ottoson, 1963; Freeman and Kendall, 1980; Coleman *et al.*, 1996; Prudic *et al.*, 2000). This is not surprising: mood correlates strongly with self-rated memory even in community populations (O'Connor *et al.*, 1990). Most psychiatrists conclude on this basis that patients' concerns about memory denote continuing psychopathology, a loss of faith in memory, or an excessive concern with normal cognitive changes (Prudic *et al.*, 2000). Others are more circumspect. Freeman *et al.* (1980) noted that ECT 'complainers', while fractionally more depressed on mood rating scales than 'non-complainers', seemed plausible and a few scored poorly on specific cognitive tests for reasons that were unclear. In similar vein, Sackeim (2000) noted that most patients report a classic temporal gradient in memory that is better explained by ECT than depression and concluded that 'attributing these subjective deficits to ongoing psychopathology or natural disease progression would seem disingenuous and defensive'. An account by one patient is especially compelling. Donahue (2000) wrote that ECT (initially unilateral and then bilateral) saved her from suicide. She felt grateful to be alive and would have ECT again if necessary but whole chunks of her life had been lost—a price she accepted but could not deny.

## Ethical issues

For patients with the capacity to consent, ECT should be administered only with their agreement. To do otherwise infringes on their right to refuse treatment. Consent must be voluntary, based on an adequate explanation of the nature of ECT, its practical implications, and side-effects, tailored to individual circumstances. Patients concerned by cardiac symptoms or memory problems, for example, need more detailed information about cardiovascular and cognitive sequelae. Verbal discussion is best supplemented by an informational brochure that patients and families can digest at leisure, modelled perhaps on the exemplary document prepared by the American Psychiatric Association (2001). Moderately depressed, cognitively intact older patients absorb and retain this sort of information quite adequately (Lapid *et al.*, 2004). A visit to the treatment suite to explain its procedures and equipment can allay patients' and relatives' concerns.

Clinicians want what is best for their patients and will advocate for ECT when its use is clearly indicated. There is a fine line, however, between persuasion and coercion. Apprehension typically settles with gentle assurance, a positive viewpoint, and attention to patients' concerns, just as with other medical and surgical procedures (McCall, 2006). Persuasion is acceptable; coercion to agree to treatment is not. Doctors and patients sometimes perceive this process quite differently. In a review of 17 reports by Rose *et al.* (2003), only half the respondents believed they had been given an adequate explanation of ECT and most had limited knowledge of actual procedures. Patients sometimes recounted giving 'consent' while heavily sedated or threatened by legal compulsion. These recollections might sometimes be false but small numbers of patients are left traumatized as a result. An account by Johnstone (1999) of the perceptions of shame and despair by 20 aggrieved ECT patients is required reading.

Some of the patients most likely to benefit from ECT are unable to consent by virtue of marked depression, psychosis, or dementia. Pointers to lack of capacity include: a refusal to speak; a rejection of general nursing and medical care; rapid forgetting of basic information about the nature and consequences of ECT; and marked ambivalence. Treatment can be applied in most jurisdictions on an involuntary basis with review by a court or tribunal. It is important to document the reasons for mandating ECT; the pros and cons of alternative treatments; patients' mental state and capacity to make to informed decisions, and family viewpoints. Except in emergencies, second opinions are encouraged. The limited research conducted to date suggests that non-consenting patients often rate their outcome as satisfactory (Wheeldon *et al.*, 1999). Patients who accept ECT passively but cannot contribute to the decision-making process are best treated involuntarily to ensure legal oversight and protection (Law-Min and Stephens, 2006).

ECT typically entails a series of treatments over a period of weeks. Mental capacity will often improve as depression and psychosis abate with the result that non-competent patients become competent and can participate in the decision to continue with treatment. Conversely, a patient made confused by ECT may lose competence for a period of time. Ethical practice requires a constant monitoring of patients' mental states, attitudes to ECT, and decisional capacity. Repeated explanations of the reasons for administering ECT and its likely benefits and side-effects may be required if patients fail to recall initial discussions.

## Attitudes to ECT

### Patients' views

Fear of ECT is widespread. In a survey of 56 Australian hospital visitors, none of whom had received ECT, many agreed that it ablated memory and rendered patients zombies (Kerr *et al.*, 1982). Psychiatrists attribute this fear to misinformation spread by popular movies and certain lobby groups (Dowman *et al.*, 2005) but, in reality, a dread of electricity is instilled in children from an early age. ECT entails loss of consciousness, electrical stimulation, and an epileptic seizure, all of which can evince anxiety.

Malcolm (1989) detailed the concerns expressed by 100 patients prior to ECT. Their fears included brain damage, memory loss, pain, being seen by strangers while unconscious, having a heart attack, and developing epilepsy. Their knowledge of ECT was rudimentary: only 16% knew that a convulsion was induced and many expected a single treatment. Older people were more stoical: 52% denied fear compared with 30% of younger ones. When the same patients were asked later what aspects most perturbed them, they nominated waiting for treatment, seeing equipment laid out, hearing staff talk in the background, breathing into an anaesthetic mask, and waking up afterwards.

In a retrospective survey, only 6% of 70 British patients rated ECT as much worse than a visit to the dentist (Benbow and Crentsil, 2004). By contrast, 7% of Australian patients said that they dreaded it and another 12% found it frightening (Kerr *et al.*, 1982). Occasional patients develop an overwhelming horror of ECT, usually after lengthy or repeated courses (Fox, 1993).

Not all patients are negatively disposed. A psychiatrist who received ECT himself described a lifting of mood and release from tearfulness, irritability, and paranoia after the first treatment. Side-effects—nausea, stiffness of the jaw, topographic disorientation, and mild memory loss—were a small price to pay in his view (A Practising Psychiatrist, 1965). Even a woman whose memory was seriously and permanently disrupted by ECT was confident that, placed in the same situation again, she would choose ECT over the agony of depression (Donahue, 2000).

Patients' views of ECT are coloured in part by their mental status. Depression brings with it fears of therapeutic nihilism. As these fears remit with treatment, opinions of ECT may become more positive (Pettinati *et al.*, 1994; Brodaty *et al.*, 2003). Favourable views post-ECT correlate with severity of mental disorder and disability pre-ECT, fewer treatment side-effects, and a perception of good care while in hospital, but not with legal status (Wheeldon *et al.*, 1999; Philpot *et al.*, 2004; Rosenquist *et al.*, 2006). This suggests that the sickest patients, who stand to derive the greatest benefit from ECT, come to perceive it most favourably.

In an intriguing meta-analysis of 16 published reports, positive views of ECT emerged most commonly from studies conducted shortly after ECT by psychiatrists using brief checklists. Studies conducted by independent investigators some time after admission using open-ended questions were much less encouraging (Rose *et al.*, 2003). This suggests that structured assessments conducted by doctors in medical environments may fail to tap patients' true perceptions.

Proposed strategies to improve acceptance of ECT include educational videos, use of ECT-experienced volunteers, minimizing time in the waiting room, and reducing exposure to technical paraphernalia (Westreich *et al.*, 1995; Koopowitz *et al.*, 2003; Parvin *et al.*, 2004). The video deployed in one study made no discernible difference to patients' knowledge, perhaps because they were too depressed to benefit, but it was greatly appreciated by families whose support is often critical (Westreich *et al.*, 1995).

### Nurses' views

Patients and families seek practical support and advice from hospital nurses whose views of ECT might shape their decision to accept or reject treatment. In an Australian survey, mental health nurses lay somewhere between psychiatrists and the general public in their ratings of ECT as a treatment of depression. Antidepressant medications, counselling, and physical activity were endorsed much more positively (Caldwell and Jorm, 2000). In an Irish survey of 593 students and professionals, more nurses than doctors rated ECT as an oppressive, damaging treatment that should be used only as a last resort (Byrne *et al.*, 2006), but exposure to ECT softened this viewpoint. In a study of 167 Welsh nurses, more of those in frequent contact with ECT patients rated it as a first line treatment of severe depression than those with no such contact (Gass, 1998).

### Families' views

Little research has been conducted of family members' attitudes to ECT, both before and after treatment. This is a deficiency since an informed, sympathetic family can do much to support patients through their illness and treatment. In the meantime, two compelling accounts have been published of relatives' battles with sceptical psychiatrists to secure ECT for a father and son, respectively, whose mental disorders had failed to respond to medications and psychotherapy. Their efforts were rewarded eventually by excellent clinical outcomes (D'Agostino, 1975; A Grateful Parent, 2005).

## Practice standards and training

### Variations in practice

Old age psychiatrists are largely convinced of ECT's value. In a survey of 230 British specialists, about 80% endorsed it as the treatment of choice of medication-resistant depressions and depressive psychoses (Benbow, 1991). This level of consensus is persuasive.

It is not expected that all psychiatrists will apply ECT using identical methods to exactly the same types of patients. Our knowledge base is still too uncertain. Even experts are divided in their views regarding electrode placement and stimulus dosing, as noted already. It is worrying, however, if practice variations stem more from ignorance and inexperience than informed differences in opinion.

In metropolitan New York, Prudic *et al.* (2001) were perturbed to find that 17% of 59 mental health facilities administered the same electrical charge to all patients; 11% of patients received outdated sine wave stimulation; 8% of facilities failed to monitor seizure duration; and 20% neglected to check patients' cognitive status. Whether these lapses detracted from patients' recoveries was unclear, but the authors concluded that 'the wide variability in how ECT is conducted undoubtedly raises public-health concerns'. Farah and McCall (1993) observed a 'Chinese menu' approach to the choice of electrode placement and stimulus dosing in their survey of 307 US psychiatrists: those who belonged to an ECT interest group were no more regular in their practices than others. Pippard (1992) was even more damning of conditions in two large adjoining health areas in southern England. ECT was administered largely by untrained and unsupervised junior doctors, equipment was often outmoded, and seizures were sometimes missed or very brief. Half of the 31 services gave serious cause for concern.

Training deficiencies are widespread. Of 160 junior doctors in England and Wales, 63% had watched an instructional video but only 53% had been supervised by an experienced psychiatrist when giving their first treatment and only 4% were routinely supervised thereafter (Duffett and Lelliott, 1998). Similar findings emerged in New South Wales, Australia, where 20% of doctors were not supervised in their first session by another medical practitioner (Halliday and Johnson, 1995).

### Clinical guidelines

Three national professional bodies have published detailed accounts of ECT's indications and contraindications; proper assessment and treatment procedures; legal and ethical issues, and training and supervision requirements (American Psychiatric Association, 2001; Royal College of Psychiatrists, 2005; Royal Australian and New Zealand College of Psychiatrists, 2005). The American Psychiatric Association stipulates that trainee psychiatrists should complete at least 10 treatments under direct supervision and then attend regular ECT review meetings. 'Privileging' to administer ECT independently requires objective evidence of safe, proficient practice that conforms to local policy. Further education might include attendance at an ECT course, a structured clinical practicum, supervised reading, and participation in quality assurance activities to identify gaps in performance and take corrective action.

A detailed checklist prepared by the Royal College of Psychiatrists' Research Unit (2005) of 'basic', 'standard', and 'ideal' policies and procedures covering all aspects of physical facilities, staff training, patient assessment and treatment, consent, and follow-up provides a template for self-appraisal in any ECT service and is highly recommended.

## Conclusions

- ECT is an effective, accepted treatment of depression. It works faster, and may be safer, than pharmacotherapy for frail, older patients but relapse rates are high once treatment stops. Continuing pharmacotherapy is mandatory. ECT works best in patients with psychomotor changes and psychotic symptoms.

- There is a place for ECT in medication-refractory cases of mania, acute schizophrenia, and catatonia.

- Electrical stimulation must always exceed seizure threshold, more for unilateral than bilateral ECT. Stimulus titration ensures that energy charges are individualized. Alternative strategies include age-based formulae. Fixed-dose, high-energy treatments are not acceptable.

- Very old patients have higher rates of cardiovascular complications, confusion, and falls. Twice weekly ECT is adequate. Benzodiazepines, anticonvulsants, and medications with anticholinergic properties should be stopped if possible.

- Cognition is often improved by ECT. Complaints of memory loss abate with time but gaps in memory may persist.

- Capacity to consent to ECT can change as treatment progresses and explanations may need to be repeated. Educational brochures and videos are encouraged.

- ECT is perceived negatively by many patients and families and great efforts must be made to address their concerns accurately and to reduce the risk of poor outcomes.

- Such a complex treatment should never be administered by untrained staff.

- Few published reports focus just on frail, aged patients. Further research is required to ensure that treatment of this vulnerable group is made as safe and effective as possible.

## References

A Grateful Parent (2005). A family member's experience with ECT. *Journal of ECT*, **21**, 199.

A Practising Psychiatrist (1965). The experience of electro-convulsive therapy. *British Journal of Psychiatry*, **111**, 365–7.

Abraham, K.R. and Kulhara, P. (1987). The efficacy of electroconvulsive therapy in the treatment of schizophrenia: a comparative study. *British Journal of Psychiatry*, **151**, 152–5.

Abramczuk, J.A. and Rose, N.M. (1979). Pre-anaesthetic assessment and the prevention of post-ECT morbidity. *British Journal of Psychiatry*, **134**, 582–7.

Abrams, R. (1997). The mortality rate with ECT. *Convulsive Therapy*, **13**, 125–7.

Abrams, R. and Taylor, M.A. (1973). Anterior bifrontal ECT: a clinical trial. *British Journal of Psychiatry*, **122**, 587–90.

Alexopoulos, G.S., Shamoian, C. J., Lucas, J., Weiser, N., and Berger, H. (1984). Medical problems of geriatric psychiatric patients and younger controls during electroconvulsive therapy. *Journal of the American Geriatrics Society*, **32**, 651–4.

American Psychiatric Association (2001). *The practice of ECT: recommendations for treatment, training and privileging*, 2nd edn. American Psychiatric Association, Washington, DC.

Bailine, S.H., Rifkin, A., Kayne, E. *et al.* (2000). Comparison of bifrontal and bitemporal ECT for major depression. *American Journal of Psychiatry*, **157**, 121–3.

Barnes, R.C., Hussein, A., Anderson, D.N., and Powell, D. (1997). Maintenance electroconvulsive therapy and cognitive function. *British Journal of Psychiatry*, **170**, 285–7.

Beale, M.D., Kellner, C.H., Pritchett, J.T., Bernstein, H.J., Burns, C.M., and Knapp, R. (1994). Stimulus dose-titration in ECT: a 2-year clinical experience. *Convulsive Therapy*, **10**, 171–6.

Benbow, S.M. (1987). The use of electroconvulsive therapy in old age psychiatry. *International Journal of Geriatric Psychiatry*, **2**, 25–30.

Benbow, S.M. (1991). Old age psychiatrists' views on the use of ECT. *International Journal of Geriatric Psychiatry*, **6**, 317–22.

Benbow, S.M. and Crentsil, J. (2004). Subjective experience of electroconvulsive therapy. *Psychiatric Bulletin*, **28**, 289–91.

Black, D.W., Bell, S., Hulbert, J., and Nasrallah, A. (1988). The importance of Axis II in patients with major depression: a controlled study. *Journal of Affective Disorders*, **14**, 115–22.

Bowley, C.J. and Walker, H.A.C. (2005). Anaesthesia for ECT. *The ECT handbook*, 2nd edn, pp. 124–35. Royal College of Psychiatrists, London.

Boylan, L.S., Haskett, R.F., Mulsant, B.H.*et al.* (2000). Determinants of seizure threshold in ECT: benzodiazepine use, anesthetic dosage, and other factors. *Journal of ECT*, **16**, 3–18.

Brodaty, H., Berle, D., Hickie, I., and Mason, C. (2001). 'Side effects' of ECT are mainly depressive phenomena and are independent of age. *Journal of Affective Disorders*, **66**, 237–45.

Brodaty, H., Berle, D., Hickie, I., and Mason, C. (2003). Perceptions of outcome from electroconvulsive therapy by depressed patients and psychiatrists. *Australian and New Zealand Journal of Psychiatry*, **37**, 196–9.

Brodaty, H., Hickie, I., Mason, C., and Prenter, L. (2000). A prospective follow-up study of ECT outcome in older depressed patients. *Journal of Affective Disorders*, **60**, 101–11.

Bruce, B.B., Henry, M.E., and Greer, D.M. (2006). Ischemic stroke after electroconvulsive therapy. *Journal of ECT*, **22**, 150–2.

Buchan, H., Johnstone, E., McPherson, K., Palmer, R.L., Crow, T.J., and Brandon, S. (1992). Who benefits from electroconvulsive therapy?: Combined results of the Leicester and Northwick Park Trials. *British Journal of Psychiatry*, **160**, 355–9.

Burd, J. and Kettl, P. (1998). Incidence of asystole in electroconvulsive therapy in elderly patients. *American Journal of Psychiatry*, **6**, 203–11.

Burke, W.J., Rubin, E.H., Zorumski, C.F.,and Wetzel, R.D. (1987). The safety of ECT in geriatric psychiatry. *Journal of the American Geriatrics Society*, **35**, 516–21.

Byrne, P., Cassidy, B., and Higgins, P. (2006). Knowledge and attitudes towards electroconvulsive therapy among health care professionals and students. *Journal of ECT*, **22**, 133–8.

Caldwell, T.M. and Jorm, A.F. (2000). Mental health nurses' beliefs about interventions for schizophrenia and depression: a comparison with psychiatrists and the public. *Australian and New Zealand Journal of Psychiatry*, **34**, 602–11.

Carlyle, W., Killick, L., and Ancill, R. (1991). ECT: an effective treatment in the screaming demented patient. *Journal of the American Geriatrics Society*, **39**, 637.

Cattan, R.A., Barry, P.P., Mead, G., Reefe, W.E., Gay, A., and Silverman, M. (1990). Electroconvulsive therapy in octogenarians. *Journal of the American Geriatrics Society*, **38**, 753–8.

Cawte, J. (1999). Mania pre-lithium. *Australian and New Zealand Journal of Psychiatry*, **33**, S7–S12.

Chanpattana, W. and Chakrabhand, M.L.S. (2001). Combined ECT and neuroleptic therapy in treatment-refractory schizophrenia: prediction of outcome. *Psychiatry Research*, **105**, 107–15.

Chanpattana, W., Chakrabhand, M.L.S., Sackeim, H.A. *et al.* (1999). Continuation ECT in treatment-resistant schizophrenia: a controlled study. *Journal of ECT*, **15**, 178–92.

Clinical Research Centre (1984). The Northwick Park ECT trial: predictors of response to real and simulated ECT. *British Journal of Psychiatry*, **144**, 227–37.

Coleman, E.A., Sackeim, H.A., Prudic, J., Devanand, D.P., McElhiney, M.C., and Moody, B.J. (1996). Subjective memory complaints prior to and following electroconvulsive therapy. *Biological Psychiatry*, **39**, 346–56.

Colenda, C.C. and McCall, W.V. (1996). A statistical model predicting the seizure threshold for right unilateral ECT in 106 patients. *Convulsive Therapy*, **12**, 3–12.

Cronholm, B. and Ottoson, J. (1960). Experimental studies of the therapeutic action of electroconvulsive therapy in endogenous depression: the role of electrical stimulation and of the seizure studied by variation of stimulus intensity and modification by lidocaine of seizure discharge. *Acta Psychiatrica et Neurologica Scandinavica*, **35**, 69–102.

Cronholm, B. and Ottosson, J,-O. (1963). The experience of memory function after electroconvulsive therapy. *British Journal of Psychiatry*, **109**, 251–8.

Currier, M.B., Murray, G.B., and Welch, C.C. (1992). Electroconvulsive therapy for post-stroke depressed geriatric patients. *Journal of Neuropsychiatry and Clinical Neurosciences*, **4**, 140–4.

D'Agostino, A.M. (1975). Depression: schism in contemporary psychiatry. *American Journal of Psychiatry*, **132**, 629–32.

Daniel, W.F. and Crovitz, H.F. (1986). Disorientation during electroconvulsive therapy. *Annals of the New York Academy of Sciences*, **462**, 293–306.

Davies, B. (1983). The first patient to receive lithium. *Australian and New Zealand Journal of Psychiatry*, **17**, 366–8.

De Carle, A. J. and Kohn, R. (2001). Risk factors for falling in a psychogeriatric unit. *International Journal of Geriatric Psychiatry*, **16**, 762–7.

Devanand, D.P., Dwork, A.J., Hutchinson, E.R., Bolwig, T.G., and Sackeim, H.A. (1994). Does ECT alter brain structure? *American Journal of Psychiatry*, **151**, 957–70.

Doessel, D.P., Scheurer, R.W., Chant, D.C., and Whiteford, H.A. (2006). Changes in private sector electroconvulsive treatment in Australia. *Australian and New Zealand Journal of Psychiatry*, **40**, 362–7.

Dolenc, T.J. and Rasmussen, K.G. (2005). The safety of electroconvulsive therapy and lithium in combination: a case series and review of the literature. *Journal of ECT*, **21**, 165–70.

Donahue, A.B. (2000). Electroconvulsive therapy and memory loss: a personal journey. *Journal of ECT*, **16**, 133–43.

Dowman, J., Patel, A., and Rajput, K. (2005). Electroconvulsive therapy: attitudes and misconceptions. *Journal of ECT*, **21**, 84–7.

Dubin, W.R., Jaffe, R., Roemer, R., Siegel, L., Shoyer, B., and Venditti, M.L. (1992). The efficacy and safety of maintenance ECT in geriatric patients. *Journal of the American Geriatrics Society*, **40**, 706–9.

Duffett, R. and Lelliott, P. (1998). Junior doctors' training in the theory and the practice of electroconvulsive therapy. *Journal of ECT*, **14**, 127–30.

Duncan, A.J., Ungvari, G.S., Russell, R.J., and Seifert, A. (1990). Maintenance ECT in very old age: case report. *Annals of Clinical Psychiatry*, **2**, 139–44.

Ende, G., Braus, D.F., Walter, S., Weber-Fuhr, W., and Henn, F.A. (2000). The hippocampus in patients treated with electroconvulsive therapy. *Archives of General Psychiatry*, **57**, 937–43.

Enns, M. and Karvelas, L. (1995). Electrical dose titration for electroconvulsive therapy: a comparison with dose prediction methods. *Convulsive Therapy*, **11**, 86–93.

Farah, A. and McCall, W.V. (1993). Electroconvulsive therapy stimulus dosing: a survey of contemporary practices. *Convulsive Therapy*, **9**, 90–4.

Fink, M., Abrams, R., Bailine, S., and Jaffe, R. (1996). Ambulatory electroconvulsive therapy: report of a task force of the Association for Convulsive Therapy. *Convulsive Therapy*, **12**, 42–55.

Flint, A.J. and Rifat, S.L. (1998). The treatment of psychotic depression in later life: a comparison of pharmacotherapy and ECT. *International Journal of Geriatric Psychiatry*, **13**, 23–8.

Folk, J.W., Kellner, C.H., Beale, M.D., Conroy, J.M., and Duc, T.A. (2000). Anesthesia for electroconvulsive therapy: a review. *Journal of ECT*, **16**, 157–70.

Fox, H.A. (1993). Patients' fear of and objection to electroconvulsive therapy. *Hospital and Community Psychiatry*, **44**, 357–60.

Fredman, B., d'Etienne, J., Smith, I., Husain, M.M., and White, P.F. (1994). Anesthesia for electroconvulsive therapy: effects of propofol and methohexital on seizure activity and recovery. *Anesthesia and Analgesia*, **74**, 75–9.

Freeman, C.P.L. and Kendall, R.E. (1980). I: Patients' experiences and attitudes. *British Journal of Psychiatry*, **137**, 8–16.

Freeman, C.P.L., Weeks, D., and Kendall, R.E. (1980). ECT: II: Patients who complain. *British Journal of Psychiatry*, **137**, 17–25.

Friedman, R.S., Mufson, M.J., Eisenberg, T.D., and Patel, M.R. (2003). Medically and psychiatrically ill: the challenge of delirious mania. *Harvard Review of Psychiatry*, **11**, 91–8.

Gagné, G.G., Furman, M.J., Carpenter, L.L., and Price, L.H. (2000). Efficacy of continuation ECT and antidepressant drugs compared to long-term antidepressants alone in depressed patients. *American Journal of Psychiatry*, **157**, 1960–5.

Gangadhar, B.N., Mayur, P.M., Janakiramaiah, N., Subbakrishna, D.K., and Rao, G.S.U. (2000). Cardiovascular response during ECT: a cross-over study across stimulus conditions. *Journal of ECT*, **16**, 177–82.

Gass, J.P. (1998). The knowledge and attitudes of mental health nurses to electro-convulsive therapy. *Journal of Advanced Nursing*, **27**, 83–90.

Godber, C., Rosenvinge, H., Wilkinson, D., and Smithies, J. (1987). Depression in old age: prognosis after ECT. *International Journal of Geriatric Psychiatry*, **2**, 19–24.

Gormley, N., Cullen, C., Walters, L., Philpot, M., and Lawlor, B. (1998). The safety and efficacy of electroconvulsive therapy in patients over age 75. *International Journal of Geriatric Psychiatry*, **13**, 871–4.

Grant, J.E. and Mohan, S.N. (2001). Treatment of agitation and aggression in four demented patients using ECT. *Journal of ECT*, **17**, 205–9.

Grover, S., Mattoo, S.K., and Gupta, N. (2005). Theories on mechanism of action of electroconvulsive therapy. *German Journal of Psychiatry*, **8**, 70–84.

Gujavarty, K., Greenberg, L.B., and Fink, M. (1987). Electroconvulsive therapy and neuroleptic medication in therapy-resistant positive-symptom psychosis. *Convulsive Therapy*, **3**, 185–95.

Halliday, G. and Johnson, G. (1995). Training to administer electroconvulsive therapy: a survey of attitudes and experiences. *Australian and New Zealand Journal of Psychiatry*, **29**, 133–8.

Hay, D.P. (1989). Electroconvulsive therapy in the medically ill elderly. *Convulsive Therapy*, **5**, 8–16.

Hermann, R.C., Dorwart R.A., Hoover, C.W., and Brody, J. (1995). Variation in ECT use in the United States. *American Journal of Psychiatry*, **152**, 869–75.

Hickie, I., Mason, C., Parker, G., and Brodaty, H. (1996). Prediction of ECT response: validation of a refined sign-based (CORE) system for defining melancholia. *British Journal of Psychiatry*, **169**, 68–74.

Holmberg, S.K., Tariot, P.N., and Challapalli, R. (1996). Efficacy of ECT for agitation in dementia: a case report. *American Journal of Geriatric Psychiatry*, **4**, 330–4.

Husain, M.M., Rush, A.J., Fink, M. *et al.* (2004). Speed of response and remission in major depressive disorder with acute electroconvulsive therapy. *Journal of Clinical Psychiatry*, **65**, 485–91.

Huuhka, M.J., Seinelä, L., Reinikainen, P., and Leinonen, E.V.J. (2003). Cardiac arrhythmias induced by ECT in elderly psychiatric patients: experience with 48-hour Holter monitoring. *Journal of ECT*, **19**, 22–5.

Johnstone, L. (1999). Adverse psychological effects of ECT. *Journal of Mental Health*, **8**, 69–85.

Kang, N. and Passmore, M.J. (2004). Successful ECT in a patient with an orbital cavernous hemangioma. *Journal of ECT*, **20**, 267–71.

Kant, R., Coffey, C.E., and Bogyi, A.M. (1999). Safety and efficacy of ECT in patients with head injury: a case series. *Journal of Neuropsychiatry and Clinical Neurosciences*, **11**, 32–7.

Kellner, C.H., Monroe, R.R., Pritchett, J., Jarrell, M.P., Bernstein, H.J., and Burns, C.M. (1992). Weekly ECT in geriatric depression. *Convulsive Therapy*, **8**, 245–52.

Kennedy, R., Mittal, D., and O'Jile, J. (2003). Electroconvulsive therapy in movement disorders: an update. *Journal of Neuropsychiatry and Clinical Neuroscience*, **15**, 407–21.

Kerr, R.A., McGrath, J.J., O'Kearney, R.T., and Price, J. (1982). ECT: misconceptions and attitudes. *Australian and New Zealand Journal of Psychiatry*, **16**, 43–9.

Koopowitz, L.R., Chur-Hansen, A., Reid, S., and Blashki, M. (2003). The subjective experience of patients who received electroconvulsive therapy. *Australian and New Zealand Journal of Psychiatry*, **37**, 49–54.

Kramer, B.A. (1999). ECT in elderly patients with schizophrenia. *American Journal of Geriatric Psychiatry*, **7**, 171–4.

Kriss, A., Blumhardt, L.D., Halliday, A.M., and Pratt, R.T.C. (1978). Neurological asymmetries immediately after unilateral ECT. *Journal of Neurology, Neurosurgery and Psychiatry*, **41**, 1135–44.

Krystal, A.D., Coffey, C.E., Weiner, R.D., and Holsinger, T. (1998). Changes in seizure threshold over the course of electroconvulsive therapy affect therapeutic response and are detected by ictal EEG ratings. *Journal of Neuropsychiatry and Clinical Neurosciences*, **10**, 178–86.

Lafferty, J.E., North, C.S., Spitznagel, E., and Isenberg, K. (2001). Laboratory screening prior to ECT. *Journal of ECT*, **17**, 158–65.

Lapid, M.I., Rummans, T.A., Pankratz, V.S., and Appelbaum, P.S. (2004). Decisional capacity of depressed elderly to consent to electroconvulsive therapy. *Journal of Geriatric Psychiatry and Neurology*, **17**, 42–46.

Law-Min, R. and Stephens, J.P. (2006). Capacity, compliance and electroconvulsive therapy (ECT): the practice of ECT among consultant psychiatrists. *Psychiatric Bulletin*, **30**, 13–15.

Lawson, J.S., Inglis, J., Delva, N.J., Rodenburg, M., Waldron, J.J., and Letemendia, F.J.J. (1990). Electrode placement in ECT: cognitive effects. *Psychological Medicine*, **20**, 335–44.

Legendre, S.A., Stern, R.A., Solomon, D.A., Furman, M.J., and Smith, K.E. (2003). The influence of cognitive reserve on memory following electroconvulsive therapy. *Journal of Neuropsychiatry and Clinical Neurosciences*, **15**, 333–9.

Lisanby, S.H., Maddox, J.H., Prudic, J., Devanand, D.P., and Sackeim, H.A. (2000). The effects of electroconvulsive therapy on memory of autobiographical and public events. *Archives of General Psychiatry*, **57**, 581–90.

Little, J.D., Atkins, M.R., Munday, J. *et al.* (2004). Bifrontal electroconvulsive therapy in the elderly: a 2-year retrospective. *Journal of ECT*, **20**, 139–41.

Little, J.D., McFarlane, J., Barton, D., and Varma, S.L. (2002). Australian and US responses to electroconvulsive therapy dosage selection. *Australian and New Zealand Journal of Psychiatry*, **36**, 629–32.

Loo, H., Galinowski, A., de Carvalho, W., Bourdel, M.C., and Poirier, M.F. (1991). Use of maintenance ECT for elderly depressed patients. *American Journal of Psychiatry*, **148**, 810.

Magid, M., Lapid, M.I., Sampson, S.M., and Mueller, P.S. (2005). Use of electroconvulsive therapy in a patient 10 days after myocardial infarction. *Journal of ECT*, **21**, 182–5.

Malcolm, K. (1989). Patients' perceptions and knowledge of electroconvulsive therapy. *Psychiatric Bulletin*, **13**, 161–5.

Manly, D.T., Oakley, S.P., and Bloch, R.M. (2000). Electroconvulsive therapy in old-old patients. *American Journal of Geriatric Psychiatry*, **8**, 232–6.

McAllister, D.A., Perri, M.G., Jordan, R.C., Rauscher, F.P., and Sattin, A. (1987). Effects of ECT given two versus three times weekly. *Psychiatry Research*, **21**, 63–9.

McCall, W.V. (2006). Refusal versus reluctance. *Journal of ECT*, **22**, 89–90.

McCall, W.V., Reid, S., and Ford, M. (1994). Electrocardiographic and cardiovascular effects of subconvulsive stimulation during titrated right unilateral ECT. *Convulsive Therapy*, **10**, 25–33.

McCall, W.V., Farah, B.A., Reboussin, D., and Colenda, C.C. (1995). Comparison of the efficacy of titrated, moderate-dose and fixed, high-dose right unilateral ECT in elderly patients. *American Journal of Geriatric Psychiatry*, **3**, 317–24.

McCall, W.V., Dunn, A., Rosenquist, P.B., and Hughes, D. (2002). Markedly suprathreshold right unilateral ECT versus minimally suprathreshold bilateral ECT: antidepressant and memory effects. *Journal of ECT*, **18**, 126–9.

McDonald, W.M. and Thompson, T.R. (2001). Treatment of mania in dementia with electroconvulsive therapy. *Psychopharmacology Bulletin*, **35**, 72–82.

McElhiney, M.C., Moody, B.J., Steif, B.L. *et al.* (1995). Autobiographical memory and mood: effects of electroconvulsive therapy. *Neuropsychology*, **9**, 501–17.

Medical Research Council (1965). Clinical trial of the treatment of depressive illness. *British Medical Journal*, **1**, 881–6.

Michael, N., Erfurth, A., Ohrmann, P., Arolt, V., Heindel, W., and Pfleiderer, B. (2003). Metabolic changes within the left dorsolateral prefrontal cortex occurring with electroconvulsive therapy in patients with treatment resistant unipolar depression. *Psychological Medicine*, **33**, 1277–84.

Mondimore, F.M., Damlouji, N., Folstein, M.F., and Tune, L. (1983). Post-ECT confusional states associated with elevated serum anticholinergic levels. *American Journal of Psychiatry*, **140**, 930–1.

Mukherjee, S., Sackeim, H.A., and Lee, C. (1988). Unilateral ECT in the treatment of manic episodes. *Convulsive Therapy*, **4**, 74–80.

Mulsant, B.H., Rosen, J., Thornton, J.E., and Zubenko, G.S. (1991). A prospective naturalistic study of electroconvulsive therapy in late-life depression. *Journal of Geriatric Psychiatry and Neurology*, **4**, 3–13.

Munk-Olsen, T., Laursen, T.M., Videbech, P., Rosenberg, R., and Mortensen, P.B. (2006). Electroconvulsive therapy: predictors and trends in utilization from 1976 to 2000. *Journal of ECT*, **22**, 127–32.

National Institute for Clinical Excellence (2003). *Guidance on the use of electroconvulsive therapy*. NICE, London.

Nelson, J.P. and Rosenberg, D.R. (1991). ECT treatment of demented elderly patients with major depression: a retrospective study of efficacy and safety. *Convulsive Therapy*, **7**, 157–65.

Ng, C., Schweitzer, I., Alexopoulus, P. *et al.* (2000). Efficacy and cognitive effects of right unilateral electroconvulsive therapy. *Journal of ECT*, **16**, 370–9.

Nobler, M.S., Sackeim, H.A., Solomou, M., Luber, B., Devanand, D.P., and Prudic, J. (1993). EEG manifestations during ECT: effects of electrode placement and stimulus intensity. *Biological Psychiatry*, **34**, 321–30.

Nobler, M.S., Sackeim, H.A., Prohovnik, I. *et al.* (1994). Regional cerebral blood flow in mood disorders, III: treatment and clinical response. *Archives of General Psychiatry*, **51**, 884–97.

Nuttall, G.A., Bowersox, M.R., Douglass, S.B. *et al.* (2004). Morbidity and mortality in the use of electroconvulsive therapy. *Journal of ECT*, **20**, 237–41.

O'Connor, D.W., Pollitt, P.A., and Roth, M. (1990). Coexisting depression and dementia in a community survey of the elderly. *International Psychogeriatrics*, **2**, 45–53.

O'Connor, M.K., Knapp, R., Husain, M. *et al.* (2001). The influence of age on the response of major depression to electroconvulsive therapy. *American Journal of Geriatric Psychiatry*, **9**, 382–90.

O'Leary, D., Gill, D., Gregory, S., and Shawcross, C. (1994). The effectiveness of real versus simulated electroconvulsive therapy in depressed elderly patients. *International Journal of Geriatric Psychiatry*, **9**, 567–71.

Olfson, M., Marcus, S., Sackeim, H.A., Thompson, J., and Pincus, H.A. (1998). Use of ECT for the inpatient treatment of recurrent major depression. *American Journal of Psychiatry*, **155**, 22–9.

Parvin, M.H., Swartz, C., and LaMontagne, B. (2004). Patient education by electroconvulsive therapy-experienced volunteer. *Journal of ECT*, **20**, 127–9.

Penney, J.F., Dinwiddie, S.H., Zorumski, C.F., and Wetzel, R.D. (1990). Concurrent and close temporal administration of lithium and ECT. *Convulsive Therapy*, **6**, 139–45.

Perera, T.D., Luber, B., Nobler, M.S., Prudic, J., Anderson, C., and Sackeim, H.A. (2004). Seizure expression during electroconvulsive therapy: relationships with clinical outcome and cognitive side effects. *Neuropsychopharmacology*, **29**, 813–25.

Petrides, G. and Fink, M. (1996). The 'half-age' stimulation strategy for ECT dosing. *Convulsive Therapy*, **12**, 138–46.

Petrides, G., Fink, M., Husain, M.M. *et al.* (2001). ECT remission rates in psychotic versus nonpsychotic depressed patients: a report from CORE. *Journal of ECT*, **17**, 244–53.

Pettinati, H.M., Stephens, S.M., Willis, K.M., and Robin, S.E. (1990). Evidence for less improvement in patients taking benzodiazepines during unilateral ECT. *American Journal of Psychiatry*, **147**, 1029–35.

Pettinati, H.M., Tamburello, T.A., Ruetsch, C.R., and Kaplan, F.N. (1994). Patient attitudes toward electroconvulsive therapy. *Psychopharmacology Bulletin*, **30**, 471–5.

Philpot, M., Collins, C., Trivedi, P., Treloar A., Gallacher, S., and Rose, D. (2004). Eliciting users' views of ECT in two mental health trusts with a user-designed questionnaire. *Journal of Mental Health*, **13**, 403–13.

Pippard, J. (1992). Audit of electroconvulsive treatment in two National Health Service Regions. *British Journal of Psychiatry*, **160**, 621–37.

Porquez, J.M., Thompson, T.R., and McDonald, W.M. (2003). Administration of ECT in a patient with an inoperable abdominal aortic aneurysm: serial imaging of the aorta during maintenance. *Journal of ECT*, **19**, 118–20.

Price, T.R.P. and McAllister, T.W. (1989). Safety and efficacy of ECT in depressed patients with dementia: a review of clinical experience. *Convulsive Therapy*, **5**, 61–74.

Prudic, J., Sackeim, H.A., and Devanand, D.P. (1990). Medication resistance and clinical response to electroconvulsive therapy. *Psychiatry Research*, **31**, 287–96.

Prudic, J., Peyser, S., and Sackeim, H.A. (2000). Subjective memory complaints: a review of patient self-assessment of memory after electroconvulsive therapy. *Journal of ECT*, **16**, 121–32.

Prudic, J., Olfson, M., Marcus, S.C., Fuller, R.B., and Sackeim, H.A. (2004). Effectiveness of electroconvulsive therapy in community settings. *Biological Psychiatry*, **55**, 301–12.

Prudic, J., Olfson, M., and Sackeim, H.A. (2001). Electro-convulsive therapy practices in the community. *Psychological Medicine*, **31**, 929–34.

Rami, L., Bernardo, M., Boget, T. *et al.* (2004). Cognitive status of psychiatric patients under maintenance electroconvulsive therapy: a one-year longitudinal study. *Journal of Neuropsychiatry and Clinical Neurosciences*, **16**, 465–71.

Ranen, N.G., Peyser, C.E., and Folstein, S.E. (1994). ECT as a treatment of depression in Huntington's disease. *Journal of Neuropsychiatry and Clinical Neurosciences*, **6**, 154–9.

Ranjkesh, F., Barekatain, M., and Akuchakian, S. (2005). Bifrontal versus right unilateral and bitemporal electroconvulsive therapy in major depressive disorder. *Journal of ECT*, **21**, 207–10.

Rao, V. and Lyketsos, C.G. (2000). The benefits and risks of ECT for patients with primary dementia who also suffer from depression. *International Journal of Geriatric Psychiatry*, **15**, 729–35.

Rasmussen, K.G., Russell, J.C., Kung, P.A., Rummans, T.A., Rae-Stuart, E., and O'Connor, M.K. (2003). Electroconvulsive therapy for patients with major depression and probable Lewy body dementia. *Journal of ECT*, **19**, 103–9.

Regestein, Q.R. and Reich, P. (1985). Electroconvulsive therapy in patients at high risk for physical complications. *Convulsive Therapy*, **1**, 101–14.

Rose, D., Wykes, T., Leese, M., Bindman, J., and Fleischmann, P. (2003). Patients' perspectives on electroconvulsive therapy: systematic review. *British Medical Journal*, **326**, 1363.

Rosenbach, M.L., Hermann, R.C., and Dorwart, R.A. (1997). Use of electroconvulsive therapy in the Medicare population between 1987 and 1992. *Psychiatric Services*, **48**, 1537–42.

Rosenquist, P.B., Dunn, A., Rapp, S., Gaba, A., and McCall, W.V. (2006). What predicts patients' expressed likelihood of choosing electroconvulsive therapy as a future treatment option. *Journal of ECT*, **22**, 33–7.

Royal Australian and New Zealand College of Psychiatrists (2005). *Electroconvulsive therapy: clinical memorandum 12*. Royal Australian and New Zealand College of Psychiatrists, Melbourne.

Royal College of Psychiatrists (2005). *The ECT handbook*, 2nd edn (ed. A.I.F. Scott). Royal College of Psychiatrists, London.

Royal College of Psychiatrists' Research Unit (2005). *Standards for the administration of ECT*. Royal College of Psychiatrists Research Unit, London.

Rubin, E.H., Kinscherf, D.A., Figiel, G.S., and Zorumski, C.F. (1993). The nature and time course of cognitive side effects during electroconvulsive therapy in the elderly. *Journal of Geriatric Psychiatry and Neurology*, **6**, 78–83.

Russ, M.J., Ackerman, S.H., Burton, L., and Shindledecker, R.D. (1990). Cognitive effects of ECT in the elderly: preliminary findings. *International Journal of Geriatric Psychiatry*, **5**, 115–18.

Russell, J.C., Rasmussen, K.G., O'Connor, M.K., Copeman, C.A., Ryan, D.A., and Rummans, T.A. (2003). Long-term maintenance ECT: a retrospective review of efficacy and cognitive outcome. *Journal of ECT*, **19**, 4–9.

Sackeim, H.A. (2000). Memory and ECT: from polarisation to reconciliation. *Journal of ECT*, **16**, 87–96.

Sackeim, H., Decina, P., Prohovnik, I., and Malitz, S. (1987). Seizure threshold in electroconvulsive therapy: effects of sex, age, electrode placement, and number of treatments. *Archives of General Psychiatry*, **44**, 355–60.

Sackeim, H.A., Prudic, J., Devanand, D.P. *et al.* (1993). Effects of stimulus intensity and electrode placement on the efficacy and cognitive effects of electroconvulsive therapy. *New England Journal of Medicine*, **328**, 839–46.

Sackeim, H.A., Luber, B., Katzman, G.P. *et al.* (1996). The effects of electroconvulsive therapy on quantitative electroencephalograms: relationship to clinical outcome. *Archives of General Psychiatry*, **53**, 814–24.

Sackeim, H.A., Prudic, J., Devanand, D.P. *et al.* (2000). A prospective, randomized, double-blind comparison of bilateral and right unilateral electroconvulsive therapy at different stimulus intensities. *Archives of General Psychiatry*, **57**, 425–34.

Sackeim, H.A., Haskett, R.F., Mulsant, B.H. *et al.* (2001). Continuation pharmacotherapy in the prevention of relapse following electroconvulsive therapy: a randomized controlled trial. *Journal of the American Medical Association*, **285**, 1299–307.

Salamero, M. (2004). Cognitive status of psychiatric patients under maintenance electroconvulsive therapy: a one-year longitudinal study. *Journal of Neuropsychiatry and Clinical Neurosciences*, **16**, 465–71.

Sartorius, A., Wolf, J., and Henn, F.A. (2005). Lithium and ECT – concurrent use still demands attention: three case reports. *World Journal of Biological Psychiatry*, **6**, 121–4.

Schwarz, T., Loewenstein, J., and Isenberg, K.E. (1995). Maintenance ECT: indications and outcome. *Convulsive Therapy*, **11**, 14–23.

Shapira, B., Lidsky, D., Gorfine, M., and Lerer, B. (1996). Electroconvulsive therapy and resistant depression: clinical implications of seizure threshold. *Journal of Clinical Psychiatry*, **57**, 32–8.

Shapira, B., Tubi, N., Drexler, N.T., Lidsky, D., Calev, A., and Lerer, B. (1998). Cost and benefit in the choice of ECT schedule: twice versus three times weekly ECT. *British Journal of Psychiatry*, **172**, 44–8.

Shiwach, R.S., Reid, W.H., and Carmody, T.J. (2001). An analysis of reported deaths following electroconvulsive therapy in Texas, 1993–1998. *Psychiatric Services*, **52**, 1095–7.

Sienaert, P., de Becker, T., Vansteelandt, K., Demyttenaere, K., and Peuskens, J. (2005). Patient satisfaction after electroconvulsive therapy. *Journal of ECT*, **21**, 227–31.

Small, J.G., Klapper, M.H., Kellams, J.J. *et al.* (1988). Electroconvulsive therapy compared with lithium in the management of manic states. *Archives of General Psychiatry*, **45**, 727–32.

Sobin, C., Sackeim, H.A., Prudic, J., Devanand, D.P., Moody, B.J., and McElhiney, M.C. (1995). Predictors of retrograde amnesia following ECT. *American Journal of Psychiatry*, **152**, 995–1001.

Sonavane, S., Borade, S., Gajbhiye, S., Shah, N., and Andrade, C. (2006). Cortical blindness associated with electroconvulsive therapy. *Journal of ECT*, **22**, 155–7.

Squire, L.R. and Slater, P.C. (1983). Electroconvulsive therapy and complaints of memory dysfunction: a prospective three-year follow-up study. *British Journal of Psychiatry*, **142**, 1–8.

Srzich, A. and Turbott, J. (2000). Nonconvulsive generalised status epilepticus following electroconvulsive therapy. *Australian and New Zealand Journal of Psychiatry*, **34**, 334–6.

Steffens, D.C., Conway, C.R., Dombeck, C.B., Wagner, H.R., Tupler, L.A., and Weiner, R.D. (2001). Severity of subcortical gray matter hyperintensity predicts ECT response in geriatric depression. *Journal of ECT*, **17**, 45–9.

Tew, J.D., Mulsant, B.H., Haskett, R.F. *et al.* (1999). Acute efficacy of ECT in the treatment of major depression in the old-old. *American Journal of Psychiatry*, **156**, 1865–70.

Thienhaus, O.J., Margletta, S., and Bennett, J.A. (1990). A study of the clinical efficacy of maintenance ECT. *Journal of Clinical Psychiatry*, **51**, 141–4.

Thornton, J.E., Mulsant, B.H., Dealy, R., and Reynolds, C.F. (1990). A retrospective study of maintenance electroconvulsive therapy in a university-based psychiatric practice. *Convulsive Therapy*, **6**, 121–9.

Tiller, J.W.G. and Ingram, N. (2006). Seizure threshold determination for electroconvulsive therapy: stimulus dose titration versus age-based estimations. *Australian and New Zealand Journal of Psychiatry*, **40**, 188–92.

Tiller, J.W.G. and Lyndon, R.W. (2003). *Electroconvulsive therapy: an Australasian guide*. Australian Postgraduate Foundation, Victoria.

Tomac, T.A., Rummans, T.A., Pileggi, T.S., and Li, H. (1997). Safety and efficacy of electroconvulsive therapy in patients over age 85. *American Journal of Geriatric Psychiatry*, **5**, 126–30.

Troller, J.N. and Sachdev, P.S. (1999). Electroconvulsive treatment of neuroleptic malignant syndrome: a review and report of cases. *Australian and New Zealand Journal of Psychiatry*, **33**, 650–9.

UK ECT Review Group (2003). Efficacy and safety of electroconvulsive therapy in depressive disorders: a systematic review and meta-analysis. *Lancet*, **361**, 799–808.

Van der Wurff, F.B., Stek, M.L., Hoogendijk, W.J.G., and Beekman, A.T.F. (2004). Discrepancy between opinion and attitude on the practice of ECT by psychiatrists specializing in old age in the Netherlands. *Journal of ECT*, **20**, 37–41.

Vanelle, J-M., Loo, H., Galinowski, A. *et al.* (1994). Maintenance ECT in intractable manic-depressive disorders. *Convulsive Therapy*, **10**, 195–205.

Van Waarde, J.A., Stolker, J.J., and van der Mast, R.C. (2001). ECT in mental retardation: a review. *Journal of ECT*, **17**, 236–43.

Wesson, M.L., Wilkinson, A.M., Anderson, D.N., and McCracken, C. (1997). Does age predict the long-term outcome of depression treated with ECT? *International Journal of Geriatric Psychiatry*, **12**, 45–51.

Westreich, L., Levine, S., Ginsburg, P., and Wilets, I. (1995). Patient knowledge about electroconvulsive therapy: effect of an informational video. *Convulsive Therapy*, **11**, 32–7.

Wheeldon, T.J., Robertson, C., Eagles, J.M., and Reid, I.C. (1999). The views and outcomes of consenting and non-consenting patients receiving ECT. *Psychological Medicine*, **29**, 221–3.

Wilkinson, A.M., Anderson, D.N., and Peters, S. (1993). Age and the effects of ECT. *International Journal of Geriatric Psychiatry*, **8**, 401–6.

Wood, D.A. and Burgess, P.M. (2003). Epidemiological analysis of electroconvulsive therapy in Victoria, Australia. *Australian and New Zealand Journal of Psychiatry*, **37**, 307–11.

Zervas, I.M., Calev, A., Jandorf, L. *et al.* (1993). Age-dependent effects of electroconvulsive therapy on memory. *Convulsive Therapy*, **9**, 39–42.

Zielinski, R.J., Roose, S.P., Devanand, D.P., Woodring, S., and Sackeim, H.A. (1993). Cardiovascular complications of ECT in depressed patients with cardiac disease. *American Journal of Psychiatry*, **150**, 904–9.

# 16

# Social work, older people, and mental health

Kathleen Bailey, Fay Brown, and Lorna Wilson

## Introduction

The role of social work with older people is continually changing. In this chapter we aim to give an overview of some of the current roles and responsibilities of social workers who work with older people with mental health needs, including people with pre-senile dementia. Since the introduction of the Care Standards Act 2000 (CSA 2000), social workers in the UK have been regulated and registered by the General Social Care Council (GSCC). The intention of the CSA 2000, set out in its codes of practice, was to create basic standards and shared values of social care, to promote development and training for workers in this field, and to provide a general process of protection for clients, their carers, and the general public.

As social workers we are trained to adhere to social work values, which include respecting diversity and promoting independence, empowerment, and the rights of the individual. However, these values are often in conflict with our social work duties as employees, governed by the policies and procedures of Local Authorities (LAs), which carry responsibility for social services. In some cases this involves challenging the limited availability of provision, and we often struggle to be creative in providing support for our clients and their carers.

Health care in the UK National Health Service (NHS) is free at the point of contact, unlike social care which often levies charges for services after assessment. Administering a service that is charged for can create practical and ethical dilemmas for the social worker, and some of these will be illustrated in the case studies that follow.

This chapter explores the impact of current legislation on older people, specifically those with mental health needs. We will also cover the care management process, delayed discharges, the varieties of service provision, out of hours services, and risk assessment.

## Legislation and social work

There is a plethora of legislation which covers the different elements of our work, but here we will look specifically at the application of the law to older people with mental health needs. (A thorough history of the law relating to social work practice may be found in Brammer (2003) and in Brayne and Carr (2003).) In this section we consider: The NHS and Community Care Act (NHS & CCA) 1990; The Mental Health Act (MHA) 1983; The National Assistance Act (NNA) 1948; The Human Rights Act (HRA) 1998; and The Mental Capacity Act (MCA) 2005.

### The NHS and Community Care Act 1990

Working with the law in relation to older people is like living in an old house that constantly needs repair and upgrading. New bits are forever being added but the house owner has to be mindful to check on what work has been put in place previously.

The NHS & CCA 1990 was introduced to collect together different legislation relating to vulnerable people in the community. Rather than replacing what had come before, it put into law a requirement to assess an individual's needs whilst being mindful of previous legislation. In practice this means assessment of a client's social, financial, physical, and mental health needs, with an emphasis on enabling clients to remain in their own home with a care plan that can address those needs, using a mixed economy of care. The 'mixed economy' means the local authorities, other statutory agencies including the NHS and housing agencies, and the voluntary and private sector. Recent years have seen the recognition of informal carers such as partners, families, and friends of the clients as providers of services.

With the information derived from the assessment, social workers have a number of options: to provide ongoing support and input, to introduce a range of services, or to refer to another agency to take the lead. Where clients are able to contribute financially to their own care there may be little or no social services input. Others, for reasons either of capacity or income, will have care packages arranged for them by social services. As people are living longer and their needs become more complex, the range of services required for them has changed. The manager of an older persons' care home commented to the director of social services that at one time their car park was filled with the cars of the residents; now it is filled with the cars of the people who work there.

### The Mental Health Act 1983

The MHA 1983 is used for patients with mental health needs who may require compulsory detention into hospital for assessment and/or treatment; or as a legal framework to support a treatment plan in the community (Table 16.1). It is primary legislation and

**Table 16.1** Detention from the community under the MHA 1983

| Section number and purpose | Maximum duration | Can patient apply to MHRT? | Can nearest relative apply to MHRT? | Will there be an automatic MHRT hearing? | Do consent to treatment rules apply? |
|---|---|---|---|---|---|
| 2: Admission for assessment | 28 days. Not renewable | Within first 14 days | No: section 23 gives them power to discharge, but see section 25 below | No | Yes |
| 3: Admission for treatment | 6 months. May be renewed for 6 months and then yearly | Within first 6 months and then in each period | No: section 23 gives them power to discharge, but see section 25 below | If one has not been held, the hospital managers refer to MHRT at 6 months and then every 3 years | Yes |
| 4: Admission for assessment in an emergency | 72 hours. Not renewable but 2nd doctor can change to section 2 | Yes. But only relevant if section 4 is converted to a section 2 | No | No | No |
| 5(2): Doctor's holding power | 72 hours. Not renewable | No | No | No | No |
| 5(4): Nurse's holding power | 6 hours. Not renewable but doctor can change to section 5(2) | No | No | No | No |
| 7: Reception into guardianship | 6 months. May be renewed for 6 months and then yearly | Within first 6 months and then in each period | No: section 23 gives them power to discharge | No | No |
| 16: Doctor reclassifies the mental disorder | For the duration of the detention | Within 28 days of being informed | Within 28 days of being informed | No | |
| 19: Transfer from guardianship to hospital | 6 months. May be renewed for 6 months and then yearly | In the first 6 months of detention and then in each period | No: section 23 gives them power to discharge, but see section 25 below | If one has not been held, the hospital managers refer to MHRT at 6 months and then every 3 years | Yes |
| 25: Restriction of discharge by nearest relative | Variable | No | Within 28 days of being informed. (No appeal if section 2) | No | |
| 29: Appointment of acting nearest relative by court | Variable | No | Within 1 year and then yearly | No | |
| 135: Warrant to search for and remove patient | 72 hours. Not renewable | No | No | No | No |
| 136: Police power in public places | 72 hours. Not renewable | No | No | No | No |

Source: Brown (2006).

can be used in the face of contradictory legislation such as the Human Rights Act 1998. However, these challenges to the MHA 1983 are recognized within the Act's Code of Practice (1999), which requires the recognition of patients' human rights as stipulated under the European Convention of Human Rights (ECHR). Therefore, a decision to use the MHA 1983 must demonstrate that the use of the mental health legislation avoided a greater harm.

Part I of the MHA 1983 clarifies the people who are covered within this legislation, who are referred to as patients. Part II covers compulsory admission to hospital and guardianship. It also specifies who is given responsibility for using the Act—doctors, the nearest relative (NR), and an approved social worker (ASW). Part V of the Act sets out the functions of the Mental Health Review Tribunal (MHRT).

The responsible medical officer (RMO), the doctor who has responsibility for a patient's treatment under the MHA, is referred to under section 34.

The NR (unlike the 'next of kin') is a person prescribed by the law, under section 26 of MHA1983. The professionals involved need to identify the correct NR, who has legal rights which can include making an application under the MHA, being informed that an application has been made, objecting to an application, and challenging the detention. Therefore, when background information is obtained about a patient, it is important for this to include their social circumstances, their relationships, and their family. There are arguments for changing the legally defined NR, who may not necessarily be suitable or likely to act in the patient's best interests (R. (on the application of E.) v Bristol City Council [2005]).

If there are concerns about the nearest relative objecting inappropriately to the use of the MHA, section 29 can be used to displace a NR. The grounds for doing so include the NR objecting unreasonably to the making of an application, or exercising their rights without due regard to the welfare of the patient or the public.

## Case study 1

Mrs Jacob, an 88-year-old woman with vascular dementia, living with her youngest daughter Eleanor, was admitted to a general hospital following a fall and had a hip replacement operation. Concerns were raised about her daughter's ability to care for her mother, as on admission Mrs Jacob had appeared physically neglected and unwashed, with dirty clothes and smelling strongly of urine. A home visit to plan for Mrs Jacob's discharge revealed a home that was cluttered and unsuitable in its current state, with a bathroom upstairs that Mrs Jacobs had been unable to reach. Eleanor was keen for her mother to return home but was unwilling to accept the support (equipment and a care package) that would be needed. On the ward, Eleanor was resistant to anyone being involved in her mother's care and would shout at her when visiting; and the staff noticed that Mrs Jacob became agitated when her daughter visited. Following an incident where Eleanor took her mother for a walk in the hospital grounds and was witnessed striking her, a multidisciplinary meeting, including an ASW and psychiatrist, was arranged. A nursing home placement was considered, to which Mrs Jacob agreed but her daughter objected. It was felt that Guardianship under the MHA should be used to support the placement. Eleanor was the NR as she was the person living with her mother providing daily care (her older sister had emigrated to Canada so could not be the NR). At a court hearing instigated by the ASW, Eleanor was displaced as the NR on the grounds that she was acting unreasonably and in a contradictory way to what the patient wanted, and Mrs Jacob moved into a nursing home. It later transpired that Eleanor had developed Pick's disease and eventually she moved into the same home as her mother.

ASWs are defined in section 145, and their duties outlined in section 13, of the MHA 1983 (Box 16.1).

The Code of Practice (1999) provides good practice guidance on how the law should be applied. In the introduction it states:

> The act does not impose a legal duty to comply with the code but as it is a statutory document, failure to follow it could be referred to in evidence in legal proceedings.

The role of the ASW is subject to review under the government agenda to amend current mental health legislation, and it is envisaged that this role will be extended to other professionals in the field of mental health. They will be known as 'approved mental health professionals' (AMHP). The role of the NR is also being revisited to recognize the changes in case law and the existence of civil partnerships (Civil Partnership Act 2005). There have been a number of documents on the key changes being proposed by the government, including plans to cover the 'Bournewood gap' (see below).

## Guardianship: section 7, MHA 1983

Guardianship is referred to in sections 7–10 of the MHA1983. Unlike other detentions in this part of the act, guardianship is about maintaining a patient in the community rather than being admitted to hospital.

> Code of Practice13.1—The purpose of guardianship is to enable patients to receive care in the community where it cannot be provided without the use of compulsory powers. It provides an authoritative framework for working with a patient, with a minimum of constraint, to achieve as independent a life as possible within the community.

---

**Box 16.1** Duty of approved social workers to make applications for admission or guardianship

13(1) It shall be the duty of an approved social worker to make an application for admission to hospital or a guardianship application in respect of a patient within the area of the local social services authority by which that officer is appointed in any case where he is satisfied that such an application ought to be made and is of the opinion, having regard to any wishes expressed by relatives of the patient or any other relevant circumstances, that it is necessary or proper for the application to be made by him.

13(2) Before making an application for the admission of a patient to hospital an approved social worker shall interview the patient in a suitable manner and satisfy himself that detention in a hospital is in all the circumstances of the case the most appropriate way of providing the care and medical treatment of which the patient stands in need.

13(3) An application under this section by an approved social worker may be made outside the area of the local social services authority by which he is appointed.

13(4) It shall be the duty of a local social services authority, if so required by the nearest relative of a patient residing in their area, to direct an approved social worker as soon as practicable to take the patient's case into consideration under subsection (1) above with a view to making an application for his admission to hospital; and if in any such case that approved social worker decides not to make an application he shall inform the nearest relative of his reasons in writing.

13(5) Nothing in this section shall be construed as authorising or requiring an application to be made by an approved social worker in contravention of the provisions of section11(4) above, or as restricting the power of an approved social worker to make any application under this Act.

---

Where it is used it must be part of the patient's overall care and treatment.

The guardianship application is addressed to the social services department; the guardian can be either social services or a person who (with the agreement of their local authority social services department) is willing to take on this role.

It provides a legal structure to support a patient who meets the criteria of the MHA so that they can receive the care they require. It is often considered for patients with an organic disorder such as dementia, but has also been successfully applied with patients with other types of mental disorders such as schizophrenia. Brenda Hoggett (1996) wrote:

> …guardianship is without teeth. There is no sanction (other than recapture) for disobeying any of the guardian's instructions …Some people, however may respond to apparent authority however toothless in fact it may be.

The powers of guardianship can be referred to as the three As:

♦ Accommodation—determining where a patient may reside, such as their own home or a care home.

- Activity—the power to require the patient to attend specified places for medical treatment, occupation, education, or training. This can include day care and outpatient appointments.
- Access—professionals involved in the client's care being granted access to the patient.

### Case study 2

Mr James was a gentleman in his late sixties with a history since his twenties of schizophrenia and of not engaging with services. He was known to hoard items of food and had been non-compliant with medication for many years. His family initiated a MHA assessment as he was denying them access to see him, and he was detained into hospital under section 2 of the MHA 1983. Discharge planning was focused on Mr James returning to his home address and on ensuring that he could continue to receive the care he needed. He agreed to the use of guardianship as he did not see it as forcing him to comply with something he disagreed with. Therefore, in relation to the three As: Accommodation—he remained in his own home; Access—the GP visited him weekly, he received a home care package and the social worker also provided regular monitoring and support; and Activity—he attended day care three times per week.

Although guardianship does not give powers to oblige an unwilling patient to take medication, this patient was influenced to do so as he had agreed to the legal framework the guardianship provided.

The concern for ASWs and social workers has always arisen around the patient's capacity to recognize the authority of the guardian. Paragraph 13.6 of the Code of Practice refers to the key elements of the care plan to include

> depending on the patient's level of "capacity", his or her recognition of the 'authority' of, and willingness to work with the guardian…

However in the revised Code of Practice (1999), it states

> …the guardian should be willing to advocate on behalf of the patient in relation to those agencies whose services are needed to carry out the care plan.

Therefore, limited capacity in a patient should not been seen as a reason not to use guardianship. The Human Rights Act 1998, Article 8 (the right to home and family life) and Article 5 (the right to liberty) are relevant to the use of guardianship; an application must demonstrate that it is in the interests of the patient to override these rights.

### Case study 3

Lurline, an 86-year-old woman with a progressive dementia lived with her daughter, who was physically disabled and known to misuse alcohol. The daughter had difficulties managing her own and her mother's daily needs and was unable to provide supervision for her. Following incidents of wandering, Lurline was detained in hospital under section 2 of the MHA 1983. She recognized that her daughter could not manage and felt she would receive more support in a care home. In a multidisciplinary meeting the psychiatric team and the social worker discussed the benefits of using the law to support Lurline's welfare. Guardianship was discussed and its use agreed, as the patient wanted to go into a home but lacked the capacity to make an independent decision and her daughter was inconsistent in her response to this decision.

### Section 117 aftercare

The law states that patients detained under sections 3, 37, 45A, 47, or 48 are to have aftercare services provided under section 117. It places a specific duty on health and social services authorities, with the cooperation of voluntary and private agencies to provide community care services to these patients. Chapter 27 of the Code of Practice also relates to the application of this section. There is no duty to charge patients for this service and thus many older people who have been detained under section 3 receive services in the community, such as care home placements, without charge. There is no government funding earmarked for aftercare under section 117 and this has meant that patients are funded from existing resources. Many local authorities limit the choice of resources available under section 117, using the same criteria as for services provided under the NHS & CCA: for example using pre-purchased beds in homes where they have block contracts.

### Practicalities of the use of the MHA 1983 with older people

There are some practical limitations to the use of the MHA with older people, particularly those with cognitive impairment: there is 'no middle ground' in the legislation that applies to work with people who are vulnerable and subject to risks while they live at home, but who do not fulfil the criteria for detention under the Act. It is not always possible to ensure that a client will accept the care that they are thought to need. Nevertheless, a formal assessment (whether or not it results in detention) under the MHA 1983 can be useful in such situations, where services have been unsuccessful in engaging with clients and all other options have been exhausted. The assessment can serve to relieve the anxiety of informal and professional carers, when risks are acknowledged and shared, ideas are exchanged, and a plan is arrived at to manage the risks as far as is possible.

Such an assessment (with two doctors and an ASW) may sometimes lead to the recognition of physical illnesses which can be treated in the community or lead to general hospital admission without use of the MHA 1983.

Alternatively, when assessment leads to admission of such a patient, the experience of receiving care from a skilled and professional team may reconcile them to the offer of care (in their own home or elsewhere) that they would formerly have refused.

An interesting group of people, exemplified by the 'Bournewood case', are those patients who are admitted informally to hospital, when their capacity to consent to the admission or to challenge it is in question.

> the Mental Health Act Commission (MHAC) describes this as 'de facto detention': the older person has no practical means of exercising his/her theoretical right to leave hospital, yet they have not been sectioned under the Act and so do not have the rights of a detained patient.

(http://www.scie.org.uk)

### Case study 4

Mr Peacock, 78 years old, has a progressive dementia and limited capacity. He is well known to the psychiatric team and has been admitted informally to a psychiatric unit to assess his nocturnal wandering and review his medication. His wife (his main carer) wants him to return home but cannot cope with the sleep deprivation caused by his wandering. Mr Peacock initially accepted being on the ward, but now he is continuingly trying to leave the building, asking staff to let him out, and standing by the front door and trying to escape. As Mr Peacock lacks capacity to consent, a MHA assessment is convened to consider whether the Act should be used to formalize his hospital stay.

In the Bournewood case, (R. v Bournewood Community and Mental Health NHS Trust Ex P.L. [1998] 3 All E.R. 289), HL, a gentleman with a learning disability, was taken into hospital and remained there as an informal patient, despite the wishes of his carers on his behalf. HL's case, and the question as to whether he had been illegally detained by the hospital, progressed through the UK courts up to the House of Lords, and finally reached the European Court of Human Rights. The judgement of the Court focused on the meanings of 'deprivation' and 'restriction' of liberty, and on the absence of procedural safeguards in UK law for patients in HL's situation. This is explored in greater detail by Jones (2006, paragraph 1–1178).

### The National Assistance Act (NAA) 1948, section 47

Section 47 of the NAA 1948 enables a community physician to apply to the magistrate's court for an order to remove to hospital an older or vulnerable person who is living in a state of neglect or squalor, or is not deemed to be receiving the care they need. Unlike the MHA 1983, it is not restricted to use with people who are experiencing a mental disorder, but it provides no legal safeguards for the patient and it is rarely used.

### The Human Rights Act (HRA) 1998

The Human Rights Act 1998 came into effect on 2 October 2000. It incorporated into UK law the articles listed under schedule 1 of the Act (see Table 16.2). When the HRA 1998 was introduced in the UK, it was recognized that there would be incompatibilities with existing legislation. The Code of Practice to the MHA 1983 (1999), recognizes the HRA 1998 as a guiding principle, subject to restrictions. A patient who wishes to invoke the HRA in order to challenge the use of the MHA 1983 can take their case to a High Court, to make a declaration of incompatibility. The courts have the power to grant awards or remedies which 'afford just satisfaction' and this can include financial awards (Sainsbury Briefing 12, December 2000).

### The Mental Capacity Act (MCA) 2005

The Mental Capacity Bill received Royal Assent in April 2005 and was implemented in April 2007. This legislation will replace Part VII of the MHA 1983 which refers to management of property and affairs of patients—in particular the Court of Protection (see Chapter 43). For people in care homes who lack capacity, the MCA has created the role of Independent Mental Capacity Advocate (IMCA).

An IMCA is someone appointed to support a person who lacks capacity but has no one to speak for them. The IMCA can make representations about a person's wishes, feelings, beliefs, and values; bring to the attention of the decision-maker all factors that are relevant to the decision; and if necessary, challenge the decision-maker on behalf of the person lacking capacity. This is particularly relevant to placements of people into care homes.

**Table 16.2** Human Rights Act 1998. European Convention on Human Rights and Fundamental Freedoms: articles

| Absolute rights[a] | Qualified rights[b] | Limited rights[c] |
| --- | --- | --- |
| Article 3: Prohibition against torture, inhuman or degrading treatment or punishment | Article 8: Right to respect for private and family life, home and correspondence | Article 2: Right to life |
| Article 4(1): Prohibition of slavery or servitude | Article 9: Freedom of thought, conscience and religion | Article 4(2): Prohibition of forced or compulsory labour |
| Article 7: Prohibition of punishment without law | Article 10: Freedom of expression | Article 5: Right to liberty |
| | Article 11: Freedom of assembly and association | Article 6(1): Right to a fair trial |

Source: Brammer (2003).

[a] High threshold but any breach is a violation of the Article.

[b] Right may be breached if: in accordance with law; breach pursues a legitimate aim; measures are proportionate.

[c] Article contains a clear statement of circumstances which permit breach of the right.

## The National Service Framework

The Department of Health introduced the concept of National Service Frameworks (NSF) through the 1999 Health Act for different categories of illness, such as cancer services, diabetes, coronary care and mental health. The NSF for Older People was published in 2001.

The NSF for Mental Health (1999) covers mental health in all age groups; but the NSF for Older People refers specifically to older

---

**Box 16.2** Service standards in the NSF for Older People

- Standard 1. Rooting Out Age Discrimination—NHS services will be provided, regardless of age, on the basis of clinical need alone. Social care services will not use age in their eligibility criteria or policies, to restrict access to available services.
- Standard 2. Person-Centred Care—NHS and social care services will treat older people as individuals and enable them to make choices about their own care. This will be achieved through the single assessment process, integrated commissioning arrangements, and integrated provision of services, including community equipment and continence services.
- Standard 3. Intermediate Care—Older people will have access to a new range of intermediate care services at home or in designated care settings, to promote their independence; by providing enhanced services from the NHS and councils to prevent unnecessary hospital admission, and effective rehabilitation services to enable early discharge from hospital and to prevent premature or unnecessary admission to long-term residential care.
- Standard 4. General Hospital Care—Older people's care in hospital will be delivered through appropriate specialist care and by hospital staff who have the right set of skills to meet their needs.

**Box 16.2** (*cont.*)

- Standard 5. Stroke—The NHS will take action to prevent strokes, working in partnership with other agencies where appropriate.
- Standard 6. Falls—The NHS, working in partnership with councils, will take action to prevent falls and reduce resultant fractures or other injuries in their populations of older people. Older people who have fallen will receive effective treatment and rehabilitation and, with their carers, receive advice on prevention through a specialized falls service.
- Standard 7. Mental Health in Older People—Older people who have mental health problems will have access to integrated mental health services provided by the NHS and councils to ensure effective diagnosis, treatment and support, for them and for their carers.
- Standard 8. The Promotion of Health and Active Life in Older Age—The health and well-being of older people will be promoted through a coordinated programme of action led by the NHS with support from councils.

Department of Health (2001)

people with mental health problems. It applies to both health and social care services, covers older people who are in hospital or their own home, in nursing homes, or intermediate care settings, and sets out eight service standards (Box 16.2).

When fully implemented, these standards should improve the availability of services, equal access, and quality of care; but in fact, despite government targets, the implementation of the NSF has been slow and variable across local authorities and health trusts.

## Care management and the assessment process

The system of care management was introduced in 1993 by the then Conservative government following the introduction of the NHS & CCA 1990. The previous model of community care services had been criticized; there were concerns that the costs of welfare services were too high (Lewis and Glennerster, 1996); and it was believed that it would be cheaper for adults to receive support in their own homes rather than moving into care homes.

The last decade has seen a dramatic expansion of services, enabling service users with a high level of need to remain at home, when previously the only option would have been a move into a care home. However, financial resources have not matched this expansion in services, and local authorities have been faced with rising expectations, higher dependency levels, and reductions in grants and budgets from central government.

### Eligibility criteria and fair access to care services

In response to these pressures, local authority provision has tended to focus on users with the highest levels of dependency and risk, leaving those with a lower level of need without provision. In order to manage the excessive demand for limited services, central government has advised LAs to develop 'eligibility criteria'.

This is a method of targeting assessment and resources to those with the greatest need. As a remedy for the unfairness and inconsistency of the previous system, the government has now set a national eligibility framework (*Fairer access to care*, Department of Health, 2002), which prioritizes risk in four categories: critical, substantial, moderate, and low. LAs set eligibility criteria to reflect the resources available.

### The care management and assessment process

Local authorities have a legal duty under section 47 of the NHS & CCA 1990 to assess a client where there appears to be a need for community care services. The eight steps of the care management process are described below.

1  Case finding: The LA has a duty to make information available to potential service users.

2  Referral: Anyone can refer a case to social services. On referral, basic information is collected on the client's needs and current circumstances.

3  Screening: Urgent cases receive a higher priority and are dealt with promptly; cases that are less urgent (according to the eligibility criteria) may have to wait for an assessment or may be referred on to other agencies.

4  Assessment: A social worker is allocated to undertake an assessment. Their role is to gather information regarding the client's current situation and history including existing support networks. The process includes identification of issues and concerns, encompassing the views of clients and carers and how these might be addressed.

5  Care planning: Having identified the service user's and carer's needs, a care plan can be written, detailing the identified needs and the type of care required to meet them.

6  Notification of assessed charge: This is a difficult area, as some believe that social care services should be free of charge, as they currently are in Scotland. A 'fairer charging assessment' must be carried out, and the service user may have to contribute to the cost of their care, or to pay the full cost, if their capital exceeds a prescribed limit. Unfortunately, some people with substantial care needs refuse to have services arranged when they know that they will have to pay for their care. Older people with mental health needs who do not recognize that they need care may see no point in paying for it. Service users who will pay the full cost of their care may prefer to arrange their care independently. This allows more flexibility and is sometimes cheaper, but the service user is dependent on the care provider, and the local authority's monitoring and safeguards may not be available. Some services are free of charge, such as short-term intermediate care, services arranged by charities or voluntary agencies, and aftercare under section 117 of the MHA 1983.

7  Purchasing and arranging care: The social worker purchases and arranges the care, choosing from options available in the statutory, voluntary, and private sectors, in the 'mixed economy'. Choice largely depends on available resources, locality, and financial restraints.

8  Monitoring and review: Once care has been provided, social workers have a duty to monitor and review the arrangements at least annually, so that the provision continues to meet the

service user's needs and any necessary adjustments can be made. A significant change in need will warrant a complete reassessment.

## Single assessment process

The single assessment process (SAP) was proposed in the NHS Plan (2000), the NSF for Older People (2001) and the NHS Improvement Plan (2004). Its aim is to standardize the assessment process across the country and to reduce the need for service users and carers to repeat the same information to a number of professionals. The emphasis is on joint working and sharing of information by professionals working in the health and social care fields. Partnership working is to begin at the strategic level, and the implementation of SAP should include GPs' surgeries, community and acute health services, local social services, primary care trusts, service user and carer groups, including voluntary organizations.

The SAP represents an upgrading of the care management process, and is intended to provide a more effective and rounded assessment, tailored (in its scale and depth) to the true level of need of the older person.

The concept of a shared, single assessment is a challenging one. Professionals need to contribute to the assessment at different stages, and to trust in the assessment information from colleagues in other organizations. Introducing the SAP requires joint working and joint training, and the development of a shared assessment tool.

The principles of SAP are good, but in reality it has proved difficult to implement; the assessments are not always shared with different professionals, so elements of it are duplicated by each professional carrying their own assessment. The four levels of the SAP are:

◆ Contact assessment: This is the point where significant needs are first suspected and described by the referrer. Information gathered at this point should identify the history of the main need, any other needs, and any possible solutions. Consent for the sharing of information is sought at this stage.

◆ Overview assessment: This examines aspects of the personal care needs, mental health and physical well-being of the person referred, their safety, their relationships, and their wishes.

◆ Specialist assessment: This assessment is required when the overview assessment has identified specific needs which are complex, unstable, and unpredictable. It is carried out by the professional who has the most appropriate expertise, and who can requisition resources to meet the need.

◆ Comprehensive assessment: Older people with multiple needs which require intensive and prolonged support with complex care packages will require a comprehensive assessment, and it is likely that a consultant (psychiatrist or geriatrician) will be involved. When all the assessments have been brought together a comprehensive summary is created.

### Case study 5

Mr Brown has lived alone in a local authority flat since the death of his wife 11 months ago. Antidepressants were prescribed 4 months ago but his compliance has been variable. A visiting relative was concerned to find him increasingly frail, low in mood, and neglecting his personal care, and contacted his GP. The GP increased his antidepressant, referred him to the local community mental health team for older people, and to the local social services team for a community care assessment. The overview assessment identified his need for a care service, for day care to reduce his isolation, and for an urgent specialist assessment by the community occupational therapist. The community psychiatric nurse (CPN) also carried out a specialist assessment, identifying some short-term memory deficits, following which the consultant psychiatrist for older adults visited Mr Brown to assess him and proposed a trial of cholinesterase drugs. Thus Mr Brown had the specialist assessments of three professionals. The comprehensive summary of these assessments led to the following care plan: twice daily home visits by carers; twice weekly visits to the local day centre; fortnightly visits by the CPN to monitor mood, medication, and general mental health; attendance at the memory clinic; additional rails and chair raisers fitted in the bathroom and lounge areas.

## Care programme approach

Following principles similar to the care management process, mental health services have the 'care programme approach' (CPA), whereby each patient in contact with mental health services has a named 'care coordinator' responsible for coordinating their care and any actions identified in their care plan. As with care management, the CPA emphasizes partnership and interagency working, quality assessment, care planning, and monitoring.

### Delayed discharges

Older people have historically been unpopular patients for admission to hospitals. Before the establishment of the NHS in 1948, voluntary hospitals (particularly those linked to medical schools) actively avoided admitting older people. As Vincent (1999) suggested 'Older people were unwelcome because they blocked beds and were not good teaching material'. Instead, these patients ended up in the old poor law infirmaries. Teaching hospital consultants were focused on 'curing' illnesses by their intervention, whereas older people tended to have chronic illnesses which were unlikely to be cured. During the Second World War many of those same consultants were redeployed to work in some of the local authority hospitals and the emergency facilities. They acquired first-hand experience of large numbers of elderly people in hospitals and some began to look in depth at the treatment of these patients and questioned the reasons why they could not be discharged. Nevertheless the problem of patients (mainly older people) who no longer need hospital treatment but have nowhere else to go has continued.

In January 2004 the Community Care Delayed Discharges Act 2003 was implemented as a means addressing the problem of 'blocked beds'. The NHS Plan 2000 had made indirect mention of the need to reduce unnecessary admissions to hospital and encourage swift and effective discharge to an appropriate setting with appropriate support. Social services were seen as the organization blocking the timely discharge of elderly people from hospital.

The Delayed Discharges Act allows reimbursement charges to be made against social services by the NHS for those patients who are fit to be discharged. This system of cross-charging was in use in countries like Sweden and Denmark to reduce the occurrence of delayed discharges.

The emphasis in the Act is on LAs to assess and arrange suitable care, in order to achieve the safe and speedy discharge of frail vulnerable people. However, research has shown that a wide range of factors contribute to delayed discharges.

## What is a delayed discharge?

The Delayed Discharges Act has given the NHS the responsibility of informing social services that the patient may be in need of community care services on discharge from hospital. Guidance on the Act states

> A delayed transfer of care occurs when a patient is ready for transfer from acute care, but is still occupying a bed designated for such care. A patient is ready for transfer when…a multidisciplinary team decision has been made that the patient is ready for transfer

Department of Health (2003–2004, p. 16)

Targets set by government attracted additional funding for initiatives to tackle this problem. An increasing range of services will allow older people to be discharged from hospital while still ensuring that they receive services appropriate for their needs. The emphasis is on partnership working, to develop long-term initiatives which will in time create stable and sustainable service provision.

The development of different schemes by health and social care has successfully reduced the delays in the acute hospitals but the delays in the non-acute hospitals do not currently attract reimbursement. It is likely that reimbursements will come into effect in all hospitals in the near future.

The Delayed Discharges Act recommends that 'those elements of a carer's assessment which relate to the patients discharge should be undertaken in the same assessment timescale….' (Delayed Discharges Act 2003, section 47).

The voluntary sector and family carers are being asked to provide more support with fewer resources. In facilitating early discharges from hospitals the voluntary sector have developed many innovative schemes, but there is now a danger that reduced funding will cause these services to fold, leaving gaps in essential services. Social workers are under pressure to move older people out of hospital, but they also have a duty to recognize those who would be put at risk by a hasty discharge from hospital.

## Case study 6

Janet Hobson lived with her husband in a sheltered housing complex for older people. She had Alzheimer's disease; she misidentified her husband, and had often wandered from her flat. Her husband contacted the CPN in a very distressed state. He described how his wife had once again not recognized him and insisted he leave the flat. He refused to leave, while trying to reason with her and she grabbed hold of his walking stick and began hitting him. This only stopped when the door bell rang and Mr Hobson could hear the district nurse calling him. As a result of this episode, the GP requested a MHA assessment, and Janet was admitted to hospital under section 2 of the MHA 1983, on the grounds that she had Alzheimer's disease, her behaviour was putting her husband and herself at considerable risk, and she lacked the capacity to consent to the admission. A week later, Mr Hobson was invited to attend a discharge planning meeting. His wife had had a stroke, which left her with very limited mobility. However, it was still planned for her to return home with a care package. Mr Hobson had a fall and fractured his hip. During his admission a case conference was convened for his wife. It was attended by his daughter.

She informed the team that her father would return home when mobile but he would not be able to continue caring for her mother due to his own frailty. Although Mrs Hobson was ready for discharge, she now needed input from a social worker to assess her and help her family identify a care home placement. She remained on the ward for a further 4 months whilst waiting for a suitable vacancy. Mrs Hobson was deemed a delayed discharge for this period. There were no reimbursement charges levied but the social worker was required to attend monthly meetings to give account of the reasons for delay.

## Ageism and equality

'Ageism' refers to prejudice and discrimination based on negative stereotypical images of older people. Karin Crawford and Janet Walker suggest that, 'Seeing a person from the perspective of their chronological age rather than from the perspective of the individual' (Crawford and Walker 2004) reinforces the experience of ageism for older people.

Standard 1 of the NSF refers specifically to rooting out age discrimination in health and social care. It is intended to improve access to services of a consistent standard across the country for all older people, and makes it clear that it is unacceptable for services to be denied to an older person due to their age. The Independence, Well-being and Choice consultation paper (Department of Health, 21 July 2005) stresses the principle that everyone should have a right to control their own lives and have choice over how their needs are met.

Older people from black and minority ethnic groups can be further disadvantaged, and experience 'double jeopardy' with the combination of ageism and racism. In residential settings, the ethnic origins of staff members do not always reflect the cultural background of the residents. Professionals must be aware of the potential for discriminatory practice, and should promote the strengths of older people by ensuring that they have equal opportunities to access appropriate services.

## Case study 7

Mrs Ivana Markovic is a 79-year-old widow, resident in the UK since the end of the Second World War, living alone in her own house. Mrs Markovic has dementia, having experienced short-term memory problems for the past 4 years. Her cognitive impairment has meant that she is losing her English language skills. Following a fall at home, she has a short admission into hospital, where it becomes clear that an interpreter is required, as she does not always understand what is said to her in English. The social worker manages to locate a care agency with care assistants who speak Serbian, and they are able to support Mrs Markovic's return home with care provided by a carer who speaks her mother tongue. The care package is gradually increased as Mrs Markovic's needs increase, but she is able to remain at home with the assistance of the professional carers who share her linguistic and cultural background.

## Intermediate care

Standard 3 of the NSF recommended the development of intermediate care services to provide alternatives to hospital when acute care is no longer required.

Intermediate care can be provided by a variety of professionals, in non-acute hospitals, in a person's own home, nursing and residential homes, and other settings. The aim of the service is to offer a time-limited period of help and rehabilitation, so as to maximize the older person's independence and reduce their need for longer-term care.

These intermediate care services should not exclude older people with mental illness; rather, 'They should provide person-centred, needs based care that holistically manages all of their physical and mental health needs…' (Department of Health, 2001).

However in practice, and in our experience, many older adults with mental health problems are excluded from most of the intermediate care services. This is due to the nature of their needs and the belief that short-term interventions cannot assist where cognitive impairment prevents clients from learning new skills.

### Integrated services and partnership working

'Partnership working between health and Social Care is a central feature of current government policy' (Glasby and Littlechild, 2004). There is a need for 'joint-ness' to prevent fragmentation; however, a number of barriers prevent close working. These include different professional values, budgets, and contractual arrangements. The removal of constraints in the system which restrict joint working entails government amendments to legislation so that money can be transferred between organizations, for more flexibility in pooled budgets and in integrated provision of services.

Joint working arrangements between health and social care and voluntary organizations are a key government priority. The more that agencies commit to integrated working the clearer it becomes that services are interdependent, and whatever action is taken in one area will have a knock-on effect in another.

## Summary of social care provision

After a full assessment and the formulation of a care plan the social worker and other professionals have the responsibility of arranging appropriate help. Here follows an overview of services that can be provided to older people.

### Sheltered housing

Sheltered housing refers to purpose-built or adapted housing that is specifically intended for disabled or older people.

The housing is usually in a scheme of flats or bungalows, with a 24-hour emergency alarm system, so that the residents can summon help when necessary; and there may also be support from an on-site or visiting warden. The amount of direct support provided will depend on the individual scheme: some offer emergency assistance, others offer more practical support.

In some areas, sheltered housing is available on the same site as residential and nursing care facilities. Older people in this sheltered accommodation can have support from on-site care staff, and if their needs change they can, without too much disruption, move into the care home facility.

However, there are limitations to sheltered housing. Older people and their relatives sometimes have unrealistic expectations, mistakenly believing that the older person will have access to help 24 hours a day. In fact the warden's responsibility is usually to alert other agencies to any problems rather than to provide help themselves. Where tenants have any health and social care needs, services from outside the housing complex will need to be organized.

Moving house can be extremely stressful, and when an older person is thinking of moving into sheltered accommodation the benefit to be gained needs to be considered very carefully. How much support will be on offer, and will extra support from outside be needed? Sometimes it is better to arrange for the extra support in the older person's present accommodation, avoiding a potentially traumatic move. For a person who has dementia, living in surroundings that are familiar may be essential to functioning independently, so any move can result in disorientation and a loss of skills.

### Domiciliary care and meals at home

A wide range of care can be provided to an older person in their own home, and the social worker should identify what package of care can maximize their independence and improve their quality of life.

Domiciliary care enables many older people to remain in their own homes. However, there are limitations. An older person with a dementing illness may be unable to recognize that they need help with daily living tasks, believing that they are still able to do everything for themselves. They may refuse to let carers into their home, or forbid them to undertake care tasks. It can be very distressing for the older person to have strangers in their home trying to help them with quite intimate tasks, and carers can be met with hostility for this reason.

Care can be provided by staff directly employed by the local authority, or by independent agencies that have a contract with the local authority. Carers receive training through the National Vocational Qualification (NVQ) system and can also be trained to a higher level by qualified nurses, giving them the skills to undertake some nursing tasks. Most care provision is made available in the daytime and evening, but some local authorities do provide care at home during the night.

In some areas there are specialist domiciliary care agencies, who have a particular interest in caring for people with mental health needs and have additional training in that area. Other agencies may specialize in caring for service users of a particular ethnic origin.

Many older people need daily assistance with preparing food. Some local authorities deliver hot meals to older people at lunch times, others organize carers to help an older person in their own home to prepare a meal.

Shopping too may be a problem. Most large supermarkets now offer delivery services, and some local authorities have contracts with particular retailers to provide a delivery shopping service. There are also specialist companies who supply and deliver frozen meals and can cater for a variety of medical or cultural dietary needs.

### Laundry service

As part of a person's care plan their domiciliary carers can provide basic assistance with washing and drying laundry, but if there is incontinence the increased volume of washing and drying may be too great to manage in this way. Most local authorities provide a service for the collection of soiled laundry from the older person's home, and the return of clean laundry on a regular basis.

## Day care

Traditionally, the purpose of the day centre was to offer a means of social interaction to older people who might be lonely and socially isolated. This is still the case, but over the last decade day centres have become increasingly multifunctional, offering a wider range of service provision to various individuals and groups in the community. Day centres vary in the times and days they are open and aim to give clients and carers a valuable break.

The specialized day services often have a higher staffing ratio, with input from professionally trained mental health staff. Some day centres are also adopting outreach schemes, whereby workers go out into the community rather than service users coming into a centre run by health staff. An outreach service is invaluable to those who find it impossible to get to a centre, as well as to carers, giving them time to go out of their home in the knowledge that that the person that they care for is being looked after.

Day hospitals are run by the NHS, offering time-limited therapeutic intervention for people in crisis, as an alternative to hospital admission, or to assist in the transition from hospital to home.

Older people also have the opportunity to attend lunch clubs. These are usually run by the voluntary sector. A mid-day meal is usually on offer, along with the opportunity for social interaction.

However, not all older people wish to attend day centres. Not everyone enjoys the idea of mixing with others in a group environment. Other obstacles are the disruptive and disorientating effect of changes in environment, and the stress for carers in getting their relative ready in the morning for the (often unpredictable) time when the transport arrives.

## Aids and adaptations

Traditionally, aids and adaptations have been focused on physical disability. More recently, developments in technology have become available for people suffering with dementia, to monitor their safety, enabling them to remain at home for longer.

Local authorities have a duty under the Chronically Sick and Disabled Persons Act (1970) to assess disability and provide appropriate aids and adaptations to improve an individual's quality of life. Assessments are usually carried out by qualified occupational therapists (OT); they are responsible for ordering and arranging any necessary equipment.

A variety of equipment can be provided in the home to make the environment safer and easier for the older person with a physical disability. For example a raised toilet seat for an older person who has difficulty sitting and standing; or a commode for those who have difficulty getting to the bathroom; and hoists and wheelchairs for people unable to move independently.

Aids are available to increase comfort and to prevent skin breakdown, such as special beds, chairs, cushions, and mattresses. For older people who have difficulty grasping objects, cutlery with larger handles or special beakers can help; lights can alert people with a hearing impairment that the doorbell is ringing. Various companies offer catalogues with a range of aids for purchase, and most areas have centres for disability where aids and equipment can be viewed and bought.

Local authorities can undertake more extensive adaptations to a person's home, such as installing a stair lift or constructing a downstairs bathroom. Disabled facilities grants are available to help meet the cost of adapting a property and are administered by local housing authorities in the UK.

As well as providing aids and equipment the OT advises on safety within the home, and is often involved jointly with social workers and other professionals in complex cases. The emphasis is on assessing risk and making the home as safe as possible without unnecessarily limiting the person's independence. Service users may lack the capacity to understand the risks and potential hazards in their own home, or to recognize that they are no longer safely able to undertake certain tasks of daily living, such as cooking. They may be advised to remove items such as rugs or clutter that could increase the risk of falls, or that the cooker should be disconnected in favour of a safer method, such as a microwave oven.

However, it is not always straightforward to provide aids and equipment for a person who has dementia, or to remove items from their home. Their current level of function may depend on familiarity; they may become disorientated if certain items are removed. Professionals have to make careful judgements about managing risk, balancing the individual's right to safety against their right to independence.

Developments in technology have made it easier to monitor the safety of older people with dementia. The term 'assistive technology' refers to any product or service designed to enable disabled people to be independent. Devices can range from very simple tools to complex hi-tech solutions. Assistive technology enables people to retain their self-reliance and confidence and can help carers to monitor at a distance the person they are caring for. For example, unobtrusive wireless sensors for gas, smoke, flood, or fire can be placed around the home to raise the alarm; other sensors can alert carers that a person with dementia has got out of their bed or chair or has left their home. There are tracking devices which use satellite technology to help trace someone who is lost, and people can be visually monitored in their own home via an internet web camera system. However, use of these technologies is controversial as they can be seen as an infringement of the person's civil liberties.

## Direct payments

The Direct Payment Act was introduced in 1996. It enables local authorities to give money to those clients assessed as requiring care for them to purchase services independently, rather than having care arranged by the LA.

Direct payments can cover all of an individual's care needs or just part of them. For example; the older person may use the money to purchase their domiciliary care, with the LA arranging respite and day care. It can be used more flexibly to include the purchasing of equipment and aids if needed.

There are, however, some restrictions. A direct payment cannot be used to purchase services which the NHS has a duty to provide, or for any permanent care home placements. Direct payments do not suit everyone. Some people do not want the burden of arranging their own care, or dealing with the financial aspects. Most LAs do offer an advisory service to help people to manage their direct payments

## Services for carers

Under the Carers & Disabled Children's Act 2000, LAs are required to offer carers an assessment of their needs, and if a need is identified then the LA has a duty to provide it. Special grants are usually available and might include money for holidays, alternative therapies, training, or even driving lessons.

The Carers Recognition & Services Act 1995 stipulates that carers have the right to ask the local authority to consider their needs alongside the needs of the person they care for. Caring for an older person with mental health needs can be challenging and exhausting, and carers often need breaks to enable them to continue their role. Local authorities can provide various respite services to meet this need. This can include arranging for the older person to go to a day centre or have a short stay in a care home. In other cases, when it is not necessary or possible for the person to leave their home, an increased care package may be arranged to replicate the carer's role and duties; or a sitting service may be provided to allow the carer to go out.

---

**Case study 8**

Dr Fisher (GP) contacts the local social services department after Kate Fellows, one of his patients, comes to see him. She is 83 years old and the sole carer to her husband, Arthur, who developed Alzheimer's disease 5 years ago. Arthur's physical health has deteriorated, with poor mobility and incontinence, and he needs full assistance with all tasks of daily living.

Mrs Fellows is exhausted; she is unable to cope any more and is not sleeping. Her husband has always been an anxious person; he does not want strangers caring for him and gets very distressed when he is left alone. With Mrs Fellows' agreement, Dr Fisher phones social services and provides basic information about the situation. A contact assessment is completed, and a social worker visits Mr and Mrs Fellows at home to carry out a specialist assessment, as it appears that Mr Fellows has complex needs. Mrs Fellows explains her situation. The social worker proposes a care package to assist Mr Fellows with his personal care needs, together with a stay in a care home to give his wife a break.

Mr Fellows is adamant that he does not want this. Mrs Fellows mentions that a neighbour who used to be a nurse has offered to care for her husband. The social worker suggests that Mr and Mrs Fellows could be provided with a direct payment of the equivalent amount of money to arrange their own care. With the direct payment, Mrs Fellows arranges for their neighbour to assist her husband with his personal care in the morning, to sit with him for 2 hours per week whilst she goes shopping, and to stay in their house whilst she goes away for a weekend break.

---

# Long-stay care: residential and nursing home care provision

In the current climate of community care many people are remaining in their own homes for longer and are more dependent on services. However, the time may come when everything possible to maintain them at home has been unsuccessful and it is no longer appropriate. The only remaining option is a move into a safer environment, where care is provided by a team of trained staff 24 hours a day.

The professionals involved must consider the risks to the older person and others if they continue to live at home. This is not always straightforward. A person with a dementing illness may lack the capacity to understand the risks involved, and may be determined to remain in their own home. As Mace and Rabins (1999) describe, for a confused person to give up their home means losing a familiar place and possessions, and cues for independent

function. The person may forget discussions that have taken place about moving into a care home, so that each time it is mentioned it is perceived as a new suggestion which they are unable to comprehend or make a reasoned decision about their situation.

When there is a conflict between what the service user and the carer want to happen, the professionals have to try to work collaboratively with them, to find a solution. This can be a long process. The voices of both the service user and the carer should be heard, and independent advocacy services can be useful in such situations. Advocacy services can be accessed by anyone; they are run by voluntary organizations or private companies, and in some areas are commissioned by the LA.

Local authorities have a duty under Part III of the National Assistance Act 1948 to provide and purchase accommodation for people who need care by virtue of age or infirmity and for whom it is not otherwise available. This act was amended by the NHS & CCA 1990 to include people who need care by reason of 'illness', rather than 'infirmity'.

Since 2002 all such homes in England, Scotland, and Wales have been known as 'care homes'. However, they are registered to provide different levels of support: as 'residential care homes' or 'care homes with nursing'. Residential homes can be run by the LA, voluntary agencies, or private companies.

In some residential homes, assistance can be available 24 hours a day to assist residents with daily living tasks. General practitioners, district nurses, and other professionals visiting as required provide support and intervention.

Nursing homes, as their title suggests, provide 24-hour care with the assistance of qualified nurses at all times. All homes providing nursing care must be registered with the District Health Authority, and by law the person in charge must be either a registered medical practitioner or a qualified nurse.

Before 2001, most people living in nursing homes were supported financially by social services. Unlike NHS services which are free of charge, support from social services is means tested. There were also many residents who paid their own fees, including the nursing component of their care. This was considered to be unfair, since nursing care in hospital or in a patient's own home is free of charge. The government remedied this discrepancy with the introduction of the Health & Social Care Act 2001. Section 49 transferred the responsibility of paying for nursing care from local authorities to the NHS. With this legislation a new assessment process was introduced to determine the proportion of 'nursing care' needed and therefore free, as opposed to the means tested 'social care' provided by the LA.

The money paid by the NHS for the nursing care component is known as the Registered Nursing Care Contribution (RNCC). There are three levels of RNCC funding ('bands'): high, medium, and low. Those needs qualifying for the high band are complex, unstable, and unpredictable, requiring frequent attention and assessment from a qualified nurse throughout the 24 hours. The medium band applies to multiple care needs that require intervention from a registered nurse on at least a daily basis. The low band applies to people whose care needs can be met with minimal input from a registered nurse.

If the assessment indicates that the need for nursing care is 'primary' (rather than 'incidental or ancillary' to the need for personal or social care) then the NHS is responsible for funding the care in its entirety (so-called 'NHS continuing care or 100% health funding').

All local and health authorities have developed their own eligibility criteria for these payments, but they have a duty to adhere to government guidance. The assessment and appeals processes are very complicated, and many legal challenges have taken place in recent years. Generally, health authorities have been criticized on the basis that their assessment process and eligibility criteria are too rigid.

All care homes are regulated by the National Care Standards Commission (NCSC), whose role is to protect vulnerable people. They have powers under the Care Standards Act 2000 to require homes to care for residents appropriately and to provide accommodation suitable for people's assessed needs. All care homes are inspected annually.

### Case study 9

Margaret Richards, aged 85 years, was widowed 10 years ago. Her son John visits his mother about once a month from his own home 100 miles away.

John visited his mother over Christmas and became concerned at her forgetfulness, her weight loss, and her inability to manage household tasks such as cooking and laundry. When he discussed these concerns with his mother she became angry, insisting that there was nothing wrong with her. He persuaded her to see her GP, who referred her to the local older persons' community mental health team, suspecting that she had developed a dementing illness.

The assessment by the psychiatrist and a social worker concluded that Mrs Richards needed help with daily living tasks (personal care, preparing meals, shopping, cleaning, and laundry); however, she would not accept this recommendation. The professionals nevertheless agreed that it would be in her best interests if she could be supported at home, so a care package was set up. Unfortunately, Mrs Richards became distressed when carers came into her home; she did not recognize who they were and would not let them assist her with personal care having always been a very private lady. She would not let them cook as she maintained she could do it herself.

Over time, her memory deteriorated and the risks to her health and safety increased. She would often go out walking inappropriately dressed for the weather and could not find her way home, being brought back by the police on numerous occasions. She was unaware of road safety, and was continuing to lose weight.

The professionals and family involved concluded that the risks had become too high, that she lacked the capacity to understand these risks, and that she needed to live in a safe environment where the care staff were skilled in dealing with dementia.

A place in a nursing home near to her son was found. This option was discussed with Mrs Richards and she reluctantly agreed to the move. The first few weeks were difficult for her, but she eventually settled. She benefited from the security and care provided and more frequent visits by her son.

## Out of hours service

The out of hours service provided by the LA, commonly called the emergency duty team (EDT), is staffed by experienced social workers and ASWs, and provides an emergency response out of usual office hours. In some areas dedicated teams exist; in other areas teams are made up of staff who work out of hours in addition to their daytime responsibilities.

An emergency is defined as a situation which has developed suddenly, unexpectedly, and needs to be dealt with urgently and

statutorily. The team provides speedy assessments that conform to statutory regulations and departmental policy. Priority is given to statutory work related to the Children Act 1989, MHA 1983 and the NHS & CC Act 1990. In addition, the Police and Criminal Evidence Act 1994 (PACE) requires the attendance at a police station by an appropriate adult (AA) if a detained person is,

> a juvenile, mentally disordered or otherwise mentally vulnerable, then a custody officer must as soon as practicable: inform the AA of the grounds for their detention, their whereabouts… [Code C, 3.15]

The EDT service can provide a social worker to act as AA when no other suitable person is available. The appropriate adult is there as an independent source of support to the communication between the police and the arrested person, advocating and raising objections where necessary.

The EDT will also respond to situations in which a vulnerable adult (who may be homeless or at risk of significant harm) cannot be left with an acceptable degree of safety until mainstream services are able to respond.

Referrals to the EDT of vulnerable older people are increasing, commonly when a carer is admitted to hospital and the person they care for needs significant intervention and support. Elderly carers are increasing in numbers and their responsibilities are substantial.

### Case study 10

Mr Jones is a 78-year-old man caring for his wife who has Parkinson's disease, diabetes, impaired vision and mobility, and moderate dementia. He has become increasingly depressed and his GP has prescribed an antidepressant. Carers who visit three times a day to assist Mrs Jones have expressed concerns about Mr Jones's weight loss and low mood. On one visit the carer assisting Mrs Jones to bed found Mr Jones tearful and shaking.

He had not given his wife her tea or medication and had not had anything himself. The on-call GP suggested Mr Jones should go into hospital, but he refused. The EDT was contacted and a MHA assessment arranged, with an ASW, the on-call psychiatrist, and another doctor (approved under section 12 of the MHA) attending. They concluded that Mr Jones needed inpatient assessment and treatment for his depression, and as he was ambivalent about this he was admitted under section 2 of the Act.

Meanwhile Mrs Jones could not be left alone. The ASW contacted their only daughter who lived 200 miles away. She was unable to come to stay, and agreed that her mother would need an emergency placement in a care home, to which Mrs Jones agreed. After contacting eight homes, the ASW found a suitable vacancy in a nursing home. Mr and Mrs Jones have a small dog who also needs care, this was arranged and funded through the NAA 1948. While the ASW was dealing with this she called a second social worker to remain with Mrs Jones, to prepare for her move to the nursing home, and to transport her there. Finally the ASW wrote a report of the events and the actions taken, to inform the appropriate daytime team, with copies for the GP and the MHA office at the hospital.

EDT work is unpredictable and often challenging. It is rarely possible to find immediate solutions and the goal has to be to maintain the person in a safe environment until the mainstream services are available. The reduction in resources country wide has reduced the options for support. The importance of clear, succinct, and timely reports cannot be overstated, to ensure that the relevant mainstream services are informed and can address the outstanding issues.

## Risk assessment/risk management

Risk is an inevitable component of life, it cannot be totally eliminated but can be monitored and strategies put in place to reduce the risks. A community care assessment will not necessarily eliminate the risk but assists in formulating a plan for managing those risks identified. This may impact on what services are provided in the best interest of the client. It is important that professionals consider whether the perceptions of risks identified by others are not influenced by their own agenda, such as for financial gain.

Risk assessment should be an integral part of any assessment. Adult abuse has been highlighted in the recent study 'No secrets' (LAC 2000; see Websites) which helped to publicize the incidence of elder abuse and has produced guidance for all those working with vulnerable adults. Until recently the abuse of older people has not been given the same focus as child abuse. Abuse can present in a number of ways including neglect, physical, sexual, financial, and psychological abuse. By formulating a risk assessment we will document risks identified and consider ways of managing these risks. This is done whilst respecting the wishes of the client and carer, incorporating local and national policies. In practice the risk assessment would include situations giving rise to the risk such as the environment, or a person's physical and mental health. The risks identified for some may include wandering, malnutrition, self-neglect, falls, and self-harm. There will also be a management plan, such as the introduction of a care package or provision of aids and other services. Finally, there is identification of the action needed and who has responsibility for implementing and monitoring the plan. The risk assessment needs to be shared with other professionals, the client, and carers where appropriate and reviewed on a regular basis. The overriding principle of the guidance is that multi-agency guidance and procedures are developed and implemented. The guidance specifies that the lead agency should be social services with a multi-agency approach.

Organizations should ensure that the guidance takes account of those who are unable to make their own decisions in terms of capacity, consent, and what might be in the person's best interest. Working in partnership with other agencies should allow recognition of and address of the abuse of vulnerable adults. Although social services have been given the lead role this does not exclude other organizations from being as involved in the identification of abuse, risk assessment, and planning to redress the impact of abuse.

Social workers have a responsibility and a duty to demonstrate that they are promoting peoples' rights and protection whilst recognizing the complexities of the situation. The expectation of the general public is that when certain risks have been identified immediate action will be taken. However, legislation limits the course of action that can be taken, as referred to earlier in this chapter.

---

### Case study 11

Frank is a 77-year-old man who lives alone in a first-floor council flat. He has a history of alcohol misuse and depression. In recent weeks he has come to the attention of the police as he has become a target of verbal abuse by local youths. The police found him slumped at the bottom of the stairs to his flat, apparently drunk and with cuts to his head. They took him to the accident and emergency unit, where (because of his low mood) he was seen by a psychiatrist and was admitted to hospital, as he was found to have a fractured skull. A referral was made to social services and an urgent case conference convened to discuss the risks of him returning to his flat. The risk assessment highlighted the following risks: falls, alcohol misuse, ongoing low mood, poor diet, poor personal hygiene, and a risk of exploitation and abuse. Frank was receptive to proposed plans to reduce these risks. These included a care package of twice daily visits to assist with washing, dressing, and preparing meals, a referral to the money management team, a home assessment with the occupational therapist, and a referral to the falls service. Day care was arranged and also a shopping service. A CPN visited Frank and monitored his mood and medication regime. Due to his vulnerability, adult protection procedures were implemented. The local police were asked to monitor the activities of the local youths and to report any concerns to the social worker. The home situation was regularly reviewed by the professionals involved in his care including his GP.

---

## Conclusion

In this chapter we have described the legislative framework relevant to older people and the assessment processes used to determine care needs, and noted the need for shared approaches and joint working between professionals. We have also considered the variety of services and resources available to older people with mental health needs, the importance of risk assessments, and the impact of risk on older people.

The case studies in this chapter are composite, and the names are fictitious.

### References and further reading

#### Books

Adams, R. (2002). *Social policy for social work*. Palgrave, Basingstoke.

Adams, R., Dominelli, L., and Payne, M. (2002). *Social work: themes, issues and critical debates*, 2nd edn. Palgrave, Basingstoke.

Banks, S. (2001). *Ethics and values in social work*. Palgrave, New York.

Brammer, A. (2003). *Social work law*. Pearson Education, Harlow.

Braye, S. and Preston-Shoot, M. (1992). *Practising social work law*, 2nd edn. Palgrave, Basingstoke.

Braye, S. and Preston-Shoot, M. (1999). *Empowering practice in social care*. Open University Press, Buckingham.

Brayne, H. and Carr, H. (2003). *Law for social workers*, 8th edn. Oxford University Press, Oxford.

Brown, R. (2006). *The approved social workers guide to mental health law*. Learning Matters, Exeter.

Crawford, K. and Walker, J. (2004). *Social work with older people*. Learning Matters, Exeter.

Cull, A.-L. and Roche, J. (2001). *The law and social work, contemporary issues for practice*. Palgrave, Basingstoke.

Dominelli, L. (2002). *Anti oppressive social work theory and practice*. Palgrave Macmillan, Basingstoke.

Dominelli, L. (2004). *Social work theory and practice for a changing profession*. Polity Press, Cambridge.

Gilbert, P. (2003). *The value of everything – social work and its importance in the field of mental health*. Russell House Publishing, Lyme Regis.

Glasby, J. and Littlechild, R. (2004). *The health and social care divide*. The Policy Press, Bristol.

Hogget, B. (1996). *Mental health law*, 4th edn. Sweet & Maxwell, London.

Hughes, B. (2000). *Older people and community care: critical theory and practice*. Open University Press, Buckingham.

Johns, R. (2003). *Using the law in social society*. Learning Matters, Exeter.

Jones, R. (2006). *Mental Health Act manual*, 10th edn. London: Sweet and Maxwell.

Kemshall, H. (2002). *Risk social policy and welfare*. Open University Press, Buckingham.

Lewis, J. & Glennerster, H. (1996). *Implementing the new community care*. Open University Press, Buckingham.

Lishman, J. (1994). *Communication in social work*. Palgrave, Basingstoke.

Lymbery, M. (2005). *Social work with older people: context, policy and practice*. Sage Publications, London.

Mace, N.L. and Rabins, P.V. (1999). *The 36-hour day. A family guide to caring for persons with Alzheimer disease, related dementing illnesses, and memory loss in later life*, 3rd edn. Johns Hopkins University Press, Baltimore, MD.

Mandelstam, M. (2005). *Community care practice and the law*, 3rd edn. Jessica Kingsley Publishers, London.

Milner, J. and O'Byrne, P. (2002). *Assessment in social work*, 2nd edn. Palgrave Macmillan, Basingstoke.

Nelson, T.D. (2004). *Ageism stereotyping and prejudice against older persons*. MIT Press, Cambridge, MA.

Parker, J. and Bradley, G. (2003). *Social work practice: assessment, planning, intervention and review*. Learning Matters, Exeter.

Pritchard, J. (2006). *Good practice with vulnerable adults*. Jessica Kingsley Publishers, London.

Thompson, N. (2001). *Anti-discriminatory practice*, 3rd edn. Palgrave, Basingstoke.

Thompson, N. (2003). *Promoting equality: challenging discrimination and oppression*, 2nd edn. Palgrave Macmillan, Basingstoke.

Tilbury, D. (2002). *Working with mental illness: a community-based approach*, 2nd edn. Palgrave, Basingstoke.

Titterton, M. (2006). *Risk & risk taking in health & social welfare*. Jessica Kingsley Publishers, London.

Vincent, J.A. (1999). *Politics power and old age*. Open University Press, Buckingham.

## Journals

Cartwright, R. (2006). Rooting out age discrimination. *Professional Social Work*, 5.

Curran, C. and Grimshaw, C. (2002). The Responsible Medical Officer under the 1983 Mental Health Act. *Open Mind*, July/August, 116.

Curran, C. and Grimshaw, C. (2006). Guide to mental Capacity Act 2005: Part 1. *Open Mind the Mental Health Magazine*, 24.

Ryan, M. (2006). Can her son be trusted. *Community Care*, 40.

Samuel, M. (2006). Vulnerable adults. *Community Care*, 10.

Smith, J. (2006). A forgotten generation. *Professional Social Work*, 10.

## Other publications

Department of Health (2000). *The NHS Plan guidance*. Department of Health, London.

Department of Health (2001). *National Service Framework for Older People*. Department of Health, London.

Department of Health (2003–2004). *SITREPS 2003–2004 definitions and guidance*. Department of Health, London.

Department of Health (2003). *The Community Care (Delayed Discharges etc) Act 2003*. Department of Health, London.

Department of Health (2004). *New agreement between NHS and voluntary sector*, ref. 2004/0339. Department of Health, London.

Department of Health (2005). *Independence well-being and choice. Our vision for the future of social care for adults in England*, gateway ref. 4930. Department of Health, London.

Department of Health (2005). *Securing better mental health for older adults*. Department of Health, London.

Health and Social Care Information Centre (2005). *Local authority personal social services statistics. Guardianship under the Mental Health Act 1983*. Health and Social Care Information Centre, Leeds.

## Websites

### Documents

Carers UK (2000). Carers UK response to Independence well-being and choice, our vision for the future of social care England. Available from: http://www.carersuk.org/policyand practice

Department of Health (1998). Partnerships in action (new opportunity for joint working between health and social services) a discussion document. Available at: http://www.dh.gov.uk/en/Publicationsandstatistics/Publications/PublicationsPolicyAndGuidance/DH_4008919

Department of Health (2000). LAC (2000)7: No secrets – guidance on developing multi-agency policies and procedures to protect vulnerable adults from abuse: guidance on developing multi-agency policies and procedures to protect vulnerable adults from abuse. Available at: http://www.dh.gov.uk/PublicationsAndStatistics/LettersAndCirculars/LocalAuthorityCirculars/AllLocalAuthorityCirculars/LocalAuthorityCircularsArticle/fs/en?CONTENT_ID=4003730&chk=pgv18R

Department of Health (2005). Independence, well-being and choice: our vision for the future of social care for adults in England. Available at: http://www.dh.gov.uk/en/Publicationsandstatistics/Publications/PublicationsPolicyAndGuidance/DH_4106477

Department of Health (2005). Involving patients and carers. Available from: http://www.dh.gov.uk/en/publicationsandstatistics/publications/index.htm

Department of Health (2006). Our health, our care, our say: a new direction for community services [see Executive Summary]. Available at: http://www.dh.gov.uk/en/Publicationsandstatistics/Publications/PublicationsPolicyAndGuidance/DH_4127453

LGA Press and Public Affairs (2005). Social care Green Paper promises to treat adults like grown-ups. Press release no SO27/05. Available at: http://www.lga.gov.uk/PressReleases.asp

Social Care Institute for Excellence (2005). Practice guide 2: assessing the mental health needs of older people. Section 8 mental health legislation. Available at: http://www.scie.org.uk/publications/practiceguides/practiceguide02/law/leg.asp

Statutory Instrument 2000 no.617 (2000). NHS Bodies & Local Authorities Partnership Arrangements Regulation. Available at: http://www.opsi.gov.uk/si/si2000/20000617.htm

### Useful websites

Action on Elder Abuse: http://www.elderabuse.org.uk/

Age Concern: http://www.ageconcern.org.uk/

Alzheimer's Disease Society: http://www.alzheimers.org.uk/

Commission for Social Care Inspection: http://www.carestandards.org.uk/

Department of Constitutional Affairs (for information on the Capacity Bill): http://www.dca.gov.uk/

Department of Health [UK]: http://www.dh.gov.uk/

Help the Aged: http://www.helptheaged.org.uk/

MIND: http://www.mind.org.uk/

National Institute for Health and Clinical Excellence (NICE): http://www.nice.org.uk/

National Institute for Mental Health in England: http://www.nimhe.org.uk/

National Statistics (statistics on older people in Britain): http://www.statistics.gov.uk/ –

Public Guardianship Office: http://www.guardianship.gov.uk/

Social Care Institute for Excellence: http://www.scie.org.uk/

The Clive Project (dementia support for younger people): http://www.thecliveproject.org.uk

The Mental Health Foundation: http://www.mentalhealth.org.uk/

The Royal College of Psychiatrists: http://www.rcpsych.ac.uk/

# 17

# Person centred care

## Dawn Brooker

How you relate to us has a big impact on the course of the disease. You can restore our personhood, and give us a sense of being needed and valued. There is a Zulu saying that is very true. "A person is a person through others". Give us reassurance, hugs, support, a meaning in life. Value us for what we can still do and be, and make sure we retain social networks. It is very hard for us to be who we once were, so let us be who we are now and realise the effort we are making to function.

Bryden (2005)

The person with Dementia or The Person with dementia?

Kitwood (1997a)

*Person centred care* means, in brief, that care is tailored to meet the needs of the individual rather than the group or the needs of the staff.

Marshall (2001)

Standard Two: *Person Centred Care*. NHS and social care services treat older people as individuals and enable them to make choices about their own care. This is achieved through the single assessment process, integrated commissioning arrangements and integrated provision of services, including community equipment and continence services.

Department of Health (2001),
National Service Framework for Older People

The term person centred care is ubiquitous in mental health services for older people. It appears in policy documents, training courses, mission statements, care planning tools, job descriptions, and information leaflets in almost every part of the UK care scene. It has been so over-used now that it actually communicates very little. As the four quotes above illustrate, person centred care means different things to different people working and writing in different contexts.

Person centred care has its origins in the work of Carl Rogers (1961) and client centred counselling and psychotherapy. The late Professor Tom Kitwood, the founder of the Bradford Dementia Group, was the first writer to use the term person centred in relation to people with dementia. Tom Kitwood provided a theoretical underpinning to the practice of person centred dementia care.

He published a continuous stream of articles in prominent journals describing his ideas on malignant social psychology; the enriched model of dementia; positive person work; and the new culture of care during the late 1980s and 1990s (Kitwood, 1987a,b, 1988, 1989, 1990a,b, 1993a,b,c, 1995a,b; Kitwood & Bredin, 1992a,b). He brought these ideas together in his best known book *Dementia reconsidered: the person comes first* (Kitwood, 1997a) which was published just before his death. In this book Kitwood said that he used the term person centred in the context of dementia care to bring together ideas and ways of working with the lived experience of people with dementia that emphasized communication and relationships. The term was intended to be a direct reference to Rogerian psychotherapy with its emphasis on authentic contact and communication.

Person centred care was part of a wider movement during the last decades of the twentieth century that proposed a new challenge to dehumanizing care practice. Within this it was recognized that older people could benefit from psychological approaches and skilled therapeutic care. The disability rights movement and the growing dissatisfaction with institutionalized care led to various codes of practice and policy documents that emphasized the rights of older people. Person centred care and the ideas that influence it continue to grow and are now an accepted part of service provision. We have person centred standards and benchmarks (Alzheimer's Society 2000; Department of Health, 2001; Baker and Edwards 2002). We now have more first-hand accounts of what it is like to live with dementia and other significant mental health problems (Mozley *et al.*, 1999; Bryden, 2005). We have practice development tools like Dementia Care Mapping to help us reflect upon the experience of formal care services from the viewpoint of the most vulnerable (Bradford Dementia Group, 2005; Brooker, 2005). We have an ever-increasing number of structured and therapeutic activity-based interventions, albeit with a variable evidence base (Cohen-Mansfield, 2005; Verkaik *et al.*, 2005). We have multi-faceted intervention models in long-term care (Finnema *et al.*, 2005; Nolan *et al.*, 2006; Brooker and Woolley, 2007). In many respects, these ideas no longer seem radical. The challenge for this century is whether it is possible to make person centred care a reality in everyday practice.

# A contemporary definition of person centred care

A few years ago I was asked to write a review on person centred dementia care (Brooker, 2004). What struck me very quickly in my reading was that there was no single accepted definition of what this much used term meant. I was also concerned that there appeared to be a growing confusion between what I understood to be person centred care from a Kitwood tradition compared with how person centred care was portrayed in the National Service Framework. The definition of person centred care is not a straightforward one. Person centred care as it relates to care services for older people has become a composite term, and any definition needs to take this into consideration. The elements of the composite can become so longwinded, however, that the definition loses focus and shape. To some it means individualized care, to others it is a value base and moral standpoint. There are people who see it as a set of techniques to work primarily with people with dementia and to others it is a phenomenological perspective and a means of communication. Person centred care has come to encompass all these elements in a short-hand phrase for what is now considered to be good-quality care for dependent older people.

In that review I summarized a contemporary definition of person centred dementia care containing four essential elements:

1 Valuing older people and those who care for them; promoting their citizenship rights and entitlements regardless of age or cognitive impairment or dependency needs.

2 Treating people as individuals; appreciating that all people have a unique history and personality, physical and mental heath, and social and economic resources and that these will affect their response to ageing and dependency.

3 Looking at the world from the perspective of the person in need of care; recognizing that each person's experience has its own psychological validity, that people act from this perspective, and that empathy with this perspective has its own therapeutic potential.

4 Recognizing that all human life, including that of older people with mental health problems, is grounded in relationships. People living with dementia and other significant mental health problems need an enriched psychosocial environment which both meets their needs for human contact and fosters opportunities for personal growth.

In order to make this definition easier to articulate these elements are summarized with the acronym VIPS:

V a moral stand point that asserts the absolute *Value* of all human lives;

I an *Individualized* approach, recognizing uniqueness;

P understanding the world from the *Perspective* of the service user;

S promotion of a positive *Social psychological milieu* in which people can experience relative well-being.

These four parts are referred to as elements of person centred care. This is in recognition of the fact that all these things can and do exist independently of each other. No one part is judged pre-eminent over another. My hypothesis is that when they are brought together, however, they define the powerful culture of a person centred approach to care. The acronym VIPS also stands for Very Important PersonS, which is an easier way of defining the outcome of person centred care for people with dementia.

As a follow on from the definition outlined above, I began to reflect upon and discuss with many people how they would know whether a care provider was working in a person centred way. These discussions and reflections eventually led to the development of the VIPS tool. The VIPS tool described six indicators for each of the elements (V, I, P, S) of person centred care. Care organizations could assess themselves against these indicators to help them to assess whether they were providing person centred care. The tool was primarily developed with care providers in long-term care services for people with dementia. It is described fully in Brooker (2007).

In this chapter, I describe the elements of the VIPS definition in relation to psychiatric services for older people and what some of the particular challenges may be in providing person centred care in this context.

# Valuing people

**Valuing older people with mental health problems:** promoting citizenship rights and entitlements regardless of age or mental health status and rooting out discriminatory practice.

Most post-industrial societies are generally ageist. Certainly on UK television, older people are the target for jokes at their expense based on stereotypes that, if they were racial, would not be allowed to be broadcast. We have increasingly dispersed family networks and complicated family structures. This means that caring directly for parents and grandparents is a real challenge. The shifting age demographics mean that there are fewer young people in society and an increasing number living into very old age. The stigma that surrounds mental health coupled together with old age and dependency, however, means that these problems are rarely talked about. Older people with mental health problems and those who care for them can become increasingly isolated and marginalized in a society that is obsessed with youth and intellectual capacity.

Across many countries, we have an increasing number of older people coupled with decreasing resources to care properly for them. All prejudices increase when resources are scarce. As the balance between older people who need care increases and the numbers of younger people and resources available for care decrease, we might predict that prejudice on the basis of age and dependency will increase.

Psychiatric services for older people exist within society and those providing these services are subject to the same prejudice as the rest of society. The lack of status and value that is attached to older people with mental health problems also extends to those who want to look after their family members and those whose employment involves caring. Giving up paid employment to care for an elderly parent is not valued by society as much as staying at home to look after a child. Likewise, the status afforded to a nurse working in a children's special care unit is much higher than the status of a nurse in an elderly care home.

Many people regard infirmity, both physical and mental, as the principal feature of old age. If infirmity equates with old age in the mind set of society, then it becomes easier to treat dependent older people as passive recipients of services who have problems to be managed rather than seeing them as active partners in care. Those responsible for creating policy, for commissioning and delivering services are part of this society and not exempt from these attitudes. Indeed, because of their greater exposure to the evidence of infirmity in later life, negative stereotypes about what it is to be old may be more strongly held.

Even within psychiatric services, patients who are elderly and the professionals who work with them often appear to have been marginalized. This marginalization is evident in the equity of service provision, resource allocation, funding for drugs, access to psychotherapy, research funding, media coverage, policy priorities, professional training and status, and the pay of care staff.

The fact that we have specialist psychiatric services for older people is in recognition that specialist skills are required to assess, diagnose, treat, and care for people with the complex set of disorders that later life can bring. Many of us working within mental health services also recognize that services for older people are sometimes seen as an add-on to what is seen by many as the main business of psychiatric services—in other words working age adults. Traditionally, psychiatric services are geared up to meet the needs of working age adults. Even the term 'working age adults' to differentiate mental health services for those in an earlier life-stage is subtly derogatory to older people. Many older people work and contribute to society long after the point of the official retirement age. Differentiating between these groups on their ability to work reinforces the notion that younger people are of use to society because of their potential to contribute whereas those in later life are classified as non-productive and therefore of less worth.

As it is unlikely that there will be a political sea change to enhance the status of older people with mental health problems, actively promoting the rights of this group has to be a fundamental component of person centred care. Unless we, as professionals, practitioners, researchers, and family members, promote the value of the people we care for and their rights to be treated as equal citizens, then we collude with the political expedient that these people do not really matter. Unless we let those in power know that this is a skilled area of work that cannot be done successfully on the cheap by staff with no training, then we are devaluing the lives of those we care for. If we devalue a person, then that is not person centred care.

If a care organization is to deliver person centred care in anything but a non-trivial manner, the rights of all people regardless of age and cognitive ability must be driven from the top down. It is the top-level leadership within a care organization that determines this. The way in which service users feel valued, or not, is determined by the overall leadership and priorities of a care organization. If older people are not a priority for the NHS then they are unlikely to be a priority for mental health and hospital trusts.

For an organization to provide person centred care to service users, it also needs to value the staff directly providing that care. If we encourage staff to adopt a person centred approach without addressing the larger organizational context, we are setting them up to fail. The practice of caring for very vulnerable people in large groups with low staffing levels can place staff in an intolerable bind when trying to provide person centred care.

Direct care workers for older people are one of the lowest paid groups in health and social care, often working in poor conditions with high risk of injury (Noelker and Ejaz, 2005). Staff turnover is high and the quality of training and supervision is generally poor.

The way in which direct care workers are treated has a direct impact on the care they provide.

There are a variety of ways in which a care organization can demonstrate its person centred value base for service users and those providing direct care. The first of these is within its mission and vision statements. An organization's mission statement spells out its reason for being and its purpose. This statement needs to include a commitment to rooting out discrimination based on age and disability. Valuing the equality of all regardless of age and cognitive disability is a difficult challenge. By highlighting this in its vision or mission statement, the organization is making public its policy of promoting the rights of all. This purpose should be clear to all members of staff at all levels from front-line to board level. It should be clear to service users and their families and to all who come into contact with the service.

To get beneath the rhetoric of equality a survey of resource allocation can highlight where rhetoric does not meet reality. Are resources and access to services truly allocated equitably regardless of age and infirmity? When comparing different age groups to whom services are provided is there equity in terms of case-loads; funding for training and professional development; skill mix; staffing ratios; access to therapies; support groups and networks?

A second important area in the provision of person centred care is in human resource management. If staff are to see communication, integrity, and nurturing important in their work then this should be their experience of how the organization relates to them as workers. Teams that see value in working together are more likely to promote a sense of shared community with service users, with less risk of scapegoating those people who do not fit in easily. Some questions that might be useful to address include the following:

- Is there a recognition of the importance of building teams that work well together and who are united in their purpose?

- What sort of induction and appraisal and reward systems exist?

- What are the terms and conditions of employment?

- How is work-place stress managed?

- Providing person centred care is emotionally labour intensive. What is done to identify when a team is in need of extra support?

- What form does extra support take? How is it accessed? How is it reviewed?

- Is there a system of debriefing and reflection following particularly stressful events? Is this the same for those working in older adults services as in services for working age adults?

A third issue in the valuing element of person centred care is whether management practices are empowering to staff delivering direct care. Staff who feel their ideas for good practice are met with enthusiasm are more likely to react positively to ideas and challenges from service users. If a 'can-do' culture exists for staff, they are more likely to promote this with service users and families. Markers of this might include clear avenues for communication that are used frequently between different levels of the organization. Without the ability to communicate effectively with each other, the basis for providing an adequate social environment is flawed. In the absence of good communication, paranoia, confusion, and anxiety flourish. This is true both for staff teams and for people in care. Staff who feel that they have been consulted over practice are more likely to institute consultation practices with families and service users. Is there an 'open door' management practice? Staff who feel that they can approach their managers if they have a problem that they cannot resolve or an idea that will improve practice, are more likely to encourage and listen to ideas from families and service users.

Having staff who are properly trained and have the opportunity to keep themselves up to date is important in providing person centred care. Psychiatric services for older people do not have a tradition of skilled care and the practices that are required to maintain it. There needs to be a recognition that this area of endeavour is skilled work that is emotionally and physically labour-intensive. Some useful questions to address might be the following:

- What is the training and education strategy?
- How are training needs identified?
- What specialist courses are available?
- How is learning supported in the workplace?
- What is the experience of students and newly qualified staff in the specialty?
- What is the level of expertise of more senior people? Have they got post-qualification experience relevant to psychiatric services for older people?
- Are there opportunities for reflective practice, supervision, and mentoring?
- When individual practitioners or staff teams are feeling out of their depth in working with a particular service user or family how is more expert help accessed?

The service environments, both physical and social, are determined by the priorities of the care organization. How good is the organization at providing supportive and inclusive physical and social environments for older people with a wide range of psychiatric disorders and concomitant physical problems? Antidiscriminatory practice means that older people with psychiatric disorders have the same rights as everyone else, but it does not mean that they do not need extra help in everyday life. For example, we would expect that those in wheelchairs have a right to enter buildings, and would provide elevators or ramps to help them to achieve this. Likewise, we would expect that a person with memory problems has the right to find their way around the building with clear signage and way-finding markers.

At a corporate level that means there should be evidence that this is taken into consideration in design briefs for buildings and fixtures and fittings. It should also ensure that all front-line staff are comfortable communicating with people with dementia. Is it policy that all staff having direct service user contact are aware of how to help someone with dementia feel at ease? Is this evidenced in staff induction and training?

Finally, in terms of the valuing element of person centred care, are continuous quality improvement mechanisms in place which are driven by knowing and acting upon needs and concerns of service users? Knowing how service users feel about the service they receive on an on-going basis is central to person centred care. In 'working age adult' mental health services, service users are increasingly being given a voice in service planning, commissioning, and training. By contrast, the voices of older people with

mental health problems are conspicuously absent. These questions may be useful:

- How does the organization know and act upon the views of service users?
- Does it undertake regular satisfaction surveys, interviews, focus groups, reference groups or observation of practice such as Dementia Care Mapping? How are these organized? How often do they occur? Whose responsibility are they? What happens to the views or decisions made at these meetings?
- Are the views of all service users regardless of level of cognitive impairment taken into account in this process, or just the most vocal?
- Are they seen as central to the decision-making process or are they just an add-on?
- Where is the voice of older service users in psychiatric commissioning?

## Person centred individualized care

**Treating people as individuals:** Appreciating that all people have a unique history and personality, physical and mental heath, and social and economic resources and that these will affect their response to mental health problems in later life.

The most concrete implication of person centred care, that sometimes becomes its whole definition, is about taking an individualized approach to assessing and meeting the needs of service users. This element of the definition encompasses all those ways of working that consider men and women with all their individual strengths and vulnerabilities, and sees their mental health problem as part of that picture rather than defining their identity. This approach again has resonance with the work of Carl Rogers for whom each client was a unique and whole person.

The UK National Service Framework (NSF) chose to focus on the individualized care element of person centred care. The aim within this standard in the NSF is about treating people as individuals and providing them with packages of care that meet their individual needs. In the more detailed Department of Health Guidance 'Mental health of older people is everybody's business' (Department of Health, 2005) the emphasis on person centred care also centres on care planning. In this context, the care plan:

supports the person to be as independent as possible in aspects of daily living but is also sensitive to meeting the needs of their disability by providing personal support when required.

Department of Health (2005, p. 31)

This is more similar to the term 'patient centred care' which is also sometimes used interchangeably with person centred care. If the intention is solely to look at a person's needs in the context of them being a patient or a resident then it is probably clearer to use the term 'individualized patient care'. Although this is clearly linked to the individualized element of person centred care, it provides a narrower focus than person centred care, in that the person can only express those individual needs that are covered by being a patient. There is a danger that by just focusing on individualized care that the person stays firmly hidden behind their disease label and that person centred care still does not occur. Although it is not possible to do person centred care without taking an individualized approach, it is possible to do individualized care that is not person centred. Inserting a problem focus into individualized care can make it difficult to continue to see the person as an individual in the round.

Kitwood (1990a,b) characterized dementia as a dialectical interplay between neurological impairment, the psychological make-up of the individual with dementia, and the social context (social psychology) in which they find themselves. This later became the enriched model of dementia, incorporating the biological, the psychological, and the social aspects of a care environment which is summarized in Box 17.1.

---

**Box 17.1** The enriched model of dementia

In the enriched model of dementia it is proposed that all of the following effect how a person with dementia acts, feels, and thinks…
Dementia = NI + H + B + P + SP
NI = Neurological Impairment
H = Health and physical fitness
B = Biography/life history
P = Personality
SP = Social Psychology

---

The 'equation' in Box 17.1 aids understanding of the unique position of each person with dementia. Each person with dementia will have a different pattern of neurological impairment, a different health profile, a unique history and personality, and a unique interplay of all this in the social aspects of their current situation. It is a person centred model rather than a biological model that has many uses in assessment and care practice. May and Edwards (in press) have used this equation as a framework for care planning.

As with the valuing element of person centred care, there are a number of indicators of the individualized element. Within a care organization, such as an NHS Trust in the UK, these indicators need to be led by those setting the clinical or care standards within the organization. These indicators are about the processes that operate to ensure that care is delivered to a high standard that focuses on individual needs.

The most obvious way in which care is individualized rests on the quality of the individual assessments and subsequent care planning. Are strengths and vulnerabilities identified across a wide range of needs and are individualized care plans in place that reflect a wide range of strengths and needs? Individualized assessment and analysis sets a basis from which therapies and interventions can be designed in order to optimize functioning and well-being. Knowing about life history, personality, lifestyle, health, cognitive support needs, and capacity are all important in producing the optimal plan of care. Other interacting factors need taking into consideration, such as level of dependency and a range of socio-economic, gender, ethnic, or cultural differences.

Are care plans reviewed on a regular basis? The needs of older people with mental health problems change over time. This is true for all of us, but when working with progressive conditions we can be particularly sure that change will occur. The pace of change will vary on an individual basis. For some the pace will be slow and insidious, so much so that it is easy to overlook subtle problems that could be remedied. For this reason it is important that there is

a fail-safe so that everyone's care plan gets looked at to ensure that it is still meeting needs. On the other hand, there will be people whose needs change very quickly, either because of the nature of their mental health problem or because of some other unstable physical health condition. Structures should be in place so that care plans can be reviewed quickly when necessary. Building good relationships with primary care and long-term care providers can help ensure that health and well-being is maintained at the optimal level. They can be useful where there are issues of significant deterioration, worsening confusion, or depression that may otherwise go unreported

There are certain processes that need to be in place to ensure that service users can maintain a sense of their own identity and minimize risks to them feeling alienated within service environments. The first of these is around personal possessions. It was not so long ago that most elderly inpatients wore hospital clothing including undergarments. People obtain much greater comfort and security from wearing clothes that look and feel familiar and using objects that are well-known. Familiar items are a touchstone in a world that feels increasingly alien to people, particularly if they have any degree of confusion. It links the present with the past, the unfamiliar with the known. If there is significant cognitive impairment, people often lose the ability to learn how to use new objects quickly whereas with old objects the patterns are well learnt. Most of us have the experience of turning on a lamp with which we are familiar without even consciously thinking about where the switch is. With a new lamp we have to stop and think. It is the latter action that becomes difficult to manage if dementia is present. Surround the person with every-day familiar items and they will be more at ease and function at a higher level.

Linked to this, it is also important that direct care workers know about individual likes, dislikes, preferences, and daily routines. If familiar objects are important, then familiar foods, drinks, music, and routines are even more so. Familiarity with day-to-day experiences helps to establish security, trust, and comfort. People with dementia are perhaps particularly vulnerable to feeling culturally isolated. If any of us are feeling vulnerable then familiar touchstones of our cultural identity, our spirituality or religion, and food and drinks and music are likely to have a calming effect. Vulnerability, anxiety, and alienation are more likely to increase if those elements are missing.

There is an increasing recognition that trying to ensure there is a familiarity in long-held routines and preferences is an important way of helping people feel at ease. Sometimes people will be able to tell us about these routines and preferences for themselves. Sometimes, they will not, which is when getting this information from family and friends can be useful. If direct care staff know food and drink preference, clothing preferences, bathing and hygiene routines, work routines, hobbies, favourite music, sports, and people, then they are more likely to be able to respond positively if the service user is in distress.

Particularly where dementia is present, the individual will find it increasingly difficult to hold on to their life stories and to be able to tell others of the defining moments that shaped their identity. In a person centred care setting, one of the tasks of caring for someone is to learn these key stories and hold this narrative for them. This can be used to improve self-esteem and to maintain an identity in the face of increasing confusion. As the capacity for engagement becomes more difficult, objects that trigger good feelings become increasingly important. Past experiences of vulnerability and trauma, particularly those that happened in childhood or teenage years, can often be relived during a dementia illness which may have emotional resonance with these past experiences. If someone has a history of being sexually abused they may find help with personal care activities particularly traumatic. Understanding a person's past history and using this knowledge in direct care is crucial to providing person centred care for people with dementia.

Some of the indicators that promote individual identity, such as ensuring people have their own personal possessions and routines or that life history is held, are very difficult to achieve when people move from home to assessment ward, to day care, and to respite. This information is often held between different services but is not communicated from one part to another. Having a system in place where this information can be gathered over time and be integrated into people's care plans is an important process in ensuring individualized person centred care.

The final indicator in individualized person centred care is having a variety of activities available that meet the interests and abilities of all service users. Boredom and lack of meaningful activity is rife in institutional care for older people generally, but particularly those with dementia who often find it difficult to initiate or sustain activities. Finding things that interest and sustain people can be a challenge. As well as knowing what is meaningful to each individual, understanding the capabilities of individuals with regard to their level of dependency and disability is important for providing suitable activities.

How this can be achieved in long-term care settings or by people living at home requires careful consideration. Who has responsibility for ensuring that service users have access to meaningful activity on a day-to-day basis? How is this provided? How is it monitored to ensure it meets the needs of individuals? In any institutional service setting, there has to be an appreciation that all staff from direct care workers through to management share in the responsibility for the provision of fun and occupation that gives meaning and structure to life and staves off boredom.

## The perspective of the service user in person centred care

**Looking at the world from the perspective of the person with the mental health problem:** Recognizing that each person's experience has its own psychological validity, that people act from this perspective, and that empathy with this perspective has its own therapeutic potential.

Person centred care is part of the phenomenological school of psychology. In this, the subjective experience of the individual is seen as the reality. The starting point for helping someone is trying to understand the world as they see it. Rogerian person centred therapeutic approaches would see entering the frame of reference of the individual and understanding the world from their point of view as key to working therapeutically. The ability to relate to a person directly, seeing them as a fellow human being, is a fundamental starting point for person centred care.

One of the challenges that faces us in old age psychiatry is trying to understand the perspective of people who are not only a great deal older than us but who may be very confused and have limited communication abilities. Putting oneself in the shoes of someone else is not an easy or trivial process. Can any of us really know what it is like to be another? The answer is no. There are ways, however, that can help us see things from the standpoint of another. Kitwood (1997c) described various ways by which dementia care practitioners could deepen their empathy toward people with dementia. These can be used in professional development and training. They include:

- listening to and reading direct accounts of the experience of those living with dementia,
- attending carefully to the actions and words of people with dementia,
- using imagination to understand the experience of dementia.

Over recent years there has been a shift in focus. This is, in part, to do with the person centred care movement itself. As people with dementia have stepped out from behind the disease label, the recognition that they have something important to say has grown. There is also a much greater acknowledgement that speaking directly on one's own behalf is deeply empowering. This trend is part of a wider movement within mental health services in the UK that care providers need to work in partnership with service users. Also, people with dementia are being assessed much earlier in the disease course. It is much more difficult to dismiss what people have to say about their experience when they are early on in their dementia.

In dementia research, phenomenological research into the early experience of Alzheimer's disease (Sabat, 2001; Clare, 2002) is now well established. Involving older people with dementia directly in the research process is promoted (Downs, 1997; Dewing, 2002). In quality of life research, self-report measures on subjective well-being (Brod *et al.*, 1999) and satisfaction with care (Mozley *et al.*, 1999) have been developed. There is now some good evidence that people with mild dementia can answer interview questions in a reliable manner and can be involved directly in the research process (Wilkinson, 2002; Hubbard *et al.*, 2003).

Similarly, in dementia care practice, engaging directly with people with dementia in a therapeutic sense is a relatively new phenomenon (Bender and Cheston, 1997). Personal accounts of living with dementia are very powerful, as the quotations from Christine Bryden used in this chapter illustrate. The UK Alzheimer's Society Living with Dementia project and the views of people with dementia worldwide (e.g. http://www.dasninternational.org) is a ready way in which we can access part of the experience of what it might be like to experience dementia.

As verbal communication becomes more difficult, attending carefully to the non-verbal behaviour or piecing together fragmented speech becomes increasingly important. The work of John Killick and Kate Allen (Killick and Allen, 2001) has been extremely influential in the UK in helping practitioners attend to the person with dementia in imaginative, creative, and reflective ways. Killick and Allen (2006) describe their work with people with advanced dementia who are near to death, based on 'coma work' principles and working using video and sound recordings paying very close attention to detail.

Like all dance partners, as care-partners in the dance with dementia, we both have to learn to listen to the music. What is happening to me, to us? What is the rhythm of our dance with dementia? Is it fast or slow? Who is in charge?

And we need to watch the musicians – the care network. Professionals, family, friends provide cues and support for our dance with dementia. And they should be watching us dance, not playing their own music!

Bryden (2005)

Another way of helping people to attend more carefully is through training them in a structured method of observation. Dementia Care Mapping (DCM) is, in part, an attempt to help care practitioners attend and observe with great care. Kitwood defined DCM thus:

DCM is a serious attempt to take the standpoint of the person with dementia, using a combination of empathy and observational skill.

Kitwood (1997a)

A number of practitioners have written about the impact of observing this way which reveals to them aspects of people's lives that they would never have noticed in their day-to-day work. Vera Bidder, a nursing assistant (Packer, 1996), described how DCM changed her empathic response to people with dementia in her care:

Shortly after the [DCM] course I became very conscious of the detractions that were still going on … I was bathing a person who was having difficulty forming a conversation. The door was flung open and the curtain pulled back. I protested, and the response was 'It's only a patient!' I was livid because it felt like it was me. I was the person having their privacy invaded. I found myself apologising to the person involved even though it wasn't my fault.

Although DCM is a way of formally observing care in the communal areas of care settings, it is evident from the feedback we receive following training courses that teaching care workers to attend more carefully to the perspective of people with dementia greatly deepens their level of empathy across all care situations.

Those who are responsible for the day-to-day management of direct care staff and clinical teams are best placed to ensure that their staff adopt the Personalized Perspectives element of person centred care. Strengths in this element are indicated by the way in which direct care staff respond to their caring role and how they demonstrate empathy with those they care for.

At a very basic level it is important to ensure that, on a day-to-day basis, service users are asked for their preferences, consent, and opinions. In order to know a person's opinion it is important that they are asked directly about this! It is surprising how often, however, this basic courtesy and social interaction does not occur, particularly in services where people are thought to have dementia. Although people may lose the capacity to make truly informed choices about abstract decisions as time goes by, the evidence is that people can make reliable decisions about long held preferences well into their dementia. Even if the capacity for understanding language is severely impaired, the non-verbal behaviour that accompanies being asked for permission or opinion will not go unnoticed and will do much to convey to the person that they are worth bothering about:

♦ In everyday practice, are people asked what they want to eat or drink, where they would like to sit, and what they need to feel comfortable?

♦ Are attempts made to discuss these sorts of issues directly with service users?

♦ Are the direct care staff good communicators generally? Do they recognize the barriers to communication due to sensory disability and have strategies to overcome these?

♦ Do they recognize the barriers to communication due to cognitive disabilities and have strategies to overcome these?

♦ When decisions need to be made that are either too complex or abstract for the service user to make an informed decision about, do staff talk to people who know them well, such as family, and who can often offer insight into their past preferences?

♦ Is this backed up by observations of the person in different situations to attempt or confirm a best estimation of their wishes?

Related to this issue is whether staff show the ability to put themselves in the position of the person they are caring for and to think about decisions from their point of view. There will be occasions where the service user is unable to fully participate and put forward their own point of view. It is important then, that staff are able to try to think things through from the view point of the service user. This may be particularly important around issues of risk assessment. There is often tremendous pressure to err on the side of caution in situations that may include some risk. Older people with mental health problems are a vulnerable group within our society and it is wholly right that those responsible for their care work to ensure their safety. Sometimes, however, older people are in danger of being kept so safe that they have no quality of life at all. There can conversely be hidden risks to emotional well-being, in the form of boredom, helplessness, depression, and giving up when physical safety is the only consideration. Often it will be up to the person's key worker or a professional to advocate on behalf of their emotional well-being.

On a day-to-day basis, is the physical environment managed to help service users feel at ease? Older people in hospitals and care homes are often at the mercy of other people controlling their physical environment. Attention may have been paid to the physical design of such facilities—they may even have won architectural awards—but unless the micro-environment is managed so that people are comfortable then such endeavour is worthless. On a day-to-day basis it is important that staff use their empathic skills to be actively aware of the people's comfort needs. Often, in institutional settings, service users may not be able to tell staff directly that they are in discomfort or they may not be able to work out for themselves how to alleviate discomfort.

Also, in people's own homes, visiting staff may interact in such a way that the person loses a sense of being in their own place. Ensuring that staff can act empathically in these situations is central to providing person centred care services.

Physical health problems can often go undetected and undiagnosed once an older person has a psychiatric diagnostic label. Are the physical health needs of people with dementia including pain assessment and sight and hearing problems given particular attention? As people may have difficulty describing symptoms of pain or sensory deficit, this has to be actively monitored by staff. Any sudden increase in the level of confusion of an older person should be treated with the suspicion that there could be a physical health problem contributing to it. Physical fitness and comfort need to be taken seriously. Poor physical health greatly intensifies the impairments caused by dementia. Pain is often undetected in people with dementia and the manifestations of the person's discomfort may be misperceived as episodes of 'challenging behaviour'. As people with dementia may have difficulty remembering episodes of pain or difficulty finding the words to describe their symptoms, the onus has to be on the carers to be proactive in this respect.

Unaddressed age-related sensory impairments such as not having the correct spectacles or functioning hearing aids often lie at the root of communication problems. If someone has poor visual perception and dysphasia due to their dementia, this only gets worse if they do not have all the help they can get from physical prostheses. Again, because of their dementia, an individual may not be able to say that they have lost their glasses or to complain that their hearing aid no longer functions. Professionals and care staff have to be vigilant on their behalf.

An area that requires particular mention here is the management of challenging behaviour. A great deal has been written about the need to understand so-called challenging behaviour from the perspective of the service user (Woods, 2001). In person centred care, 'challenging behaviour' is analysed to discover the underlying reasons for it rather than accepting it as an inevitable part of decline. As Christine Bryden (2005, p. 128) writes:

> The world goes much faster than we do, whizzing around, and we are being asked to do things, or to respond, or to play a game, or to participate in group activities. It is too fast, we want to say 'Go away, slow down, leave me alone, just go away' and maybe we might then be difficult, not cooperative. Challenging Behaviour? I believe that this is 'adaptive behaviour', where I am adapting to my care environment.

In person centred care, we try to see meaning in all behaviour and use this as a starting point of trying to help those in distress. The first step is in trying to understand the function of the behaviour for the individual and what the person is trying to tell us by the behaviour. This is particularly evident when people with dementia are in distress but cannot explain this through normal channels. Thus we might see the person act in a way that has been labelled as challenging behaviour, such as verbal or physical aggression, self-harm, shouting out, repetitive questioning, escape behaviours, paranoid behaviours, accusatory behaviours, socially inappropriate behaviours, and sexually inappropriate behaviours. These are very distressing behaviours both to the person experiencing them and to those in a caring role.

A person centred response would be to see the challenge in them as one that challenges us as a care team to find the reasons underlying the behaviour and to help the person achieve a state of well-being. In understanding the perspective of the service user and using this as part of our detailed analysis, we can then have a plan that supports personhood.

In situations where the actions of an individual service user are at odds with the safety and well-being of others, how are the rights of the individual protected? The most difficult situations in long-term care settings are when the rights of one individual are at odds with the safety and comfort of others. An example of this might arise within a housing facility where a resident who is disorientated is constantly knocking on neighbours' doors. Another example could be within a residential home where a resident has become sexually disinhibited and is making sexual advances to

others that are not welcomed. In such a situation, the initial response is that the person who is causing the problem should be removed to another facility. The problem with this response is that it may actually exacerbate the problem for the individual concerned and simply make it someone else's responsibility. In some cases, it may truly be the case that the individual's needs can be met better elsewhere because of better trained staff or higher staffing ratios. There is no simple solution to these issues; they occur with enough regularity that some mechanism for dealing with them needs to be in place *before* they occur. Usually a case conference or case review is held, and the person who may not be able to argue their own corner should have someone advocating on their behalf. In some situations this might be a social worker or a community nurse or a doctor. In other situations it might be that the organization calls on the services of a formal advocacy service.

## The person centred social-psychological environment

Recognizing that all human life is grounded in relationships and that people with mental health problems need an enriched social environment which both meets their needs for human contact and fosters opportunities for personal growth.

In providing person centred care, a supportive and nurturing social environment is the key to maintaining personhood on a day-to-day basis. Kitwood (1997a) defined personhood as:

> Personhood is a standing or status that is bestowed on one human being, by others, in the context of relationship and social being. It implies recognition, respect and trust.

Personhood can only be maintained in the context of relationships. Carl Rogers saw relationships as key to therapeutic growth and change. He highlighted the importance of the relationship and therapeutic alliance in person centred counselling. Kitwood's view of person centred care for people with dementia was that it took place in the context of relationships—*Person to person* was the title of Kitwood and Bredin's 1992 publication, which was the first book on person centred dementia care in practice. With the onset of dementia individuals are very vulnerable to their psychological defences being broken down. As the sense of self breaks down, it becomes increasingly important that the sense of self is held within the relationships that the person with dementia experiences. Bond (2001, p. 47) also includes the context of relationships within his description of personhood:

> …individuals do not function in isolation, they also have relationships with others; all human life is interconnected and interdependent.

The importance of conceptualizing older people receiving care in relationship to others has been underlined by the concept of 'relationship centred care'. Nolan *et al.* (2006) offer a useful framework for the relationships within a variety of institutional and community settings, based on developing a sense of security, continuity, belonging, purpose, achievement, and significance for older people, staff, and families. This is well articulated in the in-depth report 'My home life' (Help the Aged, 2006).

Kitwood (1997a) described personhood being undermined by a Malignant Social Psychology (MSP) of care where people with dementia experience dehumanizing interactions which includes being stigmatized, invalidated, and ignored. The impact of this on the well-being of people with dementia, who are already struggling to adapt to neurological impairment and to maintain their sense of self, is hypothesized as being psychologically damaging. Concrete examples of MSP are provided in the description of 17 types of personal detractions in DCM: descriptions of these are provided in the left-hand columns of Table 17.1.

Kitwood emphasized that episodes of MSP rarely arise from any malicious intent. Rather, they become interwoven into the care culture. This way of responding to people in care gets learnt in the same way that new staff learn to fold sheets. If you are a new health-care assistant on a hospital ward home, you learn how to communicate with patients from observing other staff. If their communication style with patients is one that is characterized by infantilization and outpacing then you will follow their lead.

The malignancy in MSP is that it eats away at the personhood of those being cared for and also it spreads from one member of staff to another very quickly. This is society's response to people with dementia generally, and it has all too often become the professional caring response. Frequent episodes of MSP undermine personhood, decrease well-being, and increase ill-being. At its worst, this leads to a radical depersonalization of people with dementia and reconfirms to wider society its belief that these people are less than human.

In a DCM evaluation all episodes of personal detractions that are observed are recorded and fed back to the care team. Once care teams become consciously aware of episodes of personal detractions and tackle them as part of a practice development process, the incidence of them often radically decreases (Brooker *et al.*, 1998).

Kitwood (1997a) also described what a positive social psychology might look like for people with dementia. If personhood is

**Table 17.1** Examples of malignant social psychology and positive person work

| Malignant social psychology | | Positive person work | |
|---|---|---|---|
| Intimidation | Making a participant fearful by using spoken threats or physical power | Warmth | Demonstrating genuine affection, care, and concern for the participant |
| Withholding | Refusing to give asked for attention, or to meet an evident need | Holding | Providing safety, security, and comfort to a participant |
| Outpacing | Providing information at a rate too fast for a participant to understand | Relaxed pace | Recognizing the importance of helping create a relaxed atmosphere |
| Infantilization | Treating a participant in a patronizing way as if they were a small child | Respect | Treating the participant as valued and recognizing their experience and age |
| Labelling | Using a label as the main way to describe or relate to someone | Acceptance | Entering into a relationship based on an attitude of acceptance |
| Disparagement | Telling a participant that they are incompetent, useless, worthless | Celebration | Recognizing, supporting, and taking delight in the participant's skills and achievements |
| Accusation | Blaming the participant for things they have done, or have not been able to do | Acknowledgement | Recognizing the participant as unique and valuing them as an individual |
| Treachery | Using trickery or deception to distract or manipulate a participant | Genuineness | Being honest and open with the participant in a way that is sensitive to their needs and feelings |
| Invalidation | Failing to acknowledge the reality of a participant | Validation | Recognizing and supporting the reality of the participant. |
| Disempowerment | Not allowing a participant to use the abilities that they do have | Empowerment | Assisting the participant to discover or employ abilities and skills |
| Imposition | Forcing a participant to do something, or denying them choice | Facilitation | Assessing levels of support required and providing it |
| Disruption | Interfering with something a participant is doing, breaking their 'frame of reference' | Enabling | Recognizing and encouraging a participant's engagement |
| Objectification | Treating a participant as if they were a lump of dead matter or an object | Collaboration | Treating the participant as a full and equal partner in what is happening |
| Stigmatization | Treating a participant as if they were a diseased object or an outcast | Recognition | Recognizing the participant's uniqueness, with an open attitude |
| Ignoring | Carrying on in the presence of a participant as if they are not there | Including | Enabling the participant to be and feel included, physically and psychologically |
| Banishment | Sending the participant away, excluding them, physically or psychologically | Belonging | Providing a sense of acceptance in a particular setting |
| Mockery | Making fun of a participant and making jokes at their expense | Fun | Using and responding to the use of fun and humour |

undermined by MSP then it should also be possible to describe the sorts of everyday interactions that would promote the maintenance of personhood. He used the term 'positive person work' to describe ten different forms of interaction that would maintain personhood. These were labelled recognition, negotiation, collaboration, play, timalation (engagement through the senses), celebration, relaxation, validation, holding, and facilitation.

In the eighth edition of DCM (DCM 8), an expanded list of descriptions of 'personal enhancers' that would enhance well-being and maintain personhood was developed (Brooker and Surr, 2005). Positive person work was used as a starting point in the development of personal enhancers. Personal enhancers are not intended to be the polar opposite of personal detractions. Rather they describe an alternative way of interacting. These are listed in the right-hand columns of Table 17.1.

In a DCM evaluation, all examples of personal enhancers are described and fed back to the care team. Again, through a process of practice development, this reinforces person centred interactions and increases the likelihood of them becoming the norm. It is not necessary to be DCM trained to recognize personal detractions or personal enhancers. They appear to be familiar aspects of care around the world. Verity and Kuhn (2007) offer many further descriptions based on personal detractions and alternative ways of responding, called put-downs and up-lifts.

Although personal detractions and personal enhancers in DCM were developed specifically in services for people with dementia, they can be observed in many other health and social care settings. A younger patient on a medical ward may experience just as many episodes of ignoring or objectification as an older person on a psychiatric assessment ward. Indeed they may experience more. MSP has a negative effect on us all, particularly when we feel anxious or vulnerable. Those with significant cognitive impairment, however, already have the disadvantage of losing their sense of self-identity and an increasing inability to make sense of why those around them are acting in this way:

> As we become more emotional and less cognitive, it's the way you talk to us, not what you say, that we will remember. We know the feeling, but don't know the plot. Your smile, your laugh and your touch are what we will connect with. Empathy heals. Just love us as we are. We're still here, in emotion and spirit, if only you could find us.
>
> Bryden (2005, p. 138)

Whether a care provider promotes the personhood of patients on a day-to day basis is largely in the hands of those responsible for the direct leadership of care facilities and clinical teams. There are some common ways in which personhood is supported or undermined.

The first is around inclusion or a sense of belonging (Nolan *et al.*, 2006). Are patients helped by staff to be included in conversations and helped to relate to others? Is there an absence of people being 'talked across'? One of the most frequently observed of all the personal detractions in DCM is ignoring. A typical example of this would be two staff members—maybe a doctor and a nurse—having a conversation, possibly about the care needs of a patient who is sitting between them, with no reference or attempt to include the patient at all. At a basic level of MSP, unless efforts are made for this not to happen, staff can treat patients they care for as if they simply are not there. In some care services patients are seen as part of the furniture—to be vacuumed around, tidied up, and polished—but not to be communicated with. In order to meet the needs of people for attachment and inclusion, staff will often need to play an active role in ensuring that patients are encouraged to take part in the social network of life. Staff have an active role in helping someone feel included on many levels. This may involve such means as using their preferred name, knowing key stories from their life and prompting their use in conversation, or physically helping them move to somewhere where they can see others and be at the centre of the action.

The second key indicator is about respect and dignity. Are all patients treated with respect? Is there an absence of service users being demeaned by 'tellings off' or labelling their shortcomings? Treating a patient with respect and courtesy indicates a powerful message that we see the person as a valued member of society and that we hold them in esteem. We enter into a relationship with someone we respect based on an attitude of acceptance and positive regard. We recognize them, remember them, and take delight in their skills and achievements. Patients are included in reviews and planning and decision-making. When there is not a culture of respect for the patients, then there is a tendency for them to be infantilized by staff, for them to be treated in a patronizing way, being told off or disparaged as if they were a naughty child. In an atmosphere of lack of respect, their shortcomings will be labelled and they may even be referred to as their labels—such as a smearer, or a shouter, or a soft diet. If people feel respected they are more likely to show respect for themselves and for those around them.

A third factor in the social environment is whether there is an atmosphere of warmth and acceptance. Warmth or an unconditional positive regard is at the heart of a supportive social psychology particularly one that helps people feel comfortable, confident, and at ease. If people do not feel welcomed and wanted by those around them then personhood shrivels. Is the service marked by smiles, genuine concern, and helpfulness? Do staff demonstrate affection, care, and concern for service users? Do they create a relaxed atmosphere by the pace of communication with service users? On the other hand is there evidence of staff not providing attention when it is asked for? Are information and choices presented at a rate that is too fast for a people to follow? Confrontation is another common response in staff teams who do not understand the nature of dementia or who are working in a culture of blame. If people feel at ease in a service setting this will be evidenced by relaxed body posture and the confidence to communicate with others.

A fourth indicator of a person centred care environment is whether patients' fears are taken seriously or whether patients are left alone for long periods in emotional distress. Validation is the recognition and the supporting of the reality of another person having particular sensitivity to the feelings and emotional state of that person. In person centred care settings there is a genuine concern to understand and acknowledge the feelings of service users. The emotional state is accepted and people are not blamed or made to feel stupid for the way they feel. If people feel that their emotional needs are respected and understood they are more likely to be in better state of emotional well-being over time. If distress is met promptly and empathically then it is likely to dissipate more quickly than if people spend long periods of time in unattended emotional distress.

A fifth indicator of a person centred care environment is whether staff help patients to be active in their own care and activity.

Enabling means identifying and encouraging someone's level of engagement within a frame of reference. It is very easy in busy care environments to take over from the older patient entirely; to feed them, to dress them, to wash them without enabling them to do the parts of these routines that they can manage for themselves. Not allowing people to use the abilities that they do have is disempowering in the extreme. The amount of support that individuals need with their own care will vary over time. The right amount of support will enable someone to feel empowered. Too little support will result in patients feeling anxious and overwhelmed. Too much support can make patients feel angry and stupid. The staff skills of facilitation—assessing the level of support required and providing the right amount—and the skill of collaboration—treating someone as a full and equal partner in what is happening, consulting, and working with them—are critical if enabling is to occur. This sort of action provides a sense of achievement.

Finally, is there evidence that service users are enabled to use regular community facilities where possible and that their lives are not led in isolation from the rest of the world? Although psychiatric services are no longer housed in walled Victorian asylums, the idea of the closed institution where people never leave the building or grounds lives on. This can particularly be the case in some nursing homes and residential units. Many people never get to put on a hat and a coat and outdoor shoes, to go on a bus or to visit the pub, shop, or place of worship. These are the activities that people take as part of ordinary life. They help us to maintain our identity and our interest in life in all its variety. Older people with mental health problems need this variety as much as anyone else. Likewise, services that support people in their own homes are often seen as a 'sitting-service' rather than a service that enables people to remain part of their community. Also, there are many nursing homes and residential homes which no-one from the local community has ever stepped into. Some places are still seen as if they have the large brick wall built around them that used to surround the old asylums. Places that encourage visitors also encourage life. There are many innovative schemes of therapists, artists, hobbyists visiting with residents. There is much that can be done by local friends and volunteers. Having a bar that is open to people from outside or a nursery or play-scheme sharing some of the communal facilities can help people maintain a sense of involvement in ordinary life and break down some of the stigma surrounding mental health problems.

## Conclusions

The term person centred care was first used by Kitwood to differentiate ways of working with people with dementia that were not framed within a biological or technical model. Understanding and expertise in the provision of person centred care have developed enormously since the term was first used. The VIPS framework does not apply just to services for people living with dementia. It applies to all who find themselves in a state of dependence and vulnerability. In other words, it applies to every single one of us. Older people with mental health problems deserve the highest standards of technical expertise. To help this section of our community feel valued as people, this expertise has to be set within the context of person centred services. We have made great strides over the past couple of decades in refining individualized assessments

and treatments, in looking at the service user's perspective, and in describing how we can support the personhood of dependent older people. What we still lack is a society that sincerely sees these issues as a worthwhile endeavour. It is the valuing element of the VIPS definition that needs addressing at a societal and political level so that health and social care resources can be utilized to enable services to maintain a person centred approach.

## References

Alzheimer's Society (2001). *Quality dementia care in care homes: person centred standards.* Alzheimer's Society, London.

Baker, C.J. and Edwards, P.A. (2002). The missing link: benchmarking person centred care. *The Journal of Dementia Care*, **10**(6), 22–23.

Bender, M.P. and Cheston, R. (1997). Inhabitants of a lost kingdom: a model for the subjective experiences of dementia. *Aging and Society*, **17**, 513–532.

Bond, J. (2001). Sociological perspectives. In *Handbook of dementia care* (ed. C. Cantley), pp. 44–61. Open University Press, Buckingham.

Bradford Dementia Group (2005). *DCM8 user's manual: the DCM method*, 8th edn. University of Bradford: Bradford.

Brod, M., Stewart, A.L., Sands, L., and Walton, P. (1999). Conceptualization and measurement of quality of life in dementia. *The Gerontologist*, **38**, 25–35.

Brooker, D. (2004). What is Person Centred Care for people with dementia? *Reviews in Clinical Gerontology*, **13**(3), 215–222.

Brooker, D. (2005). Dementia Care Mapping (DCM): a review of the research literature. *The Gerontologist*, **45**(1), 11–18.

Brooker, D. (2007). *Person centred dementia care: making services better.* Jessica Kingsley Publications, London.

Brooker, D. and Surr, C.A. (2005). *Dementia Care Mapping: principles and practice.* University of Bradford, Bradford.

Brooker, D. and Woolley, R. (2007). Enriching opportunities for people living with dementia: the development of a blueprint for a sustainable activity-based model of care. *Aging and Mental Health,* **11**, 371–383.

Brooker, D., Foster, N., Banner, A., Payne, M., and Jackson, L. (1998). The efficacy of Dementia Care Mapping as an audit tool: report of a 3-year British NHS evaluation. *Ageing and Mental Health*, **2**(1), 60–70.

Bryden, C. (2005). *Dancing with dementia: my story of living positively with dementia.* Jessica Kingsley Publishers, London.

Clare, L. (2002). We'll fight as long as we can: coping with the onset of Alzheimer's disease. *Aging and Mental Health*, **6**, 139–148.

Cohen-Mansfield, J. (2005). Nonpharmacological interventions for persons with dementia. *Alzheimer's Care Quarterly*, **6**, 129–145.

Department of Health (2001). *National Service Framework for Older People.* Department of Health, London.

Department of Health (2005). *Everybody's business: integrated mental health services for older adults, a service development guide.* Care Services Improvement Partnership (CSIP), London.

Downs, M. (1997). The emergence of the person in dementia research. *Aging and Society*, **17**, 597–607.

Dewing, J. (2002). From ritual to relationship; a person centred approach to consent in qualitative research with older people who have a dementia. *Dementia*, **1**, 157–171.

Finnema, E., Droes, R.-M., Ettema, T. *et al.* (2005). The effect of integrated emotion-oriented care versus usual care on elderly persons with dementia in the nursing home and on nursing assistants: a randomized clinical trial. *International Journal of Geriatric Psychiatry*, **20**, 330–343.

Help the Aged (2006). *My home life; quality of life in care homes.* Help the Aged, London.

Hubbard, G., Downs, M.G., and Tester, S. (2003). Including older people with dementia in research: challenges and strategies. *Aging and Mental Health*, **7**, 351–362.

Keady, J. (1996). The experience of dementia: a review of the literature and implications for nursing practice. *Journal of Clinical Nursing*, **5**, 275–288.

Killick, J. and Allen, K. (2001). *Communication and the care of people with dementia*. Open University Press, Buckingham.

Killick, J. and Allen, K (2006). The Good Sunset Project: making contact with those close to death. *Journal of Dementia Care*, **14**(1), 22–24.

Kitwood, T. (1987a). Dementia and its pathology: in brain, mind or society? *Free Associations*, **8**, 81–93.

Kitwood, T. (1987b). Explaining senile dementia: the limits of neuropathological research. *Free Associations*, **10**, 117–140.

Kitwood, T. (1988). The technical, the personal and the framing of dementia. *Social Behaviour*, **3**, 161–180.

Kitwood, T. (1989). Brain, mind and dementia: with particular reference to Alzheimer's disease. *Ageing and Society*, **9**(1), 1–15.

Kitwood, T. (1990a). The dialectics of dementia: with particular reference to Alzheimer's disease *Ageing and Society*, **10**, 177–196.

Kitwood, T. (1990b). Understanding senile dementia: a psychobiographical approach. *Free Associations*, **19**, 60–76.

Kitwood, T. (1993a). Person and process in dementia. *International Journal of Geriatric Psychiatry*, **8**(7), 541–546.

Kitwood, T. (1993b). Towards a theory of dementia care: the interpersonal process. *Ageing and Society*, **13**(1), 51–67.

Kitwood, T. (1993c). Discover the person, not the disease. *Journal of Dementia Care*, **1**(1), 16–17.

Kitwood, T. (1995a). Positive long-term changes in dementia: some preliminary observations *Journal of Mental Health*, **4**(2), 133–144.

Kitwood, T. (1995b). Building up the mosaic of good practice. *Journal of Dementia Care*, **3**(5), 12–13.

Kitwood, T. (1997a). *Dementia reconsidered*. Open University Press, Buckingham.

Kitwood, T. (1997b). The uniqueness of persons with dementia. In *State of the art in dementia care* (ed. M. Marshall). Centre for Policy on Ageing, London.

Kitwood, T. (1997c). The experience of dementia. *Aging and Mental Health*, **1**, 13–22.

Kitwood, T. and Bredin, K. (1992a). Towards a theory of dementia care: personhood and wellbeing. *Ageing and Society*, **12**, 269–287.

Kitwood, T. and Bredin, K. (1992b). *Person to person: a guide to the care of those with failing mental powers*. Gale Centre Publications, Loughton, Essex.

Marshall, M. (2001). The challenge of looking after people with dementia. *British Medical Journal*, **323**, 410–411.

May, H. and Edwards, P. *Person centred care planning: the milestones templates*. Jessica Kingsley Publications, London. (in press)

Mozley, C.G., Huxley, P., Sutcliffe, C. *et al.* (1999). 'Not knowing where I am doesn't mean I don't know what I like': cognitive impairment and quality of life responses in elderly people. *International Journal of Geriatric Psychiatry*, **14**, 776–783.

Noelker, L.S. and Ejaz, F.K. (2005). Training direct care workers for person centred care. *Public Policy and Aging Report*, **15**, 17–19.

Nolan, M., Brown, J., Davies, S., Nolan, J., and Keady, J. (2006). *The Senses Framework: improving care for older people through a relationship-centred approach*, Getting Research into Practice Series. University of Sheffield. Sheffield.

Packer, T. (1996). Shining a light on simple, crucial details. *Journal of Dementia Care*, **4**, 22–23.

Rogers, C.R. (1961). *On becoming a person*. Houghton Mifflin, Boston.

Sabat, S. (2001). *The experience of Alzheimer's disease: life through a tangled veil*. Blackwell, Oxford.

Verity, J. and Kuhn, D. (2007). *Good dementia care: a guide for direct care staff in residential settings*. Thomson Delmar, New York (in press).

Verkaik, R., Van Weert, J.C.M., and Francke, A.L. (2005). The effects of psychosocial methods on depressed, aggressive and apathetic behaviours of people with dementia: a systematic review. *International Journal of Geriatric Psychiatry*, **20**(4), 301–314.

Wilkinson, H. (2002). Including people with dementia in research: methods and motivations. In *The perspectives of people with dementia: research methods and motivations* (ed. H. Wilkinson), pp. 9–24. Jessica Kingsley Publishers, London.

Woods, R.T. (2001). Discovering the person with Alzheimer's disease: cognitive, emotional and behavioural aspects. *Aging and Mental Health*, **5**(Suppl. 1), S7–S16.

# Psychological treatments: introduction

Philip Wilkinson

In the last few years there has been increasing interest in the use of psychological treatments with older adults and an increase in research in the field. As is often the case, this increase mirrors developments in services for younger adults in which psychological interventions are, for example, now recommended in the routine management of common disorders such as schizophrenia and depressive disorder. Although psychological treatments are still far from the centre of older adult psychiatric services, clinicians working with older people need to have an awareness of the range of treatments available, their indications, and the emerging evidence base.

The use of psychological treatments with older people brings particular challenges and opportunities. One of the greatest opportunities is to link the development of psychological approaches to advances in biological treatments. Work with older people also gives clinicians the opportunity to work with creatively with older people's life experience, drawing upon patients' personal resources and those of their families. The main challenges are to demonstrate that treatments are feasible and effective with older people.

## The range of psychological treatments used with older adults

Any attempt at categorization highlights immediately the diversity of theories and methods that underlie psychological treatments and the purposes for which they have been devised. A pragmatic approach to the classification of treatments used with older adults is to separate those devised specifically for older patients (usually with dementia) from those developed with younger adults and only later used with older people (usually for depression or neurotic disorders). Therapies in the first category include reminiscence therapy, validation therapy, and reality orientation. These were some of the first treatment approaches to be formalized and evaluated, starting in the 1960s. Although many of the trials used in their evaluation have significant shortcomings by today's methodological standards, their existence represents a crucial first step in the short evolution of non-pharmacological interventions in old age psychiatry. As described in this chapter, these therapies now belong to a range of approaches that might be used with care home residents. The other treatments described in this chapter are the more prominent therapies from the second category. They are psychodynamic psychotherapy, systemic therapy, cognitive behaviour therapy, and interpersonal psychotherapy. In recent years the latter two therapies have begun to occupy an important place alongside pharmacological treatments in the management of common psychiatric disorders of old age. Table 18i.1 lists some of the therapies currently used with older people.

While categorization of psychological treatments is useful it is also liable to create false distinctions between therapies that overlap in their aims and methods. For example, in both cognitive behaviour therapy and interpersonal therapy an important goal for a depressed dementia caregiver might be to establish a new social network; although the endpoint is the same, the two therapies will employ different techniques to reach it. Both interpersonal therapy and psychodynamic therapy have a focus on interpersonal relationships but in the former this is made explicit through the use of an interpersonal inventory and, it the latter, it might be more implicit through exploration of the therapeutic relationship.

Increasingly, different psychotherapeutic approaches are used alongside each other. For example, individual therapy with a dementia caregiver might be combined with family meetings (Mittelman *et al.*, 2003). Integrative models of psychotherapy, in which methods from different therapies are blended together, are also used in the treatment of older people's personality problems. These include cognitive analytic therapy (Hepple, 2002) and dialectical behaviour therapy (Lynch *et al.*, 2007).

**Table 18i.1** Some of the psychological treatments used with older adults

| |
|---|
| Psychoanalytic and psychodynamic psychotherapy |
| Systemic therapy |
| Cognitive behaviour therapy |
| Interpersonal therapy |
| Validation therapy |
| Reminiscence therapy |
| Cognitive analytic therapy |
| Problem-solving therapy |
| Dialectical behaviour therapy |
| Cognitive stimulation therapy |

## Indications for psychological treatments with older adults

Psychological treatments might be offered to older patients or their caregivers for a number of reasons (Table 18i.2); often they will be used alongside biological and social interventions. Even if not used as distinct treatments, all of the psychotherapeutic models described in this chapter can also help the clinician to reach constructive formulations of clinical problems. As demonstrated later in this chapter, for example, systemic thinking can help to identify family factors influencing a depressed elder and psychodynamic thinking can help the clinician understand his or her own response to a challenging patient.

An interesting development is the inclusion of simple psychological interventions such as problem-solving therapy in multicomponent collaborative care interventions for depressed older adults (Hunkeler *et al.*, 2006). Trials of other therapies performed in recent years, particularly interpersonal therapy and cognitive behaviour therapy, are reviewed later in this chapter.

## Practical considerations in the use of psychological treatments with older adults

Enabling older people to access psychological treatments has always presented particular challenges; addressing these challenges is crucial in improving services. While many patients may be sufficiently fit and mobile to attend clinics independently, others may require provision of special transport or home visits by therapists. As patient transport is costly, providing treatment on a group basis, where feasible, may improve efficiency as well as providing secondary social benefits for patients. Other ways to improve patients' access to treatment include bibliotherapy (Smith *et al.*, 1997), as well as telephone and internet-based systems (NICE, 2006). It is also important to consider who will be available to support the use of a psychological intervention with an older person. As illustrated in this chapter, where patients with dementia living in care homes are concerned, interventions are best directed at paid carers rather than directly at patients themselves. Cognitive therapy with a family caregiver takes this a step further by combining training in care skills with attention to the carer's own emotions and reactions.

**Table 18i.2** Indications for psychological treatments with older adults

| |
|---|
| Patient preference, as an alternative treatment to medication, e.g. in the treatment of an anxiety disorder |
| Augmenting the effect of psychotropic medication, e.g. in the treatment of a depressive disorder |
| To avoid the use of potentially harmful medication, e.g. in managing behavioural symptoms of dementia |
| To help distressed caregivers, e.g. treating a dementia caregiver experiencing depressive and anxiety symptoms |
| To alleviate psychological problems related to ageing, e.g. to help achieve contentment and acceptance of ageing or to resolve disputes within a family brought on by the illness of an older family member |
| To provide the clinician with a psychological formulation of a patient's problems |

### Taking account of sensory and cognitive changes

Clinicians experienced in working with older people will be used to taking into account their patients' sensory and cognitive status. Sensory deficits can often be circumvented by using technical aids or by audiotaping therapy manuals for visually impaired patients. How far formal psychological treatments need to be adapted to accommodate any cognitive deficits is less clear. It is sometimes argued that discussion of adaptations risks stereotyping older people and their needs; however, it cannot be denied that in some cases impairment of memory or executive skills appears to create an impediment.

Mohlman and Gorman (2005) questioned whether executive dysfunction makes a difference to therapeutic response. To study this they rated the effects of executive dysfunction on response to cognitive behaviour therapy for generalized anxiety disorder in older adults. Their results indicated a differential response to cognitive therapy in participants with executive dysfunction: those whose executive function was poor both before and after treatment did not respond, while those whose scores improved responded quite well. This suggests that it is not simply the presence of executive dysfunction that is important but also its aetiology: those whose impairment is a result of the anxiety disorder itself may be more likely to benefit from cognitive therapy.

Less is known about the impact of memory impairment on response to psychological treatment and in particular the relationship between the severity of memory impairment and treatment response. Currently many authors recommend memory aids and other strategies to help patients retain information and skills acquired during psychotherapy. There remains a need for further empirical evaluation of these. Later in this chapter, developments in the use of cognitive behaviour therapy in the management of patients with established dementia are reviewed.

## Research into psychological treatments with older people

Psychotherapy research has both its opponents and supporters. Opponents often argue that clinical trials of psychological treatments are more likely to be flawed than trials of medication, making their conclusions less credible. In particular it is more difficult to standardize a psychological intervention and the performance of therapists (see Parry (2000) for a fuller discussion of these issues). Nonetheless, many of these problems can be addressed, and even with medication there will never be a perfect trial design. Most importantly, if adequate research into psychological treatments is not conducted then the potential beneficiaries, particularly older people, stand to lose out as agencies commissioning health care prioritize empirically supported interventions. Research trials have the added benefit of helping to refine and improve the interventions under investigation. As this chapter illustrates, certain therapies are more easily evaluated than others. In recent years the quality of psychotherapy research trials with older people has begun to improve.

Research evidence is only useful as long as it can be made relevant to patients encountered in day-to-day practice and as long as clinicians are willing to embrace it. Experienced clinicians, thinking they can predict whether their own patients will benefit from treatments, may choose not to offer empirically supported treatments.

However, reliance on clinical prediction alone may produce poorer results for patients than the more actuarial reliance on empirically based findings (Mansfield and Addis, 2001a).

## Design of psychotherapy trials

Psychological treatments, both individual and group-based, are regarded by researchers as complex interventions. That is, they are made up of a number of component interventions and their delivery is influenced by a therapist's skills. Complex interventions are, therefore, more difficult to standardize and reproduce than drug treatments. To ensure that complex interventions are fully developed and defined, a phased approach to their evaluation is recommended (Campbell *et al.*, 2000) and a framework for this process has been devised by the UK Medical Research Council (Fig. 18i.1). This framework is intended to help conceptualize the different stages in the evaluation of a complex intervention; it is not a rigidly imposed process. Many psychological interventions (for instance psychoanalytic psychotherapy) are rich in theory and have been well modelled, in keeping with the pre-clinical phase and phase I. An example of a modelling trial (phase I) is a case series of a cognitive behavioural intervention for people experiencing both depression and dementia (Scholey and Woods, 2003). Such a trial allows the intervention to be modified and refined, in preparation for a controlled evaluation. An example of a phase II exploratory study is a pilot randomized controlled trial recently completed in Oxford and Southampton, UK, in which a brief cognitive behavioural group intervention in combination with antidepressant medication was compared to medication alone in the maintenance treatment of depression in older people. The large-scale randomized controlled trials of interpersonal therapy reviewed later in this chapter (Reynolds *et al.*, 1999, 2006), are examples of definitive phase III studies. As yet, phase IV implementation studies of psychological treatments with older people are lacking.

## Interpreting psychotherapy trials

In deciding whether to offer a patient a therapy evaluated in a research trial the clinician should be guided by the following considerations (Straus and McAlister, 2004).

### The similarity of the patient to those in the study

In order for a randomized controlled trial to produce valid results as many participants as possible should complete the intervention and be monitored for the whole of the planned follow-up period. To ensure this is the case, psychological treatment trials with older adults may sometimes exclude people with significant physical illness or those living in institutions who cannot reach treatment centres; these factors, however, could be important in determining how patients respond to treatment. Biological variables in older people might influence the generalizability of findings of research trials performed with younger adults. For example, as late-life depression is associated with arteriosclerotic, inflammatory, and immune changes (Alexopoulos, 2005) it cannot be assumed that interventions shown to be efficacious with younger people will be as beneficial with older adults.

In practice the use of any intervention often relies on a trade-off between practical adaptation and possible lowering of efficacy in the face of confounders (Hepple *et al.*, 2002). However, the more that research trial methodology can be adapted to include everyday patients, the more that knowledge will be gained about the effectiveness of interventions. Therapists working with older adults should maintain a readiness to re-equip themselves in the way that surgeons need periodically to update their skills.

### The feasibility of the treatment in the clinical setting

Key questions regarding feasibility are whether there are trained therapists able to provide the intervention and how easily patients will get access to them. The shorter and easier an intervention, the

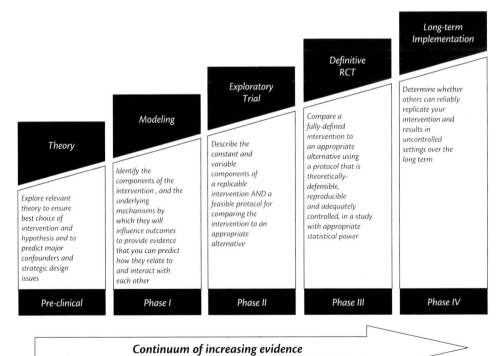

**Fig. 18i.1** Framework for trials of complex interventions. Source: *A framework for development and evaluation of RCTs for complex interventions to improve health*, Medical Research Council (2000) (http://www.mrc.ac.uk/Utilities/Documentrecord/index.htm?d=MRC003372).

more patients who stand to benefit. Difficulties might occur if all the therapists in a service are skilled in the provision of one therapy and then, on the basis of research or recommissioning, there is a call to provide a therapy of a different modality. Making a switch from providing one therapy type to another is more complex than changing prescribing practice; therapists' allegiance to a particular modality and lack of available training and supervision are common hurdles.

Use of a treatment manual can help in the delivery of a psychological treatment and also ensures that the practice of a therapy is faithful to that in a research study. This is particularly important when the terminology applied to treatments is misleading. For example the term 'reminiscence therapy' can apply to a range of therapeutic approaches with older people that involve any sort of life review and that are used both in depression and dementia (Woods, 2004). Critics of therapy manuals argue that they remove the essential individual nature of the treatment; supporters argue that although people and their problems differ, patients also have a number of clinical features in common that can be targeted by a standardized intervention (Everitt and Wessely, 2004). Therapies that lend themselves to being manualized are those that include a series of explicit strategies; those that rely more on detailed, implicit formulations than on clear strategies are harder to manualize. An important benefit of therapy manuals is that they can form the basis of dissemination and training in a new intervention (Mansfield and Addis, 2001b).

### The likely benefits of the treatment

To understand the potential benefits of a therapy to a particular patient, the clinician needs to be aware of the clinical outcomes that have been measured in a research trial. Often these are scores on symptom rating scales that might be difficult to apply directly to clinical populations. Other, more pragmatic, trial outcomes include relapse of a disorder or admission to a care home. Some therapies, for instance psychodynamic therapy, may have aims, such as developmental goals, that are not related directly to symptom severity; this makes it more difficult to find measurable outcomes to capture change. Specific outcome measures may be chosen to be relevant to a particular clinical population: later in this chapter an educational intervention with care home staff is described in which a primary outcome was prescribing rates of potentially harmful antipsychotic medication in care homes.

Once trials with relevant outcomes have been identified, the findings must be summarized in a clinically meaningful way. Here summary measures such as the 'number needed to treat' (NNT) are useful (Straus and McAlister, 2004). When a number of trials of the same intervention exist, systematic reviews give the clinician an overview of trial quality and, in some cases, a summary measure of efficacy (Everitt and Wessely, 2004).

### The patient's values

As a patient's decision to accept or decline a psychological treatment may be made on the basis of preconceived ideas about psychotherapy, the clinician should be in a position to give clear information about the nature, duration, and likelihood of benefits of treatment. Patients who are naturally more autonomous may choose a psychological intervention in preference to a drug treatment; those who prefer treatments requiring little effort may make the opposite choice. There are also mathematical models to help with this process (Straus and McAlister, 2004).

# The status of psychological treatment services for older adults

A survey of UK National Health Service psychotherapy departments showed that formal psychotherapy provision for older people was rare and that referral rates of older people to specialist psychotherapy services were low compared with younger adults. This applied especially to the older old population (Murphy, 2000). It is more difficult to determine the extent of provision within generic psychiatric services for older people. A study of the attitudes of general medical practitioners to the referral of older people with depression for psychological treatments revealed that 93% would consider referring older people for psychological treatment but only 44% had ever done so (Collins et al., 1997).

Although provision and referral rates appear to be poor, the importance of providing psychological treatments for older people is recognized by policy-makers. The UK Department of Health's document 'Securing better mental health for older adults' (Department of Health, 2005) reviewed progress on the National Service Framework for Older People published in 2001. It reported that there was still progress to be made in ensuring that older people benefited from the developments that had become available to younger people. It highlighted an ongoing need to change attitudes to older people's mental health and to improve access to specialist psychological services. The Dementia Guideline published in 2006 by the UK National Institute of Health and Clinical Excellence promotes the use of psychological treatment to help caregivers experiencing psychological distress (NICE, 2006).

Little is known of older people's understanding of and attitudes to psychological treatments. There is some evidence that many depressed older people are positively inclined towards learning behavioural strategies to help them to manage their depression and that while some might regard psychological treatment with scepticism, many can see the benefits of talking to a trained counsellor (Lawrence et al., 2006). These findings raise the question of how best to raise older people's awareness of psychological treatments.

It is often debated whether psychological treatments for older people should be provided in generic old age mental health services or in separate psychological treatment services for adults of all ages. The second model is difficult to support, however, as work with older people requires additional skills such as cognitive assessment, an understanding of physical illness and an availability to liaise with hospitals and care homes. It makes sense that the development and evaluation of treatments continue to take place within the context of integrated old age psychiatry services.

This chapter describes a number of the more prominent psychological treatment models that can be used with older people. It illustrates the diversity of methods and the steps that have been taken so far in developing and evaluating therapies for older people's particular needs.

## References

Alexopoulos, G. (2005). Depression in the elderly. *Lancet*, **365**, 1961–1970.

Campbell, M., Fitzpatrick, R., Haines, A. *et al.* (2000). Framework for design and evaluation of complex interventions to improve health. *British Medical Journal*, **321**, 694–696.

Collins, E., Katona, C., and Orrell, M.W. (1997). Management of depression in the elderly by general practitioners: referral for psychological treatments. *British Journal of Clinical Psychology*, **36**, 445–448.

Department of Health (2005). *Securing better mental health for older adults.* Available at: http://www.dh.gov.uk/en/Publicationsandstatistics/Publications/PublicationsPolicyAndGuidance/DH_4114989

Everitt, B.S. and Wessely, S. (2004). *Clinical trials in psychiatry.* Oxford University Press, Oxford.

Hepple, J. (2002). Cognitive analytic therapy. In *Psychological therapies with older people* (ed. J.N. Hepple, J. Pearce, and P.W. Wilkinson), pp. 128–160. Brunner-Routledge, Hove.

Hepple, J., Wilkinson, P., and Pearce, J. (2002). Psychological therapies with older people. An overview. In *Psychological therapies with older people* (ed. J.N. Hepple, J. Pearce, and P.W. Wilkinson), pp. 161–176. Brunner-Routledge, Hove.

Hunkeler, E.M., Katon, W., Tang, L. *et al.* (2006). Long term outcomes from the IMPACT randomised trial for depressed elderly patients in primary care. *British Medical Journal*, **332**, 259–262.

Lawrence, V., Banerjee, S., Bhugra, D. *et al.* (2006). Coping with depression in later life: a qualitative study of help-seeking in three ethnic groups. *Psychological Medicine*, **36**, 1375–1383.

Lynch, T.R., Cheavens, J.S., Cukrowicz, K.C. *et al.* (2007). Treatment of older adults with co-morbid personality disorder and depression: a dialectical behavior therapy approach. *International Journal of Geriatric Psychiatry*, **22**(2), 131–143.

Mansfield, A.K. and Addis, M.E. (2001a). Manual-based treatment. Part 2: the advantages of manual-based practice in psychotherapy. *Evidence Based Mental Health*, **4**, 100–101.

Mansfield, A.K. and Addis, M.E. (2001b). Manual-based psychotherapies in clinical practice. Part 1: assets, liabilities, and obstacles to dissemination. *Evidence Based Mental Health*, **4**, 68–69.

Mittelman, M.S., Epstein, C., and Pierzchala, A. (2003). *Counseling the Alzheimer's caregiver.* AMA Press, Chicago. IL.

Mohlman, J. and Gorman, J.M. (2005). The role of executive functioning in CBT: a pilot study with anxious older adults. *Behaviour Research and Therapy*, **43**, 447–465.

Murphy, S. (2000). Provision of psychotherapy services for older people. *Psychiatric Bulletin*, **24**, 184–187.

NICE (National Institute for Health and Clinical Excellence) (2006). *Dementia: supporting people with dementia and their carers in health and social care. Clinical guideline.* Available at: http://guidance.nice.org.uk/cg42

Parry, G. (2000). Evidence based psychotherapy: special case or special pleading? *Evidence Based Mental Health*, **4**, 35–36.

Reynolds, C.F., Frank, E., Perel, J.M. *et al.* (1999). Nortriptyline and interpersonal psychotherapy as maintenance therapies for recurrent major depression: a randomized controlled trial in patients older that 59 years. *Journal of the American Medical Association*, **281**, 39–45.

Reynolds, C.F., Dew, M.A., Pollock, B.G. *et al.* (2006). Maintenance treatment of major depression in old age. *New England Journal of Medicine*, **354**, 1130–1138.

Scholey, K.A. and Woods, B.T. (2003). A series of brief cognitive-behavioural interventions with people experiencing both dementia and depression: a description of techniques and common themes. *Clinical Psychology and Psychotherapy*, **10**, 175–185.

Smith, N.M., Floyd, M.R., Scogin, F. *et al.* (1997). Three-year follow-up of bibliotherapy for depression. *Journal of Consulting and Clinical Psychology*, **2**, 324–327.

Straus, S.E. and McAlister, F. (2004). Applying the results of trials and systematic reviews to our individual patients. *Evidence Based Mental Health*, **4**, 6–7.

Woods, B. (2004). Review: reminiscence and life review are effective therapies for depression in the elderly. *Evidence Based Mental Health*, **7**, 81.

# Psychological treatments: cognitive behaviour therapy

## Philip Wilkinson

Cognitive behaviour therapy (CBT) began to emerge as a distinct psychological treatment in the 1970s. With its roots in behaviour therapy and cognitive psychology, CBT combines a focus on conscious thought processes with attention to behavioural patterns. Initially it was developed as an intervention for depressive disorder and subsequently became a mainstay in the treatment of anxiety disorders. New applications for CBT have since emerged such that, for younger adults at least, it is now considered a core mental health intervention.

The central concept of the cognitive behavioural model is that emotional states, both positive and negative, are determined by the way in which the person processes information about the self and the world around. Negative automatic thoughts give rise to unpleasant emotional states and particular patterns of behaviour which in turn will maintain distorted thinking patterns (Beck et al., 1979). Unhelpful negative thinking patterns may be triggered by events in the outside world, but underlying them are belief systems that are often quite specific to the individual. Frequently, older people have held personal beliefs that have been functional throughout the years but which only give rise to problems in the face of negative life events or impoverished social circumstances in later life (James et al., 1999). For instance, an older lady who holds the belief 'my place is in the family' may lead a contented life for many years only to become depressed when her adult children and grandchildren move away from the area, leaving her on her own. Other beliefs held by older people may be less specific to the individual and influenced more by society and the generation. Typically these beliefs begin in childhood and are reinforced over the years; they include negative attitudes to ageing such as 'growing older is growing weaker' or 'old people must not be a burden to their families' and ideas about illness such as 'depression is shameful' (Laidlaw et al., 2004).

In CBT, information about the patient's thought patterns and underlying beliefs is used to derive a case formulation. This is combined with hypotheses about the triggers to the episode which in older people often include retirement, ill-health, and relationship strains (Thompson, 1996). The formulation, therefore, helps the therapist and patient to reach a shared understanding of why and how an episode of depression or anxiety has come about, helps them in devising therapeutic interventions, and keeps the therapy on track. This formulation-driven approach to treatment is combined with an empirically driven treatment protocol specific to the disorder in question, for instance depression or health anxiety. When cognitive behavioural interventions are used in group treatments, there is a greater emphasis on the disorder-specific formulation than on the individual formulation.

CBT is usually used as short-term treatment (up to 16 sessions) with the main focus on current symptoms and problems. It involves an active exchange of ideas between patient and therapist, with the therapist able to draw upon a range of techniques all of which aim to help the patient to modify the negative meanings that are given to situations. Negative thoughts might be tackled directly through diary monitoring or through the use of behavioural experiments. Behavioural experiments are planned activities undertaken by patients in or between cognitive therapy sessions which disconfirm existing unhelpful thoughts and provide evidence for new, more adaptive thoughts. They also provide the therapist and patient with further information about the causes of symptoms and the negative effects of behaviours that patients may have been using to try to ameliorate their distress (Bennett-Levy et al., 2004). For instance, in attempting to conceal their anxiety, socially anxious patients might employ behaviours that actually draw attention to them.

## CBT in the treatment of depression

### Trials of CBT in depression

A large body of evidence now supports the efficacy of CBT as a treatment for depression with adults of working age (NICE, 2004a). Individual CBT is as effective as antidepressants in reducing symptoms of depression and produces more enduring benefit than antidepressant treatment; it also appears to be better tolerated than antidepressants. Adding CBT to antidepressant treatment can also improve outcome in more severe depression and possibly in chronic depression. Over the last 20 years there has also been a plethora of clinical trials of CBT with older adults, but most of these have methodological shortcomings such as small sample sizes, reliance on younger media-recruited participants, absence of suitable control groups, and unspecified treatment techniques (Wilkinson, 1997). Within these small-scale trials of CBT, comparisons have included other psychotherapies in individual and group format, placebo, waiting list, and antidepressant medication (Areán and Cook, 2002). Only one randomized controlled trial exclusively with older adults met the quality standards of the NICE depression guideline reviewers, and from this trial (Thompson *et al.*, 2001) it was not possible to determine if there is a clinically significant difference between CBT and antidepressants in reducing the severity of depression.

## Content of CBT in the treatment of depression

A typical course of individual CBT for depression lasts up to 16 sessions and involves a range of therapeutic strategies (see Table 18ii.1). Behavioural strategies are used early on in treatment with the aims of making some immediate positive impact on mood and helping the patient to engage with therapy. Activity monitoring using a simple diary can show patients how inactivity worsens low mood; and that, because of negative thinking, they may be underestimating the extent to which they are managing to achieve and enjoy things. A useful behavioural experiment that demonstrates the effect of inactivity to the tired, depressed patient is to compare two strategies: retreating to bed for a long period versus engaging in an activity, whilst recording feelings, sense of mastery, and pleasure (Fennell *et al.*, 2004).

Case study 1 demonstrates the use of formulation, activity monitoring, and questioning of negative automatic thoughts in the treatment of a depressed older patient.

### Case study 1

Two years after the death of her husband, Mrs Lloyd had moved to a new city to live near her son and his family. She had always been an active and high-achieving woman and hoped to be useful to and supportive to her son and his family. However, her vision was failing due to senile macular disease which she found difficult to tolerate as it prevented her from doing the things she would wish for her family. She soon became depressed and frustrated.

In working on a case formulation with her therapist (Fig. 18ii.1), Mrs Lloyd soon recognized that she had a tendency to try to do a lot of things at once or to fuss over her son and his family in an effort to appear useful; she also tended to discount the positive statements that her son made. More recently, however, she had become less motivated with a tendency to stay in bed until late and neglect her own care; she had also become anxious before social occasions such as church meetings. The formulation also involved discussion of her earlier life experiences. She recognized the influence

**Table 18ii.1** Major cognitive behaviour therapy strategies used in the treatment of depression

| Cognitive strategies | Distraction techniques<br>Counting thoughts |
| --- | --- |
| Behavioural strategies | Monitoring activities, pleasure and mastery<br>Scheduling activities<br>Graded task assignment |
| Cognitive behavioural strategies | Identifying negative automatic thoughts<br>Questioning negative automatic thoughts<br>Behavioural experiments |
| Preventative strategies | Identifying assumptions<br>Challenging assumptions<br>Use of set-backs<br>Preparing for the future |

From Fennell (1989) with permission of M.J.V. Fennell.

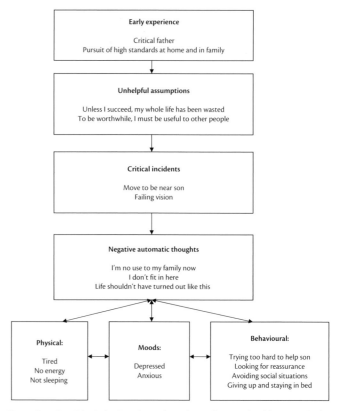

**Fig. 18ii.1** Cognitive behavioural case formulation for Mrs Lloyd (Case study 1).

of her father as she was growing up: he had always insisted that she strive to achieve the highest standards and to help others at all times. Having drawn up this formulation, Mrs Lloyd said that, for the first time, events in her life were beginning to 'connect up'.

Therapy involved identifying the activities that she could still enjoy despite her impaired vision, such as simple gardening and listening to music in the evening. She recorded her negative thoughts using a diary which enabled her to see that 'I've got into the habit of seeing the threat in every situation' (Table 18ii. 2). Sometimes she noticed that her mood was quite low when she sat down to listen to music; thought records revealed that she had a tendency then to reflect on the day with self-critical and other negative thoughts. She undertook the following behavioural experiment: having predicted that her son and his wife would be disappointed in her if she chose to entertain an old friend rather than offer to look after her grandchildren one day, she put it to the test. She observed and tackled her thoughts before and during her friend's visit and tried to limit herself to asking her son only once if they could manage without her that day. It turned out that she had an enjoyable day with her friend and discovered that this had helped her to feel more independent of her son and gave her some useful topics of conversation when she next saw him.

As Mrs Lloyd's mood improved she was able to challenge some of the assumptions that she had expressed, such as 'unless I succeed at this now, my whole life has been wasted'. She described herself as thinking straight by the end of the therapy with a more realistic and compassionate view of herself. She drew up a list of strategies to remind her how to recognize depression in the future and to manage setbacks should they occur.

**Table 18ii.2** Thought diary of Mrs Lloyd (Case study 1)

| Situation | Emotion (severity) | Negative automatic thoughts | Evidence that it's true | Evidence that it's not true | Alternative thoughts | Emotion |
|---|---|---|---|---|---|---|
| Waking up at 6 a.m. | Despondent (90%) | It's another awful day | I feel so depressed | Yes, but this is just the depression speaking | If I take one thing at a time and follow my activity schedule then I'll manage | Despondent (20%) |
| | | I shan't be able to achieve anything | I tire so easily, I should rest | If I stay in bed I'm only going to feel worse | | |
| About to visit son and his family | Sad (80%) | I'm no use to my family now | I am older and don't have the strength that I did | This is an all-or-nothing thought. When I wrote a list, I identified many ways in which they value me | There are still enough things about me that my family value | Sad (10%) |
| | Angry (30%) | Life shouldn't have turned out like this | This wasn't what I was expecting in my retirement | No-one can predict the future. It's just down to chance. This isn't going to help me to get what I want | If I take life as it comes I can make the best of it | Angry (0%) |

## Group CBT

In group CBT, psycho-educational opportunities are maximized and treatment tends to be based on an empirically derived formulation of depression rather than on individual patients' formulations. The NICE depression guideline (NICE, 2004a) concluded that there was strong evidence to suggest a clinically significant difference favouring group CBT over other group therapies in achieving remission from depression, but insufficient evidence to make comparisons with no active treatment. Although most evaluation of group CBT has been undertaken with younger adults, there are good descriptions of its use with older people (Yost *et al.*, 1986) and it is currently being evaluated as a maintenance treatment in late life depression.

## Mindfulness-based cognitive therapy

Of the recent developments in CBT for depression, one of the most fascinating and potentially useful is mindfulness-based cognitive therapy (MBCT). This method, which is based on meditation practices, has been developed with the aim of preventing the recurrence of depression. It follows on from the successful treatment at the University of Massachusetts of stress in patients with chronic pain and physical illness (Kabat-Zinn, 1990; Baer, 2003). Practising mindfulness entails becoming aware that our minds have a will of their own; that is, that our moods and actions are often governed by a stream of thoughts about past and future events. If we learn to bring our attention to an awareness of the present we will gain a better sense of control over our experience of events and ourselves (Elliston, 2001). We can choose to respond mindfully to adverse situations rather than react automatically according to an old, ingrained behaviour pattern.

The principle behind MBCT for depression is straightforward: being able mentally to step aside from a stream of thought should prevent engagement with the negative automatic thoughts that maintain depressed mood. This contrasts with traditional CBT in which the patient learns to engage with and re-evaluate their negative thoughts. This ability to switch attention away from futile thought processes is believed to be particularly helpful to sufferers of recurrent depression in whom minor dips in mood can rapidly lead to depression because of their tendency to ruminative thinking (Segal *et al.*, 2002).

Table 18ii.3 shows the structure of a MBCT course. It is usually run for a class of participants with a clear educational emphasis. Throughout the eight-session course participants learn meditation techniques, breathing exercises, and movement exercises such as yoga, and there is an expectation of daily practice of meditation. The NICE depression guideline (NICE, 2004a) states that there is some evidence with younger adults suggesting a clinically significant difference favouring MBCT for reducing the likelihood of relapse of depression after 60 weeks of follow-up, particularly in people who have had more than two episodes of depression.

**Table 18ii.3** Structure of a mindfulness-based cognitive therapy course (based on Segal *et al.* 2002)

| | |
|---|---|
| Session 1 | Understanding automatic pilot thinking: learning to move attention from thoughts to body |
| Session 2 | Dealing with barriers: learning to cope with the chatter of the mind and controlling reactions to everyday events |
| Session 3 | Mindfulness of the breath: using awareness of breathing to become more focused on the present moment |
| Session 4 | Staying present: education about depression as a package of symptoms and mindfulness as an alternative perspective |
| Session 5 | Allowing/letting be: developing an attitude of acceptance because pushing away unpleasant experience makes it worse |
| Session 6 | Thoughts are not facts: finding ways of reducing the degree of identification with thoughts and choosing whether to engage with them |
| Session 7 | How can I best take care of myself?: identifying signs of relapse and developing an action plan |
| Session 8 | Using what you have learned to deal with future moods: building in regular practice by linking to important goals and activities |

As MBCT helps patients to cease trying to solve insoluble problems it has obvious appeal as a treatment for older adults facing recurrent depression, chronic physical illness, and life stresses. Other potential benefits for older people include the support of class membership, the destigmatizing value of sharing experiences, the provision of education about depression and a method that may be easier to grasp and practise than standard CBT (Smith, 2004). Possible disadvantages, however, are that it may not be suited to people who are currently significantly depressed and those who have health anxiety who may not benefit from focusing on physical sensations.

The following statement was made by a patient summing up her experience of a MBCT course. She had joined the class having been treated with standard CBT after a traumatic bereavement and depression. She had ceased taking antidepressants after 2 years because of side-effects and although feeling generally well after CBT was still prone to episodes of sudden despair and suicidal thinking:

> We focused on breathing and body sensations, the aim being to become fully aware of the present, and get away from ruminating or yearning. Balancing *doing* with *being* is the watchword. Sitting in silence for forty minutes a day becomes enjoyable and helps!

## CBT in the management of anxiety

Following its application to the understanding of depressive disorder, the cognitive behavioural model was soon also applied in the treatment of anxiety disorders. While there is overlap between anxiety and depression in terms of symptoms and cognitions (negative predictions and a negative bias in appraising current experiences) in anxiety the negative appraisals are more selective and specific to certain situations (Beck *et al.*, 1985). The experience of anxiety may also enhance the probability of the feared event actually happening. For example, a socially anxious patient may hesitate and hold back, thereby actually undermining social performance.

The basic cognitive model of anxiety has been elaborated into a number of disorder-specific approaches. For instance, according to the cognitive model of panic disorder, sufferers misinterpret physical sensations of anxiety as signs of imminent physical catastrophe (Clark, 1986). In health anxiety patients are afraid of having an undiagnosed serious illness; they monitor and over-interpret physical symptoms and engage in safety-seeking behaviours that actually exacerbate their anxiety (Fig. 18ii.2). Patients with generalized anxiety have a number of fears about their everyday circumstances and engage in repetitive worry in an attempt to solve problems; they then worry about how their worrying is affecting them, leading to a vicious circle of anxiety (Wells, 1997).

As in the treatment of depressive disorder, CBT for anxiety is based on a case formulation of the patient's symptoms and beliefs, and draws upon a mix of thought-challenging and behavioural experiments to help the patient reappraise the threat attached to feared situations. Therapy can be provided in individual or group format. One advantage of CBT for anxious older adults is that it can help the patient to understand and manage the interaction of physical symptoms arising from anxiety and physical illness.

### Trials of CBT in anxiety

The UK National Institute for Health and Clinical Excellence concluded that CBT is an efficacious treatment for generalized anxiety disorder and panic disorder in adults of all ages (NICE, 2004b). Although there have been a number of studies evaluating CBT for anxiety specifically in older adults there are limitations to these studies so that they can only be taken as preliminary evidence of efficacy. One problem for researchers is the difficulty of recruiting older adults with pure anxiety disorders rather than anxiety co-morbid with depression; another is the high prevalence of physical illness that makes it difficult for potential subjects to enter trials or causes them to drop out. However, it is precisely these patients with both physical illness and anxiety who might stand to gain most from effective anxiety treatments. Some studies have tended to include participants with a range of anxiety symptoms but not necessarily formal diagnoses, and others have used concurrent medication but in inconsistent ways (Mohlman, 2004). However, accepting the methodological limitations of most trials, many report positive effect sizes for CBT against non-treatment controls (Nordhus and Pallesen, 2003).

Two trials that were included in the NICE review compared CBT with supportive therapies in the treatment of late life anxiety disorders. In the first (Barrowclough *et al.*, 2001) patients were aged over 55 years with diagnoses of generalized anxiety disorder, panic disorder, social phobia, and anxiety disorder not otherwise specified. Some were on stable doses of antidepressant medication. After randomization, participants received a mean number of 10 sessions of either CBT or supportive counselling. Outcomes of self-report anxiety measures at 12 months supported the efficacy of CBT, although there were many dropouts and no intention-to-treat analysis was included. In the second study (Stanley *et al.*, 1996) participants aged 55 years or more with generalized anxiety disorder received either 14 weeks of CBT or supportive psychotherapy in group format. After 6 months' follow-up both groups showed a significant improvement in outcomes, which was maintained on a range of self-report and observer-based measures. These two studies came to different conclusions about the efficacy of CBT compared with supportive counselling. The possible reasons for this difference highlight some of the difficulties in psychotherapy research: knowing whether treatments are applied similarly across different studies, and recruiting and retaining sufficient study participants to make meaningful comparisons between two potentially active treatments.

Recent trials have studied the interaction between CBT and medication in anxious older adults. Gorenstein *et al.* (2005) examined the effect of CBT in helping people keen to reduce use of benzodiazepines and other anxiolytics. Thirteen sessions of individual CBT and medication management sessions were compared with medication management alone. The CBT was based on a manual and included standard techniques of progressive muscle relaxation, breathing exercises, thought-challenging, worry strategies, problem-solving, and activity scheduling. At 6 months' follow up, controls were just as successful as CBT recipients in reducing medication but CBT completers showed significantly greater improvement on measures of anxiety, somatization, and global severity of symptoms. Again in this study there were many dropouts but the results after intention-to-treat analysis were consistent with completer analyses, although weaker. Schuurmans *et al.* (2006) investigated the efficacy of individual CBT compared with the selective serotonin reuptake inhibitor sertraline in media-recruited patients aged 60 and over with principal diagnoses of generalized anxiety disorder, panic disorder, agoraphobia, and social phobia; some were taking stable doses of benzodiazepines. CBT was of 15 sessions and consisted of relaxation, thought-challenging, and exposure based on disorder-specific models of the anxiety disorder. Despite being a well-designed trial the findings were limited because of difficulty with recruitment and dropouts leading to significant differences between the groups and loss of power. Calculation of effect sizes at 3 months showed that although both CBT and sertraline led to significant improvement in anxiety and worry compared with a waiting list control, sertraline had a stronger effect than CBT. At the present stage, therefore, there remains a need for large, adequately powered trials of CBT compared with antidepressant medication, and in combination with medication, in the treatment of late life anxiety disorders with participants who are representative of patients seen in routine clinical practice.

### Content of CBT in the treatment of health anxiety and physical illness

Figure 18ii.2 shows how CBT can be used to formulate the problems of patients with health anxiety. Treatment is aimed at identifying and reversing unhelpful thought patterns about vulnerability to illness and misinterpretation of innocuous symptoms; this can involve behavioural experiments to undo safety behaviours, such as seeking reassurance from doctors (Silver et al., 2004). Case study 2 is a summary case study of CBT in an older person with health anxiety.

### Case study 2

Mrs Woods was an 81-year-old lady living in supported accommodation. She had severe chronic obstructive pulmonary disease which restricted her to her flat. She experienced episodes of severe breathlessness and dizziness when she had not seen anyone for some time, accompanied by thoughts such as 'I'm getting a chest infection, no-one will be here to help me!' Her chest physician confirmed that her chest disease was not severe enough to account for these acute episodes. She monitored her breathing excessively from the moment she woke which in turn made her more anxious and produced hyperventilation and breathlessness. She also used her beta-agonist inhaler excessively which made her shaky and light-headed. During CBT, over a period of a few weeks, she monitored her chest symptoms and her mood. She began to recognize the symptoms of anxiety when they occurred and learned to differentiate them from symptoms of a chest infection, the anxiety having a rapid onset and being accompanied by fear, while the infection came on more slowly and was accompanied by general malaise and

a raised temperature. She recorded and challenged the negative thoughts she experienced and experimented with not resorting to extra doses of her inhaled medication. With her agreement, the warden of the establishment where she lived was also included in one treatment session so she would know how to help Mrs Woods. Her therapist provided occasional booster CBT sessions after chest infections to help her to remember her strategies.

---

This case illustrates how CBT can be used to help people with health anxiety and with their reactions to physical illness. The basis of CBT with older adults with co-morbid physical illness is to assess the way the patient has adapted to the change in physical health and to identify the meaning attached to the symptoms. For example, a person with Parkinson's disease may develop disability in excess of that determined by the actual physical disease when embarrassment caused by the tremor leads to withdrawal from social situations (Laidlaw et al., 2003). The CBT formulation can help the patient to identify this potentially remediable source of disability.

## CBT with dementia caregivers

The modification of CBT for the treatment of stressed and depressed caregivers of dementia sufferers has been an important development in recent years. Psychological symptoms are frequent in caregivers, and caregiver distress is important in determining when dementia sufferers move to institutional care. In researching interventions with caregivers, choice of appropriate outcomes is important. Concepts such as burden and strain are frequently reported, and there are a number of measures available, but increasingly the use of more clinically relevant outcomes such as caregiver depression and health-care utilization has been advocated (Black and Almeida, 2004).

Caregivers often struggle to make sense of the cognitive decline and changing behaviour of the dementia sufferer, ascribing negative meanings to them which then lead to distressing emotions (Vernooij-Dassen and Downs, 2005). This is illustrated in the following account written by a caregiver who received CBT to help him to manage symptoms associated with his wife's anxiety and the guilt he experienced when she moved into a specialist nursing home:

> My wife, Elizabeth, was diagnosed with Alzheimer's disease 4 years ago. We had been married for over 50 years. After the initial diagnosis, I tried to take care of her at home but this was very stressful indeed for both of us and after 3 years it became clear that her condition had deteriorated to such an extent that she would have to be cared for professionally, in a care home. The actual decision to send her into care was a very painful one for me and my family. After such a long life together, I had very strong guilt feelings and much stress. I was worried that she would not be looked after as well as at home and I became very fearful about visiting her. I was also concerned about my own future and the emptiness of my life alone at home.
>
> I found it impossible to explain to family and friends just how I was feeling. Instead of looking forward to the visits to my wife in the care home, I dreaded the thought of going there. I had many worries about these visits. I was worried that Elizabeth would ask me such questions as 'Where am I?' and 'Why can't I go home?' I was afraid that she would ask me to take her home, and I did not know how to deal with such a situation. It was at this point that I began to visit a cognitive therapist. From the beginning, the therapist seemed to understand my concerns. Sometimes I broke down in sessions, something I could not let myself do with my family and friends, and it was very helpful to have the therapist's understanding and sympathy. Gradually I was able

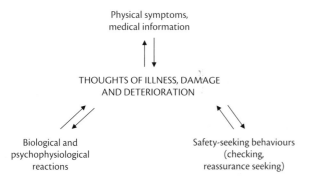

Physical symptoms, medical information

↑↓

THOUGHTS OF ILLNESS, DAMAGE AND DETERIORATION

Biological and psychophysiological reactions

Safety-seeking behaviours (checking, reassurance seeking)

**Fig. 18ii.2** Cognitive behavioural model of health anxiety, taken from Salkovskis (1992) with permission of the Royal College of Psychiatrists.

to express the emotions which previously I had hardly been able to understand myself.

The therapist told me at once that the feelings and problems I was experiencing were quite normal reactions for somebody in my position and was able to offer some explanations of the symptoms and characteristics of Alzheimer's disease. For example, he told me that while my wife's behaviour might sometimes appear normal, it was very probable that she had no real understanding of what she was saying and would certainly have no memory of any question which she might have asked me. This was an important assurance to me, because I realized that I need have no fear that I would upset her if I did not reply directly to difficult questions. The therapist persuaded me to keep this fact in my mind at each visit, and I found that it helped me very much indeed to overcome my worry about seeing my wife.

I sometimes wondered whether the method the therapist was using to confront my situation was helpful. He persuaded me to analyse my thoughts and feelings before each visit to Elizabeth and to write them down after I had returned. I was taught to question my own feelings and fears, and to rationalize the results by filling in a form which he gave me. At first I found this discipline very hard but I came to realize how valuable it was, especially when I was in a mood of despair in which feeling sorry for myself was uppermost in my mind. The habit of forcing myself to write down my thoughts and emotions helped

very much to address them and to put them into perspective. I learned to see the positive side of the situation; although my wife was in care, I was able to remember how difficult life had been for her when she was still at home and I began to notice the simple things that we could enjoy doing together in the care home.

I benefited very greatly from the therapy. My feelings of guilt about sending Elizabeth away from home are now gone, as I realize that what I had to do was in her best interests. The visits do not distress me any more and I enjoy spending time with her.

## Trials of psychological interventions with caregivers

A diverse range of psychosocial interventions has been devised to try to reduce burden, stress, and psychological morbidity amongst dementia caregivers. A systematic review of these interventions (Brodaty *et al.*, 2003) included 30 controlled studies and demonstrated marked heterogeneity in study design and sample characteristics with earlier studies being of poorer quality than more recent studies. Effect sizes were positive for psychological morbidity in three-quarters of the studies but were only statistically significant in a quarter of these (Fig. 18ii.3). Some studies also reported rates of nursing home admissions and severity of depression in the

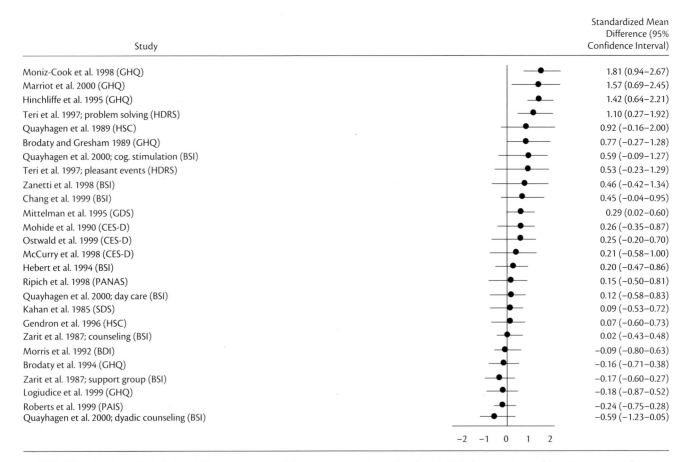

**Fig. 18ii.3** Effect sizes for psychological morbidity at most current follow-up assessment in studies of psychological interventions with caregivers, measured as standardized mean difference between treatment and control group. Abbreviations: GHQ, General Health Questionnaire; BSI, Brief Symptom Inventory; SDS, Self-rating Depression Scale; HSC, Hopkins Symptom Checklist; CES-D, Center for Epidemiological Studies Depression Scale; PANAS, Positive and Negative Affect Scale; PAIS, Psychosocial Adjustment to Illness Scale; HDRS, Hamilton Depression Rating Scale. Taken from Brodaty *et al.* (2003) with permission of Blackwell Publishing

dementia sufferer. Due to the heterogeneity of the trials, pooling of data was not feasible. In reviewing the current evidence on psychosocial interventions with dementia caregivers, the UK National Institute for Health and Clinical Excellence (NICE, 2006) concluded that there is evidence for the effectiveness of CBT on symptoms of depression and anxiety, particularly when therapy is given to caregivers with clinically significant symptoms. They also conclude that there are encouraging indications that therapy for the carer will improve the mental state of the person being cared for and delay the move to institutional care.

One of the efficacious CBT interventions is that devised by Marriott et al. (2000). This was evaluated in a randomized controlled trial comparing the CBT intervention with two control conditions of in-depth family interview only (also the initial component of the CBT intervention) and usual care only. Patients with Alzheimer's dementia and their caregivers were recruited from National Health Service community psychiatry services in Manchester. To be included in the trial caregivers needed to achieve caseness levels of symptoms on the General Health Questionnaire. Compared to the control conditions, the intervention reduced burden and brought about a greater reduction in number of cases on the General Health Questionnaire, with a 'numbers needed to treat' (NNT) of two, at 3 months' follow-up. The structure of therapy is summarized in Table 18ii.4. The aims of the intervention were: first, to help caregivers appreciate that stressful interactions can lead to disturbed behaviours in the dementia sufferer and increased distress in the caregiver; second, to help reduce stressful interactions using behaviour management techniques and calmer ways of responding; third, to reduce stress by the use of relaxation, challenging of negative automatic thoughts, and the development of the caregivers' social networks; and fourth, to help the caregivers cope with their feelings of loss. Coping skills training (sessions 12 and 13) might include, for example, helping a caregiver deal with his embarrassment when friends visit and his wife, who has dementia, becomes agitated and restless. First the therapist would explain the fact that people with dementia are susceptible to stress and noisy environments and would suggest trying to reduce this source of stress; second, the therapist introduces questioning of negative automatic thoughts to reduce the caregiver's embarrassment and shame in these situations. Other authors also stress the importance of sharing a formulation of the dementia sufferer's symptoms with the wider family so as to validate the main caregiver's role (Mittelman et al., 2003).

## Sleep problems

CBT is one of a broad range of psychological interventions to have been applied in the management of chronic sleep problems in later life. Typical components of these interventions include education about good sleep hygiene and information on normal sleeping patterns in old age. Specific cognitive strategies are used to address dysfunctional attitudes about sleep and the impact of not sleeping. For example, negative thoughts might include 'I need an unbroken night's sleep to manage the next day', or 'I must make myself sleep'. Despite a large number of trials of these interventions, only a few focus on people over 60 and are of good methodological quality; they demonstrate limited benefits of CBT (Montgomery, 2003). There appears to be some improvement in total sleep duration, maintained at 1 years' follow-up, and a reduction in night waking but no improvement in sleep onset latency. Trial participants report satisfaction with these limited improvements when compared with use of hypnotic medication. A recent trial suggests that the benefits of CBT can also be experienced by older people whose sleep problems are secondary to medical illness, and that group therapy is effective, at least in the short term (Rybarczyk et al., 2005).

## Emerging applications of CBT with older adults

### Depression and anxiety associated with memory loss

Psychological interventions for people with memory problems have two aims: to delay the progression of the memory deficit and to reduce the symptoms of anxiety and depression associated with

**Table 18ii.4** Outline of caregiver CBT intervention

| Assessment session | | Depression scores<br>Education booklet on dementia |
| --- | --- | --- |
| Sessions 1, 2, and 3 | Education sessions | Assessment of caregiver's model of illness and provision of alternative model if indicated<br>Written information on dementia, caregiver stress and availability of local services |
| Session 4 | Stress assessment | Explanation of the effects of stress and monitoring of symptoms |
| Sessions 5 and 6 | Relaxation training | Progressive relaxation and body scan taught and practised as homework |
| Sessions 7 and 8 | Managing psychological responses to stress | Explanation of role of negative automatic thoughts in stress<br>Thought records kept and challenging of negative automatic thoughts begins |
| Sessions 9 and 10 | Managing behavioural responses to stress | Tackle problems such as isolation and self-sacrificing behaviour<br>Encourage meeting of own needs |
| Session 11 | Coping skills assessment | Identify caregiver's problematic coping behaviours and thought patterns |
| Sessions 12 and 13 | Coping skills: patient behaviour management | Teach effective coping skills including use of thought challenging |
| Sessions 14 and 15 | Coping with feelings of loss | Identify feelings of loss and, where appropriate, use thought challenging to help caregiver to draw upon remaining positive aspects of relationship |

Taken with permission from therapy manual prepared by A. Marriott and C. Donaldson (unpublished) and used in trial by Marriott et al. (2000).

it by increasing the sufferer's sense of control. Therapies with the first aim include memory training and cognitive stimulation treatments targeted at improving memory and executive skills; therapies with the second aim are CBT based. People experiencing memory problems may develop unhelpful beliefs about their problems that cause symptoms, such as 'in order to engage in social activities I must remember names and faces' or 'I'm the only person who forgets things' (Kipling *et al.*, 1999). Patients with mild dementia may be able to use cognitive techniques to challenge negative automatic thoughts and to cope with challenging situations. For example, they might be assisted to challenge the self-critical and hopeless thoughts that occur when they experience episodes of memory loss. Those with more severe cognitive impairment who are unable to use these techniques might benefit from behavioural activation and scheduling pleasant events to overcome depressive withdrawal (Teri and Gallagher-Thompson, 1991). The UK National Institute for Health and Clinical Excellence conducted a systematic review of randomized controlled trials of psychological interventions for people with dementia who are experiencing depression and anxiety (NICE, 2006) but found no adequately designed trials of interventions aimed directly at sufferers; one trial was mainly with carers (teaching pleasant events scheduling and problem-solving) and the other was a service evaluation. The limits of psychological therapies in people with memory impairment and dementia are discussed in Chapter 18i.

## Psychotic symptoms

In the last few years CBT has been associated with significant advances in the understanding and treatment of psychotic symptoms in younger adults, and is now recommended as an intervention in schizophrenia. New psychological models of psychosis have been developed such as that of Garety *et al.* (2001). This proposes that adverse environmental conditions interact with a vulnerability to psychosis to trigger emotional changes and disrupt the cognitive processes of attention, perception, and judgement. Anomalous thoughts are then attributed to an external source, giving rise to delusions and hallucinations. Cognitive behavioural interventions are focused directly on delusional beliefs, beliefs about hallucinations, and other associated problems such as social anxiety (Close and Schuller, 2004). With older adults these approaches have been applied, but not formally evaluated, in the treatment of distressing visual hallucinations (Collerton and Dudley, 2004) and psychotic depression (Wilkinson and Schuller, 2003).

# Conclusions

CBT has a wide range of applications in the treatment of older adults including depressive disorder and anxiety disorders. Many components of CBT can also be applied in the routine treatment of older adults in mental health services. Helpful elements of CBT are its ability to incorporate patients' attitudes to ageing and illness and its focus on disability and physical symptoms. Outcome research has not kept pace with studies in younger adults partly due to problems of recruiting and retaining older people in clinical trials. Important areas of investigation include the role of CBT in the long-term management of depressive illness and in preventing relapse. CBT appears to be one of the more efficacious psychosocial interventions in the treatment of symptomatic dementia caregivers.

# References

Areán, P.A. and Cook, B.L. (2002). Psychotherapy and combined psychotherapy/pharmacotherapy for late life depression. *Biological Psychiatry*, **52**, 293–303.

Baer, R. (2003). Mindfulness training as a clinical intervention: a conceptual and empirical review. *Clinical Psychology Science and Practice*, **10**, 125–143.

Barrowclough, C., King, P., Colville, J., Russell, E., Burns, A., and Tarrier, N. (2001). A randomized trial of the effectiveness of cognitive-behavioural therapy and supportive counseling for anxiety symptoms in older adults. *Journal of Consulting and Clinical Psychology*, **69**, 756–762.

Beck, A.T., Rush, A.J., Shaw, B.F., and Emery, G. (1979). *Cognitive therapy of depression*. Guilford Press, New York.

Beck, A.T., Emery, G., and Greenberg, R.L. (1985). *Anxiety disorders and phobias: a cognitive perspective*. Basic Books, New York.

Bennett-Levy, J., Westbrook, D., Fennell, M., Cooper, M., Rouf, K., and Hackmann, A. (2004). Behavioural experiments: historical and conceptual underpinnings. In *Oxford guide to behavioural experiments in cognitive therapy* (ed. J. Bennett-Levy, G. Butler, M. Fennell, A. Hackmann, M. Mueller, and D. Westbrook), pp. 1–20. Oxford University Press, Oxford.

Black, W. and Almeida, O.P. (2004). A systematic review of the association between the behavioral and psychological symptoms of dementia and burden of care. *International Psychogeriatrics*, **16**(3), 295–315.

Brodaty, H., Green, A., and Koschera, A. (2003). Meta-analysis of psychosocial interventions for caregivers of people with dementia. *Journal of the American Geriatrics Society*, **51**, 657–664.

Clark, D.M. (1986). A cognitive model of panic. *Behaviour Research and Therapy*, **24**, 461–470.

Close, H. and Schuller, S. (2004). Psychotic symptoms. In *Oxford guide to behavioural experiments in cognitive therapy* (ed. J. Bennett-Levy, G. Butler, M. Fennell, A. Hackmann, M. Mueller, and D. Westbrook), pp. 245–263. Oxford University Press, Oxford.

Collerton, D. and Dudley, R. (2004). A cognitive behavioural framework for the treatment of distressing visual hallucinations in older people. *Behavioural and Cognitive Psychotherapy*, **32**, 443–455.

Elliston, P. (2001). Mindfulness in medicine and everyday life. *British Medical Journal*, **323**(2), 7322.

Fennell, M.J.V. (1989). Depression. In *Cognitive behaviour therapy for psychiatric problems: a practical guide* (ed. K. Hawton), pp. 169–234. Oxford University Press, Oxford.

Fennell, M., Bennett-Levy, J., and Westbrook, D. (2004). Depression. In *Oxford guide to behavioural experiments in cognitive therapy* (ed. J. Bennett-Levy, G. Butler, M. Fennell, A. Hackmann, M. Mueller, and D. Westbrook), pp. 205–222. Oxford University Press, Oxford.

Garety, P., Kuipers, E., Fowler, D., Freeman, D., and Bebbington, P. (2001). A cognitive model of the positive symptoms of psychosis. *Psychological Medicine*, **31**, 189–195.

Gorenstein, E.E., Kleber, M.S., Mohlman, J., DeJesus, M., Gorman, J.M., and Papp, L.A. (2005). Cognitive-behavioral therapy for management of anxiety and medication taper in older adults. *American Journal of Psychiatry*, **13**, 901–909.

James, I.A., Kendell, K., and Reichelt, F.K. (1999). Conceptualizations of depression in older people: the interaction of positive and negative beliefs. *Behavioural and Cognitive Psychotherapy*, **27**, 285–290.

Kabat-Zinn, J. (1990). *Full catastrophe living*. Piatkus, New York.

Kipling, T., Bailey, M., and Charlesworth, G. (1999). The feasibility of a cognitive behavioural therapy group for men with mild/moderate cognitive impairment. *Behavioural and Cognitive Psychotherapy*, **27**, 189–193.

Laidlaw, K., Thompson, L.W., Dick-Siskin, L., and Gallagher-Thompson, D. (2003). *Cognitive behaviour therapy with older people*. Wiley, New York.

Laidlaw, K., Thompson, L.W., and Gallagher-Thompson, D. (2004). Comprehensive conceptualization of cognitive behaviour therapy for late life depression. *Behavioural and Cognitive Psychotherapy*, **32**, 389–399.

Marriott, A., Donaldson, C., Tarrier, N., and Burns, A. (2000). Effectiveness of cognitive-behavioural family intervention in reducing the burden of care in carers of patients with Alzheimer's disease. *British Journal of Psychiatry*, **176**, 557–562.

Mittelman, M.S., Epstein, C., and Pierzchala, A. (2003). *Counseling the Alzheimer's caregiver*. AMA Press, Chicago, IL.

Mohlman, J. (2004). Psychosocial treatment of late-life generalized anxiety disorder: current status and future directions. *Clinical Psychology Review*, **24**, 149–169.

Montgomery, P. and Dennis, J. (2003). Cognitive behavioural interventions for sleep problems in adults aged 60+. *The Cochrane Database of Systematic Reviews*, 2003(1), CD003161 (available at: http://www.mrw.interscience.wiley.com/cochrane/clsysrev/articles/CD003161/frame.html).

NICE (National Institute for Health and Clinical Excellence) (2004a). *Depression: management of depression in primary and secondary care*, clinical guideline (available at: http://guidance.nice.org.uk/CG23).

NICE (National Institute for Health and Clinical Excellence) (2004b). *Anxiety: management of anxiety (panic disorder, with or without agoraphobia, and generalised anxiety disorder) in adults in primary, secondary and community care*, clinical guideline (available at: http://guidance.nice.org.uk/CG22).

NICE (National Institute for Health and Clinical Excellence) (2006). *Dementia: Supporting people with dementia and their carers in health and social care*, clinical guideline (available at: http://guidance.nice.org.uk/cg42).

Nordhus, I.H. and Pallesen, S. (2003). Psychological treatment of late-life anxiety: an empirical review. *Journal of Consulting and Clinical Psychology*, **71**, 643–651.

Rybarczyk, B., Stepanski, E., Fogg, L., Barry, P., Lopez, M., and Davis, A. (2005). A placebo-controlled test of cognitive-behavioral therapy for comorbid insomnia in older adults. *Journal of Consulting and Clinical Psychology*, **73**, 1164–1174.

Salkovskis, P. (1992). The cognitive-behavioural approach. In *Medical symptoms not explained by organic disease* (ed. F. Creed, R. Mayou, and A. Hopkins). Royal College of Psychiatrists and Royal College of Physicians of London, London.

Schuurmans, J., Comijs, H., Emmelkamp, P.M.G. *et al.* (2006). A randomized, controlled trial of the effectiveness of cognitive-behavioral therapy and sertraline versus a waitlist control group for anxiety disorders in older adults. *American Journal of Psychiatry*, **14**, 255–263.

Segal, Z.V., Williams, J.M.G., and Teasdale, J.D. (2002). *Mindfulness-based cognitive therapy for depression: a new approach to preventing relapse*. Guilford Press, New York.

Silver, A., Sanders, D., Morrison, N., and Cowey, C. (2004). Health anxiety. In *Oxford guide to behavioural experiments in cognitive therapy* (ed. J. Bennett-Levy, G. Butler, M. Fennell, A. Hackmann, M. Mueller, and D. Westbrook), pp. 81–98. Oxford University Press, Oxford.

Smith, A. (2004). Clinical uses of mindfulness training for older people. *Behavioural and Cognitive Psychotherapy*, **32**, 423–430.

Stanley, M.A., Beck, J.G., and Glassco, J.D. (1996). Treatment of generalized anxiety in older adults: a preliminary comparison of cognitive-behavioral and supportive approaches. *Behavior Therapy*, **27**, 565–581.

Teri, L. and Gallagher-Thompson, D. (1991). Cognitive-behavioral interventions for treatment of depression in Alzheimer's patients. *The Gerontologist*, **31**(3), 413–416.

Thompson, L.W. (1996). Cognitive-behavioral therapy and treatment for late-life depression. *Journal of Clinical Psychiatry*, **57**, 29–37.

Thompson, L.W., Coon, D.W., Gallagher-Thompson, D., Somner, B.R., and Koin, D. (2001). Comparison of desipramine and cognitive/behavioral therapy in the treatment of elderly outpatients with mild-to-moderate depression. *American Journal of Geriatric Psychiatry*, **9**, 225–240.

Vernooij-Dassen, M. and Downs, M. (2005). Cognitive and behavioural interventions for carers of people with dementia [Protocol]. *The Cochrane Database of Systematic Reviews*, 2005(2), CD005318 (available at: http://www.mrw.interscience.wiley.com/cochrane/clsysrev/articles/CD005318/frame.html).

Wells, A. (1997). *Cognitive therapy of anxiety disorders. a practice manual and conceptual guide*. Wiley, Chichester.

Wilkinson, P. (1997). Cognitive therapy with elderly people. *Age and Ageing*, **26**, 53–58.

Wilkinson, P. and Schuller, S. (2003). Late-onset auditory hallucinations treated with cognitive behaviour therapy. *International Journal of Geriatric Psychiatry*, **18**, 537–539.

Yost, E.B., Beutler, L.E., Corbishley, M.A., and Allender, J.R. (1986). *Group cognitive therapy: a treatment approach for depressed older adults*. Pergamon, New York.

# Psychological treatments: interpersonal psychotherapy

## Philip Wilkinson

Interpersonal psychotherapy (IPT) was originally developed as a placebo intervention for use in controlled trials of antidepressant medication, being intended to act as a high-contact but non-specific social support condition (Stuart and Robertson, 2003). Rather than being inactive, however, it proved to be efficacious and has since become a leading psychological therapy especially in the management of depressive illness. IPT is based on the straightforward observation that the origins of the depression often lie in the individual's interpersonal relationships while, at the same time, the depression itself has a negative impact on relationships. IPT is also informed by attachment, communication, and social theories. Although a person's vulnerability to depression may be biological, in IPT early experiences and unmet attachment needs are also seen as important, with episodes of illness being triggered by social pressures and disruption of interpersonal networks. Early practitioners of IPT were therefore quick to see the relevance of the model to late life depression (Sholomskas et al., 1983). The model does not ignore the biological underpinnings of depression or the role of biological treatments, it simply places the emphasis of interventions in the interpersonal domain. Having initially been developed for use in research trials, IPT remains a structured form of therapy that can be delivered in a reproducible, standardized fashion.

## IPT in the treatment of depression

### Trials of IPT in depression

IPT has been evaluated in a small number of well-designed randomized controlled trials. These trials have been reviewed by the UK National Institute of Health and Clinical Excellence (NICE, 2004) with the conclusion that IPT is more effective than placebo in the acute treatment of depression in adults of all ages when compared with usual general practitioner care. The combination of IPT and antidepressant medication is also more powerful than IPT alone, although it is not clear how the combination compares with antidepressants alone. NICE also reviewed trials of IPT as a continuation and maintenance treatment with patients who have remitted or recovered on previous treatment and concluded that there is some evidence that it is effective, especially when used in combination with antidepressant treatments.

Looking specifically at trials with older adults, NICE concluded that IPT in combination with antidepressants performed better than IPT alone but that there was insufficient evidence to determine whether IPT performed any better than antidepressants alone. There was some evidence to suggest a clinically significant difference favouring IPT plus antidepressants over medication alone on reducing the likelihood of relapse after 3 years' maintenance treatment, and a clinically significant difference favouring IPT over medication placebo on the same criterion. Since the NICE review a further major trial of maintenance IPT with older adults has been published (see below).

The defining work on IPT with older adults has been carried out at the Western Psychiatric Institute and Clinic, Pittsburgh, USA. The first major trial (Maintenance Therapies for Late Life Depression 1; MTLD1; Reynolds et al. 1999) was a randomized controlled trial with 3 years of maintenance treatment set in a research outpatient clinic with people aged 60 years and older. They had all remitted from at least their second episode of major depression having received IPT and nortriptyline as treatment in the acute phase. They were allocated to one of four maintenance treatment conditions: nortriptyline, drug placebo, IPT alone, or nortriptyline and IPT in combination. After 3 years the lowest rate of recurrence was in the group receiving combined treatment; IPT alone was more efficacious than placebo in preventing relapse, but not as much as antidepressant alone (Fig. 18iii.1). The authors observed that participants aged 70 years and over were more likely to relapse in the first year than those in the 60–69-year-old group. The combination treatment was also more likely to prevent relapse in the older participants than in the younger participants.

The next major study conducted by the Pittsburgh group focused on depressed people aged 70 years and older and compared IPT and the selective serotonin reuptake inhibitor (SSRI) paroxetine (MTLLD2; Reynolds et al. 2006). In this trial over half of the participants were in their first episode of depression, they had more co-morbid medical illnesses and more cognitive impairment (scoring at least 17 on the Mini-Mental State Examination) than those in MTLLD1. Randomization was stratified according to the number of episodes, use of augmented pharmacotherapy in the acute phase treatment, and level of cognitive impairment. Participants who had responded to acute phase therapy with paroxetine and IPT were randomly assigned to one of four maintenance treatments: paroxetine (up to 40 mg) or placebo, combined with either monthly IPT or clinical management sessions. Follow-up in this study was

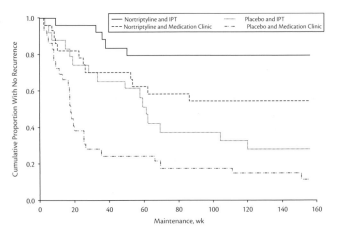

**Fig. 18iii.1** Survival analysis of the four treatment groups in MTLLD1. Taken with permission from Reynolds *et al.* (1999, p. 42). Copyright © 1999 American Medical Association. All rights reserved.

for 2 years or until the recurrence of major depression. In contrast with the findings of MTLLD1, relapse rates in MTLLD2 were no lower in those receiving the combination treatment than in those receiving antidepressant alone, and IPT without medication was no more efficacious than clinical management (Fig. 18iii.2). Not surprisingly, patients with fewer and less severe medical problems responded better to paroxetine than those with medical problems.

It is interesting to consider why patients in this study did not benefit as much from IPT as in MTLLD1. The authors speculate that the cases of late onset depression in MTLLD2 might have been more resistant to treatment, due to organic brain changes and cognitive impairment. It must also be remembered that all groups had received IPT in the acute phase of treatment so it is possible that these subjects had already gained maximum benefit from psychological treatment before entering the maintenance phase. It would also be of interest to investigate the use of IPT purely as a maintenance phase treatment.

The Pittsburgh MTLLD trials are important for a number of reasons: they are the best-designed psychotherapy trials so far

undertaken with older people; they involve long-term follow-up of patients; they begin to identify the factors that may influence treatment response; and they help to clarify the interaction between psychotherapy and antidepressant medication. The Pittsburgh group are now evaluating IPT in the treatment of older depressed people who have responded only partially to SSRI treatment.

## Content of IPT in the treatment of depression

IPT focuses on the patient's relationships in the outside world, aiming to improve them where possible or, if more appropriate, to modify the patient's reliance on unhelpful relationships. Assessment and intervention focus on the patient's styles of attachment and communication, beginning with a detailed account of interpersonal relationships. This 'interpersonal inventory' produces a full picture of current social networks and activities, previous key relationships, and quality of relationships including any disappointing aspects. Relationships reviewed include not just family and social relationships but also those with other key people such as professionals. Education on the nature of depression is given, with an emphasis on depression being an illness, and the patient is encouraged to adopt the sick role in the initial stages of therapy.

IPT follows a set structure (Fig. 18iii.3) and the plan and time frame are made explicit to the patient from the start. Once the initial sessions are completed, one or two therapeutic foci are selected. There are four possible foci in IPT: grief and loss, interpersonal role

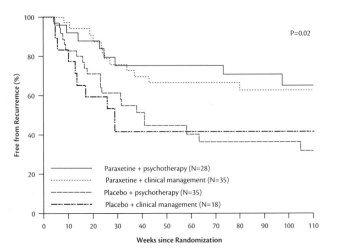

**Fig. 18iii.2** Survival analysis of the four treatment groups in MTLLD2. Taken with permission from Reynolds *et al.* (2006). Copyright © 2006 Massachusetts Medical Society. All rights reserved.

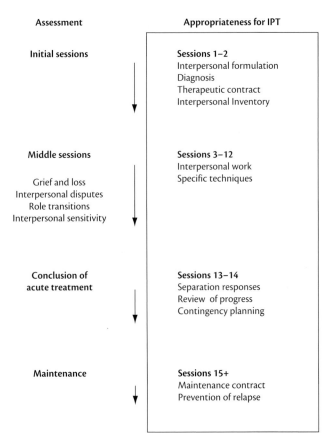

**Fig. 18iii.3** The structure of interpersonal therapy. Taken from *Interpersonal Psychotherapy: A Clinician's Guide* (ed. S. Stuart and M. Robertson). Copyright © 2003 Arnold. Reproduced by permission of Edward Arnold (Publishers) Ltd.

disputes, role transitions, and interpersonal deficits or sensitivity. The foci chosen are likely to be those most associated with hopelessness and suicidal risk; with older people those most often selected are role transition and role dispute (Miller and Reynolds, 2002). In the middle sessions of therapy the therapist uses a range of techniques to promote change in the patient's interpersonal behaviour and to help solve problems related to the chosen foci (Weissman *et al.*, 2000). Then in the concluding sessions the therapist and patient review progress together by looking again at the interpersonal inventory and problem areas before plans are made for tackling future problems. There may then be maintenance sessions for ongoing work on existing interpersonal problems or work on new problems. Further explanation of how each focus may be addressed is given below.

### Grief and loss

Grief and loss are the reactions to the death of significant people, job loss, divorce, etc.; when it gives rise to depression, grief is frequently complex or inhibited. The therapist tries to facilitate the grieving process by clarifying the nature of the relationship with the deceased and by helping the patient look for alternative supports and interests. With older adults, the grief reaction may not be for someone who has actually died but for a spouse who has become disabled or has dementia. In this case, the work may be to grieve for the loss of the healthy partner and to make necessary changes in the current social world.

### Role disputes

Role disputes are interpersonal struggles often with the partner or other family member. These disputes both contribute to depression and are made worse by the social withdrawal associated with depression. The therapist's role is to help the patient to understand his or her role in the dispute, link it with the depression, and then to take a problem-solving approach to changing aspects of the relationship. It may be that the problem can be overcome if communications are improved, or in some cases it may be that the relationship cannot be repaired. With older adults, it is often preferable to try to bolster a relationship rather than risk a significant loss late in life. Role disputes may become apparent when older people suffer physical illnesses such as cardiac disease which then impact on marital relationships.

### Role transition

Role transition means a shift in interpersonal role such as (in later life) retirement or increased dependency on an adult son or daughter after the onset of chronic illness. The therapist helps the patient to understand the link between the role transition and the depression and to look for positive as well as negative aspects of the transition in order to develop a greater sense of mastery over the new role.

### Interpersonal deficits

Interpersonal deficits (or interpersonal sensitivity) is the least validated of the four problem areas in IPT and so is usually avoided as the therapeutic focus if possible. It implies a long-term difficulty in forming interpersonal relationships and may be accompanied by a poor interpersonal network. This category will include patients with personality disorder but could also embrace those with chronic low-grade mood disorder. As with other problem areas in IPT, treatment does not focus on the early origins of the deficits but on ways of reducing social isolation, which may include identifying and reversing unhelpful patterns of relating, or improving assertiveness skills.

### Therapeutic techniques in IPT

Within the theoretical model of IPT, various therapeutic techniques can be employed to tackle the identified problems. These include education on the nature of depression, facilitation of expression of affect, behavioural methods such as problem-solving as well as cognitive strategies aimed at patients' attitudes to roles and relationships. Sometimes directive and practical interventions may also be useful in the treatment of older people, such as help with transport or finances. A difficulty that might arise in using IPT with older adults is a paucity of current relationships on which to work; in this instance the focus may need to be more on previous relationships (Frank *et al.*, 1993). Also the interpersonal inventory may take many sessions to complete if the older adult is involved in a large family of many generations with problems in a number of relationships.

### A case study

Mrs Jackson, a 65-year-old, white, married female, presented in her fourth episode of major depression, never having had any previous experience of psychotherapy. She presented with several psychosocial stressors, most prominently recent retirement. She was extremely anxious and guarded at the onset of therapy, and reported an almost complete remission of depressive symptoms in the first week. Within several weeks, however, her symptoms returned to their original severity. Mrs Jackson was quite anxious and had a difficult time engaging actively in therapy. After an initial cautious start, the educational component of IPT appeared to pay off, and she began to engage more actively. Gradually, she began talking about her difficulties adjusting to retirement. These difficulties included time management, learning to manage money, and setting boundaries on her availability for baby-sitting her grandchildren. The first five to eight sessions focused on these role transition issues.

Once Mrs Jackson began to feel somewhat better and as her trust in her therapist deepened, she began to reveal more deep-seated resentments and conflicts toward her husband. She requested that the focus shift away from her problems with retirement onto her conflicts with him. She stated that she was now willing to examine her own feelings and behaviours and work on ways to try and make life better with her husband. She grappled with many long-standing conflicts with him. Each situation that she brought to light manifested an underlying imbalance of power and control. Mrs Jackson described her husband as a benign dictator, but a dictator nonetheless. In exploring these issues in IPT, she concluded that she must try to speak up more, and to be clearer about her needs. Initially, this created more conflict as well as intense internal dissonance. She eventually began to recognize her own responsibility in allowing her husband to control even minor decisions, and she recognized it was not easy for her to assert herself. As her IPT therapist encouraged her to try alternative strategies, she was both surprised and delighted to find that her husband was more willing to share in decision-making than she thought possible. With practice, she eventually became more comfortable in this newly acquired role. Through her active participation in IPT, Mrs Jackson made healthy adjustments to retirement, and reduced the role disputes that chronically characterized her marriage. The depression that had resulted from feeling hopelessly stuck was resolved.

From Miller and Reynolds (2002) with permission of the publisher Brunner-Routledge.

In this case study the patient was experiencing a role dispute with her husband, that is a long-standing struggle over their expectations of one another. If it is felt to be unresolvable, such a situation can understandably undermine self-esteem and result in depression. In this case the patient was willing to try to renegotiate the role by first examining her own contribution to the imbalance of power. In other cases, the IPT therapist may set about to increase the struggle in order to break an impasse or simply to assist in mourning for a relationship that is actually breaking up. The therapist used a range of techniques with Mrs Jackson: detailed clarification of the problem to aid her understanding of what was happening, and communication analysis to identify communication failures and devise more effective ways of communicating. Interestingly, during IPT with older adults, an initial focus of role transition often resolves only to reveal more long-standing role disputes, often with the spouse (Miller and Reynolds, 2002).

### Maintenance IPT

When IPT is used as a maintenance therapy in depression, as in the MTLLD studies, therapy sessions may be less frequent and spread over weeks or months. The therapist aims to identify factors involved in the recurrence of depression including social deficits and long-standing patterns of interpersonal behaviour (Frank et al., 1993). Therapy is likely to involve a greater number of foci than acute phase treatment and to include a plan for identifying the early warning signs of future episodes of depression. When patients have been depressed for long periods, they need help in adapting to being a well person again, which in itself constitutes a role transition.

### Group IPT

IPT can also be provided in group format. Originally developed for the treatment of bulimia nervosa, group treatment has since been used in the treatment of depression. An advantage of the format is that it provides an 'interpersonal laboratory' in which interpersonal functioning can be observed and new ways of relating tried out (Wilfley et al., 2000). Psycho-educational aspects of treatment are strengthened and participants can join one another in applying therapeutic techniques such as decision analysis (Scocco et al., 2002). The forum can provide practical and empathic interactions between group members (Robertson et al., 2004). It may be difficult, however, to maintain an adequate focus on each participant's chosen problem area, so occasional individual sessions may be required.

## IPT in the treatment of grief

Although there is no formal agreement about when grief becomes a clinical problem and requires treatment, it is generally accepted that features warranting intervention include persistent symptoms of depression, delayed onset of grief, preoccupation with thoughts of the deceased, and distressing, intrusive thoughts related to the death. Persistent avoidance of reminders of the loss and avoidance of emotion may also suggest pathological grief. Drawing upon attachment and communication theories, IPT aims to help the grieving patient to relinquish the attachment to the lost figure, to communicate the loss to others, and to develop new attachments (Stuart and Robertson, 2003). Grief is sometimes chosen as a focus in IPT in situations where the object of attachment has not actually died but has become unavailable through separation or illness. This situation might apply, for instance, to older people caring for a spouse after a stroke or impaired by dementia. In this situation, the aim of IPT is to help the patient maximize the remaining positive aspects of the relationship, grieve for what has been lost, and support them in making the most of their social network. Severe grief reactions might also be precipitated by the loss of apparently unimportant figures because of unexpressed grief relating to losses much earlier in life (Frank et al., 1993).

## IPT in the treatment of anxiety

Depressed patients with co-morbid anxiety have often been thought to be less likely than non-anxious patients to respond to IPT, although a secondary analysis of data from two studies including the MTLLD2 study demonstrated that on most measures of co-morbid anxiety there was no effect on treatment outcomes (Lenze et al., 2003). When anxiety is present alongside depression some authors suggest certain modifications of IPT, such as provision of additional psycho-education on anxiety and the impact it can have on relationships as well as the use of cognitive behavioural strategies (Cyranowski et al., 2005). In the last few years, IPT has also been used in the management of primary anxiety disorders, including post-traumatic stress disorder and social phobia. Intuitively, IPT should help to overcome some of the social effects of anxiety such as avoidance and interpersonal sensitivity, and help older adults when anxiety disorders are triggered by retirement or traumatic events (Robertson et al., 2004).

## Conclusion

IPT is a well-established treatment used in the management of depressive illness, particularly in the United States. It has obvious applications in the treatment of depression in older people and some of the best-designed psychotherapy trials so far conducted with older people have been of IPT. Elements of IPT can be applied in the routine management of depressed patients. More work is needed to establish its efficacy with older people, including predictors of treatment response and performance in areas other than depression.

### References

Cyranowski, J.M., Frank, E., Shear, M.K. et al. (2005). Interpersonal psychotherapy for depression with panic spectrum symptoms: a pilot study. Depression and Anxiety, 21, 140–142.

Frank, E., Frank, N., Cornes, C. et al. (1993) Interpersonal psychotherapy in the treatment of late-life depression. In: New applications of interpersonal psychotherapy (ed. G.L. Klerman and M.M. Weissman). American Psychiatric Publishing, Arlington, VA.

Lenze, E.J., Mulsant, B.H., Dew, M.A. et al. (2003). Good treatment outcomes in late-life depression with comorbid anxiety. Journal of Affective Disorders, 77, 247–254.

Miller, M.D. and Reynolds, C.F.I. (2002). Interpersonal psychotherapy. In Psychological therapies with older people (ed. J. Hepple, J. Pearce, and P. Wilkinson), pp. 103–127. Brunner-Routledge, Hove.

NICE (National Institute for Health and Clinical Excellence) (2004). *Depression: management of depression in primary and secondary care*, clinical guideline (available at: http://guidance.nice.org.uk/CG23).

Reynolds, C.F., Frank, E., Perel, J.M. *et al.* (1999). Nortriptyline and interpersonal psychotherapy as maintenance therapies for recurrent major depression: a randomized controlled trial in patients older than 59 years. *Journal of the American Medical Association*, **281**, 39–45.

Reynolds, C.F., Dew, M.A., Pollock, B.G. *et al.* (2006). Maintenance treatment of major depression in old age. *New England Journal of Medicine*, **354**, 1130–1138.

Robertson, M., Rushton, P.J., Bartrum, D., and Ray, R. (2004). Group-based interpersonal psychotherapy for posttraumatic stress disorder: theoretical and clinical aspects. *International Journal of Group Psychotherapy*, **52**(4), 145–175.

Scocco, P., De Leo, D., and Frank, E. (2002). Is interpersonal psychotherapy in group format a therapeutic option in late-life depression? *Clinical Psychology and Psychotherapy*, **9**, 68–75.

Sholomskas, A.J., Chevron, E.S., Prusoff, B.A., and Berry, C. (1983). Short-term interpersonal therapy (IPT) with the depressed elderly: case reports and discussion. *American Journal of Psychotherapy*, **37**, 552–566.

Stuart, S. and Robertson, M. (2003). *Interpersonal psychotherapy. a clinician's guide*. Arnold, London.

Weissman, M.M., Markowitz, J.C., Klerman, G.L. *et al.* (2000). *Comprehensive guide to interpersonal psychotherapy*. Basic Books, New York.

Wilfley, D.E., MacKenzie, K.R., Welch, R.R., Ayres, V.E., and Weissman, M.M. (2000). *Interpersonal psychotherapy for groups*. Basic Books, New York.

# Psychological treatments: systemic interventions with older adults and their families

Eia Asen

## Introduction

As life expectancy increases, so does the number of older adults who live in couple relationships and/or with other members of the wider family. The clinical awareness of the huge significance of families for the psychological and physical well-being of older people has been relatively slow to make an impact upon family therapists and systemic practitioners. There are far too few dedicated family therapy services for older adults and their relatives. Ageism may be partially responsible for this, with the emphasis on 'saving the young', perhaps because the elderly are perceived as having lived their lives (Ivey *et al.*, 2000). However, there has been an increasing number of publications on family therapy and systemic practice with older people over the past 25 years (Herr and Weakland, 1979; Keller and Bromley, 1989; Neidhardt and Allen, 1993; Richardson *et al.*, 1994; van Amburg *et al.*, 1996; Benbow and Marriott, 1997; Tisher and Dean, 2000; Curtis and Dixon, 2005). This chapter describes the main ideas and practices of systemic family therapy, outlines guidelines for family assessments, and details specific family therapy techniques that can be used when dealing with adult patients and their families who present with psychological problems or illness in later life.

## The family and the system

The term 'systemic therapy' has replaced the more traditional term 'family therapy' as the latter appears too narrow, implying a focus only on 'the family'—whatever that is—and seemingly excluding, for example, childless couples or unattached older adults. The cultural context now is different from what it was only 50 years ago. Many different forms of committed relationships now coexist. It is not necessary to have a traditional family in order to be at the receiving end of family therapy: any relationship lends itself to a systemic approach. In fact, systemic therapy can be given to families, couples, professional systems, and even individuals (Jenkins and Asen, 1992). Why the term 'systemic'? It is possible to describe the family as a 'system' which has a variety of properties, such as hierarchies, boundaries, overt and covert conflicts between specific members, coalitions, and so on (Jackson, 1957). The family is seen as an 'open system' (von Bertalanffy, 1968) and it is part of a number of different social contexts: such as the extended family, the neighbourhood, and the cultural setting. In the systemic model individuals and families are seen as behaving according to a set of explicit and implicit rules, and it is these rules which are thought to govern interpersonal behaviours and communications (Watzlawick *et al.*, 1967). If such rules can be uncovered or discovered, and if they are believed to contribute to the presenting problems, then this has pragmatic implications for change: the rules can be questioned and challenged and new interactions can emerge. Furthermore, systems theory claims that changing just one part of the system (such as the patient's symptoms) results in changes elsewhere (for example in interactions between family members). 'Systemic therapy' addresses different levels of the system—individual, couple, family, extended family, and social setting—as well as the professional system.

In families and couples problem behaviours are sometimes so interlinked that it is impossible to distinguish between cause and effect—or what came first—as in the following frequently encountered example:

He: 'I only nag because you are so forgetful'.
She: 'But I can't remember anything if you always have a go at me'.
He: 'If you weren't upsetting me all the time I would stop nagging…'.
She: 'If you stopped nagging I wouldn't be upset and I could concentrate more and remember things…. and you wouldn't need to nag'.

Such communication exchanges can be termed 'circular': one specific 'speech act' leads to a particular response which, in turn, triggers further 'speech acts', responses, and related interactions. These recursive loops form an 'interaction pattern' in which both partners, as in the above example, can become trapped. Characteristically each person views his or her actions merely as a response to the other's responses or behaviours. It is often only possible for an outside observer to see the almost absurd circularity of some such interactions. Family systems therapy, systemic family therapy, aims to challenge and disrupt such stuck interactions and dysfunctional patterns, so that new forms of communication and interaction can emerge. Systemic work with older adults and their families aims to foster better relationships between family members, within and across generations, and to achieve more appropriate support or independence for older family members

(Richardson *et al.*, 1994). Systemic family therapy is both a specific psychological treatment method and a way of conceptualizing psychological and psychosocial disturbance. 'Thinking families' and 'thinking systems' is an important framework for any clinician involved in the assessment of older adults, their families, and the social contexts they operate in.

## The evolution of family therapy and systemic practice

Some of the early family therapy pioneers had a tendency to blame the family for the illness or problems of their offspring (Laing and Esterson, 1964) and, not surprisingly, family therapy was therefore at the outset not very popular—and particularly not with families. This parent-blaming stance was to some extent a reaction to the medical model, yet very much embedded in it: instead of genes 'causing' schizophrenia, the 'schizophrenogenic' family was blamed for causing the mental illness of one of its members. Thankfully much has changed over the past 50 years, and in the following section we shall review some of the models.

*Structural family therapy* (Minuchin *et al.* 1967; Minuchin, 1974) does not see the family as the cause but as the 'site' of the presenting problems—and also as a major resource to address these. This form of intervention is based on a normative model of family functioning, postulating that families function particularly well when certain structures prevail, such as intrafamilial hierarchies, clear boundaries, and appropriate communication patterns. Family 'structure' becomes visible through the interactions of the various sub-systems—the children, parents, or grandparents. Each family negotiates boundaries between the different generations. Grandparents, for example, are regarded as 'intrusive' if the parents find them interfering with the care of their offspring—who then can get caught up between the two generations. When parent and grandparent each demand that the child sides with the one against the other, a situation known as *triangulation* arises. Here the relative absence of boundaries between the parental and grandparental generation can contribute to family conflicts. The systemic therapist's task is to intervene so as to make the family structure approximate to the normative model of family life, with an emphasis on clearly defined boundaries and hierarchies, such as putting the grandparent in an 'appropriate' role. Techniques employed include the direct challenging of absent or rigid boundaries, 'unbalancing' the family equilibrium by temporarily joining with one member of the family against another, or setting 'homework' tasks designed to restore 'functional' hierarchies (Minuchin and Fishman, 1981). The structural approach is very active, with the systemic therapist encouraging family members to 'enact' problems in the consulting room, so that the ways in which communications become blocked or interactions get stuck can be studied '*in vivo*'. One of the therapist's jobs is to keep the 'problem' on the boil long enough for the family to find a new solution.

In *strategic systemic therapy* the focus is narrowly on the nature of the presenting symptom and the 'identified' patient. One underlying assumption is that the symptom is being maintained by the apparent 'solution'—the very behaviour(s) that seek to suppress it. For example, the 'anxious' older woman may elicit her son's overprotectiveness, a solution which may well perpetuate the problem, namely her insecurity and levels of anxiety. A structural therapist would tend to view over-protectiveness as a dysfunctional aspect of family organization and therefore challenge communication patterns which are linked to the presenting problem. Strategic therapists instead focus on the problem brought by the client or family in an attempt to solve it (Watzlawick *et al.*, 1974; Haley, 1977; Herr and Weakland, 1979). Theory has it that if the presenting problem changes, then a domino effect can be observed in other interactions and behaviours. Strategic therapists use 'reframing' as a major technique. The older adult's perceived problem is put into a different meaning-frame which provides new perspectives and leads to different communications and behaviours. For example, reframing 'forgetfulness' as the older adult's wish to give someone else a role may be a useful challenge to an entrenched belief that the older adult is incompetent or hopeless.

The *Milan systemic* approach (Boscolo *et al.*, 1987) focuses on multigenerational family patterns, looking at the struggles of different family members over several generations. It involves making elaborate hypotheses about how, for example, long-standing rivalries between a sibling group become reactivated around the time of their elderly parent's illness and how this, in turn, affects the older person's mental state. Such hypotheses lead to the designing of interventions which take into account the anticipated attempts of the family to disqualify the therapeutic interventions. In order to confirm or refute hypotheses about family process and to arrive at these interventions, the Milan team have perfected a particular interviewing technique: circular questioning (Selvini Palazzoli *et al.*, 1980). The therapist conducts the family session mostly by asking questions, seeking information about people, their differences, and the various relationships and their specific characteristics. An example of circular questioning would be to ask a person A, the grandfather for example, about his perception of aspects of the relationship between person B, grandmother, and C, grand-daughter. Talking about this in the presence of everyone inevitably produces plenty of feedback on which systemic therapists tend to base their next questions. Families and their individual members cannot help but get involved in thinking about the intricacies of their relationships with one another. A process is triggered whereby family members question each other's assumptions and behaviours and this can lead to new ways of communicating and relating.

There have been, in more recent years, some challenges to the concept of so-called 'scientific objectivity', namely the traditional view that the observer (or clinician) stands outside the process observed. *Social constructionist* theorists and practitioners (von Foerster, 1981; Gergen, 1994) focus on how the observer actively constructs what is being observed. The so-called 'reality' which therapists believe they perceive is no longer seen as being objectively 'out there': instead, reality is seen as 'invented', reflecting the therapists' own cultures and inherent belief systems. Interactions between patients, families, and clinicians reflect deeply embedded assumptions inherent in the traditional clinical discourses used to discuss experiences and relationships (Boscolo *et al.*, 1987; Atwood and Ruiz, 1993). In this sense dominant professional discourses create a 'problem-determined system' (Anderson *et al.*, 1986). If therapists view patients' experiences as evidence of illness or pathology, then these experiences can only be explored within a pathology-oriented framework. This is very limiting, particularly if the narratives in which patients and their families tell their stories or have these told (or 'storied') by others (psychiatrists, for example) do not fit these experiences (White and Epston, 1990).

*Systemic narrative therapy* attempts to help patients and their families to find new ways of making sense of their experiences and to evolve new stories, with therapy being seen as a mutually validating conversation out of which change can occur (Garland and Garland, 2001). New interviewing techniques, often referred to as therapeutic conversations, have been developed in which both family and therapist 'co-evolve' or 'co-construct' their very own ways of describing the family system, so that it no longer needs to be viewed or experienced as problematic (Jones, 1993). Such therapeutic conversations can actively challenge the contextual influences of cultural assumptions or stereotypes and beliefs, such as ageism. Roper-Hall (1993) described how this could be done when a 71-year-old widow stated that she was too old to drive. The therapist curiously inquired how the patient thought that her age made a difference and got an explanation regarding her lack of confidence. The therapist replied: 'So if you could find a way to increase your confidence, learning to drive might seem more possible?' This was followed by exploring some of the implications: 'If you did that, who would be more surprised, your older or your younger friends?' The patient seemed puzzled at first, but then started challenging her own thinking: 'Why should I be too old to drive??!' The characteristics of a post-Milan therapist are said to be those of a clinician who is 'democratic' and realistic about the possibility of change, taking non-judgemental and multipositional stances.

*Contextual family therapy* (Boszormenyi-Nagy, 1988) emphasizes the healing of relationships through growth in family commitment and trust and with the development of loyalty, fairness, and reciprocity, with great emphasis on intergenerational interventions (Anderson and Hargrave, 1990). Techniques used include life-review, using props such as family photo albums, family trees, and scrapbooks to reconsider the past and make peace with certain aspects of life to date. Involving other family members in this task brings in new perspectives and facilitates discussion. Video life reviews with older adults and their families are an effective tool in helping them to 're-story' past events with new meanings (Hargrave, 1994). These reviews have a historical and evaluative dimension and promote stronger relational ties. They also deal with transition issues such as easing everyone through difficult developmental challenges and dealing with emotional pain.

*Psycho-educational* approaches (Leff *et al.*, 1982; Kuipers *et al.*, 1992) have found their particular application in the field of adult psychiatry and especially in the work with psychotic patients and their families. These approaches tend to be used when working with the carers of mentally ill family members, teaching them about the 'illness' and its causes and the 'best' way of responding to and managing the ill person. One aim of this approach is to reduce the levels of the carers' expressed emotion and particularly the number of critical comments and amount of hostility and over-involvement they show towards the 'identified' patient. Three separate therapeutic strategies are employed to achieve this goal in working with seriously mentally ill patients and their families: (1) educational sessions for the family—teaching about the illness and the part the family can play in keeping the patient well; (2) a fortnightly relatives' group—to share experiences and solutions; and (3) family sessions. Such combined multilevel work is sadly still rather rare when it comes to treating older adults and their families. Psycho-education more often takes the form of designing interventions which alleviate carer stress, reflecting the bias towards the needs of

carers and the presumed passivity of the 'objects' of care (Richardson *et al.*, 1994).

*Brief 'solution focused'* therapy (de Shazer, 1985) is a welcome departure from pathology-dominated models, as it deliberately ignores 'problem saturated' ways of talking and focuses instead on the patterns of previous attempted solutions. The approach is based on the observation that symptoms and problems have a tendency to fluctuate. Concentrating on those times when a symptom, such as an anxiety state, is less or is not present, allows the therapist to design therapeutic strategies around the exceptions, as they form the basis of the solution. A depressed older person, for example, is sometimes more and at other times less depressed. The use of rating scales and a deliberate focus on those times when the depressive symptoms are absent leads to the identification of 'exceptions' which form the basis of the solution. Patients and their families are encouraged to amplify the solution patterns of behaviours, with the aim of driving the problem patterns into the background (George *et al.*, 1990; Iveson, 1990).

Systemic therapy has developed over the past 50 years and has now come of age. Different schools and approaches have evolved over the years, reflecting changing societal, cultural, and political priorities and landscapes. Nowadays it is fairly rare for allegedly 'pure' models to be practised, as the huge cultural variety of our clients and their families, as well as the variety of their presenting problems and the contexts within which systemic work is carried out, all require diverse and flexible responses. Post-modern systemic therapists tend to be multimodal practitioners, working in many different settings, both public and private. In the public domain, systemic practitioners tend to be part of multidisciplinary teams, and their interventions need to be part of the overall framework and approach of the team. They can contribute two distinct skills: context reading and context making.

## Context reading and context making

Understanding the request for help and the nature of the referral is usually the first step for most clinicians—whatever their theoretical orientation. The questions 'who wants help for whom (or what) and why now?' help to read the context of the referral and presenting problem. Is it actually the concerned older adult? Or is it her grown-up children? Or is it the referring social worker or psychiatrist? Problems can be contextualized at various different levels—the individual level, the level of the family or other significant relationships, the immediate social and cultural setting, the level of the professional network that is generated around the problem (and often inadvertently 'helps' to maintain it)—and the wider political context. Such multilevel context reading permits clinicians to position themselves and their teams, and helps them to consider how and with whom to start, be that the individual patient, members of the family, referring agencies, or various combinations thereof. Context reading is not a one-off activity, but an ongoing process throughout the course of therapeutic work with older adults and their families.

However, clinicians are not employed merely to read layers of context and to fashion them into plausible explanations of the presenting problem(s). Clinicians are, above all, charged with translating their understanding into clinical action, so that distress can be relieved and mental health be promoted. Systemic practitioners do this by searching for, and creating, appropriate therapeutic settings. In short, they make 'contexts for change'. Therefore, whenever systemic practitioners consider how to manage a new referral, they pose a basic question: 'what are the contexts that I need to use—or make—to address the presenting problems and issues?' This question, obscure though it may seem at first sight, opens up a multiverse of possibilities. To explain this, we can deconstruct the term 'context' into five subcategories: 'person', 'time', 'place', 'activity', and 'modality'.

The '*person context*'—the question of *who* should be present for 'sessions'—opens up many possibilities as to who should attend. It could be 'just' the older adult, it could be the couple, it could be other family members, it could include an important friend, a priest, or mullah, a neighbour, other clinicians, maybe even a manager. Many family therapists ask 'the family' to attend for the first session, but in practice they see whoever turns up. It is not uncommon for the number of clients attending the actual therapy sessions to increase over time from one person to as many as six or ten, including members of the extended family or relevant others. For example, a woman in her 80s may well turn up with a neighbour who is more involved in her well-being than members of her family. However, what can also be elicited and explored is why her own children did not come. It may be important to invite the older person and her relevant others for what could be called family *work* rather than family *therapy*—a notion which may carry connotations of blame. Other family members can be invited by letter or by a phone call explaining how and why it might be useful for them to attend. When considering *where* (the '*place context*') the family or other systemic work might best be carried out, there is also a number of options: the clinic setting, the home, on a hospital ward, in a community or religious centre, in a solicitor's office—or anywhere else that makes sense for the concerned person(s). Working in a naturalistic setting, a setting where the problem manifests itself concretely, can be more effective for some families than to confine all clinical work to neutral and impersonal clinic settings. The '*time context*' (*when*?) can be defined in terms of length, frequency, and duration of the therapeutic work. Ten or 20 minutes may be an appropriate time frame for carrying out preventive work in a general practice setting, as this is an accepted time slot and thus fits the primary care context (Asen *et al.*, 2004). At the other end of the spectrum we have 'multiproblem families', with chronic histories and entrenched interactions with multiple agencies: it is unlikely that they will respond to 60 or 90 minute sessions at monthly intervals. Here time frames for sessional work may have to be much longer, maybe a few hours, possibly with a frequency of twice or three times a week at the outset to make an impact on an otherwise stuck and lethargic system. The frequency and duration of sessions can be quite different after a few weeks: clinicians need to continuously think—and rethink—together with their patients whether the time structures created, or imposed, are still helpful. It is the joint process of continuous evaluation and revalidation that itself can contribute to healing. *How* (the '*modality context*') clinicians do what they do, depends on their training, personal experiences, and their 'self'. It has already been mentioned that in the systemic field there are now plenty of diverse schools and orientations. It would seem limited and limiting for clinicians to remain insecurely attached to just one model and proudly label themselves as a 'narrative' or 'structural' or 'solution focused' or 'social constructionist' therapist. Surely different presentations and problems, different cultural and social contexts, require different responses from clini-

cians. A therapeutic modality appropriate at the outset of a piece of clinical work may not be appropriate or effective a few weeks or months later.

This multicontextual and multimodal approach opens up new perspectives and provides choices for the clinician as well as for clients. If the contextualizing questions ('who?', 'where?', 'when?', and 'how?') are asked throughout the course of the therapeutic work, then our approach does not risk becoming stale and irrelevant. By involving our patients and their families in this questioning process, we hopefully make together relevant contexts for change, opening up, for them and us, a multiverse of new ways of seeing and experiencing. Furthermore, if clinicians are able to entertain multiple models simultaneously, systemic and non-systemic ones, then a multimodal approach can emerge, based on what the patients and their various systems require, rather than what a particular dogma requires. Multicontextual work implies that a number of different interventions are simultaneously addressed to different levels of the system: this may include work with the individual in parallel with work with the family, as well as work with the professional network and the neighbourhood.

## Systemic interventional assessments in practice

Before embarking on actual therapeutic work, it is wise to undertake a family or 'systems' assessment. Such assessments are also interventions in their own right, with many therapeutic ingredients. A systems assessment looks at the older person in relation to the wider family and the social context, evaluating how family and helpers affect the older adult and his/her illness or problem. In turn it also requires an appraisal of how the older adult's problems or illness affect the family and helpers. Systemic assessments are the basis for determining whether and how much the family can be a resource for containing or changing the presenting problems—and what interventions are indicated or not. The order in which such an assessment is carried out may vary, but the major ingredients are the same: problem identification, assessment of family relationships and communication patterns, assessment of the professional and agency network, assessment of the wider social and cultural setting.

Where assessment ends and therapy begins is often quite difficult to determine. In the field of family work this dividing line would often seem artificial: all family assessments have a potentially therapeutic function, and there is an assessment function to every therapeutic session. It could be argued that bringing the family together in front of a neutral clinician is itself a major intervention. The assessment format itself is not only designed to provide answers for the examining clinician, but also aims to generate new information for the patient and family members. For example, hearing other family members speculate about certain aspects of relationships which involve the listener, can evoke powerful thoughts and feelings, such as being misunderstood or found out, and can lead to intensive discussion and interaction. This in itself can be therapeutic because it challenges long-held beliefs and facilitates communication around issues that usually cannot be talked about openly. The sensitive clinician will know when the family resists discussing certain issues and will then make a decision as to how wise it is to probe further at that point or whether to leave this for another time.

The mnemonic PRACTICE (Christie-Seely, 1984) is an assessment tool which helps the clinician to look at problems and people in context:

P Presenting Problem

R Roles and Rules

A Affect

C Communication

T Time in family life cycle

I Illness

C Community

E Environment

## P, the Presenting Problem

The problem can be the illness itself, its result (e.g. the need for hospitalization) or the effect it has on other family members (e.g. a spouse's depression or a grandchild's behavioural problem). To elicit the relevant information the clinician asks each person about the problem and how it affects everyone:

1 How does each person see the problem?

2 Is there agreement or disagreement about what constitutes a problem? When (and by whom) was it first noticed?

3 What is the effect of the illness on each family member?

4 Who is most/least affected?

5 What is each person's explanation and expectation?

In listening to each family member's account, the clinician can highlight the effects of the problem on everyone and get family members to talk to one another directly, encouraging them to use their own problem-solving skills.

## R, Roles and Rules

Acute or chronic illness in the family can change and even reverse roles. In cases of serious acute illness, the medical care system may take over major family roles, at times conflicting with parental roles. Hospitalized older adults may find it particularly difficult having to cope with a new system of rules imposed on them which do not tally with those at home. Many families find it difficult to compete with round-the-clock nursing care that hospitals can provide, resulting in the family being tempted to leave an elderly person in hospital or a nursing home for much longer than needed. The following questions can help to clarify traditional and new family roles and rules:

1 How is the family (re-)allocating roles and functions?

2 Who is anticipating or experiencing role strains?

3 What is the power structure in the family?

4 How do family members agree about doing things differently?

5 Is the patient denying or overusing the sickness role?

6 What is the role of the helping system? How does it aid or block the family?

The clinician's task is to get the family members to talk openly about the ill person's change of role and help them consider drawing up new rules for short- and long-term survival. At times it may be necessary to convene a professional network meeting with the family to discuss and allocate appropriate roles to the various helpers and family members.

## A, Affect

It is widely known that there are considerable personal and cultural differences as to when and how much emotion people show. In many families acute or chronic illness of an older adult is frequently accompanied by an initial phase of dazed denial, followed by anxiety, hope, and fear, and not infrequently considerable resentment towards the ill member. In assessing the affective status of family members, a number of issues need to be addressed:

1 What is the predominant emotional tone in the family?

2 Is anyone controlling the family mood?

3 Who is most /least able to talk about feelings?

4 Are all family members able to express both positive and negative emotions? How appropriate is that?

5 What is the non- and para-verbal family language?

6 How has the family dealt with illness in the past?

The clinician's task is to assess as well as to facilitate the open expression of intensive emotions, and to encourage the sharing of important feelings.

## C, Communication

Clarity of communication is not only an important issue for the family but also for the medical care team. The clinician often has the task of helping his or her colleagues give clear information to the family as well as helping the family to ask important questions and get them answered:

1 Who talks to whom? Who talks for whom?

2 Who, if anybody, is the 'family switchboard'?

3 How direct is communication between family members?

4 Who blocks whom at what points?

5 What are the covert messages (para- and non-verbal)?

6 How critical or supportive are communications?

7 When does communication become confused or confusing?

The clinician can challenge a seeming conspiracy of silence regarding diagnosis. Given their age and the seriousness of their illness the elderly patient may need help in dealing with 'unfinished business' and in getting the family to consider how to make the best of the time left.

## T, Time in the family life cycle

The family life cycle provides a framework of understanding the predicament of elderly family members and gives it a historical perspective (Carter and McGoldrick, 1989; Sanborn and Bould, 1991). Retirement, widowhood, grandparenthood, illness, and dependency are the predictable stages at this point. When a young adult leaves home, this can create space for the care of an older person. How the family copes with later life transitions depends very much on the system they themselves have created over the years and how that system adjusts to losses and new demands. Successful family functioning requires flexibility in structures, roles, and responses to new challenges (Walsh, 1989) and data about past and present family functioning can be elicited:

1 Which major family transitions are imminent or have taken place?

2 What effects is illness having on the anticipated changes of the family structure?

3 How is family life going to change if the illness gets better or worse?

## I, Illness history

How families view illness varies a great deal, reflecting social and cultural values. The meanings that families attach to symptoms need to be explored by the clinician in relation to the family's personal, educational and cultural background:

1 What are the family's beliefs and fears about ageing and illness?

2 Who (if anyone) feels responsible for illness?

3 What are the beliefs about how illness is spread?

4 How have previous generations coped with old age and carer issues?

5 What are the patterns of health and illness in previous generations?

6 What is the family's experience of past and present relationships with health professionals?

## C, Community resources

Illness in older adults often requires intensive care at home or hospitalization. The family's support network will determine to what extent the patient can be managed in the home environment. There is a tendency within services to focus on the older person and their primary carer and to remain unaware of others within the care network (Curtis and Dixon, 2005). The extended family, neighbours and friends may all play an important role, so the clinician needs to evaluate the family and its social ties and support—all of which have a major influence on health:

1 Does the family want to accept the outside world or would it prefer to close ranks and cope by itself?

2 Who is perceived by whom as being potentially helpful?

3 What role could the extended family and friends play?

4 What other social support structures are available?

5 What are the family strengths? Which familiar coping strategies can be relied on? Which can't?

6 Which alternative coping strategies could be explored?

Here the clinician may wish to encourage the family to consider the 'pros' and 'cons' of accepting appropriate amounts of help from the extended family or other sources.

## E, Environmental factors

The environment within which the patient and family live is an important factor for their health: this includes housing, financial and employment situation, medical and educational facilities, religious links with the community, and, last but not least, ethnicity. Family structures and family relations are very culture dependent, and the place of older adults is influenced by diverse culture-specific concepts of authority relations, gender roles, and generational differences, the interdependence of nuclear families, visiting, and mutual aid relationships (Markides and Mindel, 1987). Families differ a great deal in how they relate to external, non-family support systems and to what extent they expect that care be provided entirely from within the family (Boyd-Franklin, 1989). What seems to make sense in one cultural context may be a sign of failure in another. Here are some questions which can help to address the social and cultural contexts within which families live:

1 What is culturally acceptable, given this family's particular ethnicity?

2 How much is the family linked with the local community?

3 Where are strong links – where does the family feel isolated?

4 What are the financial and work situations?

5 What are the housing and the neighbourhood like?

6 Does the family experience racism?

7 Which community resources are available (e.g. self-help groups, church, or other culturally relevant settings)?

The larger social, cultural, and political context all affect the health of the family. Not to take this into account in effect confirms the pathology of the individual while ignoring the 'pathological' contributions that society makes.

Older adults frequently claim that they have 'no family' or that the family is 'not important'. If clinicians unquestioningly accept this, they are likely to miss important information and lose the opportunity of using the family as a central resource. In the (often only temporary) absence of family members it is possible to undertake a 'family assessment by proxy'. This means interviewing in such a way that the views of important others are represented. Working systemically with an individual involves asking the older adult a number of questions that focus deliberately on his or her relationship with members of the family (Jenkins and Asen, 1992). This gives valuable information on how certain family issues may maintain or contribute to the present problems. Examples of such questions are as follows:

1 When you are very down, which among your family or friends is most affected?

2 Who, if anyone, do you feel isn't really bothered about you?

3 How does X respond when you are very low?

4 Who gets most irritated about you being so forgetful?

5 Of all the people who worry about you, who is the most and who is the least helpful?

This way of questioning induces thought, reflection, and self-questioning, and can often itself be 'therapeutic' in that it reveals potentially new ways of viewing one's own predicament in relation to others. This can open up new channels, particularly if such reflections are shared with other family members.

When beginning to work systemically with older adults and their families, there will initially be a problem focus, with the emphasis on getting the various members to come to some agreement as to what needs to be most urgently addressed. This can take some time since not infrequently each family member has quite a different agenda. In fact, the failure to reach consensus may well be the family's most urgent problem: one son may want to make peace and just ensure that the next year is as stress-free as possible; his sister feels the need to settle old scores and use therapy as an opportunity to tell her mother all she had not been able to tell her for the past 53 years. The elderly parents may see the purpose of family meetings as sorting out their relationship with their grandchildren and ensuring that they can see them more regularly, whereas yet another family member may be of the opinion that the elderly couple should use the sessions to tackle, once and for all, their longstanding marital problems. The clinician can feel tempted to intervene and try to rescue the situation by setting the goals or providing a focus, particularly if everyone turns to him or her for advice. Giving such advice may defuse conflicts in the short term, but is unlikely to result in the family developing its own problem-solving strategies. It is only when the immediate presenting problems have been tackled that the family can look at the more long-term issues they will have to cope with. Consequently the first few sessions may be dominated by Milan systemic circular questions (Selvini Palazzoli *et al.*, 1980), spiced with structural (Minuchin, 1974), strategic (Herr and Weakland, 1979), and solution-focused (de Shazer, 1985) techniques. During later phases of therapy contextual (Boszormenyi-Nagy, 1986), re-storying (Pocock, 1995), or relapse-prevention work (Asen and Tomson, 1992) may be more central.

## Common issues in treating older adults and their families

Iveson (1990) makes the point that three assumptions tend to inform the work of family therapists: older people's 'belongingness' (e.g. being full members of society), their responsibility for their actions, and their capacity to make choices. Therapists need to help to empower older adults rather than overprotect them. Getting the balance right is rarely easy. If we protect older people from themselves we end up making key decisions for them. If we protect them from their families or from their neighbours, we can be in danger of undermining them. Yet, if we don't, we may put them at risk. One way or another, this remains a constant dilemma for any clinician working with older adults and their families.

The next section illustrates specific issues and scenarios that can benefit from family therapy intervention.

### Illness and the ageing family

Serious illness and impending death have major effects on the family. Carer stress and exhaustion, another family member developing related symptoms, collective denial, and neglect of the older person are all symptoms of the family failing to adjust appropriately to this family crisis. Research shows that both the psychological and physical health of spouses and children of chronically ill elderly people are negatively affected, and that it is especially the female spouses of elderly male patients who are at risk (Kriegsman *et al.*, 1994). The question as to which of the offspring should be responsible for the elderly relatives can stir up considerable feelings all round. Which family member chooses—or is designated—to do the caregiving is not only related to the caregiving demands, geographical proximity, or gender, but is also influenced by family legacy (Glaberman, 1995). Children who have been exempted or excused from family responsibilities in childhood often do not get involved in the caregiving as adults when faced with responsibilities for a relative with Alzheimer's disease. Since family legacy influences who is the primary caregiver, family interventions need to address these long-term issues. It is not enough merely to focus on enabling caregivers to ask for help from relatives or on teaching them how to set limits. To help such 'unencumbered children' (Glaberman, 1995) escape from their chronic uninvolved roles may require a transgenerational, re-storying approach.

### Old business revived

Most families create, over time, their own stories or myths and the past is painted in certain ways so that points about the present can be made. Sometimes myths exist to hide shameful events or secrets. Not infrequently, when people reach the end of their lives, the time has come for them and their relatives to question some of the myths and to let out certain carefully guarded secrets. Reviving and dealing with old business in the present to improve things for more than one generation is one of the major tasks of family therapy.

---

### Case study 1

Both Mr and Mrs Brown were in their mid 80s when his depression and dementia suddenly became more serious. Mrs Brown developed cancer and their three children, all in their 40s and 50s and with their own families, became involved in their care. The older son Peter, a doctor, tried to handle the medical issues. The other son John, a lawyer, managed the legal side, and their sister Imogen, a nurse, was dispatched to deal with the practical day-to-day issues. For a few weeks this arrangement worked adequately, but gradually many old conflicts surfaced. A referral for family therapy was made by the old age psychiatrist, after a physical fight had broken out between the two brothers—in front of their parents. The first few family meetings involved only the siblings who were barely on speaking terms. Peter was accused of interfering with the treatment of both parents by constantly changing doctors, hospitals, and medication. John was charged with not handling the money matters honestly and making arrangements that benefited, above all, his own family. Imogen was blamed for siding with her mother against her father. She, in turn, accused her brothers of sticking only to their professional roles rather than getting their 'hands dirty'—and so on. Soon old unfinished business had surfaced: resentment of the two younger siblings towards their older brother who they believed had always enjoyed the privileged position of the older son and was now likely to inherit the major part of the family fortune. He pointed out that it had not been an easy position, as he had been made his mother's confidant from a very young age. In this role he had learned that she had had three major affairs which had to be kept top secret. However, somehow this so-called secret had become common knowledge though everyone seemed to subscribe to the myth that father had never found out about it. Imogen explained how she had felt totally neglected by her father and how angry she was about being asked to help out whenever it suited her parents. The initial family work consisted of six family sessions, with only the siblings present. This helped to put past and present issues into perspective and resulted in the siblings cooperating with one another—for the benefit of their parents—rather than continuing to re-enact the fights of their childhood. It was only then that two meetings in the parents' home with the whole family were convened. It turned out that father had known all along about the affairs but had been too angry to confront his wife. Many other issues were brought up, with the siblings now balanced enough not to let their own agenda interfere with the short-term management of their parents. Family work helped to develop a care plan to which all members of the family could subscribe with the minimum of conflict between the adult children. A few months later the elderly parents asked for some marital therapy 'to settle some old issues once and for all'.

## Married to the sick role

Chronic disease of older adults usually has wide-ranging effects on the family (Kriegsman *et al.*, 1994). However, at times illness can also become a 'weapon' to get at others. Repeated self-harming, for example, also contains elements of an attack on one's family. Chronic mental or physical illness can also act as 'superglue', namely holding together relationships that otherwise might fall apart. Such illness bonds are not uncommon and are often characterized by scenarios where one person is the 'patient' and the other the 'nurse'. Physical or psychological illness then become the *raison d'être* for the relationship and all parties seem to have a lot invested in keeping 'it'—the real or imaginary illness—going. For example, a woman in her late 70s who suffered a brain haemorrhage was treated as an invalid by her husband years after she had made a complete recovery. By referring continuously to her 'illness', he succeeded in making her feel helpless and dependent and she thoroughly 'learned' to doubt her own judgement. In family therapy sessions her strengths were identified and the couple were set tasks for her to increase her competence step-by-step. Over time it emerged that the major obstacle for her recovery had been her husband's resistance to letting go of the power position he had obtained as a result of her illness years ago. Given that older adults are more likely to be physically frail, there is plenty of scope for using illness in their daily battles—if need be.

### Case study 2

Mr Smith, in his 80s, was seriously diabetic and suffered frequent hypoglycaemic attacks. During these he would call for his wife and ask her to prepare a meal urgently. Mrs Smith, herself in her late 70s, suffered from what she herself called intractable back pain. She claimed that her pain was too severe to get out of bed. Mr Smith would prick his finger and take a quick blood sugar reading to verify his hypoglycaemic status and show the alarming results to his wife. Mrs Smith would then point to her 'pain-thermometer', kindly though probably unwisely fitted by one of the leading neurological hospitals in the country, which by means of a red flashing light, prominently displayed on her chest, signalled that she was 'objectively' in severe pain. Arguments between both partners would break out, each claiming to be more ill than the other and 'proving' it by referring to objective blood sugar and pain levels. At the point of referral the situation had become hopelessly stuck. Couple therapy initially focused on how each of them could survive their attacks and make themselves safe. A little later some work was done to help them understand how they had arrived at such an absurd impasse. Mrs Smith revealed that it all started some 50 years ago on the night of their wedding when Mr Smith had danced all night with his ex-girlfriend. It was soon after the honeymoon that she developed back pain ('this made me sick') and her husband patiently looked after her for years until he himself became

a 'patient'. Therapy sessions helped them to talk about how much and little they cared for one another. Some progress was made in that they changed their expectations about how much each could and should rely on the other.

## Marital therapy for octogenarians

It is never too late for couple work and a few sessions can sometimes bring about significant shifts (Carni, 1989). This may be particularly indicated when a depressed older adult lives with a very critical, if not hostile, spouse (Jones and Asen, 2000). The major issues triggering the emergence of depression or maintaining it are: past affairs (often half a century ago!); retirement after a very busy life involving a lot of travel; and over-involvement of a parent with a grown up son or daughter which fuels rivalries or produces battles over the family inheritance. Some partners never give up hope of changing the other—even if this has not proved a realistic proposition over the preceding decades. Helping people to accept the other for what he or she is may prove impossible and clinicians can challenge the couple and ask them how many years they might wish to continue to waste trying to achieve the seemingly impossible. In many respects, couple therapy for this age group is not much different from the approach one would choose with younger clients. Change is possible at any age, although the goals with older adults may be fairly modest and centre around some improvements in decision-making or certain aspects of communication. For example, the eternal complaint that 'she never listens to me' can be addressed by asking how he could be better heard or how he would have to talk so that she might find it bearable or possible to listen to him. Simple tasks, such as '4 minutes each' or 'slow motion replay' (Asen, 1995), are designed to help partners rehearse new communication patterns and facilitate better interactions between 'stuck' partners.

## Grandparenthood as antidepressant

Old age is often thought of as a time of loss—loss of friends, health, job, status, and financial security. Older adults, semi-rebelliously hovering in their 'third adolescence' between dependence and independence, do not fit easily into society. They frequently break rules and antagonize others, both inadvertently and deliberately. Their unpredictable behaviours are randomly attributed to senility or wisdom, much to the annoyance of their offspring and the continuous amusement of the grandchildren. It is frequently overlooked how much mutual benefit can be derived for grandparents and grandchildren alike by forging stronger connections between the generations. Clinicians can help to promote intergenerational work, encouraging this almost 'natural' alliance. However, this is not always unproblematic since the generation in between, namely the parents, may disapprove of the grandparental input.

### Case study 3

Jackie, a woman in her 40s, felt that her own mother Mary, aged 75, had neglected her when she was a child. However, she realized that Mary, in her role as grandmother, seemed to have a much closer relationship with her 7-year-old daughter Jodie. This brought back painful memories. Over time Jackie became increasingly rivalrous with her own mother, feeling that Jodie was being thoroughly spoilt by grandmother. Consciously or unconsciously, Jackie started blocking her mother seeing Jodie and she eventually stopped her own mother from having access to Jodie altogether. The fact that her own mother had quite distinct views of how inadequate Jackie was as a mother, further reinforced old powerful dynamics. The casualty in this conflict was Jodie, who very much missed seeing her grandmother. Family work involving the three generations proved useful, with benefits not only for Jackie and her mother, but for three if not four generations.

## Non-deliberate 'patienthood games'

The part the family plays in influencing illness is frequently underestimated: even when organic brain disease is present, the family's responses can affect the course and outcome of the condition (Davis, 1997). For example, if the grown-up children, due to their own anxieties, behave in overly responsible ways, they may soon find themselves involved in a cycle where the more they do for their parents, the more helpless the parents become, with ever-increasing demands, burden, guilt, and resentment. The vicious cycle of family overfunctioning and elderly underfunctioning can maintain or hasten symptoms labelled as senility (Walsh, 1989). After a careful assessment an over-responsible adult daughter, for example, can be assisted through family work to consider whether it might be more helpful to her father if she challenged him to do certain things by himself rather than having them done for him. Similarly an 'underinvolved' sibling may in his turn be questioned about his reluctance or inability to share the burden with the overcaring dutiful daughter.

Underestimating the skills and assets of an older adult patient is very common, but a blind acceptance of such views or beliefs makes them come true. Sometimes it may suit adult 'children' to become (over-)involved in their elderly parents' lives: perhaps to avoid issues in their own marriages, perhaps because their own children have left home and there is now a void in their lives that can be filled by fussing over someone else. Hanson (1991) has pointed out that the 'patienting process' isolates dementia sufferers, whose behaviours are constantly defined as wrong or inappropriate. Being invalidated leads the sufferers to isolate themselves further with the result that they are increasingly ignored and lose touch. Helping the family to identify the dementia sufferer's strengths and looking for exceptions to behaviours symptomatic of dementia, can result in the older adult gaining confidence and feeling useful in some domains of life.

## Indications for systemic interventions

Carpenter (1994) carried out a project in a primary health-care setting and found that almost a third of referrals of older adults mentioned marital or family problems. Grief counselling and current family and marital relationship conflicts were most often the focus for subsequent work. However, in only 9% were formal conjoint family therapy sessions conducted. Clearly, there is a need for family interventions, but the 'when' and 'what' requires some discussion. Earlier in this chapter a distinction was made between 'thinking families' and family systems therapy as a treatment modality. The former is a framework which helps the clinician to view the older adult in context and thus informs and contributes to overall treatment and management plans. In other words, 'thinking families' and 'thinking systems' is an indispensable infrastructure

for any modern clinician. Systemic therapy as a treatment modality, on the other hand, has some very specific applications, some of them described above. In addition, it may be considered in the following situations: cases of elder abuse, resistance to the elder's independence, elderly parents struggling as caregivers for dependent adult children, post-retirement issues, and when it comes to making decisions to institutionalize an elderly person.

Family systems therapy is a useful intervention in the hands of experienced clinicians who have undertaken a recognized systemic training over a number of years. Its application needs to be based on patients' needs and evidence-based research findings rather than be guided by dogmatic unsubstantiated claims. Much damage can be caused by insensitive clinicians who, for example, think it absolutely necessary to confront all painful issues immediately, whatever the risk of such an approach to the older person's health. Family systems therapy cannot be prescribed against the wishes of those meant to receive it. Meeting with the family from time to time, framed as 'discussing issues', is a low-key systemic intervention which can be more helpful than formal, ritualized 'family therapy'. Change is almost always a slow process and its pace needs to be dictated by the family rather than be forced upon it. Montalvo (1993) points out that clinical errors occur when clinicians have too narrow or too wide a focus and persist in a course of action that is not of help to the patient. His suggested remedies for lessening the possibility of error are an excellent illustration of good systemic practice and include (Montalvo 1993):

- to be alert to coexisting problems;
- to make preliminary assessments before intervening in the patient's interpersonal world;
- to establish the when and how of symptom display;
- to search for contemporary forces that maintain symptoms;
- to understand changes in decisions of the patient, the caregivers, or the providers;
- to protect the independence of the clinician's assessment.

The wider health-care system involved with older adults and their families can also be the focus of systemic intervention (Tisher and Dean, 2000). Systemic practitioners can, for example, have an important role in providing consultation to residential care homes. The physical environment, staff attitudes and morale, the organizational and management structure of the unit, and interstaff communication issues may all adversely impact on the quality of care provided (Curtis and Dixon, 2005). Addressing these issues, by facilitating discussions and identifying the strengths and resources of care home staff, is crucial to improving the context that older adults live in. Finally, the wider health-care system involved with the elderly person and family can be the focus of therapy.

In clinical practice, making a referral for 'family therapy' or 'couple counselling' is often only thought of as a last resort, rather than being an approach which could be part of the overall management plan with older adults, with diagnostic, preventive, and therapeutic aspects. Teams which have a systemic practitioner as a permanent member of staff are able to utilize different perspectives and to provide specialized inputs from different individuals and disciplines (Ross et al., 1992). Moreover, professionals working with the older adults can re-examine who their clients or patients are and consider making different 'person contexts'. It must be obvious that if the family can cope better with their elderly distressed member, then this must be better for the concerned older adult—not to mention the mental health of future generations of the very same family. And this is where systemic work with older adults can also have a useful preventive function.

# References

Anderson, H., Goolishian, H.A., and Windermand, L. (1986). Problem determined systems: toward transformation in family therapy. *Journal of Strategic and Family Therapy*, **4**, 1–13.

Anderson, W.T. and Hargrave, T.D. (1990). Contextual family therapy and older people: building trust in the intergeneration family. *Journal of Family Therapy*, **12**, 311–320.

Asen, E. and Tomson, P. (1992) *Family solutions in family practice*. Quay Publications, Lancaster.

Asen, E. (1995). *Family therapy for everyone: how to get the best out of living together*. BBC Books, London.

Asen, E., Tomson, D., Young, V., and Tomson, P. (2004). *10 Minutes for the family: systemic practice in primary care*. Routledge, London

Atwood, J. and Ruiz, J. (1993). Social constructionist therapy with the elderly. *Journal of Family Psychotherapy*, **4**, 1–31.

Benbow, S. and Marriott, A. (1997). Family therapy with elderly people. *Advances in Psychiatric Treatment*, **3**, 138–145.

Boscolo, L., Cecchin, G., Hoffman, L., and Penn, P. (1987). *Milan systemic family therapy*. Basic Books, New York.

Boszormenyi-Nagy, I.(1988). *Foundations of contextual therapy*. Brunner/Mazel, New York.

Boyd-Franklin, N. (1989). *Black families in therapy: a multisystems approach*. Guilford Press, New York.

Carni, E. (1989). To deal or not to deal with death: family therapy with three enmeshed older couples. *Family Therapy*, **16**, 60–68.

Carter, B. and McGoldrick, M. (eds) (1989). *The changing family life cycle: a framework for family therapy*, 2nd edn. Allyn and Bacon, Boston, MA.

Carpenter, J. (1994). Older adults in primary health care in the United Kingdom: an exploration of the relevance of family therapy. *Family Systems Medicine*, **12**, 133–148.

Christie-Seely, J. (ed.) (1984). *Working with families in primary care*. Preager, New York.

Curtis, A.C. and Dixon, M.S. (2005). Family therapy and systemic practice with older people: where are we now? *Journal of Family Therapy*, **27**, 43–64.

Davis, L.L. (1997). Family conflicts around dementia home-care. *Families, Systems and Health*, **15**, 85–98.

de Shazer, S. (1985). *Keys to solutions in brief therapy*. W.W. Norton, New York.

Flori, D.E. (1989). The prevalence of later life family concerns in the marriage and family therapy journal literature (1976–1985): a content analysis. *Journal of Marital and Family Therapy*, **15**, 289–297.

Garland, J. and Garland, C. (2001). *Life review in health and social care*. Brunner-Routledge, Hove.

George, E., Iveson, C., and Ratner, H. (1990). *Problem to solution*. Brief Therapy Press, London.

Gergen, K.J. (1994). *Realities and relationships: soundings in social construction*. Harvard University Press, Cambridge, MA.

Gilleard, C., Lieberman, S., and Peeler, R. (1992). Family therapy for older adults: a survey of professionals' attitudes. *Journal of Family Therapy*, **14**, 413–422.

Glaberman, J. (1995). The unencumbered child: family reputation and responsibilities in the care of relatives with Alzheimer's disease. *Family Process*, **34**, 87–99.

Haley, J. (1977). *Problem-solving therapy*. Jossey-Bass, San Francisco.

Hanson, B.G. (1991). Parts, players, and 'patienting': the social construction of senile dementia. *Family Systems Medicine*, **9**, 267–274.

Hargrave, T.D. (1994). Using video life reviews with older adults. *Journal of Family Therapy*, **16**, 259–268.

Herr, J.J. and Weakland, J.H. (1979). *Counselling elders and their families: practical techniques for applied gerontology*. Springer, New York.

Iveson, C.(1990). *Whose life? Community care of older people and their families*. BT Press, London.

Ivey, D.C., Wieling, E., and Harris, S.M. (2000). Save the young – the elderly have lived their lives; ageism in marriage and family therapy. *Family Process*, **39**, 163–175.

Jackson, D. (1957). The question of family homeostasis. *Psychiatric Quarterly Supplement*, **31**, 79–90.

Jenkins, H. and Asen, K. (1992). Family therapy without the family: a framework for systemic practice. *Journal of Family Therapy*, **14**, 1–14.

Jones, E. (1993). *Family systems therapy*. John Wiley and Sons, Chichester.

Jones, E. and Asen, E. (2000). *Systemic couple therapy and depression*. Karnac, London.

Keller, J. and Bromley, M. (1989). Psychotherapy with the elderly: a systemic model. *Journal of Psychotherapy and the Family*, **5**, 29–46.

Kriegsman, D.M.W., Penninx, B., and van Eijk, J. (1994). Chronic disease in the elderly and its impact on the family: a review of the literature. *Family Systems Medicine*, **12**, 249–267.

Kuipers, L., Leff, J., and Lam. D. (1992). *Family work for schizophrenia: a practical guide*. Gaskell, London.

Laing, R.D. and Esterson, A. (1964). *Sanity, madness and the family*. Tavistock, London.

Leff, J., Kuipers, L., Berkowitz, R., Eberlein-Vries, R., and Sturgeon, D. (1982). A controlled trial of social intervention in the families of schizophrenic patients. *British Journal of Psychiatry*, **141**, 121–134.

Markides, K.S. and Mindel, C.H. (1987). *Ageing and ethnicity*. Sage, London.

Minuchin, S. (1974). *Families and family therapy*. Tavistock, London.

Minuchin, S. and Fishman, C. (1981). *Family therapy techniques*. Harvard University Press, Cambridge, MA.

Minuchin, S., Montalvo, B., Guerney, B.G., Rosman, B.L., and Schumer, F. (1967). *Families of the slums*. Basic Books, New York.

Montalvo, B.(1993). Cautionary tales from geriatrics: eight ideas for the health provider. *Family Systems Medicine*, **11**, 89–99.

Neidhardt, E.R. and Allen, J.A. (1993). *Family therapy with the elderly*. Sage Publications, London.

Pocock, D. (1995). Searching for a better story: harnessing modern and post-modern positions in family therapy. *Journal of Family Therapy*, **17**, 149–173.

Pottle, S. (1984). Developing a network-orientated service for elderly people and their carers. In *Using family therapy* (ed. J. Carpenter and A. Treacher), pp. 149–165. Blackwell, Oxford.

Richardson, C.A., Gilleard, C., Lieberman, S., and Peeler, R. (1994). Working with older adults and their families – a review. *Journal of Family Therapy*, **16**, 225–240.

Ross, J.L., Yudin, J., and Galluzzi, K. (1992). The geriatric assessment team: a case report. *Family Systems Medicine*, **10**, 213–218.

Roper-Hall, A. (1993). Developing family therapy services with older adults. In *Using family therapy in the 90s* (ed. J. Carpenter and A. Treacher). Blackwell, Oxford.

Sanborn, B. and Bould, S. (1991). Intergenerational caregivers of the oldest old. In *Families: intergenerational and generational connections* (ed. S.K. Pfeifer and M. Sussan). Haworth Press, New York.

Selvini Palazzoli, M., Boscolo, L., Cecchin, G., and Prata, G. (1980). Hypothesizing, circularity, neutrality: three guidelines for the conductor of the session. *Family Process*, **19**, 3–12.

Tisher, M. and Dean, S. (2000). Family therapy with the elderly. *Australian and New Zealand Journal of Family Therapy*, **21**, 94–101.

van Amburg, S.M., Barber, C.E., and Zimmerman, T.S. (1996). Ageing and family therapy: prevalence of ageing issues and later life concerns in marital and family therapy literature. *Journal of Marital and Family Therapy*, **22**, 195–203.

von Bertalanffy, L. (1968). *General systems theory: foundations, development, applications*. Penguin Books, Harmondsworth.

von Foerster, H. (1981). *Observing systems*. Intersystems, Seaside, CA.

Walsh, F. (1989). The family in later life. In *The changing family life cycle: a framework for family therapy*, 2nd edn (ed. B. Carter and M. McGoldrick), pp. 312–332. Allyn and Bacon, Boston, MA.

Watzlawick, P., Jackson, D., and Beavin, J. (1967). *Pragmatics of human communication*. W.W. Norton, New York.

Watzlawick, P., Weakland, J., and Fish, R. (1974). *Change: principles of problem formation and problem resolution*. W.W. Norton, New York.

White, M. and Epston, D. (1990). *Narrative means to therapeutic ends*. W.W. Norton, New York.

# Psychological treatments: psychodynamic psychotherapy

## Jane Garner

The heart has its reasons, which reason knows not
Pascal, 1623–1662

The myth that old age psychiatry is essentially biological psychiatry fits in with Western ideas of old age which deny an emotional life to people in later years. Our wards and clinics do not have to share the age-related expectations and stereotypes of our society. A psychodynamic approach with its emphasis on the uniqueness of the patient and its understanding also of the fears and anxieties of the staff is well placed to attend to the needs of people in later life who are more diverse than a younger population, and also to address the particular feelings evoked in the people who care for them.

It is an everyday experience in clinical life for treatment plans not to work out as we had hoped or expected, e.g. the stressed wife caring for a husband with a dementia seems desperate to have her burden reduced but all attempts to provide tangible assistance are sabotaged. Each time we think we are dealing with the manifest problem, difficulties arise until the real problem is recognized—perhaps in this example the grief and rage of the spouse at the illness of the other needs to be understood before they are able to accept help. However professional we are, we recognize that different patients make us feel differently. We know the value of a confidant(e) with whom we may share private thoughts and who may help us take a different view. We recognize that in our lives we tend to repeat patterns of behaviour and relationships. We are not surprised that expectations, motivations, and factors subliminal to our awareness influence our perceptions. We know that although we cannot recall what happened to us in the first couple of years of life it nevertheless has an effect in our subsequent life. It is not a great conceptual distance to think of these everyday experiences in a psychodynamic framework. Psychoanalysis is both a technique of investigation of mental processes and a theory of treatment, although explanation and cure do not inevitably go hand in hand. Psychodynamically orientated psychotherapy is based on psychoanalytic propositions.

This chapter presents the assumptions on which the psychotherapy is based and looks at the neglect of older people in this area of clinical thinking. It details human development using a lifespan approach. The similarities and differences between work with older and younger patients are considered, along with the applicability of psychodynamic ideas not only for individual patients or groups but for the local department of old age psychiatry as a whole.

## Underlying theory

Psychodynamic theory takes a developmental perspective. Early childhood experience in interaction with innate aspects of the internal world forms our mental health. Most of our mental activities are unconscious—there is an area of emotional life outside our awareness where we put ambivalent or hostile feelings, guilt and anxiety; it is a complex area of wishes and hostility. Some of these feelings are not only descriptively unconscious but actively withheld from consciousness. This dynamically unconscious part works on the 'pleasure principle' motivated by basic instinctual urges. The conscious portion operates on the 'reality principle'. A wish-fulfilling mechanism pervades our dreams with the reality orientated part turned off with sleep: this may not be manifest but needs understanding to access the latent content. Our internal world is peopled by figures and objects from our past which nevertheless interact with the present. There may be conflict between the demands of internal figures and our present needs. Our symptoms and personality difficulties have meaning which is hidden from us. The relationship with a professional who is sensitive to these ideas may be diagnostic as well as therapeutic.

If these assumptions are accepted there is no reason why they should not also apply to older people. Freud (1905) was of a different opinion:

> The age of the patients has this much importance in determining their fitness for psychoanalytic treatment, that, on the one hand, near or above the age of fifty the elasticity of the mental processes, on which the treatment depends, is as a rule lacking – old people are no longer educable – and, on the other hand, the mass of material to be dealt with would prolong the duration of the treatment indefinitely.

It is interesting and ironic to note that Freud was 49 when he wrote this and just about to launch into the world an exciting new metapsychology. Currently no one who is over 50 or who works with older people would say that in later life ineducability is more of an issue than with younger people. In therapy some older people do extremely well and quickly. It is not necessary to reconstruct every aspect of the patient's experience, because of the length of life and history one needs to make decisions about which aspects are the most pertinent to explore and what can be safely left.

We can only speculate what it was about Freud's own time in history, his personality, and his experience that led him to such a gloomy view of late life. He seemed concerned about the specific date of his own death, how much time he had left. Perhaps he feared his own old age: his father was old enough to be his grandfather and prejudices about ageing also affect the old. There is a story that Freud's mother, Amalia, when she was 95 saw a picture of herself in the newspaper. She apparently commented 'a bad reproduction; it makes me look 100'. Actually Freud bore his own old age with some stoicism dominated as it was by an unpleasant carcinoma of the jaw; his attitude to ageing preceded that (Woodward, 1991).

Although Freud's thinking about ageing is open to refutation and criticism, his revolutionary ideas are now in expanded form being used to the benefit of older patients using the Freudian tradition of open-minded enquiry. He was a neurologist who anticipated that eventually there would be a reconciliation of neurology and psychology. Perhaps his expectations are beginning to be fulfilled. Freud's view of the organization of the mind seems to be correct in the light of modern neuroscience, although the language used is completely different (Solms, 2004). Solms is a neuropsychologist and psychoanalyst writing eloquently about the integration of the two disciplines. Although the possibility of mental life being unconscious was initially rejected on logical grounds neurobiologists now accept this, for example the patient with damage to both occipital lobes is blind consciously. When asked to guess where the light is, they may say 'I can't see', 'I don't know'. Although they cannot see they do guess well. So one does not have to be conscious of seeing to do the visual processing. There is now growing evidence of physical sequelae of psychological treatment. Perhaps there is a biological substrate for psychotherapy. The right orbital pre-frontal cortex has been suggested (Schore, 1997) as the interface for biology and psychoanalysis. Psychological treatments change functional imaging (mainly frontal) with the degree of change related to degree of clinical change. Gabbard (2000) cites the work of Finnish researchers who found psychotherapy to have a significant effect on serotonin metabolism (Viinamaki *et al.*, 1998) and of Spiegel *et al.* (1989) who found an increased lifespan in patients with metastatic breast cancer who had group therapy in comparison to those with the same diagnosis and only conventional treatment. Attachment styles too have physical sequelae, (Ciechanowski *et al.*, 2001). Perhaps it is in the borderland between disciplines where most advances in scientific therapeutics will be made.

In clinical work there is a tendency to regard some patients' problems as organically derived and others as psychogenic. In reality organic and psychogenic factors are operating in each patient: 'Even when we treat the brain with somatic treatments, we cannot bypass the mind' (Gabbard, 2001). There is fruitfulness in combining disparate literatures. To work well with older people we could usefully combine medicine, sociology, psychology, and storytelling.

Not all early analysts adhered to the idea of the inflexibility and ineducability of older people. Karl Abraham (1919) cautioned against these preconceived notions and wrote about the age of the

neurosis being more important than the age of the patient—a dictum which still stands. Carl Jung after his split with Freud went on to think more carefully about the second half of life and saw older patients. Many analysts have not specifically addressed issues of ageing but their work has then been extended by those working with this age group. For example, O'Connor (1993) and Evans (2004) have used the self-psychology of Heinz Kohut to elucidate the vulnerabilities of old age. Miesen (1993) has taken Bowlby's attachment theory, originally developed by considering small children in hospital, to understand some behaviours in older people with dementia. Hess (1989, 2004) using a perspective from Melanie Klein has written of the narcissistic tyranny some wield in old age and also emphasized the importance of loneliness in later life. An integration of psychotherapeutic theories and techniques expands the boundaries of traditional psychodynamic approaches.

## Barriers to treatment

To speak merely of 'ageism' is too simplistic for a complete description of the complex relationship we have with older people in our youth-centred society where we define age in the negative. Old age as a period of decline is a common metaphor in the West. This pervasive view of the human condition brings prejudice and stereotypes so that all that is seen are labels such as gender, race, sexual orientation, and age: individuality is lost. Older members of society are often conceived of in terms of 'the demographic time bomb' or 'a burden on the [younger] taxpayer' or 'what the hell, they are going to die soon'. These negative perceptions are mirrored in the way older people see themselves. They are less likely to be offered psychotherapy, and few seek it. This may change as the stiff-upper-lip generations are replaced by those currently in their 40s, 50s, or younger.

Early literature on the mental health of older people focused on the most impaired patients, thereby perpetuating myths about their unsuitability for psychotherapy. We tend to look for disease-based explanations of distress rather than psychological ones. The focus is on pharmacological interventions for both physical and mental health problems. One model of ageing parallels Freud's emotional-depletion view. The loss-deficit idea characterizes old age as loss of job, status, and finances, decreased social engagement and loneliness, poor health, disability, dependence, loss of cognitive skills, bereavement, and death. These aspects are important in later life but they do not apply to everyone or only apply partially—there are other aspects to consider. A different view of ageing is via a maturity model which will be discussed later. The negativity of the deficit approach—ageing is a narcissistic wound which cannot be healed—is unlikely to encourage therapists and it overemphasizes the differences between work with younger and older adults. Zivian *et al.* (1992) found that psychotherapists prefer treating younger rather than middle-aged patients and middle-aged rather than older. This was related to level of experience and knowledge of psychotherapy in later life and also to erroneous perceptions of prognosis (therapeutic nihilism). They expressed personal anxiety about growing old, a reluctance to be associated with low-status patients, and concern at limited training opportunities. Although older people have problems common to all age groups, outcome is enhanced if the therapist is not only generally well qualified but also has specialized training in working with older adults (Pinquart and Sorensen, 2001). Therapists have to deal with their own socially determined ageism as well as personal feelings, and perhaps unresolved issues with parents or grandparents. In the therapy they will have to face ideas of illness, disability, death—the patient's but also their anticipated own.

If these barriers to treatment can be overcome outcomes are good. There is increasing evidence for the effectiveness of psychoanalytic psychotherapy with older patients (Knight, 1996).

# Development, life review, mourning, and maturity

Psychoanalytic theory is a theory of *development*. The emphasis traditionally is on the first few years of life, as it is often believed that the first 5 years explain all future behaviour. Writings on the major influence of these early experiences have been expanded by schools of thought which extend development throughout life.

Carl Jung was the first modern adult developmentalist. 'Analytical Psychology', the discipline he founded after his break with Freud, was to be an extension of, not an alternative to, psychoanalysis (Bacelle, 2004). He saw personality development and an unfolding programme of universal archetypes continuing throughout life, the second half of life being governed by different principles from the first. He drew an analogy with the daily course of the sun (Jung, 1931). In the morning the rays of the sun extend outwards, the young person's life is mounting and unfolding with aims those of nature, entrenchment in the world and care of children. In the afternoon the sun draws in its rays, '…in order to illuminate itself' and 'for the ageing person it is a duty to give serious attention to himself'. This is not to be a hypochondriac or to be niggardly but for illumination of the self by focusing on culture and spirituality. In mid-life people undergo a psychological shift from developing and asserting their personality to assessing the meaning and quality of their life. The goal of life, and in therapy, is 'individuation'—identifying who you are on the basis of past, present, and future. In the afternoon of life this task supersedes the earlier task of conforming, of being a collective person. The task of the old is to look to the future as a place where you can afford to be the individual that you are. The job will not be to rush around going to lectures, seeing many patients, writing chapters. The task in later life is to discover who you are. Individuation is not about being healed from being sick but it is an attempt to be yourself, not alienated from the self, not diseased.

The worldwide archetype 'senex' is the old man who has seen enough to be content. It represents wise acceptance but also the wish to go on and learn more. Senex needs to recognize, still, the child within himself; neither are static, the inner child 'puer' needs to be used in the function of moving on. Puer and senex are potential archetypes for all; the young person too has senex within and will experience both polarities. There is a need to synthesize disparate aspects of the self (Jung, 1933).

Neo-Freudians added a sociological view to psychoanalytic theory, putting greater focus on the external world with a more interpersonal (cf. intrapersonal) model. Out of this tradition Erik Erikson, a professor of human development at Harvard University, supplemented and extended Freud's ideas which had ended in early adulthood. Development was seen to continue beyond libidinal development throughout the life cycle. He described 'Eight Ages of Man' with specific tasks to be negotiated at each (Erikson, 1959).

Cultural as well as intrapsychic factors are emphasized. The life cycle is charted through psychoanalysis and social science. The name of each of the stages indicates the conflict to be negotiated, the phase-specific task required in order to have a reasonable balance of positive attitudes. It is not a question of achievement but of balance. The negative contentions persist as a dynamic counterpart and may be stimulated by difficulties and stresses in life, by the exigencies of old age. The earlier phases of this model will be mentioned briefly.

*Basic trust vs. mistrust* is the cornerstone for future psychosocial functioning. Initially it is the trust that mother and food will be reliably available for the oral baby, not quantities of food but quality of the relationship. Subsequently that others or institutions will be sufficient for one's needs. *Autonomy vs. shame and doubt* is the stage at which autonomous will develops. The anal phase toddler is manipulating objects in his world. If he can learn self-control then self-esteem and personal pride may be developed rather than 'losing face'. *Initiative vs. guilt* is the stage at which social goals are contemplated. Guilt may be engendered by the goal set or fear of punishment of eroticised fantasies. Freud described this as the Oedipal complex. *Industry vs. inferiority* is the latency period with pleasure at producing things at school and at home but the risk is of feeling mediocre or inadequate. *Identity and role confusion* is the beginning of youth and physiological revolution. Ego identity is the integration of previous stages, there is a search for continuity and inner sameness in adolescence whilst also identifying with 'heroes' which may lead to confusion.

Subsequent junctures in Erikson's model are developmental phases in adulthood beyond Freud's stages. *Intimacy vs. isolation* is young adulthood eager for partnership and intimacy. Avoiding it may presage isolation. *Generativity vs. stagnation* is the concern for guiding the next generation including non-genital creativity. The counterpart is interpersonal impoverishment and stagnation.

There has been criticism of Erikson for ageism, suggesting he left the existential question to the end of life but actually he writes that each phase is related to all others, every strength and weakness has its precursors or derivatives in each stage. The infant has the seeds of all that is to come and the elderly person is marked by all that has been. *Ego integrity vs. despair and disgust* is the final phase described. There is no clear definition of ego integrity, but someone who possesses it accepts that his life was his own responsibility albeit set in a particular time in history. He accepts his family of origin, his position in world affairs, and his personal life to be as it had to be. Without integrity the person is beset by despair that life is too short and death is too near for a different path to be taken. The fear is of 'not being' rather than valuing 'having been'. They may be disgusted by their elderly self and others, misanthropic and contemptuous. Both young and old may feel despair at powerlessness and rage with fear of disintegration. In old age, ego despair is bitterness 'if that is all there is then it is nothing'. Out of that stance come anger, jealousy, and hatred. Ego integrity involves a preference for order and meaning, a sense of world order and spirituality. The struggle is not only about old age and death but all the previous life stage issues too. Despair is a manifestation of disintegration unconsciously repeating the despair or failure of dependency in infancy. Fear of dependency in old age is a reflection of earlier needs not being met. This elicits a terror of the future, acted out in the present. The older person has to be able to contemplate not being able to rely physically on herself for aspects of basic care which must be provided by others. Childhood experiences of dependency and how the first stage of basic trust vs. mistrust was negotiated come to the fore and assume great importance with the physical dependency of old age. If as a baby the individual had good enough experiences they will carry inside themselves a reasonably benign acceptance of the possibility of a dependent future. Those without such inner security based on earlier experiences may come to professionals with disabling symptoms of anxiety, panic, and depression (Martindale, 1989). Some severely disabled patients angrily dismiss all attempts to help claiming they can manage perfectly well without interference, whilst with others their greatest wish seems to be to have everything done for them when they could personally undertake much more, yet they complain that the care they are given is inadequate.

Other analysts have taken up the theme of continuing psychological development in adulthood and of experiences as an adult affecting future life. Colarusso and Nemiroff (1981) have presented a series of hypotheses for adult development suggesting that the nature of the developmental processes is the same in adult and child, and that it is an ongoing dynamic process, in adulthood concerned with evolution rather than formation of psychic structures. They also mention bodily change influencing development in adulthood; during ageing we gradually become aware of changes in bodily appearance and function. The biological realities of the patient's life and the mind–body relationship emphasized in work with children need to be acknowledged and spoken of in therapy. Failure to complete developmental tasks in adulthood has similar consequences in later life as the consequences of unresolved childhood conflicts. Nemiroff and Colarusso (1985) discuss 'developmental resonance' which is about all of us having a similar developmental framework so that the therapist may have an understanding of all phases of the patient's life either because they have already been there themselves or will be there at some point in the future. Throughout life disturbances in earlier stages can produce psychopathological change later interacting with phase-specific tasks. Issues dormant but present throughout life may re-emerge with force in later years.

Hildebrand (1982) drawing on the work of King (1974, 1980) has delineated particular tasks and difficulties which need to be negotiated for later life to be content. There is a fear of diminution and of loss of sexual potency, a threat of redundancy in work roles, of being replaced by younger people. After children have grown up and left home there is the need to reconsider, or even remake, the marital relationship. The person becomes aware of their own ageing, illness, and possible dependence and that what they can achieve now will be limited. The older person may feel they have failed as a parent, which Hildebrand thinks is paradoxically exacerbated in the childless. Many face loss of a partner and of intimacy. There is the need to acknowledge one's own death in terms of narcissistic loss and pain. In addition to these tasks of later life, unresolved conflicts from early stages may be reworked, perhaps appearing as 'the senescent adolescent' (Sandler, 1978). McDougall (1985) relates the metaphor of a theatrical production to observation of various aspects of the self from different ages and stages of unresolved developmental issues emerging in therapy.

Stages and phases in life are not only represented in art, literature, folk knowledge, and post-Freudian psychoanalytic literature, but they also form a framework, a developmental resonance for how life is experienced and reviewed. A mid-life awareness of mortality may prompt an appraisal of life. Thoughts of retirement may precipitate a period of self-reflection. The present is meaningful because of its connections with the past. *Life review* is not synonymous with reminiscence; it has an evaluative component aimed at resolving tensions.

The process is both intrapersonal and interpersonal (Molinari, 1999). The idea of ego integrity has a natural association with the life review process. Erikson's scheme was the main conceptual influence on Butler (1963) who developed the life review technique. He demonstrated that life review is a normal developmental task of later years. One reviews the past in order to understand the present. Older people have a propensity for life review brought about by knowledge of approaching death. The therapist facilitates and enhances this making it more deliberate and conscious (Knight, 1992).

Life review is purposeful, not to retrieve facts but to put life into perspective for self-discovery, to achieve a sense of completeness, of connectedness and coherence over the lifespan. No memory is a literal or photographic construction of what happened; it is not like a videotape. We see things through the prism of subsequent experience, personality, current situation, and the relationship with the therapist. In addition our memories are filtered through our own theories of ageing. Simple reminiscence is the recall of past experience; life review involves analysis, evaluation, and mourning. The past is surveyed reflectively with reconsideration of past experiences and their meaning. This may lead to an expanded understanding and acceptance of self and of death to come (Beadleson and Lara, 1988) as well as an enhanced sense of how any individual life is part of a larger historical and cultural circumstance. An ongoing creative meaning-making and reframing process is necessary for life review which is aimed at integrating unresolved developmental and relational aspects of experience.

In the USA the terms used for this type of work are guided autobiography and narrative gerontology. Storytelling is important; a natural means to explain actions, thoughts, and feelings in narrative form although the story may be maladaptive. It may be the telling of the tale that encourages a reluctant patient into therapy but for change and self-actualization it is the hermeneutics of life stories, the focus on new meaning to a perhaps oft repeated tale which is mutative. In the therapy it must be possible for all 'stories' to be voiced, not only those that support socially acceptable behaviour and feelings. A particular focus may be necessary in the review of a personal life and experiences but many themes present themselves: attachment style; acceptance/rebellion; independence/dependence; meaning to life; spiritual issues; ideas about death; loss and resilience; appropriate pride and esteem in the self; personal/family myths and patterns; sexuality; changing body image over the years; goals and aspirations—those met and those unachieved. Any of these themes need to be in the context of finding meaning even in the suffering old age may bring. Reflection on a life is about striving for new insights, not looking only at individual episodes of memory but how they are linked across the lifespan giving a sense of self continuous over time. The person may develop a sense of being the expert in the time in which they have lived. Coming to terms with what life has been with the personal narrative re-examined gives greater capacity to accept the present and cope with future difficulties.

The turning points in people's lives are not always those that are expected. Leonard and Burns (1999) identified predominantly role transition, an adversity, or an experience of personal growth. They questioned mid-life and older women to prioritize significant life events. Most frequently reported were not marriage or motherhood but experiences based on 'self-work' and personal growth, e.g. deciding to change lifestyle or be more independent. Those experiences were more likely in the second half of life.

A *mourning* process is a normal part of life, of life review, and therapy. Crises and losses of old age do not have to be psychologically incapacitating if they initiate a successful mourning process (Pollack, 1978). Mourning is for lost and changed parts of the self, lost others, unfulfilled hopes and aspirations. The process can liberate and release development and creativity. It is clinical experience that patients who can review aspects of life with appropriate sadness are likely to gain from the experience—those who resist looking at difficult aspects of life do less well. Suppressed mourning leading to psychological difficulties is central to psychotherapeutic work. As one acknowledges loss, paradoxically internal objects are reclaimed. Natural losses of the end of sessions and of breaks will be used in treatment. Psychotherapy to be successful involves loss (Wolf, 1977) giving up previous maladaptive, erroneous, infantile wishes and behaviour. In the same way, to move through phases of life things need to be given up. Pollack (1982) writes of mourning-liberation being the focus of work in later life. It is a universal process allowing the past to appropriately become the past and putting investment into the present and the future. Successful ageing is the ability to mourn for the self, opening up possibilities and freedoms in the years that are to come. If mourning is not achieved the patient may turn rage and despair onto herself and become depressed. For someone with sufficient internal resources the losses and traumata of ageing may be a spur to positive development, courage, and strengthening of the personality (Settlage, 1996).

Losses are important throughout life but are not the only things that happen to us. A different view of ageing is via a *maturity* model (Knight, 1992). According to this model, the healthy feel more comfortable with themselves as they age. Older people have a wealth of experience and observations accumulated over the years; experience of how people interact and interrelate, they will have expertise in particular areas; they may have lived in or with a number of different family constellations. Maturity is about inner growth coming out of awareness. Ageing happens to us but we contribute to maturity. It is not necessarily anything to do with external experiences in life but an inward journey—growing up rather than growing old.

Cicero (45 BC) wrote of a dialogue between two young men and the 84-year-old Cato who was famous for his wisdom. The young men put forward a series of negative views about old age which the old man refuted one by one, arguing that the quality of old age depends on the quality of experiences in younger age—'Blame rests with character, not with age'. Cephalus speaking to Socrates on the subject of age had earlier said something similar (Plato 4th century BC) '…for he who is of a calm and happy nature will hardly feel the pressure of age, but to him who is of an opposite disposition youth and age are equally a burden'. We are what our biological, social, cultural, and psychological past has made us, particularly how we have integrated and adapted to it. The psychological past is the most important as it defines why some falter under the pressure of physical illness, increasing isolation, age-related prejudice, financial constraints, and death of a partner while others manage and adapt. '*Quod sis esse velis*' wrote Martial, the epigrammatic poet (AD 43–104): be happy as you are. In a healthy old age this is about acceptance of what has been and what now is. It is not about striving to be young, wishing for the impossible but accepting one's life in all its complexities, that under the circumstances it was the only life one could have led also leaving oneself open to accept opportunities as they arise in the future. In this way there is a balance of 'integrity' over 'despair'.

## Similarities and differences across ages

All our patients are unique. One needs to look at the problem presented and the individual not age *per se*. Generalizations about older people should be regarded as only partial truths. Review and integration are central to progress in psychotherapy, whatever the age, and patients present the same basic human need for respect, security, self-determination. *Suitability* for treatment rests on psychological mindedness, motivation, ego strength, and the ability to enter and sustain an intensive therapeutic relationship. For a brief approach, patient and therapist need to be able to identify and adhere to a suitable focus for therapy and accept that it will end after the agreed time. In public health services, the referred patients are likely to present with multiple difficulties and too many exclusion criteria are not helpful. An assessment extended over a few sessions may be useful, seeing how the patient responds to different ideas and to the unusual situation of a private space, not only of the consulting room but also of the relationship, with examination of previously unacknowledged aspects of life and an inner world. Variables pertaining to the patient's ability to relate to another person tend to correlate with outcome.

The older patient will have accrued strengths with the passing of the years, so there may be psychological and social growth despite biological decline. Although older people may come from a generation less likely to use an emotional vocabulary, with ageing seems to come an enhanced facility to access metaphors and symbols (Barker, 1985). Meerloo (1955) writes that the approach of death leads to life review, decreased defensiveness, and easier access to the patient's unconscious. Older people also bring an increased experience of life, a greater emotional complexity, coping skills, resilience, and the capacity for delayed gratification.

The main therapeutic objective is to identify and rework sources of disturbance that have been hidden away. Connection needs to be understood between past, present, and future. All therapy makes some use of storytelling, people speaking from their own perspective discussing the history of their symptoms and themselves. This is facilitated by active listening by the therapist who will use clarification and suggestion of possible unconscious determinants. There may be multiple associations and meanings to dreams and metaphors. Repetition of metaphors and affect is meaningful (Magee, 1991) particularly if it is also expressed within the transference relationship.

The therapeutic emphasis on interiority needs to expand in old age to include *reality*. Illness and disability are a source of distress at any age. Chronic and multiple health problems are more common in older adults. Mobility may be impaired, the number of social contacts decreased, and finances restricted. These realities need to be acknowledged, as they will not be alleviated by the exploratory approach of psychotherapy, but nonetheless psychological mindedness is an important mitigating factor in dealing with adverse circumstances. All patients function within a variety of time-scales: chronological, psychological, and biological alongside the timelessness of unconscious processes (King, 1980). In addition there is the time of the social history of the patient. It is easy incorrectly to attribute cohort effects to the ageing process. Older people have had different opportunities, experiences, and concerns from later cohorts. Few staff nowadays have personal experience of the Second World War. Older people will have often had less education than younger folk. Therapists need to be sensitive to the different time perspective of people who have lived longer and had experiences in historically different socio-cultural and value systems (Kettell, 2001). The ages of patients we see in old age psychiatry services may span four decades. Some may have been raised by parents born in Victorian times, and their lives may have been affected by periods of serious economic depression and by two world wars. Over the years, modes of behaviour, social expression, and the emotional vocabulary have changed.

*Sexuality* is important throughout life and is always an aspect of dynamic psychotherapy. It is underestimated as an issue for older people (Garner and Bacelle, 2004). How sexuality is expressed or verbalized depends on the individual but is also affected by chronological age, by cohort, and by expectations of younger family members and staff. Also significant is the expectation of the person themselves who may have internalized society's idea that what is virility at 25 is lechery at 65 (Berezin, 1969). The literature on sexuality focuses on frequency, quantity rather than quality. Sexual activity can continue into extreme old age (Starr and Weiner, 1981). The complex nature of sexuality may increase with age. Physical bodies will change but in parallel with learning, experience and psychosocial development. Behaviour may become more sensual, more sophisticated. There is a need for intimate connectedness throughout life but for some the physical changes of later years provide a reason to avoid intimacy. Some therapists having internalized society's ideas about a sexless old age or having unresolved issues about parents' sexuality find it difficult to address these topics with the patient.

Some patients come to terms with their own mortality in mid-life (Jacques, 1965; Knight, 1986) so negotiating death is not a particular task for later years. For others death looms as a persecutory or depressive anxiety (Segal, 1958). Perhaps death is a longitudinal issue (Turner, 1992); that is, if one fears death when young one fears it when old. The idea that it is a particular problem for 'the old' could be seen as a projection by younger people of their fears and prejudices. Fears of death are disowned and projected into the old person by projective identification. The recipient of the projection is induced to feel it and own it as his—this also connects with the older person's own fears. Patients are seen whose fear is of 'not being'. The existential *terror* held within many of us and obscured by work and busy social relationships may come to the surface in older age, a terror of death, loneliness, and dependency. Bion (1962) writes of the 'nameless dread'. This is something imponderable. It could be death or something even worse. It is a very personal feeling in which there is no wife, no husband, no mother, no father, it is a cosmic aloneness. Relationships counteract this as do affective memories of relationships with good objects. Reawakening of early failure of dependency has been mentioned previously. There may have been an insecure attachment to mother so when mother was not present the child had terrors of not being held—literally, also not being 'held in mind'. The person's life may then have been constructed so they were not exposed to these terrors but these defensive manoeuvres face disintegration with the threat of dependency later. The repressed terror returns with the fear of falling to pieces. The therapist's task is to understand the revival of infantile terrors without infantilizing the older adult (Terry, 2006).

The defence against the dread of being abandoned to a state of utter helplessness is often a narcissistic tyranny. Hess (1987) understands the story of Shakespeare's King Lear in this way. The grandiose self is unsustainable in the face of the exigencies of old age; it is

associated with rage and contempt of others instead of the self to avoid the personal shame and humiliation of this narcissistic collapse. Shame and humiliation accompany fears of loneliness (Hess, 2004)—wanting an intimate relationship but not being perfect enough to achieve it. Klein (1963) gives a description of the dreaded loneliness in which one feels left alone with bad parts of the self, the unintegrated parts of self. We see in our services the patient who cannot be left. The terror of being on one's own without spouse, family, or friends is also a terror of being without an organizing and containing part of the self which feels lost in illness, stroke, and dementia. The person may feel driven to use others as narcissistic extensions of themselves. Sentimentality about Lear as a 'poor weak infirm and despis'd old man' may seem compassionate but it also protects the clinician from ever confronting the complex mixture of strength and frailty which we all have and which needs to be understood for change to occur. Perhaps the anxieties of age are not so different from earlier, universal anxieties—fear of loss, abandonment, and loss of autonomy but realities of later life enhance a person's fears. Anxiety about the future can be a catalyst for growth and change.

## The process of therapy

The core of dynamic therapy at any age is the relationship between the patient and the therapist. Any difference in *therapy* will be more due to the reaction of the therapist rather than process or technique. The type of *transference* has more to do with relationship experiences than with chronological age. The adult past is a source of transference (Colarusso and Nemiroff, 1981). Even parental transference may not only be from childhood but also adolescence and adult life. Transference will be more varied with an older patient, also multigenerational—at times the therapist may represent parent or grandparent, at others child or grandchild. The manifestation is varied and changing throughout the therapy. It is a rich source of information about the patient. An idealized transference is likely to cover underlying hostility, perhaps here envy of youth, holidays, a fantasized wonderful sexual life and vigour.

Each therapist's reaction to an individual patient is unique but working with older patients may evoke particular feelings. It can be difficult to maintain perspective if the only experience one has of older people is at work with patients with problems or conversely a relationship with an idealized grandparent. The therapist may have unresolved conflicts with parents. There may be a wish for admiration which interferes with recognizing the patient's needs, perhaps an unconscious wish to be needed which may encourage excessive demands from the patient. The therapist may feel the wish to protect the patient from their 'difficult' family but this prevents understanding the role the patient is playing in their own life and family and the need for them to take some responsibility for problems. If the therapist feels hostility or resentment in the relationship the patient will be kept at a distance. Unconscious reactions can reduce the therapist's availability to the patient. The therapist needs to be alert to the reality of patients' lives but also sensitive to when reality is also symbolic and being used as a way of avoiding looking at a painful psychological issue. The patient may use their age as an excuse for not changing and the therapist may use their reactions or prejudices as a 'good reason' to discharge the patient. An intense wish to discharge a patient needs to be resisted until it is understood in terms of the relationship with the therapist and the therapist's personal reactions. A *countertransference* to dependency may stimulate infantile wishes to dominate and control the parent or stimulate sadistic feelings in the unequal power relationship. It is anxiety-provoking for a therapist of any age to be confronting difficult issues of death and dependency; it will evoke fears about one's own ageing and eventual death. The therapist may be frightened of imagined escalating demands and dependency of the patient—the paradox of being controlled by the helpless (Martindale, 1989; Terry, 2006). Therapists may find an eroticized transference from this supposedly sexless older person difficult to acknowledge. Countertransference is not a problem, it is a tool in the therapy but it needs to be conscious, accepted, and understood, and it is only problematic when the therapist reacts unknowingly in response to the patient (Semel, 2006).

The relationship between the patient and therapist is also a real one and the most significant agent in therapy. The therapeutic alliance is the *sine qua non* of effective therapy. It is the collaborative working relationship which keeps the treatment going whatever the emotional ups and downs of the transference relationship. For the process to function it needs to be collaborative. The alliance forms from initial encounters and is then facilitated by reciprocal experiences. Previous poor attachment experiences can be modified. One aim of the therapeutic alliance is to provide the patient with a different, improved attachment experience.

Managing *endings* is a significant and difficult part of all therapy, especially if it is time-limited. The ending should be discussed perhaps even from the start of the work. The patient may need to grieve that time is coming to an end. The patient may feel angry at the idea of termination, but it is not helpful for positive aspects of the therapy to be totally denigrated. Knowledge of the good experiences of therapy will be a resource in times of future difficulty. The therapist working with an older patient may feel guilty at the ending linking discharge and death; the same thoughts will be with the patient. For Nemiroff and Colarusso (1985) continuation of psychotherapy represents continuation of life itself. There may need to be an existential focus on death. As there is a common general notion that a psychic life persists, it may be useful to explore the patient's ideas about life after death (Martindale, 1998). Some therapists continue to provide appointments but infrequently or else they permit the patient to return if necessary. The patient who can come back may not need to do so.

*Outcomes* are consistent with those found in younger populations. When different approaches are tested against each other outcomes are equivalent. The most important factor seems to be the working alliance between patient and therapist—the model needs to be compatible for both parties. Outcome criteria do not always do justice to the complexity of psychodynamic change. Empirical and naturalistic studies suggest good outcomes—effectiveness in real life as well as efficacy in studies (see Hepple *et al.* (2002) for discussion). There is growing evidence that psychodynamic treatment may be associated with continued improvement after termination of the therapy (Gabbard, 2001). Ideas of therapeutic change may need to be refocused for older patients (Garner, 2003). Younger patients will be able to exercise their increasing personal responsibility and autonomy on the external world. There is less opportunity for those in later life to exercise choice and take another route in life. Change may be purely internal with a new sense of acceptance and contentment. Grotjahn (1955) reported that older adults have less resistance to unpleasant insight perhaps after a lifetime's struggle with reality. Meerloo (1955) recorded an increased sense of interiority. Some older patients do well and quickly (Ardern *et al.*, 1998) motivated by a sense of urgency that this is their last chance, they need to take it and have nothing to lose.

# Dementia

The relative neglect of older people in dynamic therapy is even greater for those with a dementia, but it is important to recognize that not everything that happens to someone with dementia is organically determined. The illness trajectory is not solely determined by neurophysiology. The illness brings psychosocial problems for the patient and their relationships and an attack on personhood and identity. The introduction of antidementia drugs may paradoxically increase the need for psychotherapy. Earlier diagnosis may bring with it distress, fearfulness, and threats to close relationships. Reactions will be influenced by personality, previous history, and current psychosocial circumstances.

As the ability to spontaneously recall is lost, recognition memory persists. Implicit memory is retained longer than explicit. Affective memory remains as cognition decreases. Emotional memory is often identified as a midbrain function (Van der Kolk and McFarlane, 1996). The ability to make a relationship is retained long into the illness, enabling a therapeutic connection and alliance with an empathic therapist (Garner, 2004). Feelings and affective themes are not eliminated by dementia. There is a continuation of personality and continuity of attachment style (Magai and Cohen, 1988).

Modifications will need to be made to the practicalities of technique in middle and later stages of the disease. It may be preferable to see patients more frequently but for shorter sessions, perhaps using familiar photographs and objects. Language will be impaired but an emotional life continues without language. The patient can still have a meaningful inner world. Duffy (2006) writes of using the technique of 'therapeutic monologue' which is also used with silent adolescents or those with expressive dysphasia. The therapist speaks to the salient psychological and affective issues for the patient, being aware of and sensitive to non-verbal cues and any verbal expression, albeit difficult to follow. Work in this way may give the patient some alleviation of terror and a sense of containment and continuity for a more peaceful end.

# A psychodynamically informed service

Not everyone is suitable for psychotherapy, but all patients and staff benefit from a service which understands dynamic principles and provides opportunities for containment and reflection, understanding both the fears of the patients and also of the staff who care for them. Our health-care institutions are constructed as a form of social defence—a way of avoiding experiences of doubt, uncertainty, anxiety, and guilt (Menzies-Lyth, 1987).

Care for older patients is often custodial rather than therapeutic. Caregiving tasks need to be turned into opportunities also to interact psychotherapeutically with benefit not only to patients but also to staff who are likely then to experience less dissatisfaction and 'burn out'. Relationships will be more meaningful.

Psychotherapeutic capacities which can be applied to work in old age psychiatry include those associated with communication—for example, the capacity to listen and empathize showing an openness to the patient's emotions, capacity to make sense of the patient's experience, ability to use personal emotional response as a source of understanding, and being able to communicate such understanding to the patient. Staff need the capacity to contain anxiety and despair rather than being compelled to act, while using realistic judgement to decide when action is necessary. There needs to be some understanding of the underlying structure of guilt and persecutory anxiety. It is necessary to be able to identify idealization and a distorted perception of the staff/patient relationship, having the capacity to bear hostility and criticism without retaliation. Concepts such as therapeutic alliance, doctor/patient collaboration, transference, and countertransference apply in all our interactions with patients.

## Conclusion

Older people are offered psychotherapy significantly less often than younger ones but for those who are able to access psychotherapeutic help the outcome is comparable to that, and sometimes better than, for younger patients. Older people are often able to take the opportunity for intrapsychic and interpersonal change. Therapists need a broader perspective preserving useful elements of the traditional psychoanalytic model while also negotiating changes across the lifespan and understanding that patients have lived in a different historical context. The therapist needs to be open to reflecting on their own thoughts and prejudices about ageing. The meaning of life and death are inseparable, retrospective evaluation of one's life leading to a perspective on death.

The social and physical realities of the later years emphasize the pointlessness of the traditional arguments between biological and psychological psychiatry. Such discourse may be enjoyable but for the patient these perspectives need to converge. Distinguishing between diseases of the brain and of the mind reflects a basic ignorance of the link between the two (Damasio, 1994). The goal of psychotherapeutic intervention may be to accept biological reality with equanimity.

## References

Abraham, K. (1919). The applicability of psychoanalytic treatment to patients at an advanced age. In *Selected papers on psychoanalysis* (ed. A. Bryan and A. Strachey). Karnac, London (1988).

Ardern, M., Garner, J., and Porter, R. (1998). Curious bedfellows. *Psychoanalytic Psychotherapy*, **12**(1), 47–56.

Bacelle, L. (2004). On becoming an old man: Jung and others. In *Talking over the years: a handbook of dynamic psychotherapy with older adults* (ed. S. Evans and J. Garner), pp. 29–41. Brunner-Routledge, Hove.

Barker, P. (1985). *Using metaphors in psychotherapy*. Brunner/Mazel, New York.

Beadleson, B.M. and Lara, L.L. (1988). Reminiscence: nursing actions for the acutely ill geriatric patient. *Issues in Mental Health Nursing*, **9**(1), 83–94.

Berezin, M.A. (1969). Sex and old age. A review of the literature. *Journal of Geriatric Psychiatry*, **3**, 131–149.

Bion, W.R. (1962). The psychoanalytic study of thinking. *International Journal of Psychoanalysis*, **43**, 306–310.

Butler, R.N. (1963). The life review: an interpretation of reminiscence in the aged. *Psychiatry*, **26**, 65–76.

Cicero (45 BC). *De Senectute* [transl. Falconer W.A. (1923). *On old age.* Harvard University Press, Cambridge, MA].

Ciechanowski, P.S, Katon, W.J, Russo, J.E, and Walker, E.A. (2001). The patient-provider relationship: Attachment theory and adherence to treatment in diabetes. *American Journal of Psychiatry*, **158**(1), 29–35.

Colarusso, C.A. and Nemiroff, R.A. (1981). *Adult development: a new dimension in psychodynamic theory and practice*. Plenum, New York.

Damasio, A.R. (1994). *Descartes' error: emotion, reason and the human brain*. Grosset/Putnam, New York.

Duffy, M. (2006). Psychotherapeutic interventions for older persons with dementing disorders. In *Strategies for therapy with the elderly*, 2nd edn (ed. C.M. Brody and V.G. Semel), pp. 15–37. Springer, New York.

Erikson, E. (1959). *Identity and the life cycle*, Psychological Issues Monograph 1. International Universities Press, New York.

Evans, S. (1998). Beyond the mirror: a group analytic exploration of late life and depression. *Ageing and Mental Health*, **2**, 94–99.

Evans, S. (2004). The old self: Kohut, Winnicott and others. In *Talking over the years: a handbook of dynamic psychotherapy with older adults*. (ed. S. Evans and J. Garner), pp. 57–69. Brunner-Routledge, Hove.

Freud, S. (1905/1953). On psychotherapy. In *The standard edition of the complete psychological works of Sigmund Freud*, Vol. 6 (ed. and transl. J. Strachey), pp. 249–263. Hogarth, London.

Gabbard, G.O. (2000). A neurobiologically informed perspective on psychotherapy. *British Journal of Psychiatry*, **177**, 117–122.

Gabbard, G.O. (2001). Empirical evidence and psychotherapy: a growing scientific base. *American Journal of Psychiatry*, **158**(1), 1–3.

Garner, J. (2003). Psychotherapies and older adults. *Australian and New Zealand Journal of Psychiatry*, **37**, 537–548.

Garner, J. (2004). Dementia. In *Talking over the years: a handbook of dynamic psychotherapy with older adults* (ed. S. Evans and J. Garner), pp. 215–230. Brunner-Routledge, Hove.

Garner, J. and Bacelle, L. (2004). Sexuality. In *Talking over the years: a handbook of dynamic psychotherapy with older adults* (ed. S. Evans and J. Garner), pp. 247–263. Brunner-Routledge, Hove.

Grotjahn, M. (1955). Analytic psychotherapy with the elderly. *Psychoanalytic Review*, **42**, 419–427.

Hepple, J., Wilkinson, P., and Pearce, J. (2002). Psychological therapies with older people: an overview. In *Psychological therapies with older people: developing treatments for effective practice* (ed. J. Hepple, J. Pearce, and P. Wilkinson), pp. 161–176. Brunner-Routledge, Hove.

Hess, N. (1987). King Lear and some anxieties of old age. *British Journal of Medical Psychology*, **60**, 209–215.

Hess, N. (2004). Loneliness in old age: Klein and others. In *Talking over the years: a handbook of dynamic psychotherapy with older adults* (ed. S. Evans and J. Garner), pp. 9–27. Brunner-Routledge, Hove.

Hildebrand, P. (1982). Psychotherapy with older patients. *British Journal of Medical Psychology*, **55**, 19–28.

Jacques, E. (1965). Death and the mid life crisis. *International Journal of Psychoanalysis*, **46**, 502–514.

Jung, C.G. (1931/1979). The stages of life. In *Collected works 8* (ed. H. Read, M. Fordham, and G. Adler). Routledge and Kegan Paul, London.

Jung, C.G. (1933). *Modern man in search of a soul*. Harcourt Brace Jovanovich, New York.

Kettell, M.E. (2001). Reminiscence and the late life. Search for ego integrity: Ingmar Bergman's Wild Strawberries. *Journal of Geriatric Psychiatry*, **34**(1), 9–41.

King, P. (1974). Notes on the psychoanalysis of older patients. *Journal of Analytic Psychology*, **19**, 22–37.

King, P. (1980). The lifecycle as indicated by the nature of the transference in the psychoanalysis of the middle-aged and elderly. *International Journal of Psycho-Analysis*, **61**, 153–160.

Klein, M. (1963). On the sense of loneliness. In *Envy and Gratitude and other works*. Hogarth Press, London (1975).

Knight, B.G. (1986). *Psychotherapy with older adults*. Sage Publishing, Beverley Hills, CA.

Knight, B.G. (1992). *Older adults in psychotherapy. Case histories*. Sage Publishing, Beverley Hills, CA.

Knight, B.G. (1996). Psychodynamic therapy with older adults: lessons from scientific gerontology in *Handbook of the clinical psychology of ageing* (ed. R. Woods). Wiley, Chichester.

Leonard, R. and Burns, A. (1999). Turning points in the lives of midlife and older women. *Australian Psychologist*, **34**(2), 87–93.

McDougall, J. (1985). *Theaters of the mind*. Brunner/Mazel, New York.

Magai, C. and Cohen, C.I. (1998). Attachment style and emotion regulation in dementia patients and their relation to caregiver burden. *Journal of Gerontology*, **533**(3), 147–154.

Magee, J. (1991). Dream analysis as an aid to older adults' life review. *Journal of Gerontological Social Work*, **18**(1/2), 163–173.

Martindale, B. (1989). Becoming dependent again: the fears of some elderly persons and their younger therapists. *Psychoanalytic Psychotherapy*, **4**(1), 56–75.

Martindale, B. (1998). On ageing, dying, death and eternal life. *Psychoanalytic Psychotherapy*, **12**, 259–270.

Meerloo, J.A.M. (1955). Psychotherapy with elderly patients. *Geriatrics*, **10**, 583–587.

Menzies-Lyth, I.E.P. (1987). Containing anxiety in institutions. *Selected essays*, Vol. 1. Free Association Books, London.

Miesen, B.M.L. (1993). Alzheimer's disease, the phenomenon of parent fixation and Bowlby's attachment theory. *International Journal of Geriatric Psychiatry*, **8**, 147–153.

Mills, M.A. and Coleman, P.G. (2002). Using reminiscence and life review interventions with older people: a psychodynamic approach. *Journal of Geriatric Psychiatry*, **35**(1), 63–76.

Molinari, V. (1999). Using reminiscence and life review as natural therapeutic strategies in group therapy. In *Handbook of counselling and psychotherapy with older adults* (ed. M. Duffy), pp. 154–165. Wiley, New York.

Nemiroff, R.A. and Colarusso, C.A. (1985). *The race against time: psychotherapy and psychoanalysis in the second half of life*. Plenum, New York.

O'Connor, D. (1993). The impact of dementia: a self psychological perspective. *Journal of Gerontological Social Work*, **20**, 113–128.

Pinquart, M. and Sorensen, S. (2001). How effective are psychotherapeutic and other psychosocial interventions with older adults: a meta-analysis. *Journal of Mental Health and Aging*, **7**, 207–243.

Plato (4th century BC). *The republic* [transl. Jowett, B. (1894), Dover thrift edn (2000), p. 3].

Pollack, G.H. (1978). Process and affect: mourning and grief. *International Journal of Psychoanalysis*, **59**, 255–276.

Pollack, G.H. (1982). On ageing and psychotherapy. *International Journal of Psychoanalysis*, **63**, 275–281.

Sandler, A.M. (1978). Psychoanalysis in later life. Problems in the psychoanalysis of an aging narcissistic patient. *Journal of Geriatric Psychoanalysis*, **11**, 5–36.

Schore, A.N. (1997). A century after Freud's project: is a rapprochement between psychoanalysis and neurobiology at hand? *Journal of American Psychoanalytic Association*, **45**, 807–840.

Segal, H. (1958). Fear of death: notes on the analysis of an old man. *International Journal of Psychoanalysis*, **39**, 173–181.

Semel, V.G. (2006). Countertransference and ageism: therapist reactions to the older patient. In *Strategies for therapy with the elderly* (ed. C.M. Brody and V.G. Semel), pp. 223–235. Springer, New York.

Settlage, C.F. (1996). Transcending old age: creativity, development and psychoanalysis in the life of a centenarian. *International Journal of Psychoanalysis*, **77**, 549–564.

Solms, M. (2004). Freud returns. *Scientific American*, May, 83–88.

Spiegel, D., Bloom, J., Kraemer, H.D. *et al.* (1989). Effect of psychosocial treatment on survival of patients with metastatic breast cancer. *Lancet*, **ii**, 888–891.

Starr, B.D. and Weiner, M.B. (1981). *Sex and sexuality in the mature years*. Stein and Day, New York.

Terry, P. (2006). Terrors. *Therapy Today*, April, 8–11.

Turner, M. (1992). Individual psychodynamic psychotherapy with older adults: perspectives from a nurse psychotherapist. *Archives of Psychiatric Nursing*, **VI**(5), 266–274.

Van der Kolk, B.A. and McFarlane, A.C. (1996). The black hole of trauma. In *Traumatic stress: the effects of overwhelming experience on mind, body and society* (ed. A.C. McFarlane and L. Weisaeth), pp. 2–23, Guildford Press, New York.

Viinamaki, H., Kuikka, J., Tilhonen, J. *et al.* (1998). Change in monoamine transporter density related to clinical recovery: a case–control study. *Nordic Journal of Psychiatry*, **52**, 39–44.

Wolf, H. (1977). Loss: a central theme in psychotherapy. *British Journal of Psychology*, **50**, 11–19.

Woodward, K. (1991). *Aging and its discontents: Freud and other fictions*. Indiana University Press, Indianapolis.

Zivian, M.T., Larsen, W., Knox, J. *et al.* (1992). Psychotherapy for the elderly: psychotherapists' preferences. *Psychotherapy*, **29**(4), 668–674.

# Psychological treatments: non-pharmacological interventions in care homes

Ian A. James and Jane Fossey

## Introduction

There are approximately 410,000 older people living in care homes across the UK (Office of Fair Trading, 2005) and the majority of residents are over the age of 85 (Bajekal, 2002). Many of them have multiple physical, cognitive, and mental health difficulties, with approximately 75% of residents having dementia (MacDonald *et al.*, 2002). Thirty to forty per cent of people with dementia develop psychosis with paranoid delusions or hallucinations associated with aggression or violence (Gilley *et al.*, 1997; SIGN, 1998). The incidence of depression is high, with prevalence rates between 6% and 25% for major depression, and up to 50% for minor (Kim and Rovner, 1995; Katz and Parmalee, 1997). It is suggested, therefore, that the presentations of many of the patients referred to health services from care homes are some of the most complex that health professionals are required to treat. This is because in addition to the cognitive and psychiatric issues outlined above, one must take account of physical frailties, polypharmacy, and limited access to social facilities. Moreover residents' treatments are frequently undertaken indirectly through care staff, most of whom are often both poorly trained and poorly paid. The situation is further complicated by the lack of evidence for the efficacy of many of the pharmacological and non-pharmacological approaches used in the area, particularly in the treatment of challenging behaviours. This is the context within which health professionals are required to devise and execute treatment plans.

This chapter examines a number of the non-pharmacological treatment strategies developed for these complex settings. Owing to the fact that challenging behaviours are typically the main reason for care homes to refer to a mental health team, there will be a particular focus on these presentations in this chapter.

## Challenging behaviour (CB) presentations

Challenging behaviours include symptoms such as delusions, hallucinations, anxiety, depression, apathy, agitation, aggression, wandering, and disinhibition. These behaviours are described as 'challenging' because they are perceived to be 'unreasonable' and challenge the norms and rules of the contexts within which they occur. For example, in a care home environment, the actions of a man with dementia constantly banging on the door because he wants to go home, will often be viewed as a challenging behaviour rather than an understandable response to his distress. Likewise, a person without dementia frequently buzzing to go to the toilet during the night may also become labelled as challenging.

Challenging behaviours are common, occurring in 60–90% of people with dementia, especially in the later stages of the illness (Lykestos *et al.*, 2002; Robert *et al.*, 2005), and are associated with caregiver stress and depression (Livingston *et al.*, 1996) and an increased likelihood of admittance into long-term care (Gilley *et al.*, 2004).

Due to their high incidence and the distress associated with their occurrence, effective treatments for such problems are clearly required. Psychotropics, particularly neuroleptic medication, have typically been used to treat these problems. However, there are increasing concerns about prescribing neuroleptics for this patient group. Their use has been associated with cerebrovascular events, falls, weight gain, and accelerated cognitive decline (Ballard and Cream, 2005), while showing limited evidence of efficacy (Sink *et al.*, 2005). In the light of such concerns (Ballard and Howard, 2006) guidelines suggest that non-pharmacological interventions should generally be employed prior to the use of pharmacological treatments (NICE, 2006).

## Non-pharmacological strategies for older people

Having established a requirement for non-pharmacological approaches, one must decide which therapy to use. There is an increasing number of therapies available for older people (Tilly and Reed, 2004). It is therefore important for a therapist to have knowledge of these approaches, and the evidence base underpinning them (Livingston *et al.*, 2005; Verkaik *et al.*, 2006). Examining the effectiveness of interventions for people who are often physically frail and have dementia and/or anxiety and depression, poses particular challenges. Indeed, whilst this does not excuse poorly designed studies, it does account in some part for the lack of studies in the literature to support the large number of different interventions. Specific problems relating to conducting research in the area include difficulties administering a conceptually discrete intervention package. There is often overlap between the various forms of therapy, and many will include a mixture of environmental, orientation, and staff-training features. Hence, it is difficult to determine which aspect of the package is the change element; such confounders also mean that it is problematic to compare the various forms of therapy with each other. It is often not feasible to run double-blind studies due the rather overt nature of the interventions and difficulty in devising placebo conditions. Despite these issues, there are many published studies which can be regarded as good 'practiced-based evidence', although, admittedly, a more limited number which are good quality 'evidenced-based practice'. Table 18vi.1 provides an overview of some of the non-pharmacological approaches used with older people that have been reviewed systematically. It is relevant to

**Table 18vi 1** Non-pharmacological approaches and their evidence base

| Therapies | Systematic reviews and empirical status | Key articles |
|---|---|---|
| I: Generic therapies<br>Reality orientation: uses rehearsal and physical prompts to improve cognitive functioning related to personal orientation | A Cochrane review by Spector et al. (2000) identified six RCTs. The reviewers concluded there was evidence of improvements in terms of cognitive and behavioural features | Holden and Woods (1982), Verkaik et al. (2006) |
| Reminiscence therapy: involves discussion of past experiences individually or in a group format. Photographs, familiar objects, or sensory items used to prompt recall | A Cochrane review by Woods et al. (2005a) identified five RCTs, four containing extractable data. The reviewers reported significant results in terms of cognitions, mood, caregiver strain, and functional abilities. However, the studies were perceived to be of poor quality | Gibson (1994), Goldwasser et al. (1987), Bohlmeijer et al. (2003) |
| Validation therapy: based on the general principle of acceptance of the reality of the person and validation of his/her experience | A Cochrane review by Neal and Barton Wright (2003) identified three studies, two showing positive effects. However, the reviewers concluded there was insufficient evidence to view the approach as effective | Finnema et al., (2000), Schrijnemaekers et al. (2002) |
| Psychomotor therapy: exercises (e.g. walking and ball games) are used to target depression and behavioural difficulties | A Cochrane review by Montgomery and Dennis (2002b) examining the impact of exercise on sleep problems identified one trial that demonstrated significant effects on a range of sleep variables | Winstead-Fry and Kijek (1999), Hopman-Rock et al. (1999) |
| Multisensory stimulation: stimuli such as light, sound, and tactile sensations, often in specially designed rooms, used to increase the opportunity for communication, and improved quality of experience | A Cochrane review by Chung and Lai (2002) identified two RCTs. Despite some favourable results, the studies were so different that they could not be pooled. As such, the reviewers concluded there was insufficient evidence to view the approach as effective | Pinkney (1997), Baillon et al. (2002) |
| Cognitive stimulation therapy: derived from reality orientation, focuses on information processing rather than rehearsal of factual knowledge | Two Cochrane reviews have been conducted in this area: Clare et al. (2003) and Woods et al. (2005b). In both situations the reviewers concluded that despite positive evidence there was insufficient evidence to view the approach as effective | Cameron and Clare (2004), Meier et al. (1996) |
| Aromatherapy: use of essential oils to provide sensory experiences and interactions with staff. The oils can be administered via massage techniques or in patients' baths | A Cochrane review by Thorgrimsen et al. (2003) identified two RCTs, but only the Ballard et al. (2002) trial was reviewed. This trial, despite flaws, was viewed favourably in terms of reducing agitation and neuropsychiatric symptoms | Holmes et al. (2002), Ballard et al. (2002) |
| Music therapy: includes playing and/or listening to music as a way of generally enhancing well being. Can be used in movement therapies | A Cochrane review by Vink et al. (2003) identified five studies. However, the quality of the studies were poor. As such, the reviewers concluded there was insufficient evidence to view the approach as effective | Lord and Garner (1993), Gotell et al. (2002) |
| Environmental manipulation: use of environmental cues, signage, and appropriate building layout in order to facilitate communication, exercise, and pleasure and to reduce disorientation | A Cochrane review by Forbes et al. (2004) on the use of bright light therapy in terms of mood, sleep, and behaviour reviewed three trials. However, the quality of the studies was poor. As such, the reviewers concluded there was insufficient evidence to view the approach as effective. A Cochrane review by Price et al. (2001) on the use of environmental and social barriers to prevent wandering failed to identify suitable trials | Judd et al. (1997), Day et al. (2000) |
| II: Formulation-led approaches<br>Behavioural management techniques: based on learning theory and utilizing the antecedents and consequences of behaviour to devise and execute interventions | A systematic review by Spira and Edelstein (2006) reported 23 studies. These tended to be of poor to moderate quality, and many were single case design | Bird et al. (2002), Moniz-Cook and Bird (2003) |
| Psychotherapies: the use of cognitive behavioural therapy, interpersonal psychotherapy and other standard psychotherapeutic formats. Used with patients in early stages of dementia | NICE (2004) guidelines for depression recommend both CBT and IPT in the treatment of moderate depression. Teri et al. (1997) demonstrated the positive impact of cognitive behavioural therapy on mood and problem solving abilities in people with dementia | Teri and Gallagher-Thompson (1991), Miller and Reynolds (2002), James et al. (2003) |

note that only therapies that can be used equally for people with and without dementia are included in the table. For a comprehensive review of evidence-based psychotherapies used with older people without dementia see Mackin and Arean (2005) and Zalaquett and Stens (2006).

The first group of interventions (I) are termed 'generic', and are generally designed to promote a positive therapeutic milieu and positive well-being. It is suggested that improving people's general levels of contentment serves to improve mood, and reduces anxiety and the incidence of problematic behaviours. The second form of intervention (II) is termed 'formulation-led'. Here, typically a difficulty has already been diagnosed (depression, anxiety) or observed (agitation, shouting, wandering) and the intervention procedure is specifically targeted at the problem or its causes. These interventions routinely involve the development of a formulation to help understand the triggering and maintaining features of the problem. For example, behaviour management approaches pay particular attention to the function of the behaviour, examining in great detail the antecedents, characteristics, and consequences associated with its performance. The other formulation-based approaches often include careful observation of the behaviour, but also examine the distal features associated with the behaviour (e.g. the patient's history, personality, physical health, staff interactions, etc.). This is done in order to examine the behaviour within its widest context (Cohen-Mansfield et al., 1997).

In the following subsections interventions will be described in more detail, and further information included on their evidence base. The discussions will also include findings from non-controlled studies. As one will see, when permitting the inclusion of poorer-quality studies, more therapies become available for discussion although the evidence base supporting their use becomes correspondingly weaker. In the present context, four new forms of therapy are reviewed in addition to those outlined in Table 18vi.1.

## Use of generic psychological interventions

These forms of interventions are designed to create an atmosphere and environment aimed at promoting the well-being of residents. Many of the interventions in this category could be termed person-centred in that they are designed to (1) support the strengths of residents, (2) focus on their difficulties, and (3) foster psychological health and validate their daily experiences (see Kitwood, 1997). In this section, the generic interventions will be discussed in descending order of the strength of their evidence base. Thus initially we will discuss the more established and empirically tested therapies, and then the interventions that are often regarded as 'alternative' therapies (e.g. music therapy, aromatherapy, animal-assisted activities).

### Established generic therapies
#### Reality orientation

Reality orientation (RO) is one of the most widely used management strategies in care homes, and particularly for people with dementia. The approach attempts to orientate residents to the 'present' via the use of cues (clocks, calendars, newspapers) and/or discussion. The rationale underpinning this strategy suggests that owing to memory and orientation problems, people with dementia are often confused and this may lead to social disengagement. However, if one is able to provide cues that enable them to engage in what is happening in the 'here and now' they are able to participate in conversations in a more confident and fulfilling way.

The provision of environmental cues (e.g. signs, picture boards) also has the advantage of assisting residents with dementia to find their way around their setting. In recent years RO has become less popular as concerns have been raised about the inflexible way in which it has been practised in some services. For example, a patient who incorrectly thinks he is 25 and recently married, may get upset and even angry, if he is told repeatedly that he is actually 75 and a widower. Hence, when using this approach it is essential that one employs a sensitive, person-centred style, ensuring residents are reorientated in a validating way. In the above example, a better approach would have been to gently cue the man to the facts he is 75 and retired with a large family via the use of family photographs. Having done this, one would then be able to cue him into searching for positive and validating memories about his previous work, his children, and the joys of grandparenthood. There is debate regarding the efficacy of the approach (Verkaik et al., 2006), even in light of Spector et al.'s, (2000) favourable Cochrane review of six randomized controlled trials (RCTs). The debate centres around claims that RO can remind the participants of their deterioration (Goudie and Stokes, 1989), and it can lead to repeated confrontations with the person with dementia (Brooker, 2001). Indeed, Baines et al. (1987) found an initial lowering of mood in those attending the sessions.

### Reminiscence therapy

Reminiscence therapy (RMT) involves residents reliving past experiences, especially those that might be positive and personally significant, such as family holidays or weddings. This therapy can be used as a group therapy or with individuals. Group sessions employ activities such as art and music and often use artefacts to provide stimulation. RMT is seen as a way of increasing levels of well-being and providing pleasure and cognitive stimulation. When working with people with dementia, care staff and families are often encouraged to jointly construct historical reviews of the residents' lives (i.e. life stories). Life story work is helpful in promoting attachments between staff and residents, particularly in cases where residents have poor communication skills. There is growing evidence that RMT is an effective treatment for older people with and without dementia (see Woods et al., 2005a and Bohlmeijer et al., 2003, respectively). Indeed, the approach has many supporters (Baines et al., 1987; Gibson, 1994; Brooker and Duce, 2000) due to its flexibility and adaptability to the individual's needs (e.g. a person with severe dementia can still gain pleasure from listening to an old record).

### Cognitive stimulation therapy

Cognitive stimulation therapy (CST) has developed from RO and involves activating residents' remaining cognitive functioning through activities and presentation of information (e.g. the use of physical games, word and number games, everyday objects; see Spector et al., 2006). Recent studies show promise for this approach for people with mild to moderate dementia (Knapp et al., 2006), and also demonstrate its cost-effectiveness due to the fact that it can often be performed in a group setting. In the Spector study, the members of the group attended 7 weeks of twice weekly sessions each lasting 45 minutes. The sessions focused on diverse themes such as food, childhood, memory, etc. In comparison to a control group, those attending CST showed improvements in cognition and quality of life. Livingston et al.'s (2005) recent systematic review of six studies of various quality (e.g. Romero and Wenz, 2001; Spector et al., 2003), concluded that this approach consistently showed promise across a range of situations.

### Validation therapy

Validation therapy (VT) was developed as an 'antidote' to the perceived lack of efficacy of the RO approach with people with dementia. It was suggested by its originator, Naomi Feil, that some of the features associated with dementia such as repetition and retreating into the past were in fact active strategies to avoid stress, boredom, and loneliness and adopted by those with moderate or advanced dementia. She argued that the person with dementia can retreat into an inner reality based on feelings rather than intellect as they find their present reality too painful. VT therapists thus attempt to communicate with the person with dementia through empathizing with the feelings and hidden meanings behind their confused speech and behaviour. It is the emotional content of what is being said that is therefore more important than the person's orientation to the present. Hitch (1994) notes that VT promotes contentment, results in less negative affect and behavioural disturbance, produces positive effects, and provides the individual with insight into external reality. It is, however, suggested that therapists can become too focused on confused communication and fail to identify simple explanations such as pain or hunger. Neal and Barton Wright's (2003) Cochrane review evaluated VT's effectiveness across a number of controlled trails, employing cognitive and behavioural measures (Finnema *et al.*, 2000). They concluded that despite some positive indicators in terms of depression (Toseland *et al.*, 1997), the jury was still out with respect to its efficacy.

### Environmental modification

Modifying environments to meet the needs of residents can be effective in improving well-being and reducing unwanted behaviours for people with mild or severe dementia (Bowie and Mountain, 1997). By developing a psychosocial understanding of behaviour and its meaning for the person, the environment can be changed to meet his/her needs. The use of colour and structure in an environment can help with orientation (Gibson *et al.*, 2004). Designing an environment with a more home-like atmosphere with good lighting and some environmental stimulation can reduce unwanted and agitated behaviours (Day *et al.*, 2000). Access to safe gardens and outdoor spaces is also beneficial, and opens up the possibility of developing horticultural type therapies with residents. A comprehensive evidence base has yet to be established in this area, although a number of controlled studies (Livingston *et al.*, 2005) and a larger number of non-controlled studies have shown environment and design to be important (Judd *et al.*, 1997).

### Psychomotor therapy

Psychomotor therapy, sometimes referred to as activity therapy, is a rather varied group of action-based activities, such as dance, sport, drama, etc. It has been shown that physical exercise can have a number of health benefits for older people in care settings, such as reduction in falls, improvements in mental health and sleep (King *et al.*, 1997; Winstead-Fry and Kijek, 1999), and also an increase in older people's mood and confidence (Young and Dinan, 1994; Singh *et al.*, 2005). In addition, Alessi *et al.* (1999) found in a small-scale controlled study that daytime exercise helped to reduce daytime agitation and night-time restlessness. A study of a drama and movement group showed positive outcomes in terms of increased communication (Hokkanen *et al.*, 2003) and an earlier study showed moderate benefits in terms of relaxation and orientation (Wilkinson *et al.*, 1998). The therapeutic use of touch occurring

with activity programmes has also been found to reduce disruptive vocalizations (Woods *et al.*, 2004). Despite these findings, two of the three better quality controlled trials conducted in the area failed to find significant differences in terms of depression and apathy when compared with treatment as usual (Hopman-Rock *et al.*, 1999) and low 'activity' sessions (Dröes, 1991). However, the third study (Montgomery and Dennis, 2002b) showed a positive impact of exercise on a range of sleep variables.

### Multisensory therapy

Multisensory approaches usually involve using an activity room which has been designed to provide several types of sensory stimulation, such as light (often in the form of fibre optics which can move and be flexible), texture (cushions and vibrating pads), smell, and sound. The use of these resources is tailored to the individual person and therefore all of the forms of stimulation are not necessarily used in one session. Some of the reported benefits for those with more advanced dementia include a reduction in aggressive behaviours, apathy, and depression and an increase in interaction and signs of well-being (van Weert *et al.*, 2005a,b). However, individuals differ in their response to this treatment, with some studies failing to find an effect and some obtaining a negative one. The latter findings highlight the need for individualized assessments and planning (Hope, 1998). It is also possible to bring sensory experiences into the daily lives of people with dementia through the use of interesting and stimulating decoration, colour schemes, and textures in the environment and the selection of personal care items, such as toiletries, which are scented (Wenbourn, 2003). Chung and Lai's (2002) Cochrane review of this therapy stated that overall the findings were, as yet, inconclusive. However, more recently, Verkaik *et al.*'s, (2006) review has suggested that multisensory approaches are particularly effective in the treatment of apathy and depression both in care and in the community.

## Alternative generic therapies

The next group of interventions are frequently viewed as alternative therapies. As in other areas of health care, alternative therapies are gaining currency, but to date there is limited evidence relating to their efficacy (Marshall and Hutchinson, 2001). This issue is gradually being addressed and a review of the most popular forms of alternative therapies is provided below.

### Aromatherapy

Aromatherapy is one of the fastest developing forms of complementary therapies (Burns *et al.*, 2002). It appears to have several advantages over the widely used pharmacological treatments employed in care settings. It has a positive image and its use aids interaction while providing a sensory experience. It is well-tolerated in comparison to neuroleptic or other sedative medication. The essential oils used also have the advantage that there are several routes of administration such as inhalation, bathing or massage, or topical application in a cream. The two main essential oils used in aromatherapy for dementia are extracted from lavender and lemon balm. There have been positive results from recent controlled trials which have shown significant improvements in agitation symptoms with excellent compliance and tolerability (Ballard *et al.*, 2002; Holmes *et al.*, 2002). It is relevant to note, however, that Thorgrimsen *et al.*'s (2003) review stated that there were flaws in both of these controlled studies, and thus the findings must be treated with caution.

### Music therapy

Several studies have reported benefits gained by people with dementia from music therapy (Killick and Allan, 1999; Wood, 2007) and a review of the literature (Sherratt *et al.*, 2004) suggests that music provides a medium for meaningful activity. The therapy may involve the person engaging in a musical activity, or merely listening to songs or compositions. For example, Lord and Garner (1993) showed increased levels of well-being, better social skills, and improvements in autobiographical memory in a group of residents interacting with music. Such improvements were not observed in a comparison group engaged in other activities. There have also been reported improvements in depressive symptoms through participation in reminiscence-focused music groups (Ashida, 2002), and improvements in communication and irritability when engaged in structured playing of music (Suzuki *et al.*, 2004). In addition, the use of background music and singing has been shown to increase communication between people with dementia and their carers (Gotell *et al.*, 2002). The poor quality of studies has been noted in Cochrane review (Vink *et al.*, 2003) and limits the supporting evidence for this type of intervention. Nevertheless, it can still be considered useful in some individual cases for reducing unwanted behaviour and improving communication.

### Art therapy

Art is used in many care settings, with therapists employing both observational and interactive methodologies (drama, model making, and drawing and painting). In terms of the latter, drawing and painting can provide residents with the opportunity for self-expression, a means of non-verbal communication, opportunities for deriving a sense of achievement and occupation, and the chance to exercise some choice in terms of colours or themes. Art therapy can be tailored to an individual's level of ability and avoids a confrontation of cognitive losses. It is also a medium in which people may have the opportunity to explore new skills (Mottram, 2003) and thereby enhance their self-esteem. In the case of people with dementia, art therapy has been shown to provide meaningful stimulation and improve social interaction and levels of self-esteem (Killick and Allan 1999). One of the few quality studies in the area was a controlled study investigating the effects of drama and movement on depression in groups of day-hospital attendees (Wilkinson *et al.*, 1998). Despite some favourable indicators, no significant findings were observed in terms of depression compared with those receiving treatment as usual.

### Animal-assisted activities

Animals introduced into nursing homes as regular visitors or as home-pets have been shown to have positive effects, including reducing blood pressure, strain, tension, and loneliness and increasing life expectancy (Farkas, 1997). Short-term interactions with dogs have been shown to increase social interaction with, and between, older people with mental impairment (Brunmeier *et al.*, 1986; Greer *et al.*, 2001). The presence of a dog can decrease social isolation and agitation in people with Alzheimer's disease in the daytime (McCabe *et al.*, 2002) and during 'sundowning hours' (Churchill *et al.*, 1999). It can also lead to greater alertness, increased non-verbal communication (smiling), and physical contact (Batson *et al.*, 1998). In the longer term, use of a companion animal by people with Alzheimer's disease can lead to less verbal aggression and anxiety (Fritz *et al.*, 1996). Studies of the presence of other types of animal have also demonstrated benefits. For example, the presence of a fish tank in a dining area has been shown to reduce physically aggressive behaviours and enhance the nutritional intake of home residents with dementia (Edwards and Beck, 2004). The welfare of the animal must be a key consideration, with thought being given to practical and hygiene issues and the animal's own emotional reactions to potentially stressful situations. However, these concerns can be addressed with careful planning and adherence to well-developed guidelines of which there are examples from the UK and USA (Delta Society, 1996; Dono and Ormerod, 2005).

### Using dolls and toys

The use of dolls and toys in care settings is not new (Libin and Cohen-Mansfield, 2004), but has only recently been studied in a systematic manner (James *et al.*, 2005; Mackenzie *et al.*, 2006a,b). Investigations have involved the introduction of dolls and teddy bears into care homes following a standard format (Mackenzie *et al.*, 2006b). Typically, staff are given information and guidelines on their use prior to their introduction (Mackenzie *et al.*, 2007). The findings from these investigations have been favourable for both residents and staff (James *et al.*, 2006b; Mackenzie *et al.*, 2006a,b,c). For example, following the introduction of dolls into two homes for the elderly mentally ill, the researchers found that 69% of care staff reported improvement in residents' well-being. Specifically, they noted improvements in residents' interaction with staff; interaction with other residents; level of activity; happiness/contentment; amenability to care interventions and agitation. As with many interventions, careful planning is needed to address practical aspects and problems that may arise with this approach (i.e. dolls being mislaid, disputes over ownership, etc.). However, if such aspects are attended to, therapeutic benefits are attainable.

## Use of formulation-led interventions

In this section we describe interventions that are targeted at specific presentations involving the development of formulations of the triggers and maintaining features in relation to individual residents' difficulties. First we will investigate some standard psychotherapeutic approaches (cognitive behaviour therapy (CBT), interpersonal therapy (IPT)) whose use is limited to those with mild impairment. We will then go on to discuss therapies that can be used with all presentations, even with cases of severe dementia (behaviour therapy (BT) and needs-led frameworks). It is relevant to note that the function of the formulation differs with respect to these two broad types of therapy. CBT and IPT formulations are designed to help 'patients' gain a better understanding of their problems. In contrast, BT and the needs-led frameworks employ formulations often as vehicles to enable staff to gain a better understanding of residents' difficulties. This is particularly important, because in cases of severe dementia it is the staff who are required to carry out the interventions. For this reason, we call BT and needs-led therapies 'staff-centred, person-focused' approaches.

## Standard psychotherapies

Over the last 10 years there has been an increasing interest in applying CBT and IPT to people with cognitive impairment. Teri and Gallagher-Thompson (1991) reported positive findings from a clinical trial of CBT with people in the early stages of Alzheimer's disease. Teri *et al.* (1997) also conducted a quality RCT teaching community patients with dementia to engage in pleasurable events and to problem solve. Both conditions significantly improved mood in comparison to a control group. Single case and group CBT has also been used by other researchers with some favourable results (Koder, 1998; Kipling *et al.*, 1999). Interpersonal therapy, as the name suggests, examines the person's distress within an interpersonal context. In this sense, there is a great deal of overlap with the person-centred work of Kitwood (1997) and Stokes (2000). It uses a specific framework whereby a patient's distress is conceptualized through one of four domains—interpersonal disputes, interpersonal/ personality difficulties, bereavement, transitions/life events. There is good empirical evidence for this form of treatment with older people (Miller and Reynolds, 2002); it has only recently been applied in the area of dementia (James *et al.*, 2003).

### Staff-centred, person-focused approaches

Even though these approaches can be employed with a range of presentations, they have been specifically designed to be used in situations where patients have poor communication skills and/or poor insight. For this reason they are to be suitable for working with people with severe dementia.

#### Behaviour therapy (BT)

Traditionally, BT has been based on principles of conditioning and learning theory, using strategies aimed at suppressing or eliminating problematic behaviours. More recently, positive programming methodologies (La Vigna and Donnellan, 1986) have employed non-aversive methods in helping to develop more functional behaviours. Moniz-Cook *et al.* (1998) suggest that behaviour analysis is often the starting point of most other forms of therapeutic intervention in this area. Behaviour therapy requires a detailed assessment period in which the triggers, behaviours, and reinforcers (i.e. the antecedents, behaviour, and consequences (ABC)) are identified and their relationships made clear. The therapist will often use some kind of chart or diary to gather information about the manifestations of a behaviour and the sequence of actions leading up to it. Interventions are then based on the analysis of these results. Emerson (1998) suggests focusing on three key features when designing an intervention: taking account of a person's preferences; changing the context in which the behaviour takes place; and using reinforcement strategies and schedules that reduce the behaviour.

The efficacy of BT has been demonstrated in the context of dementia in a number of studies (Burgio and Fisher, 2000). For example, there is evidence of successful reductions in wandering, incontinence and other forms of stereotypic behaviours (Bakke, 1997). While Meares and Draper (1999), Bird *et al.* (1995), and Rapp *et al.* (1992) present case studies testifying to the efficacy of BT, they all note that the behaviours had diverse causes and maintaining factors, and propose that behavioural interventions must be tailored to individual cases. Spira and Edelstein (2006) have undertaken a systematic review of the use of BT with people with dementia and reported optimistic findings. However, they noted that few of the 23 articles meeting their inclusion criteria could be regarded as 'quality' studies.

#### Needs-led therapies

Currently there are a number of conceptual models that examine challenging behaviours (CB) in terms of people's needs (James, 1999; Cohen-Mansfield, 2000; James *et al.*, 2006a; NICE, 2006). These frameworks typically involve obtaining two types of information: (1) background features (history, pre-morbid personality and coping style, cognitive status, mental health status, physical health status, environmental and contextual status) and (2) a comprehensive description of the CB episode—these are the verbal and non-verbal signs displayed by the person during the challenging episode. By putting these two types of information together, one is in a stronger position to accurately identify the person's needs (see Fig. 18vi.1).

The needs-based models highlight the fact that CBs are usually not unpredictable random actions, rather they are rational activities with a high degree of predictability. Indeed, CBs are frequently manifestations of residents' attempts to cope in situations they are misperceiving or are confused by. For example, consider the case of Mrs W. She was referred, by her GP, because of '… repeated episodes of physical aggression towards staff with no apparent triggers'. However, on examining the behaviour more closely, undertaking a functional analysis, and gathering background information, a clear pattern emerged (see Fig. 18vi.1).

The figure outlines how background information can be utilized to identify underlying causes and the needs of a person with CB, thus informing the intervention. Therefore, it is suggested that if one can understand enough about the circumstances in which the behaviours are occurring, the therapist is in a better position to work with the staff to prevent it happening in the future. In order to be confident that one has identified the needs of the person with dementia, the therapist must collect information from a wide range of sources. Key informants are family and staff, as they are able to provide information about background issues and the specifics of the CB episodes. It takes skill on the part of the therapist to gather this information in a sensitive and helpful manner from carers (Ballard *et al.*, 2001; Knocker, 2002). In addition to collecting information, it is vital that the staff play an active role in the formulation process. This will give them a sense of ownership of the formulation, and they are more likely to take an active role in the intervention phase. The following guidelines were used in Fossey *et al.*'s (2006) care home study:

- Enlist the staff's help in collecting the information. Support them in doing this, because developing a formulation is usually a new approach for most of them. Clear guidance from the therapist ensures that the staff are generating and identifying utilizable information from the appropriate sources.

- Once sufficient data have been collected, it is recommended that the therapist organizes a brain-storming session in order to formulate the resident's CB. It is helpful to clarify the goals of the session, which are usually: (1) to generate hypotheses regarding the needs of the person with dementia; (2) to explain how the resident's behaviours might relate to his/her needs (e.g. when the identified need is believed to be loneliness, one is then required to explain why he/she is communicating this via aggression); (3) to identify what pieces of information are still required in order to have a better understanding of the situation (e.g. GP notes, medical files); (4) to produce a set of practical interventions that enable the resident to meet his/her needs in a less problematic manner.

- The style of the above session should be friendly, open and interactive. Indeed, the therapist should encourage staff participation, particularly the views of the care assistants who do the majority of the hands-on care.

Despite needs-led strategies currently being one of the most popular approaches (Cohen-Mansfield, 2000), there are few studies

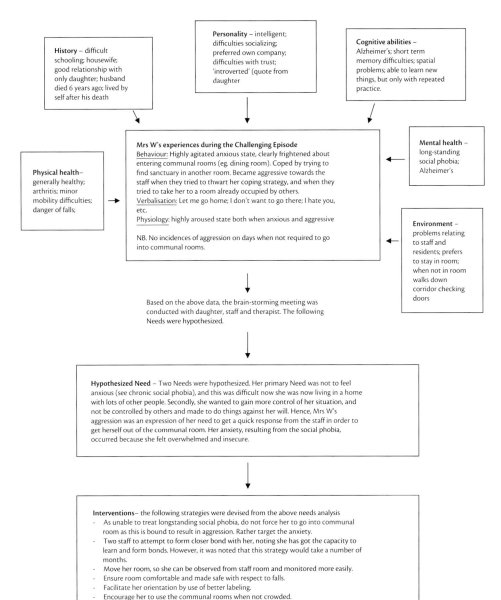

**History** – difficult schooling; housewife; good relationship with only daughter; husband died 6 years ago; lived by self after his death

**Personality** – intelligent; difficulties socializing; preferred own company; difficulties with trust; 'introverted' (quote from daughter

**Cognitive abilities** – Alzheimer's; short term memory difficulties; spatial problems; able to learn new things, but only with repeated practice.

**Mental health** – long-standing social phobia; Alzheimer's

**Physical health** – generally healthy; arthritis; minor mobility difficulties; danger of falls;

**Mrs W's experiences during the Challenging Episode**
Behaviour: Highly agitated anxious state, clearly frightened about entering communal rooms (eg. dining room). Coped by trying to find sanctuary in another room. Became aggressive towards the staff when they tried to thwart her coping strategy, and when they tried to take her to a room already occupied by others.
Verbalisation: Let me go home; I don't want to go there; I hate you, etc.
Physiology: highly aroused state both when anxious and aggressive

NB. No incidences of aggression on days when not required to go into communal rooms.

**Environment** – problems relating to staff and residents; prefers to stay in room; when not in room walks down corridor checking doors

Based on the above data, the brain-storming meeting was conducted with daughter, staff and therapist. The following Needs were hypothesized.

**Hypothesized Need** – Two Needs were hypothesized. Her primary Need was not to feel anxious (see chronic social phobia), and this was difficult now she was now living in a home with lots of other people. Secondly, she wanted to gain more control of her situation, and not be controlled by others and made to do things against her will. Hence, Mrs W's aggression was an expression of her need to get a quick response from the staff in order to get herself out of the communal room. Her anxiety, resulting from the social phobia, occurred because she felt overwhelmed and insecure.

**Interventions** – the following strategies were devised from the above needs analysis
- As unable to treat longstanding social phobia, do not force her to go into communal room as this is bound to result in aggression. Rather target the anxiety.
- Two staff to attempt to form closer bond with her, noting she has got the capacity to learn and form bonds. However, it was noted that this strategy would take a number of months.
- Move her room, so she can be observed from staff room and monitored more easily.
- Ensure room comfortable and made safe with respect to falls.
- Facilitate her orientation by use of better labeling.
- Encourage her to use the communal rooms when not crowded.

**Fig. 18vi.1** Factors used to formulate Mrs W's challenging behaviour.

demonstrating their efficacy. Even the studies that have employed it with good results did this as part of a package of treatments (Fossey *et al.*, 2006) and thus one must be cautious in attributing the success to any single feature. However, a recent clinical audit from a team using the formulation-based approach has demonstrated encouraging results in a case series format ($n = 40$) (Wood-Mitchell *et al.*, 2007).

## Staff training

As demonstrated above, staff are a vital piece of the jig-saw in delivering good care in homes. de Vugt *et al.* (2004), using a longitudinal design, showed that caregiving management strategies were associated with incidences and types of behavioural problems. For example, impatience, irritation, or anger of the caregiver with residents was more likely to result in greater resident agitation.

In a number of European countries, such as Norway and the Netherlands, most staff require qualifications prior to obtaining jobs in care homes. This is not the situation in the UK or the USA, and the majority of people working in our homes have not received any recognized form of training. This is evident in the lack of knowledge and skill of many of the staff, and is also reflected in the status and pay afforded to them. The profile of staff training requirements has been raised recently owing to the emphasis on non-pharmacological interventions (Department of Health, 2005), and also because there is evidence that a number of CBs result from poor practice. For example, night-time agitation/sleep disturbance is commonly caused by staff waking residents; aggression is associated with poor interactions between staff and residents during personal care activities (Moniz-Cook and Bird, 2003).

The methods of staff education have been varied and have involved broad-ranging teaching programmes (Beck *et al.*, 1999), specific skills training (Burgio *et al.*, 2002), and the use of reflective practice tools such as dementia care mapping (DCM). The latter is an observational framework to assess the activity and level of well-being from a resident's standpoint, and provide information about caregiver interactions—from which action plans for care improvement can be developed (Bradford Dementia Group,1997). The DCM tool also acts as an audit of person-centred practice and has been used with positive results in some studies and had a more equivocal impact in others. The fact that it can be both an intervention and outcome evaluation can make its true worth difficult to assess, but it has good face validity and is generally well received by practitioners (Brooker, 2005).

In general, evidence shows that staff can be trained to deliver better care (Smyer *et al.*, 1992; Rovner *et al.*, 1996; Moniz-Cook *et al.*, 1998; Opie *et al.*, 2002; Schrijnemaekers *et al.*, 2002), but the effects do not tend to generalize across care activities and they tend to fade with time. Owing to concerns about the limited long-term impact of training, it appears that employing training interventions alone may not the best use of clinical time unless the training is supported by continued supervision and organizational development.

Of late, a number of studies have attempted to improve the status of care by intervening at the organizational level. For example, relatives have been encouraged to work alongside staff and get involved in care planning, delivery, and review. The results have been mixed, with family members having difficulties in sustaining their involvement (Gaugler *et al.*, 2004; Train *et al.*, 2005). On balance the organizational studies show limited evidence of sustained improvement in culture, attitudes, or the quality of care (Aylward *et al.*, 2003).

## Summary

Having reviewed many of the treatments currently available, it is worth noting the commonalities between the various interventions. Indeed, in many of the studies the treatments employed similar mechanisms of change, often promoting activities, cognitive stimulation, and person-centred approaches. From our perspective, and an examination of the modus operandi of many of the treatments presented, good communication skills and an ability to interact positively are key to those studies that have demonstrated positive effects. This is because many residents in care homes find it an isolating experience, due to a combination of the losses experienced (social networks, familiar environment and routines) and cognitive (memory and orientation) problems resulting from dementia. Therefore, when a therapist or staff member engages with residents using activities, photographs, music, an animal, doll, massage, etc., their level of interpersonal contact rises considerably. For many residents this will result in an increase in mood and well-being. It is also our view that the formats provided within the various approaches provide staff with specific structures that aid the ability of the staff to communicate. This feature was particularly evident in the studies using dolls (James *et al.*, 2005), in which staff reported that the dolls gave them a focus of conversation. It is relevant to note that in the above study many staff admitted that they often found speaking to people with dementia difficult.

The present review has also shown that there is a general move towards more person-centred and staff-centred foci of care. Through the use of such perspectives, greater attempts are now made to understand the individual's experience of his/her problem within an intrapsychic, interpersonal, and environmental context (Bond and Corner, 2001). It is this perspective which leads to a further shared feature with respect to the interventions: that is the systemic perspective. Onishi *et al.* (2006), in a large survey of three different types of Japanese care facilities, found that the incidences and forms of problematic behaviours differed across settings. The carers' abilities to cope with the behaviours also varied. From their findings, the researchers suggested that such systemic knowledge of the resilience of such settings was crucial in determining the appropriateness of placements and transfers. Therefore, it is clearly important to recognize how the context of the relationships of a person with dementia with their family and caregivers affects both the individual and their caregivers. Such a view emphasizes the need to work with all of the systems involved in the resident's care (families, professional carers, organizations, etc.). Indeed, care staff and families are integral to the treatment strategies and are essential in obtaining valid and reliable information and constructing appropriate formulations and interventions. It is evident therefore that carer/staff training is an integral part of most treatment programmes. Despite the relevance of this issue, there remain relatively few 'quality' studies in the area (eg. Moniz-Cook *et al.*, 1998; Proctor *et al.*, 1999; Marriot *et al.*, 2000; see also Cohen-Mansfield *et al.*, 1997). Clearly the area of training and support is important and worthy of further work, and such studies need to be large and sufficiently powered, with robust designs that include follow-up methods. The latter issue is given particular emphasis in the NICE guidelines on dementia (NICE, 2006), with specific mention of the need to develop and deliver person-centred educational programmes. Finally, it is evident from this review that the evidence base underpinning non-pharmacological interventions is growing, but to date remains somewhat equivocal with respect to most of the approaches being used in our care homes.

## References

Alessi, C.A., Yoon, E.J., Schnelle, J.F., al-Samarrai, N.R. and Cruise, P.A. (1999). A randomized trial of a combined physical activity and environmental intervention in nursing home residents: do sleep and agitation improve? *Journal of the American Geriatric Society*, **47**(7), 784–791.

Ashida, S. (2002). The effect of reminiscence music therapy sessions on changes in depressive symptoms in elderly persons with dementia. *Journal of Music Therapy*, **37**, 170–182.

Aylward, S., Stolee, P., Keat, N., and Johncox, V. (2003). Effectiveness of continuing education in long term care: a literature review. *Gerontologist*, **43**, 259–271.

Baillon, S., van Diepen, E., and Prettyman, R (2002). Multi-sensory therapy in psychiatric care. *Advances in Psychiatric Treatment*, **8**, 444–452.

Baines, S., Saxby, P. and Ehlert, K. (1987). Reality orientation and reminiscence therapy: a controlled crossover study of elderly confused people. *British Journal of Psychiatry*, **151**, 222–231.

Bajekal, M. (2002). *Health Survey for England 2000: care homes and their residents*. The Stationary Office, London.

Baker, R., Holloway, J., and Holkamp, C. (2003). Effects of multi-sensory stimulation for people with dementia. *Journal of Advanced Nursing*, **43**(5), 465–477.

Bakke, B. (1997). Applied behaviour analysis for behavioural problems in Alzheimer's disease. *Geriatrics*, **52**(Suppl. 12), 40–43.

Ballard, C. and Cream, J. (2005). Drugs used to relieve behavioural symptoms in people with dementia or an unacceptable chemical cosh? *International Psychogeriatrics*, **17**(1), 4–12.

Ballard, C. and Howard, R. (2006). Neuroleptic drugs in dementia: benefits and harm. *Nature Reviews Neuroscience*, **7**, 492–500.

Ballard, C.G., O'Brien, J., James, I. and Swann, A. (2001) *Dementia: management of behavioural and psychological symptoms*. Oxford University Press, Oxford.

Ballard, C.G., O'Brien, J.T., Reichelt, K., and Perry, E.K. (2002). Aromatherapy as a safe and effective treatment for the management of agitation in severe dementia: the results of a double-blind, placebo-controlled trial with Melissa. *Journal of Clinical Psychiatry*, **63**, 553–558.

Batson, K., McCabe, B.W., Baun, M.M., and Wilson, C.A. (1998). The effects of a therapy dog on socialisation and physiological indicators of stress in persons diagnosed with Alzheimer's disease. In *Companion animals in human health* (ed. C.C. Wilson and D.C. Turner). Sage, Thousand Oaks, CA.

Beck, C., Ortigara, A., Mercer, S., and Shue, V. (1999). Enabling and empowering certified nursing assistants for quality dementia care. *International Journal of Geriatric Psychiatry*, **14**, 197–212.

Bird, M., Alexopoulos, P., and Adamowicz, J. (1995). Success and failure in five case studies: use of cued recall to ameliorate behaviour problems in senile dementia. *International Journal of Geriatric Psychiatry*, **10**, 305–311.

Bird, M., Llewellyn-Jones, R., Smithers, H., and Korten, A. (2002). *Psychosocial approaches to challenging behaviour in dementia: a controlled trial*, Report to the Commonwealth Department of Health and Ageing. CDHA, Canberra.

Bohlmeijer, E., Smit, F., and Cuipers, P. (2003). Effects of reminiscence and life review on late-life depression: a meta-analysis. *International Journal of Geriatric Psychiatry*, **18**, 1088–1094.

Bond, J. (2001). Sociological perspectives. In *A handbook of dementia care* (ed. C. Cantley), pp. 44–61. Open University Press, Buckingham.

Bond, J. and Corner, L. (2001). Researching dementia: are there unique methodological challenges for health services research? *Ageing and Society*, **21**, 95–116.

Bowie, P. and Mountain, G. (1997). The relationship between patient behaviour and environmental quality for the dementing. *International Journal of Geriatric Psychiatry*, **12**, 718–723.

Bradford Dementia Group (1997). *Evaluating dementia care: the DCM method*, 7th edn. Bradford University, Bradford.

Brooker, D. (2001). Enriching lives: evaluation of the Extracare activity challenge. *Journal of Dementia Care*, **9**(3), 33–37.

Brooker, D. (2005). Dementia care mapping: a review of the research literature. *The Gerontologist*, **45**(Suppl. 1), 11–18.

Brooker, D. and Duce, L. (2000). Wellbeing and activity in dementia: a comparison of group reminiscence therapy, structured goal-directed group activity and unstructured time. *Aging and Mental Health*, **4**(4), 354–358.

Brunmeier, C., McArthur, M., Baun, M., and Bergstrom, N. (1986). *The effects of a dog on the social interaction of mentally impaired institutionalised elderly*. University of Nebraska Medical Centre College of Nursing, Omaha.

Burgio, L. and Fisher, S. (2000). Application of psychosocial interventions for treating behavioural and psychological symptoms of dementia. *International Psychogeriatrics*, **12**, 351–358.

Burgio, L.D., Stevens, A., Burgio, K.L., Roth, D.L., Paul, P., and Gerstle, J. (2002). Teaching and maintaining behaviour management skills in the nursing home. *The Gerontologist*, **42**, 487–496.

Burns, A., Byrne, J., Ballard, C., and Holmes, C. (2002). Sensory stimulation in dementia: an effective option for managing behavioural problems. *British Medical Journal*, **325**, 1312–1313.

Burns, I. Cox, H., and Plant, H. (2000). Leisure or therapeutics? Snoezelen and the care of older persons with dementia. *International Journal of Nursing Practice*, **6**, 118–126.

Cameron, M.H. and Clare, L. (2004). Cognition-based interventions for people with mild cognitive impairment. *Cochrane Database of Systematic Reviews*, 2004 Issue 2, art no. CD004745. John Wiley and Sons, Ltd Chichester, UK. DOI: 10.1002/14651858.CD004745.pub2.

Churchill, M., Safaoui, J., McCabe, B., and Baun, M. (1999). Using a therapy dog to alleviate the agitation and desocialisation of people with Alzheimer's disease. *Journal of Psychosocial Nursing and Mental Health Services*, **37**, 16–22.

Chung, J.C.C. and Lai, C.K.Y. (2002). Snoezelen for dementia. *Cochrane Database of Systematic Reviews*, 2002, Issue 4, art. no. CD003152. DOI: 10.1002/14651858.CD003152.

Clare, L., Woods, R.T., Moniz-Cook, E.D., Orrell, M., and Spector, A. (2003). Cognitive rehabilitation and cognitive training for early-stage Alzheimer's disease and vascular dementia. *Cochrane Database of Systematic Reviews*, 2003, Issue 4, art. no. CD003260. DOI: 10.1002/14651858.CD003260.

Cohen-Mansfield, J. (2000). Use of patient characteristics to determine non-pharmacological interventions for behavioural and psychological symptoms of dementia. *International Psychogeriatrics*, **12**(1), 373–380.

Cohen-Mansfield, J., Werner, P., Culpepper, W.J. and Barkley, D. (1997). Evaluation of an in-service training programme on dementia and wandering. *Journal of Gerontological Nursing*, **23**, 40–47.

Day, K., Carreon, D. and Stump, C. (2000). Therapeutic design of environments for people with dementia: a review of the empirical research. *The Gerontologist*, **40**, 397–416.

Delta Society (1996). *Human–animal health connections in animal assisted therapy: standards of practice*. Delta Society, Bellevue, WA.

de Vugt, M., Stevents, F., Aalten, P. *et al.* (2004). Do caregiver management strategies influence patient behaviour in dementia. *International Journal of Geriatric Psychiatry*, **19**(1), 85–92.

Department of Health (2005). Written Ministerial Statement on the expansion of independent nurse prescribing and introduction of pharmacists independent prescribing. DoH, London (www.dh.gov.uk/en/Publicationsandstatistics).

Dono, J.-A. and Ormerod, E. (2005). Older people and pets: a comprehensive guide. SCAS, Oxford.

Dröes, R.M. (1991). Effecten van psychosociale behandelingsvormen bij SDAT-patiente. [The effects of psychosocial treatment methods in SDAT patients]. In *Beweging. Over psychosociale hulpverlening aan demente ouderen [Psychosocial care for demented elderly]*. Utrecht: De Tijdstroom.

Edwards, N. and Beck, A.M. (2004). Using aquariums in managing Alzheimer's disease: influence on resident nutrition and behaviours and improving staff morale. *10th International Conference on Human–Animal Interactions, People and Animals: A Timeless Relationship*, Glasgow, Scotland, 6–9 October 2004. International Association of Human-Animal Interaction Organizations, Glasgow.

Emerson, E. (1998). Working with people with challenging behaviour. In *Clinical psychology and people with intellectual disabilities* (ed. E. Emerson, C. Hatton, J. Bromley, and A. Caine), pp. 127–153. John Wiley and Sons, Chichester.

Farkas, M. (1997). A cold nose can warm the heart. *Michigan Health & Hospitals*, **33**, 38.

Finnema, E. (2000). *Emotion-oriented care in dementia. a psychosocial approach*. Regenboog, Groningen.

Finnema, E., Dröes, R.M., Kooij, C.H., *et al.* (1998). The design of a large-scale experimental study into the effect of emotion oriented care on demented elderly and professional carers in nursing homes. *Archives of Gerontological Geriatrics*, Suppl. 6, 193–200.

Finnema, E., Droes, R.M., Ribbe, M., and Van Tilburg, W. (2000). The effects of emotion-oriented approaches in the care for persons suffering from dementia: a review of the literature. *International Journal Geriatric Psychiatry*, **15**(2), 141–61.

Forbes, D., Morgan, D.G., Bangma, J., Peacock, S., and Adamson, J. (2004). Light therapy for managing sleep, behaviour, and mood disturbances in dementia. *Cochrane Database of Systematic Reviews* 2004, Issue 2, art. no. CD003946. DOI: 10.1002/14651858.CD003946.pub2.

Fossey, J., Ballard, C.G., Juszczak, E. *et al.* (2006). Effect of enhanced psychosocial care on antipsychotic use in nursing home residents with severe dementia: cluster randomised trial. *British Medical Journal*, **332**, 756–758.

Fritz, C.L., Farver, T.B., Hart, L.A., and Kass, P.H. (1996). Companion animals and the psychological health of Alzheimer patients' caregivers. *Psychological Reports*, **78**(2), 467–481.

Gatz, M., Fiske, A., Fox L. *et al.* (1998). Empirically validated psychological treatments for older adults. *Journal of Mental Health and Ageing*, **4**, 9–46.

Gaugler, J.E., Anderson, K.A., Zarit, S.H., and Pearlin, L.I. (2004). Family involvement in nursing homes: effects on stress and well-being. *Aging and Mental Health*, **8**, 65–75.

Gibson, F. (1994). What can reminiscence contribute to people with dementia? In *Reminiscence reviewed: evaluations, achievements, perspectives* (ed. J. Bornat), pp. 46–60. Open University Press, Buckingham.

Gibson, M.C., MacLean, J., Borrie, M., and Geiger, J. (2004). Orientation behaviors in residents relocated to a redesigned dementia care unit. *American Journal of Alzheimer's Disease and Other Dementias*, **19**, 45–49.

Gilley, D.W., Wilson, R.S., Beckett, L.A., and Evans, D.A. (1997). Psychotic symptoms and physically aggressive behaviour in Alzheimer's disease. *Journal of the American Geriatrics Society*, **45**, 1074–1079.

Gilley, D.W., Bienias, J.L., Wilson, R.S., Bennett, D.A., Beck, T.L., and Evans, D.A. (2004). Influence of behavioral symptoms on rates of institutionalization for persons with Alzheimer's disease. *Psychological Medicine*, **34**, 1129–1135.

Goldwasser, A.N., Auerbach, S.M., and Harkins, S.W. (1987). Cognitive, affective, and behavioural effects of reminiscence group therapy on demented elderly. *International Journal of Ageing and Human Development*, **25**(3), 209–222.

Gotell, E., Brown, S., and Ekman, S. (2002). Caregiver singing and background music in dementia care. *Western Journal of Nursing Research*, **24**, 195–216.

Goudie, F. and Stokes, G. (1989). Understanding confusion. *Nursing Times*, **85**, 35–37.

Greer, K.L., Pustay, K.A., Zaun, T.C., and Coppens, P. (2001). A comparison of the effects of toys versus live animals on the communication of patients with dementia of the Alzheimer's type. *Clinical Gerontologist*, **24**, 157–182.

Hermans, D.G., Htay, U. Hla, and McShane, R. (2006). Non-pharmacological interventions for wandering of people with dementia in the domestic setting. *Cochrane Database of Systematic Reviews* 2007, Issue 1. art. no. CD005994. DOI: 10.1002/14651858.CD005994.pub2.

Hitch, S. (1994). Cognitive therapy as a tool for the caring elderly confused person. *Journal of Clinical Nursing*, **3**, 49–55.

Hokkanen, L., Rantala, L., Remes, A.-M., Harkonen, B., Viramo, P., and Winblad, I. (2003). Dance/movement therapeutic methods in management of dementia. *Journal of the American Geriatrics Society*, **51**(4), 576–7.

Holden, U. and Woods, R.T. (1982). *Reality orientation: psychological approaches to the confused elderly*. Churchill Livingstone, Edinburgh.

Holmes, C., Hopkins, V., Hensford, C., MacLaughlin, V., Wilkinson, D., and Rosenvinge, H. (2002). Lavender oil as a treatment for agitated behaviour in severe dementia: a placebo controlled study. *International Journal of Geriatric Psychiatry*, **17**(4), 305–308.

Hope, K. (1998). The effects of multi sensory environments with older people with dementia. *Journal of Psychiatric and Mental Health Nursing*, **5**, 377–385.

Hopman-Rock, M., Staats, P.G., Takm, E.C.P.M., and Dröes, R.M. (1999). The effects of psychomotor activation program for use in groups of cognitively impaired people in homes for the elderly. *International Journal Geriatric Psychiatry*, **14**, 633–642.

Howard, R., Ballard, C., O'Brien, J., and Burns, A. (2001). Guidelines for the management of agitation in dementia. *International Journal Geriatric Psychiatry*, **16**, 714–717.

James, I.A. (1999). Using a cognitive rationale to conceptualise anxiety in people with dementia. *Behavioural and Cognitive Psychotherapy*, **27**(4), 345–351.

James, I.A., Postma, K., and Mackenzie, L. (2003). Using an IPT conceptualisation to treat a depressed person with dementia. *Behaviour and Cognitive Psychotherapy*, **31**(3), 451–456.

James, I.A., Reichelt, F.K., Morse, R., and Mackenzie, L. (2005). The therapeutic use of dolls in dementia care. *Journal of Dementia Care*, **13**(3), 19–21.

James, I.A, Stephens, M., Mackenzie, L., and Roe. P. (2006a). Dealing with challenging behaviour through an analysis of need: the Colombo approach. In *On the move: walking not wandering* (ed. M. Marshall). Hawker Publications.

James, I.A., Mackenzie, L., and Mukaetova-Ladinska, E. (2006b). Doll use in care homes for people with dementia. *International Journal of Geriatric Psychiatry*, **21**, 1093–1098.

Judd, S., Marshall, M., and Phippen, P. (1997) *Design for dementia*. Hawker, London.

Katz, I.R. and Parmalee, P.A. (1997). Overview. In *Depression in long term and residential care* (ed. R.L. Rubenstein and M.P. Lawton). Springer, New York.

Killick, J. and Allan, K. (1999). The arts in dementia care: tapping a rich resource. *Journal of Dementia Care*, **7**, 35–38.

Kim, E. and Rovner, B.W. (1995). Epidemiology of psychiatric disturbance in nursing homes. *Psychiatric Annals*, **25**, 409–412.

King, A.C., Oman, R.F., Brassington, G.S., Bliwise, D.L., and Haskell, W.L. (1997). Moderate-intensity exercise and self-rated quality of sleep in older adults: a randomized controlled trial. *Journal of the American Medical Association*, **277**(1), 32–37.

Kipling, T., Bailey, M., and Charlesworth, G. (1999). The feasibility of a cognitive behavioural therapy group for men with a mild/moderate cognitive impairment. *Behavioural and Cognitive Psychotherapy*, **27**, 189–193.

Kitwood, T. (1997). *Dementia reconsidered: the person comes first*. Open University Press, Buckingham.

Knapp, M., Thorgrimsen, L., Patel, A. *et al.* (2006). Cognitive stimulation therapy for people with dementia: cost-effectiveness analysis. *British Journal of Psychiatry*, **188**, 574–580.

Knocker, S. (2002). Just how far have we really come? *Journal of Dementia Care*, **10**(1), 8–9.

Koder, D. (1998). Treatment of anxiety in the cognitively impaired elderly: can CBT help? *International Psychogeriatrics*, **10**(2), 173–182.

La Vigna, G. and Donnellan, A. (1986). *Alternative to punishment: solving behaviour problems with non-aversive strategies*. Irvington, New York.

Libin, A. and Cohen-Mansfield, J. (2004). Therapeutic robocat for nursing home residents with dementia: preliminary enquiry. *American Journal of Alzheimer's Disease and Other Dementias*, **19**, 111–116.

Livingston, G., Manela, M., and Katona, C. (1996). Depression and other psychiatric morbidity in carers of elderly people living at home. *British Medical Journal*, **312**, 153.

Livingston, G., Johnston, K., Katona, C., Paton, J., and Lyketsos, C. (2005). Systematic review of psychological approaches to the management of neuropsychiatric symptoms of dementia. *American Journal of Psychiatry*, **162**(11), 1996–2021.

Lord, T. and Garner, E. (1993). Effects of music on Alzheimer patients. *Perceptual and Motor Skills*, **76**, 451–455.

Lyketsos, C., Veiel, L.L., Baker, A., and Steele, C. (1999). A randomised controlled trial of bright light therapy for agitated behaviours in dementia patients residing in longterm care. *International Journal of Geriatric Psychiatry*, **14**, 520525.

Lykestos, C.G., Lopez, O., Jones, B., Fitzpatrick, A., Breitner, J., and Dekosky, S. (2002). Prevalence of neuropsychiatric symptoms in dementia and mild cognitive impairment. *Journal of the American Medical Association*, **288**, 1457–1483.

McCabe, B., Baun, M., Speich, D., and Agrawal, S. (2002). Resident dog in an Alzheimer's unit. *Western Journal of Nursing Research*, **24**, 684–696.

MacDonald, A.J.D., Carpenter, G.I., Box, O., Roberts, A., and Sahu, S. (2002). Dementia and use of psychotropic medication in non 'elderly mentally infirm' nursing homes in south east England. *Age and Ageing*, **31**, 58–64.

Mackenzie, L., Wood-Mitchell, A., and James, I.A. (2006a). Thinking about dolls. *Journal of Dementia Care*, **14**(2), 16–17.

Mackenzie, L., James, I.A., Morse, R., Mukaetova-Ladinska, E., and Reichelt, F.K. (2006b). A pilot study on the use of dolls for people with dementia. *Age and Ageing*, **35**(4), 441–444.

Mackenzie, L., Wood-Mitchell, A., and James, I.A. (2006c). *Guidelines on the use of dolls in care settings*. Centre for the Health of the Elderly, Newcastle General Hospital, Newcastle upon Tyne.

Mackenzie, L., Wood-Mitchell, A., and James, I.A. (2007). Guidelines on using dolls. *Journal of Dementia Care*, **15**(1), 26–27.

Mackin, R.S. and Arean, P.A. (2005). Evidence-based psychotherapeutic interventions for geriatric depression. *Psychiatric Clinics of North America*, **28**, 805–820.

Marriott, A., Donaldson, C., Tarrier, N., and Burns, A. (2000). Effectiveness f cognitive—behavioural family intervention in reducing the burden of care in carers of patients with Alzheimer's disease. *British Journal of Psychiatry*, **176**, 557–562.

Marshall, M. and Hutchinson, S. (2001). Responses of family caregivers and family members with Alzheimer's disease to an activity kit: an ethnographic study. *Journal of Advanced Nursing*. **35**(4), 488–496.

Meares, S. and Draper, B. (1999). Treatment of vocally disruptive behaviour of multifactorial aetiology. *International Journal of Geriatric Psychiatry*, **14**, 285–290.

Meier, D., Eemimi-Funfschilling, D., Monsch, A.U., and Stanhelin, H.B. (1996). Kognitives Kompetenztraining mit Patienten im Anfangsstadium einer Demenz [Cognitive competence training with patients in the early stages of dementia]. *Zeitschrift fur Gerntopsychologie*, **9**, 207–217.

Miller, M. and Reynolds, C.F. (2002). Interpersonal psychotherapy. In *Psychological therapies with older people* (ed. J. Hepple, J. Pearce, and P. Wilkinson). Brunner-Routledge, London.

Moniz-Cook, E.D. and Bird, M. (2003). Sensory stimulation and dementia: cause of behavioural and psychological symptoms of dementia needs to be established first. *British Medical Journal*, **326**, 661.

Moniz-Cook, E., Agar, S., Silver, M. *et al.* (1998). Can staff training reduce carer stress and behavioural disturbance in the elderly mentally ill? *International Journal of Geriatric Psychiatry*, **13**, 149–158.

Montgomery, P. and Dennis, J. (2002a). Bright light therapy for sleep problems in adults aged 60+. *Cochrane Database of Systematic Reviews*, 2002, Issue 2, art. no. CD003403. DOI: 10.1002/14651858. CD003403.

Montgomery, P. and Dennis, J. (2002b). Physical exercise for sleep problems in adults aged 60+. *Cochrane Database of Systematic Reviews*, Issue 4, art. no. CD003404. DOI: 10.1002/14651858.CD003404.

Mottram, P. (2003). Art therapy with clients who have dementia. *Dementia*, **2**, 272–277.

Neal, M. and Barton Wright, P. (2003). Validation therapy for dementia. *Cochrane Database of Systematic Reviews*, 2003, Issue 3, art. no. CD001394. DOI: 10.1002/14651858.CD001394.

NICE (2004). *Depression: management of depression in primary and secondary care*, Clinical guideline 23 (http://guidance.nice.org.uk/cg23).

NICE (2006). *Dementia: supporting people with dementia and their carers*, Clinical Guideline 42 (http://guidance.nice.org.uk/cg42).

Office of Fair Trading (2005) *Care homes for older people in the UK: a market study*. Office of Fair Trading, London.

Onishi, J., Suzuki, Y., Umegaki, H. *et al.* (2006). Behavioral, psychological and physical symptoms in group homes for older adults with dementia. *International Psychogeriatrics*, **18**(1), 76–86.

Opie, J., Doyle, C., and O'Connor, D.W. (2002). Challenging behaviours in nursing home residents with dementia: a randomised controlled trial of multidisciplinary interventions. *International Journal of Geriatric Psychiatry*, **17**, 6–13.

Pinkney, L. (1997). A comparison of the snoezelen environment with a music relaxation group with senile dementia. *British Journal of Occupational Therapy*, **60**, 209–212.

Price, J.D., Hermans, D.G., and Grimley Evans, J. (2001). Subjective barriers to prevent wandering of cognitively impaired people. *Cochrane Database of Systematic Reviews*, 2001, Issue 1, art. no. CD001932. DOI: 10.1002/14651858.CD001932.

Proctor, R., Powell, H.S., Burns, A. *et al.* (1998a). An observational study to evaluate the impact of a specialist outreach team on the quality of care in nursing and residential homes. *Ageing and Mental Health*, **2**(3), 232–238.

Proctor, R., Powell, H.S., Tarrier, N., and Burns, A. (1998b). The impact of training and support and stress among care staff in nursing and residential homes for the elderly. *Journal of Mental Health (UK)*, **7**(1), 59–70.

Proctor, R., Burns, A., Powell, H.S. *et al.* (1999). Behavioural management in nursing and residential homes: a randomised control trial. *Lancet*, **354**, 26–29.

Rapp, M.F., Flint, A.J., Herrmann, N., and Proulx, G.B. (1992). Behavioural disturbances in the demented elderly: phenomenology, pharmacotherapy and behavioural management. *Canadian Journal of Psychiatry*, **37**, 651–657.

Robert, P.H., Verhey, F.R., Byrne, E.J. *et al.* (2005). Grouping for behavioral and psychological symptoms in dementia: clinical and biological aspects. Consensus paper of the European Alzheimer disease consortium. *European Psychiatry*, **20**, 490–496.

Romero, B. and Wenz, M. (2001) Self-maintenance therapy in Alzheimer's disease. *Neuropsychological Rehabilitation*, **11**, 333–355.

Rovner, B.W., Steele, C.D., Shmuely, Y., and Folstein, N.F. (1996). A randomised trial of dementia care in nursing homes. *Journal of the American Geriatric Society*, **44**, 7–13, 91–92.

Schrijnemaekers, V., Vanrossum, E., Candel, M. *et al.* (2002). Effects of emotion oriented care on elderly people with cognitive impairment and behavioural problems. *International Journal of Geriatric Psychiatry*, **17**, 926–937.

Sherratt, K., Thornton, A., and Hatton, C. (2004) Music interventions for people with dementia: a review of the literature. *Aging and Mental Health*, **8**, 3–12.

SIGN (Scottish Intercollegiate Guidelines Network) (1998). *Interventions in the management of behavioural and psychological aspects of dementia*. SIGN, Edinburgh.

Singh, N., Stavrinos, T.M., Scarbek, Y. *et al.*(2005). A randomized controlled trial of high versus low intensity weight training versus general practitioner care for clinical depression in older adults. *Journals of Gerontology Series A: Biological Sciences and Medical Sciences*, **60**, 768–776.

Sink, K.M., Holden, F.H., and Yaffe, K. (2005). Pharmacological treatment of neuropsychiatric symptoms of dementia: a review of the evidence. *Journal of the American Medical Association*, **293**(5), 596–608.

Smyer, M., Brannon, D., and Cohn, M. (1992). Improving nursing-home care through training and job re-design. *Gerontologist*, **32**, 327–333.

Spector, A., Orrell, M., Davies, S., and Woods, B. (2000). Reality orientation for dementia. *Cochrane Database of Systematic Reviews*, 2000, Issue 3, art. no. CD001119. DOI: 10.1002/14651858.CD001119.pub2.

Spector, A., Orrell, M., Davies, S., and Woods, R.T. (2002b). Reminiscence therapy for dementia (Cochrane Review). *The Cochrane Library*, Update Software, Issue 4. Oxford.

Spector, A., Thorgrimsen, L., Woods, B. *et al.* (2003). Efficacy of an evidence-based cognitive stimulation programme for people with dementia: randomised controlled trial. *British Journal of Psychiatry*, **183**, 248–254.

Spector, A., Thorgrimsen, L., Woods, B., and Orrell, M. (2006). *Making a difference: an evidence-based group programme to offer cognitive stimulation therapy (CST) to people with dementia*. Hawker Publications, London.

Spira, A. and Edelstein, B. (2006). Behavioral interventions for agitation in older adults with dementia: an evaluative review. *International Psychogeriatrics*, **18**(2), 195–225.

Stokes, G. (2000). *Challenging behaviour in dementia: a person-centred approach*. Speechmark, Bicester.

Suzuki, M., Kanamori, M., Watanabe, M. *et al.* (2004). Behavioral and endocrinological evaluation of music therapy for elderly patients with dementia. *Nursing and Health Sciences*, **6**, 11–18.

Teri, L. and Gallagher-Thompson, D. (1991). Cognitive-behavioral interventions for treatment of depression in Alzheimer's patients. *Gerontologist*, **31**(3), 413–416.

Teri, L., Logsdon, R.G., Uomoto, J., and McCurry, S.M. (1997). Behavioural treatment of depression in dementia patients: a controlled clinical trial. *Journals of Gerontology Series B: Psychological Sciences and Social Sciences*, **52**(4), 159–166.

Thompson, C. and Spilsbury, K. (1998). Support for carers of people with Alzheimer's type dementia. *Cochrane Database of Systematic Reviews*,1998, Issue 3. art. no. CD000454. DOI: 10.1002/14651858. CD000454.

Thompson, C.A.., Spilsbury, K., and Barnes, C. (2003). Information and support interventions for carers of people with dementia. *Cochrane Database of Systematic Reviews*, Issue 2, DOI: 10.1002/14651858. CD004513.pub2.

Thorgrimsen, L., Spector, A., Wiles, A., and Orrell, M. (2003). Aroma therapy for dementia. *Cochrane Database of Systematic Reviews*, 2003, Issue 3, art. no. CD003150. DOI: 10.1002/14651858.CD003150.

Tilly, J. and Reed, P. (2004). *Evidence on interventions to improve quality of care for residents with dementia in nursing and assisted living facilities*. Alzheimer's Association, Washington, DC.

Toseland, R.W., Diehl, M., Freeman, K., Manzaneres, T., Naleppa, M., and McCallion, P. (1997). The impact of validation group therapy on nursing home residents with dementia. *Journal of Applied Gerontology*, **16**, 31–50.

Train, G., Nurock, S., Kitchen, G., Manela, M., and Livingston, G. (2005). A qualitative study of the views of residents with dementia, their relatives and staff about work practice in long term care settings. *International Psychogeriatrics*, **17**, 237–251.

van Weert, J.C., van Dulmen, A.M., Spreeuwenberg, P.M., Ribbe, M.W., and Bensing, J.M. (2005a). Behavioral and mood effects of snoezelen integrated into 24-hour dementia care. *Journal of the American Geriatrics Society*, **53**, 24–33.

van Weert, J.C., van Dulmen, A.M., Spreeuwenberg, P.M., Ribbe, M.W., and Bensing, J.M. (2005b). Effects of snoezelen, integrated in 24 h dementia care, on nurse-patient communication during morning care. *Patient Education and Counseling*, **58**, 312–326.

Verkaik, R., van Weert, J., and Francke, A. (2006). The effects of psychosocial methods on depressed, aggressive and apathetic behaviours of people with dementia: a systematic review. *International Journal of Geriatric Psychiatry*, **20**, 301–314.

Vernooij-Dassen, M. and Downs, M. (2005). Cognitive and behavioural interventions for carers of people with dementia. *Cochrane Database of Systematic Reviews*, 2005, Issue 2, art. no. CD005318. DOI: 10.1002/14651858.CD005318.

Viggo Hansen, N., Jørgensen, T., and Ørtenblad, L. (2004). Massage and touch for dementia. *Cochrane Database of Systematic Reviews*, 2006, Issue 4, art. no. CD004989. DOI: 10.1002/14651858.CD004989.pub2.

Vink, A.C., Birks, J.S., Bruinsma, M.S., and Scholten, R.J.P.M. (2003). Music therapy for people with dementia. *Cochrane Database of Systematic Reviews*, 2003, Issue 4, art. no. CD003477. DOI: 10.1002/14651858. CD003477.pub2.

Wenbourn, J. (2003). Using a sensory approach to improve well-being. *Nursing and Residential Care*, **5**, 431–432.

Wilkinson, N., Srikumar, S., Shaw, K., and Orrell, M. (1998) Drama and movement therapy in dementia: a pilot study. *Arts in Psychotherapy*, **25**(3), 195–207.

Winstead-Fry, P. and Kijek, J. (1999). An integrative review and meta-analysis of therapeutic touch research. *Alternative Therapies in Health and Medicine*, **5**, 58–67.

Wood, S. (2007). Chalfont Lodge Choir: heart of a home community. *Journal of Dementia Care*, **15**(1), 22–25.

Wood-Mitchell, A., Mackenzie, L., Stephenson, M. James, I.A. (2007) Treating challenging behaviour in care settings: audit of a community service using the Neuropsychiatric Inventory. *National PSIGE Conference Edition*, Nottingham, UK.

Woods, B., Spector, A., Jones, C., Orrell, M., and Davies., S. (2005a). Reminiscence therapy for dementia. *Cochrane Database of Systematic Reviews*, 2005, Issue 2, art. no. CD001120. DOI: 10.1002/14651858. CD001120.pub2.

Woods, B., Spector, A.E., Prendergast, L., and Orrell, M. (2005b). Cognitive stimulation to improve cognitive functioning in people with dementia (Protocol). Cochrane Database of Systematic Reviews, 2005, Issue 4, art. no. CD005562. DOI: 10.1002/14651858.CD005562.

Woods, D.L., Rapp, C.G., and Beck, C.E. (2004). Escalation/de-escalation patterns of behavioral symptoms of persons with dementia. *Aging and Mental Health*, **8**(2), 126–32.

Young, A. and Dinan, S. (1994). *ABC of sports medicine: fitness for older people. British Medical Journal*, **309**, 331–334.

Zalaquett, C. and Stens, A. (2006). Psychosocial treatments for major depression and dysthymia in older adults: a review of the research literature. *Journal of Counseling and Development*, **84**(2), 192–201.

# SECTION III

# Psychiatric services

# 19

# Principles of service provision in old age psychiatry

## Tom Dening

## Introduction

The principles and practice of mental health services for older people occupy the vital middle ground between what we know scientifically about mental disorders in old age and how this knowledge can make a difference to the lives of individual older people. Old age psychiatry is perhaps unusual among medical specialities in that it has grown up with a strong sense of how services should be organized and provided. This has derived from two influences—first, recognition of the limited resources available and, second, appreciation of epidemiological and public-health issues among some of its main founders.

The scope of this chapter is of necessity broad. Some important topics, for example memory clinics and care homes, are covered in separate chapters in this book. Much of the material quoted derives from the United Kingdom (more specifically, from England) but many of the issues are general and applicable worldwide.

## History

It is generally accepted that old age psychiatry originated in the UK. The earliest traces of the speciality are to be found in the early 1940s (Hilton, 2005a). Before the Second World War, there was virtually no interest in older people's mental or physical health issues, most conditions being assumed to be degenerative, 'senile', and not amenable to treatment. By the early 1940s, there were large numbers of older people with mental disorders in hospitals like the Royal Edinburgh Hospital and Tooting Bec, in London. Felix Post, at first working in Edinburgh and encouraged by Professor Henderson, published one of the first clinical studies of mental disorders in old age (Post, 1944). Aubrey Lewis, in London, was also highly influential, for example addressing the Annual Meeting of the Royal Medico-Psychological Association in 1945 (Lewis, 1946) and being active through the Mental Health Standing Advisory Committee of the new National Health Service (Hilton, 2005a).

Several accounts are available of further developments of old age psychiatry (e.g. Arie, 1989, Shulman and Arie, 1991). Important advances included seminal clinical studies, especially those by Felix Post (e.g. Post, 1962; and his textbook, Post, 1965) and Martin Roth (1955). These provided evidence that not all mental disorders could be ascribed to senility and opened the possibility of offering effective treatments for certain disorders, especially affective states. Services dedicated to older people began to open in a patchy fashion across Britain (e.g. Arie, 1970). The common interests of psychiatrists working in this area led first to the formation of an informal gathering, followed by an official group within the Royal College of Psychiatrists in 1973 and then a full Specialist Section in 1978. Old age psychiatry was recognized by the UK Department of Health as a separate speciality in 1989. Numbers of consultant old age psychiatrists have continued to rise, the most recent estimate for England being 508 (http://www.ic.nhs.uk/pubs/nhsstaff).

For several years, the development of old age psychiatry proceeded apart from that of geriatric medicine, despite the obvious overlap in clientele. The reasons for this were complex, not least a dismissive attitude of the physicians. More common ground was reached by a joint Royal Colleges document on the care of older people with mental illness, produced in 1989, more recently updated (Royal College of Psychiatrists/Royal College of Physicians, 1998). Another area which lagged behind the developing clinical services has been policy. Until the publication of *Services for Mental Illness Related to Old Age* (Department of Health and Social Security, 1972), there had been no conceptual progress for over 20 years (Hilton, 2005b).

Developments in other countries have been influenced to varying degrees by the UK experience. Patterns of service reflect national factors such as the nature of the healthcare system, the degree to which old age psychiatrists are generalists or dementia specialists, and of course the level of resources in the individual country. Snowdon and Arie (2005) have described service developments and also the establishment of national and international organizations for old age psychiatry. Particularly influential has been the International Psychogeriatric Association (IPA), founded in 1982. A recent survey by the World Psychiatric Association (Camus *et al.*, 2003) found that 40 out of 48 countries responding provided some specific mental health services for older people and 13 of these countries recognized old age psychiatry as a separate speciality. Over 20 countries had at least one academic chair in old age psychiatry. The World Health Organization Atlas records 51% of 185 countries as having a national mental health programme for older people (http://www.who.int/mental_health/evidence/atlas). Many of the countries that do not are in Africa or the Middle East.

## Principles and values

One of the strengths of old age psychiatry, besides its consideration of epidemiological factors, has been a keen interest in the values underlying its practice. For example, Arie and Jolley (1982) listed five principles: flexibility; responsiveness and availability; non-hierarchical use of staff; domiciliary assessment; and willingness to collaborate with other services and agencies. The list has been amended in various places but the most general statements of values are to be found in series of consensus statements, jointly issued by the World Health Organization and the Geriatric Psychiatry Section of the World Psychiatric Association.

Altogether, there are four consensus statements, concerning psychiatry of the elderly (WHO, 1996), organization of care (WHO, 1997), education (WHO, 1998), and reducing stigma and discrimination against older people with mental disorders (WHO, 2002). Of these, that on organization of services has probably been the most influential and it is the most relevant to this chapter. As well as setting out seven underlying principles (forming the acronym CARITAS; see Table 19.1), the document describes the various types of care that may be provided and the components of specialist services.

**Table 19.1** Principles of care in old age psychiatry

| Good quality care for older people with mental health problems is: |
| --- |
| Comprehensive |
| Accessible |
| Responsive |
| Individualized |
| Transdisciplinary |
| Accountable |
| Systemic |
| A **comprehensive** service should take into account all aspects of the patient's physical, psychological, and social needs and wishes and be patient-centred |
| An **accessible** service is user-friendly and readily available, minimizing the geographical, cultural, financial, political, and linguistic obstacles to obtaining care |
| A **responsive** service is one that listens to and understands the problems brought to its attention and acts promptly and appropriately |
| An **individualized** service focuses on each person with a mental health problem in her/his family and community context. The planning of care must be tailored for and acceptable to the individual and family, and should aim wherever possible to maintain and support the person within her/his home environment |
| A **transdisciplinary** approach goes beyond traditional professional boundaries to optimize the contributions of people with a range of personal and professional skills. Such an approach also facilitates collaboration with voluntary and other agencies to provide a comprehensive range of community-orientated services |
| An **accountable** service is one that accepts responsibility for assuring the quality of the service it delivers and monitors this in partnership with patients and their families. Such a service must be ethically and culturally sensitive |
| A **systemic** approach flexibly integrates all available services to ensure continuity of care and coordinates all levels of service providers including local, provincial, and national governments and community organizations |

World Health Organization/World Psychiatric Association (1997).

## Health policy and old age psychiatry

### United Kingdom

In England, the main policy initiative relevant to old age psychiatry is the *National Service Framework for Older People* (NSF OP; Department of Health, 2001a) but there are other important policies and areas of legislation of relevance to older people. These include the *National Service Framework for Mental Health* (NSF MH; Department of Health, 1999), guidance on dementia care (National Collaborating Centre for Mental Health, 2006), anti-dementia drugs (NICE, 2007), the National Suicide Prevention Strategy, the Mental Health Bill, and the Mental Capacity Act 2005. Legal and mental capacity issues are, however, discussed elsewhere in this book. Overall government policy for older people is set out as *Opportunity Age*, from the Department of Work and Pensions (http://www.dwp.gov.uk/opportunity_age/).

The NSF OP set out eight standards across a range of health issues for older people. Of these, standard 7 relates specifically to mental health, though it is clear that all the other standards are in some way relevant to people with mental health problems. Standard 7 has a particular focus on dementia and depression, as the commonest disorders. It describes service models for specialist services and includes illustrative care pathways. Its stated aim is 'To promote good mental health in older people and to treat and support those older people with dementia and depression' and the standard is that 'Older people who have mental health problems have access to integrated mental health services, provided by the NHS and councils to ensure effective diagnosis, treatment and support, for them and their carers'.

The NSF MH, published 2 years earlier, focused on mental health for adults of working age, but it is evident that some of its proposals also apply to older people. It has seven standards, which cover mental health promotion, primary care and access to services, services for people with severe mental illness, carers, and preventing suicide.

The NSF OP was generally well received but, in contrast to the NSF MH, there were no specific financial resources for service developments. The actions and milestones were criticized as they do not relate to clinical standards or outcomes for patients, but focus more on the establishment of local agreements and protocols (Alzheimer's Society, 2002). There was concern that the absence of specific targets for older people's mental health would lead to neglect by commissioners. There was also a sense that the mental health standard of the NSF OP did not contain sufficient vision to set a direction for future services. As ever, there was a risk of older people's mental health issues falling between the wider mental health agenda, on the one hand, and the wider old people's agenda on the other. Subsequent experience has borne out several of these concerns. Suggestions that the age boundary between working age and older people's mental health services should be blurred (Philp and Appleby, 2005) so that patients are assigned to services on the basis of need have caused some anxiety among old age psychiatrists who wonder if this may be a threat to the speciality as a whole.

The most recent vision for service development is contained in *Everybody's Business* (Care Services Improvement Partnership, 2005a), which is a service development guide produced in collaboration with the Department of Health. It aims to build upon the service models of the NSF OP and describes the foundations and key elements of a comprehensive older people's mental health service.

**Table 19.2** Everybody's business: key elements of comprehensive mental health services for older people

| | |
|---|---|
| Foundations for developing a comprehensive older adult mental health service | Involving service users and carers |
| | Health promotion |
| | Assessment and care planning |
| | Developing culturally appropriate services |
| | Workforce development |
| | A whole systems approach to commissioning integrated services |
| | Leadership: champions, managers, and leaders |
| Primary and community care | Primary care |
| | Home care |
| | Day services |
| | Housing |
| | Assistive technology and telecare |
| | Care in residential settings |
| Intermediate care | Integrated community mental health teams |
| Care for people in the general hospital | Memory assessment services |
| Other specialist mental health services | Psychological therapies |
| | Inpatient care |
| Special groups | Younger people with dementia |
| | Older people with learning disabilities |
| | Mental health care for older prisoners |

The sections of the guide are listed in Table 19.2. The guide takes a broad perspective on the responsibilities for good services and summarizes much current good practice. It is intended to inform a national service mapping exercise of older people's mental health services (http://www.opmhmapping.org.uk/) and this will also form the basis of health and social care inspection and quality monitoring as conducted by the Healthcare Commission and the Commission for Social Care Inspection. The main guide is supplemented by additional material on http://www.everybodysbusiness. org.uk/. The main limitations are that the guidance concentrates on service organization and does not say much about the use of evidence-based treatments and, as with the NSF, there are no identified resources to ensure that developments really take place. The Royal College of Psychiatrists has produced a similar document, *Raising the Standard* (Faculty of Old Age Psychiatry, 2006), which includes some potentially helpful service standards.

During recent years, there have been several non-governmental contributions towards the agenda of how older people's mental health services should develop. Kerslake *et al.* (2003) surveyed 26 local authorities and NHS Trusts in relation to progress on standard 7 of the NSF OP, and found that while 75% had a strategic plan there were widespread gaps in provision, notably in intermediate care, supported housing, and long-term care. Bowers *et al.* (2005) published a report entitled *Moving Out of the Shadows*, which arose from a collaboration between the Older People's Programme, Better Government for Older People, and Help the Aged. In it, they reviewed progress on the NSF OP, and suggested necessary elements for developing whole-system, integrated service strategies for older people's mental health services.

In the field of dementia, the UK has benefited from a network of several Dementia Services Development Centres (DSDCs). These are based on the structure of the original DSDC, established in Stirling by Mary Marshall in 1989. They have a four-fold agenda—information, training, research, and service development. Independent of service provider organizations, they have formed collaborations with universities, and indeed most are located in academic departments. The model has attracted interest in other countries, notably in northern Europe. Although several DSDCs have struggled to attract stable funding, they have nonetheless contributed at many levels, including influencing policy makers. DSDCs form part of a community of mutual interest, centred on social and person centred (as opposed to biomedical) approaches to dementia care, which also includes the Bradford Dementia Group and the *Journal of Dementia Care*. In the north of England, the Northern Dementia Collaborative has adopted the model of health collaboratives used in other conditions, notably cancer, to ensure that consumer views are combined with best practice across a region.

Commissioning of services for older people has been a particular frustration for old age psychiatrists and their teams because of the contrast between their own enthusiasm and a marked lack of interest and urgency from health and social care commissioners. Towards this end, the National Mental Health Partnership (2005), a group of NHS Mental Health Trusts, produced a standards-based framework for commissioning services. The framework has nine standards, including health promotion, primary care, crisis intervention, community teams, intermediate and inpatient care, liaison across the care system, specialist placements, suicide prevention, and support to carers.

Two non-government (voluntary sector) organizations, the Mental Health Foundation and Age Concern, jointly established an Inquiry into Mental Health and Well-Being in Later Life (MHILLI; http://www.mhilli.org/). This is a 3-year, UK-wide project with aims that include: raising awareness of this much neglected issue; empowering older people; creating an evidence base; influencing policy and planning; improving services; and providing a good model of partnership and UK-wide working. It has an interesting methodology, with a commissioned literature review being used to set questions for as wide a range of participants as possible. The first review concerned health promotion (Lee, 2006), to be followed by a review of practice and services.

These recent contributions in particular emphasize a need for older people's mental health services to be *integrated*, though the term integration is imprecise and can be applied in various ways, e.g. in terms of budgets, organizations, commissioning, and/or teams. Lingard and Milne (2004) surveyed the current state of integration among community mental health teams for older people across England and provided various resources, including a checklist for agencies to assess their own progress on integration.

The UK has four different legislatures, so the NSF OP is not applicable across the other countries of the UK. Wales is at present consulting on its version of the NSF OP, which broadly has the same eight standards as the English version. The Welsh mental health standard reads as follows:

> Older people who have a high risk of developing mental health problems and others with related diagnosis have access to primary prevention and integrated services to ensure timely and appropriate assessment, diagnosis, treatment and support for them and their carers.

The Welsh NSF OP contains more action points than for England, and several of these are more specific and relate to clinical activity, not just the establishment of local agreements.

In Scotland and Northern Ireland, there are not currently any national policies for older people's mental health.

### International perspectives

A detailed discussion of mental health policy in other countries is beyond the scope of this chapter. Draper *et al.*, (2005) and Burns *et al.* (2005) include several accounts of psychogeriatric or dementia services in various countries, and several of these contributions outline national policies. The state of affairs is variable across the world, though there is global awareness of the impact of ageing populations. Several countries have produced a national plan for dementia (e.g. Australia, Ireland, France), though progress in implementation has been variable. Other countries are committed to producing one, e.g. Mexico, The Netherlands, Spain. Other countries, such as Germany and Japan, have put more emphasis on reforming social and long-term care insurance policies.

The World Health Organization has a Mental Health Policy Project (http://www.who.int/mental_health/policy/MHPolicy_factsheet.pdf), aimed at encouraging those 40% of countries which do not have a national mental health policy (for any age groups) to develop suitable programmes. However, disappointingly, there is no specific guidance on older people's mental health, and the document on organization of mental health services (WHO, 2003) does not mention older people at all.

Where they do exist, policies are more likely to relate to dementia as such, rather than the broader remit of old age psychiatry since, as mentioned above, not all countries have extensive coverage in the speciality. There are both strengths and weaknesses in focusing on dementia. Dementia is of course a massive economic issue (estimated total annual costs in UK may be as high as £17 billion; Bosanquet, 2001) but excluding other mental disorders in older people may be disadvantageous—it is only to easy to overlook the needs of depressed older people.

The economic importance of dementia has attracted the interest of the Organisation for Economic Co-operation and Development (OECD), which recently published a survey of dementia care in nine of its member countries (Moise *et al.*, 2004). This report summarizes epidemiological, clinical, and policy issues in dementia, as well as providing an analysis of its economic impact and costs in the nine countries. Table 19.3 lists the shared principles that underlie the organization of dementia care services internationally, a list that could apply to mental health problems in general. The concluding section of the report discusses the service needs of people

**Table 19.3** Common policy principles in relation to dementia

| |
|---|
| Remain at home as long as possible—delay institutionalization |
| Support carers in order to achieve this |
| Patients need as much control over their care as possible, but recognize limitations due to cognitive impairment (e.g. in relation to having the capacity to make informed choices) |
| Coordination of services at local level where possible |
| Institutional care, when required, should be as home-like as possible |
| Equate service provision with need |
| Early diagnosis should be encouraged |

Organisation for Economic Co-operation and Development (Moise *et al.*, 2004).

with dementia, how to support carers, which interventions are effective, and what the future may bring, especially whether there will be adequate resources to support dementia care.

## The nature and scope of old age psychiatry services

It is hard to set precise limits for what constitutes the activity of old age psychiatry, since mental health problems in older people may be encountered and dealt with in various settings, not just those specifically designated for the purpose. Indeed, most interactions will be in social care settings, such as day centres or home care services, or in primary care, where most common disorders, such as depression, frequently present. However, the contributions of social care and primary care are discussed in Chapters 16 and 20.

There are also variations as to the boundaries of specialist services. In some countries, especially if old age psychiatry is not a recognized speciality, this work may be undertaken by general psychiatrists, geriatric physicians, or neurologists. Some services limit themselves to dementia, while others have a more comprehensive basis.

Incidentally, terminology is a considerable problem in this area. First, there is the problem of what to call the client group itself: 'the aged' or 'the elderly' are not currently favoured, and it is probably preferred to use the term 'older people'. This is not without problems. It may be asked 'older than whom?' Different ages are used for the start of this period, as low as 50 in some policy documents. The commonest cut-off is 65, but this creates a heterogeneous group spanning more than one generation. People aged 65 are often free of health problems, so there are attempts to define those at most risk (e.g. 'frail elderly') or of more advanced years (e.g. the 'oldest old'), though several definitions exist for both of these concepts.

Then there are problems as to how to name the speciality. In the UK 'psychogeriatrics' has largely been superseded by 'old age psychiatry' as its practitioners have emphasized their links with the rest of psychiatry. However, in the NHS as a multidisciplinary service, there is a tendency to talk about 'mental health' rather than 'psychiatry' as the latter hints at medical patronage. Outside of health settings, it is now fashionable to speak of 'mental well-being', as even 'mental health' is seen as too 'medical'. In North America, the relevant speciality is 'geriatric psychiatry', though this is often a rather different activity from UK old age psychiatry, as the integral links with community teams are not always present to the same degree. Blazer (2000) criticized geriatric psychiatry in the USA for moving away from the principles of comprehensive, interdisciplinary assessment and therapy, and tending to abandon frail, very old people in favour of those nearer 65 with less complex needs. Enough sophistry! I have generally used the term 'older people' and I am using 'old age psychiatry' and 'older people's mental health services' somewhat interchangeably.

However, despite these problems of terms and boundaries, the following section is mainly about the model of old age psychiatry that has developed from the influences discussed above. It considers the elements of a comprehensive specialist mental health service for older people, including evidence to support current practice. The current shape of services owes much to the energy and innovation of early old age psychiatrists, but over the last 10–15 years there has been increasing attention to more formal evaluations of services (Banerjee and Dickinson, 1997), including randomized controlled trials (RCTs) and, more recently, several systematic reviews (e.g. Draper, 2000; Bartels *et al.*, 2002, 2003; Van Citters and Bartels, 2004; Draper and Low, 2005a,b).

# Essential components of old age psychiatry services

## Community mental health teams

The NSF OP suggests that core members of the specialist mental health service should include consultant old age psychiatrists, community mental health nurses, clinical psychologists, occupational therapists, and social workers (Department of Health, 2001a). However, the additional input of untrained staff, such as health or social care assistants, can also be invaluable, and adequate administrative support is essential. There should also be agreed working and referral arrangements with other professionals, such as physiotherapists and dieticians. Most community mental health teams would aim for this structure, though variations are often seen in practice. Most frequently, one or more professional group may be lacking—often clinical psychology as there is a lack of practitioners working with old people. Quite often, too, there may just be a single consultant psychiatrist for a team, and the consultant may work somewhat detached from the team, perhaps taking separate referrals but also having other commitments elsewhere, for example to inpatient units.

Teams characteristically cover an agreed sector, which may be defined geographically or else by which general practices refer to the team. In the UK, teams usually deal with the full range of mental disorders, not solely dementia. There will be an agreed route of referral, with most referrals in practice coming from primary care, but also from other sources, including social services, residential homes and sometimes directly from families. Patients appear reluctant to refer themselves, even to teams with open referral policies.

Teams are of variable size, often smaller in rural areas. Within a larger team, there is scope for some subdivision of responsibilities or for specialization. For example, each member of the team may be linked to an individual GP surgery or have links with one or more residential or nursing homes in the patch. Or they may develop special roles, such as monitoring patients on antidementia drugs.

Leadership in teams is a commonly discussed theme, but there are several aspects to how a team is led. For example, the team will be managed as part of the service to which it belongs; the staff in it will be line managed; they will also have their own professional group hierarchies, which may include supervision of their clinical work; and there may a designated team leader, whose role will include such matters as chairing the referral allocation meeting. As well as this, consultant psychiatrists are often expected to provide clinical leadership to the team, though this is a complex construct. It seems to include a commitment to be involved in the assessment and management of the more complicated cases and to act as one of the main conduits between the community team and other parts of the service, especially inpatient care.

There is accumulating evidence that community mental health teams for older people offer effective interventions. One of the first evaluations of the impact of a community team was by O'Connor *et al.* (1991) who found that early intervention led to *increased* admissions to long-term care within a 2-year period for people with dementia living alone. This may have reflected that this group were in fact living in conditions of high risk and relative neglect.

More recently, Callahan *et al.* (2006) found that an interdisciplinary team working collaboratively with primary care provided significant improvements in the quality of care and in behavioural and psychological symptoms of dementia among primary care patients and their caregivers.

However, most RCTs of interventions by community mental health teams have concentrated on depression (Draper and Low, 2005a). Of these, four out of six reported that the team input was more effective than the control intervention, findings supported by data from several uncontrolled studies.

There is a general consensus that assessment and management should take place at home where possible, rather than, say, in outpatient clinics. It has been demonstrated that initial assessments by non-medical members of the multidisciplinary team can be effective (Collighan *et al.*, 1993). Case management, in various forms, often known in the UK as the 'care programme approach', is an effective way of ensuring that patients are kept in contact with the service. Care management seems to be effective at keeping people with dementia at home for longer periods (Challis *et al.*, 2002) and in general outcomes seem to be better for team management approaches than for simply providing consultations and advice (Woods *et al.*, 2003). It is accepted that specialist teams for older people are more effective at managing depression in older people than general adult mental health teams, though this has not been formally evaluated (Draper and Low, 2005a).

As regards the specific role of psychiatry, consultant domiciliary visits are probably best targeted at more complex cases: studies of the outcome of consultant home visits are not easy to interpret because of this (Orrell and Katona, 1998). Home-based practice lessens the rate of failed appointments and also may cost less than running an outpatient clinic (Anderson and Aquilina, 2002; Aquilina and Anderson, 2002). However, many old age psychiatrists continue to hold outpatient clinics in addition to seeing patients at home. Such clinics may be very useful for following up relatively mobile patients, often those with functional disorders. For example, monitoring certain patients on lithium treatment may be efficiently managed this way (Head and Dening, 1998).

Thus, community mental health teams for older people are well established in various countries, and there is good evidence to support this style of service. There remain several issues where further research evidence would be helpful. For example, there are no recent studies of crisis intervention services for older people (Ratna, 1982), and there are no studies that evaluate the outcomes from different members of the multidisciplinary team.

As has been emphasized in Chapter 4, numbers of older people in developing countries, and consequently numbers of people with dementia, are increasing more sharply than in the developed world. This, combined with the limited resources that may be available for mental health services, requires new methods of case finding and service provision (e.g. Shaji *et al.*, 2002). Services need to have realistic goals, they should be based on careful mapping of all local resources that may be supportive of older people, and they can work through general health workers with suitable brief training (Dening and Shaji, 2005).

## Memory clinics

Memory clinics are discussed in Chapter 21. They have proved popular with old age psychiatrists, who are now responsible for most of those held in the UK (Lindesay et al, 2002), particularly as a means of assessing for treatment with antidementia drugs and of monitoring patients on such treatment. The assessment of mild cognitive impairment is another task for which memory clinics are well suited (Phipps and O'Brien, 2002). There is a balance to be struck between the extent of the investigations performed by a memory clinic and its ability to respond to referrals. Certainly some psychiatrists have struggled with the rigour of their clinic protocols, leading to long waiting lists for assessment, and critics have argued that memory clinics may divert scarce resources from more valuable integrated community-based care (Pelosi *et al.*, 2006). From the academic aspect, memory clinics are probably the most effective means of recruiting patients for trials of new drugs, and they can provide rich sources of longitudinal data that have done much to illuminate the variable natural history of dementia.

## Day hospitals

Day hospitals (often referred to in the USA as 'partial hospitalization programs') are regarded as a key component of old age psychiatry services, though their efficacy is often called into question. In the UK, day hospitals are generally distinguished from day centres, the latter being run by social care providers or the voluntary sector, whereas day hospitals are part of the health service. There are therefore differences in the types of staffing to be found in each type of facility. Day hospitals are more likely to focus on assessment and therapeutic activities, and are generally looking to discharge patients elsewhere, either after an agreed period of attendance or once a suitable outcome has been achieved. Day centres do not have the same emphasis on assessment, activities are generally diversionary rather than therapeutic, and indefinite attendance is not usually a problem. An important difference, certainly in the UK, is that day hospitals, as part of the National Health Service, do not charge for attendance, and often transport is easier to arrange (though sometimes equally unreliable!). In practice, however, there is considerable overlap. Indeed, *higher* levels of disability may be found in day centres than day hospitals (Audit Commission, 2000). Critics of day hospitals have pointed out a lack of therapeutic activities, inability to move patients on to other facilities, and a lack of evidence that day hospitals prevent hospital admissions (Fasey, 1994).

Day hospitals themselves are quite variable, especially depending on the relative proportions of patients with functional disorders and dementia. Many organize for these groups to attend largely on separate days as the type of programme appropriate to each may be quite different. Some day facilities cater for patients with long-term severe mental illness and, again, this group have different needs from patients being treated for shorter episodes of depression. And most day hospitals will have a small number of patients whose exact diagnosis is difficult to pinpoint but whose personalities are so difficult that they do not fit into ordinary day centres. In rural areas, because of distance and travelling time, it may be necessary to hold the day hospital in different localities on different days, which means that on each day there will be a more heterogeneous group of patients.

A national survey of day hospitals, coordinated by the Royal College of Psychiatrists, confirmed that there is wide diversity in the style and use of day hospital facilities across the UK (Audini *et al.*, 2001). The majority of old age psychiatrists had access to day hospitals, over half the patients (56%) had dementia, and there were variations in treatments offered and lengths of stay.

This diversity stimulated the formation of a day hospital network to encourage communication and share experiences between day hospital providers.

Thus, given the mixed nature of day hospitals, and the heterogeneity of patients attending, it is scarcely surprising that the simple question 'Do day hospitals work?' is virtually unanswerable. Different patients will be aiming at different outcomes, so using simple outcome measures could miss significant benefits. There are relatively few studies of outcomes from day hospital attendance. The only RCT (Ashaye *et al.*, 2003) was not primarily about outcomes but was an evaluation of a standardized needs assessment (CANE; Orrell and Hancock, 2004). However, both groups, i.e. those assessed by the CANE and the controls, showed improvements in unmet needs and Health of the Nation Outcome Scale (HoNOS 65+) scores over a 3-month period, even though physical dependency and behavioural problems increased. Other studies provide evidence that day hospitals are effective in improving mental health outcomes, especially for depression (e.g. Mackenzie *et al.*, 2006). There is a distinct lack of comparisons between day hospitals and either inpatient or community treatment, so their role in providing acute care is so far unresolved. It is more likely, however, that day hospitals are a useful adjunct to discharge from inpatient care, rather than in preventing admissions (Howard, 1994). Certainly, despite indications of their effectiveness, a more robust evidence base for day hospitals is needed (Hoe *et al.*, 2005).

## Respite care

Respite care comprises a mixture of activities, aimed at giving caregivers temporary opportunities to be away from the patient in order to reduce their stress and to delay or prevent nursing home admission. There are broadly three types of respite, including short residential placements, day care, and home care (Royal College of Psychiatrists, 2005a). Nowadays, short-stay respite care is generally provided in residential and nursing homes rather than in hospitals. Respite care may be planned or offered in a crisis or at the request of the carer.

Several evaluations of respite care were conducted in the 1980s and 1990s to see if the service was effective at delaying or avoiding admission to long-term care (reviewed by Melzer *et al.*, 1999) but there is no conclusive evidence in terms of direct benefits to patients, relief of carer burden, or delay in admission to long-term care. However, carers do use respite care when it is available and they often describe high levels of satisfaction with it. They may often express a wish either for more respite or for more flexible arrangements (Homer and Gilleard, 1994). In practice, it seems as though respite care may be used by some carers to help them keep the patient at home for longer whereas, for others, respite care functions as a stepping stone on the way to long-term care. Sometimes, perhaps, respite care is offered when what is needed is really long-term care, in which situation it may be regarded as a form of rationing. However, overall, it does appear that providing respite in various forms, in partnership with other agencies, is a legitimate activity for old age psychiatry services.

## Support to carers

Old age psychiatry was perhaps one of the first areas where carer issues were first recognized, e.g. Argyle *et al.*, 1985). Carers of people with dementia seem to have particularly high levels of stress and lower levels of satisfaction with services than other carers (e.g. Philp *et al.*, 1995; Bedford *et al.*, 1996). Consequently, assessments of patients also routinely include assessment of their carers' mental state and coping resources. Indeed, in the UK, the Carers Act 2000 entitles carers to their own separate assessments.

Most services provided for patients will also directly or indirectly benefit carers, the simplest example being that treating the patient's symptoms will make life more tolerable for the carer. Many of the services for people with dementia, for example day care or the management of difficult behaviour, are often aimed primarily at improving matters for the carer. Respite care is provided to give carers a much-needed break. A recent meta-analysis has shown that psychosocial interventions for carers of people with dementia can be effective across a range of outcomes (Brodaty *et al.*, 2003).

As well as this, there is considerable interest in supporting carers (especially carers of people with dementia) through educational and other means. At the most basic level, this includes carer support groups, where carers can provide mutual support by sharing experiences and passing on skills they have learned from their own roles. More formal programmes have been developed and evaluated (Mittelman *et al.*, 1996; Brodaty *et al.*, 1997), which comprise various elements, such as improving carers' knowledge of mental health problems and teaching exercises to deal more effectively with challenging behaviours. Less intensive carer education programmes are commonly provided, but these have not so far been shown to be as effective in reducing carer stress.

Carers also have an important role to play in the formal and informal education of personnel training in old age psychiatry and other professional groups; and they can provide a valuable independent perspective in the evaluation of mental health services (Melzer *et al.*, 1996; Dening and Lawton, 1998). They are often the most passionate and effective lobbyists on behalf of people with dementia especially.

## Inpatient care

In general, wards for older patients are separate from those for adults under 65. Experience of wards for mixed ages is that they disadvantage older people who may be relatively neglected in the face of demands placed by younger, psychotic, and disturbed patients. Perhaps surprisingly, the evidence from a small number of studies of older patients on general psychiatry wards suggests that clinical outcomes are acceptable, but in most of these studies an old age psychiatrist was attached to the unit (Draper and Low, 2005a). It is also customary to separate dementia and functional illness, since experience suggests that depressed patients find the presence of patients with dementia and behaviour problems quite difficult to bear.

Although joint assessment wards with geriatric medicine were at one time recommended, they are now uncommon. Various factors have contributed to this, but it appears that geriatric physicians are more comfortable with a responsive psychiatric liaison service and geriatric psychiatrists are satisfied if there is adequate access to medical and diagnostic facilities for their physically unwell patients. It can, however, leave something of a lottery as to whether a person with dementia lands up in a medical or a psychiatric bed. Certainly there is evidence that the mental health of older people with depression or cognitive impairment does not benefit from admissions to general medical wards (Cole, 1993), and patients with depression fare better in psychiatric rather than general wards (Norquist *et al.*, 1995).

Inpatient care for dementia has changed more radically in recent years than that for functional disorders. The most obvious change is the large decrease in long-stay hospital beds for dementia. The amount of respite care provided in hospital has also decreased. Second, early psychogeriatric services used to designate beds for dementia assessment, the idea being to generate a comprehensive care plan which could be followed through in the community. However, it has become clear that such assessment is more appropriately carried out in the community, and acute dementia beds are now used for particularly difficult behavioural problems. A third change is that there was a vogue for 'challenging behaviour units', which proposed to offer intensive behavioural treatments for the most agitated and aggressive individuals. However, as behavioural disturbance is by far the most common reason for psychiatric admission in dementia, it seems pointless to designate some units in this way. In practice too, challenging behaviour units were often ineffective, and generally the concept has been abandoned.

Published evidence certainly suggests that good links between inpatient units and their respective community teams are beneficial for patients. Community follow-up, including outpatient attendance and community psychiatric nurse visits, reduces readmission for patients with depression (Philpot *et al.*, 2000). Longer lengths of stay in hospital are also associated with fewer readmissions, but the relationship between length of stay and other outcomes is less clear (Draper, 2000). Uncontrolled studies of inpatient treatment suggest quite good treatment outcomes both for depression and for behavioural and psychological symptoms in dementia (BPSD) (Draper and Low, 2005b).

Long-term psychogeriatric beds were provided in much greater numbers in the past, with considerable criticism of the care provided in long-stay wards in old hospitals. In recent years, studies have examined outcomes in newer, purpose-built facilities or among patients discharged from hospital to community settings. Generally, patients discharged to community settings do better than those who remain in hospital, with greater staff satisfaction (Wills and Leff, 1996; Trieman *et al.*, 1999), but it remains unclear if this applies to those with the most severe behaviour disorders (Draper and Low, 2005b).

## Consultation-liaison psychiatry

There is ample evidence to demonstrate that older people in general hospitals have high levels of psychiatric morbidity, especially dementia and depression. For most old age psychiatry services, patients in general hospital beds form a high proportion of the total of cases referred, about one-third being a typical figure. This important topic is discussed in Chapter 22. From the point of view of this section, it is worth noting how various models of consultation and liaison have developed. Mental health liaison nurses seem an effective way of assessing and managing many cases, as well as forming close links with their general nursing colleagues, but it is clear that more evidence is required as to how these services should be most effectively provided (Baldwin *et al.*, 2004). Commitment from geriatric medicine is also required to develop a successful service, and the recent joint document *Who Cares Wins* (Royal College of Psychiatrists, 2005b) is welcome in this regard. Service development in the UK is currently somewhat hampered by uncertainty about the commissioning arrangements—that is, whether liaison services should be funded from the mental health or the general hospital budget. This is amplified by the separation of general medical and mental health services into different organizations (Holmes *et al.*, 2003).

## Relationships to other agencies

There are several key relationships to consider, several of which are discussed more detail in other chapters of this book. They include working with social services (Chapter 16), primary care (Chapter 20), other branches of medicine (Chapter 22), non-government agencies, and residential and nursing homes (Chapter 23).

### Working with primary care

Given that most older people live in the community and that the large majority of referrals to old age psychiatry services come from primary care, this working relationship is extremely important in any consideration of how services should develop. As mentioned above, most old age psychiatry services operate on a sectorized basis, the boundaries usually determined by those of general practices. Individual members of the multidisciplinary team often relate to individual surgeries within the local area, so as to improve mutual understanding and working relationships, for example attending practice team meetings on a regular basis.

Whilst it is important to emphasize that most cases of dementia reside in the community, from the point of view of the individual general practitioner, dementia is not that common a condition. An average GP, with a list size of around 2000 and an average age distribution, will see just one or two new cases a year and will have around 14 cases at various stages of dementia (Iliffe and Drennan, 2001). However, because of the more episodic nature of depression, GPs will encounter cases of depression more often. It is therefore probably more realistic to improve GPs' performance in this area by means of improved support rather than expecting them to radically increase their knowledge of dementia and other conditions. Turner *et al.* (2004) argued that, for dementia, educational support for GPs should concentrate on epidemiological knowledge, disclosure of the diagnosis, and management of behaviour problems. Other relevant support could include computerized information to improve prescribing; introduction of standardized assessments of mood and cognition as part of routine health checks; development of care pathways and guidelines for referral and treatment; and ready access to advice from the specialist mental health service.

There is good evidence from RCTs to support various forms of collaboration between primary care and old age psychiatry services. For example, Llewellyn-Jones *et al.* (1999) found that a multifaceted shared care intervention improved depression in a group of older people in various residential settings, including self-care units. The multicentre IMPACT study (Unutzer *et al.*, 2002), including 1800 people aged 60 and over, reported significant improvements in depression from a joint intervention coordinated by a depression case manager. The PEARLS programme (Ciechanowski *et al.*, 2004), a community-integrated, home-based treatment for depression, significantly reduced depressive symptoms and improved health status for chronically medically ill over 60s with minor depression and dysthymia. Other evidence suggests that physically ill patients can benefit from joint interventions aimed at treating depression (Flaherty *et al.*, 1998; Schrader *et al.*, 2005).

The organizational relationships with primary care are also important. In England, health funding is allocated through a network of Primary Care Trusts (PCTs), which commission health services on behalf of their local populations. PCTs are the providers of primary care, and in some cases they may be the providers of the local specialist mental health services too. PCTs are responsible for the implementation of the NSF OP and for mental health, and so they are obliged to work with specialist services and other agencies in the drawing up of local protocols, care pathways, guidelines, and so forth.

### Working with social care

Most formal care for people with dementia in the UK is provided through social care, rather than health. Services are either commissioned by local authority social services departments or purchased directly by clients. The NHS and social services departments are encouraged to work closely together towards integrated commissioning and service provision to improve efficiency and responsiveness (Hughes *et al.*, 2001; Reilly *et al.*, 2003). Many mental health trusts in England now have partnerships with social services, including seconded social work staff, and in the future health and social care may merge into care trusts.

In England, the cornerstone for care services is the single assessment process (SAP), as introduced by the NSF. This has several tiers, from an initial basic assessment to more detailed specialist assessments. Several versions are available, including different specialist assessments (Orrell and Hancock, 2004). The SAP considers various aspects including the user's view of the problem, clinical background, mental health assessment, social situation, and safety issues. Carers are identified and may be offered their own assessment. Assessment and active care management should promote older people's independence by preventing deterioration and managing crises (Challis *et al.*, 2002). Social care provision for people with functional mental disorders as opposed to dementia is often underdeveloped or such individuals find they do not meet local eligibility criteria for services to be provided.

### Working with consumers

Older people vary greatly, ranging from active and independent to distinctly frail and needing significant care and support. People born more recently are often more conscious of their entitlements and are more assertive in dealing with services. Public services are now encouraging a stronger voice from consumers. Carers have contributed to developing services for some time (Dening and Lawton, 1998), but only more recently have older service users, including those with dementia, been actively engaged (Barnett, 2000; Allan, 2001). Volunteer peer support services for older people with mental health problems, aimed at promoting recovery, are an interesting new development, but the concept requires further evaluation (Briscoe *et al.*, 2005).

Genuine user and carer input requires resources, as it takes time and patience to get older people together in order to ascertain their views. Nonetheless, their participation in service development, management, and evaluation can be invaluable. Consumers are supported by a strong voluntary sector, especially the national Alzheimer's organizations for people with dementia, but Age Concern and the Mental Health Foundation also take an interest in functional disorders.

## Special areas
### Gender

Women live longer than men, the ratio of women to men increasing with advanced age. They are more likely to be bereaved and to live alone. Depression is commoner in women at all ages. Women are more likely to be spouse carers than men. Most older people presenting to health and social care are women, so this area may legitimately be regarded as a feminist issue.

In contrast, older men are in a declining section of the population and may have difficulty finding male company and support in such facilities as day centres. They are more likely to be supported by a co-resident carer, which greatly reduces their risk of moving into institutional care (Banerjee *et al.*, 2003). Suicide rates are, however, higher among older men.

### Black and minority ethnic groups

Just about all countries of the world have significant numbers of people from different ethnic and cultural backgrounds. Developed countries often have large numbers of people who have immigrated from elsewhere, for various reasons including looking for work or to escape persecution. In general, minority ethnic groups have a younger age profile than the majority population but even so significant numbers of older people may be involved. For example, there are now nearly 250,000 individuals aged 60 plus from minority ethnic groups living in the UK. Such groups vary greatly in their access to material and social resources. Indian elderly persons are less likely to experience multiple deprivations, with similar levels to White older people. However just under half of older Pakistanis and Bangladeshis, two-fifths of older Black Caribbean and a quarter of Irish elders experience medium or high levels of deprivation (Evandrou, 2000).

Levels of deprivation affect the well-being of minority ethnic elders. Some illnesses are more common among specific groups, e.g. hypertension and stroke among African-Caribbean people and diabetes among South Asians. Rates of dementia and depression may be high in certain groups (Livingston *et al.*, 2001), though the excess of dementia in people of African-Caribbean origin is probably of vascular aetiology rather than due to immigration *per se*. Minority groups may be reluctant to acknowledge the existence of mental disorders and therefore may not see psychiatric services as appropriate to their needs (Marwaha and Livingston, 2002). Future services need to be culturally appropriate, ensuring accessibility for all including those who do not have English as their first language (Patel *et al.*, 1998, Sadavoy *et al.*, 2004).

### Rural areas

Rural areas present particular challenges to older people's mental health services, but they are important as often the proportion of older people in rural communities is higher than elsewhere. In some parts of the world, rural areas are extremely remote or at great distances from centres of population. Studies of rural health and social care consistently highlight certain themes, such as poor access to assessment and diagnostic services, sparse public facilities such as daytime activities or paid caregivers, and difficulties with isolation compounded by poor and expensive transport. All of these apply to people with dementia or other mental health problems, and to their carers. Other obstacles, such as denial of illness and uncooperative or absent family members, seem to be more frequent in rural settings (Teel, 2004) although, conversely, satisfaction with local doctors and health services seems to be higher (Farmer *et al.*, 2005).

A few studies have examined the circumstances of rural older people, mainly with dementia, in relation to the care they receive. Innes *et al.* (2005) found that certain aspects of rural life in Scotland balanced to some extent the gaps in services, and a Canadian study (Bedard *et al.*, 2004) found that rural caregivers did not experience higher levels of burden even though rural patients had a higher level of behavioural disturbance. In north Wales, carers received most essential services even though levels of services were low, but the main problems were a lack of crisis support and a reluctance to accept long-term care when it was needed (Wenger *et al.*, 2002).

Rural health care is perhaps more likely to require novel approaches to providing services (Chalifoux *et al.*, 1996). Some work has used family and care staff focus groups to identify ways of providing accessible services (Morgan *et al.*, 2002). Small, flexible day centres can be valued and effective, though there are attendant problems about storing and transporting records and materials, and about effective supervision and management of staff (Gibson and Whittington, 1995). Training programmes for caregivers that have been designed to be transportable may be useful (Hepburn *et al.*, 2003) and advances in telecommunications have obvious potential to reach people in remote places (Sumner, 2001), though some issues such as funding of equipment, confidentiality, and ethical conduct of teleconsultations are not fully worked out (Goins *et al.*, 2001). Nonetheless, there is still a need for new ideas, perhaps making more use of generic services or everyday environments such as supermarkets and hairdressers, to provide flexible and effective support to patients and carers.

### Prisons

There are significant numbers of older people among the inmates of prisons and special hospitals. Indeed, in England and Wales the prison population is ageing more rapidly than the wider community, with about 1700, mainly male, prisoners aged over 60 by 2004 (HM Chief Inspector of Prisons, 2004). Identification and treatment of mental disorders in prisoners is often difficult but may be readily overlooked in older prisoners, as they are less disruptive. Many prisoners are in unsuitable conditions with only limited facilities to support them after release. The same applies to patients in special hospitals, who may remain detained longer than necessary because there are no alternatives (Yorston, 1999; Fazel *et al.*, 2001). Whether there should be a subspeciality of old age forensic psychiatry remains open to debate (Nnatu *et al.*, 2005). Aspects of crime in relation to old age psychiatry are discussed further in Chapter 40.

### Learning disabilities

People with learning disabilities have higher rates of early onset dementia than the general population. They may also be excluded from consideration by mainstream health and social facilities. Current UK policy (Department of Health, 2001b) emphasizes the need for people with learning disabilities to access normal services wherever possible. Building on this, the Foundation for People with Learning Disabilities (2002) developed an extensive programme of work, Growing Older with Learning Disabilities (GOLD), which ranges from issues of healthy ageing to the services required for dementia and palliative care for people with learning disabilities.

In general, however, specialist services for people with learning disabilities cover the whole age range, and people who develop dementia continue to be served by facilities with expertise in learning disabilities. In future, there will need to be more closely defined working arrangements between primary care, learning disabilities services, and older people's mental health services.

### Gay and lesbian older people

Gay and lesbian older people may have significant difficulties as social attitudes towards gay and lesbian relationships have been much less tolerant in the past. Also gay and lesbian partners are not necessarily recognized as the next of kin by statutory services and this may cause considerable distress. Few older people's services are targeted towards the needs of this group (Warner *et al.*, 2003).

### Very old people

Definitions of the 'oldest old' or 'very old people' are variable and the thresholds have increased over time with growing numbers of people aged 90 plus. Several cohort studies of very old people and centenarians have been conducted (e.g. Samuelsson *et al.*, 1997; Baltes and Mayer, 1999). Only 25–30% of centenarians live independently; most are in residential or nursing home care.

With great age, the epidemiology of common illnesses changes. Circulatory diseases become an increasingly common cause of death, but the age-specific incidence and mortality rates of most cancers decline beyond the age of 90. With regard to mental health, centenarians scored lower on cognitive tests and were more likely to feel useless and that life was routine, not exciting (Martin *et al.*, 1992). Variable estimates of the prevalence of dementia in centenarians have been reported. Although prevalence studies of dementia suggest that there may be a survivor effect at extreme old age, incidence studies show an increasing incidence of dementia in the population up to at least the age of 90, making this unlikely (Matthews *et al.*, 2005).

Within the everyday practice of old age psychiatry, there is a noticeable increase in the age of many of the patients referred, with consequent increases in medical co-morbidity, physical disability, and complex social care needs. This underscores the importance of providing mental health services for very old people that are comprehensive, interdisciplinary, and allied to provision of physical health care (Blazer, 2000). There is a clear need for the policy and research agendas to address the needs of this group (Dening and Gabe, 2000).

### Elder abuse

The mistreatment of older people is considered in more detail in Chapter 39. From the point of old age psychiatry services, there are perhaps two main issues. One of these is a concern with the frequency that abuse of older patients can occur in institutional settings including hospitals. There is a sad catalogue of hospital inquiries (e.g. Commission for Health Improvement, 2000, 2003), which highlight similar themes, such as geographical isolation, low staffing levels, lack of training, lack of nursing leadership, and lack of clinical governance. Hopefully, action plans (e.g. Care Standards Improvement Partnership, 2005b) will address these issues, though adequate financial resources are required as well as exhortations to do better.

The other issue for old age psychiatry services is to participate as part of the multi-agency, interdisciplinary response to cases that arise in all settings. This may include various roles, such as psychiatric assessment of the victim and/or the perpetrator, assessments of mental capacity, especially when financial abuse is suspected, and participating in vulnerable people's procedures. In England, policy is set out in the document *No Secrets* (Department of Heath, 2000).

## Quality and evaluation of services

Quality is a complex concept with more than one definition. However, in this section the term is used to address questions of how well services function and how this can be measured. 'How well' implies that services can be 'good' or 'bad', that they can be better or worse than other services, and that some kinds of standards are in operation. These standards may be explicit or implicit, they may internally generated or imposed from outside, and they may be absolute or relative. Increasingly, 'evidence' is required to demonstrate quality, and mere assertions and descriptions are less acceptable, as they may not reflect what is happening in practice. Service quality is of interest for different reasons to different groups—obviously, to patients and carers, but also professionals, their employers, funding bodies such as health authorities, insurers, and governments, and the public at large. Large-scale failures of quality are of course of media interest too.

Perhaps until the introduction of managerial approaches to health care in the 1980s, issues of quality were largely addressed subjectively. But, perhaps along with the importation of other business concepts, an emphasis on quality seems to have begun around that time, initially in the form of quality assurance and clinical audit, followed by total quality management and related concepts. In the UK, an inquiry into poor practice at a paediatric cardiac surgery unit in the late 1990s changed the direction of the agenda and introduced the concept of clinical governance.

Clinical governance may be defined as 'a framework through which [healthcare] organizations are accountable for continuously improving the quality of their services and safeguarding high standards of care by creating an environment in which excellence in clinical care will flourish' (Scally and Donaldson, 1998). As it relates to quality within all the clinical activities of a service, clinical governance has a very broad scope and contains many domains, some of which are listed in Table 19.4; see also James *et al.* (2005) for a more detailed discussion of clinical governance in relation to mental health. Clearly, these are crucial activities for old age psychiatry services.

**Table 19.4** Topics within the scope of clinical governance

| |
|---|
| Clinical policies |
| Clinical procedures |
| Protocols, guidelines, shared care agreements |
| Risk management and patient safety |
| Poor performance and disciplinary procedures |
| Incident reporting |
| Complaints |
| Patient advocacy and liaison |
| Clinical audit/clinical effectiveness |
| Medicines management and prescribing guidance |
| Clinical record keeping |
| Compliance with relevant legislation, e.g. Mental Health Act |
| Leadership and team working |
| Training and education |
| Appraisal and mentoring |

It is generally accepted that effective clinical governance requires active clinical involvement in order to make a real impact in raising standards at the point of service delivery, but there is often a tension with the needs of managers and funding organizations to impose their agenda or their own targets and standards. The extent to which this occurs may vary in different countries, with the UK having a strong top-down emphasis, despite the protestations of government that it runs a devolved National Health Service. Currently, the scope of clinical governance seems to be evolving into a wider remit of 'healthcare governance' which also encompasses such matters as financial risks to health service organizations.

How does an old age psychiatry service demonstrate its commitment to (improving) quality? As I have suggested, active clinical involvement is essential. There is usually an external agenda of government and/or local targets but, nonetheless, most services will have areas where they wish to focus their energies. Most initiatives aimed at raising standards seem to do so by reducing variations between practitioners and therefore much of the quality agenda is about moving towards more standardized procedures, driven where possible by protocols and guidelines. This is not unique to old age psychiatry, nor too is a tendency to look at processes along 'the patient's journey'.

Thus, a mixture of initiatives, both local and national, may be applied to promote quality and evaluation in this way. Important stages in the patient's journey in relation to specialist mental health services include the following:

1 Referral criteria. Ensuring that the service sees those patients who are in most need within a reasonable time-scale needs collaboration with referrers, especially primary care. Agreeing thresholds not only for referral but also for discharge from a specialist service is an important way of controlling the caseloads of team members.

2 Standardized assessments. The single assessment process, set out in the NSF OP, underlines the importance of making comprehensive and standard assessments. Several versions of comprehensive assessment are available, such as the Camberwell Assessment of Need for the Elderly (CANE; Orrell and Hancock, 2004), but there are also many standard rating scales available for more specific purposes, such as assessment of cognition or of mood (compiled by Burns et al., 2003).

3 Guidelines and protocols for treatment. Clinical guidelines are systematically developed statements to assist clinicians and patients in making decisions about appropriate treatment for specific conditions. Protocols are written plans specifying the procedures to be followed in providing care for a particular condition. Integrated care pathways are locally agreed summaries of practice, based on the best available evidence, for a specific condition or patient group. A care pathway may therefore be the application of a guideline in a practical situation. Clinical guidelines so far available to inform old age psychiatry tend to concentrate on dementia rather than other mental disorders (Burns et al., 2002) and they vary as to how systematically derived they are. Guidelines and protocols may cover the whole management of a condition or they may emphasis specific aspects of treatment, e.g. the use of antidementia drugs or psychological treatments.

4 Care management. As mental health problems in old age often require input from a range of professionals and from different agencies, ways of recording, storing, and sharing information are extremely important in ensuring a quality service. In the UK, this is provided through the care programme approach (CPA), which uses standard documentation and provides a comprehensive record that can be regularly updated and shared with patients and carers. Integrating different systems of care management has been the biggest challenge to successful joint working between health and social services. There is obvious potential to use electronic versions of the CPA so that the same patient data can be readily available to different professionals at different sites. Whether electronic notes will abolish all paper records remains to be seen.

5 Outcomes. In theory at least, measuring outcomes should be the gold standard for quality, as it has more direct relevance to patients than do the proxy alternatives of structure and process that are usually measured instead. However, outcome measurement has long been a problem for mental health and this is especially so in old age psychiatry, where often 'bad' outcomes such as death or institutionalization may actually follow episodes of very high-quality care. Alastair Macdonald (2005) has argued eloquently for the routine measurement of outcomes, using such scales as the Health of the Nation Outcome Scales for Older People (HoNOS65+; Burns et al., 1999). Attaining this goal should be enhanced by the introduction of a national clinical electronic record system.

Evaluation of services takes various forms. Research plays a part in this, but health services research may be complex and costly. As mentioned above, RCTs are relatively rare. It is impossible for an individual service to investigate most aspects of service delivery in this way. Instead, a range of approaches are used, of which clinical audit and surveys are probably the most important. Clinical audit is a tool to measure the way in which things are being done assessed against agreed standards, leading to a cycle of making the necessary changes and then reauditing. Clinical audit is ubiquitously practised but enthusiasm for it varies markedly between practitioners. The selection of topics for audit may be both 'top-down' (imposed) or 'bottom-up' (chosen) and this may create tensions. There may be limited administrative resources to support the work and the evidence that audit leads to better outcomes for patients is predictably thin.

Other approaches to measuring and improving service quality include diverse internal activities, such as complaints reporting and investigations of untoward incidents. These may suggest obvious improvements in local policies or procedures. Comparative data are now gathered across organizations in the UK, though difficulties in interpretation mean that such data are more often used to allocate resources or plan services (for example bed numbers) than as comparators of quality. External inspections by outside bodies, such as the Healthcare Commission or the Mental Health Act Commission, in the UK, also provide a lot information on the quality of services, much of which is publicly accessible.

In recent years there has been increased emphasis on the contribution of consumers in the evaluation of health care. 'Consumers' includes patients, carers, and the wider public, though it is usually just the first two groups who are involved in service evaluation. In old age mental health, carers often act as proxies for patients, especially for people with dementia, but it is important to recognize that the interests of patients and carers do not necessarily coincide (Dening and Lawton, 1998).

Some organizations will have user and carer input at board level, which enables consumers to influence planning and policy as well as evaluation. Consumers should certainly be represented in local clinical governance processes, for example on clinical governance committees. Patients and carers can play an important part in clinical audit, for example in the selection of topics for audit, in the gathering of data, and in deciding what action needs to be taken when the information is available. More often, in practice, patients and carers may be involved in surveys, for example of their satisfaction with particular parts of the service (wards, clinics etc.) or with particular treatments.

Quality, therefore, is a concept both simple and complex. A commitment to quality must run through an old age psychiatry service. This includes keeping abreast of developments in the field and applying them appropriately to the local context, and having an inquisitive and critical attitude in measuring how the service performs and how it may be continually improved. It remains the case that service quality arises from the practitioners who provide the service, and without their energy, enthusiasm, and enterprise, purely 'top-down' or managerial approaches to quality will not be successful.

## Resources and rationing

Across the world, resources available for older people's mental health services are limited, but in varying ways. In developing countries, access to any form of health care may be a problem, but in a developed country there may be limited access to magnetic resonance scans or antidementia drugs. Available resources depend on such factors as the national health budget for the country, the allocation of health spending within the total budget, attitudes to providing services for older people and/or those with mental health problems, and the ways in which decisions about rationing are made. The main influence on the total amount appears to be gross domestic product (GDP), which correlates quite well despite some variations between countries. Political and cultural factors are probably more influential than empirical evidence in determining national levels of spending.

Three main factors determine how money is allocated within health, namely efficiency (including cost-effectiveness), equity, and political considerations (Musgrove 1999). Efficiency includes clinical effectiveness, for example as demonstrated by RCTs, but also cost-effectiveness and benefit (Maynard, 2001). In the UK, the National Institute for Health and Clinical Excellence (NICE) considers cost-effectiveness in decisions about public funding for new treatments.

Equity is a complex concept (Culyer, 2001), though it does not necessarily mean equality of access or treatment. A sense of fairness, of justice, of equivalent access to advice and treatment should be fundamental to the way that most publicly funded services are organized, and so therefore to mental health services for older people in almost any part of the world. Not all systems rate equity so highly, so that in private insurance-funded systems, issues of individuality and choice might be seen as more important.

The notion of *need* is central to equity, as equity is about the level of funding or service to provide for a given level of need but, unfortunately, there is no single agreed definition of need (Culyer, 2001). For example, equity may be considered at a macro (population) level or a micro (individual) level; there are differences between

equity of health status and equity of health care. Should needs meet with the same response, or should responses be proportionate to needs? If so, where do costs fit in to the decision process? Equity may be applied in relation to geographical area, age, social/cultural background, and the nature of the disability or disease. It can also refer to the spread and ease of access to services as well as the appropriateness of services for particular groups.

How can the needs of different diagnostic and care groups can be validly compared.? Do some tasks have priority over others: for example does saving a life have a greater claim than offering care over a period of time for someone with a disability? Various measures are proposed, the most widely known being quality-adjusted life years (QALYs), but all of them have problems. Such measures are often ageist as they take into account the life expectancy after the intervention. Another real practical problem for mental health is how to decide between two approaches to equity, namely maximizing patient welfare with the available budget versus giving priority to those in most need (Griffiths *et al.*, 2000).

As well as these problems, health equity neglects other forms of socio-economic inequality, although socio-economic factors are probably the biggest determinant of health inequality. This suggests that health equity is not an end in itself but represents a utilitarian goal (Lindbladh *et al.*, 1998).

### Rationing

There will always be an excess of need (or demand) for health care above the resources available, so decisions will be taken about the allocation of spending and of the care available to patients. One definition of rationing is a 'failure to offer care or the denial of care from which patients would benefit' (Maynard, 1999). Mechanic (1995) distinguishes between explicit and implicit forms of rationing. Recently, explicit rationing has grown with fixed budgets and the development of eligibility criteria and rating systems based on the values given to certain outcomes. Managed care in the USA is probably the most developed such system. Methods of determining 'core services' or including the public voice in places such as Oregon and New Zealand have received attention (e.g. Cumming, 1997; New, 1998).

However, in practice, most rationing follows a more mixed course and at all levels people seem reluctant to take really hard decisions. For example, in the UK budgets are set centrally but then the responsibility for them is devolved to local level, with obvious potential risks for efficiency and equity (Sheldon and Smith 2000). In part, this may reflect politicians' wishes not to be held directly responsible for unpopular decisions.

It remains debatable who should take decisions about tough choices. Some regard the issue as an empirical one, that better research will eventually guide us to the correct choices (Williams 2001), while others (e.g. Mechanic 1995) argue that attempts at explicit rationing are unstable as they simply focus conflict and dissatisfaction. It may be useful to arrive at a consensus of 'medically futile treatment' that prolongs survival at all costs, irrespective of any quality of life (Zucker and Zucker 1997) or to agree limits on the infinite quest for perfect health (Callahan, 1998), but these issues remain controversial.

If rationing is not explicit, then much of the burden falls upon clinicians, who often have reservations about the task (Weinstein, 2001). Despite this, Mechanic (1995) argues largely for implicit rationing, ultimately depending on the discretion of professionals informed by practice guidelines, outcomes research, and other relevant information. Rationing remains a contentious topic, with various stakeholders vying for influence but minimal responsibility. Allocation of healthcare funding is determined by a mixture of influences, and rationing reflects these, though at a more micro level.

### Funding and old age psychiatry

Despite strong arguments for equity, older people with mental health problems are often disadvantaged in the allocation of funding, especially by a lack of advocacy and political influence, and by age discrimination, in particular the use of age as a rationing criterion.

Using age as a criterion on which to base rationing decisions has been both proposed (e.g. Daniels, 1988; Shaw, 1994) and opposed (e.g. Rivlin, 1995; Evans, 1997; Clarke, 2001). The arguments include, among others, the 'long innings' argument and concerns about the expense of treating old people using resources that could be better used elsewhere. The first argument is fallacious as it is clearly wrong to esteem the lives of all younger people above those of all older people simply on the basis of their chronological age; and the second argument overlooks the fact that most health spending on older people is not for high-tech acute treatment but for less intensive support for chronic conditions like dementia or arthritis (Rivlin, 1995). Perhaps also society has special duties and obligations towards older people to ensure that their needs for care are met (Jecker and Pearlman, 1989)—it is often stated that the quality of society can be ascertained from how it treats its older people. In addition, age discrimination equates to a form of gender discrimination, given the longer life expectancy of women (Jecker, 1991).

Overall, government policy opposes using age as an eligibility criterion. As mentioned above, 'rooting out age discrimination' is the first among eight standards in the English NSF for Older People (Department of Health, 2001a). It states that 'National Health services will be provided, regardless of age, on the basis of clinical need alone. Social care services will not use age in their eligibility criteria or policies, to restrict access to available services'. Thus, using age as an explicit criterion is not allowed, though it is harder to tell if age is still being used covertly.

Funding may be inequitable for other reasons, for example, as in the USA, where there is an emphasis upon acute episodes of care rather than long-term needs and reimbursement for mental disorders is paid at a lower rate than for physical illness. These factors influence how and where patients present with various types of complaint (Callahan, 2001). Setting priorities for mental health may require different assumptions from those underpinning acute care, for example that it is a legitimate goal of medicine to offer services to people for relief of pain and suffering or to provide prolonged care even if they cannot be cured (Callahan, 1994, 1999). The actual allocation of resources depends on how competing principles such as efficiency, equity, local consumer views, and local availability of skills and treatments are resolved at a local level (Rosenheck, 1999).

Another example of inequity in funding applies to long-term care for older people in England. Despite the recommendations of a government-appointed Royal Commission (1999) that all long-term care for older people should be provided free of charge, the Department of Health in England has introduced a system where nursing care is provided without charge, but other forms of care are means tested and charged for. This discriminates against people with dementia or other mental health problems as they are not in receipt of care which meets the official definition of nursing care.

## Specialist training and research in old age psychiatry

One important sign of a robust speciality is the development of specialist training programmes and their recognition by official bodies. For old age psychiatry, this has closely matched the development of older people's mental health services. Various curricula and training guidelines have been developed since the late 1970s but formal criteria for training in old age psychiatry were first adopted in the UK in 1989, followed by programmes in the USA, Canada, and Australasia (Draper, 2003).

The European Association of Geriatric Psychiatry, in collaboration with the World Health Organization and the World Psychiatric Association Section of Psychiatry of the Elderly, has published a consensus curriculum of skill-based objectives for specialist training in old age psychiatry (Gustafson *et al.*, 2003). The curriculum comprises 22 areas of competence and learning objectives. These include clinical skills such as recognition of mental health problems, history taking, and physical examination; relevant areas of knowledge including ageing and the mental disorders of old age; treatment, management, and care as well as the organization of services. There are some rather specific domains, including end-of-life issues and elder abuse. The last few areas of competence in the list are also general topics, such as prevention, teaching, knowledge management, and research. The curriculum is likely to help the development of old age psychiatry programmes in countries where this is under consideration, though the areas of competence are not operationally defined and the curriculum does not provide much guidance as to how they should be assessed.

Another problem is that the curriculum relates to old age *psychiatry* and not other mental health professions. There is considerable scope for developing nursing skills, not just in relation to drug treatments and prescribing (Voyer and Martin, 2003). In the USA, particularly because of poor recruitment to geriatric psychiatry programmes, the emphasis has been more multidisciplinary. Also, the need for adequate training and research activity as an integral part of service developments has been more strongly argued by American authors (Halpain *et al.*, 1999; Jeste *et al.*, 1999; Bartels, 2003). Halpain *et al.* (1999) provided estimates of the numbers of various professional groups that would be needed within the next decade or more, for example up to 5000 geriatric psychiatrists with 400–500 academic psychiatrists. These authors also made suggestions as to how late-life mental disorders should be part of wider health and public education, as well as for students (Halpain *et al.*, 2005) and in speciality programmes. Jeste *et al.* (1999) described an 'upcoming crisis in geriatric mental health' characterized by inadequate research infrastructure, health funding, trained personnel, and healthcare delivery systems. They argued for a strategic research agenda in this area to stimulate interest, funding, training, and service development. Bartels (2003), reporting to the President's New Freedom Commission on Mental Health, identified 10 major policy issues, which were grouped into three overarching themes: access and continuity of services; quality; and workforce and caregiver capacity. Each of these was used to make specific policy recommendations, including such measures as outreach and integrated services, service coordination, [combating] stigma and cultural sensitivity, implementation of evidence-based practices, increasing numbers of providers, and enhancing caregiver and peer support services.

For the future, we can expect to see recognized training curricula becoming established in more countries. In those countries with recognized old age psychiatry programmes, in keeping with general educational trends, there will be more emphasis on acquiring specific competencies, replacement of formal examinations with other forms of assessment, and active moves towards more multidisciplinary teaching and learning in both basic and specialist training.

## Challenges and future issues

### Population change

It is generally accepted that the biggest challenge to services for old people across the world is posed by demographic change and the ageing population. This takes different forms in different countries. At present, the developed countries of Europe, Japan, and North America have the highest percentages of people aged 65 and over in their populations. Over the next 20–30 years, numbers of older people will continue to increase but the greatest increase will be in the numbers of very old people, those aged 85 and above.

In contrast, developing countries have lower percentages of old people but in general their populations are ageing at a faster rate. That is, numbers of people aged over 65 will increase by a greater proportion than in Europe or North America; and, as certain countries (China, India, Indonesia, for example) have very large total populations, the absolute numbers of older people in these countries will grow very rapidly. Thus, the number of people with dementia in developing countries will soon, if it does not already, exceed the number in the developed world.

These changes affect mental health and old age psychiatry in several ways. Obviously, there will be more old people with mental health problems, including an estimated 32 million people with dementia by 2025 (Prince and Trebilco, 2005). Levels of other forms of illness and disability will also rise, and where the numbers of very old people are growing rapidly this will mean more complex co-morbidity of physical and mental disorders. At the same time, an increasing proportion of retired people will affect the national economy, especially if the working age population is not expanding. This has both economic and workforce effects on the resources that are available for the health and social services available to older people.

### Scientific advances

It is of course impossible to predict what scientific discoveries may influence the future course of mental disorders in old age. At present, no single development seems likely to have a startling impact upon conditions such as Alzheimer's disease. Better general health may affect dementia and depression too, though this is difficult to demonstrate. The future availability of pre-symptomatic diagnosis of dementia would have an impact upon the demand for services. Clinicians will become adept at using currently available treatments more efficiently. For example, perhaps Alzheimer's disease may respond better to a combination of several treatments, rather than a single drug such as a cholinesterase inhibitor. It will, however, be difficult to do RCTs to investigate combined treatments as large numbers of patients will be required. In the treatment of depression and psychotic illnesses, improved use of newer antidepressant, mood-stabilizing, and antipsychotic drugs, together with use of combined treatments, will bring better outcomes with fewer side-effects for many patients.

In the immediate future, however, it is most likely that older people will be most helped by the more effective provision of services. Simple routes of referrals, prompt and efficient assessments, access to specialized treatment when needed, care and support at home wherever possible, all backed up by effective care coordination, are all elements of good services that are supported by evidence. In keeping with trends across the whole of medicine (and indeed, society in general), it can predicted that the voice of patients and carers as consumers will become more powerful and this too will influence the type of services available and how they are provided.

The quality of services can also be improved by the application of information and communications technology, in various ways, such as improved access to information for users and carers through the Internet to the application of (often simple) devices in the individual's home to provide prompts and reminders or to activate alarms. Technology is likely to be used increasingly to provide contact with services across long distances, for example in rural areas. Finally, the potential of electronic care records is yet to be fully realized as systems are only now being established, but it is probable that individuals will take a much more active role in their health care by taking responsibility for the record. This could transform the current relationship between consumers and providers of services.

### Boundaries

As described above, old age psychiatry arose in response to a set of circumstances, including neglect and excessive use of institutional care. In most instances, service developments have been led by service providers, especially psychiatrists, and this has been criticized for leading to undue emphasis on clinical issues as opposed to the wider social context (Finch, 2004). It is true that a more rational approach would be to start at the level of public-health, with commissioners leading an integrated framework of health and social services, but the reality is usually that mental health services for older people are often neglected in favour of more 'glamorous' areas, so the role of providers as champions of the agenda is far from finished.

Old age psychiatry has usually kept certain boundaries, providing services for all patients above a specified age (usually 65), with some variations, e.g. whether or not they cater for younger patients with dementia (Royal College of Psychiatrists, 2000) or older patients with schizophrenia or other severe mental illness who have been cared for by rehabilitation services. These boundaries are currently under challenge. Sixty-five has been a convenient age as it is the UK retirement age for men and also it is around this age that the prevalence and incidence of dementia start to rise sharply. However, there are now proposals to increase the retirement age, and it can also be argued that it is ageist to provide a service that is defined by a criterion of a certain age. Certainly many people of pensionable years do not regard themselves as old and may resent being referred to old age services simply because they are (say) 66.

If the age criterion is abandoned, there may be pressure on old age psychiatry services to concentrate on dementia, with functional illnesses remaining the province of general adult psychiatry. There are some problems with this. One of the most important skills of old age psychiatrists is the differential diagnosis between dementia and other forms of mental disorder. They are also expert in assessing the complex interplay between multiple factors like cognitive disorder, mood disturbance, physical illness, and medication. These issues are almost always relevant in older patients, even those who have had episodes of psychiatric disorder in earlier life, as it is often subtle changes in presentation that indicate the emergence of a new problem. These are not the core skills of most general adult psychiatrists, so it seems retrograde to assert that old age psychiatry should not treat functional illness for the sake of political correctness. Furthermore, this line of thinking ignores the way in which older people are often neglected or even terrorized in mixed age settings, where the attention is often on the most disturbed and aggressive individuals.

Thus, in the view of this author, older people with mental health problems of all kinds are likely to benefit from age-based specialist services. There is clearly room for flexibility—reaching a given age should be a prompt for considering which service may be preferred or may be more appropriate, rather than a rigidly applied rule. It is well accepted that clear processes are needed to manage the process of transition from working age to old age mental health services. These must be equitably applied, otherwise there is a risk of favouritism or the dumping of inconvenient patients on the new service.

Other boundary issues will be important in shaping the future of old age psychiatry. These include relationships with other old age specialists, primary care, and social care. In developed countries such as the UK, where the numbers of very old people are increasing rapidly, this means that many new patients will have increasingly complicated medical histories with several physical problems and complex lists of drugs. This will require closer working relationships with geriatric medicine to ensure that patients receive adequate physical assessment as well as treatment of mental health problems.

As regards primary care, it is to be hoped that general practitioners can be helped to be more confident about making diagnoses in older people, and probably that they will gradually assume most of the responsibility for cholinesterase treatments for dementia. In England, social care teams are now often integrated with primary care teams, and there may be teams aimed at preventing inappropriate admissions to hospital. This may have implications for specialist community mental health teams, which may be encouraged to merge with the generic older peoples' teams. This is probably better in theory than in practice: such initiatives usually lead to the relative neglect of mental health issues, especially people with functional disorders who do not fall easily into the 'vulnerable elderly at risk' models that are used in such work. Perhaps a model of service delivery based on tiers of ascending order of complexity needs to be negotiated and established (Draper *et al.*, 2006). Such a model already operates with child and adolescent mental health services in the UK.

Lastly, an obvious trend in old age mental health services has been the significant decrease in the amount of care directly provided by specialist services. This includes the large reduction in inpatient beds, starting with long-stay beds for people with dementia but more recently in bed numbers generally, and also reductions in day hospital places and respite care. At the time of writing, in the UK, this trend shows no sign of abating. This has two main implications. The first is that much less psychiatric work is done in mental hospital settings and much more on a consultative basis in other premises—people's homes, day centres, care homes, and general hospitals. In general, this is to be welcomed, as it seems a better use of scarce mental health skills and can be used to reach a greater number of people who need assessment and treatment. The second implication is perhaps that the future may not include inpatient care at all. While this would fit with certain political directions, it would be highly unfortunate to lose the capacity to carry out clinical and behavioural assessments of older people in specialist facilities. Who else would relish the challenge of psychotically depressed suicidal patients with complex medical problems, or someone with dementia and noisy, aggressive behaviour?

## Comment

Thus, there are plenty of problems and challenges facing old age psychiatry and its position seems under some pressure at present. In a time of change, we are constantly reminded that nothing is for ever. But there are some areas in which to be confident. There will be no shortage of mental health need among older people and there will always be a need for skilled specialist advice in dealing with complex or difficult problems. There are sound empirical arguments for specialist services in this area, and they have a good track record of delivering good services with limited resources. Old age psychiatrists and their teams remain well placed to meet the challenges of this most interesting area of clinical work for the foreseeable future.

## References

Allan, K. (2001). *Communication and consultation: exploring ways for staff to involve people with dementia in developing services.* Policy Press, Bristol.

Alzheimer's Society (2002). *Let's make it happen.* Alzheimer's Society, London.

Anderson, D.N. and Aquilina, C. (2002). Domiciliary clinics I: effects on non-attendance. *International Journal of Geriatric Psychiatry*, **17**, 941–944.

Aquilina, C. and Anderson, D. (2002). Domiciliary clinics II: a cost minimisation analysis. *International Journal of Geriatric Psychiatry*, **17**, 945–949.

Argyle, N., Jestice, S., and Brook, C.P. (1985). Psychogeriatric patients: their supporters' problems. *Age and Ageing*, **14**, 355–360.

Arie, T. (1970). The first year of the Goodmayes psychiatric service for old people. *Lancet*, **ii**, 1179–1182.

Arie, T. (1989). Martin Roth and the 'Psychogeriatricians'. In *Contemporary themes in psychiatry: a tribute to Sir Martin Roth* (ed. K. Davison and A. Kerr), pp. 231–238. Gaskell, London.

Arie, T. and Jolley, D. (1982). Making services work: organisation and style of psychogeriatric services. In *The psychiatry of late life* (ed. R. Levy and F. Post), pp. 222–251. Blackwell, Oxford.

Ashaye, O.A., Livingston, G., and Orrell, M. (2003). Does standardised needs assessment improve the outcome of psychiatric day hospital care for older people? *Aging and Mental Health*, **7**, 195–199.

Audini, B., Lelliott, P., Banerjee, S., Goddard, C., Wattis, J., and Wilson, K. (2001). *Old age psychiatric day hospital survey.* Royal College of Psychiatrists Research Unit, London.

Audit Commission (2000). *Forget me not: mental health services for older people.* Audit Commission, London.

Baldwin, R., Pratt, H., Goring, H., Marriott, A., and Roberts, C. (2004). Does a nurse-led mental health liaison service for older people reduce psychiatric morbidity in acute general medical wards? A randomised controlled trial. *Age and Ageing*, **33**, 472–478.

Baltes, P.B. and Mayer, K.U. (eds) (1999). *The Berlin Aging Study: aging from 70 to 100*. Cambridge University Press, Cambridge.

Banerjee, S. and Dickinson, E. (1997). Evidence-based health care in old age psychiatry. *International Journal of Psychiatry in Medicine*, **27**, 283–292.

Banerjee, S., Murray, J., Foley, B., Atkins, L., Schneider, J., and Mann, A. (2003). Predictors of institutionalisation in people with dementia. *Journal of Neurology Neurosurgery and Psychiatry*, **74**, 1315–1316.

Barnett, E. (2000). *Including the person with dementia in designing and delivering care: 'I need to be me!'*. Jessica Kingsley, London.

Bartels, S.J. (2003). Improving the system of care for older adults with mental illness in the United States: findings and recommendations for the President's New Freedom Commission on Mental Health. *American Journal of Geriatric Psychiatry*, **11**, 486–497.

Bartels, S.J., Dums, A.R., Oxman, T.E. *et al.*(2002). Evidence-based practices in geriatric mental health care. *Psychiatric Services*, **53**, 1419–1431.

Bartels, S.J., Dums, A.R., Oxman, T.E. *et al.* (2003). Evidence-based practices in geriatric mental health care: an overview of systematic reviews and meta-analyses. *Psychiatric Clinics of North America*, **26**, 971–990.

Bedard, M., Koivuranta, A., and Stuckey, A. (2004). Health impact on caregivers of providing informal care to a cognitively impaired older adult: rural versus urban settings. *Canadian Journal of Rural Medicine*, **9**, 15–23.

Bedford, S., Melzer, D., Dening, T. *et al.* (1996). What becomes of people with dementia referred to community mental health teams? *International Journal of Geriatric Psychiatry*, **11**, 1051–1056.

Blazer, D. (2000). Psychiatry and the oldest old. *American Journal of Psychiatry*, **157**, 1915–1924.

Bosanquet, N. (2001). The socioeconomic impact of Alzheimer's disease. *International Journal of Geriatric Psychiatry*, **16**, 249–253.

Bowers, H., Eastman, M., Harris, J., and Macadam, A. (2005). *Moving out of the shadows: a report on mental health and wellbeing in later life*. Help and Care Development, London.

Briscoe, J., Orwin, D., Ashton, L., and Burdett, J. (2005). *Being there: a peer support service for older adults with mental illness*. Health Research Council of New Zealand, Auckland.

Brodaty, H., Gresham, M., and Luscombe, G. (1997). The Prince Henry Hospital dementia caregivers' training programme. *International Journal of Geriatric Psychiatry*, **12**, 183–192.

Brodaty, H., Green, A., and Korschera, A. (2003). Meta-analysis of psychosocial interventions for caregivers of people with dementia. *Journal of the American Geriatrics Society*, **51**, 657–64.

Burns, A., Beevor, A., Lelliott, P. *et al.* (1999). Health of the Nation Outcome Scales for Older People (HoNOS65+). *British Journal of Psychiatry*, **174**, 424–427.

Burns, A., Dening, T., and Lawlor, B. (2002). *Clinical guidelines in old age psychiatry*. Dunitz, London.

Burns, A., Lawlor, B., and Craig, S. (2003). *Assessment scales in old age psychiatry*, 2nd edn. Dunitz, London.

Burns, A., O'Brien, J., and Ames, D. (2005). *Dementia*, 3rd edn. Hodder Arnold, London.

Callahan, C.M. (2001). Geriatric psychiatry from a geriatrician's viewpoint. *Psychiatric Bulletin*, **25**, 149–150.

Callahan, C.M., Boustani, M.A., Unverzagt, F.W. *et al.* (2006). Effectiveness of collaborative care for older adults with Alzheimer disease: a randomized controlled trial. *Journal of the American Medical Association*, **295**, 2148–2157.

Callahan, D. (1994). Setting mental health priorities: problems and possibilities. *Milbank Quarterly*, **72**, 451–470.

Callahan, D. (1998). *False hopes: why America's quest for perfect health is a recipe for failure*. Simon and Schuster, New York.

Callahan, D. (1999). Balancing efficiency and need in allocating resources to care of persons with serious mental illness. *Psychiatric Services*, **50**, 664–666.

Camus, V., Katona, C., de Medonça Lima, C.A. *et al.* (2003). Teaching and training in old age psychiatry: a general survey of the World Psychiatric Association member societies. *International Journal of Geriatric Psychiatry*, **18**, 694–699.

Care Services Improvement Partnership (2005a). *Everybody's business: integrated mental health services for older adults: a service development guide*. CSIP, London.

Care Services Improvement Partnership (2005b). *Moving on: key learning from Rowan Ward*. CSIP, London.

Chalifoux, Z., Neese, J.B., Buckwalter, K.C., Litwak, E., and Abraham, I.L. (1996). Mental health services for rural elderly: innovative service strategies. *Community Mental Health Journal*, **32**, 463–480.

Challis, D., von Abendorff, R., Brown, P., Chesterman, J., and Hughes, J. (2002). Care management, dementia care and specialist mental health services: an evaluation. *International Journal of Geriatric Psychiatry*, **17**, 315–325.

Ciechanowski, P., Wagner, E., Schmaling, K. *et al.* (2004). Community-integrated home-based depression treatment in older adults: a randomized controlled trial. *Journal of the American Medical Association*, **291**, 1569–1577.

Clarke, C.M. (2001). Rationing scarce life-sustaining resources on the basis of age. *Journal of Advanced Nursing*, **35**, 799–804.

Cole, M.G. (1993). The impact of geriatric medical services on mental state. *International Psychogeriatrics*, **5**, 91–101.

Collighan, G., Macdonald, A., Herzberg, J., Philpot, M., and Lindesay, J. (1993). An evaluation of the multidisciplinary approach to psychiatric diagnosis in elderly people. *British Medical Journal*, **306**, 821–824.

Commission for Health Improvement (2000). *Investigation into the North Lakeland NHS Trust*. CHI, London.

Commission for Health Improvement (2003). *Investigation into matters arising from care on Rowan Ward, Manchester Mental Health and Social Care Trust*. The Stationery Office, London.

Culyer, A.J. (2001). Equity – some theory and its policy implications. *Journal of Medical Ethics*, **27**, 275–283.

Cumming, J. (1997). Defining core services: New Zealand experience. *Journal of Health Services Research and Policy*, **2**, 31–37.

Daniels, N. (1988). *Am I my brother's keeper? An essay on justice between the young and old*. Oxford University Press, New York.

Dening, T. and Gabe, R. (2000). Disability and contact with services in very old people. *Reviews in Clinical Gerontology*, **10**, 291–309.

Dening, T. and Lawton, C. (1998). The role of carers in evaluating mental health services for older people. *International Journal of Geriatric Psychiatry*, **13**, 863–870.

Dening, T. and Shaji, K.S. (2005). Psychogeriatric service delivery with limited resources. In *Psychogeriatric service delivery: an international perspective* (ed. B. Draper, P. Melding, and H. Brodaty), pp. 327–344. Oxford University Press, Oxford.

Department of Health (1999). *National Service Framework for Mental Health*. Department of Health, London.

Department of Health (2000). *No secrets*. Department of Health, London.

Department of Health (2001a). *National Service Framework for Older People*. Department of Health, London.

Department of Health (2001b). *Valuing people: a new strategy for learning disability for the 21st century*. Department of Health, London.

Department of Health and Social Security (1972). *Services for mental illness related to old age*. HMSO, London.

Draper, B. (2000). The effectiveness of old age psychiatry services. *International Journal of Geriatric Psychiatry*, **15**, 687–703.

Draper, B. (2003). Training in old age psychiatry. *International Journal of Geriatric Psychiatry*, **18**, 683–685.

Draper, B. and Low, L.F. (2005a). Evidence-based psychogeriatric service delivery. In *Psychogeriatric service delivery: an international perspective* (ed. B. Draper, P. Melding, and H. Brodaty), pp. 75–123. Oxford University Press, Oxford.

Draper, B. and Low, L.F. (2005b). What is the effectiveness of acute hospital treatment of older people with mental disorders? *International Psychogeriatrics*, **17**, 539–555.

Draper, B., Melding, P., and Brodaty, H. (eds) (2005). *Psychogeriatric service delivery: an international perspective*. Oxford University Press, Oxford.

Draper, B., Brodaty, H., and Low, L.F. (2006). A tiered model of psychogeriatric service delivery: an evidence-based approach. *International Journal of Geriatric Psychiatry*, **21**, 645–653.

Evandrou, M. (2000). Social inequalities in later life. *Population Trends*, **101**, 11–18.

Evans, J.G. (1997). The rationing debate: rationing health care by age: the case against. *British Medical Journal*, **314**, 822–825.

Faculty of Old Age Psychiatry (2006). *Raising the standard: specialist services for older people with mental illness*. Royal College of Psychiatrists, London.

Farmer, J., Hinds, K., Richards, H., and Godden, D. (2005). Urban versus rural populations' view of health care in Scotland. *Journal of Health Service Research and Policy*, **10**, 212–219.

Fasey, C. (1994). The day hospital in old age psychiatry: the case against. *International Journal of Geriatric Psychiatry*, **9**, 519–523.

Fazel, S., Hope, T., O'Donnell, I., and Jacoby, R. (2001). Hidden psychiatric morbidity in elderly prisoners. *British Journal of Psychiatry*, **179**, 535–539.

Finch, J. (2004). *Evaluating mental health services for older people*. Radcliffe, Abingdon.

Flaherty, J.H., McBride, M., Marzouk, S. *et al.* (1998). Decreasing hospitalization rates for older home care patients with symptoms of depression. *Journal of the American Geriatrics Society*, **46**, 31–38.

Foundation for People with Learning Disabilities (2002). *Today and tomorrow: the report of the Growing Older with Learning Disabilities (GOLD) programme*. Foundation for People with Learning Disabilities, London.

Gibson, F. and Whittington, D. (1995). *Day care in rural areas*, Social Care Research Report 7. Joseph Rowntree Foundation, York.

Goins, R.T., Kategile, U., and Dudley K.C. (2001). Telemedicine, rural elderly, and policy issues. *Journal of Aging and Social Policy*, **13**, 53–71.

Griffiths, S., Reynolds, J., and Hope, T. (2000). Priority setting in practice. In *The global challenge of health care rationing* (ed. A. Coulter and C. Ham), pp. 203–213. Open University Press, Buckingham.

Gustafson, L., Burns, A., Katona, C. *et al.* (2003). Skill-based objectives for specialist training in old age psychiatry. *International Journal of Geriatric Psychiatry*, **18**, 686–693.

Halpain, M.C., Harris, M.J., McClure, F.S., and Jeste, D.V. (1999). Training in geriatric mental health: needs and strategies. *Psychiatric Services*, **50**, 1205–1208.

Halpain, M.C., Jeste, D.V., Trinidad, G.I., Wetherell, J.L., and Lebowitz, B.D. (2005). Intensive short-term research training for undergraduate, graduate, and medical students: early experience with a new national-level approach in geriatric mental health. *Academic Psychiatry*, **29**, 58–65.

Head, L. and Dening, T. (1998). Lithium in the over-65s: who is taking it and who is monitoring it? *International Journal of Geriatric Psychiatry*, **13**, 164–171.

Hepburn, K.W., Lewis, M., Sherman, C.W., and Tornatore, J. (2003). The Savvy Caregiver Program: developing and testing a transportable dementia family caregiver training program. *Gerontologist*, **43**, 908–915.

Hilton, C. (2005a). The origins of old age psychiatry in Britain in the 1940s. *History of Psychiatry*, **16**, 267–289.

Hilton, C. (2005b). The clinical psychiatry of late life in Britain from 1950 to 1970: an overview. *International Journal of Geriatric Psychiatry*, **20**, 423–428.

HM Chief Inspector of Prisons (2004). '*No problems – old and quiet': older prisoners in England and Wales*. HM Inspectorate of Prisons, London.

Hoe, J., Ashaye, K., and Orrell, M. (2005). Don't seize the day hospital! Recent research on the effectiveness of day hospitals for older people with mental health problems. *International Journal of Geriatric Psychiatry*, **20**, 694–698.

Holmes, J., Bentley, K., and Cameron, I. (2003). A UK survey of psychiatric services for older people in general hospitals. *International Journal of Geriatric Psychiatry*, **18**, 716–721.

Homer, A.C. and Gilleard, C.J. (1994). The effect of inpatient respite care on elderly patients and their carers. *Age and Ageing*, **23**, 274–276.

Howard, R. (1994). The day hospital in old age psychiatry: the case in favour. *International Journal of Geriatric Psychiatry*, **9**, 525–529.

Hughes, J., Stewart, K., Challis, D., Darton, R., and Weiner, K. (2001). Care management and the care programme approach: towards integration in old age mental health services. *International Journal of Geriatric Psychiatry*, **16**, 266–272.

Iliffe, S. and Drennan, V. (2001). *Primary care and dementia*. Jessica Kingsley, London.

Innes, A., Blackstock, K., Mason, A., Smith, A., and Cox, S. (2005). Dementia care provision in rural Scotland: service users' and carers' experiences. *Health and Social Care in the Community*, **13**, 354–365.

James, A., Worrall, A., and Kendall, T. (eds) (2005). *Clinical governance in mental health and learning disability services: a practical guide*. Gaskell, London.

Jecker, N.S. (1991). Age-based rationing and women. *Journal of the American Medical Assocaition*, **266**, 3012–3015.

Jecker, N.S. and Pearlman, R.A. (1989). Ethical constraints on rationing medical care by age. *Journal of the American Geriatrics Society*, **37**, 1067–1075.

Jeste, D.V., Alexopoulos, G.S., Bartels, S.J. *et al.* (1999). Consensus statement on the upcoming crisis in geriatric mental health: research agenda for the next 2 decades. *Archives of General Psychiatry*, **56**, 848–853.

Kerslake, A., Moultrie, K., and Parsons, M. (2003). *The shape of future care for older people with mental health needs*. Institute of Public Care, Oxford.

Lee, M. (2006). *Promoting mental health and well-being in later life*. Age Concern/Mental Health Foundation, London.

Lewis, A. (1946). Ageing and senility: a major problem of psychiatry. *Journal of Mental Science*, **92**, 150–170.

Lindbladh, E., Lytttkens, C.H., Hanson, B.S., and Ostergren, P.O. (1998). Equity is out of fashion? An essay on autonomy and health policy in the individualized society. *Social Science and Medicine*, **46**, 1017–1025.

Lindesay, J., Marudkar, M., van Diepen, E., and Wilcock, G. (2002). The second Leicester survey of memory clinics in the British Isles. *International Journal of Geriatric Psychiatry*, **17**, 41–47.

Lingard, J. and Milne, A. (2004). *Integrating older people's mental health services: community mental health teams – a commentary and resource document*. Department of Health, London.

Livingston, G., Leavey, G., Kitchen, G., Manela, M., Sembhi, S., and Katona, C. (2001). Mental health of migrants – the Islington study. *British Journal of Psychiatry*, **179**, 361–366.

Llewellyn-Jones, R.H., Baikie, K.A., Smithers, H., Cohen, J., Snowdon, J., and Tennant, C.C. (1999). Multifaceted shared care intervention for late life depression in residential care: randomised controlled trial. *British Medical Journal*, **319**, 676–682.

Macdonald, A. (2005). Evaluation of service delivery. In *Psychogeriatric service delivery: an international perspective* (ed. B. Draper, P. Melding, and H. Brodaty), pp. 309–326. Oxford University Press, Oxford.

Mackenzie, C.S., Rosenberg, M., and Major, M. (2006). Evaluation of a psychiatric day hospital program for elderly patients with mood disorders. *International Psychogeriatrics*, **18**, 631–641.

Martin, P., Poon, L.W., Clayton, G.M., Lee, H.S., Fulks, J.S., and Johnson, M.A. (1992). Personality, life events and coping in the oldest-old. *International Journal of Aging and Human Development*, **34**, 19–30.

Marwaha, S. and Livingston, G. (2002). Stigma, racism or choice. Why do depressed ethnic elders avoid psychiatrists? *Journal of Affective Disorders*, **72**, 257–265.

Matthews, F., Brayne, C., and MRC Cognitive Function and Ageing Study Investigators (2005). The incidence of dementia in England and Wales: findings from the five identical sites of the MRC CFA study. *Public Library of Science Medicine*, **2**, e193.

Maynard, A. (1999). Rationing health care: an exploration. *Health Policy*, **49**, 5–11.

Maynard, A. (2001). Ethics and health care 'underfunding'. *Journal of Medical Ethics*, **27**, 223–227.

Mechanic, D. (1995). Dilemmas in rationing health care services: the case for implicit rationing. *British Medical Journal*, **310**, 1655–1659.

Melzer, D., Bedford, S., Dening, T. *et al.* (1996). Carers and the monitoring of psychogeriatric community teams. *International Journal of Geriatric Psychiatry*, **11**, 1057–1061.

Melzer, D., Pearce, K., Cooper, B., and Brayne, C. (1999). Epidemiologically based needs assessment: Alzheimer's disease and other dementias. In *Health care and needs assessment: the epidemiologically based needs assessment reviews – first series update* (ed. A. Stevens *et al.*), pp. 235–248. Radcliffe, Abingdon.

Mittelman, M.S., Ferris, S.H., Shulman, E., Steinberg, G., and Levin, B. (1996). A family intervention to delay nursing home placement of patients with Alzheimer disease. A randomized controlled trial. *Journal of the American Medical Association*, **276**, 1725–1731.

Moise, P., Schwarzinger, M., Um, M-Y., and the Dementia Experts Group (2004). *Dementia care in 9 OECD countries: a comparative analysis*, OECD Working Paper no. 13. OECD, Paris.

Morgan, D.G., Semchuk, K.M., Stewart, N.J., and D'Arcy, C. (2002). Rural families caring for a relative with dementia: barriers to use of formal services. *Social Science and Medicine*, **55**, 1129–1142.

Musgrove, P. (1999). Public spending on health care: how are different criteria related? *Health Policy*, **47**, 207–223.

National Collaborating Centre for Mental Health (2007). *Dementia: A NICE–SCIE Guideline on supporting people with dementia and their carers in health and social care*. British Psychological Society/Gaskell, London.

National Institute for Health and Clinical Excellence (2006). *NICE technology appraisal guidance 111: Donepezil, galantamine, rivastigmine (review) and memantine for the treament of Alzheimer's disease*. NICE, London.

National Mental Health Partnership (2005). *Commissioning and developing mental health services for older people: a briefing paper for policy makers, commissioners and service providers*. NMHP, London.

New, B. (ed.) (1998). *Rationing: talk and action in health care*. BMJ Publishing Group, London.

Nnatu, I.O., Mahomed, F., and Shah, A. (2005). Is there a need for elderly forensic services? *Medicine Science and Law*, **45**, 154–160.

Norquist, G., Wells, K.B., Rogers, W.H. *et al.* (1995). Quality of care for depressed elderly patients hospitalized in the specialty psychiatric units or general medical wards. *Archives of General Psychiatry*, **52**, 695–701.

O'Connor, D.W., Pollitt, P.A., Brook, C.P., Reiss, B.B., and Roth, M. (1991). Does early intervention reduce the number of elderly people with dementia admitted to institutions for long term care? *British Medical Journal*, **302**, 871–875.

Orrell, M. and Hancock, G. (2004). *CANE: Camberwell Assessment of Need for the Elderly*. Gaskell, London.

Orrell, M. and Katona, C. (1998). Do consultant home visits have a future in old age psychiatry? *International Journal of Geriatric Psychiatry*, **13**, 355–357.

Patel, N., Mirza, N.R., Lindblad, P., Amstrup, K., and Samaoli, O. (1998). *Dementia and minority ethnic older people: managing care in the UK, Denmark and France*. Russell House, London.

Pelosi, A.J., McNulty, S.V., and Jackson, G.A. (2006). Role of cholinesterase inhibitors in dementia care needs rethinking. *British Medical Journal*, **333**, 491–493.

Philp, I. and Appleby, L. (2005). *Securing better mental health for older adults*. Department of Health, London.

Philp, I., McKee, K.J., Meldrum, P. *et al.* (1995). Community care for demented and non-demented elderly people: a comparison study of financial burden, service use, and unmet needs in family supporters. *British Medical Journal*, **310**, 1503–1506.

Philpot, M., Drahman, I., Ball, C., and Macdonald, A. (2000). The prognosis of late-life depression in two contiguous old age psychiatry services: an exploratory study. *Aging and Mental Health*, **4**, 72–78.

Phipps, A.J. and O'Brien, J.T. (2002). Memory clinics and clinical governance – a UK perspective. *International Journal of Geriatric Psychiatry*, **17**, 1128–1132.

Post, F. (1944). Some problems arising from a study of mental patients over the age of 60 years. *Journal of Mental Science*, **90**, 554–565.

Post, F. (1962). *The significance of affective symptoms in old age: a follow up study of 100 patients*, Maudsley Monograph no. 10. Oxford University Press, Oxford.

Post, F. (1965). *The clinical psychiatry of late life*. Pergamon, Oxford.

Prince, M. and Trebilco, P. (2005). Mental health services for older people: a developing countries perspective. In *Psychogeriatric service delivery: an international perspective* (ed. B. Draper, P. Melding, and H. Brodaty), pp. 33–53. Oxford University Press, Oxford.

Ratna, L. (1982). Crisis intervention in psychogeriatrics: a two-year follow-up study. *British Journal of Psychiatry*, **141**, 296–301.

Reilly, S., Challis, D., Burns, A., and Hughes, J. (2003). Does integration really make a difference? A comparison of old age psychiatry services in England and Northern Ireland. *International Journal of Geriatric Psychiatry*, **18**, 887–893.

Rivlin, M.M. (1995). Protecting elderly people: flaws in ageist arguments. *British Medical Journal*, **310**, 1179–1182.

Rosenheck, R.A. (1999). Principles for priority setting in mental health services and their implications for the least well off. *Psychiatric Services*, **50**, 653–658.

Roth, M. (1955). The natural history of mental disorder in old age. *Journal of Mental Science*, **101**, 281–301.

Royal College of Psychiatrists/Royal College of Physicians (1998). *The care of older people with mental illness: specialist services and medical training*. Royal College of Psychiatrists/Royal College of Physicians, London.

Royal College of Psychiatrists (2000). *Services for younger people with Alzheimer's disease and other dementias*. Royal College of Psychiatrists, London.

Royal College of Psychiatrists (2005a). *Forgetful but not forgotten: assessment and aspects of treatment of people with dementia by a specialist old age psychiatry service*. Royal College of Psychiatrists, London.

Royal College of Psychiatrists (2005b). *Who care wins: improving the outcome for older people admitted to the general hospital*. Royal College of Psychiatrists, London.

Royal Commission on Long Term Care (1999). *With respect to old age: long term care – rights and responsibilities*. The Stationery Office, London.

Sadavoy, J., Meier, R., and Ong, A.Y. (2004). Barriers to access to mental health services for ethnic seniors: the Toronto study. *Canadian Journal of Psychiatry*, **49**, 192–199.

Samuelsson, S.M., Alfredson, B.B., Hagberg, B. *et al.* (1997). The Swedish Centenarian Study: a multi-disciplinary study of five consecutive cohorts at the age of 100. *International Journal of Aging and Human Development*, **45**, 223–253.

Scally, G. and Donaldson, L.J. (1998). Clinical governance and the drive for quality improvement in the new NHS in England. *British Medical Journal*, **317**, 61–65.

Schrader, G., Cheok, F., Hordacre, A.L., Marker, J., and Wade, V. (2005). Effect of psychiatry liaison with general practitioners on depression in recently hospitalised cardiac patients: a randomised controlled trial. *Medical Journal of Australia*, **182**, 272–276.

Shaji, K.S., Arun Kishore, N.R., Lal, K.P., and Prince, M. (2002). Revealing a hidden problem: an evaluation of a community dementia case-finding program from the Indian 10/66 dementia research network. *International Journal of Geriatric Psychiatry*, **17**, 222–225.

Shaw, A.B. (1994). In defence of ageism. *Journal of Medical Ethics*, **20**, 188–191.

Sheldon, T.A. and Smith, P.C. (2000). Equity in the allocation of health care resources. *Health Economics*, **9**, 571–574.

Shulman, K. and Arie T. (1991). UK survey of psychiatric services for the elderly: direction for developing services. *Canadian Journal of Psychiatry*, **36**, 169–175.

Snowdon, J. and Arie, T. (2005). A history of psychogeriatric services. In *Psychogeriatric service delivery: an international perspective* (ed. B. Draper, P. Melding, and H. Brodaty), pp. 3–20. Oxford University Press, Oxford.

Sumner C.R. (2001). Telepsychiatry: challenges in rural aging. *Journal of Rural Health*, **17**, 370–373.

Teel, C.S. (2004). Rural practitioners' experiences in dementia diagnosis and treatment. *Aging and Mental Health*, **8**, 422–429.

Trieman, N., Leff, J., and Glover, G. (1999). Outcome of long stay psychiatric patients resettled in the community: a prospective cohort study. *British Medical Journal*, **319**, 13–16.

Turner, S., Iliffe, S., Downs, M. *et al.* (2004). General practitioners' knowledge, confidence and attitudes in the diagnosis and management of dementia. *Age and Ageing*, **33**, 461–467.

Unutzer, J., Katon, W., Callahan, C.M. *et al.* (2002). Collaborative care management of late-life depression in the primary care setting: a randomized controlled trial. *Journal of the American Medical Association*, **288**, 2836–2845.

Van Citters, A.D. and Bartels, S.J. (2004). A systematic review of the effectiveness of community-based mental health outreach services for older adults. *Psychiatric Services*, **55**, 1237–1249.

Voyer, P. and Martin, L.S. (2003). Improving geriatric mental health nursing care: making a case for going beyond psychotropic medications. *International Journal of Mental Health Nursing*, **12**, 11–21.

Warner, J.P., Wright, L., Blanchard, M., and King, M. (2003). The psychological health and quality of life of older lesbians and gay men: a snowball sampling pilot study. *International Journal of Geriatric Psychiatry*, **18**, 754–755.

Weinstein, M.C. (2001). Should physicians be gatekeepers of medical resources? *Journal of Medical Ethics*, **27**, 268–274.

Wenger, G.C., Scott, A., and Seddon, D. (2002). The experience of caring for older people with dementia in a rural area: using services. *Aging and Mental Health*, **6**, 30–38.

Williams, A. (2001). How economics could extend the scope of ethical discourse. *Journal of Medical Ethics*, **27**, 251–255.

Wills, W. and Leff, J. (1996). The TAPS project. 30: quality of life for elderly mentally ill patients – a comparison of hospital and community settings. *International Journal of Geriatric Psychiatry*, **11**, 953–963.

Woods, R.T., Wills, W., Higginson, I.J., Hobbins, J., and Whitby, M. (2003). Support in the community for people with dementia and their carers: a comparative outcome study of specialist mental health service interventions. *International Journal of Geriatric Psychiatry*, **18**, 298–307.

WHO (1996). *Psychiatry of the elderly: a consensus statement*. World Health Organization/World Psychiatric Association, Geneva.

WHO (1997). *Organization of care in psychiatry of the elderly: a technical consensus statement*. World Health Organization/World Psychiatric Association, Geneva.

WHO (1998). *Education in psychiatry of the elderly: a technical consensus statement*. World Health Organization/World Psychiatric Association, Geneva.

WHO (2002). *Reducing stigma and discrimination against older people with mental disorders: a technical consensus statement*. World Health Organization/World Psychiatric Association, Geneva.

WHO (2003). *Organization of services for mental health*. World Health Organization, Geneva.

Yorston, G. (1999). Old age forensic psychiatry. *British Journal of Psychiatry*, **174**, 193–195.

Zucker, M.B. and Zucker, H.D. (eds) (1997). *Medical futility and the evaluation of life-sustaining interventions*. Cambridge University Press, Cambridge.

# 20

# Clinical practice: primary care of older people with mental illness

Helen J. Graham and Louise Robinson

The general practitioner (GP) gives personal, primary, and continuing care to individuals, families, and a practice population, irrespective of age, sex, and illness. His or her aim is to make early diagnoses and to include and integrate physical, psychological, and social factors into considerations about health and illness; he or she will undertake the continuing management of patients with chronic, recurrent, or terminal illnesses, and will know how and when to intervene, through treatment, prevention, and education.

This concept of care (Leewenhorst Statement 1974, quoted in Taylor and Taylor, 1988) gives GPs a unique involvement with the full range of health problems of older people in the context of their families and the community. GPs are familiar with most aspects of mental illness in older patients, much of which is ill-defined and is interwoven with the complexities of the many personal, social, and medical problems of this age group. Good primary care also involves the rational use of hospital-based resources which is achieved through the GP's role as a 'gate-keeper' to specialist services. Conversely, effective specialist care involves the cooperation of the GP.

## The delivery of primary health care and general practitioner services

In the UK, GP services are an integral part of the National Health Service (NHS) in which GPs practise as independent contractors. The population is required to register with a general practice and each patient is allocated by the practice to the list of a named GP. Each practice determines its locality boundaries and only accepts patients who reside within this area. Patients remain registered with a practice unless application is formally made to change to a different practice. The long-term trend to large multiple-partner practices in the UK has increased the number of partnerships of five or more GPs from 18 to 32% of the total from 1991 to 2005, while single-handed GPs account for only 21% of all practices (RCGP, 2006a). Two-thirds of GP premises are owner-occupied, 21% are rented from the private sector, and 16% are health centre premises (RCGP, 2005).

GPs increasingly work with a range of healthcare professionals to form the primary healthcare team which may include practice nurses,

community nurses, nurse practitioners, health visitors, practice managers, administrative staff, counsellors, and psychiatric nurses. Team working is essential in order to manage the complex demands placed on general practice which are partly due to caring for an increasingly ageing population with chronic and multiple health problems. The greater emphasis on preventative care, the transfer of clinical responsibility for some chronic diseases from secondary to primary care, and the shift in service provision in order to deliver care closer to patients' homes has contributed to these demands (Department of Health, 2006a).

The Health Act 1999 made provision for Primary Care Trusts (PCTs) to be established nationally, each serving a local population of between 60,000 and 150,000 patients (HMSO, 1999). Trusts are charged with planning, securing, and improving primary and community health services in their area, developing services for the locality, and implementing clinical governance (quality control mechanisms). In England, from 2005, general practices have had the opportunity to undertake practice-based commissioning through the formation of consortia of local practices which work together to develop innovative ways of developing and contracting clinical patient services (RCGP, 2006b). An indicative budget is negotiated which allows flexibility in the commissioning of patient care from hospitals and community services and in managing prescribing costs, but which excludes mental health services (Department of Health, 2006b).

The implementation of a new General Practice Contract in 2004 has fundamentally changed the way in which primary practitioners work in the UK. The contract defines essential primary care services and optional enhanced services that are additionally remunerated. Also it links achievements in clinical and non-clinical quality to financial rewards, through a Quality and Outcomes Framework derived from evidence-based care (NHS Confederation, 2006). The system encourages the delivery of optimum care in 10 clinical domains, with emphasis on chronic diseases (Lester *et al.*, 2006). The new contract established a formal role for the GP with a special clinical interest to run locality specialist clinics in accordance with the health needs of the population. Its overall aim is to bring clinical services closer to patients (RCGP, 2006c). Guidance has been produced for a range of appropriate specialist services such as mental illness, diabetes, and palliative care (Department of Health, 2006c) although the evidence base for the cost-effectiveness of such services has yet to be developed (Kernick and Mannion, 2005). Additional funding is allocated to practices in areas of high deprivation and aims to support inner-city practices. An Index of Multiple Deprivation has been devised based on domains of deprivation such as low income, health deprivation and disability, barriers to housing and services, living environment deprivation, employment deprivation, and crime (Department of Health, 2005a).

Increasing patient demand for out-of-hours care and a national commitment to explicit standards of care defined in a set of National Service Frameworks (Department of Health, 1999a) led to the development of a range of innovative primary care services. In addition to registration with a local GP, patients may use primary care walk-in centres which are located in public places such as supermarkets and railway stations, although older people consult less often in these settings and are under-represented in those attending walk-in centres (Salisbury and Munro, 2002). Patients have access to first-level health advice through a nation-wide direct access telephone service, known as NHS Direct. The centres are staffed with 24-hour availability by nurses who advise on self-care using computer-based decision pathways, GP or specialist referral, or the use of local services. Since 2004, statutory responsibility for ensuring the provision of out-of-hours care has been transferred from GPs to local PCTs. General practices have a choice of electing to provide practice-based 24-hour care 7 days a week, sharing the workload with colleagues through an out-of-hours 'cooperative', or of opting out of the provision of out-of-hours care and transferring responsibility to the PCT. Out-of-hours cooperatives are based in emergency centres and provide care for populations of up to 1 million. In a study of patients of all ages who received out-of-hours care, initially half received telephone advice by a doctor or nurse, one-third attended a primary care centre, and one-quarter were visited at home. However, for patients aged over 65, about half of all out-of-hours calls resulted in a home visit, and of these, those aged over 75 had a hospital admission rate which was seven times that of infants (Salisbury et al., 2000). The integration of social workers into the cooperatives facilitates urgent assessments of patients under the Mental Health Act and emergency admission to residential care.

# Epidemiology of general practice care of older people

The list size for a general practice in the UK in 2005 is just over 6000 for an average partnership, and corresponds to an average workload for each doctor of approximately 1700 patients (RCGP, 2006a). The list may be 'personal' as in a single-handed practice or 'combined' where patients are free to consult any doctor in a group practice. A full-time GP with an average list size can expect to care for approximately 140 patients aged 65–74 (8.1%), 95 patients aged over 75 (5.6%) and about 30 (1.8%) aged over 85 years (Department of Health, 2004).

Consultation patterns based on the General Practice Research Database for 1992–1998 showed that the mean age-standardized consultation rate for patients of all ages was 3.85 (3.01 for males and 4.71 for females) and that the consultation rates for those aged over 65 years showed an upward trend (Fleming and Ross, 1999; Rowlands and Moser, 2002). In 2004, the General Household Survey reported an average annual consultation rate for persons aged over 65 years of six for men and seven for women, in addition to an annual average of three to four consultations with a practice nurse (Office for National Statistics, 2005). Older people have fewer patient-initiated visits and are more likely to attend for follow-up of established disease. There is a trend for general practice consultations to take place in the surgery (86%) compared to those in the home (4%) or by telephone (10%). The average consultation time for patients of all ages is 13.3 minutes, with older patients tending to consult for longer than younger age groups (RCGP, 2005). General practitioner contact rates are 17% higher for elderly people living in communal establishments and 8% higher in older people living alone than those living in standard accommodation (McNeice and Majeed, 1999). To compensate for this additional workload, GPs receive weighted capitation fees for patients aged over 65 years. Consultation patterns, however, in older patients with mental illness compared to those without mental illness show that people with dementia are low users of health services, consult their GP less frequently, and are more likely to have seen a community nurse, while those with depression are high users of community medical services, and are more likely to have seen a community nurse (Nelson et al., 2002).

## Screening of older people

The reservoir of unreported illness in elderly patients assessed at home (Williamson et al., 1964) has been demonstrated in many general practice-based studies, and led to the opinion that opportunistic case finding or screening is more appropriate to the needs of older patients. Another approach would be to focus care on 'at risk' groups of elderly people. Non-consulters have been studied in detail to discover whether they are an 'at-risk' population. Of patients aged over 75 years who had not consulted their GP in the previous year, just over 50% who were visited needed action for simple and remediable conditions (Williams, 1984). By contrast, other studies found few unreported problems and concluded that non-consulters constituted a health elite (Ebrahim et al., 1984). Selected screening of elderly patients to identify those most 'at risk' was pioneered by Barber et al. (1980) with patients aged over 70 who were sent a postal questionnaire enquiring about medico-social problems. This eliminated 20% of patients with no 'at-risk' factors. The remainder were seen by their GP, of whom 91% were found to have problems requiring attention. Freer (1987) recommended opportunistic consultation-based screening of elderly patients using a modification of Barber's questionnaire, and found that fewer than 30% of screened patients required follow-up. Evidence for the benefits of screening in studies using controlled trials is equivocal (Tulloch and Moore, 1979; Hendricksen et al., 1984; Vetter et al.,1984), although the evidence suggested that there were vulnerable groups of older people who should be screened. These included: people aged 75 years and over; those who live alone; older people recently bereaved; those recently discharged from hospital; those requiring home help and community services; those asking for residential care; those planning to give up their homes for any other reason (Bergmann and Jacoby, 1983); those who have moved home within the last 2 years; and the divorced or separated (Taylor et al., 1983).

In the UK 1990 New Contract, whole-population screening for the over 75s was introduced (Health Departments of Great Britain, 1989) but in a large randomized controlled trial it was shown to confer little or no benefit to quality of life or health outcomes (Fletcher *et al.*, 2004). The over-75s health checks were dropped from the 2006 General Practice contract and replaced by managed care for targeted patient groups (Lester *et al.*, 2006). The National Service Framework for Older People (Department of Health, 2001) recommended a single assessment process that would combine a brief contact assessment by a GP or primary care nurse using a case-finding approach and a social welfare review by social services, but this recommendation has not been widely accepted (Iliffe and Orrell, 2006).

## Monitoring chronic disease and the provision of coordinated care in older people

The Quality and Outcomes Framework of the 2006 NHS contract rewards GPs for the provision of high-quality care using a series of evidence-based indicators in specified clinical domains which include: diabetes, coronary heart disease, chronic obstructive pulmonary disease, heart failure, epilepsy, hypothryroidism, asthma, atrial fibrillation, chronic renal failure, stroke and transient ischaemic attacks, mental illness, dementia, cancer and palliative care, learning disabilities, and smoking (Department of Health, 2006c). Because the incidence of most of these conditions increases with age, care tends to be focused on older patients and can be delegated to practice nurses or nurse practitioners.

The Quality and Outcomes Framework requires practices to produce patient disease registers to demonstrate the percentage of registered patients diagnosed with specified chronic conditions. Psychiatric disorders include: dementia, depression, learning disability, and mental illness defined as schizophrenia, bipolar disorder and other psychoses. The following indicators are used: patients with dementia and mental illness should have a care review during the previous 15 months; patients with depression should have an assessment of the severity at the outset of treatment using an assessment tool validated for primary care, and, if on lithium therapy, should have a record of serum lithium levels within the previous 6 months, and serum creatinine and thyroid levels within the previous 15 months (Department of Health, 2006c). The palliative care indicator requires a register of patients considered to be in need of palliative or supportive care if their death in the next 12 months can be reasonably predicted. The palliative care register should include cancer and non-cancer patients for whom there should be regular multidisciplinary case reviews at least 3-monthly and which should consider the needs of carers. Of the 1% of the population dying each year, about one-third will suffer from frailty and dementia and have multiple organ failure. An individual GP can expect six or seven deaths annually of patients suffering from dementia, frailty, and multiple co-morbidity (Gold Standards Framework, 2006).

## The detection and diagnosis of mental illness in older patients

The possibility of early detection of psychiatric disorder was explored in studies of general practice patients aged 65 years and over in Newcastle upon Tyne (Bergmann, 1981). The research team encouraged early referral of patients by their GPs. This produced a referral rate of 2.8% in the practice population aged 65 years and over. An epidemiological approach using a screening questionnaire with the same population found a total prevalence of psychiatric morbidity estimated at 21.9%. The conclusion drawn was that GPs referred only those who were very ill, and that, generally, the proportion of known cases was very low.

With regard to screening for mental illness in primary care, there is currently insufficient evidence to recommend for or against routine screening for dementia in older adults (Boustani *et al.*, 2003). This study showed that some screening tests have good sensitivity but only fair specificity in detecting dementia. A recent Cochrane Review found substantial evidence that the use of screening instruments for depression had minimal impact on the detection, management, and outcome of the illness (Gilbody *et al.*, 2005). However, screening for depression in patients who have concurrent chronic physical illness such as diabetes and cardiovascular disease is an effective strategy but only within a collaborative care system (National Institute for Clinical Excellence, 2004). This recommendation has been incorporated into the Quality and Outcomes Framework for depression.

# The epidemiology of mental illness in general practice

The prevalence of mental illness in the community in the UK is difficult to establish because of variations in screening criteria and the populations screened. Prevalence figures have probably changed little since the results of the study based in Newcastle upon Tyne, on patients aged 65 years and over who lived at home (Kay *et al.*, 1964). This study showed that a GP with a list of 2000 patients, of whom 300 are aged 65 years and over, could expect: 30 (10%) with an organic brain syndrome; 93 (31%) with a functional disorder of whom 78 (26%) would suffer from an affective disorder; six (1.9%) with schizophrenia, paraphrenia, and paranoid states; and a further eight (2.6%) with other disorders such as mental subnormality, marked personality deviations, or hypochondriasis. National morbidity statistics from general practice show that dementia is associated with an annual incidence of 1.6 new patients per GP, an annual prevalence of 3.6 patients consulting, and an annual workload of 7.4 consultations per GP (RCGP, 1995).

Medical services deal only with the visible tip of the 'iceberg' of mental illness and handicap. By contrast with the prevalence figures noted above, GP consultations in people over 65 were only 2% (affective psychosis), 0.4% (schizophrenia and paranoid states), and 7% (neurotic disorders) (RCGP, 2001). The prevalence of depression in older people in nursing and residential care is recognised to be two to four times greater than for those living independently in the community with rates ranging from 20% to 45% (Jongenelis *et al.*, 2004).

Research into the outcome of untreated depression has yielded conflicting results. Episodes of untreated or non-recognized depression in adults of all ages had similar outcomes to treated cases; however, this may not be so in moderate to severe depression (Goldberg *et al.*, 1998). Diagnostic difficulties for GPs in the detection of depression include lack of clear diagnostic criteria and the time constraints of an average doctor–patient consultation in which a complex mix of medical, psychological, and social problems have to be addressed.

# The presentation of mental illness in general practice

Psychiatric problems in elderly patients present commonly to the GP in a variety of ways.

## Affective disorders

Patients who suffer from affective disorders may present with mood change, anxiety, irritability, negativity, changes in appetite, concentration and sleep patterns, physical symptoms, and low energy. Frequent surgery attendances for multiple unexplained symptoms suggest hypochondriasis and possible anxiety and depression. Older patients are more likely than younger patients to present with somatic symptoms when they are psychologically unwell. The multiple pathology of advancing age encourages somatization, especially when associated with underlying mood disturbance. Patients' problems may be presented by relatives who express anxiety over changed behaviour, observed mood swings, or reduced social responsiveness. Sometimes it is the GP who detects depression through a patient's apparent mood changes over successive consultations, or through casual requests for treatment.

Examples of common presentations include:

◆ A depressed 87-year-old feels 'out-of-sorts' and wants a 'tonic'.

◆ 'Stronger sleeping tablets' are requested through the receptionist by an elderly housebound patient who lives alone and who insists that previous medication no longer works. On visiting, the patient is found to be lonely and depressed.

◆ Repeated requests by an ambulant patient 'to do away with me because I'm a burden to everyone' suggests an underlying depression.

Older patients are probably likely to consult at times of major life events (Murphy, 1982) especially those associated with loss, notably bereavement, but also moving home and loss of function and independence (for example, through strokes (House, 1987), myocardial infarction, or amputation), makes older patients particularly likely to present at such times. Grief, stress, and emotional pain associated with these events, or their anniversaries, may lead to obvious sadness and depression, exacerbation of coexistent disease, or an increase in psychosomatic symptoms, particularly those which reflect illness in the 'lost' relative. The history in Case 1 is illustrative.

---

### Case 1

An 80-year-old widow consulted with exacerbation of long-standing tinnitus and a feeling of being 'drained'. She added that the following day was the anniversary of her husband's death and she would visit the cemetery. She left without treatment commenting that she felt better for talking as she always felt so alone.

---

Major personal illness, physical deterioration (Murphy, 1982), an inability to perform activities of daily living (Iliffe *et al.*, 1993), and acquired brain injury (RCP, 2005) are associated with concomitant depression, as are viral infections (especially influenza) and frequent falls (Vetter and Ford, 1989). Excessive alcohol intake can mask depression, although Dewar and Jones (1990) demonstrated in their community survey that heavy consumption tended to be in those with least physical, mental, and social disability. Social problems may signify underlying mental illness through requests for rehousing, for help with marital or family relationships, or through failure to cope with day-to-day activities.

## Acute confusional states

Emergency calls to older patients with acute delirium are generally made at the request of alarmed relatives or neighbours. They are usually associated with acute physical illness and nearly always require emergency admission of the patient for investigation. Common acute causes in general practice are pneumonia, urinary tract infections, severe congestive cardiac failure, dehydration, drug toxicity (e.g. Case 2), and metabolic causes such as diabetic ketoacidosis. Subacute presentation can occur with a subdural haematoma following a recent fall which may not be mentioned by the patient.

---

### Case 2

An 84-year-old sufferer from Parkinson's disease who was well controlled on levodopa suddenly became confused with visual hallucinations. Careful inspection of his medication found that he had been prescribed a double dose of levodopa in error. Omission of the tablets for 3 days before resuming the lower dose resulted in remission.

---

## Psychotic illness

Older patients with delusions, hallucinations, and persecutory ideas are more likely to suffer from depressive illness, although a minority will have schizophrenia or paraphrenia. Visual hallucinations also occur in Lewy body dementia. The GP may detect ideas of reference, or paranoia, often involving neighbours, when conversing with the patient. Sometimes, inconsistencies in the history will alert the GP to a delusional state, as illustrated in Cases 3 and 4.

---

### Case 3

A 68-year-old patient who lived alone and was independent in self-care requested repeated home visits for recurrent ill-defined abdominal pains which had been diagnosed as irritable bowel syndrome. She attributed each episode of pain to her noisy next-door neighbours whose voices, heard through the adjoining wall, accused her of various misdemeanours. The story seemed convincing until it was observed that she lived in an end of terrace house and had no neighbours on the side she described as noisy. She was subsequently diagnosed as suffering from paraphrenia, and responded to treatment with thioridazine.

---

### Case 4

An 87-year-old woman who lived alone as a lodger in a family house developed persecutory ideas about her landlady who, she thought, wanted to get rid of her. She imagined people in her living room who sometimes tried to take her away. She also confused day with night. The landlady asked her GP to visit because she was wandering around the house at night. She had lost 13 kg in weight, and had a haemoglobin of 8 g per 100 ml. Further investigation found no active physical disease, and her anorexia and weight loss were attributed to a paranoid psychotic illness which subsequently improved on trifluoperazine.

---

## Behaviour disorders and personality changes

General practice contains a small number of older patients who are eccentric, or who have difficult or aggressive personalities. Sometimes reclusive patients pose problems of non-concordance particularly if they are ill and refusing help from neighbours and the primary healthcare team. Unravelling the ethical implications of these situations is challenging, particularly when patients with no demonstrable cognitive impairment or mental illness fully accept the consequences of their decisions to refuse care, or to live in unhygienic or unheated homes. A psychiatric opinion can be useful to the GP in differentiating between mental illness and personality disorders, particularly if use of statutory procedures such as Section 47 of the National Assistance Act 1948 is being considered.

### Dementia: making a diagnosis

The diagnosis of dementia can be delayed by the insidiousness of the symptoms and the perceptions of both lay and professional people that this may be normal ageing (Bamford *et al.*, 2004). Although general practice is often the first point of contact for patients with dementia, GPs are often reluctant to use brief cognitive tests and to question relatives of patients who appear to be demented for fear of causing distress (O'Connor *et al.*, 1993), and miss the opportunity of identifying cases by not responding to symptoms, behaviours, and other events that may be indicators of dementia (Boise *et al.*, 2004). A high index of suspicion and a proactive approach using diagnostic guidelines increases the diagnostic yield and facilitates appropriate selection for referral (Van Hout *et al.*, 2000). Although the early recognition and the diagnosis of dementia by GPs is variable, and widespread underdetection is reported (England, 2006), it has been shown that the majority of GPs felt confident in making the diagnosis (Turner *et al.*, 2004). Studies of educational interventions to help increase the detection rates by GPs have demonstrated that decision support software and practice-based workshops significantly improved detection rates (Downs *et al.*, 2006).

Unreliable histories, a dishevelled appearance, failure to recognize the doctor after years of interactive personal care, non-concordance with treatment in a previously compliant patient, hoarding of medication, and poor coping ability at home all suggest dementia. Suspicions of family carers recorded in patients' notes help prompt further evaluation at subsequent contacts, and aid earlier diagnosis (Bamford *et al.*, 2007). Indirect presentation of a demented patient is common, and is the cue for the GP to take constructive action. Relatives or neighbours may consult, expressing concern about a patient's increasing memory loss, reduced social responsiveness, unaccounted financial expenditure, or vulnerability to fraud. A deteriorating home situation may be described in which forgetfulness leads to domestic disasters such as flooding, gas leaks, kitchen fires from burnt out cooking utensils, or security problems with unlocked doors and windows. Key workers, such as receptionists or community pharmacists, may report difficulties in patients' management of repeat prescribing. The community nurse may observe disorientation of a patient visited for other needs, or a health visitor may report a family crisis precipitated by failure to cope with a person suffering from undiagnosed dementia, as illustrated in Case 5.

### Case 5

A young mother with a 5-month-old baby was visited at home by her health visitor who noted post-natal depression. Before the birth, the mother had been so concerned about her father's memory loss that without seeking advice she had taken him in to live in their two-bedroom, local authority rented flat. The strain of caring for her baby and her confused father in overcrowded conditions proved too difficult. Referral of her father to the department of old age psychiatry confirmed the diagnosis of Alzheimer's dementia. Attendance by the father at a day centre, and rehousing of the family led to remission of the young mother's depression.

## Management of the patient with suspected dementia

The initial assessment includes a careful history from the patient, the carer, and information from the patient's notes. It is usually possible to differentiate the slow progression of Alzheimer's dementia from the sudden deterioration in memory or coping ability of multi-infarct dementia which is often associated with a history of stroke or transient ischaemic episodes. A search for a reversible cause of dementia at the initial assessment is important. A history of a recent fall suggests the possibility of a subdural haematoma and, if suspected, immediate referral to a geriatrician or neurologist should be made for an urgent CT brain scan (Case 6). A review of medication, to include drugs prescribed within the practice and by emergency medical or specialist services, may identify incorrect dosage which is causing intellectual impairment. Sedatives, tranquillizers, antiparkinsonian agents, and hypotensives are among offending drugs. Adjustment or withdrawal of these will clarify the diagnosis. Depression masquerading as dementia ('pseudo-dementia') should be considered and, if suspected, a trial of antidepressants is indicated. Normal pressure hydrocephalus, hypothyroidism presenting as dementia, syphilis, hypercalcaemia, and vitamin deficiencies as the cause of, rather than result of, dementia are rarities in practice. A physical examination of the patient, particularly to detect anaemia, cardiac disorders, neurological evidence of previous stroke, and undiagnosed malignancy, is essential. Baseline investigations to include a full blood count, erythrocyte sedimentation rate, biochemistry, thyroid function tests, and syphilis serology provide a good medical evaluation prior to further assessment, although results are more likely to detect coexistent medical pathology than to aid the differential diagnosis of dementia. The correction of iron- or vitamin-deficient anaemias, the control of cardiac arrhythmias, and treatment of hypothyroidism is good medical practice, but there is a risk of the GP diverting clinical interest into 'medicalization of the patient' rather than confronting the management of the underlying dementia.

The main decision to be taken at this stage is whether to refer the patient for further assessment and management. This depends on local service provision, and whether the patient lives alone or with a family or carers who are available, able, and willing to provide care. Exploring the feelings of patients and carers, and consideration of available options, supplemented by an assessment of the patient's needs by a community nurse, provides sound preparation before taking decisions. The advantages of early referral to an old age psychiatry service include: early confirmation of the diagnosis without duplication of investigations in general practice; ease of planning appropriate support services, including day care; greater carer satisfaction through reassurance that the problem has been thoroughly addressed; and the early familiarity with the home situation by professional staff in order to facilitate management of future crises. If the patient can be accompanied by a carer who can confirm the history, referral to an old age psychiatry outpatient department, multidisciplinary assessment clinic, or memory clinic is the preferred approach of some clinicians. Others recommend an initial specialist domiciliary visit to the patient in the presence of relatives to supplement the presentation of the problem, and allow discussion of a suitable care plan, liaising with the local authority social services care coordinator. As a consequence of increased emphasis on community services, specialist 'outreach' clinics in old age psychiatry have been established in some general practices. These are more convenient than hospital outpatient visits and less distressing for both patient and carer. Despite the need to inform patients and their families sensitively and accurately of a diagnosis of dementia, disclosure rates vary considerably. A recent systematic review revealed that carers were told the diagnosis more frequently than patients and there was considerable use of euphemistic terms by health professionals (Bamford *et al.*, 2004).

### Case 6

The warden of a sheltered housing unit requested a GP to visit an 81-year-old female resident who had been 'going down-hill' mentally for the past few weeks with memory loss, intermittent confusion, incontinence, and difficulty with self-care. The patient had a past history of atrial fibrillation and transient ischaemic episodes from cerebral emboli, and had been commenced on warfarin. The warden recalled a fall 6 weeks earlier, after which the patient had been examined at hospital and reassured that no injury had occurred. Re-referral for further investigation resulted in the detection of chronic bilateral subdural haematomas on CT scan, with no cerebral atrophy. Following surgery, her confusion cleared. Despite only partial recovery of memory, she was again able to cope alone.

### Long-term management of patients with dementia

Together with their old age psychiatry colleagues, GPs, as leaders of the primary healthcare team, are responsible for coordinating and directing the long-term clinical management of patients with dementia. Local authority social services are responsible for the social care and support of the patient. Care should be tailored to the needs and circumstances of individual patients and carers, and should be multifactorial in approach. The aims of care are: to provide relevant information on prognosis, care options, and legal issues; to treat underlying medical conditions or disability; to recognize personal and social needs; to ensure regular risk assessment and carer support; to manage behavioural and relationship problems; and to ensure, where possible, that the patient remains in their preferred place of care (Robinson *et al.*, 2004).

The success of maintaining the patient at home depends on the quality of the relationship with carers and on identifying and addressing carers' needs (Department of Health, 1990). Forty-two per cent of the supporters of older people living alone were prepared to accept permanent residential care for them, compared with only 5% of the supporters who had been living with the old person for 50 years or more. The likelihood of being supported when one is demented is increased if one has been living with a person for a very long time—an average of 36 years in the review by Bergmann and Jacoby (1983). Carers of people with dementia face particular stresses in comparison with other caregiving groups, experiencing increased social isolation and greater detrimental effects on their physical and emotional well-being (Ory *et al.*, 1999; Clark and King, 2003).

Regular visits by the community psychiatric nurse, the community nurse, and a named GP, regardless of whether the patient lives alone or with carers, provides a multidisciplinary approach and facilitates coordination between primary and secondary care. It is important to identify the individual needs of carers and how they can contribute, whilst respecting their limitations and recognizing which services can supplement care. Support services include: local authority social services for home care assistants, meals-on-wheels, clubs and carer support groups, advice on financial benefits, respite care; physiotherapy or occupational therapy for aids and adaptations; the voluntary sector for sitting services and contact with self-help groups such as the Alzheimer's Society. When a patient lives alone dependence on services will be greater. The aim should be to provide daily contact with the home. If a patient living alone suffers from severe dementia, it may be necessary to abandon community care after a short trial and arrange for admission to residential care. The introduction of an Admiral Nursing Service, specialist nurses with expertise in dementia care and support (Greenwood and Walsh, 1995), may lead to more seamless care. However, current evidence shows little difference in patient or carer outcomes between families receiving this specialist service and those supported by existing community teams (Woods *et al.*, 2003).

Distressing problems arising with progression of dementia, include sleep disturbance, behavioural problems, such as wandering, swallowing difficulties, incontinence, and immobility. For behavioural problems, non-pharmacological interventions are recommended above pharmacological ones (Howard *et al.*, 2001), but evidence on their effectiveness is lacking (Robinson *et al.*, 2006). The prescription of a night tranquillizer such as chlormethiazole, one to two capsules, helps nocturnal disturbance or, at lower doses, to control daytime agitation. However, neuroleptic drugs should be used carefully due to a lack of evidence concerning long-term efficacy and the increased morbidity and mortality risks associated with their use (Ballard and O'Brien, 1999). Advice on regular toileting to encourage continence and, if incontinence is a problem, the provision of aids such as pads, pants, and protective mattress sheets are available through the community nursing services. Referral to the community physiotherapist and occupational therapist for assessment, including provision of aids and appliances, will assist with problems of mobility.

Treatment of medical conditions coexisting with dementia should be continued, if supervision is available, until a decision is made for palliative care. However, hypertension treatment in patients with vascular dementia may no longer be needed as blood pressure has been shown to decline with the onset of dementia (den Heijer *et al.*, 2003; Qui *et al.*, 2004; Pettiti *et al.*, 2005). Prescribing of cholinesterase inhibitors to people with moderate dementia is recommended (National Institute for Clinical Excellence, 2001) in order to reduce the rate of deterioration. The use of shared care protocols (O'Brien *et al.*, 2001) provides a framework for GPs to continue prescribing such drugs once a specialist decision to initiate treatment has been made.

### Social care

In comparison with the intended service-led provision (Department of Health, 1990), the 1993 community care reforms placed increased emphasis on care at home with local authority social services assuming responsibility for assessing patients' care and social needs.

This enabled older people to live in their own home through the provision of day care, domiciliary care, and respite care.

The recent White Paper on health and social care '*Our health, our care, our say—a new direction for community services*' aims to improve the current provision of community care through increasing the choices available to users of these services and creating more integrated services (Department of Health, 2006a). Initiatives include a personal health and social care plan in a patient's records to integrate health and social care provision and the establishment of joint health and social care teams. People who require social care can opt to receive payments directly and purchase services themselves. The introduction of practice-based commissioning will give GPs direct responsibility for joint commissioning and may lead to more innovative integrated care models in the community (Department of Health, 2006b).

Welfare benefits provide some financial remuneration for people with a chronic illness and their family carers. They include: Disability Living Allowance with care and mobility components for those aged under 65 years; Attendance Allowance if aged over 65 with special rules if terminally ill; Housing Benefit; Invalid Care Allowance for carers aged between 16–65 who are spending at least 35 hours weekly caring for a severely disabled person; Income Support; and Council Tax benefits (Department of Social Security, 2000). The Orange Badge scheme of parking concessions allows people with severe mobility impairment or their carers to park close to the places they want to reach, and is available also to those with severe memory impairment.

### Legal and ethical issues

The GP is well placed to provide sensitive and timely discussion of legal and financial matters, including information or advice about seeking 'power of attorney' and 'lasting power or attorney' (LPA) (see Chapter 43). These are legal documents authorized through a solicitor, which allow a person (the donor) to give another (the attorney), the responsibility to act on the donor's behalf in relation to property and financial affairs. An advance directive, or living will, allows the patient to set out their wishes about future treatment and life-saving interventions should he or she develop irreversible cognitive impairment or other advanced disease (Doyal, 1995). In a recent study, only 11% of people with dementia had made a living will (Mitchell *et al.*, 2004). The organization EXIT advises that patients should inform their GP of their decision to make an advance directive, and a copy of the statement should be filed with their health records.

The Mental Capacity Act 2005 provides a statutory framework for acting and making decisions on behalf of adults who lack the mental capacity to do so for themselves. The code of practice associated with the Act provides guidance on good practice for those acting under the terms of the Act. It contains: (1) guidance on how to assess capacity, (2) a statutory framework for an advance directive, and (3) advice on how to manage patient decisions, once the advance directive is applied (Department of Constitutional Affairs, 2006). The Act will also see the introduction of a new formal power of attorney, lasting power of attorney (LPA) which will replace the provision for existing enduring powers of attorney (EPA), although the latter will remain valid if executed before the implementation of the new Act. LPAs will extend the areas in which donors can authorize others to make decisions on their behalf to include health care and medical treatment, i.e. any matter of personal welfare in addition to financial affairs. The Act will establish an Independent Mental Capacity Advocate (IMCA) service which will provide representation and support for individuals who lack capacity but who have no one else to support them when major decisions are being made about their lives.

### The demented patient who lives alone

Providing primary care services for older demented patients who live alone poses special problems, and may only be possible through the goodwill of neighbours. If access to the home is unreliable, arrangements should be made with neighbours to hold emergency keys. Neighbours are reassured by contact with the GP and by discussion about when to request help. If there is no available supervision from the family carers or the community nurse, the taking of medication can be simplified by use of a 'Dosett' box in which medication is placed into daily dosage compartments dispensed on a weekly basis by a pharmacist. Single demented patients may cause concern over security, and personal road and home safety. The local police welcome information about these vulnerable residents and this is particularly encouraged if there is a local neighbourhood security scheme. When eventually these patients require admission to a protected environment, a residential care or nursing care home is more appropriate than a sheltered housing unit where the need to become familiar with new surroundings whilst still living independently is liable to accentuate confusion (see Case 7).

---

### Case 7

An 84-year-old woman with dementia who had no relatives lived alone with difficulty. The social services arranged admission to a nearby sheltered housing unit. Within a short time she appeared more confused, her room became squalid, she roamed the streets, and was frequently returned by the police. She developed paranoid behaviour, attacked several residents, and was formally admitted to hospital under Section 2 of the Mental Health Act. She was subsequently transferred to a nursing home for the elderly mentally infirm. It would have been more appropriate to have admitted her there directly from her own home after careful assessment, rather than into sheltered housing.

---

## Caring for the carers. The role of the general practitioner

General practitioners have a vital role in supporting carers. The majority of carers perceive that of all health service employees, GPs have the greatest power to improve their lives (Carers Association, 1998). A survey of elderly dependants living in the community found the following effects on carers: one-quarter felt their health to be adversely affected; one-quarter felt their social life was impaired; one-sixth felt their family life had suffered; and almost one-fifth, especially daughters, reported unbearable stress (Kings Fund Carers Unit, 1989; Jones and Peters, 1992).

The 2006 General Practitioner Contract has encouraged a more proactive approach in supporting carers. Practices are rewarded for implementing a management system that includes a protocol for the identification of carers and a mechanism for the referral of carers for social services assessment in accordance with the Carers

(Equal Opportunities) Act 2004 (Department of Health, 2005b). Practice staff who support carers should have access to a regularly updated directory of local services covering NHS, local authority, and voluntary and private sector provision, to include self-help and support groups, and they should encourage patients and carers to participate in these. Information given to carers should include Internet websites which provide information on mental illness and self-help and carers' support groups (Alzheimer's Society, 2006; Institute of Psychiatry, 2006). At a personal level, carers expect realistic information about dementia, the implications of the diagnosis and its prognosis, and how to make best use of available facilities (Department of Health 1999b). Services should be adapted to the individual circumstances of the carer and the patient, with regard to differing racial, cultural, and religious backgrounds. The carer should be accepted as a contributing member of the care team, and effective communication with carers should be encouraged through discussion and the keeping of clear, concise records. For housebound patients, a shared care record will maintain continuity and improve communication. The shared record is held in the home and everyone involved in the care of the patient should be invited to contribute to it regularly.

The mental and physical health of carers is paramount if community care is to be a realistic, long-term possibility. Usually the carer and the carer's family are registered with the same practice as the patient. As it is the family who bear the major burden of caring for elderly people, the GP is the pivotal support for the family unit. The GP's role should include offering advice to carers on their personal health, acknowledging the carers' crucial contributions and the problems they experience, and giving emotional support by counselling the carer on their attitudes and expectations. The stress experienced by carers who look after demented elderly patients has been shown to lead to psychiatric morbidity in addition to common physical problems such as tiredness, musculoskeletal strains, and insomnia caused by the heavy physical demands of care (Ory *et al.*, 1999). Carers of people with psychiatric disorders, particularly women carers, have an increased risk of depression (Livingston *et al.*, 1996). Referral to the community nurse to teach the practical skills needed for home nursing and to reassure carers that they are doing the job well will alleviate the physical strain. Vigilance by the GP in detecting early signs of strain or poor coping will help to avert crises.

How well a carer copes depends on her personality, her health, and the quality of the pre-morbid relationship with the dependent person (Anderson, 1987). The experience of families who care for people with dementia has been likened to 'coping with a living death' (Woods, 1989). Recognition of the importance to the carer of clinging to memories, and of maintaining the appearance of the patient as a mark of her success in the carer's role, will improve morale and self-esteem.

## Respite care

Carers are at risk of increasing isolation and exhaustion through the intensity of their 24-hour responsibility. To prevent this and to delay institutionalization, the GP should emphasize the value of relief care on: a daily basis, with day centres or sitting services; and in the long term by the rotation of care with other family members or through planned regular admissions to respite beds in residential care or hospital. The GP should be prepared to advise carers and families on respite care, and offer information on the range of options and the referral process appropriate to the patient's level of dependency. Respite care is appropriate when the carer is ill or needs a break. For support in the home, domiciliary care may be offered by voluntary organizations or home care agencies such as Counsel and Care, the Alzheimer's Society, and local authority social services. Families and carers are reassured to know that voluntary organizations are regulated and required to work to specific care standards. Short-term care can be arranged in residential care homes for patients who are mobile and only mildly confused, or short-term care in nursing homes or hospitals should be arranged if the patient needs nursing, is seriously confused, or is doubly incontinent. If the patient is self-funding, private care arrangements are made, but if financial assistance is needed, referral for a community care assessment should be made to the local authority social services by the carer or GP well before the planned admission date (see Chapter 16). Patients are assessed against eligibility criteria for funded care. When a patient requires nursing care or supervision, or needs multidisciplinary assessment and rehabilitation, admission to hospital or nursing home is the responsibility of the NHS. Since April 2004, the NHS and local authority councils have been required to identify people who are likely to require short-stay respite care, and to agree arrangements for their management. They may refer the patient to the local home coordinator or lead nurse for the PCT, who will advise about local arrangements.

Although respite admission provides an opportunity for multidisciplinary assessment of the patient, and may delay institutionalization, it does not seem to reduce the overall burden on the carer (Eccles *et al.*, 1998). Heavily dependent patients may need regular admissions, for example, for 2 out of every 6 weeks, to ease the strain on the carer. Relatives appreciate the opportunity of visiting the home or hospital beforehand to gain confidence in the staff and the surroundings. Otherwise, the family may have reservations about delegating care to staff who are less familiar with the patient's condition than they are themselves.

Disadvantages of respite care for the carer include the difficulties of visiting patients in hospital or nursing homes; feelings of sadness, loneliness, or even guilt on being separated from their relative; and the possibility of institutional cross-infections. Some carers, however, refuse offers of help, or indeed any support. Others may stoically underplay the strain of caring, and deny the seriousness of the illness in their relative. The outlook in such situations is poor. The GP, however, should be aware of possible underlying depression in the carer as an explanation of this behaviour. The history in Case 8 illustrates this.

### Case 8

A 68-year-old married woman who had refused help in the care of her demented husband was admitted to hospital after taking an overdose of sleeping tablets. On recovery, she was found to be depressed. She commented that she could think of no other solution to the burden of coping with her sick husband. Her depression responded well to antidepressants, and she eventually agreed to her husband attending a day centre.

## Situations which require hospital admission

A point may be reached when the carer is no longer willing, or able, to cope. Increasing debility of the patient outstrips the tolerance of the carer and is particularly likely to occur when sleep disturbance, incontinence, and general immobility are problems (Sanford, 1975). The patient then requires long-term care. It is important to be aware of elder abuse, which may be a symptom of strain in the carer (see Chapter 39). If this is suspected, the GP should refer the patient to social services for an assessment, and perhaps for transfer to a place of safety in hospital or residential care.

Acute admissions mostly occur when there is unexpected illness in the carer, or when a mildly demented patient who lives alone suffers a self-limiting illness which, under normal circumstances, would not require admission. In some areas 'Hospital at Home' schemes are available, and these may be more appropriate. They provide comprehensive nursing at home for people who would traditionally have been cared for in hospital. Out-of-hours emergency calls by relatives who infrequently visit a mildly demented patient living alone, and insist that 'something must be done' before their return home, is not an uncommon crisis, and may express their own guilt.

## General practitioners and specialist services

General practice acts as a filter to specialist medical services. Although referral rates are influenced by factors such as the clinical skills and interests of doctors, the availability of specialist services, and patients' expectations, variation is substantial with a 25-fold difference between those who refer the most and the least. Much of the variation in mental health services has been shown to be associated with the population demographics, population morbidity, and the effect of provider differences within secondary care (Melzer et al., 1999). The restructuring of the NHS has brought about a shift of resources from hospital to community, with community-based specialist mental health teams now being widespread in the UK. Locality commissioning of specialist services by PCTs or practice-based commissioning influences the development of healthcare strategies for local populations. The range of services include primary care based specialist clinics, community mental health centres, community 'shifted' outpatient or 'outreach' clinics, and domiciliary visiting by a psychiatrist or community psychiatric nurse (Goldberg and Jackson, 1992; RCGP, 1993). Community care is popular with patients and allows the GP to be involved with patient management. However, in a study of specialist outreach clinics there was no increased interaction between specialists and GPs (Bailey et al., 1994).

Community psychiatric nurses in general practice have been identified as providing primarily patient support and patient assessment in 46% and 13% of referrals, respectively (Briscoe and Wilkinson, 1989). Domiciliary visiting may be arranged directly at the request of the GP and a hospital- or community-based specialist, or may be incorporated into a practice-based outreach clinic for patients who cannot attend hospital or the surgery on medical grounds and who need diagnosis or treatment. They are costly in time and resources, and it is questionable whether the same management outcome could be achieved by telephone consultation between the GP and the specialist. Domiciliary consultations can be helpful in the following situations: the assessment of patients in difficult home circumstances; unwillingness of patients or carers to take up care recommendations; initial evaluation of a patient recently presenting with significant memory impairment; assessment under the Mental Health Act; or, clarification of the appropriateness of care by an old age psychiatrist or geriatrician where

symptom overlap occurs (see Case 9). Referral to a geriatrician is indicated if, in addition to psychiatric symptoms, the patient is acutely ill, especially if confused or if life-threatening physical illness is present.

---

**Case 9**

A woman of 83 years who has lost contact with her family lives alone in a bed-sit flat. Another lodger, a 48-year-old unemployed man who drinks excessively, repeatedly requests visits from the GP because of his concern over her deteriorating health and the need for her to be rehoused. She suffers from maturity onset diabetes (apparently controlled by diet), iron deficiency anaemia, and episodes of congestive cardiac failure with fluctuating levels of confusion. Her accommodation is filthy and her appearance neglected, yet she shops regularly for her pension and food for herself and the other lodger. She has refused a home care assistant and meals on wheels. Social services report that she is capable of making her own decisions, but are concerned about possible physical abuse by the lodger. Admissions to the geriatric unit for acute illness have resulted in self-discharge before psychiatric assessment could be arranged. At a routine visit, her GP notes her poor performance on mental testing and arranges a domiciliary visit by a psychiatrist, who considers that she has only minimal mental impairment. She agrees to visits by the community psychiatric nurse and to attend the psychiatric day unit for further assessment.

---

## Hospital communication

The success of a patient's rehabilitation following hospital discharge depends on the adequacy and timing of information provided to the GP at the time of discharge. Initial notification by telephone or facsimile (fax) in advance is more likely to encourage an early home visit by the GP than if only a letter is sent. Prompt discharge letters should include information on the patient's care needs, particularly in relation to community services and carer support, medication, general condition, and follow-up requirements. Sending discharge letters with patients to be handed to the GP is unreliable, especially when patients have poor mobility, live alone, or suffer memory loss. Williams and Fitton (1990), in a study of the causes of readmission of older patients, found that lack of discharge information to the GP was three times more common than failure of the GP to visit a recently discharged patient after notification. Good specialist communication from outpatient departments and day-hospitals is essential for continuity of care (RCP, 1994). First attendances, discharges, and a change in the treatment or condition of a patient should be reported, as should annual progress of patients attending for long-term care. Letters should summarize the findings at consultation, an assessment and management plan, and have educational value for the GP (Westerman et al., 1990).

When patients are discharged or managed as outpatients, effective liaison between hospital staff and GPs is essential, especially when patient medication is initiated or changed. For patients under consultant supervision, medication should normally be prescribed in hospital and dispensed in the hospital pharmacy for not less than 14 days at discharge, or after referral to and treatment in outpatients. In situations where the consultant requests that the GP should continue treating, the consultant should give the GP timely notification of the patient's diagnosis and details of the drug therapy.

The doctor who signs the prescription has legal responsibility for the consequences of drug treatment, and must not prescribe without adequate clinical information. It is therefore unacceptable for hospital staff to expect GPs to do so (Department of Health, 1991).

## Intermediate care

The development of rehabilitation and care schemes which are intermediate between acute hospital care and long-term institutional care has led to a range of alternative provision termed intermediate care. Such services are designed to maximize independence and prevent unnecessary hospital admissions. The National Service Framework for Older People (Department of Health, 2001) has set clear targets for the future expansion of intermediate care services. Most schemes offer short-term interventions (1–6 weeks) and involve cooperative working with other agencies including PCTs, local authority social services, and the voluntary and private sectors. For acute care, recent developments aim to bridge the divide between hospital trusts and local authorities. Examples include innovative services such as 'hospital at home' or 'supported discharge' schemes in which the patient is discharged early from hospital and supported by intensive home nursing. 'Rapid response' services may be available to maintain acutely ill patients at home. There is evidence that hospital at home is acceptable to both patients and carers and provides care as effectively as does hospital admission (Wilson *et al.*, 1999). However, the cost-effectiveness of intermediate care schemes in general remains uncertain (Jones *et al.*, 1999; Steiner *et al.*, 2001) and the availability of hospital at home schemes is variable (Corrado, 2000). An alternative to acute hospital admission is the use of small community hospitals or nursing homes, in which inpatient care is provided by GPs and their multidisciplinary teams who usually have recourse to specialist advice. This is a useful option when insufficient home care or community support makes continuing home care untenable, particularly when mentally impaired patients require acute generalist care or rehabilitation. Continuing care schemes, rehabilitation, and palliative care may be provided by community outreach teams or by domiciliary and occupational therapy services as alternatives to day hospital or inpatient care.

## Home care services and residential care

The trend towards increased home care provision by local authority social services and independent sector organizations has allowed people to remain in their own homes for longer than was previously possible before admission to a residential care home or nursing care facility. Intensive home care services and increased contact hours by care staff have contributed to improvements in the quality of life and independence of older people (NHS Health and Social Care Information Centre, 2006). The GP has a coordinating role and acts as a point of contact for community care staff. The decision to transfer a patient into residential care is difficult and should only be taken after all possible community support services in the home have been explored with the patient's relatives and the community planning team. The latter consists of community nurses, social services, and, in patients with complex needs, the community matron employed by the local PCT. Patients or their relatives seeking admission to a home are advised to discuss the situation with the community nurses caring for the patient and with the patient's GP before requesting assessment for a nursing home placement.

Nursing homes lie predominantly within the independent sector and are subject to registration with the NHS (see Chapter 23). There has been a downward trend in the number of general and mental nursing homes with a slight increase in the proportion of beds available for people with mental illness. Of the total number of occupied nursing home beds, 82% are occupied by people aged 65 and over, and two-fifths by people aged 85 and over. On average, general nursing homes have 35 registered beds and mental nursing homes 31 beds, although homes vary enormously in size. Medical care in nursing homes may be provided by an attending medical officer appointed by the home, or by a local general practice under contract for the provision of general medical care to include regular visits to the home, out-of-hours care, and preventive services such as annual influenza immunization. Only 7% of nursing homes have a resident medical practitioner (Department of Health, 2002). Patients in residential care homes register with a local GP and have access to general medical care in the same way as the general population.

Studies have shown that in the population living in residential care, there is a high prevalence of physical dependency and depression; and even higher prevalence rates of up to 70% for dementia (Nelson *et al.*, 2002). This results in high rates of consultation, prescribing, and referral for the attending GP, with the workload for patients in nursing homes being double that for other patients over the age of 74 years (Carlisle, 1999). Few depressed patients in residential care receive appropriate management. The outcome of depression in residents can be improved by enhancing the clinical skills of GPs and care staff, and by providing depression-related health education and activity programmes (Llewellyn-Jones *et al.*, 1999).

### Terminal illness at home

A GP can expect an average of 20 deaths from their list each year, of which about one-quarter will be at home (Gold Standards Framework, 2006). Most of these will be among older patients, some of whom will suffer from mental illness. In the UK, over 40% of people with dementia die in the community (McCarthy *et al.*, 1997). It is the GP who coordinates their care, both for those who die at home, and, in the time preceding admission, for those who die in hospital or hospice care. About 70% of elderly people with dementia die from bronchopneumonia, a finding confirmed on post-mortem (Burns *et al.*, 1990) whilst cardiovascular disease, pulmonary embolus, septicaemia, and renal failure account for the remainder of deaths.

When a patient with dementia becomes ill with a respiratory infection, the GP should discuss the poor prognosis with relatives and discover their preferences and their knowledge of their relative's wishes for the preferred place of care. Wherever the patient is cared for and whatever the mental status, the principles of good terminal care apply. These include: mouth care, the control of distressing symptoms such as pain or constipation; the involvement of community nurses and specialist palliative care services; and attention to the need for emotional and practical support for both patients and their families. People with dementia and their families require more input from healthcare and social services prior to death than do people with terminal cancer (McCarthy *et al.*, 1997). In the USA, specialist units similar to hospices have been introduced for people with dementia. These have been shown to be more effective clinically and economically than traditional long-term care (Volicer *et al.*, 1994). However, such examples of specialist care for people with dementia are rare in the UK. The National Institute for Health and Clinical Excellence has recommended the use of care pathways to improve the quality of care at the end of life (Ellershaw, 1997; Thomas, 2003). These care pathways contain detailed guidance on how to transfer the principles of specialist palliative care as given in hospices to other settings in which patients are cared for during their last few days of life. Practices are required to maintain a palliative care register and regularly to review the listed patients as indicated in the Quality and Outcomes Framework (NHS Confederation, 2006).

Death from dementia is not unexpected, and in theory the carer of a person with dementia has time to adjust to the prognosis of this fatally progressive disease. Nevertheless, the intensity and intimacy of caring leaves the main carer bereft of a role after a patient's death. The carer's expected sense of relief may be overshadowed by a bereavement, and they will require much consolation and counselling; yet such support from primary care is not always forthcoming. Although bereavement support has recently been advocated as an area of prevention in primary care, practices are divided over whether such support should be proactive or reactive (Harris and Kendrick, 1998).

## Prescribing in general practice

Prescribing of antidepressants and atypical antipsychotics has been gradually rising over the past 5 years and has resulted in an increase in the overall cost of drugs used for mental health, despite a slight reduction in the cost of serotonin reuptake inhibitors (Prescription Pricing Authority, 2005). In a study of patients aged over 65, 13% were taking antidepressants (Nelson, *et al.*, 2002). This increase in prescribing of antidepressants cannot be explained by an increased incidence or prevalence of depression seen in general practice (Munoz-Arroyo *et al.*, 2006) and it may reflect the increased prescribing of serotonin reuptake inhibitors (Hollingshurst *et al.*, 2005). Most patients who are managed in general practice have mild to moderate depression, for whom the prescribing of antidepressants is not indicated (National Institute for Clinical Excellence, 2004). In a large cross-sectional community survey, people with dementia were more likely to be taking antipsychotics, and people with depression were most likely to be taking both antidepressants and hypnotics or anxiolytics compared to other groups (Nelson *et al.*, 2002).

The prescribing of hypnotics in general practice is a particular problem. Pressure from elderly patients and their carers or residential home staff to prescribe hypnotics should be resisted as the elderly are at risk of becoming ataxic and confused, and liable to fall and injure themselves (British National Formulary, 2006). The use of benzodiazepines should be questioned because of their potential for physical and psychological dependence, and tolerance. Hypnotics should be considered only for short-term use when insomnia is severe, disabling, or causing extreme distress, and, if prescribed, should only be given in short courses of 2–4 weeks, preferably using small doses of drugs with short half-lives such as chlormethiazole and temazepam (Swift, 1993).

In 2006, UK medicine legislation allowed extended prescribing in primary care by practice-based and community nurses who have received special training and are entered onto a special register maintained by the Nursing and Midwifery Council. They may prescribe any licensed medicine for any condition with the exception of controlled drugs although they are accountable for their prescribing to their employers. All primary care prescribers are encouraged to prescribe generic rather than proprietary drugs in order to contain costs, and this has resulted in a national generic prescribing rate of 80% (RCGP, 2006d). Practices with patients who live more than a mile (2.5 km.) from a retail pharmacy can apply to be a dispensing practice, enabling them to have an on-site dispensary and to issue medication to patients directly. General practices commonly prescribe from an electronic practice formulary compiled with the advice of the local PCT pharmacist who may provide prescribing guidelines for groups of drugs. When a specialist doctor asks a GP to prescribe a specialist drug for a patient who is referred back from specialist to primary care, the GP should be provided with information and support on its usage, although he or she is not obliged to prescribe the drug if they do not feel confident about doing so.

When prescribing for depression in elderly patients, the choice of antidepressant should be based on the individual patient's requirements and should consider the presence of concomitant disease, existing therapy, suicide risk, and previous response to antidepressant therapy. Low doses should be used for initial treatment in older people, and patients should be monitored for hyponatraemia (British National Formulary, 2006). However, GPs tend not only to prescribe subtherapeutic doses of antidepressants (Orrell *et al.*, 1995) but also seem reluctant to treat for the recommended minimum of at least 1 year. Patients who have had two or more depressive illnesses or have experienced functional impairment should be prescribed antidepressants for 2 years (National Institute for Clinical Excellence, 2004).

Prescribing for elderly patients requires caution to allow for the increased susceptibility to commonly used drugs and the likelihood of multiple medication. Good GP care in the prescribing of drugs for older patients involves:

- review of the appropriateness of medication and of dosage at the time of the initial prescription and in continuing therapy;

- ensuring that the patient and carer understand the purpose and nature of the medication;

- the prescribing of lower drug doses, generally starting at 50% of the dose prescribed to younger adults;

- prescribing simple regimes with full and clear instructions of how and when to take medication—statements such as 'take as required', 'PRN', and 'as instructed by the physician' should be avoided for regular medication;

- checking the labelling of medicine containers for legibility taking account of the patient's visual acuity;

- the maintenance of clear documentation of prescribed drugs and any changes in them. For the patient this might be with a repeat prescription card, computer printout, or 'tablet timetable'; for the practice, it should be documented on the patient's records including the electronic record; and with the hospital if the patient has shared care;

- an efficient repeat prescribing system with a clear practice policy on the frequent review of prescriptions.

Routine repeat prescribing should be avoided for certain groups of elderly patients:

◆ the acutely ill;

◆ those who are depressed. Instead, clinical review should be undertaken at the renewal of each monthly prescription;

◆ those with impaired renal, hepatic, or cardiac function, who should be monitored for systems deterioration and the dosage adjusted accordingly;

◆ those with a history of heavy alcohol intake;

◆ those with dementia. They should not be prescribed any drugs unless they can be supervised by a carer or community nurse;

◆ those who are withdrawing from antidepressants or long term anxiolytics. The withdrawal should be done slowly and the patient seen frequently over 2–3 months to detect early relapse of depression. Patients taking benzodiazepines or chlormethiazole require stepwise, monitored dose reduction over several weeks or sometimes months before stopping to prevent withdrawal symptoms (British National Formulary, 2006).

## The use of computers as an aid to efficient prescribing

The monitoring of prescribing in general practice has been improved by the use of computerized prescribing systems and electronic patient records. This facilitates repeat prescribing, allows monitoring of potential drug interactions and allergies, and simplifies patient medication review. Modern computer systems run background checks when prescriptions are written to ensure that necessary blood tests and monitoring have been performed. If they have been overlooked, the computer system alerts the prescriber. For example, when patients are taking lithium the computer will check that lithium levels, thyroid function, and renal tests have been undertaken. Over 75% of all prescriptions in general practice are issued without patient consultation as repeat prescriptions for those taking long-term medication. Guidance on medicines management under the Quality and Outcomes Framework is that patients who are prescribed four or more medicines should have an annual medicines review (Department of Health, 2006c).

An electronic prescription service has been introduced throughout England with access by GPs' surgeries, community pharmacies, and appliance contractors. This has the potential to allow healthcare professionals to access information on medication that has been dispensed to patients they see. The service enables electronic prescriptions to be generated, transmitted, received, and, once dispensed by the pharmacist, sent to the reimbursement agency, the Prescription Pricing Authority. A repeat dispensing system has been introduced which enables patients taking medication on repeat prescription to by-pass their GP and obtain the prescription directly from their pharmacist until a medication review is due by their GP. The aim of the service is to streamline the prescription process, provide greater convenience for patients and carers, reduce the repeat prescribing burden for GPs, and through the involvement of the pharmacist improve accuracy in dispensing (NHS, 2005a).

## The use of computerized patient lists for screening, audit, and research

The use of computers for patient registration, practice management, and prescribing (Fig. 20.1) is universal in UK general practice.

Electronic patient records are used to enter medical histories and consultations, and to transfer clinical investigation data from local hospital laboratories. Screening and the monitoring of disease and disability can be undertaken using the computerized registration details of patients, although these are limited by the input of clinical details (Fig 20.2).

Electronic patient registers are compiled using sources of data from electronic patient records, and these have superseded the previous card indexed age–sex registers. Software programs can search patient lists by defined characteristics such as year of birth, socioeconomic information, therapeutic treatment, or clinical diagnosis from coded data input. The READ coding system based on the International Classification of Diseases (Department of Health, 1993) is used in UK general practice. Therapeutic searches are commonly used to compile disease registers. For example, a search using the names of commonly prescribed antidepressant drugs is more likely to identify patients treated for depression than would the use of 'depression' as the key search word.

The National Programme for IT has launched a service for the NHS which holds basic information such as patient name, address, and date of birth. Known as the Patient Demographic Service, it is used for the electronic transfer of patient information between general practices, community trusts, hospitals, and laboratories with the aim of bringing about a process of seamless care and paperless clinical practice. The system has recently been extended to the direct booking of hospital outpatient appointments by GPs, known as the 'choose and book' scheme and incorporates strong measures to safeguard the security of clinical and personal data (NHS, 2005b). Most computer systems have a disease prevention display, adjusted for the patient's age and sex, and decision support tools as an aid to defining clinical problems, managing continuing problems, and initiating opportunistic health promotion. Electronic reminders or 'Post-it notes' are displayed on the screen during the consultation and prompt the clinician to pursue useful management strategies (Sullivan and Wyatt, 2006). Although Health Authorities have computer links with primary care, hold centralized patient registration data and forward medical records when patients change practice, and despite advances in information technology, there are still problems with the maintenance of accurate primary care age–sex registers. Inaccuracies in the age–sex register increase with the age of the population, due to increased mortality, and turnover in patient registrations associated with population movement. Failure to notify the practice of these changes leads to list inflation in which patients (known as 'ghost' patients) are wrongly included on the practice register. The implications of such errors in health screening programmes, population surveys, and research is considerable in terms of time expenditure and the accuracy of denominator values used in epidemiological studies.

# Research opportunities–methodological issues

General practice provides a wealth of opportunities for research. To achieve a whole-population approach in epidemiological surveys or in studies of community care it is worth considering the potential of general practice. Advantages include: the possibility of a more accurate database compared to the electoral register; a personal

**Full Report**

| Mrs. Marjorie Robertson | 02/11/1915 | Female | NHS13456 | Applied |

**Address**
12 View Hill London SE22 ORG

**Communication numbers**
Telephone - home            0171 567 1234

**Problems**

| | | |
|---|---|---|
| Atrial Fibrillation | Started: 14/07/2000 | Ended: |
| Depression - management of | Started: 14/04/2000 | Ended: |
| Heart failure | Started: 15/12/1999 | Ended: |
| Currently Relevant | Started: 03/01/1996 | Ended: |

**Allergy and Intolerance**

| | | | |
|---|---|---|---|
| 27/04/1995 | Allergy | Moderate | PENICILLIN V tabs 250mg |

**Medical History**

| | |
|---|---|
| 26/06/2000 | [V]Fitting or adjustment of cardiac pacemaker |
| 14/05/2000 | Atrial fibrillation and flutter |
| 04/05/2000 | Palpitations |
| 14/04/2000 | O/E - depressed |
| 06/12/1999 | Home visit elderly assessment |

**Repeat Masters**

| | | | |
|---|---|---|---|
| DIGOXIN tabs 125micrograms ONCE DAILY | Until: 15/11/2000 | Last issued: 15/08/2000 | Number of issues: 1 of 12 |
| SERTRALINE tabs 50mg ONCE DAILY | Until: 15/11/2000 | Last issued: 15/08/2000 | Number of issues: 1 of 6 |
| WARFARIN SODIUM tabs 3mg EVERY DAY | Until: 03/10/2000 | Last issued: 15/08/2000 | Number of issues: 1 of 6 |

**Acute and Repeat Issue Therapy**

| | | | |
|---|---|---|---|
| 17/02/2000 | issued   CO-AMILOFRUSE tabs 2.5mg+20mg | Supply: (30) tablet(s) | IN THE MORNING |

**Consultation**

| | | |
|---|---|---|
| 26/06/2000 | Discharge details | |
| 25/05/2000 | Letter from Outpatients | |
| 14/05/2000 | Surgery consultation | Dr. Jack Kerrush |
| 04/05/2000 | Surgery consultation | Dr. Jack Kerrush |
| 14/04/2000 | Out of hours, Practice | Dr. William Preston |
| 15/12/1999 | Acute visit | Miss Ellie Nabule |
| 06/12/1999 | Clinic | Miss Ellie Nabule |

**Blood pressure**

| | | |
|---|---|---|
| 04/05/2000 | BP 190/110 | recall due: |
| 06/12/1999 | BP 180/105 | recall due: |

**Referrals and Requests**
11/05/2000   Refer for Palpitations at Cardiology department
by: Dr. Jack Kerrush

**Fig. 20.1** Computer display in a GP's surgery: sample medical history and therapy history. (Reproduced from the Vision GP computer programme by kind permission of INPS.)

approach to the patient through the GP which results in higher response rates; access to the patient's medical records; and the GP's personal knowledge and contact with patients which facilitates data collection and interpretation of results. Criteria for the selection of suitable practices include: efficient practice organization; a computerized age–sex register with Health Authority links; good liaison with hospital services, and, if possible, the use of training practices where there is a commitment to high standards of care, audit, and research. The question of whether to involve multiple small practices or one large group practice should be considered along with the demographic balance of the practice populations. This avoids the use of skewed population samples and ensures the recruitment of sufficient patient numbers.

Having enlisted the cooperation of an interested general practice, it is essential to gain consent from participating GPs and, at the outset, to visit the practice to explain the project to all staff. The acceptability of protocols, letters, questionnaires, and pilot studies should be confirmed with staff before seeking approval from local research ethics committee. Establishing a link with a key practice administrator and a GP from each practice facilitates effective organization. It is recommended practice, according to the requirements of the Data Protection Act, 1998, that researchers should obtain the consent of the patient or subjects before the practice is able to release their contact details to the research team. In communicating with patients, it is essential to provide information on the research project and its potential benefits. The identity of the research clinician and their relationship with the practice should be explained. Patients appreciate a choice of venue for an interview, usually the preferences range between home, the surgery, or the hospital. The researcher should provide an identity card, a letter of introduction from the link GP, and a contact telephone number for security reasons and to reassure patients, relatives, and neighbours. Where door-to-door surveys are being carried out it is essential to inform the local police because neighbours will rightly be highly

---

**Full Report**

---

**Mrs. Marjorie Robertson**                    22/07/1921        Female        4628081042

**Address**

**Communication numbers**
Telephone - home

**Problems**
Osteoarthritis                              Started: 12/09/2001        Ended:
Chest Infections                            Started: 05/10/2000        Ended:
Chronic Obstructive Pulmonary Disease       Started: 11/01/2000        Ended:
Currently Relevant                          Started: 30/10/1995        Ended:

**Advice Given**
14/08/1996  Advice to patient - subject        Advice                                          GENERAL

**Agencies**
14/08/1996  Domiciliary services                                                    Dr. Jim Kelly

**Diet**
14/08/1996  Diet - patient initiated            Eating habits: Good Type of diet:

**Exercise**
14/08/1996  Exercise grading Moderate X2 WEEKLY KCH OSTEOPOROSIS CLASS              Dr. Jim Kelly

**Hearing (over 75 years)**
14/08/1996  O/E - hearing tested-8th nerve Treatment being received WEARS AID       Dr. Jim Kelly

**Mental cognitive**
14/08/1996  O/E - state of mind Referral

**Mental emotional state**
14/08/1996  O/E - state of mind Referral                                           Dr. Jim Kelly

**Mobility level**
14/08/1996  Mobile outside with aid Mobile outside with aid

**Physical health**
14/08/1996  Geriatric health exam, Treatment being received OSTEOPOROSIS C/O KCH   Dr. Jim Kelly

**Sleep pattern**
14/08/1996  [D]Sleep disturbances Satisfactory                                     Dr. Jim Kelly

**Vision in the elderly**
14/08/1996  Ophthalmological monitoring Satisfactory C/O OPTICIAN                  Dr. Jim Kelly

**New Registration Consultation**
14/08/1996  New patient screen            Seen by: Dr. G Adam          Clinician: Dr. S Woods

**Over 75 years check**
14/08/1996  Geriatric screening           Seen by: Dr. Jim Kelly       Clinician: Dr. H Tegner

**Urinalysis - Glucose**
14/08/1996  Urine test for glucose Nil

**Urinalysis - Protein**
14/08/1996  Urine test for glucose Nil

**Allowances received - Elderly**
14/08/1996  OAP PENSION

**Carers - elderly**
14/08/1996  Domiciliary services MANAGES ALL OWN DOMESTIC CHORES & GARDEN

**Foot care**
14/08/1996  Feet examination ATTENDS THE SURGERY

**Next of kin - elderly**
14/08/1996  Relation: Other relative MRS VERONICA CASE - DAUGHTER IN LAW

**Optician last seen**
14/08/1996  Seen by optician                    1994

**Risk factors - elderly**
14/08/1996  Risk factors: Yes HYPERTENSION (TREATED) - OSTEOPOROSIS

**Hygiene - elderly**
14/08/1996  Geriatric health exam, Hygeine Home: Good Personal: Good

**Fig. 20.2** Computer display in a GP's surgery: sample health assessment record. (Reproduced from the Vision GP computer programme by kind permission of INPS.)

suspicious. There is usually a long lead-in time when setting up research and the actual interviewing, so a check on a patient's health status should be made by practice staff prior to visiting so as to avoid the distress of including acutely ill or recently deceased subjects. A common problem when interviewing in the community is how to respond to patients' requests for medical advice. As the interviewer is not providing general medical care, any difficulties should with the patient's consent be referred to the patient's doctor. Patients may alert practices when surveys involve questions of a medical nature. The success of research in general practice depends on respect for the relationship between the patient, the neighbourhood, and the GP.

On completion of the research, feedback to the general practices involved helps to integrate the results with the clinical needs of patients, and to foster a sense of purpose and satisfaction. It is courteous to acknowledge the contributions of participating practices in papers submitted for publication. Indeed, if a GP has personally collected research data, joint authorship should be considered. This will provide a sense of goodwill which may lead to further fruitful collaboration with general practice.

## References

Alzheimer's Society (2006). *Caring for someone with dementia* (http://www.alzheimers.org.uk/Caring_for_someone_with_dementia; accessed 21 August 2006).

Anderson, R. (1987). The unremitting burden on carers. *British Medical Journal*, **294**, 73–4.

Bailey, J.J., Black, M.E., and Wilkin, D. (1994). Specialist outreach clinics in general practice. *British Medical Journal*, **308**, 1083–6.

Ballard, C. and O'Brien, J. (1999). Treating behavioural and psychological signs in Alzheimer's disease: the evidence for current pharmacological treatments is not strong. *British Medical Journal*, **319**,138–9.

Bamford, C., Lamont, S., Eccles, M., Robinson, L., May, C., and Bond, J. (2004). Disclosing a diagnosis of dementia: a systematic review. *International Journal of Geriatric Psychiatry*, **19**(2), 151–69.

Bamford, C., Eccles, M., Steen, N., and Robinson, L. (2007). Can primary care record review facilitate diagnosis of dementia? *Family Practice*, **24**(2), 108–16.

Barber, J.H., Wallis, J.B., and McKeating, E. (1980). A postal screening questionnaire in preventive geriatric care. *Journal of the Royal College of General Practitioners*, **30**, 49–51.

Bergmann, K. (1981). Geronto-psychiatric prevention. In *Epidemiology and prevention of mental illness in old age*, Proceedings of the Nordic Geronto-Psychiatric Symposium, Silkeborg (ed. G. Magnusson, J. Neilson, and J. Buch), pp. 87–92.

Bergmann, K. and Jacoby, R. (1983). The limitation and possibilities of community care for the elderly demented. In *Elderly people in the community: their service needs*, Ch. 8, pp. 141–67. HMSO, London.

Boise, L., Neal, M.B., and Kaye, J. (2004). Dementia assessment in primary care: results from a study in three managed care systems. *The Journals of Gerontology Series A: Biological Sciences and Medical Sciences*, **59**, M621–M626.

Boustani, M., Peterrson, B., Hanson, L., Harris, R., and Lohr, K. (2003). Screening for dementia in primary care: a summary of the evidence for the US Preventative Services Task Force. *Annals of Internal Medicine*, **138**, 927–37.

Briscoe, M. and Wilkinson, G. (1989). General practitioners' use of community psychiatric nursing services: a preliminary survey. *Journal of the Royal College of General Practitioners*, **39**, 412–14.

British National Formulary (2006). *British National Formulary*, No. 51, Ch. 4 Central nervous system, pp. 173–9, 195–206. British Medical Association and Royal Pharmaceutical Society of Great Britain, London (http://www.bnf.org).

Burns, A., Jacoby, R., Luthert, P., and Levy, R. (1990). Cause of death in Alzheimer's disease. *Age and Ageing*, **19**, 341–4.

Carers Association (1998) *Ignored and invisible? Carers experience of the NHS*. Carers National Association, London.

Carlisle, R. (1999) Do nursing home residents use high levels of general practice services? *British Journal of General Practice*, **49**, 645–6.

Clark, P. and King, K. (2003). Comparison of family caregivers; stroke survivors vs. persons with Alzheimer's disease. *Journal of Gerontological Nursing*, **29**(2), 45–53.

Corrado, O.J. (2000) Caring for older hospital-at-home patients. *Age and Ageing*, **29**, 97–8.

den Heijer, T., Skoog, I., Oudkerk, M. *et al.* (2003). Association between blood pressure levels over time and brain atrophy in the elderly. *Neurobiology and Aging*, **24**, 307–13.

Department of Constitutional Affairs (2007). *Mental Capacity Act, 2005. Code of practice*. London, The Stationary Office (http://www.dca.gov.uk/menincap/legis.htm#codeofpractice).

Department of Health (1990). *Caring for people – community care in the next decade and beyond*. Department of Health Publications, London.

Department of Health (1991). *Responsibilities of prescribing between hospital and general practice*. Department of Health Publications, London.

Department of Health (1993). *A national thesaurus of clinical terms in Read Codes*. NHS Executive, HMSO, London.

Department of Health (1999a). *Saving lives: our healthier nation*. The Stationery Office, London.

Department of Health (1999b). *Caring about carers: a national strategy for carers*. Department of Health Publications, London.

Department of Health (2001). *National Service Framework for Older People* (http://www.dh.gov.uk/en/Publicationsandstatistics/Publications/PublicationsPolicyAndGuidance/DH_4003066; accessed 21 August 2006).

Department of Health (2002). *Community care statistics 2001. Private nursing homes, hospitals and clinics*, Bulletin 2002/09. Department of Health, London (http://www.dh.gov.uk/en/PublicationsAndStatistics/Statistics/StatisticalWorkAreas/statisticalsocialcare/; accessed 10 May 2007).

Department of Health (2004). *General and personal medical services statistics, England and Wales. 30th September 2004. GMS & PMS combined national statistics tables*. Department of Health Publications, London (http://www.dh.gov.uk/en/Publicationsandstatistics/Statistics/StatisticalWorkAreas/Statisticalworkforce; accessed 10 May 2007).

Department of Health (2005a). *Resource allocation: weighted capitation*, 5th edn. The Stationery Office, London.

Department of Health (2005b). *Carers and Disabled Children Act 2000 and Carers (Equal Opportunities) Act 2004 combined policy guidance* (http://www.dh.gov.uk/en/Publicationsandstatistics/Publications/PublicationsPolicyAndGuidance/DH_4118023; accessed 10 May 2007).

Department of Health (2006a). *Our health, our care, our say: a new direction for community services. Health and social care working together in partnership* (http://www.dh.gov.uk/en/Policyandguidance/Organisationpolicy/Modernisation/Ourhealthourcareoursay/index.htm; accessed 10 May 2007).

Department of Health (2006b). *Practice based commissioning: achieving universal coverage* (http://www.dh.gov.uk/en/Publicationsandstatistics/Publications/PublicationsPolicyAndGuidance/DH_4127125; accessed 10 May 2007).

Department of Health (2006c). *The new GMS contract 2006/7*. The Stationery Office, London.

Department of Social Security (2000). *A catalogue of leaflets, posters and information*. Benefits Agency, Manchester.

Dewar, R. and Jones, D. (1990). *Determinants of alcohol consumption in the elderly: a community survey*, British Geriatrics Society, Autumn Meeting Abstracts. British Geriatrics Society, London.

Doyal, L. (1995). Advance directives. *British Medical Journal*, **310**, 612–13.

Downs, M., Turner, S., Bryans, M. *et al.* (2006). Effectiveness of educational interventions in improving detection and management of dementia in primary care: cluster randomised controlled study. *British Medical Journal*, **332**, 692–5.

Ebrahim, S., Hedley, R., and Sheldon, M. (1984). Low levels of ill health among elderly non-consulters in general practice. *British Medical Journal*, **289**, 1273–5.

Eccles, M., Clarke, J., Livingston, M., Freemantle, N., and Mason, J. (1998). North of England evidence based guidelines development project: guideline for the primary care management of dementia. *British Medical Journal*, **317**, 802–8.

Ellershaw, J., Foster, A., Murphy, D., Shea, T., and Overill, S. (1997). Developing an integrated pathway for the dying patient. *European Journal of Palliative Care*, **4**, 203–7.

England, E. (2006). Improving the management of dementia. *British Journal of General Practice*, **332**, 681–2.

Fleming, D.M. and Ross, A.M. (1999). *Weekly returns service report for 1998*. Birmingham Research Unit of the Royal College of General Practitioners (RCGP), Birmingham.

Fletcher, A.E., Price, G.M., Ng, E.S.W. *et al.* (2004). Population based multi-dimensional assessment of older people in UK general practice: a cluster- randomised factorial trial. *Lancet*, **364**,1667–77.

Freer, C.B. (1987). Consultation-based screening of the elderly in general practice: a pilot study. *Journal of the Royal College of General Practitioners*, **37**, 455–6.

Gilbody, S.M., House, A.O., and Sheldon, T. (2005). Screening and case finding for depression. *Cochrane Database of Systematic Reviews*, Issue 4, CD002792.

Goldberg, D. and Jackson, G. (1992). Interface between primary care and specialist mental health care. *British Journal of General Practice*, **42**, 267–8.

Goldberg D., Privett, M., Utson, B. *et al.* (1998). The effects of detection and treatment on the outcome of major depression in primary care: a naturalistic study in 15 cities. *British Journal of General Practice*, **49**,1840–4.

Gold Standards Framework (2006). *Palliative care and the GMC contract. Prognostic indicator guidance* (http://www.goldstandardsframework.nhs.uk/content/gp_contract/QOF_Introduction_Paper_1.pdf; accessed 10 May 2007).

Greenwood, M. and Walsh, K. (1995). Supporting carers in their own right. *Journal of Dementia Care*, **3**, 14–16.

Harris, T. and Kendrick, T. (1998). Bereavement care in general practice: a survey in South Thames Region. *British Journal of General Practice*, **48**, 1560–4.

Health Departments of Great Britain (1989). *General practice in the National Health Service: the 1990 contract*, Appendix A, pp. 19–20. Health Departments of Great Britain, London.

Hendricksen, C., Lund, E., and Stromgard, E. (1984). Consequences of assessment and intervention among elderly people; a three year randomised controlled trial. *British Medical Journal*, **289**, 1522–4.

HMSO (Her Majesty's Stationery Office) (1999). *The Health Act 1999*. Office of Public Sector Information, HMSO, London (http://www.opsi.gov.uk/legislation; accessed 29 August 2006).

Hollingshurst, S., Kessler, D., Peters, T., and Gunnell, D. (2005). Opportunity cost of antidepressant prescribing in England: analysis of routine data. *British Medical Journal*, **330**, 999–1000.

House, A. (1987). Depression after stroke. *British Medical Journal*, **294**, 76–8.

Howard, R., Ballard, C., O'Brien, J., and Burns, A., on behalf of the UK and Ireland Group for Optimization of Management in Dementia. (2001). Guidelines for the management of agitation in dementia. *International Journal of Geriatric Psychiatry*, **16**(7), 714–17.

Iliffe, S. and Orrell, M. (2006). Identifying unmet health needs in older people. *British Journal of General Practice*, **56**, 404–6.

Iliffe, S., Gallivan, S., Haines, A. *et al.* (1993). Assessment of elderly people in general practice–4: depression and functional disability. *British Journal of General Practice*, **43**, 371–4.

Institute of Psychiatry (2006). *Mental health information for friends, family and carers* (http://www.mentalhealthcare.org.uk; accessed 29 August 2006).

Jones, D.A. and Peters, T J. (1992). Caring for elderly dependants: effects on the carers' quality of life. *Age and Ageing*, **21**, 421–8.

Jones, J., Wilson, A., Parker, H. *et al.* (1999). Economic evaluation of hospital at home versus hospital care: cost minimisation analysis of data from randomised controlled trial. *British Medical Journal*, **319**, 1547–50.

Jongenelis, K., Pot, A.M., Eisses, A.M., Beekman, A.T., Kluiter, H., and Ribbe, M.W. (2004). Prevalence and risk indicators of depression in elderly nursing home patients: the AGED study. *Journal of Affective Disorders*, **83**, 135–42.

Kay, D.W., Beamish, P., and Roth, M. (1964). Old age mental disorders in Newcastle upon Tyne. *British Journal of Psychiatry*, **110**, 146–58.

Kernick, D. and Mannion, R. (2005). Developing an evidence base for intermediate care delivered by GPs with a special interest. *British Journal of General Practice*, **55**, 908–10.

Kings Fund Carers Unit (1989). *Doctors, carers and general practice*. MSD Foundation, London.

Lester, H., Sharp, D.J., Hobbs, F.D.R., and Lakhani, M. (2006). The Quality Outcomes Framework of the GMS contract. *British Journal of General Practice*, **56**, 245–6.

Livingston, G., Manela, M., and Katona, C. (1996). Depression and other psychiatric morbidity in carers of elderly people living at home. *British Medical Journal*, **312**,153–6.

Llewellyn-Jones, R.H., Baikie, K.A., Smithers, H. *et al.* (1999). Multifaceted shared care intervention for late life depression in residential care: randomised controlled trial. *British Medical Journal*, **319**, 676–82.

McCarthy, M., Addington-Hall, J., and Altmann, D. (1997). The experience of dying with dementia: a retrospective study. *International Journal of Geriatric Psychiatry*, **12**, 404–9.

McNeice, R. and Majeed, A. (1999). Socio-economic differences in general practice consultation rates in patients aged 65 and over: prospective cohort study. *British Medical Journal*, **319**, 26–98.

Melzer, D., Watters, L., Paykel, E., Singh, K., and Gormley, N. (1999). Factors explaining the use of psychiatric services by general practices. *British Journal of General Practice*, **49**, 887–91.

Mitchell, S., Kiely, D., and Hamel, M. (2004). Dying with advanced dementia in the nursing home. *Archives of Internal Medicine*, **164**, 321–6.

Munoz-Arroyo, R., Sutton, M. and Morrison, J. (2006). Exploring potential explanations for the increase in antidepressant prescribing in Scotland using secondary analyses of routine data. *British Journal of General Practice*, **56**, 423–8.

Murphy, E. (1982). Social origins of depression in old age. *British Journal of Psychiatry*, **141**, 135–42.

National Institute for Clinical Excellence (2001). *Guidance on the use of donezepil, risostigmine and galantamine for the treatment of Alzheimer's disease*, Guidance No. 19. National Institute for Health and Clinical Excellence, Wetherby (http://www.nice.org.uk; accessed 23 August 2006).

National Institute for Clinical Excellence (2004). *Depression: management of depression in primary and secondary care*, Clinical Guidelines 23, Guidance No 19. National Institute for Health and Clinical Excellence, Wetherby (http://www.nice.org.uk; accessed 23 August 2006).

Nelson, T., Livingston, G., Knapp, M., Manela, M., Kitchen, G., and Katona, C. (2002). Slicing the health service cake: the Islington study. *Age and Aging*, **31**, 445–50.

NHS (2005a) *Connecting for health. The electronic prescription service* (http://www.connectingforhealth.nhs.uk/eps; accessed 23 August 2006).

NHS (2005b). *Choose and book: ensuring a secure environment for your patients' information* (http://www.chooseandbook.nhs.uk/staff/whatis; accessed 23 August 2006).

NHS Confederation (2006). *Revisions to the GMC contract 2006/7*. NHS Employers and General Practitioner Committee, British Medical Association, London (http://www.nhsemployers.org/primary/; accessed 21 August 2006).

NHS Health and Social Care Information Centre (2006). *Community care statistics 2005: referral, assessments and packages of care for adults, England*. The Information Centre, Knowledge for Care, Leeds (http://www.ic.nhs.uk/pubs/commcare05adultsengsum; accessed 29 August 2006).

O'Brien, J., Robinson, L., and Fairbairn, A. (2001). Proposed shared care protocol between primary and secondary care for the ongoing management of those on anti-dementia medication. *Journal of Primary Care Psychiatry*, **7**(3), 111–13.

O'Connor, D.W., Fertig, A., Grande, M.J. *et al.* (1993). Dementia in general practice: the practical consequences of a more positive approach to diagnosis. *British Journal of General Practice*, **43**, 185–8.

Office for National Statistics (2005). *General Household Survey 2004*. National Statistics Online http://www.statistics.gov.uk/StatBase; accessed 29 August 2006).

Orrell, M., Collins, C., Shergill, S., and Katona, C. (1995). The management of depression in the elderly by general practitioners. Part (i) – The use of anti-depressants. *Family Practice*, **12**(1), 5–11.

Ory, M., Hoffman, R. R., Yee, J., Tennstedt, S., and Schulz, R. (1999). Prevalence and impact of caregiving: a detailed comparison between dementia and non-dementia caregivers. *Gerontology*, **39**, 177–85.

Pettiti, D., Crooks, V., Buckwalter, J., and Chiu, V. (2005). Blood pressure levels before dementia. A*rchives of Neurology*, **62**, 112–16.

Prescription Pricing Authority (2005). *Prescribing review – drugs used in mental health* (http://www.ppa.org.uk//news/pact-092005.htm; accessed 10 May 2007).

Qui, C., von Strauss, E., Winblad, B., and Fratiglioni, L. (2004). Decline in blood pressure over time and risk or dementia: a longitudinal study from the Kungsholmen Project. *Stroke*, **35**(8), 1810–15.

RCGP (Royal College of General Practitioners), Office of Population Censuses and Surveys, Department of Health and Social Security (1995). *Morbidity statistics from general practice: fourth national 1991–1992*. Her Majesty's Stationery Office, London.

RCGP (2001). *Royal College of General Practitioners Birmingham Research Unit. Weekly returns service. Annual prevalence report*. Royal College of General Practitioners, Birmingham.

RCGP (Royal College of General Practitioners) (1993). *Shared care of patients with mental health problems. Report of a Joint Royal College Working Group*, Royal College of Psychiatrists and Royal College of General Practitioners Occasional Paper 60. Royal College of General Practitioners.

RCGP (Royal College of General Practitioners) (2005). *General Practice in the UK: a basic overview*, Information Sheet No. 4. Royal College of General Practitioners, London.

RCGP (Royal College of General Practitioners) (2006a). *Profile of UK practices*, Information Sheet No. 2. Royal College of General Practitioners, London.

RCGP (Royal College of General Practitioners) (2006b). *Practice management in the UK*, Information Sheet. Royal College of General Practitioners. London.

RCGP (Royal College of General Practitioners) (2006c). *General practitioners with special interests*, Information Sheet. Royal College of General Practitioners, London.

RCGP (Royal College of General Practitioners) (2006d). *Prescribing in primary care* (http://www.rcgp.org.uk/pdf/ISS_INFO_10_MARCH06.pdf; accessed 10 May 2007).

RCP (Royal College of Physicians) (1994). *Geriatric day hospitals. Their role and guidelines for good practice*. Royal College of Physicians of London, London.

RCP (Royal College of Physicians) (2005). *Use of antidepressant medication in adults undergoing recovery and rehabilitation following acquired brain injury*, National Guidelines No. 4. Royal College of Physicians, London.

Robinson, L. (2004). Dementia. In *World Health Organisation guide to mental and neurological health in primary care – a guide to mental and neurological ill health in adults, adolescents and children* (ed. R. Jenkins *et al.*). The Royal Society for Medicine, London.

Robinson, L., Hutchings, D., Corner, L. *et al.* (2006). Wandering in dementia: a systematic literature review of the effectiveness of non-pharmacological interventions to prevent wandering in dementia and evaluation of the ethical implications and acceptability of their use. *Health Technology Assessment*, **10**(26).

Rowlands, S. and Moser, K. (2002) Consultation rates from the General Practice Research Database. *British Journal of General Practice*, **52**, 658–60.

Salisbury, C., Trivella, M., and Bruster, S. (2000). Demand for and supply of out of hours care from general practitioners in England and Scotland: observational study based on routinely collected data. *British Medical Journal*, **320**, 618–21.

Salisbury, C. and Munro J. (2002). Walk-in centres in primary care: a review of the international literature. *British Journal of General Practice*, **53**, 53–9.

Sanford, J.R. (1975). Tolerance of debility in elderly dependants by supporters at home: its significance for hospital practice. *British Medical Journal*, **3**, 471–3.

Steiner, A., Walsh, B., Pickering, R.M. *et al.* (2001). Therapeutic nursing or unblocking beds? A randomised controlled trial of a post-acute intermediate care unit. *British Medical Journal*, **322**, 453–60.

Sullivan, F. and and Wyatt, J.C. (2006). *ABC of health informatics*. BMJ Books, Blackwell Publishing, Oxford.

Swift, C.G. (1993). Sleep and sleep problems in elderly people. *ABC of sleep disorders*, pp. 37–40. BMJ Publishing Group, London.

Taylor, J. and Taylor, D. (1988). *The assessment of general medical training in general medical practice*, pp. 10–11. University of York, York.

Taylor, R., Ford, G., and Barber, H. (1983). *The elderly at risk: a critical review of problems and progress in screening and case finding*. Age Concern Research Unit, London.

Thomas, K. (2003). *Caring for the dying at home. Companions on a journey*. Radcliffe Medical Press. Oxford.

Tulloch, A.J. and Moore, V.L. (1979). A randomized controlled trial of geriatric screening and surveillance in general practice. *Journal of the Royal College of General Practitioners*, **29**, 733–42.

Turner, S., Illiffe, S., Downs, M. *et al.* (2004). *Age and Ageing*, **33**, 461–7.

Van Hout, H., Vernooij-Dassen, M., Poels, P., Hoefnagels, W., and Grol, R. (2000). Are general practitioners able to accurately diagnose dementia and identify Alzheimer's disease? A comparison with an outpatient memory clinic. *British Journal of General Practice*, **50**, 311–12.

Vetter, N.J., and Ford, D. (1989). Anxiety and depression scores in elderly fallers. *International Journal of Geriatric Psychiatry*, **4**, 159–63.

Vetter, N.J., Jones, D.E., and Victor, C.R. (1984). Effect of health visitors working with elderly patients in general practice: a randomised controlled trial. *British Medical Journal*, **288**, 369–72.

Volicer, L., Collard, A., Hurley, A. *et al.* (1994). Impact of special care units for patients with advanced Alzheimer's disease on patient discomfort and costs. *Journal of the American Geriatrics Society*, **42**, 597–603.

Westerman, R.F., Hull, F.M., Bezemar, P.D., and Gort, G. (1990). A study of communication between general practitioners and specialists. *British Journal of General Practice*, **40**, 445–9.

Williams, E (1984). Characteristics of patients aged over 75 not seen during one year in general practice. *British Medical Journal*, **300**, 159–61.

Williams, I.E., and Fitton, F. (1990). General practitioner response to elderly patients discharged from hospital. *British Medical Journal*, **300**, 159–61.

Williamson, J., Stokoe, I.H., Gray, S. *et al.* (1964). Old people at home: their unreported needs. *Lancet*, **1**, 1117–20.

Wilson, A., Parker, H., Wynn, A. *et al.* (1999). Randomised controlled trial of effectiveness of Leicester hospital at home scheme compared with hospital care. *British Medical Journal*, **19**, 1542–6.

Woods, R.T. (1989). *Alzheimer's disease: coping with a living death*. Souvenir Press, London.

Woods, R., Wills, W., Higginson, I., Hobbins, J., and Whitby, M. (2003). Support in the community for people with dementia and their carers: a comparative outcome study of specialist mental health service interventions. *International Journal of Geriatric Psychiatry*, **18**, 298–307.

# 21

# Memory clinics

James Lindesay

## Introduction

Specialist memory clinics have a relatively short history. The first to bear this name were set up in the USA in the mid-1970s, with the specific aim of attracting patients in the earlier stages of dementia, who at that time were not being referred to any specialist service (Fraser, 1992). They provided assessment, treatment, and advice, and from the outset there was an explicit focus on research, particularly treatment trials. Although the main interest of these clinics was in dementia, they were called 'memory clinics' in order to avoid the stigma associated with this disorder, and to focus attention on memory impairment as an important early sign. Until the mid-1990s there was a steady if modest growth of such clinics in the USA and elsewhere in the developed world, usually set up in academic centres by interested professionals with particular research and educational interests. They were not at this time perceived as an essential element of service provision for people with dementia; for example, in 1993 a survey in the UK identified only 20 active memory clinics (Wright and Lindesay, 1995). This state of affairs changed dramatically with the licensing of the first cholinesterase inhibitor drug (donepezil) for Alzheimer's disease in 1997. Faced with the challenge of responding to a rise in referrals of people with memory complaints in search of treatment, old age psychiatry services have adopted the memory clinic model as a means of providing the necessary diagnostic assessment and therapeutic monitoring. A second UK memory clinic survey carried out in 1999 found 58 operational clinics, with evidence of others in the process of being established (Lindesay et al., 2002). The new clinics set up after 1997 were typically based in mainstream old age psychiatry services, were focused mainly on diagnostic assessment and monitoring of drug treatment, and were smaller and less involved in activities such as research and teaching than the traditional memory clinics. They were, however, similar to the traditional clinics in terms of being multiprofessional, and aiming to carry out detailed assessments of patients, using similar standardised instruments and investigations. As the UK National Service Framework (NSF) for Older People (Department of Health, 2001) makes clear, memory clinics are now increasingly regarded as a core component of a comprehensive old age psychiatry service.

## What is a memory clinic?

There has never been an explicit agreed model of what a memory clinic is, or of how it should function, and the evidence suggests that a wide range of services now operate under this label (Lindesay et al., 2002). However, within this diversity, there is an important common theme. Most memory clinics are primarily concerned with the early assessment and diagnosis of dementia, and the subsequent provision of appropriate treatment, care, information, and support to patients in the mild to moderate stages of the illness (Luce et al., 2001). It is this focus on the particular needs of people early in the course of dementia (and their families) that distinguishes the memory clinic from all the other components of a comprehensive dementia care service, and determines how it is staffed, where it is located, and what it does. Phipps and O'Brien (2002) provide a generic specification for a memory clinic focusing on mild cognitive impairment, and suggest some quality standards against which its performance can be measured. An important implication of this focus on early dementia is that memory clinic patients typically retain capacity and judgement, and the clinical relationship is therefore much more of an equal partnership than is usual in conventional old age psychiatry services, where a benign paternalism is often unavoidable.

## The memory clinic team

Like the old age psychiatry services with which they are now often linked, memory clinics have a multidisciplinary ethos. In many instances, the memory clinic team is simply a number of individuals from the district psychogeriatric service coming together in a particular place at a particular time, to assess a particular group of referrals to that service. There may also be staff support from other parts of the local health and social services, or additional members resourced by funding allocated to specific patient groups seen in the memory clinic, for example those on antidementia drugs, or those with young onset dementia. A memory clinic cannot function without a core team of a doctor (psychiatrist, physician, neurologist), a nurse, and appropriate clerical and administrative support (Bullock and Qizilbash, 2002; Jolley et al., 2006). Other professionals who may have regular sessional input into a memory clinic include: clinical psychologists/neuropsychologists; speech and language therapists; occupational therapists; and support workers from voluntary sector organizations such as the Alzheimer's Society. Students and trainees from any or all of these professional groups may be attached to the memory clinic for a period of time, and contribute to its functioning. Depending on local interest and resources, other professionals such as social workers, pharmacists, and dieticians may be involved with the clinic on a regular basis, but they are more likely to be consulted *ad hoc* when the need arises (Jolley *et al.*, 2006).

Where should memory clinic patients be seen and assessed? Unlike mainstream old age psychiatry services, there is no principle of domiciliary assessment, and many memory clinics are located in hospital- or community-based outpatient facilities. This is probably because for the mildly cognitively impaired patient group, the limitations of assessing individuals away from their domestic environments are fewer, and are offset by the benefits of better assessment facilities, faster patient throughput, and less staff time spent in travelling. Of course, it may be apparent on referral or initial assessment that a home assessment is desirable or necessary, and there should be an option to provide this. Ideally, the memory clinic setting will be welcoming, comfortable, and free from distractions. It should be possible to interview patients and any family members/informants both together and separately if need be. There should also be facilities for the team to meet before or after the clinic to present cases, make care plans, and discuss problems. This staff meeting is also an important element of the educational function of the memory clinic (see below).

## Assessment and diagnosis

Detailed patient assessment is at the heart of a memory clinic's activities. However, the nature and content of this assessment will be determined to a great extent by the types of patient that are referred to it, and it is important to be clear what the referral criteria are. For example, a policy of open (self-) referral typically results in a much lower yield of dementia cases than referral by general practitioners (GPs) (Kelly *et al.*, 1995), and may not represent an efficient use of resources. Dementia care protocols in the UK now explicitly involve primary care in the initial assessment and screening of dementia, and should be linked to specialist memory clinic referral. Other factors that will have a bearing on the nature of the assessment and therefore the skills and resources required include the age of the patients (elderly only, or all ages), the ethnic and linguistic make-up of the local population, and the inclusion or otherwise of specific patient groups: for example, those with learning disabilities, alcoholic brain damage, or head injury. It may be that some groups will be better served by a specialist memory clinic, e.g. those with learning disabilities (Hassiotis *et al.*, 2003). Occasionally patients are referred for whom, from the information provided, it is apparent that an urgent response is required. Memory clinics need to decide if they are in a position to take such cases on; if not, there need to be arrangements in place to transfer them to local psychiatric or medical services as appropriate. Some clinics operate a triage process, in which all patients (or a selected group) are seen and assessed shortly after referral by a member of staff to identify those in whom the likely cause of the cognitive complaint is a functional psychiatric disorder such as depression or anxiety, and who can be directed to more appropriate sources of help and support.

The key components of the patient assessment are: clinical history; mental state examination; neuropsychological assessment; physical examination; laboratory investigations; neuroimaging; and functional and social assessment. These are discussed in detail elsewhere in this textbook, but a few points of relevance to the memory clinic population may be added here.

Regarding the clinical history, it should be emphasized that an informant history, ideally from a close family member, remains essential. Despite the fact that the patient may appear only mildly cognitively impaired and be able to give a good account of themselves, it is important that the story is corroborated. Some aspects of the disorder, for example subtle changes in personality or behaviour, may not be apparent to the patient, and some issues, such as alcohol abuse, may not be disclosed by them. Informants may also be in a better position to provide details of any relevant family medical or psychiatric history. All patients should therefore be asked to bring with them somebody who knows them well, and who can act as an informant.

When assessing the patient's mental state, it is important to look for evidence of depression or anxiety, as these are a common cause of subjective cognitive inefficiency, particularly in younger adults, and may result in a memory clinic referral. It should not be forgotten, however, that depression and anxiety may also accompany the onset of cognitive impairment in dementia. If a patient is significantly depressed or anxious, it may be necessary to treat this before proceeding with the cognitive assessment. A number of validated scales are available to assist with this aspect of the assessment, e.g. the Geriatric Depression Scale (Yesavage *et al.*, 1983) and the Beck Depression Inventory (Beck *et al.*, 1961) for depression, and Geriatric Anxiety Inventory (GAI; Pachana *et al.*, 2006) for anxiety. The Cornell Depression Scale (Alexopoulos *et al.*, 1998) and the Rating Anxiety in Dementia (RAID) scale (Shankar *et al.*, 1999) have been developed for use in patients with dementia. Psychotic symptoms may also occur in the early stages of dementia, and need to be enquired after. Significantly disturbed behaviour usually results in patients being referred to agencies other than memory clinics, but mild or intermittent episodes may be reported by carers at the clinic assessment. More common in this patient group are concerns about loss of initiative, apathy, social withdrawal, and lapses in judgement or decorum. Most patients attending a memory clinic have good awareness of and insight into their difficulties, but it is important to assess this formally; some patients may be denying their problems or attempting to conceal them. The Neuropsychiatric Inventory (NPI; Cummings *et al.*, 1994) is a useful screen for non-cognitive symptoms in dementia that is based on carers' observations. If memory clinics run by non-psychiatric specialities such as neurology do not include some form of psychiatric evaluation as a routine part of their assessment, they will miss functional psychiatric diagnoses (Hejl *et al.*, 2003).

All patients should receive a standardized neuropsychological assessment as part of their evaluation. A full, formal assessment by a trained neuropsychologist, deploying a battery of well-chosen validated, norm-based, educationally and culturally appropriate tests, will provide very useful information regarding differential diagnosis and localization of impairments. However, in many areas, memory clinics will not be able to call routinely upon this service; in these circumstances clinic staff will need to become familiar with one of the simplified test batteries available, such as the CAMCOG (Roth *et al.*, 1988) or the Alzheimer's Disease Assessment Scale (ADAS; Rosen *et al.* 1984), that assess a wide range of cognitive domains. A number of well-validated computerized test batteries are also available (e.g. CANTAB; Morris *et al.*, 1987; Wesnes *et al.*, 1999), but have yet to find a routine place in clinical assessment. In some clinics, speech and language therapists provide a valuable additional element to the neuropsychological assessment (Stevens and Ripich, 1999).

Physical examination and laboratory investigations are an essential component of patient assessment, to exclude treatable causes for dementia, and to identify any physical co-morbidity that may have an impact on mental functioning. Depending on the local dementia care protocols, this aspect of the assessment may have already been carried out prior to memory clinic referral, but it is necessary to see copies of any test results, and advisable to repeat the cardiovascular and neurological examinations.

Structural neuroimaging is an important element of the patient assessment in many clinics, and in some it is carried out routinely. It is still arguable as to whether MRI or CT scanning is preferable in this patient group (see Chapter 13); however, unless you examine the scans yourself, the key factor determining their utility will be the quality of the radiologist's report. It is well worth discussing with your local radiology department what information you want from the scan, and what it is able to provide.

Although the focus of a memory clinic is on diagnostic assessment, it is also essential to evaluate the patient's functional abilities and their personal and social circumstances. The caregiver is the most reliable source of information about these, in terms of activities of daily living (Rogers *et al.*, 1994). A number of standardized functional assessment scales are available, for example the Dependency Scale (Stern *et al.*, 1994), the Functional Assessment Staging Tool (FAST; Riesberg, 1988), the Assessment of Motor and Process Skills (AMPS; Fisher *et al.*, 1992), and the Bristol Activities of Daily Living Scale (BADLS; Bucks *et al.*, 1996). No one of these scales is demonstrably superior in this patient group, and all suffer from floor effects when cognitive impairment is mild and functioning largely unimpaired. If significant functional limitations are identified, this would be an indication for a further domiciliary assessment of a patient's disabilities and needs. A key component of the functional assessment is an assessment of risk, both to the patient and to others. Even a mild degree of cognitive impairment may expose the individual to significant risks of harm, particularly if they live alone or are still at work. If the patient is still driving, part of the risk assessment is to determine whether or not they are safe to continue doing so (see Chapter 44.). In a similar vein, it may be necessary to assess the patient's legal competence to consent to treatment, manage their assets, make a will, embark on marriage, and live where they choose (Jolley *et al.*, 2006) (see Chapters 41–43)

The family and other carers are the key elements of the patient's support network, and no assessment is complete without a review of their capacities and needs (Department of Health, 1999). Carers may have health problems of their own, or they may need to go out to work or look after young families; any or all of these may limit their ability to provide effective care and supervision as the patient's dementia progresses. A number of scales to assess carer strain are available (e.g. Zarit *et al.*, 1960; Greene *et al.*, 1982). In many cases, memory clinic patients have engaged with a service before there is significant functional impairment, so there is a valuable opportunity through regular follow-up to anticipate and prevent disruptive and distressing crises.

The aim of assessment is to arrive at a diagnosis and a management plan for the patient (see below). Sometimes, however, this is not possible, or the patient is found to have a mild cognitive impairment (MCI) not amounting to a diagnosis of dementia (see Chapter 26). In such cases, further non-routine investigations such as functional SPECT scanning or EEG may be helpful, but it may be necessary to wait and repeat the assessment in 6–12 months, to determine if there has been any progression. It is important that this group is followed up, because patients with MCI who present to memory clinics have a higher rate of conversion to dementia than do those identified in population-based surveys (Petersen *et al.*, 1999; Larrieu *et al.*, 2002). One study has suggested that most patients attending a memory clinic have a stable diagnosis by the time they had been seen four times over a period of 2 years (O'Neill *et al.*, 1992); however, a few individuals with MCI may require follow-up for longer than this. Significant rates of progression to dementia have also been reported in memory clinic patients deemed cognitively normal at initial assessment (Visser *et al.*, 2000; Edwards *et al.*, 2004).

Following patient assessment and discussion of the findings, a report of these should be prepared and sent to the referring agency and the patient's GP if different. This report should also include details of any care plan that has been agreed. Where appropriate, it may also be useful for the patient to have a copy of this report (Department of Health, 2000).

## Management

Management begins with the diagnosis, and the disclosure of that diagnosis to the patient and the family. In the case of dementia, this raises some important issues (Pinner, 2000). If the cognitive impairment is severe, there is little to be gained from telling the patient, but most patients seen in a memory clinic retain significant levels of capacity and judgement; they will understand the diagnosis and its implications, and will be able to make use of that information in making plans for the future. The great majority of patients wish to be told the diagnosis, and there does not appear to be any lasting harm as a result (Pinner and Bouman, 2003). The presumption therefore must be that the patient should be told, and that they and the family should be supported as appropriate. A good place to start is with the patient's own perceptions of the problem. It should not be assumed that everyone attending a memory clinic is prepared for the worst; in the study by Pinner and Bouman (2003) only 28% of the patients had any insight that they might have dementia. Similarly, we should not expect patients and their families to share our level of understanding (Werner, 2001); it is not uncommon after a careful disclosure and explanation of the diagnosis of Alzheimer's disease for the patient to respond: 'Thank God it's not dementia, doctor'. The disclosure of a diagnosis such as dementia is a process, not an event; there is a great deal of information to be imparted and the implications of this thought through. The patient and the family will need every opportunity to return and ask questions: 'How long have I got?', 'What can be done?', 'Is it hereditary?', 'Can I still drive?', 'Will vitamins/crosswords/exercise/diet help?', 'What about this alternative treatment I've found on the Internet?', 'How do I get into a drug trial?'. None of these questions is easy to answer, but all must be responded to honestly and sympathetically if a good and therapeutic alliance is to be maintained.

It should not be forgotten that the diagnosis of dementia also has important implications for the person closest to the patient (usually the spouse), who suddenly finds themselves wearing the label of 'carer', with all that this implies. They should be given the opportunity to meet with the local voluntary sector support worker if one is attached to the clinic, or provided with contact details for the local or national Alzheimer's Society if not. This provides a valuable contact that is independent from the patient, and at one remove from the clinic, to which they can turn for support and advocacy. They are also entitled to a formal assessment of their own needs by social services. The wider family may also have concerns of their own, particularly if there is a family history of dementia. First-degree relatives of the patient face a difficult choice in deciding whether or not to have their own cognitive function assessed, and may need some advice about this (Werner and Heinik, 2004). Regarding genetic testing, in over 95% of families there is no test that can identify which individuals will go on to develop dementia, and genotyping, even for *APOE* status, will not be helpful (Sadovnik, 2002). If there is a very strong family history, or links to a known pedigree, individuals should be referred on to the local genetic counselling service, where there are the skills and resources to manage their needs effectively.

One of the important reasons for disclosure of the diagnosis is that the patient cannot give informed consent to treatment in ignorance of it. The clinical management of the various forms of dementia are discussed elsewhere in this book, and will not be repeated here. For patients with diagnoses other than dementia, there are various options. Depending on resources and caseloads, memory clinic staff may wish to manage conditions such as depression and anxiety themselves, or they may refer them back to the GP with advice on management, or on to the appropriate adult or old age psychiatric service. The GP should be informed of any uncorrected vascular risk factors identified during the memory clinic assessment (hypertension, hyperlipidaemia, hypercholesterolaemia, raised blood glucose, etc.)

Resources permitting, memory clinics may also be in a position to provide a number of non-pharmacological interventions. Many memory clinics run groups for both patients and carers, and while the primary function of these may be to provide a supportive network, some explicitly address 'coping with forgetfulness', helping individuals to develop strategies to minimize the effect of their impaired memory (e.g. Zarit *et al.*, 2004). Three approaches to memory training appear to be associated with some evidence of efficacy: the facilitation of residual explicit memory (e.g. memory training); enhancement of learning through preserved implicit memory (e.g. expanding rehearsal, vanishing cues, and errorless learning); and compensation for deficits using prosthetic support (e.g. training patients to use external memory aids) (De Vreese *et al.*, 1999; Grandmaison and Simard, 2003). It appears that intact metamemory (awareness of the memory problem) is an important determinant of the efficacy of these strategies (Clare *et al.*, 2005), and this is more likely to be preserved in the mild-to-moderate stages of Alzheimer's disease seen in memory clinic patients. Patients and families can also be helped to overcome the frustration and distress that often accompanies and aggravates memory failure. In cases where language is impaired early in the course of the disorder, a speech and language therapist may be able to provide some useful strategies to improve communication (Stevens and Ripich, 1999).

'Assistive technology' is a term used to describe the various prostheses (some simple, some extremely sophisticated) that are now being developed and marketed in increasing numbers for people with dementia and their families, to provide support in the areas of recall, safety, communication, and enhancement of leisure (Woolham, 2006). A comprehensive non-commercial database of available products can be found at http://www.atdementia.org.uk.

## Information

The provision of information to the patient and the family begins even before they have been seen, with details about the clinic, where it is, their appointment details, who should come along, and what they can expect when they attend. Written notification of the appointment should be followed up with a telephone reminder a day or two before. After assessment of the patient comes the critical issue of disclosure and discussion of the diagnosis (see above). In support of this, there is now a wealth of good-quality material about dementia available in libraries, bookshops, on the Internet, and from groups such as the Alzheimer's Society (their factsheets are available at: http://www.alzheimers.org.uk/Facts_about_dementia/factsheets.htm). The clinician's task is to direct people to reliable sources of information and, importantly, to respond to any queries arising from it. At the time of diagnosis, it is also necessary to inform any patient who is still driving of their obligation to inform the DVLA and their insurers, unless the clinician is of the opinion that they should stop driving immediately.

Information will also need to be provided about the various treatment options open to the patient, and the possible benefits and risks associated with these. It is also useful to provide more general health education, as the dementing patient's compromised brain is very vulnerable to the adverse toxic, metabolic, and hypoxic effects of episodes of physical ill-health. 'Healthy heart' advice is important, since cardiovascular and cerebrovascular disease have many risk factors in common. In the present state of knowledge, there is no reason to discourage moderate consumption of alcohol, unless the patient has a past history of alcohol abuse.

The need for information will continue throughout the course of the patient's illness, as the problems and the challenges change. Patients' and carers' groups are a good means of identifying and addressing this need, and meetings may be organized around a rolling programme of topics identified by the members. Popular subjects include: information about dementia (to back up that provided in written material), legal and financial issues, keeping healthy, relaxation, alternative therapies, and updates on research.

## Support

As should be apparent from the preceding sections, the provision of both practical and emotional support to patients and their families is critical at all stages of their journey. Every contact with the memory clinic is an opportunity to give information and support, and to identify and address any new or unmet needs. By this means, clinics are providing much more than simply 'treatment monitoring' when they review patients on cholinesterase inhibitor drugs. One of the key means by which memory clinics can support their patients is by ensuring they have effective links with other services and agencies, so that as the dementia progresses emerging problems and new needs can be effectively addressed. Sometimes this may be formalized in terms of protocols or service agreements, but more often these links are maintained by ground-level networking between health and social care professionals. An efficient flow and exchange of information between service elements is vital, and this may well include the patient and their family, either by means of receiving copies of their care plan and clinical correspondence or by patient- and carer-held records (Simpson *et al.*, 2006).

# Research and teaching

New approaches to the drug treatment of Alzheimer's disease and other dementias require evaluation in clinical populations, as do the many psychosocial and other interventions currently being proposed for early stage dementia. While the function of memory clinics has now developed considerably from their origins as research settings, they still have much to offer in this respect. Many of the patients and carers are highly motivated to participate in research projects, particularly treatment trials, and if the dementia is relatively mild, there are fewer issues concerning informed consent for such studies. Over time, a valuable working partnership between patients, their families, and researchers can be created, to the benefit of all (Smith *et al.*, 1998). Information and feedback is crucial to this; once again, the patients' and carers' groups are an excellent venue for researchers to present their plans and report their findings. Another advantage that memory clinics offer the researcher is that routine data collection is often more complete and systematic than in other parts of the service, and lends itself to both descriptive and outcome research projects, and to audit (Jolley *et al.*, 2006). A common core data set for memory clinics would enable comparisons between services and collaborative pooling to increase statistical power. This has yet to be formalized, but it should be feasible to derive such a minimum data set from routine clinical practice in most clinics (Bullock and Qizilbash, 2002; Lindesay *et al.*, 2002) (Table 21.1). Clinics involved in studies requiring the post-mortem harvesting of brains will need to ensure that they have systems in place to maintain contact with their patients beyond the point at which they might normally be transferred to another part of the service. There will also need to be procedures for those who die at weekends, or at a distance from the clinic.

Memory clinics are well placed to provide training in the assessment and care of dementia to a wide range of professions at all levels from undergraduate through post-graduate to senior staff wishing to enhance or update their skills. Some longer-term training attachments to the clinic may significantly expand its workforce. Memory clinics can become the local centres of excellence for dementia, and develop or contribute to educational activities for other groups such as staff working in acute medical settings, or nursing homes. Through their links with voluntary sector groups and contacts with the media, they can also have a role in public education about dementia. Finally, the educational needs of the

**Table 21.1** A minimum data set for memory clinics (adapted from Bullock and Qizilbash, 2002)

| | | | | | |
|---|---|---|---|---|---|
| Demographic | Age/date of birth | | | Blood pressure | |
| | Gender | | | Radial pulse (rate, rhythm) | |
| | Place of residence (alone/with family/assisted/ nursing home) | | | Carotid bruit | |
| | | | | Cardiac murmur | |
| | Caregiver and level of contact | | Other assessments | Baseline/follow-up | Cognitive (MMSE) |
| | Address and other contact details | | | | Non-cognitive (NPI) |
| | Years of education | | | | Functional (e.g. Dependency Scale) |
| | Occupation: | What? | | | Global (CDR, GDS) |
| | Driver? | In work/retired | | | |
| History | Onset: | When? Sudden/gradual? | Caregiver burden | Time spent in supervision, care provision. Screen for caregiver burden (e.g. Zarit) | |
| | Family history: | Who (parents, siblings, others)? | | | |
| | | What (possible/probable dementia, CVA, other)? | Other investigations | Computed tomography/MRI Laboratory screening tests: | U&Es, LFTs, TFTs, FBC, glucose, B$_{12}$/folate, VDRL, autoantibodies |
| | Medical history: | Cardiovascular (angina, MI, dysrhythmias) | Diagnosis | Dementia: | Possible/probable Alzheimer's |
| | | Cerebrovascular (stroke, TIA) | | | Vascular dementia |
| | | Hypertension | | | Dementia with Lewy bodies |
| | | Diabetes mellitus | | | Frontotemporal dementia (frontal/temporal variants) |
| | | Significant head injury | | | Mixed |
| | | Cancer treated | | | Other |
| | | Epilepsy/fits | | | |
| | | Falls | | Mild cognitive impairment | |
| | | Tobacco use | | Other: | Depression |
| | | Alcohol use | | | Anxiety |
| | | Past psychiatric history | | | Learning disability |
| | | Medication (current, recent past) | | | Hypothyroid |
| | | | | | Vitamin B$_{12}$ deficiency |
| Physical examination | Height | | | | Head injury |
| | Weight | | | | Alcohol abuse |

Abbreviations: CVA, cardiovascular accident; MI, myocardial infarction; TIA, transient ischaemic attack; MMSE, Mini-Mental State Examination; NPI, Neuropsychiatric Inventory; CDR, Clinical Dementia Rating; GDS, Global Deterioration Scale; U&Es, urea and electrolytes; LFTs, liver function tests; TFTs, thyroid function tests; FBC, full blood count; VDRL, Venereal Disease Research Laboratory test.

memory clinic staff themselves should not be forgotten; everyone should be engaged in a programme of continuing professional and personal development.

## The effectiveness of memory clinics

To date, most of the literature on memory clinics has been descriptive, and there has been little formal evaluation of their functioning. It appears that users of memory clinics (patients, carers, GPs) appreciate the diagnostic service, although there is room for improvement regarding the clarity of information and advice given (van Hout *et al.*, 2001; Foreman *et al.*, 2004; Gardner *et al.*, 2004). One study asked family members about the 'good and bad surprises' associated with their experience of a memory clinic, as a means of identifying possible areas for improvement (Wackerbarth, 2001). In general, good surprises related to process expectations (e.g. emotional support, provider attitudes, treatment availability, quality of the assessment), whereas bad surprises related to outcome expectations (e.g. diagnosis, family reactions). Concerns have been expressed about the equity of service provision, particularly to non-English speakers in English-speaking countries (LoGiudice *et al.*, 2001; Lovestone and Murray, 2001), and it is likely that there are other socio-economic factors limiting accessibility. Outcome studies are few and far between; one focusing on psychosocial outcomes of carers found that while the provision of counselling, education, and referral to support services was associated with improved health-related quality of life, there were no changes in caregivers' psychological morbidity, burden, or knowledge of dementia (LoGiudice *et al.*, 1999). With regard to the treatment function of memory clinics, there is a small but growing literature on cholinesterase inhibitor therapy in real-world clinical practice as opposed to RCTs, examining outcomes such as mortality (Lopez-Pousa *et al.*, 2006) and patterns of symptom response (Behl *et al.*, 2006). It is not known to what extent memory clinics are cost-effective compared to other models of service, but this has not prevented organizations such as the UK National Institute for Health and Clinical Excellence (NICE, 2005) from voicing approval of their development.

## Conclusions

In the past, memory clinics have been criticized as costly, research-oriented luxuries, focusing on mild cases of dementia with few if any significant support needs (Pelosi *et al.*, 2006). This is to ignore the point that mild dementia progresses to severe dementia, and there is much that can be done in the early stages to prepare patients and families, and to anticipate and prevent some of the later problems. The move of the memory clinic from the academic margins towards the heart of old age psychiatry service provision has occurred in response to therapeutic advances, and further developments will only reinforce the need for early diagnosis, treatment, and support. The challenge for all dementia services in the coming years will be to match levels of provision to the projected growth in the numbers of individuals affected.

## References

Alexopoulos, G.S., Abrams, R.C., Young, R.C., and Shamoian, C.A. (1988). Cornell scale for depression in dementia. *Biological Psychiatry*, **23**, 271–84.

Beck, A.T., Ward, C.H., Mendelson, M., Mock, J.E., and Erbaugh, J. (1961). An inventory for measuring depression. *Archives of General Psychiatry*, **4**, 561–71.

Behl, P., Lanctot, K.L., Streiner, D.L., Guimont, I., and Black, S.E. (2006). Cholinesterase inhibitors slow decline in executive functions, rather than memory, in Alzheimer's disease: a 1-year observational study in the Sunnybrook dementia cohort. *Current Alzheimer Research*, **3**, 147–56.

Bucks, R.S., Ashworth, D.L., Wilcock, G., and Siegfried, K. (1996). Assessment of activities of daily living in dementia: development of the Bristol activities of daily living scale. *Age and Ageing*, **25**, 113–20.

Bullock, R. and Qizilbash, N. (2002). Memory clinics- a guide to implementation and evaluation. In *Evidence-based dementia practice* (ed. N. Qizilbash, L.S. Schneider, H. Chui *et al.*), pp. 828–43. Blackwell Publishing, Oxford.

Clare, L., Markova, I., Verhey, F., and Kenny, G. (2005). Awareness in dementia: a review of assessment methods and measures. *Aging and Mental Health*, **9**, 394–413.

Cummings, J.L., Mega, M., Gray, K., Rosenberg-Thompson, S., Carusi, D.A., and Gornbein, J. (1994). The Neuropsychiatric Inventory: comprehensive assessment of psychopathology in dementia. *Neurology*, **44**, 2308–14.

Department of Health (1999). *Caring about carers. A national strategy for carers.* HMSO, London.

Department of Health (2000). *The NHS Plan.* Department of Health, London.

Department of Health (2001). *National service framework for older people.* Department of Health, London.

De Vreese, L., Neri, M., Foiravanti, M. *et al.* (1999). Memory rehabilitation in Alzheimer's disease: a review of progress. *International Journal of Geriatric Psychiatry*, **16**, 794–809.

Edwards, E.R., Lindquist, K., and Yaffe, K. (2004). Clinical profile and course of cognitively normal patients evaluated in memory disorders clinics. *Neurology*, **11**, 639–42.

Fisher, A.G., Liu, Y., Velozo, C.A., and Pan, A.W. (1992). Cross-cultural assessment of process skills. *American Journal of Occupational Therapy*, **46**, 876–85.

Foreman, P., Gardner, I., and Davis, S. (2004). Multidisciplinary memory clinics: what is important to caregivers and clients? *International Journal of Geriatric Psychiatry*, **19**, 588–9.

Fraser, M. (1992). Memory clinics and memory training. In *Recent advances in psychogeriatrics 2* (ed. T. Arie), pp. 105–16. Churchill Livingstone, London.

Gardner, I., Foreman, P., and Davis, S. (2004). Cognitive, dementia, and memory service clinics: opinions of general practitioners. *American Journal of Alzheimer's Disease and Other Dementias*, **19**, 105–10.

Grandmaison, E. and Simard, M. (2003). A clinical review of memory stimulation programs in Alzheimer's disease. *Journal of Neuropsychiatry and Clinical Neuroscience*, **15**, 130–44.

Greene, J.G., Smith, R., Gardiner, M., and Timbury, G.C. (1982). Measuring behavioural disturbance of elderly patients in the community and its effect on relatives: a factor analytic study. *Age and Ageing*, **11**, 121–6.

Hassiotis, A., Strydom, A., Allen, K., and Walker, Z. (2003). A memory clinic for older people with intellectual difficulties. *Aging and Mental Health*, **7**, 418–23.

Hejl, A.M., Hording, M., Hasselbalch, E., Dam, H., Hemmingsen, R., and Waldemar, G. (2003). Psychiatric morbidity in a neurology-based memory clinic: the effect of systematic psychiatric evaluation. *Journal of the American Geriatrics Society*, 51, 1773–8.

Jolley, D., Benbow, S.M., and Grizzell, M. (2006). Memory clinics. *Postgraduate Medical Journal*, **82**, 199–206.

Kelly, C.A., Harvey, R.J., Nicholl, C.G., Stevens, S.J., and Pitt, B.M.N. (1995). Specialist memory clinics: the experience of the Hammersmith Hospital. *Facts and Research in Gerontology*, 25–30.

Larrieu, S., Letenneur, L., Orgoozo, J.M. *et al.* (2002). Incidence and outcome of mild cognitive impairment in a population-based prospective cohort. *Neurology*, **26**, 1594–9.

Lindesay, J., Marudkar, M., van Diepen, E., and Wilcock, G. (2002). The second Leicester survey of memory clinics in the British Isles. *International Journal of Geriatric Psychiatry*, **17**, 41–7.

LoGiudice, D., Waltrowicz, W., Brown, K., Burrows, C., Ames, D., and Flicker, L. (1999). Do memory clinics improve the quality of life of carers? A randomized pilot trial. *International Journal of Geriatric Psychiatry*, **14**, 626–32.

LoGiudice, D., Hassett, A., Cook, R., Flicker, L., and Ames, D. (2001). Equity of access to a memory clinic in Melbourne? Non-English speaking background of attenders are more severely demented and have increased rate of psychiatric disorders. *International Journal of Geriatric Psychiatry*, **16**, 327–34.

Lopez-Pousa, S., Olmo, J.G., Franch, J.V. et al. (2006). Comparative analysis of mortality in patients with Alzheimer's disease treated with donepezil or galantamine. *Age and Ageing*, **35**, 365–71.

Lovestone, S. and Murray, D. (2001). Acetylcholinesterase treatment-modelling potential demand and auditing practice. *International Journal of Geriatric Psychiatry*, **16**, 1136–42.

Luce, A., McKeith, I., Swann, A., Daniel, S., and O'Brien, J. (2001). How do memory clinics compare with traditional old age psychiatry services? *International Journal of Geriatric Psychiatry*, **16**, 837–45.

Morris, R.G., Evenden, J.L., Sahakian, B.J., and Robbins, T.W. (1987). Computer-aided assessment of dementia: comparative studies of neuropsychological deficits in Alzheimer-type dementia and Parkinson's disease. In *Cognitive neurochemistry* (ed. S.M. Stahl, S.D. Iverson, and E.C. Goodman). Oxford University Press, Oxford.

NICE (National Institute for Health and Clinical Excellence) (2005). *Appraisal consultation document. Donepezil, rivastigmine, galantamine and memantine for the treatment of Alzheimer's disease* (http://www.nice.org.uk).

O'Neill, D., Surmon, D.J., and Wilcock, G.K. (1992). Longitudinal diagnosis of memory disorders. *Age and Ageing*, **21**, 393–7.

Pachana, N.A., Byrne, G.J., Siddle, H., Koloski, N., Harley, E., and Arnold, E. (2006). Development and validation of the Geriatric Anxiety Inventory. *International Psychogeriatrics*, **29**, 1–12.

Pelosi, A.J., McNulty, S.V., and Jackson, G.A. (2006). Role of cholinesterase inhibitors in dementia care needs rethinking. *British Medical Journal*, **333**, 491–3.

Petersen, R.C., Smith, G.E., Waring, S.C., Ivnik, R.J., Tangalos, E.G., and Kokmen, E. (1999). Mild cognitive impairment: clinical characterization and outcome. *Archives of Neurology*, **56**, 303–8.

Phipps, A.J. and O'Brien, J.T. (2002). Memory clinics and clinical governance – a UK perspective. *International Journal of Geriatric Psychiatry*, **17**, 1128–32.

Pinner, G. (2000). Truth-telling and the diagnosis of dementia. *British Journal of Psychiatry*, **176**, 514–15.

Pinner, G. and Bouman, W.P. (2003). Attitudes of patients with mild dementia and their carers towards disclosure of the diagnosis. *International Psychogeriatrics*, **15**, 279–88.

Riesberg, B. (1988). Functional Assessment Staging (FAST). *Psychopharmacology Bulletin*, **24**, 653–5.

Rogers, J.C., Holm, M.B., and Goldstein, G. (1994). Stability and change in functional assessment of patients with geropsychiatric disorders. *American Journal of Occupational Therapy*, **48**, 914–18.

Rosen, W.G., Mohs, R.C., and Davies, K.L. (1984). A new rating scale for Alzheimer's disease. *American Journal of Psychiatry*, **141**, 1356–64.

Roth, M., Huppert, F.A., Tym, E., and Mountjoy, C.Q. (1988). *CAMDEX: The Cambridge Examination for Mental Disorders of the Elderly*. Cambridge University Press, Cambridge.

Sadovnik, A.D. (2002). Genetic counselling. In *Evidence-based dementia practice* (ed. N. Qizilbash, L.S. Schneider, H. Chui et al.), pp. 795–800. Blackwell Publishing, Oxford.

Shankar, K.K., Walker, M., Frost, D., and Orrell, M.W. (1999). The development of a valid and reliable scale for rating anxiety in dementia. *Aging and Mental Health*, **3**, 39–49.

Simpson, R., Wakefield, P., Spiers, N., Jagger, C., and Lindesay, J. (2006). Carer-held records for dementia: a controlled trial. *International Psychogeriatrics*, **18**, 259–68.

Smith, A., King, F., Hindley, N., Barnetson, L., Barton, J., and Jobst, K.A. (1998). The experience of research participation and the value of diagnosis in dementia: Implications for practice. *Journal of Mental Health*, **7**, 309–21.

Stern, Y., Albert, S., Sano, M. et al. (1994). Assessing patient dependence in Alzheimer's disease. *Journal of Gerontology*, **49**, M216–M222.

Stevens, S. and Ripich, D. (1999). The role of the speech and language therapist. In *Diagnosis and management of dementia: a manual for memory disorders teams* (ed. G.K. Wilcock, R.S. Bucks, and K. Rockwood), pp. 137–57. Oxford University Press, Oxford.

van Hout, H.P., Vernooij-Dassen, M.J., Hoefnagels, W.H., and Grol, R.P. (2001). Measuring the opinions of memory clinic users: patients, relatives and general practitioners. *International Journal of Geriatric Psychiatry*, **16**, 846–51.

Visser, P.J., Verhey, F.R., Ponds, R.W., Cruts, M., Van Broeckhoven, C.L., and Jolles, J. (2000). Course of objective memory impairment in non-demented subjects attending a memory clinic and predictors of outcome. *International Journal of Geriatric Psychiatry*, **15**, 363–72.

Wackerbarth, S. (2001). Using 'good and bad surprises' to guide improvement efforts: insights from a memory assessment clinic. *The Joint Commission Journal on Quality Improvement*, **27**, 362–8.

Werner, P. (2001). Correlates of family care-givers' knowledge about Alzheimer's disease. *International Journal of Geriatric Psychiatry*, **16**, 32–8.

Werner, P. and Heinik, J. (2004). Intentions of first-degree relatives of patients with Alzheimer's disease to seek a cognitive status examination. *International Journal of Geriatric Psychiatry*, **19**, 479–86.

Wesnes, K.A., Hildebrand, K., and Mohr, E. (1999). Computerized cognitive assessment. In *Diagnosis and management of dementia: a manual for memory disorders teams* (ed. G.K. Wilcock, R.S. Bucks, and K. Rockwood), pp. 124–36. Oxford University Press, Oxford.

Woolham, J. (ed.). (2006). *Assistive technology in dementia care: developing the role of technology in the care and rehabilitation of people with dementia – current trends and perspectives*. Hawker Publications, London.

Wright, N. and Lindesay, J. (1995). A survey of memory clinics in the British Isles. *International Journal of Geriatric Psychiatry*, **10**, 379–85.

Yesavage, J.A., Brink, T.L., Rose, T.L., and Lunn, O. (1983). Development and validation of a geriatric depression screening scale: a preliminary report. *Journal of Psychiatric Research*, **17**, 37–49.

Zarit, S.H., Reever, K.E., and Bach-Peterson, J. (1960). Relatives of the impaired elderly: correlates of 'feelings of burden'. *Gerontologist*, **20**, 649–55.

Zarit, S.H., Femia, E.E., Watson, J., Rice-Oeschger, L., and Kakos, B. (2004). Memory club: a group intervention for people with early-stage dementia and their care partners. *Gerontologist*, **44**, 262–9.

# 22

# Liaison old age psychiatry

## John Holmes

The last 5 years have seen an increase in interest in liaison psychiatry services for older people in the UK. This is not surprising, since specialist liaison psychiatry services exist for adults of working age in many places, yet most patients in general hospitals, where liaison psychiatry services operate, are aged 65 years or older. This chapter sets out the case of need for specific liaison psychiatry services for older people, discusses what services look like and what they do, and advises on how services can be established successfully.

## Introduction

Two-thirds of general hospital beds in the UK are occupied by people aged 65 years or older (Department of Health, 2001; Scottish Office, 2001). Older people are found almost everywhere in the general hospital; care of the elderly departments by definition have older patients in their beds, but general medical wards, general surgery, orthopaedics, respiratory wards, cardiology, and many other specialities also look after older people. Figure 22.1 shows the distribution of non-elective admissions of older people to a range of specialities in a large teaching hospital, and demonstrates that, apart from paediatrics and obstetrics, the care of older people is core business for most medical and surgical specialities.

Why should this be of interest to psychiatrists? There are five reasons: (1) the prevalence of mental health problems in the general hospital setting is higher than in community settings; (2) these mental health problems independently predict poor outcomes; (3) the management of mental health problems in older people in this setting is often suboptimal; (4) referrals from general hospitals comprise 25% of referrals received by old age psychiatry services; (5) the prevalent older people's mental health service model in the UK does not adequately meet the challenge of optimizing management and improving outcomes (Working Group of the Faculty of Old Age Psychiatry, 2005).

## How common are mental health problems in older people in the general hospital?

Attempting to determine the prevalence of mental health problems in general hospital settings is fraught with problems because of the high number of potential biases, as follows:

- **The hospital setting**. The prevalence of depression, dementia, and delirium will be different in different areas of the hospital.

Older people on orthopaedic wards have much higher levels of delirium than the general medical setting because of the higher levels of risk factors for delirium in the older trauma population. The case mix of physical problems can vary from day to day on a general medical or surgical ward, leading to fluctuations in the prevalence of associated mental health problems, whereas areas dealing with single conditions (such as coronary care units or stroke wards) are likely to have more consistent prevalences.

- **Case-finding** can be difficult. For example, many people in hospital report depressive symptoms, but when viewed in the context of their physical illness, levels of distress, and the fact that general hospital wards seem designed to produce melancholy, the use of symptom checklists may lead to over-diagnosis of formal depressive episodes when many people have adjustment disorders that will resolve spontaneously on discharge or as their physical problem resolves (Winrow and Holmes, 2005). Delirium waxes and wanes in severity, meaning that studies examining participants frequently over several days will find higher rates of delirium than those looking only once. Delirium shares many features with dementia but has a different aetiology and time-course, and delirium commonly occurs superimposed on dementia; perhaps this is why some researchers have not differentiated between the two and have simply measured cognitive impairment, which can also be present in depression. And of course, it is perfectly possible to have depression and dementia together, yet most case-finding instruments (for example the Geriatric Mental State Schedule (Gurland et al., 1976)) have only a single diagnostic output, usually based on a hierarchical system where organic diagnoses over-ride functional ones.

- **Recruitment**. Studies excluding the 30% of patients in general medical wards who lack the capacity to consent to participation (Raymont et al., 2004) will fail to recognize the dementia and delirium that have produced this incapacity. The timing of recruitment is also important, since length of hospital stay is positively skewed, meaning that recruitment of participants after one week in hospital will miss those who have already been discharged or died.

- **Sampling methods**. People with specific conditions such as hip fracture present at a rate manageable by researchers, meaning that recruitment to a prevalence study can be comprehensive. In contrast, a busy medical assessment unit can turn over its entire

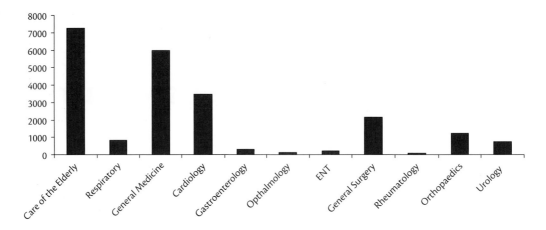

**Fig. 22.1** The distribution of emergency admissions of older people within a general hospital over a 1-year period.

population in a couple of days, requiring a large number of researchers (bringing issues of inter-rater reliability) or a suitable method of randomly sampling for potential participants.

Despite these problems, a systematic review (Working Group of the Faculty of Old Age Psychiatry, 2005) has revealed 97 studies that met pre-defined quality criteria (out of a total of 576 studies). These 97 studies reveal a large amount of evidence for higher levels of depression, dementia, and delirium in a variety of hospital settings than found in the community. Alcohol misuse and anxiety are also present, as is schizophrenia, though at rates no higher than in community surveys. Further details are found in Table 22.1. There are some notable absences; we appear to know very little about somatization disorders in older people in this setting (Wijeratne *et al.*, 2003), although personal experience suggests that they certainly exist, and there is little evidence available on self-harm in older people, though one study suggests that older people comprise 2.7% of the self-harm population presenting to accident and emergency departments (Horrocks *et al.*, 2003). Much of the stroke literature is not exclusive to older people, but there are high levels of delirium, dementia, and depression reported in people after stroke (Ferro *et al.*, 2002; Merino and Hachinski, 2002; Turner-Stokes and Hassan, 2002). We are also beginning to appreciate that mental health problems exist in other previously unresearched conditions, such as chronic obstructive pulmonary disease (Yohannes *et al.*, 2000).

If the prevalence figures are to be believed, then some 60% of older people in a typical general hospital have a mental health problem, either associated with a physical problem or as the sole reason for presentation. This represents a third of the total number of occupied beds in that hospital, meaning that the general hospital is providing inpatient care to about six times as many older people with mental health problems than the local mental health services do.

## The impact on outcomes

Having established that mental health problems are common in older people in general hospitals, we now turn to the effect on outcomes. This leads to the question of which outcomes and for whom. Individual patients may be interested in their survival, independence, and quality of life. Carers want to know about the level of carer burden and strain. Clinicians will share the aims of their patients but will also be interested in quality of care. Health service commissioners and managers, whilst aware of the importance of the above, are also concerned about financial and organizational costs. However, as with determining prevalence, carrying out research in this area has several pitfalls. Outcome studies in this setting must first have all the features of a good prevalence study, detailed above. Then they need to address the following:

◆ **Timing of recruitment.** Because of the changing nature of exposure to different risks at different times of a hospital admission, and the skewed length of stay, an inception cohort study with a common time of recruitment early in the admission is required. This, however, brings ethical issues related to allowing enough

**Table 22.1** The prevalence of mental health problems in older people in general hospitals

| Dliagnosis | No. of studies | Total no. of participants | Mean sample size | Prevalence range (%) | Mean prevalence (%) |
|---|---|---|---|---|---|
| Depression | 47 | 14,632 | 311 | 5–58 | 29 |
| Delirium | 31 | 9601 | 309 | 7–61 | 20 |
| Dementia | 17 | 3845 | 226 | 5–45 | 31 |
| Cognitive impairment | 33 | 13,882 | 421 | 7–88 | 22 |
| Anxiety | 3 | 1346 | 449 | 1–34 | 8 |
| Schizophrenia | 4 | 1878 | 376 | 1–8 | 1.4 |
| Alcohol misuse | 4 | 1314 | 329 | 1–5 | 3 |

time for informed consent to be sought. Additionally, the severity of physical illness may preclude entry into a research study at a common inception point.

- **Confounding variables**. There are many variables that can affect outcome in the general hospital population. These include age, gender, severity and number of physical illnesses, pre-admission abilities of activities of daily living, social support, being cared for by a specialist team, what type of anaesthetic is used during surgery, and many others. Add to these dementia, delirium, and depression, and indeed delirium superimposed on dementia which may have a particularly bad prognosis (Andrew *et al.*, 2006), and we have a complex data set to acquire and analyse.

- **Sample size and analysis**. Whereas studies of prevalence can be carried out with relatively small numbers since the three main conditions being examined are common, the large number of confounding variables for outcomes means that a much larger sample size is required. For example, in order to determine the impact of psychiatric illness in an orthopaedic population with 90% power and a *P*-value of 0.05, a sample size of 660 is required (Holmes and House, 2000a). The correct statistical methods are also important; for endpoints such as discharge, death, readmission, and institutionalization, survival analysis (using a Cox proportional hazards model) is usually the most appropriate technique, with identical follow-up periods for all participants to ensure equal exposure to risks and adequate accounting for those participants who have died as they are no longer at risk of other outcomes.

With this is mind a further systematic review of outcomes in this population has been carried out (Working Group of the Faculty of Old Age Psychiatry, 2005). This found 27 studies meeting pre-defined quality criteria. Findings were mixed, with many studies reporting no impact on outcomes such as mortality, length of stay, and independence. Heterogeneity of case-determining instruments, outcomes measured, duration of follow-up, and statistical techniques means that a meta-analysis of these studies is not feasible. It is noteworthy that only three studies had sample sizes larger than the 660 suggested by the above power calculation, meaning that the likelihood of a type II statistical error is high; that is, that an important effect may have not reached the statistical significance it may have done with a larger sample. This is borne out by the fact that the larger studies in this review show robust adverse effects for depression, delirium, dementia, and unspecified cognitive impairment on mortality, length of hospital stay, institutionalization, physical dependence, and general health status. This means that as well as being common, mental health problems in older people in general hospitals are independent predictors of poor outcomes that are of interest to patients, carers, clinicians, commissioners, and managers.

## Why are outcomes so bad?

There are several possible factors contributing to poor outcomes. The index mental health problem itself may bring worse outcomes, no matter how well it is managed. However, there is evidence to suggest that management of mental health problems in older people in the general hospital setting is far from optimal, and that this suboptimal management may itself contribute to adverse outcomes. There are several possible explanations:

- Mental health problems are poorly detected. General ward staff are not tuned in to mental health problems, and do not routinely screen for them in the same way that they screen for physical problems, for example by taking temperatures, pulse rate, and blood pressure. Where mental health problems are identified in older people it is usually through their behaviour—or more accurately, perceived misbehaviour such as aggression, wandering, interfering with other patients, and refusing medication (Atkin *et al.*, 2005). In the hip fracture population, where the delirious are in the majority, rates of detection by clinicians are half those of researchers (Gustafson *et al.*, 1991) and in the broader medical population detection rates are only between 32% and 67% (Inouye, 1994). The same is true of depression, with as few as 10% of cases being identified in routine care (Cole and Bellavance, 1997). One description of older people referred to a liaison psychiatry service for assessment of mood found that 40% had a delirium as the cause of their mood symptoms (Farrell and Ganzini, 1995).

- Physical care needs are prioritized over mental health needs. The focus is on physical interventions for physical problems, with mental health problems not seen as life-threatening. Even when staff have the time to talk to a confused patient, they are uncomfortable doing so and would rather tidy up the ward (Atkin *et al.*, 2005). In some cases, mental health needs are ignored completely in the expectation that they will go away spontaneously (Holmes *et al.*, 2002).

- General hospital staff lack the knowledge and skills to manage mental health problems. This leads to treatment rates for depression as low as 25% (Holmes and House, 2000a), to an over-reliance on psychotropic medication in delirium rather than techniques such as de-escalation and environmental manipulation (Holmes *et al.*, 2003b), and to wide variations in the choice of medication, dose, and route of administration with some doctors prescribing doses that are well above British National Formulary maxima and that could be described as poisonous rather than therapeutic (Hally and Cooney, 2005). These are all staff who have been through training programmes that are supposed to equip them for their future careers, yet examination of the content of many of these training programmes reveals a paucity of mental health experience and training, with what training there is often being questionable—one focus group participant revealed that their mental health experience consisted of 4 weeks in a day hospital where they played bingo, did exercises, and threw a ball at each other (Atkin *et al.*, 2005), hardly helpful when having to manage complex problems in a general hospital setting. This means that the skill-mix on general wards does not address mental health needs adequately (Norquist *et al.*, 1995).

- Mental health services are seen as slow to respond. Referrals are not made as they will slow down the discharge process at a time when there is marked pressure on hospital beds and lengths of hospital stay are reducing (Holmes *et al.*, 2002). Only 5% of old age psychiatrists surveyed felt that their service was generally able to respond to general hospital referrals within one working day, and 60% felt that a response time of five or more days was a realistic target (Holmes *et al.*, 2003a).

- There are low referral rates from particular specialities. Consultant old age psychiatrists considered that there were several medical and surgical specialities that had inappropriately low referral rates, including orthopaedics, general surgery, and neurology (Holmes *et al.*, 2003a), the former a particular worry given the extremely high prevalence and adverse impact of mental health problems in the hip fracture population (Holmes and House, 2000a,b).

Despite these problems, general nursing staff and other colleagues often recognize that they are not adequately trained to manage older people with mental health problems; they feel that they are doing their patients a disservice, and that similar mismanagement of physical problems would not be tolerated (Atkin *et al.*, 2005).

Overarching all of this is the organizational and managerial structure of the National Health Service, particularly in England and Wales, where providers of acute hospital care and mental health care sit in different organizations with different organizational objectives and what seems like a silo mentality. If the attitudes of general hospital staff are reflected by their own managers, the lack of ownership of older people with mental health problems in the general hospital setting could be a further reason why outcomes for this group are so poor. This is reflected at a higher level too; at the time of writing a search of the English Department of Health website reveals only two hits for delirium, one of the commonest conditions found in older people in general hospitals.

It seems therefore that there are deficiencies at several stages contributing to poor outcomes, including at level of the individual practitioner and at an organizational level too. We will next consider how these deficiencies can be addressed.

## Improving outcomes

There have been several intervention studies in physically ill older people with mental health problems, but few of high quality. For example, a Cochrane Review has revealed only one randomized controlled trial for the treatment of depression in this population (Gill and Hatcher, 2000). Examination of the multicomponent intervention studies to reduce the incidence and severity of delirium reveals that most of the interventions could simply be described as good nursing and medical care (Cole, 2004), for example ensuring that patients are hydrated, nourished, and have optimal sensory input. However, if the reasons for poor outcomes explored above are to be believed, there needs to be a mechanism for addressing deficits in knowledge, skills, and attitudes of a wide range of health-care professionals, as well as enabling the routine delivery of mental health care by mental health professionals in the general hospital setting. This is echoed by nursing colleagues, who want help to be able to identify and manage less complex mental health problems. They also feel that better signposting to old age psychiatry services would also help them, with clear referral routes, a more rapid response, direct access to a mental health professional for telephone advice on management, any member of the ward team able to refer for an old age psychiatry assessment, and more ward-based follow-up and review by mental health staff. General nurses also identified a group of patients with complex physical and mental health-care needs that would be best met in an environment where they were working side by side with mental health nurses on the same ward, and noted that such a resource would be invaluable for training (Atkin *et al.*, 2005). This means that part of the answer to the problem of mental health problems in general hospitals is likely to lie in the configuration and activity of old age psychiatry service rather than antidepressants or antipsychotics alone.

It is now time to examine the kind of input that old age psychiatry services provide to general hospitals, to see if it meets the requirements of our nursing colleagues. Before we do this, we need to consider the types of service model that could possibly operate, together with the pros and cons of each model. We also need to understand the meaning of the two terms, consultation and liaison, in this context.

## Consultation or liaison?

As a trainee psychiatrist I found that any referral originating in the general hospital setting was called a liaison referral, and colleagues would talk about liaison activity when talking about their responses to these referrals. The response entailed a visit to the referring ward, scrutiny of the notes, discussion with whichever clinicians were available, assessment of the patient, and the writing of a management plan in the medical notes. Sometimes further discussion with ward staff would take place. However, it was not unusual to find few clinicians to speak to, particularly as many assessments were carried out late in the day on the way home, meaning that little true liaison took place. It was also often difficult to clarify exactly what question the referrer had in mind, and to obtain further relevant information about the patient and their circumstances. In addition, recommendations made in medical notes were not often followed, something that was not often appreciated as few patients were followed up on the ward. A more correct term for this type of work is consultation, a model that relies on general hospital staff to detect mental health problems, refer on a case-by-case basis and follow the advice offered, and we have already highlighted deficits in these areas.

What are the alternatives? One possibility is a true liaison approach, where the service is more proactive, working collaboratively with general hospital colleagues to train and educate them so that they are confident in the basics of the management of the common mental health problems they come across, and so they know who, when, and where to refer. The response to referrals is more prompt, and a frequent presence on general wards allows for the delivery of mental health care (including brief psychological therapies) routinely, including opportunities for modelling good care to general staff. This has much more potential to improve outcomes, and in particular to challenge the negative attitudes to older people with mental health problems that seem to be at the heart of the problem. The liaison approach requires a consultation service operating in the background, able to respond to referrals received, so these services are known as consultation-liaison services in some parts of the world. Table 22.2 shows the pros and cons of consultation and liaison.

Liaison psychiatry services already exist in the UK for adults of working age, with 93 funded consultant posts (Swift and Guthrie, 2003), a specialist Faculty of Liaison Psychiatry of the Royal College of Psychiatrists, and training with specialist accreditation. They have developed despite the lack of a robust evidence base for their effectiveness (Ruddy and House, 2005). The same specialist services and training do not exist for old age psychiatry, despite the English National Service Framework for Older People (Department of Health, 2001) calling for action to root out age discrimination in the National Health Service. Some liaison psychiatry services for adults of working age see older people, often solely after self-harm or in emergencies, but this is far from universal (Ruddy and House, 2003).

**Table 22.2** The differences between consultation and liaison for the general hospital setting

| Consultation | Liaison |
|---|---|
| Reactive | Proactive |
| Low cost | Higher cost |
| Professionally isolated | Collaboration with other professions |
| General hospital referrals a low priority | General hospital referrals a high priority |
| Slow response to referrals | Rapid response to referrals |
| Low review rates | Frequent review rates |
| Some poor quality referrals | Fewer poor referrals |
| Poor adherence to recommendations | Improved adherence to recommendations |
| No influence on practice of general hospital staff | Influences practice of general hospital staff |
| Mental health managerially separate from general services | Mental health managerially integrated with general services |

Adapted from Working Group of the Faculty of Old Age Psychiatry (2005).

## Models of liaison

Most old age psychiatry services offer the consultation model to general hospitals, although many old age psychiatrists would prefer to offer a liaison model (Holmes *et al.*, 2003a). Possible models providing general hospital input are discussed below.

### The standard sector model

This is currently the prevalent service model, providing comprehensive mental health services for a population of older people defined either by geography or general practitioner. General hospital input is on a consultation basis and referrals are usually seen by medical staff, although other members of the community mental health team may visit people already on their caseload. In order to access this service, referrers need to know which sector service to refer to and how to make contact. Old age psychiatry services are increasingly based away from general hospital settings, so there may be inefficiencies in travelling and parking built into this model. However, there is good communication about clinical cases within the community team, and continuity of care is perceived to be better. Response to general hospital referrals can be slow, particularly as referrals of people in the community are seen as more at risk and so are prioritized (Holmes *et al.*, 2002). Review of patients does not often happen. Because several different psychiatrists from different sectors and of different grades can potentially respond to referrals, opinions and advice offered may not be consistent, providing a potential source of confusion to general hospital colleagues. This model also assumes that the psychiatrist is in the best position to assess and offer advice, although there are occasions when input from other mental health professionals may be much more appropriate. Opportunities for teaching and training are limited with this model.

### The enhanced sector model

Where this model operates, a community mental health team receives additional staffing (usually nursing) ring-fenced to provide input to the general hospital. This creates more opportunities for non-medical assessments and more reviews, and continuity of care is good. However, most limitations of the standard sector model apply, and staff time intended for general hospital work may be eroded by pressures of work in the community.

### Outreach from mental health wards

With the outreach model, staff from mental health wards provide input to general hospital wards. This is usually on a consultation basis, although often staff will review a patient who has been transferred from the psychiatric ward to the general hospital ward, or who is about to be transferred the other way. There is the potential for training and education with this model, but it does depend on psychiatric ward staff not being needed on their own ward, and psychiatric ward staff are as busy as their general hospital colleagues. For this model to work at all, the psychiatric ward needs to be on the general hospital site and this is not necessarily the case in many places. The response to a referral may be slow when an urgent assessment is necessary.

### The liaison mental health nurse

Here, a specialist mental health nurse is based in the general hospital and provides a responsive liaison mental health service to general hospital wards. Referrals are seen quickly, and more patients are reviewed to monitor their mental state and check that advice is being followed. Some patients may subsequently need a psychiatric review, with the nurse acting at least in part as a triage point. This means that there should be access to a psychiatrist as part of this model. A particular benefit of this model is the possibility of offering advice on the non-pharmacological management of difficult behaviour. A liaison nurse has time for teaching and training, although the hierarchical nature of general hospital professionals may mean that some professional groups may be difficult for the nurse to access. However, through good training programmes, protocols for screening and treating can be developed with general hospital staff as true partners. Interfaces with the other old age psychiatry services (and in particular the community mental health teams) need to be clarified and agreed so that continuity of care can be delivered, albeit through more than one health-care professional. Many liaison nurses work in isolation and this leads to a high workload and the possibility of burnout.

### The liaison psychiatrist

An old age liaison psychiatrist has dedicated time for general hospital work. Their activity is similar to that of the liaison mental health nurse, with a rapid response to referrals and an emphasis on teaching and training. A medical background brings an understanding of the complexity of some medical problems but there may be less expertise in the area of behavioural management. As with the liaison nurse, interfaces and communication with other parts of the service are important, and increasing workloads can lead to burnout. Both the liaison nurse and liaison psychiatrist operate in a unidisciplinary way, unlike mental health services in most settings.

### The shared care ward

In this model, a ward on the general hospital site has psychiatric and general nurses, psychiatrists, physicians, and therapy staff who work together delivering care to patients with both physical and mental health-care needs that would otherwise fall between services. It is an add-on to other services, having a small bed base (12 to 16 beds are adequate) but is able to cope with complex care needs presented by, for example, someone with an agitated delirium, and is also able to provide a haven for those detained under the Mental Health Act who can then receive the psychiatric care that they require in the general hospital. The shared care ward can act as a training resource for many staff, who are able to learn new knowledge and skills from colleagues of other disciplines whilst working side by side with them. Existing examples of shared care wards are varied, but those that are successful have clear admission and discharge criteria and are explicitly not used to accommodate patients waiting for placement. Systematic evaluations of effectiveness are, however, lacking, due in part to the complexity of the evaluation and the low numbers of patients an individual ward will admit over time.

## The hospital mental health team

In this, the most complete model of true liaison, a multidisciplinary team with a similar professional mix to a community mental health team (psychiatrists, mental health nurses, clinical psychologists, social workers, occupational therapists, etc.) works with the general hospital population as its sector, with a large and transient population. Individual team members can build up affiliations with particular parts of the general hospital, and can call upon the specialist skills of other team members as appropriate. Teaching and training of general hospital staff are core business for a hospital mental health team, resulting in the ward staff taking ownership and responsibility for mental health problems on that ward and providing the basics of management, with specialist referral to the mental health team as required. There is a single point of access and referrals are responded to promptly (often the same day). There is also the possibility of introducing staff support in areas where stress is high, such as in intensive care. As with other liaison models, good communication is important. The hospital mental health team is the model of care recommended for old age psychiatry services in England (Department of Health and Care Services Improvement Partnership, 2005).

## Other teams and disciplines

In some places, teams exist to provide specialist input for specific psychiatric illnesses in older people. Examples include accelerated discharge teams for people with dementia. These teams are usually organized in a similar way to a hospital mental health team but are not designed to offer a comprehensive service. Clinical psychologists also work in general hospitals but do not often work along with other mental health professions (Holmes *et al.*, 2002).

## The older person's liaison mental health outpatient clinic

Where a hospital mental health team is established, it will come across some patients for whom brief follow-up after hospital discharge is required, such as someone with an adjustment disorder or resolving delirium. Also, older people can present with somatization disorder (Sheehan *et al.*, 2003) and with intertwined physical and psychiatric problems that are not severe enough to warrant admission to hospital but require specialist assessment and treatment. Because of this it may be worth establishing a specialist liaison clinic, similar to those existing for adults of working age, where the specialist skills of the liaison practitioner can be harnessed.

# The UK picture

In the UK the predominant model for providing old age psychiatry input to general hospitals is the traditional sector model, used by 73% of old age psychiatrists surveyed, and of the liaison models only the liaison nurse was the model used in any great number (14%) (Holmes *et al.*, 2003a). However, many old age psychiatrists surveyed to establish this provision were unhappy with their own services for older people in general hospitals, with most preferring a liaison model (liaison psychiatrist, liaison nurse, or hospital mental health team) if they were given the choice. Table 22.3 shows comments from survey respondents about the influences on their choice of preferred models.

These comments are both interesting and informative. They remind us that some health-care professionals see any change as a

**Table 22.3** Reasons influencing choice of model for input into the general hospital

| Choosing the traditional sector model | It's the service I inherited. I believe this traditional sector model is still most appropriate for community referrals. I cannot provide a full liaison service |
| --- | --- |
| | Keeps the patients within our own community mental health teams so not having to liaise with yet another set of professionals who are not well known to us |
| | Continuity of care |
| | Why change? |
| | Liaison… although I see it as very important is still an unpaid hobby and development area |
| | A sense that the patients in hospital are being looked after, the patient living alone and unwell seems more worthy |
| | If a patient is in a hospital bed they are already in a place of safety |
| Choosing a liaison model | The educational part of liaison is missing |
| | Complexity of patient problems needs a multidisciplinary team approach and that needs to be based in the District General Hospital not visiting occasionally |
| | Dedicated team can influence the atmosphere in medical wards and over time change practice and attitudes |
| | Patients get a bad deal |
| | We suffer from fairly concrete opposition from the general hospital trust and some of the geriatric physicians to setting up joint services—the general attitude is that anyone with a psychiatric label should be put in a corner and ignored—almost universal on surgical and orthopaedic wards |

From Holmes et al. (2002).

threat, and that there are many barriers to developing liaison-style services. Not only are older people with mental health problems in general hospital wards not owned by general hospital staff, it seems that many old age psychiatrists also do not wish to own them, believing them to be perfectly safe where they are. However, if we are happy with the status quo then we must also be happy with the continuation of the poor outcomes experienced by older people mentioned earlier in this chapter, and that seems to be letting them down badly.

So, what evidence is there that introducing a liaison service can help? Unfortunately there is little high-quality evidence to show us that the introduction of a liaison service can make a difference to outcomes. The evaluation of the efficacy and effectiveness of a liaison service requires a large, multicentre, randomized controlled trial. The unit of randomization should be at the level of the hospital to avoid the control group receiving care from a group of staff already educated by the liaison team. Such an evaluation is complex and not as scientific as a straightforward randomized controlled trial of a drug. It is also expensive and perceived by research funders to be high risk. The best evidence that there is comes from the USA, where a controlled study of the impact of a liaison service suggests that the introduction of a liaison psychiatry screen–treat intervention reduced the overall median length of stay of a hip fracture population by 2 days and produced a cost benefit (Strain *et al.*, 1991). There are doubts over the generalizability of one single study in an orthopaedic setting, perhaps explaining the low uptake of liaison services in the UK. A systematic review of the effectiveness of services does, however, suggest that the liaison approach is beneficial (Draper, 2000).

Despite this, liaison psychiatry services for older people have existed in a policy vacuum. Where they do exist, it has been due to opportunistic developments by individual enthusiasts rather than because of policy directives. The lack of joint working by providers of physical care and psychiatric care and their commissioners does not help. Neither does the fact that liaison psychiatry work is not costed or counted at an organizational level, with no changes in income streams for increases or decreases in activity. It is also unclear whose responsibility it is to fund liaison psychiatry—is it the general hospital or is it the primary care commissioners? All parties, including the mental health provider services, seem to perceive this crucial activity as a potential diversion of their scarce resources. There is no direct link to NHS performance indicators that health-care providers are measured by, and specifically no link at all to the performance indicators of mental health providers. This is particularly important since the organization that benefits most from a liaison service is not the mental health provider (trust or equivalent organization) that provides the service but the general hospital provider trust in which the service sits. This is a difficult message to get across to some managerial colleagues, and only a whole-systems view can resolve the problem.

## What an old age liaison service should do

There are several domains to a liaison service's activity. These are mentioned in detail elsewhere (Working Group of the Faculty of Old Age Psychiatry, 2005), but essentially consist of the following:

- Clinical activity
  - the prompt assessment, diagnosis, and management of referred older people, including all those who have self-harmed;

- risk assessment and risk moderation;
- incorporation of advice and treatments into care plans;
- regular review to monitor response to treatment and adherence to advice;
- engagement with carers and relatives;
- arranging suitable psychiatric aftercare (including transfer to a psychiatric setting where appropriate).
- Educational and promotional activity
  - provide educational programmes to improve detection and management of common psychiatric disorders in the general hospital setting;
  - develop treatment protocols and care pathways in conjunction with general hospital colleagues to improve ownership and uptake;
  - develop training posts within the service for a range of disciplines;
  - raise awareness of the importance of mental health and challenge and reduce stigma;
  - advocacy for vulnerable groups.
- Operational activity
  - develop operational policies and clinical governance structures;
  - establish clear lines of management for all professionals;
  - use clear signposting for referrers, including a single point of access;
  - record clinical and service related data for audit purposes;
  - work collaboratively with general hospital colleagues to develop shared objectives and outcomes.

In order to deliver the above, liaison practitioners need a certain set of knowledge, skills, and attitudes. Most important are the clinical knowledge skills required to assess complex cases in what can feel like an alien and sometimes hostile setting. These skills may be difficult to obtain, and many liaison practitioners have had to learn their clinical skills on the job, there being no other route of acquisition. Excellent written and oral communication skills are necessary, both to carry out and communicate the findings of clinical assessments and management plans and to deliver teaching and training that is accessible to all. The excellent liaison practitioner will be able to develop a relevant curriculum for the general hospital team and will not only impart their knowledge but promote good communication skills, along with a sense of their enthusiasm for the work. Leadership skills are important, and many liaison practitioners find themselves championing the cause of mental health to many. Good negotiating skills are useful when issues such as funding arise. One less recognized but equally important skill is that of diplomacy; sometimes it is necessary to stay calm and politely point out that mistakes have been made rather than resort immediately to a complaints procedure. This is particularly important since liaison psychiatry is a long game with few quick wins, and shifting staff attitudes can take years rather than months or weeks in some parts of the hospital.

## The liaison curriculum

If teaching general hospital staff is a key component of liaison psychiatry activity, then what is to be taught? There are several important areas to cover.

### The general approach

Those with psychiatric conditions are people too, and should be treated as such. A holistic, person centred approach should be the cornerstone of the liaison curriculum, with dignity and respect promoted to all staff. Talking to people with a mental health problem is a particular skill that will need to be taught.

### Specific conditions

Dementia, delirium, and depression are the commonest mental health problems found in general hospitals and all qualified staff should be competent in their management as applied to their own practice. Staff should understand that, for example, someone who is depressed lacks motivation and energy due to their depression and is not simply being lazy. Alcohol misuse, anxiety, and substance abuse are also important. All mental health problems, such as schizophrenia, can be found in general hospitals and staff should be aware of the basics of management.

### Problem behaviours

The most obvious is the challenging behaviour associated with agitated dementia and delirium, and an introduction to de-escalation techniques will be necessary. Staff need to understand that someone with dementia who wanders round the ward is likely to be looking for something purposefully rather than deliberately misbehaving. Motivational techniques can be helpful in some patients, and staff (particularly rehabilitation staff) will benefit from knowing about these.

### Psychotropic medications

Information about the effects and side-effects of common medication is useful, together with the basic modes of action and speed of onset of effectiveness. Mood stabilizers and depot antipsychotics may be stopped in hospital, and staff need to know that they should be restarted or a liaison psychiatry opinion sought.

### Legal issues

There is increasing awareness of issues of capacity and consent in the general hospital setting, from consent for major surgical procedures through to discharge planning. Every health-care professional should be aware that consent is an issue for their daily practice, and be conversant with the law relating to capacity and consent in their particular legislature. General hospital staff are particularly confused by mental health legislation, and this should be a component of any liaison curriculum.

## Steps towards establishing a liaison service

Despite the potential barriers to service development, several places in the UK have successfully established liaison psychiatry services for older people. The final part of this chapter examines the steps necessary to establish and perpetuate a successful liaison psychiatry service for older people.

### Assessment of need

It is necessary to provide evidence that a service is required. Establish how many older people with mental health problems there are likely to be in your local general hospital, assuming the prevalences in Table 22.1 are correct, and link that to what is known about the poor outcomes. Draw on the experience of patients and carers; the local branch of the Alzheimer's Society will have people with adverse experiences of general hospital care. What national policies may be relevant? The Internet is a useful resource of policy and related documents to brief you. Become a salesperson to get your message across.

### Scoping the project

Who are the key stakeholders and what motivates them? What are their must-dos and how can you link to them? You will need to engage a wide range of supporters across health, social care, and voluntary agencies who will all need briefing about why they should support you. Look for opportunities to change, including sources of funding that are briefly available for pilot or similar projects. What capacity is there for change, and are there reorganizations of services that you can link with?

### Mapping the process

What will your service look like? A range of factors influence this, including hospital size, geography, current service resourcing and provision, and local opinion. Think of it as an evolutionary process if resources are scant at the moment. Use national standards for staffing of services (Faculty of Old Age Psychiatry, 2006). What is already there that can be built on? A single liaison nurse can be used as the foundations for a larger multidisciplinary team. What blocks to progress are there? Individual clinicians may be unsympathetic to your cause, in which case sell it to them better or if that fails find a way around them. Find out where others have been successful and collaborate rather than reinventing the wheel.

### Service design

This includes the design of clinical pathways that cross interfaces, together with services to ensure the optimal working of these pathways. An operational policy will be needed, together with support systems to deliver the policy. Decisions about paperwork are required—which trust's medical records are written in and by whom? Which trust logo is on the letterhead? Line management of clinicians and administrative staff will be required, and this can be from the general hospital management structure or from the mental health provider. IT systems and support will be needed, and decisions about which organization's IT systems (both hardware and software) will be used by the service; there are advantages and disadvantages to using either the mental health provider's or the general hospital's IT systems (which will inevitably be incompatible with each other). Developing and delivering the educational curriculum may require liaison with local and national education and training bodies.

### Implementation

Establishing a liaison service is complex and requires senior managerial input for project management if it is to succeed. The vision and aims of the service should be shared with clinical and managerial teams involved (both in the general hospital and the mental health provider organization), so that teams understand what is happening and sign up to the new arrangements. A robust communications strategy will ensure the sharing of relevant clinical information so that appropriate follow-up can be arranged. Should the service be launched incrementally and rolled out gradually to different areas of the hospital, or is it a big bang launch, everything starting at the same time? The decision on the launch may be closely related to recruitment; if there are only a few people who are likely to meet your person specification the slower, incremental launch with ongoing recruitment may be better. Don't forget accommodation; a base in the general hospital will allow the service to run at peak efficiency.

## Evaluation

Once you have established a service you will be expected to show that it works. Although evaluation is a complex process, and outcomes are subject to influence by a large number of confounding factors, it is still possible to show that the service is having an effect. One thing that is always seen is an increase in referrals, resulting in more older people accessing specialist mental health assessment and treatment, and all liaison services should prospectively harvest these data since no-one else will do it for them. Outcomes examined should be measured in individual patients and carers, for example through a satisfaction questionnaire. Similar tools can be used with general ward staff so that it can be demonstrated that the service is well received and perceived as helpful. As well as these qualitative approaches, it is possible to obtain hard outcome measures such as length of stay for those patients coded by patient administration system databases as having a primary or secondary mental health problem; although coding may not be particularly accurate and probably underestimates the level of mental health problems, this is not likely to be systematically biased. It is worth bearing in mind that patients referred to the service are, by definition, likely to have an increased length of stay compared with those not referred. Other areas to measure may include delayed transfers of care, psychotropic prescriptions (pharmacy colleagues may be able to help with this), and referrals to community teams and other mental health services for follow-up after discharge. Teaching activity should be recorded, and its impact measured by regular checks on the knowledge and skills of general hospital staff. Audit cycles can repeatedly report rapid responses to referrals and prompt written communications with relevant teams. A successful evaluation process needs to be built in to the day-to-day working of the liaison service, and should be linked to the performance management process.

## Sustainability and spread

A successful evaluation is one good way of attaining sustainability, but it is important not to be complacent. Key stakeholders will move on to other posts, bringing new people you will have to sell your service to. Difficult issues may arise, and it is important to be open and honest rather than papering over the cracks. Succession strategies are vital in what are usually small teams, and enthusing trainees in all professions is one way of ensuring successful succession. Keep asking 'Can we do it better?'; strive for improvement and be flexible within resources. Liaison can be lonely so find a network of like-minded people and get support and new ideas from them. Tell others what you do and they may come to you for ideas too.

## Conclusion

This chapter has highlighted some of the challenges for research and service development in a complex and until recently under-recognized area. Mental health problems are common in older people in general hospitals, and the poor outcomes they experience ought to be a rallying call for better services and a clearer understanding of the effectiveness of liaison services. The information in this chapter is intended to stimulate more interest in the area, and to spark discussions about different service models that make things better for older people in general hospitals.

## Further reading

Draper, B. and Melding, P. (eds) (2001). *Geriatric consultation liaison psychiatry*. Oxford University Press, Oxford.

Royal College of Psychiatrists (2005). *Who cares wins. Improving the outcome for older people admitted to the general hospital*, Report of a Working Group for the Faculty of Old Age Psychiatry. Royal College of Psychiatrists. London.

## References

Andrew, M., Freter, S., and Rockwood, K. (2006). Prevalence and outcomes of delirium in community and non-acute care settings in people without dementia: a report from the Canadian Study of Health and Aging. *BMC Medicine*, **4**(1), 15.

Atkin, K., Holmes, J., and Martin, C.L. (2005). Provision of care for older people with co-morbid mental illness in general hospitals: general nurses' perceptions of their training needs., *International Journal of Geriatric Psychiatry*, **20**(11), 1081–1083.

Cole, M.G. (2004). Delirium in elderly patients. *American Journal of Geriatric Psychiatry*, **12**(1), 7–21.

Cole, M.G. and Bellavance, F. (1997). Depression in elderly medical inpatients: a meta-analysis of outcomes. *Canadian Medical Association Journal*, **157**(8), 1055–1060.

Department of Health (2001). *National Service Framework for Older People*. Department of Health, London.

Department of Health and Care Services Improvement Partnership (2005). *Everybody's business. Integrated mental health services for older adults: a service development guide*. Department of Health and Care Services Improvement Partnership, London.

Draper, B. (2000). The effectiveness of old age psychiatry services. *International Journal of Geriatric Psychiatry*, **15**(8), 687–703.

Faculty of Old Age Psychiatry (2006). *Raising the standard: specialist services for older people with mental illness*. Royal College of Psychiatrists, London.

Farrell, K.R. and Ganzini, L. (1995). Misdiagnosing delirium as depression in medically ill elderly patients. *Archives of Internal Medicine*, **155**(22), 2459–2464.

Ferro, J.M., Caeiro, L., and Verdelho, A. (2002). Delirium in acute stroke. *Current Opinion in Neurology*, **15**(1), 51–55.

Gill, D. and Hatcher, S. (2000). Antidepressants for depression in medical illness. *Cochrane Database of Systematic Reviews* 2000, Issue 4, Art. No. CD001312. DOI: 10.1002/14651858.CD001312.pub2.

Gurland, B., Copeland, J., Sharpe, L., and Kelleher, M. (1976). The geriatric mental status interview (GMS). *International Journal of Aging and Human Development*, **7**(4), 303–311.

Gustafson, Y., Brannstrom, B., Norberg, A., Bucht, G., and Winblad, B. (1991). Underdiagnosis and poor documentation of acute confusional states in elderly hip fracture patients. *Journal of the American Geriatrics Society*, **39**(8), 760–765.

Hally, O. and Cooney, C. (2005). Delirium in the hospitalised elderly: an audit of NCHD prescribing practice. *Irish Journal of Psychological Medicine*, **22**(4), 133–136. 2005.

Holmes, J. and House, A. (2000a). Psychiatric illness predicts poor outcome after surgery for hip fracture: a prospective cohort study. *Psychological Medicine*, **30**, 921–929.

Holmes, J. and House, A.O. (2000b). Psychiatric illness in hip fracture. Systematic review. *Age and Ageing*, **29**(6), 537–546.

Holmes, J., Bentley, K., and Cameron, I. (2002). *Between two stools: psychiatric services for older people in general hospitals.* University of Leeds, Leeds.

Holmes, J., Bentley, K., and Cameron, I. (2003a). A UK survey of psychiatric services for older people in general hospitals. *International Journal of Geriatric Psychiatry*, **18**(8), 716–721.

Holmes, J., Millard, J., Greer, D., and Silcock, J. (2003b). Trends in psychotropic drug use in older people in general hospitals. *Pharmaceutical Journal*, **271**(7272), 584–586.

Horrocks, J., Price, S., House, A., and Owens, D. (2003). Self-injury attendances in the accident and emergency department: clinical database study. *British Journal of Psychiatry*, **183**(1), 34–39.

Inouye, S.K. (1994). The dilemma of delirium: clinical and research controversies regarding diagnosis and evaluation of delirium in hospitalized elderly medical patients. *American Journal of Medicine*, **97**(3), 278–288.

Merino, J.G. and Hachinski, V. (2002). Stroke-related dementia. *Current Atherosclerosis Reports*, **4**(4), 285–290.

Norquist, G., Wells, K.B., Rogers, W.H., Davis, L.M., Kahn, K., and Brook, R. (1995). Quality of care for depressed elderly patients hospitalized in the specialty psychiatric units or general medical wards. *Archives of General Psychiatry*, **52**(8), 695–701.

Raymont, V., Bingley, W., Buchanan, A. *et al.* (2004). Prevalence of mental incapacity in medical inpatients and associated risk factors: cross-sectional study. *Lancet*, **364**(9443), 1421–1427.

Ruddy, R. and House, A. (2003). A standard liaison psychiatry service structure? A study of the liaison psychiatry services within six strategic health authorities. *Psychiatric Bulletin*, **27**(12), 457–460.

Ruddy, R. and House, A. (2005). Meta-review of high-quality systematic reviews of interventions in key areas of liaison psychiatry. *British Journal of Psychiatry*, **187**, 109–120.

Scottish Office (2001). *Adding life to years. Report of the expert group on healthcare of older people.* Scottish Office Health Department, Edinburgh.

Sheehan, B., Bass, C., Briggs, R., and Jacoby, R. (2003). Somatic symptoms among older depressed primary care patients. *International Journal of Geriatric Psychiatry*, **18**(6), 547–548.

Strain, J.J., Lyons, J.S., Hammer, J.S. *et al.* (1991). Cost offset from a psychiatric consultation-liaison intervention with elderly hip fracture patients. *American Journal of Psychiatry*, **148**(8), 1044–1049.

Swift, G. and Guthrie, E. (2003). Liaison psychiatry continues to expand: developing services in the British Isles. *Psychiatric Bulletin*, **27**(9), 339–341.

Turner-Stokes, L. and Hassan, N. (2002). Depression after stroke: a review of the evidence base to inform the development of an integrated care pathway. Part 1: Diagnosis, frequency and impact. *Clinical Rehabilitation*, **16**(3), 231–247.

Wijeratne, C., Brodaty, H., Hickie, I., Wijeratne, C., Brodaty, H., and Hickie, I. (2003). The neglect of somatoform disorders by old age psychiatry: some explanations and suggestions for future research. *International Journal of Geriatric Psychiatry*, **18**(9), 812–819.

Winrow, A. and Holmes, J. (2005). Old age medical patients screening positive for depression. *Irish Journal of Psychological Medicine*, **22**(4), 124–127.

Working Group of the Faculty of Old Age Psychiatry (2005). *Who cares wins: improving the outcome for older people admitted to the general hospital.* Royal College of Psychiatrists, London.

Yohannes, A.M., Baldwin, R.C., and Connolly, M.J. (2000). Depression and anxiety in elderly outpatients with chronic obstructive pulmonary disease: prevalence, and validation of the BASDEC screening questionnaire. *International Journal of Geriatric Psychiatry*, **15**(12), 1090–1096.

# 23

# Mental health in care homes for older people

## Tom Dening and Alisoun Milne

This chapter aims to outline the context, prevalence, nature, and management of mental health problems amongst older people living in residential or nursing care. Specifically, it will offer an overview of: the development of the care home sector; its regulation and funding; a profile of care home residents; their physical and mental health; and an outline of the key services and treatments that are available to those with mental health problems. The main focus of the chapter is the UK, but with reference to other countries where appropriate. Hospital care is excluded as it rarely provides long-term care; and support for older people with lifelong mental illness is discussed in Chapter 33. By way of setting the scene, we begin with an introduction to the background and development of care home provision in the UK.

## Care homes

### Care homes in the UK

Long-term care in the UK has developed based on a fundamental distinction between health care—care provided to 'the sick and infirm'—and social care—care for the 'frail and old' (Dudman, 2006). The former have historically been served by the National Health Service where care is free at the point of delivery; the latter via local authority social services departments where care has been, and continues to be, means tested. Concerns about the rising costs of NHS long-term care in the 1970s and 1980s coupled with changes to the funding of care home provision, resulted in a substantial reduction of NHS provision and a significant growth in the number of homes, particularly in the independent sector.

Care homes are categorized by the type of care they provide, nursing or personal, and also by the nature of the provider—social services, independent, or voluntary sector. Residential care homes provide personal care with activities of daily living such as washing, dressing, and giving medication. Nursing homes tend to provide care for people with higher dependency needs, including those who need nursing-related support or regular medical attention; for example, stoma care or the management of tube feeding. Some homes provide 'specialist care' for particular groups, most notably older people with a mental illness. Until recently some NHS hospitals provided free continuing care for a small proportion of very frail older people, including those with severe dementia. However, most 'continuing care' patients are now placed in nursing homes;

some of these are NHS run although in some cases the NHS buys places in private nursing homes (Dudman, 2006). In 2004, the Healthcare Market Review estimated that there were around 485,000 places in care homes in the UK (see Table 23.1), a significant decrease from a peak of 575,000 in 1996 (Laing & Buisson, 2006). There are a total of 13,500 residential and nursing care homes for older people in the UK (Laing & Buisson, 2006). Around 5% of the population aged over 65 resides in a care home, a figure comparable to many other developed countries (Organisation for Economic Co-operation and Development, 2005).

As the figures show, most care is provided by independent care homes. Over the past 20 years there has been a significant shift in the balance of provision from the public to the private sector (Office of Fair Trading, 2005). Figure 23.1 illustrates the transformation of care services from a predominantly public sector activity in the mid-1970s to a predominantly private sector activity now. The total value of the care home market in 2005 was estimated at £11.7 billion; private sector operators accounted for £7.6 billion (Laing & Buisson, 2006).

Overall, homes are also becoming larger. One-third of care home providers in the private and voluntary sectors have three or more homes, and there is a trend towards a greater concentration of provision in fewer larger homes (Laing & Buisson, 2006). Most UK care homes have between 20 and 30 places, although there is considerable variation in size; homes ranging from two or three places to over 100 (Commission for Social Care Inspection (CSCI), 2005). Residential care homes tend to be smaller than nursing homes with 24 compared to 44 beds on average. Most beds in local authority

**Table 23.1** Care home places in the UK

| Category of care | No. of places |
|---|---|
| Private nursing care | 164,000 |
| Private residential care | 182,000 |
| Voluntary nursing care | 15,000 |
| Voluntary residential care | 49,700 |
| Public provision (NHS and local authority) | 74,600 |
| Total | 485,300 |

Source: Laing & Buisson (2006).

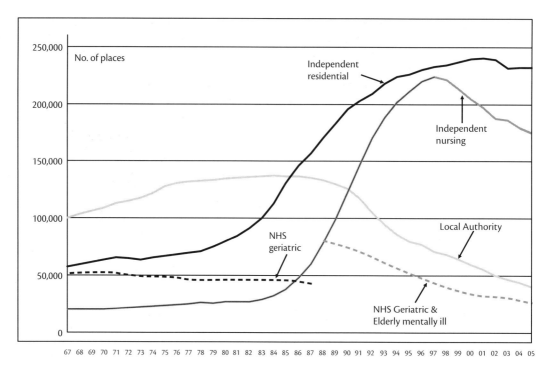

**Fig. 23.1** Nursing and residential care places for the elderly and physically disabled by sector, UK, April 1967–2005. (From Laing & Buisson, 2006.)

and voluntary sector care homes are single rooms; percentages are lower in the private sector and nursing homes (Netten *et al.*, 2001). About 50% have en suite facilities and over three-quarters have washbasins. Homes have an average occupancy rate of 92% or above.

The availability of residential care varies considerably on a geographical basis. In England, there are an average of 55 residential places per 1000 people over 65, but one in ten councils have fewer than 38/1000 whilst the same proportion have more than 70. This difference is more pronounced for nursing homes, with the top 10% of councils having three times the number of places as the bottom 10% (CSCI, 2005). In terms of specialist mental health provision, fewer than half of UK care homes are specifically registered to care for people with dementia (PWD) (Laing & Buisson, 2006), though in practice a higher proportion must have residents with dementia. Shortages in providing care for PWD have been widely noted in national studies; it has been identified as a particular challenge in London and the southeast of England (Wanless, 2006). Lack of locally available care can result in people being placed away from their local area (CSCI, 2005).

### Demand for care homes

Demand for, and provision of, care home places has been subject to considerable change over the last 20 years (Owen and National Care Homes Research and Development Forum (NCHRDF), 2006). Until 1993 there was a rapid expansion in the care home market particularly—as noted above—in the independent sector (Netten *et al.*, 2001). Since the mid-1990s, demand has been falling and there has been a steady decline in care home places. Between 2003 and 2005, 20,000 (5%) beds were lost in England (CSCI, 2005) and between 2000 and 2005, 148 care homes closed in Scotland (Care Commission, 2004). Closures affect smaller homes disproportionately.

This pattern is a consequence of a set of intersecting demand and supply side factors. Supply side factors include: insufficient local authority funding, recruitment problems especially of nursing staff, high running costs, and cost implications of national minimum standards (Netten *et al.*, 2001). In particular, many homes are unable to raise the funds necessary to do structural work required by the registering authority, the Commission for Social Care Inspection (CSCI). Those issues which have reduced demand for care home places are primarily an emphasis on community-based care, enhanced expectations of family carers, and the development of alternative models of long-term support.

The potential impact of extra care housing (ECH)[1] is particularly notable. Although we lack systematic evidence, several studies suggest that ECH residents show a reduction in health-care need, improved function, greater independence and autonomy, and a better quality of life than their care home counterparts (Helen Ogilvy Associates, 1999; ExtraCare Charitable Trust, 2007). ECH may also reduce the incidence and duration of admission to hospital (Laing & Buisson, 2006) and evidence from other European countries suggests that it directly contributes to lower demand for care home placement (Coolen and Weekers, 1998). In Denmark, for example, the number of places in homes halved between 1987 and 2003; in Holland only 4% (150,000) of people aged over 55 spend any length of time in a care home (de Klerk, 2004). That its costs are comparable with those of care homes is additionally relevant (Laing & Buisson, 2006).

---

[1] Extra care housing is housing with support and care provided in addition. There is more than one kind of ECH; it a concept rather than a type of housing. Extra care housing can be owned, rented, part owned and part rented, or leasehold.

Housing with care is emerging as the predominant choice of older people across mainland Europe and is increasingly popular in the UK (Brooks *et al.*, 2003; ExtraCare Charitable Trust, 2007). Its developing capacity to provide effective support to PWD—as well as those who are physically frail—is of particular note. Existing evidence suggests that people who develop dementia after they have moved into ECH continue to be supported; placing people who already have dementia tends not to work as well (Vallelly *et al.*, 2006). In 2003 there were estimated to be between 12,000 and 24,000 extra care units in England as well as 23,700 sheltered housing units (Laing & Buisson, 2006; Vallelly *et al.*, 2006). The recent Wanless social care review recommended that the current 'very low level' of provision be significantly increased to accommodate future demand (Wanless, 2006).

Whatever the potential of alternative models, it is important to acknowledge the impact of the projected growth in the UK population aged 85 and over from 1.1 million in 2004 to 4.2 million in 2051. The compression of morbidity amongst the 'oldest old', multiple frailties, and the prevalence of dementia combine to make a significant increase in demand for care home provision very likely. Growth may need to be as much as 150%, or an additional 680,000 places (Wittenberg *et al.*, 2004). This would require an increase in spending from £12.9 billion in 2000 to £53.9 billion in 2051.

## The profile of care home residents

Although the proportion of older people living in care homes is small, the lifetime risk of being in residential care is considerable. As might be expected, the chance of being admitted to a home increases with age; for the 65–74 age group, 0.9% of the population resides in care homes, compared with 4.3% between the ages of 75 and 84 and 20.7% of those aged 85 and over (Laing & Buisson, 2006). Women residents tend to be older, with an average age of 85.6 years, compared with 83.2 for men (Milne and Williams, 2000). People admitted to nursing homes are slightly younger than those admitted to residential care (Netten *et al.*, 2001).

Bebbington *et al.* (2001) identified several characteristics common to care home residents. Typically they are over 80 years, female, have previously lived alone, are poor or dependent solely on benefits, and have multiple disabilities or long-standing illness. Women are twice as likely to live in a care home as men; they occupy 80% of registered beds in nursing homes for elderly mentally ill (EMI) patients (Melzer *et al.*, 1999; Netten *et al.*, 2002). Factors that protect against admission are: availability of informal support, adequate income, and living in a housing environment which is adapted to accommodate enhanced levels of disability (Milne *et al.*, 2001; Dening and Milne, 2005).

Currently, there are relatively few ethnic minority elders in long-term care in the UK. In 2001 only 1.2% of those surveyed were from an ethnic minority (Bebbington *et al.*, 2001).

In the USA data indicate that higher rates of residential care occur in the majority White population; this appears also to be true in Britain. This may reflect the fact that the demographic profile of minority populations is younger and also that long-term care—if accessed at all—tends to be provided specifically for older people from that minority (Milne and Chryssanthopoulou, 2005).

People admitted to nursing homes have higher levels of dependency than those admitted to residential care (Bebbington *et al.*, 2001). In one study, over 90% of nursing home residents were classified as 'severely disabled', compared with 70% in residential

care, with the prevalence of severe disability significantly higher among women than in men (Bajekal, 2002). Overall, 57% of women and 48% of men need help with one or more 'self-care' tasks such as dressing or washing (Office of Fair Trading, 2005). It is important to note that across the sector it is people with dementia who dominate the care home population.

Most people enter a care home because they can no longer live independently for reasons of physical and/or mental illness. A recent report (Office of Fair Trading, 2005) identified physical ill-health as the primary reason in 69% of cases, mental health in 43% of cases, for 42% the cause was functional disablement, and carer stress was cited by 38%. Lack of motivation (22%) and the unsuitability of the person's own home (15%) were also significant reasons. For most, admission is a consequence of multiple difficulties. Bebbington *et al.* (2001) found that over half of the admissions to residential care came from hospital; this rose to two-thirds for nursing home admissions.

Although moving into a care home is a major life decision, it is often taken when people have very little information, when they are under pressure to make a quick decision, and when they are feeling ill or frail (Office of Fair Trading, 2005). Although many older people would rather not move into a care home, it is important to recognize that those who have made the move can identify advantages with their new home, including the safe environment, the care they receive, and the company of others (Boaz *et al.*, 1999). This process of adjustment also emerged in interviews undertaken with people with dementia who had recently moved into a care home (Moriarty and Webb, 2000).

## Quality of life and quality of care

Improving the quality of care in care homes is a primary goal of both policy and practice, one which is facilitated by a better understanding of quality of life (QoL) in care homes and supported by a coherent system of regulation (discussed in the following section). The authors focus on people with dementia (PWD) as they are the majority of residents and present the greatest challenge to care staff.

Assessing QoL amongst care home residents is a difficult task. It is a complex construct, which is variously measured and evaluated. A range of scales exist, several of which have been specifically developed for work with people with dementia. Probably the most widely studied measure in PWD is the Quality of Life in Alzheimer's Disease Scale (QoL-AD; Logsdon *et al.*, 1999). It has 13 items, including physical and mental health, personal relationships, finances, and overall life quality, and it can be completed by caregivers or patients, even those with fairly severe dementia (Hoe *et al.*, 2005).

A persistent challenge in evaluating QoL is that there are often differences between observer (staff) ratings and residents' own responses. This appears to be a consequence of a difference in emphasis: a recent study found that residents' QoL scores were most affected by the presence of depression and anxiety, whereas staff ratings were more associated with dependency and behaviour problems (Hoe *et al.*, 2006). Caregiver ratings seem to be particularly affected by their own attitudes towards dementia care (Winzelberg *et al.*, 2005). Thus, it may be argued that a full picture of QoL requires a combination of measures, incorporating observations of residents as well as the views of residents, carers, and staff (Gaugler *et al.*, 2004; Sloane *et al.*, 2005).

Despite the difficulties associated with measurement, evidence to date suggests that QoL in care homes is largely determined by the existence of mental health problems and subjective well-being (e.g. Samus *et al.*, 2005; Smallbrugge *et al.*, 2006). Systematic assessment of residents' needs, and consideration of whether or not they have been met, has been suggested as a means of improving QoL (Hancock *et al.*, 2006). The Camberwell Assessment of Need for the Elderly (CANE; Orrell and Hancock, 2004) has been used towards this end. Addressing well-being has also been highlighted (Bergland and Kirkevold, 2001).

Limited consensus also exists in relation to the linked concept of quality of care. First, as with QoL, there are multiple perspectives to be accommodated. Second, the components of 'care' include those elements that are provided within the home as well as those offered by external sources, such as medical care and social support. Third, good quality care depends on a range of micro level (satisfied staff) and macro level (financial stability of the provider) factors and their interaction; this make its assessment complex and multi-faceted. An important contribution to this field has been the development of Dementia Care Mapping, an observational approach where items recording residents' activity can be combined to calculate a dementia care index score (Ballard *et al.*, 2001a). Its person centred basis, relatively widespread use in care settings, and its validity make it a popular and reliable tool to assess and enhance quality of care (Fossey *et al.*, 2002).

As might be expected, evidence about the quality of care in homes is mixed. Some of the variation between studies results from methodological differences. For example, studies adopting a 'checklist' approach (e.g. Tune and Bowie, 2000) tend to reach more positive conclusions than those using direct observations (e.g. Ballard *et al.*, 2001a). Although there is a limited literature on residents' own views, one study interestingly found that the emphasis on 'homeliness' in care homes did not produce greater resident satisfaction than the 'institutional' setting of a long-stay hospital ward (Higgs *et al.*, 1998). Train *et al.* (2005a) found that the main theme identified by residents was a need to be able to make choices.

Certain specific aspects of care also need to be considered in assessing the quality of care. These include prescribing patterns and covert administration of medication, physical restraint, electronic tagging, and abuse. Elder abuse is addressed elsewhere in the book (Chapter 39) and concerns about excessive or inappropriate prescribing are discussed below. Physical restraints, including clothing, cot sides, or chairs, are still worryingly prevalent and, because of staff attitudes to risk, it can be difficult to reduce even in planned interventions (Sullivan-Marx *et al.*, 1999). Although electronic tagging has been advocated in certain circumstances to prevent wandering and to facilitate a more open environment it has been criticized for emphasizing technology and control instead of working towards better, more individualized care (e.g. Hughes and Louw, 2002). Administering medication concealed in food or beverages appears to be a widespread practice in care homes (Treloar *et al.*, 2000; Kirkevold and Engedal, 2005). As a number of residents with severe dementia may lack the capacity to consent, or withhold their consent, to treatment this measure may occasionally be necessary, but it is concerning when it becomes routine, has not been the subject of discussion among the care team or with the patient's family, and is not documented.

Much remains to be done in this developing area. Further research may provide greater consensus about what constitutes a robust and reliable assessment of quality of care and which measures are useful for particular settings and purposes. A more enlightened view of assessing risks among residents can lead to reduced use of restraint (Counsel and Care, 2001). There is considerable scope for work on residents' views, especially people with dementia (Barnett, 2000; Kane *et al.*, 2003). There is not only an emerging research agenda but widespread public and policy recognition of the need to improve care (Owen and NCHRDF, 2006). The contribution of care standards to this process is the focus of the following section.

# Regulating the care home sector

In the last few years there have been major changes in the regulatory arrangements for care homes, with new legislation aimed at improving the standards of care provided by all care services. In England and Wales this has been enacted through the Care Standards Act 2000, in Scotland through the Regulation of Care (Scotland) Act 2001, and in Northern Ireland through the Health and Personal Social Services Act (Northern Ireland) 2001.

One of the key aims of the legislation has been the introduction of national minimum standards across the UK (Department of Health, 1999, 2002). The standards apply to seven key areas: choice of home, health and personal care, daily life and social activities, complaints and protection, environment, staffing and management, and administration. Regulatory bodies are established in each country to apply and monitor these standards—in England, the Commission for Social Care Inspection (CSCI); in Wales, the Care Standards Inspectorate; and in Scotland, the Care Commission. Inspections take place once or twice a year; the inspector rates the care home against each standard on a scale of 1–4. Where there are weaknesses these need to be addressed by the provider; the ultimate sanction is withdrawal of the home's registration. Regular reviews of social care provision, including care home inspections, are published. CSCI does not cover NHS provision, which is at present the responsibility of the Healthcare Commission. Proposed legislation in 2008 will allow these two bodies to merge into the Social Care and Health Inspectorate.

## Trends in the quality of residential care services

Since 2002/03—when care homes in England were first inspected by CSCI—there is evidence that the quality of residential care has improved. In 2004/05, an average of 72% of standards in care homes for older people were met compared to 59% in 2002/03. Further, 22% met at least 90% of all standards compared with 7% in 2002/03. In general, nursing homes performed better than residential care homes. There is, however, no evidence that homes providing specifically for PWD (so-called EMI homes, from the antiquated term 'elderly mentally infirm') provide better quality care than non-EMI homes (Reilly *et al.*, 2006). CSCI inspections indicate that residential care provided by the voluntary sector significantly out-performed similar services in the other sectors; council-run services 'performed the poorest overall' in part due to a lack of investment in the fabric of the buildings (Commission for Social Care Inspection, 2005). There is UK-wide geographical variation suggesting that the quality of care an older person receives is significantly influenced by where they live; this is particularly so for specialist homes for people with dementia.

In England, homes performed best in relation to the standards on arranging introductory visits; personal space; establishing links with the community; rights; and autonomy and choice. Three priority areas emerged as key areas for improvement in reports from England and Scotland: managing medication appropriately and safely; operating safe working practices, e.g. not keeping bleach next to residents' food; and recruitment practices, especially Criminal Records Bureau and Protection of Vulnerable Adults checks. Ensuring that residents have appropriate care plans is also an important marker of overall care quality: those homes that did so were more likely to be judged as meeting residents' needs effectively (CSCI, 2005). For residents with dementia, certain factors were important for well-being: the reassurance of daily routine; privacy, dignity and choice; contact with family and friends; and the availability of pleasurable activities (Care Commission, 2004).

## Staffing

In England, there are approximately 450,000 people working in care homes (Meyer, 2006). They are almost exclusively female, often work part time, and tend to be low paid. Turnover and vacancy rates are variable across the country, with some areas having major difficulties in recruitment and retention; homes routinely employ staff whose first language is not the same as the residents. It is estimated that only 20% of care assistants in local authority or private sector homes have even a basic care qualification, this being despite an policy goal that at least 50% of care staff would have a minimum qualification by the end of 2005 (Laing & Buisson, 2006; Centre for Policy on Ageing, 2001). In the UK, staffing quality is regulated by means of the minimum standards for care services but also by the establishment of a General Social Care Council (for England, with equivalent bodies for Scotland, Wales, and Northern Ireland) to regulate the training and conduct of social care staff. National minimum standards specifically address 'staffing levels' and 'skill mix'. These must be 'appropriate to meet the assessed needs of the residents', the size, the layout, and the purpose of the home.

Inadequate staffing levels are also a significant problem: in residential homes there is approximately one full-time member of care staff for every three places and one part-time worker for every 2.5 places (Netten et al., 2001). Dual-registered and nursing homes have higher levels of full-time staffing, with one full-time member of care staff for just over every two places, but they have similar levels of part-time staff as residential homes. About a third of nursing posts in nursing homes are filled by registered nurses (Royal College of Nursing, 2004) and a lack of qualified nursing staff is a frequent reason for care home closures (Netten et al., 2001). Paradoxically, requirements for higher levels of staffing and training may have contributed to a reduction in specialist homes for older people with mental health problems (Wanless, 2006).

Recruitment and retention of care home staff, both qualified and unqualified, is a major issue, especially in areas where the cost of living is high, for example in Greater London and southeast England (Robinson and Banks, 2005). Many consider that this problem will only be coherently addressed if wages for care home staff are significantly increased; a shift that can be ill-afforded by the care home sector at present.

## Funding issues

International comparisons show that funding for long-term care is a major issue across the world. No country has a fully funded social care insurance scheme for long-term care and the affordability and sustainability of current funding arrangements are dependent on the state of national economies (Glendinning et al., 2004). The cost of residential and nursing home care is means tested and divided between the state and the individual. Over the last three decades there have been significant changes to the funding of long-term care. In the 1970s a quarter of older people in residential care homes in England were funded by the NHS but by 1995 this figure was just 10% (Netten et al., 2001). This is partly due to a distinction between 'nursing care'—paid for by the NHS—and 'personal care'—means tested and partially or wholly paid for by the individual. This distinction is not made in Scotland where all long-term care is state funded. At the time of writing, the English Department of Health is consulting on proposals for a national, rather than a local, approach to eligibility for NHS funded health and nursing care.

Across the UK, around two-thirds of care home residents are publicly funded, in full or partially (Netten et al., 2001). There are marked geographical differences in whether people are self-funding; not surprisingly this is commoner in prosperous areas such as southeast England. Private spending on residential and home care by older people is estimated at over £3.5 billion a year (Laing & Buisson, 2006).

Average fees across the UK are £496 per week for nursing homes and £345 per week for residential homes (Laing & Buisson, 2006), although London and the southeast are more expensive. Overall, fees for residential care have increased substantially in recent years whilst the number of people in care has remained largely constant. Self-funders often pay significantly higher fees than those funded by the local authority for similar services and amenities, effectively subsidising the cost of care for those who are publicly funded (Office of Fair Trading, 2005). Furthermore, they are often admitted at lower levels of dependency (Department of Health, 2006).

Funding for long-term care is a persistent problem. Overall, 60% (this figure includes care for younger adults with disabilities or chronic illness as well as older people) of all local authority expenditure is committed to residential and nursing care despite policy commitment to reduced use of institutional care and to investment in community-based services (Wanless, 2006). In 2004/05 total spending by English local authorities on care homes was around £4.5 billion; £3 billion on residential care and £1.4 billion on nursing care. In addition, NHS spending on nursing care in care homes was around £550 million. Local authorities frequently claim that central government funding is chronically inadequate, yet government maintains that councils have sufficient funds. This discrepancy may arise from the historical basis of allocations, which no longer reflect the high levels of dependency present in the current care home population (Social Policy Ageing and Information Network, 2005). The introduction of a national single assessment process may help to address this issue by looking at the complexity of need rather than how much the local authority is able to pay (Department of Health, 2001).

The boundary between free nursing care and means tested social care is one of the most contested aspects of this terrain. In 2003, the Health Service Ombudsman criticized the NHS for being overly restrictive in its eligibility criteria for (free) 'nursing care' in care homes. NHS organizations have since been reviewing local policies, and reimbursing residents who were wrongly charged for nursing care. The arena is complex, confusing, and inequitable; it also works to the particular disadvantage of less articulate users and their families. The Office of Fair Trading (2005) found that a quarter of care home residents in the UK had 'fee related terms that are either unclear or unfair'. As a consequence care homes are now obliged to provide details of prices *prior* to the older person moving in.

## The health of care home residents

### Physical health

Care home residents are a frail group, with high levels of physical and mental health conditions. Chronic illnesses and disabilities are common, frequently with evidence of unmet need or inadequate care. For example, although about 80% of residents have some degree of hearing impairment, care staff only recognize the problem in a minority of cases and provision of hearing aids is consequently low (Cohen-Mansfield and Taylor, 2004). In another study, around 9% of residents had diabetes but fewer than half were regularly reviewed by a GP or practice nurse (Taylor and Hendra, 2000). Even fewer (less than 10%) are reviewed in specialist clinics (Sinclair *et al.*, 1997). Complications of diabetes are common, and one study found over half the diabetic residents were in pain on admission (Travis *et al.*, 2004). Cancer is also underdiagnosed in some homes, possibly more so in rural areas (Dobalian *et al.*, 2003).

Multiple physical problems and/or co-morbidity with mental disorders are common. Medical conditions and associated disability are the main reasons underlying admission to care homes, rather than non-specific frailty or social needs. In one UK study of 16,000 residents, over half had dementia, stroke, or other neurodegenerative disease, 78% had at least one form of mental impairment, 71% were incontinent, and 76% needed help with mobility or were immobile (Bowman *et al.*, 2004). Overall, 27% were immobile, confused, and incontinent. There is considerable overlap between residential and nursing homes as to the levels of disability and physical dependency. This may result from changes in residents' physical health after admission to the home (Rothera *et al.*, 2003), but there may also be inconsistencies in the assessments made before admission. It also calls into question the validity of the distinction between residential and nursing care.

### Pain

It is beyond the scope of this chapter to discuss all the major physical problems in detail but certain issues are worth highlighting, especially those that impact upon mental health. Pain is common, from arthritis and pressure areas especially. Although reported prevalence rates vary widely, depending on how the presence of pain is ascertained and the sample under consideration, half or more of care home residents have been identified as experiencing one or more painful conditions. Pain can often make individuals restless, agitated, or even depressed. Cipher and Clifford (2004), in a study of factors contributing to quality of life among residents, found that pain frequently underlay behavioural disturbances and depression, and thereby indirectly affected activities of daily living. People who are already depressed are perhaps more sensitive to pain and are more likely to complain of it (Parmelee *et al.*, 1991). Residents with dementia may be less likely to indicate that they are in pain and consequently may not be offered analgesia as frequently as more communicative residents (Nygaard and Jarland, 2005). A randomized controlled trial found that agitated residents with dementia were more likely to spend time in social interaction and positive activities, and less time in distress, when they were given regular doses of paracetamol than when they received placebo (Chibnall

*et al.*, 2005). Thus, improved pain management may benefit the health and quality of life of residents with dementia.

Better understanding and improved management of pain in residents with dementia requires wider use of pain rating scales, including those with non-verbal items (such as facial expression) that can be used for patients with language impairment. There is also a need for exploration of the relevance of pain in different forms of dementia since, for example, patients with vascular dementia are prescribed analgesics more frequently than those with Alzheimer's disease (Scherder *et al.*, 2005).

### Mobility and falls

Mobility problems are common in the care home population and most residents have some limitation of mobility (Bowman *et al.*, 2004; Williams *et al.*, 2005). Thapa *et al.* (1995) examined risk factors for falls among 282 residents in 12 homes. Individual independent risk factors were: being aged 75 or over, impaired functional ability, balance problems, a fall in the preceding 90 days, and behaviour problems. The presence of all five risk factors was associated with a 10-fold risk of falling. Psychotropic medication also had an independent effect, approximately doubling the risk, and accounting for 36% of the attributable risk of falling in those residents receiving such medication. Although antipsychotic drugs are probably a key causal factor, selective serotonin reuptake inhibitors also increase the risk of falling and causing injury (Arfken *et al.*, 2001). The presence of dementia approximately doubles the risk of sustaining a significant injury (van Doorn *et al.*, 2003).

Various attempts have been made to improve mobility and reduce the rate of serious falls. MacRae *et al.* (1996) evaluated a 12-week walking programme, which led to increases in endurance and distance walked but did not affect other measures, such as overall quality of life or numbers of falls. The use of hip protectors does not seem to reduce the rate of hip fractures in nursing homes (Parker *et al.*, 2006). Two randomized controlled trials of multifactorial falls prevention programmes both had modestly encouraging but non-significant findings in favour of the interventions (Ray *et al.*, 1997; Dyer *et al.*, 2004).

### Nutrition and fluids

Concern is often expressed about poor standards of nutrition in care homes. Food may be poorly presented or unappetizing, the environment may be uncongenial, special diets (for religious observance or medical conditions) may be unavailable, and residents often have conditions which may affect their ability to feed themselves or to swallow their food. In a US study of 407 people with dementia in 45 assisted living facilities and nursing homes, 54% had low food intake and 51% had low fluid intake (Reed *et al.*, 2005). Staff monitoring of residents, having meals in a public dining area, and the presence of non-institutional features were each associated with higher food and fluid intake. Some homes have paid considerable attention to the eating environment, for example ensuring that mealtimes are undisturbed by televisions, visitors, and domestic bustle, and that food is served in a family style rather than as in an industrial canteen (Nijs *et al.*, 2006).

The use of feeding tubes (percutaneous endoscopic gastrostomy, or PEG, tubes) in care home residents is variable across the world but is especially prevalent in the USA, perhaps for defensive reasons. Over one-third of severely cognitively impaired residents in the USA, more than 63,000 people, had feeding tubes (Mitchell *et al.*, 2003). Certainly clinical factors, such as dysphagia and history of stroke, increase the likelihood of tube placement, but other, non-clinical, variables appear to be significant also including the person's ethnic origin and the nature and location of the nursing home (Gessert *et al.*, 2000; Mitchell *et al.*, 2003). Feeding tubes do not prolong survival in dementia and may be associated with significant complications (Mitchell *et al.*, 1997; Murphy and Lipman, 2003). The persistence of the practice is a matter for concern, especially as well-planned palliative care interventions can be effective in reducing the use of feeding tubes (Monteleoni and Clark, 2004).

## End of life care

The mortality rate amongst care home residents can be expected to be high, given their advanced years and the prevalence of serious health problems. The baseline 1-year survival rate for people in UK care homes is 66% overall; it is 59% in nursing homes where the median survival is about 18 months (Rothera *et al.*, 2002). Care home residents are often admitted to hospital, notably for medical illnesses such as infections and heart failure (Bowman *et al.*, 2001). Godden and Pollock (2001) compared emergency hospital admissions among care home residents with those for older people living in the community, and found higher risks of admission for all diagnoses (relative risk = 1.4) and especially for injuries and fractured neck of femur (relative risk = 4). Care home residents also had a higher risk of dying in hospital, especially within 48 hours of admission (relative risk = 3.6).

Deaths often occur in care homes, with about 20% of deaths in the UK occurring in nursing or residential homes (National Council for Palliative Care, 2006). Outcomes of emergencies, such as cardiac arrest, in care homes are very poor, and it has been argued that there is little point in providing cardiopulmonary resuscitation in most long-term care settings (Conroy *et al.*, 2006). Deaths are, however, usually heralded by more gradual decline, often with increased utilization of health-care services (Bercovitz *et al.*, 2005), and changes in symptoms and mental states of residents are often seen in the last months of life. For example, residents with dementia have been reported to show increased verbal agitation but reduced verbal interactions with others, and they may be more liable to be restrained (Allen *et al.*, 2005). Depression is often overlooked and undertreated during the last months of life (Evers *et al.*, 2002), though whether depressive symptoms are actually increased during the last months of life is debatable (Cuijpers, 2001). Risk scores calculated from clinical data can predict the risk of mortality within 6 months (Mitchell *et al.*, 2004a) and thus may help to reduce the frequency of inappropriate transfers to hospitals (Lamberg *et al.*, 2005).

Management of dying patients in care homes, especially those with dementia, varies considerably and is often inadequate (Mitchell *et al.*, 2004b). For example, compared with people dying of cancer, dementia patients are more likely to be tube fed or to have unnecessary physical investigations (Mitchell *et al.*, 2004c), though whether this would be so outside the USA is as yet untested. A strong case has often been made for better palliative care in care homes (Katz and Peace, 2003) or for increased use of hospice facilities (Hanson *et al.*, 2005). Establishing specialist palliative care units for people with dementia has also been proposed (Hughes *et al.*, 2005) though it would seem more appropriate to improve the overall quality of end of life care in nursing homes rather than expect very frail residents to move to an unfamiliar setting. Where death is expected, care home staff are well placed to provide good care, especially if they are adequately trained and supported to do so (Munn *et al.*, 2006). For a more comprehensive discussion of palliative care in dementia, the reader is referred to Hughes (2006).

## Dementia

The prevalence of dementia in care homes is high; a recent large UK study identified 62% of residents as having dementia (Matthews and Dening, 2002). The rate was slightly higher in women but did not increase significantly with age, perhaps reflecting the threshold of impairment at which people enter long-term care. If residents with dementia have greater mortality than those without, then the total burden of dementia may be greater than this cross-sectional figure suggests. The prevalence of dementia is fairly consistent across different types of care home, so even homes that are not registered as 'dementia care homes' have a majority of residents with significant cognitive impairment (Macdonald *et al.*, 2002). It may therefore be argued that dementia care is actually the main business of long-term care for older people. Unfortunately, staff assessments of the presence of dementia may be inaccurate (Sørensen *et al.*, 2001) or influenced by staff attitudes to dementia (Macdonald and Woods, 2005), and there may be perverse incentives not to identify it, as this could result in a more expensive placement being required (Macdonald and Dening, 2002).

Many residents with dementia have behaviour disturbances, especially activity disturbances (agitation), aggression, psychosis, and depressed mood, with reported prevalences of such behaviour problems as high as 80–90% (Brodaty *et al.*, 2001; Margallo-Lana *et al.*, 2001). Perhaps of particular concern are self-harming behaviours, which may be active, such as scratching oneself or punching objects (de Jonghe-Rouleau *et al.*, 2005) or passive, for example refusal to take food or drink (Draper *et al.*, 2003). Overall, behaviour problems are liable to persist over one or more years (Ballard *et al.*, 2001b), and whilst some problems resolve they are often replaced by other forms of challenging behaviour.

Although dementia itself is viewed as a progressive and irreversible condition, evidence suggests that care home admission does not hasten health-related decline, at least in the short term. In fact as a consequence of identifying and treating hitherto unknown medical conditions and good nutrition the overall health of some demented residents may improve. Buttar *et al.* (2003) found that, of those patients with severe cognitive impairment, 14% showed improvements in the 6 months following admission, apparently due to better and more regular diet, treatment of physical illnesses, and antidepressant treatment. Furthermore, whilst some people with dementia are physically frail, a significant number—who tend to be admitted as a consequence of behavioural problems such as aggression or wandering—are relatively robust. In fact Magaziner *et al.* (2005) found that newly admitted nursing home residents with dementia were more physically fit and had lower rates of mortality than residents without dementia. Although other studies (e.g. Landi *et al.*, 1998) have found an association between severe dementia and mortality, this probably results from limited use of medical services and medication for this population. It may also reflect a 'palliative care approach' with less aggressive treatment of people with dementia (Burton *et al.*, 2001).

## Interventions for dementia

It is usually recommended that non-pharmacological interventions for behaviour problems in dementia are considered ahead of drug treatments, as they are less likely to have serious side-effects. Several reviews have examined the management of challenging behaviour in dementia, with some concentrating specifically on care homes (Allen-Burge et al., 1999; Camp et al., 2002; Snowden et al., 2003; Landreville et al., 2006). This subject is discussed in Chapter 18vi of this book.

There have rightly been concerns about excessive prescribing of psychotropic drugs, especially antipsychotics, to older people in care homes. Numerous studies over the last decade have shown that high proportions of residents receive antipsychotics. For example, Waite (2002) lists seven studies, totalling over 3500 residents, where, overall, about a quarter were receiving neuroleptics. Most of these patients had dementia, though a proportion had other mental disorders, notably schizophrenia (Snowdon et al., 2005). Antipsychotics have many side-effects, for example sedation, impaired mobility, and increased risk of stroke. There is a small but significant increased risk of death with atypical antipsychotics compared to placebo (Schneider et al., 2005) and conventional antipsychotics also have similar risks (Wang et al., 2005). Furthermore, there are concerns that antipsychotics are used as a convenient substitute for good-quality care. The issue regularly attracts media and political attention. In the USA, prescribing was restricted by the Omnibus Budget Reconciliation Act of 1987 (often known as OBRA 87). This did lead to lower levels of prescribing but with little evidence of improved outcomes for residents (Hughes and Lapane, 2005).

Antipsychotics are, however, only modestly effective in treating behavioural and psychotic symptoms in dementia. A Cochrane Review (Ballard et al., 2006) concluded that risperidone and olanzapine were effective in reducing aggression and risperidone was effective in reducing psychotic symptoms but, because of the high levels of adverse events, they should only be used if there was marked risk or severe distress. In practice too, effectiveness appears to be limited as high levels of psychiatric symptoms persist in nursing homes despite treatment (Draper et al., 2001). Withdrawing patients from antipsychotics is usually well tolerated and adverse effects on behaviour are less common than might be expected (Cohen-Mansfield et al., 1999) though sleep disturbance may be a problem (Ruths et al., 2004).

Prescribing of antipsychotics remains controversial. Not all studies have concluded that prescribing in care homes is inappropriate (Macdonald et al., 2002) or associated with increased mortality (Suh and Shah, 2005); this seems to reflect lack of consensus as to what the proper indications are. In some places, antipsychotic usage has fallen while antidepressants have been used more (e.g. Nygaard et al., 2004), but elsewhere the use of antipsychotics has increased modestly, probably reflecting more residents with schizophrenia rather than increased prescribing to people with dementia (Lindesay et al., 2003). In the USA, the trend in antipsychotic prescribing has recently been upwards again (Briesacher et al., 2005), and there is currently more emphasis on improving quality of care rather than simply controlling prescribing (Hughes and Lapane, 2005). Criteria for assessing the appropriateness of prescribing have been advocated (Oborne et al., 2002) and various interventions, such as training and support for care home staff (Schmidt et al., 1998; Fossey et al., 2006), and clinical pharmacist input (Furniss et al., 2000; Lane et al., 2004), can be effective in reducing inappropriate prescribing. The challenge is how to make such experimental interventions part of routine practice.

Other types of medication have been evaluated in treating behaviour problems in dementia, and this literature is reviewed elsewhere in the book. Relatively few studies have looked specifically at care home residents. A randomized controlled trial of divalproex (800 mg per day for 6 weeks) did not show any benefit in the treatment of agitation (Tariot et al., 2005). In a randomized controlled trial of propranolol (mean dose 106 mg per day for 6 weeks), agitation, aggression, and anxiety were significantly reduced in the treatment group (Peskind et al., 2005). An open label study of rivastigmine (3–12 mg per day for a total of 52 weeks) found stable cognitive function and improved behavioural symptoms (Aupperle et al., 2004), and a cross-over study of opioid treatment for agitation in severe dementia also reported positive findings (Manfredi et al., 2003). Most of these studies have methodological shortcomings, most often small numbers, so the findings should be regarded as provisional.

## Depression

The importance of depression in residential and nursing homes was first convincingly demonstrated over 20 years ago (Mann et al., 1984) in a study which found that 38% of a sample of over 400 residents were depressed. Depression was particularly associated with: visual impairment and incontinence, increased dependency, problem behaviours such as wandering and aggression, having been admitted from one's own home, and belonging to a minority religion. A follow-up study after 3.6 years (Ames et al., 1988) found that two-thirds of the residents had died but, of those surviving, only 17% had recovered from depression. Interventions for depression were often difficult to implement and their outcomes were not particularly successful (Ames, 1990). Since then, several studies have reported prevalence rates ranging from 20% to 52%, and at least five studies have examined factors that may be associated with depression (Jones et al., 2003; Chow et al., 2004; Eisses et al., 2004; Gruber-Baldini et al., 2005; Lin et al., 2005). Although there is incomplete agreement between them, most reported that functional impairment appears to be an important independent risk factor for depression. Other associations include physical health variables, such as pain, dysphagia, and heart disease; psychological variables, such as loneliness and neuroticism; and social variables. Depression appears to be more common in for-profit homes and in contexts where residents do not have public funding support.

Assessment of depression in care homes may be difficult for various reasons, and depression is often not recognized by care staff (Bagley et al., 2000). One primary challenge is in diagnosing depression in residents with severe dementia—indeed, prevalence studies often exclude up to a third of residents for this reason. Further, care staff may lack the knowledge and skills to recognize depression, especially if the main symptoms are changes in behaviour, such as aggressive behaviour or disruptive vocalization (Dwyer and Byrne, 2000; Menon et al., 2001; Bartels et al., 2003a). There may also even be financial disincentives to recognize the presence of mental disorders (Snowdon, 2005). These combined findings have led to the suggestion that residents with dementia should be routinely screened for depression (Cohen et al., 2003).

Identifying depression is important as it has a potent effect on well being (Smallbrugge et al., 2006) and is implicated in suicides and attempted suicides in both care home residents and the community-based elderly population (Scocco et al., 2006). It is not clear whether rates are higher in care homes. The course of depression in homes is not well understood, but Payne et al. (2002) found that although 20% of residents were depressed on admission only 7.5% of these were still depressed 12 months later. However, the annual attack rate for depression was 26%, though most of the new episodes resolved within 6 months or less, possibly because of the availability of adequate treatment. Bruce et al. (2002) reported that 71% of their sample of 73 (out of a total of 539) residents with major depression were experiencing their first episode, and that most of these episodes lasted more than 2 months. In general, more longitudinal studies are needed: we simply do not know if we are dealing with a relatively mild and transient phenomenon or the onset of severe, enduring, and disabling symptoms.

In treating depression, serotonin reuptake inhibitors are prescribed more commonly than tricyclics. When tricyclic antidepressants are used, it is often for indications other than depression, such as insomnia, pain, or itching (Borson et al., 2002). The treatment offered is often not adequate, for example subtherapeutic doses of antidepressants or being offered anxiolytics and hypnotics instead (Brown et al., 2002). Nonetheless, prescribing of antidepressants has increased dramatically in several countries, in part due to concerns about antipsychotics but probably also in recognition of the importance of treating depression (Arthur et al., 2002; Datto et al., 2002). Unfortunately, prescribing may be influenced as much by the characteristics of the home as by the clinical needs of residents (Lapane and Hughes, 2004).

Other psychosocial interventions, including care staff training (Eisses et al., 2005) and interventions aimed at secondary prevention (Cuijpers and van Lammeren, 2001), often show encouraging results including better recognition of depression, but it is difficult to demonstrate positive outcomes in terms of lower levels of depression. A randomized controlled trial of a three-pronged shared care intervention (Llewellyn-Jones et al., 1999) did show modest improvements in depression scores but successful studies are limited.

## Other mental health problems

Although dementia and depression are the commonest mental health problems in care home populations, other disorders may be present too. Sleep disorders are discussed in Chapter 36. Anxiety symptoms are also common, though their severity varies, and anxiety may be symptomatic of other disorders, such as depression or physical illness. Smallbrugge et al. (2005) found that, in a sample of over 300 patients, 5.7% had anxiety disorders, 4.2% had subthreshold anxiety disorders, and nearly 30% had anxiety symptoms. Anxiety disorders were associated with health-related variables, notably depression and stroke. There is a lack of treatment studies for anxiety disorders.

The number of people with severe long-term mental illnesses, such as schizophrenia and bipolar disorder, has risen in many developed countries, especially since the closure of large psychiatric hospitals. Irrespective of diagnosis, whether an individual is living in the community or in a home is predicted by more severe symptoms, cognitive impairment, greater functional impairment,

more aggression, and unmarried status (Bartels et al., 1997). Positive symptoms in schizophrenia are often persistent and seem to be related to verbal aggression (Bowie et al., 2001). Such patients often fit poorly into conventional nursing home environments and other models of care, e.g. separate units or supported community living, may be preferable (Dencker and Gottfries, 1991; Bartels et al., 2003b). Depla et al. (2003) reviewed six Dutch programmes that employed various means to cater for older people with chronic mental illnesses. Overall, the favoured model was deploying psychiatric staff to work with care home staff, rather than having a psychiatric unit within the home or the home itself employing its own psychiatrically trained staff.

## Improving care for residents
### Care home staff

Care home staff are a vital human resource; their attitudes and behaviour have a profound influence on the quality of care in a home and on the lived experiences of residents. As noted earlier, staffing levels are often inadequate and there are few accurate data regarding 'appropriate skill mix' despite this being a national minimum standard. Investment in training is also variable; its availability and quality uneven (Meyer, 2006). As raising levels of qualified staff is a primary route to improving care—and is also a minimum standard—this is a key concern. Some individual homes and care home organizations have developed training strategies whilst others pay it little attention; the not-for-profit sector tends to have a more positive approach to staff training (Centre for Policy on Ageing, 2001).

Although working in care homes is often physically and emotionally demanding, quite high levels of job satisfaction have been reported (Brodaty et al., 2003a) and satisfaction is closely related to staff attitudes, especially a person centred approach in the home (Zimmerman et al., 2005). Nonetheless, the most prevalent perceptions among care staff of people with dementia tend to be negative, e.g. that they are anxious, unpredictable, and have little control over their behaviour (Brodaty et al., 2003a) and staff perceive that levels of behavioural disturbance among residents have increased over time (Train et al., 2005b).

Most of the literature on training for care staff is not specifically focused on mental health issues, and few studies have used experimental designs to examine the impact of staff training on mental health outcomes. Ray et al. (1993), in a non-randomized controlled trial, found that an educational intervention led to a 72% reduction in days of antipsychotic prescribing compared to 13% in the control group, as well as a decrease in the use of physical restraints. Proctor et al. (1999) employed a training and education intervention, aimed at improving care planning skills. Residents in the intervention group had significantly improved scores for depression and cognitive impairment but not for behaviour ratings and activities of daily living, indicating that improved care planning did benefit residents. Moxon et al. (2001), in an uncontrolled evaluation of an educational approach to the detection and management of depression, reported improved ability of care staff to detect depression and reduction of depressive symptoms in seven out of eight residents who were studied in detail. Teri et al. (2005) performed a small randomized controlled trial to evaluate a dementia-specific programme (STAR; Staff Training in Assisted living and Residences), with positive results, both for residents' outcomes and staff satisfaction. Other interventions that involve family caregivers as well as staff have been evaluated, again with favourable outcomes (McCallion *et al.*, 1999; Ducharme *et al.*, 2005; Specht *et al.*, 2005). Various resources are available to support training for care home staff, including books (e.g. Conn *et al.*, 2001), training manuals, CD-ROMs, and other resources (e.g. Powell, 2000; Sawdon, 2006).

These findings are consistent with other studies of educational interventions (Nolan and Keady, 1996) that show a range of beneficial outcomes in the short term. However, to have a persistent and longer-term effect the learning has to be embedded into the culture and practice of the home; this may be difficult if staff turnover is rapid. Involvement of managers in training is crucial to promoting continuity. Active forms of learning with ongoing supervision have been identified as more effective than more traditional didactic teaching (Meyer, 2006). A key problem relates to which agency should provide resources for training. As it is an agenda which is partly the responsibility of the care home, the commissioning or funding agency, and the umbrella organizations tasked with delivering the government's commitment to raising standards, this issue is not always clear.

## General health care

The provision of general practice support to homes is uneven and there are often concerns about the quality of service provided. Reductions in long-stay hospital beds have transferred significant additional responsibility to primary care. One study estimated that the additional workload equated to 160 full-time general practitioners (Kavanagh and Knapp, 1998). Development of primary care to support care homes has been piecemeal (Audit Commission, 2000). A minority of homes, more often nursing or larger homes may pay GPs directly for their services to residents (Glendinning *et al.*, 2002). Even if they do not have such a contract, they may encourage residents to register with a particular surgery close to the care home, limiting individual choice (Jacobs, 2003). Other homes try to maintain continuity of GP care resulting in residents being registered with a number of different practices, some of which may be some distance away. Where there is a more formal arrangement with GPs, regular medical sessions may be held, though the existence of such a contract is no guarantee of this occurring. There is at present limited evidence about the relative effectiveness of different models of GP work in care homes.

As regards the quality of primary care, Fahey *et al.* (2003) found that nursing home residents fared worse than people living in their own homes on several explicit quality indicators. They were less likely to be prescribed beneficial drugs (beta-blockers after myocardial infarction), more likely to receive potentially harmful drugs (antipsychotics and laxatives), and less likely to have their blood pressure monitored in the presence of either heart disease or diabetes. Other evidence has shown that continuity in out of hours medical cover leads to more appropriate management and fewer admissions to hospital (Bellelli *et al.*, 2001). Among health professionals, district (community) nurses are the most frequent visitors to care homes (Goodman *et al.*, 2005), but their expectations are often rather different from those of care staff and examples of true collaboration are limited.

Access to specialist services is also variable, both in terms of community-based specialists such as pharmacists and continence advisers (Peet *et al.*, 1996) and hospital-based services such

as geriatricians. A controlled trial of a pharmacy intervention in Australia reduced the use of all classes of drugs by 15%, with significant cost savings and no differences in morbidity or survival (Roberts *et al.*, 2001). As mentioned above, care home residents are at higher risk of requiring hospital admission than older people living in the community, and their outcomes in hospital are also worse, with higher rates of death during admission.

How can matters be improved? There is evidence that actively managed primary care, with access to interdisciplinary team support can be effective in reducing hospital admissions, with no adverse effects on mortality (Joseph and Boult, 1998). An integrated approach to health care, led by primary care and utilizing standardized comprehensive assessments of residents, has been advocated (e.g. Black and Bowman, 1997; Bowman *et al.*, 1999; Royal College of Physicians, 2000). Different models of primary care support to care homes need to be evaluated against one another. Further, a balance needs to be struck between one local practice providing regular input to a home, and the rights of residents to choose their own GPs or remain registered with practices they have often been with for many years.

## Mental health services and care homes

Support in managing mental health problems from specialist psychiatric teams is valued by most care homes, although many feel that additional input should be provided (Audit Commission, 2002). Advice regarding diagnosis and pharmacological management is generally more available than advice about behavioural or psychological approaches (Reichman *et al.*, 1998). A review of the literature (Bartels *et al.*, 2002) found three main models of mental health service delivery: psychiatrist-centred, nurse-centred, and multidisciplinary interventions. Although most studies suggested that mental health services are effective in improving clinical outcomes and reducing the need for hospitalization, relatively few controlled trials have been conducted. The least effective model appeared to be a traditional consultation service, and multidisciplinary interventions that combine clinical advice with staff training and education appear the most promising. Presumably, however, they are also more expensive to provide.

There are relatively few controlled trials of mental health service interventions. Rovner *et al.* (1996) evaluated a dementia care programme (AGE; Activities, Guidance for psychotropic medications, and Educational rounds). At 6-month follow-up the intervention group had lower levels of behavioural disorders and were receiving less psychotropic medication and physical restraint. Ballard *et al.* (2002) found that a psychiatric liaison service, delivered through weekly nurse visits, led to significant reductions in neuroleptic prescribing, GP contacts, and psychiatric hospital admissions, although there were no significant changes in well being or psychological and behavioural symptoms. Opie *et al.* (2002) used a range of interventions, including psychosocial strategies, nursing approaches, psychotropic medication, and pain management. Although there were improvements in symptoms, these were seen in all residents and not confined to the treatment group, suggesting a general and non-specific effect of the interventions upon the participating homes. Brodaty *et al.* (2003b) compared three interventions: psychogeriatric case management, specialist psychogeriatric consultation to GPs, and standard care. Although symptoms of depression and psychosis improved in all three groups there were no significant differences, again indicating a powerful non-specific effect for such interventions. Kotynia-English *et al.* (2005) evaluated systematic screening and early clinical intervention of all residents for depression and other forms of psychiatric morbidity, but found that this made no significant difference to health outcomes at 12 months.

Overall, it appears that mental health service involvement with care homes is beneficial to residents, but no single model is convincingly the most effective. The mechanisms by which interventions work are obscure and non-specific (Hawthorne) effects are commonly observed (Rosewarne *et al.*, 1997). Perhaps these findings are unsurprising as residents and their difficulties are not homogeneous and so a range of interventions will be required in practice. Growing interest and awareness of the importance of this area has led to guidance from the American Geriatrics Society and the American Association for Geriatric Psychiatry (2003a,b). In the UK, the National Care Homes Research and Development Forum was established in 2003 (Owen and NCHRDF, 2006) to improve networking between researchers and practitioners in the field, and the International Psychogeriatric Association has also recently established a task force on mental health services in nursing homes.

# Conclusions

Residents of care homes are a significant proportion of the population of older people. In many countries, there is a high chance of any individual spending the latter part of their life in a care home, and many of us will die in one. Because of the frail nature of residents, especially the high prevalence of dementia and communication challenges, their needs are easy to overlook. Mental health problems are very common, and have attracted some practice and research attention. Thus there is some evidence as to what is effective and what may be harmful in care home settings. Mental health services have an important part to play in support of care home staff and primary care, though the most effective and efficient way of using specialist mental health input has not yet been adequately demonstrated. It is to be hoped that future work will emphasize the perspectives of residents themselves and will concentrate on interventions that improve the quality of residents' lives and the quality of the care they receive.

## References

Allen, R.S., Burgio, L.D., Fisher, S.E., Hardin, J.M., and Shuster, J.L. (2005). Behavioral characteristics of agitated nursing home residents with dementia at the end of life. *Gerontologist*, **45**, 661–666.

Allen-Burge, R., Stevens, A.B., and Burgio, L.D. (1999). Effective behavioral interventions for decreasing dementia-related challenging behavior in nursing homes. *International Journal of Geriatric Psychiatry*, **14**, 213–232.

American Geriatrics Society and American Association for Geriatric Psychiatry (2003a). Consensus statement on improving the quality of mental health care in US nursing homes: management of depression and behavioral symptoms associated with dementia. *Journal of the American Geriatrics Society*, **51**, 1287–1298.

American Geriatrics Society and American Association for Geriatric Psychiatry (2003b). The American Geriatrics Society and American Association for Geriatric Psychiatry recommendations for policies in support of quality mental health care in US nursing homes. *Journal of the American Geriatrics Society*, **51**, 1298–1304.

Ames, D. (1990). Depression among elderly residents of local-authority residential homes: its nature and the efficacy of intervention. *British Journal of Psychiatry*, **156**, 667–675.

Ames, D., Ashby, D., Mann, A.H., and Graham, N. (1988). Psychiatric illness in elderly residents of Part III homes in one London borough: prognosis and review. *Age and Ageing*, **17**, 249–256.

Arfken, C.L., Wilson, J.G., and Aronson, S.M. (2001). Retrospective review of selective serotonin reuptake inhibitors and falling in older nursing home residents. *International Psychogeriatrics*, **13**, 85–91.

Arthur, A., Matthews, R., Jagger, C., and Lindesay, J. (2002). Factors associated with antidepressant treatment in residential care: changes between 1990 and 1997. *International Journal of Geriatric Psychiatry*, **21**, 54–60.

Audit Commission (2000). *Forget me not: mental health services for older people*. Audit Commission, London

Audit Commission (2002). *Forget me not: developing mental health services for older people in England*. Audit Commission, London.

Aupperle, P.M., Koumaras, B., Chen, M., Pabinowicz, A., and Mirski, D. (2004). Long-term effects of rivastigmine treatment on neuropsychiatric and behavioral disturbances in nursing home residents with moderate to severe Alzheimer's disease: results of a 52-week open-label study. *Current Medical Research and Opinion*, **20**, 1605–1620.

Bagley, H., Cordingley, L., Burns, A. *et al.* (2000). Recognition of depression by staff in nursing and residential homes. *Journal of Clinical Nursing*, **9**, 445–450.

Bajekal, M. (2002). *Health survey for England 2000: care homes and their residents*. The Stationery Office, London.

Ballard, C., Fossey, J., Chithramohan, R. *et al.* (2001a). Quality of care in private sector and NHS facilities for people with dementia: cross sectional study. *British Medical Journal*, **323**, 426–427.

Ballard, C.G., Margallo-Lana, M., Fossey, J. *et al.* (2001b). A 1-year follow-up study of behavioral and psychological symptoms in dementia among people in care environments. *Journal of Clinical Psychiatry*, **62**, 631–636.

Ballard, C., Lowell, I., James, I. *et al.* (2002). Can psychiatric liaison reduce neuroleptic use and reduce health service utilization for dementia patients residing in care facilities? *International Journal of Geriatric Psychiatry*, **17**, 140–145.

Ballard, C., Waite, J., and Birks, J. (2006). Atypical antipsychotics for aggression and psychosis in Alzheimer's disease. *Cochrane Database of Systematic Reviews* 2006, Issue 1, Art. No. CD003476. DOI: 10.1002/14651858.CD003476.pub2.

Barnett, E. (2000). *Including the person with dementia in designing and delivering care: 'I need to be me!'* Jessica Kingsley, London.

Bartels, S.J., Mueser, K.T., and Miles, K.M. (1997). A comparative study of elderly patients with schizophrenia and bipolar disorder in nursing homes and the community. *Schizophrenia Research*, **30**, 181–190.

Bartels, S.J., Moak, G.S., and Dums, A.R. (2002). Models of mental health services in nursing homes: a review of the literature. *Psychiatric Services*, **53**, 1390–1396.

Bartels, S.J., Horn, S.D., Smout, R.J. *et al.* (2003a). Agitation and depression in frail nursing home elderly patients with dementia: treatment characteristics and service use. *American Journal of Geriatric Psychiatry*, **11**, 231–238.

Bartels, S.J., Miles, K.M., Dums, A.R., and Levine, K.J. (2003b). Are nursing homes appropriate for older adults with severe mental illness? Conflicting consumer and clinician views and implications for the Olmstead decision. *Journal of the American Geriatrics Society*, **51**, 1571–1579.

Bebbington, A., Darton, R., and Netten, A. (2001). *Care homes for older people, volume 2: admissions, needs and outcomes*. Personal Social Services Research Unit, University of Kent, Canterbury.

Bellelli, G., Frisoni, G.B., Barbisoni, P., Boffelli, S., Rozzini, R., and Trabucchi, M. (2001). The management of adverse clinical events in nursing homes: a 1-year survey study. *Journal of the American Geriatrics Society*, **49**, 915–925.

Bercovitz, A., Gruber-Baldini, A.L., Burton, L.C., and Hebel, J.R. (2005). Healthcare utilization of nursing home residents: comparison between decedents and survivors. *Journal of the American Geriatrics Society*, **53**, 2069–2075.

Bergland, A. and Kirkevold, M. (2001). Thriving – a useful theoretical perspective to capture the experience of well-being among frail elderly in nursing homes? *Journal of Advanced Nursing*, **36**, 426–432.

Black, D. and Bowman, C. (1997). Community institutional care for frail elderly people. *British Medical Journal*, **315**, 441–442.

Boaz, A., Hayden, C, and Bernard, M. (1999). *Attitudes and aspirations of older people: a review of the literature*. Department of Social Security, London.

Borson, S., Scanlan, J.M., Doane, K., and Gray, S. (2002). Antidepressant prescribing in nursing homes: is there a place for tricyclics? *International Journal of Geriatric Psychiatry*, **17**, 1140–1145.

Bowie, C.R., Moriarty, P.J., Harvey, P.D., Parrella, M., White L., and Davis K.L. (2001). Aggression in elderly schizophrenic patients: a comparison of nursing home and state hospital residents. *Journal of Neuropsychiatry and Clinical Neurosciences*, **13**, 357–366.

Bowman, C., Johnson, M., Venables, D., Foote, C., and Kane, R.L. (1999). Geriatric care in the UK: aligning services to needs. *British Medical Journal*, **319**, 1119–1122.

Bowman, C., Whistler, J., and Ellerby M. (2004). A national census of care home residents. *Age and Ageing*, **33**, 561–566.

Bowman, C.E., Elford, J., Dovey, J., Campbell, S., and Barrowclough, H. (2001). Acute hospital admissions from nursing homes: some may be avoidable. *Postgraduate Medical Journal*, **77**, 40–42.

Briesacher, B.A., Limcangco, M.R., Simoni-Wastila, L. *et al.* (2005). The quality of neuroleptic prescribing in nursing homes. *Archives of Internal Medicine*, **165**, 1280–1285.

Brodaty, H., Draper, B., Saab, D. *et al.* (2001). Psychosis, depression and behavioural disturbances in Sydney nursing home residents: prevalence and predictors. *International Journal of Geriatric Psychiatry*, **16**, 504–512.

Brodaty, H., Draper, B., Low, L.F. (2003a). Nursing home staff attitudes towards residents with dementia: strain and satisfaction with work. *Journal of Advanced Nursing*, **44**, 583–590.

Brodaty, H., Draper, B., Millar, J. *et al.* (2003b). Randomized controlled trial of different models of care for nursing home residents with dementia complicated by depression or psychosis. *Journal of Clinical Psychiatry*, **64**, 63–72.

Brooks, L., Abarno, T., and Smith, M. (2003) *Care and support in very sheltered housing*. Counsel and Care, London.

Brown, M.N., Laplace, K.L., and Luisi, A.F. (2002). The management of depression in older nursing home residents. *Journal of the American Geriatrics Society*, **50**, 69–76.

Bruce, M.L., McAvay, G.J., Raue, P.J. *et al.* (2002). Major depression in elderly home health care patients. *American Journal of Psychiatry*, **159**, 1367–1374.

Burton, L.C., German, P.S., Gruber-Baldini, A.L., Hebel, J.R., Zimmerman, S., and Magaziner, J. (2001). Medical care for nursing home residents: differences by dementia status. *Journal of the American Geriatrics Society*, **49**, 142–147.

Buttar, A.B., Mhyre, J., Fries, B.E., and Blaum, C.S. (2003). Six-month cognitive improvement in nursing home residents with severe cognitive impairment. *Journal of Geriatric Psychiatry and Neurology*, **16**, 100–108.

Camp, C.J., Cohen-Mansfield, J., and Capezuti, E.A. (2002). Use of non-pharmacologic interventions among nursing home residents with dementia. *Psychiatric Services*, **53**, 1397–1401.

Care Commission (2004). *A review of the quality of care homes in Scotland 2004*. Care Commission, Dundee.

Centre for Policy on Ageing (2001). *CPA briefings: residential care and older people*, http://www.cpa.org.uk/policy/briefings/residential_care_and_older_people.pdf.

Chibnall, J.T., Tait, R.C., Harman, B., and Luebbert, R.A. (2005). Effect of acetaminophen on behavior, well-being, and psychotropic medication use in nursing home residents with moderate-to-severe dementia. *Journal of the American Geriatrics Society*, **53**, 1921–1929.

Chow, E., Kong, B., Wong, M. *et al.* (2004). The prevalence of depressive symptoms among elderly Chinese private nursing home residents in Hong Kong. *International Journal of Geriatric Psychiatry*, **19**, 734–740.

Cipher, D.J. and Clifford, P.A. (2004). Dementia, pain, depression, behavioral disturbances, and ADLs: toward a comprehensive conceptualization of quality of life in long-term care. *International Journal of Geriatric Psychiatry*, **19**, 741–748.

Cohen, C.I., Hyland, K., and Kimhy, D. (2003). The utility of mandatory depression screening of dementia patients in nursing homes. *American Journal of Psychiatry*, **160**, 2012–2017.

Cohen-Mansfield, J. and Taylor, J.W. (2004). Hearing aid use in nursing homes, part 1: prevalence rates of hearing impairment and hearing aid use. *Journal of the American Medical Directors Association*, **5**, 283–288.

Cohen-Mansfield, J., Lipson, S., Werner, P., Billig, N., Taylor, L., and Woosley, R. (1999). Withdrawal of haloperidol, thioridazine, and lorazepam in the nursing home: a controlled double-blind study. *Archives of Internal Medicine*, **159**, 1733–1740.

Coolen, J. and Weekers, S. (1998). Long term care in the Netherlands: public funding and private provision within a universalistic welfare state. In *Rights and realities: comparing new developments in long term care for older people* (ed. C. Glendinning). Policy Press, Bristol.

Commission for Social Care Inspection (2005). *The state of social care in England 2004/05*. Commission for Social Care Inspection, London.

Conn, D.K., Herrmann, N., Kaye, A., Rewilak, D., and Schogt, B. (eds) (2001). *Practical psychiatry in the long-term care facility*. Hogrefe and Huber, Seattle.

Conroy, S.P., Luxton, T., Dingwall, R., Harwood, R.H., and Gladman, J.R. (2006). Cardiopulmonary resuscitation in continuing care settings: time for a rethink? *British Medical Journal*, **332**, 479–482.

Counsel and Care (2001). *Residents taking risks: minimising the use of restraint – a guide for care homes*. Counsel and Care, London.

Cuijpers, P. (2001). Mortality and depressive symptoms in inhabitants of residential homes. *International Journal of Geriatric Psychiatry*, **16**, 131–138.

Cuijpers, P. and van Lammeren, P. (2001). Secondary prevention of depressive symptoms in elderly inhabitants of residential homes. *International Journal of Geriatric Psychiatry*, **16**, 702–708.

Datto, C.J., Oslin, D.W., Streim, J.E., Scheinthal, S.M., DiFilippo, S., and Katz, I.R. (2002). Pharmacologic treatment of depression in nursing home residents: a mental health services perspective. *Journal of Geriatric Psychiatry and Neurology*, **15**, 141–146.

De Jonghe-Rouleau, A.P., Pot, A.M., and de Jonghe, J.F. (2005). Self-injurious behaviour in nursing home residents. *International Journal of Geriatric Psychiatry*, **20**, 651–657.

De Klerk, M.M.Y. (2004). *Care and housing for vulnerable elderly: report on the elderly 2004*. Social and Cultural Planning Office, The Hague.

Dencker, K. and Gottfries, C. (1991). The closure of a major psychiatric hospital: can psychiatric patients in long-term care be integrated into existing nursing homes? *Journal of Geriatric Psychiatry and Neurology*, **4**, 149–156.

Dening, T.R. and Milne, A. (2005). Providing residential and nursing home care. In *Menopause, postmenopause and ageing* (ed. L. Keith), pp. 98–105. Royal Society of Medicine, London.

Department of Health (1999). *Fit for the future? National required standards for residential and nursing homes for older people*. The Stationery Office, London.

Department of Health (2001). *National Service Framework for Older People*. Department of Health, London.

Department of Health (2002). *Care homes for older people, national minimum standards*. The Stationery Office, London.

Department of Health (2006). *Our health, our care, our say: a new direction for community services*. Department of Health, London.

Depla, M.F., Pols, J., de Lange, J., Smits, C.H., de Graaf, R., and Heeren, T.J. (2003). Integrating mental health care into residential homes for the elderly: an analysis of six Dutch programs for older people with severe and persistent mental illness. *Journal of the American Geriatrics Society*, **51**, 1275–1279.

Dobalian, A., Tsao, J.C., and Radcliff, T.A. (2003). Diagnosed mental and physical health conditions in the United States nursing home population: differences between urban and rural facilities. *Journal of Rural Health*, **19**, 477–483.

Draper, B., Brodaty, H., Low, L.F. *et al.* (2001). Use of psychotropics in Sydney nursing homes: associations with depression, psychosis, and behavioral disturbances. *International Psychogeriatrics*, **13**, 107–120.

Draper, B., Brodaty, H., Low, L.F., and Richards, V. (2003). Prediction of mortality in nursing home residents: impact of passive self-harm behaviors. *International Psychogeriatrics*, **15**, 187–196.

Ducharme, F., Lévesque, L., Lachance, L., Giroux, F., Legault, A., and Préville, M. (2005). 'Taking Care of Myself': efficacy of an intervention programme for caregivers of a relative with dementia living in a long-term care setting. *Dementia*, **4**, 23–47.

Dudman, J. (2006). The state of play: care homes in the UK today. In *My home life: quality of life in care homes – a review of the literature* (ed. T. Owen and National Care Home Research and Development Forum). Help the Aged, London.

Dwyer, M. and Byrne, G.J. (2000). Disruptive vocalization and depression in older nursing home residents. *International Psychogeriatrics*, **12**, 463–471.

Dyer, C.A., Taylor, G.J., Reed, M., Dyer C.A., Robertson, D.R., and Harrington, R. (2004). Falls prevention in residential care homes: a randomised controlled trial. *Age and Ageing*, **33**, 596–602.

Eisses, A.M., Kluiter, H., Jongenelis, K, Pot, A.M., Beekman, A.T., and Ormel, J. (2004). Risk indicators of depression in residential homes. *International Journal of Geriatric Psychiatry*, **19**, 634–640.

Eisses, A.M., Kluiter, H., Jongenelis, K, Pot, A.M., Beekman, A.T., and Ormel, J. (2005). Care staff training in detection of depression in residential homes for the elderly: randomised trial. *British Journal of Psychiatry*, **186**, 404–409.

Evers, M.M., Samuels, S.C., Lantz, M., Khan, K., Brickman, A.M., and Marin, D.B. (2002). The prevalence, diagnosis and treatment of depression in dementia patients in chronic care facilities in the last six months of life. *International Journal of Geriatric Psychiatry*, **17**, 464–472.

ExtraCare Charitable Trust (2007). http://www.hcl.uk.com/test/extracare/

Fahey, T., Montgomery, A.A., Barnes, J., and Protheroe, J. (2003). Quality of care for elderly residents in nursing homes and elderly people living alone: controlled observational study. *British Medical Journal*, **326**, 580–583.

Fossey, J., Lee, L., and Ballard, C. (2002). Dementia Care Mapping as a research tool for measuring quality of life in care settings: psychometric properties. *International Journal of Geriatric Psychiatry*, **17**, 1064–1070.

Fossey, J., Ballard, C., Juszczak, E. *et al.* (2006). Effect of enhanced psychosocial care on antipsychotic use in nursing home residents with severe dementia: cluster randomised trial. *British Medical Journal*, **332**, 756–758.

Furniss, L., Burns, A., Craig, S.K., Scobie, S., Cooke, J., and Faragher, B. (2000). Effects of a pharmacist's medication review in nursing homes. *British Journal of Psychiatry*, **176**, 563–567.

Gaugler, J.E., Leach, C.R., and Anderson, K.A. (2004). Correlates of resident psychosocial status in long-term care. *International Journal of Geriatric Psychiatry*, **19**, 773–780.

Gessert, C.E., Mosier, M.C., Brown, E.F., and Frey, B. (2000). Tube feeding in nursing home residents with severe and irreversible cognitive impairment. *Journal of the American Geriatrics Society*, **48**, 1593–1600.

Glendinning, C., Jacobs, S., Alborz, A., and Hann, M. (2002). A survey of access to medical services in nursing and residential homes in England. *British Journal of General Practice*, **52**, 545–548.

Glendinning, C., Davies, B., Pickard, L., and Comas-Herrera, A. (2004). *Funding long-term care for older people: lessons from other countries*. Joseph Rowntree Foundation, York.

Godden, S. and Pollock, A.M. (2001). The use of acute hospital services by elderly residents of nursing and residential care homes. *Health and Social Care in the Community*, **9**, 367–374.

Goodman, C., Robb, N., Drennan, V., and Woolley, R. (2005). Partnership working by default: district nurses and care home staff providing care for older people. *Health and Social Care in the Community*, **13**, 553–62.

Gruber-Baldini, A.L., Zimmerman, S., Williams, C.S., Reed, P.S., Gill, K.S., and Preisser, J.S. (2005). Characteristics associated with depression in long-term care residents with dementia. *Gerontologist*, **45**(Special Issue 1), 50–55.

Hancock, G.A., Woods, R., Challis, D., and Orrell, M. (2006). The needs of older people with dementia in residential care. *International Journal of Geriatric Psychiatry*, **21**, 43–49.

Hanson, L.C., Reynolds, K.S., Henderson, M., and Pickard, C.G. (2005). A quality improvement intervention to increase palliative care in nursing homes. *Journal of Palliative Medicine*, **8**, 576–584.

Helen Ogilvy Associates (1999). *Evaluation of Fairfield Court*. Anchor Trust, London.

Higgs P., Macdonald, L., Macdonald, J., and Ward, M. (1998). Home from home: residents' opinions of nursing homes and long-stay wards. *Age and Ageing*, **27**, 199–205.

Hoe, J., Katona, C., Roch, B., and Livingston, G. (2005). Use of the QOL-AD for measuring quality of life in people with severe dementia – the LASER-AD study. *Age and Ageing*, **34**, 130–135.

Hoe, J., Hancock, G., Livingston, G., and Orrell, M. (2006). Quality of life of people with dementia in residential care homes. *British Journal of Psychiatry*, **188**, 460–464.

Hughes, C.M. and Lapane, K.L. (2005). Administrative initiatives for reducing inappropriate prescribing of psychotropic drugs in nursing homes: how successful have they been? *Drugs and Aging*, **22**, 339–351.

Hughes, J.C. (ed.). (2006). *Palliative care in severe dementia*. Quay, London.

Hughes, J.C. and Louw, S. (2002). Electronic tagging of people who wander. *British Medical Journal*, **325**, 847–848.

Hughes, J.C., Robinson, L., and Volicer, L. (2005). Specialist palliative care in dementia: specialised units with outreach and liaison are needed. *British Medical Journal*, **330**, 57–58.

Jacobs, S. (2003). Addressing the problems associated with general practitioners' workload in nursing and residential homes: findings from a qualitative study. *British Journal of General Practice*, **53**, 113–119.

Jones, R.N., Marcantonio, E.R., and Rabinowitz, T. (2003). Prevalence and correlates of recognized depression in US nursing homes. *Journal of the American Geriatrics Society*, **51**, 1404–1409.

Joseph, A. and Boult, C. (1998). Managed primary care of nursing home residents. *Journal of the American Geriatrics Society*, **46**, 1152–1156.

Kane, R.A., Kling, K.C., Bershadsky, B. *et al.* (2003). Quality of life measures for nursing home residents. *Journal of Gerontology A: Biological Sciences and Medical Sciences*, **58**, 240–248.

Katz, J. and Peace, S. (eds) (2003). *End of life in care homes: a palliative care approach*. Oxford University Press, Oxford.

Kavanagh, S. and Knapp, M. (1998). The impact on general practitioners of the changing balance of care for elderly people living in institutions. *British Medical Journal*, **317**, 322–327.

Kirkevold, Ø. and Engedal, K. (2005). Concealment of drugs in food and beverages in nursing homes: cross sectional study. *British Medical Journal*, **330**, 20–22.

Kotynia-English, R., McGowan, H., and Almeida, O.P. (2005). A randomized trial of early psychiatric intervention in residential care: impact on health outcomes. *International Psychogeriatrics*, **17**, 475–485.

Laing & Buisson (2006). *Care of elderly people: market survey 2005*. Laing & Buisson, London.

Lamberg, J.L., Person, C.J., Kiely, D.K., and Mitchell, S.L. (2005). Decisions to hospitalize nursing home residents dying with advanced dementia. *Journal of the American Geriatrics Society*, **53**, 1396–1401.

Landi, F., Gambassi, G., Lapane, K.L. *et al.* (1998). Comorbidity and drug use in cognitively impaired elderly living in long-term care. *Dementia and Geriatric Cognitive Disorders*, **9**, 347–356.

Landreville, P., Bédard, A., Verrault, R. *et al.* (2006). Non-pharmacological interventions for aggressive behavior in older adults living in long-term care facilities. *International Psychogeriatrics*, **18**, 47–73.

Lane, C.J., Bronskill, S.E., Sykora, K. *et al.* (2004). Potentially inappropriate prescribing in Ontario community-dwelling older adults and nursing home residents. *Journal of the American Geriatrics Society*, **52**, 861–866.

Lapane, K.L. and Hughes, C.M. (2004). Which organizational characteristics are associated with increased management of depression in US nursing homes? *Medical Care*, **42**, 992–1000.

Lin, L.C., Wang, T.G., Chen, M.Y., Wu, S.C., and Portwood, M.J. (2005). Depressive symptoms in long-term care residents in Taiwan. *Journal of Advanced Nursing*, **51**, 30–37.

Lindesay, J., Matthews, R., and Jagger, C. (2003). Factors associated with antipsychotic drug use in residential care: changes between 1990 and 1997. *International Journal of Geriatric Psychiatry*, **18**, 511–519.

Llewellyn-Jones, R.H., Baikie, K.A., Smithers, H., Cohen, J., Snowdon, J., and Tennant, C.C. (1999). Multifaceted shared care intervention for late life depression in residential care: randomised controlled trial. *British Medical Journal*, **319**, 676–682.

Logsdon, R.G., Gibbons, L.E., McCurry S.M. *et al.* (1999). Quality of life in Alzheimer's disease: patient and caregiver reports. *Journal of Mental Health and Aging*, **5**, 21–32.

McCallion, P., Toseland, R.W., and Freeman, K. (1999). An evaluation of a family visit education program. *Journal of the American Geriatrics Society*, **47**, 203–214.

Macdonald, A.J. and Dening, T.R. (2002). Dementia is being ignored in NHS and social care. *British Medical Journal*, **324**, 548.

Macdonald, A.J. and Woods, R.T. (2005). Attitudes to dementia and dementia care held by nursing staff in UK 'non-EMI' care homes: what difference do they make? *International Psychogeriatrics*, **17**, 383–391.

Macdonald, A.J., Carpenter, G.I., Box, O., Roberts, A., and Sahu, S. (2002). Dementia and the use of psychotropic medication in non-'elderly mentally infirm' nursing homes in south east England. *Age and Ageing*, **31**, 58–64.

MacRae, P.G., Asplund, L.A., Schnelle, J.F., Ouslander, J.G., Abrahamse, A., and Morris, C. (1996). A walking program for nursing home residents: effects on walk endurance, physical activity, mobility, and quality of life. *Journal of the American Geriatrics Society*, **44**, 175–180.

Magaziner, J. Zimmerman, S., Gruber-Baldini, A.L. *et al.* (2005). Mortality and adverse health events in newly admitted nursing home residents with and without dementia. *Journal of the American Geriatrics Society*, **53**, 1858–1866.

Manfredi, P.L., Breuer, B., Wallenstein, S., Stegmann, M., Bottomley, G., and Libow, L. (2003). Opioid treatment for agitation in patients with advanced dementia. *International Journal of Geriatric Psychiatry*, **18**, 700–705.

Mann, A.H., Graham, N., and Ashby, D. (1984). Psychiatric illness in residential homes for the elderly: a survey in one London borough. *Age and Ageing*, **13**, 257–265.

Margallo-Lana, M., Swann, A., O'Brien, J. *et al.* (2001). Prevalence and pharmacological management of behavioural and psychological symptoms of dementia amongst dementia sufferers living in care environments. *International Journal of Geriatric Psychiatry*, **16**, 39–44.

Matthews, F.E and Dening, T.R. (2002). Prevalence of dementia in institutional care. *Lancet*, **360**, 225–226.

Melzer, D., McWilliams, B., Brayne, C., Johnson, T., and Bond, J. (1999). Profile of disability in elderly people: estimates from a longitudinal population study. *British Medical Journal*, **318**, 1108–1111.

Menon, A.S., Gruber-Baldini, A.L., Hebel, J.R. *et al.* (2001). Relationship between aggressive behaviors and depression among nursing home residents with dementia. *International Journal of Geriatric Psychiatry*, **16**, 139–146.

Meyer, J. (2006). Keeping the workforce fit for purpose. In *My home life: quality of life in care homes – a review of the literature* (ed. T. Owen and National Care Home Research and Development Forum). Help the Aged, London.

Milne, A. and Chryssanthopoulou, C. (2005). Dementia caregiving in Black and Asian populations: reviewing and refining the research agenda. *Journal of Community and Applied Social Psychology*, **15**, 319–337.

Milne, A. and Williams, J. (2000). Meeting the mental health needs of older women: taking social inequality into account. *Ageing and Society*, **20**, 699–723.

Milne, A., Hatzidimitriadou, E., Chryssanthopoulou, C., and Owen, T. (2001). *Caring in later life: reviewing the role of older carers*. Help the Aged, London.

Mitchell, S.L., Kiely, D.K., and Lipsitz, L.A. (1997). The risk factors and impact on survival of feeding tube placement in nursing home residents with severe cognitive impairment. *Archives of Internal Medicine*, **157**, 327–332.

Mitchell, S.L., Teno, J.M., Roy, J., Kabumoto, G., and Mor, V. (2003). Clinical and organizational factors associated with feeding tube use among nursing home residents with advanced cognitive impairment. *Journal of the American Medical Association*, **290**, 73–80.

Mitchell, S.L., Kiely, D.K., Hamel, M.B., Park, P.S., Morris, J.N., and Fries B.F. (2004a). Estimating prognosis for nursing home residents with advanced dementia. *Journal of the American Medical Association*, **291**, 2734–2740.

Mitchell, S.L., Kiely, D.K., and Hamel, M.B. (2004b). Dying with advanced dementia in the nursing home. *Archives of Internal Medicine*, **164**, 321–326.

Mitchell, S.L., Morris, J.N., Park, P.S., and Fries, B.E. (2004c). Terminal care for persons with advanced dementia in the nursing home and home care settings. *Journal of Palliative Medicine*, **7**, 808–816.

Monteleoni, C. and Clark, E. (2004). Using rapid-cycle quality improvement methodology to reduce feeding tubes in patients with advanced dementia: before and after study. *British Medical Journal*, **329**, 491–494.

Moriarty, J. and Webb, S. (2000). *Part of their lives: community care for older people with dementia*. Policy Press, Bristol.

Moxon, S., Lyne, K., Sinclair, I., Young, P., and Kirk, C. (2001). Mental health in residential homes: a role for care staff. *Ageing and Society*, **21**, 71–93.

Munn, J.C., Hanson, L.C., Zimmerman, S., Sloane, P.D., and Mitchell, C.M. (2006). Is hospice associated with improved end-of-life care in nursing homes and assisted living facilities? *Journal of the American Geriatrics Society*, **54**, 490–495.

Murphy, L.M. and Lipman, T.O. (2003). Percutaneous endoscopic gastrostomy does not prolong survival in patients with dementia. *Archives of Internal Medicine*, **163**, 1351–1353.

National Council for Palliative Care (2006). *Introductory guide to end of life care in care homes*. Department of Health, London.

Netten, A., Bebbington, A., Darton, R., and Forder, J. (2001). *Care homes for older people. Volume 1: Facilities, residents and costs*. Personal Social Services Research Unit, University of Kent, Canterbury.

Netten. A., Darton. R, and Curtis, L. (2002). *Self funded admissions to care homes*, Research Report 159. Department of Work and Pensions, London.

Nijs, A.N., de Graaf, C., Kok, F.J., and van Staveren, W.A. (2006). Effect of family style mealtimes on quality of life, physical performance, and body weight of nursing home residents: cluster randomised controlled trial. *British Medical Journal*, **332**, 1180–1183.

Nolan, M. and Keady, J. (1996). Training in long-term care: the road to better quality. *Reviews in Clinical Gerontology*, **6**, 333–342.

Nygaard, H.A. and Jarland, M. (2005). Are nursing home patients with dementia diagnosis at increased risk for inadequate pain treatment? *International Journal of Geriatric Psychiatry*, **20**, 730–737.

Nygaard, H.A., Ruths, S., Straand, J., and Naik, M. (2004). Not less but different: psychotropic drug utilization trends in Norwegian nursing homes during a 12-year period. The Bergen District Nursing Home (BEDNURS) Study. *Aging Clinical and Experimental Research*, **16**, 277–282.

Oborne, C.A., Hooper, R., Li, K.C., Swift, C.G., and Jackson, S.H. (2002). An indicator of appropriate neuroleptic prescribing in nursing homes. *Age and Ageing*, **31**, 435–439.

Office of Fair Trading (2005). *Care homes for older people in the UK, a market study*. Office of Fair Trading, London.

Opie, J., Doyle, C., and O'Connor, D.W. (2002). Challenging behaviour in nursing home residents with dementia: a randomized controlled trial of multidisciplinary interventions. *International Journal of Geriatric Psychiatry*, **17**, 6–13.

Organisation for Economic Co-operation and Development (2005). *Long-term care for older people*. OECD, Paris.

Orrell, M. and Hancock, G. (2004). *CANE: Camberwell Assessment of Need for the Elderly*. Gaskell, London.

Owen, T. and National Care Home Research and Development Forum (eds) (2006). *My home life: quality of life in care homes – a review of the literature*. Help the Aged, London.

Parker, M.J., Gillespie, W.J., and Gillespie, L.D. (2006) Effectiveness of hip protectors for preventing hip fractures in elderly people: systematic review. *British Medical Journal*, **332**, 571–574.

Parmelee, P.A., Katz, I.R., and Lawton, M.P. (1991). The relation of pain to depression among institutionalized aged. *Journal of Gerontology*, **46**, 15–21.

Payne, J.L., Sheppard, J-M., Steinberg, M., *et al.* (2002). Incidence, prevalence, and outcomes of depression in residents of a long-term care facility with dementia. *International Journal of Geriatric Psychiatry*, **17**, 247–253.

Peet, S.M., Castleden, C.M., McGrother, C.W., and Duffin, H.M. (1996). The management of urinary incontinence in residential and nursing homes for older people, *Age and Ageing*, **25**, 139–143.

Peskind, E.R., Tsuang, D.W., Bonner, L.T. *et al.* (2005). Propranolol for disruptive behaviors in nursing home residents with probable or possible Alzheimer disease: a placebo-controlled study. *Alzheimer Disease and Associated Disorders*, **19**, 23–28.

Powell, J. (2000). *Care to communicate: helping the older person with dementia*. Hawker, London.

Proctor, R., Burns, A., and Powell, H.S. *et al.* (1999). Behavioural management in nursing and residential homes: a randomised controlled trial. *Lancet*, **354**, 26–29.

Ray, W.A., Taylor, J.A., Meador, K.G. *et al.* (1993). Reducing antipsychotic drug use in nursing homes: a controlled trial of provider education. *Archives of Internal Medicine*, **153**, 713–721.

Ray, W.A., Taylor, J.A., Meador, K.G. *et al.* (1997). A randomized trial of a consultation service to reduce falls in nursing homes. *Journal of the American Medical Association*, **278**, 557–562.

Reed, P.S., Zimmerman, S., Sloane, P.D., Williams, C.S., and Boustani, M. (2005). Characteristics associated with low food and fluid intake in long-term care residents with dementia. *Gerontologist*, **45**(Special Issue 1), 74–80.

Reichman, W.E., Coyne, A.C., Borson, S. *et al.* (1998). Psychiatric consultation in the nursing home: a survey of six states. *American Journal of Geriatric Psychiatry*, **6**, 320–327.

Reilly, S., Abendstern, M., Hughes, J., Challis, D., Venables, D., and Pedersen, I. (2006), Quality in long-term care homes for people with dementia: an assessment of specialist provision. *Ageing and Society*, **26**, 649–668.

Roberts, M.S., Stokes, J.A., King, M.A. *et al.* (2001). Outcomes of a randomized controlled trial of a clinical pharmacy intervention in 52 nursing homes. *British Journal of Clinical Pharmacology*, **51**, 257–265.

Robinson, J. and Banks, P. (2005). *The business of caring: Kings Fund inquiry into care services for older people in London*. Kings Fund, London.

Rosewarne, R., Bruce, A., and McKenna, M. (1997). Dementia programme effectiveness in long-term care. *International Journal of Geriatric Psychiatry*, **12**, 173–182.

Rothera, I., Jones, R., Harwood, R., Avery, A., and Waite, J. (2002). Survival in a cohort of social services placements in nursing and residential homes: factors associated with life expectancy and mortality. *Public Health*, **116**, 160–165.

Rothera, I., Jones, R., Harwood, R., Avery, A., and Waite, J. (2003). Health status and assessed need for a cohort of older people admitted to nursing and residential homes. *Age and Ageing*, **32**, 303–309.

Rovner, B.W., Steele, C.D., Shmuely, Y., and Folstein, M.F. (1996). A randomized trial of dementia care in nursing homes. *Journal of the American Geriatrics Society*, **44**, 7–13.

Royal College of Nursing (2004). *RCN care home survey 2004: impact of low fees for care homes in the UK*. Royal College of Nursing, London.

Royal College of Physicians, Royal College of Nursing, and British Geriatrics Society. (2000). *The health and care of older people in care homes: a comprehensive interdisciplinary approach*. Royal College of Physicians, London.

Ruths, S., Straand, J., Nygaard, H.A., Bjorvatn, B., and Pallesen, S. (2004). Effect of antipsychotic withdrawal on behavior and sleep/wake activity in nursing home residents with dementia: a randomized, placebo-controlled, double-blinded study. *Journal of the American Geriatrics Society*, **52**, 1737–1743.

Samus, Q.M., Rosenblatt, A., Steele, C. *et al.* (2005). The association of neuropsychiatric symptoms and environment with quality of life in assisted living residents with dementia. *Gerontologist*, **45**(Special Issue 1), 19–26.

Sawdon, J. (2006). *Connect with us: a resource for care home managers developing services for people with dementia*. Dementia North, Northumbria University, Newcastle upon Tyne.

Scherder, E., Oosterman, J., Swaab, D. *et al.* (2005). Recent developments in pain in dementia. *British Medical Journal*, **330**, 461–646.

Schmidt I., Claesson, C.B., Westerholm, B., Nilsson, L.G., and Svarstad, B.L. (1998). The impact of regular multidisciplinary team interventions on psychotropic prescribing in Swedish nursing homes. *Journal of the American Geriatrics Society*, **46**, 77–82.

Schneider, L.S., Dagerman, K.S., and Insel, P. (2005). Risk of death with atypical antipsychotic drug treatment for dementia: meta-analysis of randomized placebo-controlled trials. *Journal of the American Medical Association*, **294**, 1934–1943.

Scocco, P., Rapattoni, M., and Fantoni, G. (2006). Nursing home institutionalization: a source of *eustress* or *distress* for the elderly? *International Journal of Geriatric Psychiatry*, **21**, 281–287.

Scocco, P., Rapattoni, M., Fantoni, G. *et al.* (2006). Suicidal behaviour in nursing homes: a survey in a region of north-east Italy. *International Journal of Geriatric Psychiatry*, **21**, 307–311.

Scottish Executive (2001). *Regulation of Care (Scotland) Act 2001*. Scottish Executive, Edinburgh.

Sinclair, A.J., Allard, I., and Bayer, A. (1997). Observations of diabetes care in long-term institutional settings with measures of cognitive function and dependency. *Diabetes Care*, **20**, 778–784.

Sloane, P.D., Zimmerman, S., Williams, C.S., Reed, P.S., Gill, K.S., and Preisser, J.S. (2005). Evaluating the quality of life of long-term care residents with dementia. *Gerontologist*, **45**(Special Issue 1), 37–49.

Smallbrugge, M., Pot, A.M., Jongenelis, L., Beekman, A.T., and Eefsting, J.A. (2005). Prevalence and correlates of anxiety among nursing home patients. *Journal of Affective Disorders*, **88**, 145–153.

Smallbrugge, M., Pot, A.M., Jongenelis, L., Gundy, C.M., Beekman, A.T., and Eefsting, J.A. (2006). The impact of depression and anxiety on well being, disability and use of health care services in nursing home patients. *International Journal of Geriatric Psychiatry*, **21**, 325–332.

Snowden, M., Sato, K., and Roy-Byrne, P. (2003). Assessment and treatment of nursing home residents with depression or behavioral symptoms associated with dementia: a review of the literature. *Journal of the American Geriatrics Society*, **51**, 1305–1317.

Snowdon J. (2005). The role of psychogeriatric services in long-term residential care settings. In *Psychogeriatric service delivery: an international perspective* (ed. B. Draper, P. Melding, and H. Brodaty), pp. 213–233. Oxford University Press, Oxford.

Snowdon, J., Day, S., and Baker, W. (2005). Why and how antipsychotic drugs are used in 40 Sydney nursing homes. *International Journal of Geriatric Psychiatry*, **20**, 1146–1152.

Social Policy Ageing and Information Network (2005). *What price care in old age? Three years on from SPAIN's 'Underfunding of social care' paper, what has changed?* SPAIN, London.

Sørensen, L., Foldspang, A., Gulmann, N.C., and Munk-Jørgensen, P. (2001). Assessment of dementia in nursing home residents by nurses and assistants: criteria validity and determinants. *International Journal of Geriatric Psychiatry*, **16**, 615–621.

Specht, J.K., Park, M., Maas, M.L., Reed, D., Swanson, E., and Buckwalter, K.C. (2005). Interventions for residents with dementia and their family and staff caregivers: evaluating the effectiveness of measures of outcomes in long-term care. *Journal of Gerontological Nursing*, **31**, 6–14.

Suh, G.H. and Shah, A. (2005). Effect of antipsychotics on mortality in elderly patients with dementia: a 1-year prospective study in a nursing home. *International Psychogeriatrics*, **17**, 429–441.

Sullivan-Marx, E.M., Strumpf, N.E., Evans, L.K., Baumgarten, M., and Maislin, G. (1999). Predictors of continuing physical restraint use in nursing home residents following restraint reduction efforts. *Journal of the American Geriatrics Society*, **47**, 342–348.

Tariot, P.N., Raman, R., Jakimovich, L. *et al.* (2005). Divalproex sodium in nursing home residents with possible or probable Alzheimer disease complicated by agitation: a randomized, controlled trial. *American Journal of Geriatric Psychiatry*, **13**, 942–949.

Taylor C. and Hendra, T. (2000). The prevalence of diabetes mellitus and quality of diabetic care in residential and nursing homes: a postal survey. *Age and Ageing*, **29**, 447–450.

Teri, L., Huda, P., Gibbons, L., Young, H., and van Leynseele, J. (2005). STAR: a dementia-specific training program for staff in assisted living residences. *Gerontologist*, **45**, 686–693.

Thapa, P.B., Gideon, P., Fought, R.L., and Ray, W.A. (1995). Psychotropic drugs and risk of recurrent falls in ambulatory nursing home residents. *American Journal of Epidemiology*, **142**, 202–211.

Train, G.H., Nurock, S.A., Manela, M., Kitchen, G., and Livingston, G.A. (2005a). A qualitative study of the experiences of long-term care for residents with dementia, their relatives and staff. *Aging and Mental Health*, **9**, 119–128.

Train, G.H., Nurock, S., Kitchen, G., Manela, M., and Livingston, G.A. (2005b). A qualitative study of the views of residents with dementia, their relatives and staff about work practices in long-term care settings. *International Psychogeriatrics*, **17**, 237–251.

Travis, S.S., Buchanan, R.J., Wang, S., and Kim, M. (2004). Analyses of nursing home residents with diabetes at admission. *Journal of the American Medical Directors Association*, **5**, 320–327.

Treloar, A., Beats, B., and Philpot, M. (2000). A pill in the sandwich: covert medication in food and drink. *Journal of the Royal Society of Medicine*, **93**, 408–411.

Tune, P. and Bowie, P. (2000). The quality of residential and nursing home care for people with dementia. *Age and Ageing*, **29**, 325–328.

Vallelly, S., Evans, S., Fear, T., and Means, R. (2006). *Opening doors to independence*. Housing 21, London.

Van Doorn, C., Gruber-Baldini, A.L., Zimmerman, S. *et al.* (2003). Dementia as a risk factor for falls and fall injuries among nursing home residents. *Journal of the American Geriatrics Society*, **51**, 1213–1218.

Waite, J. (2002). Keep taking the medicine? *Age and Ageing*, **31**, 423–425.

Wang, P.S., Schneeweiss, S., Avorn, J. *et al.* (2005). Risk of death in elderly users of conventional vs. atypical antipsychotic medications. *New England Journal of Medicine*, **353**, 2335–2341.

Wanless, D. (2006). *Securing good care for older people: taking a long term view*. Kings Fund, London.

Williams, S.W., Williams, C.S., Zimmerman, S. *et al.* (2005). Characteristics associated with mobility limitation in long-term care residents with dementia. *Gerontologist*, **45**(Special Issue 1), 62–67.

Winzelberg, G.S., Williams, C.S., Preisser, J.S., Zimmerman, S., and Sloane, P.D. (2005). Factors associated with nursing assistant quality-of-life ratings for residents with dementia in long-term care facilities. *Gerontologist*, **45**(Special Issue 1), 106–114.

Wittenberg, R., Comas-Herrera, A., Pickard, L., and Hancock, R. (2004). *Future demand for long term care in the UK: a summary of projections of long term care finance for older people to 2051*. Joseph Rowntree Foundation, York.

Zimmerman, S., Williams, C.S., Reed, P.S., et al. (2005). Attitudes, stress, and satisfaction of staff who care for residents with dementia. *Gerontologist*, **45**(Special Issue 1), 96–105.

# 24

# Good design for dementia means a better building for everyone

## Mary Marshall and Gareth Hoskins

This chapter presents a rationale for good design for people with dementia, explains what this means, and discusses some of the challenges associated with achieving it. It then examines a case study: the consultation and planning process and the actual building of a nursing home in Edinburgh. The brief for this nursing home specified that although the home was not intended solely for people with dementia, the design throughout should be suitable for their needs. Given that the majority of people in most nursing homes have dementia, this is entirely appropriate.

## Why is good design important for people with dementia?

Over the last 10 years the social approach to understanding dementia has gained greater respect, and is increasingly seen as an essential part of the process of both assessment and intervention. In brief, it suggests that a lot of what we see in someone with dementia, and a lot of what they experience, is a result of the interaction between the damage to their brain and their social and built environment. Thus the way we treat people with dementia is fundamental, as is the place they live. Kitwood (1997) is perhaps the most lucid exponent of the impact on people with dementia of their social and built environment; he describes the failure to understand this as subjecting them to a 'malignant social psychology'.

The International Classification of Functioning, Disability and Health, known as ICF, was endorsed by the World Health Organization in 2001. The components of the ICF are the health condition itself (which affects and is affected by bodily functions and structures); activities; and social participation. These in turn affect and are affected by environmental factors and personal factors. Rather than seeing the medical and social models as in opposition to each other, the ICF is based on an integration of both (section 5). This chapter is firmly based on the conviction that we must integrate the medical and social models if we are to serve people with dementia effectively.

The capacity of the built environment to disable people with impairments (at least as far as wheelchair users are concerned) is clearly well understood in the UK. This understanding resulted in the Disability Discrimination Act of 1995, which was fully implemented in 2004. There is a plethora of design guides and guidance to ensure that buildings are fully accessible to people with physical conditions affecting their mobility, reach, grip, sight, and hearing. The ageism inherent in the disability access world means that mobility problems are widely understood and their design requirements are implemented, since it is the younger people with mobility impairments who are the most articulate. It is now generally understood that people have 'impairments', and it is the social and built environment that cause the 'disability'. However, this is much less well understood where cognitive impairments are concerned.

## Compensating for the impairments of old age

To understand the design requirements of people with dementia it is necessary to understand the impairments for which the design must compensate.

First to consider are the impairments of ageing, since most people with dementia are older people. As people age, they are likely to develop impaired mobility, sight, and hearing. Most older people are able to manage these impairments because they understand that they have them and they learn how to compensate for them. This understanding and learning is much harder for people with dementia.

For example, mobility problems for older people require buildings to be without steps, to have shorter distances between essential rooms, and to have handrails. Sight problems in old age may include generally impaired vision (often exacerbated by conditions such as tunnel vision), loss of the ability to see three dimensions, and decrease in colour sensitivity. From the age of 50 people begin to experience heightened sensitivity to glare. The eyes of people aged over 70 are three times slower to adapt to changes in light levels, which is an important consideration when people go from room to room, or from outside to inside. They are likely to need three times the usual level of illumination to perform tasks. Koncelik (2003) reminds us that thinking about colour and light in buildings is fraught with 'design mysticism and myth'. For example, it is believed that some colours make people calmer or other colours cheer them up. However, there is no solid evidence of any relationship between colour and behaviour, and older people have increasing difficulty in differentiating colours anyway.

Hearing is very poorly understood in relation to design. As we get older we experience selective high-frequency hearing loss (presbyacusis) which impairs our ability to discriminate between sounds such as conversation and background noise. Hiatt (1995) asserts that noise for people with dementia is the equivalent of stairs for people in wheelchairs. Noise quickly becomes overwhelming. Many buildings for older people actually amplify and mix sounds instead of reducing them. Hard surfaces and many different sources of noise such as vacuum cleaners, dishwashers, radios, televisions, clattering trolleys and cutlery, make it very difficult for older people to concentrate on what they want to hear.

The reason for emphasizing these impairments of old age is that people with dementia lose the ability to conceptualize what their problem is, and to work out how to deal with it. M. Powell Lawton, the father of environmental gerontology, wrote about 'environmental press' (Lawton, 1987), by which he meant that the more disabled we are, the more we are victims of the buildings in which we live or spend our days, because we are powerless to do anything about them.

## Compensating for the impairments of dementia

In simple terms the impairments of most people with dementia are: impaired memory, impaired learning, and impaired reasoning. Many people with dementia also experience very high levels of stress, which further reduces their functioning and their ability to deal with their built environment. A lot of unnecessary disability (or 'excess disability' as it is sometimes called) is caused by environments which are experienced as hostile by people with dementia.

*Impaired memory* affects people's ability to recall where they are, and instead they may try to understand a building in relation to their longer-term memory. For a person with dementia it is difficult to make sense of modern buildings in terms of buildings they knew 50 years ago, given the extraordinarily strange environments that are our hospitals and care homes. It is even harder if they think they are at work or at school. For staff, it is challenging to make environments feel like home and be 'age-appropriate', since most staff will have little idea of what homes were like when the 85-year-olds they care for were setting up house as young adults.

*Impaired learning* will affect people's ability to learn that they have a visual or hearing impairment. It will be hard for them to learn their way around a building: some people with dementia will learn a route if they repeat it often enough; others will never do so.

*Impaired reasoning* will affect the ability to work out what a problem is and what to do about it. People with dementia will often not understand that they could see better if they put the light on, or hear better if they turned off all the other noise; they will not make sense of stairs, when they are unable to see depth. They will struggle to work out where things are, or how to operate equipment such as taps, or shower controls, or modern cookers.

## How do we compensate for these impairments?

There are two ways of approaching designing for dementia. One is by applying a set of principles to a building and its interior design. The other is to use a checklist. The first is obviously preferable since a checklist will never be comprehensive, but it would seem that a combination of both is helpful to most people. There is now a substantial literature on designing for dementia (Calkins, 1988; Cohen and Weisman, 1991; Cohen and Day, 1993; Netten, 1993; Brawley, 1997; Judd *et al.*, 1998; Cantley and Wilson, 2003; Utton, 2006). Also,

dementia has been included in a few of the design guides for older people generally (Centre for Accessible Environments, 1998). Although research is patchy (Day *et al.*, 2000), there is a well-established international consensus both on principles and on useful design features. These have been summarized in Judd *et al.* (1998) and a slightly modified version is given below.

The consensus on *principles* is that design should:

◆ compensate for impairments
◆ maximize independence
◆ enhance self-esteem and confidence
◆ demonstrate care for staff
◆ be orientating and understandable
◆ welcome relatives and the local community
◆ allow control of stimuli.

The consensus on design *features* includes:

◆ small size
◆ familiar, domestic, homely in style
◆ plenty of scope for ordinary activities (e.g. unit kitchens, washing lines, garden sheds)
◆ unobtrusive concern for safety
◆ different rooms for different functions
◆ age-appropriate furniture and fittings
◆ safe outside space
◆ single rooms big enough for lots of personal belongings
◆ good signage and multiple cues where possible, e.g. sight, smell, sound
◆ use of objects rather than colour for orientation
◆ enhancement of visual access
◆ control of stimuli, especially noise.

These design recommendations ought to be part of any guidance relating to the Disability Discrimination Act. They are relevant for anybody with a cognitive impairment for whatever reason. They should be part of guidance on domestic as well as public buildings and should, at the very least, be required of any health or care facility. All of us are cognitively impaired at some times, such as when we are very tired and stressed (often at airports or stations), or when we are ill or on medication. If all buildings were designed with cognitive impairment in mind they would be helpful to the general public as well as to people with specific cognitive impairments. There are many terms for this concept of designing for all of us, at all times, whatever temporary or permanent impairments we have: *barrier-free design, design for life, lifetime homes*, and so on.

However, there are many challenges in designing for people with dementia, and we address some of them below.

## Challenges

### A place to work

Buildings for people with dementia are usually also the workplace of staff and there can be a real tension between these two demands. Nevertheless Marshall (2005) has argued that good design for dementia can make life easier for staff. People with dementia in hospitals and care homes need to have a space that they can make sense of, where they can find their way and get around easily and safely, and where they feel that their own individuality is reinforced. This generally means that the space needs to be like home—their home, where they maintain familiar routines and activities and do pretty much what they want, when they want—as they would do at home.

On the other hand, staff need a building that makes their job as easy as possible. They want spaces that can be kept clean, where infection control is easy, where they can keep the patients or residents clean, and deal quickly with incontinence. They need to feel that the people they are caring for are safe. They also need private space, space to shower and rest, a place to meet and learn, and somewhere to do their paperwork without interruption.

## A place which reassures relatives

Relatives have their own needs in terms of the design of the buildings in which the person they care about is living, either temporarily or permanently. They should feel proud about the look of the place, so they do not feel too guilty when they visit. They need to feel confident that their relative or friend with dementia is safe. They need spaces that allow them to do things such as make a cup of tea with their relative, or to go for a walk in the garden, or to be comfortable together in private.

There can be really problematic conflicts between the needs of people with dementia and the needs of their relatives. For example, relatives may feel better about a home that looks like a hotel, even though it is totally confusing for the person with dementia. Staying in hotels in the UK was only for very privileged people until recently, and most very old people will have had very little experience of such an environment. Relatives may not be happy to have the older person's bedroom full of old and scruffy furniture and much-loved objects, even when these are very reassuring for the person concerned. Relatives may not be happy with apparently unsafe features such as kitchens for residents/patients, or easily accessible outside space.

Technology will play an increasing part in keeping people with dementia safe without impairing their quality of life. Examples include kitchen cookers with hidden switches so they only work when staff are present, and induction cookers which only warm the contents of the pan, and not the hotplate. Global Positioning Systems (GPS) will be used increasingly to locate people who are lost outside the home or ward. Passive infrared devices can alert staff to patients or residents who are at risk if they get up in the night. Of course not all risks can be eliminated. Staff need to talk this principle through with relatives, when they explain their approach to risk assessment and say what they have done to minimize risk without compromising quality of life.

## Costs and compromises

Good buildings for people with dementia are often seen as more expensive, although this may just reflect the need to improve on the general run of buildings for older people. If we designed all buildings to be dementia-friendly then the tensions about costs would be reduced. Features that are particularly cost-sensitive are small-scale and open-plan. It needs to be clearly understood that although the initial costs of an appropriate building may be high, the long-term costs of a disabling building may be higher. For example, a unit caring for more than eight people with dementia will result in more confusion amongst them, as they struggle to learn who all the staff and fellow residents are, struggle to find their way around a larger unit, struggle with the extra noise and turmoil created by larger numbers, and fail to eat because of the noise and other over-stimulation in the dining rooms.

Gardens are often simply patches of grass because the budget has been trimmed of anything else. This has a real impact on people with dementia who walk a lot, and on all residents who need to be outside to receive the necessary vitamin D from sunlight. The majority of residents and patients in long-stay units are deficient in vitamin D. Pollock (2001) provides good guidance on designing gardens for exercise and activity.

Naturally there are compromises to be made but they should be made in the full knowledge of their impact. A lounge which is not adjacent and visible from the bedrooms will mean that people cannot find it. A large dining room will mean more noise. When people sitting in the lounge or dining room cannot see where the toilet is, there will be greater restlessness and anxiety, and more incontinence.

## Normal activities

Normal everyday activities are the main 'therapy' for people with dementia, and making sure that they are familiar and failure-free is important. But providing a building which makes it easy to undertake normal activities such as cooking, cleaning, hanging out the washing, going for a walk, gardening, and so on is not easy, for a number of reasons. These activities can be seen as risky, although they need not be if they are designed carefully in a way that puts the staff in control where appropriate.

Fire risk and infection control are often given as the reasons why normal activities cannot take place. Good design can minimize both. If fire officers are involved at an early stage in the design and understand the rationale, they can make adjustments such as extra suppressants, and relocated fire doors, and occasionally some relaxation of the regulations. The same applies to infection control.

The risk of depression in care homes is rarely considered, but it is very high and must in some part be related to the extremes of boredom experienced by many residents and patients. The aphorism 'boredom is the equivalent of bedsores for people with dementia' is worth bearing in mind. Impaired memory makes it imperative that people with dementia are helped to undertake familiar activities which make sense to them in terms of their past.

## Designing for a progressive condition

People with dementia are not a homogeneous group. This is a progressive condition with a highly fluctuating course. People with dementia explain that they can be well one day and very impaired the next, they can be better in the morning than in the afternoon. Their brain damage can increase over time and their mental and physical health can deteriorate. People who are relatively unimpaired experience less 'environmental press' in the sense that they are more able to understand and control buildings, and they can manage in buildings with less visual access. They do not, for example, have to see a recognizable door of a room to find it, whereas those who are more impaired will not find a room unless they can see it.

People who are less impaired will find ways of learning where their bedroom is, whereas people who are more impaired will need individually tailored signage on the door. There is no uniformly successful form of individual door signage: some people will recognize themselves in photographs, some will like a number (perhaps that of their own house), others will need a three-dimensional object. Person-centred staff will demonstrate this philosophy in the care they take to find the most effective item for each resident/patient.

People with different degrees of impairment will need different degrees of surveillance. Very anxious people with dementia need the reassurance of seeing their relative or a staff member at all times. Other people need to be watched because they can hurt themselves or others with their behaviour.

'Wandering' is a good example of behaviour with design implications (Marshall and Allan 2006). Traditionally 'wandering' was seen as a result of brain damage and the design requirement was to have 'safe wandering paths'. Today a more considered view is emerging, which suggests that people walk a lot for very different reasons, and that on the whole walking is a healthy occupation which should be encouraged. The focus should be on making it a positive and safe experience. This requires space to walk inside and outside with places to rest and things to see on the way. Some people walk because they are lost, or searching for a particular room (often the toilet); so enabling design is very helpful, especially if it is familiar and reassuring too.

Challenging behaviour tends to be interpreted as behaviour which makes life difficult for staff and other residents, whereas people who are withdrawn and silent tend to be ignored. There is increasing understanding nowadays that behaviour is a means of communication which we need to understand and respond to. Buildings can and should play their part in helping people with this kind of challenging behaviour by providing appropriate stimulation and opportunities for relevant activities.

## Different lifestyles

That people with dementia need a place that feels familiar is obvious, but how to achieve it, given their very different life histories, is not. Culturally appropriate design is going to be the next big challenge as the members of minority groups grow older. A person who spent their formative years in a village in Bangladesh will need a very different design from someone who spent them in a pre-war Polish village. Even within the British population there are major differences. If we were designing for an upper middle class British group we might want to use white tablecloths and good silverware in the dining room. We might not have a kitchen alongside the dining room so that people could do kitchen chores. If we were designing for a group of people from a poor inner-city community or from a remote rural area we might think about having an outside WC, and a kitchen which was highly visible. The décor of the two units would be very different.

In the UK we seem unable to see cultural differences within our indigenous communities because we cannot confront issues of class. We also often fail to confront issues of gender. This is particularly important for some minority ethnic groups where men and women need separate spaces. The same applies in some indigenous British communities such as Scottish fishing villages, where mixing socially is rare and for special occasions only, and men would not expect to have to participate in kitchen chores. They would certainly want a men-only space.

Some people experienced terrible trauma in their formative years, especially if they were in occupied Europe. They may be extremely anxious and need to have an obvious escape route at all times. Anything which resembles an institution may be very frightening.

How do we resolve the design needs arising from different life histories and cultures? For some groups the design required may be so different that they need special buildings, or additional facilities such as different toilets, or space for worship. It is, however, unlikely that numbers will be such that this is possible for most people. We will continue to mix people with dementia from all sorts of cultural and class backgrounds. If we do this we should make it easy for staff and relatives to modify spaces. In some instances it may be possible to have differences between lounges (not a word used by the upper middle classes, who would be happier with 'sitting' or 'living' rooms). And it is always possible to make individual bedrooms very different. There is a dearth of literature about successful culturally appropriate design, but Bennett (2000) is an exception. She is an Australian architect who has written about designing for Japanese people with dementia, and for indigenous Australian communities.

## Complex needs

We are becoming increasingly aware of the design needs of people with dementia who also have conditions such as learning disability, or alcohol problems, or some other progressive disorder such as multiple sclerosis, Parkinson's disease, or Huntington's disease. Some people with dementia will be blind, from birth or later; some will likewise be deaf. Younger people with early onset dementia will need an age-appropriate ambience. People with alcohol-related brain damage may have particular design requirements. Usually they too are younger, and may have had a life in the forces or in homeless accommodation, so their concept of 'home' will not be a domestic environment. Special equipment for people with complex needs will put a strain on efforts to make a familiar space—acutely so, when people with dementia need terminal care. Then they may need extra space for equipment, especially beds and hoists, and their rooms very quickly cease to be personal and familiar. Meeting these many different complex needs would be easier if all rooms were bigger initially.

## Short and long stay

Some people need short-term care, if there has been a crisis at home, to give their carers a break, or because their condition needs urgent attention outwith their home, perhaps because their behaviour has become particularly challenging. They present a design challenge because there may be insufficient time or information to provide for their specific requirements. They need a place that seems familiar, understandable, and full of cues right away. This often means redundant cueing since it will be impossible beforehand to know what will suit them. Thus a bedroom door might have a number, their name, a photograph and a doorknocker to differentiate it, only one of which will make sense to them. For anyone with dementia it is important to make the toilet door highly visible but it is especially important for people who do not have time to learn at all. To be highly visible, a toilet door will be painted red or yellow (the colour most easily recognized as colour differentiation fails); it will have a large pictorial symbol and word sign on it, about 4 feet from the floor; and it will have a prominent landmark nearby such as a small cupboard or a striking picture.

It is different for permanent residents/patients. As far as the building allows, their spaces can be fully adapted to their needs. Furniture, pictures, objects, décor, and signage can all be modified to suit the individual and their background. Pollock (2003) has written a useful book on the design of interiors.

There is very little literature on the design of day hospitals or day centres for people with dementia. This must, in part, be because there are many approaches to day settings. Some are small, family size groupings who stay together all day. Others are larger and divide into groups for different activities. The design guidance for residential settings applies equally to day care, and some of it is easier to implement. For example, it is easier to achieve unobtrusive surveillance through the use of large alcoves for different activities. They make more sense in a day setting, where there is less need for the place to look like home. Indeed many men who go to day care think they are going out to work or to a club.

## Adapting a flat or house

Designing housing for older people should take account of all the requirements of dementia, since many of the tenants will arrive with dementia or will develop it while they live there. It is more challenging to modify existing houses and flats. If the person with dementia has lived in the same place for a long time, the learning about what is where and how it works may be very well-established. If they are moving into a new house or flat, various modifications can make that learning easier. These include: making the bathroom door more visible and removing cupboard doors or installing glass-fronted cupboards, so that people can see what is inside. (This is a lot more effective than covering the house in sticky labels.) Sometimes safety devices will be needed: devices which turn cookers off if the pan is too hot, or which switch on the light to the toilet when the person enters. The front door may need attention, in order to discourage the person with dementia from going out. The solution varies hugely from person to person. For some, a 'no-entry' sign will work; for others a curtain; door magnets can activate a verbal warning during the night, or can alert a neighbour or community alarm service. There are useful books on these technologies such as Marshall (2000) and Woolham (2005).

## Increasing numbers

As the post-war baby bulge is ageing, there will be dramatic increases in the numbers of older people and people with dementia in addition to the continuing smaller increases resulting from greater longevity. The buildings being constructed today are expected to last for at least 30 years, and they will need to serve an increasingly demanding and well-informed cohort of people.

## Delivering theory in day-to-day practice

The creation of such responsive environments is not solely an issue for designers and architects, who need to understand how particular environments can be organized to give positive assistance to people with impairments. Indeed, as previously noted, there is already (within the UK) a legislative requirement to provide for those with impairment. There is also a good base of understanding and guidance on the design of environments for people with cognitive impairments, but this has yet to find its way into most 'disability design' materials.

The challenge of achieving responsive designed environments is often complicated by more fundamental issues which hamper the full implementation of acknowledged best practice. Often these are cultural or economic issues. Society's attitudes towards the value of elderly people and their care result in funding provisions that are inadequate and incapable of providing quality environments.

The budgetary constraints imposed within the care sector in the UK can clearly be seen to produce buildings of a lower quality than examples across northern Europe. These buildings compare poorly in their basic standards of construction and therefore lifespan; and in their quality of environment, scale of facility, and incorporation of simple design considerations. The creation of better environments for older people and people with dementia does not depend only on the knowledge and understanding possessed by the designers of these environments. It also depends, crucially, on changing the funding mechanisms and institutional attitudes which regard design with suspicion, and as a costly luxury, rather than understanding it as a long-term benefit for those in care.

Good design is not simply a question of style or taste. It arises from the careful synthesis of many interrelated factors, such as fitness for purpose, layout, integration with surroundings, sense of place, construction methods, and value for money.

Well-designed health-care buildings can have a positive effect, not just in terms of the quality of life and the spirits and health of residents. They can reduce stress in carers and staff, have a positive effect on staff performance and retention, and provide better long-term value for money.

## Developing an exemplar—a model for providing improved care

These fundamental issues have been central to the development and design of an exemplar project—the provision of new elderly care homes in Edinburgh, funded through public sources (the City of Edinburgh Council (CEC) and NHS Lothian).

This exemplar project was commissioned in 2003 with the initial aim of developing a design-focused brief for a new elderly care home within the city. This home was to be developed and constructed as an 'exemplar' on a first site, then the project (and in particular the brief) would form the 'model' for a series of new homes on sites across the city. The project was the outcome of an architectural competition, by which a design team was selected from a group of practices with acknowledged experience of designing for dementia.

In line with *A City for All Ages* (City of Edinburgh Council, 2000), the city's strategy for the care of its elderly population, key considerations were that the brief should:

- ◆ seek to create an environment that looked beyond the 'minimum care standards' of provision;

- ◆ explore how such provision could cater for the prevalence of dementia within the growing elderly population (whilst the home was not expected to care solely for residents with dementia, the fact that up to 70% of people now in care homes have symptoms of dementia made this a key consideration);

- ◆ identify how the particular requirements for those with dementia could be met within a 'standard' care home, to ensure continuity of care as people's condition progresses;

- ◆ explore how the particular requirements of the different cultural groups within this population might be appropriately accommodated;

- ◆ provide new facilities that would be long-lasting in their quality of construction and would incorporate best practice in energy efficiency and environmental sustainability.

## An inclusive and consultative approach to developing a brief

A noteworthy aspect of the project was the way in which the 'model' brief for the new homes was created. It was not a brief centred solely around an accommodation schedule drawn up by an estates department or a commissioning body. Rather, the brief was developed over a period of thorough consultation in which the architectural team was partnered with a group of residents drawn from existing residential homes across the city. The aim of this consultative process was to develop a brief that was realistic and resident-focused, based upon a thorough understanding of the day-to-day issues facing those receiving and those providing care. The method used was to engage in consultative research into the quality and experience of life in residential homes, and into their mode of operation; to develop out of this a series of fundamental principles; and to use these principles to lead the design of the new accommodation.

Facilitated by Senior Action Group Edinburgh and the architectural team through funding from CEC, a series of visits and assessments of a wide range of existing homes across Lothian was carried out. Linked with these visits, a number of consultation meetings were held, not only with residents but with all interested people including relatives, carers, nursing staff, catering staff, managers, day care groups, and social workers involved in the day-to-day operation of the homes. As well as drawing opinion and comment from these events, the architectural team worked shadow shifts with care assistants to get a 'hands on' understanding of the day-to-day operation and activities within the homes.

Importantly, a period of 4 months was set aside within the project programme to enable the combined 'design team' to develop the brief through a number of clear stages, as follows:

- researching and reviewing existing 'local' care accommodation;

- gathering opinion and comment from users on the life and operation of these facilities;

- researching and reviewing examples of care provision from other countries;

- clarifying advantages and disadvantages, from the examples reviewed and from user feedback;

- out of the synthesis of all this information, creating a series of aspirational principles to guide the atmosphere and organization of the new homes;

- establishing an outline of accommodation requirements, guided by the key principles identified through the steps above.

At the completion of each of these stages the findings were reviewed with a 'project steering group' composed of residents and of staff from the CEC Social Work Department representing the different services that would be involved in the resulting home (Fig. 24.1).

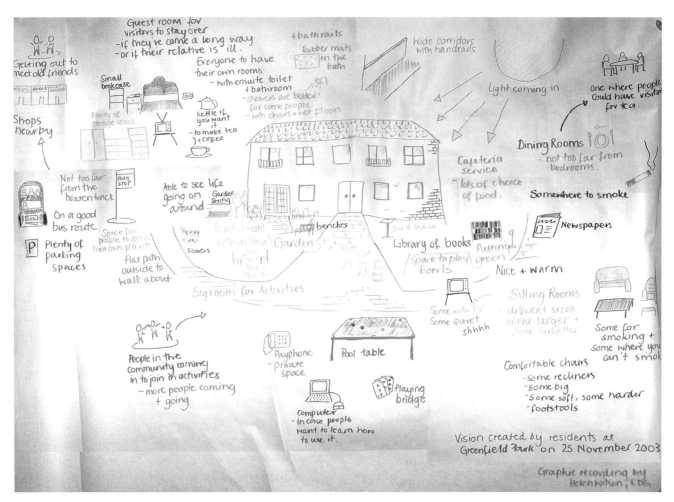

**Fig. 24.1** 'Briefing' drawing prepared by residents.

## Findings and design brief recommendations

This gathering of information from design guidance, existing facilities, feedback from users and staff, and the experience of other countries highlighted the following key points. They range from large-scale issues such as the siting of the home, down to the matters which determine the personal experience of an individual.

One important question was how dementia-friendly design could be integrated in a practicable manner into the design of a general care home. This is particularly important in ensuring that residents in a home who develop dementia can remain there, cared for within a familiar environment, and amongst a group of known fellow residents.

### Choice of site and relationship to the 'outside world'

Through a combination of funding constraints and the limited availability of sites large enough to accommodate the size of care home currently seen as the standard (i.e. 40–60 beds), new homes are often built in peripheral areas where land prices are relatively low. Often this means that homes are situated alongside inappropriate neighbouring uses, or in areas with little activity and few public transport links. Often people who have lived most of their lives in urban locations find themselves relatively isolated at a peripheral site.

> **Briefing recommendation**: Potential sites should be carefully reviewed in terms of the appropriateness of adjacent uses, and should have proximity to existing public transport links, facilities, and amenities to take advantage of potential access and interaction with the wider community outside the home.

### Site fit and 'place making'

The 'standard models' used by many providers mean that homes are often built with little consideration as to how these generic layouts might relate to the specific character or shape of individual sites. Many homes we visited had poor outlooks and took little advantage of the orientation or shape of their site to create considered external spaces. As a result many homes have an introverted and isolated feel about them, marooned within unused areas of grass. Such standard approaches miss out on some of the passive benefits that can be gained, for example, from a home being sited alongside a street, where the residents are able to watch the activities of everyday life outside the home.

Many standard care homes would fail to meet the requirements of 'Designing Places', the Scottish Executive's Planning Policy Guidance (Scottish Executive, 2001), which sets out fundamental aspects of the environment that should be considered by any development.

> **Briefing recommendation**: The layout and organization of the home on the site should take account of issues of site access, levels, orientation, views, and characteristics. The relationship of the home with adjacent properties, boundaries, and streets should enable engagement with surrounding communities and create well-considered and usable external spaces.

### Economics vs. size

Many of the new-build homes in the UK are relatively large, generally accommodating between 40 and 60 residents. Many residents commented that this resulted in places that felt too large and institutional, and that the number of 'unknown faces' was overwhelming. In the staff's view, the high ratio of residents to staff and the scale of such homes limited the time that they could spend in engaging individually with residents.

In fact the UK is one of the few countries that provide care for older people through this large scale of facility. Examples across Scandinavia and Europe tended towards smaller-scale facilities (usually accommodating around 20 residents), which are then further split into smaller domestic sized groups.

> **Briefing recommendation**: Whilst it was acknowledged that at 60 beds, the proposed homes were larger than might ideally be provided, CEC's strategic funding for the provision of 240 beds over the city (for which this project was to be the guide) had already been established on the basis of this scale of units as the most economically viable. In setting their funding model, however, CEC had recognized the need for a higher level of capital funding to provide homes of better quality than the 'minimum standard', and had allowed for this. It was agreed that the overall 60 bed home should be broken down into smaller units of a maximum of 10 people each, and preferably fewer if feasible.

### Domestic feel vs. scale of building

A 'domestic feel' is often one of the main aspirations in a care home, in an attempt to create some sense of familiarity for the residents. In many of the 'standard models' for care homes there appears, however, to be a striving for a domestic *appearance*, rather than an understanding of what it is that makes a home or house feel domestic. Instead of breaking down these large-scale buildings into appropriately scaled 'dwellings', precedence is given to the operational requirements of running a home. This results in single linked floor plans which adopt the domestic language of the mass house builders, so producing the ubiquitous 'style' of the standard UK care home. The style is that of the monster bungalow—an over scaled mass of building, with the superficial appearance of a bungalow, but thereby losing all clarity of circulation and movement and quality of day lighting for those within.

> **Briefing recommendation**: Achieving a feeling of domesticity was agreed as a fundamental principle for the home. However, this should be achieved through a qualitative consideration of the scale, layout, and feel of the internal environment, and the breaking down of the overall scale of the units within the home, rather than through attempting to wrap the home in an over-scaled appearance of a domestic building.

### Staffing provision vs. size of living groups

Staffing levels are often determined more by the available revenue than by the care needs of the residents. Fundamental aspects of designing a higher-quality care environment for residents, such as breaking down the overall scale of a home into several smaller units, tend to be resisted by operators who are more interested in the minimum number of staff needed to 'oversee' residents.

> **Briefing recommendation**: It was agreed that staffing levels and operating costs should be carefully reviewed, to recognize the benefits to care resulting from smaller-scale groupings of residents.

### Enabling familiarity and individuality

Residents benefit from an environment that is familiar and which allows them to maintain a sense of individuality and independence. Such an environment aids understanding, assists residents' ability to manage every day, and reduces stress.

Creating an environment of this kind is, however, one of the main challenges for designers.

A sense of individuality rests on one's control of one's own environment, and on one's ability to undertake everyday activities safely. Elderly care accommodation invariably caters for people of varying degrees of ability. People with dementia who have reached the stage of needing full-time care may have impaired ability to carry out daily activities safely without help. If so, it is vital to provide that help, through either technological or carer assistance, so that the person can continue to engage in their familiar and reassuring activities.

In institutional care, concerns about safety generally prevent residents from undertaking such simple tasks as making a cup of tea for themselves. Likewise, meals are usually provided centrally in larger communal areas, and so some of the most basic of everyday activities such as cooking are removed from the daily personal ritual of the residents. Whilst many homes provide a range of activities for their residents, there is much less opportunity for individuals to pursue their own particular interests themselves. Reasons given for this are that staff are not available to supervise, or that a space suitable for the particular interest cannot be found. Homes focus on group activities such as music, crafts, and games, but it is the simple everyday tasks such as washing-up, serving meals, or cleaning a room that provide the basic sense of continuity and of familiarity.

Residents often bring small personal items such as ornaments, mementos, and photographs with them when they move into a home. It should be simple to allow residents also to bring their familiar pieces of furniture, to make their individual rooms their own. Often, however, this simple means of improving someone's environment is hampered by lack of space, or by the operator's insistence, for ease of handling, on the use of institutional beds or seats. In a bedroom meeting the minimum care standard of 12.5 m², there is barely room for any item of a resident's furniture (Fig. 24.3(a)).

**Briefing recommendation**: The project should explore the scale and organization of individual rooms to establish an optimum size for allowing residents to personalize their own rooms by bringing large items of furniture, and to enable greater use of these spaces. Individual rooms should allow double beds, sitting areas, and provision for a tea-making area for more able residents.

It was acknowledged that this would require a larger area per room than the 'minimum standard' of 12.5 m², and that this would require a higher level of funding. The appropriate balance in terms of higher cost and an improved, larger scale of room should be assessed in consideration of the long-term benefits in quality of the care environment and adaptability.

### Ease of orientation and way-finding

The clarity, simplicity, and ease with which a person with cognitive impairments can orientate themselves and find their way around where they live is fundamental to creating a good care environment. Many existing homes—both conversions and new builds—have extremely circuitous routes between bedroom spaces and living spaces. Bedrooms may end up being considerable distances from communal spaces; they may even be on a different floor from the place that people are trying to get to; and certain residents may become isolated. Fire escape requirements can lead to fire doors being sited without thought of their effect on day-to-day traffic in the home; so they block views between spaces and hamper the ease of movement around the home.

All these issues can increase the anxiety, stress, and confusion experienced by a person in the home.

**Briefing recommendation**: The design of the home should provide a clearly understandable environment to allow residents to move and find their way around easily, and for staff to operate effectively. The designer should liaise closely with the fire department and building control to minimize the intrusion of fire safety measures in order to maintain as domestic a feel as possible. Views to the outside and way-finding signals should be incorporated throughout to help residents orientate themselves and recognize their surroundings.

### Integration of special needs and challenging behaviour

A key question that came out of the consultation exercise, important both for residents and staff, was how particular special needs could be appropriately accommodated within a care home. Should a home have a dedicated unit for people with dementia, particularly those with more challenging behaviour? Their specific needs can be a source of distress to other residents, and a source of demand for increased levels of supervision and care. But there was another view expressed: that people already in a care home who gradually develop dementia cope better by remaining within their existing care environment than by being moved into specialized accommodation. The continuity of the place that has become familiar avoids the stress and upset of being moved to new accommodation; the friendships established amongst fellow residents and the support of recognizable staff make some compensation for their cognitive decline.

**Briefing recommendation**: Rather than provide a separate unit for special needs, the entire home should be designed to achieve a high level of awareness of the needs of people with dementia, so as to enable them to remain within the familiarity of established residential groups. However, in order to make this workable, the design should also accommodate a variety of shared spaces with a close relationship between these spaces and individual rooms, to allow staff easily and quickly to take an upset or confrontational resident into another environment, away from the main group.

### Centralized vs. dispersed meal provision

Whilst some residents enjoyed the 'event' of going from their own living areas to a centralized communal dining area, it was on the whole considered to be a negative experience. It seemed to be driven more by the ease of providing a service than by thoughts of the residents' perspective on enjoyment of a meal. More dispersed dining spaces, linked to smaller group living areas, were felt by most residents to be more enjoyable; and staff on the whole felt that this arrangement was better for residents with dementia who became anxious in a more communal environment. It may not be practicable or safe for meals to be prepared at these dispersed dining areas, among the residents. But bringing the meals to these areas, serving them, even engaging residents in this process, was thought to be a positive contribution to the sense of recognizable everyday routines.

**Briefing recommendation**: meals should be provided in small 'family sized' dining and kitchen areas within each of the smaller residential groups. Each dining area should be provided with a kitchenette to allow meals to be served within the residents' own 'house' and for residents to be encouraged to take part either at mealtimes or in activities around the kitchen area. The finishes within the dining/kitchen area should be domestic and not institutional.

## Multistorey living and lifts

It is commonly thought that care homes should ideally be on a single level to eliminate barriers and ensure ease of movement. The majority of homes visited, however, were on two or more floors, generally as a result of the limitation of site size that cannot accommodate the large footprint required by a single-storey home. Residents were generally not particularly concerned about living on floors above ground level, as most people spend much of their lives either in flats in multistorey buildings or in houses often over two storeys. The residents' concerns focused more on the provision and maintenance of lifts. Often there is only one lift within a multi-level home. This means that travelling between floors for meals, activities, or access to the outside is slow. Worse, if the lift breaks down, people can be stranded on their particular floor, particularly if their mobility is impaired.

**Briefing recommendation**: Homes can be provided over two floors, but preferably not more than two, to avoid potential isolation of residents. In doing so each floor should have adequate support, and communal spaces should be provided on both levels to ensure that residents can access all facilities. It is also important that any home provided over two floors should have at least two lifts, firstly to reduce waiting time for travel between levels and, more importantly, to ensure that residents are not stranded in the event of breakdown.

## Communal spaces, day spaces, activities, and the individual

The opportunity to get out of your room to meet other people, to go for a walk, or for a change of place is extremely important for residents' well-being. The provision of space for activities is important for any care home. Unfortunately, the cost of providing such space often means that provision is limited, or that spaces have to double up with other uses. Frequently lounges, dining areas, and day-care provision have to share their space in this way. Because time is needed to change the set up of rooms, especially in preparing for mealtimes, there is an inbuilt disincentive to making them available for other activities.

Whilst on the whole we found a reasonable provision of space for group activities, there was generally little choice for residents who wanted to pursue other activities, or who simply wanted to be out of their room without necessarily taking part in a wider group.

**Briefing recommendation**: In breaking down the scale of the overall home to form smaller 'family sized' groupings of residents, it is important to provide a range of smaller shared spaces associated with each of these. This allows residents to carry out day-to-day activities within their familiar group. A range of spaces, from a separate day room to a dining/kitchen and other smaller sitting spaces, give residents the opportunity to find individual space away from the others in the group.

Importantly for residents with dementia, this range of communal areas allows active spaces to be positioned at strategic intervals throughout the home both to assist recognition and orientation and to provide focuses of activity when walking through the home.

## Access to and use of garden space

Access to the outside or to garden spaces was found to be surprisingly limited over the range of homes visited. Some attention is usually given to the areas around the main entrance. However, poor planning of the site and layout often resulted in overshadowed gardens, in characterless external spaces which lacked access and were neglected, unusable, or infrequently used. There were other homes where gardens or external courtyards had been provided, but these too had relatively low use, because of difficult access or poor maintenance.

**Briefing recommendation**: External spaces and garden areas should be seen, provided and designed as carefully considered extensions of the internal environment. Such spaces can act positively both for encouraging residents to move safely out into the fresh air and for providing an attractive and stimulating outlook from internal spaces.

## General quality of internal environments—light, views, scale of spaces

The quality of the internal environment in care homes varies enormously. Many homes created by the conversion of existing (often Victorian) houses are poor in their access and ease of movement (Fig. 24.3(b)), particularly when new extensions have been linked to existing spaces. But they usually have much better quality of daylight, wider views, and more internal space simply because of the size of the original windows and rooms. Many new-build homes on the other hand have a clearer overall organization, but their size has dictated very deep plan arrangements, and their windows are often small (because they cost more to build than does a brick external wall). These forces result in badly lit, oppressive interior spaces.

**Briefing recommendation**: A home should be organized to make best use of the particular qualities of its site and should take into account orientation, views, and outlook. The scale and configuration of the home and the relationship of the internal and external environment should ensure that all spaces, particularly residents' bedrooms, have a pleasant outlook. Large windows should be positioned carefully throughout to provide good daylight—not just in rooms but importantly also in circulation and communal areas.

## General build quality and long-term sustainability

Often, as a result of cost limitations and the short-termist attitude towards building quality, many standard care homes are poorly constructed and use poor materials both externally and internally. In an attempt to maximize the internal area, many homes are built with little thought of their external appearance, other than minimizing cost. Internal finishes are often basic. This results in homes with poor acoustics, which can appear tired very quickly. The maintenance and refurbishment costs are higher in the long term than they would have been if more initial capital expenditure had been made. With this general approach to minimizing capital costs, little consideration is given to issues of sustainability and energy awareness that should produce a long-term payback to revenue costs and future flexibility and adaptability.

**Briefing recommendation**: The internal fabric of the home should use good standards of materials and workmanship, with particular attention to acoustics between residents' rooms. In providing a higher level of materials and finish than in 'standard' homes, the finishes should also not be overly driven by the demands of institutional cleaning regimes. More domestic types of finish (particularly floor finishes) should be considered.

Externally, the design of the home should try to draw on its surroundings to create some sense of place or character that might make the home more memorable for its residents, and allow it to contribute positively to its surrounding environment.

The design of the home should use all basic forms of energy conservation in its means of construction, from good insulation, day-lighting,

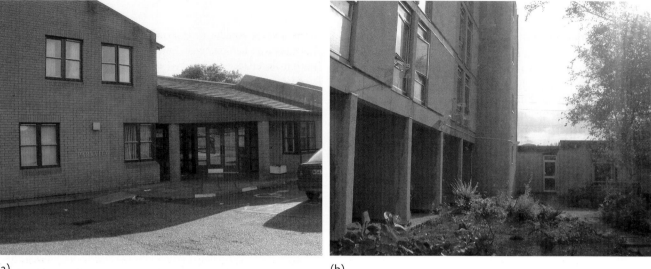

(a)

(b)

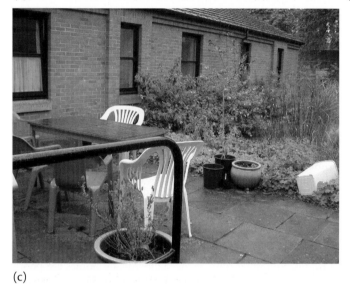

(c)

**Fig. 24.2** (a)–(c) Poor examples of nursing homes.

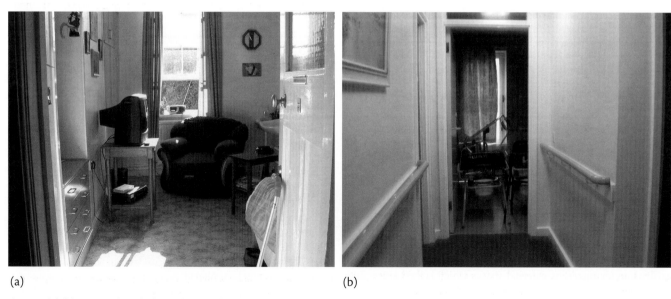

(a)

(b)

**Fig. 24.3** (a), (b) Interiors of poorly designed nursing homes.

and rainwater harvesting to minimize running costs and water usage, to natural ventilation to provide a more 'healthy' internal environment.

## Accommodation and quality of environment

Out of these guiding principles the joint design team of architects, residents, and CEC Social Work established a detailed schedule of accommodation. The linking of principles to accommodation requirements was the key step in this process. It provided a narrative which described the nature and feel of the particular areas (something often overlooked in commissioning), and it determined the size of spaces (generally considerably larger than the 'minimum care standards'), that would be needed to achieve the aspirations enshrined in the principles.

The acknowledged importance of 'space' (appropriate area) in the new home can be clearly seen through a comparison with a standard third-party provider care home accommodating the same number of residents:

- standard 60-bed care home, c. 2800–3000 m$^2$,
- CEC exemplar care home (60 beds), 3516 m$^2$.

The combination of larger space, additional areas, and more facilities results in a home which is approximately 18% larger than the usual provision. Whilst this reflects the intended improvement in quality of environment and care, the larger overall area presents two problems:

- It clearly results in a bigger building. The design and configuration of the layout need to be handled carefully if the problems of scale and poor orientation identified through the consultation exercise are to be avoided.
- A building with a larger area and additional facilities has higher capital construction costs. Broadly speaking, the scale of existing new-build care homes has evolved through a combination of the economics of the funding allowed per resident and the spatial requirements of providing a service. Whilst the increased area of the exemplar home enables many of the desirable aspects of the care environment identified through the consultation process to be addressed, it results in a capital construction cost that is beyond the scope of the current funding mechanisms for elderly care provision.

The first of these can be dealt with through careful design. But the fact that current funding levels limit the quality of care environment that can be achieved presents a more fundamental problem. In the case of the CEC project, the long-term benefits to the city's elderly residents were recognized, and additional funding was found to allow the home to be built. A widespread extension of this approach to building homes for older people would require a fundamental review of policy on funding for care.

## Exploring layouts and the importance of place

Whilst the principles established for the CEC project are to act as a 'standard' for the series of new homes to be built, one of these principles is that the design of each home should take careful account of its site, and maximize the advantages of its particular situation and qualities. All the homes share elements of their accommodation, but each should have a very clear sense of individuality and place, arising from its relationship to its particular site.

The next stage in the development of the exemplar project was to consult closely with the residents' group and staff groups to test out how various configurations of the accommodation on the proposed site might work.

This first project was to be built on an inner city site at the edge of Lochend Park in Edinburgh. The site was bounded on two sides by busy roads fronted by housing and a small number of shops, and on its other two by parkland with views to mature woodland and to the distant Salisbury Craggs to the south. A floodlit football pitch sat within the park immediately adjacent to the site.

A number of different configurations were explored in relation to:

- entry and access (clarity of front door, management of car parking and servicing, ease of access to public transport);
- the boundaries of the site, and outside activity along the street edges and park (including the pros and cons of the activity and noise generated by the adjacent football pitch);
- orientation in terms of daylight, views, and outlook (including the possible benefits to energy usage and sustainability);
- numbers of storeys (the overall footprint on the site set against availability of garden space for residents);
- different ways of disposing the 60 beds into living units (clusters, individual houses, courtyard blocks, etc.);
- location, scale, and numbers of garden spaces and their relationship to building(s);
- existing topography of site (i.e. the best use and fit with the varying slopes and levels across the site).

Each of the possible configurations was explored through a combination of drawings, diagrams and three-dimensional study models (Fig. 24.4(a–d)). This enabled the benefits or disadvantages of each to be clearly demonstrated, understood, and discussed by the groups. Finally, agreement was reached on the configuration that best met the criteria that had been established in the brief.

## The preferred option—a simple and understandable diagram

The preferred option is for a simple, clear layout, which arranges the residential accommodation along the edge of the site and links these spaces by a 'street' of communal and support spaces which form a 'buffer' to the adjacent football pitch. The simplicity and clarity of the overall diagram, and the way in which this layout is shaped to take advantage of the different aspects of the Lochend site, will, we hope, create an environment for residents and staff that is as clear, understandable, and as easy to move around in as possible (Fig. 24.5(a)).

The design acknowledges that this is a big building and does not try to allude to domesticity through 'dressing up' the building as a monster bungalow. Instead, the diagram makes a clear distinction between what is (and should be) the relatively private living spaces and the more public or larger-scale group, activity, and support spaces. The 60 beds are divided into three units each with 20 people. Rather than attempt to give the entire care home a domestic scale, it is the three units that have been designed clearly as large individual houses. Each has two floors, with 10 people on each floor. Each floor is further divided, by the arrangement of the floor plan, into two groups of four and six.

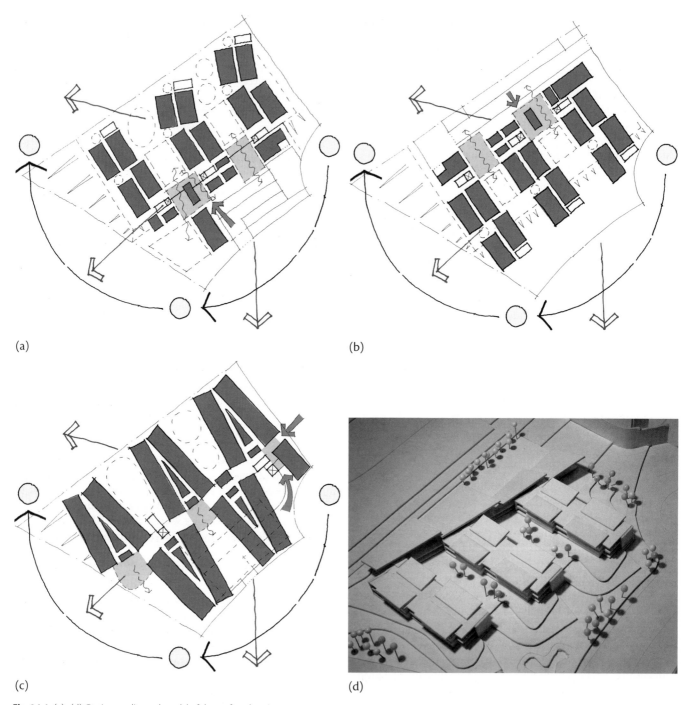

(a)

(b)

(c)

(d)

**Fig. 24.4** (a)–(d) Option studies and model of the preferred option.

The three 'houses' each have their own 'front door' from which residents can step out into the linear street that connects them. The houses are arranged as fingers reaching out from the street to create and contain a series of safe, interlinked garden spaces orientated towards the south. This configuration of the gardens and the external routes, and the orientation of the overall complex, allow good levels of daylight into the houses and the street.

The street forms a safe, enclosed route that runs diagonally across the full width of the site and combines the practical question of creating internal links between the three houses with the more experiential themes that came out of the consultation exercise. The street provides a clear route for people to walk along, with activities and views both along its length and at either end (Fig. 24.5(b)). At one end is the main entrance to the complex, opening out from a courtyard off the main road; the far end of the street culminates in a communal activity space, with views out across the park. Different activity spaces, seating niches, and window bays opening out on to garden areas, are arranged along the length of the street.

The internal street continues on to end in a series of new day-care spaces located at the junction between the entrance to the site and the pavement edge. The day spaces provide dedicated accommodation for people who come in from outside to receive day care in the home. This arrangement overcomes the problem of displacement of residents from their own territory, and creates a place where residents can 'go to' from the home. They can meet those who have come in for the day, if they choose, and they can walk down the street where it runs alongside the main road and look out onto the activity of the road and the adjacent shops.

The design also incorporates spaces for a hairdresser, library, computer/study room, and café (linked to the central kitchen.

The 'front doors' on each floor of the three houses open out on to the street. A lift is provided at these entrance points to make sure that residents on the upper floor have ease of access between the two levels of the complex. A link balcony connects between the houses and other first-floor activity spaces along this upper level of the street. The consultation review highlighted a desire by the residents to go out of their homes to take part in activities, whilst also recognizing than the frailty or impairments of many residents might prevent them from doing so. Therefore the street is designed deliberately as a much more open, larger scale, glassy enclosure than the more domestic format of the houses. This provides a semipublic space to which people can go, out of the front door of their house and into the more street-like environment. Here they can meet friends or relatives, and take part in communal or public activities, whilst remaining within the overall safety of the wider home.

## The houses—creating appropriately domestic environments

As described above, each of the three houses extends over two floors. Each of these floors is divided into space for groups of four and six people, in order to create small family sized groups. Each person has their own *en suite* bedroom with views to one of the courtyard gardens, but each group also has a range of shared living spaces (Fig. 24.6(a)):

- A living room near the 'front door' of the house where residents can watch others passing by in the home's 'street', and where they can welcome visitors without taking them (as with any everyday house) too far into the more private areas of their home.

- A kitchen/diner on a domestic and familiar scale, where the group of residents have their meals, rather than in the typical communal dining rooms found in many standard homes. Though the meals are prepared in a central 'back of house' kitchen they are brought to and served from domestic-scale kitchens in each of the houses, around a traditional dining room table (Fig. 24.6(b)).

- A smaller sitting space overlooking the woodland garden, to provide residents with an alternative space to sit in, separate from both the kitchen/diner and the living room.

These shared spaces are placed at either end and at the centre of each house to provide 'breaks' along their length. These split the overall length of each floor into smaller more easily understood groups of rooms, and provide breathing spaces of daylight, activity, and views along the length of the hall running through each house.

The doorways into the different spaces within each house are treated in different ways to aid recognition and understanding for residents:

- activity spaces are kept as open and as visible as possible from the main routes;

- shared toilets are positioned to be clearly visible from activity spaces;

- bedroom doors are highlighted and given additional space, both for manoeuvring wheelchairs and for placing familiar objects and signage to help residents to recognize their rooms;

- support spaces, such as cleaners' cupboards etc are deliberately located out of the way and played down, to minimize confusion;

- fire stairs and doorways at either end are purposely located to one side of the main route through each house. The activity of day-to-day life is given prominence, so that residents are not faced with fire doors with signage telling them to 'push for exit'.

The most private area of the home, a person's bedroom, is seen as the key to creating a strong sense of familiarity and reducing stress.

## The bedroom—appropriately scaled spaces for individual needs

One of the most important outcomes of the consultation process was the recognition that the 'minimum care standard' of 12.5 m² for a bedroom, the standard adopted for economic reasons by many new-build care homes, is quite inadequate as living space for someone in long-term care.

The design of the bedroom is at the heart of the provision of a high-quality care environment for people, particularly those with impairments such as dementia. Unlike an ordinary domestic bedroom, bedroom spaces in residential care are used for long periods through the day. Some residents find it very hard to adjust to large groups of unknown people (the other residents and staff), others simply want some privacy away from others. To these people, the bedroom provides the only refuge. In most homes, the evening meal is provided quite early (between 4.30 and 5.30 p.m.), and is followed by little in the way of structured activity for residents in the evening. Consequently, many residents retire to their bedrooms early and spend much of their evening in these rooms.

Even where lounges or visitors rooms are provided, many residents (and their visitors) prefer to use their bedroom for visits rather than sit in rooms shared with other residents. The minimum care standard bedroom does not provide adequate space to combine more than one comfortable chair, bedside table, and bed for the resident, taking into account the space needed by staff for providing care and for cleaning the room. Visitors are reduced to perching in ranks along the edge of the resident's bed, and the idea of creating a more familiar environment with items of the resident's own furniture is simply not achievable. Because of restrictions on space and concerns about safety it is generally not possible for residents to make any refreshments for relatives or friends in their room, and this again restricts opportunities for interaction and individuality. These small cramped rooms are often made more claustrophobic through poor day-lighting and ventilation.

An important part of the resident's room is the *en suite* bathroom, generally about 3.5 m² in size. The design of these spaces is

(a)

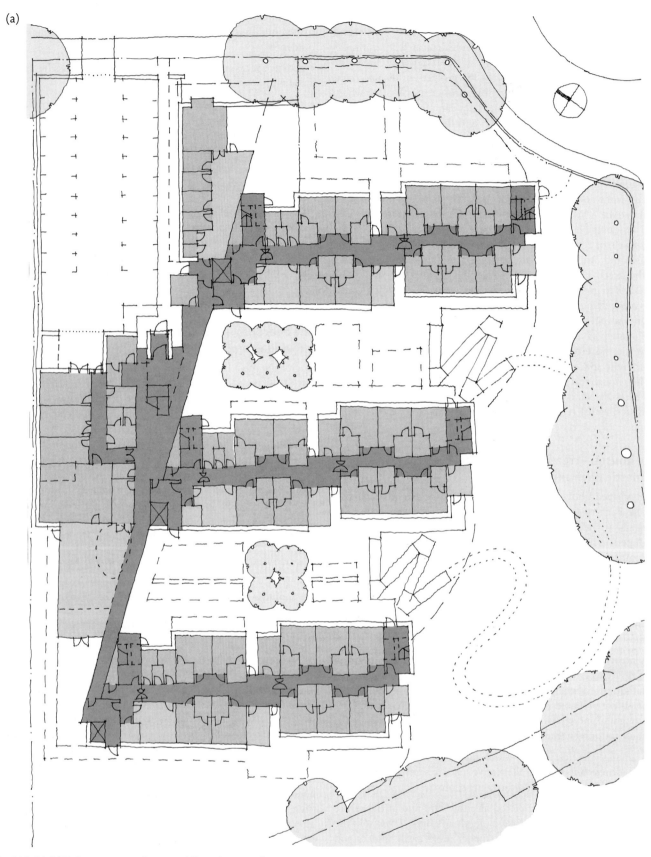

**Fig. 24.5** (a), (b) Basic arrangement diagram and illustrative street view.

(b)

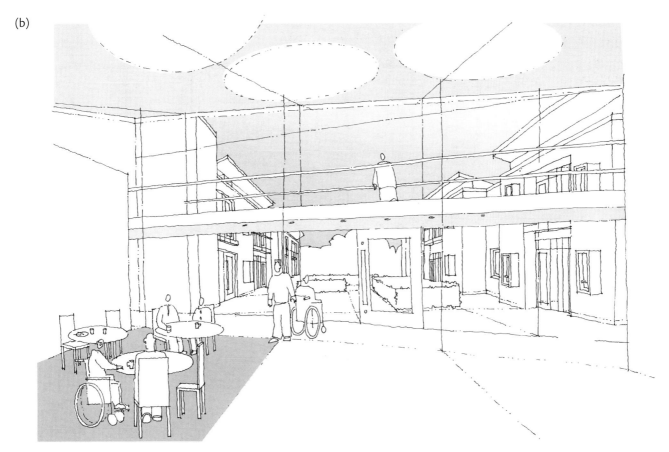

**Fig. 24.5** (Continued)

focused on the requirements for assistance and handling, and they tend not to have any daylight, to make no allowance for individuality, for use as a place for relaxation, or for taking time over 'getting yourself ready for going out'.

In response to these needs, the exemplar design provides significantly larger individual rooms, with bedroom/living spaces of 18 m$^2$ and *en suites* of 5.5 m$^2$ (Fig. 24.7).

These larger rooms are designed to create different areas which allow residents to bring their own furniture and to arrange it as they wish, to make as familiar an environment as possible, whilst also providing plenty of space for staff to assist them. With this additional space, the rooms can be configured to provide an entry area which, with more able residents, can incorporate a small tea bar, a dressing area, an area for their bed, and importantly, an area for seats and a small table for entertaining visitors. Both the bed area and the sitting area have large windows with opening lights that are easy for residents to operate, to ensure good daylight and ventilation and to enhance the feeling of space. The ceiling of the room is split, with a lower ceiling over the bed which enhances the definition between the bed area and the sitting area. This also, from a more practical point of view, provides a space in which a recessed track for a hoist can easily be retrofitted if required.

The *en suite* bathrooms are configured to ensure that the toilet is visible from the bed space, to make it easier for residents to locate and use the facilities. The larger space allows a greater ease of movement around the room (either with aids or with someone assisting), whilst also allowing for the incorporation of more domestic items of furniture such as shelves and storage units, to make the room more personal and less utilitarian. The economics of the available budget did not allow the bathrooms to be configured on an external wall to provide a window. The bathrooms have therefore been provided with concealed artificial day lighting, to create an illusion of daylight and improve the 'feel' of these otherwise internal spaces.

## Building the exemplar

Building work was completed in June 2007 (Fig. 24.8). In trying to create first a brief and then an actual building that seeks to improve the quality of the care environment for elderly people, the City of Edinburgh Council and the team involved have come under very public criticism. This came primarily from private providers, who objected to the eventual build cost being higher than that of a standard care home for a similar number of residents. The point overlooked in these criticisms was that the whole aim of the new home was to respond to the findings of the consultative process. In addressing the fundamental issues identified by the consultation process, the design has sought to:

♦ provide considerably larger areas both for activities and to enable individuals to live in a dignified manner;

(a)

(b)

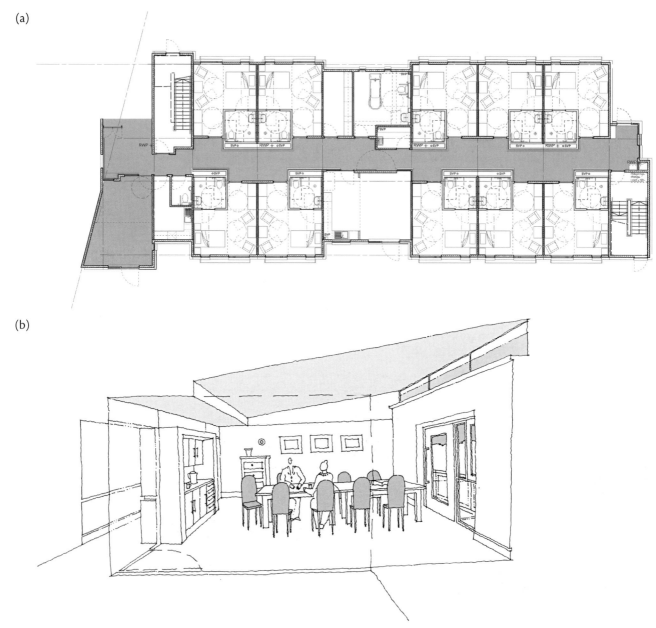

**Fig. 24.6** (a) and (b) Ten-person 'house' layout and illustrative view of shared dining kitchen spaces.

◆ create a clear, understandable, and familiar environment for elderly people, particularly for those with cognitive impairments;

◆ engage with and take advantage of the qualities of the site to create an individual and recognizable 'place' for residents;

◆ incorporate a good standard and quality of basic construction methods and materials to ensure increased lifespan of the home;

◆ incorporate well-informed thinking on sustainability, so as to address issues of running costs and flexibility.

Our understanding of the built environment and how it can positively affect people with dementia will continue to evolve. As more people live longer, this understanding should become a widely recognized and accepted part of planning for the everyday care of older people. In the meantime, however, it is hoped that the CEC Exemplar Project will raise the awareness of residents' needs, of the inadequacy of many 'standard' care homes, and of the fundamental issues that need to be addressed in relation to their basic design and construction. In this way, we hope to raise the quality of the care environment provided in the UK.

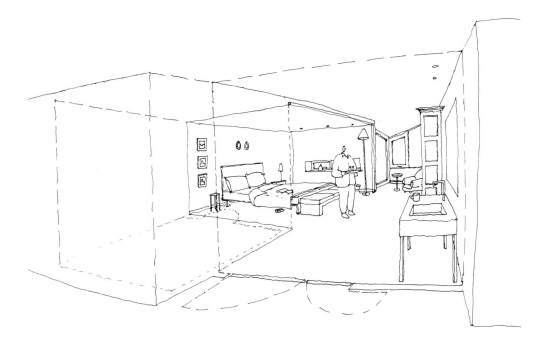

**Fig. 24.7** Illustrative view of 'increased area' bedroom.

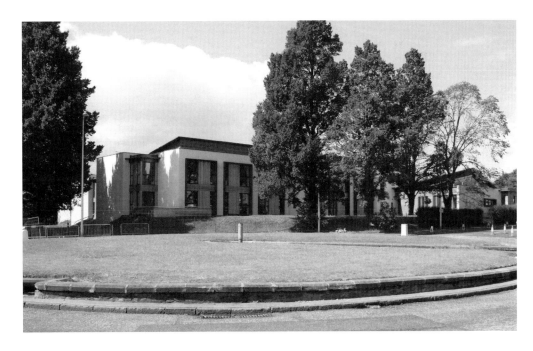

**Fig. 24.8** Illustrative view of final design.

## References

Bennett, K. (2000). Designing for cultural diversity: an Australian view. In *Just another disability: making design dementia friendly, conference proceedings of the European Conference, 1–2 October 1999, Mackintosh School of Architecture, Glasgow* (ed. S. Stewart and A. Page). Just Another Disability, Glasgow.

Brawley, E.C. (1997). *Designing for Alzheimer's disease*. John Wiley & Sons, New York.

Calkins, M.P. (1988). *Design for dementia: planning environments for the elderly and the confused*. National Health Publishing, Owing Mills, MD.

Cantley, C. and Wilson, R.C. (2003). *Put yourself in my place: designing and managing care homes for people with dementia*. Policy Press, Bristol.

Centre for Accessible Environments (1998). *The design of residential care and nursing homes for older people*. Centre for Accessible Environments, London.

City of Edinburgh Council (2000). *A city for all ages action plan. Edinburgh's joint plan for older people*. City of Edinburgh Council Corporate Services, Edinburgh.

Cohen, U. and Day, K. (1993). *Contemporary environments for people with dementia*. Johns Hopkins University Press, Baltimore, MD.

Cohen, U. and Weisman G.D. (1991). *Holding on to home: designing environments for people with dementia.* Johns Hopkins University Press, Baltimore, MD.

Day, K., Carreon, D., and Stump, C. (2000). The therapeutic design of environments for people with dementia: a review of the empirical research. *The Gerontologist*, **40**(4), 397–416.

Hiatt, L.G. (1995). Understanding the physical environment. *Pride Institute Journal of Long Term Care*, **4**(2), 12–22.

Judd, S., Marshall, M., and Phippen, P. (1998). *Design for dementia.* Hawker Publications, London.

Kitwood, T. (1997). *Dementia reconsidered: the person comes first.* Open University Press, Buckingham.

Koncelik, J.A. (2003). The human factors of aging and the micro-environment: personal surroundings, technology and product development. In *Physical environments and aging: critical contributions of M. Powell Lawton to theory and practice* (ed. R.J. Scheidt and P.G. Windley), pp. 117–134. Haworth Press, Binghampton, NY.

Lawton, M.P. (1975). *Planning and managing housing for the elderly.* John Wiley and Sons, New York.

Marshall, M. (ed.) (2000). *ASTRID, a social and technological response to meeting the needs of individuals with dementia and their carers.* Hawker Publications, London.

Marshall, M. (2005). Helping staff and patients with dementia through design. In *Dementia* (ed. A. Burns, J. O'Brian, and D. Ames). Hodder Arnold, London.

Marshall, M. and Allan, K. (eds) (2006). *Dementia: walking not wandering. Fresh approaches to understanding and practice.* Hawker Publications, London.

Neeten, A. (1993). *A positive environment.* Ashgate Publishing, Aldershot.

Pollock, A. (2001). *Designing gardens for people with dementia.* Dementia Services Development Centre, Stirling.

Pollock, R. (2003). *Designing interiors for people with dementia.* Dementia Services Development Centre, Stirling.

Pollock, R. (2006). *Designing lighting for people with dementia.* Dementia Services Development Centre, Stirling.

Scottish Executive (2001). *Designing places. A policy statement for Scotland* (http://www.scotland.gov.uk/library3/planning/dpps-00.asp).

Utton, D. (2006). *Designing homes for people with dementia.* Journal of Dementia Care, London.

World Health Organization (2001). International Classification of Impairments, Disabilities and Handicaps (ICIDH). *Fifty-fourth World Health Assembly, Geneva, 14–22 May 2001* (resolution WHA54.21).

Woolham, J. (ed.) (2005). *Developing the role of technology in the care and rehabilitation of people with dementia – current trends and perspectives.* Hawker Publications, London.

# SECTION IV

# Specific disorders

# 25

# Epidemiology of the dementias of old age

Laura Fratiglioni, Eva von Strauss, and Chengxuan Qiu

## Introduction

Dementia is a clinical syndrome characterized by multiple cognitive deficits severe enough to interfere with daily functioning, including social and professional activities (American Psychiatric Association, 1987). Cognitive decline, which is a central component of the dementia process, comprises deteriorative changes in memory and at least one of the other cognitive domains, such as aphasia, apraxia, or disturbances in executive functioning. Alzheimer's disease (AD) is the most common cause of dementia in the elderly, accounting for 60–70% of all dementia cases (Fratiglioni and Rocca, 2001).

Dementia has become a relevant issue from both scientific and public health perspectives due to the worldwide phenomenon of ageing populations. In 1990, 26 nations had more than 2 million elderly citizens aged 65 years and older, and the projections indicate that an additional 34 countries will join the list by 2030 (Kinsella and Velkoff, 2002). Developed countries, which have already seen a dramatic increase in numbers of people over 65 years of age, will experience a progressive ageing of the elderly population itself. Due to the exponential increase of incidence and prevalence of dementia with increasing age, dementia has become one of the most common diseases in the elderly, and a major cause of disability, institutionalization, and death (Agüero-Torres et al., 1998, 1999, 2001).

In the last decades, an increasing amount of attention from the scientific community has focused on dementia in general and on specific dementing disorders. Epidemiology is one of the leading research areas, with the ultimate objective being to develop preventative strategies. Prevention is traditionally divided into three levels: primary, secondary, and tertiary prevention. Primary prevention aims to reduce the incidence of the disease by eliminating or treating specific risk factors that may decrease the risk or delay the development of the disease. Secondary prevention aims to reduce the prevalence of the disease by preventing the progression of the disease from the initial phase to a complete clinical picture or by shortening its duration. Tertiary prevention aims to reduce the impact of complications of long-term disease and disability, and consists of measures aimed at evaluating care, minimizing suffering, and maximizing potential years of useful life. This chapter deals with the occurrence and primary prevention of dementia and AD.

## Occurrence

The occurrence of a disease in a specified population is commonly described by two measures: prevalence and incidence. Prevalence refers to the proportion of people affected by the disease in a defined population at a given point in time, whereas incidence is defined as the number of new cases that occur during a specified period of time in a population at risk for developing that disease. The prevalence is determined by both incidence and disease duration. The disease-specific mortality rate can be used, too, as a measure of incidence provided that the case-fatality rate is high and that the survival duration of the disease is short and constant (Gordis, 2000). The case-fatality rate refers to the percentage of persons with a specified disease who die as a result of that illness within a given period. The disease-specific mortality refers to the probability of dying from a certain disease in a defined population and time period, and it is determined by incidence and case-fatality rate.

## Prevalence

There are a large number of community-based prevalence studies concerning dementia and AD across continents. Meta-analysis has been utilized to obtain more precise estimates of dementia prevalence (Jorm et al,. 1987; Ritchie and Kildea, 1995; Fratiglioni et al., 1999; Lobo et al., 2000). Despite different inclusion criteria, these meta-analyses result in strikingly similar estimates of dementia prevalence (Fratiglioni and Rocca, 2001). The prevalence is very low before 60 years of age, and increases exponentially with advanced age (Fig. 25.1). Age-specific prevalence rates are estimated to be approximately 1% in subjects aged 60–64 years, 1.5% at 65–69 years, 3% at 70–74 years, 6% at 75–79 years, 13% at 80–84 years, 24% at 85–89 years, 34% at 90–94 years, and 45% at the most advanced ages of 95 years and older. A study based on the Delphi consensus method estimated that the global dementia prevalence among old people aged 60+ was 3.9%, and regional prevalence figures were 1.6% in Africa, 3.9% in Eastern Europe, 4.0% in China, 4.6% in Latin America, 5.4% in Western Europe, and 6.4% in North America (Ferri et al., 2005). Currently, more than 24 million people in the world have dementia and this number will double in 20 years (Wimo et al., 2003; Ferri et al., 2005).

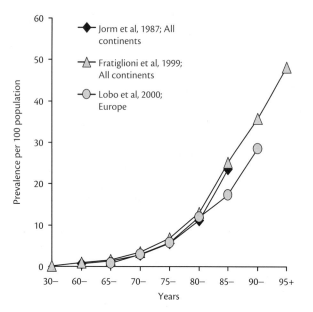

**Fig. 25.1** Age-specific prevalence rates of dementia (per 100 population) from all continents and Europe.

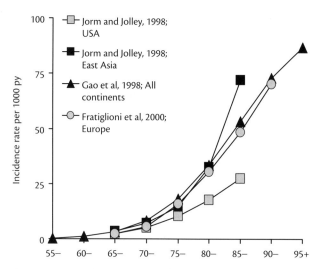

**Fig. 25.2** Age-specific incidence rates of dementia (per 1000 person-years at risk) from different regions and all continents.

With respect to dementia subtypes, the pooled data of 11 European population-based studies show that, among people aged 65 years and older, the age-standardized prevalence is 6.4% for all-cause dementia, 4.4% for AD, and 1.6% for vascular dementia (Lobo *et al.*, 2000). Similar to dementia in general, prevalence rates of both AD and vascular dementia increase exponentially with advancing age up to 90 years. Of all dementia cases, AD and vascular dementia account for 54% and 16%, respectively. Previous studies showed higher proportions of vascular dementia in East Asia, but more recent studies have not confirmed this pattern (Fratiglioni and Rocca, 2001). A multicentre investigation in China showed that the prevalence was 3.5% for AD and 1.1% for vascular dementia in persons aged 65 years and older, and the proportions of dementia subtypes were comparable with those reported from Western countries (Zhang *et al.*, 2005).

## Incidence

In the last two decades numerous incidence studies have been published. Three meta-analyses have reported estimates of dementia incidence in all continents, and from different regions of the world (Gao *et al.*, 1998; Jorm and Jolley, 1998; Fratiglioni *et al.*, 2000a). These analyses show a similar pattern of the age-specific incidence of dementia, i.e. incidence rates increase almost exponentially with age (Fig. 25.2). The incidence rates of dementia by age groups are approximately 1 (per 1000 person-years) in people aged 60–64 years, 2–3 in those aged 65–69, 6–8 in those aged 70–74, 11–18 in those aged 75–79, 20–30 in those aged 80–84, 30–50 in those aged 85–89, and 70–75 in those aged 90 and older. Of all incident dementia cases in Europe, AD accounts for 60–70% and vascular dementia accounts for 15–20%.

There are inconsistent findings with respect to whether the incidence of dementia continues to increase even in more advanced ages. Whether dementia incidence reaches a plateau at a certain age is a relevant issue for projecting the burden of the disease as well as for understanding its aetiology. A consistently exponential increase in dementia incidence with increasing age suggests that the disease is an inevitable consequence of ageing, whereas a convergence to or a decline at a certain age may suggest that the very old population has

reduced vulnerability, owing perhaps to genetic or environmental factors (Miech *et al.*, 2002). Pooled data from early studies in Europe suggested a decline in AD incidence mainly among elderly men (Andersen *et al.*, 1999). The Cache County Study further found that the incidence of dementia and AD increased with age, peaked, and then started to decline at extreme old ages for both men (over 93 years) and women (over 97 years) (Miech *et al.*, 2002). However, some meta-analyses and recent studies in Europe provide no evidence for the potential decline in the incidence of dementia and AD among the oldest old groups (Fratiglioni *et al.*, 2000a; Matthews and Brayne, 2005; Ravaglia *et al.*, 2005a). The apparent decline found in some studies may be an artefact of the poor response rates, survival effects, and the nature of populations previously sampled in these very old age groups (Matthews and Brayne, 2005).

The incidence rates of dementia are quite similar in the younger-old age group (e.g. younger than 75 years) throughout different continents, but substantial variations are reported among the older ages (Fratiglioni *et al.*, 1999). The incidence rates of dementia and AD are reported to be lower in North America than in Europe and Asia; these variations may be mostly due to differences in the study design and case ascertainment. In addition, the pooled data from eight European studies suggest a geographical dissociation across Europe, with higher incidence rates being found among the oldest-old of northwestern countries than among southern countries (Fratiglioni *et al.*, 2000a). Methodological differences, rather than different regional distributions of possible risk factors for dementia, may be responsible for this pattern. To assess possible geographical variations in dementia incidence among five areas in England and Wales characterized by different vascular risk patterns, a recent study used identical methodology and found no evidence of variation in incidence rates (Matthews and Brayne, 2005).

## Mortality

The malignant nature of AD was first suggested in the follow-up study of the community sample aged 65 years and older in Shanghai, China, in which AD was found to increase the risk of dying by three-fold, compared with a four-fold impact of cancer (Katzman *et al.*, 1994). This finding is reinforced by pooled data and population-based follow-up studies, which show that persons with dementia have a two to five times higher risk of dying than non-demented people (Baldereschi *et al.*, 1999; Jagger *et al.*, 2000; Helmer *et al.*, 2001; Noale *et al.*, 2003; Gühne *et al.*, 2006). Indeed, follow-up studies have consistently shown that dementia shortens life expectancy, with the median survival time of those with dementia ranging from 2 to 4 years after the diagnosis, depending on the age of onset and other demographic features (Agüero-Torres *et al.*, 1999; Witthaus *et al.*, 1999; Helmer *et al.*, 2001; Wolfson *et al.*, 2001). The proportion of deaths attributable to dementia increases with advanced ages, with dementia accounting for approximately one-third of deaths in persons aged 85 years and older (Aevarsson *et al.*, 1998; Tschanz *et al.*, 2004). Despite dementia being widely regarded as a leading cause of death, death certificates usually grossly underreport dementia (Jin *et al.*, 2004), even when multiple causes of death are taken into account (Beard *et al.*, 1996; Ganguli and Rodriguez, 1999). In a US-wide study, dementia mortality rates were heavily dependent on the methods used to ascertain the causes of death. When the diagnosis of dementia was made following an informant interview, the mortality rate for dementia was doubled compared with making the diagnosis from a review of local medical records. This rate was 5–9 times greater than the frequency with which dementia was even mentioned on death certificates and 15–17 times greater than the rate at which dementia was certified as the underlying cause of death (Lanska, 1998). Based on the data from the East Boston study, it was estimated that 7.1% of all deaths in the USA in 1995 were attributable to AD, placing AD as the third leading cause of death (Ewbank, 1999).

# Primary prevention

The dementias are multifactorial disorders, in which genetic and non-genetic factors as well as their interactions contribute to their initiation, clinical expression, and progression. Identifying the influential factors has relevant implications for the understanding of pathological mechanisms as well as for the development of preventative strategies against dementia. The aetiological studies have so far mostly focused on dementia in general and AD in particular; studies concerning vascular dementia and other forms of dementia are limited. In this part of the chapter, we summarize the major findings concerning aetiology and primary prevention of dementia in general and specifically AD.

Several aetiological hypotheses for dementia and AD have been proposed (Table 25.1). It is well known that genetic susceptibility plays a part in both familial and sporadic forms of AD. Mutations in the amyloid precursor protein gene and homologous presenilin-1 and -2 genes account for most cases of familial AD (Blennow *et al.*, 2006). The apolipoprotein E gene (*APOE*) ε4 allele is the only established susceptibility gene for AD. Of the non-genetic factors, increasing evidence from multidisciplinary studies supports different aetiological hypotheses for dementia and for AD as well. First, the vascular hypothesis implies that vascular risk factors and vascular disorders occurring over a life course may be involved in the pathogenesis and clinical expression of dementia including Alzheimer-type dementia (Qiu *et al.*, 2005; Chui, 2006). Second, the psychosocial hypothesis states that an active and socially integrated lifestyle in middle age or late life may protect against or delay the onset of dementia by providing reserve and reducing psychological stress (Fratiglioni *et al.*, 2004). In addition, the inflammatory hypothesis is based essentially on the observation that neuritic plaques in the brain are associated with inflammatory proteins, suggesting that inflammatory mechanisms may play a role in processes leading to neurodegeneration. Finally, other mechanisms such oxidative stress and exposure to toxic agents may also contribute to the pathogenetic processes of the dementias.

## A life-course approach

The life-course approach considers biological and social factors acting during early life, middle age, and late life as relevant for the development of dementia in late life. This approach seeks to identify time windows when exposures have their greatest effect on outcome and to determine whether accumulative exposures could have integrative or additive effects over the life course (Kuh and Ben-Shlomo, 2004; Whalley *et al.*, 2006). Thus, the risk of dementia in late life may not be determined in any single time period of the lifespan, rather, it may be a result of complex interactions of genetic susceptibility, biological factors, and environmental exposures experienced over the life course. For example, the reserve hypothesis proposes that compensations in some aspects of brain structure and function could buffer the effects of neuropathology such that the greater the reserve, the more severe pathological changes are needed to cause clinically functional impairment (Stern, 2006). It is suggested that the reserve can be conceived as the sum of its lifetime input (Richards and Deary, 2005). In support of the life-course approach in exploring the aetiology of the disease, evidence is accumulating that the genetic and non-genetic factors over the lifespan can influence the risk of dementia in late life. In addition, the life-course approach model introduces the relevant concept of 'time period [or window] at exposure', which might be highly relevant for chronic disorders with a long latent period such as dementia and AD (Fratiglioni and Rocca, 2001). A certain factor might increase the risk of the disease if a subject is exposed during a specific time period, whereas the same factor may show an effect of reducing the risk of the disease in another life period, due to differential interactions with other risk factors or due to selective survival. For instance, uncontrolled high blood pressure in middle age is a risk factor for late life dementia, whereas low blood pressure in very old people is related to dementia development, suggesting that a proper level of blood pressure may be imperative for the very old to maintain cerebral perfusion and to reduce dementia risk (Qiu *et al.*, 2005; Ruitenberg *et al.*, 2005).

## Major risk and protective factors

### Demographic features
#### Age and sex

Age is the most consistent and significant risk factor for dementia and AD. The prevalence and incidence of dementia and AD rise almost exponentially with advancing age. Both rates double every 5 years from the age of 65 to 85 (Figs 25.1 and 25.2). Higher prevalence and incidence rates of AD and dementia among women than men have been found in numerous cross-sectional and longitudinal studies. The pooled follow-up data from Europe confirm the gender-specific pattern (Launer *et al.*, 1999; Fratiglioni *et al.*, 2000a). However, the gender difference was not found by some studies from North America (Bachman *et al.*, 1993; Rocca *et al.*, 1998; Kawas *et al.*, 2000). The higher incidence of dementia in women may be due to different mechanisms (Fratiglioni *et al.*, 1997; Fratiglioni and Rocca, 2001): (1) men who survive up to advanced ages may become more resistant against dementia; (2) men are more frequently exposed to multiple risk factors such as head trauma and occupational

**Table 25.1** Putative risk and protective (in italic) factors for dementia and AD throughout the life course and by the underlying aetiological hypotheses

| Aetiological hypothesis | At birth | Childhood and early adulthood | Middle age | Old age |
| --- | --- | --- | --- | --- |
| Genetic | Familial aggregation<br>*APOE ε4 allele* | Familial aggregation | | |
| Vascular | | | Smoking<br>Alcohol intake<br>Obesity<br>Hypertension<br>Dyslipidaemia<br>*Antihypertensive therapy* | Smoking<br>Alcohol intake<br>High/low BP<br>Diabetes mellitus<br>Clinical/silent stroke<br>Heart disease<br>Dyslipidaemia<br>Hyperhomocysteinaemia<br>*Antihypertensive therapy* |
| Psychosocial | | Low education<br>Low SES | Depression<br>*Physical activity*<br>*Mentally stimulating activity* | Depression<br>*Social network*<br>*Leisure activity* |
| Inflammatory | | | Inflammatory markers | Inflammatory markers<br>*NSAIDs*<br>*HRT* |
| Toxic and oxidative stress | | | Head trauma<br>Aluminium<br>Occupational toxics | Head trauma<br>Deficiency in vitamins<br>A, E, C, B$_{12}$, and folate<br>*Dietary factors* |

Abbreviations: AD, Alzheimer's disease; *APOE*, apolipoprotein E gene; BP, blood pressure; HRT, hormone replacement therapy; NSAIDs, non-steroidal anti-inflammatory drugs; SES, socio-economic status.

toxics, which may lead to earlier occurrence of dementia; and (3) oestrogen level is higher among elderly men than elderly women, which may partially protect men against dementia.

### Education, occupation, and socio-economic status (SES)

The Shanghai Study first reported an association of low education with increased age-specific prevalence of dementia and AD (Zhang *et al.*, 1990). This finding was replicated in numerous prevalence surveys (Schmand *et al.*, 1997; De Ronchi *et al.*, 1998) and prospective cohort studies (Evans *et al.*, 1997b; Qiu *et al.*, 2001; Di Carlo *et al.*, 2002). The high correlation of education with SES has been examined by relating both factors simultaneously to dementia risk, but an independent association was detected only with education (Evans *et al.*, 1997b; Ravaglia *et al.*, 2002; Karp *et al.*, 2004). The reserve hypothesis is proposed to interpret this association as education enhancing the neural reserve (Katzman, 1993) or stimulating functional compensations (Stern, 2006). Individuals with higher reserve may need more Alzheimer-type lesions or cerebrovascular pathological changes than those with lower reserve to express the clinical syndrome of dementia (Wilson *et al.*, 2003). Indeed, education may play different roles in dementia and may have more than one role at the same time. Education may not only be an indicator of cognitive stimulation, but also an indicator of early life circumstances (Moceri *et al.*, 2000), a surrogate of intelligence quotient (Whalley *et al.*, 2000), and an indicator of SES (Karp *et al.*, 2004). Finally, an alternative interpretation is that subjects with less education are more likely to be clinically diagnosed as having dementia at an earlier neuropathological stage than more highly educated persons (Qiu *et al.*, 2001).

Having manual work, especially in manufacturing industry, as the principal lifetime occupation has been related to AD and dementia in some studies (Fratiglioni *et al.*, 1993; Stern *et al.*, 1994;

Bonaiuto *et al.*, 1995; Qiu *et al.*, 2003a), suggesting a possible implication for occupational exposures in dementia. Occupational exposure to heavy metals such as aluminium and mercury has been suggested, but not strongly confirmed, as a risk factor (Mutter *et al.*, 2004; Perl and Moalem, 2006). In addition, occupational exposure to extremely low-frequency magnetic fields has been shown to be related to dementia (Sobel *et al.*, 1995; 1996; Feychting *et al.*, 2003; Hakansson *et al.*, 2003; Qiu *et al.*, 2004a), but these findings warrant further verification.

### Genetic susceptibility

#### Familial aggregation

First-degree relatives of AD patients have a higher lifetime risk of developing AD than the general population or relatives of non-demented subjects (Devi *et al.*, 2000; Green *et al.*, 2002). Familial aggregation has been reported for both early and late onset AD (Fratiglioni *et al.*, 1993). It is also likely that the combined effect of genetic and environmental factors contributes to the phenomenon of familial aggregation. Twin studies provide an opportunity to address this issue by comparing concordance rates among monozygotic twins, who share both the genes and the early life environment, to the concordance rates among dizygotic twins, who share only approximately 50% of the genes and early life environment. In the Swedish Twin Registry, the heritability of AD is estimated to be 58%, whereas other variance may be attributable to non-genetic factors (Gatz *et al.*, 2006).

#### The APOE ε4 allele

The *APOE* ε4 allele is the only established genetic factor for both early and late onset AD. The *APOE* ε4 allele is a susceptibility gene that increases the risk of AD, but even homozygotic carriers of the ε4 allele do not necessarily develop the disease, whereas individuals without the ε4 allele may have AD. The effect of the ε4 allele decreases with increasing age (Farrer *et al.*, 1997), and after the age of 75 years 15–20% of AD cases are attributable to the *APOE* genotype (Evans *et al.* 1997a; Qiu *et al.*, 2004b). Familial aggregation of dementia and AD can only be partially explained by *APOE* polymorphism, implying that other genetic factors may be active and need to be detected (Huang *et al.*, 2004).

## Vascular risk factors

### Smoking

Experimental and epidemiological data have suggested that nicotine may exert a protective effect against Parkinson's disease (Ross and Petrovitch, 2001), which may be true for other neurodegenerative diseases in the elderly. Earlier studies seem to support this hypothesis as a decreased risk of AD was detected among smokers (Fratiglioni and Wang, 2000). However, this result was probably due to survival bias as smokers are proportionally less numerous among prevalent cases (Wang *et al.*, 1999; Hill *et al.*, 2003; Tyas *et al.*, 2003). When incident cases were examined, the protective effect of smoking on AD was no longer present (Wang *et al.*, 1999; Doll *et al.*, 2000). By contrast, some prospective studies even found a significantly increased risk of AD associated with cigarette smoking (Tyas *et al.*, 2003; Aggarwal *et al.*, 2006), especially among non-carriers of the *APOE* ε4 allele (Ott *et al.*, 1998; Merchant *et al.*, 1999). Thus, in contrast to the initial hypothesis of a protective effect, cigarette smoking actually appears to be a risk factor for dementia and AD.

### Alcohol consumption

The relationship between use of alcohol and risk of dementia largely depends on the amount of alcohol consumed. Heavy use of alcohol causes 'alcoholic dementia', a specific form of dementia. In addition, use of alcohol may increase the risk of vascular dementia (Yoshitake *et al.*, 1995). In the Kungsholmen Project, alcohol abuse was related to prevalent AD (Fratiglioni *et al.*, 1993), but light to moderate alcohol consumption was associated with reduced incidence of dementia and AD (Huang *et al.*, 2002). Several other studies also reported an association of moderate wine drinking with lower risk of dementia (Orgogozo *et al.*, 1997; Elias *et al.*, 1999; Ruitenberg *et al.*, 2002), leading to the hypothesis that moderate alcohol intake may protect against dementia. These findings are in line with the studies indicating a J-shaped curve between alcohol intake and cognitive performance (Elias *et al.*, 1999; Stampfer *et al.*, 2005) as well as between alcohol consumption and cardiovascular disease (Sacco *et al.*, 1999). However, the role of moderate alcohol intake in dementia remains controversial, as the inverse association may be due to information bias, healthy lifestyle confounding, different exposure assessments, or outcome misclassification. In contrast, the deleterious effect of high alcohol consumption emerges clearly from a recent study where heavier drinkers at middle age had a more than three-fold increased risk of dementia in late life, especially among those carrying the *APOE* ε4 allele (Anttila *et al.*, 2004).

### High serum cholesterol

An association between mid-life elevated cholesterol and increased risk of late-life AD is reported in some studies (Notkola *et al.*, 1998; Kivipelto *et al.*, 2002; Whitmer *et al.*, 2005b), but not confirmed by others (Kalmijn *et al.*, 2000; Tan *et al.*, 2003). Controversial findings are also reported when serum cholesterol is examined in late life. A large-scale cross-sectional study in France shows that hyperlipidaemia is related to increased risk of dementia, especially non-Alzheimer type dementia (Dufouil *et al.*, 2005). However, several

cohort studies with a relatively short period of follow-up found no association of late-life total cholesterol level with the risk of AD and dementia (Li *et al.*, 2004; Hayden *et al.*, 2006), or even found an association of high total cholesterol with decreased AD risk (Kuusisto *et al.*, 1997; Romas *et al.*, 1999; Reitz *et al.*, 2004; Mielke *et al.*, 2005). Several cross-sectional and case–control studies have reported statin use to be associated with a lower prevalence of AD (Jick *et al.*, 2000; Hajjar *et al.*, 2002; Rockwood *et al.*, 2002; Rodriguez *et al.*, 2002). Statins are cholesterol-lowering agents that work by inhibiting 3-hydroxy-3-methylglutaryl coenzyme A reductase or by other mechanisms (DeKosky, 2005). However, prospective cohort studies and clinical trials have generally not replicated these findings (Heart Protection Study Collaborative Group, 2002; Li *et al.*, 2004; Rea *et al.*, 2005; Zandi *et al.*, 2005).

### Blood pressure

As the most powerful risk factor for cerebrovascular disease, hypertension might also be expected to be a risk factor for dementia, especially vascular dementia (Posner *et al.*, 2002). However, since the first report from the Gothenburg study (Skoog *et al.*, 1996), evidence has been accumulating that hypertension or high blood pressure may be a risk factor even for AD (Launer, 2002). Neuropathological studies have linked hypertension to the neurodegenerative markers in the brain (Sparks *et al.*, 1995; Petrovitch *et al.*, 2000; Roher *et al.*, 2003), suggesting that long-term high blood pressure may play a causal role in AD by involving the neurodegenerative process or causing brain atrophy (Korf *et al.*, 2004). Alternatively, clinical or silent cerebral ischaemic lesions caused by hypertension may interact with neurodegenerative lesions to produce a dementia syndrome in subjects not having sufficient neurodegenerative damage to express dementia (Snowdon *et al.*, 1997; Esiri *et al.*, 1999).

The relationship between blood pressure and dementia and AD seems to be age-dependent (Petitti *et al.*, 2005; Qiu *et al.*, 2005). Several studies provide substantial evidence of the association of mid-life high blood pressure with increased risk of late-life dementia and AD (Launer *et al.*, 2000; Kivipelto *et al.*, 2001; Whitmer *et al.*, 2005b); such an association may be independent of *APOE* genotype and other vascular risk factors (Kivipelto *et al.*, 2002). In very old people (e.g. over 75 years), however, the effect of high blood pressure is much weaker and the deleterious effect may be present only for very high systolic pressure (e.g. >180 mm Hg) (Guo *et al.*, 1999b; Qiu *et al.*, 2003c). By contrast, at this advanced age, low blood pressure seems to predict the risk of AD and dementia (Ruitenberg *et al.*, 2001; Qiu *et al.*, 2003c; Verghese *et al.*, 2003a). As dementia has a long latent period, low blood pressure may be a sign of impending illness rather than a cause of the disease. However, a few studies with more than 6 years of follow-up confirm such an association (Morris *et al.*, 2001; Qiu *et al.*, 2003c; Verghese *et al.*, 2003a), suggesting that low blood pressure in late life may be involved in the development or clinical expression of dementia and AD (Qiu *et al.*, 2005; Ruitenberg *et al.*, 2005).

### Antihypertensive therapy

Longitudinal studies show that use of antihypertensive drugs is associated with reduced risk of cognitive decline (Murray *et al.*, 2002; Hajjar *et al.*, 2005) and dementia (Guo *et al.*, 1999a; in t'Veld *et al.*, 2001a; Yasar *et al.*, 2005; Khachaturian *et al.*, 2006). However, five large-scale randomized clinical trials have yielded mixed results. First, the Medical Research Council's trial indicates that treating moderate hypertension with diuretics does not influence cognitive functioning in any direction (Prince *et al.*, 1996). Second, the SHEP trial found that active treatment with thiazide diuretics reduced the risk of cardiovascular events, but not of cognitive impairment and dementia (SHEP Cooperative Research Group, 1991). However, reanalysis of the database suggested that differential dropout rates between treatment and placebo groups might have obscured the ability of appraising a potential effect of antihypertensive treatment against cognitive decline and dementia (Di Bari *et al.*, 2001). Third, the Syst-Eur trial, in which patients with isolated systolic hypertension were treated by a calcium-channel blocker, showed that active therapy reduced dementia risk by 50% over a 2-year period (Forette *et al.*, 1998). Following the termination of the initial trial, all participants were continued on active therapy for another 2 years; the extended trial confirmed that long-term antihypertensive therapy reduces dementia risk by 55% (Forette *et al.*, 2002). Fourth, the PROGRESS trial aimed to examine whether the blood pressure-lowering regimen reduced the risk of recurrent stroke, dementia, and cognitive decline in persons with a history of cerebrovascular disease. This trial found that the therapeutic regimen did not affect the overall risk of dementia, but did reduce the risk of 'dementia with recurrent stroke' and of 'cognitive decline with recurrent stroke' (Tzourio *et al.*, 2003). Finally, the SCOPE study compared candesartan with usual antihypertensive regimens in reducing the risk of cardiovascular events, cognitive decline, and dementia among elderly patients with mild to moderate hypertension. After 4 years' follow-up, no significant difference in dementia incidence and cognitive decline was found between the two groups (Lithell *et al.*, 2003).

### Vascular diseases

#### Diabetes mellitus

The increased risk of both vascular and degenerative dementias among persons with diabetes is reported in several longitudinal studies (Leibson *et al.*, 1997; Brayne *et al.*, 1998; Ott *et al.*, 1999; Luchsinger *et al.*, 2001; Arvanitakis *et al.*, 2004; Xu *et al.*, 2004; Akomolafe *et al.*, 2006), and confirmed by a systematic review (Biessels *et al.*, 2006). Borderline diabetes or impaired glucose tolerance is also linked to an increased risk of dementia and AD in very old people (Xu *et al.*, 2007). Such an association may reflect a direct effect of hyperglycaemia on neurodegenerative changes in the brain (Peila *et al.*, 2002; Korf *et al.*, 2006) or an effect of hyperinsulinaemia (Luchsinger *et al.*, 2004a) or due to the diabetes-related co-morbidities such as hypertension and dyslipidaemia.

#### Cerebrovascular disease

Multiple cerebral infarcts, recurrent and strategic stroke are the main risk factors for post-stroke dementia (Leys *et al.*, 2005). Even clinically silent strokes and cerebral white matter lesions detected on brain imaging are associated with increased risk of dementia and cognitive decline (Vermeer *et al.*, 2003; Liebetrau *et al.*, 2004; Prins *et al.*, 2004). The *APOE* ε4 allele does not account for the relation of stroke to dementia, although the allele is known to be a risk factor for both disorders (Zhu *et al.*, 2000). However, the role of stroke in Alzheimer-type dementia remains under debate. Some studies report an association between stroke and the development of AD and cognitive decline (Honig *et al.*, 2003; Hayden *et al.*, 2004; Reitz *et al.*, 2006). As mentioned earlier, cerebrovascular lesions and neurodegenerative changes may be coincident processes causing additive damage to the ageing brain (Snowdon *et al.*, 1997; Esiri *et al.*, 1999).

#### Heart disease

Cardiovascular disease is associated with an increased incidence of dementia and AD in the cohort of Cardiovascular Health Study,

with the highest risk being seen in people with peripheral arterial disease (Newman *et al.*, 2005), suggesting that extensive peripheral atherosclerosis is a risk factor for AD (Hofman *et al.*, 1997; Beeri *et al.*, 2006). In addition, other heart diseases may be independently related to an increased risk of dementia such as atrial fibrillation (Ott *et al.*, 1997) and heart failure (Polidori *et al.*, 2006; Qiu *et al.*, 2006; Lavery *et al.*, 2007). In the Kungsholmen Project, heart failure was associated with an increased risk of dementia and AD of more than 80%, but proper use of antihypertensive drugs might partially counteract this increased risk (Qiu *et al.*, 2006).

### Dietary factors

#### Obesity

Obesity has been intensively investigated in relation to dementia risk. From these studies, a lifespan-dependent pattern emerges such that a mid-life higher body mass index (BMI) is a risk factor for dementia and AD, whereas an accelerated decline in BMI during late life may anticipate the occurrence of dementia (Gustafson, 2006). A higher BMI at the age of around 50 years was related to increased risk of dementia 20–25 years later (Kivipelto *et al.*, 2005; Rosengren *et al.*, 2005; Whitmer *et al.*, 2005a). But this was not confirmed in the cohort of Japanese-American men; instead, a greater decline in BMI approximately 10 years prior to dementia was detected (Stewart *et al.*, 2005). In line with this finding, some follow-up studies of elderly people suggest that accelerated decline in BMI is associated with subsequent development of AD (Buchman *et al.*, 2005; Johnson *et al.*, 2006). Low BMI in late life may be related to a higher risk for AD developing over a subsequent 5–6-year period (Nourhashemi *et al.*, 2003). Thus, low BMI and weight loss can be interpreted as markers for pre-clinical AD, particularly when measured 6–10 years prior to the clinical diagnosis.

#### Anti-oxidant vitamins

A diet rich in fruits, vegetables, anti-oxidants, and flavonoids benefits health in general, but it remains uncertain whether such a dietary pattern is helpful for the prevention of AD (Dai *et al.*, 2006). Some follow-up studies have reported a decrease in AD risk associated with increasing dietary or supplementary intake of vitamins E and C (Engelhart *et al.*, 2002b; Morris *et al.*, 2002; Zandi *et al.*, 2004). Further, two recent studies concluded that higher adherence to a 'Mediterranean diet' (i.e. a dietary pattern with higher intake of fish, fruits, and vegetables rich in anti-oxidants) is associated with reduced risk of AD independent of vascular pathways (Scarmeas *et al.*, 2006a,b). However, dietary or supplemental vitamin E intake in either middle age or late life was not associated with the risk of AD (Masaki *et al.*, 2000; Luchsinger *et al.*, 2003; Laurin *et al.*, 2004). Furthermore, plasma levels of vitamins A and E were not associated with AD and cognitive decline in the Rotterdam Study (Engelhart *et al.*, 2005). Finally, randomized clinical trials with relative short-term use of vitamin E supplementation fail to show any effect against cognitive impairment, although long-term use (e.g. ≥15 years) could be neuroprotective (Petersen *et al.*, 2005; Kang *et al.*, 2006).

#### Vitamin B$_{12}$, folic acid, and homocysteine

Mixed results are reported on the association of vitamin B$_{12}$ and folate with dementia (Luchsinger and Mayeux, 2004). Two longitudinal studies suggested an inverse association of low serum vitamin B$_{12}$ and folate with increased risk of dementia and AD (Wang *et al.*, 2001; Maxwell *et al.*, 2002). Experimental studies support the hypothesis of a protective effect of folate against cognitive deterioration (Morris, 2003). However, a Cochrane Systematic

Review and randomized clinical trials concluded that folic acid and vitamin $B_{12}$ supplementations have no benefits on cognition, although folate plus vitamin $B_{12}$ are effective in reducing serum homocysteine (Malouf et al., 2003; Eussen et al., 2006). Hyperhomocysteinaemia is a known risk factor for cardiac and cerebrovascular diseases. Thus, homocysteine may contribute to dementia through vascular mechanisms or neurotoxic effects. An association between high serum homocysteine and increased risk of dementia and cognitive decline is suggested in several cohort studies (Seshadri et al., 2002; Ravaglia et al., 2005b; Schafer et al., 2005), but not confirmed by others (Morris et al., 2003b; Luchsinger et al., 2004b). Further, a pilot study suggested that high-dose B vitamins (folic acid, $B_{12}$, and $B_6$) that reduce homocysteine levels may slow AD progression (Aisen et al., 2003), but a recent controlled clinical trial does not support the hypothesis that homocysteine lowering with B vitamins improves cognitive performance (McMahon et al., 2006).

### Unsaturated fats and fish

Fatty acids could be involved in the development of dementia through various mechanisms such as atherosclerosis and inflammation (Kalmijn, 2000). An association of high intake of saturated fats with elevated risk of AD and cognitive decline is suggested by some prospective studies (Kalmijn et al., 1997; Morris et al., 2003a; Laitinen et al., 2006), but not by others (Barberger-Gateau et al., 2002). A diet high in polyunsaturated and fish-related fats is known to be associated with a low risk of vascular disease (Kris-Etherton et al., 2001); thus, it may be plausible to extend the beneficial effects to the prevention of dementia. In support of this hypothesis, high intake of fish and n3 polyunsaturated fatty acid has been associated with a decreased risk of AD and dementia (Barberger-Gateau et al., 2002; Morris et al., 2003a; Huang et al., 2005). In the Framingham cohort, a high level of plasma docosahexaenoic acid was associated with a lower risk of AD and dementia (Schaefer et al., 2006), and the consumption of more than two servings of fish per week also was associated with a 50% reduced risk of AD. Plasma docosahexaenoic acid was significantly correlated with fish intake in this cohort. By contrast, in the Rotterdam study cohort, neither high intake of total and saturated fats nor low intake of polyunsaturated fatty acids was associated with the risk of dementia and its main subtypes (Engelhart et al., 2002a).

## Clustering of vascular factors and disorders

Vascular risk factors often coexist in the elderly and they operate through common pathological mechanisms. Several studies have consistently shown that the risk of AD and dementia increases with increasing number of vascular risk factors (Kalmijn et al., 2000; Luchsinger et al., 2005; Mitnitski et al., 2006; Kivipelto et al., 2006). Different vascular risk scores have been developed to quantify the risk of dementia and AD associated with the clustering of multiple vascular risk factors. The risk scores provide reasonable estimation of the probability of having dementia some years later, and may identify high-risk individuals even in mid-life (Kivipelto et al., 2006). However, the implementation of such scores in clinical practice is still limited by the low predictive values.

## Inflammation

### Serum inflammatory markers

Some community-based studies have examined the relation of inflammatory markers to dementia. Serum levels of C-reactive protein (CRP) in mid-life are associated with an increased risk of both Alzheimer and vascular dementias, suggesting that inflammatory markers may reflect both peripheral disease and cerebral mechanisms related to dementia, and that these processes are measurable for a long time before dementia is manifested (Schmidt et al., 2002). Two cohort studies also found an association of serum inflammatory markers (e.g. CRP and interleukin-6) measured at old ages with increased incidence of dementia (van Exel et al., 2003; Engelhart et al., 2004). Of the inflammatory markers, CRP seems to be the most promising marker for identifying persons at risk for dementia and cognitive decline. It remains unknown, however, if lowering levels of inflammatory markers could reduce the risk of dementia.

### Non-steroidal anti-inflammatory drugs (NSAIDs)

The use of NSAIDs is associated with lower AD risk in several observational studies, including some prospective investigations (Stewart et al., 1997; in t'Veld et al., 2001b; Landi et al., 2003; Cornelius et al., 2004). A systematic review of observational studies confirmed that use of NSAIDs for more than 2 years has a greater benefit against AD and dementia (Etminan et al., 2003; Szekely et al., 2004), supporting the hypothesis that long-term treatment with NSAIDs is required to obtain a possible protective effect against dementia. However, it cannot be ruled out that the beneficial effect may result from various forms of bias in these studies (de Craen et al., 2005). The major clinical trial of anti-inflammatory prevention on AD has been suspended due to increased risk of cardiovascular events among the treatment group (ADAPT Research Group, 2006).

## Psychosocial factors

### Social network

Evidence from longitudinal observational studies suggests that a poor social network or social disengagement is associated with cognitive decline and dementia (Bassuk et al., 1999; Fratiglioni et al., 2000b, 2004). The risk for dementia is increased in old people with increasing social isolation and less frequent and unsatisfactory contacts with relatives and friends (Fratiglioni et al., 2000b). Rich social networks imply better social support leading to better access to resources and material goods. Rich social networks also provide affective and intellectual stimulation that can influence different health outcomes through behavioural, psychological, and physiological pathways (Seeman and Crimmins, 2001).

### Leisure activities

A systematic review found seven observational studies reporting lower risk of dementia, AD, or both in subjects with greater engagement in mentally stimulating activities (Fratiglioni et al., 2004). Due to the long pre-clinical phase in dementia (Bäckman et al., 2001), reverse causality cannot be ruled out. Most studies have adjusted for cognitive performances at the time of activity assessment and leisure activities are assessed at least 3 years before dementia diagnosis, and some reports are based on intervals longer than 5 years (Wang et al., 2002; Verghese et al., 2003b). The Swedish Twin Registry suggests that participation in a greater number of leisure activities during early and middle adulthood, especially intellectual–cultural activities, is significantly associated with lower risk of AD and dementia (Crowe et al., 2003). Low social engagement in late life and a decline in social engagement from middle age to late life are also associated with a double risk of developing dementia (Saczynski et al., 2006). Different types of activities have been examined, including travelling, knitting, and gardening (Fabrigoule et al., 1995), dancing, playing board games, and musical instruments (Verghese et al., 2003b), and reading, social visits, cultural activities, and watching specific television programmes

(Crowe *et al.*, 2003). Due to the cultural and individual differences in choosing specific activities, some researchers summarize mentally stimulating activities into a composite score. For example, a cognitive activity score that involves participation in seven common activities with information processing as a central component was associated with a reduced risk of AD after controlling for demographics as well as for *APOE* ε4 allele, medical conditions, and depressive symptoms (Wilson *et al.*, 2002b,c). In the Kungsholmen Project, a four-grade score to characterize the mental, social, and physical components of each activity was developed by both researchers and a sample of elderly people; high scores in two or all of the three components were associated with a substantial reduction in the risk of dementia occurring 6 years later (Karp *et al.*, 2006). Clearly, different leisure activities require use of different cognitive components and further research is needed to better understand the cognitive load of different activities.

### Physical activity

In a systematic review of longitudinal observational studies, physical activities were found to be related to a lower risk of dementia and AD in six of nine studies (Fratiglioni *et al.*, 2004). Exercise is also associated with a reduced risk of dementia and AD (Larson *et al.*, 2006). In the Kungsholmen Project, the physical component presenting in various leisure activities, rather than any specific physical exercise or sport, was related to a decreased dementia risk (Karp *et al.*, 2006). In addition, low-intensity activity such as walking may reduce the risk of dementia and cognitive decline (Abbott *et al.*, 2004; Weuve *et al.*, 2004). Recently, a strong protective effect of regular physical activity at middle age against dementia detected 20 years later was reported, especially for persons with the *APOE* ε4 allele (Rovio *et al.*, 2005). The possible benefits of physical training on cognition have been evaluated in several small randomized controlled trials, but the effects of short-term training programs are equivocal (Churchill *et al.*, 2002). As it may take years to achieve high levels of physical fitness, brief periods of exercise may not have substantial benefits on cognitive processes, but could still be effective in that subset of cognitive domains that are more sensitive to the age-related decrements. This is supported by meta-analysis and randomized controlled intervention studies (Kramer *et al.*, 1999; Colcombe and Kramer, 2003).

### Other factors

#### Hormone replacement therapy

Oestrogen therapy has been linked to a lower risk of dementia in numerous observational studies. Initial case–control studies, followed by prospective cohort studies, show a dose–response relationship with greater protection for a longer duration of exposure (Tang *et al.*, 1996; Kawas *et al.*, 1997; Waring *et al.*, 1999; Zandi *et al.*, 2002). Potential biological mechanisms for such beneficial effects include vascular, cholinergic, and anti-oxidant processes. However, cohort studies and clinical trials of oestrogen therapy have failed to confirm any protective effect (Seshadri *et al.*, 2001; Kang *et al.*, 2004). For instance, in the Women's Health Initiative Memory Study, oestrogen therapy alone did not reduce the incidence of probable dementia and mild cognitive impairment; instead, the therapy increased the risk for both endpoints combined (Shumaker *et al.*, 2004; Espeland *et al.*, 2004). Furthermore, a doubly increased risk for both dementia and mild cognitive impairment is found when treatments with oestrogen and oestrogen plus progestin are taken into account. Thus, many questions about hormonal therapy

and dementia risk remain unsolved. In particular, we still do not know if either perimenopausal initiation of therapy that is more consistent with observational studies or other dosages and forms of oestrogen (e.g. estradiol) would have a neuroprotective effect (Craig *et al.*, 2005).

### Traumatic brain injury

Traumatic brain injury has been extensively investigated as a possible risk factor for AD, but the findings remain controversial (Starkstein and Jorge, 2005). In the early 1990s, a meta-analysis of seven case–control studies reported an increased AD risk associated with head injury with loss of consciousness in males, but not in females (Mortimer *et al.*, 1991). This finding was replicated by another meta-analysis of case–control studies more than 10 years later (Fleminger *et al.*, 2003). Some longitudinal studies found no association of head trauma with AD risk (Launer *et al.*, 1999; Mehta *et al.*, 1999), whereas others found an increased AD risk associated with only severe head injury (Schofield *et al.*, 1997; Plassman *et al.*, 2000). In addition, a synergistic effect of head injury with *APOE* ε4 allele on AD risk is suggested in some studies (Mayeux *et al.*, 1995), but not confirmed by others (Mehta *et al.*, 1999; Guo *et al.*, 2000). Traumatic brain injury may increase β-amyloid in cerebrospinal fluid (Nicoll *et al.*, 1995; Emmerling *et al.*, 2000) or reduce brain reserve (Katzman, 2004). Despite the biological plausibility, the association of head trauma with AD risk as well as the influence of *APOE* genotype on the association needs further investigation.

### Depression

Several studies have reported an association between a history of depression and elevated risk of later development of dementia and AD (Wilson *et al.*, 2002a; Green *et al.*, 2003; Modrego and Ferrandez, 2004; Andersen *et al.*, 2005; Dal Forno *et al.*, 2005), but it remains uncertain whether depression is a pre-clinical symptom or a pure risk factor for dementia (Jorm, 2001; Ganguli *et al.*, 2006). A recent meta-analysis reported a double risk of dementia in depressed subjects from both case–control and cohort studies (Ownby *et al.*, 2006). As the interval between diagnoses of depression and AD is positively related to an increased risk of later developing AD, the authors concluded that, rather than a prodrome, depression may be a risk factor for AD.

### Gene–environment interaction

The Rotterdam Study showed an interaction of *APOE* ε4 and atherosclerosis in the aetiology of AD (Hofman *et al.*, 1997). The *APOE* ε4 allele in combination with stroke also substantially increases the risk of sporadic and familial AD (Zhu *et al.*, 2000; Rippon *et al.*, 2006). In the Kungsholmen Project, the *APOE* ε4 allele interacts with high systolic and low diastolic pressure to greatly increase the risk of AD, and the use of antihypertensive drugs could counteract the combined risk effect of the *APOE* ε4 allele and high systolic pressure on AD (Qiu *et al.*, 2003b). The CAIDE study suggests that *APOE* genotype may modify the relation of mid-life alcohol consumption to the risk of dementia, as high alcohol intake was associated with an increased risk of dementia only among carriers of the *APOE* ε4 allele (Anttila *et al.*, 2004). Although possible interactions between genetic predisposition and non-genetic factors in modifying AD and dementia risk have been suggested, these reports are still too limited to be able to trace any conclusions.

**Table 25.2** Scientific evidence supporting risk and protective (in italic) factors of dementia and AD by different aetiological hypotheses

| Aetiological hypotheses | Evidence | | |
|---|---|---|---|
| | **Insufficient** | **Limited** | **Moderate or strong** |
| Genetic | | | *APOE* ε4 allele[1]<br>Familial aggregation |
| Vascular | High cholesterol<br>Cigarette smoking<br>Obesity<br>*Dietary factors (e.g. fish and vegetables)* | Late life very high BP<br>Late life low BP<br>Heart disease<br>Silent stroke<br>*Moderate alcohol intake* | Diabetes mellitus<br>Mid-life high BP<br>Clinical stroke<br>Atherosclerosis<br>*Antihypertensive drugs* |
| Psychosocial | Depression<br>Low SES | *Mid-life physical activity*<br>*Late life social network* | Low education<br>*Late life mentally stimulating activities and physical activity* |
| Inflammatory | Inflammatory markers<br>*HRT* | *NSAIDs* | |
| Toxic and oxidative stress | Folate and vitamins B₁₂, A, E, and C deficiency<br>Occupational exposure to toxics<br>*Antioxidants* | Head trauma | |

Abbreviations: AD, Alzheimer's disease; *APOE*, apolipoprotein E gene; BP, blood pressure; HRT, hormone replacement therapy; NSAIDs, non-steroidal anti-inflammatory drugs; SES, socio-economic status.

[1] The *APOE* ε4 allele is the only aetiological factor with strong evidence for AD.

## Scientific evidence: summary and conclusions

Following an initiative of the Swedish Council on Technology Assessment in Health Care (SBU, 2006), specific criteria to summarize the scientific evidence concerning risk and protective factors for dementia were proposed and implemented. Similar to criteria adopted for other diseases, these criteria integrate the internal validity with basic causal criteria to weight the study quality. A four-grade evidence score is developed by integrating the number and proportion of studies reporting a specific association with the quality index; the scientific evidence is considered strong when several articles with a high quality index have consistently reported the same finding, moderate evidence also includes high-quality reports but the finding is supported by a limited number of studies, or the quality is moderate but compensated by several positive reports, limited evidence is defined by a limited number of medium-quality studies, and insufficient evidence consists of reports with some methodological uncertainty independent of number of published studies. Based on these criteria, Table 25.2 summarizes the current scientific evidence, in which the single risk or protective factor is listed according to the underlying biological mechanisms. The genetic, vascular, and psychosocial hypotheses are supported by moderate or strong evidence. Whereas implementing preventive strategies targeting the genetic susceptibility is limited, the other two hypotheses can easily lead to prevention programmes.

## Preventive strategies

On the basis of the evidence supporting the risk and protective factors for dementia and AD as summarized in Table 25.2, at the moment it seems possible to delineate two preventive strategies against the dementias:

1 An optimal control of vascular risk factors in both middle and late life. Several explanations have been proposed for vascular risk factors such as hypertension, diabetes, cerebrovascular disease, and heart disease being involved in the pathogenesis of Alzheimer-type dementia (Iadecola and Gorelick, 2003; Casserly and Topol, 2004): (a) coincidence of vascular factors and AD pathology in the elderly; (b) precipitating effect of cerebrovascular disease; (c) interactive effect of Alzheimer-type and vascular lesions; and (d) misclassification of mixed dementia as AD. Although the mechanisms linking vascular risk factors to AD are not fully understood, prevention is possible as most vascular risk factors and diseases are modifiable or amenable to prevention and treatment (Fratiglioni *et al.*, 2006). For primary prevention, controlling high blood pressure in middle age, avoiding mid-life obesity, and appropriately treating diabetes are the major intervention actions. Furthermore, intervention studies have demonstrated that diabetes can be prevented by changing lifestyles with regard to dietary habits and physical activities (Knowler *et al.*, 2002; Lindström *et al.*, 2006). Some studies also show that people who maintain tight control over their blood glucose levels tend to score better on tests of cognitive function than those with poorly controlled diabetes. Thus, it is anticipated that these intervention measures targeting diabetes could also reduce the risk of dementia. Finally, to postpone clinical expression of the dementia syndrome in old people, preventing recurrent cerebrovascular disease as well as maintaining sufficient cerebral perfusion by adequately managing heart failure and avoiding very low blood pressure seems to be critical.

2 An active and socially integrated lifestyle in young adulthood and old age. Extensive social networks and active engagement or regular participation in intellectually stimulating activities significantly lower the risk of AD and other forms of dementia. This effect may be due to an increased 'cognitive reserve', the ability to cope with or compensate for the neuropathological changes associated with dementia (Bennett *et al.*, 2006), or due to other mechanisms such as reduced psychosocial stress and vascular damage (Fratiglioni *et al.*, 2004). Physical exercise may reduce the risk of brain damage from atherosclerosis, but the relevance

of physical activity itself remains subject to debate, as most physical activities also include social and mental components. Complex leisure activities with all three components of physical, mental, and social activities seem to have the most beneficial effect (Karp *et al.*, 2006). It is likely that a mentally and socially integrated lifestyle in late life could postpone the onset of clinical dementia and AD. Indeed, even delaying the onset of dementia by 5 years would halve dementia prevalence and substantially decrease the number of dementia cases in the community, which will confer great beneficial effect at both the individual and the societal levels.

In summary, there is increasing evidence to suggest that vascular risk factors and vascular disorders substantially contribute to the development of cognitive impairment and dementia. Adequately managing vascular factors and diseases may be one of the promising preventive measures against dementia and cognitive decline. In addition, a more extensive social network, social engagement, physical activity, and mentally stimulating activity are relevant for preserving cognitive function and for delaying the onset of dementia in the elderly population. The most effective strategy to achieve this goal may be to encourage people to practise these preventive measures over the life course including early adulthood, middle age, and later in life. Active use of these intervention strategies should improve dramatically the chances of retaining a highly functional brain in late life.

## References

Abbott, R.D., White, L.R., Ross, G.W., Masaki, K.H., Curb, J.D., and Petrovitch, H. (2004). Walking and dementia in physically capable elderly men. *Journal of the American Medical Association*, **292**, 1447–53.

ADAPT Research Group (2006). Cardiovascular and cerebrovascular events in the randomized, controlled Alzheimer's Disease Anti-inflammatory Prevention Trial (ADAPT). *PLoS Clinical Trials*, **1**, e33, doi:10.1371/journal.pctr.0010033.

Aevarsson, O., Svanborg, A., and Skoog, I. (1998). Seven-year survival rate after age 85 years: relation to Alzheimer disease and vascular dementia. *Archives of Neurology*, **55**, 1226–32.

Aggarwal, N.T., Bienias, J.L., Bennett, D.A. *et al.* (2006). The relation of cigarette smoking to incident Alzheimer's disease in a biracial urban community population. *Neuroepidemiology*, **26**, 140–6.

Agüero-Torres, H., Fratiglioni, L., Guo, Z., Viitanen, M., von Strauss, E., and Winblad, B. (1998). Dementia is the major cause of functional dependence in the elderly: 3-year follow-up data from a population-based study. *American Journal of Public Health*, **88**, 1452–6.

Agüero-Torres, H., Fratiglioni, L., Guo, Z., Viitanen, M., and Winblad, B. (1999). Mortality from dementia in advanced age: a 5-year follow-up study of incident dementia cases. *Journal of Clinical Epidemiology*, **52**, 737–43.

Agüero-Torres, H., von Strauss, E., Viitanen, M., Winblad, B., and Fratiglioni, L. (2001). Institutionalization in the elderly: the role of chronic diseases and dementia. Cross-sectional and longitudinal data from a population-based study. *Journal of Clinical Epidemiology*, **54**, 795–801.

Aisen, P.S., Egelko, S., Andrews, H. *et al.* (2003). A pilot study of vitamins to lower plasma homocysteine levels in Alzheimer disease. *American Journal of Geriatric Psychiatry*, **11**, 246–9.

Akomolafe, A., Beiser, A., Meigs, J.B. *et al.* (2006). Diabetes mellitus and risk of developing Alzheimer disease: results from the Framingham Study. *Archives of Neurology*, **63**, 1551–5.

American Psychiatric Association (1987). *Diagnostic and statistic manual of mental disorders*, 3rd edn, revised (DSM-III-R), pp. 97–163. American Psychiatric Association, Washington, DC.

Andersen, K., Launer, L.J., Dewey, M.E. *et al.* (1999). Gender differences in the incidence of AD and vascular dementia: The EURODEM Studies. EURODEM Incidence Research Group. *Neurology*, **53**, 1992–7.

Andersen, K., Lolk, A., Kragh-Sorensen, P., Petersen, N.E., and Green, A. (2005). Depression and the risk of Alzheimer disease. *Epidemiology*, **16**, 233–8.

Anttila, T., Helkala, E.L., Viitanen, M. *et al.* (2004). Alcohol drinking in middle age and subsequent risk of mild cognitive impairment and dementia in old age: a prospective population based study. *British Medical Journal*, **329**, 539.

Arvanitakis, Z., Wilson, R.S., Bienias, J.L., Evans, D.A., and Bennett, D.A. (2004). Diabetes mellitus and risk of Alzheimer disease and decline in cognitive function. *Archives of Neurology*, **61**, 661–6.

Bachman, D.L., Wolf, P.A., Linn, R.T. *et al.* (1993). Incidence of dementia and probable Alzheimer's disease in a general population: the Framingham Study. *Neurology*, **43**, 515–19.

Bäckman, L., Small, B.J., and Fratiglioni, L. (2001). Stability of the preclinical episodic memory deficit in Alzheimer's disease. *Brain*, **124**, 96–102.

Baldereschi, M., Di Carlo, A., Maggi, S. *et al.* (1999). Dementia is a major predictor of death among the Italian elderly. The Italian Longitudinal Study on Aging. *Neurology*, **52**, 709–13.

Barberger-Gateau, P., Letenneur, L., Deschamps, V., Peres, K., Dartigues, J.F., and Renaud, S. (2002). Fish, meat, and risk of dementia: cohort study. *British Medical Journal*, **325**, 932–3.

Bassuk, S.S., Glass, T.A., and Berkman, L.F. (1999). Social disengagement and incident cognitive decline in community-dwelling elderly persons. *Annals of Internal Medicine*, **131**, 165–73.

Beard, C.M., Kokmen, E., Sigler, C., Smith, G.E., Petterson, T., and O'Brien, P.C. (1996). Cause of death in Alzheimer's disease. *Annals of Epidemiology*, **6**, 195–200.

Beeri, M.S., Rapp, M., Silverman, J.M. *et al.* (2006). Coronary artery disease is associated with Alzheimer disease neuropathology in APOE4 carriers. *Neurology*, **66**, 1399–404.

Bennett, D.A., Schneider, J.A., Tang, Y., Arnold, S.E., and Wilson, R.S. (2006). The effect of social networks on the relation between Alzheimer's disease pathology and level of cognitive function in old people: a longitudinal cohort study. *Lancet Neurology*, **5**, 406–12.

Biessels, G.J., Staekenborg, S., Brunner, E., Brayne, C., and Scheltens, P. (2006). Risk of dementia in diabetes mellitus: a systematic review. *Lancet Neurology*, **5**, 64–74.

Blennow, K., de Leon, M.J., and Zetterberg, H. (2006). Alzheimer's disease. *Lancet*, **368**, 387–403.

Bonaiuto, S., Rocca, W.A., Lippi, A. *et al.* (1995). Education and occupation as risk factors for dementia: a population-based case-control study. *Neuroepidemiology*, **14**, 101–9.

Brayne, C., Gill, C., Huppert, F.A. *et al.* (1998). Vascular risks and incident dementia: results from a cohort study of the very old. *Dementia and Geriatric Cognitive Disorders*, **9**, 175–80.

Buchman, A.S., Wilson, R.S., Bienias, J.L., Shah, R.C., Evans, D.A., and Bennett, D.A. (2005). Change in body mass index and risk of incident Alzheimer disease. *Neurology*, **65**, 892–7.

Casserly, I. and Topol, E. (2004). Convergence of atherosclerosis and Alzheimer's disease: inflammation, cholesterol, and misfolded proteins. *Lancet*, **363**, 1139–46.

Chui, H.C. (2006). Vascular cognitive impairment: today and tomorrow. *Alzheimer's & Dementia*, **2**, 185–94.

Churchill, J.D., Galvez, R., Colcombe, S., Swain, R.A., Kramer, A.F., and Greenough, W.T. (2002). Exercise, experience and the aging brain. *Neurobiology of Aging*, **23**, 941–55.

Colcombe, S. and Kramer, A.F. (2003). Fitness effects on the cognitive function of older adults: a meta-analytic study. *Psychological Science*, **14**, 125–30.

Cornelius, C., Fastbom, J., Winblad, B., and Viitanen, M. (2004). Aspirin, NSAIDs, risk of dementia, and influence of the apolipoprotein E ε4 allele in an elderly population. *Neuroepidemiology*, **23**, 135–43.

Craig, M.C., Maki, P.M., and Murphy, D.G. (2005). The Women's Health Initiative Memory Study: findings and implications for treatment. *Lancet Neurology*, **4**, 190–4.

Crowe, M., Andel, R., Pedersen, N.L., Johansson, B., and Gatz, M. (2003). Does participation in leisure activities lead to reduced risk of Alzheimer's disease? A prospective study of Swedish twins. *The Journals of Gerontology Series B: Psychological Sciences and Social Sciences*, **58**, P249–P255.

Dai, Q., Borenstein, A.R., Wu, Y., Jackson, J.C., and Larson, E.B. (2006). Fruit and vegetable juices and Alzheimer's disease: the Kame Project. *American Journal of Medicine*, **119**, 751–9.

Dal Forno, G., Palermo, M.T., Donohue, J.E., Karagiozis, H., Zonderman, A.B., and Kawas, C.H. (2005). Depressive symptoms, sex, and risk for Alzheimer's disease. *Annals of Neurology*, **57**, 381–7.

de Craen, A.J., Gussekloo, J., Vrijsen, B., and Westendorp, R.G. (2005). Meta-analysis of nonsteroidal anti-inflammatory drug use and risk of dementia. *American Journal of Epidemiology*, **161**, 114–20.

DeKosky, S.T. (2005). Statin therapy in the treatment of Alzheimer disease: what is the rationale? *American Journal of Medicine*, **118**(Suppl. 12A), 48–53.

De Ronchi, D., Fratiglioni, L., Rucci, P., Paternico, A., Graziani, S., and Dalmonte, E. (1998). The effect of education on dementia occurrence in an Italian population with middle to high socioeconomic status. *Neurology*, **50**, 1231–8.

Devi, G., Ottman, R., Tang, M.X., Marder, K., Stern, Y., and Mayeux, R. (2000). Familial aggregation of Alzheimer disease among whites, African Americans, and Caribbean Hispanics in northern Manhattan. *Archives of Neurology*, **57**, 72–7.

Di Bari, M., Pahor, M., Franse, L.V. *et al.* (2001). Dementia and disability outcomes in large hypertension trials: lessons learned from the systolic hypertension in the elderly program (SHEP) trial. *American Journal of Epidemiology*, **153**, 72–8.

Di Carlo, A., Baldereschi, M., Amaducci, L. *et al.* (2002). Incidence of dementia, Alzheimer's disease, and vascular dementia in Italy. The ILSA Study. *Journal of the American Geriatrics Society*, **50**, 41–8.

Doll, R., Peto, R., Boreham, J., and Sutherland, I. (2000). Smoking and dementia in male British doctors: prospective study. *British Medical Journal*, **320**, 1097–102.

Dufouil, C., Richard, F., Fievet, N. *et al.* (2005). APOE genotype, cholesterol level, lipid-lowering treatment, and dementia: the Three-City Study. *Neurology*, **64**, 1531–8.

Elias, P.K., Elias, M.F., D'Agostino, R.B., Silbershatz, H., and Wolf, P.A. (1999). Alcohol consumption and cognitive performance in the Framingham Heart Study. *American Journal of Epidemiology*, **150**, 580–9.

Emmerling, M.R., Morganti-Kossmann, M.C., Kossmann, T. *et al.* (2000). Traumatic brain injury elevates the Alzheimer's amyloid peptide A beta 42 in human CSF. A possible role for nerve cell injury. *Annals of the New York Academy of Sciences*, **903**, 118–22.

Engelhart, M.J., Geerlings, M.I., Ruitenberg, A. *et al.* (2002a). Diet and risk of dementia: does fat matter? The Rotterdam Study. *Neurology*, **59**, 1915–21.

Engelhart, M.J., Geerlings, M.I., Ruitenberg, A. *et al.* (2002b). Dietary intake of antioxidants and risk of Alzheimer disease. *Journal of the American Medical Association*, **287**, 3223–9.

Engelhart, M.J., Geerlings, M.I., Meijer, J. *et al.* (2004). Inflammatory proteins in plasma and the risk of dementia: the Rotterdam study. *Archives of Neurology*, **61**, 668–72.

Engelhart, M.J., Ruitenberg, A., Meijer, J. *et al.* (2005). Plasma levels of antioxidants are not associated with Alzheimer's disease or cognitive decline. *Dementia and Geriatric Cognitive Disorders*, **19**, 134–9.

Esiri, M.M., Nagy, Z., Smith, M.Z., Barnetson, L., and Smith, A.D. (1999). Cerebrovascular disease and threshold for dementia in the early stages of Alzheimer's disease. *Lancet*, **354**, 919–20.

Espeland, M.A., Rapp, S.R., Shumaker, S.A. *et al.* (2004). Conjugated equine estrogens and global cognitive function in postmenopausal women: Women's Health Initiative Memory Study. *Journal of the American Medical Association*, **291**, 2959–68.

Etminan, M., Gill, S., and Samii, A. (2003). Effect of non-steroidal anti-inflammatory drugs on risk of Alzheimer's disease: systematic review and meta-analysis of observational studies. *British Medical Journal*, **327**, 128.

Eussen, S.J., de Groot, L.C., Joosten, L.W. *et al.* (2006). Effect of oral vitamin B-12 with or without folic acid on cognitive function in older people with mild vitamin B-12 deficiency: a randomized, placebo-controlled trial. *American Journal of Clinical Nutrition*, **84**, 361–70.

Evans, D.A., Beckett, L.A., Field, T.S. *et al.* (1997a). Apolipoprotein E epsilon4 and incidence of Alzheimer disease in a community population of older persons. *Journal of the American Medical Association*, **277**, 822–4.

Evans, D.A., Hebert, L.E., Beckett, L.A. *et al.* (1997b). Education and other measures of socioeconomic status and risk of incident Alzheimer disease in a defined population of older persons. *Archives of Neurology*, **54**, 1399–405.

Ewbank, D.C. (1999). Deaths attributable to Alzheimer's disease in the United States. *American Journal of Public Health*, **89**, 90–2.

Fabrigoule, C., Letenneur, L., Dartigues, J.F., Zarrouk, M., Commenges, D., and Barberger-Gateau, P. (1995). Social and leisure activities and risk of dementia: a prospective longitudinal study. *Journal of the American Geriatrics Society*, **43**, 485–90.

Farrer, L.A., Cupples, L.A., Haines, J.L. *et al.* (1997). Effects of age, sex, and ethnicity on the association between apolipoprotein E genotype and Alzheimer disease. A meta-analysis. *Journal of the American Medical Association*, **278**, 1349–56.

Ferri, C.P., Prince, M., Brayne, C. *et al.* (2005). Global prevalence of dementia: a Delphi consensus study. *Lancet*, **366**, 2112–17.

Feychting, M., Jonsson, F., Pedersen, N.L., and Ahlbom, A. (2003). Occupational magnetic field exposure and neurodegenerative disease. *Epidemiology*, **14**, 413–19.

Fleminger, S., Oliver, D.L., Lovestone, S., Rabe-Hesketh, S., and Giora, A. (2003). Head injury as a risk factor for Alzheimer's disease: the evidence 10 years on; a partial replication. *Journal of Neurology, Neurosurgery, and Psychiatry*, **74**, 857–62.

Forette, F., Seux, M.L., Staessen, J.A. *et al.* (1998). Prevention of dementia in randomised double-blind placebo-controlled Systolic Hypertension in Europe (Syst-Eur) trial. *Lancet*, **352**, 1347–51.

Forette, F., Seux, M.L., Staessen, J.A. *et al.* (2002). The prevention of dementia with antihypertensive treatment: new evidence from the Systolic Hypertension in Europe (Syst-Eur) study. *Archives of Internal Medicine*, **162**, 2046–52.

Fratiglioni, L. and Rocca, W. (2001). Epidemiology of dementia. In *Handbook of neuropsychology: aging and dementia* (ed. F. Boller and S.F. Cappa), pp.193–215. Elsevier Science, Amsterdam.

Fratiglioni, L. and Wang, H.X. (2000). Smoking and Parkinson's and Alzheimer's disease: review of the epidemiological studies. *Behavioural Brain Research*, **113**, 117–20.

Fratiglioni, L., Ahlbom, A., Viitanen, M., and Winblad, B. (1993). Risk factors for late-onset Alzheimer's disease: a population-based, case-control study. *Annals of Neurology*, **33**, 258–66.

Fratiglioni, L., Viitanen, M., von Strauss, E., Tontodonati, V., Herlitz, A., and Winblad, B. (1997). Very old women at highest risk of dementia and Alzheimer's disease: incidence data from the Kungsholmen Project, Stockholm. *Neurology*, **48**, 132–8.

Fratiglioni, L., De Ronchi, D., and Agüero-Torres, H. (1999). Worldwide prevalence and incidence of dementia. *Drugs & Aging*, **15**, 365–75.

Fratiglioni, L., Launer, L.J., Andersen, K. *et al.* (2000a). Incidence of dementia and major subtypes in Europe: A collaborative study of population-based cohorts. Neurologic Diseases in the Elderly Research Group. *Neurology*, **54**, S10–S15.

Fratiglioni, L., Wang, H.X., Ericsson, K., Maytan, M., and Winblad, B. (2000b). Influence of social network on occurrence of dementia: a community-based longitudinal study. *Lancet*, **355**, 1315–19.

Fratiglioni, L., Paillard-Borg, S., and Winblad, B. (2004). An active and socially integrated lifestyle in late life might protect against dementia. *Lancet Neurology*, **3**, 343–53.

Fratiglioni, L., Qiu, C., and Palmer, K. (2006). Commentary on 'vascular cognitive impairment: today and tomorrow'. Vascular cognitive impairment: time for prevention? *Alzheimer's & Dementia*, **2**, 202–4.

Ganguli, M. and Rodriguez, E.G. (1999). Reporting of dementia on death certificates: a community study. *Journal of the American Geriatric Society*, **47**, 842–9.

Ganguli, M., Du, Y., Dodge, H.H., Ratcliff, G.G., and Chang, C.C. (2006). Depressive symptoms and cognitive decline in late life: a prospective epidemiological study. *Archives of General Psychiatry*, **63**, 153–60.

Gao, S., Hendrie, H.C., Hall, K.S., and Hui, S. (1998). The relationships between age, sex, and the incidence of dementia and Alzheimer disease: a meta-analysis. *Archives of General Psychiatry*, **55**, 809–15.

Gatz, M., Reynolds, C.A., Fratiglioni, L. *et al.* (2006). Role of genes and environments for explaining Alzheimer disease. *Archives of General Psychiatry*, **63**, 168–74.

Gordis, L. (2000). *Epidemiology*, 2nd edn, pp. 42–4. W.B. Saunders Company, Philadelphia.

Green, R.C., Cupples, L.A., Go, R. *et al.* (2002). Risk of dementia among white and African American relatives of patients with Alzheimer disease. *Journal of the American Medical Association*, **287**, 329–36.

Green, R.C., Cupples, L.A., Kurz, A. *et al.* (2003). Depression as a risk factor for Alzheimer disease: the MIRAGE Study. *Archives of Neurology*, **60**, 753–9.

Gühne, U., Matschinger, H., Angermeyer, M.C., and Riedel-Heller, S.G. (2006). Incident dementia cases and mortality. Results of the Leipzig Longitudinal Study of the Aged (LEILA75+). *Dementia and Geriatric Cognitive Disorders*, **22**, 185–93.

Guo, Z., Fratiglioni, L., Zhu, L., Fastbom, J., Winblad, B., and Viitanen, M. (1999a). Occurrence and progression of dementia in a community population aged 75 years and older: relationship of antihypertensive medication use. *Archives of Neurology*, **56**, 991–6.

Guo, Z., Viitanen, M., Winblad, B., and Fratiglioni, L. (1999b). Low blood pressure and incidence of dementia in a very old sample: dependent on initial cognition. *Journal of the American Geriatrics Society*, **47**, 723–6.

Guo, Z., Cupples, L.A., Kurz, A. *et al.* (2000). Head injury and the risk of AD in the MIRAGE study. *Neurology*, **54**, 1316–23.

Gustafson, D. (2006). Adiposity indices and dementia. *Lancet Neurology*, **5**, 713–20.

Hajjar, I., Schumpert, J., Hirth, V., Wieland, D., and Eleazer, G.P. (2002). The impact of the use of statins on the prevalence of dementia and the progression of cognitive impairment. *The Journals of Gerontology Series A: Biological Sciences and Medical Sciences*, **57**, M414–M418.

Hajjar, I., Catoe, H., Sixta, S. *et al.* (2005). Cross-sectional and longitudinal association between antihypertensive medications and cognitive impairment in an elderly population. *The Journals of Gerontology Series A: Biological Sciences and Medical Sciences*, **60**, 67–73.

Hakansson, N., Gustavsson, P., Johansen, C., and Floderus, B. (2003). Neurodegenerative diseases in welders and other workers exposed to high levels of magnetic fields. *Epidemiology*, **14**, 420–6.

Hayden, K.M., Pieper, C.F., Welsh-Bohmer, K.A., Breitner, J.C., Norton, M.C., and Munger, R. (2004). Self- or proxy-reported stroke and the risk of Alzheimer disease. *Archives of Neurology*, **61**, 982.

Hayden, K.M., Zandi, P.P., Lyketsos, C.G. *et al.* (2006). Vascular risk factors for incident Alzheimer disease and vascular dementia: the Cache County study. *Alzheimer Disease and Associated Disorders*, **20**, 93–100.

Heart Protection Study Collaborative Group (2002). MRC/BHF Heart Protection Study of cholesterol lowering with simvastatin in 20,536 high-risk individuals: a randomised placebo-controlled trial. *Lancet*, **360**, 7–22.

Helmer, C., Joly, P., Letenneur, L., Commenges, D., and Dartigues, J.F. (2001). Mortality with dementia: results from a French prospective community-based cohort. *American Journal Epidemiology*, **154**, 642–8.

Hill, G., Connelly, J., Hebert, R., Lindsay, J., and Millar, W. (2003). Neyman's bias re-visited. *Journal of Clinical Epidemiology*, **56**, 293–6.

Hofman, A., Ott, A., Breteler, M.M. *et al.* (1997). Atherosclerosis, apolipoprotein E, and prevalence of dementia and Alzheimer's disease in the Rotterdam Study. *Lancet*, **349**, 151–4.

Honig, L.S., Tang, M.X., Albert, S. *et al.* (2003). Stroke and the risk of Alzheimer disease. *Archives of Neurology*, **60**, 1707–12.

Huang, T.L., Zandi, P.P., Tucker, K.L. *et al.* (2005). Benefits of fatty fish on dementia risk are stronger for those without APOE ε4. *Neurology*, **65**, 1409–14.

Huang, W., Qiu, C., Winblad, B., and Fratiglioni, L. (2002). Alcohol consumption and incidence of dementia in a community sample aged 75 years and older. *Journal of Clinical Epidemiology*, **55**, 959–64.

Huang, W., Qiu, C., von Strauss, E., Winblad, B., and Fratiglioni, L. (2004). APOE genotype, family history of dementia, and Alzheimer disease risk: a 6-year follow-up study. *Archives of Neurology*, **61**, 1930–4.

Iadecola, C. and Gorelick, P.B. (2003). Converging pathogenic mechanisms in vascular and neurodegenerative dementia. *Stroke*, **34**, 335–7.

in 't Veld, B.A., Ruitenberg, A., Hofman, A., Stricker, B.H., and Breteler, M.M. (2001a). Antihypertensive drugs and incidence of dementia: the Rotterdam Study. *Neurobiology of Aging*, **22**, 407–12.

in 't Veld, B.A., Ruitenberg, A., Hofman, A. *et al.* (2001b). Nonsteroidal anti-inflammatory drugs and the risk of Alzheimer's disease. *New England Journal of Medicine*, **345**, 1515–21.

Jagger, C., Andersen, K., Breteler, M.M. *et al.* (2000). Prognosis with dementia in Europe: a collaborative study of population-based cohorts. Neurologic Diseases in the Elderly Research Group. *Neurology*, **54**, S16–S20.

Jick, H., Zornberg, G.L., Jick, S.S., Seshadri, S., and Drachman, D.A. (2000). Statins and the risk of dementia. *Lancet*, **356**, 1627–31.

Jin, Y.P., Gatz, M., Johansson, B., and Pedersen, N.L. (2004). Sensitivity and specificity of dementia coding in two Swedish disease registries. *Neurology*, **63**, 739–41.

Johnson, D.K., Wilkins, C.H., and Morris, J.C. (2006). Accelerated weight loss may precede diagnosis in Alzheimer disease. *Archives of Neurology*, **63**, 1312–17.

Jorm, A.F. (2001). History of depression as a risk factor for dementia: an updated review. *Australian and New Zealand Journal of Psychiatry*, **35**, 776–81.

Jorm, A.F. and Jolley, D. (1998). The incidence of dementia: a meta-analysis. *Neurology* **51**, 728–33.

Jorm, A.F., Korten, A.E., and Henderson, A.S. (1987). The prevalence of dementia: a quantitative integration of the literature. *Acta Psychiatrica Scandinavica*, **76**, 465–79.

Kalmijn, S. (2000). Fatty acid intake and the risk of dementia and cognitive decline: a review of clinical and epidemiological studies. *Journal of Nutrition, Health & Aging*, **4**, 202–7.

Kalmijn, S., Launer, L.J., Ott, A., Witteman, J.C., Hofman, A., and Breteler, M.M. (1997). Dietary fat intake and the risk of incident dementia in the Rotterdam Study. *Annals of Neurology*, **42**, 776–82.

Kalmijn, S., Foley, D., White, L. *et al.* (2000). Metabolic cardiovascular syndrome and risk of dementia in Japanese-American elderly men. The Honolulu-Asia aging study. *Arteriosclerosis, Thrombosis, and Vascular Biology*, **20**, 2255–60.

Kang, J.H., Weuve, J., and Grodstein, F. (2004). Postmenopausal hormone therapy and risk of cognitive decline in community-dwelling aging women. *Neurology*, **63**, 101–7.

Kang, J.H., Cook, N., Manson, J., Buring, J.E., and Grodstein, F. (2006). A randomized trial of vitamin E supplementation and cognitive function in women. *Archives of Internal Medicine*, **166**, 2462–8.

Karp, A., Kåreholt, I., Qiu, C., Bellander, T., Winblad, B., and Fratiglioni, L. (2004). Relation of education and occupation-based socioeconomic status to incident Alzheimer's disease. *American Journal of Epidemiology*, **159**, 175–83.

Karp, A., Paillard-Borg, S., Wang, H.X., Silverstein, M., Winblad, B., and Fratiglioni, L. (2006). Mental, physical and social components in leisure activities equally contribute to decrease dementia risk. *Dementia and Geriatric Cognitive Disorders*, **21**, 65–73.

Katzman, R. (1993). Education and the prevalence of dementia and Alzheimer's disease. *Neurology*, **43**, 13–20.

Katzman, R. (2004). Luigi Amaducci memorial award winner's paper 2003. A neurologist's view of Alzheimer's disease and dementia. *International Psychogeriatrics*, **16**, 259–73.

Katzman, R., Hill, L.R., Yu, E.S. *et al.* (1994). The malignancy of dementia. Predictors of mortality in clinically diagnosed dementia in a population survey of Shanghai, China. *Archives of Neurology*, **51**, 1220–5.

Kawas, C., Resnick, S., Morrison, A. *et al.* (1997). A prospective study of estrogen replacement therapy and the risk of developing Alzheimer's disease: the Baltimore Longitudinal Study of Aging. *Neurology*, **48**, 1517–21.

Kawas, C., Gray, S., Brookmeyer, R., Fozard, J., and Zonderman, A. (2000). Age-specific incidence rates of Alzheimer's disease: the Baltimore Longitudinal Study of Aging. *Neurology*, **54**, 2072–7.

Khachaturian, A.S., Zandi, P.P., Lyketsos, C.G. *et al.* (2006). Antihypertensive medication use and incident Alzheimer disease: the Cache County Study. *Archives of Neurology*, **63**, 686–92.

Kinsella, K. and Velkoff, V.A. (2002). The demographics of aging. *Aging Clinical and Experimental Research*, **14**, 159–69.

Kivipelto, M., Helkala, E.L., Laakso, M.P. *et al.* (2001). Midlife vascular risk factors and Alzheimer's disease in later life: longitudinal, population based study. *British Medical Journal*, **322**, 1447–51.

Kivipelto, M., Helkala, E.L., Laakso, M.P. *et al.* (2002). Apolipoprotein E ε4 allele, elevated midlife total cholesterol level, and high midlife systolic blood pressure are independent risk factors for late-life Alzheimer disease. *Annals of Internal Medicine*, **137**, 149–55.

Kivipelto, M., Ngandu, T., Fratiglioni, L. *et al.* (2005). Obesity and vascular risk factors at midlife and the risk of dementia and Alzheimer disease. *Archives of Neurology*, **62**, 1556–60.

Kivipelto, M., Ngandu, T., Laatikainen, T., Winblad, B., Soininen, H., and Tuomilehto, J. (2006). Risk score for the prediction of dementia risk in 20 years among middle aged people: a longitudinal, population-based study. *Lancet Neurology*, **5**, 735–41.

Knowler, W.C., Barrett-Connor, E., Fowler, S.E. *et al.* (2002). Reduction in the incidence of type 2 diabetes with lifestyle intervention or metformin. *New England Journal of Medicine*, **346**, 393–403.

Korf, E.S., White, L.R., Scheltens, P., and Launer, L.J. (2004). Midlife blood pressure and the risk of hippocampal atrophy: the Honolulu Asia Aging Study. *Hypertension*, **44**, 29–34.

Korf, E.S., White, L.R., Scheltens, P., and Launer, L.J. (2006). Brain aging in very old men with type 2 diabetes: the Honolulu-Asia Aging Study. *Diabetes Care*, **29**, 2268–74.

Kramer, A.F., Hahn, S., Cohen, N.J. *et al.* (1999). Ageing, fitness and neurocognitive function. *Nature*, **400**, 418–19.

Kris-Etherton, P., Daniels, S.R., Eckel, R.H. *et al.* (2001). Summary of the scientific conference on dietary fatty acids and cardiovascular health: conference summary from the nutrition committee of the American Heart Association. *Circulation*, **103**, 1034–9.

Kuh, D. and Ben-Shlomo, Y. (2004). *A life course approach to chronic disease epidemiology*, 2nd edn, pp. 1–14. Oxford University Press, New York.

Kuusisto, J., Koivisto, K., Mykkanen, L. *et al.* (1997). Association between features of the insulin resistance syndrome and Alzheimer's disease independently of apolipoprotein E4 phenotype: cross sectional population based study. *British Medical Journal*, **315**, 1045–9.

Laitinen MH, Ngandu T, Rovio S, et al. (2006). Fat intake at midlife and risk of dementia and Alzheimer's disease: a population-based study. *Dementia and Geriatric Cognitive Disorders*, **22**, 99–107.

Landi, F., Cesari, M., Onder, G., Russo, A., Torre, S., and Bernabei, R. (2003). Non-steroidal anti-inflammatory drug (NSAID) use and Alzheimer disease in community-dwelling elderly patients. *American Journal of Geriatric Psychiatry*, **11**, 179–85.

Lanska, D.J. (1998). Dementia mortality in the United States. Results of the 1986 National Mortality Followback Survey. *Neurology*, **50**, 362–7.

Larson, E.B., Wang, L., Bowen, J.D. *et al.* (2006). Exercise is associated with reduced risk for incident dementia among persons 65 years of age and older. *Annals of Internal Medicine*, **144**, 73–81.

Launer, L.J. (2002). Demonstrating the case that AD is a vascular disease: epidemiologic evidence. *Ageing Research Reviews*, **1**, 61–77.

Launer, L.J., Andersen, K., Dewey, M.E. *et al.* (1999). Rates and risk factors for dementia and Alzheimer's disease: results from EURODEM pooled analyses. EURODEM Incidence Research Group and Work Groups. European Studies of Dementia. *Neurology*, **52**, 78–84.

Launer, L.J., Ross, G.W., Petrovitch, H. *et al.* (2000). Midlife blood pressure and dementia: the Honolulu-Asia aging study. *Neurobiology of Aging*, **21**, 49–55.

Laurin, D., Masaki, K.H., Foley, D.J., White, L.R., and Launer, L.J. (2004). Midlife dietary intake of antioxidants and risk of late-life incident dementia: the Honolulu-Asia Aging Study. *American Journal of Epidemiology*, **159**, 959–67.

Lavery, L., Bilt, J.V., Chang, C.C., Saxton, J.A., and Ganguli, M. (2007). The association between congestive heart failure and cognitive performance in a primary care population of elderly adults: the Steel Valley Seniors Survey. *International Psychogeriatrics*, **19**, 215–25.

Leibson, C.L., Rocca, W.A., Hanson, V.A. *et al.* (1997). Risk of dementia among persons with diabetes mellitus: a population-based cohort study. *American Journal of Epidemiology*, **145**, 301–8.

Leys, D., Henon, H., Mackowiak-Cordoliani, M.A., and Pasquier, F. (2005). Poststroke dementia. *Lancet Neurology*, **4**, 752–9.

Li, G., Higdon, R., Kukull, W.A. *et al.* (2004). Statin therapy and risk of dementia in the elderly: a community-based prospective cohort study. *Neurology*, **63**, 1624–8.

Liebetrau, M., Steen, B., Hamann, G.F., and Skoog, I. (2004). Silent and symptomatic infarcts on cranial computerized tomography in relation to dementia and mortality: a population-based study in 85-year-old subjects. *Stroke*, **35**, 1816–20.

Lindström, J., Ilanne-Parikka, P., Peltonen, M. *et al.* (2006). Sustained reduction in the incidence of type 2 diabetes by lifestyle intervention: follow-up of the Finnish Diabetes Prevention Study. *Lancet*, **368**, 1673–9.

Lithell, H., Hansson, L., Skoog, I. *et al.* (2003). The Study on Cognition and Prognosis in the Elderly (SCOPE): principal results of a randomized double-blind intervention trial. *Journal of Hypertension*, **21**, 875–86.

Lobo, A., Launer, L.J., Fratiglioni, L. *et al.* (2000). Prevalence of dementia and major subtypes in Europe: A collaborative study of population-based cohorts. Neurologic Diseases in the Elderly Research Group. *Neurology*, **54**, S4–S9.

Luchsinger, J.A. and Mayeux, R. (2004). Dietary factors and Alzheimer's disease. *Lancet Neurology*, **3**, 579–87.

Luchsinger, J.A., Tang, M.X., Stern, Y., Shea, S., and Mayeux, R. (2001). Diabetes mellitus and risk of Alzheimer's disease and dementia with stroke in a multiethnic cohort. *American Journal of Epidemiology*, **154**, 635–41.

Luchsinger, J.A., Tang, M.X., Shea, S., and Mayeux, R. (2003). Antioxidant vitamin intake and risk of Alzheimer disease. *Archives of Neurology*, **60**, 203–8.

Luchsinger, J.A., Tang, M.X., Shea, S., and Mayeux, R. (2004a). Hyperinsulinemia and risk of Alzheimer disease. *Neurology*, **63**, 1187–92.

Luchsinger, J.A., Tang, M.X., Shea, S., Miller, J., Green, R., and Mayeux, R. (2004b). Plasma homocysteine levels and risk of Alzheimer disease. *Neurology*, **62**, 1972–6.

Luchsinger, J.A., Reitz, C., Honig, L.S., Tang, M.X., Shea, S., and Mayeux, R. (2005). Aggregation of vascular risk factors and risk of incident Alzheimer disease. *Neurology*, **65**, 545–51.

Malouf, R., Grimley Evans, J., and Areosa Sastre, A. (2003). Folic acid with or without vitamin B12 for cognition and dementia. *Cochrane Database of Systematic Reviews* 2003, Issue 4, Art. No. CD004514. DOI: 10.1002/14651858.CD004514.

Masaki, K.H., Losonczy, K.G., Izmirlian, G. *et al.* (2000). Association of vitamin E and C supplement use with cognitive function and dementia in elderly men. *Neurology*, **54**, 1265–72.

Matthews, F. and Brayne, C. (2005). The incidence of dementia in England and Wales: findings from the five identical sites of the MRC CFA Study. *PLoS Med*, **2**, e193.

Maxwell, C.J., Hogan, D.B., and Ebly, E.M. (2002). Serum folate levels and subsequent adverse cerebrovascular outcomes in elderly persons. *Dementia and Geriatric Cognitive Disorders*, **13**, 225–34.

Mayeux, R., Ottman, R., Maestre, G., *et al.* (1995). Synergistic effects of traumatic head injury and apolipoprotein-ε4 in patients with Alzheimer's disease. *Neurology*, **45**, 555–7.

McMahon, J.A., Green, T.J., Skeaff, C.M., Knight, R.G., Mann, J.I., and Williams, S.M. (2006). A controlled trial of homocysteine lowering and cognitive performance. *New England Journal of Medicine*, **354**, 2764–72.

Mehta, K.M., Ott, A., Kalmijn, S. *et al.* (1999). Head trauma and risk of dementia and Alzheimer's disease: The Rotterdam Study. *Neurology*, **53**, 1959–62.

Merchant, C., Tang, M.X., Albert, S., Manly, J., Stern, Y., and Mayeux, R. (1999). The influence of smoking on the risk of Alzheimer's disease. *Neurology*, **52**, 1408–12.

Miech, R.A., Breitner, J.C., Zandi, P.P., Khachaturian, A.S., Anthony, J.C., and Mayer, L. (2002). Incidence of AD may decline in the early 90s for men, later for women: The Cache County study. *Neurology*, **58**, 209–18.

Mielke, M.M., Zandi, P.P., Sjogren, M. *et al.* (2005). High total cholesterol levels in late life associated with a reduced risk of dementia. *Neurology*, **64**, 1689–95.

Mitnitski, A., Skoog, I., Song, X. *et al.* (2006). A vascular risk factor index in relation to mortality and incident dementia. *European Journal of Neurology*, **13**, 514–21.

Moceri, V.M., Kukull, W.A., Emanuel, I., van Belle, G., and Larson, E.B. (2000). Early-life risk factors and the development of Alzheimer's disease. *Neurology*, **54**, 415–20.

Modrego, P.J. and Ferrandez, J. (2004). Depression in patients with mild cognitive impairment increases the risk of developing dementia of Alzheimer type: a prospective cohort study. *Archives of Neurology*, **61**, 1290–3.

Morris, M.C., Scherr, P.A., Hebert, L.E., Glynn, R.J., Bennett, D.A., and Evans, D.A. (2001). Association of incident Alzheimer disease and blood pressure measured from 13 years before to 2 years after diagnosis in a large community study. *Archives of Neurology*, **58**, 1640–6.

Morris, M.C., Evans, D.A., Bienias, J.L. *et al.* (2002). Dietary intake of antioxidant nutrients and the risk of incident Alzheimer disease in a biracial community study. *Journal of the American Medical Association*, **287**, 3230–7.

Morris, M.C., Evans, D.A., Bienias, J.L. *et al.* (2003a). Dietary fats and the risk of incident Alzheimer disease. *Archives of Neurology*, **60**, 194–200.

Morris, M.C., Evans, D.A., and Bienias, J.L. *et al.* (2003b). Consumption of fish and n-3 fatty acids and risk of incident Alzheimer disease. *Archives of Neurology*, **60**, 940–6.

Morris, M.S. (2003). Homocysteine and Alzheimer's disease. *Lancet Neurology*, **2**, 425–8.

Mortimer, J.A., van Duijn, C.M., Chandra, V. *et al.* (1991). Head trauma as a risk factor for Alzheimer's disease: a collaborative re-analysis of case-control studies. EURODEM Risk Factors Research Group. *International Journal of Epidemiology*, **20**(Suppl. 2), S28–S35.

Murray, M.D., Lane, K.A., Gao, S. *et al.* (2002). Preservation of cognitive function with antihypertensive medications: a longitudinal analysis of a community-based sample of African Americans. *Archives of Internal Medicine*, **162**, 2090–6.

Mutter, J., Naumann, J., Sadaghiani, C., Schneider, R., and Walach, H. (2004). Alzheimer disease: mercury as pathogenetic factor and apolipoprotein E as a moderator. *Neuroendocrinology Letters*, **25**, 331–9.

Newman, A.B., Fitzpatrick, A.L., Lopez, O. *et al.* (2005). Dementia and Alzheimer's disease incidence in relationship to cardiovascular disease in the Cardiovascular Health Study cohort. *Journal of the American Geriatrics Society*, **53**, 1101–7.

Nicoll, J.A., Roberts, G.W., and Graham, D.I. (1995). Apolipoprotein E ε4 allele is associated with deposition of amyloid beta-protein following head injury. *Nature Medicine*, **1**, 135–7.

Noale, M., Maggi, S., Minicuci, N. *et al.* (2003). Dementia and disability: impact on mortality. The Italian Longitudinal Study on Aging. *Dementia and Geriatric Cognitive Disorders*, **16**, 7–14.

Notkola, I.L., Sulkava, R., Pekkanen, J. *et al.* (1998). Serum total cholesterol, apolipoprotein E ε4 allele, and Alzheimer's disease. *Neuroepidemiology*, **17**, 14–20.

Nourhashemi, F., Deschamps, V., Larrieu, S., Letenneur, L., Dartigues, J.F., and Barberger-Gateau, P. (2003). Body mass index and incidence of dementia: the PAQUID study. *Neurology*, **60**, 117–19.

Orgogozo, J.M., Dartigues, J.F., Lafont, S. *et al.* (1997). Wine consumption and dementia in the elderly: a prospective community study in the Bordeaux area. *Revue Neurologique*, **153**, 185–92.

Ott, A., Breteler, M.M., de Bruyne, M.C., van Harskamp, F., Grobbee, D.E., and Hofman, A. (1997). Atrial fibrillation and dementia in a population-based study. The Rotterdam Study. *Stroke*, **28**, 316–21.

Ott, A., Slooter, A.J., Hofman, A. *et al.* (1998). Smoking and risk of dementia and Alzheimer's disease in a population-based cohort study: the Rotterdam Study. *Lancet*, **351**, 1840–3.

Ott, A., Stolk, R.P., van Harskamp, F., Pols, H.A., Hofman, A., and Breteler, M.M. (1999). Diabetes mellitus and the risk of dementia: The Rotterdam Study. *Neurology*, **53**, 1937–42

Ownby, R.L., Crocco, E., Acevedo, A., John, V., and Loewenstein, D. (2006). Depression and risk for Alzheimer disease: systematic review, meta-analysis, and metaregression analysis. *Archives of General Psychiatry*, **63**, 530–8.

Peila, R., Rodriguez, B.L., Launer, L.J. (2002). Type 2 diabetes, APOE gene, and the risk for dementia and related pathologies: The Honolulu-Asia Aging Study. *Diabetes*, **51**, 1256–62.

Perl, D.P. and Moalem, S. (2006). Aluminum and Alzheimer's disease, a personal perspective after 25 years. *Journal of Alzheimer's Disease*, **9**, 291–300.

Petersen, R.C., Thomas, R.G., Grundman, M. *et al.* (2005). Vitamin E and donepezil for the treatment of mild cognitive impairment. *New England Journal of Medicine*, **352**, 2379–88.

Petitti, D.B., Crooks, V.C., Buckwalter, J.G., and Chiu, V. (2005). Blood pressure levels before dementia. *Archives of Neurology*, **62**, 112–16.

Petrovitch, H., White, L.R., Izmirilian, G. *et al.* (2000). Midlife blood pressure and neuritic plaques, neurofibrillary tangles, and brain weight at death: the HAAS. Honolulu-Asia aging Study. *Neurobiology of Aging*, **21**, 57–62.

Plassman, B.L., Havlik, R.J., Steffens, D.C. *et al.* (2000). Documented head injury in early adulthood and risk of Alzheimer's disease and other dementias. *Neurology*, **55**, 1158–66.

Polidori, M.C., Mariani, E., Mecocci, P., and Nelles, G. (2006). Congestive heart failure and Alzheimer's disease. *Neurological Research*, **28**, 588–94.

Posner, H.B., Tang, M.X., Luchsinger, J., Lantigua, R., Stern, Y., and Mayeux, R. (2002). The relationship of hypertension in the elderly to AD, vascular dementia, and cognitive function. *Neurology*, **58**, 1175–81.

Prince, M.J., Bird, A.S., Blizard, R.A., and Mann, A.H. (1996). Is the cognitive function of older patients affected by antihypertensive treatment? Results from 54 months of the Medical Research Council's trial of hypertension in older adults. *British Medical Journal*, **312**, 801–5.

Prins, N.D., van Dijk, E.J., den Heijer, T. *et al.* (2004). Cerebral white matter lesions and the risk of dementia. *Archives of Neurology*, **61**, 1531–4.

Qiu, C., Bäckman, L., Winblad, B., Agüero-Torres, H., and Fratiglioni, L. (2001). The influence of education on clinically diagnosed dementia incidence and mortality data from the Kungsholmen Project. *Archives of Neurology*, **58**, 2034–9.

Qiu, C., Karp, A., von Strauss, E., Winblad, B., Fratiglioni, L., and Bellander, T. (2003a). Lifetime principal occupation and risk of Alzheimer's disease in the Kungsholmen project. *American Journal of Industrial Medicine*, **43**, 204–11.

Qiu, C., Winblad, B., Fastbom, J., and Fratiglioni, L. (2003b). Combined effects of APOE genotype, blood pressure, and antihypertensive drug use on incident AD. *Neurology*, **61**, 655–60.

Qiu, C., von Strauss, E., Fastbom, J., Winblad, B., and Fratiglioni, L. (2003c). Low blood pressure and risk of dementia in the Kungsholmen project: a 6-year follow-up study. *Archives of Neurology*, **60**, 223–8.

Qiu, C., Fratiglioni, L., Karp, A., Winblad, B., and Bellander, T. (2004a). Occupational exposure to electromagnetic fields and risk of Alzheimer's disease. *Epidemiology*, **15**, 687–94.

Qiu, C., Kivipelto, M., Agüero-Torres, H., Winblad, B., and Fratiglioni, L. (2004b). Risk and protective effects of the APOE gene towards Alzheimer's disease in the Kungsholmen project: variation by age and sex. *Journal of Neurology, Neurosurgery, and Psychiatry*, **75**, 828–33.

Qiu, C., Winblad, B., and Fratiglioni, L. (2005). The age-dependent relation of blood pressure to cognitive function and dementia. *Lancet Neurology*, **4**, 487–99.

Qiu, C., Winblad, B., Marengoni, A., Klarin, I., Fastbom, J., and Fratiglioni, L. (2006). Heart failure and risk of dementia and Alzheimer disease: a population-based cohort study. *Archives of Internal Medicine*, **166**, 1003–8.

Ravaglia, G., Forti, P., Maioli, F. *et al.* (2002). Education, occupation, and prevalence of dementia: findings from the Conselice study. *Dementia and Geriatric Cognitive Disorders*, **14**, 90–100.

Ravaglia, G., Forti, P., Maioli, F. *et al.* (2005a). Incidence and etiology of dementia in a large elderly Italian population. *Neurology*, **64**, 1525–30.

Ravaglia, G., Forti, P., Maioli, F. *et al.* (2005b). Homocysteine and folate as risk factors for dementia and Alzheimer disease. *American Journal of Clinical Nutrition*, **82**, 636–43.

Rea, T.D., Breitner, J.C., Psaty, B.M. *et al.* (2005). Statin use and the risk of incident dementia: the Cardiovascular Health Study. *Archives of Neurology*, **62**, 1047–51.

Reitz, C., Luchsinger, J.A., Tang, M.X., Manly, J., and Mayeux, R. (2006). Stroke and memory performance in elderly persons without dementia. *Archives of Neurology*, **63**, 571–6.

Reitz, C., Tang, M.X., Luchsinger, J., Mayeux, R. (2004). Relation of plasma lipids to Alzheimer disease and vascular dementia. *Archives of Neurology*, **61**, 705–14.

Richards, M. and Deary, I.J. (2005). A life course approach to cognitive reserve: a model for cognitive aging and development? *Annals of Neurology*, **58**, 617–22.

Rippon, G.A., Tang, M.X., Lee, J.H., Lantigua, R., Medrano, M., and Mayeux, R. (2006). Familial Alzheimer disease in Latinos: interaction between APOE, stroke, and estrogen replacement. *Neurology*, **66**, 35–40.

Ritchie, K. and Kildea, D. (1995). Is senile dementia 'age-related' or 'ageing-related'?–evidence from meta-analysis of dementia prevalence in the oldest old. *Lancet*, **346**, 931–4.

Rocca, W.A., Cha, R.H., Waring, S.C., and Kokmen, E. (1998). Incidence of dementia and Alzheimer's disease: a reanalysis of data from Rochester, Minnesota, 1975–1984. *American Journal of Epidemiology*, **148**, 51–62.

Rockwood, K., Kirkland, S., Hogan, D.B. *et al.* (2002). Use of lipid-lowering agents, indication bias, and the risk of dementia in community-dwelling elderly people. *Archives of Neurology*, **59**, 223–7.

Rodriguez, E.G., Dodge, H.H., Birzescu, M.A., Stoehr, G.P., and Ganguli, M. (2002). Use of lipid-lowering drugs in older adults with and without dementia: a community-based epidemiological study. *Journal of the American Geriatrics Society*, **50**, 1852–6.

Roher, A.E., Esh, C., Kokjohn, T.A. *et al.* (2003). Circle of Willis atherosclerosis is a risk factor for sporadic Alzheimer's disease. *Arteriosclerosis, Thrombosis, and Vascular Biology*, **23**, 2055–62.

Romas, S.N., Tang, M.X., Berglund, L., and Mayeux, R. (1999). APOE genotype, plasma lipids, lipoproteins, and AD in community elderly. *Neurology*, **53**, 517–21.

Rosengren, A., Skoog, I., Gustafson, D., and Wilhelmsen, L. (2005). Body mass index, other cardiovascular risk factors, and hospitalization for dementia. *Archives of Internal Medicine*, **165**, 321–6.

Ross, G.W. and Petrovitch, H. (2001). Current evidence for neuroprotective effects of nicotine and caffeine against Parkinson's disease. *Drugs & Aging*, **18**, 797–806.

Rovio, S., Kåreholt, I., Helkala, E.L. *et al.* (2005). Leisure-time physical activity at midlife and the risk of dementia and Alzheimer's disease. *Lancet Neurology*, **4**, 705–11.

Ruitenberg, A., Skoog, I., Ott, A. *et al.* (2001). Blood pressure and risk of dementia: results from the Rotterdam study and the Gothenburg H-70 Study. *Dementia and Geriatric Cognitive Disorders*, **12**, 33–9.

Ruitenberg, A., van Swieten, J.C., Witteman, J.C. *et al.* (2002). Alcohol consumption and risk of dementia: the Rotterdam Study. *Lancet*, **359**, 281–6.

Ruitenberg, A., den Heijer, T., Bakker, S.L. *et al.* (2005). Cerebral hypoperfusion and clinical onset of dementia: the Rotterdam Study. *Annals of Neurology*, **57**, 789–94.

Sacco, R.L., Elkind, M., Boden-Albala, B. *et al.* (1999). The protective effect of moderate alcohol consumption on ischemic stroke. *Journal of the American Medical Association*, **281**, 53–60.

Saczynski, J.S., Pfeifer, L.A., Masaki, K. *et al.* (2006). The effect of social engagement on incident dementia: the Honolulu-Asia Aging Study. *American Journal of Epidemiology*, **163**, 433–40.

SBU (Statens Beredning för Medicinsk Utvärdering) (2006). *Demenssjukdomar: en systematisk litteraturöversikt* [in Swedish], pp. 22–9, SBU, Stockholm.

Scarmeas, N., Stern, Y., Mayeux, R., and Luchsinger, J.A. (2006a). Mediterranean diet, Alzheimer disease, and vascular mediation. *Archives of Neurology*, **63**, 1709–17.

Scarmeas, N., Stern, Y., Tang, M.X., Mayeux, R., and Luchsinger, J.A. (2006b). Mediterranean diet and risk for Alzheimer's disease. *Annals of Neurology*, **59**, 912–21.

Schaefer, E.J., Bongard, V., Beiser, A.S. *et al.* (2006). Plasma phosphatidylcholine docosahexaenoic acid content and risk of dementia and Alzheimer disease: the Framingham Heart Study. *Archives of Neurology*, **63**, 1545–50.

Schafer, J.H., Glass, T.A., Bolla, K.I., Mintz, M., Jedlicka, A.E., and Schwartz, B.S. (2005). Homocysteine and cognitive function in a population-based study of older adults. *Journal of the American Geriatrics Society*, **53**, 381–8.

Schmand, B., Smit, J., Lindeboom, J. *et al.* (1997). Low education is a genuine risk factor for accelerated memory decline and dementia. *Journal of Clinical Epidemiology*, **50**, 1025–33.

Schmidt, R., Schmidt, H., Curb, J.D., Masaki, K., White, L.R., and Launer, L.J. (2002). Early inflammation and dementia: a 25-year follow-up of the Honolulu-Asia Aging Study. *Annals of Neurology*, **52**, 168–74.

Schofield, P.W., Tang, M., Marder, K. *et al.* (1997). Alzheimer's disease after remote head injury: an incidence study. *Journal of Neurology, Neurosurgery, and Psychiatry*, **62**, 119–24.

Seeman, T.E. and Crimmins, E. (2001). Social environment effects on health and aging: integrating epidemiologic and demographic approaches and perspectives. *Annals of the New York Academy of Sciences*, **954**, 88–117.

Seshadri, S., Zornberg, G.L., Derby, L.E., Myers, M.W., Jick, H., and Drachman, D.A. (2001). Postmenopausal estrogen replacement therapy and the risk of Alzheimer disease. *Archives of Neurology*, **58**, 435–40.

Seshadri, S., Beiser, A., Selhub, J. *et al.* (2002). Plasma homocysteine as a risk factor for dementia and Alzheimer's disease. *New England Journal of Medicine*, **346**, 476–83.

SHEP Cooperative Research Group (1991). Prevention of stroke by antihypertensive drug treatment in older persons with isolated systolic hypertension. Final results of the Systolic Hypertension in the Elderly Program (SHEP). *Journal of the American Medical Association*, **265**, 3255–64.

Shumaker, S.A., Legault, C., Kuller, L. *et al.* (2004). Conjugated equine estrogens and incidence of probable dementia and mild cognitive impairment in postmenopausal women: Women's Health Initiative Memory Study. *Journal of the American Medical Association*, **291**, 2947–58.

Skoog, I., Lernfelt, B., Landahl, S. *et al.* (1996). 15-year longitudinal study of blood pressure and dementia. *Lancet*, **347**, 1141–5.

Snowdon, D.A., Greiner, L.H., Mortimer, J.A., Riley, K.P., Greiner, P.A., and Markesbery, W.R. (1997). Brain infarction and the clinical expression of Alzheimer disease: the Nun Study. *Journal of the American Medical Association*, **277**, 813–17.

Sobel, E., Davanipour, Z., Sulkava, R. *et al.* (1995). Occupations with exposure to electromagnetic fields: a possible risk factor for Alzheimer's disease. *American Journal of Epidemiology*, **142**, 515–24.

Sobel, E., Dunn, M., Davanipour, Z., Qian, Z., and Chui, H.C. (1996). Elevated risk of Alzheimer's disease among workers with likely electromagnetic field exposure. *Neurology*, **47**, 1477–81.

Sparks, D.L., Scheff, S.W., Liu, H., Landers, T.M., Coyne, C.M., and Hunsaker, J.C. (1995). Increased incidence of neurofibrillary tangles (NFT) in non-demented individuals with hypertension. *Journal of the Neurological Sciences*, **131**, 162–9.

Stampfer, M.J., Kang, J.H., Chen, J., Cherry, R., and Grodstein, F. (2005). Effects of moderate alcohol consumption on cognitive function in women. *New England Journal of Medicine*, **352**, 245–53.

Starkstein, S.E. and Jorge, R (2005). Dementia after traumatic brain injury. *International Psychogeriatrics*, **17**(Suppl. 1), S93–S107.

Stern, Y. (2006). Cognitive reserve and Alzheimer disease. *Alzheimer Disease and Associated Disorders*, **20**, S69–S74.

Stern, Y., Gurland, B., Tatemichi, T.K., Tang, M.X., Wilder, D., and Mayeux, R. (1994). Influence of education and occupation on the incidence of Alzheimer's disease. *Journal of the American Medical Association*, **271**, 1004–10.

Stewart, R., Masaki, K., Xue, Q.L. *et al.* (2005). A 32-year prospective study of change in body weight and incident dementia: the Honolulu-Asia Aging Study. *Archives of Neurology*, **62**, 55–60.

Stewart, W.F., Kawas, C., Corrada, M., and Metter, E.J. (1997). Risk of Alzheimer's disease and duration of NSAID use. *Neurology*, **48**, 626–32.

Szekely, C.A., Thorne, J.E., Zandi, P.P. *et al.* (2004). Nonsteroidal anti-inflammatory drugs for the prevention of Alzheimer's disease: a systematic review. *Neuroepidemiology*, **23**, 159–69.

Tan, Z.S., Seshadri, S., Beiser, A. *et al.* (2003). Plasma total cholesterol level as a risk factor for Alzheimer disease: the Framingham Study. *Archives of Internal Medicine*, **163**, 1053–7.

Tang, M.X., Jacobs, D., Stern, Y. *et al.* (1996). Effect of oestrogen during menopause on risk and age at onset of Alzheimer's disease. *Lancet*, **348**, 429–32.

Tschanz, J.T., Corcoran, C., Skoog, I. *et al.* (2004). Dementia: the leading predictor of death in a defined elderly population: the Cache County Study. *Neurology*, **62**, 1156–62.

Tyas, S.L., White, L.R., Petrovitch, H. *et al.* (2003). Mid-life smoking and late-life dementia: the Honolulu-Asia Aging Study. *Neurobiology of Aging*, **24**, 589–96.

Tzourio, C., Anderson, C., Chapman, N. *et al.* (2003). Effects of blood pressure lowering with perindopril and indapamide therapy on dementia and cognitive decline in patients with cerebrovascular disease. *Archives of Internal Medicine*, **163**, 1069–75.

van Exel, E., de Craen, A.J., Remarque, E.J. *et al.* (2003). Interaction of atherosclerosis and inflammation in elderly subjects with poor cognitive function. *Neurology*, **61**, 1695–701.

Verghese, J., Lipton, R.B., Hall, C.B., Kuslansky, G., and Katz, M.J. (2003a). Low blood pressure and the risk of dementia in very old individuals. *Neurology*, **61**, 1667–72.

Verghese, J., Lipton, R.B., Katz, M.J. *et al.* (2003b). Leisure activities and the risk of dementia in the elderly. *New England Journal of Medicine*, **348**, 2508–16.

Vermeer, S.E., Prins, N.D., den Heijer, T., Hofman, A., Koudstaal, P.J., and Breteler, M.M. (2003). Silent brain infarcts and the risk of dementia and cognitive decline. *New England Journal of Medicine*, **348**, 1215–22.

Wang, H.X., Fratiglioni, L., Frisoni, G.B., Viitanen, M., and Winblad, B. (1999). Smoking and the occurrence of Alzheimer's disease: cross-sectional and longitudinal data in a population-based study. *American Journal of Epidemiology*, **149**, 640–4.

Wang, H.X., Wahlin, A., Basun, H., Fastbom, J., Winblad, B., and Fratiglioni, L. (2001). Vitamin B(12) and folate in relation to the development of Alzheimer's disease. *Neurology*, **56**, 1188–94.

Wang, H.X., Karp, A., Winblad, B., and Fratiglioni, L. (2002). Late-life engagement in social and leisure activities is associated with a decreased risk of dementia: a longitudinal study from the Kungsholmen project. *American Journal of Epidemiology*, **155**, 1081–7.

Waring, S.C., Rocca, W.A., Petersen, R.C., O'Brien, P.C., Tangalos, E.G., Kokmen, E. (1999). Postmenopausal estrogen replacement therapy and risk of AD: a population-based study. *Neurology*, **52**, 965–70.

Weuve, J., Kang, J.H., Manson, J.E., Breteler, M.M., Ware, J.H., and Grodstein, F. (2004). Physical activity, including walking, and cognitive function in older women. *Journal of the American Medical Association*, **292**, 1454–61.

Whalley, L.J., Starr, J.M., Athawes, R., Hunter, D., Pattie, A., and Deary, I.J. (2000). Childhood mental ability and dementia. *Neurology*, **55**, 1455–9.

Whalley, L.J., Dick, F.D., and McNeill, G. (2006). A life-course approach to the aetiology of late-onset dementias. *Lancet Neurology*, **5**, 87–96.

Whitmer, R.A., Gunderson, E.P., Barrett-Connor, E., Quesenberry, C.P., Jr, and Yaffe, K. (2005a). Obesity in middle age and future risk of dementia: a 27 year longitudinal population based study. *British Medical Journal*, **330**, 1360.

Whitmer, R.A., Sidney, S., Selby, J., Johnston, S.C., and Yaffe, K. (2005b). Midlife cardiovascular risk factors and risk of dementia in late life. *Neurology*, **64**, 277–81.

Wilson, R.S., Barnes, L.L., Mendes de Leon, C.F. *et al.* (2002a). Depressive symptoms, cognitive decline, and risk of AD in older persons. *Neurology*, **59**, 364–70.

Wilson, R.S., Bennett, D.A., Bienias, J.L. *et al.* (2002b). Cognitive activity and incident AD in a population-based sample of older persons. *Neurology*, **59**, 1910–4.

Wilson, R.S., Mendes De Leon, C.F., Barnes, L.L. *et al.* (2002c). Participation in cognitively stimulating activities and risk of incident Alzheimer disease. *Journal of the American Medical Association*, **287**, 742–8.

Wilson, R., Barnes, L., and Bennett, D. (2003). Assessment of lifetime participation in cognitively stimulating activities. *Journal of Clinical and Experimental Neuropsychology*, **25**, 634–42.

Wimo, A., Winblad, B., Agüero-Torres, H., and von Strauss, E. (2003). The magnitude of dementia occurrence in the world. *Alzheimer Disease and Associated Disorders*, **17**, 63–7.

Witthaus, E., Ott, A., Barendregt, J.J., Breteler, M., and Bonneux, L. (1999). Burden of mortality and morbidity from dementia. *Alzheimer Disease and Associated Disorders*, **13**, 176–81.

Wolfson, C., Wolfson, D.B., Asgharian, M. *et al.* (2001). A reevaluation of the duration of survival after the onset of dementia. *New England Journal of Medicine*, **344**, 1111–16.

Xu, W.L., Qiu, C.X., Wahlin, A., Winblad, B., and Fratiglioni, L. (2004). Diabetes mellitus and risk of dementia in the Kungsholmen project: a 6-year follow-up study. *Neurology*, **63**, 1181–6.

Xu, W.L., Qiu, C.X., Winblad, B., and Fratiglioni, L. (2007). The effect of borderline diabetes mellitus on the risk of dementia and Alzheimer disease. *Diabetes*, **56**, 211–16.

Yasar, S., Corrada, M., Brookmeyer, R., and Kawas, C. (2005). Calcium channel blockers and risk of AD: the Baltimore Longitudinal Study of Aging. *Neurobiology of Aging*, **26**, 157–63.

Yoshitake, T., Kiyohara, Y., Kato, I. *et al.* (1995). Incidence and risk factors of vascular dementia and Alzheimer's disease in a defined elderly Japanese population: the Hisayama Study. *Neurology*, **45**, 1161–8.

Zandi, P.P., Carlson, M.C., Plassman, B.L. *et al.* (2002). Hormone replacement therapy and incidence of Alzheimer disease in older women: the Cache County Study. *Journal of the American Medical Association*, **288**, 2123–9.

Zandi, P.P., Anthony, J.C., Khachaturian, A.S. *et al.* (2004). Reduced risk of Alzheimer disease in users of antioxidant vitamin supplements: the Cache County Study. *Archives of Neurology*, **61**, 82–8.

Zandi, P.P., Sparks, D.L., Khachaturian, A.S. *et al.* (2005). Do statins reduce risk of incident dementia and Alzheimer disease? The Cache County Study. *Archives of General Psychiatry*, **62**, 217–24.

Zhang, M.Y., Katzman, R., Salmon, D. *et al.* (1990). The prevalence of dementia and Alzheimer's disease in Shanghai, China: impact of age, gender, and education. *Annals of Neurology*, **27**, 428–37.

Zhang, Z.X., Zahner, G.E., Roman, G.C. *et al.* (2005). Dementia subtypes in China: prevalence in Beijing, Xian, Shanghai, and Chengdu. *Archives of Neurology*, **62**, 447–53.

Zhu, L., Fratiglioni, L., Guo, Z. *et al.* (2000). Incidence of dementia in relation to stroke and the apolipoprotein E ε4 allele in the very old. Findings from a population-based longitudinal study. *Stroke*, **31**, 53–60.

# 26

# Mild cognitive impairment

John T. O'Brien

## Introduction

Mild cognitive impairment has become a generally accepted term to describe a condition or conditions where subjects have recognizable degrees of objective cognitive impairment which fall short of current standardized definitions for either a dementia syndrome in general or for particular disorders such as Alzheimer's disease, dementia with Lewy bodies, or frontotemporal dementia. However, whether mild cognitive impairment remains a discrete syndrome, part of a continuum with normal ageing, or the early expression of various forms of progressive neurological problems that have yet to manifest themselves fully remains an uncertain and controversial area which is often the subject of heated debate. Whilst some widely accepted definitions of mild cognitive impairment syndromes have emerged, it is important to note that there are as yet no internationally agreed diagnostic criteria, and mild cognitive impairment does not, as yet, appear in international classifications such as DSM-IV (APA, 1994) or ICD-10 (WHO, 1992).

This chapter will summarize some of the key issues surrounding the historical development of mild cognitive impairment, some of the conceptual issues related to the use of the term as a diagnosis, summarize what is known regarding clinical features, pathophysiology, prognosis, and therapeutics, and outline current clinical practice in the area. There are difficulties with terminology in this area, and for the purposes of this chapter mild cognitive impairment(s) will be used when referring to a more general description of mild pre-dementia syndromes and Mild Cognitive Impairment (MCI) when referring to the more specific syndrome described by Petersen and colleagues and detailed below.

## Historical and conceptual development

### Cognitive impairment and normal ageing

An age-related decline in cognitive function has long been recognized and has been demonstrated in several longitudinal studies of ageing. In particular, age-related changes predominantly affect certain cognitive domains or components more than others. For example, at a global cognitive level intelligence is often divided into crystallized intelligence, which represents the accrual of information over time, and fluid intelligence, which reflects the ability to acquire or use new information. Crystallized intelligence, which is measured by tasks involving vocabulary and knowledge-based abilities, tends to be relatively preserved with age. In contrast, fluid intelligence, which is assessed by tasks such as problem solving and speed of performance, tends to show an age-related decline (Schaie, 1989). More discrete cognitive functions such as memory also show specific age-related differences. For example, semantic memory, or memory regarding knowledge of facts about the world, is well preserved with ageing whilst declarative memory (representing the ability to learn new information) tends to decline with age. The rate at which cognition declines with age is highly variable, with some subjects showing little age-related decline and others quite a substantial drop, but with most people showing relatively stable cognitive function until around the age of about 60 (Hertzog and Schaie, 1988).

There continues to be a debate about whether dementia represents a continuum with normal ageing (a case often championed by epidemiologists) or a distinct and separate disease process (Brayne and Calloway, 1988). Where those with mild cognitive impairments should be positioned is clearly inextricably linked with this debate. Since mild cognitive impairment in general, or MCI in particular, represents a state which falls short of dementia, in the continuum model it would simply be viewed as a milder degree of cognitive and functional disturbance than dementia, and would remain on a continuum with both 'normal' age-related changes and with dementia. However, even if one accepts that dementia is a distinct disease from normal ageing, this still leaves the status of MCI unclear. In this case, it could either represent part of a continuum with 'normal' ageing (as before), or else be viewed as a separate 'subsyndromal' disorder with discrete clinical features and outcome. The latter is more in keeping with the traditional medical or clinical view, whilst the former is often the conceptual model adopted by those working in the fields of epidemiology and psychology. At the outset it is important to be clear that neither model may be right or wrong, and just as light can be viewed as a particle or a wave, both views of MCI may have validity in certain circumstances. A parallel often used is that of hypertension. Whilst blood pressure is undeniably normally distributed in a population, there are certain cut-offs (with definitions which can change over time in the light of new research evidence) which define a distinct group as 'hypertensive' or 'hypotensive'. Although recognizably part of a continuum, the validity for defining such subgroups at various levels of blood pressure comes from the fact that they have a distinct outcome and prognosis (for example, a certain risk of developing cardiovascular and cerebrovascular disease) and for which certain interventions have proven efficacy in reducing this risk. Similarly, even if one adopts the continuum view of mild cognitive impairment and dementia, there may still be merits in recognizing particular subgroups that are valid in terms of having a particular prognosis and/or therapeutic response.

## Definitions of pre-dementia syndromes

Those who champion the cause of people with mild cognitive impairments as having a separate syndrome refer to its distinct clinical features, outcome, pathophysiology, and therapeutics which are detailed later in this chapter. However, the description and characterization of syndromes of cognitive impairment which fall short of dementia is not new. Definitions of dementia have remained reasonably constant over the last few decades and generally require deficits in memory and one or more other higher cortical functions, together with evidence of decline from pre-morbid functioning which results in impairment in social and/or occupational functioning. The very nature of defining dementia in this way means that there will be those with cognitive difficulties which fall short of this definition, either because their cognitive deficit does not involve memory, because they involve one rather than two cognitive domains, or because cognitive deficits are insufficient to cause social and/or occupational functioning. There have been several attempts over the last 40 years to try to categorize and define such mild cognitive impairments.

One of the earliest attempts to define 'subclinical' cognitive problems was Kral's notion of 'benign senescent forgetfulness' (BSF) (Kral, 1962) which referred to patients in a nursing home setting subjectively complaining of a particular difficulty with recall without clear objective evidence of impairment. Kral was later able to distinguish this group from those with malignant forgetfulness (which would now be called dementia) who did have objective impairment in terms of differences in outcome—the malignant group have a much higher mortality at follow-up. One problem with more widespread investigation or adoption of Kral's concept of BSF was the lack of standardized criteria to define people with the condition. More formal diagnostic criteria for 'age associated memory impairment' (AAMI) were proposed by Crook and colleagues on behalf of the National Institute of Mental Health (Crook *et al.*, 1987). They defined AAMI as changes in older (aged over 50) people comprising subjective complaints of memory loss verified by a decrement of memory of at least one standard deviation below means established for younger adults. By its very definition, referencing memory in older people to that of younger subjects, AAMI sought to capture what many consider to be those with normal age-related changes as having an 'abnormal' syndrome. This over-inclusiveness was one of the main criticisms of AAMI (O'Brien and Levy, 1992), though a second important one, as articulated by Levy (1994) was that there was no reason to consider that cognitive decline in later life should solely be confined to memory. In collaboration with the International Psychogeriatric Association and the World Health Organization, an alternative concept of 'ageing associated cognitive decline' (AACD) was proposed (Levy, 1994) with two main differences from AAMI; firstly, the deficits had to be referenced to norms for older and not younger subjects and, secondly, a wider range of cognitive functions could be affected

including attention, learning, thinking, language, and visuospatial function in addition to memory. As would be expected, AACD targeted a more severe state of impairment within a larger AAMI group (Richards *et al.*, 1999). The concept of 'cognitive impairment no dementia' (CIND) has been developed within the framework of the Canadian Study of Health and Ageing, and describes older people from an epidemiological sample who have a cognitive impairment that falls short of dementia (Graham *et al.*, 1997), which was associated with functional impairment and may represent an underlying physical problem. The concept was to some extent validated by the poor outcome of this group, in terms of a two-fold risk of loss of independence and a three-fold risk of developing dementia at 5-year follow-up (Tuokko *et al.*, 2003).

However, such attempts to categorize disorders of mild cognitive impairment are not reflected in current international classifications systems. For example, in DSM-IV (APA, 1994) the condition of 'age-related cognitive decline' is included in the chapter of 'conditions that may be a focus for clinical attention' rather than the main diagnostic chapters and defines the condition as 'an objectively identified decline in cognitive functioning, consequent to the ageing process, that is within normal limits given the person's age'. It states that the category should only be considered after it has been determined that the cognitive impairment is not attributable to a specific mental disorder. The only other mild cognitive syndrome referred to is 'mild neurocognitive disorder' which refers to an impairment in two or more areas of cognition which is due to a medical disorder. ICD-10 (WHO, 1992) described 'mild cognitive disorder', which refers to a disorder of memory, learning, and concentration often accompanied by mental fatigue; it must be documented by formal neuropsychological testing and can be attributable to cerebral disease or systemic disease.

The more recent, and currently the most widely used, concept of MCI developed from the work of Petersen and colleagues at the Mayo Clinic, who undertook a series of careful longitudinal studies on older people with cognitive problems (Petersen *et al.*, 1999; Petersen, 2004). Although it is apparent that MCI represents yet another in a long line of attempts to define a subclinical cognitive syndrome, it has gained much wider acceptance than previous concepts to the extent that it has recently been the focus of large-scale therapeutic randomized controlled studies. MCI has gained such acceptance largely because of the strength of the evidence base supporting it as a syndrome, which had been lacking for previous concepts which had only rarely been the focus of research attention. For this reason, the rest of the chapter focuses more specifically on MCI.

## Is MCI a discrete syndrome or early dementia?

A separate, though related, conceptual issue to whether or not milder cognitive impairments are part of normal ageing is whether they represent a discrete syndrome (or syndromes) in their own right or whether they should be viewed as an early phase of an underlying (and as yet undiagnosed) progressive dementia. This may seem an obvious and trivial issue, yet it fundamentally affects how one views MCI and strongly influences approaches to diagnosis and management. For example, if MCI is seen as a discrete syndrome then there need to be rigorous attempts to define the syndrome, validate diagnostic criteria for MCI, investigate and determine its neurobiology, and develop appropriate therapeutic strategies to prevent subsequent 'progression' to different forms of dementia.

However, if it is felt to be the early stage in a progressive degenerative process, then the focus should be on trying to establish the nature of that underlying neurological process at the earliest possible opportunity. In this instance, recognizing and managing MCI as a discrete syndrome would potentially be a major obstacle to this process.

## Diagnostic criteria

The original diagnostic criteria were produced by Petersen *et al.* (1999) and focused on what has become know as the amnestic (or memory) form of MCI; they are reproduced in Table 26.1. While these have been widely adopted, there is still no consensus in the field regarding a single set of criteria for MCI, though the broad criteria were recommended for use by an international consensus group (Winblad *et al.*, 2004). The need for a subjective memory complaint has been questioned, for as with dementia there are likely to be subjects who have definite cognitive impairments but do not complain of these. Do such subjects have MCI or not? Similarly, is corroboration by an informant an essential part of diagnosis; if so what happens when there is no informant? To what extent are potential co-morbid conditions that may be associated with cognitive disturbance excluded? What degree of objective memory impairment is necessary, and how is this to be assessed—on one single test, or several; at one single time point, or at two or more? In the literature, most studies on MCI have adopted a cut-off of 1.5 standard deviations or less to define those with MCI. However, as pointed out by Negash *et al.* (2005), most investigators do not appear to realize that this cut-off was not actually the one used by the Mayo group in their original description to define the concept, it merely represented the mean memory impairment which they demonstrated in those defined as MCI. As such, Negash *et al.* (2005) emphasize the importance of assessment of the memory complaint and objective measure of dysfunction in the context of the individual, in other words not just what is statistically less than normal, but what is less than normal performance for the particular individual. This will be particularly important for those of either high or low intelligence or level of education. However, whilst making excellent clinical sense, it could be argued that such a departure from a strict cut-off will represent a further difficulty in reliably applying such criteria in different centres, especially in a research context.

MCI criteria require general cognitive function to be 'essentially' normal. This can allow those with MCI to have minor impairments, but if they had significant impairments in a second cognitive domain then they may well fulfil criteria for dementia. The need for clinical judgement rather than the use of cut-off scores is again highlighted in this regard by the Mayo Clinic group (Negash *et al.*, 2005). Activity of daily living (ADL) performance is generally well preserved, but in a comparison of subjects with MCI compared with older subjects without MCI, minor functional impairments can be demonstrated, albeit falling well short of those seen in people with dementia (Petersen, 2004). The final issue of not being demented hinges also on this assessment of ADL combined with assessment of whether two or more cognitive domains are affected. It is also important to note here that in the assessment of those with MCI and early dementia certain clinical dementia rating scales are often used, such as the Clinical Dementia Rating Scale (CDR) (Hughes *et al.*, 1982). Whilst these scales are helpful, they do not directly map to a diagnosis, which can be a source of confusion. For example, a CDR of 0.5 (labelled in the scale as 'questionable dementia') can be compatible with either the clinical syndrome of MCI or early Alzheimer's disease.

**Table 26.1** Amnestic type of mild cognitive impairment

| |
|---|
| Memory complaint, preferably corroborated by an informant |
| Memory impairment relative to age-matched and education-matched healthy people |
| Essentially preserved general cognitive function |
| Largely intact activities of daily living |
| Not clinically demented |

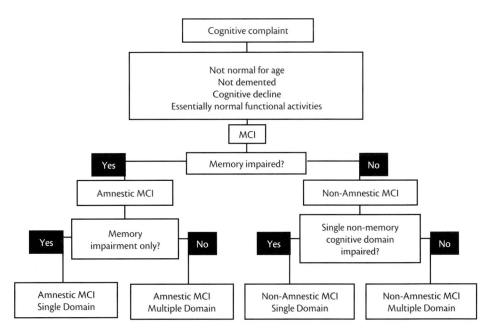

**Fig. 26.1** Criteria for mild cognitive impairment (from Petersen, 2004).

Recognizing that memory is not the only cognitive domain affected in those with mild cognitive impairments, the concept of MCI has more recently been broadened to include other subtypes, particularly 'non-amnestic' MCI (Petersen, 2004; Winblad *et al.*, 2004), in a move reminiscent of the way AAMI broadened out to the AACD concept a decade earlier. In this scheme (Fig. 26.1) MCI is divided into amnestic, where memory is impaired, and non-amnestic, where it is not, and then each subtype is further divided into whether a single or more than one cognitive domain is affected, giving four main types of MCI (amnestic single domain, amnestic multidomain, non-amnestic single domain, non-amnestic multi-domain). The arguments for such subdivision are: (1) this reflects the clinical reality of how patients present; and (2) the clinical syndromes will or may have different outcomes in terms of disease progression. As an approach to diagnosis this is illustrated in Fig. 26.2(a) which illustrates a situation where different clinical syndromes are illustrated as having a distinct courses. As can be seen, whilst amnestic MCI may be particularly helpful in predicting Alzheimer's disease, non-amnestic and non-cognitive types might have less in the way of positive predictive power in that they will potentially represent early stages of a multitude of different underlying pathologies. The extent to which this is true remains uncertain, due to a lack of detailed longitudinal studies involving non-amnestic MCI. However, one may consider other classifications of MCI, such as those based on aetiology. As such, one might consider degenerative MCI as being largely due to early Alzheimer-type pathology and map in most cases to the clinical type of amnestic MCI. Vascular MCI, which has been the subject of relatively little research attention would reflect a pattern of largely attentional and executive impairment with relatively well-preserved memory in the presence of associated cortical and/or subcortical vascular changes on imaging (O'Brien *et al.*, 2003). As such, it would be expected to predominantly manifest as non-amnestic MCI. This different approach to early diagnosis is shown in Fig. 26.2(b). Here different 'prodromal' syndromes representing the early stages of the different underlying pathologies may be defined on a much broader basis than just cognition. So, for example, one might have

a clinical syndrome suggestive of early cerebrovascular cognitive impairment, one suggestive of early frontotemporal disease, and one suggestive of early Lewy body disease. These would then represent the clinical entities which would be of interest for further assessment and follow-up, rather than cognitive-based paradigms. Which of these approaches will ultimately have the greatest clinical utility remains to be seen.

## The validity of MCI as a disorder

Whether a constellation of features describing a syndrome really represent a distinct disorder or not has exercised much of psychiatric nosology over the years, and nowhere is this more pertinent than when discussing MCI. It is generally recognized that a disorder cannot be so classified until it meets certain criteria, such as those laid down by Kendell (1989). These criteria are listed in Table 26.2. MCI fits some of these criteria better than others. A syndrome has been identified, sufficient to be the focus of therapeutic studies, but international consensus on criteria has not been obtained, unlike for the common causes of dementia. Perhaps the weakest point is the establishment of a point of rarity from the related syndromes of dementia or normal ageing, though if dementia can be distinguished from normal ageing using criteria for dementia, then arguably MCI can be distinguished from both by using the appropriate criteria shown in Table 26.1. MCI has been shown to have a distinct course (outlined below) and arguably this represents the strongest

**Table 26.2** Kendell's (1989) criteria for classification as a 'disease'

| |
|---|
| Identification of a particular syndrome (a set of correlated symptoms with a set time course) |
| Demonstration of a point of rarity, or boundary, from related syndromes |
| A distinct course of a treatment or outcome |
| Family or genetic studies, showing that the syndrome 'breeds true' |
| Association with a fundamental underlying abnormality (for example, on laboratory tests) |

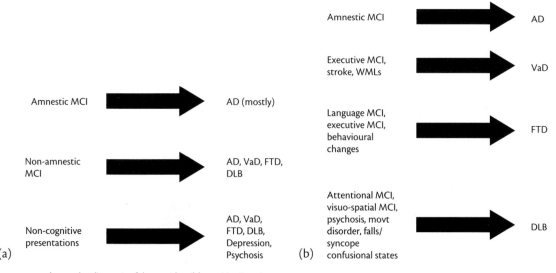

**Fig. 26.2** Different approaches to the diagnosis of those with mild cognitive impairments.

grounds for considering it a separate disorder. Treatment response also appears different from dementia, and whilst a specific abnormality associated with MCI has not been shown, many studies have suggested neurobiological changes, whether at autopsy or in terms of brain imaging, which are different from those seen in normal ageing and dementia. On this basis, Petersen and O'Brien (2006) strongly argue that MCI fulfils criteria for clinical validity to a much greater extent than many currently well-accepted psychiatric disorders, and that there is a compelling case for the inclusion of MCI, especially amnestic MCI, in future classifications such as DSM-V (due in 2012) and ICD-11.

## Reliability and validity of diagnosis

However, despite these arguments, some have cast doubt over the reliability and validity of the syndrome of MCI, largely based on findings from longitudinal population-based epidemiological studies. One difficulty is that the definitions for MCI were developed in a clinic setting and based on a full and detailed psychiatric/neurological examination of individual subjects. As such, direct translation to epidemiological sampling studies is inherently difficult, if not impossible. Most studies have been forced to use a variety of adaptations of the MCI criteria to fit with already existing data sets and have shown a prevalence amongst older people of between 3% and 19%, with incidence of 8–58 per 1000 per year (Gauthier et al., 2006). The risk of developing dementia has varied between 11% and 33% over 2 years, but more importantly findings have demonstrated that up to 50% of those with MCI at a baseline assessment appear to return to normal a year later (Ritchie et al., 2001; Ganguli et al. 2004). Whilst some consider that such studies argue against the validity of the syndrome, others feel this represents the fact that many factors affect cognitive performance in older people apart from underlying brain dysfunction, including education, psychiatric co-morbidity, genetics, hormonal changes, and the use of drugs including anticholinergics. Since many of these factors, and their influence, can change over time it may be why many cases of MCI are reversible in community settings (Gauthier et al., 2006). In contrast, it can be argued that those referred to memory clinics and other specialized centres are unlike the general population in that they are actually seeking services for a perceived memory problem which is likely to have been persistent enough to have prompted referral.

## Clinical features

The primary feature of those with MCI is clearly cognitive impairment, most usually but not always in memory. Petersen et al. (1999) describe that the distinction between control subjects and subjects with MCI was in the area of memory, while other cognitive functions were comparable, though as subjects were defined by having a memory impairment there is considerable circularity here. When the subjects with MCI were compared with the patients with very mild Alzheimer's disease, memory performance was similar, but patients with Alzheimer's disease were more impaired in other cognitive domains as well. Activities of daily living skills and functional abilities are largely intact in MCI subjects, part of the reason that they do not meet criteria for dementia, yet detailed study shows that those with MCI do have significant but mild impairments, especially in instrumental (rather than basic) ADLs

(Petersen, 2004). Neuropsychiatric features have been investigated and are more common in those with MCI than controls. Feldman et al. (2004) studied over 1000 subjects with MCI using the Neuropsychiatric Inventory, finding some neuropsychiatric symptoms in the majority (59%). In a more detailed analysis of a much smaller group of 28 MCI subjects, Hwang et al. (2004) found the most common symptoms in the MCI group were dysphoria (39%), apathy (39%), irritability (29%), and anxiety (25%). There were significant differences in apathy, dysphoria, irritability, anxiety, agitation, and aberrant motor behaviour between the MCI and control groups. In contrast, only delusions were significantly less common in MCI compared with mild Alzheimer's subjects. It is clear that MCI, even though defined cognitively, has more than just cognitive symptoms.

## Pathophysiology

### Neuroimaging changes

Neuroimaging has frequently been used as a tool to investigate brain changes in different dementias, and so has naturally been applied to those with MCI to try to seek and understand what, if any, neurobiological changes can be determined. Structural neuroimaging changes in Alzheimer's disease include generalized brain atrophy with specific involvement of the entorhinal cortex and hippocampus, with increased rates of atrophy on serial imaging. Reduced hippocampal and/or entorhinal cortex volume, together with increased rates of atrophy on serial magnetic resonance (MR), have also been shown to be predictive of the subsequent development of dementia (Rusinek et al., 2003). Since the amnestic form of MCI bears a close relationship to Alzheimer's disease, it might be expected that imaging changes in MCI may be similar to those in Alzheimer's disease. This has indeed been shown to be the case, with people with MCI showing evidence of mild hippocampal atrophy compared with older controls, though not with such severe changes as those with established Alzheimer's disease. Some studies have found that the entorhinal cortex is a better discriminator between those with MCI and normal controls than the hippocampus (Du et al., 2001), whilst others have found both structures to be equally helpful (Xu et al., 2000). Studies investigating other imaging changes, such as MR spectroscopy have also shown changes. Kantarci et al. (2000) found that myoinositol/creatinine ratios were increased in MCI subjects relative to normal controls, and in those with AD relative to those with MCI. However, N-acetylaspartate (NAA)/creatinine ratios did not differ between MCI and controls, but were reduced in AD. Since myoinositol reflects glial activity, it was suggested that this may be a more useful marker earlier in the disease process than NAA which is usually thought to reflect neuronal integrity. Ackl et al. (2005) showed regionally specific spectroscopic changes between MCI and Alzheimer's disease. MCI subjects showed reduced NAA in the hippocampus of both MCI and AD,    parietal reductions only in the AD group. Using a technique allowing whole-brain quantification of NAA, Falini et al. (2005) showed that both structural and metabolic findings of those with MCI were mid-way between those of healthy volunteers and those in established Alzheimer's disease. As such, results of structural and spectroscopic MR studies to date support the view that MCI has neurobiological changes consistent with the transitional state between normal ageing and dementia, in this case Alzheimer's disease.

Similarly, both single photon emission computed tomography (SPECT) and positron emission tomography (PET) studies have generally shown hypoperfusion in those with MCI in areas such as the posterior parietal cortex and posterior cingulate areas which are shown to be affected in early Alzheimer's disease (Chetelat *et al.*, 2005; Pakrasi and O'Brien, 2005). In keeping with the structural imaging findings, functional imaging changes are somewhere between those seen in normal ageing and Alzheimer's disease. Studies of amyloid burden using Pittsburgh compound-B, which have already been undertaken in Alzheimer's disease (Klunk *et al.*, 2004), are ongoing in MCI and results indicate abnormalities in some people with MCI, though whether PET changes accurately predict conversion to dementia is unclear.

## Pathological studies

Detailed pathological studies of large numbers of subjects with MCI prospectively assessed during life are not available. Initial studies on small numbers of subjects have suggested that individuals with MCI show an increased burden of tau pathology in terms of medial temporal lobe tangles (Mitchell *et al.*, 2002) whilst amyloid load in the entorhinal cortex is intermediate between normal subjects and those with Alzheimer's disease (Mufson *et al.*, 1999; Bennett *et al.*, 2002, 2005). Vascular pathology can also be an important cause of cognitive impairments (O'Brien *et al.*, 2003) and Bennett *et al.* (2005) showed that cerebrovascular disease, in addition to neurodegenerative pathology, was associated with MCI in the Nun Study. Lewy body pathology was rarer, but still present in 8% of MCI cases. Others, from an imaging perspective, have also emphasized that vascular changes in the white matter are likely to be an important component of MCI (DeCarli *et al.*, 2001; Medina *et al.*, 2006), though their role and possible interaction with degenerative pathology in the clinical expression of MCI requires further clarification.

## Neurochemistry

A central feature of many dementias, especially Alzheimer's disease and dementia with Lewy bodies, is of a substantial cholinergic deficit. Mufson *et al.* (2002) reported a 38% loss of cholinergic neurons from the nucleus basalis of Meynert in those with MCI, similar to the reduction seen in early Alzheimer's disease (43%). In contrast, DeKosky and colleagues found evidence of increased cholinergic activity, with preserved choline acetyltransferase activity in the hippocampus and frontal cortex of older people with MCI (DeKosky *et al.*, 2002). They suggested that this up-regulation may reflect a compensatory mechanism in the face of declining cognitive ability. This is supported by other work suggesting that cells remaining in the nucleus basalis have enhanced metabolic activity in MCI, but not AD (Dubelaar *et al.*, 2006) and such a compensation has also been seen in some functional MRI (fMRI) studies which have paradoxically shown increased areas of activation in those with MCI compared with both normal controls and those with AD (Dickerson *et al.*, 2005). Studies investigating synaptic proteins have shown some changes which may reflect loss of dendritic plasticity in MCI (Counts *et al.*, 2006). In summary, neurochemical changes suggestive of transmitter and synaptic alterations have been demonstrated in MCI, though unlike the pathological findings in which MCI is a 'halfway' point between normal ageing and Alzheimer's disease, they suggest some degree of compensatory up-regulation, presumably in a attempt to overcome the decline in neuronal functioning consequent on the increased burden of pathology.

## Genetic and other biomarkers

Genetic associations of MCI appear similar to Alzheimer's disease, with increased rates of *APOE* ε4 reported which may predict future cognitive decline (Farlow *et al.*, 2004). Other biomarkers have also been investigated. For example, Alzheimer's disease has been associated with raised levels of tau (especially phosphorylated tau) and reduced levels of β-amyloid in CSF. Several studies have identified similar changes in those with MCI, albeit to a lesser extent than is seen in Alzheimer's disease. In a large and comprehensive study, Hansson *et al.* (2006) showed that MCI cases who had pathological CSF (low levels of β-amyloid and raised levels of total and phosphorylated tau) were at significantly greater risk of progression to Alzheimer's disease. Rates were 27% per year if CSF was abnormal compared to 1% per year if CSF was normal.

# Prognosis

Petersen *et al.* (1999) described the first and still the largest study of approximately 220 people (mean age 79 years) who fulfilled Mayo Clinic criteria for amnestic MCI and were then followed for 3 to 6 years. Subjects progress to dementia at a rate of approximately 12% per year, in contrast to a normal older cohort who develop dementia at a rate of 1–2% per year. Moreover, over the course of 6 years 80% had converted to dementia, suggesting the original MCI group did indeed represent a population at very high risk of subsequent dementia (Negash, 2005). Most subjects developed Alzheimer's disease. In a comprehensive review Bruscoli and Lovestone (2004) identified 19 longitudinal studies of MCI and found an overall rate of conversion of 10% per year, but with large differences between studies. The main factor accounting for the variability was the source of subjects, with self-selected clinic attendees having the highest conversion rate. Within studies they found that poor performance on cognitive testing at baseline predicted conversion with a high degree of accuracy, including that subjective and objective evidence of cognitive decline did predict conversion to dementia, with such subjects forming a good group to select for disease modification studies. As well as a poorer cognitive outcome, MCI is also associated with increasing mortality (Bennett *et al.*, 2002). Overall, therefore, a substantial body of evidence supports MCI as representing a high-risk group of those destined to develop dementia, in particular Alzheimer's disease.

The outcome of non-amnestic forms of MCI has not been well investigated. Within the Canadian Study for Health and Ageing Wentzel *et al.* (2001) followed those with presumed vascular cognitive impairment without dementia (vascular CIND) and found that of 149 participants, 46% developed dementia after 5 years, suggesting that vascular CIND was certainly not a benign condition. Boeve *et al.* (2004) studied 21 cases of dementia with Lewy bodies who had initially presented as MCI. Perhaps surprisingly, ten had originally presented as amnestic MCI, six as single non-memory domain MCI, four with multiple domain MCI with amnesia, and one with multiple domain MCI without amnesia. REM sleep behaviour disorder (RBD) has been described as a predictor of Parkinson's disease and has a strong association with dementia with Lewy bodies. In their sample, 11 MCI cases also had RBD (loss of normal muscle atonia during REM sleep, with patients 'acting out' their dreams and often reported by carers). Of these, ten of the eleven (91%) subsequently developed dementia with

Lewy bodies. Patients with mild cognitive impairments after stroke are also at increased risk of subsequently developing dementia, with rates of 25% at 2 years reported (Altieri *et al.*, 2004). However, improvements are also seen in some subjects (Ballard *et al.*, 2003). The syndrome of mild cognitive impairment of frontotemporal type has been described in a small case series by de Mendonca *et al.* (2004) who found that a combination of clinical features (apathy, disinhibition, irritability), cognitive impairments (in attention, initiation, and conceptual thinking), and neuroimaging (frontal atrophy) predicted six out of seven patients who subsequently developed frontotemporal dementia within a 2-year period. Further work is necessary on the long-term outcome of non-amnestic forms of MCI, though the evidence to date also suggests high rates of conversion to dementia.

## Predictors of conversion to dementia

Several predictors of conversion to dementia in those with MCI have been described, including severity and nature of baseline cognitive performance (particularly impaired episodic recall), older age, possession of particular genotype (*APOE* ε4), presence of functional impairments (Peres *et al.*, 2006), and particular imaging changes including volume loss in the hippocampus and entorhinal cortex (Stoub *et al.*, 2005), increased rates of whole brain atrophy on serial scanning (Jack *et al.*, 2005), and hypometabolism/hypoperfusion on functional imaging (de Leon *et al.*, 2001) as well as the CSF biomarkers referred to earlier. It has been reported that multidomain amnestic MCI has a higher conversion rate (50% over 3 years) than pure amnestic MCI (20%) (Tabert *et al.* 2006). However, all of these predictors, whilst highly significant at a group level, cannot predict with much certainty whether or not an individual with MCI will develop dementia. Until more definitive biological or other predictors can be defined, they are unlikely to be clinically applicable to individual patients though they will remain a keen focus of research attention.

## Therapeutics and management

Clinically, patients with MCI will often have been referred by their GP to old age psychiatry, neurology, or memory clinic services with cognitive problems, with the main question being whether or not they have an early dementia. Clearly, the first step is a full and thorough assessment of the nature of the problem, its duration, extent, and effects on everyday functioning. As with the assessment of those with dementia, a full history from patient and informant as well as mental state, physical, and cognitive examination will be needed together, in most cases, with screening laboratory investigations, including blood tests and often neuroimaging. Common presentations of MCI include those with functional psychiatric illness, particularly depression, which is strongly associated with both subjective memory complaints and objective evidence of impairment (O'Brien *et al.*, 2004), anxiety and stress, concurrent physical ill-health, and concurrent medication. Obviously, if particular causes are found for MCI, then it would then be viewed as secondary (either to psychiatric illness, physical ill-health, or medication) and as with the management of delirium, the primary treatment should be aimed at alleviating the cause of the cognitive impairment. Once these other problems have been excluded, and assuming the person does not meet the criteria for dementia, then if MCI criteria are met then the most clinically pragmatic action is to use this 'label' as a working diagnosis.

Individual clinicians will then vary considerably as to what they tell patients, with some suggesting such cases should be viewed as part of the general population and treated as if they were normal, others that they should be informed they have a mild cognitive problem and that they are at an increased risk of developing dementia in the future. The latter is the standard practice in many old age psychiatry services and memory clinics and information sheets for those with MCI have been developed. Often, such patients are actually very relieved to be told they are not suffering from a dementing illness, though this news has to be tempered with information that they are still at substantially higher risk than the general population of subsequently developing dementia. Often such cases are managed with a combination of information and support, and regular review (for example, annually) which has been suggested as good practice by the American Academy of Neurology (Knopman *et al.*, 2001) and recent NICE guidelines for Dementia (nice.org.uk). Support and memory remediation and training groups for those with MCI and their carers are being developed. Carers of those with MCI may demonstrate caregiver burden (Garand *et al.*, 2005) so, as with people with dementia, may also require particular intervention. There has been much interest in cognitive training, since low educational ability and reduced engagement in mentally stimulating activities has been shown in population studies to be a predictor of subsequent dementia. Cognitive training strategies have been shown to have some benefits with normal older people (Ball *et al.*, 2002) and effects have also been reported in those with MCI, though not yet in randomized controlled trials. Other management strategies for those with MCI are largely based on knowledge of risk factors and consist of treatment of concurrent disorders, control of vascular risk factors, and advice and support regarding cognitive difficulties.

Specific pharmacological therapeutic strategies for MCI are currently lacking as the first wave of clinical studies aimed at symptomatic drug treatment for amnestic MCI have largely been negative. Salloway *et al.* (2004) reported a study of 270 MCI subjects randomized to donepezil or placebo for 42 days. There was no significant different between groups on primary outcome measures, though some of the secondary outcomes tended to favour donepezil. Petersen *et al.* (2005) reported results from the Memory Impairment Study which showed no significant difference in progression from amnestic MCI to Alzheimer's disease in those allocated to vitamin E or donepezil compared to placebo over a 3-year period. Differences in favour of donepezil were reported at 12 months but were non-significant at the main primary endpoint of 3 years. Intriguingly, there was an interaction with genotype in secondary analysis in that *APOE* ε4 carriers, a subgroup, did have a reduced rate of conversion to dementia when treated with donepezil. There have been two studies of galantamine reported in abstract form which have largely been negative in terms of clinical effect, though in one substudy which included serial MRI, galantamine slowed the rate of whole brain atrophy compared to placebo in some subgroups. However, an unexpected finding was of an increased mortality in the galantamine-treated MCI group (though mortality rates in the placebo group were unusually low), leading to a recent Cochrane Review to recommend against prescription of galantamine for those with MCI because of no clear benefit but risk of harm (Loy and Schneider, 2006).

# Conclusion

Despite a large body of research, MCI remains a somewhat difficult and controversial area. The subtype of amnestic MCI is best defined, and represents a clinically important group who are at high risk of progressing to dementia, usually Alzheimer's disease. In terms of clinical application, it is important to remember that the original MCI descriptions, now validated by follow-up studies, were based on the careful clinical assessment of objective cognitive impairment in the individual patient, rather than by rigidly applying a strict cut-off on a cognitive test score. Although the conceptual and nosological status of MCI in general, and particularly non-amnestic forms of MCI, remains to be fully defined, the concept has already proved useful in terms of defining a high-risk population for the future development of dementia and as a target for therapeutic studies. The fact that studies to date have been negative should not deter research for therapies aimed at delaying the onset and/or progression of dementia. Before these are applied to the general population, it is very likely that the first group of subjects to be selected for such studies will be those with MCI, or future refinements of the syndrome.

# References

Ackl, N., Ising, M., Schreiber, Y.A., Atiya, M., Sonntag, A., and Auer, D.P. (2005). Hippocampal metabolic abnormalities in mild cognitive impairment and Alzheimer's disease. *Neuroscience Letters*, **384**, 23–8.

Altieri, M., Di Piero, V., Pasquini, M. *et al.* (2004). Delayed poststroke dementia: a 4-year follow-up study. *Neurology*, **62**, 2193–97.

APA (1994). *Diagnostic and statistical manual of mental disorders*, 4th edn. American Psychiatric Association, Washington, DC.

Ball, K., Berch, D.B., Helmers, K.F. *et al.* (2002). Effects of cognitive training interventions with older adults: a randomized controlled trial. [see comment] *Journal of the American Medical Association*, **288**, 2271–81.

Ballard, C., Rowan, E., Stephens, S., Kalaria, R., and Kenny, R.A. (2003). Prospective follow-up study between 3 and 15 months after stroke: improvements and decline in cognitive function among dementia-free stroke survivors >75 years of age. [see comment] *Stroke*, **34**, 2440–44.

Bennett, D.A., Wilson, R.S., Schneider, J.A. *et al.* (2002). Natural history of mild cognitive impairment in older persons. *Neurology*, **59**, 198–205.

Bennett, D.A., Schneider, J.A, Bienias, J.L., Evans, D.A., and Wilson, R.S. (2005). Mild cognitive impairment is related to Alzheimer disease pathology and cerebral infarctions. *Neurology*, **64**, 834–41.

Boeve, B.F., Ferman, T.J., Smith, G.E. *et al.* (2004). Mild cognitive impairment preceding dementia with Lewy bodies. *Neurology*, **62**, A86–A87.

Brayne, C. and Calloway, P. (1988). Normal ageing, impaired cognitive function, and senile dementia of the Alzheimer's type: a continuum? *Lancet*, **1**, 1265–7.

Bruscoli, M. and Lovestone, S. (2004). Is MCI really just early dementia? A systematic review of conversion studies. *International Psychogeriatrics*, **16**, 129–40.

Chetelat, G., Eustache, F., Viader, F. *et al.* (2005). FDG-PET measurement is more accurate than neuropsychological assessments to predict global cognitive deterioration in patients with mild cognitive impairment. *Neurocase*, **11**, 14–25.

Counts, S.E., Nadeem, M., Lad, S.P., Wuu, J., and Mufson, E.J. (2006). Differential expression of synaptic proteins in the frontal and temporal cortex of elderly subjects with mild cognitive impairment. *Journal of Neuropathology and Experimental Neurology*, **65**, 592–601.

Crook, T., Bahar, H., and Sudilovsky, A. (1987). Age-associated memory impairment: diagnostic criteria and treatment strategies. *International Journal of Neurology*, **21–22**, 73–82.

de Leon, M.J., Convit, A., Wolf, O.T. *et al.* (2001). Prediction of cognitive decline in normal elderly subjects with 2-[(18)F]fluoro-2-deoxy-D-glucose/poitron-emission tomography (FDG/PET). *Proceedings of the National Academy of Sciences of the USA*, **98**, 10966–71.

de Mendonca, A., Ribeiro, F., Guerreiro, M., and Garcia, C. (2004). Frontotemporal mild cognitive impairment. *Journal of Alzheimer's Disease*, **6**, 1–9.

DeCarli, C., Miller, B.L., Swan, G.E., Reed, T., Wolf, P.A., and Carmelli, D. (2001). Cerebrovascular and brain morphologic correlates of mild cognitive impairment in the National Heart, Lung, and Blood Institute Twin Study. *Archives of Neurology*, **58**, 643–7.

DeKosky, S.T., Ikonomovic, M.D., Styren, S.D. *et al.* (2002). Upregulation of choline acetyltransferase activity in hippocampus and frontal cortex of elderly subjects with mild cognitive impairment. [comment] *Annals of Neurology*, **51**, 145–55.

Dickerson, B.C., Salat, D.H., Greve, D.N. *et al.* (2005). Increased hippocampal activation in mild cognitive impairment compared to normal aging and AD. *Neurology*, **65**, 404–11.

Du, A.T., Schuff, N., Amend, D. *et al.* (2001). Magnetic resonance imaging of the entorhinal cortex and hippocampus in mild cognitive impairment and Alzheimer's disease. *Journal of Neurology, Neurosurgery and Psychiatry*, **71**, 441–7.

Dubelaar, E.J., Mufson, E.J., ter Meulen, W.G., Van Heerikhuize, J.J., Verwer, R.W., and Swaab, D.F. (2006). Increased metabolic activity in nucleus basalis of Meynert neurons in elderly individuals with mild cognitive impairment as indicated by the size of the Golgi apparatus. *Journal of Neuropathology and Experimental Neurology*, **65**, 257–66.

Falini, A., Bozzali, M., Magnani, G. *et al.* (2005). A whole brain MR spectroscopy study from patients with Alzheimer's disease and mild cognitive impairment. *Neuroimage*, **26**, 1159–63.

Farlow, M.R., He, Y., Tekin, S., Xu, J., Lane, R., and Charles, H.C. (2004). Impact of APOE in mild cognitive impairment. *Neurology*, **63**, 1898–901.

Feldman, H., Scheltens, P., Scarpini, E. *et al.* (2004). Behavioral symptoms in mild cognitive impairment. *Neurology*, **62**, 1199–201. [Erratum appears in *Neurology*, 2004, **63**(4), 764.]

Ganguli, M., Dodge, H.H., Shen, C., and DeKosky, S.T. (2004). Mild cognitive impairment, amnestic type: an epidemiologic study. *Neurology*, **63**, 115–21.

Garand, L., Dew, M.A., Eazor, L.R., DeKosky, S.T., and Reynolds, C.F., 3rd (2005). Caregiving burden and psychiatric morbidity in spouses of persons with mild cognitive impairment. *International Journal of Geriatric Psychiatry*, **20**, 512–22.

Gauthier, S., Reisberg, B., Zaudig, M. *et al.* (2006). Mild cognitive impairment. *Lancet*, **367**, 1262–70.

Graham, J.E., Rockwood, K., Beattie, B.L. *et al.* (1997). Prevalence and severity of cognitive impairment with and without dementia in an elderly population. *Lancet*, **349**, 1793–6.

Hansson, O., Zetterberg, H., Buchhave, P., Londos, E., Blennow, K., and Minthon, L. (2006). Association between CSF biomarkers and incipient Alzheimer's disease in patients with mild cognitive impairment: a follow-up study. *Lancet Neurology*, **5**, 228–34.

Hertzog, C. and Schaie, K.W. (1988). Stability and change in adult intelligence: 2. Simultaneous analysis of longitudinal means and covariance structures. *Psychology and Aging*, **3**, 122–30.

Hughes, C.P., Berg, L., Danziger, W.L., Coben, L.A., and Martin, R.L. (1982). A new clinical scale for the staging of dementia. *British Journal of Psychiatry*, **140**, 566–72.

Hwang, T.J., Masterman, D.L., Ortiz, F., Fairbanks, L.A., and Cummings, J.L. (2004). Mild cognitive impairment is associated with characteristic neuropsychiatric symptoms. *Alzheimer Disease and Associated Disorders*, **18**, 17–21.

Jack, C.R., Jr, Shiung, M.M., Weigand, S.D. *et al.* (2005). Brain atrophy rates predict subsequent clinical conversion in normal elderly and amnestic MCI. *Neurology*, **65**, 1227–31.

Kantarci, K., Jack, C.R., Jr, Xu, Y.C. *et al.* (2000). Regional metabolic patterns in mild cognitive impairment and Alzheimer's disease: A 1H MRS study. *Neurology*, **55**, 210–17.

Kendell, R.E. (1989). Clinical validity. *Psychological Medicine*, **19**, 45–55.

Klunk, W.E., Engler, H., Nordberg, A. *et al.* (2004). Imaging brain amyloid in Alzheimer's disease with Pittsburgh Compound-B. *Annals of Neurology*, **55**, 306–19.

Knopman, D.S., DeKosky, S.T., Cummings, J.L. *et al.* (2001). Practice parameter: diagnosis of dementia (an evidence-based review). Report of the Quality Standards Subcommittee of the American Academy of Neurology. [see comment] *Neurology*, **56**, 1143–53.

Kral, V. (1962). Senescent forgetfulness: benign and malignant. *Canadian Medical Association Journal*, **86**, 257–60.

Levy, R. (1994). Aging-associated cognitive decline. *International Psychogeriatrics*, **6**, 63–8.

Loy, C. and Schneider, L. (2006). Galantamine for Alzheimer's disease and mild cognitive impairment. *Cochrane Database of Systematic Reviews* 2006, Issue 1, Art. No. CD001747. DOI: 10.1002/14651858. CD001747.pub3.

Medina, D., DeToledo-Morrell, L., Urresta, F. *et al.* (2006). White matter changes in mild cognitive impairment and AD: A diffusion tensor imaging study. *Neurobiology of Aging*, **27**, 663–72.

Mitchell, T.W., Mufson, E.J., Schneider, J.A. *et al.* (2002). Parahippocampal tau pathology in healthy aging, mild cognitive impairment, and early Alzheimer's disease. *Annals of Neurology*, **51**, 182–9.

Mufson, E.J., Chen, E.Y., Cochran, E.J., Beckett, L.A., Bennett, D.A., and Kordower, J.H. (1999). Entorhinal cortex beta-amyloid load in individuals with mild cognitive impairment. *Experimental Neurology*, **158**, 469–90.

Mufson, E.J., Ma, S.Y., Dills, J. *et al.* (2002). Loss of basal forebrain P75(NTR) immunoreactivity in subjects with mild cognitive impairment and Alzheimer's disease. *Journal of Comparative Neurology*, **443**, 136–53.

Negash, S., Geda, Y.E., and Petersen, R.C. (2005) In *Dementia* (ed. A. Burns, J.T. O'Brien, and D. Ames), pp. 338–46. Hodder, London.

O'Brien, J.T. and Levy, R. (1992). Age associated memory impairment. *British Medical Journal*, **304**, 5–6.

O'Brien, J.T., Erkinjuntti, T., Reisberg, B. *et al.* (2003). Vascular cognitive impairment. *Lancet. Neurology*, **2**, 89–98.

O'Brien, J.T., Lloyd, A., McKeith, I., Gholkar, A., and Ferrier, N. (2004). A longitudinal study of hippocampal volume, cortisol levels, and cognition in older depressed subjects. *American Journal of Psychiatry*, **161**, 2081–90.

Pakrasi, S. and O'Brien, J.T. (2005). Emission tomography in dementia. *Nuclear Medicine Communications*, **26**, 189–96.

Peres, K., Chrysostome, V., Fabrigoule, C., Orgogozo, J.M., Dartigues, J.F., and Barberger-Gateau, P. (2006). Restriction in complex activities of daily living in MCI: impact on outcome. *Neurology*, **67**, 461–6.

Petersen, R.C. (2004). Mild cognitive impairment as a diagnostic entity. *Journal of Internal Medicine*, **256**, 183–94.

Petersen, R.C. and O'Brien, J.T. (2006). Mild cognitive impairment should be considered for DSM-V. *Journal of Geriatric Psychiatry and Neurology*, **19**(3), 147–54.

Petersen, R.C., Smith, G.E., Waring, S.C., Ivnik, R.J., Tangalos, E.G., and Kokmen, E. (1999). Mild cognitive impairment: clinical characterization and outcome. *Archives of Neurology*, **56**, 303–8.

Petersen, R.C., Thomas, R.G., Grundman, M. *et al.* (2005). Vitamin E and donepezil for the treatment of mild cognitive impairment. *New England Journal of Medicine*, **352**, 2379–88.

Richards, M., Touchon, J., Ledesert, B., and Richie, K. (1999). Cognitive decline in ageing: are AAMI and AACD distinct entities? *International Journal of Geriatric Psychiatry*, **14**, 534–40.

Ritchie, K., Artero, S., and Touchon, J. (2001). Classification criteria for mild cognitive impairment: a population-based validation study. *Neurology*, **56**, 37–42.

Rusinek, H., De Santi, S., Frid, D. *et al.* (2003). Regional brain atrophy rate predicts future cognitive decline: 6-year longitudinal MR imaging study of normal aging. *Radiology*, **229**, 691–6.

Salloway, S., Ferris, S., Kluger, A. *et al.* (2004). Efficacy of donepezil in mild cognitive impairment: a randomized placebo-controlled trial. *Neurology*, **63**, 651–7.

Schaie, K.W. (1989). Perceptual speed in adulthood: cross-sectional and longitudinal studies. *Psychology and Aging*, **4**, 443–53.

Stoub, T.R., Bulgakova, M., Leurgans, S. *et al.* (2005). MRI predictors of risk of incident Alzheimer disease: a longitudinal study. *Neurology*, **64**, 1520–4.

Tabert, M.H., Manly, J.J., Liu, X. *et al.* (2006). Neuropsychological prediction of conversion to Alzheimer disease in patients with mild cognitive impairment. *Archives of General Psychiatry*, **63**, 916–24.

Tuokko, H., Frerichs, R., Graham, J. *et al.* (2003). Five-year follow-up of cognitive impairment with no dementia. *Archives of Neurology*, **60**, 577–82.

Wentzel, C., Rockwood, K., MacKnight, C. *et al.* (2001). Progression of impairment in patients with vascular cognitive impairment without dementia. *Neurology*, **57**, 714–16.

WHO (1992). The ICD-10 classification of mental and behavioural disorders. World Health Organization, Geneva.

Winblad, B., Palmer, K., Kivipelto, M. *et al.* (2004). Mild cognitive impairment – beyond controversies, towards a consensus: report of the International Working Group on Mild Cognitive Impairment. *Journal of Internal Medicine*, **256**, 240–6.

Xu, Y., Jack, C.R., Jr, O'Brien, P.C. *et al.* (2000). Usefulness of MRI measures of entorhinal cortex versus hippocampus in AD. *Neurology*, **54**, 1760–7.

# Clinical aspects of dementia: living with dementia

Peter J. S. Ashley

## Introduction

D-Day (dementia-day) came at the start of the 21st century; at least for me—25 July 2000 to be precise. But the run up to D-Day started in 1997—let me explain.

In 1997, as a hardworking Group Technical Director of a computer graphics and media company, the time had come for my wife (Ann) and I to take our annual holiday. As was our practice each year we set aside 14 days for relaxation in the 'luxury' of a five-star hotel with warm weather, sand, and sea, on this occasion, in the Dominican Republic. Little did we realize that this was to be our last real holiday. My only memory of the holiday was of the third day when exhausted, delirious, semiconscious, and hallucinating I was confined to bed. My wife tells me that the local hotel doctor failed to diagnose the cause of my problems through lack of knowledge and local hospital support facilities.

Having spent the rest of the holiday in bed my wife managed to get me back home. My GP organized admission to the infectious diseases unit at a hospital in Liverpool[1] leading eventually to a diagnosis of Legionnaires' disease. With severe pneumonia and liver failure, and of course Legionnaires' disease (which wasn't diagnosed at that time), the hospital staff worked tirelessly to ensure that I made it. When eventually the laboratory tests came through I was on the road to what I thought was recovery but which in the event proved to be quite the opposite.

Discharge for anticipated convalescence took place to my home and into the care of my wife, only to be followed by a period of chronic fatigue and depression. Months passed during which both my physical and mental condition worsened and in spite of many outpatient visits to see my consultants in Liverpool, no explanation could be found for my continued deterioration in health.

My GP suggested trying an SSRI to combat my increasing depression. Fortunately my next-door neighbour, a senior consultant psychiatrist, suggested a referral to our large local Mental Health Trust hospital[2] where it was later proposed that I enter as an inpatient initially for a period of a few weeks, but which on and off turned out to be most of 1998 and 1999.

During this period numerous tests were made and therapies tried including a wide spectrum of drugs and seven sessions of ECT. Weekends at home took place occasionally and it was during one such weekend that I tried quite seriously to take my own life; something I was to repeat later that year but less seriously, more as a desperate cry for help. Clearly the general hospital accident and emergency department had to work hard on the first occasion to ensure my survival but minimal support was necessary on the second.

My treatment continued both as an inpatient and outpatient at the mental health hospital. Whilst at home one evening I complained of pains in my arms and chest which, after having been 'blue lighted' to hospital by ambulance, turned out to be a full blown heart attack. Again medical teams came to my rescue but I was left with the possibility of surgery (although my consultant cardiologist subsequently decided against this)—I continued to suffer from angina.

I was to have another severe cardiac incident on millennium eve, 31 December 1999. When reminded of this I can visualize myself with others in the cardiac ward all with oxygen masks strapped to our faces—amusing now with hindsight but a pitiful sight at the time.

As my apparent mental condition was getting no better, memory, particularly short term, was bad and I was still having visual and occasional auditory hallucinations; in spring 2000 my consultant psychiatrist decided to refer me to the Neurological Department of Manchester Royal Infirmary Trust to see a professor of neurology and his research team.

What followed is a series of events over a 3-month period which led up to D-Day!

Extensive cognitive evaluation was undertaken by the team headed by a consultant physiologist which in itself proved quite exhausting—physical testing and a broad battery of blood testing, EEGs under varying conditions, MRI and SPECT scans, and then on subsequent visits these were repeated.

On 25 July 2000 an early morning visit had been arranged at the request of a senior consultant. After the usual opening informalities the consultant said in as sympathetic way as is possible, addressing both myself and my wife, 'Mr Ashley do you wish me to tell you our conclusions?'. 'Yes' said I, 'please be absolutely open with us'. 'Mr Ashley you have Lewy body syndrome.' 'Do you mean dementia?' was my reply. 'Yes; we call it DLB, Dementia with Lewy Bodies'.

---

[1] http://www.rlbuht.nhs.uk/content/default.asp?web=228&sub=446&page=1270 formally prior to 2001 at Aintree.

[2] http://www.5boroughspartnership.nhs.uk/ formally Warrington Community Care Mental Health Trust.

We then had a very unemotional conversation, were taken through all the test results including the MRI and SPECT scans, asked if we had any other questions, and a follow-up appointment was finally set up.

## Living with dementia

After leaving the consulting rooms my wife and I stopped in the hospital café had a cup of tea and then drove home numb with shock. It wasn't until the late afternoon whilst sitting out on our patio that the full force of the diagnosis hit home. We cried with each other for hours and in the ensuing days we started to come to terms with the diagnosis which, on reflection, we'd half expected as the investigations proceeded. I had a terminal illness with unbelievable consequences not only for me but for my wife and family.

Words just cannot explain the mental 'contortions' we both went through during the following days. From being a person with a high level of intelligence, having a responsible job from which I had to retire prematurely some years previously when originally diagnosed with some form of mental illness, to becoming someone who was to turn into a 'vegetable'. Needing a wife who would have to increasingly dedicate much of her time to my welfare. The realization of the total impact this would have on those plans we had for the future and a happy retirement. The enormous effect it would have on our three daughters and their families. Our friends, how would they react; would we have time for them or would they have time for us?

More than anything, what was DLB how would it develop, and over what time duration? Who was available to advise and help; it clearly wasn't just a medical problem, it had social consequences as well. Our 40 years of married life would now be under great strain. How could we continue to demonstrate our continuing love for each other—would it survive the strain?

And then there were our grandchildren; I wouldn't see them growing up—I most probably wouldn't recognize them. What would they think of a grandfather who was unable to show them signs of affection and love?

Days turned into weeks, weeks into months in this tortuous hell of mourning.

In the meantime my consultants were taking a different view, looking at ways by which some type of respite could be achieved. According to NHS policy the family of the three cholinesterase drugs which were available were only available to those diagnosed with Alzheimer's disease not 'other dementias' of which DLB was one. With tremendous efforts on their part they were able, after 3 months, to get me on a trial of rivastigmine (Exelon), and it became evident to me that the greatest benefit could be obtained from the maximum dose of 12 mg daily. I was once again admitted to mental health hospital to be 'weaned' on to the medication. Three milligrams at first to ensure that I could tolerate the potential side-effects of nausea and stomach problems. Whilst some occurred, I was determined that the process continue, so the next highest dose was tried. With increased tolerance as time went by, the dosage progression continued at home until, after 3 months, I was on the maximum dose with no side-effects at all.

It was now 6 months after D-Day and my whole attitude changed, virtually overnight: my depression lifted greatly; I could think positively instead of negatively; I would talk quite openly to others about my condition; and if stigma surrounded mental illness or more particularly dementia, I would have none of it. Rivastigmine was no doubt just starting to have some effect but the whole process whereby other people, especially the medical profession, rallied round to fight my cause was the major catalyst in what I believe to be a minor miracle. As I've often said in subsequent presentations, I refer to this as my 'Resurrection'.

I am not saying all was suddenly well. My short-term memory had become markedly worse, hallucinations were with me most of the time, tremor was becoming a major problem, I was losing the ability to coordinate some of my basic motor functions. From being a reasonable pianist and organist I was barely able to play a tune on the piano with one finger let alone 'ten'; my writing was becoming poor but my power to think logically and to reason let alone articulate my thoughts was still as good as ever.

I was determined to put those working skills to the test and this I started with a vengeance in about January 2001.

From being the technical director of a company which produced graphic computer and communication systems which had, to a great extent, pre-dated the arrival of the Internet, I was able to use the developing web to my advantage.

I used the Internet to thoroughly seek for information on dementia and especially DLB. I looked up, and made contact with, some of the country's leading experts in the field and wrote to them. I investigated areas of support both for both myself and my wife who was obviously my major carer (care partner) and undertook various other activities which I will now cover in more detail.

During this research I came across the UK Alzheimer's Society (http://www.alzheimers.org.uk) and joined as a member in 2001. This provided access to a wide range of information and facilities and with the encouragement of Harry Cayton (the then Chief Executive, later the National Director for Patients and the Public, Department of Health) and the late Brian Roycroft, the Chairman, I agreed that my name be put forward for nomination as a Trustee of the Society. Following my formal appointment at the annual general meeting I took my place on the Council, and turned out to be the first person with dementia in the world to be appointed to a society/association's governing body.

This success was to spur me on; to increase my feeling of worth and to act as a counter to the disease. I shouldn't minimize the problems that arose, mobility was poor; however, my wife was able to help with this. My short-term memory was bad and with increasing parkinsonian-like tremors, writing was now virtually impossible. However, with my technical background I was able to identify a voice recorder[3] which would record for 22 hours with an excellent sound sensitivity. This machine has become an absolute lifeline to me as I record every meeting, conference, and important conversation, later transferring the resulting files onto my computer, and I have an indexed memory of nearly everything that takes place in my daily life. There's not a day goes by when I don't use the machine, and I'd go so far as saying it's better than relying on one's 'normal' memory. Whilst a pair of Duracell® AAA batteries supposedly last 660 hours, I must have become one of their best customers for the supply of this product.

The use of computers might have become a problem, but again, using my technical skills and harnessing appropriate software

---

3  Olympus DM1 http://www.olympus.co.uk/consumer/2581_DM-1.htm

products, this has been minimized. Whilst my keyboard skills are poor, with the aid of software such as voice recognition[4] I'm able to cope.

At the time of writing this chapter I have two workstations networked together, one laptop linked by wireless, one PDA also linked by wireless, my voice recording system, and two mobile telephones linked into everything. Not forgetting my home telephone system from which I can also record conversations.

Membership of the UK Alzheimer's Society provided a wide range of opportunities both to learn more about my condition, the subject of dementia in general, and to broaden my network of contacts not only with others having similar conditions to my own, but with professionals.

I was asked first by branches of the Society to talk to members about 'Living with Dementia'[5], this broadened as time went by to include presentations on radio[6] and later on promotional videos.

Through the Society I became aware of the work of Alzheimer Europe (http://www.alzheimer-europe.org) and Alzheimer's Disease International (ADI; http://www.alz.co.uk) and was asked to give plenary presentations at their conferences in Maastricht and Barcelona[7] respectively. Since that time I've given plenary or workshop presentations at most of their conferences. One notable exception being the ADI Conference in the Dominican Republic where, for obvious reasons, I was somewhat reluctant to return. I must stress, however, that valiant work is being untaken in that country in support of people with dementia and their carers, headed by Dr Daisy Acosta and others.[8]

Various professional bodies had expressed interest in the work I was doing and I was asked by all three manufacturers of the cholinesterase drugs to give presentations to their members of staff and client groups comprising leading consultants. This occurred both in the UK and in Ireland.

In 2002 I was approached by Alzheimer Ireland (http://www.alzheimer.ie) (I have since become a member) to undertake a series of lectures throughout their country, and also to give interviews on radio and TV. Notable among these was an appearance on the RTE 'Late, Late Show' a chat-show screened throughout the whole of Ireland, with a large viewing audience.

I was particularly honoured to be invited to address the International Psychogeriatric Association (IPA; http://www.ipa-online.org) and be their guest, together with my wife, at their annual conference in Budapest where I had the opportunity of meeting some of the world's leading experts in the field of dementia; people who have enabled me to understand more fully my own condition and that of others. Real friendships were established and have been maintained to the present day.

We learn from each other for, as I say, those of us with dementia are the real experts, *we see the world from the inside out whilst the professionals only see our world from the outside in*. We need each other, for without the ongoing research into the genesis of the condition, no progress can be made. However, those of us who are able

to explain our innermost feelings with a dementia condition, can only aid the progress of finding solutions for treatment and, eventually, one hopes, some form of cure.

I had established in my mind that the '*use it or lose it*' philosophy had merit, and in 2002 the opportunity arose for people to apply to become non-executive directors of various NHS Trusts. For some time I'd followed the fortunes of the Mental Health Trust where I was treated, and so decided to apply for such a position, as the Trust was about to extend over five areas instead of the one. As a backstop I also applied for a similar position with our local Primary Care Trust. Much to my surprise I was short-listed for both and, whilst it wasn't mandatory or even ethical to ask an applicant to declare his medical condition, the Mental Health Trust was bound to know; although clearly this hadn't featured in their considerations to short-list.

Interviews took place, and at each I formally declared on a voluntary basis my medical condition. I was given a fair hearing but after a short time had elapsed I was contacted by the chairman of the new Mental Health Trust and told that I had not been successful because only one non-executive was being appointed from my area, but not to be dejected as I might be getting some positive news from the Primary Care Trust (PCT).

On 1 April 2002 I became a non-executive director (NED) of Warrington Primary Care Trust[9] and served successfully in that capacity for 4½ years until September 2006 when a major reorganization of PCTs took place.

Warrington PCT remained in being as it was within a unitary authority, and I, along with the Chairman and all six NEDs, applied for reappointment; only two of the original NEDs were re-elected.

I, along with many other Chairs and NEDs have complained that the re-election process was not even handed and was politically motivated—our voices have been ignored.[10]

The NHS is becoming a disaster area, with mental health a major victim. Politicians will naturally argue otherwise, but those of us in the front line, and particularly patients, know otherwise.

During the past 5 years (7 years since diagnosis) I have been privileged to sit on various Department of Health and NHS Boards and groups where I hope to have made a contribution towards better conditions for people with mental health problems and more particularly dementia. I name a few, some of which are still active:

- the working group on patient choice
- the National Diagnostics Leadership Board
- the ministerial advice board (former minister John Hutton) on the National Programme for Information Technology (NPfIT) (now Connecting for Health, CfH)
- Electronic Social Care Records Implementation Board (ESCR)
- Care Services Improvement Partnership (CSIP) (northwest), Co-Chair Mental Health and Older People's Board
- Royal College of Psychiatrists working group on dementia
- National Institute for Health and Clinical Excellence (NICE)/ Social Care Institute for Excellence (SCIE) dementia guideline development group, etc.

[4] IBM ViaVoice Version 10 http://www-306.ibm.com/software/voice/viavoice/

[5] A title I generally adopted to describe my presentations.

[6] Peter White interviews on BBC Radio 4 'You and yours'.

[7] Web cast can be found at http://webcasts.prous.com/alzheimer2002/program.asp

[8] http://www.alzheimer.com.do/index.htm

[9] http://www.warrington-health.nhs.uk/

[10] http://www.hsj.co.uk/healthservicejournal/Login.do (you will need to set up a password to access this).

I am particularly proud of the work we have done in drawing up what we all believe to be the definitive guideline for dementia[11] in the UK; a model which will be copied elsewhere in the world.

The guideline group was the first of its kind co-sponsored by both health and social care which is so appropriate in the management of dementia.

The group comprised 28 members:

◆ professors or other medical professionals, 11

◆ professors or other social care professionals, 5

◆ professionals from the National Collaborating Centre for Mental Health and Health Economists, 9

◆ carers, 2

◆ person with dementia (myself), 1.

Over 2½ years the group worked hard to produce a series of documents and associated tools which can be best summarized by the main subheading to the full (391-page) guideline:

Dementia–The NICE-SCIE guideline on supporting people with dementia and their carers in health and social care.

I would certainly recommend readers of this chapter to read the full guideline or, if that is not possible, some or all of the related publications:

◆ Dementia: quick reference guide

◆ Dementia: understanding NICE guidance

◆ Dementia: implementation advice

◆ Dementia: costing report

◆ Dementia: costing template

◆ Dementia: supplementary costing report and template

◆ Dementia: audit criteria

◆ Dementia: presenter slides

## Important notes

At the start of this chapter I made reference to the fact that the cholinesterase drugs weren't generally available for those with dementia other than Alzheimer's—this is still the case and I understand this will not be reviewed by the NICE Technical Appraisals Committee before 2008.

Just prior to the completion of the Dementia Guideline the NICE Technical Appraisals Committee reviewed the availability of cholinesterase drugs for Alzheimer's and after several appeals ruled that now only limited availability would be given to those a with moderate or moderate to severe diagnosis (Mini-Mental State Examination ≤ 20 or ≥10).[12] The drug memantine was also included in this appraisal.

NICE required the Dementia Guideline Development Group to include this in their guideline. The majority of the guideline members were opposed to this but as they felt it would be a waste of all the other good work contained therein, we had reluctantly to agree.

Back in 2001 Dr Nori Graham (now Honorary President of ADI) suggested that I might be interest in joining a then embryonic Internet organization called DASN (Dementia Advocacy and Support Network). The intention was that people anywhere within the world with a diagnosis of early stage dementia could offer mutual support via a bulletin board communication network running under Yahoo[13] and also via an associated website;[14] the name was subsequently changed to DASNI to reflect its international membership, and in recent years carers have also been given the opportunity of joining.

The current membership is some 300 and I, along with others, run a small board of management or directors. In addition to the bulletin board and the website we have chat-rooms (text only) staged at various times each day hosted by one of our members. Some of us, with appropriate facilities, also operate one-to-one voice conferences over Sky.Pe.[15] The membership is predominantly North American but there are members in many other countries; the current President is Australian and the former one Canadian. DASNI has formed a close association with ADI and from time to time its members give joint presentations.

With the aggressive nature of most dementias, interplay between members can get quite volatile at times, but the entire organization is mastering its problems and is now set to grow from strength to strength.

A new planned organization is under early discussion by the management board whereby stronger links will be forged with likeminded bodies in different countries, but this has yet to be finalized.

Since my diagnosis in 2000 (D-Day) I have preached that people with dementia need to be empowered to run their lives for as long as they are able. We cannot quantify the value that we place upon our carers and care partners, nor the professionals who minister to our every need but our *independence must not be taken away from us too soon*.

The following are the words of an American friend of mine, Dr Richard Taylor, diagnosed with early stage dementia, most likely to be Alzheimer's disease, and a member of DASNI. They encapsulate some of the thoughts that pass through his mind and which are shared by many of us. Richard's words are quoted verbatim and with his full permission:

Tell me Richard: do you want us to pull you out of bed, strip off your clothes, drag you down the hall, and force you in the shower …or do you want to get up, take off your own clothes, walk down the hall and let us help you take a shower? But what if I don't want to take a shower because I don't think I need one? What if I'm afraid and don't want strangers to touch me or see me naked and why can't I tell you this?

Do you want to eat breakfast at 7:00 a.m. or 9:00 a.m.? But what if I don't like to eat breakfast, period?

Do you want to walk down the hall now or when I can find time later on today? But of course you must walk down the hall before the end of my shift. But what if I don't feel like walking now and I don't want

---

[11]  NICE/SCIE Dementia Guideline: http://www.nice.org.uk/guidance/cg42

[12]  http://www.nice.org.uk/guidance/TA111

[13]  http://health.groups.yahoo.com/group/DASN/

[14]  http://www.dasninternational.org/

[15]  http://www.skype.com/

to give up the basic right of walking down the hall when and if I want to, whenever I want to? Richard, do you want to live at home and run the risk of falling down and probably starving to death on the bathroom floor, or do you want to move into nursing home? But what if I don't fall down and I am afraid of nursing homes? Do you want to visit with your grand-daughter with me always in the room watching, or do you want to not see her? But what if I love my grand daughter but you always butt in when I am playing with her? But what if this makes me feel like a prisoner in a sexual predator prison?

Do you want to buy this pair of underwear or that pair of underwear—you have a choice. But what if I don't want to wear underwear? What if I don't want to wear a bra? What if I don't want to dress like you or like I did a couple of years ago?

The more you are like me the fewer choices you get!

That's the rule in our culture. Even if tragically you don't even know it yourself, you need to be fixed, confined, cared for, protected, and taken care of.

What about my feelings of being restricted, treated as a child, demeaned, frustrated, entrapped? Nonsense, you are just paranoid.

Even near death, even in death I am a full and whole person. I am not ¾ of a person, ½ of a person or ¼ of person, 1/73rd of a person. Every moment of my life I am a whole person. Why do individuals younger than me constantly use themselves as the reference point for what is a whole person and what is a damaged person, a disabled person, a person who has stopped evolving as a human being and started to deteriorate as a human being, someone who is less and less and less and less than complete as a human being? Someone who wants and needs to be fixed so they can be more like their caretakers? Why don't people appreciate the fact I am still one of them! Just not exactly like one of them—slightly different but basically the same.

Because they don't know what it is like to be me? Mostly they don't want to know until it happens to them. What about the professionals who serve people with dementia, old-old people, people with cognitive disorders, people who are not living in the same perceived world as are their carers and professional carers? What is their reference point to 'fix' us, to help us—to make us whole again? What is their goal? To make us more like them for as long as possible, and if that's not possible to keep us from acting up or out, or being in pain? What about working with and for me? What about devoting your life to first understanding and appreciating me and the 600,000 me's who have early onset Alzheimer's in the early stage, or the 6 million of us who have dementia, probably of the Alzheimer's type, or, or …? Who is trying to help us be all we can be for as long as we can be? Who wants to help enable us to be as much as we want, as much as we can, as much as we should?

Too many well intended people inadvertently disable us through restrictive practices, rules and regulations. No risks = a well-lived life in a nursing home. Says who? The residents or most all the other non-residents; are regulations written to protect us also causing us never to be challenged? Never having to figure something out for ourselves? Never allowing us to go as far out on a limb as we want? Unless we have been declared legally incompetent (and even that classification I have my doubts about), we still have a right to life, liberty and the pursuit of happiness, and we are paying you to help us continue to exercise those rights to the extent we want to exercise them. How many residents helped write the rules? Who asked them what, when? Who interviews staff before they are hired? Who evaluates my care and the services delivered to me? When do I start counting as someone instead of something? 'Person centred care is the answer', trumpet carers and professionals. 'Giving you choices is what you need and want. We know!' Who decides what choices we may and may not make is the real question. Giving different choices is not the same as deciding

which services you get to make a choice about. Can I skip bathing for a week? What about eating? When I don't want to get out of bed—what are my choices?

I am not living in a nursing home. I have dementia, probably of the Alzheimer's type. Even now as I live at home loving, well intended carers and professionals are starting to disable, and neglect spending time in enabling me to be all I want to be, all I can be. There is a clear sameness between the ways older people are perceived and treated and the way people with dementia are treated. Neither group needs, nor deserves, to be treated in those ways! Please stop acting those ways around me, with me. Please take the time to know who I am today. What are my wants and needs? What do I believe about the world around me and in me? Stop worrying about the why's of my life unless you are an unemployed psychologist or a researcher with a grant to find out what's wrong with me, and how can it be fixed.

First listen to me. Know me as best you can through my eyes (some call it empathy). Appreciate me as a whole person. Relate to me as an equal. I am losing my ability to make choices about who and what I am, how I act and react. Yours are still all intact. Please make choices for yourself which support me feeling good about myself, continually evolving into someone who has a purpose, finds meaning in life, enjoys being alive.

'Richard' ©Richard Taylor PhD, January 2007

We need *carers not keepers*, another phrase of mine used in most of my presentations. When I go to see my doctor or consultant they talk to me and not across me to my carer. When my carer takes me to my day centre she/he doesn't tell me to say thank you—I will do if I want to.

These and many others are points that have been embodied in our NICE/SCIE dementia guideline; these are points that I and others ensured were included in the Mental Capacity Act 2005[16] when the initial drafting took place. As a member of the Alzheimer Europe working group on Advanced Directives these are points that were given careful consideration in its drafting.[17]

There follows a summary of an article written by Joanne McDonnell (née Schofield) and myself in the *Journal of Dementia Care*, **10**(2), pp. 20–22 (Mar/Apr 2002)[18]:

Peter Ashley has Lewy body dementia. Joanne Schofield is a clinical manager. Together they have a mission: to encourage others in Peter's situation to make choices and plan for their future care. In this article they set out principles and practical issues, arguing for greater awareness among professionals.

Each Monday. I go to my day centre,[19] to attend the early onset dementia group at the Mental Health Hospital in Winwick, Warrington, the same hospital I entered as an inpatient back in 1997; this is the best day of my week for I'm with my own friends, my real friends, people like me. The staff are totally dedicated, the salt of the earth, the NHS are trying to close it. No way should this be allowed to happen. On Saturday I attend a similar group in Warrington run by the social services department.

---

16  http://www.opsi.gov.uk/acts/acts2005/20050009.htm
17  http://www.alzheimer-europe.org/?lm2=DD1048476B10
18  http://www.careinfo.org/cgi-bin/articles.pl
19  The Beckett Day Centre: http://www.5boroughspartnership.nhs.uk/txt_page.asp?sitemap_id=231

Some say I'm unique in the way I've managed to handle my condition—*not so*. I know others around the world who have been as successful.

To what do I attribute the apparent slow decline in my condition, for decline there is and I know it?

- Constant support of my wife and family.
- The cholinesterase drug rivastigmine (Exelon).
- A relatively high IQ before diagnosis.
- The adoption of the work ethic.

- Use it or lose it
- Being a born fighter with a positive attitude.
- All my friends both professional and non-professional.
- The early diagnosis by highly talented and dedicated consultants.
- Continuing support from my consultants, support workers, registered mental nurses, and care assistants.

**I am living with dementia, NOT dying from dementia.**

© Peter J. S. Ashley, January 2007

# Clinical aspects of dementia: the syndrome of dementia

Alan Thomas

Dementia is not a disease but a major clinical syndrome, of which amnesia is the hallmark and the most well known and, usually, prominent feature. When someone with a possible dementia is referred to a clinician, the clinician should proceed through a two-stage process. First he or she should determine whether or not the patient has the features of the dementia syndrome. Second, if the patient does have a dementia, the clinician should attempt to decide which possible cause of dementia the patient is suffering from. This second stage should not be regarded as merely an interesting exercise in classification, as it has important management, prognostic, and therapeutic implications. Not only may rarer treatable causes of dementia, such as normal pressure hydrocephalus or hypothyroidism, be detected but accurate recognition of the dementia subtype is also important. Both typical (McKeith *et al.*, 1992) and atypical antipsychotic drugs (Ballard *et al.*, 1998) can prove harmful and even fatal to people with dementia with Lewy bodies (DLB); appropriate treatments can slow the advance of vascular dementia (VaD); and, of course, there are now licensed treatments available for Alzheimer's disease (AD). The assessment process is described in detail elsewhere (Chapter 10) and here we will focus on the current clinical criteria for diagnosing the dementia syndrome.

## The dementia syndrome

The concept of dementia has developed from a poorly described chronic organic brain condition to the present operationally defined syndrome of ICD-10 (WHO, 1992) and DSM-IV (APA, 1994). These criteria are summarized in Table 27ii.1. Both of these manuals require evidence of multiple cognitive deficits, which must include memory impairment, accompanied by some evidence of a decline in functioning. Typical deficits, in addition to the amnesia, include disorientation, aphasia, apraxia, and agnosia (these are dealt with in Chapter 27iii). These higher cortical deficits must represent a change and occur in clear consciousness (i.e. not occur only during a delirium). ICD-10 adds that the cognitive symptoms and related impairments need to have been present for 6 months in order to make a confident diagnosis of dementia. Previously dementia was regarded as a chronic and irreversible condition, but the present criteria hedge around this subject with ICD-10 now saying this is 'usually' the case and DSM-IV demanding it only for its 'dementia of the Alzheimer's type' criteria. A study of the very

similar DSM-IIIR criteria (APA, 1987) showed them to have very good inter-rater reliability, with kappa scores of up to 0.7 (Baldereschi *et al.*, 1994) but there are some conceptual and practical issues which need to be considered.

## Conceptual problems

The placing of memory impairment at the core of the dementia syndrome, and especially the emphasis on it characteristically involving problems with new learning at its onset, ties it very closely to AD and it is arguably something of a self-fulfilling prophecy to then find AD as the commonest cause of dementia. Were executive dysfunction, for example, made the central and mandatory feature of dementia the proportion with VaD would be higher and those with dementia due to neurodegenerative disease correspondingly lower. However, amnesia is the most easily recognized and described cognitive deficit, and consequently the major cause of referral, and it is unlikely that those with significant deficits elsewhere will have entirely normal memory function. The problem of the requirement for clear consciousness has been highlighted by the recognition of DLB (see Chapter 27v) in which fluctuation in consciousness is a characteristic feature (McKeith *et al.*, 2005). However, fluctuation is also common in vascular dementia (Hachinski *et al.*, 1975) and occurs in AD too (Robertson *et al.*, 1998). As alluded to above, the previous concept of dementia being irreversible or progressive is not entirely abandoned in the current diagnostic criteria but is likely to be so soon. Not only are some dementias, including AD, clearly static for periods but the cholinesterase inhibitors can now symptomatically reverse (at least for short periods) the dementia syndrome in some people, especially those with AD and DLB. Also the criteria do not recognize mixed dementia, which is increasingly recognized to account for a substantial proportion of cases.

## Practical problems

The two major differential diagnoses to be excluded when considering whether cognitive impairment is due to a dementia are depression and delirium. Two kinds of problem can arise at initial assessment. First there may be co-morbidity (e.g. delirium often occurs together with dementia) and the contribution of each to the cognitive impairment may not be revealed for some time, until the delirium is fully resolved. Each cause then needs to be dealt with in

**Table 27ii.1** The dementia syndrome (ICD-10 and DSM-IV)

| |
| --- |
| Multiple cognitive deficits (which must include amnesia) |
| Functional impairment |
| Clear consciousness |
| Change from previous level |
| Long duration (> 6 months) |

its own right until the situation becomes clearer. Second there can be real difficulty distinguishing the cause at initial presentation. Some cases of delirium are 'subacute' and grumble on for a long period as their underlying cause persists (see Chapter 28) whilst severe depression in the elderly may manifest itself as marked cognitive impairment (so-called 'depressive pseudodementia'; see Chapter 29ii). Careful monitoring should clarify the situation with time, but making a confident diagnosis at first presentation is best avoided in such cases.

Sometimes, especially in memory clinics specializing in assessing possible early dementia, a patient is confirmed to have multiple cognitive deficits on testing but does not show any functional impairment in their daily living; such individuals need monitoring but would not, as yet, fulfil diagnostic criteria for dementia. Similarly, patients are sometimes seen with a clear deficit in only one cognitive domain; again they would not meet dementia criteria but need monitoring as often they will progress to multiple deficits with functional impairment (i.e. dementia) over time. The criterion in ICD-10 that the deficits must have been present for at least 6 months is usually fulfilled without difficulty. Occasionally the claim is made that deficits have only been present for a few months. This may credibly be the case in a VaD where the impairment began

with a stroke, and the commonly used diagnostic criteria for VaD recognize this. In those without such a sudden onset such a claim is more likely to represent lack of awareness or denial about the true duration of onset of the illness, and in such cases the severity of current impairments often strongly suggest a longer duration. In practice the more practical approach is to look for evidence of chronicity of illness and the absence of delirium.

## References

APA (American Psychiatric Association) (1987). *Diagnostic and statistical manual of mental disorders*, 3rd edn, revised (DSM-IIIR). APA, Washington, DC.

APA (American Psychiatric Association) (1994). *Diagnostic and statistical manual of mental disorders*, 4th edn (DSM-IV). APA, Washington, DC.

Baldereschi, M., Amato, M.P., Nencini, P. *et al.* (1994). Cross-national interrater agreement on the clinical diagnostic criteria for dementia. WHO-PRA Age-Associated Dementia Working Group, WHO-Program for Research on Aging, Health of Elderly Program. *Neurology*, **44**, 239–42.

Ballard, C., Grace, J., McKeith, I., and Holmes, C. (1998). Neuroleptic sensitivity in dementia with Lewy bodies and Alzheimer's disease. *Lancet*, **351**, 1032–3.

Hachinski, V.C., Iliff, L.D., Zilhka, E. *et al.* (1975). Cerebral blood flow in dementia. *Archives of Neurology*, **32**, 632–7.

McKeith, I., Fairbairn, A., Perry, R., Thompson, P., and Perry, E. (1992). Neuroleptic sensitivity in patients with senile dementia of Lewy body type. *British Medical Journal*, **305**, 673–8.

McKeith, I.G., Dickson, D.W., Lowe, J. *et al.* (2005). Diagnosis and management of dementia with Lewy bodies: third report of the DLB Consortium. *Neurology*, **65**, 1863–72.

Robertson, B., Blennow, K., and Gottfries, C.G. (1998) Delirium in dementia. *International Journal of Geriatric Psychiatry*, **13**, 49–56.

WHO (1992). *International classification of diseases and health related problems* (ICD-10). Geneva, World Health Organization.

# Clinical aspects of dementia: Alzheimer's disease

## Alan Thomas

Alois Alzheimer wrote his original report (Alzheimer, 1907) on a 51-year-old woman (Auguste D) who had suffered an illness involving cognitive impairment and other symptoms including delusions and hallucinations. At post-mortem he described the principal neuropathological features, senile plaques and neurofibrillary tangles, of what we now call Alzheimer's disease. This eponymous term was coined by Kraepelin and was initially restricted to a pre-senile degenerative dementia. After several decades it was conceded that older people with identical symptomatology and pathological features had the same disease and, in fact, formed the great majority of cases. Thus today Alzheimer's disease (AD) refers to a characteristic clinical syndrome which usually occurs in later life and which is associated with the neuropathological findings described in detail in Chapter 5.

## Alzheimer's disease and the dementia syndrome

### Diagnostic criteria for Alzheimer's disease

#### ICD-10 and DSM-IV criteria

Having confirmed a patient has the dementia syndrome (see Chapter 27ii) then the next stage is to try and establish the cause. Since AD causes over 50% of all dementia it has come to be regarded almost as the model for dementia. As such there is still a tendency to diagnose AD by default rather than by the positive identification of the clinical syndrome described below. Table 27iii.1 shows the current diagnostic criteria for AD. ICD-10 and DSM-IV both require that dementia due to AD has an insidious onset and a gradual progression. AD cannot be diagnosed if there is a sudden onset or if there are neurological signs indicating focal brain damage or if the dementia can be explained by other brain or systemic diseases.

Applying these criteria requires a systematic and thorough assessment: a full history (including from an informant), mental state examination, cognitive examination, physical assessment (including neurological examination), and investigations. The latter are important because alternative causes include both systemic diseases, e.g. vitamin $B_{12}$ deficiency and hypothyroidism, and brain diseases, e.g. normal pressure hydrocephalus and stroke. A list of suggested investigations is given in Table 27iii.2.

### NINCDS–ADRDA Criteria

Both the ICD-10 and DSM-IV criteria for AD are closely related to the more rigorous NINCDS–ADRDA (National Institute of Neurological and Communicative Disorders and Stroke–Alzheimer's Disease and Related Disorders Association) criteria (McKhann et al., 1984). These are the widely used research criteria for AD and are shown in the Appendix. The McKhann criteria have three levels of certainty for AD diagnosis: definite AD, probable AD, and possible AD. Definite AD can only be diagnosed at post-mortem where tissue evidence confirms AD in someone already recognized as having probable AD. To make a diagnosis of probable AD requires multiple cognitive deficits (including memory) which progressively worsen and occur without disturbance of consciousness in someone with a dementia syndrome. The probable AD diagnosis also requires basic cognitive testing, e.g. the Mini-Mental State Examination (MMSE) (Folstein et al., 1975), to demonstrate the deficits and some confirmation of these by other neuropsychological tests. The criteria also set age limits of between 45 and 90 for the onset of the dementia because of potential difficulties in interpreting cognitive tests in people over 90. There are also similar exclusion criteria to ICD-10 and DSM-IV in that there must be no disturbance of consciousness and no systemic or brain diseases that could explain the impairment. Where all these criteria cannot be met clinically, e.g. a fluctuating course or sudden onset, then a diagnosis of possible AD should be made. The NINCDS–ADRDA criteria have been shown to have a sensitivity and specificity for AD of over 80% (Burns et al., 1990e; McKeith et al., 2000a) and very good inter-rater reliability (Farrer et al., 1994).

### Differential diagnosis

In practice the exclusion criteria for AD regarding apoplectic onset and focal signs specified above usually exclude people who have had a stroke, although other causes, e.g. head trauma or tumour, will also be excluded. Where there is evidence of cerebrovascular disease which is thought likely to contribute to the dementia (usually evidence of stroke clinically or on neuroimaging) then both ICD-10 and DSM-IV state that a double diagnosis of AD and vascular dementia (VaD) should be made (although many clinicians will refer to this as a 'mixed dementia'). Ideally such a double diagnosis should be made when there is clear evidence of each disease

**Table 27iii.1** Diagnostic criteria for Alzheimer's disease (ICD-10 and DSM-IV)

| |
|---|
| Fulfil criteria for dementia syndrome |
| Insidious onset |
| Gradual progression |
| No focal neurological signs |
| No evidence for a systemic or brain disease sufficient to cause dementia |

process contributing to the dementia, e.g. someone with AD who subsequently has a stroke and suddenly declines cognitively. However, in clinical practice a more pragmatic decision will often be made based on evidence for both AD and VaD such that a single pure diagnosis cannot confidently be made. The diagnosis of VaD is dealt with in detail in Chapter 27iv.

The other major differential diagnosis for the dementia syndrome in the elderly is dementia with Lewy bodies (DLB), which is covered in Chapter 27v. In the revised consensus criteria for DLB (McKeith *et al.*, 2005) it can be diagnosed confidently (probable DLB) in the presence of at least two of the three core features (recurrent visual hallucinations, fluctuation, and spontaneous parkinsonism) or one core feature plus one supportive feature (neuroleptic sensitivity, REM sleep behaviour disorder, dopaminergic abnormalities in the basal ganglia on functional neuroimaging). However, when only one of these core or supportive features is found possible DLB may be diagnosed (McKeith *et al.*, 2005), although subjects may meet criteria for possible AD (McKhann *et al.*, 1984) as well. Fluctuation can occur in AD (particularly in moderate and severe dementia) and visual hallucinations are also found (see below), so the presence of these features does not necessarily preclude a diagnosis of AD. The situation will often become clearer over time, e.g. the development of parkinsonism, but in any case serious consideration should be given to treating

**Table 27iii.2** Recommended investigations in dementia and Alzheimer's disease

| |
|---|
| Full blood count |
| Erythrocyte sedimentation rate or viscosity |
| Urea, creatinine and electrolytes (including calcium) |
| Liver function tests |
| Thyroid function tests |
| Vitamin B$_{12}$ and folate |
| Syphilis serology |
| Blood glucose |
| Cholesterol |
| Mid-stream specimen of urine |
| Chest X-ray |
| ECG |
| EEG (mild diffuse slowing) |
| CT/MR scan of head (may be normal, or show generalized atrophy or focal atrophy in medial temporal lobe) |
| Single photon emission tomography (SPET) scan—useful in selected cases (bilateral symmetric temporo-parietal hypoperfusion) |

such people with cholinesterase inhibitors. Apart from cognition, symptoms such as delusions, hallucinations, apathy, and agitation are likely to improve (McKeith *et al.*, 2000a,b).

In younger patients frontotemporal dementia should be considered, especially if frontal features are prominent, e.g. primitive reflexes, disinhibition, or marked apathy. This is dealt with in Chapter 27vi. Sometimes other rarer causes of dementia, e.g. hypothyroidism or normal pressure hydrocephalus, may be found in someone with apparent AD. However, it should be remembered that conditions such as hypothyroidism and mild B$_{12}$/folate deficiency are common and their presence on screening does not necessarily indicate they are solely responsible for the cognitive difficulties. A concomitant diagnosis of AD may still apply, and whether such a decision is correct will reveal itself when the other possible cause of the dementia is treated.

## Summary

The diagnosis of AD is a two-stage process. First clinical evidence for the dementia syndrome is gathered, and depression and delirium are excluded, and then the presentation is examined to see if it fits the above AD criteria of insidious onset and gradual progression in the absence of other possible causes. The two main other causes to consider in the elderly are VaD and DLB. Usually a careful assessment allows such distinctions to be made, but sometimes the clinician needs to wait patiently for further evidence as the disease progresses. Such distinctions are important because depression and delirium clearly merit a different kind of treatment from any cause of dementia and, as outlined in Chapter 27ii, the three major causes of dementia also carry different treatment implications.

# Clinical features of Alzheimer's disease

## Cognitive symptoms

These are central to the concept of dementia and AD and are dealt with in detail elsewhere (see Chapters 3 and 11). Here we will just describe the key symptoms and their progression as they are usually encountered in AD in clinical practice. (Note: here we will use aphasia and dysphasia synonymously, although strictly speaking the former refers to complete impairment of language and the latter to partial impairment. The same applies *mutatis mutandis* to apraxia/dyspraxia, alexia/dyslexia, and agraphia/dysgraphia.)

## Amnesia

Memory impairment is the classic presenting complaint for AD although other symptoms, e.g. apathy, subtle personality changes and dysphasia, are often found early in the illness too. The amnesia typically presents with a history of misplacing and losing objects, forgetting appointments or repeatedly asking the same question. At this early stage working memory (for example, the ability to repeat back a few words or a list of numbers) is relatively unimpaired. However, the ability to recall such words or numbers a few minutes later is significantly impaired because the earliest deficits in AD are in the process of encoding or laying down new information in the memory stores. This probably results from damage to the hippocampal formation, which is the site of the earliest pathological damage in AD. This failure to lay down new memories can be demonstrated more clearly by tests in which a patient is read a short story and asked to recall it (logical memory tests) or when a long list of words are read and repeated attempts are made to learn the list, e.g. the Rey Auditory Verbal Learning Test. Impairment in new learning also leads to the characteristic disorientation in time and place that is prominent even in early AD.

In the early stage of AD the recall of previously learned information remains good, showing that memory retrieval processes remain intact. This pattern results in the characteristic pattern of a failure of new learning (no memory for recent events) combined with clear memories of events earlier in life. As the disease progresses the memory impairment broadens to include retrieval of older memories and these are typically lost according to Ribot's law (more recent information is lost before more remote events) so the patient appears to live in the ever more distant past. As well as these losses in episodic memory (personally related events occurring in a specific situation) there are accompanying losses in semantic memory (facts and vocabulary) and visuospatial memory (remembering pictures, faces).

### Aphasia (dysphasia)

Deficits in cortical language production are usually present if they are searched for in the early stages of AD. The earliest manifestation is in word-finding difficulties in which the patient struggles from time to time to find the correct words to complete sentences. Attempts to cover this up by using circumlocutions are common and may be cleverly executed by brighter subjects so the deficits are hidden. At this time there is also usually an impairment in the naming of objects (nominal aphasia) which will initially be for the names of less common items rather than the more common objects which are frequently tested, e.g. pen or glasses. Thus pointing at objects in the room, e.g. a video recorder, or parts of objects, e.g. the winder on a watch, may show some nominal aphasia which would not otherwise be revealed. As the AD progresses these deficits worsen and problems in the comprehension of language develop (receptive dysphasia) and expression of language shows syntactical errors and simplification of sentence structure. Verbal perseveration, in which the patient repeats the same answer to consecutive questions, may now occur too. The development of these deficits has serious consequences as the patient now increasingly struggles to understand what is going on around him and to communicate his confusion and distress clearly to others. It should not be assumed that a concurrent loss of all understanding occurs as patients may still be sensitive to emotional and other non-verbal cues.

As the dementia becomes severe then marked poverty of the content of speech develops, with the repetition of short simple sentences on favourite themes and, eventually, mutism may occur. Some patients babble meaningless sounds or repeat words and phrases they hear (echolalia). Progression in language deterioration is not inevitable and many patients remain superficially fluent. They maintain a social discourse which can deceive the unwary about the true extent of their cognitive impairment. Careful attention to their language comprehension and production, however, will invariably reveal a pattern of language impairment including the above deficits.

### Apraxia (dyspraxia)

Dyspraxia is the failure to carry out complex motor tasks due to deficits in the higher cortical control of movement; not because of damage to the peripheral sensory or motor systems or in coordination. It typically occurs with cortical deficits in the dominant (usually left) parietal lobe but as with other cognitive symptoms in dementia dysfunction in other areas is usually present too. Ideomotor apraxia is the form usually elicited and refers to the inability of the patient to carry out a motor task to command. Examples include: asking a patient to wave; demonstrate how he brushes his teeth; or show how she combs her hair. Other common 'dyspraxias' sought by the clinician are dressing dyspraxia and constructional dyspraxia. Strictly speaking these are not dyspraxias as they are not necessarily due primarily to higher motor failure. Dressing dyspraxia refers to the common difficulty patients have in putting their clothes on correctly due to faulty visuospatial processing, which results in them being unable to orientate their body properly in relation to their clothing. It is usually taken to indicate right (non-dominant) parietal lobe damage. Constructional dyspraxia refers to the failure to adequately reproduce a two- (or three-) dimensional drawing, e.g. a star or a clock, or to the similar failure to assemble blocks into the required model. Like dressing, such tasks actually involve multiple cognitive domains (visual, spatial, sensory, motor) but failure is usually taken to indicate right (non-dominant) parietal damage. All these dyspraxias have dire consequences for the patient's ability to carry out many activities of daily living. Cooking, cleaning, and general housework require the ability to carry out motor sequences, as do more basic activities such as eating and using the toilet. Failure in such domains is not primarily due to memory but to dyspraxic losses. Relatives may misunderstand why someone who appears healthy apart from an apparently mild memory impairment should struggle in such areas and explaining the global nature of dementia can help them understand the true situation.

### Agnosia

Agnosia is the failure to correctly interpret a sensory input in the presence of an intact sensory system and it is common in AD. It is due to cortical damage and can occur in any sensory modality, though visual agnosia is the form usually met in clinical practice. In visual agnosia a patient sees an object but does not recognize it. Perhaps the most well known is prosopagnosia in which the patient fails to recognize a familiar face and when the face is that of a relative it can be very distressing for all concerned. Other common agnosias include failure to recognize objects around the house, e.g. mistaking the kettle for the teapot or the dustbin for the toilet, and these too can have serious consequences for the patient.

### Frontal-executive dysfunction

Damage to the frontal lobes leads to inflexibility in thinking and difficulties in problem-solving, planning, and correctly sequencing behaviour. This is a complex area, but one which should nonetheless be tested during assessment of dementia. It is dealt with in more detail in Chapter 11. Proverbs have traditionally been used to test how concrete and inflexible someone's reasoning is, but they are often very difficult to interpret. 'Similarities and differences' tests involve asking the patient what two objects (e.g. table and chair; shoe and boot) have in common and how they differ. Again these can be difficult to interpret but some attempt should be made, especially in someone who appears frontally impaired (e.g. markedly disinhibited). Easier to interpret are verbal fluency tests of frontal lobe function. These involve asking the patient to name as many objects as they can in a category in 1 minute (e.g. fruit or animals) or asking them to generate as many words as they can think of beginning with the same letter in 1 minute (e.g. F, A and S in 'the FAS test'). As a rough guide a normal subject should produce more than 15 words for each in a minute and less than 10 is clearly abnormal. A third kind of frontal test involves testing the subject's ability to shift from one item to another, and this reveals perseverative problems. A sequence of alternating shapes or numbers may be written and the patient asked to continue the sequence. Motor perseveration can be demonstrated using the Luria two-step or three-step tests (in which the subject is asked to copy the examiner in alternately opening and closing the hand or making a fist then an edge and then a palm, respectively). In someone who shows any of these 'frontal' features it is particularly important to examine for 'primitive reflexes' (see below).

### Other cognitive deficits

Corresponding to the above deficits in spoken language are impairments in reading (dyslexia) and writing (dysgraphia) which can be often identified with simple tests in AD using pen, paper, and reading material. Acalculia (more accurately anarithmetria) is the loss of the ability to do simple sums and can similarly be tested for in a straightforward way. Right/left disorientation may be detected by asking the patient to obey commands such as 'point to the left ear with the right forefinger'.

## Non-cognitive symptoms

### Psychotic symptoms

As mentioned above, in his original report Alois Alzheimer (1907) described both delusions and hallucinations in his patient Auguste D and the emphasis in diagnosis on the cognitive symptoms of dementia can distract from the fact that psychotic symptoms are very common. Table 27iii.3 gives summary estimates of the monthly prevalence in clinical settings (that is, hospital inpatients and day patients, outpatients, and other clinic patients) in AD of the most important non-cognitive symptoms derived from the research presented below; lifetime rates will be much higher. Accurately eliciting these mental state phenomena can be difficult in people with dementia and the figures quoted below are derived from interviews with informants, who may over-rate some symptoms (e.g. depression) compared with trained observers (Burns *et al.*, 1990c). The rates of all the psychotic symptoms vary widely depending on, amongst other things, how the phenomena are defined, which patients are sampled, and the time frame over which the survey is conducted. Also it is worth noting that many of the studies were conducted before the accurate recognition of DLB was possible, which has a much higher rate of psychosis, and so the figures for AD are likely to be inflated a little by an admixture of DLB patients.

**Table 27iii.3** Approximate monthly prevalence of non-cognitive symptoms in Alzheimer's disease

| Psychotic | Delusions, 30% |
| | Misidentifications, 30% |
| | Hallucinations, 20% |
| Mood | Depression, 25% |
| | Euphoria, <1% |
| | Anxiety, 30–50% |
| Behavioural | Apathy, 70% |
| | Agitation, 30% |
| | Wandering, 20% |
| | Physical aggression, 20% |
| | Verbal aggression, 40% |

### Delusions

Delusional beliefs are common, can be very distressing to carers, and may contribute to early institutionalization. They are often understandable as attempts by the patient to make sense of his or her situation, and include beliefs that objects have been stolen, a spouse is unfaithful, or that intruders have been in the house. These beliefs commonly have a paranoid flavour and tend to lack the complexity and systemization of the delusions seen in schizophrenia. The delusions are often short-lived and can therefore be difficult to distinguish from confabulations. For hospital patients the prevalence of delusions in published studies varies from about 25% (Cooper *et al.*, 1991) to about 50% (Hirono *et al.*, 1998). Burns *et al.* (1990a) studied a sample of AD patients in a catchment area and found 16% to have delusions at some point in their illness and 11% to have had them in the previous 12 months. This figure is lower than most studies looking at clinically derived samples. Ballard and Walker (1999) systematically reviewed the literature and found a mean prevalence of delusions of 31% in all clinical settings and 23% in community settings. Burns *et al.* (1990a) found delusions were three times more prevalent in men.

### Misidentification syndromes

Misidentification syndromes are sometimes called delusional misidentifications and might be better termed symptoms than syndromes. They are very common in AD occurring in about 23–30% of sufferers at some time and in about 19% during a single year (Rubin *et al.*, 1988, Burns *et al.*, 1990b). They have been classified as delusions and as hallucinations depending on how the phenomena are understood. For example, the common assertion by a demented patient that someone else has been in the house, when their family denies such a possibility, could be a paranoid delusional belief or a visual hallucination. In practice it is often not possible to clarify the experience well enough to determine the exact form of the psychotic experience. Another common kind of misidentification is the conviction that a relative or friend is someone else (which may be a Capgras symptom if the misidentified person is accepted as looking exactly the same as their 'double', though this may be difficult to tease out in AD). Commonly a spouse is misidentified as a son or daughter or vice versa, but sometimes the patient believes the misidentified person is a stranger and this may provoke a strong reaction. Other symptoms include beliefs that people or events on the television are occurring in the living room and the misidentification of the patient's own image in the mirror as another person ('mirror sign'). Wrongly believing strangers to have been in the house appears to be the commonest form of misidentification, being found in 12–17%; misidentifying people occurs in about 12%; misidentifying images from the television is found in 6–12%; and misidentifying a mirror image occurs in about 4–7% (Rubin *et al.*, 1988; Burns *et al.*, 1990b). Overall, studies show misidentification occurs in 30% of people with AD (Ballard and Walker, 1999). Like delusions, these misidentification syndromes appear to be more likely to occur in men (Burns *et al.*, 1990b).

### Hallucinations

Hallucinations are less common than delusions and misidentification syndromes. However, study figures here may be underestimates reflecting an unavoidable bias in the way in which the symptoms are rated. The scores are informant based and informants will probably be unaware of the full extent of someone else's internal hallucinatory experiences whilst it seems reasonable to believe that delusions and misidentifications are almost certain to reveal themselves. Visual hallucinations are commoner than auditory hallucinations, and whilst olfactory, gustatory, and tactile hallucinations also occur in AD, they are much rarer. Studies in clinical settings have found prevalence rates for all hallucinations of between 10% (Mega *et al.*, 1996) and 40% (Gilley *et al.*, 1997) in AD. In their systematic review Ballard and Walker (1999) found mean prevalence rates of 21% for all hallucinations (14% for visual hallucinations and 7% for auditory hallucinations) in clinical settings.

### Management of psychotic symptoms in AD

Pharmacological and non-pharmacological interventions may both be of benefit. In addition to dealing with general health matters, especially with sensory deficits which may be exacerbating hallucinations, increasing the general level of stimulation, e.g. by arranging day care or attendance at a day centre, may be of benefit to someone who has hallucinations or misidentifications. Other interventions can include playing soothing music, using video tapes of familiar figures in conversation, and removing the mirror for someone with the mirror sign.

Several studies have evaluated whether drug treatments are effective for psychosis in dementia but there is controversy about the risk:benefit ratio of these drugs in AD and in dementia in general. Antipsychotic drugs have been prescribed empirically for a long time but the 'typical' antipsychotics are likely to produce adverse effects in these vulnerable patients. Most studies have been small or used broad outcome measures such as behavioural change rather than focusing on specific symptoms. However, several larger randomized trials of atypical antipsychotics have been reported, and these, together with the smaller trials, have been subject to systematic review (Sink *et al.*, 2005; Ballard *et al.*, 2006). The conclusions were that there is modest evidence for the efficacy of risperidone and olanzapine for treating psychosis and aggression in dementia but this benefit needs to be weighed against the approximately 1.5-fold increase in mortality on these agents. Thus it is reasonable to conclude their use should be restricted to those who are severely disturbed or seriously aggressive. There is little evidence that typical antipsychotics are efficacious for treating behavioural disturbance in dementia, although haloperidol may be beneficial and evidence suggests increases in mortality are associated with these agents too, perhaps at higher rates than for atypicals (Wang *et al.*, 2005).

However, it is important to note that evidence for other classes of medication is even weaker. Although antidepressants (especially trazadone), mood stabilizers (previously carbamazepine was widely used but more recently sodium valproate has become commonly prescribed), and benzodiazepines have been and still are widely used for a range of behavioural disturbances in AD, there is no consistent evidence from randomized trials to support such prescribing practice (Sink *et al.*, 2005). The best evidence, perhaps unsurprisingly in treating people with dementia, is for antidementia drugs (cholinesterase inhibitors and to a lesser extent memantine) (Sink *et al.*, 2005).

Whilst helpful, such summaries of evidence hide many of the difficulties in interpreting the studies. For example, all the atypical studies were carried out in nursing homes in people with moderate or severe dementia (MMSE scores of less than 15), raising the issue of whether these findings can be generalized to less cognitively impaired and physically frail patients; patients able to enter randomized studies are less psychotic and disturbed than many patients encountered in clinical practice; and it is difficult to interpret what changes of a few points on rating scales mean in clinical practice.

Against the modest benefit for antipsychotics in AD and the limited availability of alternatives the treating psychiatrist has to balance the evidence for harm. Regulatory bodies in different countries have issued warnings about an increased risk of death and cerebrovascular adverse events in people with dementia taking antipsychotics, e.g. the Committee for the Safety of Medicines in the United Kingdom (2004) and the US Food and Drug Administration (2005). A difficulty for clinicians has been that many of the data have not been publicly available; consequently in a meta-analysis on the risk of death with atypical antipsychotics of 15 eligible trials 9 were unpublished, with the authors extracting data from abstracts presented at research meetings (Schneider *et al.*, 2005). They reported a statistically significant increase of about 50% in mortality in patients taking atypical antipsychotics but identified a similar increase in those on haloperidol. Comparisons with typical antipsychotics are difficult due to the lack of randomized evidence, but a retrospective cohort study of 22,890 elderly subjects taking typical and atypical antipsychotics found the former group to have a higher mortality (Wang *et al.*, 2005). Another concern has been whether the use of antipsychotics hastens cognitive decline in dementia (McShane *et al.*, 1997) and one randomized trial suggests this might be the case (Ballard *et al.*, 2005). Overall it is clear that there are reasons for concern about the use of antipsychotics in dementia, with their use increasing mortality and cerebrovascular events and possibly worsening cognition. There is also no doubt that they are over-prescribed, given the modest benefits they appear to confer, and their use should probably be confined to those with persistent and severe psychosis and associated agitation or aggression.

In such patients it is prudent to begin with a non-pharmacological approach, although the evidence for such interventions is very weak (Livingston *et al.*, 2005) (see Chapter 18vi for details). If this approach fails and the behaviour remains problematic then a cholinesterase inhibitor should be considered because these drugs appear to have the best risk:benefit ratio. If this option is not available (prescribing restrictions make this difficult in many countries) then recourse to an atypical antipsychotic (in low dose) will be necessary and because of the risks discussed above clinicians should explain their reasons for such treatment to patients and, if appropriate, their next of kin.

### Mood changes

Alterations in mood are also extremely common in dementia, with depression being the most common. Here we are concerned with depression occurring during established AD; the relationship of depression to AD as a risk factor is considered below and the concept of 'depressive pseudodementia' is dealt with in Chapter 29ii.

One problem is what is meant by the term 'depression'. Even separating studies looking at depressed mood, depressive symptoms, and depressive syndromes still leaves enormous variability with rates varying from 0–87% for depressed mood (Knesevich *et al.*, 1983; Merriam *et al.*, 1988); from 0–89% for all depressive symptoms (Wragg and Jeste, 1989); and from 0–30% for depressive syndromes (Burns *et al.*, 1990c; Teri and Wagner, 1991). These rates vary because different populations are sampled, different instruments are used, and different raters make the rating. Problems in the assessment of depressive symptoms also occur because apathy can easily be mistaken for depression whilst many depressive symptoms, e.g. poor appetite, weight loss, and sleep disturbance, are also common features of dementia itself.

In a review of studies examining depressive syndromes diagnosed using standardized criteria Ballard *et al.* (1996) found major depression to occur in 21% of dementia sufferers in clinical settings and 13% in the community. No clear association between depression and the severity of dementia has been found, with some studies showing depression to be more common in milder dementia and others showing the opposite.

Depression decreases the quality of life of dementia sufferers, may reduce the duration of survival (Burns *et al.*, 1991c) and would therefore appear to be important to treat. However, depression and depressive symptoms are usually short-lived in dementia and pharmacotherapy is not without risks, as elderly people with dementia are very prone to adverse effects. Simple social interventions, e.g. befriending or a day centre, should be considered and drug treatment used only if the depression is severe or prolonged.

Selective serotonin reuptake inhibitors (SSRIs) (Lyketsos *et al.*, 2003; Nyth *et al.*, 1992), moclobemide (Roth *et al.*, 1996), and tricyclic antidepressants (TCAs) (Petracca *et al.*, 1996) have all been shown to alleviate depression in dementia. However, the quality of most reported studies is poor and a systematic review for the Cochrane Collaboration did not find clear evidence for the efficacy of antidepressants in dementia (Bains *et al.*, 2002). Further large studies are needed to clarify this important issue. TCAs should be avoided because they worsen cognitive impairment and have higher drop-out rates (Taragano *et al.*, 1997) and SSRIs are safe, even in cardiac disease (Glassman *et al.*, 2002) and are therefore the initial drug treatment of choice.

Elevation of mood in dementia is much less common and less frequently studied than depression. Burns *et al.* (1990c) found only one patient (out of 178) who reported manic symptoms and only six who had any observable evidence of mania. Other studies have reported higher rates of euphoria (Wragg and Jeste, 1989). Anxiety has been much less studied than even euphoria in dementia but, consistent with clinical experience, it is common with studies finding a rate ranging from 30% (Mendez *et al.*, 1990) to 50% (Patterson *et al.*, 1990).

## Behavioural symptoms

Changes in behaviour are common and an estimate of the monthly prevalence of some of the most important disturbances is given in Table 27iii.3.

### Apathy

Apathy is diminished motivation, and manifests itself as a listlessness in which the patient has lost the drive to engage in activities. It is often confused with low mood and anhedonia, which is a loss of ability to enjoy previously pleasurable activities. Although they all may be present together they are not the same phenomenon (Levy *et al.*, 1998). The distinction is important, because carers often think someone with AD is depressed when he has apathy as a part of his dementia. Apathy is probably the most common behavioural change in AD and Mega *et al.* (1996) detected apathy in 72% of outpatients with AD. Apathy is common early in AD and typically becomes more severe as the cognitive impairment worsens.

At presentation apathy is frequently a complaint given by relatives who often misunderstand it as laziness and become frustrated by it. Explaining that apathy is a feature of dementia can remove this misunderstanding and the tension it brings. Although there are no licensed treatments available at the present time for apathy there is evidence that the cholinesterase inhibitors are especially effective in treating this symptom and they may be considered as an intervention (McKeith *et al.*, 2000).

### Overactivity

A number of overlapping phenomena involving overactive behaviour are commonly found in AD. The most well known are agitation, which may be defined as painful inner tension associated with excessive motor activity (American Psychiatric Association, 1994), and wandering. However, other 'aberrant motor behaviours' are recognized and sometimes measured, e.g. rummaging in drawers and repeatedly taking clothes on and off. All such overactive behaviours tend to become more common with increasing severity of the dementia. Wandering is found in about 20% of people with AD (Burns *et al.*, 1990d) and the only other available figures for overactive behaviours are for agitation, which is found in about 30% of people with AD (Cohen *et al.*, 1993). Several drugs may help such behaviours, and while low-dose antipsychotics are the most widely prescribed, carbamazepine may also be helpful (Tariot *et al.*, 1998).

### Aggression

Aggression is a major problem in dementia. It is common, and when present causes great distress to the carers and is a common reason for admission to hospital and transfer to residential care. It is open to different definitions, and even when verbal aggression (shouting, swearing) is distinguished from physical aggression (punching, kicking, biting, pushing, pinching, etc.) there is still much scope for differences of opinion in each category about what constitutes aggression. Burns *et al.* (1990d) defined aggression narrowly as behaviour liable to cause physical injury to others and still found 20% of their AD subjects to have aggression. Broader definitions naturally lead to higher figures, and verbal aggression is usually found to be two to three times more common than physical aggression. Burns *et al.* (1990d) found aggression to be much more common in male sufferers of AD. They also found that it became more common with increasing cognitive impairment, rising from 8% in mild AD to 24% in severe AD. Treatment of aggression is fraught with the same problems as that for psychosis and studies not unreasonably frequently assess both problems together (as psychosis may be causing aggressive behaviour). Thus there is evidence for benefit from using atypical antipsychotics (Sink *et al.*, 2005) but the risks of such medication need to be considered. An initial report of benefit from carbamazepine in aggression (at about 300 mg a day) (Tariot *et al.*, 1998) has not been supported by a subsequent study (Olin *et al.*, 2001) and all four randomized trials of sodium valproate for agitation/aggression have failed to demonstrate benefit from active treatment (e.g. Sink *et al.*, 2005; Tariot *et al.*, 2005).

## Neurovegetative symptoms

### Sleep

Sleep disturbance is another common feature of dementia which can have devastating consequences for carers. It may take the form of frequent waking, reduced sleep quality, or a disturbance to circadian rhythms. The well-recognized day–night reversal was found to occur in 28% of patients in one study (Reisberg *et al.*, 1987) and all forms of sleep disturbance have been found in between 45% and 70% of AD patients (Rabins *et al.*, 1982; Merriam *et al.*, 1988). To reduce the strain from sleep disturbance the spouse may sleep in another bed or in another room and psychotropic medication (hypnotics and antipsychotics) is frequently prescribed. Sleep deprivation can eventually lead to exhaustion for the spouse if it persists, especially when it is associated with night wandering. Respite care can then be of great help, although placement in residential care may finally be needed.

### Eating

Difficulties with feeding are common in dementia. These tend to progress from initial problems using cutlery with associated spillage of food through to complete dependence on others for feeding. In addition there may be specific problem behaviours related to eating. Some patients refuse food whilst others stuff food rapidly and clumsily into their mouths. The latter binge eating is common, occurring in 10% of people with AD (Burns *et al.*, 1990d) and this figure is constant for all severities of dementia. It may be part of a wider Kluver–Bucy syndrome, although the full syndrome is rare (Burns *et al.*, 1990d).

### Sexual disinhibition

Sexual disinhibition is also a feature of the Kluver–Bucy syndrome and is another problem which causes great distress to carers. It occurs in about 7% of dementia sufferers but unlike binge eating it is rare in mild dementia and increases markedly with dementia severity (Burns *et al.*, 1990d).

## Personality changes

Alterations in personality are ubiquitous in dementia and changes in personality are inseparable from some of the above behavioural changes, e.g. apathy and sexual disinhibition. However, it is important to note they do occur very early in AD and 75% of people with mild AD show personality changes (Rubin *et al.*, 1987). These may precede the cognitive deficits and are often subtle in form, but none the less they are frequently recognized and commented upon by carers. Such information should be cautiously interpreted, as family and friends are often too closely involved to be able to comment accurately and dispassionately and may either exaggerate or deny any changes. As the AD progresses these initially subtle personality alterations tend to become more evident.

Personality changes not included in the above section on behavioural changes are suspiciousness and disengagement. Suspiciousness is common, and was found in 25% of AD subjects (Patterson and Bolger, 1994). It may or may not eventually consolidate into frank paranoid delusions and can cause great friction as repeated accusations are made about the motives and behaviour of well-meaning carers and relatives. Disengagement refers to the detached state of emotional indifference seen often in AD which is associated with a loss of rapport with other people. The patient is no longer concerned about the feelings of others or affected by their attention or lack of it. Such disengagement can be upsetting to relatives and needs to be distinguished from the low mood of depression.

## Physical symptoms

### Neurological

Early in AD neurological examination is usually normal. Focal neurological signs suggest a vascular dementia or other cause of focal damage whilst extrapyramidal signs indicate DLB. Primitive reflexes, however, may occur early in AD although their frequency increases as the dementia worsens. Burns *et al.* (1991a) found the snout reflex was easily the most common, occurring in 41% of their clinical sample. The grasp reflex was identified in 7% and the palmomental in 2.5%. As the disease progresses non-specific changes occur in both gait and balance and myoclonic jerks and other seizures may develop. In the late stage bilateral non-focal signs (e.g. upgoing plantars) may be seen.

### Incontinence

Urinary incontinence is a common and well-recognized feature of AD and has been found in 48% of AD subjects (Burns *et al.*, 1990d), though this figure disguises its strong association with disease severity. Incontinence was found in only 8% of those with mild AD but in 94% of patients with severe AD (Burns *et al.*, 1990d). This association has important implications in diagnosis, as incontinence early in a dementia is characteristic of other dementias, especially frontotemporal dementia and normal pressure hydrocephalus. Thus the presence of urinary incontinence early in a dementia should lead to a more serious search for possible causes other than AD. It is also vital to consider and exclude other causes of incontinence. Urinary tract infections, especially in women, are a common finding and may be the cause of the incontinence, rather than the dementia. Also the incontinence may result from poor mobility or failure to find the toilet in a strange environment (e.g. when someone has just been admitted to an inpatient unit).

### General physical changes

AD is associated with a general physical deterioration in which the patient loses weight and develops a stooped posture associated with instability and gait abnormalities. Weight loss may be an intrinsic feature of the disease process or secondary to the progressive impairments, which can result in an inadequate consumption of food and fluids. Cronin-Stubbs *et al.* (1997) demonstrated that older people with AD lost weight at over three and a half times the rate of healthy age-matched controls, a rate of weight loss more severe than in elderly people with cancer. Weight loss was found to be more rapid in earlier stages of the disease, suggesting it is at least in part due directly to the disease process. Whatever the cause this marked weight loss is likely to contribute to the high mortality of AD.

## Summary

Whilst cognitive symptoms are central to the diagnosis of AD, non-cognitive symptoms are arguably of more importance in management. Psychotic and mood symptoms are very common, a cause of distress to both patients and carers, and, in many cases, treatable in their own right. The behavioural disturbances, accompanying personality changes and neurovegetative symptoms are also much more common than is usually recognized and all place great strain on carers. Psychosocial interventions are usually necessary, whilst some of these (apathy, agitation, aggression, sleep disturbance) may respond to pharmacological treatment. The physical symptoms in AD remind us it is a debilitating condition requiring ongoing assessment and long-term palliative care.

# Aetiology of Alzheimer's disease

Identifying risk factors for AD is important for two main reasons. Identification of risk factors and protective factors enables potentially new treatments or public health interventions to be developed. Second these aetiological factors may throw light on the pathogenesis of AD, stimulating new research which can further our understanding of the disease process leading to new treatment opportunities. Table 27iii.4 summarizes our present state of knowledge about the aetiological factors involved in AD.

## Demographic risk factors

### Age

It is easily forgotten that old age is the most important risk factor for AD as its prevalence rises rapidly after 60, approximately doubling every 5 years. But for how long does such a rise continue? It is still not clear whether the increase continues indefinitely (so everyone would develop AD if they lived long enough) or tails off. There is evidence the prevalence of dementia plateaus for people in their 90s and may even drop in the very old (Ritchie and Kildea, 1995). However, incidence studies are a better measure of whether age itself is a causal factor in AD and dementia, and a meta-analysis of such studies found the incidence of both AD and dementia continues to increase with increasing age up to the age of 98, although the rate of acceleration does slow down (Gao et al., 1998). Studies of centenarians are clearly difficult to perform but Blansjaar et al. (2000) identified all people over 100 in an area of Holland and managed to assess 15 of these 17 individuals. All were found to be demented, with 12 having a moderate to severe dementia.

### Sex

It is well recognized that AD is more common in women, but is female gender an independent risk factor? It could simply be that women live longer than men and consequently are at higher risk or live longer with the illness. Such possibilities might confound prevalence but not incidence studies. One meta-analysis found women to have a higher incidence of AD than men but not a higher incidence of dementia in general (Gao et al., 1998). Another meta-analysis found that women tend to have a higher incidence in very old age

but not in the younger old (Jorm and Jolley, 1998) whilst a pooled analysis of four large prospective studies again found women to be at increased risk for AD and for those over 90 the women's rate was three times higher (Andersen et al., 1999). If further research supports such a sex-related risk then it could be related to post-menopausal changes in oestrogens or to an interaction of sex with apolipoprotein E (*APOE*) genotype (Gao et al., 1998).

### Ethnicity

Some studies show the incidence of AD differs in different parts of the world, and in a meta-analysis Jorm and Jolley (1998) found dementia and AD to have a higher incidence in Europe than in East Asia. However, the way in which dementia is diagnosed shows significant differences even within the same culture, and such differences are likely to be more marked between different cultures and probably dwarf any real differences that may be present. Studies are needed in which identical methods are applied in a range of countries to determine whether real variations are present. One such cohort study, using identical assessment methods in Nigeria and Indianapolis (African-Americans), reported an increased incidence of dementia and AD in the African-Americans (Hendrie et al., 2001). The reason for this difference is not known.

## Genetic risk factors

### Family history

It has long been recognized that AD is more common in families of probands, and 25–50% of people with AD have an affected relative. A meta-analysis showed that those with a first-degree relative (parent, sibling, child) with AD had a 3.5-fold increase in their risk of developing AD (Van Duijn et al., 1991). Generally those with an early onset of the disease (before 65 years) show a stronger familial risk, although they account for less than 5% of all AD cases; conversely the increased risk is very much reduced for those whose relatives develop AD in very old age. However, genes still appear to make a substantial contribution to risk because a large twin study in Sweden following an 'elderly' (age range 52–98) cohort over 5 years estimated that 48% of the variation in risk of developing AD was due to genetic risk (Pedersen et al., 2004). A number of important genes, which account for some of the genetic contribution, have been identified and are mentioned briefly below (see Chapter 7 for details).

### Down's syndrome

Virtually all people with Down's syndrome have the neuropathological features of AD by the age of 40 years (Mann et al., 1986) and this is due to them having a extra copy of the amyloid precursor protein gene located on chromosome 21. However, the prevalence of dementia in people with Down's is much less than 100% even by age 50, although it is clearly markedly elevated for age (Zigman et al., 1996). The reason for this discrepancy between pathology and function is not understood, and complex interactions between maternal age and frequency of the *APOE* ε4 allele (see below) have been proposed. In addition the added difficulties of making an accurate clinical diagnosis in this group is likely to contribute to the variable findings.

### Apolipoprotein E polymorphism

Apolipoprotein E (ApoE) is a plasma protein involved in lipid transport and its gene is located on chromosome 19 (19q13.2). It has three common alleles, ε2, ε3 and ε4, which in the normal population

**Table 27iii.4** Aetiological factors in Alzheimer's disease

| | |
|---|---|
| Established risk factors | Age<br>Family history<br>Down's syndrome<br>Apolipoprotein ε4 allele<br>Autosomal dominant mutations |
| Probable risk factors | Depression<br>Hypertension<br>Head injury |
| Possible risk factors | Female gender<br>Low intelligence/education<br>Diabetes<br>Smoking<br>Aluminium |
| Possible protective factors | Anti-inflammatory medication<br>Oestrogen<br>Apolipoprotein ε2 allele<br>High intelligence/education |

(in Caucasians) have allele frequencies of about 7%, 77%, and 16% respectively (Zannis *et al.*, 1993). Many studies have shown the ε4 allele to be much more common in AD subjects, occurring in 30–50% (Roses, 1996). A recent meta-analysis found age-adjusted odds ratios for AD of 2.6 for ε2/ε4 heterozygotes, 3.2 for ε3/ε4, and 14.9 for ε4/ε4 homozygotes (Farrer *et al.*, 1997). Thus *APOE* ε4 alleles have a dose-dependent effect in increasing the risk for AD. Other studies have demonstrated the increased risk conferred by *APOE* ε4 is related to it bringing forward the time of onset of AD (Roses, 1996). However, these striking findings need to be put in context. Up to 50% of those who are homozygous for ε4 and who live beyond 90 do not develop AD and about two-thirds of those who develop AD have no ε4 allele (Henderson *et al.*, 1995). It should also be noted there is evidence the ε2 allele may be protective as Farrer *et al.* (1997) found an odds ratio for AD of 0.6 for the combined ε2/ε2 and ε2/ε3 genotypes.

### Autosomal dominant gene mutations

Three genetic loci have been identified with mutations conferring an autosomal dominant pattern of inheritance for AD with almost complete penetrance. These are mutations in the amyloid precursor protein gene on chromosome 21, in the presenilin-1 gene on chromosome 14 and in the presenilin-2 gene on chromosome 1. All are associated with early onset AD (before 65 years) and account for less than 2% of all AD cases (Farrer *et al.*, 1997); they do not seem to be present in even the majority of early onset familial AD cases (Cruts *et al.*, 1998). Their importance lies in the clues they are giving about the pathogenesis of AD. For example, these mutations all lead to an excessive production of the pathogenetic long-chain form of the amyloid beta protein (Aβ42) (Hardy, 1997) and the presenilin-1 protein may be an important enzyme (gamma secretase) involved in producing this Aβ42 protein (De Strooper *et al.*, 1999; Saftig *et al.*, 1999).

### Other gene mutations

It is clear the above genes do not account for all of the genetic contribution to AD, and researchers are busy trying to identify further important genes. Two genes on chromosome 12 have been proposed as risk factors for AD: the low-density lipoprotein receptor-related gene (Kang *et al.*, 1997) and the alpha-2 macroglobulin gene (Liao *et al.*, 1998). Each of these is of interest as they produce proteins which could play an important role in the pathogenesis of AD, but research findings are presently inconsistent for these and other genes less frequently associated with an increased AD risk.

### Intelligence and education as risk factors

There is evidence that people with lower intelligence and educational attainments have an increased risk of developing AD. Some studies (though not all) have shown that people with a lower level of education have a higher rate of AD or cognitive impairment (Stern *et al.*, 1994b; White *et al.*, 1994; Farmer *et al.*, 1995). The most obvious explanations for such findings are that cognitive tests, e.g: the MMSE, are sensitive to education and so poorly educated people cross the thresholds more easily and better educated people are more able to compensate for their disease impairments and so present later or not all if death supervenes. Consistent with this, one functional neuroimaging study showed regional cerebral blood flow to be lower in the parietal and temporal lobes in better educated subjects compared with more poorly educated subjects who had been matched for the severity of their dementia, indicating

they had more advanced disease (Stern *et al.*, 1992). However, it appears such parsimonious explanations (intelligent people compensate better and cognitive tests are insensitive to education) may not suffice as there is evidence that low pre-morbid intelligence, which is correlated with low education, directly influences the pathogenesis of AD. An epidemiological study, which has followed a group of nuns for many years, has shown not only that those nuns with lower verbal ability in early life (a proxy measure of intelligence) had poorer cognitive functioning and a higher rate of AD but that at post-mortem all of those with neuropathological evidence of AD had low verbal ability (Snowdon *et al.*, 1996). Therefore high intelligence may not just delay presentation through compensatory mechanisms but may actually protect against the pathological process of AD itself.

### Depression as a risk factor

It is generally agreed that depression is often a prodromal feature of AD, so that those early in their dementing process can appear initially to have a depression. But is depression an independent risk factor for developing dementia or AD? Several case–control and cohort studies have examined this in the last few years and a thorough meta-analysis, identifying studies in which a specific diagnosis of depression was made (rather than depressive symptoms), found 20 good-quality published studies indicating any history of depression conferred a doubling of the risk of developing AD [odds ratios of 2.03 (1.73–2.38) for case–control studies and 1.90 (1.55–2.33) for cohort studies] (Ownby *et al.*, 2006). This provides strong support for depression as a risk factor and its effects could be mediated by its association with high cortisol levels and hypothalamic–pituitary–adrenal axis activation as animal studies have shown such features to be related to hippocampal atrophy (O'Brien, 1997). Alternatively increased vascular pathology associated with depression (Alexopoulos *et al.*, 1997) could provide the link as vascular factors are linked with increased AD (see below).

### Vascular risk factors

Over recent years the debate about the relationship of AD to VaD has been complicated or clarified (depending on one's point of view) by evidence that vascular disease may directly contribute to the pathology of AD. In fact this is far from a new idea as in his original paper Alois Alzheimer (Alzheimer, 1907) described vascular pathology at post-mortem in Auguste D. Both apolipoprotein E and homocysteine (discussed elsewhere) are also vascular risk factors and may exert their pathogenic effects in AD via vascular disease. There is good evidence for hypertension as a risk factor for AD. A prospective study examining the effects of blood pressure on dementia found that hypertension 10 and 15 years earlier increased the rate of AD (Skoog *et al.*, 1996) and a treatment study, which examined whether treating systolic hypertension in the elderly would reduce the rate of dementia and AD, found that treatment produced a 50% reduction in dementia (mainly AD) over 2 years (Forette *et al.*, 1998) with this reduction continuing to 4 years in an open label extension study (Forette *et al.*, 2002). However, another study failed to find any reduction in dementia risk or cognitive decline overall over 4 years, using an ACE inhibitor with or without a diruretic to lower blood pressure, although they did find a reduction in dementia in the post-stroke group (Tzourio *et al.*, 2003); a further study using an angiotensin receptor antagonist to lower blood pressure found no reduction in dementia risk or cognitive decline (Lithell *et al.*, 2003). The benefits of reduction of blood pressure on dementia risk are therefore unclear at the current time.

Elevated cholesterol in mid-life, an established risk factor for coronary heart disease and stroke disease, has been associated with an increased risk of developing dementia in cohort studies (Kivipelto *et al.*, 2001; Whitmer *et al.*, 2005b). Reduction of cholesterol using statins has been proposed to modify AD through several mechanisms in addition to cholesterol lowering, including antioxidative effects, inhibition of butryl cholinesterase, and increasing the trafficking of amyloid precursor protein (Darvesh *et al.*, 2004) and two cross-sectional analyses have reported a reduction in dementia in people taking statins (Jick *et al.*, 2000; Wolozin *et al.*, 2000). However, concern was expressed about 'bias by indication' in these studies (that is, healthier, better-educated people are more likely to take statins) and this view is supported by the finding in a 5-year prospective study that, whilst statin use was inversely associated with dementia, use in patients without dementia did not reduce incident dementia risk (Zandi *et al.*, 2005). Further caution about the potential benefits of statin use in reducing AD and dementia arises from the findings in two large randomized placebo controlled trials of two different statins [simvastatin in the Heart Protection Study (Heart Protection Study Collaborative Group, 2002) and pravastatin in the PROSPER study (Shepherd *et al.*, 2002)] which both failed to find any benefits of statin use on cognitive function or in reducing dementia risk.

Other vascular risk factors which may increase the risk of AD are the metabolic factors of obesity and diabetes. Diabetes has also been found to increase the risk of dementia in general (relative risk 1.9) and, more specifically, AD (relative risk 1.9) (Ott *et al.*, 1999) and obesity in mid-life has also been linked with an increased risk of dementia (Whitmer *et al.*, 2005a) and both dementia and AD [odds ratio (OR) 2.4] (Kivipelto *et al.*, 2005). However, the benefits of weight reduction and improved glucose control need investigation. Such vascular risk factors may be additive in effect because combining obesity with hypertension and high cholesterol led to a much larger combined risk (OR 6.2) (Kivipelto *et al.*, 2005) and in another prospective study (over 5.5 years) diabetes, smoking, hypertension, and heart disease all increased the risk of AD but their additive effect was much stronger, increasing the risk by over three-fold (Luchsinger *et al.*, 2005).

## Head injury as a risk factor

A meta-analysis of case–control studies of head injury (with loss of consciousness) showed it to be associated with an 80% increase in risk of AD (Mortimer *et al.*, 1991). These early studies used retrospective assessments from relatives, raising the risk of recollection bias, and studies using medical records of head injury have shown no association (Williams *et al.*, 1991; Breteler *et al.*, 1995). Head injury has been shown to increase amyloid-beta protein deposits in the brain, demonstrating a plausible mechanism for a link between head injury and AD (Roberts *et al.*, 1991). It is therefore interesting to note that Mayeux *et al.* (1995) found head injury is only a risk factor for AD in people with the *APOE* ε4 allele.

## Other possible risk factors

### Metals

Studies some years ago showed increased aluminium in the brains of subjects with AD and that aluminium is neurotoxic (Crapper

*et al.*, 1973; Trapp *et al.*, 1978). This led to the suggestion that it may play a role in the causation of AD, and epidemiological studies found higher rates of AD in areas with high aluminium content in the drinking water (Doll, 1993). However, other studies did not confirm these early findings and it is clear that aluminium is neither necessary nor sufficient to cause AD (Walton, 1991). More recently attention has switched to other metals which are found in high quantities in the brain; abnormalities in metal homeostasis, especially zinc and copper, occur in AD and may increase oxidative damage and the formation of amyloid-beta plaques (Maynard *et al.*, 2005). Consistent with this, in a small randomized trial in AD the metal protein attenuating compound (MPAC) clioquinol, which buffers zinc and copper, led to less deterioration in more severely ill patients (Ritchie *et al.*, 2003), but this drug has serious optic side-effects and further trials using other compounds are needed.

### Smoking

One meta-analysis of case–control studies found smokers had a 20% reduction in AD (Graves *et al.*, 1991). A plausible mechanism is that smoking increases nicotinic receptors in the cortex and this could counteract the cholinergic deficit in AD; the role of nicotine as a potential neuroprotective agent in AD has received support from the finding that nicotine treatment reduces deposition of amyloid-beta in mice (Hellstrom-Lindahl *et al.*, 2004). However, a prospective study found the opposite, with smokers having twice the risk of AD (Ott *et al.*, 1998) and a more recent meta-analysis examining both case–control and prospective cohort studies reported conflicting findings, with case–control studies suggesting smoking was protective but cohort studies linking smoking with an increase in AD (Almeida *et al.*, 2002).

### Homocysteine, vitamin B$_{12}$, and folate

Cognitive impairment is associated with deficiencies in folate and vitamin B$_{12}$. Homocysteine is an amino acid intermediary in methionine metabolism and its blood levels increase with deficiencies in folate and B$_{12}$ because its elimination is dependent on these vitamins; the risk of cognitive impairment and dementia associated with their deficiencies may be related to raised homocysteine levels. Some case–control studies have reported high homocysteine levels in AD (Clarke *et al.*, 1998; McCaddon *et al.*, 1998) and high homocysteine levels predict cognitive decline (McCaddon *et al.*, 2001) and have been reported to be a risk factor for the development of dementia, including AD (Seshadri *et al.*, 2002). However, a prospective study of homocysteine and cognitive impairment found no relationship between them (Kalmijn *et al.*, 1999) and systematic reviews of intervention studies found no evidence for any benefit on cognition or dementia using B$_{12}$ with and without folate (Malouf and Areosa Sastre, 2003; Malouf *et al.*, 2003).

### Oestrogen

A series of systematic reviews and meta-analyses of cohort and case–control studies (Yaffe *et al.*, 1998; Leblanc *et al.*, 2001; Nelson *et al.*, 2002) have reported oestrogen use to be associated with a reduction in the risk of developing AD of 29% to 34%. However, randomized trials (e.g. Henderson *et al.* 2000; Mulnard *et al.*, 2000; Wang *et al.*, 2000) have failed to find any clinically meaningful evidence of benefit in treating patients with mild to moderate AD with oestrogen. A large primary prevention trial, the WHIMS trial (the Women's Health Initiative Memory Study), examined the possible benefit of hormone replacement therapy (HRT)/oestrogen replacement therapy (ERT) in reducing the frequency of or time of onset of dementia in post-menopausal women, but adverse outcomes led to both arms being terminated early (treatment led to increased rates of stroke, coronary heart disease, venous thromboembolism, and breast carcinoma). The use of unopposed oestrogen over 7 years was associated with a non-significant increased risk of dementia, hazard ratio 1.49 (95%CI 0.83–2.66) (Shumaker et al., 2004), and treatment with combined oestrogen and progestin over 4 years led to a doubling of dementia risk, hazard ratio 2.05 (95%CI 1.21–3.48) (Hays et al., 2003). Combining these two groups, there was a highly clinically and statistically significant increase in dementia in women taking HRT, hazard ratio 1.76 (95%CI 1.19–2.60) (Shumaker et al., 2004). It appears that oestrogen use is a risk factor for AD and dementia rather than a protective factor.

### Protective factors: anti-inflammatory medication

A review of case–control studies has suggested that arthritis, non-steroidal anti-inflammatory drugs (NSAIDs), and steroids are protective factors for AD, reducing the risk by about 50% (McGeer et al., 1996). This fits with current views that AD is associated with an inflammatory response in the brain because senile plaques are associated with prominent astrocytosis and microglial activation (Dickson et al., 1988) and proinflammatory cytokines are increased in the brain in AD subjects (Wood et al., 1993). A dampener for enthusiasm about the role of inflammation in AD is that all randomized controlled trials using anti-inflammatory drugs, including ibuprofen, prednisolone, naproxen, and COX inhibitors, in established AD have been negative (Aisen et al., 2000, 2003; Imbimbo, 2004; Reines et al., 2004).

### Protective effects of vitamins and anti-oxidants

Oxidative stress is thought to be important in the development of dementia and neurons are especially vulnerable to oxidative stress because the brain has a high oxygen consumption and a lack of anti-oxidant enzymes, e.g. superoxide dismutase (SOD-1), compared with other organs (Esposito et al., 2002) and is more dependent on dietary anti-oxidants including tocopherols, ascorbic acid, carotenoids, vitamin A, and flavonoids. Although using vitamins as anti-oxidants has been frequently cited as protective for AD, cross-sectional and cohort studies have reported mixed findings on the possibility of nutritional and/or supplementary dietary anti-oxidants reducing the risk of dementia (Engelhart et al., 2002, 2005; Morris et al., 2002; Tabet et al., 2002; Larrieu et al., 2004). The only randomized trial of vitamin E supplementation in AD (in moderately impaired subjects) reported that after adjustment for baseline MMSE (but not before) vitamin E delayed time to a composite endpoint by 230 days (Sano et al., 1997). However, there were no differences in a range of secondary outcome measures including the Alzheimer's Disease Assessment Scale cognitive subscale (ADAS-Cog) and MMSE. A larger randomized trial of 769 subjects compared progression to possible or probable AD in subjects with amnestic mild cognitive impairment (Petersen et al., 2005). Subjects were randomized to vitamin E (2000 IU), donepezil (10 mg), or placebo for 3 years and no difference in outcome was observed, casting doubt on the benefits of anti-oxidant treatment in preventing or slowing the development of AD.

### Protective effects of alcohol

Although case–control studies show no association in general between alcohol and AD (Graves et al., 1991) a prospective study found wine drinking was protective for AD, reducing the risk by 80% for moderate drinkers compared with non-drinkers (Orgogozo et al., 1997). A mechanism for this protection could involve the anti-oxidant properties of red wine specifically rather than the alcohol itself. However, one prospective study found an association between heavy alcohol consumption and dementia (Saunders et al., 1991), and another reported that both high and no alcohol consumption in mid-life led to an increase in mild cognitive impairment and possibly dementia (Anttila et al., 2004) suggesting there may be a U-shaped relationship between alcohol consumption and dementia risk.

### Summary

There is clear evidence that age and family history are major risk factors for AD. A few key genes have been identified which are causal in some early-onset cases (presenilin-1, presenilin-2, and amyloid precursor protein) and contribute in late onset cases (apolipoprotein E). Down's syndrome is the only other well-recognized risk factor and this is mediated via amyloid precursor protein. Beyond this the best current evidence supports depression, hypertension, and head injury as risk factors for AD. There is no conclusive evidence for other risk factors but there is current interest in obesity, diabetes, and other vascular factors.

## Prognosis of Alzheimer's disease

Until recently no specific treatments were available for AD and so, unlike most other psychiatric disorders, studies of prognosis were largely of the natural history of the condition. However, the introduction of the cholinesterase inhibitors (see Chapter 27viii) has now changed this, and in future the effects of these new treatments on prognosis must be considered.

### The natural history of Alzheimer's disease

Every old age psychiatrist is familiar with the considerable variability in the pattern, progress, and outcome of AD. All the studies following the natural history of the disease bear this out as they show substantial variations in symptomatology and rates of decline. The practical consequence of this for the clinician is that it makes it very difficult to give accurate predictions to patients or their families about the likely progress of the disease after the diagnosis has been made. Following the introduction of the cholinesterase inhibitors there has been a trend towards earlier diagnosis, which introduces further difficulties because the disease is being picked up at a time before current clinical and research experience has been acquired. Furthermore, we know little about the effects of the drugs themselves in the longer term, which makes prognostic predictions even more perilous in patients on these treatments.

However, patients and relatives will continue to seek information on prognosis, and two of the most common outcomes of interest are time to institutionalization in some form of residential care and time to death. Knopman et al. (1988) examined time from diagnosis to institutionalization and found that for patients with mild AD 12% were in nursing homes by 1 year and 35% by 2 years. For those severely affected at outset the figures were 39% at 1 year and 62% at 2 years. Whilst helpful, such figures disguise the fact that certain kinds of symptom (agitation, wandering, aggression, and sleep disturbance) tend to precipitate much earlier institutionalization. These behaviours, which are very distressing for all concerned, are major predictors of early institutionalization (Haupt and Kurz, 1993; Bianchetti *et al.*, 1995). Time from diagnosis to death is highly variable, with the mean length of survival from diagnosis ranging from 1 year up to 16 years. This is highly dependent on how early the diagnosis is made, although certain other factors, for example age at onset, are also important (see below under Predicting rates of decline). However, studies do give a fairly consistent median survival of 5 to 6 years (Walsh *et al.*, 1990; Heyman *et al.*, 1996). Unsurprisingly, the mildest patients at outset tend to show the longest times to both institutionalization and death.

The cause of death in AD can be difficult to determine. As with other chronic diseases in the elderly many people will die with the disease rather than from it. Since AD is associated with marked weight loss and physical decline (Cronin-Stubbs *et al.*, 1997) it is clearly at least a contributory factor to death in many people with advanced disease, although frequently AD is not even mentioned on the death certificate (Burns *et al.*, 1990f). Whether AD directly causes death is less certain, although it seems plausible as some sufferers do simply fade away without any other obvious cause of death occurring. Many others develop an infection or other complications of immobility and physical debilitation and die of some combination of causes.

## Measuring rates of decline

Two kinds of instrument (global rating scales and cognitive scales) have been used to try and measure the rate of decline in AD. The global measures, e.g. the Clinical Dementia Rating Scale (CDR; Hughes *et al.*, 1982), tend to change very slowly over a few years and so are not useful measures of change clinically. The cognitive scales do show significant changes over the course of a year. Some of these are in common use and a knowledge of the research figures may help a clinician to see how rapidly any patient is declining compared with these norms and thus could help clarify the prediction of progress and outcome, although the substantial variability should always be borne in mind. The annual rate of change in the MMSE (Folstein *et al.*, 1975) is about 2.5 points a year for moderately affected patients, with higher rates for more severely affected patients and lower rates for milder cases (Salmon *et al.*, 1990). Two larger instruments are the CAMCOG [the cognitive component of the Cambridge Mental Disorders of the Elderly (CAMDEX)] and ADAS-Cog. Burns *et al.* (1991b) used the CAMCOG to follow the progress of 110 AD patients. They found a drop of about 12 points in the first year (maximum score 107 with 80/79 as the cut-off for dementia). This included change in every main subsection, but many of the scores were already near the floor at baseline and this instrument appears less useful in more advanced dementia. A couple of studies have used ADAS-Cog (maximum score 70) and have shown an annual rate of change of 8 to 9 points (Kramer-Ginsberg *et al.*, 1988; Yesavage *et al.*, 1988).

## Predicting rates of decline

Within the rough framework of the above figures for rates of decline and time to institutionalization and death are there any clinical features which can help sharpen the prediction in individual cases? The severity of the dementia is predictive in that the more severe the dementia the more rapid the rate of decline

(Morris *et al.*, 1993). Consistent with this, decline is nonlinear, being slower at the milder stage but accelerating as the dementia progresses (Teri *et al.*, 1995). Age of onset is also a recognized predictor of deterioration, with early onset dementias showing more rapid cognitive and functional decline (Jacobs *et al.*, 1994; Teri *et al.*, 1995).

Other factors which have been investigated without a clear conclusion include sex, level of education, *APOE* genotype, oestrogen, and NSAIDs.

Extrapyramidal symptoms appear to predict more rapid deterioration in AD, though results are complicated by the likely mixing together in earlier studies of patients with AD and DLB (Miller *et al.*, 1991). However, a more recent study in a purer AD group also found that extrapyramidal symptoms were associated with greater functional decline and more rapid institutionalization, although there was no association with cognitive decline (Lopez *et al.*, 1997). A number of studies have found psychotic symptoms to predict more rapid deterioration, although when groups have been matched for severity of AD at outset the findings have been mixed. Some studies have found psychosis does still predict rate of decline (Chui *et al.*, 1994; Stern *et al.*, 1994a) but others have not found this (Reisberg *et al.*, 1986; Chen *et al.*, 1991). One longitudinal study has not found depression to predict decline (Lopez *et al.*, 1990) but, unsurprisingly, it has been shown to be associated with greater impairment on activities of daily living (Pearson *et al.*, 1989). Both psychotic and depressive symptoms are clinically important, regardless of whether they predict deterioration, because they increase the suffering of the patients and their carers and, as discussed above, they should be treated in their own right.

## The effects of drug treatment on prognosis

Antipsychotic drugs appear to worsen cognitive decline in dementia (McShane *et al.*, 1997; Ballard *et al.*, 2005) and are associated with increased mortality (Schneider *et al.*, 2005). They have also been shown to adversely affect patients with DLB (Ballard *et al.*, 1998; Dickson *et al.*, 1988; McKeith *et al.*, 1992). It appears that whilst these widely prescribed drugs do show benefits in the short term for specific symptoms (as shown above) there is a danger they may worsen patient status overall. The evidence suggests they should only be used with caution, as outlined earlier, and they need close monitoring and regular review with the aim of discontinuing treatment after 4–6 months to reduce the longer-term risks.

What about cholinesterase inhibitors? At the outset here we should remind ourselves these drugs clearly improve the prognosis of AD in the short term for the 50–60% who respond to them (see Chapter 27 viii). Patients enjoy improved cognitive function, a reduction in disturbed behaviour, and important gains in function in everyday life, and such benefits continue for several years on treatment. It remains unclear whether or not these drugs slow down the disease process itself. While theoretically they might modify the disease, as cholinergic stimulation may reduce the phosphorylation of tau (a key stage in tangle formation), no reliable data exist for a disease-slowing effect at present.

## Summary

The pattern and progression of AD is highly variable. Predictors of decline are greater severity of illness and early age of onset, which both predict a more rapid course, and extrapyramidal and psychotic symptoms, which probably do so too. Whilst antipsychotic drugs are of benefit in the short-term in treating some non-cognitive symptoms their long-term use may worsen the prognosis; cholinesterase inhibitors, on the other hand, improve prognosis in the short term but their effects in the longer term on the disease are unclear.

## References

Aisen, P.S., Davis, K.L., Berg, J.D. *et al.* (2000). A randomized controlled trial of prednisone in Alzheimer's disease. Alzheimer's Disease Cooperative Study. *Neurology*, **54**, 588–93.

Aisen, P.S., Schafer, K.A., Grundman, M. *et al.* (2003). Effects of rofecoxib or naproxen vs placebo on Alzheimer disease progression: a randomized controlled trial. *Journal of the American Medical Association*, **289**, 2819–26.

Alexopoulos, G.S., Meyers, B.S., Young, R.C., Campbell, S., Silbersweig, D., and Charlson, M. (1997). 'Vascular depression' hypothesis. *Archives of General Psychiatry*, **54**, 915–22.

Almeida, O.P., Hulse, G.K., Lawrence, D., and Flicker, L. (2002). Smoking as a risk factor for Alzheimer's disease: contrasting evidence from a systematic review of case-control and cohort studies. *Addiction*, **97**, 15–28.

Alzheimer, A. (1907). Uber eine eigenartig Erkrankung der Hirnrinde. *Allgemeine Zeitschrift für Psychiatrie und Psychisch-gerichtliche Medizin*, **64**, 146–8.

American Psychiatric Association (1994). *Diagnostic and statistical manual of mental disorders*, 4th edn. American Psychiatric Association, Washington, DC.

Andersen, K., Launer, L.J., Dewey, M.E. *et al.* (1999). Gender differences in the incidence of AD and vascular dementia: The EURODEM Studies. EURODEM Incidence Research Group. *Neurology*, **53**, 1992–7.

Anttila, T., Helkala, E.L., Viitanen, M. *et al.* (2004). Alcohol drinking in middle age and subsequent risk of mild cognitive impairment and dementia in old age: a prospective population based study. *British Medical Journal*, **329**, 4.

Bains, J., Birks, J.S., and Dening, T.R. (2002). Antidepressants for treating depression in dementia. *Cochrane Database of Systematic Reviews* 2002, Issue 4. Art. No. CD003944. DOI: 10.1002/14651858.CD003944.

Ballard, C.G. and Walker, M. (1999). Neuropsychiatric aspects of Alzheimer's disease. *Current Psychiatry Reports*, **1**, 49–60.

Ballard, C.G., Bannister, C., and Oyebode, F. (1996). Depression in dementia sufferers. *International Journal of Geriatric Psychiatry*, **11**, 507–15.

Ballard, C., Grace, J., McKeith, I., and Holmes, C. (1998). Neuroleptic sensitivity in dementia with Lewy bodies and Alzheimer's disease. *Lancet*, **351**, 1032–3.

Ballard, C., Margallo-Lana, M., Juszczak, E. *et al.* (2005). Quetiapine and rivastigmine and cognitive decline in Alzheimer's disease: randomised double blind placebo controlled trial. *British Medical Journal*, **330**, 874.

Ballard, C., Waite, J., and Birks, J. (2006). *Atypical antipsychotics for aggression and psychosis in Alzheimer's disease*. Art. No. CD003476. DOI: 10.1002/14651858.CD003476.pub2 (http://www.cochrane.org/reviews/en/ab003476.html).

Bianchetti, A., Scuratti, A., Zanetti, O. *et al.* (1995). Predictors of mortality and institutionalization in Alzheimer disease patients 1 year after discharge from an Alzheimer dementia unit. *Dementia*, **6**, 108–12.

Blansjaar, B.A., Thomassen, R., and Van Schaick, H.W. (2000). Prevalence of dementia in centenarians. *International Journal of Geriatric Psychiatry*, **15**, 219–25.

Breteler, M.M., De Groot, R.R., Van Romunde, L.K., and Hofman, A. (1995). Risk of dementia in patients with Parkinson's disease, epilepsy, and severe head trauma: a register-based follow-up study. *American Journal of Epidemiology*, **142**, 1300–5.

Burns, A., Jacoby, R., and Levy, R. (1990a). Psychiatric phenomena in Alzheimer's disease. I: Disorders of thought content. *British Journal of Psychiatry*, **157**, 72–6, 92–4.

Burns, A., Jacoby, R., and Levy, R. (1990b). Psychiatric phenomena in Alzheimer's disease. II: Disorders of perception. *British Journal of Psychiatry*, **157**, 76–81, 92–4.

Burns, A., Jacoby, R., and Levy, R. (1990c). Psychiatric phenomena in Alzheimer's disease. III: Disorders of mood. *British Journal of Psychiatry*, **157**, 81–6, 92–4.

Burns, A., Jacoby, R., and Levy, R. (1990d). Psychiatric phenomena in Alzheimer's disease. IV: Disorders of behaviour. *British Journal of Psychiatry*, **157**, 86–94.

Burns, A., Luthert, P., Levy, R., Jacoby, R., and Lantos, P. (1990e). Accuracy of clinical diagnosis of Alzheimer's disease. *British Medical Journal*, **301**, 1026.

Burns, A., Jacoby, R., Luthert, P., and Levy, R. (1990f). Cause of death in Alzheimer's disease. *Age and Ageing*, **19**, 341–4.

Burns, A., Jacoby, R., and Levy, R. (1991a). Neurological signs in Alzheimer's disease. *Age and Ageing*, **20**, 45–51.

Burns, A., Jacoby, R., and Levy, R. (1991b). Progression of cognitive impairment in Alzheimer's disease. *Journal of the American Geriatrics Society*, **39**, 39–45.

Burns, A., Lewis, G., Jacoby, R., and Levy, R. (1991c). Factors affecting survival in Alzheimer's disease. *Psychological Medicine*, **21**, 363–70.

Chen, J.Y., Stern, Y., Sano, M., and Mayeux, R. (1991). Cumulative risks of developing extrapyramidal signs, psychosis, or myoclonus in the course of Alzheimer's disease. *Archives of Neurology*, **48**, 1141–3.

Chui, H.C., Lyness, S.A., Sobel, E., and Schneider, L.S. (1994). Extrapyramidal signs and psychiatric symptoms predict faster cognitive decline in Alzheimer's disease. *Archives of Neurology*, **51**, 676–81.

Clarke, R., Smith, A.D., Jobst, K.A., Refsum, H., Sutton, L., and Ueland, P.M. (1998). Folate, vitamin B12, and serum total homocysteine levels in confirmed Alzheimer disease. *Archives of Neurology*, **55**, 1449–55.

Cohen, D., Eisdorfer, C., Gorelick, P. *et al.* (1993). Psychopathology associated with Alzheimer's disease and related disorders. *Journal of Gerontology*, **48**, M255–M260.

Committee for the Safety of Medicines (2004). CEM/CMO/2004/1 (see http://www.info.doh.gov.uk/doh/embroadcast.nsf/vwDiscussionAll/3D8DBB48B26FF90280256E520045977A).

Cooper, J.K., Mungas, D., and Verma, M. (1991). Psychotic symptoms in Alzheimer's disease. *International Journal of Geriatric Psychiatry*, **6**, 721–6.

Crapper, D.R., Krishnan, S.S., and Dalton, A.J. (1973). Brain aluminum distribution in Alzheimer's disease and experimental neurofibrillary degeneration. *Transactions of the American Neurological Association*, **98**, 17–20.

Cronin-Stubbs, D., Beckett, L.A., Scherr, P.A. *et al.* (1997). Weight loss in people with Alzheimer's disease: a prospective population based analysis. *British Medical Journal*, **314**, 178–9.

Cruts, M., Van Duijn, C.M., Backhovens, H. *et al.* (1998). Estimation of the genetic contribution of presenilin-1 and -2 mutations in a population-based study of presenile Alzheimer disease. *Human Molecular Genetics*, **7**, 43–51.

Darvesh, S., Martin, E., Walsh, R., and Rockwood, K. (2004). Differential effects of lipid-lowering agents on human cholinesterases. *Clinical Biochemistry*, **37**, 42–9.

De Strooper, B., Annaert, W., Cupers, P. *et al.* (1999). A presenilin-1-dependent gamma-secretase-like protease mediates release of Notch intracellular domain. *Nature*, **398**, 518–22.

Dickson, D.W., Farlo, J., Davies, P., Crystal, H., Fuld, P., and Yen, S.H. (1988). Alzheimer's disease. A double-labeling immunohistochemical study of senile plaques. *American Journal of Pathology*, **132**, 86–101.

Doll, R. (1993). Review: Alzheimer's disease and environmental aluminium. *Age and Ageing*, **22**, 138–53.

Engelhart, M.J., Geerlings, M.I., Ruitenberg, A. *et al.* (2002). Dietary intake of antioxidants and risk of Alzheimer disease. *Journal of the American Medical Association*, **287**, 3223–9.

Engelhart, M.J., Ruitenberg, A., Meijer, J. *et al.* (2005). Plasma levels of antioxidants are not associated with Alzheimer's disease or cognitive decline. *Dementia and Geriatric Cognitive Disorders*, **19**, 134–9.

Esposito, E., Rotilio, D., Di Matteo, V., Di Giulio, C., Cacchio, M., and Algeri, S. (2002). A review of specific dietary antioxidants and the effects on biochemical mechanisms related to neurodegenerative processes. *Neurobiology of Aging*, **23**, 719–35.

Farmer, M.E., Kittner, S.J., Rae, D.S., Bartko, J.J., and Regier, D.A. (1995). Education and change in cognitive function. The Epidemiologic Catchment Area Study. *Annals of Epidemiology*, **5**, 1–7.

Farrer, L.A., Cupples, L.A., Blackburn, S. *et al.* (1994). Interrater agreement for diagnosis of Alzheimer's disease: the MIRAGE study. *Neurology*, **44**, 652–6.

Farrer, L.A., Cupples, L.A., Haines, J.L. *et al.* (1997). Effects of age, sex, and ethnicity on the association between apolipoprotein E genotype and Alzheimer disease. A meta-analysis. APOE and Alzheimer Disease Meta Analysis Consortium. *Journal of the American Medical Association*, **278**, 1349–56.

Folstein, M.F., Folstein, S.E., and McHugh, P.R. (1975). 'Mini-mental state'. A practical method for grading the cognitive state of patients for the clinician. *Journal of Psychiatric Research*, **12**, 189–98.

Forette, F., Seux, M.L., Staessen, J.A. *et al.* (1998). Prevention of dementia in randomised double-blind placebo-controlled Systolic Hypertension in Europe (Syst-Eur). trial. *Lancet*, **352**, 1347–51.

Forette, F., Seux, M.L., Staessen, J.A. *et al.* (2002). The prevention of dementia with antihypertensive treatment: new evidence from the Systolic Hypertension in Europe (Syst-Eur) study. *Archives of Internal Medicine*, **162**, 2046–52.

Gao, S., Hendrie, H.C., Hall, K.S., and Hui, S. (1998). The relationships between age, sex, and the incidence of dementia and Alzheimer disease: a meta-analysis. *Archives of General Psychiatry*, **55**, 809–15.

Gilley, D.W., Wilson, R.S., Beckett, L.A., and Evans, D.A. (1997). Psychotic symptoms and physically aggressive behavior in Alzheimer's disease. *Journal of the American Geriatrics Society*, **45**, 1074–9.

Glassman, A.H., O'Connor, C.M., Califf, R.M. *et al.* (2002). Sertraline treatment of major depression in patients with acute MI or unstable angina. *Journal of the American Medical Association*, **288**, 701–9.

Graves, A.B., Van Duijn, C.M., Chandra, V. *et al.* (1991). Alcohol and tobacco consumption as risk factors for Alzheimer's disease: a collaborative re-analysis of case-control studies. EURODEM Risk Factors Research Group. *International Journal of Epidemiology*, **20**, S48–S57.

Hardy, J. (1997). Amyloid, the presenilins and Alzheimer's disease. *Trends in Neurosciences*, **20**, 154–9.

Haupt, M. and Kurz, A. (1993). Predictors of nursing home placement in patients with Alzheimer's disease. *International Journal of Geriatric Psychiatry*, **8**, 741–6.

Hays, J., Ockene, J.K., Brunner, R.L. *et al.* (2003). Effects of estrogen plus progestin on health-related quality of life. *New England Journal of Medicine*, **348**, 1839–54.

Heart Protection Study Collaborative Group (2002). MRC/BHF Heart Protection Study of cholesterol lowering with simvastatin in 20,536 high-risk individuals: a randomised placebo-controlled trial. *Lancet*, **360**, 7–22.

Hellstrom-Lindahl, E., Court, J., Keverne, J. *et al.* (2004). Nicotine reduces A beta in the brain and cerebral vessels of APPsw mice. *European Journal of Neuroscience*, **19**, 2703–10.

Henderson, A.S., Easteal, S., Jorm, A.F. *et al.* (1995). Apolipoprotein E allele epsilon 4, dementia, and cognitive decline in a population sample. *Lancet*, **346**, 1387–90.

Henderson, V.W., Paganini-Hill, A., Miller, B.L. *et al.* (2000). Estrogen for Alzheimer's disease in women: randomized, double-blind, placebo-controlled trial. *Neurology*, **54**, 295–301.

Hendrie, H.C., Ogunniyi, A., Hall, K.S. *et al.* (2001). Incidence of dementia and Alzheimer disease in 2 communities: Yoruba residing in Ibadan, Nigeria, and African Americans residing in Indianapolis, Indiana. *Journal of the American Medical Association*, **285**, 739–47.

Heyman, A., Peterson, B., Fillenbaum, G., and Pieper, C. (1996). The consortium to establish a registry for Alzheimer's disease (CERAD). Part XIV: Demographic and clinical predictors of survival in patients with Alzheimer's disease. *Neurology*, **46**, 656–60.

Hirono, N., Mori, E., Yasuda, M. *et al.* (1998). Factors associated with psychotic symptoms in Alzheimer's disease. *Journal of Neurology, Neurosurgery and Psychiatry*, **64**, 648–52.

Hughes, C.P., Berg, L., Danziger, W.L., Coben, L.A., and Martin, R.L. (1982). A new clinical scale for the staging of dementia. *British Journal of Psychiatry*, **140**, 566–72.

Imbimbo, B.P. (2004). The potential role of non-steroidal anti-inflammatory drugs in treating Alzheimer's disease. *Expert Opinion on Investigational Drugs*, **13**, 1469–81.

Jacobs, D., Sano, M., Marder, K. *et al.* (1994). Age at onset of Alzheimer's disease: relation to pattern of cognitive dysfunction and rate of decline. *Neurology*, **44**, 1215–20.

Jick, H., Zornberg, G.L., Jick, S.S., Seshardi, S., and Drachman, D.A. (2000). Statins and the risk of dementia. *Lancet*, **356**, 1627–31.

Jorm, A.F. (2001). History of depression as a risk factor for dementia: an updated review. *Australian and New Zealand Journal of Psychiatry*, **35**, 776–81.

Jorm, A.F. and Jolley, D. (1998). The incidence of dementia: a meta-analysis. *Neurology*, **51**, 728–33.

Kalmijn, S., Launer, L.J., Lindemans, J., Bots, M.L., Hofman, A., and Breteler, M.M. (1999). Total homocysteine and cognitive decline in a community-based sample of elderly subjects: the Rotterdam Study. *American Journal of Epidemiology*, **150**, 283–9.

Kang, D.E., Saitoh, T., Chen, X. *et al.* (1997). Genetic association of the low-density lipoprotein receptor-related protein gene (LRP), an apolipoprotein E receptor, with late-onset alzheimer's disease. *Neurology*, **49**, 56–61.

Kivipelto, M., Helkala, E.L., Laakso, M.P. *et al.* (2001). Midlife vascular risk factors and Alzheimer's disease in later life: longitudinal, population based study. *British Medical Journal*, **322**, 1447–51.

Kivipelto, M., Ngandu, T., Fratiglioni, L. *et al.* (2005). Obesity and vascular risk factors at midlife and the risk of dementia and Alzheimer disease. *Archives of Neurology*, **62**, 1556–60.

Knesevich, J.W., Martin, R.L., Berg, L., and Danziger, W. (1983). Preliminary report on affective symptoms in the early stages of senile dementia of the Alzheimer type. *American Journal of Psychiatry*, **140**, 233–5.

Knopman, D.S., Kitto, J., Deinard, S., and Heiring, J. (1988). Longitudinal study of death and institutionalization in patients with primary degenerative dementia. *Journal of the American Geriatrics Society*, **36**, 108–12.

Kramer-Ginsberg, E., Mohs, R.C., Aryan, M. *et al.* (1988). Clinical predictors of course for Alzheimer patients in a longitudinal study: a preliminary report. *Psychopharmacology Bulletin*, **24**, 458–62.

Larrieu, S., Letenneur, L., Helmer, C., Dartigues, J.F., and Barberger-Gateau, P. (2004). Nutritional factors and risk of incident dementia in the PAQUID longitudinal cohort. *Journal of Nutrition, Health and Aging*, **8**, 150–4.

Leblanc, E.S., Janowsky, J., Chan, B.K., and Nelson, H.D. (2001). Hormone replacement therapy and cognition: systematic review and meta-analysis. *Journal of the American Medical Association*, **285**, 1489–99.

Levy, M.L., Cummings, J.L., Fairbanks, L.A. *et al.* (1998). Apathy is not depression. *Journal of Neuropsychiatry and Clinical Neurosciences*, **10**, 314–19.

Liao, A., Nitsch, R.M., Greenberg, S.M. *et al.* (1998). Genetic association of an alpha2-macroglobulin (Val1000Ile). polymorphism and Alzheimer's disease. *Human Molecular Genetics*, **7**, 1953–6.

Lithell, H., Hansson, L., Skoog, I. *et al.* (2003). The Study on Cognition and Prognosis in the Elderly (SCOPE): principal results of a randomized double-blind intervention trial. *Journal of Hypertension*, **21**, 875–86.

Livingston, G., Johnston, K., Katona, C., Paton, J., Lyketsos, C.G., and Old Age Task Force of the World Federation of Biological Psychiatry (2005). Systematic review of psychological approaches to the management of neuropsychiatric symptoms of dementia. *American Journal of Psychiatry*, **162**, 1996–2021.

Lopez, O.L., Boller, F., Becker, J.T., Miller, M., and Reynolds, C.F.D. (1990). Alzheimer's disease and depression: neuropsychological impairment and progression of the illness. *American Journal of Psychiatry*, **147**, 855–60.

Lopez, O.L., Wisnieski, S.R., Becker, J.T., Boller, F., and Dekosky, S.T. (1997). Extrapyramidal signs in patients with probable Alzheimer disease. *Archives of Neurology*, **54**, 969–75.

Luchsinger, J.A., Reitz, C., Honig, L.S., Tang, M.X., Shea, S., and Mayeux, R. (2005). Aggregation of vascular risk factors and risk of incident Alzheimer disease. *Neurology*, **65**, 545–51.

Lyketsos, C.G., Delcampo, L., Steinberg, M. *et al*. (2003). Treating depression in Alzheimer disease: efficacy and safety of sertraline therapy, and the benefits of depression reduction: the DIADS. *Archives of General Psychiatry*, **60**, 737–46.

McCaddon, A., Davies, G., Hudson, P., Tandy, S., and Cattell, H. (1998). Total homocysteine in senile dementia of Alzheimer type. *International Journal of Geriatric Psychiatry*, **13**, 235–9.

McCaddon, A., Hudson, P., Davies, G., Hughes, A., Williams, J.H. and Wilkinson, C. (2001). Homocysteine and cognitive decline in healthy elderly. *Dementia and Geriatric Cognitive Disorders*, **12**, 309–13.

McGeer, P.L., Schulzer, M., and McGeer, E.G. (1996). Arthritis and anti-inflammatory agents as possible protective factors for Alzheimer's disease: a review of 17 epidemiologic studies. *Neurology*, **47**, 425–32.

McKeith, I., Fairbairn, A., Perry, R., Thompson, P., and Perry, E. (1992). Neuroleptic sensitivity in patients with senile dementia of Lewy body type. *British Medical Journal*, **305**, 673–8.

McKeith, I., Ballard, C., O'Brien, J. *et al*. (2000a). Predictive accuracy of clinical diagnostic criteria for dementia with Lewy bodies: a prospective neuropathological validation study. *Neurology*, **54**, 1050–8.

McKeith, I., Del Ser, T., Spano, P. *et al*. (2000b). Efficacy of rivastigmine in dementia with Lewy bodies: a randomised, double-blind, placebo-controlled international study. *Lancet*, **356**, 2031–6.

McKeith, I.G., Ballard, C.G., Perry, R.H. *et al*. (2000c). Prospective validation of consensus criteria for the diagnosis of dementia with Lewy bodies. *Neurology*, **54**, 1050–8.

McKeith, I.G., Dickson, D.W., Lowe, J. *et al*. (2005). Diagnosis and management of dementia with Lewy bodies: third report of the DLB Consortium. *Neurology*, **65**, 1863–72.

McKhann, G., Drachman, D., Folstein, M., Katzman, R., Price, D., and Stadlan, E.M. (1984). Clinical diagnosis of Alzheimer's disease: report of the NINCDS-ADRDA Work Group under the auspices of Department of Health and Human Services Task Force on Alzheimer's Disease. *Neurology*, **34**, 939–44.

McShane, R., Keene, J., Gedling, K., Fairburn, C., Jacoby, R., and Hope, T. (1997). Do neuroleptic drugs hasten cognitive decline in dementia? Prospective study with necropsy follow up. *British Medical Journal*, **314**, 266–70.

Malouf, R. and Areosa Sastre, A. (2003). Vitamin B12 for cognition. *Cochrane Database of Systematic Reviews* 2003, Issue 3, Art. No. CD004394. DOI: 10.1002/14651858.CD004394.

Malouf, R., Grimley Evans, J., and Areosa Sastre, A. (2003). Folic acid with or without vitamin B12 for cognition and dementia. *Cochrane Database of Systematic Reviews* 2003, Issue 4, Art. No. CD004514. DOI: 10.1002/14651858.CD004514.

Mann, D.M., Yates, P.O., Marcyniuk, B., and Ravindra, C.R. (1986). The topography of plaques and tangles in Down's syndrome patients of different ages. *Neuropathology and Applied Neurobiology*, **12**, 447–57.

Mayeux, R., Ottman, R., Maestre, G. *et al*. (1995). Synergistic effects of traumatic head injury and apolipoprotein-epsilon 4 in patients with Alzheimer's disease. *Neurology*, **45**, 555–7.

Maynard, C.J., Bush, A.I., Masters, C.L., Cappai, R. and Li, Q.X. (2005). Metals and amyloid-beta in Alzheimer's disease. *International Journal of Experimental Pathology*, **86**, 147–59.

Mega, M.S., Cummings, J.L., Fiorello, T., and Gornbein, J. (1996). The spectrum of behavioral changes in Alzheimer's disease. *Neurology*, **46**, 130–5.

Mendez, M.F., Martin, R.J., Smyth, K.A., and Whitehouse, P.J. (1990). Psychiatric symptoms associated with Alzheimer's disease. *Journal of Neuropsychiatry and Clinical Neurosciences*, **2**, 28–33.

Merriam, A.E., Aronson, M.K., Gaston, P., Wey, S.L., and Katz, I. (1988). The psychiatric symptoms of Alzheimer's disease. *Journal of the American Geriatrics Society*, **36**, 7–12.

Miller, T.P., Tinklenberg, J.R., Brooks, J.O.D., and Yesavage, J.A. (1991). Cognitive decline in patients with Alzheimer disease: differences in patients with and without extrapyramidal signs. *Alzheimer Disease and Associated Disorders*, **5**, 251–6.

Morris, J.C., Edland, S., Clark, C. *et al*. (1993). The consortium to establish a registry for Alzheimer's disease (CERAD). Part IV. Rates of cognitive change in the longitudinal assessment of probable Alzheimer's disease. *Neurology*, **43**, 2457–65.

Morris, M.C., Evans, D.A., Bienias, J.L. *et al*. (2002). Dietary intake of antioxidant nutrients and the risk of incident Alzheimer disease in a biracial community study. *Journal of the American Medical Association*, **287**, 3230–7.

Mortimer, J.A., Van Duijn, C.M., Chandra, V. *et al*. (1991). Head trauma as a risk factor for Alzheimer's disease: a collaborative re-analysis of case-control studies. EURODEM Risk Factors Research Group. *International Journal of Epidemiology*, **20**, S28–S35.

Mulnard, R.A., Cotman, C.W., Kawas, C. *et al*. (2000). Estrogen replacement therapy for treatment of mild to moderate Alzheimer disease: a randomized controlled trial. Alzheimer's Disease Cooperative Study. *Journal of the American Medical Association*, **283**, 1007–15.

Nelson, H.D., Humphrey, L.L., Nygren, P., Teutsch, S.M., and Allan, J.D. (2002). Postmenopausal hormone replacement therapy: scientific review. *Journal of the American Medical Association*, **288**, 872–81.

Nyth, A.L., Gottfries, C.G., Lyby, K. *et al*. (1992). A controlled multicenter clinical study of citalopram and placebo in elderly depressed patients with and without concomitant dementia. *Acta Psychiatrica Scandinavica*, **86**, 138–45.

O'Brien, J.T. (1997). The 'glucocorticoid cascade' hypothesis in man. Prolonged stress may cause permanent brain damage. *British Journal of Psychiatry*, **170**, 199–201.

Olin, J.T., Fox, L.S., Pawluczyk, S., Taggart, N.A., and Schneider, L.S. (2001). A pilot randomized trial of carbamazepine for behavioral symptoms in treatment-resistant outpatients with Alzheimer disease. *American Journal of Geriatric Psychiatry*, **9**, 400–5.

Orgogozo, J.M., Dartigues, J.F., Lafont, S. *et al*. (1997). Wine consumption and dementia in the elderly: a prospective community study in the Bordeaux area. *Revue Neurologique*, **153**, 185–92.

Ott, A., Slooter, A.J., Hofman, A. *et al*. (1998). Smoking and risk of dementia and Alzheimer's disease in a population-based cohort study: the Rotterdam Study. *Lancet*, **351**, 1840–3.

Ott, A., Stolk, R.P., Van Harskamp, F., Pols, H.A., Hofman, A., and Breteler, M.M. (1999). Diabetes mellitus and the risk of dementia: the Rotterdam Study. *Neurology*, **53**, 1937–42.

Ownby, R.L, Crocco, E., Acevedo, A., Vineeth, J., and Loewenstein, D. (2006). Depression and risk for Alzheimer disease: systematic review, meta-analysis and metaregression analysis. *Archives of General Psychiatry*, **63**, 530–8.

Patterson, M.B. and Bolger, J.P. (1994). Assessment of behavioral symptoms in Alzheimer disease. *Alzheimer Disease and Associated Disorders*, **8**, 4–20.

Patterson, M.B., Schnell, A.H., Martin, R.J., Mendez, M.F., Smyth, K.A., and Whitehouse, P.J. (1990). Assessment of behavioral and affective symptoms in Alzheimer's disease. *Journal of Geriatric Psychiatry and Neurology*, **3**, 21–30.

Pearson, J.L., Teri, L., Reifler, B.V., and Raskind, M.A. (1989). Functional status and cognitive impairment in Alzheimer's patients with and without depression. *Journal of the American Geriatrics Society*, **37**, 1117–21.

Pedersen, N.L., Gatz, M., Berg, S., and Johansson, B. (2004). How heritable is Alzheimer's disease late in life? Findings from Swedish twins. *Annals of Neurology*, **55**, 180–5.

Petersen, R.C., Thomas, R.G., Grundman, M. *et al.* (2005). Vitamin E and donepezil for the treatment of mild cognitive impairment. *New England Journal of Medicine*, **352**, 2379–88.

Petracca, G., Teson, A., Chemerinski, E., Leiguarda, R., and Starkstein, S.E. (1996). A double-blind placebo-controlled study of clomipramine in depressed patients with Alzheimer's disease. *Journal of Neuropsychiatry and Clinical Neurosciences*, **8**, 270–5.

Rabins, P.V., Mace, N.L., and Lucas, M.J. (1982). The impact of dementia on the family. *Journal of the American Medical Association*, **248**, 333–5.

Reines, S.A., Block, G.A., Morris, J.C. et al. (2004). Rofecoxib: no effect on Alzheimer's disease in a 1-year, randomized, blinded, controlled study. *Neurology*, **62**, 66–71.

Reisberg, B., Ferris, S.H., Shulman, E. *et al.* (1986). Longitudinal course of normal aging and progressive dementia of the Alzheimer's type: a prospective study of 106 subjects over a 3.6 year mean interval. *Progress in Neuro-Psychopharmacology and Biological Psychiatry*, **10**, 571–8.

Reisberg, B., Borenstein, J., Salob, S.P., Ferris, S.H., Franssen, E., and Georgotas, A. (1987). Behavioral symptoms in Alzheimer's disease: phenomenology and treatment. *Journal of Clinical Psychiatry*, **48**, 9–15.

Ritchie, C.W., Bush, A.I., MacKinnon, A. *et al.* (2003). Metal-protein attenuation with iodochlorhydroxyquin (clioquinol). targeting Abeta amyloid deposition and toxicity in Alzheimer disease: a pilot phase 2 clinical trial. *Archives of Neurology*, **60**, 1685–91. [Erratum in *Archives of Neurology* 2004 **61**(5), 776.]

Ritchie, K. and Kildea, D. (1995). Is senile dementia 'age-related' or 'ageing-related'?–evidence from meta-analysis of dementia prevalence in the oldest old. *Lancet*, **346**, 931–4.

Roberts, G.W., Gentleman, S.M., Lynch, A., and Graham, D.I. (1991). beta A4 amyloid protein deposition in brain after head trauma. *Lancet*, **338**, 1422–3.

Roses, A.D. (1996). Apolipoprotein E alleles as risk factors in Alzheimer's disease. *Annual Review of Medicine*, **47**, 387–400.

Roth, M., Mountjoy, C.Q., and Amrein, R. (1996). Moclobemide in elderly patients with cognitive decline and depression: an international double-blind, placebo-controlled trial. *British Journal of Psychiatry*, **168**, 149–57.

Rubin, E.H., Morris, J.C., and Berg, L. (1987). The progression of personality changes in senile dementia of the Alzheimer's type. *Journal of the American Geriatrics Society*, **35**, 721–5.

Rubin, E.H., Drevets, W.C., and Burke, W.J. (1988). The nature of psychotic symptoms in senile dementia of the Alzheimer type. *Journal of Geriatric Psychiatry and Neurology*, **1**, 16–20.

Saftig, P., Hartmann, D., and De Strooper, B. (1999). The function of presenilin-1 in amyloid beta-peptide generation and brain development. *European Archives of Psychiatry and Clinical Neuroscience*, **249**, 271–9.

Salmon, D.P., Thal, L.J., Butters, N., and Heindel, W.C. (1990). Longitudinal evaluation of dementia of the Alzheimer type: a comparison of 3 standardized mental status examinations. *Neurology*, **40**, 1225–30.

Sano, M., Ernesto, C., Thomas, R.G. *et al.* (1997). A controlled trial of selegiline, alpha-tocopherol, or both as treatment for Alzheimer's disease. The Alzheimer's Disease Cooperative Study. *New England Journal of Medicine*, **336**, 1216–22.

Saunders, P.A., Copeland, J.R., Dewey, M.E. *et al.* (1991). Heavy drinking as a risk factor for depression and dementia in elderly men. Findings from the Liverpool longitudinal community study. *British Journal of Psychiatry*, **159**, 213–16.

Schneider, L.S., Dagerman, K.S., and Insel, P. (2005). Risk of death with atypical antipsychotic drug treatment for dementia: meta-analysis of randomized placebo-controlled trials. *Journal of the American Medical Association*, **294**, 1934–43.

Seshadri, S., Beiser, A., Selhub, J. *et al.* (2002). Plasma homocysteine as a risk factor for dementia and Alzheimer's disease. *New England Journal of Medicine*, **346**, 476–83.

Shepherd, J., Blauw, G.J., Murphy, M.B. *et al.* (2002). Pravastatin in elderly individuals at risk of vascular disease (PROSPER): a randomised controlled trial. *Lancet*, **360**, 1623–30.

Shumaker, S.A., Legault, C., Kuller, L. *et al.* (2004). Conjugated equine estrogens and incidence of probable dementia and mild cognitive impairment in postmenopausal women: Women's Health Initiative Memory Study. *Journal of the American Medical Association*, **291**, 2947–58.

Sink, K.M., Holden, K.F. and Yaffe, K. (2005). Pharmacological treatment of neuropsychiatric symptoms of dementia: a review of the evidence. *Journal of the American Medical Association*, **293**, 596–608.

Skoog, I., Lernfelt, B., Landahl, S. *et al.* (1996). 15-year longitudinal study of blood pressure and dementia. *Lancet*, **347**, 1141–5.

Snowdon, D.A., Kemper, S.J., Mortimer, J.A., Greiner, L.H., Wekstein, D.R., and Markesbery, W.R. (1996). Linguistic ability in early life and cognitive function and Alzheimer's disease in late life. Findings from the Nun Study. *Journal of the American Medical Association*, **275**, 528–32.

Stern, Y., Alexander, G.E., Prohovnik, I., and Mayeux, R. (1992). Inverse relationship between education and parietotemporal perfusion deficit in Alzheimer's disease. *Annals of Neurology*, **32**, 371–5.

Stern, Y., Albert, M., Brandt, J. *et al.* (1994a). Utility of extrapyramidal signs and psychosis as predictors of cognitive and functional decline, nursing home admission, and death in Alzheimer's disease: prospective analyses from the Predictors Study. *Neurology*, **44**, 2300–7.

Stern, Y., Gurland, B., Tatemichi, T.K., Tang, M.X., Wilder, D., and Mayeux, R. (1994b). Influence of education and occupation on the incidence of Alzheimer's disease. *Journal of the American Medical Association*, **271**, 1004–10.

Tabet, N., Mantle, D., Walker, Z., and Orrell, M. (2002). Endogenous antioxidant activities in relation to concurrent vitamins A, C, and E intake in dementia. *International Psychogeriatrics*, **14**, 7–15.

Taragano, F.E., Lyketsos, C.G., Mangone, C.A., Allegri, R.F., and Comesana-Diaz, E. (1997). A double-blind, randomized, fixed-dose trial of fluoxetine vs. amitriptyline in the treatment of major depression complicating Alzheimer's disease. *Psychosomatics*, **38**, 246–52.

Tariot, P.N., Erb, R., Podgorski, C.A. *et al.* (1998). Efficacy and tolerability of carbamazepine for agitation and aggression in dementia. *American Journal of Psychiatry*, **155**, 54–61.

Tariot, P.N., Raman, R., Jakimovich, L. *et al.* (2005). Divalproex sodium in nursing home residents with possible or probable Alzheimer disease complicated by agitation: a randomized, controlled trial. *American Journal of Geriatric Psychiatry*, **13**, 942–9.

Teri, L. and Wagner, A.W. (1991). Assessment of depression in patients with Alzheimer's disease: concordance among informants. *Psychology and Aging*, **6**, 280–5.

Teri, L., Mccurry, S.M., Edland, S.D., Kukull, W.A., and Larson, E.B. (1995). Cognitive decline in Alzheimer's disease: a longitudinal investigation of risk factors for accelerated decline. *Journals of Gerontology. Series A: Biological Sciences and Medical Sciences*, **50A**, M49–M55.

Trapp, G.A., Miner, G.D., Zimmerman, R.L., Mastri, A.R., and Heston, L.L. (1978). Aluminum levels in brain in Alzheimer's disease. *Biological Psychiatry*, **13**, 709–18.

Tzourio, C., Anderson, C., Chapman, N. *et al.* (2003). Effects of blood pressure lowering with perindopril and indapamide therapy on dementia and cognitive decline in patients with cerebrovascular disease. *Archives of Internal Medicine*, **163**, 1069–75.

US Food and Drug Administration (2005). *FDS: public health advisory: deaths with antipsychotics in elderly patients with behavioural disturbances.* USFDA, Rockville, MD.

Van Duijn, C.M., Clayton, D., Chandra, V. *et al.* (1991). Familial aggregation of Alzheimer's disease and related disorders: a collaborative re-analysis of case-control studies. EURODEM Risk Factors Research Group. *International Journal of Epidemiology*, **20**, S13–S20.

Walsh, J.S., Welch, H.G., and Larson, E.B. (1990). Survival of outpatients with Alzheimer-type dementia. *Annals of Internal Medicine*, **113**, 429–34.

Walton, L. (1991). *Alzheimer's disease and the environment*. Royal Society of Medicine Press, London.

Wang, P.N., Liao, S.Q., Liu, R.S. *et al.* (2000). Effects of estrogen on cognition, mood, and cerebral blood flow in AD: a controlled study. *Neurology*, **54**, 2061–6.

Wang, P.S., Schneeweiss, S., Avorn, J. *et al.* (2005). Risk of death in elderly users of conventional vs. atypical antipsychotic medications. *New England Journal of Medicine*, **353**, 2335–41.

White, L., Katzman, R., Losonczy, K. *et al.* (1994). Association of education with incidence of cognitive impairment in three established populations for epidemiologic studies of the elderly. *Journal of Clinical Epidemiology*, **47**, 363–74.

Whitmer, R.A., Gunderson, E.P., Barrett-Connor, E., Quesenberry, C.P., Jr, and Yaffe, K. (2005a). Obesity in middle age and future risk of dementia: a 27 year longitudinal population based study. *British Medical Journal*, **330**, 1360.

Whitmer, R.A., Sidney, S., Selby, J., Johnston, S.C., and Yaffe, K. (2005b). Midlife cardiovascular risk factors and risk of dementia in late life. *Neurology*, **64**, 277–81.

Williams, D.B., Annegers, J.F., Kokmen, E., O'Brien, P.C., and Kurland, L.T. (1991). Brain injury and neurologic sequelae: a cohort study of dementia, parkinsonism, and amyotrophic lateral sclerosis. *Neurology*, **41**, 1554–7.

Wolozin, B., Kellman, W., Ruosseau, P., Celesia, G.G., and Siegel, G. (2000). Decreased prevalence of Alzheimer disease associated with 3-hydroxy-3-methyglutaryl coenzyme A reductase inhibitors. *Archives of Neurology*, **57**, 1439–43.

Wood, J.A., Wood, P.L., Ryan, R. *et al.* (1993). Cytokine indices in Alzheimer's temporal cortex: no changes in mature IL-1 beta or IL-1RA but increases in the associated acute phase proteins IL-6, alpha 2-macroglobulin and C-reactive protein. *Brain Research*, **629**, 245–52.

Wragg, R.E. and Jeste, D.V. (1989). Overview of depression and psychosis in Alzheimer's disease. *American Journal of Psychiatry*, **146**, 577–87.

Yaffe, K., Sawaya, G., Lieberburg, I., and Grady, D. (1998). Estrogen therapy in postmenopausal women: effects on cognitive function and dementia. *Journal of the American Medical Association*, **279**, 688–95.

Yesavage, J.A., Poulsen, S.L., Sheikh, J., and Tanke, E. (1988). Rates of change of common measures of impairment in senile dementia of the Alzheimer's type. *Psychopharmacology Bulletin*, **24**, 531–4.

Zandi, P.P., Sparks, D.L., Khachaturian, A.S. *et al.* (2005). Do statins reduce risk of incident dementia and Alzheimer disease? The Cache County Study. *Archives of General Psychiatry*, **62**, 217–24.

Zannis, V.I., Kardassis, D., and Zanni, E.E. (1993). Genetic mutations affecting human lipoproteins, their receptors, and their enzymes. *Advances in Human Genetics*, **21**, 145–319.

Zigman, W.B., Schupf, N., Sersen, E., and Silverman, W. (1996). Prevalence of dementia in adults with and without Down syndrome. *American Journal of Mental Retardation*, **100**, 403–12.

# Appendix 1

## NINCDS–ADRDA criteria for clinical diagnosis of Alzheimer's disease.

I   The criteria for the clinical diagnosis of PROBABLE Alzheimer's disease include: dementia established by clinical examination and documented by the Mini-Mental Test, Blessed Dementia Scale, or some similar examination, and confirmed by neuropsychological tests; deficits in two or more areas of cognition; progressive worsening memory and other cognitive functions; no disturbance of consciousness; onset between ages 40 and 90, most often after age 65; and absence of systemic disorders or other brain diseases that in and of themselves could account for the progressive deficits in memory and cognition.

II  The diagnosis of PROBABLE Alzheimer's disease is supported by: progressive deterioration of specific cognitive functions such as language (aphasia), motor skills (apraxia), and perception (agnosia); impaired activities of daily living and altered patterns of behaviour; family history of similar disorders, particularly if confirmed neuropathologically; and laboratory results of: normal lumbar puncture as evaluated by standard techniques; normal pattern or non-specific changes in EEG, such as increased slow-wave activity, and evidence of cerebral atrophy on CT with progression documented by serial observation.

III Other clinical features consistent with the diagnosis of PROBABLE Alzheimer's disease, after exclusion of causes of dementia other than Alzheimer's disease, include: plateaus in the course of progression of the illness; associated symptoms of depression, insomnia, incontinence, delusions, illusions, hallucinations, catastrophic verbal, emotional, or physical outbursts, sexual disorders, and weight loss; other neurological abnormalities in some patients, especially with more advanced disease and including motor signs such as increased muscle tone, myoclonus, or gait disorder; seizures in advanced disease; and CT normal for age.

IV  Features that make the diagnosis of PROBABLE Alzheimer's disease uncertain or unlikely include: sudden, apoplectic onset; focal neurological findings such as hemiparesis, sensory loss visual field deficits, and incoordination early in the course of the illness; and seizures or gait disturbances at the onset or very early in the course of the illness.

V   Clinical diagnosis of POSSIBLE Alzheimer's disease: may be made on the basis of the dementia syndrome, in the absence of other neurological, psychiatric, or systemic disorder sufficient to cause dementia, and in the presence of variation in the onset, in the presentation, or in the clinical course: may be made in the presence of a second systemic or brain disorder sufficient to produce dementia, which is not considered to be the cause of the dementia; and should be used in research studies when a single, gradually progressive severe cognitive deficit is identified in the absence of other identifiable cause.

VI  Criteria for diagnosis of DEFINITE Alzheimer's disease are: the clinical criteria for probable Alzheimer's disease and histopathological evidence obtained from a biopsy or autopsy.

VII Classification of Alzheimer's disease for research purpose should specify features that may differentiate subtypes of the disorder, such as: familial occurrence; onset before age 65; presence of trisomy-21; and coexistence of other relevant conditions such as Parkinson's disease.

# Clinical aspects of dementia: vascular and mixed dementia

Robert Stewart

'Vascular dementia' has attracted substantially less research attention to date than Alzheimer's disease. This may be because it falls between traditional clinical specialities, being seen as the province of stroke researchers by those interested in dementia and vice versa. A more fundamental reason is that establishing its validity as a 'diagnosis' has been persistently elusive. Because psychiatric diagnoses are usually derived from a clinician's subjective judgement applied to a person's subjective experiences (and/or their behaviour reported by a close other, and/or an interpretation of their score on a brief structured questionnaire), there is ample room for variability in their application. Consequently, a major objective of psychiatric research has been to standardize the process of diagnosis so that the findings from one research group can be understood by another. Ideally these findings should also be understood by a clinician; however, research diagnoses are developed to maximize reliability rather than validity and, particularly when restrictive, can drift a considerable distance from those routinely applied in clinical practice. Sometimes diagnostic systems fail to keep up with accumulating knowledge about a clinical condition, or fail to reflect changing presentations. Vascular dementia is a good example of this failure.

## Dementia—lumping or splitting

Because psychiatric symptoms co-occur in a variety of combinations, with few that can be truly said to be pathognomonic of a particular disorder, there is fertile ground for disagreement about how to group symptoms into 'diagnoses'. Dementia researchers, like those in many other fields of research, are often themselves categorized into 'lumpers' or 'splitters' based on whether they prefer, respectively, to consider cases within a single category (accepting the problem of heterogeneity in causal mechanisms and clinical presentations), or within a number of subcategories (accepting a degree of overlap between these). Naturally, neither position reflects the truth, and a considerable amount of effort has probably been wasted in debate between the two camps. Physicists have been happy for a long time to accept that light exists as both a wave and a particle, so there is no particular reason why dementia cannot be viewed, at least within the research arena, as both single and multiple conditions.

## Definitions of vascular dementia

Changing fashions for 'lumping' or 'splitting' of dementia are fundamental to the problems underlying vascular dementia as a diagnosis. Throughout the first half of the 20th century, later onset ('senile') dementia was viewed as an inevitable consequence of ageing and, since atherosclerosis was a popular substrate for ageing, most dementia was assumed to be 'vascular'. Seminal post-mortem studies in the 1960s and early 1970s challenged this by demonstrating the importance of Alzheimer pathology—previously assumed only to underlie rare early onset ('pre-senile') syndromes. However, it was evident that multiple cerebral infarctions were also responsible, and a second 'diagnosis' of multi-infarct dementia arose, later to be subsumed under the broader category of vascular dementia.

One of the first criteria for vascular dementia to come into widespread use in research settings was the Hachinski Ischemic Scale. Interestingly this was never intended for this purpose and was only briefly described in the original report (Hachinski *et al.*, 1975). It was devised simply by scaling 13 features of 'arteriosclerotic psychosis' from a widely read textbook (Mayer-Gross *et al.*, 1969). Some features refer to the course of the dementia (e.g. abrupt onset, stepwise deterioration, fluctuation), some to symptoms (e.g. nocturnal confusion, depression, somatic complaints), and some to the likely presence of or risk for cerebrovascular disease (e.g. history of strokes or hypertension, focal neurological signs). No attempt was made to validate the instrument or to investigate its scaling properties or the validity of the different weights given to some items. Despite this, it was found to have the highest inter-rater reliability in an independent evaluation of case identification instruments for vascular dementia (Chui *et al.*, 2000). This is probably because it seeks to ascertain whether significant cerebrovascular disease is present in the context of dementia, rather than whether it is causally related.

Considering the standard current classification systems, DSM-IV criteria require the presence of dementia and either focal neurological signs/symptoms, or evidence of cerebrovascular disease judged to be aetiologically related (American Psychiatric Association, 1994). A requirement for an early stepwise course of decline was dropped between DSM-IIIR and DSM-IV. ICD-10 criteria are stricter, requiring both evidence of focal brain damage and evidence of cerebrovascular disease judged to be aetiologically related, as well as an uneven distribution of cognitive deficits.

Probably the most widely used criteria in research settings are those developed in a 1991 workshop of the neuroepidemiology branch of the National Institute of Neurological Disorders and Stroke and the Association Internationale pour la Recherche et l'Enseignement en Neurosciences (NINDS–AIREN; Román *et al.*, 1993). A diagnosis of vascular dementia using NINDS–AIREN criteria rests on evidence of cerebrovascular disease (both clinical and from neuroimaging), and an observed relationship between cerebrovascular disease and dementia (such as an onset within 3 months of an acute stroke or an abrupt deterioration in cognitive functioning, or a fluctuating or stepwise deterioration).

The system of subdividing dementia based on assumed underlying causation has therefore persisted into current diagnostic schedules. However, there have been several changes over the subsequent 30–40 years, with relevance to vascular dementia, suggesting that a reappraisal should at least be considered:

◆ *Changing cohorts.* Older people dying in the 1960s lived through times when there was little opportunity to prevent or control cerebrovascular disease. More severe and florid pathology would have been observed at post mortem than would be expected (in developed nations) today. People with dementia known to clinical services are now frequently in their ninth and tenth decades. Mixed pathology is much more likely to be present and the majority will have at least mild levels of cerebrovascular disease which may be coincidental or, at least, not a sole causal factor.

◆ *Advances in neuropathology.* Early studies predominantly focused on multiple cortical infarctions. Other more subtle forms of cerebrovascular pathology, such as lacunar infarction, white matter disease, vascular amyloid deposition, and microangiopathy, have subsequently been highlighted. These may increase the risk of dementia but may not, in isolation, be sufficient to cause the clinical presentation; instead, a combination of pathological processes may be necessary.

◆ *Advances in neuroimaging.* Clinical diagnostic criteria for multi-infarct or vascular dementia have traditionally relied on a history of vascular risk factors, a history suggestive of recurrent strokes, and evidence on clinical examination of neurological deficits indicative of cortical stroke. Subsequent technological advances now allow *in vivo* identification of subclinical changes such as white matter hyperintensities and alterations in patterns of perfusion and connectivity. However, these are all common in unaffected people in old age and cannot be assumed to be causal.

## Problems with 'vascular dementia' as a diagnosis

Dementia is poorly represented by traditional diagnostic categories. The validity of vascular dementia as a diagnosis rests on the demonstration of a discrete syndrome (dementia) with a clear primary cause ('vascular'), and with good clinical and clinico-pathological reliability. These criteria are challenged in several respects:

◆ The clinical course of dementia (i.e. 'stepwise' versus 'gradual' deterioration) has been found to be a poor predictor of pathological findings (Fischer *et al.*, 1990).

◆ Dementia following clinical stroke frequently shows a gradual deterioration and has been found to occur without further infarction in many, if not the majority of, cases (Tatemichi *et al.*, 1994; Kokmen *et al.*, 1996).

◆ Risk factors for stroke have been found to be risk factors not only for vascular dementia but also for clinical Alzheimer's disease (Stewart, 1998).

◆ Dementia in community samples is frequently associated with mixed rather than discrete pathology (Holmes *et al.*, 1999). Cerebrovascular disease has been found to be rarely associated with dementia in the absence of Alzheimer pathology (Hulette *et al.*, 1997).

◆ Research diagnostic criteria poorly reflect underlying pathology. Although cerebrovascular pathology is likely to be present in cases with a previous diagnosis of vascular dementia, it is also frequently present in people with other clinical diagnoses (Holmes *et al.*, 1999).

◆ Clinical diagnostic criteria for vascular dementia have poor inter-rater reliability (Lopez *et al.*, 1994; Chui *et al.*, 2000). Higher agreement is found where criteria simply estimate the degree of cerebrovascular disease in the context of dementia (Hachinski *et al.*, 1975). Much lower agreement is found where a judgement is required as to whether the dementia was caused by cerebrovascular disease. Different diagnostic schedules also show poor agreement with each other (Chui *et al.*, 2000).

◆ Operational definitions of dementia have been criticized for focusing excessively on memory impairment and for poorly reflecting cognitive impairment relating to vascular disease which more often affects non-memory domains such as executive function (Bowler and Hachinski, 2000).

## Should dementia be subclassified?

A fundamental problem with the traditional subcategorization of dementia (which underlies many of the unsatisfactory findings for vascular dementia listed above) is that each subcategory assumes a single underlying cause. Common sense suggests that this is very unlikely to be true in the majority of late onset cases, where mixed pathology is likely to be responsible. The principal reason that the system has persisted is that it has been felt to have some utility in Alzheimer's disease research. If risk factors for a particular pathological process are to be identified, there is some rationale for excluding people with evidence of any other pathology. This can be readily carried out for Alzheimer's disease since levels of vascular pathology can be reasonably approximated (and screened out) by clinical examination or neuroimaging. The same is not true for vascular dementia since Alzheimer pathology cannot (yet) be quantified *in vivo*. The only means of defining 'pure' vascular dementia is, having established a temporal relationship between stroke episodes and cognitive decline, to exclude those with evidence of gradual decline in between strokes. This process relies heavily on retrospective and potentially inaccurate information. If pure and mixed disorders cannot be accurately defined, is there any sense in continuing to apply diagnostic labels which assume this to be the case? Furthermore, the utility of defining Alzheimer's disease as a diagnosis of exclusion has also been called into question. The problem is that the exclusion of people with potentially significant vascular disease not only reduces the generalizability of a case sample, but also introduces bias if the same exclusion criteria are not applied to control groups.

## Implications of the diagnostic problem

If vascular dementia as a diagnosis poorly reflects underlying pathology and relies on a differentiation from Alzheimer's disease which involves a large degree of subjective judgement and 'guesswork', then research that attempts to apply these criteria is fraught with methodological shortcomings. Prevalence studies will be difficult to interpret if between-site equivalence cannot be assumed. Furthermore, any observed between-site differences in prevalence (or in the proportion of dementia which is defined as 'vascular') may simply reflect underlying differences in stroke incidence. Case–control studies become difficult if all cases have evidence of cerebrovascular disease by definition (or if it is absent or minimal in the case of Alzheimer's disease) since they will differ from controls in many respects through selection bias, resulting in spurious positive or negative findings. Implications for clinical trials are also substantial and will be discussed later.

One of the most important consequences of the 'diagnosis problem' has been that the role of vascular factors in dementia has been underestimated until relatively recently. If vascular factors are not often associated with dementia in isolation (i.e. other coexisting pathology is required), this does not mean that they are not important risk factors. The following sections will review some of the evidence for this and discuss potential causal pathways, before considering potential implications for the treatment and prevention of dementia.

## Does vascular dementia exist? Specific syndromes

If vascular dementia and Alzheimer's disease are not clearly distinguishable disorders, the continued usefulness of a subcategorizing diagnostic system is questionable. However, this only applies to age groups where overlapping pathology is likely. People who develop dementia relatively early—for example, in their seventh decade or younger—are much more likely to have a single underlying pathology which can reasonably be guessed. It may therefore still be appropriate to subcategorize dementia in cases with younger onset. Furthermore, there are particular syndromes within the 'vascular dementia' category which can reasonably be considered as discrete diagnoses. These include genetic disorders such as 'cerebral autosomal dominant arteriopathy with subcortical infarcts and leucoencephalopathy' (CADASIL). This is a familial disorder manifesting as recurrent strokes (most often lacunar infarcts) usually in the fourth to sixth decades, occurring in the absence of vascular risk factors and associated in most cases with a subcortical dementia and pseudobulbar palsy. The principal underlying pathology is an abnormality in basal smooth muscle cells, predominantly in the media of small cerebral arteries, and underlying mutations have been successfully identified in the Notch3 gene on chromosome 19 (Joutel et al., 1997). Other syndromes of familial vascular dementia have been described (Table 27iv.1) and it is likely that, as with Alzheimer's disease, further discrete disorders exist which may be explained by specific mutations.

**Table 27iv. 1** Examples of specific vascular dementia syndromes

| | |
|---|---|
| Genetic disorders | Sickle cell disease |
| | CADASIL |
| | Hereditary cerebral haemorrhage with amyloidosis—Dutch and Icelandic types |
| | Familial British dementia with amyloid angiopathy |
| | Homocystinuria |
| | Fabry's disease |
| | Hereditary endotheliopathy with retinopathy, nephropathy, and stroke (HERNS) |
| | Mitochondrial myopathy, encephalopathy, lactic acidosis and stroke-like episodes (MELAS) |
| | Strategic infarct dementia |
| Conditions associated with cerebrovascular pathology and secondary dementia | Subdural haematoma |
| | Systemic lupus erythematosus |
| | Polyarteritis nodosa |
| | Buerger's disease |
| | Polycythaemia rubra vera |
| | Neurosyphilis |

As well as genetic disorders, cases of dementia have been described which appear to have been caused by specific single 'strategic' infarctions, most often within thalamic structures (Tatemichi et al., 1992b), and which may also be considered as discrete diagnoses. In addition several non-cardiovascular disorders which may cause secondary dementia do so through their effects on the vasculature (Table 27iv.1), although such disorders cause only a very small proportion of dementia cases.

## How common is dementia after stroke?

Difficulties in applying diagnostic criteria for vascular dementia should not obscure the importance of vascular disorders as risk factors for dementia. Prospective studies have found prevalence rates of around 20–30% for dementia 3 months after an acute stroke (Tatemichi et al., 1992a). The Framingham Study estimated a two-fold increased risk over a 10-year period (Ivan et al., 2004), and this has been found to remain raised over at least two decades after an index stroke (Kokmen et al., 1996). A recent study suggested a stronger association with cognitive impairment in the absence of dementia (Srikanth et al., 2004), but this may reflect differences in deciding the point at which mild cognitive impairment is distinguished from dementia (i.e. when it is believed to be affecting activities of daily living) in the context of a previous stroke. Selective mortality (in people with stroke who are at risk of developing dementia) is likely to be a diluting factor and may explain a stronger association in younger compared to older people (Ivan et al., 2004).

## What are the risk factors for post-stroke dementia?

Although strategic infarct dementia syndromes have been described (Tatemichi et al., 1992b), population-based studies have yet to demonstrate a clear association between stroke location and risk of dementia, for example with respect to arterial territories of cortical infarctions (Censori et al., 1996; Pohjasvaara et al., 1998; Desmond et al., 2000) and the location (or number) of lacunar infarctions (Loeb et al., 1992). Other factors which have been identified as associated with risk of dementia following stroke (albeit not always consistently between studies) are increased age, lower levels of education, previous stroke disease, and vascular risk factors such as diabetes, recent smoking, and atrial fibrillation (Censori *et al.*, 1996; Pohjasvaara *et al.*, 1998; Barba *et al.*, 2000; Desmond *et al.*, 2000). The role of blood pressure level is uncertain: most report no association but one study found that risk of dementia was associated with lower blood pressure and orthostatic changes (Pohjasvaara *et al.*, 1998). Disorders associated with hypoxia and ischaemia (such as seizures, arrhythmias, and pneumonia) have also been found to be associated with higher risk of dementia after stroke (Moroney *et al.*, 1996).

Although prospective studies following a major stroke have been important in understanding dementia associated with cerebrovascular disease, they may not be generalizable to situations where multiple smaller infarctions have occurred. A different design of study investigated factors associated with dementia in a sample of people all of whom had multiple cerebral infarctions (Gorelick *et al.*, 1993). Independent risk factors were: increased age, lower educational attainment, previous myocardial infarction, recent smoking, and lower systolic blood pressure. CT findings associated with dementia were: more severe stroke, left cortical infarction, and diffuse enlargement of the lateral ventricle suggesting cerebral atrophy (Gorelick *et al.*, 1992).

## What are the clinical features of post-stroke dementia?

As has been mentioned earlier, many cases of dementia following stroke appear to follow an Alzheimer-like clinical course and to occur without further episodes of infarction (Tatemichi *et al.*, 1994; Kokmen *et al.*, 1996; Honig *et al.*, 2003). Pre-stroke cognitive decline has been found in many cases (Kase *et al.*, 1998), and appears to be associated with atrophic changes on neuroimaging rather than early cerebrovascular disease (Pohjasvaara *et al.*, 1999). In addition, not only does stroke predict cognitive impairment but cognitive impairment is also associated with a raised risk of future stroke (Ferucci *et al.*, 1996), and dementia following stroke predicts further stroke episodes (Moroney *et al.*, 1997). Taken together this evidence suggests that there is a close (although potentially complex) interrelationship between stroke and primary degenerative changes underlying many cases of apparent vascular dementia, and that the stroke itself may be a relatively late event in an ongoing process of insidious cognitive decline. A more recent study found that the clinical picture shifted from one consistent with Alzheimer's disease over the first 2 years after a stroke to a more classic 'vascular dementia' picture over years 2–4 (Altieri *et al.*, 2004). This is consistent with a process in which the stroke episode precipitates dementia in people with pre-existing Alzheimer pathology. Those without this vulnerability maintain their cognitive function initially, but remain at risk of further strokes and of dementia occurring at a later stage as a result of these.

## Vascular risk factors and dementia

Although clinical stroke is strongly associated with dementia, it does not appear to be the initiating event for cognitive decline in many cases. A large body of evidence suggests that some risk factors for cerebrovascular disease may also be risk factors for dementia—both due to Alzheimer's disease and vascular dementia, as estimated clinically.

### Hypertension

Hypertension, a powerful risk factor for cerebrovascular disease, has received particular attention (Stewart, 1999). However, it is only relatively recently that results of prospective studies have begun to clarify the relationship between blood pressure and dementia. It has been repeatedly found that raised blood pressure in mid-life predicts cognitive impairment 10–15 years later (Elias *et al.*, 1993; Launer *et al.*, 1995; Skoog *et al.*, 1996; Kilander *et al.*, 1998). However, dementia tends to be associated with lower blood pressure in cross-sectional studies of older age groups (Guo *et al.*, 1996), including post-stroke dementia as mentioned earlier.

### Hyperlipidaemia

Raised lipid levels have received less attention than blood pressure as risk factors for dementia and results are also conflicting. Some studies, predominantly from Scandinavian populations, have suggested that raised mid-life total cholesterol is associated with later dementia (Notkola *et al.*, 1998; Kivipelto *et al.*, 2001, 2002, 2005). However, others have found over shorter periods of follow-up that higher total cholesterol levels are associated with lower risk of dementia (Mielke *et al.*, 2005) or show no association at all (Reitz *et al.*, 2004).

### Diabetes and metabolic syndrome

Type 2 (non-insulin-dependent) diabetes has also been found to be a risk factor for dementia, both vascular dementia and Alzheimer's disease (Ott *et al.*, 1999; Peila *et al.*, 2002), particularly in those receiving or requiring insulin treatment (Ott *et al.*, 1999). Selective mortality is likely to be an important factor, reducing the co-occurrence of the two conditions, which may explain some negative findings (MacKnight *et al.*, 2002). Strong interactions were reported between hypertension and diabetes as predictors of cognitive impairment in the Framingham Study (Elias *et al.*, 1997). However, much of the effect of diabetes on risk of dementia appears to be independent of cerebrovascular disease and may involve other non-vascular pathways or common underlying factors (Stewart and Liolitsa, 1999). Several studies have also reported associations between risk of dementia and the pre-diabetic state of insulin resistance or 'metabolic syndrome', either estimated through vascular risk factor clustering (Kalmijn *et al.*, 2000) or directly measured hyperinsulinaemia (Luchsinger *et al.*, 2004). One study, however, found that both low and high insulin were associated with later dementia (Peila *et al.*, 2004).

### Other vascular risk factors

Other vascular factors associated with dementia include ECG evidence of ischaemia (Prince *et al.*, 1994) and atrial fibrillation (Ott *et al.*, 1997), as well as measures of peripheral and carotid atherosclerosis (Hofman *et al.*, 1997). Early reports that smoking might be protective against AD appear to have arisen because of biased recall and effects on mortality. More recent findings from larger populations have suggested that smoking is, if anything, a risk factor for all types of dementia (Ott *et al.*, 1998; Luchsinger *et al.*, 2005), although this effect may be restricted to particular subgroups (Ott *et al.*, 1998). Several studies have found that people who are more physically active have a lower risk of dementia (Yoshitake *et al.*, 1995; Laurin *et al.*, 2001; Rovio *et al.*, 2005), which may or may not be mediated through effects on the vasculature. A large amount of attention has focused on dietary risk or protective factors for dementia. With many measures to choose from and a sizeable risk of type 1 statistical error, it is difficult to draw firm conclusions; however, there are several reports that an atherogenic diet is associated with increased risk (Kalmijn *et al.*, 1997; Luchsinger *et al.*, 2002). Some studies have suggested that mid-life obesity is a risk factor for dementia (Gustafson *et al.*, 2003), although others with shorter follow-up periods have found the opposite (Nourhashemi *et al.*, 2003).

# Mechanisms of association

What is becoming increasingly apparent is that people at increased risk for stroke are also at increased risk for dementia, whether this is defined clinically as vascular dementia (i.e. with evidence of significant co-morbid cerebrovascular disease) or Alzheimer's disease. The apparent associations with Alzheimer's disease do not appear to be explained by missed infarctions (Ott *et al.*, 1999), or dementia with primary vascular pathology misclassified as Alzheimer's disease (Hulette *et al.*, 1997) although the wide variety of cerebrovascular pathology and the limited ability of even a detailed neuropathological assessment to identify potentially relevant cerebrovascular pathology means a direct contribution from cerebrovascular disease remains a possible explanation. An explanation is more likely to lie in links between vascular disease and Alzheimer's disease. These may involve four possible pathways which need not be mutually exclusive.

## Interactions at a pathological level

There are numerous possible ways in which vascular processes may induce or accelerate Alzheimer pathology (Stewart, 1998). These include amyloid deposition as a response to ischaemia, links through inflammatory pathways, blood–brain barrier disturbance secondary to cerebrovascular disease, and, for diabetes, abnormal protein glycosylation secondary to prolonged hyperglycaemia. These processes predict that people with vascular disease will have higher levels of Alzheimer pathology—a hypothesis which is difficult to test except in the rare instances where neuropathological follow-up has been carried out in people without dementia. An early study found increased Alzheimer pathology associated with hypertension or coronary artery disease in people without previous dementia (Sparks *et al.*, 1995, 1996). Elevated mid-life blood pressure was also associated with decreased brain volume and Alzheimer pathology in a cohort study with a relatively large pathological follow-up (Petrovitch *et al.*, 2000). The same study also found associations between diabetes and increased Alzheimer pathology (Peila *et al.*, 2002), although associations were found with a protective rather than atherogenic lipid profile (Launer *et al.*, 2001), a finding which requires further clarification.

## Clinical/symptomatic interactions

As well as acting directly on the progression of Alzheimer pathology, vascular disorders may also accelerate the onset of symptomatic dementia at relatively early stages of co-morbid Alzheimer's disease. In a US study of elderly nuns who were screened in late life and followed to post-mortem, a lower level of Alzheimer pathology was observed in association with dementia if infarction was also present, suggesting that the infarction had accelerated the onset (Snowdon *et al.*, 1997). Similar findings were observed in the Oxford OPTIMA study where early Alzheimer pathology was associated with much greater cognitive impairment if cerebrovascular disease was also present (Esiri *et al.*, 1999). In another study using a community-derived sample, significant interactions were found between the presence of cerebral amyloid angiopathy and Alzheimer pathology in their association with previous level of cognitive impairment (Pfeifer *et al.*, 2002).

A possible reason for these findings is that memory impairment secondary to early Alzheimer's disease may be more likely to be noticed as 'dementia' if other cognitive domains are also affected. White matter disease may be important in this respect, since subtle disruption of fronto-subcortical pathways may result in impaired executive function. White matter hyperintensities on magnetic resonance imaging are common in older age groups and are associated with vascular risk factors, particularly hypertension (Breteler *et al.*, 1994b). Although they are more common in dementia and, across a population, are associated with relative cognitive impairment (Breteler *et al.*, 1994a), at an individual level they may be severe without any apparent clinical manifestations (Fein *et al.*, 1990). They do not therefore appear to be sufficient in themselves to cause dementia but may precipitate this in the presence of other pathology such as early Alzheimer's disease.

## Common underlying factors

An association between vascular disease and Alzheimer's disease may be explained by a common underlying risk factor. Both vascular status and dementia have causal processes operating across the lifecourse with ample opportunity for interaction at many stages (Table 27iv.2); most research fails or is unable to take this into consideration and is potentially limited by focusing at a very late stage on long-term evolving processes. Vascular risk factors such as hypertension and diabetes are commonly classified as 'environmental' risk factors for dementia. However they are known to have a substantial familial aetiology and it is possible that common genetic factors explain some of their association with Alzheimer's disease (Stewart and Liolitsa, 1999; Lovestone, 1999). Lifestyle factors such as diet, physical activity, and personality could also potentially underlie later associations.

## Effects of Alzheimer's disease on the vasculature

It is possible that Alzheimer's disease induces or exacerbates cerebrovascular pathology. Even long-duration prospective studies cannot conclusively demonstrate the direction of causation if pathological processes begin one or two decades before clinical symptoms become manifest. Deposition of amyloid occurs in cerebral blood vessels as well as the brain parenchyma in Alzheimer's disease and this 'amyloid angiopathy' is associated with both cerebral haemorrhage and small infarctions (Olichney *et al.*, 2000). Abnormalities in capillary structure have also been reported in Alzheimer's disease (de la Torre and Mussivand, 1993). It is therefore possible that the presence of Alzheimer's disease may exacerbate or accelerate vascular pathology, or render the brain more vulnerable to further insults. Early cognitive decline may also affect factors such as diet, exercise, and adherence to prescribed medication which in turn may influence the risk of cerebrovascular events.

**Table 27iv. 2** A life-course model of the relationship between vascular factors and dementia

| | |
|---|---|
| Infancy and childhood | Genetic factors determining later vascular risk and cognitive impairment<br>Environmental stressors affecting both vascular risk (e.g. blood pressure, proneness to obesity) and cognitive function (level of attainment in childhood and/or vulnerability to later neurodegeneration) |
| Early adulthood | Level of 'attained' cognitive function set determining risk of later impairment ('reserve')<br>Socio-economic status influencing vascular risk profile, and risk behaviour (smoking, diet, physical activity) |
| Mid-life | Vascular risk factors becoming manifest (hypertension, obesity, dyslipidaemia)<br>Possible subtle early cognitive changes secondary to vascular damage; also very early Alzheimer and vascular pathological changes<br>Continuing manifestation of lifestyle-related risk factors (diet, smoking, exercise) |
| Late life | Impact of clinical cerebrovascular disease (stroke, transient ischaemic attack) on cognitive function<br>Co-occurring or consequent Alzheimer's disease<br>Metabolic changes associated with frailty (e.g. weight loss, decline in blood pressure) possibly exaggerated in pre-clinical and clinical dementia<br>Chronic effects of raised vascular risk (e.g. diminished blood pressure reactivity)<br>Selective mortality (survivors with vascular risk factors potentially at lower risk due to other unknown protective factors) |

# Changes in vascular risk profile prior to dementia

As described earlier, the relationship between vascular risk factors and dementia appears to depend on the length of time which has elapsed between the two measurement points. Factors such as raised blood pressure, raised cholesterol, and increased body mass index are most likely to be identified as risk factors for dementia in studies with at least 15–20 years' follow-up. Studies with a shorter duration of follow-up often fail to demonstrate an association, or find that the association is in the opposite direction to that anticipated. There is increasing recognition that dementia is accompanied by physical changes which are detectable at a pre-clinical stage. Severe weight loss is a well-recognized feature of late stage dementia; however, more subtle weight change is identifiable prior to the onset of the clinical disorder (Barrett-Connor *et al.*, 1996; Nourhashemi *et al.*, 2003; Stewart *et al.*, 2005) and is already accelerating at that time (Stewart *et al.*, 2005). Blood pressure also declines prior to the onset of clinical dementia (Skoog *et al.*, 1996; Qiu *et al.*, 2004; Petitti *et al.*, 2005), which may or may not be a marker of the same underlying process (e.g. effects of neurodegeneration on metabolic balance). Interestingly, changes in cholesterol levels prior to dementia appear to follow a different pattern with a relatively early decline (Stewart *et al.*, 2007). A decline in cholesterol may be a marker of processes (for example an inflammatory event) accompanying initial pathological changes rather than later neuronal loss.

# Vascular risk factors and dementia treatment—clinical implications

What implications does current research have for clinicians? In theory these should be numerous since vascular disease is one of few potentially modifiable risk factors for dementia. However, although research attention is increasing in this area, there is woefully little direct evidence, at present, for any intervention to prevent or treat dementia through modifying vascular risk. Despite this, there are particular issues which can be addressed to some extent.

## Treatment of dementia through modifying vascular risk

If vascular disease were to cause dementia through damaging the brain directly, or through accelerating the progression of Alzheimer pathology, then it is likely that these processes would continue to contribute to the progression of disease after diagnosis. Interventions to halt or slow the progression of vascular disease could therefore be expected at least to prevent further cognitive decline, and possibly even improve cognitive function. However, there has been little research into potential interventions. Even for aspirin, only one randomized trial has been published: a pilot study of 70 patients with multi-infarct dementia randomized to aspirin or no additional treatment over 3 years (Meyer *et al.*, 1989). Improvement in cognitive scores and cerebral blood flow was noted over the first 2 years in the treatment group. However, the protocol did not involve a placebo and participants were not blind to their allocation. Another study found that men at high risk of cardiovascular disease who had received warfarin or aspirin (as part of a randomized double-blind trial) had better cognitive function at the end of a 5-year trial period than those receiving placebo (Richards *et al.*, 1997). Cognitive assessment was not carried out at the start of the trial, but since allocation was randomized and groups were similar in many other respects it is likely that this represents an effect of the intervention. The association with higher cognitive scores was principally in those receiving aspirin rather than warfarin. Finally, one recent trial reported a beneficial effect of atorvastatin on progression of Alzheimer's disease (Sparks *et al.*, 2005), although it is not certain whether this effect was due to vascular or other effects of this cholesterol-lowering agent. Furthermore, the findings were equivocal at 12 months' follow-up and it should be borne in mind that other statin trials have failed to show any benefit on cognitive decline prior to dementia (as discussed further below). Apart from drug treatments, other lifestyle changes may have an impact. There is trial evidence, for example, of a benefit of aerobic against anaerobic exercise on cognitive function in sedentary men (Kramer *et al.*, 1999). Important questions, such as the effects of glycaemic control in people with co-morbid dementia and diabetes, remain unanswered.

## Prevention of stroke in dementia

It is therefore uncertain whether modification of vascular risk in people with established dementia has an impact on the course of cognitive decline. However, there is also little evidence at present that such measures are contraindicated. The prescription of aspirin or the treatment of hypertension in a patient with dementia and cerebrovascular disease might be carried out not only in the hope of preventing further cognitive decline but also to prevent stroke. Complex ethical issues surround the question of how intensively to treat co-morbid disease in individuals with clinical dementia, particularly when the latter is at an advanced stage. In addition, although there may be no upper age limit for stroke prevention (Staessen *et al.*, 2000), the effectiveness of interventions such as control of blood pressure has not been adequately assessed in the context of co-morbid multiple infarctions and dementia. However, it is important to bear in mind that while some may consider an acute fatal stroke to be a preferable alternative to end-stage dementia, a non-fatal episode may lead to a lengthy period of disability and suffering which might have been prevented. It is now accepted that intensive screening for preventable risk factors should take place in people with single or recurrent strokes. There is no good reason why people who happen to have dementia should be excluded from that process, although an undoubted issue with 'vascular dementia' has been the problem of 'falling between stools' and the risk for people with this diagnosis receiving suboptimal attention from both stroke and dementia services.

### Treatment of dementia in people who have cerebrovascular disease

Although there is no good research evidence to suggest that 'vascular dementia' and 'Alzheimer's disease' can be adequately separated as distinct disorders, the persistence of the two diagnoses in clinical parlance has led to their application in clinical trials and, hence, to determine treatment 'eligibility'. Although there is some trial evidence for a beneficial effect of acetyl-cholinesterase inhibitors in people with 'vascular dementia', this is most evident for the sub-group with potentially mixed disease (Erkinjuntti *et al.*, 2002). People with 'pure' vascular dementia have been very hard to identify, and the lack of detectable cognitive decline in the placebo group over the course of a standard trial means that treatment effects are hard to demonstrate. The danger is that difficulties encountered in applying diagnostic criteria (which are predictable given the lack of evidence to support their applicability) will lead to limited enthusiasm for further trials in people with cerebrovascular disease and dementia. Recommended indications for future treatments will be limited to Alzheimer's disease alone because of a lack of evidence in other 'disorders'. If dementia with cerebrovascular disease is classified as 'vascular' in clinical practice then people with Alzheimer's disease may fail to receive treatment on the basis of co-morbidity. Since the likelihood of co-morbidity is influenced by gender, socio-economic status, and ethnicity, important inequalities in access may result (Stewart 2001a,b).

## Vascular risk factors and dementia— implications for prevention of dementia

The implications of current research for the prevention of dementia are substantial, whether vascular risk factors directly induce dementia pathology or accelerate the onset of the clinical syndrome. However, effects may be difficult to demonstrate in conventional clinical trials because of the potentially long period over which risk factors exert their action, and the changed relationships between levels of risk factors and dementia closer to the clinical onset of the latter. Furthermore, most interventions may be well established as beneficial for other reasons (e.g. preventing cardiac

disease and stroke), so that it may not be possible ethically to have a placebo group, or to retain a double-blind placebo comparison, for a sufficient time period to test an impact on dementia incidence. All of these issues may explain the largely negative results of antihypertensive agents: of trials to date, most have found no effect on incidence of dementia or cognitive decline (Prince *et al.*, 1996; Starr *et al.*, 1996; Lithell *et al.*, 2003; Tzourio *et al.*, 2003). In a subgroup analysis of the PROGRESS study, an effect was found of an ACE inhibitor and a diuretic on cognitive decline and dementia in people with recurrent stroke over the follow-up period (Tzourio *et al.*, 2003), and a further analysis showed an effect on slowing the progression of white matter lesions (Dufouil *et al.*, 2005). Only one trial has conclusively demonstrated an effect on dementia incidence (Forette *et al.*, 1998), which was sustained in open-label follow-up (Forette *et al.*, 2002). To date this is the only trial of a calcium channel blocker, and the apparent effect on dementia incidence might represent a property of this group of agents rather than an effect of blood pressure lowering. With respect to cholesterol lowering, three trials of statins have found no effect on cognitive function or decline (Santanello *et al.*, 1997; Heart Protection Study Collaborative Group, 2002; Shepherd *et al.*, 2002); however, the recent trial findings of a possible effect of atorvastatin (which has different lipid solubility) on cognitive decline in people with dementia (Sparks *et al.*, 2005), may indicate that further research is required.

As has been discussed earlier, although high blood pressure is a risk factor for dementia, blood pressure is frequently lower than average by the time clinical dementia has developed. A concern obviously arises that over-zealous correction of blood pressure may itself be a risk factor for dementia (for example, through episodes of hypoperfusion, and ischaemia or infarction in critical 'water-shed' zones). However currently there is little evidence to support this. Blood pressure is observed to be progressively lower at increasingly advanced stages of dementia (Guo *et al.*, 1996), suggesting that it is a secondary phenomenon and/or a marker of general physical frailty. One observational study of patients with multi-infarct dementia (Meyer *et al.*, 1986) suggested that a better clinical course occurred if systolic blood pressure remained within the 'upper limits of normal' (that is 135–150 mmHg) compared with lower levels. However, it cannot be concluded whether this observation was explained by blood pressure treatment, factors associated with the dementia, or co-morbid disease.

## What is vascular dementia?

Vascular disease has long been recognized as an important cause of dementia. Current evidence supports this, even though vascular disorders are frequently not a single cause in isolation but instead interact with other neuropathological processes. Renewed recognition of this and of the potential for prevention or treatment of dementia has resulted in welcome but long-overdue research interest and advice for those affected (e.g. http://www.alzheimers.org. uk/VascularDementia/index.htm). Vascular dementia as a research field is therefore alive and well. The question remains what to do with the diagnosis. Its continued usefulness is doubted even by those with whose names it is most closely associated. However, there is uncertainty as to what should replace it. 'Vascular cognitive impairment' has been suggested in order to move away from a memory-focused view of dementia (Bowler and Hachinski, 2000; O'Brien *et al.*, 2003), although this reflects a recognition of the issue and a direction for future research rather than a diagnostic category. Indeed, the most recent consensus guidelines concerning the optimal design of further research in this area (Hachinski *et al.*, 2006) sensibly do not attempt to impose diagnostic criteria in the absence of an evidence base. However, the name itself still assumes that cerebrovascular disease can be separated out and identified as a single underlying cause of cognitive impairment. For epidemiological research, cognitive decline (deterioration in cognitive test scores over time) is becoming a more favoured outcome measure over 'dementia'. However, this is difficult to apply clinically because of the wide variety of cognitive test batteries (and lack of consensus on which ones to use), because of uncertainty as to what is 'normal' fluctuation in performance, and because clinical judgements often need to be made without the luxury of a follow-up period. An alternative, at least for clinical purposes, is to consider dementia as the principal diagnosis (expanding criteria if necessary to include those with significant impairment in non-memory domains) and to include vascular disease as one of several potential predisposing, precipitating, or maintaining factors. This approach is at least in keeping with the tradition of the diagnostic formulation and with the reality of multiple, interacting, and overlapping disorders (and causes for disorders) in older age groups.

## References

Altieri, M., Di Piero, V., Pasquini, M. *et al.* (2004). Delayed poststroke dementia: a 4-year follow-up study. *Neurology*, **62**, 2193–2197.

American Psychiatric Association (1994). *Diagnostic and statistical manual of mental disorders*, 4th edn. American Psychiatric Association, Washington, DC.

Barba, R., Martínez-Espinosa, S., Rodríguez-Garcia, E., Pondal, M., Vicancos, J., and Del Ser, T. (2000). Poststroke dementia: clinical features and risk factors. *Stroke*, **31**, 1494–1501.

Barrett-Connor, E., Edelstein, S.L., Corey-Bloom, J., and Wiederholt, W.C. (1996). Weight loss precedes dementia in community-dwelling older adults. *Journal of the American Geriatrics Society*, **44**, 1147–1152.

Bowler, J.V. and Hachinski, V. (2000). Criteria for vascular dementia: replacing dogma with data. *Archives of Neurology*, **57**, 170–171.

Breteler, M.M.B., van Amerongen, N.M., van Swieten, J.C. *et al.* (1994a). Cognitive correlates of ventricular enlargement and cerebral white matter lesions on magnetic resonance imaging. *Stroke*, **25**, 1109–1115.

Breteler, M.M.B., van Swieten, J.C., Bots, M.L. *et al.* (1994b). Cerebral white matter lesions, vascular risk factors, and cognitive function in a population-based study: the Rotterdam Study. *Neurology*, **44**, 1246–1252.

Censori, B., Manara, O., Agostinis, C. *et al.* (1996). Dementia after first stroke. *Stroke*, **27**, 1205–1210.

Chui, H.C., Mack, W., Jackson, J.E. *et al.* (2000). Clinical criteria for the diagnosis of vascular dementia. *Archives of Neurology*, **57**, 191–196.

de la Torre, J.C. and Mussivand, T. (1993). Can disturbed brain microcirculation cause Alzheimer's disease? *Neurological Research*, **15**, 146–153.

Desmond, D.W., Moroney, J.T., Paik, M.C. *et al.* (2000). Frequency and clinical determinants of dementia after ischemic stroke. *Neurology*, **54**, 1124–1131.

Dufouil, C., Chalmers, J., Coskun, O. *et al.* (2005). Effects of blood pressure lowering on cerebral white matter hyperintensities in patients with stroke: the PROGRESS (Perindopril Protection Against Recurrent Stroke Study) Magnetic Resonance Imaging Substudy. *Circulation*, **112**, 1644–1650.

Elias, M.F., Wolf, P.A., D'Agostino, R.B., Cobb, J., and White, L.R. (1993). Untreated blood pressure level is inversely related to cognitive functioning: the Framingham Study. *American Journal of Epidemiology*, **138**, 353–364.

Elias, P.K., Elias, M.F., D'Agostino, R.B. *et al.* (1997). NIDDM and blood pressure as risk factors for poor cognitive performance. *Diabetes Care*, **20**, 1388–1395.

Erkinjuntti, T., Kurz, A., Gauthier, S. *et al.* (2002). Efficacy of galantamine in probable vascular dementia and Alzheimer's disease combined with cerebrovascular disease: a randomised trial. *Lancet*, **359**, 1283–1290.

Esiri, M.M., Nagy, Z., Smith, M.Z., Barnetson, L., and Smith, A.D. (1999). Cerebrovascular disease and threshold for dementia in the early stages of Alzheimer's disease. *Lancet*, **354**, 919–920.

Fein, G., Van Dyke, C., Davenport, L. *et al.* (1990). Preservation of normal cognitive functioning in elderly subjects with extensive white-matter lesions of long duration. *Archives of General Psychiatry*, **47**, 220–223.

Ferucci, L., Guralnik, J.M., Salive, M.E. *et al.* (1996). Cognitive impairment and risk of stroke in the older population. *Journal of the American Geriatrics Society*, **44**, 237–241.

Fischer, P., Gatterer, G., Marterer, A., Simanyi, M., and Danielczyk, W. (1990). Course characteristics in the differentiation of dementia of the Alzheimer type and multi-infarct dementia. *Acta Psychiatrica Scandanavica*, **81**, 551–553.

Forette, F., Seux, M.-L., Staessen, J.A. *et al.* (1998). Prevention of dementia in randomised double-blind placebo-controlled Systolic Hypertension in Europe (Syst-Eur) trial. *Lancet*, **352**, 1347–1351.

Forette, F., Seux, M.-L., Staessen, J.A. *et al.* (2002). The prevention of dementia with antihypertensive treatment. New evidence from the Systolic Hypertension in Europe (Syst-Eur) study. *Archives of Internal Medicine*, **162**, 2046–2052.

Gorelick, P.B., Chatterjee, A., Patel, D. *et al.* (1992). Cranial computerised tomographic observations in multi-infarct dementia. *Stroke*, **23**, 804–811.

Gorelick, P.B., Brody, J., Cohen, D. *et al.* (1993). Risk factors for dementia associated with multiple cerebral infarcts. *Archives of Neurology*, **50**, 714–720.

Guo, Z., Viitanen, M., Fratiglioni, L., and Winblad, B. (1996). Low blood pressure and dementia in elderly people: the Kungsholmen Project. *British Medical Journal*, **312**, 805–808.

Gustafson, D., Rothenberg, E., Blennow, K., Steen, B., and Skoog, I. (2003). An 18-year follow-up of overweight and risk of Alzheimer disease. *Archives of Internal Medicine*, **163**, 1524–1528.

Hachinski, V.C., Iliff, L.D., Zilhka, E. *et al.* (1975). Cerebral blood flow in dementia. *Archives of Neurology*, **32**, 632–637.

Hachinski, V., Iadecola, C., Petersen, R.C. *et al.* (2006). National Institute of Neurological Disorders and Stroke–Canadian Stroke Network vascular cognitive impairment harmonization standards. *Stroke*, **37**, 2220–2241.

Heart Protection Study Collaborative Group (2002). MRC/BHF Heart Protection Study of cholesterol lowering with simvastatin in 20,536 high-risk individuals: a randomised placebo-controlled trial. *Lancet*, **360**, 7–22.

Hofman, A., Ott, A., Breteler, M.M.B. *et al.* (1997). Atherosclerosis, apolipoprotein E, and prevalence of dementia and Alzheimer's disease in the Rotterdam Study. *Lancet*, **349**, 151–154.

Holmes, C., Cairns, N., Lantos, P., and Mann, A. (1999). Validity of current clinical criteria for Alzheimer's disease, vascular dementia and dementia with Lewy bodies. *British Journal of Psychiatry*, **174**, 45–50.

Honig, L.S., Tang, M.-X., Albert, S. *et al.* (2003). Stroke and the risk of Alzheimer disease. *Archives of Neurology*, **60**, 1707–1712.

Hulette, C., Nochlin, D., McKeel, D. *et al.* (1997). Clinical-neuropathological findings in multi-infarct dementia: a report of six autopsied cases. *Neurology*, **48**, 668–672.

Ivan, C.S., Seshadri, S., Beiser, A. *et al.* (2004). Dementia after stroke: the Framingham Study. *Stroke*, **35**, 1264–1268.

Joutel, A., Vahedi, K., Corpechot, C. et al. (1997). Strong clustering and stereotyped nature of Notch3 mutations in CADASIL patients. *Lancet*, **350**, 1511–1515.

Kalmijn, S., Launer, L.J., Ott, A., Witteman, J.C.M., Hofman, A., and Breteler, M.M.B. (1997). Dietary fat intake and the risk of incident dementia in the Rotterdam Study. *Annals of Neurology*, **42**, 776–782.

Kalmijn, S., Foley, D., White, L. et al. (2000). Metabolic cardiovascular syndrome and risk of dementia in Japanese-American elderly men. *Arteriosclerosis, Thrombosis & Vascular Biology*, **20**, 2255–2260.

Kase, C.S., Wolf, P.A., Kelly-Hayes, M., Kannel, W.B., Beiser, A., and D'Agostino, R.B. (1998). Intellectual decline after stroke: the Framingham Study. *Stroke*, **29**, 805–812.

Kilander, L., Nyman, H., Boberg, M., Hansson, L., and Lithell, H. (1998). Hypertension is related to cognitive impairment. A 20-year follow-up of 999 men. *Hypertension*, **31**, 780–786.

Kivipelto, M., Helkala, E.-L., Laakso, M.P. et al. (2001). Midlife vascular risk factors and Alzheimer's disease in later life: longitudinal, population based study. *British Medical Journal*, **322**, 1447–1451.

Kivipelto, M., Helkala, E.-L., Laakso, M.P. et al. (2002). Apolipoprotein E e4 allele, elevated midlife total cholesterol level, and high midlife systolic blood pressure are independent risk factors for late-life Alzheimer disease. *Annals of Internal Medicine*, **137**, 149–155.

Kivipelto, M., Nganda, T., Fratiglioni, L. et al. (2005). Obesity and vascular risk factors at midlife and the risk of dementia and Alzheimer's disease. *Archives of Neurology*, **62**, 1556–1560.

Kokmen, E., Whistman, J.P., O'Fallon, W.M., Chu, C.P., and Beard, C.M. (1996). Dementia after ischemic stroke: a population-based study in Rochester, Minnesota (1960–1984). *Neurology*, **19**, 154–159.

Kramer, A.F., Hahn, S., Cohen, N.J. et al. (1999). Ageing, fitness and neurocognitive function. *Nature*, **400**, 418–419.

Launer, L.J., Masaki, K., Petrovitch, H., Foley, D., and Havlik, R.J. (1995). The association between midlife blood pressure levels and late-life cognitive function. *Journal of the American Medical Association*, **274**, 1846–1851.

Launer, L.J., White, L.R., Petrovitch, H., Ross, G.W., and Curb, J.D. (2001). Cholesterol and neuropathologic markers of AD. A population-based autopsy study. *Neurology*, **57**, 1447–1452.

Laurin, D., Verreault, R., Lindsay, J., MacPherson, K., and Rockwood, K. (2001). Physical activity and risk of cognitive impairment and dementia in elderly persons. *Archives of Neurology*, **58**, 498–504.

Lithell, H., Hansson, L., Skoog, I. et al. (2003). The Study on Cognition and Prognosis in the Elderly (SCOPE): principal results of a randomized double-blind intervention trial. *Journal of Hypertension*, **21**, 875–886.

Loeb, C., Gandolfo, C., Croce, R., and Conti, M. (1992). Dementia associated with lacunar infarction. *Stroke*, **23**, 1225–1229.

Lopez, O.L., Larumbe, M.R., Becker, J.T. et al. (1994). Reliability of NINDS-AIREN clinical criteria for the diagnosis of vascular dementia. *Neurology*, **44**, 1240–1245.

Lovestone, S. (1999). Diabetes and dementia: is the brain another site of end-organ damage? *Neurology*, **53**, 1907–1909.

Luchsinger, J.A., Tang, M.-X., Shea, S., and Mayeux, R. (2002). Caloric intake and the risk of Alzheimer disease. *Archives of Neurology*, **59**, 1258–1263.

Luchsinger, J.A., Tang, M.-X., Shea, S., and Mayeux, R. (2004). Hyperinsulinemia and risk of Alzheimer disease. *Neurology*, **63**, 1187–1192.

Luchsinger, J.A., Reitz, C., Honig, L.S., Tang, M.X., Shea, S., and Mayeux, R. (2005). Aggregation of vascular risk factors and risk of incident Alzheimer disease. *Neurology*, **65**, 545–551.

MacKnight, C., Rockwood, K., Awalt, E., and McDowell, I. (2002). Diabetes mellitus and the risk of dementia, Alzheimer's disease and vascular cognitive impairment in the Canadian Study of Health and Aging. *Dementia and Geriatric Cognitive Disorders*, **14**, 77–83.

Mayer-Gross, W., Slater, E., and Roth, M. (1969) *Clinical psychiatry*, 3rd edn. Bailliere, Tindall & Carsell, London.

Meyer, J.S., Judd, B.W., Tawaklna, T., Rogers, R.L., and Mortel, K.F. (1986). Improved cognition after control of risk factors for multi-infarct dementia. *Journal of the American Medical Association*, **256**, 2203–2309.

Meyer, J.S., Rogers, R.L., McClintic, K., Mortel, K.F., and Lofti, J. (1989). Randomized clinical trial of daily aspirin therapy in multi-infarct dementia. *Journal of the American Geriatrics Society*, **37**, 549–555.

Mielke, M.M., Zandi, P.P., Sjogren, M. et al. (2005). High total cholesterol levels in late life associated with a reduced risk of dementia. *Neurology*, **64**, 1689–1695.

Moroney, J.T., Bagiella, E., Desmond, D.W., Paik, M., Stern, Y., and Tatemichi, T.K. (1996). Risk factors for incident dementia after stroke. Role of hypoxic and ischaemic disorders. *Stroke*, **27**, 1283–1289.

Moroney, J.T., Bagiella, E., Tatemichi, T.K., Paik, M., and Stern, Y. (1997). Dementia after stroke increases the risk of long-term stroke recurrence. *Neurology*, **48**, 1317–1325.

Notkola, I.-L., Sulkava, R., Pekkanen, J. et al. (1998). Serum total cholesterol, apolipoprotein E 4 allele, and Alzheimer's disease. *Neuroepidemiology*, **17**, 14–20.

Nourhashemi, F., Deschamps, V., Larrieu, S., Letenneur, L., Dartigues, J.-F., and Barberger-Gateau, P. (2003). Body mass index and incidence of dementia: the PAQUID study. *Neurology*, **60**, 117–119.

O'Brien, J.T., Erkinjuntti, T., Reisberg, B. et al. (2003). Vascular cognitive impairment. *Lancet Neurology*, **2**, 89–98.

Olichney, J.M., Hansen, L.A., Lee, J.H., Hofsetter, C.R., Katzman, R., and Thal, L.J. (2000). Relationship between severe amyloid angiopathy, apolipoprotein E genotype, and vascular lesions in Alzheimer's disease. *Annals of the New York Academy of Sciences*, **903**, 138–148.

Ott, A., Breteler, M.M.B., de Bruyne, M.C., van Harskamp, F., Grobbee, D.E., and Hofman, A. (1997). Atrial fibrillation and dementia in a population-based study. *Stroke*, **28**, 316–321.

Ott, A., Slooter, A.J.C., Hofman, A. et al. (1998). Smoking and the risk of dementia and Alzheimer's disease in a population-based cohort study: the Rotterdam Study. *Lancet*, **351**, 1840–1843.

Ott, A., Stolk, R.P., van Harskamp, F., Pols, H.A.P., Hofman, A., and Breteler, M.M.B. (1999). Diabetes mellitus and the risk of dementia. *Neurology*, **53**, 1937–1942.

Peila, R., Rodriguez, B.L., and Launer, L.J. (2002). Type 2 diabetes, APOE gene, and the risk for dementia and related pathologies: the Honolulu-Asia Aging Study. *Diabetes*, **51**, 1256–1262.

Peila, R., Rodriguez, B.L., White, L.R., and Launer, L.J. (2004). Fasting insulin and incident dementia in an elderly population of Japanese-American men. *Neurology*, **63**, 228–233.

Petitti, D.B., Crooks, V.C., Buckwalter, J.G., and Chiu, V. (2005). Blood pressure levels before dementia. *Archives of Neurology*, **62**, 112–116.

Petrovitch, H., White, L.R., Izmirilian, G. et al. (2000). Midlife blood pressure and neuritic plaques, neurofibrillary tangles, and brain weight at death: the Honolulu Asia Aging Study. *Neurobiology of Aging*, **21**, 57–62.

Pfeifer, L.A., White, L.R., Ross, G.W., Petrovitch, H., and Launer, L.J. (2002). Cerebral amyloid angiopathy and cognitive function: the HAAS autopsy study. *Neurology*, **58**, 1629–1634.

Pohjasvaara, T., Erkinjuntti, T., Ylikoski, R., Hietanen, M., Vataja, R., and Kaste, M. (1998). Clinical determinants of poststroke dementia. *Stroke*, **29**, 75–81.

Pohjasvaara, T., Mäntylä, R., Aronen, H.J. et al. (1999). Clinical and radiological determinants of prestroke cognitive decline in a stroke cohort. *Journal of Neurology, Neurosurgery and Psychiatry*, **67**, 742–748.

Prince, M., Cullen, M., and Mann, A. (1994). Risk factors for Alzheimer's disease and dementia: a case-control study based on the MRC elderly hypertension trial. *Neurology*, **44**, 97–104.

Prince, M.J., Bird, A.S., Blizard, R.A., and Mann, A.H. (1996). Is the cognitive function of older patients affected by antihypertensive treatment? Results from 54 months of the Medical Research Council's treatment trial of hypertension in older adults. *British Medical Journal*, **312**, 801–804.

Qiu, C., von Strauss, E., Winblad, B., and Fratiglioni, L. (2004). Decline in blood pressure over time and risk of dementia: a longitudinal study from the Kungsholmen Project. *Stroke*, **35**, 1810–1815.

Reitz, C., Tang, M.-X., Luchsinger, J., and Mayeux, R. (2004). Relation of plasma lipids to Alzheimer disease and vascular dementia. *Archives of Neurology*, **61**, 705–714.

Richards, M., Meade, T.W., Peart, S., Brennan, P.J., and Mann, A.H. (1997). Is there any evidence for a protective effect of antithrombotic medication on cognitive function in men at risk of cardiovascular disease? Some preliminary findings. *Journal of Neurology, Neurosurgery and Psychiatry*, **62**, 269–272.

Román, G.C., Tatemichi, T.K., Erkinjuntti, T. *et al.* (1993). Vascular dementia: diagnostic criteria for research studies: Report of the NINDS-AIREN International Workshop. *Neurology*, **43**, 1609–1611.

Rovio, S., Kareholt, I., Helkala, E.-L. *et al.* (2005). Leisure-time physical activity at midlife and the risk of dementia and Alzheimer's disease. *Lancet Neurology*, **4**, 705–711.

Santanello, N.C., Barber, B.L., Applegate, W.B. *et al.* (1997). Effect of pharmacologic lipid lowering on health-related quality of life in older persons: results from the Cholesterol Reduction in Seniors Program (CRISP) Pilot Study. *Journal of the American Geriatrics Society*, **45**, 8–14.

Shepherd, J., Blauw, G.J., Murphy, M.B. *et al.* (2002). Pravastatin in elderly individuals at risk of vascular disease (PROSPER): a randomized controlled trial. *Lancet*, **360**, 1623–1630.

Skoog, I., Lernfelt, B., Landahl, S. *et al.* (1996). 15-year longitudinal study of blood pressure and dementia. *Lancet*, **347**, 1141–1145.

Snowdon, D.A., Greiner, L.H., Mortimer, J.A., Riley, K.P., Greiner, P.A., and Markesbery, W.R. (1997). Brain infarction and the clinical expression of Alzheimer disease. *Journal of the American Medical Association*, **277**, 813–817.

Sparks, D.L., Scheff, S.W., Liu, H., Landers, T.M., Coyne, C.M., and Hunsaker, J.C. (1995). Increased incidence of neurofibrillary tangles (NFT) in non-demented individuals with hypertension. *Journal of the Neurological Sciences*, **131**, 162–169.

Sparks, D.L., Scheff, S.W., Liu, H. *et al.* (1996). Increased density of senile plaques (SP), but not neurofibrillary tangles (NFT), in non-demented individuals with the apolipoprotein E4 allele: comparison to confirmed Alzheimer's disease patients. *Journal of the Neurological Sciences*, **138**, 97–104.

Sparks, D.L., Sabbagh, M.N., Connor, D.J. *et al.* (2005). Atorvastatin for the treatment of mild to moderate Alzheimer Disease. *Archives of Neurology*, **62**, 753–757.

Srikanth, V.K., Anderson, J.F.I., Donnan, G.A. *et al.* (2004). Progressive dementia after first-ever stroke: a community-based follow-up study. *Neurology*, **63**, 785–792.

Staessen, J.A., Gasowski, J., Wang, J.G. *et al.* (2000). Risks of untreated and treated isolated systolic hypertension in the elderly: meta-analysis of outcome trials. *Lancet*, **355**, 865–872.

Starr, J.M., Whalley, L.J., and Deary, I.J. (1996). The effects of antihypertensive treatment on cognitive function: results from the HOPE study. *Journal of the American Geriatrics Society*, **44**, 411–415.

Stewart, R. (1998). Cardiovascular factors in Alzheimer's disease. *Journal of Neurology, Neurosurgery and Psychiatry*, **65**, 143–147.

Stewart, R. (1999). Hypertension and cognitive decline. *British Journal of Psychiatry*, **174**, 286–287.

Stewart, R. (2001a). Applications of cholinesterase inhibitors. *Lancet*, **358**, 73–74.

Stewart, R. (2001b). NICE guidelines and the treatment of Alzheimer's disease: evidence-based medicine may be discriminatory. *British Journal of Psychiatry*, **179**, 367

Stewart, R. and Liolitsa, D. (1999). Type 2 diabetes mellitus, cognitive impairment and dementia. *Diabetic Medicine*, **16**, 93–112.

Stewart, R., Masaki, K., Xue, Q.-L. *et al.* (2005). A 32-year prospective study of change in body weight and incident dementia: the Honolulu-Asia Aging Study. *Archives of Neurology*, **62**, 55–60.

Stewart, R., Xue, Q.-L., White, L.R., and Launer, L.J. (2007). 26-year change in total cholesterol levels and incident dementia. The Honolulu-Asia Aging Study. *Archives of Neurology*, **64**, 103–107.

Tatemichi, T.K., Desmond, D.W., Mayeux, R. *et al.* (1992a). Dementia after stroke: baseline frequency, risks and clinical features in a hospitalised cohort. *Neurology*, **42**, 1185–1193.

Tatemichi, T.K., Desmond, D.W., Prohovnik, I. *et al.* (1992b). Confusion and memory loss from capsular genu infarction: a thalamocortical disconnection syndrome? *Neurology*, **42**, 1966–1979.

Tatemichi, T.K., Paik, M., Bagiella, E. *et al.* (1994). Risk of dementia after stroke in a hospitalised cohort: results of a longitudinal study. *Neurology*, **44**, 1885–1891.

Tzourio, C., Anderson, C., Chapman, N. *et al.* (2003). Effects of blood pressure lowering with perindopril and indapamide therapy on dementia and cognitive decline in patients with cerebrovascular disease. *Archives of Internal Medicine*, **163**, 1069–1075.

Yoshitake, T., Kiyohara, Y., Kato, I. *et al.* (1995). Incidence and risk factors of vascular dementia and Alzheimer's disease in a defined elderly Japanese population: the Hisayama Study. *Neurology*, **45**, 1161–1168.

# Clinical aspects of dementia: dementia in Parkinson's disease and dementia with Lewy bodies

Rupert McShane

Although Alzheimer's disease is the commonest form of neurodegenerative disorder, Lewy body pathology is much more common than previously thought. Its clinical importance lies in the fact that it is associated with typical features, which will often be missed unless the patient and caregiver are specifically asked. This matters both clinically and economically: such patients are preferential responders to cholinesterase inhibitors, decline faster, have higher cost of care needs, and can be treated more cost-effectively than patients with Alzheimer's disease.

## What are Lewy bodies?

Lewy bodies (LBs) are the neuronal inclusion bodies which, when accompanied by the characteristic clinical syndrome of tremor, rigidity, and bradykinesia, define idiopathic Parkinson's disease. In Parkinson's disease they are typically found in the pigmented neurons of the substantia nigra and locus ceruleus and in the neurons of the cholinergic nucleus basalis of Meynert, but LB pathology in other areas (e.g. the olfactory bulb, the amygdala, the dorsal nucleus of the vagus) usually occurs first. Similar inclusions are also present in multisystem atrophy and amyotrophic lateral sclerosis (motor neuron disease). This family of conditions has been termed 'the alpha-synucleinopathies' because in each of them the characteristic pathology includes abnormal aggregations of alpha-synuclein. Aggregated, filamentous alpha-synuclein is a major constituent of LBs, Lewy neurites, and neuraxonal spheroids. Other constituents of LBs include ubiquitin and neurofilament. The predilection areas for the formation of cortical LBs are the cingulate, parahippocampal gyrus, insula cortex, and temporal and frontal neocortex. The finding that many cases of autosomal dominant, single gene, familial Alzheimer's disease (AD) have LBs in the amygdala and elsewhere suggests that alpha-synuclein aggregation can be precipitated either directly or as a distal consequence of abnormalities of amyloid processing (Lippa *et al.*, 1998).

## Epidemiology

Lewy body pathology is more common than is identified clinically. Population-based clinical studies of those over 65 years typically find rates of clinical dementia with Lewy bodies (DLB) of 0.1%, though this may be much higher in those over 75 years (3.3%) (Rahkonen *et al.*, 2003) and is higher in clinical studies of those with dementia (0–30.5%) (Zaccai *et al.*, 2005). Prospective cohort studies find that 7–14% of people dying without dementia or cognitive impairment have LB pathology (Bennett *et al.*, 2006). In brain bank series of patients with dementia, 20% of cases have LB pathology in the brainstem and as many as 50–60% of those with AD also have alpha-synuclein aggregations in the amygdala (Hamilton, 2000). An epidemiologically based study of the elderly found LBs in about 40% (Zaccai *et al.*, 2006)

James Parkinson's original description suggested that intellectual function is 'uninjured' in the shaking palsy which came to bear his name. However, half the cases described by Friederich Lewy in his 1923 monograph on the neuropathology of PD had dementia and the rate of dementia in clinical PD of 24 to 31% (Aarsland *et al.*, 2005a) is at least two to five times that expected in age-matched controls. Longitudinal studies suggest that most patients with PD who survive will eventually develop dementia (Aarsland *et al.*, 2003). The relative risk of incident dementia in a given year is approximately 1.7 times that of controls (Marder *et al.*, 1995).

## A brief history of DLB

DLB is a disease with a short history of rather intense debate about its nosological status. Japanese neuropathologists were the first to describe the presence of 'cortical LBs' (Okazaki *et al.*, 1961; Kosaka *et al.*, 1976), and the recognition that cortical LBs might be associated with dementia and a characteristic clinical syndrome led to a more widespread interest. Consensus was reached rather quickly on the clinical but not the neuropathological criteria for DLB (McKeith *et al.*, 1996). The main stumbling block then was that there was a lack of consensus on the neuropathological evaluation of AD. This was important because most (approximately 95%) cases with the clinical syndrome have at least some non-neuritic plaques and many have a few tangles. Were these cases of a Lewy body variant of AD? The introduction of a routine method for assessing tangles (NIA Reagan) cleared the way for the third revision of the consensus criteria (McKeith *et al.*, 2005). Here, the emphasis has shifted slightly from the question of 'What pathology predicts dementia?' to 'What pathology predicts the syndrome within dementia?'. One reason for this shift is that a simple equation between the presence of cortical LBs and dementia is not possible: a few ubiquitinated cortical LBs are found in most cases of PD without dementia (Hughes *et al.*, 1993); whether LBs occur more commonly in those with dementia may depend on details of the neuropathological staining method (Zaccai *et al.*, 2006); and many of the cases of late AD with alpha-synuclein aggregations restricted to the amygdala do not have the features regarded as characteristic of clinical DLB syndrome.

This iterative process of getting the best match between clinical symptoms and neuropathology has good clinical face validity and utility. The fact that it is tautological—since neuropathological criteria can only be validated against the clinical syndrome, which can only be validated against neuropathological criteria—means that it is likely that there will be some cases in which the same disease process is occurring but which do not meet either clinical or neuropathological criteria. Ultimately this will only matter if a treatment directed at this process becomes available.

A further taxonomic issue has assumed more importance recently: the distinction between dementia occurring in established Parkinson's disease of at least a year's duration (Parkinson's disease dementia; PDD), and that where the dementia and parkinsonism occur at approximately the same time (DLB). One practical reason for this distinction, which was introduced in the 1996 criteria (McKeith *et al.*, 1996), was the demands of drug licensing. Since DLB had not gained wide acceptance as a distinct disease entity, particularly in the USA, it was not possible to market any compounds for its treatment. By contrast, both dementia and PD were clearly established entities. A further scientific reason lay in the debate over the significance of AD pathology, which was unresolved at the time. The result of this split was that a cholinesterase inhibitor (rivastigmine) has been licensed for the treatment of PDD but not DLB (see below).

Whilst there may be subtle differences in the neuropathology associated with the two clinical syndromes of PDD and DLB, there are no major differences between the two in cognitive profile, attentional performance, neuropsychiatric features, sleep disorders, autonomic dysfunction, type and severity of parkinsonism, neuroleptic sensitivity, and responsiveness to cholinesterase inhibitors (McKeith *et al.*, 2004; Thomas *et al.*, 2005)

The boundary between mild cognitive impairment and dementia is of relevance to DLB and PD as well as to AD. Most patients with PD have subtle cognitive impairment. This is characterized by slowed thinking (the so-called 'bradyphrenia' of subcortical dementia), and deficits in visuospatial function, in shifting attention, and in executive function. Whether these deficits reach the point where the patient can be considered to have dementia depends on the threshold adopted for the definition of functional, social, or occupational impairment (which is currently part of the definition of dementia). Inter-rater reliability of this is not good in patients with relatively mild cognitive impairment (MCI). The utility of the concept of 'DLB MCI' or 'PD MCI' will largely depend on whether the associated symptoms need treating and are treatable. Some patients with Lewy body pathology, and who have hallmark features needed for DLB diagnosis (see below), may not meet dementia criteria and yet their symptoms, such as their visual hallucinations, may respond well to cholinesterase inhibitor treatment.

## Clinical diagnosis

The diagnosis of PDD is probably the easiest of all dementias: a patient with established PD who develops dementia has PDD unless there are other explanations (e.g. a stroke). By contrast, the diagnosis of DLB requires much more clinical attention to detail.

The third revision of the consensus clinical criteria for DLB (McKeith *et al.*, 2005) (Box 27v.1) extends that of 1996 to include REM sleep behaviour disorder, imaging evidence of dopaminergic neuronal loss, and neuroleptic sensitivity.

Most validation studies of the 1996 criteria (see McKeith *et al.*, 2004) found that patients meeting these criteria were very likely to have LBs (specificities of approximately 80%). The main weakness of the criteria was that they failed to pick up a significant number of cases which turned out to have LBs. Reported sensitivities were very variable, with an average of 60%, though they reached 80% in a prospective study from Newcastle (McKeith *et al.*, 2000a). One reason for the poor sensitivities was possibly that features such as fluctuating attention and hallucinations were obscured when the overall level of cognitive decline, or of AD pathology, was severe. Another was that LB pathology may sometimes develop only late in dementia, long after the defining clinical symptoms have been assessed. In other cases, the burden of pathology may have been so slight as to not influence the clinical picture. As described above, the solution has lain in the alteration and standardization of neuropathological criteria. However, this means that there are not yet any studies assessing how well the new clinical criteria perform. The main hope is that the sensitivity will be improved.

---

**Box 27v.1** Consensus criteria for probable dementia with Lewy bodies

Two of the following three:
- Fluctuating cognition with pronounced variations in attention and alertness
- Recurrent visual hallucinations that are typically well formed and detailed
- Spontaneous features of parkinsonism

OR one of the above PLUS one of the following:
- REM sleep behaviour disorder
- Severe neuroleptic sensitivity
- Low dopamine transporter uptake in basal ganglia demonstrated by SPECT or PET imaging

# The core features of DLB

## Visual hallucinations

Visual hallucinations are present in 60–70% of cases of DLB. The visual hallucinations are typically of people or animals which often disappear when attention is directly focused on the presumed image. Some patients complain of seeing smoke or fire, or water on surfaces. Detailed, formed visual hallucinations are often preceded by visual illusions or vivid dreams. The illusions commonly take the form of seeing faces or animals in the detailed textures of patterns on furniture, or in trees.

Patients with isolated visual hallucinations or psychosis in the absence of cognitive impairment are at increased risk of developing dementia (Ostling *et al.*, 2006). Similarly, patients with PD who develop hallucinations are more likely to develop dementia (Stern *et al.*, 1993). Whilst they may be made worse by all antiparkinsonian medication, careful enquiry will generally elicit the presence of hallucinations before starting such medication. The link between Charles Bonnet syndrome (CBS) and DLB is uncertain since there are no substantial neuropathological studies of CBS. CBS is generally thought of as the association of persistent visual hallucinations with visual impairment, in the absence of intellectual impairment. However, advanced age is a consistently reported risk factor for CBS and detailed neuropsychology suggests that most cases have at least mildly impaired cognitive function (Pliskin *et al.*, 1996). Although poor eyesight makes hallucinations in DLB worse, it probably does not affect whether or not they occur in dementia (McShane *et al.*, 1995).

Visual hallucinations are a marker of more severe cholinergic deficit in DLB and PDD (Perry *et al.*, 1990). They respond particularly well to treatment with cholinesterase inhibitors. For example, in clinical trials rivastigmine produced a good cognitive and functional response (McKeith *et al.*, 2000b; Burn *et al.*, 2006). Although delusions also respond to rivastigmine, the aetiology of delusions may be different from that of hallucinations since up-regulation of the post-synaptic muscarinic receptor is associated with delusions but not hallucinations (Ballard *et al.*, 2000b).

## Fluctuation

It has been suggested in jest that 'dementia with LBs' is a misnomer and the condition should be termed 'delirium with LBs' because fluctuation in attention is a core part of the syndrome of DLB and of delirium. Assessing the severity and frequency of fluctuation is not easy. At a simple level, the amplitude can be assessed by asking the caregiver to give examples of what the patient can do when at their best and when at their worst. The Oxford Project to Investigate Memory and Ageing, found that a simple question about brief fluctuations ('Are there brief periods during 24 hours when he seems much worse and then times when he is quite clear?') was a much better discriminator of those with pathological DLB from AD than a question about longer fluctuations ('Are there episodes lasting days or weeks when his thinking seems quite clear and then becomes muddled?'). However, it is probably better to use a more structured approach routinely. The One Day Fluctuation Assessment Scale (Walker *et al.*, 2000a) rates items such as attention, drowsiness, episodes of incoherence, falls, and fluctuation. The Mayo Fluctuations Composite Scale suggests that the presence of three of the following four features may be most discriminating: daytime drowsiness and lethargy, daytime sleep of two or more hours, staring into space for long periods, and episodes of disorganized speech (Ferman *et al.*, 2004). These scales have yet to be neuropathologically validated.

Computerized assessment has shown that patients with clinical DLB have marked fluctuations in reaction times over the course of a simple 90 s task. The approach has been validated by showing that second-to-second reductions in EEG activity coincided with periods of slowed reaction times (Walker *et al.*, 2000b). Rivastigmine (McKeith *et al.*, 2000b) and donepezil (Rowan *et al.*, 2007) also reduce this fluctuation, implying it is due to a cholinergic deficit. This may be via thalamic projections.

Fluctuation is also a common sequela of levodopa treatment in PD, is related to the availability of levodopa and is reduced by catechol-*O*-methyl transferase inhibitors such as entacopone. However, many patients with DLB with fluctuations are not taking levodopa, either because they do not have sufficient parkinsonism to warrant it, or because the levodopa exacerbates their hallucinations.

## Parkinsonism

Just as 'cerebral reserve' often prevents cognitive impairment becoming immediately apparent, parkinsonism does not occur until 60% of the dopaminergic neurons in the substantia nigra are lost or dopamine levels in the basal ganglia fall by 80%. Interestingly, subtle extrapyramidalism in the elderly, non-demented population predicts the onset of dementia rather than PD (Richards *et al.*, 1993). Parkinsonism is not an invariable feature of DLB at presentation. Indeed, its absence is the commonest reason for clinicians to miss the diagnosis of DLB.

The pattern of parkinsonism in DLB is similar to the subtype commonly seen in late onset PD—postural instability gait disorder. Unilateral signs and tremor are less common. An impassive expression (facial masking), often associated with a rather staring expression due to a low blink rate, and bradykinesia are more common. Indeed, presentation of PD with bilateral features or facial masking predicts the onset of dementia and of visual hallucinations (Stern *et al.*, 1993). The tremor is often not pronounced, and caregivers occasionally report that it improves as cognitive function worsens. Presumably, the worsening cholinergic deficit acts in the same way as giving an anticholinergic drug such as procyclidine.

## REM sleep behaviour disorder

Vivid dreams in DLB are sometimes associated with REM sleep behaviour disorder. In this condition the normal mechanisms which inhibit muscle activity in REM sleep break down and patients start to act out their dreams (Boeve *et al.*, 1998). As an isolated symptom, RBD is associated with impaired olfaction (Fantini *et al.*, 2006) and is a common harbinger of the development of a clinical alpha-synucleinopathy (Iranzo *et al.*, 2006). Disorder of REM sleep can also be associated with cataplexy, a symptom which is commonly misdiagnosed as being of vascular origin.

## Neuroleptic sensitivity

A profound adverse reaction to neuroleptics is commonly seen in patients with DLB. It may take the form of worsened confusion as well as an abrupt worsening of parkinsonism (McKeith *et al.*, 1992). It occurs both with typical and atypical neuroleptics, though more with the former, and may be more prevalent in DLB than in PD. This may be due to a greater failure in DLB than in PD of post-synaptic dopamine receptor up-regulation in response to the pre-synaptic dopaminergic deficit. Neuroleptic D2 antagonists thus occupy a greater proportion of post-synaptic dopamine receptors in DLB than PD (Piggott *et al.*, 1999). Interestingly, neuroleptic sensitivity does not seem to occur in dementia patients who do not have LB pathology (e.g. patients with pure AD) (Aarsland *et al.*, 2005b) and neuroleptics may be associated with more severe tangle formation in DLB (Ballard *et al.*, 2005)

### Dopaminergic imaging

The dopaminergic deficits in DLB may turn out to be useful diagnostically since patients with DLB have reduced density of pre-synaptic dopamine reuptake protein in the posterior putamen (see Fig. 27v.1). This can be visualized using cocaine-analogue ligands and single photon emission computed tomography (SPECT) imaging (Walker *et al.*, 1999). The technique gave sensitivity for the distinction between DLB and AD of 78% against clinical criteria using [123]I-radiolabelled 2β-carbomethoxy-3β-(4-iodophenyl)-*N*-(3-fluoropropyl) nortropane (FP-CIT) (O'Brien *et al.*, 2004). As a result of a phase III trial of 326 dementia patients, which produced similar results (sensitivity 77.7% and specificity 90.4% for

distinguishing DLB from non-DLB dementia) this investigation now has a licence (McKeith *et al.*, 2007). However, its incremental value over and above the clinical criteria, and its cost-effectiveness, have yet to be established.

### Supporting features

The consensus criteria also include a variety of clinical features which, while not necessary for the diagnosis, are supportive:

◆ repeated falls and syncope

◆ transient, unexplained loss of consciousness

◆ severe autonomic dysfunction, e.g. orthostatic hypotension, urinary incontinence

◆ hallucinations in other modalities

◆ systematized delusions

◆ depression

◆ relative preservation of medial temporal lobe structures on CT/MRI scan

◆ generalized low uptake on SPECT/positron emission tomography (PET) perfusion scan with reduced occipital activity

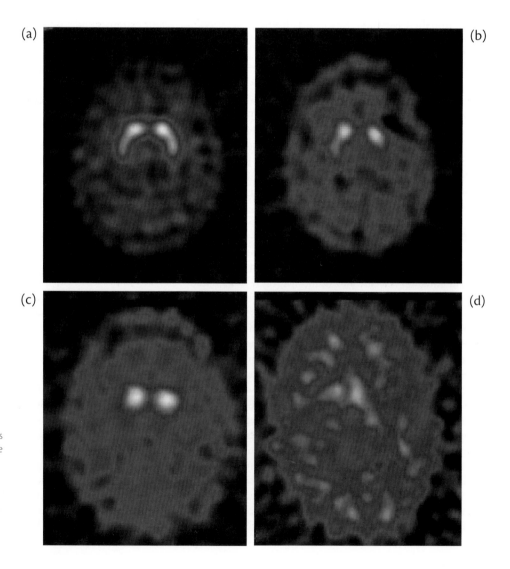

(a)    (b)    (c)    (d)

**Fig. 27v.1** Normal (a) and abnormal (b)–(d) FP-CIT SPECT images in subjects with dementia. (b) Asymmetric uptake in the putamen with near normal on one side (type 1). (c) Greatly reduced putamen uptake bilaterally (type 2). (d) Uptake is virtually absent (type 3). (Taken from McKeith *et al.* 2007, with permission.) See Plate 9 for a colour version of this figure.

- abnormal (low uptake) [123]I-*meta*-iodobenzylguanidine (MIBG) myocardial scintigraphy
- prominent slow wave activity on EEG with temporal lobe transient sharp waves.

Impaired olfactory function is also more common in neuropathological DLB than other dementias (McShane *et al.*, 2001; Olichney *et al.*, 2005). Forced-choice tests of olfactory recognition can be easily and cheaply used in the clinic to distinguish clinically between mild DLB and mild AD (Williams *et al.*, 2006), and further research will establish whether they may merit wider use.

The neuropsychological profile of patients with DLB differs from that of patients with AD in several ways. The visuospatial deficits seen in DLB are more marked than expected for overall level of cognitive function and are associated with the presence of visual hallucinations. Memory function, particularly recognition memory, is better preserved than in AD. Deficits of attention are common and associated with fluctuation. Verbal fluency and executive function are also impaired. A ratio of praxis score to memory function has been found to distinguish cases with DLB from AD with specificity of 98% and sensitivity of 33% (or 84% and 63% depending on the cut-off point used) (Ballard *et al.*, 1999).

Structural imaging may reveal a degree of atrophy of the medial temporal lobes, and the hippocampal gyrus in particular, which is less than expected for the level of cognitive impairment (Barber *et al.*, 2000). SPECT imaging with HMPAO and a new muscarinic ligand show occipital hypoperfusion, and alterations in occipital muscarinic acetylcholine receptors (Colloby *et al.*, 2006). As with the established link between LB pathologies in the anterior and inferior temporal lobe (Harding *et al.*, 2002), this may underpin the pathophysiology of visual hallucinations.

# The management of DLB

## What to tell the patient and carer

In explaining the diagnosis, a simple explanation of the condition as 'an overlap between Alzheimer's and Parkinson's' is more likely to be useful than detailed explanations of the taxonomy of DLB.

The fluctuating nature of the attentional deficits can be perplexing for caregivers, particularly because periods of high functioning indicate that such abilities have not been irretrievably lost. However, this can be a useful lead in to a discussion about the maximum potential benefit of medication that can reasonably be expected. A simple explanation for the attentional deficits is that the patient runs out of the 'steam' needed for thinking, because of the cholinergic deficit. The more the patient tries to resolve the muddle, the less they can build up the necessary head of steam to think clearly.

In patients with dementia who have lost insight, it is usually unhelpful for their caregivers to contradict any delusional ideas. However, insight into the illusory nature of hallucinations is very often retained in DLB, particularly in the early stages. In such cases, reassurance that the patient's eyes or imagination are 'playing tricks' with them is useful. An explanation of the progression from vivid dreams, through illusions and plucking at the sheets or picking imaginary threads from the floor, to formed '*de novo*' hallucinations often helps caregivers to make sense of their experience. Since poor eyesight can make visual hallucinations worse it is sensible to maximize the patient's visual acuity. Cataract extraction early in the course may retard the development of hallucinations. Increasing the power and number of light bulbs in the room where the patient typically sits may help since hallucinations are usually more prominent in low lighting and in the evening. Furniture and curtains with patterns which are likely to provoke the visual illusions can be covered or replaced with monochromatic material. Paradoxically, illusions are less likely to occur in a new or moderately stimulating environment than in a familiar environment where there is little to occupy the patient's mind. Patients rarely hallucinate when their attention is taken by visitors but are often found doing so when guests arrive, who are then frequently able to helpfully describe the patient's experiences.

Sometimes it is necessary to advise families about the need to give the patient with bradyphrenia more time to respond or to carry out tasks. The difficulty that the patient has in rapid shifting of attention means that family members should try not to speak more than one at a time or interrupt each other. When this sort of communication occurs in the interview, it can be helpful to point this out gently so that the family understand what is being referred to.

The main target symptoms for drug treatment are parkinsonism, visual hallucinations, delusions, and agitation. An important question in the drug management of DLB, or of psychiatric complications in PD, is not *which* drug to use, but whether to use *any* drug. Reassurance can sometimes be sufficient and it is sometimes better to start by withdrawing drugs than introducing new ones. One suggested scheme is to withdraw antiparkinsonian drugs from the psychotic PD patient in the following order: anticholinergic, selegeline, dopamine agonists, levodopa. The need for antihypertensives should also be reviewed since they can exacerbate the fluctuating hypotension caused by autonomic dysfunction in DLB and PDD (Londos *et al.*, 2000).

## Drug management

The first-line management of the cognitive impairment, psychosis, and agitation of DLB and PDD is a cholinesterase inhibitor (ChEI). Such treatment is cost-effective (National Collaborating Centre for Mental Health, 2006), in part because the cost of care of dementia patients with parkinsonism is greater than that of those with AD (Murman *et al.*, 2003; Bostrom *et al.*, 2006), in part because treatments successfully targeting hallucinations will be cost-effective (Herrmann *et al.*, 2006), and in part because patients with DLB or PDD are more likely to respond to a ChEI than those with AD (Van Der Putt *et al.*, 2006).

In the only large randomized trial of a ChEI in DLB, rivastigmine alleviated a *post-hoc* defined cluster of symptoms (visual hallucinations, delusions, anxiety, and apathy) (McKeith *et al.*, 2000b). Of those taking active drug 60% had a 30% reduction in symptom scores, compared to 30% on placebo. Rivastigmine has also been shown to be sufficiently beneficial for cognitive function, activities of daily living function, and behavioural and psychological symptoms in PDD that licenses for rivastigmine for the treatment of PDD were awarded by the US Food and Drug Administration (FDA) and the European Medicines Agency (EMEA) (Emre *et al.*, 2004).

Although patients should be warned of the possible gastrointestinal side-effects such as loss of appetite, nausea, and diarrhoea, clinical experience suggests that these are less likely to occur in those with more severe dementia. There is a small risk of worsening tremor as a result of ChEI treatment (Thomas *et al.*, 2005).

Levodopa-exacerbated hallucinations are less common when ChEIs are co-prescribed. Therefore, one strategy to improve parkinsonism in DLB or in psychotic patients with PD, is to prescribe as high a dose of ChEI as the side-effects (usually nausea) allow, and then introduce levodopa.

Drugs which relieve psychosis and agitation often cause parkinsonism, and vice versa. There is a risk of neuroleptic sensitivity even with atypical neuroleptics, of which there are no placebo controlled trials in DLB. A controlled trial of olanzapine for psychosis in PD was stopped early because of worsening parkinsonism (Goetz et al., 2000). Open label studies, and those in AD, suggest that among the atypical neuroleptics parkinsonism is least likely to occur with clozapine or quetiapine and more likely with risperidone and olanzapine. Olanzapine may be especially likely to exacerbate confusion.

As with AD, depression may be the presenting feature of DLB. It needs to be distinguished from the apathy and bradyphrenia of DLB, which may respond to a ChEI. Clinicians differ on whether they would prescribe a ChEI or a selective serotonin reuptake inhibitor (SSRI) first, but most are agreed that SSRIs are preferable to tricyclic antidepressants because they are less likely to exacerbate the cholinergic deficits, constipation, and postural hypotension of DLB.

## References

Aarsland, D., Andersen, K., Larsen. J.P., Lolk, A., and Kragh-Sorensen, P. (2003). Prevalence and characteristics of dementia in Parkinson disease: an 8-year prospective study. Archives of Neurology, 60, 387–92.

Aarsland, D., Zaccai, J., and Brayne, C. (2005a). A systematic review of prevalence studies of dementia in Parkinson's disease. Movement Disorders, 20, 1255–63.

Aarsland, D., Perry, R., Larsen, J.P. et al. (2005b). Neuroleptic sensitivity in Parkinson's disease and parkinsonian dementias. Journal of Clinical Psychiatry, 66, 633–7.

Ballard, C., Ayre, G., O'Brien, J. et al. (1999). Simple standardised neuropsychological assessments aid in the differential diagnosis of dementia with Lewy bodies from Alzheimer's disease and vascular dementia. Dementia and Geriatric Cognitive Disorders, 10, 104–8.

Ballard, C., O'Brien, J., Barber, B. et al. (2000a). Neurocardiovascular instability, hypotensive episodes, and MRI lesions in neurodegenerative dementia. Annals of New York Academy of Science, 903, 442–5.

Ballard, C., Piggott, M., Johnson, M. et al. (2000b). Delusions associated with elevated muscarinic binding in dementia with Lewy bodies. Annals of Neurology, 48, 868–76.

Ballard, C.G., Perry, R.H., McKeith, I.G., and Perry, E.K. (2005). Neuroleptics are associated with more severe tangle pathology in dementia with Lewy bodies. International Journal of Geriatric Psychiatry, 20, 872–5.

Barber, R., Ballard, C., McKeith, I.G., Gholkar, A., and O'Brien, J.T. (2000). MRI volumetric study of dementia with Lewy bodies. Neurology, 54, 1304–9.

Bennett, D.A., Schneider, J.A., Arvanitakis, Z. et al. (2006). Neuropathology of older persons without cognitive impairment from two community-based studies. Neurology, 66, 1837–44.

Boeve, B.F., Silber, M.H., Ferman, T.J. et al. (1998). REM sleep behavior disorder and degenerative dementia: an association likely reflecting Lewy body disease. Neurology, 51, 363–70.

Bostrom, F., Jonsson, L., Minthon, L., and Londos, E. (2006). Patients with Lewy body dementia use more resources than those with Alzheimer's disease. International Journal of Geriatric Psychiatry, Dec 29 [Epub ahead of print].

Burn, D., Emre, M., McKeith, I. et al. (2006). Effects of rivastigmine in patients with and without visual hallucinations in dementia associated with Parkinson's disease. Movement Disorders, 21, 1899–907.

Colloby, S.J., Pakrasi, S., Firbank, M.J. et al. (2006). In vivo SPECT imaging of muscarinic acetylcholine receptors using (R,R) 123I-QNB in dementia with Lewy bodies and Parkinson's disease dementia. Neuroimage, 33, 423–9.

Emre, M., Aarsland, D., Albanese, A. et al. (2004). Rivastigmine for dementia associated with Parkinson's disease. New England Journal of Medicine, 351, 2509–18.

Fantini, M.L., Postuma, R.B., Montplaisir, J., and Ferini-Strambi, L. (2006). Olfactory deficit in idiopathic rapid eye movements sleep behavior disorder. Brain Research Bulletin, 70, 386–90.

Ferman, T.J., Smith, G.E., Boeve, B.F. et al. (2004). DLB fluctuations: specific features that reliably differentiate from AD and normal aging. Neurology, 62, 181–7.

Goetz, C.G., Blasucci, L.M., Leurgans, S., and Pappert, E.J. (2000). Olanzapine and clozapine: comparative effects on motor function in hallucinating PD patients. Neurology, 55, 789–94.

Hamilton, R.L. (2000). Lewy bodies in Alzheimer's disease: a neuropathological review of 145 cases using alphasynuclein immunohistochemistry. Brain Pathology, 10, 378–84.

Harding, A.J., Broe, G.A., and Halliday, G.M. (2002). Visual hallucinations in Lewy body disease relate to Lewy bodies in the temporal lobe. Brain, 125, 391–403.

Herrmann, N., Lanctot, K.L., Sambrook, R. et al. (2006). The contribution of neuropsychiatric symptoms to the cost of dementia care. International Journal of Geriatric Psychiatry, 21, 972–6.

Hughes, A.J., Daniel, S.E., Blankson, S., and Lees, A.J. (1993). A clinicopathologic study of 100 cases of Parkinson's disease. Archives of Neurology, 50, 140–8.

Iranzo, A., Molinuevo, J.L., Santamaria, J. et al. (2006). Rapid-eye-movement sleep behaviour disorder as an early marker for a neurodegenerative disorder: a descriptive study. Lancet Neurology, 5, 572–7.

Kosaka, K., Oyanagi, S., Matsushita, M., and Hori, A. (1976). Presenile dementia with Alzheimer-, Pick- and Lewy-body changes. Acta Neuropathologica Berlin, 36, 221–33.

Lippa, C.F., Fujiwara, H., Mann, D.M. et al. (1998). Lewy bodies contain altered alpha-synuclein in brains of many familial Alzheimer's disease patients with mutations in presenilin and amyloid precursor protein genes. American Journal of Pathology, 153, 1365–70.

Londos, E., Passant, U., and Gustafson, L. (2000). Blood pressure and drug treatment in clinically diagnosed Lewy body dementia and Alzheimer's disease. Archives of Gerontology and Geriatrics, 30, 35–46.

McKeith, I., Fairbairn, A., Perry, R., Thompson, P., and Perry, E. (1992). Neuroleptic sensitivity in patients with senile dementia of Lewy body type. British Medical Journal, 305, 673–8.

McKeith, I.G., Galasko, D., Kosaka, K. et al. (1996). Consensus guidelines for the clinical and pathological diagnosis of Dementia with Lewy Bodies (DLB): report of the Consortium on DLB International Workshop. Neurology, 47, 1113–24.

McKeith, I.G., Ballard, C.G., Perry, R.H. et al. (2000a). Prospective validation of consensus criteria for the diagnosis of dementia with Lewy bodies. Neurology, 54, 1050–8.

McKeith, I., Del Ser, T., Spano, P. et al. (2000b). Efficacy of rivastigmine in dementia with Lewy bodies: a randomised, double-blind, placebo-controlled international study. Lancet, 356, 2031–6.

McKeith, I., Mintzer, J., Aarsland, D. et al. on behalf of the International Psychogeriatric Association Expert Meeting on DLB (2004). Dementia with Lewy bodies. Lancet Neurology, 3, 9–28.

McKeith, I.G., Dickson, D.W., Lowe, J. et al. (2005). Diagnosis and management of dementia with Lewy bodies: third report of the DLB Consortium. Neurology, 65(12), 1863–72.

McKeith, I., O'Brien, J., Walker, Z. et al. (2007). Sensitivity and specificity of dopamine transporter imaging with 123I-FP-CIT SPECT in dementia with Lewy bodies: a phase III, multicentre study. Lancet Neurology, 6(4), 305–13.

McShane, R., Gedling, K., Reading, M., McDonald, B., Esiri, M.M., and Hope, T. (1995). Prospective study of relations between cortical Lewy bodies, poor eyesight and hallucinations in Alzheimer's disease. Journal of Neurology, Neurosurgery and Psychiatry 59, 185–8.

McShane, R.H., Nagy, Z., Esiri, M.M. et al. (2001). Anosmia in dementia is associated with Lewy bodies rather than Alzheimer's pathology. Journal of Neurology, Neurosurgery and Psychiatry, 70, 739–43.

Marder, K., Tang, M.X., Cote, L., Stern, Y., and Mayeux, R. (1995). The frequency and associated risk factors for dementia in patients with Parkinson's disease. *Archives of Neurology*, **52**, 695–701.

Murman, D.L., Kuo, S.B., Powell, M.C., and Colenda, C.C. (2003). The impact of parkinsonism on costs of care in patients with AD and dementia with Lewy bodies. *Neurology*, **61**, 944–9.

National Collaborating Centre for Mental Health (2006). Dementia: supporting people with dementia and their carers in health and social care. *National Clinical Practice Guideline*, No 42, Appendix 17 (http://www.nice.org.uk/guidance/cg42/guidance/pdf/English).

O'Brien, J.T., Colloby, S., Fenwick, J. *et al.* (2004). Dopamine transporter loss visualized with FP-CIT SPECT in the differential diagnosis of dementia with Lewy bodies. *Archives of Neurology*, **61**(6), 919–25.

Okazaki, H., Lipkin, L.E., and Aronson, S.M. (1961). Diffuse intracytoplasmic ganglionin inclusion (Lewy type). associated with progressive dementia and quadraparesis in flexion. *Journal of Neuropathology and Experimental Neurology*, **20**, 237–44.

Olichney, J.M., Murphy, C., Hofstetter, C.R. *et al.* (2005). Anosmia is very common in the Lewy body variant of Alzheimer's disease. *Journal of Neurology, Neurosurgery and Psychiatry*, **76**, 342–7.

Ostling, S., Palsson, S.P., and Skoog, I. (2006). The incidence of first-onset psychotic symptoms and paranoid ideation in a representative population sample followed from age 70–90 years. Relation to mortality and later development of dementia. *International Journal of Geriatric Psychiatry*, Nov. 20 [Epub ahead of print].

Perry, E.K., Marshall, E., Perry, R.H. *et al.* (1990). Cholinergic and dopaminergic activities in senile dementia of Lewy body type. *Alzheimer's Disease and Associated Disorders*, **4**, 87–95.

Piggott, M.A., Perry, E.K., Marshall, E.F. *et al.* (1998). Nigrostriatal dopaminergic activities in dementia with Lewy bodies in relation to neuroleptic sensitivity: comparisons with Parkinson's disease. *Biological Psychiatry*, **44**, 765–74.

Piggott, M.A., Marshall, E.F., Thomas, N. *et al.* (1999). Striatal dopaminergic markers in dementia with Lewy bodies, Alzheimer's and Parkinson's diseases: rostrocaudal distribution. *Brain*, **122**(8), 1449–68.

Pliskin, N.H., Kiolbasa, T.A., Towle, V.L. *et al.* (1996). Charles Bonnet syndrome: an early marker for dementia? *Journal of American Geriatric Society*, **44**, 1055–61.

Rahkonen, T., Eloniemi-Sulkava, U., Rissanen, S., Vatanen, A., Viramo, P., and Sulkava, R. (2003). Dementia with Lewy bodies according to the consensus criteria in a general population aged 75 years or older. *Journal of Neurology, Neurosurgery and Psychiatry*, **74**, 720–4.

Richards, M., Stern, Y., and Mayeux, R. (1993). Subtle extrapyramidal signs can predict the development of dementia in elderly individuals. *Neurology*, **43**, 2184–8.

Rowan, E., McKeith, I.G., Saxby, B.K. *et al.* (2007). Effects of donepezil on central processing speed and attentional measures in Parkinson's disease with dementia and dementia with Lewy bodies. *Dementia and Geriatric Cognitive Disorders*, **23**, 161–7.

Stern, Y., Marder, K., Tang, M.X., and Mayeux, R. (1993). Antecedent clinical features associated with dementia in Parkinson's disease. *Neurology*, **43**, 1690–2.

Thomas, A.J., Burn, D.J., Rowan, E.N. *et al.* (2005). A comparison of the efficacy of donepezil in Parkinson's disease with dementia and dementia with Lewy bodies. *International Journal of Geriatric Psychiatry*, **20**, 938–44.

Van Der Putt, R., Dineen, C., Janes, D., Series, H., and McShane, R. (2006). Effectiveness of acetylcholinesterase inhibitors: diagnosis and severity as predictors of response in routine practice. *International Journal of Geriatric Psychiatry*, **21**, 755–60.

Walker, M.P., Ayre, G.A., Cummings, J.L. *et al.* (2000a). The Clinician Assessment of Fluctuation and the One Day Fluctuation Assessment Scale. Two methods to assess fluctuating confusion in dementia. *British Journal of Psychiatry*, **177**, 252–6.

Walker, M.P., Ayre, G.A., Perry, E.K. *et al.* (2000b). Quantification and characterisation of fluctuating cognition in dementia with Lewy bodies and Alzheimer's disease. *Dementia and Geriatric Cognitive Disorders*, **11**, 327–35.

Walker, Z., Costa, D.C., Ince, P., McKeith, I.G., and Katona, C.L. (1999). In-vivo demonstration of dopaminergic degeneration in dementia with Lewy bodies. *Lancet*, **354**, 646–7.

Williams, S., Williams, J., Combrinck, M., and McShane, R. (2006). Olfactory testing distinguishes dementia with Lewy bodies (DLB). from Alzheimer's disease in mild dementia. *Alzheimer's & Dementia: the Journal of the Alzheimer's Association*, **2**(3, Suppl.), S267–S268.

Zaccai, J., McCracken, C., and Brayne, C. (2005). A systematic review of prevalence and incidence studies of dementia with Lewy bodies. *Age and Ageing*, **34**, 561–6.

Zaccai, J., Brayne, C., and Ince, P. (2006). Alpha-synucleinopathy in a multicenter population-based elderly cohort – MRC cognitive Function and Ageing Study: Associations with in-life cognitive data. *Alzheimer's & Dementia: the Journal of the Alzheimer's Association*, **2**(3, Suppl.), S561–S562.

# Clinical aspects of dementia: frontotemporal dementia

Florence Pasquier, Vincent Deramecourt, and Florence Lebert

Frontotemporal dementia (FTD) is characterized clinically by progressive changes in social, behavioural, and language function. The highest incidence of FTD is between 50 and 60 years of age, although it sometimes occurs much earlier and late onset FTD has been reported. FTD is the second commonest cause of degenerative dementia in patients aged 65 years or less, after Alzheimer's disease (AD) (Ratnavalli et al., 2002), and it accounts for about 5% of late onset dementia (Pasquier et al., 1999a). Since its initial description, especially by Arnold Pick, it has commonly been considered difficult to distinguish from AD and it remains underdiagnosed and often misdiagnosed as AD (Mendez et al., 1993; Knopman et al., 2005) since it may fulfil the current criteria of probable AD (McKhann et al., 1984; Varma et al., 1999). About 40% of FTD cases are not diagnosed (Rosso et al., 2003b), and those who are are often diagnosed after some delay (Pasquier et al., 2004).

## History of FTD: evolution of concepts and terminology

Arnold Pick described six patients with circumscribed atrophies (Pick, 1892, 1901a,b, 1904, 1906), more than a century ago. Not all of them had what we now call Pick's disease. Two had Alzheimer's disease, one had a stroke, and one had general paresis. Two pathological hallmarks of focal brain atrophies were described by Alois Alzheimer in 1911 (Alzheimer, 1910–1911): achromatic neuronal ballooning (Pick cells) and intraneuronal argentophilic inclusion bodies (Pick bodies) without senile plaques or tangles. Difficulties with translation contributed to the long-lasting confusion between Pick's atrophy (non-specific circumscribed atrophy) and Pick's disease (with specific histological features) (Pasquier and Petit, 1997) and to this day difficulties remain in relating the range of pathological changes in FTD to different patterns of clinical presentation. Lars Gustafson, a psychiatrist in Lund, Sweden observed patients with degenerative dementia whose behaviour differed from that of typical patients with AD and Neary and colleagues from Manchester, UK published similar cases at the same period (Neary et al., 1986). The Lund and Manchester groups both emphasized the frequency of these dementias and the reliability of the clinical distinction from Alzheimer's disease. An international conference on 'frontal lobe degeneration of non-Alzheimer type' was held in Lund in 1992 covering all aspects of the subject and an entire issue of Dementia was dedicated to this update in 1993. In April 1994 the Lund and Manchester groups published a consensus on 'clinical and neuropathological criteria for frontotemporal dementia' (Brun et al., 1994). The core diagnostic features included behavioural disorders of insidious onset and slow progression, affective symptoms, speech disorders, intact abilities to negotiate the environment (spatial orientation and praxis preserved), and investigations (neurological, neuropsychological, EEG, and imaging) suggestive of an impairment of the anterior part of the brain. The clinical diagnostic criteria were validated and showed a substantial inter-rater reliability ($k = 0.75$, as good as the NINCDS–ADRDA for AD) and a good validity (sensitivity 85%, specificity 97%, positive predictive value 96.5%, negative predictive value 95.5) (Lopez et al., 1999). More recently, the accuracy of the ante-mortem diagnosis of FTD (34 out of 433 cases) was found still to be moderately sensitive (85%) but highly specific (99%) (Knopman et al., 2005). An update and extension of the Lund and Manchester criteria was published in 1998 (Neary et al., 1998). According to this revision, FTD is one of three clinical presentations of frontotemporal lobar degeneration (FTLD), together with progressive non-fluent aphasia (PNFA) and semantic dementia (SD, i.e. fluent aphasia and associative agnosia). The generic term FTLD refers to the common neuropathological feature, i.e. the circumscribed progressive degeneration of the frontotemporal lobes.

A working group then recommended that, from a clinical perspective, these cases be referred to collectively as FTD (McKhann et al., 2001) although this group acknowledged that this term includes groups of patients whose pathological conditions and genetic mechanisms are heterogeneous, because, at least at present, the association of these distinct pathological and genetic entities cannot be correlated with distinct clinical symptoms. Thus FTD may refer to all presentations of FTLD or to one of three main variants (the frontal variant, fv-FTD) with the other two variants (SD and PNFA) being designated as temporal variants of FTD, tv-FTD).

# Epidemiology of frontotemporal dementia.

## Prevalence and incidence

Community-based studies of early onset dementia (i.e. less than 65 years of age) in England reported that 13.8% of cases with dementia in London in the 30–64 years age group were FTD (32.3% were AD) (Harvey *et al.*, 1998) and in Cambridge (Ratnavalli *et al.*, 2002) 15.7% had FTD and 25% had AD. Only one study provided indications on the incidence of FTD: in Rochester, Minnesota, it was found to be 2.2 for ages 40 to 49, 3.3 for ages 50 to 59, and 8.9 for ages 60 to 69 (Knopman *et al.*, 2004). For comparison, the corresponding rates for Alzheimer's disease were 0.0, 3.3, and 88.9. There is a drop in the relative frequency of FTD after an onset age of 70 years (Barker *et al.*, 2002).

## Age

FTDs are pre-senile dementias, with a median age of onset between 45 and 60 years. Patients with FTD (mean age, 57.5 years) and SD (59.3 years) had an earlier age at onset than patients with PNFA (63.0 years) in the large US–German cohort (Johnson *et al.*, 2005). In a representative sample of 85-year-olds ($n = 451$) in Sweden, 14 individuals (3%) fulfilled criteria for fv-FTD, more than previously expected in this age group. A moderate to severe frontal atrophy was found on CT scan in all cases (Gislason *et al.*, 2003). Nine of them did not fulfil criteria for dementia.

## Sex

Although there is no overall sex preponderance in FTD (Rosso *et al.*, 2003b), in the US–German cohort there were significantly more men diagnosed as having FTD (63.5%) and SD (66.7%) than PNFA (39%).

## Risk factors

A retrospective case–control study showed that head trauma was associated with an odds ratio of 3.3 (95% confidence interval 1.3–8.1). Thyroid disease was also associated with a 2.5 times increased risk of FTD but this was not significant after adjustment. (Rosso *et al.*, 2003a). This may be related to experimental studies showing that splicing of tau mRNA variants is regulated by thyroid hormone. Abnormalities of thyroid hormone levels are common in FTD (38%) (Rosso *et al.*, 2003a).

## Genetics

This is addressed in detail in Chapter 7 and so will only be summarized here. About 40% of FTD patients have a positive family history of dementia (at least one first-degree relative with dementia before the age of 80 years, or identification of a mutation) of whom half have an autosomal dominant pattern of inheritance (Rosso *et al.*, 2003b). The incidence of FTD is increased ten-fold in the first-degree relatives of FTD patients compared with the incidence of FTD in the population, without clustering of other dementia (Grasbeck *et al.*, 2005).

The first report of genetic linkage in an FTD pedigree was to chromosome 17 (Wilhelmsen *et al.*, 1994). A number of groups have replicated this linkage to chromosome 17q21–22 in other pedigrees and the term 'FTD and parkinsonism linked to chromosome 17' (FTDP-17) was adopted to describe the clinical and pathological spectrum. Mutations in the tau gene (microtubule-associated protein tau, *MAPT*) have been identified in some of these families (34 different mutations so far (Zarranz *et al.*, 2005), but a number

of these families show neither tau mutations nor tau deposition on neuropathological assessment, suggesting that there may be a second gene involved that is located close to the tau gene. A tau mutation is found in 5.9–17.6% of FTD populations, in 25–32% of patients with a positive family history, in only 4% of cases without a family history (Stanford *et al.*, 2004), in more than half of cases in the presence of tau pathology, and in almost all cases in familial FTD with tauopathy. Recently, a mutation in the gene coding for progranulin (*PGRN*), a growth factor involved in multiple physiological and pathological processes including development, wound repair, inflammation, and tumourigenesis has been identified (Baker *et al.*, 2006; Cruts *et al.*, 2006).

Mutations on chromosome 3 (*FTD3*) have also been described (Skibinski *et al.*, 2005) in a large family from Denmark. Tau inclusions were found in neurons and some glial cells in the absence of beta-amyloid deposits (Yancopoulou *et al.*, 2003). The presence of filamentous tau protein suggests a possible link between tau and the mutation on chromosome 3 (Yancopoulou *et al.*, 2003). Hereditary FTD has also been associated with amyotrophic lateral sclerosis in some families, and this form has shown linkage to another genetic locus: chromosome 9q21–q22 (Hosler *et al.*, 2000). Tau pathology seems absent or sparse but ubiquitin inclusions are found.

Genetic counselling is difficult in FTD because of the clinical heterogeneity, misdiagnoses, and loss of family history. In addition, not all the mutations have been reported in families with clear autosomal dominant inheritance.

# Clinical features

FTD based on international clinical criteria (Neary *et al.*, 1998) includes a progressive behavioural disorder with insidious onset, affective symptoms, language disorder, frontal executive dysfunction with preserved spatial orientation, and selective frontotemporal atrophy or hypoperfusion/hypometabolism. The absence of severe amnesia is debatable (Graham *et al.*, 2005), but the absence of visuospatial and perceptual symptoms is reliable (Hodges *et al.*, 2004). The clinical features are summarized in Box 27vi.1. However, behaviour is not always the first complaint expressed either by the patient or the informant in FTD, and language disorders are not always the first complaint of patients with PNFA or SD (Pijnenburg *et al.*, 2004).

## Behavioural (or frontal) variant of FTD (fv-FTD)

The clinical features are so characteristic that the diagnosis may be made on the basis of an interview with a close relative even after the patient's death (Barber *et al.*, 1995). Behavioural and affective changes (change of character and disordered social conduct) are the dominant features initially and throughout the disease course. Contrary to AD, behavioural changes precede or are associated with cognitive decline, and memory impairment is rarely the first symptom reported by the family, who typically consider it of secondary importance compared to the behavioural disorder. The most frequently reported first symptom is a loss of interest, often attributed to depression, although families usually recognize that patients do not show sadness or feelings of worthlessness or guilt (Pasquier *et al.*, 1999b). Other frequent symptoms are disinhibition, anxiety, language disorders (including unaccustomed use of coarse words), changes in eating and drinking habits, and behavioural dyscontrol (restlessness, rituals, etc.). Socially disruptive behaviours may lead to arrest and even prosecution (Miller *et al.*, 1997).

**Box 27vi.1** Clinical diagnostic criteria of frontotemporal lobar degeneration (after Neary *et al.,* 1998)

## List 1: The clinical diagnostic features of FTD: clinical profile

Character change and disordered social conduct are the dominant features initially and throughout the disease course. Instrumental functions of perception, spatial skills, praxis, and memory are intact or relatively well preserved.

### I. Core diagnostic features

Insidious onset and gradual progression
Early decline in social interpersonal conduct
Early impairment in regulation of personal conduct
Early emotional blunting
Early loss of insight

### II. Supportive diagnostic features

1. Behavioural disorder
   Decline in personal hygiene and grooming
   Mental rigidity and inflexibility
   Distractibility and impersistence
   Hyperorality and dietary changes
   Perseverative and stereotyped behaviour
   Utilization behaviour
2. Language and speech
   Altered speech output: aspontaneity and economy of speech; pressure of speech
   Stereotypy of speech
   Echolalia
   Perseverations
   Mutism
3. Physical signs
   Primitive reflexes
   Incontinence
   Akinesia, rigidity and tremor
   Low and labile blood pressure
   Bulbar palsy, muscular weakness and wasting, and fasciculations are features associated motor neuron disease present in some patients
4. Investigation
   Neuropsychology: significant impairment on frontal lobe tests in the absence of severe amnesia, aphasia, or perceptuospatial disorders.
   EEG: normal, despite clinically evident dementia
   Brain imaging (structural and/or functional): predominant frontal and/or anterior temporal abnormality

## List 2: The clinical diagnostic features of progressive non-fluent aphasia: clinical profile

Disorder of expressive language is the dominant feature initially and throughout the disease course. Other aspects of cognition are intact or relatively well preserved.

### I. Core diagnostic features

Insidious onset and gradual progression
Non-fluent spontaneous speech with at least one of the following: agrammatism, phonemic paraphasias, anomia

### II. Supporting diagnostic features

1. Speech and language
   Stuttering or oral apraxia
   Impaired repetition
   Alexia, agraphia
   Early preservation of word meaning
   Late mutism
2. Behaviour
   Early preservation of social skills
   Late behavioural changes similar to FTD
3. Physical signs: late contralateral primitive reflexes, akinesia, rigidity and tremor
4. Investigations
   Neuropsychology: non-fluent aphasia in the absence of severe amnesia or perceptuospatial disorder
   EEG: normal or minor asymmetric slowing
   Imaging (structural and/or functional): asymmetric abnormality predominantly affecting dominant (usually left) hemisphere

## List 3: The clinical diagnostic features of semantic aphasia and associative agnosia: clinical profile

Semantic disorder (impaired understanding of word meaning and/or object identity) is the dominant feature initially and throughout the disease course. Other aspects of cognition, including autobiographic memory, are intact or relatively well preserved.

### I. Core diagnostic features

1. Insidious onset and gradual progression
2. Language disorder characterized by:
   Progressive, fluent, empty spontaneous speech
   Loss of word meaning, manifest by impaired naming and comprehension
   Semantic paraphasia and/or
3. Perceptual disorder characterized by:
   Prosopagnosia
   Agnosia associative
4. Preserved perceptual matching and drawing reproduction
5. Preserved single-word repetition
6. Preserved ability to read aloud and write to dictation orthographically regular words

### II. Supportive diagnostic features

1. Speech and language
   Pressure of speech
   Idiosyncratic word usage
   Absence of phonemic paraphasias
   Surface dyslexia and dysgraphia
   Preserved calculation
2. Behaviour
   Loss of sympathy and empathy
   Narrowed preoccupations
   Parsimony
3. Physical signs: absent or late primitive reflexes
4. Investigations
   Neuropsychology: profound semantic loss, manifest in failure of word comprehension and naming and/or face and object recognition. Preserved phonology and syntax, and elementary perceptual processing, spatial skills, and day-to-day memorizing
   EEG: normal

> **Box 27vi.1** (*cont.*)
>
> Imaging (structural and/or functional): predominant anterior temporal abnormality (symmetric or not)
>
> ## List 4: Features common to clinical syndromes of FTLD (extension of lists 1 to 3)
>
> ### III. Supportive features
>
> Onset before 65 years: positive family history of similar disorder in first-degree relative. Bulbar palsy, muscular weakness and wasting, fasciculations (associated motor neuron disease present in a minority of patients)
>
> ### IV. Diagnostic exclusion features
>
> 1. Historical and clinical. Abrupt onset with ictal event, head trauma related to onset, early and severe amnesia, spatial disorientation, logoclonic festinant speech with loss of train of thought, myoclonus, corticospinal weakness, cerebellar ataxia, choreoathetosis
> 2. Investigations. Brain imaging: predominant post-central structural or functional deficit, multifocal lesions on CT or MRI. Laboratory tests indicating brain involvement of metabolic or inflammatory disorder such as MS, syphilis, AIDS and Herpes simplex encephalitis
>
> ### V. Relative diagnostic exclusion features
>
> Typical history of chronic alcoholism, sustained hypertension, history of vascular disease (e.g. angina, claudication)

Sociopathic acts include unsolicited sexual acts, traffic violations, physical assaults, and other unacceptable behaviours. About 10% of patients with FTD exhibit a dramatic change in their self as defined by changes in political, social, religious (Miller *et al.*, 2001), or musical (Geroldi *et al.*, 2000) values, usually correlated with a selective non-dominant frontal dysfunction. Right-sided FTD is associated with socially undesirable behaviour (criminal behaviour, aggression, loss of job, alienation from family/friends, financial recklessness, sexually deviant behaviour, and abnormal response to spousal crisis) (Mychnack *et al.*, 2001).

### Behaviour

A behavioural frontotemporal dysfunction assessment scale validated on patients at the mild stage [Mini-Mental State Examination (MMSE) > 18] helps to distinguish between FTD, AD, and vascular dementia (VaD) (Lebert *et al.*, 1998). The items of the structured interview are classified into four classes: self-monitoring dyscontrol, self-neglect, self-centred behaviour, and affective behaviour (Box 27vi.2). A score of 1 is given for the class if at least one symptom is present and it reflects a substantive change from the patient's pre-morbid state and not a long-standing character trait. A total score of 3 or more gives a sensitivity of 100%, a specificity of 93%, and a diagnostic accuracy of FTD of 97% (Lebert *et al.*, 1998). The assessment of neuropsychiatric symptoms with other standardized scales or inventories can also be useful to distinguish dementia patients with FTD and AD (Levy *et al.*, 1996; Kertesz *et al.*, 1997, 2000; Swartz *et al.*, 1997b; Mendez *et al.*, 1998; Hirono *et al.*, 1999; Bozeat *et al.*, 2000a).

FTD patients frequently have an increase in appetite, with a loss of social graces, and they may eat quickly. They have a frequent altered food preference for sweet foods, and significant weight gain occurs in more than 30% of FTD patients. Stereotypical behaviours are more complex in FTD than in AD (Nyatsanza *et al.*, 2003) and some of them are more common in FTD than in AD: counting/clock watching; consistently choosing the same leisure activity or hobby; repetitively eating the same food; and rigid adherence to routine (Nyatsanza *et al.*, 2003). Delusions are reported but hallucinations are rare. Although patients typically do not complain about sleep disturbance they are frequently observed lying quietly awake at night and have hypersomnia during the day.

> **Box 27vi.2** Frontotemporal Behavioral Scale (BFS) (Lebert *et al.*, 1998)
>
> ### I. Self-monitoring dyscontrol
>
> Changes of food taste (e.g. has developed new preference for sweets)
> Hyperorality (eats excessively, puts inedible things in mouth)
> Alcohol abuse (new appetite for alcohol)
> Verbal disinhibition (makes remarks without social awareness, loss of social tact)
> Behavioural disinhibition (behaves without social awareness, without tact)
> Irritability (becomes easily irritable without reason)
> Inappropriate emotional reacting (laughs or cries without any change of affective context or mood changes)
> Restlessness (becomes physically overactive at any time, unable to stay in the same place for a long time)
>
> ### II. Self-neglect (decline in personal hygiene and grooming)
>
> Not washing, dirtiness, neglect of personal hygiene
> Neglect of clothing, lack of harmonization of clothing
> Lack of hair care
>
> ### III. Self-centred behaviour
>
> Apathetic (lacks initiative, needs to be stimulated to initiate things, tendency to sleep unless stimulated)
> Perseverative, stereotyped behaviour (ritualistic preoccupations, becomes anxious about money, food, tobacco, times of meals, etc.)
> Perseverative thoughts, inflexibility
> Hypochondriasis (somatic complaints)
> Social neglect (lack interest in social activities)
> Selfishness, self-centredness, lack of empathy or concern for others, and loss of feelings of embarrassment
>
> ### IV. Affective disorders
>
> Elation (elated at any time)
> Apparent sadness (at any time, the face is unexpressive)
> Flat affect (affective indifference, especially for family members)
> Emotionalism (heightened tendency to cry more frequently, more easily, or more vigorously because of precipitating circumstances: thoughts [about family, illness, sad events]; expression of sympathy, arrival or departure of visitors, presence of strangers, inability to perform a task, watching television [scenes of tragedy, war, etc.]; listening to music)

At interview, FTD patients with sociopathic acts are aware of their behaviour and know that it is wrong, but cannot prevent themselves from acting impulsively (Mendez *et al.*, 2005b). They claim subsequent remorse, but they do not act on it or show concern for the consequences.

Loss of insight is a core diagnostic criterion for FTD. FTD patients may recognize behavioural change or cognitive deficits (such as memory difficulties), but do not see any problem with these changes, although they may have lost their job, have financial difficulties, or be separated from their spouse and children. It differs from the unawareness of disease (anosagnosia) observed in AD. In a study comparing questionnaires completed by patients and first-degree relative informants on the current personality of the patients, patients with FTD exaggerated positive qualities, and minimized negative qualities. Informants completed a second questionnaire retrospectively, describing subjects' personalities before disease onset. The self-reports of patients with FTD most closely matched their pre-morbid personalities suggesting a failure to update their self-image after disease onset (Rankin *et al.*, 2005b).

## Cognition

At early stages, brief global ratings, such as the MMSE, are normal but more detailed cognitive batteries, such as the Dementia Rating Scale (Mattis, 1976), are more sensitive to early disease. Before becoming too apathetic, patients are usually compliant during such testing, although they manifest an 'economy of effort' and tend to provide 'don't know'-type responses. Responses can be rapid and impulsive or very delayed, and sometimes logorrhoea may be difficult to control. The striking feature, when formally testing patients, is the dissociation between severe alteration in personality and behaviour and breakdown in social competence, and the relative preservation of cognitive skills. Most studies comparing FTD patients with AD patients have matched for overall dementia severity with the MMSE, and found significantly worse performance among AD patients on verbal anterograde memory tests, non-language measures such as visual construction, non-verbal memory, and calculation. A comparison of the pattern of cognitive deficits in autopsy-confirmed FTD and AD patients showed that patients with FTD performed significantly worse than patients with AD on letter and category fluency tests (sensitive to frontal lobe dysfunction), but significantly better on the Mattis Dementia Rating Scale memory subscale, block design test, and clock drawing test (sensitive to medial temporal and parietal association cortices) (Rascovsky *et al.*, 2002).

Most FTLD patients are not obviously amnesic. They are able to provide autobiographical information and behave as if they had 'absent-mindedness' and 'faulty attention' rather than primary amnesia. They do not forget personally relevant events such as mealtimes. However, they are impaired on formal testing. The pattern of cognitive decline differs from that of AD: memory performance benefits from cues and from the provision of multiple-choice alternative responses; FTD patients have better encoding, and demonstrate a slower forgetting rate than AD patients. This suggests a deficit of retrieval strategies more than a storage problem (Pasquier *et al.*, 2001). However, severe memory impairment does occur in FTD: about 10% of patients with FTD from the brain banks of Cambridge (UK) and Sydney, showed this pattern (Graham *et al.*, 2005), with no noticeable behavioural change initially in half

the subjects. All of them developed behavioural features and the initial diagnosis of AD was revised to FTD in half of them.

A defective performance on the classical 'frontal lobe' (executive) tasks, such as tests of abstraction, planning, mental flexibility (Stroop test, trail making test), sorting tests (Wisconsin Card Sorting test), logical arrangement of images, or verbal fluency, is not specific for FTD. Moreover, these tests may be performed in the normal range in the early stage of the disease. AD and FTD patients both show executive dysfunction and confabulation, but FTD patients confabulate more than AD patients on memories of personal past episodes and personal plans (Nedjam *et al.*, 2004).

Patients with fv-FTD have difficulties in recognizing facial emotions, including anger, sadness, and disgust, fear and contempt—a deficit that may contribute to their impaired social skills (Lavenu *et al.*, 1999; Lavenu and Pasquier, 2005). Impairment is most pronounced in the recognition of negative emotions (Rosen *et al.*, 2002; Fernandez-Duque and Black, 2005). Besides facial recognition, deficits in the recognition of emotion involve other modalities such as vocal emotion (Keane *et al.*, 2002). Using the Interpersonal Reactivity Index—a measure of cognitive and emotional empathy—completed by first-degree relatives of patients, levels of empathy are lower in FTD than in AD and normal controls (Rankin *et al.*, 2005a), with a disruption of cognitive empathy but not of the emotional component of empathy.

FTD patients have an impaired theory of mind (Gregory *et al.*, 2002): they have impaired ability to interpret social situation and ascribe mental states to others, which is interpreted as one component of widespread executive deficits (Snowden *et al.*, 2003).

Language tends to be grammatically correct without paraphasias. However, there is often economy of output. Hypophonia and marked loss of prosody may be evident. Perseveration, echolalia, and stereotypies occur in the course of the disease and mutism ensues in the final stages.

## Temporal variant of FTD (tv-FTD): semantic dementia (SD)

Semantic dementia presents with progressive loss of vocabulary affecting expressive and receptive language in the context of fluent speech production. The patients show anomia, impairment in single word comprehension, and impoverished semantic knowledge with preservation of phonology, syntax, visuospatial abilities, and day-to-day (episodic) memory (Snowden *et al.*, 1989; Hodges *et al.*, 1992). Aware of their difficulties, patients with SD may, complain of 'loss of words'. Some authors have described a left temporal variant of FTD with mainly language disorders (Seeley *et al.*, 2005), and a right temporal variant of FTD with mainly prosopagnosia changes (Joubert *et al.*, 2004).

## Behaviour

The only behaviours that differ significantly between fv-FTD and tv-FTD on behavioural scales are apathy, greater in fv-FTD, and sleep disorders, which are more frequent in tv-FTD (Liu *et al.*, 2004). Depression is also more frequent in tv-FTD than in fv-FTD (Bozeat *et al.*, 2000a; Liu *et al.*, 2004), a finding that may be explained by the better insight that patients with tv-FTD have into some of their symptoms.

Both fv-FTD and SD groups show significantly lower levels of empathy than either AD patients or normal controls, but patients with SD show disruption of both emotional and cognitive empathy, whereas fv-FTD patients show only disruption of cognitive empathy (Rankin et al., 2005a). Social avoidance occurs more often in fv-FTD and social seeking in SD (Snowden et al., 2001).

Patients with SD characteristically show a narrowing of interests and often become preoccupied with a single activity, which they pursue assiduously. This contrasts with the general loss of interest and purposelessness of behaviour in fv-FTD. Patients with semantic dementia are more likely to establish repetitive behavioural routines and to clockwatch, and they show greater emotional insightfulness, as defined by demonstration of distress, anxiety, or concern when confronted by their difficulties. They manifest unusual preoccupation for money and parsimony.

Lack of emotional response is pervasive in fv-FTD, whereas it is more selective in semantic dementia affecting particularly the capacity to show fear. Semantic loss may explain the lack of awareness of danger in patients with SD: these patients no longer have conceptual knowledge about the potentially adverse properties of objects (e.g. boiling water) or situations (e.g. crossing a busy road). Loss of emotional insight and absence of the feelings of disgust favours fv-FTD, whereas presence of insight and the capability of showing disgust favours SD (Snowden et al., 2001).

### Cognition

Patients with SD ask for the meaning of everyday vocabulary and may display strange reactions and feelings when confronted with common words. Although they have no difficulties in day-to-day (episodic) memory, and are well oriented until late in the course of the disease, they often show deficits in formal neuropsychological testing, especially involving verbal material. Their breakdown in semantic representations underlying language comprehension is shown by a breakdown in naming tests such word–picture matching (single word comprehension), the pyramid and palm tree test, and a category fluency test. Assessment of language shows semantic paraphasias, and surface dyslexia or dysgraphia (difficulties with reading or spelling irregular words).

They have good recognition memory (if perceptually identical) for objects or faces, but they appear to be affected by a peculiar form of autobiographical amnesia, involving older memories more than recent ones (Snowden et al., 1996a; Piolino et al., 2003; Hou et al., 2005). Also in the case of non-autobiographical remote memory they appear to show a 'reverse' temporal gradient, with better retrieval of recent famous names (Hodges and Graham, 1998). This finding has been attributed to the relative sparing of the hippocampal formation, which according to some models is not only responsible for memory acquisition, but also for the storage of recent memories. On the other hand, the severe disruption of temporal neocortex would be responsible for the loss of semantic memory, as well as of remote autobiographical knowledge.

Because of the multimodal semantic memory impairment, patients have impaired identification of sounds (Bozeat et al., 2000b) objects, place and monuments, odours, etc. (associative agnosia). They have normal performances in tests of attention, executive functions (Perry and Hodges, 2000), non-verbal problem-solving (progressive matrices), and perceptual and spatial abilities.

### Progressive non-fluent aphasia (PNFA)

PNFA is the most common variety of primary progressive aphasia (PPA), a syndrome described as a progressive language impairment

without dementia for at least 2 years (Mesulam, 2001). Subsequently, some behavioural changes similar to FTD may develop. In PNFA, the predominant impairment is a profound disturbance of expressive language, accompanied by left perisylvian atrophy and anterior insular hypometabolism leading to mutism, but even those patients who are mute may have relatively well-preserved memory and visuospatial orientation and function surprisingly well in the community in contrast to aphasia in AD, which is usually superimposed on memory and visuospatial loss.

### Behaviour

There is no behaviour change initially. Later, changes similar to those of fv-FTD may occur. However, self-neglect and bland affect are unusual.

### Cognition

They exhibit non-fluent spontaneous speech which is laborious and characterized by agrammatism, phonemic paraphasias, and a lack of words. Confrontation naming may be better than expected when listening to the spontaneous speech. Repetition is impaired. Numerous phonemic paraphasias occur in oral and written language, even if written production is less impaired than oral output. Reading aloud is affected but comprehension (in all modalities) is preserved for a long time.

It is difficult to demonstrate the integrity of non-language domains in primary progressive aphasia because most neuropsychological tests of memory, reasoning, and attention require language competence for their performance. One study tested reasoning and cognitive flexibility non-verbally in patients with PPA using a modified version of the visual verbal test. Patients with PPA and normal controls performed similarly, detecting commonalities among objects and shifting from one sorting principle to another. In contrast, both AD and FTD patients were significantly impaired on both measures (Wicklund et al., 2004).

Memory of day-to-day events is retained well and patients cope well with the skills of everyday life. Patients have good performance on semantic memory tests, except when verbal memory output is required. Category fluency is less affected than letter fluency.

## Physical examination

Physical signs are generally limited to the presence of primitive reflexes. FTD can be associated with clinical manifestation of an extrapyramidal disorder or motor neuron disease (MND). Limb rigidity is reported in fv-FTD but not in semantic dementia (Snowden et al., 2001).

## Investigations

### Imaging in FTD

Standard neuropsychological tests and conventional brain imaging techniques [MRI and single photon emission computed tomography (SPECT)] may not be sensitive to the early changes in FTD (Pasquier et al., 1997; Gregory et al., 1999). Over time, however, abnormalities in the anterior part of the brain develop in all patients and examples are given in Chapter 13.

### Structural imaging

Structural imaging commonly shows atrophy of the frontal lobes and the anterior part of the temporal lobes. Predominant temporal atrophy on neuroimaging was reported in 40% of cases and was asymmetric in 72%, but in patients with frontotemporal atrophy asymmetry was seen in only 25% (Rosso *et al.*, 2003b). Atrophy of the hippocampus in FTD is less severe than in AD, but atrophy of the entorhinal cortex is equally severe (Frisoni *et al.*, 1999). Although atrophy of the corpus callosum is not specific to any degenerative dementia, the pattern of atrophy is different among patients with FTD (anterior quarter), PSP (middle-anterior quarter), and AD (posterior quarter) (Yamauchi *et al.*, 2000).

Increasing severity of atrophy occurs with increasing disease duration, but severity of atrophy is not related to pathological subtype (Kril *et al.*, 2005). Frontal, limbic, and temporal regions are affected early in the disease and temporal lobe atrophy is the best predictor of disease duration.

### Functional imaging

Positron emission tomography (PET) shows decreased resting glucose metabolism levels in frontal and temporal cortices in FTD, contrasting with a decrease in parietal, posterior cingulate, and temporal regions in AD, and in frontal area only in FTD-MND (Jeong *et al.*, 2005). SPECT supports the diagnosis of FTD when it shows an uptake decrease in frontal and temporal regions only, although it is not specific.

Functional imaging indicates an apathetic syndrome associated with a prevalent dorsolateral and frontal medial hypometabolism, whereas the disinhibited syndrome demonstrates a selective hypometabolism in interconnected limbic structures (the cingulate cortex, hippocampus/amygdala, and accumbens nucleus) (Franceschi *et al.*, 2005).

### CSF biomarkers

Although a low level of tau in the CSF is never seen in AD and is observed in a third of neuropathologically confirmed FTD (Grossman *et al.*, 2005), CSF biomarkers are not yet reliable diagnostic markers for FTD, since tau levels vary widely. This is probably because of the large spectrum of histopathologies contributing to the disease. Phospho tau has been shown to differentiate AD from non-AD groups of dementia, especially from FTD (Hampel and Teipel, 2004), but not consistently (Verbeek *et al.*, 2005). Tau phosphorylated at threonine 231 (p-tau231) may show excellent differentiation between AD and FTD, whereas serine 181 (p-tau181) enhances accurate differentiation between AD and dementia with Lewy bodies (Hampel and Teipel, 2004).

### Electroencephalography

EEG was thought to be normal in FTD and thus a normal EEG in dementia was considered as a marker for FTD (Brun *et al.*, 1994). However, even though seizures are rare in FTD, compared to AD, some mutations on chromosome 17 are associated with early seizures (Sperfeld *et al.*, 1999), and a quantitative EEG study found differences between AD and FTD (Lindau *et al.*, 2003).

## Differential diagnosis

In most cases, it is easy to distinguish between AD and FTD (Pasquier, 2005). Information from close relatives can distinguish between the two diseases (Barber *et al.*, 1995): FTD presents with progressive changes in social conduct in the context of good cognitive skills, preserved spatial orientation, or progressive language disorders;

AD usually starts with anterograde episodic memory deficits, or, more rarely, with visual or visuospatial disorders in the context of preserved social skills. FTD occurs in the pre-senium (usually before the age of 65 years), whereas most cases of AD begin after the age of 65 years. The presence of impaired orientation and apraxia increases the likelihood of a patient having AD, while the presence of problem-solving difficulty increases the likelihood of a patient having FTD. Imaging shows only anterior cerebral abnormalities in FTD more or less spreading posteriorly. Changes located in the posterior part of the brain with no continuity with anterior changes exclude the diagnosis of FTD, but predominant changes in the anterior part of the brain can be observed in confirmed AD.

Perhaps the most difficult differential diagnosis of FTD is VaD, mainly the subcortical ischaemic subtype, because both have apathy and irritability as key features. In VaD, disinhibition and physical neglect are frequent symptoms (just like in FTD), whereas emotionalism is much more common in VaD. In FTD lack of concern or bland affect are more frequent than emotionalism. MRI is a crucial tool for the differential diagnosis, looking for evidence of cerebrovascular disease and an important issue in the management of patients is the control of vascular risk factors in VaD.

Patients with dementia with Lewy bodies may present early executive and language dysfunction or behavioural or affective states that suggest FTD (Bonner *et al.*, 2003). But cognitive fluctuations, hallucinations, and REM sleep disorders are not symptoms of FTD, although hallucinations have been described in families with FTD with the recently described progranulin mutation.

Other neurodegenerative diseases may also present with symptoms suggestive of FTD. However, subcortical dementias, e.g. due to Huntington's disease, usually have other characteristic features (see Chapter 27vii). Progressive supranuclear palsy (PSP) may present with frontal lobe symptoms before the parkinsonian features appear and the supranuclear palsy occurs. Similarly, overlap exists between FTD and MND, both clinically and pathologically. A significant minority of patients with FTD develop MND (Bak and Hodges, 1999).

It is also important to note that many symptoms in FTD may suggest the presence of a mental illness other than dementia, but criteria for full psychiatric syndromes are rarely met. Apathy, loss of interest, and change in eating behaviour may be interpreted as depression but FTD patients do not experience sadness or guilt, do not show pessimism and suicidal thinking, and in fact show a surprising lack of concern about themselves. FTD patients may have stereotypical movements with compulsive behaviours suggestive of obsessive–compulsive disorders. However, patients have no distressing feelings of internal or psychic tension, anxiety, or depression (Mendez *et al.*, 2005a). Disinhibition, and hyperactivity may be suggestive of a manic episode, but again other characteristic symptoms of mania, e.g. grandiose thinking and elated mood, tend not to occur.

## Natural history

### Progression of behaviour

Behavioural changes progress whatever the presentation (Marczinski *et al.*, 2004). Some changes, such as restlessness or eating disorders and hyperorality, are long-lasting. Verbal disinhibition decreases together with a reduction of speech, evolving toward mutism. All patients become increasingly apathetic.

## Progression of cognitive changes

At first, FTD typically manifests with behavioural changes and relatively stable global cognition. Cognitive decline occurs later, with the mean MMSE decreasing by 2.3 points in 2 years in one study (Pasquier et al., 1999b). However, important individual variations occurred and 21 patients (30%) could not perform the MMSE after this period. After a 5-year follow-up the mean annual decline of the MMSE score was found to be 0.9 ± 1.4 in FTD patients with a mean MMSE score at first visit of 24.5 ±11.5 (Pasquier et al., 2004). Other studies have reported a larger annual decline in MMSE score, probably because the drop in responses below a score of 18 was not taken into account (Roberson et al., 2005).

## Progression of physical signs

Weight gain occurs initially but weight loss occurs when apathy prevents overeating. Difficulty with swallowing is frequent and may be alarming because of the inappropriate hyperorality. Extrapyramidal features, mainly rigidity, are almost constant, and hemiparesis is relatively frequent in asymmetrical cases. A minority of patients develop MND. Low blood pressure, cold extremities, hypotension, and other dysautonomic disorders occur. Seizures are infrequent. Patients with FTD often die suddenly, even before the terminal stage of the disease, and the cause of this is often not identified. This may be related to dysautonomia, and choking was the direct cause of premature death in more than 13% of patients (Pasquier et al., 2004).

## Survival

Although FTD is often thought to have a shorter course than AD it is not clear this is the case because there is a longer delay before first symptoms and diagnosis in FTD than in AD (Pasquier et al., 2004).

In one study the mean duration of FTD was estimated at 8 years (2–20 years) (Snowden et al., 1996b) and in a series of 552 consecutive patients followed up for 5.5 years, the mean duration of the disease was 2 years longer in fv-FTD (n = 73) than in AD (n = 479) patients, probably because at entry mean age was 10 years younger, and mean MMSE score was 5 points higher in FTD than in AD. But when adjusted for age, sex, and level of education, survival rate did not differ significantly (Pasquier et al., 2004).

## Neuropathology

Unlike other dementia syndromes, notably Alzheimer's disease, FTD encompasses considerable pathological heterogeneity. This is dealt with in detail in Chapter 5 and is summarized in Fig. 27vi.1. There are two main types of pathology.

A first type is characterized by *tau deposition* in neurons or glial cells, or both; it comprises several subvariants: those with classic argyrophilic, tau-positive intraneuronal Pick bodies (Pick's disease); those with tau gene mutations (FTDP-17), and diffuse tau-positive neuronal and astrocytic immunoreactivity; those characterized by tau-positive astrocytic plaques and ballooned achromatic neurons (corticobasal degeneration); those with tufted astrocytes and tangles (PSP), and those with tau-positive argyrophilic grain disease. Patients with tau-positive pathology tend to be older than those without tau pathology (Hodges et al., 2004).

A second type (FTLD-U) is characterized by the presence of cytoplasmic *ubiquitin-only-positive, tau- and alpha-synuclein-negative* neuronal cytoplasmic inclusions and dystrophic neurites in frontal and temporal cortices, and hippocampus. When similar pathological changes are accompanied by histological features of MND, the term FTLD-MND is used. The latter pathological changes may be found in patients with or without clinical evidence of MND.

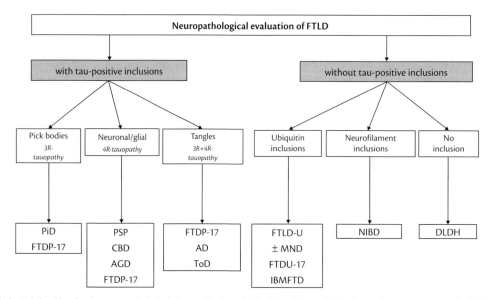

**Fig. 27vi.1** Neuropathological algorithm for the neuropathological characterization of FTD. Abbreviations: 3R/4R, three or four repeat tauopathy; PiD, Pick disease; FTDP-17, frontotemporal dementia with parkinsonism linked to chromosome 17 (tau mutation); PSP, progressive supranuclear palsy; CBD, corticobasal degeneration; AGD, argyrophylic grain disease; AD, Alzheimer's disease; ToD, tangle-only dementia; FTLD-U, frontotemporal lobar degeneration with ubiquitin inclusions; MND, motor neuron disease; FTDU-17, familial frontotemporal dementia with ubiquitin inclusion linked to chromosome 17 (progranulin mutation); IBMFTD, familial inclusion body myopathy with Paget disease and frontotemporal dementia (valosin containing protein mutation); NIBD, neurofilament intermediate body disease; DLDH, dementia lacking distinctive histology

# Neurochemistry

The neurochemical pathology of FTD is discussed in Chapter 6 but the main neurobiological change reported in FTD is a serotonergic deficit and this appears to be more post-synaptic than pre-synaptic (Sparks and Markesbery, 1991; Procter *et al.*, 1999; Franceschi *et al.*, 2005). Low brain levels of serotonin are associated with symptoms of anxiety, depression, quarrelsome behaviours, and impulsive aggression (aan het Rot *et al.*, 2006; Wrase *et al.*, 2006).

There is clinical evidence of basal ganglia dopamine dysfunction in some FTD (extrapyramidal symptoms), and a PET study has shown decreased pre-synaptic dopamine transporter in the putamen and caudate of FTD patients.

In contrast to AD the cholinergic system is spared: intact acetylcholine levels, cortical choline acetyltransferase, and post-synaptic muscarinic receptor binding, and preservation of neurons in the nucleus basalis of Meynert (Huey *et al.*, 2006).

# Treatments

The paucity of pharmacologic trials for FTD is probably due to a combination of the illness only recently being clinically defined and the failure to recognize FTD patients. Currently the treatments used for FTD are based on medications used to treat the behavioural symptoms in other conditions. This strategy has limitations, since different physiological processes may underlie similar clinical symptoms.

## Serotonergic treatments

Serotonergic treatments have been most studied, but only two double-blind randomized controlled trials are available. The first, a cross-over, study of 10 patients, reported that treatment with 40 mg of paroxetine for 6 weeks did not improve behavioural symptoms and was associated with a worsening of some memory tasks, compared to placebo (Deakin *et al.*, 2004). The worsened cognition may reflect the anticholinergic effects of higher-dose paroxetine (Huey *et al.*, 2006). Most open-label studies of selective serotonin reuptake inhibitors (SSRIs), however, have shown an improvement of behaviour (Swartz *et al.*, 1997a; Lebert and Pasquier, 1999; Chow, 2003; Ikeda *et al.*, 2004). SSRIs have also been used in open trials with benefit on stereotyped behaviours with fluvoxamine (Ikeda *et al.*, 2004) and stereotypical movements with sertraline (Mendez *et al.*, 2005a).

The second randomized study was of 300 mg/day of trazodone, also in a 6-week cross-over trial, in 26 patients [mean MMSE score 20.8 + 8.3, mean Neuropsychiatric Inventory (NPI) score 53 + 17.9 at baseline] (Lebert *et al.*, 2004; Lebert, 2006). Trazodone is an atypical serotonergic agent with moderate serotonin reuptake inhibition and a serotonergic (5-HT1A, 5-HT1C, and 5-HT2) antagonist effect with an active metabolite [*meta*-chlorophenyl-piperazine (*m*-CPP)] which is a direct serotonin receptor agonist. It is also an adrenergic alpha-1 (post-synaptic), alpha-2 (pre-synaptic), and H1 histamine blocker. There was a large and significant decrease of the NPI score with trazodone (mean 18.22 versus 1.1 points with placebo). A decrease of more than 50% in the NPI score was observed in 10 patients on trazodone. The improvement was mainly based on the improvement in four items of the NPI scale—eating disorders, agitation, irritability, and depression/dysphoria. There was no change on the MMSE score and trazodone

was well tolerated. The placebo-controlled trial was followed by an open label extension study for more than 2 years (116 weeks) of 300 mg/day trazodone (Lebert, 2006). The mean NPI score between baseline and final assessment decreased by 20.5 + 9.5 points and no patient had an increase in final NPI score. This indicates that trazodone may be effective in reducing behavioural symptoms in FTD in the long term, and the magnitude of efficacy from trazodone may be higher than that from other serotonergic agents. Delusions, aggression, anxiety, and irritability decreased significantly with 150 mg/day of trazodone; 300 mg were necessary to decrease depression, disinhibition, and aberrant motor behaviour (Lebert and Pasquier, 1999).

Since trazodone differs from other serotonergic agents in two aspects—the 5-HT2a antagonist effect and an agonist effect related to its metabolite *m*-CPP—and the 5-HT2a receptors are mainly present in frontal regions and decreased in FTD, drugs with 5-HT2a receptor actions have a good rationale for pharmacological research in FTD (Lebert, 2006). A meta-analysis of antidepressant medication in FTD patients has been performed (Huey *et al.*, 2006) and, consistent with these data, concluded that serotonergic treatments improve the behavioural but not the cognitive symptoms in FTD.

## Other treatments

A within-subjects, double-blind, placebo-controlled procedure investigated the effects of a single dose of methylphenidate (40 mg) and showed that it 'normalized' the decision-making behaviour of patients such as they became less risk taking on medication, although there were no significant effects on other aspects of cognitive function. Moreover, there was no normal subjective and autonomic response to methylphenidate seen in elderly subjects (Rahman *et al.*, 2006). A case report showed a significant behavioural improvement, whereas at the same time slowing on quantitative EEG was partially normalized (Goforth *et al.*, 2004).

Selegiline (Moretti *et al.*, 2002) and moclobemide (Adler *et al.*, 2003) improved affect, behaviour, and speech in open label trials in a small number of subjects, but patients with FTD treated with cholinesterase inhibitors showed an increase in aggressiveness and agitation (Moretti *et al.*, 2003) and hypersensitivity of FTD patients to neuroleptics has been reported (Pijnenburg *et al.*, 2003).

The α-2 adrenoreceptor antagonist idazoxan was found to produce dose-dependent improvements in performance, particularly on neuropsychological tests sensitive to frontal lobe dysfunction (Coull *et al.*, 1996) and piracetam was associated in some FTD patients with a worsening of behaviour including hyperphagia and carbohydrate craving, irritability, impulsiveness, and disinhibition (Moretti *et al.*, 2003).

An observational study on a limited number of women, found a positive association between oestrogen replacement therapy (ERT) and FTD: 70% of women diagnosed with FTD were treated with ERT at the time of their evaluation versus 20% of women with AD and 24% in the general population (Levine and Hewett, 2003).

## Non-pharmacological treatment

Language disorders need intervention from speech therapists, and they may also be able to help with difficulties in swallowing. Information to caregivers on support groups, and social support are necessary. Patients should be advised not to drive and efforts made to prevent hyperphagia and excessive alcohol consumption.

# References

aan het Rot, M., Moskowitz, D.M., Pinard, G., and Young, S.N. (2006). Social behaviour and mood in everyday life: the effects of tryptophan in quarrelsome individuals. *Journal of Psychiatry and Neuroscience*, **31**, 253–262.

Adler, G., Teufel, M., and Drach, L.M. (2003). Pharmacological treatment of frontotemporal dementia: treatment response to the MAO-A inhibitor moclobemide. *International Journal of Geriatric Psychiatry*, **18**, 653–655.

Alzheimer, A. (1910–1911). Über eigenartige Krankheitsfälle des späteren Alters. *Zeitschrift für die Gesamte Neurologie und Psychiatrie*, **4**, 356–385.

Bak, T.H. and Hodges, J.R. (1999). Cognition, language and behaviour in motor neurone disease: evidence of frontotemporal dysfunction. *Dementia and Geriatric Cognitive Disorders*, **10**(Suppl. 1), 29–32.

Baker, M., Mackenzie, I.R., Pickering-Brown, S.M. *et al.* (2006). Mutations in progranulin cause tau-negative frontotemporal dementia linked to chromosome 17. *Nature*, **442**, 916–919.

Barber, R., Snowden, J.S., and Craufurd, D. (1995). Frontotemporal dementia and Alzheimer's disease: retrospective differentiation using information from informants. *Journal of Neurology, Neurosurgery and Psychiatry*, **59**, 61–70.

Barker, W.W., Luis, C.A., Kashuba, A. *et al.* (2002). Relative frequencies of Alzheimer disease, Lewy body, vascular and frontotemporal dementia, and hippocampal sclerosis in the state of Florida Brain Bank. *Alzheimer Disease and Associated Disorders*, **16**, 203–212.

Bonner LT, Tsuang DW, Cherrier MM, *et al.* (2003). Familial dementia with Lewy bodies with an atypical clinical presentation. *Journal of Geriatrics Psychiatry and Neurology* 16:59–64.

Bozeat, S., Gregory, C.A., Lambon Ralph, M.A., and Hodges, J.R. (2000a). Which neuropsychiatric and behavioural features distinguish frontal and temporal variants of frontotemporal dementia from Alzheimer's disease. *Journal of Neurology, Neurosurgery and Psychiatry*, **69**, 178–186.

Bozeat, S., Lambon Ralph, M.A., Patterson, K., Garrard, P., and Hodges, J.R. (2000b). Non-verbal semantic impairment in semantic dementia. *Neuropsychologia*, **38**, 1207–1215.

Brun, A., Englund, E., Gustafson, L. *et al.* (1994). Clinical and neuropathological criteria for frontotemporal dementia. *Journal of Neurology, Neurosurgery and Psychiatry*, **57**, 416–418.

Chow, T.W. (2003). Frontotemporal dementias: clinical features and management. *Seminars in Clinical Neuropsychiatry*, **8**, 58–70.

Coull, J.T., Sahakian, B.J., and Hodges, J.R. (1996). The alpha(2) antagonist idazoxan remediates certain attentional and executive dysfunction in patients with dementia of frontal type. *Psychopharmacology (Berlin)*, **123**, 239–249.

Cruts, M., Gijselinck, I., van der Zee, J. *et al.* (2006). Null mutations in progranulin cause ubiquitin-positive frontotemproal dementia linked to chromosome 17q21. *Nature*, **442**, 920–924.

Deakin, J.B., Rahman, S., Nestor, P.J., Hodges, J.R., and Sahakian, B.J. (2004). Paroxetine does not improve symptoms and impairs cognition in frontotemporal dementia: a double-blind randomized controlled trial. *Psychopharmacology (Berlin)*, **172**, 400–408.

Fernandez-Duque, D. and Black, S.E. (2005). Impaired recognition of negative facial emotions in patients with frontotemporal dementia. *Neuropsychologia*, **43**, 1673–1687.

Franceschi, M., Anchisi, D., Peltai, O. *et al.* (2005). Glucose metabolism and serotonin receptors in the frontotemporal lobe degeneration. *Annals of Neurology*, **57**, 216–225.

Frisoni, G.B., Laasko, M., Beltramello, A. *et al.* (1999). Hippocampal and entorhinal cortex atrophy in frontotemporal dementia and Alzheimer's disease. *Neurology*, **52**, 91–100.

Geroldi, C., Metitieri, T., Binetti, G., Zanetti, O., Trabucchi, M., and Frisoni, G.B. (2000). Pop music and frontotemporal dementia. *Neurology*, **55**, 1935–1936.

Gislason, T.B., Sjogren, M., Larsson, L., and Skoog, I. (2003). The prevalence of frontal variant frontotemporal dementia and the frontal lobe syndrome in a population based sample of 85 year olds. *Journal of Neurology, Neurosurgery and Psychiatry*, **74**, 867–871.

Goforth, H.W., Konopka, L., Primeau, M. *et al.* (2004). Quantitative electroencephalography in frontotemporal dementia with methylphenidate response: a case study. *Clinical EEG and Neuroscience*, **35**, 108–111.

Graham, A., Davies, R., Xuereb, J. *et al.* (2005). Pathologically proven frontotemporal dementia presenting with severe amnesia. *Brain*, **138**, 597–605.

Grasbeck, A., Horstmann, V., Nilsson, K., Sjobeck, M., Sjostrom, H., and Gustafson, L. (2005). Dementia in first-degree relatives of patients with frontotemporal dementia. A family history study. *Dementia and Geriatric Cognitive Disorders*, **19**, 145–153.

Gregory, C.A., Serra-Mestres, J., and Hodges, J.R. (1999). Early diagnosis of the frontal variant of frontotemporal dementia: how sensitive are standard neuroimaging and neuropsychologic tests? *Neuropsychiatry, Neuropsychology, and Behavioral Neurology*, **12**, 128–135.

Gregory, C., Lough, S., Stone, V. *et al.* (2002). Theory of mind in patients with frontal variant frontotemporal dementia and Alzheimer's disease: theoretical and practical implications. *Brain*, **125**, 752–764.

Grossman, M., Farmer, J., Leight, S. *et al.* (2005). Cerebrospinal fluid profile in frontotemporal dementia and Alzheimer's disease. *Annals of Neurology*, **57**, 721–729.

Hampel, H. and Teipel, S.J. (2004). Total and phosphorylated tau proteins: evaluation as core biomarker candidates in frontotemporal dementia. *Dementia and Geriatric Cognitive Disorders*, **17**, 350–354.

Harvey, R.J., Rossor, M.N., Skelton-Robinson, M., and Garralda, E. (1998). Young onset dementia: epidemiology, clinical symptoms, family burden, support and outcome. Available at http://dementia.ion.ucl.ac.uk

Hirono, N., Mori, E., Tanimukai, S. *et al.* (1999). Distinctive neurobehavioral features among neurodegenerative dementias. *Journal of Neuropsychiatry and Clinical Neurosciences*, **11**, 498–503.

Hodges, J.R. and Graham, K.S. (1998). A reversal of the temporal gradient of for famous person knowledge in semantic dementia: implications for the neural organisation of long-term memory. *Neuropsychologia*, **36**, 803–825.

Hodges, J.R., Patterson, K., and Oxbury, S.E.F. (1992). Semantic dementia: progressive fluent aphasia with temporal lobe atrophy. *Brain*, **115**, 1783–1806.

Hodges, J.R., Davies, R.R., Xuereb, J.H. *et al.* (2004). Clinicopathological correlates in frontotemporal dementia. *Annals of Neurology*, **56**, 399–406.

Hosler, B.A., Siddique, T., Sapp, P.C. *et al.* (2000). Linkage of familial amyotrophic lateral sclerosis with frontotemporal dementia to chromosome 9q21-q22. *Journal of the American Medical Association*, **284**, 1664–1669.

Hou, C.E., Miller, B.L., and Kramer, J.H. (2005). Patterns of autobiographical memory loss in dementia. *International Journal of Geriatric Psychiatry*, **20**, 809–815.

Huey, E.D., Putman, K., and Grafman, J. (2006). A systematic review of neurotransmitter deficits and treatments in frontotemporal dementia. *Neurology*, **66**, 17–22.

Ikeda, M., Shigenobu, K., Fukuhara, R. *et al.* (2004). Efficacy of fluvoxamine as a treatment for behavioral symptoms in frontotemporal lobar degeneration patients. *Dementia and Geriatric Cognitive Disorders*, **17**, 117–121.

Jeong, Y., Park, K.C., Cho, S.S. *et al.* (2005). Pattern of glucose hypometabolism in frontotemporal dementia with motor neuron disease. *Neurology*, **64**, 734–736.

Johnson, J.K., Diehl, J., Mendez, M.F. *et al.* (2005). Frontotemporal lobar degeneration: demographic characteristics of 353 patients. *Archives of Neurology*, **62**, 925–930.

Joubert, S., Felician, O., Barbeau, E. *et al.* (2004). Progressive prosopagnosia. Clinical and neuroimaging results. *Neurology*, **63**, 1962–1965.

Keane, J., Calder, A.J., Hodges, J.R., and Young, A.W. (2002). Face and emotion processing in frontal variant frontotemporal dementia. *Neuropsychologia*, **40**, 655–665.

Kertesz, A., Davidson, W., and Fox, H. (1997). Frontal Behavioral Inventory: diagnostic criteria for frontal lobe dementia. *Canadian Journal of Neurological Sciences*, **24**, 29–36.

Kertesz, A., Nadkarni, N., Davidson, W., and Thomas, A.W. (2000). The Frontal Behavioral Inventory in the differential diagnosis of frontotemporal dementia. *Journal of the International Neuropsychological Society*, **6**, 460–468.

Knopman, D.S., Petersen, R.C., Edland, S.D., Cha, R.H., and Rocca, W.A. (2004). The incidence of frontotemporal lobar degeneration in Rochester, Minnesota, 1990 through 1994. *Neurology*, **62**, 506–508.

Knopman, D.S., Boeve, B.F., Parisi, J.E. et al. (2005). Antemortem diagnosis of frontotemporal lobar degeneration. *Annals of Neurology*, **57**, 480–488.

Kril, J.J., Macdonald, V., Patel, S., Png, F., and Hallyday, G.M. (2005). Distribution of brain atrophy in behavioral variant frontotemporal dementia. *Journal of the Neurological Sciences*, **232**, 83–90.

Lavenu, I. and Pasquier, F. (2005). Perception of emotion on faces in frontotemporal dementia and Alzheimer's disease. A longitudinal study. *Dementia and Geriatric Cognitive Disorders*, **19**, 37–41.

Lavenu, I., Pasquier, F., Lebert, F., Petit, H., and Van der Linden, M. (1999). Perception of emotion in frontotemporal dementia and in Alzheimer's disease. *Alzheimer Disease and Associated Disorders*, **13**, 96–101.

Lebert, F. (2006). Behavioral benefits of trazodone are sustained for the long term in frontotemporal dementia. *Therapy*, **3**, 93–96.

Lebert, F. and Pasquier, F. (1999). Trazodone in the treatment of behaviour in frontotemporal dementia. *Human Psychopharmacology – Clinical and Experimental*, **14**, 279–281.

Lebert, F., Pasquier, F., Souliez, L., and Petit, H. (1998). Frontotemporal behavioral scale. *Alzheimer Disease and Associated Disorders*, **12**, 335–339.

Lebert, F., Stekke, W., Hasenbroekx, C., and Pasquier, F. (2004). Frontotemporal dementia: a randomised, controlled trial with trazodone. *Dementia and Geriatric Cognitive Disorders*, **17**, 355–359.

Levine, A.J. and Hewett, L. (2003). Estrogen replacement therapy and frontotemporal dementia. *Maturitas*, **45**, 83–88.

Levy, M.L., Miller, B.L., Cummings, J.L., Fairbanks, L.A., and Craig, A. (1996). Alzheimer disease and frontotemporal dementias. Behavioral distinctions. *Archives of Neurology*, **53**, 687–690.

Lindau, M., Jelic, V., Johansson, S.-E., Andersen, C., and Wahlund, L.-O. (2003). Quantitative EEG abnormalities and cognitive dysfunctions in frontotemporal dementia and Alzheimer's disease. *Dementia and Geriatric Cognitive Disorders*, **15**, 106–114.

Liu, W., Miller, B.L., Kramer, J.H. et al. (2004). Behavioral disorders in the frontal and temporal variants of frontotemporal dementia. *Neurology*, **62**, 742–748.

Lopez, O.L., Litvan, I., Catt, K.E. et al. (1999). Accuracy of four clinical diagnostic criteria for the diagnosis of neurodegenerative dementias. *Neurology*, **53**, 1292–1299.

McKhann, G., Drachman, D., Folstein, M., Katzman, R., Price, D., and Stadlan, E.M. (1984). Clinical diagnosis of Alzheimer's disease: report of the NINCDS-ADRDA Work Group under the auspices of the Department of Health and Human Services Task Force on Alzheimer's disease. *Neurology*, **34**, 939–944.

McKhann, G.M., Albert, M.S., Grossman, M., Miller, B., Dickson, D., and Trojanowski, J.Q. (2001). Clinical and pathological diagnosis of frontotemporal dementia. Report of the Work Group on Frontotemporal Dementia and Pick's Disease. *Archives of Neurology*, **58**, 1803–1809.

Marczinski, C.A., Davidson, W., and Kertesz, A. (2004). A longitudinal study of behavior in frontotemporal dementia and primary progressive aphasia. *Cognitive and Behavioral Neurology*, **17**, 185–190.

Mattis, S. (1976). Mental status examination for organic mental syndrome in the elderly patients. In *Geriatric psychiatry: a handbook for psychiatrists and primary care physicians* (ed. L. Bellak and T.B. Karasu), pp. 77–101. Grune & Stratton, New York.

Mendez, M.F., Selwood, A., Mastri, A.R., and Frey, W.H. (1993). Pick's disease versus Alzheimer's disease: a comparison of clinical characteristics. *Neurology*, **43**, 289–292.

Mendez, M.F., Perryman, K.M., Miller, B.L., and Cummings, J.L. (1998). Behavioral differences between frontotemporal dementia and Alzheimer's disease: a comparison on the BEHAVE-AD rating scale. *International Psychogeriatrics*, **10**, 155–162.

Mendez, M.F., Shapira, J.S., and Miller, B.L. (2005a). Stereotypical movements and frontotemporal dementia. *Movement Disorders*, **20**, 742–745.

Mendez, M.F., Chen, A.K., Shapira, J.S., and Miller, B.L. (2005b). Acquired sociopathy and frontotemporal dementia. *Dementia and Geriatric Cognitive Disorders*, **20**, 99–104.

Mesulam, M.M. (2001). Primary progressive aphasia. *Annals of Neurology*, **49**, 425–432.

Miller, B.L., Darby, A., Benson, D.F., Cummings, J.L., and Miller, M.H. (1997). Aggressive, socially disruptive and antisocial behaviour associated with fronto-temporal dementia. *British Journal of Psychiatry*, **170**, 150–155.

Miller, B.L., Seeley, W.W., Mychack, P., Rosen, H.R., Mena, I., and Boone, K. (2001). Neuroanatomy of the self: evidence from patients with fronto-temporal dementia. *Neurology*, **57**, 817–821.

Moretti, R., Torre, P., Antonello, R.M., Cazzato, G., and Bava, A. (2002). Effects of selegiline on fronto-temporal dementia: a neuropsychological evaluation. *International Journal of Geriatric Psychiatry*, **17**, 391–392.

Moretti, R., Torre, P., Antonello, R.M., Cazzato, G., and Bava, A. (2003). Frontotemporal dementia: paroxetine as a possible treatment of behavior symptoms. A randomized, controlled, open 14-month study. *European Neurology*, **49**, 13–19.

Mychnack, P., Kramer, J.H., Boone, K.B., and Miller, B.L. (2001). The influence of right frontotemporal dysfunction on social behavior in frontotemporal dementia. *Neurology*, **56**(Suppl. 4), S11–S15.

Neary, D., Snowden, J.S., Bowen, D.M. et al. (1986). Neuropsychological syndromes in presenile dementia due to cerebral atrophy. *Journal of Neurology, Neurosurgery and Psychiatry*, **49**, 163–174.

Neary, D., Snowden, J.S., Gustafson, L. et al. (1998). Frontotemporal lobar degeneration. A consensus on clinical diagnostic criteria. *Neurology*, **51**, 1546–1554.

Nedjam, Z., Devouche, E., and Dalla Barba, G. (2004). Confabulation, but not executive dysfunction discriminate AD from frontotemporal dementia. *European Journal of Neurology*, **11**, 728–733.

Nyatsanza, S., Shetty, Y., Gregory, C., Lough, S., Dawson, K., and Hodges, J.R. (2003). A study of stereotypic behaviours in Alzheimer's disease and frontal and temporal variant frontotemporal dementia. *Journal of Neurology, Neurosurgery and Psychiatry*, **74**, 1398–1402.

Pasquier, F. (2005). Telling the difference between frontotemporal dementia and Alzheimer's disease. *Current Opinion in Psychiatry*, **18**, 628–632.

Pasquier, F. and Petit, H. (1997). Frontotemporal dementia: its rediscovery. *European Neurology*, **38**, 1–6.

Pasquier, F., Lavenu, I., Lebert, F., Jacob, B., Steinling, M., and Petit, H. (1997). The use of SPECT in a multidisciplinary memory clinic. *Dementia and Geriatric Cognitive Disorders*, **8**, 85–91.

Pasquier, F., Lebert, F., and Petit, H. (1999a). Organisation des centres de la mémoire et perspectives. *Revue Neurologique (Paris)*, **155**(Suppl. 4), S83–S92.

Pasquier, F., Lebert, F., Lavenu, I., and Guillaume, B. (1999b). The clinical picture of frontotemporal dementia: diagnosis and follow-up. *Dementia and Geriatric Cognitive Disorders*, **10**(Suppl. 1), 10–14.

Pasquier, F., Grymonprez, L., Lebert, F., and Van der Linden, M. (2001). Memory impairment differs in frontotemporal dementia and Alzheimer's disease. *Neurocase*, **7**, 161–171.

Pasquier, F., Richard, F., and Lebert, F. (2004). Natural history of frontotemporal dementia: comparison with Alzheimer's disease. *Dementia and Geriatric Cognitive Disorders*, **17**, 253–257.

Perry, R.J. and Hodges, J.R. (2000). Differentiating frontal and temporal variant frontotemporal dementia from Alzheimer's disease. *Neurology*, **54**, 2277–2284.

Pick, A. (1892). Über die Beziehungen der senilen Hirnatrophie zur Aphasie. *Prager Medizinische Wochenschrift*, **17**, 165–167.

Pick, A. (1901a). Senile Hirnatrophie als Grundlage von Hederscheinungen. *Wiener Klinische Wochenschrift*, **14**, 403–404.

Pick, A. (1901b). Uber Symptomenkomplexe bedingt durch die Kombination sub-corticaler Herdaffekionen mit seniler Hirnatrophie. *Wien Klinische Wochenschrift*, 1121.

Pick, A. (1904). Zur Symptomatologie der linksseitigen Schlafenlappenatrophie. *Monatschrift für Psychiatrie und Neurologie*, **16**, 378–388.

Pick, A. (1906). Über einen weiteren Symptomencomplex im Rahmen der Demenita Senilis, bedingt durch umschriebene starkere Hirnatrophie (gemischte Apraxie). *Monatschrift für Psychiatrie und Neurologie*, **19**, 97–108.

Pijnenburg, Y.A., Sampson, E.L., Harvey, R.J., Fox, N.C., and Rossor, M.N. (2003). Vulnerability to neuroleptic side effects in frontotemporal lobar degeneration. *International Journal of Geriatric Psychiatry*, **18**, 67–72.

Pijnenburg, Y.A.L., Gillissen, F., Jonker, C., and Scheltens, P. (2004). Initial complaints in frontotemporal lobar degeneration. *Dementia and Geriatric Cognitive Disorders*, **17**, 302–306.

Piolino, P., Desgranges, B., Belliard, S. *et al.* (2003). Autobiographical memory and autonoetic consciousness: triple dissociation in neurodegenerative diseases. *Brain*, **126**, 2203–2219.

Procter, A.W., Qurne, M., and Francis, P.T. (1999). Neurochemical features of frontotemporal dementia. *Dementia and Geriatric Cognitive Disorders*, **10**(Suppl. 11), 80–84.

Rahman, S., Sahakian, B.J., Hodges, J.R., Rogers, R.D., and Robbins, T.W. (1999). Specific cognitive deficits in mild frontal variant frontotemporal dementia. *Brain*, **122**, 1469–1493.

Rahman, S., Robbins, T.W., Hodges, J.R. *et al.* (2006). Methylphenidate ('Ritalin') can ameliorate abnormal risk-taking behavior in the frontal variant of frontotemporal dementia. *Neuropsychopharmacology*, **31**, 651–658.

Rankin, K.P., Kramer, J.H., and Miller, B.L. (2005a). Patterns of cognitive and emotional empathy in frontotemporal lobar degeneration. *Cognitive and Behavioral Neurology*, **18**, 28–36.

Rankin, K.P., Baldwin, E., Pace-Savitsky, C., Kramer, J.H., and Miller, B.L. (2005b). Self awareness and personality change in dementia. *Journal of Neurology, Neurosurgery and Psychiatry*, **76**, 632–639.

Rascovsky, K., Salmon, D.P., Ho, G.J. *et al.* (2002). Cognitive profiles differ in autopsy-confirmed frontotemporal dementia and AD. *Neurology*, **58**, 1801–1808.

Ratnavalli, E., Brayne, C., Dawson, K., and Hodges, J.R. (2002). The prevalence of frontotemporal dementia. *Neurology*, **58**, 1615–1621.

Roberson, E.D., Hesse, J.H., Rose, K.D. *et al.* (2005). Frontotemporal dementia progresses to death faster than Alzheimer disease. *Neurology*, **65**, 719–725.

Rosen, H.J., Perry, R.J., Murphy, J. *et al.* (2002). Emotion comprehension in the temporal variant of frontotemporal dementia. *Brain*, **125**, 2286–2295.

Rosso, S.M., Landweer, E.-J., Houterman, M., Donker Kaat, L., van Duijn, C.M., and van Swieten, J.C. (2003a). Medical and environmental risk factors for sporadic frontotemporal dementia: a retrospective case-control study. *Journal of Neurology, Neurosurgery and Psychiatry*, **74**, 1574–1576.

Rosso, S.M., Kaat, L.D., Baks, T. *et al.* (2003b). Frontotemporal dementia in The Netherlands: patients characteristics and prevalence estimates from a population-based study. *Brain*, **126**, 2016–2022.

Seeley, W.W., Bauer, A.M., Miller, B.L. *et al.* (2005). The natural history of temporal variant frontotemporal dementia. *Neurology*, **64**, 1384–1390.

Skibinski, G., Parkinson, N.J., Brown, J.M. *et al.* (2005). Mutations in the endosomal ESCRTIII-complex subunit CHMP2B in frontotemporal dementia. *Nature Genetics*, **37**, 806–808.

Snowden, J.S., Goulding, P.J., and Neary, D. (1989). Semantic dementia: a form of circumscribed cerebral atrophy. *Behavioural Neurology*, **2**, 167–182.

Snowden, J.S., Griffiths, H.L., and Neary, D. (1996a). Semantic-episodic memory interactions in semantic dementia: implications for retrograde memory function. *Cognitive Neuropsychology*, **13**, 1101–1137.

Snowden, J.S., Neary, D., and Mann, D.M.A. (1996b). *Fronto-temporal lobar degeneration: fronto-temporal dementia, progressive aphasia, semantic dementia*. Churchill Livingston, New York.

Snowden, J.S., Bathgate, D., Varma, A., Blackshaw, A., Gibbons, Z.C., and Neary, D. (2001). Distinct behavioural profiles in frontotemporal dementia and semantic dementia. *Journal of Neurology, Neurosurgery and Psychiatry*, **70**, 323–332.

Snowden, J.S., Gibbons, Z.C., Blackshaw, A. *et al.* (2003). Social cognition in frontotemporal dementia and Huntington's disease. *Neuropsychologia*, **41**, 688–701.

Sparks, D.L. and Markesbery, W.R. (1991). Altered serotoninergic and cholinergic synaptic markers in Pick's disease. *Archives of Neurology*, **48**, 796–799.

Sperfeld, A.D., Collatz, M.B., Baier, H. *et al.* (1999). FTDP-17: an early-onset phenotype with parkinsonism and epileptic seizures caused by a novel mutation. *Annals of Neurology*, **46**, 708–715.

Stanford, P.M., Brooks, W.S., Teber, E.T. *et al.* (2004). Frequency of tau mutations in familial and sporadic frontotemporal dementia and other tauopathies. *Journal of Neurology*, **251**, 1098–1104.

Swartz, J.R., Miller, B.L., Lesser, I.M., and Darby, A.M. (1997a). Frontotemporal dementia: treatment response to serotonin selective reuptake inhibitors. *Journal of Clinical Psychiatry*, **58**, 212–216.

Swartz, J.R., Miller, B.L., Lesser, I.M. *et al.* (1997b). Behavioral phenomenology in Alzheimer's disease, frontotemporal dementia, and late-life depression: a retrospective analysis. *Journal of Geriatric Psychiatry and Neurology*, **10**, 67–74.

Varma, A.R., Snowden, J.S., Lloyd, J.J., Talbot, P.R., Mann, D.M.A., and Neary, D. (1999). Evaluation of the NINCDS-ADRDA criteria in the differentiation of Alzheimer's disease and frontotemporal dementia. *Journal of Neurology, Neurosurgery and Psychiatry*, **66**, 184–188.

Verbeek, M.M., Pijnenburg, Y.A., Schoonenboom, N.S., Kremer, B.P.H., and Scheltens, P. (2005). Cerebrospinal fluid tau levels in frontotemporal dementia. *Annals of Neurology*, **58**, 657–657.

Wicklund, A.H., Johnson, N., and Weintraub, S. (2004). Preservation of reasoning in primary progressive aphasia: further differentiation from Alzheimer's disease and the behavioral presentation of frontotemporal dementia. *Journal of Clinical and Experimental Neuropsychology*, **26**, 347–355.

Wilhelmsen, K.C., Lynch, T., Pavlou, E., Higgins, M., and Nygaard, T.G. (1994). Localization of disinhibition–dementia–parkinsonism– amyotrophy complex to 17q21–22. *American Journal of Human Genetics*, **55**, 1159–1165.

Wrase, J., Reimold, M., Puls, I., Kienast, T., and Heinz, A. (2006). Serotonergic dysfunction: brain imaging and behavioral correlates. *Cognition and Affective Behavioral Neurosciences*, **6**, 53–61.

Yamauchi, H., Fukuyama, H., Nagahama, Y. *et al.* (2000). Comparison of the pattern of atrophy of the corpus callosum in frontotemporal dementia, progressive supranuclear palsy, and Alzheimer's disease. *Journal of Neurology, Neurosurgery and Psychiatry*, **69**, 623–629.

Yancopoulou, D., Crowther, R.A., Chakrabarti, L., Gydesen, S., Brown, J.M., and Spillantini, M.G. (2003). Tau protein in frontotemporal dementia linked to chromosome 3 (FTD-3). *Journal of Neuropathology and Experimental Neurology*, **62**, 878–882.

Zarranz, J.J., Ferrer, I., Lezcano, E. *et al.* (2005). A novel mutation (K317M) in the MAPT gene causes FTDP and motor neuron disease. *Neurology*, **64**, 1578–1585.

# Clinical aspects of dementia: neurological dementias

Andrew Graham

## Introduction

Dementia with onset in old age is usually due to underlying neuro-degeneration; most commonly, Alzheimer's disease (AD). Other neurodegenerative causes of late onset dementia include Parkinson's disease dementia or dementia with Lewy bodies (PDD/DLB) and, more rarely, frontotemporal dementia (FTD). These conditions, in which dementia tends to be the presenting or predominant feature, and neurodegenerative pathology is the cause, are often referred to as the *primary* dementias and are covered independently in Chapters 27iii, 27v, and 27vi. But dementia can also arise as a complication of a range of other neurological and general medical conditions, generally accompanied by other, non-cognitive abnormalities. This varied group of illnesses gives rise to what are known as the *secondary* dementias.

The majority of secondary dementias are due to underlying general medical conditions where dementia is accompanied by a range of manifestations in other systems. Perhaps the most important is vascular disease: vascular cognitive impairment and vascular dementia form a separate topic and are covered in Chapter 27iv. Alternative general medical causes of a secondary dementia include conditions such as hypothyroidism, vitamin $B_{12}$ deficiency, congestive cardiac failure, chronic obstructive pulmonary disease, and many others. In all these situations the diagnosis may be suggested by general medical assessment and investigations. Although less commonly encountered than the primary dementias, such secondary dementias are an important topic within the psychiatry of old age, not least because some of them are at least partially *reversible*. By contrast, despite decades of research, the primary dementias remain essentially incurable, and the only available treatments are supportive and symptomatic.

In other secondary dementias the underlying medical disorder primarily affects the brain, with few if any manifestations in other organ systems. Such secondary dementias are sometimes referred to as the 'neurological' dementias, and it is this group of conditions which form the focus of this chapter. The label covers an exceptional range of conditions, all of which are much less common than either the primary dementias or the general medical causes of a secondary dementia. A comprehensive survey of the field is therefore beyond the scope of this chapter, which aims instead to summarize the key features of a representative selection of neurological dementias: idiopathic normal pressure hydrocephalus; Huntington's disease; multiple sclerosis; autoimmune limbic encephalitis; and prion disease.

## Idiopathic normal pressure hydrocephalus

### Overview

Hydrocephalus is an umbrella term for the abnormal accumulation of cerebrospinal fluid (CSF) within the cranium, whether due to defective CSF production, flow, or absorption. The two main types are *obstructive hydrocephalus*, where there is a structural barrier to flow of CSF through the ventricular system, and *communicating hydrocephalus*, where the defect is inadequate absorption of CSF by the arachnoid granulations. Hydrocephalus secondary to overproduction of CSF is rare. Communicating hydrocephalus may in turn be classified as either *primary* or *secondary*. In secondary communicating hydrocephalus, the defect in CSF absorption is due to a well-established cause of damage to the arachnoid granulations, for example as a result of meningitis, subarachnoid haemorrhage, or significant head injury. In primary communicating hydrocephalus, no such cause is apparent.

A confusion of terms can sometimes arise at this point. In 1965 Adams and colleagues published a description of three cases in which patients with ventriculomegaly, gait disturbance, dementia, and urinary incontinence were helped by the insertion of a ventricular shunt (Adams *et al.*, 1965). All three patients had CSF opening pressures within the normal range, and in two of the three cases no secondary underlying cause for the hydrocephalus could be found. The paper was entitled 'Symptomatic occult hydrocephalus with "normal" cerebrospinal fluid pressure – a treatable syndrome', and subsequently it was suggested that this type of shunt-responsive primary, or idiopathic communicating hydrocephalus should be termed 'idiopathic normal pressure hydrocephalus', or INPH. However, this label is controversial—intracranial pressure (ICP) in INPH is in fact on average slightly higher than normal, with frequent superadded pulses of slightly increased pressure known as B waves. For this reason, some authors have suggested the alternative label 'idiopathic adult hydrocephalus syndrome'.

### Pathophysiology

The pathophysiology of INPH is incompletely understood. CSF dynamics are clearly disturbed, with a high resistance to CSF outflow, slightly raised intracranial pressure, increased B waves, an increased aqueductal stroke volume, and ventriculomegaly. However, the underlying cause for this disturbance is unknown, as is the mechanism by which these CSF pressure abnormalities affect the brain and result in clinical symptoms. A leading theory is that the symptoms of INPH are due to a complex interaction between a disturbance of CSF dynamics and cerebrovascular small vessel disease, resulting in low-grade cerebral ischaemia of periventricular white matter. This view is supported by both PET (Momjian *et al.*, 2004) and microdialysis studies (Agren-Wilsson *et al.*, 2005), the latter study also showing that this low-grade ischaemia is improved by removal of CSF.

## Epidemiology

Accurate figures for the incidence and prevalence of INPH are difficult to ascertain. In a Bavarian door-to-door community-based survey of 982 people older than 65 years the population prevalence of INPH was 0.4%, compared to a prevalence of 0.7% for PD (Trenkwalder *et al.*, 1995). In this study, the diagnosis of INPH was made clinically, but subsequently supported by CT scanning in all cases. In a recent survey of six Swedish neurosurgical centres, the number of shunt insertions performed was between three and six operations per 100,000 adults per year, of which about 30% were for INPH and 20% for secondary NPH (Tisell *et al.* 2005). These figures suggest that INPH is an uncommon but not insignificant cause of dementia in old age.

## Clinical features

The diagnosis of INPH rests first of all on clinical suspicion. The cardinal feature is disturbance of balance and gait, which almost always precedes the development of other symptoms and worsens insidiously over months and years. Patients walk with a mildly broad-based, small-stepped gait, and locomotion is impaired to a degree out of all proportion to the examination findings on the couch or bed. For this reason the gait disturbance is sometimes termed a gait apraxia, or frontal gait apraxia (because of its presumed localization). The gait disturbance is also symmetrical, and although minor extrapyramidal features may be found on examination, the presentation is quite distinct from that of idiopathic Parkinson's disease. Cognitive impairment is present in the majority of patients with INPH by the time of diagnosis, with up to 60% of patients scoring less than 25/30 on the Mini-Mental State Examination (MMSE). The profile of cognitive impairment is generally classified as 'subcortical', with pronounced slowness of thought, difficulty in sustaining, dividing, and switching attention, and difficulties in planning. However, simple screening tests are generally unable to discriminate between the profiles of cognitive impairment associated with INPH and AD. Finally, urinary urgency, frequency, and incontinence are common but non-specific features.

## Investigations

A CT or MRI brain scan should be performed in any patient with clinical features suggestive of INPH. The first aim of neuroimaging is to exclude any structural lesion, and the second is to look for supporting evidence for INPH. Enlargement of the ventricles is a cardinal feature of INPH, and is traditionally assessed by calculation of Evan's ratio, the ratio of the greatest width of the frontal horns of the lateral ventricles to the maximum internal width of the skull. An Evan's ratio greater than 0.3 suggests significant

ventriculomegaly, but other features are also important: for example, disproportionate widening of the temporal horns of the lateral ventricles, or flattening of the cortical sulci superiorly. In patients in whom significant ventriculomegaly is accompanied by marked cortical atrophy or signs of extensive cerebrovascular disease ventriculomegaly may simply represent loss of brain tissue rather than INPH.

If there is supporting evidence for INPH on neuroimaging, the next step is typically specialist referral to either neurology or neurosurgical services. The aim at this stage is to secure the diagnosis clinically before proceeding to further, more invasive tests and a decision about surgery. Important alternative diagnoses to exclude would be AD and PD; significant vascular disease; and common neurological disorders of old age such as cervical spondylotic myelopathy, lumbar canal stenosis, or a polyneuropathy. Exclusion of these possibilities rests largely on clinical assessment, but occasionally imaging of the spine or nerve conduction studies may be necessary. If CT is the only form of neuroimaging available, an MRI of the brain will also be required to confidently rule out subtle secondary causes of hydrocephalus such as aqueduct stenosis. Based on the combination of clinical features and imaging abnormalities consensus clinical diagnostic criteria for possible and probable INPH have recently been developed (Relkin *et al.* 2005), and are summarized in Table 27vii.1 below.

**Table 27vii.1** Diagnostic criteria for probable and possible idiopathic normal pressure hydrocephalus (INPH) (adapted from Relkin *et al.*, 2005)

|  | **Probable INPH** | **Possible INPH** |
|---|---|---|
| History | Must include:<br><br>Insidious onset<br>Onset > 40 years<br>Minimum duration 3–6 months<br>Progression<br>No antecedent event<br>No other general medical or neurological diagnosis that could explain ventricular enlargement | Subacute or undetermined onset<br>Onset after childhood<br>Duration < 3 months or indeterminate<br>May be antecedent event or other general medical or neurological diagnosis that could explain ventricular enlargement, but not causally related (in the opinion of the clinician) |
| Clinical | Must include:<br>Gait/balance disturbance, plus impairment in cognition, urinary function, or both | Incontinence and/or cognitive impairment in the absence of an observable gait or balance disorder<br>Gait disturbance or dementia alone |
| Imaging | Must include:<br>Ventricular enlargement (Evan's index > 0.3), not attributable to atrophy or congenital enlargement<br>No macroscopic obstruction to CSF flow | Ventricular enlargement consistent with hydrocephalus<br>May be associated with significant cerebral atrophy or structural lesion, but not causally related (in the opinion of the clinician) |
| Physiological | Must include:<br>CSF opening pressure in the range 7–24.5 cm $H_2O$ | CSF opening pressure measurement not available or outside the range for probable INPH |

## Assessment prior to shunting

If specialist assessment confirms the diagnosis of INPH, the next step is to decide if surgery (the placement of a ventricular shunt) will be of benefit. This usually involves further invasive investigations, either to measure aspects of CSF dynamics directly or to simulate the result of a shunt by removing a volume of CSF. The most widely used investigation is probably the CSF tap test, where 40–50 ml of CSF is withdrawn by lumbar puncture with assessment of gait and cognition before and afterwards. Unfortunately, while this test has a reasonable specificity and positive predictive value (i.e. a positive result is a good predictor of a response to shunting), it has a low sensitivity and negative predictive value (i.e. a negative result does not exclude a response to shunting). For this reason, some neurosurgical centres advocate a prolonged trial of CSF removal, usually involving the placement of a lumbar catheter and the steady drainage of CSF (approximately 10 ml/hour) over 72 hours. There is certainly some evidence that external lumbar CSF drainage is more sensitive in predicting response to shunting than a simple tap test, but at the expense of a hospital stay and the risk of catheter-related complications, including infection. For these reasons, lumbar CSF drainage is not a routine investigation in most centres.

Alternatively, CSF dynamics may be measured directly. Twenty-four hour intracranial pressure monitoring often reveals abnormalities that indicate poor cerebral compliance, such as the presence of low-amplitude B waves (as mentioned above). However, studies suggest that the presence or absence of B waves has a poor correlation with response to shunting. A more comprehensive assessment of CSF dynamics can be obtained by CSF infusion testing, in which saline is infused into the subarachnoid space through a lumbar puncture needle while CSF pressure is continuously recorded via a second lumbar puncture needle placed at a different level. In most patients the pressure rises constantly and then reaches a plateau. From the baseline pressure, plateau pressure, and infusion rate the resistance to CSF absorption can be calculated. At present, CSF infusion measurements suffer from the same problem as drainage studies when it comes to predicting a response to shunting, namely a good specificity but poorer sensitivity. However, sophisticated analysis of the infusion data and refinements of the technique may improve its sensitivity in the future.

## Shunt insertion and outcome

The usual procedure in patients with INPH selected for surgery is placement of a ventriculo-peritoneal (VP) shunt. The range of available shunt systems is wide and preferences vary from centre to centre. Shunts are coupled to a valve, which may be flow-regulated or differential pressure-regulated, and modern devices allow the reading and adjustment of valve settings after implantation. Data from the UK Shunt Registry do not show any significant differences in the shunt revision rates between the various valve systems, although the management of complications such as over-drainage (causing a low-pressure subdural haematoma) is obviously made much easier by an adjustable valve (Zemack and Romner, 2002).

There is no doubt that the nature and magnitude of the benefit obtained by shunting is controversial. The most recent Cochrane Review concluded that 'there is no evidence to indicate whether placement of a shunt is effective in the management of NPH' (Esmonde and Cooke, 2002). The authors of this systematic review draw attention to the lack of placebo-controlled trials of shunt insertion in INPH, although of course ethical approval, recruitment, blinding, and follow-up for any such trial would all represent considerable challenges. In non-placebo-controlled studies up to 60% of patients demonstrate improvement after shunting (Hebb and Cusimano, 2001), but it is uncertain whether this benefit is sustained in the long term. Unfortunately, out of the key triad of impairments in INPH dementia is the feature least likely to respond to shunting (Savolainen et al., 2002; Poca et al., 2004), although the earlier a shunt is placed the higher the likelihood of a good outcome. Importantly, improvement appears to be independent of age (Marmarou et al., 2005).

### Key points: INPH

♦ INPH is an uncommon, but potentially reversible cause of dementia in old age.

♦ INPH should be excluded in patients with the classical triad of gait impairment, dementia, and urinary incontinence.

♦ Assessment comprises CT or MRI brain imaging followed by referral to specialist neurology or neurosurgery services.

♦ CSF removal or CSF dynamic testing are usually required before making a decision on suitability for shunt insertion.

♦ Gait impairment is the feature most likely to improve after shunting; the milder the dementia, the better the chance of a good outcome.

# Huntington's disease

## Overview

Huntington's disease (HD) is an inherited, autosomal dominant neurodegenerative disorder resulting from an unstable expansion of a CAG trinucleotide repeat in the gene coding for the protein huntingtin on chromosome 4. The normal repeat number is between 6 and 35, and expansions of 40–44 repeats or greater lead to HD with 100% penetrance. The clinical features of HD usually emerge in early adulthood, but both juvenile and late onset presentations are well recognized. HD is commonly associated with prominent psychiatric symptoms, and when it presents in old age the clinical syndrome may be atypical. The family history may also be obscured by factors such as death from other causes in an affected parent or sibling before clinical features of HD are manifest; missing or 'hidden' relatives with unrecognized HD, particularly relatives who committed suicide; and non-paternity. Up to 10% of cases of HD may represent new mutations. For old age psychiatrists, an appreciation of the wide range of clinical features in HD is therefore important to avoid a missed or delayed diagnosis. The only assessment that definitively excludes HD is genetic testing.

## Epidemiology

HD is one of the commonest inherited neurodegenerative illnesses, with a prevalence in most Western European countries of between 4 and 8 per 100,000 (Harper, 1986). Lower prevalences are seen in certain other countries (e.g. Finland) and ethnic groups (e.g. Afro-Caribbean populations), but essentially HD is found worldwide. The peak age of onset is between 35 and 44 years, but HD can present at any age. Both sexes are affected equally.

## Clinical features

HD classically presents with the combination of a movement disorder and a frontal dementia. The initial movement disorder is typically involuntary (chorea, athetosis, or dystonia), progressing to an akinetic-rigid state later. However, some patients with late onset HD may present with an akinetic-rigid syndrome and minimal chorea, causing diagnostic confusion (Reuter et al., 2000). Other physical clues to the diagnosis include oculomotor abnormalities (e.g. slowed voluntary saccades and impersistence of gaze).

The range of psychiatric and cognitive symptoms reported in HD is wide. The commonest psychiatric disturbance is depression, affecting 40–50% of patients with HD during the course of their illness. The suicide rate in HD is reported to be four to six times higher than in the general population and in one early cohort of HD patients suicide accounted for over 2% of deaths (Schoenfeld et al., 1984). Anxiety and obsessive–compulsive symptoms are also frequently reported. Psychosis is less common, but up to 10% of patients show psychotic symptoms at some stage in their illness, usually poorly systematized paranoia with behavioural changes such as aggression and irritability. An early age of onset may be associated with an increased risk of psychosis, and psychiatric disturbance can occasionally be the presenting feature of HD in younger patients (Lovestone et al., 1996). Frank auditory hallucinations of the type seen in schizophrenia are rare.

Cognitively, patients with HD show prominent deficits on tests of attention, semantic verbal fluency, processing speed, and executive function. Performance on tests of memory can be poor, but the profile of problems (recall affected more than recognition), suggests difficulties with retrieval rather than encoding. Cognitive impairment can also be detected prior to diagnosis in gene-positive individuals at risk for the development of HD (Lawrence et al., 1998a,b).

## Investigations

MRI in patients with HD may show generalized cortical atrophy or specific caudate atrophy. Genetic testing for the CAG expansion is now a routine procedure, but because of the significant implications of a positive test for the patient and their family, referral to clinical genetics services for counselling prior to testing is generally recommended.

## Treatment and outcome

There is no cure for HD. Neuropsychiatric symptoms may all be treated with conventional medications, but many HD patients have an increased sensitivity to side-effects. Longitudinal studies show a steady decline in cognitive function, with progressive functional disability and eventual death after an interval ranging from 10 to 30 years.

## Key points: Huntington's disease

- HD is an inherited, autosomal dominant neurodegenerative condition that most usually presents with the combination of a frontal dementia and involuntary movement disorder.

- Late onset HD is well described and may present atypically, for example as an akinetic-rigid syndrome. Sometimes the family history is obscured or lacking.

- HD can only be completely excluded by genetic testing. Because of the implications of a positive test it may be wise to involve clinical genetics services prior to making a diagnosis.

- There is no cure for HD, although survival may be prolonged in some patients.

# Multiple sclerosis

## Overview

Multiple sclerosis (MS) is a chronic, relapsing and remitting or progressive disease of the central nervous system that is increasingly recognized to involve both inflammatory/demyelinating and neurodegenerative processes. A variety of presentations are recognized, with relapsing and remitting, secondarily progressive, and primary progressive forms. MS may be associated with a variety of neuropsychiatric symptoms and cognitive deficits, but cross-sectional studies have shown little correlation between cognitive impairment and either disease duration or physical disability. Cognitive impairment may occasionally be the presenting or only manifestation of MS (Zarei et al., 2003).

## Epidemiology

The prevalence of MS varies widely according to geography and ethnic group, with the highest rates to be found in populations of northern European descent. In a longitudinal study over 15 years in Olmstead County, Minnesota, the prevalence of MS was determined to be 177 per 100,000 of the adult population (Mayr et al., 2003); in a similar longitudinal study in Cambridge, UK, the prevalence was 152 per 100,000 (Robertson et al., 1996). Disease onset is typically between the ages of 15 and 50 years, but later onset is well recognized (Polliack et al., 2001). Alternatively, patients with a previous clinically isolated syndrome or an established diagnosis of MS may present to old age psychiatry services decades later with a dementia, raising the question as to whether the dementia is secondary to their pre-existing demyelinating disease.

## Clinical features

Acute inflammatory/demyelinating attacks in MS may affect any site within the CNS, potentially giving rise to an enormous breadth of clinical manifestations. A prototypical site for attacks is the optic nerve, resulting in the syndrome of acute optic neuritis. In this condition, visual loss develops in an eye over hours or days, accompanied by pain on eye movements. Fundoscopy may show unilateral disc swelling acutely, replaced later by optic disc pallor. Visual loss then plateaus, and improves partially or completely over subsequent weeks. The patient may be left with a very subtle deficit that is only evident on careful examination (for example, normal visual acuity but reduced colour vision in that eye), or show Uhtoff's phenomenon: a temporary return of symptoms in the eye when subjected to a stress such as a change in temperature, physical exertion, or an intercurrent illness. It is important to note that a temporary exacerbation of symptoms in this way does not constitute a relapse. Other sites commonly affected in MS include the brainstem and spinal cord.

The disease course in MS is extremely variable. Most commonly, the initial pattern is of attacks affecting different sites in the CNS at different times but good recovery between attacks (relapsing–remitting MS). However, after a period of years recovery after attacks tends to be less complete, leading to a gradual accumulation of fixed disability, followed later by steady deterioration irrespective of the frequency or severity of acute attacks (secondarily progressive MS). Occasionally, patients follow a steadily progressive course from the onset of their disease (primary progressive MS). It is tempting to assume that reducing the frequency or severity of acute attacks would retard the progression of disability in MS, but unfortunately this is not necessarily the case. Increasingly, evidence suggests that neurodegeneration is taking place alongside inflammatory/demyelinating changes from an early stage (Chard *et al.*, 2002).

A wide range of neuropsychiatric and cognitive disorders are seen in patients with MS. The most common neuropsychiatric problems are mood disorders (euphoria, which may become mania, or depression); psychosis is rare, but recognized. Cognitively, impairment is generally most marked on tests of attention, processing speed, and executive function, followed by impairment on tests of verbal memory (recall more so than recognition). Language functions are generally better preserved, and frank aphasia secondary to MS is rare. In keeping with the presumed frontal/subcortical basis of this profile of deficits, possibly the best predictor of cognitive impairment in MS is bilateral frontal lobe atrophy (Benedict *et al.*, 2002).

### Investigations

The key investigation in suspected MS is an MRI scan, typically showing multiple high-signal white matter lesions. However, high-signal white matter lesions are a common enough finding in old age, and may be non-specific or reflect small-vessel disease. Features that might specifically suggest demyelination include an ovoid shape to the lesions, enhancement after contrast in acute lesions, and involvement of the corpus callosum, brainstem, and cerebellum; recent diagnostic criteria specify the profile of expected MRI abnormalities in MS very closely (McDonald *et al.*, 2001; Polman *et al.*, 2005). Other supportive investigation results include unilateral or bilateral delay on visual evoked potentials (VEPs) and positive oligoclonal bands in CSF (but not serum) at lumbar puncture. Assessment of suspected MS and access to these secondary investigations will usually require referral to local neurology services.

### Treatment and outcome

There is no curative treatment for MS. A short course of corticosteroids may speed recovery from acute relapses, but has no impact on the development of later disability. For patients with frequent disabling relapses, disease-modifying treatments are now available. The beta-interferons and glatiramer acetate reduce relapse rates by approximately a third; agents in development such as CAMPATH 1-H may reduce relapse rates by up to two-thirds. However, once again the impact of these treatments on the development of eventual disability remains to be shown, and all may be associated with significant side-effects. Given the frontal/subcortical profile of deficits in dementia associated with MS it might be expected that cognitive rehabilitation would be of benefit, but systematic studies in this area are lacking.

### Key points: multiple sclerosis

◆ MS may be associated with a variety of cognitive and psychiatric disturbances including dementia.

◆ MS is an uncommon cause of dementia in old age, but might be suspected in a patient with a clinically isolated syndrome or established MS in middle life who later goes on to develop a frontal-subcortical pattern of cognitive impairment.

◆ The key test in suspected MS is an MRI scan, but distinguishing between demyelination and vascular disease in old age can be difficult and specialist assessment and/or secondary investigations (evoked potentials and CSF examination) are likely to be required for a definite diagnosis

## Limbic encephalitis/Hashimoto's encephalopathy

### Overview

A range of disorders are now recognized in which CNS dysfunction is accompanied by evidence of circulating tissue- or system-specific autoantibodies. In some of these disorders the abnormal antibody response is secondary to an underlying medical condition and in others no underlying condition can be found. Although uncommon, antibody-mediated CNS disorders are potentially treatable and may present with psychiatric symptoms or cognitive impairment but little else. For these reasons it is important that old age psychiatrists are aware of the variety of presentations that may result from such conditions, and the clues that should prompt further investigation and referral.

### Limbic encephalitis

The term limbic encephalitis refers to a range of conditions in which there is relatively selective inflammation or dysfunction of the limbic system (the hippocampus, amygdala, hypothalamus, and insular and cingulate cortex). Patients show subacute development of memory impairment, confusion, and/or altered mental status, typically accompanied by seizures and high-signal changes in the medial temporal lobes on MRI, but not all features are present in every individual. An important cause of limbic encephalitis is Herpes simplex encephalitis, the commonest cause of infective viral encephalitis in the UK, but non-infective causes are increasingly recognized (see below).

The earliest descriptions of limbic encephalitis emphasized its association with underlying cancer, although the neurological syndrome may precede the presentation of the tumour by months or even years (Corsellis *et al.*, 1968). A wide variety of paraneoplastic antibodies associated with different cancers have now been described (see Table 27vii.2), suggesting an immune mechanism, but the targets of these antibodies are generally non-specific, it is by no means clear that the antibodies detected are pathogenic, and the response to immune treatment is often disappointing (Voltz, 2002). The mainstay of management is therefore generally treatment of the underlying cancer.

However, recent work shows that in other patients limbic encephalitis may be a primary autoimmune illness caused by highly specific antibodies to voltage-gated potassium channels (VGKCs)

**Table 27vii.2** Subgroups of paraneoplastic limbic encephalitis (adapted from Voltz, 2002)

| Antibody | Common underlying cancers | Sex distribution | Common clinical features |
|---|---|---|---|
| Anti-Hu | SCLC | M > F | Additional PEM/SN |
| Anti-Ta/Ma2 | Testicular seminoma | M > F | Subacute, brainstem |
| ANNA-3 | SCLC | M = F | Additional PEM/SN |
| Anti-CRMP5/CV2 | SCLC, thymoma | F > M | Subacute, severe |

SCLC, small cell lung cancer; PEM/SN, paraneoplastic encephalomyelitis/sensory neuropathy.

(a) 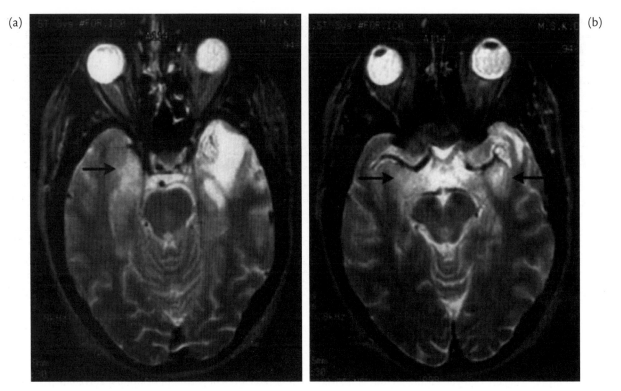 (b)

**Fig. 27vii.1** MRI findings in paraneoplastic limbic encephalitis (reproduced with permission from Gultekin *et al.* 2000). Note the bright signal (arrows in (a) and (b)) in the medial aspect of the temporal lobes. In (a) the more intense signal in the left temporal lobe corresponds to oedema after a brain biopsy.

(Thieben *et al.*, 2004; Vincent *et al.*, 2004). Such patients rarely show an underlying cancer, with the exception of occasional cases of thymoma. The evidence for a pathogenic role for the antibodies in VGKC-associated limbic encephalitis is much more compelling than for paraneoplastic limbic encephalitis, and symptoms may be at least partly responsive to immune treatment with intravenous immunoglobulin, plasma exchange, or high-dose steroids. The timing of treatment is also important. If treatment is delayed, irreversible medial temporal lobe atrophy may develop, and so it is important to identify and treat such patients as early as possible in the course of their disease.

The spectrum of clinical symptoms associated with anti-VGKC antibodies continues to expand, with both purely psychiatric and purely cognitive presentations reported (Parthasarathi *et al.*, 2006). This can make the diagnosis of atypical cases difficult. However, there are a number of clues that may suggest a diagnosis of typical VGKC-associated limbic encephalitis. Hyponatraemia is common, as are seizures, with the hyponatraemia preceding the introduction of anti-epileptic medication. Both the low sodium and the seizures may be resistant to treatment. Where neuropsychological assessment is possible, dysfunction of episodic memory is striking. On investigation, many patients show abnormal high signal in the temporal lobes and focal temporal abnormalities on EEG. Typical MRI findings in patients with paraneoplastic and VGKC-associated limbic encephalitis are illustrated in Figs 27vii.1 and 27vii.2.

CSF examination findings are usually non-specific, showing at most a modest lymphocytosis. The incidence of VGKC-associated limbic encephalitis in old age is unknown, but the majority of patients reported to date have presented in mid-life or later.

Suspicion of the diagnosis should prompt an early neurological referral.

## Hashimoto's encephalopathy

The association of a subacute encephalopathy with autoimmune thyroid disease was first reported by Brain and colleagues (Brain *et al.*, 1966). A solitary patient was described with cognitive impairment, agitation, tremor, hallucinations, and fluctuating confusion on the background of proven Hashimoto's thyroiditis and strongly positive antithyroid microsomal and antithyroglobulin antibodies—a combination that was subsequently termed Hashimoto's encephalopathy. A recent comprehensive literature review identified 85 patients with this constellation of features, suggesting that this is not a chance association, and noted an almost universal improvement in the patients' condition following steroid treatment (Chong *et al.*, 2003). However, it remains uncertain whether the antithyroid antibodies are actually pathogenic or simply an incidental marker of immune dysfunction. For this reason, neutral terms such as 'steroid-responsive encephalopathy' or 'steroid-responsive encephalopathy associated with Hashimoto's thyroiditis' have been proposed.

## Key points: limbic encephalitis/Hashimoto's encephalopathy

◆ Autoimmune limbic encephalitis is a condition in which there is relatively selective inflammation or dysfunction of the limbic system, leading to subacute memory impairment, confusion, and (often) seizures, associated with medial temporal lobe abnormalities on MRI.

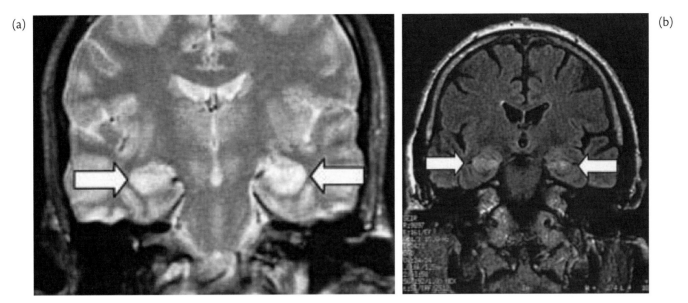

**Fig. 27vii.2** MRI findings in autoimmune limbic encephalitis (reproduced with permission from Vincent *et al.*, 2004). (a) T$_2$-weighted MRI showing bilateral hippocampal signal change (arrows) at disease onset. (b) FLAIR coronal MRI revealing signal change affecting anterior temporal lobe structures including each hippocampus (arrows).

◆ Paraneoplastic limbic encephalitis is most usually due to underlying small cell lung cancer.

◆ Patients with VGKC-associated limbic encephalitis may show prominent hyponatraemia and seizures that are resistant to treatment.

◆ An encephalopathy may also be seen in association with autoimmune thyroiditis and strongly positive antithyroid antibodies, and is often exquisitely responsive to steroid treatment.

# Prion diseases

## Overview

The prion diseases are a group of disorders in which fulminant spongiform neurodegeneration results in a rapidly progressive and ultimately fatal dementia. The pathogenic process involves conversion of a normal cell surface protein, termed cellular prion protein or PrP$^C$, into an abnormally folded and protease-resistant isoform (PrP$^{Sc}$). This abnormally folded protein is then deposited in the brain: whether it is the conversion or the deposition of PrP$^{Sc}$ that gives rise to the subsequent neurodegeneration is still a matter for debate. Approximately 15% of cases are familial, secondary to a mutation in the prion protein gene (*PRNP*), but the majority of cases are sporadic. Pathological classification of sporadic cases depends on two factors: first, the pattern of polymorphisms at codon 129 of the *PRNP* gene, which may be methionine–methionine (MM), methionine–valine (MV), or valine–valine (VV); and second, the size of the protease-resistant core fragment of the PrP$^{Sc}$ protein. In the most commonly applied classificatory system, two sizes of core are recognized (1 and 2), giving rise to six possible combinations of genotype and fragment size (MM1; MM2; MV1; MV2; VV1; VV2) (Parchi *et al.*, 1999). These genotype/isotype combinations are in turn associated with distinct clinical phenotypes of prion disease (see Table 27vii.3). This tidy classification is unfortunately upset by the increasing recognition that patients may show different prion isotypes in different brain regions, leading for example to mixed MM1/2 disease.

## Epidemiology

The commonest form of human prion disease is classical sporadic Creutzfeldt–Jakob disease (CJD), which has an approximate annual incidence of 1–2 per million population. There is little or no variation in incidence across geographical boundaries or ethnic groups.

## Clinical features

Inherited prion disease is an important cause of early onset dementia (Finckh *et al.*, 2000), but not of dementia in old age. Recognized genetic abnormalities include point mutations in the C-terminal domain, premature STOP codon mutations, and insertion of additional octapeptide repeats in the N-terminal domain. In the largest kindred of familial CJD yet described, originating from southeast England, the causative mutation is a six-octapeptide repeat (6-OPRI). The age of onset in this particular family has invariably been below the age of 55 years, with death by 65 years, and a very wide spectrum of presentations in affected family members is described (Mead *et al.*, 2006). In other kindreds with point mutations the age of onset is older, but even so familial prion disease is unlikely to present to old age psychiatry services.

Sporadic CJD, however, is well described in patients over the age of 65. In one series of 300 patients with pathologically proven prion disease the oldest age at onset was 91 years, although obviously this represents an extreme case (Parchi *et al.*, 1999). The disorder is characterized by relentlessly progressive cognitive decline, typically associated with pyramidal, extrapyramidal, and cerebellar dysfunction of varying degrees together with an involuntary movement disorder (usually myoclonus). If onset is in middle life or later (>50 years), sporadic CJD most commonly presents with the classic combination of a rapidly progressive dementia with myoclonus, but alternative presentations include progressive cortical blindness (the Heidenhain variant), or a progressive cerebellar syndrome

**Table 27vii.3** Classification of sporadic Creutzfeldt–Jakob disease according to molecular phenotype (adapted from Parchi et al., 1999)

| Molecular phenotype | Previous classification | Frequency (%) | Duration (months) | Prominent clinical features | Typical EEG (periodic sharp wave complexes) |
|---|---|---|---|---|---|
| MM1/MV1 | (1) Classical sporadic CJD; (2) Heidenhain variant | 70 | 3.9 | (1) Rapidly progressive dementia with myoclonus; (2) prominent visual impairment (in up to 40%) | Common |
| VV2 | Ataxic variant | 16 | 6.5 | Ataxia at onset; dementia later | Uncommon |
| MV2 | Kuru variant | 9 | 17.1 | Ataxia plus dementia at onset; may be extrapyramidal or psychiatric features later; extended survival (>2 years) in some patients | Uncommon |
| MM2—thalamic | Thalamic variant | 2 | 15.6 | Ataxia plus dementia; insomnia, and psychomotor hyperactivity | Uncommon |
| MM2—cortical | – | 2 | 15.7 | Progressive dementia | Uncommon |
| VV1 | – | 1 | 15.3 | Progressive dementia | Uncommon |

(the Brownell–Oppenheimer variant). The prognosis in later onset sporadic CJD is uniformly poor, often involving progression to akinetic mutism and death within months.

Extraordinarily, although PrP$^{Sc}$ is not a conventional infectious agent, prion diseases are transmissible from human to human by exposure to affected body tissues or fluids. Iatrogenic CJD can be contracted from PrP$^{Sc}$-contaminated human-derived growth hormone, dura mater extracts used in neurosurgical procedures, corneal grafts, and EEG depth electrodes. However, iatrogenic CJD often presents many years after exposure, typically with a rapidly progressive cerebellar syndrome rather than dementia with myoclonus, and this can lead to a delay in recognition and diagnosis.

Transmission may even take place across species, which has lead in turn to one of the most worrying UK public health disasters of recent decades. Scrapie, an endemic encephalopathic illness of sheep and goats in the UK (but not other countries such as New Zealand), has long been recognized to be a prion disease but was never previously thought to be transmissible to humans. Then, during the 1980s and early 1990s the UK saw an epidemic of a novel prion disease of cattle termed bovine spongiform encephalopathy, or BSE. The initial cause of the BSE epidemic was probably the transmission of abnormal prion protein to cattle when nervous tissue from scrapie-affected sheep found its way into cattle feed. Once this 'species barrier' had been jumped, matters were compounded when nervous tissue from affected cattle was in turn incorporated into feed for their brethren. Eventually the total number of cattle definitely diagnosed with BSE in the UK was nearly 200,000, but the true number is likely to have been much higher; an additional 4 million asymptomatic cattle aged >30 months were also slaughtered in an effort to halt the epidemic.

Despite these measures, it is estimated that over 600,000 cattle affected with BSE entered the human food chain (Anderson et al., 1996). It was not long before patients with a novel type of CJD were recognized, often with purely psychiatric symptoms in the initial stages (Bateman et al., 1995; Britton et al., 1995). The mean age of onset in variant CJD (vCJD) has to date been much earlier than for classical sporadic CJD, but old age psychiatrists should not be complacent—of the first 100 patients with vCJD, the oldest was aged 74 years (Spencer et al., 2002). One of the key differences

between sporadic CJD and vCJD is that tissues outside the nervous system can be affected. The BSE prion protein is hypothesized to enter the body through the gut, and PrP$^{Sc}$ deposition can be seen in lymphoid tissue at a variety of sites including the appendix (Hilton et al., 1998) and the tonsils. This also means that vCJD can potentially be transmitted between humans by exposure to affected non-nervous tissue, including blood transfusion (Llewelyn et al., 2004; Peden et al., 2004). Although the annual incidence appears to be declining, the eventual extent of the human vCJD problem remains a matter of speculation. To date (August 2007), 166 cases of definite or probable vCJD have been reported in the UK, of whom 161 have died (with pathological confirmation of the diagnosis in 112 patients) (http://www.cjd.ed.ac.uk/figures.htm; accessed 22/8/07). Finally, until recently all clinical cases of vCJD in the UK have been methionine–methionine homozygous at codon 129 of *PRNP*, with the exception of 1 patient with probable iatrogenic vCJD who carried an MV genotype. No clinical cases to date have carried a VV genotype, but a recent retrospective study looking for prion protein reactivity in appendix tissue found three positive cases (from over 12,000 samples), two of whom were VV homozygous. It is therefore possible that vCJD-infected individuals with a valine homozygous codon 129 *PRNP* genotype have a prolonged incubation, and will result in a 'second wave' of cases after an unknown time period (Ironside et al., 2006).

### Investigations

MRI may be entirely normal in all forms of CJD, especially early in the course of the disease, but subtle imaging abnormalities are increasingly recognized. Some patients with sporadic CJD show high signal in the caudate nuclei, while vCJD may be associated with high signal in the pulvinar nucleus of the thalamus (see Fig. 27vii.3). This 'pulvinar sign' now forms part of the diagnostic criteria for vCJD, although it is not entirely specific and has also been described in conditions such as Wernicke–Korsakoff syndrome and paraneoplastic limbic encephalitis (Doherty et al., 2002; Mihara et al., 2005).

The EEG is often abnormal, classically with periodic sharp wave complexes (PSWCs; seen in sporadic CJD but not vCJD). At lumbar puncture, CSF constituents are normal, with negative oligoclonal bands, but a raised CSF 14–3–3 protein may be found. A recent

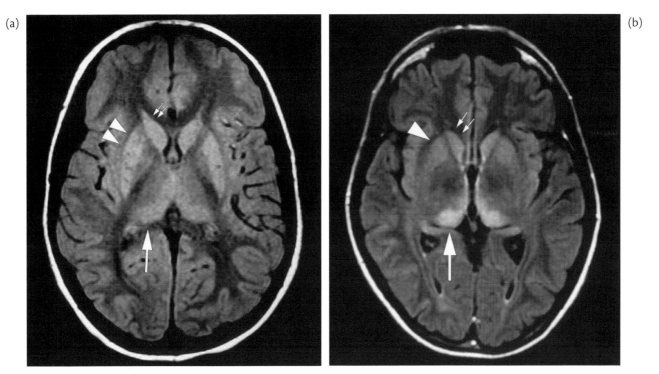

**Fig. 27vii.3** MRI findings in sporadic and variant Creutzfeldt–Jakob disease (reproduced with permission from Summers *et al.*, 2004). (a) FLAIR sequence in sporadic CJD, showing hyperintensity of all deep grey matter nuclei, with the putamen (arrowheads) and caudate (small double arrows) brighter than the pulvinar (large arrow). (b) FLAIR sequence in variant CJD, showing hyperintensity of all deep grey matter nuclei of the opposite pattern, with the pulvinar (large arrow) brighter than the putamen (arrowhead) and caudate (small double arrows).

comprehensive study of investigation results in 2451 patients with pathologically confirmed prion disease suggests that the most important determinants of abnormal results are age at onset, disease duration, and molecular subtype (Collins *et al.*, 2006). For example, the probability that the EEG will show PSWCs increases with patient age but decreases with disease duration. Similarly, disease duration of >12 months reduces the chance of a positive CSF 14–3–3 result. Regarding molecular biology, patients presenting with classical sporadic CJD and predominant cortical involvement (likely MM1 and MV1 subtypes) are more likely to show PSWCs on EEG, while patients presenting with ataxia and predominant subcortical involvement are more likely to show basal ganglia abnormalities on MRI. Overall, a single negative test cannot exclude prion disease and combinations of investigations are recommended.

The key test in familial prion disease is obviously sequencing of the *PRNP* gene. The gold standard in sporadic cases is tissue biopsy with demonstration of abnormal accumulations of PrP^Sc; in sporadic CJD this means brain biopsy, but in vCJD (where lymphoid tissue outside of the CNS is also affected), tonsillar biopsy may be diagnostic. In the UK, advice on the investigation and management of patients with suspected prion disease can be obtained through regional neurology services or the National Prion Clinic.

### Key points: prion disease

- Prion disease is an uncommon cause of dementia in old age.

- The form of prion disease most likely to present to old age psychiatrists is classical sporadic CJD, with the combination of a rapidly progressive dementia and myoclonus.

- Positive investigations in prion disease include abnormal signal change on MRI, PSWCs on EEG, and 14–3–3 protein in the CSF, but the yield of these tests depends on the age of onset, disease duration, and underlying molecular subtype.

- Definitive diagnosis can only be achieved by tissue biopsy, or in familial cases sequencing of the *PRNP* gene.

- The prognosis in late onset classical sporadic CJD is uniformly poor, with deterioration and death in months. There is currently no effective treatment.

### References

Adams, R.D., Fisher, C.M. *et al.* (1965). Symptomatic occult hydrocephalus with 'normal' cerebrospinal fluid pressure. A treatable syndrome. *New England Journal of Medicine*, **273**, 117–26.

Agren-Wilsson, A., Eklund, A. *et al.* (2005). Brain energy metabolism and intracranial pressure in idiopathic adult hydrocephalus syndrome. *Journal of Neurology, Neurosurgery and Psychiatry*, **76**(8), 1088–93.

Anderson, R.M., Donnelly, C.A. *et al.* (1996). Transmission dynamics and epidemiology of BSE in British cattle. *Nature*, **382**(6594), 779–88.

Bateman, D., Hilton, D. *et al.* (1995). Sporadic Creutzfeldt–Jakob disease in a 18-year-old in the UK. *Lancet*, **346**(8983), 1155–6.

Benedict, R.H., Bakshi, R. *et al.* (2002). Frontal cortex atrophy predicts cognitive impairment in multiple sclerosis. *Journal of Neuropsychiatry and Clinical Neuroscience*, **14**(1), 44–51.

Brain, L., Jellinek, E.H. *et al.* (1966). Hashimoto's disease and encephalopathy. *Lancet*, **2**(7462), 512–14.

Britton, T.C., al-Sarraj, S. *et al.* (1995). Sporadic Creutzfeldt-Jakob disease in a 16-year-old in the UK. *Lancet*, **346**(8983), 1155.

Chard, D.T., Griffin, C.M. *et al.* (2002). Brain atrophy in clinically early relapsing-remitting multiple sclerosis. *Brain*, **125**(2), 327–37.

Chong, J.Y., Rowland, L.P. *et al.* (2003). Hashimoto encephalopathy: syndrome or myth? *Archives of Neurology*, **60**(2), 164–71.

Collins, S.J., Sanchez-Juan, P. *et al.* (2006). Determinants of diagnostic investigation sensitivities across the clinical spectrum of sporadic Creutzfeldt–Jakob disease. *Brain*, **129**(9), 2278–87.

Corsellis, J.A., Goldberg, G.J. *et al.* (1968). Limbic encephalitis and its association with carcinoma. *Brain*, **91**(3), 481–96.

Doherty, M.J., Watson, N.F. *et al.* (2002). Diffusion abnormalities in patients with Wernicke encephalopathy. *Neurology*, **58**(4), 655–7.

Esmonde, T. and Cooke, S. (2002). *Shunting for normal pressure hydrocephalus (NPH)*. Art. No. CD003157. DOI: 10.1002/14651858. CD003157 (http://www.cochrane.org/reviews/en/ab003157.html).

Finckh, U., Muller-Thomsen, T. *et al.* (2000). High prevalence of pathogenic mutations in patients with early-onset dementia detected by sequence analyses of four different genes. *American Journal of Human Genetics*, **66**(1), 110–17.

Gultekin, S.H., Rosenfeld, M.R. *et al.* (2000). Paraneoplastic limbic encephalitis: neurological symptoms, immunological findings and tumour association in 50 patients. *Brain*, **123**, 1481–94.

Harper, P.S. (1986). The prevention of Huntington's chorea. *Journal of the Royal College of Physicians of London*, **20**(1), 7–14.

Hebb, A.O. and Cusimano, M.D. (2001). Idiopathic normal pressure hydrocephalus: a systematic review of diagnosis and outcome. *Neurosurgery*, **49**(5), 1166–84.

Hilton, D.A., Fathers, E. *et al.* (1998). Prion immunoreactivity in appendix before clinical onset of variant Creutzfeldt–Jakob disease. *Lancet*, **352**(9129), 703–4.

Ironside, J.W., Bishop, M.T. *et al.* (2006). Variant Creutzfeldt–Jakob disease: prion protein genotype analysis of positive appendix tissue samples from a retrospective prevalence study. *British Medical Journal*, **332**, 1186–8.

Lawrence, A.D., Hodges, J.R. *et al.* (1998a). Evidence for specific cognitive deficits in preclinical Huntington's disease. *Brain*, **121**, 1329–41.

Lawrence, A.D., Weeks, R.A. *et al.* (1998b). The relationship between striatal dopamine receptor binding and cognitive performance in Huntington's disease. *Brain* **121**(7), 1343–55.

Llewelyn, C.A., Hewitt, P.E. *et al.* (2004). Possible transmission of variant Creutzfeldt–Jakob disease by blood transfusion. *Lancet*, **363**(9407), 417–21.

Lovestone, S., Hodgson, S. *et al.* (1996). Familial psychiatric presentation of Huntington's disease. *Journal of Medical Genetics*, **33**(2), 128–31.

McDonald, W.I., Compston, A. *et al.* (2001). Recommended diagnostic criteria for multiple sclerosis: guidelines from the International Panel on the diagnosis of multiple sclerosis. *Annals of Neurology*, **50**(1), 121–7.

Marmarou, A., Bergsneider, M. *et al.* (2005). The value of supplemental prognostic tests for the preoperative assessment of idiopathic normal-pressure hydrocephalus. *Neurosurgery*, **57**(3, Suppl.), S17–S28 [discussion ii–v].

Mayr, W.T., Pittock, S.J. *et al.* (2003). Incidence and prevalence of multiple sclerosis in Olmsted County, Minnesota, 1985–2000. *Neurology*, **61**(10), 1373–7.

Mead, S., Poulter, M. *et al.* (2006). Inherited prion disease with six octapeptide repeat insertional mutation–molecular analysis of phenotypic heterogeneity. *Brain*, **129**(9), 2297–317.

Mihara, M., Sugase, S. *et al.* (2005). The pulvinar sign in a case of paraneoplastic limbic encephalitis associated with non-Hodgkin's lymphoma. *Journal of Neurology, Neurosurgery and Psychiatry*, **76**(6), 882–4.

Momjian, S., Owler, B.K. *et al.* (2004). Pattern of white matter regional cerebral blood flow and autoregulation in normal pressure hydrocephalus. *Brain*, **127**(5), 965–72.

Parchi, P., Giese, A. *et al.* (1999). Classification of sporadic Creutzfeldt-Jakob disease based on molecular and phenotypic analysis of 300 subjects. *Annals of Neurology*, **46**(2), 224–33.

Parthasarathi, U.D., Harrower, T. *et al.* (2006). Psychiatric presentation of voltage-gated potassium channel antibody-associated encephalopathy. Case report. *British Journal of Psychiatry*, **189**, 182–3.

Peden, A.H., Head, M.W. *et al.* (2004). Preclinical vCJD after blood transfusion in a PRNP codon 129 heterozygous patient. *Lancet*, **364**(9433), 527–9.

Poca, M.A., Mataro, M. *et al.* (2004). Is the placement of shunts in patients with idiopathic normal-pressure hydrocephalus worth the risk? Results of a study based on continuous monitoring of intracranial pressure. *Journal of Neurosurgery*, **100**(5), 855–66.

Polliack, M.L., Barak, Y. *et al.* (2001). Late-onset multiple sclerosis. *Journal of the American Geriatrics Society*, **49**(2), 168–71.

Polman, C.H., Reingold, S.C. *et al.* (2005). Diagnostic criteria for multiple sclerosis: 2005 revisions to the McDonald Criteria. *Annals of Neurology*, **58**(6), 840–6.

Relkin, N., Marmarou, A. *et al.* (2005). Diagnosing idiopathic normal-pressure hydrocephalus. *Neurosurgery*, **57**(3, Suppl.), S4–S16.

Reuter, I., Hu, M.T. *et al.* (2000). Late onset levodopa responsive Huntington's disease with minimal chorea masquerading as Parkinson plus syndrome. *Journal of Neurology, Neurosurgery and Psychiatry*, **68**(2), 238–41.

Robertson, N., Deans, J. *et al.* (1996). Multiple sclerosis in south Cambridgeshire: incidence and prevalence based on a district register. *Journal of Epidemiology and Community Health*, **50**(3), 274–9.

Savolainen, S., Hurskainen, H. *et al.* (2002). Five-year outcome of normal pressure hydrocephalus with or without a shunt: predictive value of the clinical signs, neuropsychological evaluation and infusion test. *Acta Neurochirurgica*, **144**(6), 515–23 [discussion 523].

Schoenfeld, M., Myers, R.H. *et al.* (1984). Increased rate of suicide among patients with Huntington's disease. *Journal of Neurology, Neurosurgery and Psychiatry*, **47**(12), 1283–7.

Spencer, M.D., Knight, R.S. *et al.* (2002). First hundred cases of variant Creutzfeldt-Jakob disease: retrospective case note review of early psychiatric and neurological features. *British Medical Journal*, **324**(7352), 1479–82.

Summers, D.M., Collie, D.A. *et al.* (2004). The pulvinar sign in variant Creutzfeldt–Jakob disease. *Archives of Neurology*, **61**, 446–7.

Thieben, M.J., Lennon, V.A. *et al.* (2004). Potentially reversible autoimmune limbic encephalitis with neuronal potassium channel antibody. *Neurology*, **62**(7), 1177–82.

Tisell, M., Hoglund, M. *et al.* (2005). National and regional incidence of surgery for adult hydrocephalus in Sweden. *Acta Neurologica Scandinavica*, **112**(2), 72–5.

Trenkwalder, C., Schwarz, J. *et al.* (1995). Starnberg trial on epidemiology of Parkinsonism and hypertension in the elderly. Prevalence of Parkinson's disease and related disorders assessed by a door-to-door survey of inhabitants older than 65 years. *Archives of Neurology*, **52**(10), 1017–22.

Vincent, A., Buckley, C. *et al.* (2004). Potassium channel antibody-associated encephalopathy: a potentially immunotherapy-responsive form of limbic encephalitis. *Brain*, **127**(3), 701–12.

Voltz, R. (2002). Paraneoplastic neurological syndromes: an update on diagnosis, pathogenesis, and therapy. *Lancet Neurology*, **1**(5), 294–305.

Zarei, M., Chandran, S. *et al.* (2003). Cognitive presentation of multiple sclerosis: evidence for a cortical variant. *Journal of Neurology, Neurosurgery and Psychiatry*, **74**(7), 872–7.

Zemack, G. and Romner, B. (2002). Adjustable valves in normal-pressure hydrocephalus: a retrospective study of 218 patients. *Neurosurgery*, **51**(6), 1392–400 [discussion 1400–2].

# Clinical aspects of dementia: specific pharmacological treatments for Alzheimer's disease

Gordon Wilcock

## Introduction

A number of treatment approaches for Alzheimer's disease (AD) have been explored over the years, but it was not until the emergence of the cholinergic hypothesis of AD that a rational approach to treatment, specifically targeted at the neurochemical pathology of AD, came to the fore. Reports in the mid-1970s of substantial reductions in the levels of enzymes responsible for the synthesis of acetylcholine (Bowen *et al.*, 1976; Davies and Maloney, 1976; Perry *et al.*, 1977) led to the hypothesis that it might be possible to develop therapeutic strategies similar to the levodopa treatment approach to Parkinson's disease. This has been reviewed by Francis *et al.* (1999). It subsequently became clear that a number of other neurotransmitter abnormalities are present in the brain in AD, and these have also formed the basis for therapeutic hypotheses, and at least one of these, based upon glutamate modulation, underpins another approach to treatment.

Early attempts to treat the cholinergic deficit with lecithin and choline (i.e. precursor loading) produced disappointing results. However, the development of compounds that were effective as cholinesterase inhibitors (ChEIs)—thereby preserving the smaller amounts of acetylcholine being produced in the Alzheimer brain—showed sufficient promise for extensive clinical evaluation to be undertaken, and several of these compounds have now been licensed for a number of years, and funded—despite controversy in some quarters about the magnitude of their clinical benefit. Even though these are modest, in the eyes of many they have proved a major step forward in the pharmacological treatment of people with mild to moderate AD, and in the case of memantine, also in severe AD.

In addition to treatment strategies based upon the neurochemical pathology in Alzheimer's disease, and which produce mainly symptomatic relief, other approaches have targeted the fundamental pathology of AD, i.e. the production of the beta-amyloid protein and the neurofibrillary tangle. Some of these are now in clinical evaluation, and for some strategies phase III clinical trials are under way. There have been, in addition, a number of alternative approaches that may prove to be helpful in AD, but which, if successful, may work through a more general neuroprotective mechanism rather than an antiplaque or antitangle strategy. Examples include the use of anti-oxidative treatments, and the increasing recognition of the role of neurotrophic factors, such as nerve growth factor (NGF). The latter has stimulated interest in exploring a potential role for neurotrophins and similar molecules as neuroprotective agents in AD. This chapter will provide an overview of the present position of these different therapeutic strategies.

## Cholinesterase inhibitors

Pharmacological studies of ChEIs show that they have a number of different properties, e.g. they can be competitive or non-competitive inhibitors, can vary in the degree of reversibility of their action, and so on. Initially it was felt that these features might affect their clinical utility, but in general, for those that have received a licence, there is little to choose between them on the basis of their pharmacological features. Tacrine was the first cholinomimetic compound to undergo an extensive clinical evaluation programme, and to gain subsequent approval for its use in some, but not all, countries. Its modest efficacy, albeit limited by its side-effect profile, was clearly established for periods of up to 30 weeks in three pivotal studies (Davis *et al.*, 1992; Farlow *et al.*, 1992; Knapp *et al.*, 1994). This proved that there were modest benefits for some people with mild to moderate AD in terms of dose-related improvement in cognition and in a global evaluation of a person's well-being and quality of life. A related compound, velnacrine, was shown to have similar efficacy, but had an unacceptable side-effect profile and did not receive a licence. Tacrine was prescribed for some 300,000 or so patients worldwide, but arguably its main benefit lies in the fact that it paved the way for the second generation of ChEIs which have lower toxicity. These include donepezil, rivastigmine, and galantamine, amongst others.

The value of ChEIs for the treatment of AD has been contentious (Courtney *et al.*, 2004; Kaduszkiewicz *et al.*, 2005; Pelosi *et al.*, 2006). Most of the reservations have concentrated on clinical trial design and the interpretation of the results, the findings of more negative trials, and concern that resources have been diverted to fund the drugs that could be better spent in other forms of care. The trial reported by Courtney *et al.* (2004), the AD2000 study, demonstrated more disappointing results than industry-funded trials and its authors also criticized the interpretation of many of the more positive studies. However, this study is itself regarded by many as also methodologically flawed, e.g. on account of inappropriate selection criteria, and its power—it was originally designed to recruit 3000 subjects but managed to report on only 565 subjects. Despite these and other criticisms, it was surprising that the results did favour active treatment with donepezil over placebo for some outcome measures, even though the magnitude of the benefit was relatively small. This further emphasizes the need for improved trial methodology.

## Specific cholinesterase inhibitors

### Donepezil

Donepezil was licensed in the UK in February 1997, and in many parts of Europe was the first available treatment for mild to moderately severe AD. Its efficacy was assessed in accordance with regulatory requirements, across a range of modalities, including cognition, global functioning, and ability to undertake activities of daily living (ADL). There have also been trials to assess its efficacy in controlling the neuropsychiatric manifestations of AD. This drug has probably been the most extensively evaluated of the currently available compounds, and has accumulated significant exposure within the various clinical studies, as have galantamine and rivastigmine. One of the early pivotal studies evaluated the use of donepezil at either 5 mg or 10 mg against placebo, over a 6-month period, in some 473 patients (Rogers *et al.*, 1998). The main endpoints were an improvement in cognition as shown on the Alzheimer 's Disease Assessment Scale cognitive subscale (ADAS-Cog; Rosen *et al.*, 1984) and a general overall clinical assessment using a semistructured instrument, i.e. Clinician's Interview Based Impression of Change with caregiver input (the CIBIC-Plus), a global assessment measure, which allowed an overall impression of change in four major functional domains: general, cognition, behavioural, and ADL. A quarter of the patients taking the higher, 10 mg, dose improved by 7 points or more on the ADAS-Cog (cf. 8% on placebo), indicating they had benefited by at least a 6–12 months' gain in cognitive function when this was compared with their baseline level. On the more general CIBIC-Plus measure, 10% of those on placebo improved compared with 25% receiving donepezil. A responder analysis showed that four patients would need to be treated to gain an improvement in terms of a 4-point change in the ADAS-Cog, compared with eight for an improvement on the CIBIC-Plus (Allen, 1999). There is also some evidence of a continued treatment effect with long-term therapy (Evans *et al.*, 2000). Open study has extended the duration of experience with donepezil to 240 weeks (Rogers *et al.*, 2000); however, it needs to be remembered that such studies are unblinded continuations of shorter double-blinded randomized controlled trials, and need to be treated with caution as all sorts of biases can creep in, for example selective dropping out of those with a poor response, rendering objective interpretation of the results difficult. However, they are of some value as long-term placebo-controlled studies cannot be undertaken. They would be unethical since they would deprive subjects of the only available effective treatment for long periods if they were allocated to the placebo group.

### Rivastigmine

Like the other ChEIs, rivastigmine has been shown to be modestly effective in all three major domains of AD—namely, cognition, activities of daily living, and global functioning—in 30–50% of treated patients, depending upon which domain is being reported (Corey-Bloom *et al.*, 1998; Schneider *et al.*, 1998; Rösler *et al.*, 1999). It is important to appreciate that, as with all ChEIs, the benefits may include *improvement* in cognition or well-being, or *stabilization* of the symptomatic deterioration. Some evidence for the latter has been claimed in open-label extension studies. Rivastigmine also significantly inhibits butyrylcholinesterase as well as acetylcholinesterase, which may make an important contribution to its efficacy.

### Galantamine

As well as reversibly and competitively inhibiting acetylcholinesterase this also modulates nicotinic acetylcholine receptors which may prove to be of additional clinical relevance, because activation of pre-synaptic nicotinic receptors has been shown to increase the release of acetylcholine, and also of other neurotransmitters, such as glutamate, that are deficient in AD. A number of studies of galantamine (Raskind *et al.*, 2000; Tariot *et al.*, 2000; Wilcock *et al.*, 2000) have confirmed its efficacy and tolerability in those patients with mild to moderate AD. During a 6-month, placebo-controlled study, galantamine was shown to alleviate caregiver burden in AD, indicating that the cognitive and functional benefits of galantamine for the patient are translated into beneficial effects on caregiver burden (Wilcock and Lilienfeld, 2000). The time that caregivers needed to spend supervising or assisting patients with AD was reduced by up to 1 hour a day.

### Other cholinesterase inhibitors

There are a number of other compounds under review, including metrifonate and various physostigmine analogues. At the time of writing, these are not available to the clinician, and they will not be discussed further.

## General properties of cholinesterase inhibitors

### Practical prescribing considerations

As described above, there is reliable evidence that ChEIs are effective in a significant proportion of people with mild to moderate AD and probably in severe AD too (see below), and that this is represented in some people by an improvement in cognition, functional ability, etc. Moreover, in some it would appear that treatment with a ChEI stabilizes that person's symptoms for a variable period. As there is no means of determining who will, or will not, respond to such treatment, a 3-month trial of efficacy would seem justifiable in most people who meet the entry criteria. Some would advocate a longer trial period, i.e. a minimum of 6 months, and there will indeed be some patients for whom it is impossible to determine benefit after a shorter trial.

In general, two to three times as many people in the active treatment arms of studies meet the accepted criteria for efficacy compared with those in the placebo arm, and this ratio is approximately mirrored by the adverse event profile. The latter is mainly what would be expected from cholinergic enhancement, with gastrointestinal tract symptoms being especially prominent. Most of the adverse events experienced occur during the initial, early titration phase of treatment. These events are usually short-lived, and can be successfully treated in most cases with an appropriate antiemetic. Many patients require no treatment, and the majority are free of adverse events, or experience only minimal symptoms. The number of patients discontinuing treatment because of adverse events is fewer in clinical practice than in the clinical trials.

Their potential for adverse interactions with other drugs is to some extent dependent upon their mechanism of action, including selectivity and the reversibility of receptor binding characteristics. This includes some of those used in anaesthetic practice, and possibly others such as ranitidine and cimetidine, although neither of these has proved a significant problem in practice. The side-effect profile and potential for interactions compares favourably with frequently used drugs in elderly patients, such as many of the antidepressants and neuroleptics. Caution should be exercised, however, in those patients with reversible airways disease or in some cardiac conditions such as conduction defects or significant bradycardia as they may increase vagal tone. Choosing the appropriate patients for treatment requires careful consideration.

When should treatment be stopped in those in whom there has been a favourable response? This is a difficult question, to which only a pragmatic response can be given. Wherever possible, protocols allowing an objective assessment of response in a number of domains should be employed, but in clinical practice it is rarely possible to undertake such a comprehensive approach. Nevertheless, some attempt at objectivity is worthwhile, and for many people this may mean the use of a simple general test of cognition, such as the Mini-Mental State Examination (MMSE), coupled with a global measure formed from the relative's, or other caregiver's, opinion and supplemented by the clinical notes made at earlier consultations. Whenever it looks as if a patient is deteriorating, a phased withdrawal of treatment may reveal whether or not there is still benefit; if the benefit is judged worthwhile, the treatment should be restarted.

In January 2001 in the UK the National Institute for Clinical Excellence (NICE, 2001) published guidance for the general use of donepezil, rivastigmine, and galantamine in the treatment of AD, which superseded previous advice. They confirmed that these drugs should be made available in the UK as part of the NHS as one component in the management of people with mild to moderate AD. It was suggested that they should be made available to those with an MMSE score above 12, in whom a specialist clinician had made the diagnosis of probable AD, using tests of cognitive, global, and behavioural functioning, in addition to assessment of activities of daily living. The guidance indicated that compliance should be taken into account, and that in many cases this would need a relative or careworker who was sufficiently in contact with the patient to be able to monitor compliance. Although it was suggested that treatment should be initiated in a consultant or specialist clinic, it was accepted that in due course general practitioners might take over prescribing but, if so, under a shared-care protocol with clear treatment endpoints. NICE indicated that an assessment should be made between 2 and 4 months after reaching the maintenance dose of the drug, and that continued treatment should be prescribed only where there had been an improvement or no deterioration in the MMSE score, together with evidence of global improvement on the basis of behavioural and functional assessment. NICE further suggested that, once the medication regime is stabilized, there should be reassessments approximately every 6 months, and that

the drug should be continued only while the patient's MMSE score remains above 12, and that the patient's global, functional, and behavioural condition suggests that the drug is continuing to have a worthwhile effect. When the MMSE score falls below 12 points, the guidance indicated that the treatment would normally be discontinued, but it did not make this an absolute requirement. The NICE guidance also indicated that the 6-monthly review should probably be undertaken by a specialist clinic.

This guidance in the UK was welcomed by most working in the field, and also by many of the families of patients. However, more recently (2006) NICE have revised their opinion and are recommending that treatment should only be available to those with moderate dementia secondary to AD, i.e. that the benefits of ChEIs are not adequate to justify funding in people with mild dementia, by which they mean those with an MMSE score above 20. This decision was upheld after appeal, and has caused considerable dismay, and some would say outrage, and a judicial review, sought by the Alzheimer's society in 2007 left the evidence unchanged. They have also called for further research into this area, e.g. to identify appropriate starting and stopping rules for treatment, and to provide robust and relevant data on both short- and long-term outcomes. Their next scheduled review is due to commence in September 2008.

### Non-cognitive symptoms

There is also an emerging picture that ChEIs may help with the management of non-cognitive symptoms in people with AD. Neuropsychiatric symptoms and loss of functional ability are the main drivers for admission of a person with dementia to an institution, they increase the cost of their care, and are also the main cause of stress in caregivers. Several reports have confirmed the benefits of ChEIs in modifying neuropsychiatric symptoms (Levy et al., 1999; Trinh et al., 2003).

This is important in light of the adverse event profile of other treatments to modify these symptoms. In particular, neuroleptics cause parkinsonism, sedation, postural hypotension, falls, and sedation. More recently some of the atypical neuroleptics have been linked to a higher incidence of stroke and cerebrovascular conditions. All three licensed ChEIs have been shown in clinical trials to have benefits in a range of neuropsychiatric symptoms, including delusions, hallucinations, anxiety, and motor agitation. The benefits of ChEI therapy on functional impairment were found to be worthwhile in 90% of trials included in a meta-analysis, which also confirmed that there was no difference in benefit between the different drugs (Cummings and Masterman, 1998). Collectively this evidence supports a link (even though it may be an indirect effect) between non-cognitive symptoms and functional ability and the cholinergic system. Such benefits may have pharmaco-economic implications, i.e. reduction in cost of treatment, but before funding can be justified, it will be necessary to confirm this preliminary evidence in properly conducted, randomized and placebo-controlled clinical trials.

### Use in more severe dementia

As well as requiring a fairly secure diagnosis of probable AD, at present the indication for ChEIs prescription is only for those patients with mild to moderately severe dementia, but this may change as the outcomes of trials in more severely demented subjects are assessed by regulatory and funding bodies, although this may involve an uphill struggle. One recent study examined the benefits to people with AD living in nursing homes (Winblad et al., 2006).

It included 95 patients who were assigned to the donepezil arm and 99 patients assigned to placebo during the 6-month study. Those treated with donepezil improved more on cognition and activities of daily living at 6 months after initiation of treatment compared with baseline than did the control subjects. The adverse events profile was comparable between groups with most being transient, and mild or moderate in severity. It is very difficult to assess what results like this mean in relation to quality of life for more severely affected patients, but they suggest that treatment with this group of drugs may be beneficial.

### Long-term use of cholinesterase inhibitors

ChEIs have mainly been evaluated in relatively short-term trials, up to 6 months in duration, and their acceptance by licensing authorities has been influenced by these studies. Most of the longer-term trials have been open-label continuation studies because of the ethical problems of withholding an effective treatment from people with AD in a placebo arm, when it is known that many would benefit from their prescription. The absence of a placebo arm in these studies makes their interpretation difficult, and the use of historical data from earlier naturalistic non-treated cohorts, or data extrapolated from shorter study periods, is fraught with bias.

In clinical practice patients and their caregivers frequently report continued benefit for periods of up to 18 months or 2 years, and in some cases benefit seems to be maintained for even longer, verified by temporary withdrawal of treatment or reduction in dose. This evidence is of course subjective and may be subject to many biases, but must have some weight, and those who appear to sustain longer-term benefit will probably continue to receive the benefit of the doubt.

Patients often appear to maintain their improvement for a month or so after drug is discontinued. Whether this is the result of drug levels being maintained in the brain for longer than expected, or whether there is some other more fundamental explanation is unknown. However, the latter is a possibility and has led to the suggestion that these compounds may have a disease-modifying effect on the pathology, rather than just acting at a symptomatic level. Indeed there are pre-clinical data that support this possibility. It has been shown that muscarinic receptor stimulation has an effect on the processing of amyloid precursor protein (APP) from which the amyloidogenic peptide is produced, such that APP processing is directed more down the non-amyloidogenic cleavage pathway (Nitsch et al., 1992). The pre-clinical evidence for the concept of neuroprotection at a cellular level has been reviewed recently and is more than a little convincing (Francis et al., 2005).

There is also clinical evidence from some, but not all, neuroimaging studies which may imply that these drugs could have a neuroprotective effect, which in turn would support the concept of the potential benefit of longer-term treatment. For example, in a prospective cohort study of 54 AD patients receiving donepezil, and 93 control subjects, who underwent MRI on two occasions at a 1-year interval (Hashimoto et al., 2005), the rate of hippocampal atrophy was significantly less among the treated patients (mean annual rate of atrophy 3.82%; SD 2.84%) compared with the control subjects (mean annual rate of atrophy 5.04%; SD 2.54%). Similar neuroprotection was reported in a study of 26 minimal to mild AD patients in whom brain grey matter density changes were quantified over 20 weeks, using voxel-based morphometry in which the authors report that rivastigmine, but not donepezil or galantamine, preserved baseline cortical grey matter density (Venneri et al., 2005); from these data

they suggest that dual cholinesterase inhibition, i.e. inhibition of both acetylcholinesterase and butyrylcholinesterase, is required for this effect. However, this is a very small study over a short time span and needs replication in larger numbers over longer periods. Nevertheless, these data do add to that suggestion that ChEIs *may* have neuroprotective properties.

## Cholinergic agonists

A number of cholinergic agonists, mainly muscarinic receptor agonists, have been evaluated as treatments for AD. In general, the benefit and adverse event profile has proved disappointing. However, there is some evidence that these agents (e.g. xanomeline, a selective muscarinic agonist) may improve behavioural difficulties such as vocal outbursts and psychotic symptoms (Bodick et al., 1997).

## Memantine

Glutamate modulation has been explored as a possible therapeutic strategy for AD and other dementias. Memantine is one such drug that may work through this mechanism. It blocks N-methyl-D-aspartate (NMDA) receptor channels in the resting state, and has been investigated in large clinical trials in both AD and vascular dementia. It is one of the few compounds so far investigated in more severe dementias, and is currently licensed for the treatment of moderate to severe dementia caused by AD.

A trial (Reisberg et al., 2003) which was conducted specifically in patients with moderate to severe AD in a 28-week double-blind, parallel-group study revealed that global ability ratings at endpoint favoured the memantine-treated group, but just failed to reach the 5% level of significance in the intention-to-treat (ITT) analysis, although it achieved significance in the analysis of observed cases at week 28 ($P = 0.03$). Performance on the activities of daily living scale was similar in both groups at baseline, but at week 28 there was significantly less deterioration in the memantine-treated group.

Three of the other outcome measures showed changes in favour of memantine: the Severe Impairment Battery which measures cognitive impairment in advanced AD (Panisset et al., 1994; Schmitt et al., 1997); the Functional Assessment Staging scale (Sclan & Reisberg, 1992); and the Resource Utilisation in Dementia instrument assessing caregiver burden and AD-related health economic data (Wimo et al., 1998). In addition, memantine was well tolerated.

The relatively benign adverse event profile of memantine has led to evaluation of its potential for modifying difficult behaviour in people with dementia, just as mentioned above in relation to the ChEIs. Early evidence is beginning to emerge (Gauthier et al., 2005) and it is beginning to be used off-licence for this indication. These authors analysed the total and individual domain scores in the Neuropsychiatric Inventory (NPI) (Cummings et al., 1994) in the ITT populations of two randomized controlled studies involving memantine (Reisberg et al., 2003; Tariot et al., 2004) and concluded that there was a beneficial effect in these patients with moderate to severe AD, especially in agitation and aggression.

There has been much interest in combining memantine with a ChEI and evaluating the impact of the combination of these complementary approaches in the management of AD. In a randomized, double-blind, placebo-controlled clinical trial of 404 patients with moderate to severe AD and MMSE scores of 5 to 14, who were already receiving stable doses of donepezil, co-treatment with memantine resulted in significantly better outcomes than placebo. This was true for measures of cognition, activities of daily living, global outcome, and behaviour, and the combination was well tolerated (Tariot *et al.*, 2004).

## Other approaches not specifically directed at the cholinergic system or basic neuropathology of Alzheimer's disease

A considerable number of potential treatment strategies have been developed that fit into this category. Some of the more recent or controversial approaches are included below.

### Ginkgo biloba

There has been a lot of controversy about the use of Ginkgo biloba. This is made from extracts of the leaves of the maidenhair tree, and has long been in use in China for a number of different indications, but more recently for cognitive enhancement. It has many potential active ingredients and mechanisms of action. The difficulty in identifying and evaluating the active ingredients is likely to cause problems with the regulatory authorities were it to be submitted for such approval. A recent Cochrane Review (Birks and Evans 2002) concluded that it appears to be safe in use with no excess side-effects compared with placebo. Many of the early trials used unsatisfactory methods, were small, and publication bias cannot be excluded. Although there was some evidence of improvement in cognition and function associated with ginkgo, the three more modern trials showed inconsistent results. There is need for a large trial using modern methodology and permitting an ITT analysis to provide robust estimates of the size and mechanism of any treatment effects.

### Oestrogen replacement treatment

The use of oestrogen replacement treatment in AD remains controversial. There is epidemiological evidence that women of post-menopausal age taking oestrogen preparations may have a reduced or delayed risk of developing dementia (e.g. Tang *et al.*, 1996). This led to the hope that it may be a useful adjunctive treatment in those who have already contracted the disease. However, two recent studies, albeit on relatively small numbers of people with AD, and for a relatively short period, have failed to show any significant benefit (Henderson *et al.*, 2000; Wang *et al.*, 2000).

More recently a negative outcome has been reported from an analysis of a trial based upon the Women's Health Initiative (WHI) in the US. Oestrogen plus progestin therapy increased the risk for probable dementia in post-menopausal women aged 65 years or older. In addition, oestrogen plus progestin therapy did not prevent mild cognitive impairment, which in many cases is pre-clinical AD, in these women. Furthermore, there was an increased risk of cerebrovascular and cardiovascular disease, carcinoma, and thromboembolism with this approach. These findings, coupled with previously reported WHI data, support the conclusion that the risks of oestrogen plus progestin outweigh the benefits (Rapp *et al.*, 2003; Shumaker *et al.*, 2003).

### Anti-oxidant therapy

This has also been explored in AD based upon the premise that cellular respiration produces oxygen derivatives and other free radicals which may be particularly harmful to specific intracellular structures, especially those that are rich in lipids. Under normal circumstances, these radicals are rapidly dealt with by intracellular mechanisms. However, neurons are known to have reduced levels of one important major anti-oxidant, glutathione, whilst they may have a higher level of oxidative stress related to the very high oxygen consumption of the brain. Whether this is specifically relevant to AD itself, or if harmful, has a more general effect upon the background level of neuronal numbers and function, is unclear. The best known anti-oxidant in relation to Alzheimer's disease is vitamin E, and one study (Sano *et al.*, 1997) provided some evidence that the use of vitamin E in high doses may slow the progression of AD in those who are moderately severely affected. However, the literature presents confusing evidence. In a recent trial of vitamin E and donepezil in people with mild cognitive impairment, many of whom have 'pre-clinical' AD, the result for the vitamin E component was clearly negative in terms of preventing or slowing the onset of AD (Petersen *et al.*, 2005), which has implications for the treatment of established disease.

### Anti-inflammatory drugs

Evidence that an inflammatory process may be present in the brain in AD (e.g. the association of a number of acute-phase protein markers and cytokines in and around the typical plaques), was one reason for the exploration of anti-inflammatory compounds as therapeutic agents. The other reason is the apparent protection conferred by anti-inflammatory compounds noted in some of the longitudinal studies of ageing. This phenomenon is now well described in the literature, and has stimulated trials of anti-inflammatory drugs in those with the disease. Limited early trials, (e.g. Rogers *et al.*, 1993), suggested a possible slowing of the disease process in some subjects with mild to moderate AD, and the outcome of further studies is awaited. Experience with steroids, e.g. prednisone, has, however, proved disappointing. In a double-blind, randomized control trial of prednisone in 138 subjects over a 12-month period there was no difference in outcome measures between the treated and the placebo arms of the study, but there was a suggestion that those receiving prednisone declined behaviourally (Aisen *et al.*, 2000). More recently a study comparing a selective COX-2 non-steroidal anti-inflammatory drug against a non-selective drug also came up with a negative outcome (Aisen *et al.*, 2003).

However, the explanation for these negative results seems to lie in the choice of drug. It transpires that despite the abundant evidence for an inflammatory component to the pathology of AD, some members of one class of the anti-inflammatory agents have an effect that is independent of their anti-inflammatory properties. This is an ability to modulate beta-amyloid production (see below), and is not a class effect, i.e. it is only vested in some members of the class, and also is not a property of steroids such as prednisone (Weggen *et al.*, 2001, 2003; Eriksen *et al.*, 2003).

## Strategies designed to rectify the underlying cellular pathology in Alzheimer's disease

More fundamental therapeutic strategies have also been under development, some of which are moving into the phase of early clinical evaluation. These include attempts to try and prevent the deposition of amyloid precursor protein, or accelerate its removal once it has been deposited. Some of these approaches rely upon knowledge gained from our understanding of the genetic contributions to AD, particularly those affecting the presenilin genes, and involve preventing potentially harmful cleavage of the amyloid precursor protein molecule by specific proteases. Other anti-amyloid approaches include attempts to try and reduce the damage that it may cause once it has been deposited.

## Immunotherapy for Alzheimer's disease

One exciting approach has been the theory, gained from experiments with transgenic mice, that it may be possible to generate antibodies against the amyloid-beta (Aβ) peptide, which will lead to clearance of amyloid from the brain or prevent its formation from the peptide.

The seminal work of Schenk et al. (1999) caused much excitement. They reported that monthly inoculation of transgenic mice, engineered to produce cerebral human Aβ, with a preparation of Aβ and an adjuvant, led to high anti-Aβ antibody levels and an attenuation of brain amyloid deposition. They also showed a favourable impact on brain amyloid levels when the inoculations were started at an age when there was already considerable amyloid deposition. This was followed by a report that passive administration of mouse monoclonal antibodies against Aβ produced a similar outcome (Bard et al., 2000). The most likely mechanism appeared to be enhanced clearance of amyloid by the microglial/macrophage system, and in a direct imaging paradigm it was shown that administration of antibodies directly onto the brain surface removed pre-existing amyloid deposits (Bacskai et al., 2001).

There are, however, two other possible modes of action to explain this amyloid-lowering effect. Some have postulated that little antibody actually penetrates the blood–brain barrier, and that the amyloid-lowering properties of the antibodies lie more in trapping the Aβ in the bloodstream (DeMattos et al., 2001, 2002). The latter in effect becomes a 'peripheral sink', and evidence is accumulating to support this contention. The third possibility was considered before either of the other two, and suggests that binding of the antibody to the Aβ reduced or prevented its ability to form amyloid fibrils (Solomon, 2001). It is probable that all three mechanisms play a part, and also possible that there are other mechanisms too, as yet unidentified. If these findings represent what is happening in the human brain affected by AD, the deposition of amyloid becomes a matter of the balance between its production and removal, and not just a matter of overproduction of a harmful protein, as was previously considered to be the case by many working in the field. Despite this, it is important not to forget that these hypotheses are predicated upon a genetically engineered mouse model of amyloid accumulation, which may not be the same as AD in the human context.

Based upon this and other relevant data, Elan and Wyeth established a trial of an amyloid vaccine in 2001, which included 375 subjects. Unfortunately about 6% of the subjects developed an aseptic meningoencephalitis and the trial had to stop prematurely. Nevertheless, it provided some useful information. Autopsy on one of the subjects who died confirmed that their brain had much less amyloid than expected, compared to brains from control subjects at a comparable stage of the disease, thus mirroring the transgenic mouse data (Nicoll et al., 2003). Only a preliminary and partial analysis of the clinical data is available, mainly because of the early termination, but this suggested that 20 subjects who generated an antibody response experienced some decline in the rate of progres-sion of their symptoms in one centre (Hock et al., 2003), whilst a later report which included a larger number of subjects found more minor benefits, although the authors concluded that immunotherapy may be useful in AD (Gilman et al., 2005). Other studies are now under way which will eventually clarify the place of this approach to treating people with AD.

## Reducing Aβ production

Aβ is the product of one form of cleavage of amyloid precursor protein (APP) which involves secretase enzymes. Under normal circumstances most APP is first cleaved by β-secretase and then by α-secretase, which does not lead to Aβ accumulation. In AD, it seems that much APP is cleaved by γ-secretase rather than α-secretase, releasing the 42 amino acid peptide that is the basis of amyloid accumulation. There has been much interest in exploring inhibitors or modulators of both β- and γ-secretases as a means of preventing amyloid deposition.

Preliminary reports indicate that treatment with a γ-secretase inhibitor may have a beneficial effect on plasma and CSF Aβ levels, but these are early studies (Siemers et al., 2006) and more definitive data are needed, especially as inhibiting γ-secretase may adversely affect its physiological function in other tissues. More is known about one of the γ-secretase modulators, R-Flurbiprofen, which rather than inhibiting the enzyme activity affects the cleavage pattern by allosteric modulation, such that shorter peptide moieties are produced which do not go on to produce Aβ. Although developed from a non-steroidal anti-inflammatory agent, it has no anti-inflammatory or COX-2 impact, nor the adverse event profile of these drugs. This has been evaluated in a phase II study, and is now in phase III evaluation in two trials including mild AD patients.

This randomized double-blind study evaluated 12 months' treatment with 400 mg b.i.d., 800 mg b.i.d. or placebo in 207 subjects with mild to moderate AD. In a pre-specified analysis, there was a statistically significant interaction between treatment group and baseline disease severity, indicating that an analysis of the two groups combined was not appropriate, and that mild and moderate groups should be analysed separately. At entry, approximately one-third of subjects had moderate AD as defined by a MMSE score of 19 or less and two-thirds had mild AD as defined by a MMSE of 20 to 26 inclusive. The primary endpoints of cognitive (ADAS-cog) and functional (ADCS-ADL and CDR-sb) decline over 12 months, comparing 800 mg b.i.d. versus placebo in the mild disease group, showed a trend toward slowing of cognitive decline, and a statistically significant benefit in activities of daily living ($P = 0.03$) and global function ($P = 0.04$). The effect sizes for mild subjects receiving 800 mg b.i.d. ranged from 34–45%, meaning that the decline in cognition and function in subjects taking 800 mg b.i.d. was 34–45% less than the decline in subjects taking placebo. Effects were greater for patients achieving high drug concentration in plasma. The effect sizes for mild patients who achieved high drug concentrations in plasma ranged from 36–62%. There was no evidence of benefit for those subjects with moderate disease severity at baseline receiving 800 mg b.i.d., nor for mild or moderate subjects receiving 400 mg b.i.d.

At the end of this study, over 80% of eligible patients were enrolled into a 1-year follow-on treatment study in which placebo patients were randomized into one of the two treatment groups, and treated patients continued their stable dose. Treatment groups remained blinded to patient/investigator. Patients taking the 800 mg b.i.d. dose continued to show benefit in cognition, ADL, and global function in the follow-on study (Wilcock *et al.*, 2006). Ultimately, we will learn from the phase III trials whether or not this strategy is an effective disease-modifying, as opposed to symptom-modifying, treatment for AD.

## Preventing production of neurofibrillary tangles

The other main pathological lesion in AD is neurofibrillary tangles. These are formed intracellularly through the hyperphosphorylation of microtubule-associated proteins, especially tau. It is possible that strategies to dephosphorylate tau or to reduce the level of abnormal phosphorylation might also be beneficial, and these are also under exploration, e.g. lithium.

## Neurotrophic factors

Finally, there is considerable interest in the use of neurotrophic substances (i.e. naturally occurring peptides or proteins) to protect neurons from damage or to augment their natural plasticity. As far as the latter is concerned, nerve growth factor (NGF) is the most likely candidate. A small number of patients have been treated with intracerebroventricular NGF in Sweden, with modest, if any, real benefit. However, the dosing pattern and quantity of NGF delivered may not have been optimal and further work in this field is necessary. It is probable that intraparenchymal delivery of NGF into the region of the basal nucleus of Meynert, where most of the cholinergic cells that are important in AD reside, will be more efficacious than intracerebroventricular delivery, and may also avoid some of the adverse events associated with delivery into the CSF. The outcome of a small-scale phase I trial of NGF gene therapy has recently been reported. Fibroblasts genetically modified to produce NGF were transplanted into the forebrain in eight subjects, six of whom were studied for a mean of 22 months. Cognitive evaluation suggested some slowing of the rate of decline, and PET studies showed an increase in cortical 18-fluorodeoxyglucose after treatment. Autopsy on one subject suggested robust growth responses to NGF treatment (Tuszynski *et al.*, 2005). Further studies are required to explore this concept further, but even if successful, it is unlikely that treatment requiring neurosurgical intervention will become standard. A successful outcome is more likely to accelerate the search for NGF mimetics that can be administered by other routes.

In conclusion, we have advanced a long way since the earliest studies with cholinergic drugs, e.g. physostigmine and tacrine. Not only is symptomatic treatment a reality, albeit at a modest level and only for some patients, but disease-modifying, i.e. neuroprotective, treatments may be on the horizon. There is considerable hope for the future.

## References

Aisen, P.S., Davis, K.L., Berg, J.D. *et al.* (2000). A randomized controlled trial of prednisone in Alzheimer's disease. *Neurology*, **54**, 588–93.

Aisen, P.S., Schafer, K.A., Grundman, M. *et al.* (2003). Effects of rofecoxib or naproxen vs placebo on Alzheimer disease progression: a randomized controlled trial. *Journal of the American Medical Association*, **289**, 2819–26.

Allen, H. (1999). Anti-dementia drugs. [editorial] *International Journal of Geriatric Psychiatry*, **14**, 239–43.

Bacskai, B.J., Kajdasz, S.T., Christie, R.H. *et al.* (2001). Imaging of amyloid-beta deposits in brains of living mice permits direct observation of clearance of plaques with immunotherapy. *Nature Medicine*, **7**, 369–72.

Bard, F., Cannon, C., Barbour, R. *et al.* (2000). Peripherally administered antibodies against amyloid beta-peptide enter the central nervous system and reduce pathology in a mouse model of Alzheimer disease. *Nature Medicine*, **6**, 916–19.

Birks, J., and Grimley Evans, J. (2002). Ginkgo biloba for cognitive impairment and dementia(Cochrane Review). *The Cochrane Database of Systematic Reviews*, Issue 4, Art. No. CD003120. DOI:10.1002/14651858.CD003120.

Bodick, N.C., Offen, W.W., Levey, A. I. *et al.* (1997). Effects of xanomeline, a selective muscarinic receptor agonist, on cognitive function and behavioral symptoms in Alzheimer's disease. *Archives of Neurology*, **54**, 465–73.

Bowen, D.M., Smith, C.B., White, P., *et al.* (1976). Neurotransmitter-related enzymes and indices of hypoxia in senile dementia and other abiotrophies. *Brain*, **99**, 459–96.

Corey-Bloom, J., Anand, R., Veach, J. and the ENA 713 B352 Study Group (1998). A randomised trial evaluating the efficacy and safety of ENA 713(rivastigmine tartrate), a new acetylcholinesterase inhibitor, in patients with Alzheimer's disease. *International Journal of Geriatric Psychopharmacology*, **1**, 55–65.

Courtney, C., Farrell, D., Gray, R. *et al.* (2004). Long-term donepezil treatment in 565 patients with Alzheimer's disease (AD2000): randomised double-blind trial. *Lancet*, **363**, 2105–15.

Cummings, J.L. and Masterman, D.L. (1998). Assessment of treatment-associated changes in behavior and cholinergic therapy of neuropsychiatric symptoms in Alzheimer's disease. *Journal of Clinical Psychiatry*, **59**(Suppl. 13), 23–30.

Cummings, J.L., Mega, M., Gray, K., Rosenberg-Thompson, S., Carusi, D.A., and Gornbein, J. (1994). The Neuropsychiatric Inventory: comprehensive assessment of psychopathology in dementia. *Neurology*, **44**, 2308–14.

Davies, P. and Maloney, A.J.F. (1976). Selective loss of central cholinergic neurones in Alzheimer's disease. *Lancet*, **ii**, 1403.

Davis, K.L., Thal, L.J., Gamzu, E.R. *et al.* (1992). A double-blind, placebo-controlled multicenter study of tacrine for Alzheimer's disease. *New England Journal of Medicine*, **327**, 1253–9.

DeMattos, R.B., Bales, K.R., Cummins, D.J., Dodart, J.C., Paul, S.M., and Holtzman, D.M.(2001). Peripheral anti-A beta antibody alters CNS and plasma A beta clearance and decreases brain A beta burden in a mouse model of Alzheimer's disease. *Proceedings of the National Academy of Sciences USA*, **98**, 8850–5.

DeMattos, R.B., Bales, K.R., Cummins, D.J., Paul, S.M., and Holtzman, D.M. (2002). Brain to plasma amyloid-beta efflux: a measure of brain amyloid burden in a mouse model of Alzheimer's disease. *Science*, **295**, 2264–7.

Eriksen, J.L., Sagi, S.A., Smith, T.E. *et al.* (2003). NSAIDs and enantiomers of flurbiprofen target gamma-secretase and lower Abeta 42 *in vivo*. *Journal of Clinical Investigation*, **112**, 440–9.

Evans, M., Ellis, A., Watson, D., and Chowdhury, T. (2000). Sustained cognitive improvement following treatment of Alzheimer's disease with donepezil. *International Journal of Geriatric Psychiatry*, **15**, 50–3.

Farlow, M., Gracon S.I., Hershey L.A., *et al.* (1992). A controlled trial of tacrine in Alzheimer's disease. The Tacrine Study Group. *Journal of the American Medical Association*, **268**, 2523–9.

Fillit, H., Weinreb, H., Cholst, I. *et al.* (1986). Observations in a preliminary open trial of estradiol therapy for senile dementia-Alzheimer's type. *Psychoneuroendocrinology*, **11**, 337–45.

Francis, P.T., Palmer, A.M., Snape M., and Wilcock G.K. (1999). The cholinergic hypothesis of Alzheimer's disease: a review of progress. *Journal of Neurology, Neurosurgery and Psychiatry*, **66**, 137–47.

Francis, P.T., Nordberg, A., and Arnold, S.E. (2005). A preclinical view of cholinesterase inhibitors in neuroprotection: do they provide more than symptomatic benefits in Alzheimer's disease? 1. *Trends in Pharmacological Science*, **26**, 104–11.

Gauthier, S., Wirth, Y., and Mobius, H.J. (2005). Effects of memantine on behavioural symptoms in Alzheimer's disease patients: an analysis of the Neuropsychiatric Inventory (NPI) data of two randomised, controlled studies. *International Journal of Geriatric Psychiatry*, **20**, 459–64.

Gilman, S., Koller, M., Black, R.S. *et al.* (2005). Clinical effects of Abeta immunization (AN1792) in patients with AD in an interrupted trial. *Neurology*, **64**, 1553–62.

Hashimoto, M., Kazui, H., Matsumoto, K., Nakano, Y., Yasuda, M., and Mori, E. (2005). Does donepezil treatment slow the progression of hippocampal atrophy in patients with Alzheimer's disease? *American Journal of Psychiatry*, **162**, 676–82.

Henderson, V.W., Paganini-Hill, A., Miller, B.L. *et al.* (2000). Estrogen for Alzheimer's disease in women. Randomized, double blind, placebo-controlled trial. *Neurology*, **54**, 295–301.

Hock, C., Konietzko, U., Streffer, J.R. *et al.* (2003). Antibodies against beta-amyloid slow cognitive decline in Alzheimer's disease. *Neuron*, **38**, 547–54.

Kaduszkiewicz, H., Zimmermann, T., Beck-Bornholdt, H.P., and van den Bussche, B.H. (2005). Cholinesterase inhibitors for patients with Alzheimer's disease: systematic review of randomised clinical trials. *British Medical Journal*, **331**, 321–7.

Knapp, J.M., Knopman, D.S., Soloman P.R. *et al.* (1994). A 30-week randomized controlled trial of high-dose tacrine in patients with Alzheimer's disease. The Tacrine Study Group. *Journal of the American Medical Association*, **271**, 985–91.

Levy, M.L., Cummings, J.L., and Kahn-Rose, R. (1999). Neuropsychiatric symptoms and cholinergic therapy for Alzheimer's disease. *Gerontology*, **45**(Suppl. 1), 15–22.

NICE (2001). *Technology appraisal guidance no. 19*. National Institute for Clinical Excellence, London.

National Institute for Health and Clinical Excellence (2006). *NICE technology appraisal guidance 111: Donepezil, galantamine, rivastigmine (review) and memantine for the treatment of Alzheimer's diesease*. NICE, London.

Nicoll, J.A.R., Wilkinson, D.G., Holmes, C., Steart, P., Markham, H., and Weller, R. (2003). Neuropathology of human Alzheimer's disease after immunisation with amyloid beta-peptide: a case report. *Nature Medicine*, **9**, 448–52.

Nitsch, R.M., Slack, B.E., Wurtman, R.J., and Growdon, J.H. (1992). Release of Alzheimer amyloid precursor derivatives stimulated by activation of muscarinic acetylcholine receptors. *Science*, **258**, 304–7.

Ohkura, T., Isse, K., Akazawa, K., Hamamoto, M., Yaoi, Y., and Hagino, N. (1995). Long-term estrogen replacement therapy in female patients with dementia of the Alzheimer type: 7 case reports. *Dementia*, **6**, 99–107.

Panisset, M., Roudier, M., Saxton, J., and Boller, F. (1994). Severe impairment battery. A neuropsychological test for severely demented patients. *Archives of Neurology*, **51**, 41–5.

Pelosi, A.J., McNulty, S.V., and Jackson, G.A. (2006). Role of cholinesterase inhibitors in dementia care needs rethinking. *British Medical Journal*, **333**, 491–3.

Perry, E.K., Gibson, P.H., Blessed, G. *et al.* (1977). Neurotransmitter enzyme abnormalities in senile dementia. Choline acetyl-transferase and glutamic acid decarboxlyase activities in necropsy brain tissue. *Journal of Neurological Science*, **34**, 247–65.

Petersen, R.C., Thomas, R.G., Grundman, M. *et al.* (2005).Vitamin E and donepezil for the treatment of mild cognitive impairment. *New England Journal of Medicine*, **352**, 2379–88.

Rapp, S.R., Espeland, M.A., Shumaker, S.A. *et al.* (2003). Effect of estrogen plus progestin on global cognitive function in postmenopausal women: the Women's Health Initiative Memory Study: a randomized controlled trial. *Journal of the American Medical Association*, **289**, 2663–72.

Raskind, M.A., Peskind, E.R., Wessel, T., and Yuan, W. (2000). Galantamine in Alzheimer's disease: a six-month randomised, placebo-controlled trial with a 6-month extension. *Neurology*, **54**, 2261–8.

Reisberg, B., Doody, R., Stoffler, A., Schmitt, F., Ferris, S., and Mobius, H.J. (2003). Memantine in moderate-to-severe Alzheimer's disease. *New England Journal of Medicine*, **348**, 1333–1341.

Rogers J., Kirby, L.C., Hempelman, S.R. *et al.*(1993). Clinical trial of indomethacin in Alzheimer's disease. *Neurology*, **43**, 1609–11.

Rogers, S.L., Farlow, M.R., Doody, R.S., Mohs, R., and Friedhoff, L.T. (1998). A 24-week,double-blind, placebo-controlled trial of donepezil in patients with Alzheimer's disease. Donepezil Study Group. *Neurology*, **50**, 136–45.

Rogers, S.L., Doody, R.S., Pratt, R.D., and Ieni, J.R. (2000). Long-term efficacy and safety of donepezil in the treatment of Alzheimer's disease: final analysis of a US multicentre open-label study. *European Neuropsychopharmacology*, **10**, 195–203.

Rosen, W.G., Mohs, R.C., and Davis K.L. (1984). A new rating scale for Alzheimer's disease. *American Journal of Psychiatry*, **141**, 1356–64.

Rösler, M., Anand, R., Cicin-Sain, A. *et al.* (1999). Efficacy and safety of rivastigmine in patients with Alzheimer's disease: international randomised controlled trial. *British Medical Journal*, **318**, 633–8.

Sano, M., Ernesto, C., Thomas, R.G. *et al.* (1997). A controlled trial of selegiline, alpha-tocopherol, or both as treatment for Alzheimer's disease. The Alzheimer's Disease Co-operative Study. *New England Journal of Medicine*, **336**, 1216–22.

Schenk, D., Barbour, R., Dunn, W *et al.* (1999). Immunization with amyloid-beta attenuates Alzheimer-disease-like pathology in the PDAPP mouse. [see comments] *Nature*, **400**, 173–7.

Schmitt, F.A., Ashford, W., Ernesto, C. *et al.* (1997).The severe impairment battery: concurrent validity and the assessment of longitudinal change in Alzheimer's disease. The Alzheimer's Disease Cooperative Study. *Alzheimer Disease and Associated Disorders*, **11**(Suppl. 2), S51–S56.

Schneider, A., Anand, R., and Farlow, M. (1998). Systematic review of the efficacy of rivastigmine for patients with Alzheimer's disease. *International Journal of Geriatric Psychopharmacology*, **1**(Suppl. 1), S26–S34.

Sclan, S.G. and Reisberg, B. (1992). Functional assessment staging (FAST) in Alzheimer's disease: reliability, validity, and ordinality. *International Psychogeriatrics*, **4**(Suppl. 1), 55–69.

Shumaker, S.A., Legault, C., Rapp, S.R. *et al.* (2003). Estrogen plus progestin and the incidence of dementia and mild cognitive impairment in postmenopausal women: the Women's Health Initiative Memory Study: a randomized controlled trial. *Journal of the American Medical Association*, **289**, 2651–62.

Siemers, E.R., Quinn, J.F., Kaye, J. *et al.* (2006). Effects of a gamma-secretase inhibitor in a randomized study of patients with Alzheimer disease. *Neurology*, **66**, 602–4.

Solomon, B. (2001). Immunotherapeutic strategies for prevention and treatment of Alzheimer's disease. *DNA Cell Biology*, **20**, 697–703.

Tang, M.X., Jacobs, D., Stern Y. *et al.* (1996). Effect of oestrogen during menopause on risk and age at onset of Alzheimer's disease. *Lancet*, **348**, 429–32.

Tariot, P.N., Solomon, P.R., Morris, J.C. *et al.* (2000). A 5-month, randomized, placebo-controlled trial of galantamine in AD. *Neurology*, **54**, 2269–76.

Tariot, P.N., Farlow, M.R., Grossberg, G.T., Graham, S.M., McDonald, S., and Gergel, I. (2004). Memantine treatment in patients with moderate to severe Alzheimer disease already receiving donepezil: a randomized controlled trial. *Journal of the American Medical Association*, **291**, 317–24.

Trinh, N.H., Hoblyn, J., Mohanty, S., and Yaffe, K. (2003). Efficacy of cholinesterase inhibitors in the treatment of neuropsychiatric symptoms and functional impairment in Alzheimer disease: a meta-analysis. *Journal of the American Medical Association*, **289**, 210–216.

Tuszynski, M.H., Thal, L., Pay, M. *et al.* (2005). A phase 1clinical trial of nerve growth factor gene therapy for Alzheimer disease. *Nature Medicine*, **11**, 551–5.

Venneri, A., McGeown, W.J., and Shanks, M.F. (2005). Empirical evidence of neuroprotection by dual cholinesterase inhibition in Alzheimer's disease. *Neuroreport*, **16**, 107–10.

Wang, P.N., Liao, S.Q., Liu, R.S. *et al.* (2000). Effects of estrogen on cognition, mood, and cerebral blood flow in AD: a controlled study. *Neurology*, **54**, 2061–6.

Weggen, S., Eriksen, J.L., Das, P. *et al.* (2001). A subset of NSAIDs lower amyloidogenic Abeta42 independently of cyclooxygenase activity. *Nature*, **414**, 212–16.

Weggen, S., Eriksen, J.L., Sagi, S.A. *et al.* (2003). Evidence that nonsteroidal anti-inflammatory drugs decrease amyloid beta 42 production by direct modulation of gamma-secretase activity. *Journal of Biological Chemistry*, **278**, 31831–7.

Wilcock, G.K. and Lilienfeld, S. (2000). Galantamine alleviates caregiver burden in Alzheimer's disease: a 6-month placebo-controlled study. *World Alzheimer Congress July 2000, Washington, DC* (unpublished poster presentation).

Wilcock, G.K., Lilienfeld, S., and Gaens, E. (2000). Efficacy and safety of galantamine in patients with mild to moderate Alzheimer's disease: multi-centre randomised controlled trial. *British Medical Journal*, **321**, 1445–9.

Wilcock, G., Black, S., Haworth, J. *et al* (2006). Efficacy and safetyof MPC-7869 (R-flurbiprofen), a selective Ab42-lowering agent, in Alzheimer's disease(AD): results of a 12-month phase 2 trial and 1-year follow-on study. *Alzheimer's and Dementia*, **2**(Suppl. 1), S81.

Wimo, A., Wetterholm, A.L., Mastey, V., and Winblad, B. (1998). Evaluation of the healthcare resource utilisation and caregiver time in anti-dementia drug trials. In *Health economics of dementia* (ed. A. Wimo, B. Jonsson, G. Karlsson, and B. Winblad), pp. 465–99. John Wiley, Chichester.

Winblad, B., Kilander, L., Eriksson, S. *et al.* (2006). Donepezil in patients with severe Alzheimer's disease: double-blind, parallel-group, placebo-controlled study. *Lancet*, **367**, 1057–65.

# Clinical aspects of dementia: the management of dementia

Jane Pearce

## Introduction

Dementia is a progressive disorder with continually changing implications for management. While patterns of progression are variable, and change in the contextual factors may be unpredictable, some future needs can be anticipated. The core principles of management are: maximizing adaptation, maintaining function, taking due account of risks, and planning for the future at each stage of the disorder. Changes in the carers' state of health and personal resources, and other stressors in their lives, will be important for the well-being of the patient.

With increasing dependence on others, the person with dementia may come under the care of different services and in new environments. Their family will be faced with difficult decisions: How will I know when the time has come for him or her to go into nursing care? How long can she stay at home? Are these reasonable risks? However, moves to new environments and new staff bring new risks, some of which might be subtle and non-technical; for example the quality of knowledge about the person as an individual can become degraded. This may not only affect quality of daily life but might impede decision-making about future emotive and significant changes in emphasis of care. How do we spot the signs that the time has come for a shift from adaptive to palliative care? Symptoms in late stage dementia are comparable to those in patients with the late stages of cancer but strategies to manage symptoms of pain and low mood are required for longer periods.

Information-sharing is a central part of management. The professional has an early primary task to establish with the patient his or her consent for assessment and treatment. Although most research has focused on the disclosure of diagnosis, much of the resulting management will revolve around the non-technical aspects of dementia. Helping patients establish their values for their future care and constructive involvement of significant others are other early tasks. Work may be needed to maximize people's capacity to recognize the importance of key people in their lives now that they have dementia. This needs to be done before they can give consent to involving these people in information exchange and planning. Friends, family, and formal helpers or carers may well have been concerned with the effects of the person's changing capacities and may have been making delicate decisions about how much and how soon to intervene before professional help was sought.

Sensitivity to the pre-existing responsibilities, relationships, and feelings of these 'important others' requires active management in parallel. Family members' own experiences and values will influence the way in which they wish to be involved and the capacities they bring to the emotive and challenging matters such as risk, restriction of liberty, conflict of interests, and the demands of end-of-life decisions. Poor communication or failure to adapt to changed roles may lead to inferior outcomes for the patient.

This chapter will therefore consider the engagement of the patient and family or other carers in collaborative planning for management. It will also discuss specific management issues including the broad principles and current evidence base for the management of behavioural and psychological symptoms. Other specific issues discussed will include best practice in information-sharing, approaches to maintaining daily pleasurable activity, communication, interventions with families, and issues for palliative care. This chapter will not cover the specific pharmacological treatments for Alzheimer's disease (see Chapter 27viii).

## Assessment

A process of assessment and reassessment is the basis of management since dementia is a progressive condition. Assessment covers the presenting problem(s), current functional ability of the patient, any risks of harm to self or to others, the patient's social circumstances, and the ability of the caregiver to provide the type of care needed. It is also necessary to screen for concurrent physical and psychological conditions. While it is necessary to take a broad approach because of the range of effects that dementia has, it is crucial to focus on specific areas in order to ensure that, where there are interventions of known efficacy, these are applied.

### Definition of presenting problems and current functional ability

In the present chapter we focus on the collection of information: a precise description of the presenting problems, their nature, and history of their onset is required. There are a number of behavioural and psychological symptoms of dementia which lead to morbidity in patients and carers. Behaviours include agitation and restlessness, physical aggression, sleep disturbance, screaming or shouting, disinhibition, inappropriate control of continence or expression of sexuality, abnormal patterns of eating, and wandering or shadowing people. Psychological symptoms include low mood, anxiety, hallucinations, delusions, misidentifications, and apathy.

A functional assessment is important in order to establish the patient's strengths and weaknesses, and standardized assessment tools are helpful to track changes. Functional activity reflects motor, perceptual skills (including visual), cognitive abilities, and general well-being. It is generally thought of as having two main aspects: firstly basic activities of daily living (BADL) such as self-care and self-maintenance skills (washing, bathing, dressing, maintaining continence, eating, transferring, grooming); secondly the more complex skills that relate to the roles adults perform in order to live independently in the community—the instrumental activities of daily living (IADL). The latter include social and occupational activities that are multifaceted and require organizational and planning skills. Carers can find it helpful to be involved in assessments of strengths and weaknesses, as well as monitoring using standardized rating scales.

## Risk assessment

Risks are common in dementia, and systematic consideration of risk may therefore be valuable. Risk assessment refers to a method of weighing the probability of the range of outcomes that might arise (Vinestock, 1996). Relevant questions are:

◆ Is there a risk of harm?

◆ If so, what sort of harm, to whom, and what is the likely severity?

◆ How likely is it to happen?

◆ How immediate is the risk and how long will it last?

◆ What factors contribute to the risk?

◆ How can these factors be modified or managed?

In dementia there are risks of harm occurring both to the patient and to others. Risk will change with the progression of the disorder and therefore should be reviewed regularly. Risks to self may result from specific behaviours, from diminished mastery of the environment, and through vulnerability from the actions of others. Risk related to psychiatric disorder, such as the risk of deliberate self-harm, also needs to be considered. Alcohol misuse may already be an aetiological factor for the dementia, but forgetfulness may also lead social drinkers to lose control and thus compound the cognitive losses. Inability or unwillingness to accept help when needed for nutrition and other basic daily needs can result in poor physical health and well-being. Wandering can result in falling or getting lost in unsafe areas. Falls are significantly more common in dementia, and occur particularly to people who have relatively well-preserved functional capability. They are associated with the use of medication, wandering, and current acute confusion and may indicate the need for a greater level of supervision (CHSR, 1998). There is a particular risk of falls in dementia with Lewy bodies (McKeith *et al.*, 2005).

The dependency needs associated with dementia, and the consequent potential for emotional stress on caregivers, can make the person with dementia more vulnerable to physical, emotional, financial, or sexual abuse and exploitation from those on whom he or she depends (APA, 1997). Particular vigilance may be indicated where carers are poorly supported, where there is misuse of alcohol, or where there are pre-existing relationship problems. Complicating factors include the dementia sufferer's limited ability to protest and, sometimes, their reluctance to receive outside help.

Risk to others may be posed by aggressive behaviours, for example in the context of personal care or when carers act to stop the person wandering out at night. Verbal aggression is the commonest form and the longest lasting in the course of dementia. Serious aggression is rare but aggressive resistance and physical aggression are most prevalent among people with more severe dementia and may persist until death (Keene *et al.*, 1999). The presence of delusions is an important association with physical violence (Deutsch *et al.*, 1991). Indicators of increased risk of dangerous aggression include conflict with others, a previous episode of serious aggression, sudden changes in the environment as well as psychiatric co-morbidity (Hindley and Gordon, 2000).

Other sources of hazards in the patient's own environment include fire risks from inappropriate use of electrical appliances and smoking habits, public health risks from failure to handle refuse and household hygiene, and risks of affray from accusations of theft and trespass made to people around. The risk associated with accidents from driving is considered elsewhere in Chapter 44.

## Screening for concurrent physical and psychological illness

In the person with dementia presentation of physical illness may be masked by lack of complaints about typical symptoms (McCormick *et al.*, 1994). Behavioural change may be the most evident feature. Hence at times of change in well-being, function, or behaviour screening for common conditions by physical examination, blood, and urine tests can be indicated. Common aetiologies include acute infections, electrolyte imbalance, metabolic imbalance, heart failure, and the side-effects of medication (since patients with dementia are prone to adverse effects and are frequently taking multiple medications including those with anticholinergic side-effects). Some physical symptoms such as nocturnal dyspnoea and sleep disturbance may trigger behavioural problems; dysuria may trigger inappropriate exposure of genitals or constipation may trigger inappropriate defaecation. A source of pain or physical discomfort may trigger noise-making or agitation, aggression, or sleep disturbance. Liaison with geriatricians may be important in informing decisions about useful pathways of investigation.

Finally it is important to consider co-morbidity with psychiatric disorder. Where behaviours are aggressive or agitated it is particularly important to look actively for signs of psychosis and depression (CHSR, 1998). Anxiety disorders are common, particularly in mild dementia, but may be obscured by cognitive symptoms (Wands *et al.*, 1990; Ballard *et al.*, 1994). It is suggested that there are subgroups of anxious patients with dementia: autonomic and situational anxiety; anxiety with depression; and anxiety with psychotic symptoms (Ballard *et al.*, 1996b). Depressive disorder is also common and the prevalence is higher in nursing homes (Ballard *et al.*, 1996a). Patients' responses to enquiry about symptoms and signs of depression or anxiety can be affected by dementia-related impairment in concentration, memory, and judgement.

Depression reduces communication skills and performance on independent activities of daily living (Fitz and Teri, 1994). The depression may therefore be misidentified as a primary progression of the dementia. Secondly, classic descriptions helpfully remind us that 'depressive ideas are fragmentary and transient' and that the 'mood change is short lived and shallow' particularly in more severe dementia (Roth, 1955). Thirdly, biological symptoms may be obscured by features of dementia affecting eating, sleeping, and motor activity. However, where there is a personal or family history of depression or recent adverse events such as bereavement or relocation, the likelihood of depression being present is increased (CHSR, 1998). Carers' observations of recent changes in activity and behaviour will often be useful. The validity of utilizing a carer observation-based assessment for depression in dementia is demonstrated in the Cornell Scale (a rating scale devised for monitoring the progress of depression in dementia; Alexopoulos *et al.*, 1988). Carers assess the behaviour in five domains of function, namely mood-related signs, behavioural disturbance, physical signs, cyclic functions, and ideational disturbance.

### Carer assessment

Assessment of the social circumstances includes reviewing the caregiver's ability to provide the type of care needed, current use of formal carer services, and the quality and adequacy of the caregiver's own social and family support systems. Changes in carers' state of health and personal resources, and other stressors in their lives, should be assessed. Physical illness in carers may also be important and may too be masked, for example being rationalized as stress or exhaustion. Symptoms may be minimized because of the concerns they have about the consequences for the person for whom they care.

## General principles of management

### Management plans

A management plan should address support, adaptation, and adjustment related to functional decline and progressive cognitive loss, the social context of living, and requirements of carers, and take account of any risks that have been identified (core management). For the functional impairments the early needs will be in the domain of information, advice, and monitoring. Useful areas include advice on developing structure and routine in daily life, the adoption of memory aids, reduction in complexity of tasks and activities, optimizing communication, together with guidance on basic self-care such as nutrition, sleep, and exercise. General management plans should be regularly reviewed and updated in the light of the changing capacities of the patient, changes for carers, and should be forward looking. While patterns of progression are variable and change in the contextual factors may be unpredictable, some future needs can be anticipated.

When specific problems are present, targeted interventions with clear goals and regular monitoring to evaluate effectiveness and to detect any adverse consequences are used. Where interventions are complex, and in particular where potential risks occur, priorities for intervention must first be established. The risk management should be shared with the patient, carers, and other workers. Differences of opinion need to be talked through and, when decisions are made, the basis of these should be made clear and understandable.

Often several agencies will be involved when plans are more complex and monitoring of service provision is therefore important (SSI, 1997). Have the promised services been delivered and has the patient accepted or refused them? Where risk remains high despite attempts to ameliorate it, compulsion may become necessary. Guardianship under the Mental Health Act may offer

an appropriate framework, for example enabling careworkers to enter a person's home despite initial barriers. Hospital admission may be used to enable further assessment and development of a care plan and to provide periods of more intensive evaluation with trained staff available throughout the 24 hours. The Mental Health Act provisions may be needed for admission when community interventions are unsuccessful, particularly when patients are unable to recognize their need for care and actively refuse help.

### Collaborative care

Integration of care is clinically recognized as important. A network of care may include primary care, social and personal care services, and mental health teams. Services may include domiciliary care, day care, or residential care. Unless there are specific reasons why not, the patient and their family member (or friend) who is most closely involved in their care should be part of the network. Identifying the friends and family members who should be part of the network is an important task. Thought should be given to how involvement in planning and information sharing can be maximized for the patient with sensitivity to the responsibilities, relationships, and feelings that are involved. Obtaining consent and agreement as to what and how information will be shared is an early goal in management. There may at times be valid reasons for not involving the patient in the care planning. However, there is evidence to demonstrate that people with dementia can participate in family meetings (Jeffery, 1987; Benbow *et al.*, 1993). Specific techniques to facilitate communication are described below. For people with dementia who live alone the home carer often becomes one of the most significant relationships in their life. The home carer may become important in expressing the voice of the patient and in giving the 'user view' (SSI, 1997). Their participation in care reviews is therefore very important.

Not all people with a dementia will be under specialist mental health services and primary care may play a key role. When there is use of specialist mental health services, the care programme approach (CPA) has to be applied (Department of Health, 1990). The CPA requires that the patient has a key worker, that there is full assessment of health and social needs, that a care plan is agreed with the patient and his or her main carers, and that a record is made of unmet needs. Liaison needs to be especially good when risks are present so that all involved share and understand the concerns, detect increases in risk, and know who to communicate with about such changes. Liaison with primary care can help ensure that the forgetful person continues to receive health promotion, e.g. care for chronic illnesses, treatment of osteoporosis, managing stroke risk factors, and access to influenza vaccination.

### Carer and family involvement

It is not only the carer–patient relationship that is affected in dementia (Garwick *et al.*, 1994): the carer's own relationships with other family members such as adult children and siblings may also be affected. Ripple effects occur in families as the change in one set of relationships has implications for other relationships. Sometimes the family may be able to serve as an important buffering for a carer and the level of stress he or she carries. Nodal points in the illness such as decisions whether a person with dementia should move to another residence can be a point of crisis within a family. Management of emotion to enhance mutual support can be valuable, and consistency and continuity of family support networks is a predictor for lower caregiver burden. Carer needs are dealt with elsewhere and are a central part of the management of dementia.

When dementia is of early onset the immediate impact on family relationships may include children still living at home. There may be shifts in family relationships with increased closeness to the caregiving parent, sadness at the loss of the affected parent, and needs for more support and genetic counselling (Harvey, 1998). Children also experience frustration on seeing that their parent's practical needs are not appropriately met and may want training for themselves in coping with challenging behaviour.

Younger patients are relatively more likely to have frontotemporal and alcohol-related dementias and hence they more commonly experience focal symptoms such as dysphasia and behavioural disturbance (Seltzer and Sherwin, 1983; Harvey, 1998). These can be disruptive of family relationships and associated with carer stress. The potential for carer stress is increased also because of the impact of dementia on lifestyle in a younger family with adults holding work and child-raising roles. Sexual relationships may also be more disrupted, with extremes both of loss of sexual intimacy and also, in a minority, of abnormal increase in sexual drive. In dementia in Down's syndrome the earlier the age of presentation the higher the frequency of behavioural and personality change (Holland *et al.*, 2000). Here the family unit may involve older carers and precipitate the need for changes in established caring relationships.

Consideration also has to be given to the wide range of family structures among different ethnic groups and to the wide variation of family groupings within cultures. The notion that ethnic minorities have high levels of family integration is as simplistic as are assumptions about family roles and duties of care among ethnic minorities.

## Specific management issues and interventions

### Engaging the patient

The primary care team is important in identifying dementia and initiating contact with health and other services. The primary care response to presented problems is shaped by the patient's response to their illness as well as by their family members' concerns and expectations. Referral may result from the concerns of people other than the patient and a route to assessment should be found that an individual is most comfortable with. There may be a range of barriers to accepting referral, particularly where denial or lack of insight is present. Difficulties can also arise when the initial symptomatology is disruptive of relationships or includes paranoia or anxiety. Mental health teams can support the primary care team in the pre-referral stage.

A preliminary risk assessment may be useful if there is considerable reluctance on the part of a patient or over-zealous concern by friends or neighbours. GP guidelines may be helpful in the pre-referral phase advising on indicators of the presence of dementia (CHSR, 1998) and preliminary physical investigation (Haines and Katona, 1992). Firstly the guidance suggests that history of loss of function is more indicative of dementia than is the complaint of subjective memory impairment. The four domains of instrumental activities of daily living significantly associated with cognitive impairment are: managing medication, using the telephone, coping with a budget, and using transportation. Secondly it is recommended

that formal cognitive testing is used to enhance clinical judgement since the GP's clinical judgment alone compares unfavourably with the use of formal cognitive testing in the diagnosis of dementia. Evidence-based guidelines support the usual clinical practice of non-use of compulsion; it is unusual to use mental health legislation to overcome practical difficulties or lack of cooperation with investigations (Royal College of Psychiatrists, 1995).

A common point of concern or interest between patient and referrer needs to be established. Bridges may be built through attention on a physical health focus for some, through the investigation offered by a memory clinic for others, while for other people assessment of cognitive function may only be possible once a community psychiatric nurse has built up the person's trust and confidence. A variety of routes of referral and venues for first consultations are needed in order to provide flexibility and sensitivity to what the patient is willing to accept. Additional barriers may exist for ethnic minority users; training community ethnic group liaison and link workers may open routes to services.

Standard services for dementia in older populations are inadequate to meet the needs of younger people with dementia, and specialist services are recommended (Royal College of Psychiatrists and Alzheimer's Society, 2006). Given generic dementia service provisions, patients with younger onset dementia use fewer community services but more institutional care. Financial implications may also be more serious for patients with younger onset dementia since both the patient's and the spouse's work may be required in order to support the family. Opportunities and earning potential are threatened by the dementia, and the loss of one's job may in turn affect pension rights. Moreover, the need for care may mean that both the patient's and the carer's jobs may be threatened. In contrast where onset is later, patients will already be adjusted to living on a pension without paid employment.

Standard service settings designed for the majority may also fail to meet the needs of patients from ethnic minority groups. However, intra-ethnic group variation is greater than inter-ethnic group variation and the experiences of people with dementia and their carers show that the important issues for service providers to consider are language, religious belief and observance, cultural practices (including food and personal care practices), and social support and coping mechanisms; but these issues, it is argued, are applicable to all individuals with dementia, independent of apparent ethnicity. Promotion of cultural competence in service provision should not be relegated to an ethnic minority agenda (Iliffe and Manthorpe, 2004).

Despite this there are some specific issues to be considered in meeting needs appropriately. Dementia contributes to loss of the second language and reversion to mother tongue may confound accuracy of diagnosis. In addition to educational and cultural factors, incorrect assumptions about literacy, and the misunderstanding of certain concepts can result in overestimating cognitive loss while missing other functional reasons for deterioration in a person's function (Bhatnagar and Frank, 1997). Some members of ethnic minorities may suffer greater disability from cognitive impairment because of poorer physical health, disadvantaged economic circumstances, or social isolation (Manthorpe and Hettiaratchy, 1993). A subgroup may have been exposed to trauma arising from social upheaval, prior displacement (especially among refugees), and other adverse circumstances that are related to migration. They may feel more isolated from their own community, in particular from younger generations who cannot share their memories. The losses of dementia (in particular loss of control and autonomy) may also trigger the re-emergence of past traumatic experiences (Miesen and Jones, 1997).

Ethno-sensitive care therefore requires more than provision of translation services. Liaison workers educated in mental health may play a helpful role when services do not have staff from the similar ethnic background.

## Information-sharing

Involvement of patients in information exchange and decision-making at all stages of their illness is good practice and the value of maintaining a truthful relationship with a patient is part of professional practice. At the outset of assessment it is helpful to seek permission for disclosure to family or carers.

Disclosure of the diagnosis is the most studied area of information-sharing in dementia. There is evidence that health professionals have been reluctant to tell patients that their diagnosis is of dementia (Bamford et al., 2004). Research indicates that patients generally would like to know about the diagnosis and prognosis of dementia (Turnbull et al., 2003). For some, withholding of diagnosis is distressing and a study of carers has identified that both uncertain diagnosis and late diagnosis is unhelpful to patients (Bamford et al., 2004). When their reactions to the diagnosis were sought, patients frequently offer positive views, including opportunities for advance planning, and benefit from understanding what is happening to them (Beattie et al., 2004; Carpenter, 2004). The skills required of professionals in diagnostic disclosure are similar to those used in other serious illnesses such as cancer. Diagnostic disclosure is not a one-off event, and patient-led discussion is applicable with adjustment and compensation for the current level of cognitive impairment.

Carers may sometimes attempt to steer their relative away from such discussion and it is important to consider whether discussion of the diagnosis should be carried out jointly with a carer or alone with the patient. Family members may be reluctant to have their relative learn the truth despite indicating that they would like to be told if it were themselves developing the illness (Maguire et al., 1996; Barnes et al., 1997; Bamford et al., 2004). This is one of many difficult decisions with which carers and family members become involved in dementia. It is suggested that carers should think about a range of questions in deciding whether or not to tell the person the truth. Examples of useful questions are 'Will not telling the truth make things more difficult in the long run?' 'If the situation were reversed would you want to know the truth?' (Alzheimer's Society, 2005, pp. 64–73). In some instances there will be personal health implications for the family, such as in Huntington's disease when genetic counselling should be offered for family members. Where an argument has been made that disadvantages of disclosing the diagnosis are thought to outweigh advantages, this should be clearly recorded in the patient's notes.

Following discussion of diagnosis patients should be helped to use the information positively. Specific pharmacological treatments for the dementia should be considered. A detailed account of these treatments is given elsewhere in this book and will not be repeated here (see previous sections of Chapter 27).

A collaborative approach to decision-making should continue. For example, patients should be helped to plan for their own interests and autonomy (including organizing finances, choices of medication, which family and friends to involve, and making advanced directives for future health care). Helping people to identify their values is thought to assist them in thinking about, and making, health-care choices. An example of a tool to assist is the Values History Form (Institute for Ethics, University of New Mexico). This invites a person to think in a structured way about the beliefs, preferences, and values that matter most to him or her personally in making health-care choices. How do we feel about our overall health? What personal relationships in our lives are important to us? How do we feel about independence or dependence? About pain, illness, dying, and death? What are our goals for the future? The discussion of such considerations could be helpful to carers and family in future when participating in difficult decisions. Narrative-based approaches can also be helpful by building up and recording stories about the 'Person'. These can inform care decisions when consent and capacity are compromised, for example in decisions as to the use of assistive technology such as electronic tagging to reduce risks (Astell, 2006).

Carers need to be informed of diagnosis and what to expect in the future. They need to be informed about what services and interventions can help. When carers are asked about their experiences in relation to diagnosis they talk of the importance of information and support being available to them and the affected person after they know the diagnosis (Hughes et al., 2002; Alzheimer's Society, 2005). They also describe distress in the context of a wide range of difficult decisions both before and after the diagnosis of dementia is made. There are decisions to be made about what behaviours are acceptable, taking over control, how much risk-taking is right. Many of these are more difficult because of the ways in which they are tied up with the well-being of the carer themselves. There are problems for carers in balancing their own needs with those of the person with dementia. Further difficulties arise where there are pre-existing ambivalent relationships, current ambivalence, and the presence of paranoia (for example leading to accusations or misidentification of the carer). Family carers are helped in their caring roles through shared decision-making with the professionals and other supporters.

## Maximizing communication

Communication can be affected early on in dementia with receptive or expressive dysphasias. The pragmatics of language (turn-taking and topic management) may also be affected. Reduced ability to communicate has an impact on relationships as well as on the well-being of the patient and the early stages of management. Specific attention to compensating for functional language loss is relevant to everyone involved. Steps taken will include attempting to use a calm and organized environment which is free of distractions; sensory input, both hearing and vision, should be maximized and clear initiation of conversation may be established by use of face-to-face contact or touch; the matters to be discussed should be simplified and presented one idea at a time. Orientation to the topic of conversation may help, as well as written prompts and reminders. Gesture may remain intact and may be helpful. The person, or those who know him or her well, can help determine in which way they can be assisted if they get stuck. For example, does sentence completion help or make things worse? Reassurance and support for frustration needs to be given when this occurs.

Speech and language therapists can be of help in providing more information about communication skills and deficits and in giving advice on maximizing current skills. Helpful techniques include vocabulary access by semantic and/or phonemic cueing, circumlocution, and gesture. Communication strategies have been demonstrated to reduce professional and family carer stress (Ripich, 1994). Validation therapy is an approach to communication which acknowledges and supports the feelings of a disorientated person in whatever reality they experience rather than grounding them in the here and now (Neal and Barton Wright, 2003).

## Maintaining function through pleasurable activities

Loss of opportunity to engage in pleasurable and rewarding activities is important both for the individual and for carers since such losses contribute to a vicious cycle of less communication, lower mood, less participation in any activity, and increased dependence on others. As the disease progresses there needs to be an on-going process of finding activities within the person's ability, and a structured approach can be helpful. Carers who are aware of appropriate and enjoyable activities enjoy an improved sense of efficacy and reduced feelings of burden (Teri and Logsdon, 1991).

There may also be a preventive role; for example in residential settings the combination of structured exercise and conversation (but not either alone) may reduce deterioration in mobility (Cott et al., 2002). In addition there is evidence that attention to the social, environmental, and cultural aspects of meal times as well as enhanced menus can play a role in prevention of weight loss (Keller et al., 2003; Manthorpe and Watson, 2003).

## Managing behavioural and psychological symptoms

Here we will deal with broad principles for managing the range of behavioural and psychological symptoms of dementia. A unified approach is justified because there is frequently overlap in presenting features and some common therapeutic interventions.

The management is based on further assessment for and intervention of a range of possible contributory factors. These might lie in the nature of the dementia, in the environment (including those involved in trying to do the supporting), and in the individual who is affected by his or her dementia. Further assessment to identify concurrent physical health problems, sources of physical discomfort (like constipation or pain), and medication side effects will include physical examination and blood tests. Possible concurrent psychological contributory factors (symptoms such as worry, anxiety, and paranoia) should be sought as well as an understanding of the person's characteristic reactions to their circumstances. Habitual ways of reacting to events and everyday life may have been modified by the dementia as well as by the reactions of those around him or her. The availability, nature, and quality of relationships with others as well as their current ability to cope with the needs of the person with dementia will shape behaviour patterns. The characteristics of the care environment should also be considered, for example physical space, comfort, and adaptations to promote independence. Simple interventions including distraction, reassurance, managing physical ailments, space, or good lighting can be effective.

More specific psychosocial interventions in institutional settings have been studied (Opie et al., 1999). Enriched environments (using artefacts, tape-recordings, paintings, etc.) designed to create 'natural' or 'homelike' settings may be used to reduce agitation, aggression, and wandering into others' rooms. Use of colour or curtains to obscure door handles or mirrors by doors may reduce frequency of using doors to exit safe areas. Activity programmes with trained volunteers may reduce aggressive incidents in patients whose wandering occurs in the context of boredom and inactivity. Similarly recordings of preferred music, family members' voices, sensory stimulation, and simple exercise may result in reductions in verbally disruptive behaviours. Dementia-related sleep changes can be helpfully addressed by behavioural techniques, such as caregiver sleep hygiene education and daily walking (McCurry et al., 2005).

When symptoms are persistent, interventions for specific behavioural problems can utilize the structure of the ABC analysis of behaviour (Stokes, 1990). Analysis is made through observation of the Antecedents and Consequences of each problem Behaviour. While in principle antecedent activities should be avoided, frequently these are unavoidable. For example the use of the toilet or bathing may be associated with aggression. Given the difficulty of new learning in patients with dementia, it is suggested that environmental factors and the behaviours of caregivers should be changed. In a community-based randomized controlled study a family carers' 'behavioural management strategy' resulted in a reduction in aggression nearing a significant level (Gormley et al., 2001). This study is of particular interest because carers were able to develop skills in behavioural analysis and were able to devise interventions themselves. Structured, systematically applied, and time-limited interventions carried out under the supervision of professionals have so far been shown to have benefit on affective symptoms (contentment, interest, and improved facial expression), but limited benefit for disruptive behaviour (Teri et al., 1997; Beck et al., 2005).

A recent systematic review has looked at the current evidence for all the psychologically based therapies of neuropsychiatric symptoms in dementia (Livingston et al., 2005). Behavioural management techniques centred on individual behaviours and psycho-educational interventions centred on caregivers' behaviours (individual rather than group intervention) are effective interventions and have lasting benefits. Snoezelen and music therapy can be effective within the treatment session but have no maintained benefits (Koger and Brotons, 2000; Baker et al., 2001; Chung and Lai, 2002). Training for caregivers in behavioural techniques has inconsistent outcomes. Evidence of efficacy is not available for a number of other therapeutic activities (including reality orientation, physical exercise, socialization, and interactive contact or touch). There is a small amount of evidence to commend further study of cognitive stimulation therapy and reminiscence therapy.

If psychosocial or behavioural interventions have limited success, the use of medication may be appropriate. Where any medication is used, particular note should be made of side-effect profiles and potential to worsen confusion, increase the risk of falls, or reduce mobility. Provision should be made for supervision of correct and safe administration.

## Psychosis and aggression

Aggression, agitation, and hallucinations are common in dementia, and although they will often be transient they are correlated with entry into institutional care (Ballard et al., 1991). Current evidence from systematic reviews suggests that the efficacy of typical antipsychotics is limited, and adverse effects are common in the management of psychotic symptoms, aggression, and other behavioural problems (Sink *et al.*, 2005; Ballard *et al.*, 2006). There is evidence of efficacy of the atypical antipsychotics risperidone and olanzapine in reducing aggression and risperidone in reducing psychosis. Risperidone and olanzapine are associated with risks of serious adverse cerebrovascular events and extrapyramidal side-effects which may outweigh the benefits, especially when used in the longer term (Schneider *et al.*, 2005). A clinical decision to use antipsychotics should therefore take into account the risks to patient and carers of the symptoms, the levels of distress, and potentially adverse medication effects. Patients who have stabilized on antipsychotics and are free from behavioural disturbances may not relapse when antipsychotics are withdrawn (Ballard *et al.*, 2004). There are associations between antipsychotic use and poorer prognosis in the dementia (McShane *et al.*, 1997). Neuroleptics should not be used where Lewy body disease is suspected because of the neuroleptic sensitivity syndrome (McKeith *et al.*, 1995).

There is now an accumulating body of evidence in mild to moderate dementia indicating the effectiveness of cholinesterase inhibitors in the non-cognitive symptoms of dementia. Donepezil is associated with reducing psychotic symptoms and a number of behavioural symptoms; there is an indication of effectiveness of galantamine on both 'functional ability' and behaviour (Tariot *et al.*, 2000) and of rivastigmine in the management of associated symptoms in Alzheimer's disease (Anand *et al.*, 2000). Rivastigmine is effective in reducing apathy, anxiety, and hallucinations in Lewy body disease (McKeith *et al.*, 2000).

## Agitation

The herb *Salvia officinalis* has a historical reputation for calming agitation, and this has been upheld by the one small RCT (Akhondzadeh *et al.*, 2003). Trazodone may be considered and one small RCT showed reduced agitation when accompanied by depressive symptoms (Sultzer *et al.*, 2001). Mood stabilizers are not licensed in the UK to treat agitation in dementia. There is some RCT evidence to indicate some beneficial effect of carbamazepine on agitation in severe dementia (Tariot, 1998). Significant adverse effects, including sedation and ataxia, and a range of drug interactions limit its use. There is an absence of evidence to recommend the use of sodium valproate for agitation and related behaviours (Lonergan and Luxenberg, 2004). From the studies available there is no evidence of efficacy at low dose and unacceptable adverse effects at higher dose.

## Sleep disturbance

Sleep disturbance that has not been responsive to practical sleep hygiene interventions may warrant the short-term use of hypnotics. There is no evidence to support the use of melatonin in sleep disturbance in dementia (Serfaty *et al.*, 2002; Singer *et al.*, 2003). There are insufficient data to recommend bright-light therapy for sleep disturbance or agitation (Ancoli-Israel *et al.*, 2003; Fontana Gasio *et al.*, 2003).

## Anxiety

In early dementia, treatment of anxiety with non-pharmacological methods such as relaxation and anxiety management is possible. The actual content of any fears and concerns can be explored. For example, is there fear of losing control or losing the affections of others, or is there experience of stress due to impaired social functioning? Some individuals may be helped by discussion of their memory loss in detail; akin to the way they might discuss their loss of ability to mobilize independently (Knight, 1986). Patient groups, particularly in the early stages of dementia, may be helpful by providing peer support and may assist with coping and problem-solving (Birnie, 1997). Individual psychodynamic work may be considered, again starting early in dementia when facilitation of emotional outlet and grieving for losses can be a realistic goal (Hausman, 1992), although there is no clear evidence to support this.

Anxiolytic medication may be indicated for short periods when anxiety is associated with agitation, or for carrying out a particular procedure such as tooth extraction. However, the use of these may be limited by the side-effects of sedation, worsening confusion, and risk of falls.

## Depression

Treatment of depression is covered in detail elsewhere in this book (see Chapter 29ii). Cognitive and behavioural strategies have been described for managing depression in dementia (Teri and Gallagher-Thompson, 1991). Cognitive strategies are more applicable in mild dementia. Daily thought records can be kept by the patient, and negative thoughts can be challenged in treatment sessions. In this way a number of depressive features such as worthlessness and sleep disturbance can be addressed. A behavioural model is applicable in more severe dementia. The carer tracks their relative's mood and the frequency (and duration) of pleasurable activities. Caregiver training is then used to increase the relative's pleasurable experiences and decrease behavioural disturbances that interfere with opportunities for pleasurable experience (Teri, 1994). The efficacy of behavioural treatment to improve mood has been demonstrated in controlled studies (Teri *et al.*, 1997; Proctor *et al.*, 1999).

It is unclear whether pharmacological treatments work as well in people with dementia as in non-demented older people. The Cochrane Review draws attention to the paucity of research and consequent weak support for the effectiveness of newer antidepressants in depression in dementia (Bains *et al.*, 2002). Careful evaluation of each patient on antidepressant medication is therefore important, and treatment is perhaps best reserved for those with more severe or persistent symptoms. Consideration should also be given to the side-effect profiles of antidepressants, including effects on cognitive function. In practice this means choosing a selective serotonin reuptake inhibitor (SSRI) rather than a tricyclic agent because of the greater tolerability, kinder side-effect profile, and reduced risk of arrhythmias on SSRIs (Glassman, 1998).

## Working with carers and family

It is important for the patient that his or her family and friends adapt to the changes brought about by dementia. Even a family that functions well in terms of its ability to communicate, solve problems, and adapt can be challenged by the changes in function that result from dementia. Providing relevant knowledge may be all that is required for such a family in order for them to be able to adapt their usual ways of communicating about problems and to develop their own solutions. In other cases a family's failed solution to difficulties can be viewed as the problem and can be directly tackled through family problem-focused interventions (Herr and Weakland, 1979). Times of crisis (for example the death of a husband carer) can also present families with tasks that they do not have the resources to tackle. At such times conflicts of interest (for example between siblings over finances or priorities) may arise. Poor communication or failure to adapt to changed roles may also lead to inferior outcomes for the patient. Family interventions may be helpful in these situations (Ratna and Davies, 1984). There is evidence to suggest that brief psychotherapy has no benefit for the dementia sufferer but it may provide some benefits for the carer by improving their reactions to some of the symptoms (Burns *et al.,* 2005).

Where there is a pre-existing history of poor family adaptation and function, dementia may become the latest chapter of a long-term struggle for all concerned (Knight, 1986). Family therapy may be helpful in this situation. Issues of abuse or neglect may also be addressed through family therapy (Goldstein, 1990) and carer stress can usefully be approached using family therapy models (Gilleard *et al.,* 1992).

Family teams who work with older patients and their families have documented their work with patients who have dementia. There is evidence that family interventions may be successfully applied and helpful and that dementia does not preclude using these techniques (Benbow *et al.,* 1993). A variety of models may be applicable for families containing a member with dementia. Models described have included family problem-solving (Bonjean, 1989), systemic (Benbow *et al.,* 1993), and behavioural (Marriott *et al.,* 2000).

A number of useful ideas can be taken from family therapy and applied in everyday work with care networks or within the family groupings around the older person with dementia (Pearce, 2002). For example, a family meeting to decide how to share care, solve a current problem, or simply to impart information and education can be useful. A family forum can also provide an opportunity for professionals to observe family interaction and to assess family coping strategies. It can also provide everyone present with an opportunity to be heard and to face conflicts between family members' own needs and those of the index patient. Emotions of guilt and hostility are common, as are the reactions of avoidance and distancing; these are often associated with tension within relationships.

## Managing later stages

The progression of the disease is associated with the need for others to assume greater levels of responsibility for the person's functioning and with progression through different services and environments. The quality of knowledge about patients as individuals can become degraded. We have already referred to the benefits of narrative-based and values-based assessment, and at this stage use of previously collated narrative about the person can counter this loss when more care is either delivered by professionals or involves an institution. Environmental aspects of care are considered elsewhere in this book (Chapter 24). There are a number of aspects of the environment that will influence their appropriateness for an individual patient's needs. Variables include the physical quality, hygiene, space, and privacy offered by the accommodation as well as social aspects of the environment such as access to appropriate social stimulation and support. In general, simplification,

availability of activity and company, together with provision of necessary safety, are positive features of care environments (Lawton *et al.,* 1989). In institutional settings one needs to consider whether the staff are adequately trained to meet the individual patient's needs in addition to managing the demands from other patients. Commitment to and knowledge of working with dementia is relevant as is the staff's ability to adapt to change with the progression of the disease (Rovner *et al.,* 1996). Staff may or may not have the skills, knowledge, and senior supervision to engage in interventions. Qualities of good care in dementia services are described as 'person centred care' and include promotion of comfort and meeting the need for attachment and feelings of inclusion; meaningful occupation and maintenance of personal identity have been suggested as the key components of psychosocial care in dementia (Kitwood, 1997).

The later stages include terminal care with a resulting shift in emphasis from adaptation to palliative care. General principles from palliative care can usefully be applied (Post and Whitehouse, 1995). Terminal care involves an interdisciplinary approach attending to both the patient's and the family's needs. Palliative measures, limited medical intervention, and non-aggressive treatment of infections may be appropriate but must be combined with a consideration of ethical issues. An important aspect of reassessment is to identify the time for shifts in the balance of care plans to include palliative principles.

Patients with dementia lived on average 8½ years in the 11-year longitudinal study of Hope *et al.* (2001), two-thirds dying in a debilitated state. Seventy-six per cent had spent a mean period of 18 months in an institution prior to death. Over half were hypophagic, a third were unable to walk, and three-quarters were incontinent of urine. In a retrospective study of the experience of dying with dementia the most frequent symptoms in addition to cognitive loss in the last year of life were urinary incontinence, pain, low mood, constipation, and the loss of appetite (McCarthy *et al.,* 1997). These symptoms are comparable to those in patients with cancer but dementia patients suffered them for longer periods. The high frequency of reports both of pain and of low mood in the last year of life requires further research. This finding is consistent with clinical experience and reminds us of the importance of developing appropriate strategies of management.

Carer and family needs in this stage include positive affirmation and good communication with staff in long-term care settings. Those family and friends who have previously been key carers might experience a variety of emotional and moral dilemmas. Carers may need to be given permission to withdraw at this stage (Bonnel, 1996). Their personal thoughts and wishes that the person might die should be recognized. Validation of the past caring is important but may not be offered by long-term care settings which did not know the sufferer or carer personally during the preceding stages of the illness. A communication strategy at this stage requires that one determines what the family's expectations are about the roles, if any, that they want to take in planning, the support they need for this, and about the type of feedback they are hoping for from the care staff.

Again family members may suffer distress when participating in decision-making on behalf of their affected relative. Many decisions in the later stages are emotive such as feeding, nutrition, and treatment of potentially fatal events. Professional attitudes and priorities may be at variance with those of family and adequate dialogue without dominance of the more medical values at the expense of those of carers is necessary (Coetzee *et al.*, 2003). Clear information on the consequences of possible intervention and alternatives should be provided, together with encouragement to explore the values and desires of family members as well as the perceptions of the values and desires of the sufferer (Eggenberger and Nelms, 2004). Adequate dialogue between carers, family, and professionals should take values and evidence into account as well as the impact of emotion and distress arising within the predicament. Such deliberations combine knowledge, reflection, and life experience with social, emotional, and ethical capacities, and demand reasoning of a kind described for millennia under the concept of wisdom (Edmondson and Pearce, 2006). Wise practice on the part of professionals can enhance their support of both the person with dementia and his or her carers in demanding decisions.

## References

Akhondzadeh, S., Noroozian, M., Mohammadi, M., Ohadinia, S., Jamshidi, A.H., and Khani, M. (2003). *Salvia officinalis* extract in the treatment of patients with mild to moderate Alzheimer's Disease: a double blind, randomised and placebo-controlled trial. *Journal of Clinical Pharmacology and Therapeutics*, **28**, 53–9.

Alexopoulos, G., Abrams, R.C., Young, R.C., and Shamoian, C.A. (1988). Cornell scale for depression in dementia. *Biological Psychiatry*, **23**, 271–84.

Alzheimer's Society (2005). *Making difficult decisions*. Alzheimer's Society, London.

Anand, R., Messina, J., and Hartman, R. (2000). Dose-response effect of rivastigmine in the treatment of Alzheimer's Disease. *International Journal of Geriatric Psychopharmacology*, **2**, 68–72.

Ancoli-Israel, S., Martin, J.L., Gehrman, P. *et al.* (2003). Effect of light on agitation in institutionalized patients with severe Alzheimer's disease. *American Journal of Geriatric Psychiatry*, **11**(2), 194–203.

APA (American Psychiatric Association) (1997). Practice guideline for the treatment of patients with Alzheimer's disease and other dementias of late life. *American Journal of Psychiatry*, **154**(Suppl.), 1–39.

Astell, J.A. (2006). Technology and personhood in dementia care. *Quality in Ageing*, **7**, 15–26.

Aurer, S.R., Monteiro, J., Turossian, C., Sinaiko, E., Boksyg, J., and Reisbert, B. (1996). The treatment of behavioural symptoms in dementia: Haloperidol, thiordazine and fluoxetine: a double blind, placebo-controlled eight month study. *Neurobiology of Aging*, **17**, 652.

Bains, J., Birks, J.S., Dening, T.R. (2002). Antidepressants for treating depression in dementia. *Cochrane Database of Systematic Reviews* 2002, Issue 4. Art. No.: CD003944. DOI: 10.1002/14651858.CD003944.

Baker, R., Bell, S., Gibson, S., Holloway, J. *et al.* (2001). A randomised controlled trial of the effects of multisensory stimulation (MSS) for people with dementia. *British Journal of Clinical Psychology*, **40**(1), 81–96.

Ballard, C.G., Chithiramohan, R.N., Bannister, C., Handy, S., and Todd, N. (1991). Paranoid features in the elderly with dementia. *International Journal of Geriatric Psychiatry*, **6**, 155–7.

Ballard, C.G., Mohan, R.N.C., Patel, A., and Graham, C. (1994). Anxiety disorder in dementia. *Irish Journal of Psychiatry*, **11**, 108–9.

Ballard, C.G., Bannister, C., and Oyebode, F. (1996a). Depression in dementia sufferers. *International Journal of Geriatric Psychiatry*, **11**, 507–15.

Ballard, C.G., Boyle, A., Bowler, C., and Lindesay, J. (1996b). Anxiety disorders in dementia sufferers. *International Journal of Geriatric Psychiatry*, **11**, 987–90.

Ballard, C.G., Thomas, A., Fossey, J. *et al.* (2004). A 3-month, randomised, placebo-controlled, neuroleptic discontinuation study in 100 people with dementia: the neuropsychiatric inventory median cutoff is a predictor of clinical outcome. *Journal of Clinical Psychiatry*, **65**(1), 114–19.

Ballard, C., Waite, J., Birks, J. (2006). Atypical antipsychotics for aggression and psychosis in Alzheimer's disease. *Cochrane Database of Systematic Reviews* 2006, Issue 1, Art. No. CD003476. DOI: 10.1002/14651858. CD003476.pub2.

Bamford, C., Lamont, S., Eccles, M., Robinson, L., May, C., and Bond, J. (2004). Disclosing a diagnosis of dementia: a systematic review. *International Journal of Geriatric Psychiatry*, **19**, 151–69.

Barnes, R.C. (1997). Telling the diagnosis to patients with Alzheimer's disease: relatives should act as proxy for patient. *British Medical Journal*, **314**, 375–6.

Beattie, A., Daker-White, G., Gilliard, J., and Means, R. (2004). 'How can they tell?' A qualitative study of the views of younger people about their dementia and dementia care services. *Health and Social Care in the Community*, **12**, 359–68.

Beck, C.K., Vogelpohl, T.S., Rasin, J.H. *et al.* (2005). Effects of behavioural interventions on disruptive behaviour and affect in demented nursing home residents. *Nursing Research*, **51**(4), 219–28.

Benbow, S.M., Marriott, A., Morley, M., and Walsh, S. (1993). Family therapy and dementia: review and clinical experience. *International Journal of Geriatric Psychiatry*, **8**, 717–25.

Bhatnagar, K. and Frank, J. (1997). Psychiatric disorders in elderly from the Indian sub-continent living in Bradford. *International Journal of Geriatric Psychiatry*, **12**, 907–12.

Birnie, J. (1997). A memory group for older adults. *PSIGE Newsletter*, **59**, 30–3.

Bonjean, M.J. (1989). Solution focussed psychotherapy with families caring for an Alzheimer's patient. *Journal of Psychotherapy and the Family*, **5**, 197–210.

Bonnel, W.B. (1996). Not gone and not forgotten: a spouse's experience of late-stage Alzheimer's disease. *Journal of Psychosomatic Nursing*, **34**, 23–7.

Burns, A., Guthrie, E., Marino-Francis, F. *et al.* (2005). Brief psychotherapy in Alzheimer's disease. *British Journal of Psychiatry*, **187**, 143–7.

Carpenter, B. (2004). Disclosing a dementia diagnosis: a review of opinion and practice, and a proposed research agenda. *Gerontologist*, **44**, 149–58.

CHSR (Centre for Health Services Research and Department of Primary Care) (1998). *The primary care management of dementia: north of England evidence-based guideline development project*. CHSR, Newcastle.

Chung, J.C.C. and Lai, C.K.Y. (2002). Snoezelen for dementia. *Cochrane Database of Systematic Reviews* 2002, Issue 4, Art. No. CD003152. DOI: 10.1002/14651858.CD003152.

Coetzee, R.H., Leask, S.J., and Jones, R.J. (2003). The attitudes of carers and old age psychiatrists towards the treatment of potentially fatal events in end-stage dementia. *International Journal of Geriatric Psychiatry*, **18**, 169–73.

Cott, C.A., Dawson, P., Sidani, S., and Wells, D. (2002). The effects of a walking/talking program on communication, ambulational and functional status in residents with Alzheimer's disease. *Alzheimer's Disease and Associated Disorders*, **16**, 81–7.

Department of Health (1990). *The Care Programme approach*. Health circular-HC (90)23/LASSL(90)11. Department of Health, London.

Deutsch, L.H., Bylsma, F.W., Rovner, B.W., Steele, C., and Folstein, M.F. (1991). Psychosis and physical aggression in probable Alzheimer's disease. *American Journal of Psychiatry*, **148**, 1159–63.

Edmondson, R. and Pearce, J. (2006). The practice of health care: wisdom as a model. *Medicine, Health Care and Philosophy*, **10**, 233–44.

Eggenberger, S.K. and Nelms, T.P. (2004). Artificial hydration and nutrition in advanced Alzheimer's disease: facilitating family decision-making. *Journal of Clinical Nursing*, **13**, 661–7.

Fitz, A.E. and Teri, L. (1994). Depression, cognition and functional ability in patients with Alzheimer's disease. *Journal of the American Geriatrics Society*, **42**, 186–91.

Fontana Gasio, P., Krauchi, K., Cajochen, C. *et al.* (2003). Dawn-dusk simulation light therapy of disturbed circadian rest-activity cycles in demented elderly. *Experimental Gerontology*, **38**, 207–16.

Garwick, A.W., Detzner, D., and Boss, P. (1994). Family perceptions of living with Alzheimer's disease. *Family Process*, **33**, 327–40.

Gilleard, C., Lieberman, S., and Peeler, R. (1992). Family therapy for older adults: a survey of professionals' attitudes. *Journal of Family Therapy*, **14**, 413–22.

Glassman, A.H. (1998). Cardiovascular effects of antidepressant drugs: updated. *Journal of Clinical Psychiatry*, **59**(Suppl. 15), 13–18.

Goldstein, M.Z. (1990). The role of mutual support groups and family therapy for caregivers of demented elderly. *Journal of Geriatric Psychiatry*, **23**, 117–28.

Gormley, N., Lyons, D., and Howard, R. (2001). Behavioural management of aggression in dementia: A randomised controlled trial. *Age and Aging*, **30**, 141–5.

Haines, A. and Katona, C. (1992). In *Dementia in old age* [clinical guidelines], Royal College of General Practitioners Occasional Paper 58, pp. 62–6. Royal College of General Practitioners, London.

Harvey, R.J. (1998). *Young onset dementia: epidemiology, clinical symptoms, family burden, support and outcome*. Dementia research centre, UCL London (http://www.dementia.ion.ucl.ac.uk/).

Hausman, C. (1992). Dynamic psychotherapy with elderly demented patients. In *Care-giving in dementia: research and applications* (ed. G. Jones and B.L. Miesen), pp. 181–98. Routledge, London.

Herr, J.J. and Weakland, J.H. (1979). *Counselling elders and their families: practical techniques for applied gerontology*. Springer, New York.

Hindley, N. and Gordon, H. (2000). The elderly, dementia, aggression and risk assessment. *International Journal of Geriatric Psychiatry*, **15**, 254–9.

Holland, A.J., Hon, J., Huppert, F.A., and Stevens, F. (2000). Incidence and course of dementia in people with Down's syndrome: findings from a population-based study. *Journal of Intellectual Disability Research*, **44**, 138–46.

Holmes, C., Hopkins, V., Hensford, C., MacLaughlin, V., Wilkinson, D., and Rosenvinge, H. (2002). Lavender oil as a treatment for agitated behaviour in severe dementia: a placebo controlled study. *International Journal of Geriatric Psychiatry*, **17**(4), 305–8.

Hope, T., Keene, J., Fairburn, C.G., and Jacoby, R. (2001). Death and dementia. *International Journal of Geriatric Psychiatry*, **16**, 969–74.

Hughes, J.C., Hope, T., Reader, S., and Rice, D. (2002). Dementia and ethics: the views of informal carers. *Journal of the Royal Society of Medicine*, **95**, 242–6.

Iliffe, S. and Manthorpe, J. (2004). The debate on ethnicity and dementia: from category fallacy to person-centred care? *Aging and Mental Health*, **8**, 283–92.

Institute for Ethics, University of New Mexico *Values history form* (http://hsc.unm.edu/ethics/advdir/vhform_eng.shtml).

Jeffery, D. (1987). Should you involve an older person about whom there is an issue of cognitive competence in family meetings? *PSIGE Newsletter*, **24**, 8–11.

Keene, J., Hope, T., Fairburn, C.G., Jacoby, R., Gedling, K., and Ware, C.J. (1999). Natural history of aggressive behaviour in dementia. *International Journal of Geriatric Psychiatry*, **14**, 541–8.

Keller, H.H., Gibbs, A.J., Boudreau, L.D., Goy, R.E., Pattillo, M.S., and Brown, H.M. (2003). Prevention of weight loss in dementia with comprehensive nutritional treatment. *Journal of the American Geriatrics Society*, **51**(7), 945–52.

Kitwood, T. (1997). The experience of dementia. *Aging and Mental Health*, **1**, 13–22.

Knight, B. (1986). *Psychotherapy with older adults*. Sage, Beverly Hills, CA.

Koger, S.M. and Brotons, M. (2000). Music therapy for dementia symptoms. *Cochrane Database Systematic Review* 2000 (3), CD001121.

Lawton, M.P., Brody, E.M., and Saperstein, A.R. (1989). A controlled study of respite services for caregivers of Alzheimer's patients. *Gerontologist*, **29**, 8–16.

Livingston, G., Johnston, K., Katona, C. *et al.* (2005). Systematic review of psychological approaches to the management of neuropsychiatric symptoms of dementia. *American Journal of Psychiatry*, **162**, 1996–2021.

Lonergan, E.T. and Luxenberg, J. (2004). Valproate for agitation in dementia. *Cochrane Database of Systematic Reviews* 2004, Issue 2, Art. No. CD003945. DOI: 10.1002/14651858.CD003945.pub2.

McCarthy, M., Addington-Hall, J., and Altmann, D. (1997). The experience of dying with dementia: a retrospective study. *International Journal of Geriatric Psychiatry*, **12**, 404–9.

McCormick, W.C., Kukull, W.A., van Belle, G., Bowen, J.D., Teri, L., and Larsen, E.B. (1994). Symptom patterns and comorbidity in the early stages of Alzheimer's disease. *Journal of the American Geriatrics Society*, **42**, 517–21.

McCurry, S.M., Gibbons, L.E., Logsdon, R.G., Vitiello, M., and Teri, L. (2005). Training caregivers to change the sleep practices of patients with dementia: the NITE-AD project. *Journal of the American Geriatrics Society*, **51**, 1455–60.

McKeith, I.G., Harrison, R.W.S., and Ballard, C.G. (1995). Neuroleptic sensitivity to risperidone in Lewy body dementia. *Lancet*, **346**, 699.

McKeith, I.G., Grace, J.B., Walker, S. *et al.* (2000). Rivastigmine in the treatment of dementia with Lewy bodies: preliminary findings from an open trial. *International Journal of Geriatric Psychiatry*, **15**, 387–92.

McKeith, I.G., Dickson, D.W., Lowe, J. *et al.* (2005). Diagnosis and management of dementia with Lewy bodies: third report of the DLB Consortium. *Neurology*, **65**, 1863–72.

McShane, R., Keene, J., Gedling, K., Fairburn, C., Jacoby, R., and Hope, T. (1997). Do neuroleptic drugs hasten cognitive decline in dementia? Prospective study with necroscopy follow up. *British Medical Journal*, **314**, 266–70.

Maguire, C.P., Kirby, M., Coen, R., Coakley, D., Lawlor, B., and O'Neill, D. (1996). Family members' attitudes towards telling the patient with Alzheimer's disease their diagnosis. *British Medical Journal*, **313**, 529–30.

Manthorpe, J. and Hettiaratchy, P. (1993). Ethnic minority elders in the UK. *International Review of Psychiatry*, **5**, 171–8.

Manthorpe, J. and Watson, R. (2003). Poorly served? Eating and dementia. *Journal of Advanced Nursing*, **41**, 162–9.

Marriott, A., Donaldson, C., Tarrier, N., and Burns, A. (2000). Effectiveness of cognitive-behavioural family intervention in reducing the burden of care in carers of patients with Alzheimer's disease. *British Journal of Psychiatry*, **176**, 557–62.

Miesen, B.M.L. and Jones, G. (1997). Psychic pain resurfacing in dementia. From new to past trauma. In *Past trauma in later life* (ed. L. Hunt, M. Marshall, and C. Rowlings), pp. 142–54. Jessica Kingsley, London.

Neal, M. and Barton Wright, P. (2003). Validation therapy for dementia. *Cochrane Database of Systematic Reviews* 2003, Issue 3, Art. No. CD001394. DOI: 10.1002/14651858.CD001394.

Opie, J., Rossewarne, R. and O'Connor, D.W. (1999). The efficacy of psychosocial approaches to behaviour disorders in dementia: a systematic literature review. *Australian and New Zealand Journal of Psychiatry*, **33**, 789–99.

Pearce, J. (2002). Systemic therapy. In *Psychological therapies with older people* (ed. J. Hepple), pp. 76–102. Brunner-Routledge, Hove.

Post, S.G. and Whitehouse, P.J. (1995). Fairhill guidelines on ethics of the care of people with Alzheimer's disease: a clinical summary. *Journal of the American Geriatric Society*, **43**, 1423–9.

Proctor, R., Burns, A., Powell, H.S. *et al.* (1999). Behavioural management in nursing and residential homes: a randomised controlled trial. *Lancet*, **354**, 26–9.

Ratna, L. and Davies, J. (1984). Family therapy with the elderly mentally ill. Some strategies and techniques. *British Journal of Psychiatry*, **145**, 311–15.

Ripich, D.N. (1994). Functional communication with AD patients: a caregiver training program. *Alzheimer Disease and Associated Disorders*, **8**, 95–109.

Roth, M. (1955). The natural history of mental disorder in old age. *Journal of Mental Science*, **101**, 281–301.

Rovner, B.W., Steele, C.D., Shmuely, Y., and Folstein, M.F. (1996). A randomised trial of dementia care in nursing homes. *Journal of the American Geriatrics Society*, **44**, 7–13.

Royal College of Psychiatrists (1995). *Consensus statement on the assessment and investigation of an elderly person with suspected cognitive impairment by a specialist old age psychiatry service*, Council Report CR 49. Royal College of Psychiatrists, London.

Royal College of Psychiatrists and Alzheimer's Society (2006). *Services for younger people with Alzheimer's disease and other dementias*, Council Report CR135. Royal College of Psychiatrists, London.

Schneider, L.S., Dagerman, K.S., and Insel, P. (2005). Risk of death with atypical antipsychotic drug treatment for dementia: meta-analysis of randomised placebo-controlled trials. *Journal of American Medical Association*, **19**, 1934–43.

Seltzer, B. and Sherwin, I. (1983). A comparison of clinical features of early and late onset primary degenerative dementia. *Archives of Neurology*, **40**, 143–6.

Serfaty, M., Kennell-Webb, S., Warner, J., Blizard, R., and Raven, P. (2002). Double blind randomised placebo controlled trial of low dose melatonin for sleep disorders in dementia. *International Journal of Geriatric Psychiatry*, **17**(12), 1120–7.

Singer, C., Tactenberg, R.E., Kaye, J. *et al.* (2003). A multicentre, placebo-controlled trial of melatonin for sleep disturbance in Alzheimer's disease. *Sleep*, **26**(7), 893–901.

Sink, K.M., Holden, K.F., and Yaffe, K. (2005). Pharmacological treatment of neuropsychiatric symptoms of dementia: a review of the evidence. *Journal of American Medical Association*, **293**, 596–608.

SSI (Social Services Inspectorate) (1997). *Older people with mental health problems living alone. Anybody's priority?* Department of Health, London.

Stokes, G. (1990). *Common problems with the elderly confused: screaming and shouting.* Winslow Press, Bicester.

Sultzer, D.L., Gray, K.F., Gunay, I., Wheatley, M.V., and Mahler, M.E. (2001). Does behavioural improvement with haloperidol or trazodone treatment depend on psychosis or mood symptoms in patients with dementia? *Journal of the American Geriatrics Society*, **49**(10), 1294–300.

Tariot, P.N., Erb, R., Podgorski, C.A. *et al.* (1998). Efficacy and tolerability of carbamazepine for agitation and aggression in dementia. *American Journal of Psychiatry*, **155**, 54–61.

Tariot, P.N., Solomon, P.R., Morris, J.C., Kershaw, P., Lilienfeld, S., and Ding, C. (2000). A 5-month, randomised, placebo-controlled trial of galantamine in AD: the USA-10 Study Group. *Neurology*, **54**, 2269–76.

Teri, L. (1994). Behavioral treatment of depression in patients with dementia. *Alzheimer Disease and Associated Disorders*, **8**, 66–74.

Teri, L. and Gallagher-Thompson, D. (1991). Cognitive-behavioural interventions for treatment of depression in Alzheimer's patients. *The Gerontologist*, **31**, 413–16.

Teri, L. and Logsdon, R.G. (1991). Identifying pleasant activities for Alzheimer's Disease patients: the Pleasant Events Schedule-AD. *The Gerontologist*, **31**, 124–7.

Teri, L. Logsdon, R.G., Uomoto, J.M., and McCurry, S.M. (1997). Reducing excess disability in dementia patients: training caregivers to manage patient depression. *Journal of Gerontology*, **52**, 159–66.

Turnbull, Q., Wolf, A.M., and Holroyd, S. (2003). Attitudes of elderly subjects toward 'truth telling' for the diagnosis of Alzheimer's disease. *Journal of Geriatric Psychiatry and Neurology*, **16**, 90–3.

Vinestock, M. (1996). Risk assessment. 'A word to the wise'? *Advances in Psychiatric Treatment*, **2**, 3–10.

Wands, K., Merskey, H., Hachinski, V.C., Fishman, M., Fox, F., and Boniferro, M. (1990). A questionnaire investigation of anxiety and depression in early dementia. *Journal of the American Geriatrics Society*, **36**, 535–8.

# Delirium

## Jenny Hogg

## Introduction

Delirium (acute confusional state) is a clinical syndrome which commonly affects the elderly with an acute medical illness. Whilst rates vary from study to study, it would seem to affect approximately 30% of hospital inpatients aged over 65 years, but in the community the prevalence is found to be lower at approximately 1–2% rising steeply with age to 14% in those over 85 years, but even this may be an underestimate (Folstein *et al.*, 1991; Rahkonen *et al.*, 2001). Despite being the most common psychiatric condition affecting hospital inpatients, it is predominantly managed by general physicians and geriatricians, many of whom have had no specific training to recognize or deal with it and its consequences.

Delirium is characterized by an abrupt global impairment of cognitive processes including thinking, remembering, and perceiving. There are attention abnormalities with a decreased awareness of environment and self. There is a defective ability to extract, process, and retain information. The person's grasp of situations is faulty and there is a diminished capacity to act in the customary purposeful, sustained, and goal-directed manner. Symptoms usually fluctuate, being more prominent at night. The person may display hyperactive or hypoactive behaviour, or a mixture of the two. There must be a precipitating medical or physical cause.

## Historical perspective

Outside medical circles the term 'delirium' has been used metaphorically to denote any form of mental aberration, including uncontrollable excitement or emotion. To some extent this wider meaning persists to the present day. Delirium is derived from the Latin words '*de*' meaning 'out of' and '*lira*' meaning the 'furrow', which produced the now obsolete English verb 'delire', meaning to go wrong, to go astray from reason, to rave, to wander in mind, or to be delirious or mad (Murray, 1897; Hart, 1936).

The clinical constellation of a symptomatic acute mental disorder associated with fever, which featured cognitive and behavioural disturbance as well as disruption of sleep, which improved when the fever improved, was recognized 2500 years ago by Hippocrates and his peers. They made the distinction between this syndrome (delirium) and mental illness of unknown cause (dementia) (Lipowski, 1990).

Sadly some 2000 years later the syndrome of delirium is often undiagnosed as clinicians fail to appreciate the distinction so eloquently described in ancient times.

## Diagnostic criteria and assessment tools for delirium

The main diagnostic criteria for delirium in current use are defined in the fourth edition of the *Diagnostic and Statistical Manual of Mental Disorders* (DSM-IV), which are similar to the International Classification of Diseases 10 (ICD-10) criteria, and to those in the recent UK guidelines (Potter and George, 2006). These state that in order to make the diagnosis of delirium a patient must show each of the features 1–4 listed in Table 28.1.

There have been numerous bedside assessments for the specific diagnosis of delirium, although in practice these are rarely used by physicians and junior medical staff, the diagnosis usually being reached on clinical grounds. The most commonly used diagnostic tool is the Confusion Assessment Method (CAM) (see Table 28.2). It is designed to be used by non-psychiatrists and can be used by trained nursing staff. It has been shown to be sensitive, specific, and reliable in the detection of delirium (Inouye *et al.*, 1990).

### Subsyndromal delirium

Subsyndromal delirium is a term which can be applied to patients possessing one or more, but not all of the symptoms of delirium. The risk factors are identical to those for delirium and, as one may guess, the outcome for such patients is intermediate between those with no diagnostic features of delirium and those with the full-blown syndrome. Patients with subsyndromal delirium require identification and clinical attention in line with management of delirium in order to achieve the best outcome (Levkoff *et al.*, 1996; Cole *et al.*, 2002).

## Making the diagnosis of delirium

Delirium is underdiagnosed for a variety of reasons and may be unrecognized by doctors and nurses in up to two-thirds of cases (Foreman and Milisen, 2004) This is a cause of great concern as delirium is present in at least 10% of acute unselected medical admissions in a typical hospital in the UK (George *et al.*, 1997),

**Table 28.1** Features for diagnosis of delirium

| | |
|---|---|
| 1 | Disturbance of consciousness (i.e. reduced clarity of awareness of the environment) with reduced ability to focus, sustain or shift attention |
| 2 | A change in cognition (such as memory deficit, disorientation, language disturbance) or the development of a perceptual disturbance that is not better accounted for by a pre-existing or evolving dementia |
| 3 | The disturbance develops over a short period of time (usually hours to days) and tends to fluctuate during the course of the day |
| 4 | There is evidence from the history, physical examination, or laboratory findings that the disturbance is caused by the direct physiological consequences of a general medical condition, substance intoxication or substance withdrawal |

**Table 28.2** Confusion Assessment Method (CAM). The diagnosis of delirium requires the presence of features 1 and 2 and either 3 or 4

| | |
|---|---|
| 1 | Acute onset and fluctuating course: This feature is usually obtained from a family member or nurse and is shown by positive responses to the following questions: Is there any evidence of an acute change in the patient's mental status form baseline? Did the abnormal behaviour fluctuate during the day, i.e. come and go, or increase or decease in severity? |
| 2 | Inattention: This feature is shown by a positive response to the question: Did the patient have difficulty focusing attention, for example, being easily distractible, or having difficulty keeping track of what was being said? |
| 3 | Disorganized thinking: Was the patient's thinking disorganised or incoherent, such as rambling or irrelevant conversation, unclear or illogical flows of ideas, or unpredictable switching from subject to subject? |
| 4 | Altered level of consciousness: This feature is shown by any answer other than alert to the following question: Overall how would you rate this person's level of consciousness? [Alert (normal); vigilant (hyperalert); lethargic (drowsy, easily aroused); stupor (difficult to arouse); coma (unrousable)] |

with a further 15% of the elderly developing the delirium syndrome during their hospital stay (Inouye *et al.*, 1999).

There are often problems with making the diagnosis from the beginning of the patient's illness. The initial assessment is undertaken by either the accident and emergency doctors or in the general practice setting. As cases of delirium come to light acutely, and often during the evening or night, the patient's usual GP is not always available. Many patients already have a diagnosis of a dementia, and the acute confusion observed is often assumed to be the patient's norm, especially if the patient is unaccompanied during their assessment. Once admitted to hospital the patient is usually under the care of a non-geriatrician. Non-geriatricians have rarely received training in any aspects of old age psychiatry and will often only recognize the hyperactive phenotype of delirium. There may be an under-appreciation of the importance of making a diagnosis due to the lack of specific medical treatment and unawareness of the clinical consequences, which will be discussed later in this chapter. Unless nursing staff are specifically questioned the physician may remain unaware of nocturnal problems with the patient or may assume it is the patient's usual behaviour. The patient may not have the opportunity to be assessed by a multidisciplinary team and the case may only come to light when there are problems discharging the patient. This is a particular problem with patients living in residential care as the carers who know the patient best in terms of activities of daily living rarely visit during the hospital stay. In medical units operating an unselected admissions policy an old age psychiatry liaison service is vital, especially for dealing with this type of scenario. In many hospitals the nursing teams on general medical wards have received training in the area of delirium by their liaison team and have the opportunity to refer to the team themselves. There are now a few specialist dual-care units around the country where patients with delirium can be admitted for assessment and management by a multidisciplinary team. Such teams will usually consist of a geriatrician, old age psychiatrist, nurses with both mental health and physical health training, occupational therapists, physiotherapists, and psychologists. Currently, however, the majority of hospitals rely solely on a liaison model or a consultation model. In hospital settings, the diagnosis should be considered in all elderly patients who have cognitive impairment, both at presentation or during their inpatient stay.

A key factor in diagnosis is obtaining a good pre-morbid history from a close relative or carer. A baseline assessment of cognitive function in all elderly patients is useful, and many units now perform

a routine Abbreviated Mental Test Score (Jitapunkul *et al.*, 1991) on all admissions to the acute medical unit as part of an admission pro forma or may use the Mini-Mental State Examination (MMSE; Folstein *et al.*, 1975). Repeating such ratings at intervals during the inpatient stay may highlight the fluctuations in cognition which characterize the delirious patient. Patients with dementia will usually have a more fixed cognitive impairment. Serial cognitive assessment is particularly useful in detecting the 15% of elderly admissions who will develop a delirium during their stay, and as delirium is more common in those with dementia changes in cognitive test scores may provide valuable information about a developing delirium in these high-risk patients too. Pre-morbid baseline information is especially helpful in this group, particularly if obtained from a carer or relative.

## Differential diagnosis of delirium

The main differential diagnoses of delirium are dementia and depression. As all three conditions are common in the elderly hospitalized population, it is hardly surprising to find the patient may have two or three of these conditions to a greater or lesser degree.

Dementia is the main risk factor for developing delirium. It is thought that up to two-thirds of cases of delirium have co-existent dementia (Inouye, 1997; Cole, 2004). To a lesser degree depression (Gustafson *et al.*, 1988; Foreman, 1989) has been identified as a risk factor for delirium.

Delirium is distinguished from dementia by several features. The most important is the mode of onset. Delirium develops over hours to days whereas dementia usually commences gradually over months or years.

Fluctuations in mental state typically occur frequently and rapidly, within minutes or hours, in delirium, but in dementia changes occur gradually. Although more subtle rapid cognitive fluctuations do occur in dementia with Lewy bodies (DLB), cognitive fluctuations are a key diagnostic feature (see Chapter 27v). Arousal levels are also abnormal in delirium, the patient being either hyperaroused or somnolent, and psychomotor activity is increased or decreased along with these changes. Delusions and hallucinations are more common in delirium than in dementia of the Alzheimer's type and vascular dementia. In DLB hallucinations are common, and other features of this condition such as parkinsonism should be sought to aid the diagnosis. These patients are prone to delirium-like episodes, and if the frequency and severity of hallucinations suddenly increase this should be suspected. DLB is therefore an important differential diagnosis in unexplained delirium. Vascular dementia of the multi-infarct type is characterized by step-wise deteriorations of cognitive function. Occasionally one of these step wise changes can cause an abrupt change in the patient's mood or personality, particularly if the new lesion is in the frontal lobe. This can manifest in a similar way to a hyperactive delirium and can be very difficult to differentiate. Other acute lesions causing apathy and poor volition can similarly be difficult to separate from the hypoactive type of delirium. Depression may also be mistaken for the hypoactive type of delirium. Patients may present to hospital with a relatively minor illness but because of their failure to engage with staff, poor nutritional intake, and lack of volition to attend to their own personal hygiene, delirium is suspected. Often the dilemma can be resolved with a good pre-morbid account, which will usually describe a gradual rather than sudden onset of such symptoms. The problem with distinguishing the two can arise because of difficulties in establishing this, particularly if the patient lives alone with no close relatives or friends. The two diagnoses can usually be separated by performing cognitive testing and observing for cognitive fluctuations and by observing the mood which is more constantly low in depression but typically fluctuates in delirium. Similarly mania can occasionally be mistaken for a hyperactive delirium. Again the history is important as this will usually reveal a gradual acceleration of the person's heightened mood over days to weeks rather than the more precipitous changes in mood seen in delirium.

Thus the key to arriving at a diagnosis of delirium is the history. The patient is often unable to give a lucid history so it is imperative that a history is taken from a relative or carer. Careful questioning about the patient's usual cognition, physical abilities, and continence is vital, as often the acute medical condition causing the delirium is minor and may need to be looked for carefully if the diagnosis is suspected.

## Clinical types of delirium

There are three phenotypes of delirium, hyperactive (classical), hypoactive, and mixed.

The hyperactive or 'florid' type, despite being the least common type, is the most frequently diagnosed. These patients often display signs of increased sympathetic activity including tachycardia, sweating, dilated pupils, flushed face, and increased blood pressure. They are restless and repeatedly seek reassurance from staff. They will often interfere with other patients' belongings, causing distress. Fellow patients with acute medical illnesses find these patients difficult to share a room with. They are often kept awake all night, and by day find it difficult to relax as they are fearful the delirious patient will fall. The hyperactive group certainly are a high falls risk

as they will often pace the ward with poor appreciation of danger from, for example, wet floors and obstacles. Although they may usually use a walking aid, they will often leave it behind and grasp onto walls and pieces of hospital furniture, many of which are on wheels. Such patients require a high level of observation in order to prevent falls, and are probably best managed on specialist units in cubicles. Sadly there is a lack of such accommodation in most hospitals.

About a third of patients with delirium have the 'hypoactive' type. Such patients are underdiagnosed as they do not cause the upheaval on the ward their hyperactive peers do. Classically the patient has poor oral intake and can be recognized on the ward slumped over their meal tray with food falling out of their mouth. They may fall asleep mid-way through a conversation with their relatives. These patients require vigilance to avoid pressure damage, malnutrition, and dehydration. They often require intravenous fluids, special mattresses, and intravenous medication. Often one may see the untouched morning medication pot in the afternoon, which contains the vital antibiotics required to treat the underlying medical illness. These patients often require feeding and supervision to take their medications. Despite often only modest rises in infection and inflammatory markers, it may be wisest to choose intravenous antibiotics to ensure adequate delivery, as this may well speed up recovery, reduce hospital length of stay, and therefore minimize the complications described above.

The most common phenotype of delirium is the mixed type which affects almost half of all cases. As its name suggests, the patient will fluctuate between hyperactivity and hypoactivity. The former is often only evident at night, and careful questioning of the night nursing staff is often needed to make the diagnosis. By day, these patients can seem ready to go home, and indeed may often demand discharge as they lack insight and recollection of the previous night's events. Behaviour and sleep charts are useful in this situation as they will highlight such problems to both the daytime nursing and medical staff as well as the patient and relatives. Sensitive handling of such a situation is required, and it is worth involving close relatives at an early stage so they may help persuade their loved one it is too early for home. Sadly with current bed pressures such patients are often discharged too early, and require readmission. This is an unhappy consequence for the patient and their family and care must be taken in planning such a patient's discharge to avoid this.

## Causes of delirium

To attribute delirium to a 'cause' one must be able to relate the acute confusion to an observed factor which is known to cause confusion, and then see improvement following treatment or cessation of the factor responsible (Francis *et al.*, 1990).

We now recognize that delirium not only occurs with fever and infection but can occur in many other physical health problems. Several researchers have analysed the causes of delirium in hospital admissions. Findings are similar from most studies. One series (George *et al.*, 1997) is representative of the delirium experience in most district general hospitals in the UK. This found that the major causes were infection (one-third), stroke (one-tenth), and medication (one-tenth). Other causes are detailed in Table 28.3. Several patients (25%) had more than one contributory factor.

**Table 28.3** Causes of delirium in 171 sequential medical admissions

| Cause | Number of cases | % of cases |
|---|---|---|
| Infection | 73 | 34 |
| Chest | 40 | |
| Urinary | 25 | |
| Other | 8 | |
| Stroke | 24 | 11 |
| Drugs (analgesics, hypnotics, sedatives, and anticholinergics) | 24 | 11 |
| Myocardial infarction | 11 | 5 |
| Fractures | 10 | 5 |
| Hip | 7 | |
| Other | 3 | |
| Carcinoma | 10 | 5 |
| Fluid and electrolyte imbalance | 9 | 4 |
| Heart failure | 8 | 4 |
| Diabetes (hyper- or hypoglycaemia) | 7 | 3 |
| Peripheral vascular disease/gangrene | 6 | 3 |
| Alcohol withdrawal | 6 | 3 |
| Gastrointestinal bleed | 5 | 2 |
| Respiratory failure | 5 | 2 |
| Pulmonary embolus | 4 | 2 |
| Anaemia | 4 | 2 |
| Perforation of duodenal ulcer | 2 | 1 |
| Subdural haematoma | 2 | 1 |
| Brain tumour | 1 | 0.5 |
| Miscellaneous | 6 | 3 |
| Total | 217[a] | |

[a] Forty-two patients (25%) had two or more equally contributing causes.

# Predisposing and precipitating factors for delirium

Researchers in the field of delirium have looked at the factors which are common to those patients presenting with delirium. In the elderly delirium is rarely caused by a single factor. It is usually a composite of the mental and physical vulnerability of the patient and the severity of the physical insults. As one may expect, the more vulnerable the patient, the easier it is for that patient to develop delirium. Predisposing factors have been shown in many studies to be increasing age, pre-existing dementia, severity of illness, metabolic and electrolyte imbalance, the use of psychoactive medications, and a previous episode of delirium (Gustafson *et al.*, 1988; Rockwood, 1989; Rogers *et al.*, 1989; Francis *et al.*, 1990; Schor *et al.*, 1992). Similarly other studies have identified risk factors for those who develop delirium during their hospital stay. These factors include visual impairment, increasing severity of illness, cognitive impairment, and dehydration (Inouye *et al.*, 1993). The more factors present the higher the risk of developing a delirium. Other studies (Schor *et al.*, 1992) have identified in addition male sex, fracture on admission, and neuroleptic and narcotic use, and although this study failed to identify medications with anticholinergic effects as a risk factor, a further study

(Han *et al.*, 2001) showed that exposure to such medications is associated with a subsequent increase in the severity of delirium symptoms.

Iatrogenic factors which may precipitate a delirium in susceptible persons, such as those with baseline factors described above, have also been identified (Inouye *et al.*, 1996). These include use of physical restraints, malnutrition, more than three new medications added, and use of a bladder catheter.

# Prevention of delirium during a hospital stay

With this in mind one can see how attempts can be made to reduce the incidence of delirium in hospital patients. Some authors suggest that delirium could be prevented in up to a third of patients who develop delirium during their hospital stay (Inouye *et al.*, 1999; Marcantonio *et al.*, 2001). One group of patients who lend themselves to this type of research are those sustaining a fractured neck of the femur. This group of patients represent a frail elderly group who often share the baseline characteristics described above which predispose to delirium. Several studies have shown that delirium develops in between 35% and 65% of such cases without any preventative measures (Gustafson *et al.*, 1988).

The interventions shown to be of particular value in the population with a fractured neck of the femur included avoidance of peri-operative hypotension, post-operative hypoxaemia, prompt surgical intervention (within 24 hours where possible), use of spinal anaesthesia (as opposed to general anaesthesia), and more aggressive use of blood transfusion (Gustafson *et al.*, 1991). Nursing interventions shown to be of use include orientation to time, place, and situation, correction of sensory deficits, and increased continuity of care (Williams *et al.*, 1985). Later work has shown that a geriatrician consultation with optimization of pre-existing medical conditions can help further (Marcantonio *et al.*, 2001). In this study not only was the incidence of delirium reduced, but in those who developed delirium the duration and severity was reduced.

A more difficult group to study are elderly patients presenting to an acute medical unit. The incidence of delirium at presentation to hospital is higher than in the population with a fractured neck of the femur, although the two groups share many other features. In those without delirium at presentation, the rates of developing delirium during a hospital stay can be reduced from 15% to 10% with a multicomponent intervention programme (Inouye *et al.*, 1999). These interventions included the following protocols: *orientation* (communication boards, reorientation to environment, getting to know staff), *therapeutic activities* (discussion of current events, structured reminiscence, word games), *non-pharmacological sleep* (warm drinks, relaxation tapes, music, back massage, restoration of day/night pattern), *sleep enhancement* (noise reduction at night, schedule adjustments, e.g. of medication and procedures), and *early mobilization* (ambulation or bed/chair-based exercises three times a day, minimal use of immobilizing equipment, e.g. bladder catheters, physical restraints). For those with specific problems a visual protocol, hearing protocol, and dehydration protocol were used as appropriate. Although this research was done in the USA, it should be transferable to clinical practice elsewhere, and the new UK guidelines (Potter and George, 2006) embrace many of these interventions.

## Orientation

Unfortunately many acute units in the UK seem unable to accommodate patients in the same location for the length of their hospital stay. Patients can be moved around the hospital in excess of four times during their admission, and it is little wonder they become disorientated. The elderly patient with a simple urinary tract infection is often first in line to be boarded from a medical ward to a surgical ward to make way for a patient perceived to be more medically unwell, with little regard for the possible sequel of a delirium (Mattice, 1989).

## Therapeutic activities

The use of cognitive stimulation is helpful in preventing delirium. Many relatives will unwittingly engage in this activity with their loved one, but there are often short visiting hours on wards, with patients frequently complaining that the hospital day feels very long. Good access to newspapers, reading books, and the television is of help as well as more structured activities with therapy and ward staff. Patients will often enjoy interaction with other patients but it will often take members of staff to introduce patients to each other to 'break the ice'. Chronic short staffing can be a barrier to activities such as word games, structured reminiscence, and daily discussions of current events. In units where such activities occur there is a higher level of satisfaction and lower degree of boredom described by the patients.

## Sleep interventions

Hospitals are noisy places, especially at night. Many patients are unused to sharing a room with anyone and hence may have difficulties falling asleep and maintaining sleep due to background noises such as a fellow patient snoring. Sleep deprivation has been shown as a risk factor in the development of delirium, hence the need to ensure a refreshing night's sleep. Ward staff should ensure that patients are as relaxed as possible by nightfall and know not only where the toilet facilities are but how to summon assistance if needed. The balance between adequate lighting to ensure patients do not sustain a fall on visiting the bathroom and darkness to assist patients to fall asleep and maintain sleep is a tricky one. It may be useful to establish which patients regularly use the bathroom during the night and position them on the ward accordingly. Patients known to be noisy at night may benefit from a cubicle, but as cubicle accommodation is a premium in the UK this is not always possible.

## Early mobilization

For patients who are independently ambulant this is easily achievable. The target population, however, often use a mobility aid such as a walking frame, stick(s), or crutches. Many patients fail to bring their mobility aid to hospital when acutely admitted which further hampers the aim of early mobilization. Asking family members to bring such equipment in at an early stage is useful, especially if the admission falls over a weekend, as physiotherapy staff are not generally available for mobility assessments over this period in the UK.

A detailed history of the patient's usual mobility is of great use, and attempts to maintain it will not only assist in prevention of delirium but will also facilitate discharge.

Patients may have been catheterized on admission because of continence problems or to monitor fluid balance. This should be reviewed and the catheter removed at the earliest possible opportunity. The initial decision to catheterize should be made carefully by senior staff unless the patient is in urinary retention or is critically unwell. Cot sides and other forms of physical restraint should be avoided where possible (Evans and Strumpf, 1989; Lofgreen et al., 1989; Sullivan-Marx, 1994).

# Management of the patient with delirium
## Initial clinical management of delirium

As mentioned earlier in this chapter the key to diagnosing delirium lies in establishing an acute change in cognition and behaviour. Often this information is only available from relatives and carers. In parallel with investigating the baseline status of the patient the clinician must perform appropriate medical investigations. In light of the information known about the likely causes of delirium there are certain investigations required for all patients presenting with an acute confusion. Often the frail elderly fail to display the classical signs of, for example, a chest infection, such as fever, cough, increased sputum production, and dyspnoea. Instead they may present with anorexia and somnolence with new pressure damage. Minimum investigations for cases of delirium should include thorough clinical examination and review of medications including those purchased 'over the counter'. Blood tests should include full blood count, glucose, urea and electrolytes, corrected calcium, liver function and thyroid function tests, inflammatory markers (for example C-reactive protein), urinary dipstick, and if appropriate mid-stream urinary specimen. If sepsis is suspected blood cultures should be done as well as arterial blood gases for lactate levels and hypoxia. A chest X-ray and 12-lead ECG should be performed in most cases. Investigations requiring disruption, such as a trip to the X-ray department should be performed at an appropriate time unless clinically urgent. Waking a patient for a 'routine' chest X-ray at 3 a.m. should be avoided where possible. If the cause is still unclear a rectal examination may be warranted, as faecal impaction is a known cause of delirium especially in the advanced dementia group.

Prompt treatment with appropriate fluids, antibiotics, and oxygen via the route which is the most likely to ensure adequate delivery but minimize distress is the optimum. If the patient is excessively somnolent, adequate fluids and medications via the oral route are unlikely to be achieved and the intravenous route should be used. If the patient is hyperactive and wandersome then the intravenous route may be hazardous and prolonged one-to-one attention to get medication and fluids delivered is probably the best choice. Subcutaneous fluids overnight may also be effective. Accurate recording of medications being taken rather than delivered to the bedside is imperative. Similarly, accurate fluid and nutritional intake is an important factor in the recovery of the patient.

Although the hyperactive form of delirium seems the most problematic, it is in fact the hypoactive form which carries a worse prognosis. Such patients need very strict attention to nutrition and fluid balance as they are prone to malnutrition and dehydration. Due to their relative immobility they are highly prone to hypostatic pneumonias, pressure damage, and deep vein thrombosis. The attending physicians and nursing staff need to be aware of these potential problems. Prompt use of pressure-relieving mattresses, prophylactic low-molecular weight heparin, interventions such as nasogastric feeding tubes, and low threshold for antibiotics at the earliest sign of chest infection are vital to promote a good outcome.

Problems in dealing with the hyperactive form of delirium are slightly different. Whilst sharing the problems of nutrition and fluid balance, this group are highly prone to falls. Patients with delirium who fall and fracture the neck of their femur do very badly. Judicious use of hip protectors may help, but often these patients may need one-to-one nursing during their worst phase. These patients are also susceptible to oversedation. Overzealous staff can be too hasty with a second or third dose of sedative which may cause the patient to become virtually comatose, putting them at similar risks to their hypoactive peers.

### Supportive and behavioural management of delirium

It is humbling to read an adaptation of Barrough's account of the management of delirium, first published in 1583:

> Treatment had to involve attention to the patient's needs: if he was troubled by the light, he had to be placed in a dark room. Moreover, 'let his dearest friends come to him, and let them sometime speake gently and softly unto him, and sometimes rebuke him sharply'. His diet had to be light. The patient had to be left undisturbed, since 'per-turbations of the mind do hurt frenetick [delirious] persons exceed-ingly'. Sleep needed to be ensured by the use of appropriate medications such as opium or henbane, taking care not to oversedate the patient, as this could turn the 'frenesie [hyperactive form of delirium] into a lethargie [hypoactive form of delirium] whereby you may cause him to sleepe so, that you can awake him no more'.

> from Lipowski (1990)

Clearly there is much sense in the above narrative. In the 21st century patients with delirium are in some ways managed less well than they were some 500 or so years ago. They are housed in busy, noisy wards with care performed by complete strangers. They frequently move beds within a ward or move to other wards around the hospital with yet more strangers dealing with their personal care. Interventions including urinary catheterization and the use of physical restraints have been shown to be detrimental to patients at risk of developing delirium. Intuitively it would follow that those already with delirium would tolerate such interventions badly.

Most non-delirious in-patients complain about poor sleep due to excessive night-time noise. Patients with delirium need their sleep even more and are often in hospital for much longer with further sleep deprivation than those without delirium.

The new delirium guidelines (Potter and George, 2006) encapsulate all aspects of good supportive practice. Whilst acknowledging that the most important aspect of management is to treat the underlying cause there are areas which can be improved on to facilitate a smooth recovery. The guidelines are summarized below.

Ensure:

◆ Lighting levels are appropriate for the time of day.

◆ Regular and repeated (at least three times daily) cues to improve personal orientation.

◆ Use of clocks and calendars to improve orientation.

◆ Hearing aids and spectacles should be available as appropriate and in good working order.

◆ Continuity of care from nursing staff.

◆ Encouragement of mobility and engagement in activities and with other people.

◆ Approach and handle patients gently.

◆ Elimination of unexpected and irritating noise (e.g. pump alarms).

◆ Regular analgesia, e.g. paracetamol.

◆ Encouragement of visits from family and friends who may be able to help calm the patient.

◆ Explain the cause of the confusion to relatives. Encourage family to bring in familiar objects and pictures from home and participate in rehabilitation.

◆ Fluid intake to prevent dehydration (use subcutaneous fluids if necessary).

◆ Good diet, fluid intake, and mobility to prevent constipation.

◆ Adequate CNS oxygen delivery (use supplemental oxygen to keep saturation above 95%).

◆ Good sleep pattern (use milky drinks at bedtime, exercise during the day).

Avoid:

◆ Inter- and intra-ward transfers.

◆ Use of physical restraint.

◆ Constipation.

◆ Anticholinergic drugs where possible and keep drug treatment to a minimum.

◆ Catheters where possible.

## Medications and delirium

### Current medications

It is known that medication often has a central role in the causation of delirium, and may be the only cause in about 10% of all cases (George *et al.*, 1997). Patients in the community, particularly those in 24-hour care, are often commenced on medication for a particular symptom, and although ideally their medication should be reviewed regularly in the light of their current behaviours, this rarely happens unless the patient presents to the GP with a problem that is linked to that medication.

In any elderly patient presenting to hospital, but especially for those with delirium, it is important to evaluate the patient's medication list. Often the patient and their relatives have little recollection of why a particular drug was commenced. Drugs acting on the central nervous system should receive particular attention, as studies have shown these drugs are the most incriminated in cases of delirium. Patients with dementia presenting with a delirium are often on a neuroleptic such as risperidone, olanzapine, or quetiapine; particularly if the patient has a hypoactive form of delirium these should be omitted and reintroduced only if necessary. Conversely if the patient is on a cholinesterase inhibitor (for example donepezil, rivastigmine, or galantamine) this should not be stopped as the effects may be devastating on the patient's baseline function once the delirium has settled. The other group of agents to be scrutinized carefully are the opiates. Patients frequently present on tramadol, for example, which may have originally been started following a fracture or other specific injury. Careful evaluation of pain is needed and in many cases such medications can be withdrawn successfully.

### Medications to treat delirium

Because of the fluctuant nature of delirium, the patient who is somnolent by day may be extremely active at night. Often the most junior doctor is called through the night to prescribe something to 'calm the patient down'. Such doctors are often ill-prepared to handle the request and may prescribe either a large dose of sedative (partly due to the high doses suggested in the text books and formularies), or when a smaller dose is prescribed they may not put a time frame on when the dose can be repeated so the patient may receive several doses within a short space of time. The following day the damage is often evident with the patient being found almost comatose barely protecting their own airway. Many hospitals now have a junior doctors' handbook to address this issue and training is delivered on the subject of night sedation at an early stage.

In parallel to the training of junior doctors on this subject, nursing training, especially for those on night shift, is of use. If the patient can be supported on the ward through the night with measures such as warm milky drinks, relative quiet, and if possible a single cubicle then a better outcome will be achieved in the long run.

Sometimes despite supportive measures sedation is required for the safety of the patient, other patients, and staff. The medication chosen is usually haloperidol, in small doses starting at 0.5 mg at 2-hourly intervals if the patients fail to settle. A maximum of 5 mg per day is recommended. If the oral route is impossible the haloperidol can be given intramuscularly at a dose of 1–2 mg. Haloperidol is used as it is the only medication which has been studied in any depth and it has the advantage of being relatively free of anticholinergic properties.

In the recent UK delirium guidelines (Potter and George, 2006) lorazepam is recommended for specific groups of patients namely those with Parkinson's disease and those with DLB. It is used in doses of 0.5–1 mg orally which can be given at 2-hourly intervals and if the patient fails to settle up to a maximum of 3 mg per day. This is in preference to haloperidol which is known to markedly worsen the motor symptoms of parkinsonism. There is a paucity of literature on drug treatment of delirium. This is probably due to the inherent difficulty in conducting a large randomized trial owing to the fact that delirium is diverse and has numerous causes. There have been small trials conducted in various subgroups of patients, such as those with AIDS (Breitbart et al., 1996). This trial compared haloperidol, chlorpromazine, and lorazepam in a double-blind design. The outcomes showed haloperidol and chlorpromazine to be equally effective, but use of lorazepam was limited by side-effects. As this group of patients were highly specific and of a much younger age range it is unlikely the findings are directly transferable to the more typical delirium population.

As the cholinergic system seems heavily involved in the aetiology of delirium in some cases, it is little wonder clinicians have pondered the potential benefits of the cholinesterase inhibitors in delirium. One case report (Wengel et al., 1998) suggests that the cholinesterase inhibitor donepezil caused a dramatic improvement in symptoms of delirium in a patient with mild Alzheimer's disease, but there are certainly no randomized controlled trials to date to recommend this as a definitive treatment.

## Role of the electroencephalogram (EEG) in delirium

In the literature, there are numerous references to the EEG changes seen in delirium. These are the increase in slow-wave activity and the slowing and disruption of the normal alpha rhythm (Romano and Engel, 1944).

Whilst some comment that the EEG is widely accepted as a valuable ancillary laboratory procedure for diagnosis and serial evaluation of delirium (Koponen, 1991), this tool is rarely used routinely in the UK. The practicalities of routine EEG examination for delirious patients seem prohibitive. As discussed earlier in this chapter, important features of management of delirium include avoidance of disturbing and distressing interventions. As neurology services in the UK tend to be located in tertiary referral centres this investigation for many would require an ambulance trip. The EEG is used as a research tool in delirium and also when the diagnosis is in doubt. Of special value is its use when the differential includes conditions such as Creutzfeldt–Jakob disease and non-convulsive status epilepticus.

## Communication in delirium

### Communication with patients

Patients who have had an episode of delirium often recall their experience as frightening or they will feel they 'lost' the time during which they had their worst symptoms. Some patients do retain some insight, especially those without dementia, and it is important to ensure that the patient is communicated with during their stay.

It is well recognized that sensory impairment (especially vision and hearing) is a risk factor for the development of delirium, and intuitively one would suppose that the ability to communicate adequately would be important in the recovery period. Patients may have lucid periods during their delirium and one should opportunistically use these times to reassure the patient and orientate them to their location and condition.

It seems unproductive and cruel to dwell on previous evening's behaviours with the patient. One often overhears relatives doing this very thing and understandably the patient feels anxious, upset, and scared of the evening ahead. A quiet word with relatives early on in the admission can be helpful. When patients are ready for discharge it can be useful to explain to them that they have had an episode of delirium and what the identified cause was (if known). They should be warned it may recur but the best advice for them is to seek their GP earlier rather than later if they are feeling unwell. Timely antibiotics may avert a further delirium and this information should be conveyed to the GP and relatives as well.

### Communication with relatives and carers

There are three phases of communication with relatives and carers which need to be completed for a satisfactory outcome.

The first phase is the fact-finding and tentative diagnostic phase. Information initially needs to flow from the relatives and carers to hospital staff. This includes details of home situation, usual activities of daily living, usual medications, and mobility. This information can be gleaned over the phone if necessary, although a face-to-face meeting is preferable. More sensitive is the information regarding the patient's usual cognitive abilities. Relatives and carers will often say 'they were fine' when asked about memory and awareness of personal risk. One often needs to probe more deeply to ensure they have not been attributing 'leaving the gas on' or 'failing to lock the door' to 'well it's their age isn't it doctor?' One may often uncover evidence that there has been a decline in cognitive ability and sometimes just asking the questions can enable relatives to see that they have been failing to acknowledge it. Judicious questioning on the four factors identified in the study that looked at which instrumental activities of daily living (IADL) are related to cognitive impairment independent of age, sex, and education, namely telephone use, use of transport, responsibility for medication intake, and handling finances may help clarify the presence of a pre-existing cognitive decline (Barberger-Gateau et al., 1992).

The second phase involves informing the relatives and carers about delirium. They often find seeing their loved one distressed and agitated very upsetting and require appropriate counselling. Often they will become angry with ward staff as a way of expressing their feelings, and may appear unduly irate, particularly if belongings of the patient have become lost or misplaced. The best way to counsel the relatives and carers is usually to remove them from the immediate bed area into a quiet room. Asking them what information they have been given is a good way to start the conversation. Letting them tell their version of events from 'being aware of something being wrong' to the present moment is both informative and therapeutic for the relative. Encouraging junior medical staff and nursing staff to observe this meeting is often very helpful for all concerned. Meeting relatives is a cause of much anxiety with junior doctors, especially if they are unsure of the facts and have witnessed the relative being assertive with the nursing staff. Seeing how their seniors handle the situation is invaluable training from both a knowledge angle and an interpersonal skills angle.

Gentle explanation of what delirium is and what can be expected in terms of recovery then needs to be delivered. This needs to be carefully considered. No longer is it acceptable to assure relatives that delirium is a transient phenomenon with no lasting effects. On the contrary, delirium carries a significant morbidity and mortality of its own when other factors such as severity of illness are controlled for. The amount of information given at this time may be brief as the delirium may have come as a complete shock to relatives. In cases where the index delirium is the first sign of any abnormal cognitive behaviour, information needs to be given with an assurance that follow-up will be planned with an appropriate person. Ideally this should be a psychogeriatrician, but where this is not readily available a geriatrician with an interest in this field may be a reasonable alternative. If the patient has had mild problems prior to the index delirium, the diagnosis will usually be that of a mild dementia. Again specialist follow up with psychogeriatric colleagues is recommended (Potter and George, 2006).

The relatives and carers need to be reassured that the course of delirium is fluctuant. If the patient has a good day which is then followed by two bad days they may assume the worst. They need advice on how best they can help the patient. Suggesting they bring a few photographs or perhaps a favourite ornament may be of help. If the patient is not eating or drinking well it may be helpful for them to visit at mealtimes to assist with feeding. Playing simple card games and talking about yesteryear may help improve distress. Where appropriate, advice on conversation can be of use. Delirious patients often believe they are back in the past and constant correction is rarely helpful. Steering conversation away from such topics, with gentle reorientation is of use.

Relatives and carers will appreciate the time given to this conversation even if they become upset during it. It is of value to have a member of the nursing staff present as often this will help improve relationships on the ward. Relatives often feel they must 'stick up for their parent's rights' and this often comes across as intimidating and aggressive to junior nursing and medical staff. These staff members may unwittingly display negative body language which further exacerbates the problem. Probing gently into some of the verbal complaints can be done at this meeting if appropriate.

The third phase involves a discussion of the future. Families often want to know what to expect in the short, medium, and longer term. Clearly this will depend on many factors including age and co-morbidity and the severity of the acute physical illness which caused the delirium, which are all patient specific. It should be emphasized that the presence of delirium will add a further complication, hampering the acute recovery, as it has been shown that delirium is an independent prognostic determinant of hospital outcomes (Inouye et al., 1998).

The medium-term prognosis used to be thought of as good. Providing the patient recovered from the initial illness the delirium was thought to be completely reversible. Studies from the last two decades suggest that this is no longer the case (for more details see below). It is best to suggest to relatives that the majority of the features of delirium improve with time and that the time span can vary from days to weeks. In many cases features of the delirium can extend beyond discharge, lasting up to and beyond 6 months.

In the longer term, delirium may herald the arrival of dementia. Long-term follow-up of delirium survivors show an excess incidence of dementia.

Clear transcription of conversations with relatives is very important. In subsequent clinic appointments it is unlikely that the clinician will recall exactly what was said and what the specific worries and fears of the patient and relatives were. It is useful to inform the GP of the content of such conversations as they will often be the first port of call if further difficulties arise. If mild and previously unrecognized cognitive impairment is uncovered during the hospital stay this too needs to be conveyed to the GP. Issues such as non-compliance with medications may need to be addressed in different ways by the primary care team in light of this information.

## Prognosis of delirium

With the exception of researchers in the field of delirium, it was thought until recently that delirium was a transient reversible syndrome with a good prognosis. Many general physicians still believe this to be the case, although as already alluded to in the previous section, the evidence overwhelmingly points to delirium being a marker for physical and cognitive decline and increased mortality.

### Physical health aspects of the prognosis of delirium

In the past, relatives and carers would be confidently told the cognitive state of the patient with delirium would return to normal almost as quickly as it had become impaired. The attending physician would concentrate chiefly on discussing the prognosis of the (causative) medical condition and its severity, rather than the accompanying delirium. In some ways this was understandable.

Many physicians have had no post-graduate training in psychiatric conditions and feel out of their comfort zone when discussing such matters. In the 1980s and 1990s numerous studies showed that delirium was an independent risk factor in poor outcomes from hospital admission. This message has been poorly received and acknowledged by general medical physicians. It is astonishing that a condition affecting at least 10% of medical admissions should be so misunderstood.

The differences in prognosis of those with and those without delirium begins at the onset of the delirium, and persists through hospital stay and discharge until death. Various endpoints have been used by researchers to demonstrate this.

Hospital mortality was featured in one of the first studies (Rabins and Folstein, 1982). Although the authors did show an excess hospital mortality, subsequent studies, which perhaps controlled more carefully for severity of illness and presence of dementia, did not reach statistical significance (Francis *et al.*, 1990; Levkoff *et al.*, 1992; George *et al.*, 1997; O'Keeffe and Lavan, 1997; Inouye *et al.*, 1998).

Increased length of hospital stay of delirious versus non-delirious patients has not been statistically proven as yet, but there is certainly a trend. This work is fraught with statistical difficulties, as many of the controls develop incidental delirium during their hospital stay.

Other factors such as the development of complications of hospitalization, for example urinary incontinence, falls, and pressure damage, were more likely to occur in the delirious (Gustafson *et al.*, 1988; O'Keeffe and Lavan, 1997).

Excess functional decline in those patients with delirium compared with those without has been demonstrated at 3 and 6 months post-hospital discharge by one group (Murray *et al.*, 1993), whilst other researchers have shown that such differences may take some time to be apparent. At 3 months one group found no difference at all (Pompei *et al.*, 1994) and although Francis *et al.*'s (1990) study showed no statistical difference in functional decline at 6 months' follow-up, at 2 years a statistical difference was observed between the functional abilities of the groups (Francis and Kapoor, 1992).

There are higher readmission rates amongst those with delirium (George *et al.*, 1997) and significantly increased rates of long-term institutionalization evident as early as 6 months post-discharge (Francis and Kapoor, 1992; O'Keeffe and Lavan, 1997; Inouye *et al.*, 1998).

In the longer term there is an excess mortality in patients who have had an episode of delirium than those with a similar physical illness without delirium. This was found at 6 and 12 months' follow-up in one study (George *et al.*, 1997) and in follow-up to 3 years in another (Rockwood *et al.*, 1999).

The cause for these poor physical outcomes remains unclear. Researchers have strived to reduce possible bias by matching patients carefully with controls, yet still these differences exist. For example, when dementia patients with a delirium are matched to dementia patients without delirium the physical differences and increased mortality remain.

## Mental health aspects of prognosis of delirium

Aspects of prognosis which concern relatives the most are behaviour and cognition. Anecdotally, relatives may describe a previous episode of delirium from which the patient never fully recovered. There is some evidence that a substantial proportion of cases of delirium are unresolved at discharge, and in about half of the cases there are persistent symptoms at 1 month. Even by 6 months not all the new symptoms of delirium had disappeared (Levkoff *et al.*, 1992; George *et al.*, 1997; Marcantonio *et al.*, 2000, 2003; Kiely *et al.*, 2004).

It is now known that delirium does have long-term cognitive implications, even for those deemed to have recovered from their delirium. Follow up of patients in several studies have shown accelerated decline in cognition, compared with controls matched for cognitive function at baseline (Koponen and Riekkinen, 1989; Francis and Kapoor, 1992; Rockwood *et al.*, 1999; Dolan *et al.*, 2000; Rahkonen *et al.*, 2000; McCusker *et al.*, 2001; Jackson *et al.*, 2004). It is not just those with dementia who show an accelerated decline. For example those with delirium who had cognitive testing scores in the normal range at discharge had higher than expected rates of dementia when followed for 2 years.

In 1959, Engel and Romano suggested that delirium and dementia may be different aspects of a similar process in which delirium may induce irreversible brain damage. They based their hypothesis on the EEG findings of slowing in delirium. They proposed a mechanism of impaired cerebral metabolism, ranging from decreased ability to synthesize neurotransmitters to eventual cell death (Engel and Romano, 1959). Other researchers suggest that delirium may induce long term or even permanent cognitive decline, which is manifested by functional decline (Murray *et al.*, 1993).

Alternatively, delirium may be a marker of dementia. Acute physical illness may uncover a brain which is operating on low reserves of neurotransmitter activity, with little ability to cope with the increased demands. When put under stress the brain no longer copes and the concept of 'acute brain failure' occurs (Francis and Kapoor, 1992).

Knowledge of the prognosis of delirium has increased over the last two decades. This knowledge now needs to be disseminated amongst acute care physicians and geriatricians in order for patients to be best managed. The development of new guidelines (Potter and George, 2006), and incorporation of delirium into the undergraduate and post-graduate curricula may help to address this.

# Neuropathophysiology of delirium

There are thought to be three factors involved in the pathogenesis of delirium at the cellular level. These include neurotransmitters, glucocorticoids, and cytokines.

## The role of neurotransmitters in the pathogenesis of delirium

One major hypothesis is that a deficiency of the neurotransmitter acetylcholine plays a key role in the pathogenesis of delirium. This is supported by the following statements from the works of several researchers (Tune *et al.*, 1981; Golinger *et al.*, 1987; Trzepacz, 1994; Mach *et al.*, 1995; Flacker *et al.*, 1998; Han *et al.*, 2001; Trzepacz and van der Mast R, 2002; Roche, 2003):

♦ Delirium can be induced in susceptible individuals by anticholinergic drugs.

♦ Patients on anticholinergic drugs have higher rates of delirium.

♦ Medications used to treat myasthenia gravis, an autoimmune condition with antibodies directed against the neuromuscular acetylcholine receptors, can reverse delirium caused by anticholinergic drugs.

- Cholinesterase inhibitors improve some of the symptoms of delirium even in cases not related to anticholinergic medication.

- Serum anticholinesterase activity is known to be raised in patients with delirium.

- Delirium is associated with a reduction in the cerebral oxidative metabolism, with subsequent reduction of neurotransmitter levels.

- Hypoxia seems to disproportionately affect synthesis of cerebral acetylcholine, as it would seem this neurotransmitter pathway is particularly sensitive to low oxygen levels.

These statements are not without some contention. A small study of older nursing home residents showed serum anticholinergic activity was raised during illness and declined following recovery. This effect was observed in those with and without delirium, and was not observed to be related to changes in medication (Flacker and Lipsitz, 1999). This work followed previous studies which have questioned the hypothesis that reduced cholinergic neurotransmission is the main pathophysiological precipitant of delirium. These authors challenge the assumption that serum anticholinergic activity is a stable patient characteristic, resulting from their medications or their metabolites. If this were true they argue that manipulation of medication could prevent delirium, which is clearly not the case. Epidemiological studies of delirium have not shown anticholinergic medications to be statistically associated with delirium in either medical or post-operative patients (Francis and Kapoor, 1992; Schor et al., 1992; Marcantonio, 1994). These authors suggest that raised serum anticholinergic activity and delirium may arise from the same endogenous trigger, rather than the raised activity being the causative factor for the other.

Other neurotransmitters and iatrogenic agents which stimulate or inhibit neurons can contribute to delirium. Dopaminergic activity is intimately involved with cholinergic activity, the former appearing to have a regulatory control on the latter (Trzepacz and van der Mast, 2002). Agents interfering with this balance can precipitate delirium. The majority of agents used to treat Parkinson's disease can precipitate delirium, for example levodopa and the dopamine agonists. Dopamine antagonists, including antipsychotics such as haloperidol, can treat symptoms of delirium.

Serotonin may play an important role in the development of delirium. The 'serotonin syndrome' characterized by confusion, restlessness, tremor, and diaphoresis, shares many of the features seen in hyperactive delirium.

Unfortunately trying to study a particular neurotransmitter in isolation is a difficult task. In most areas of the brain there are numerous pathways which use different transmitters. It may be that the balance between various neurotransmitters is lost in delirium rather than any particular one being either present in excess or deficient.

Other neurotransmitters may have a role, but the evidence is less well developed. These include norepinephrine, gamma-aminobutyric acid, glutamate, and melatonin. Some believe that these other neurotransmitters have an effect on delirium by interfering with the cholinergic/dopaminergic balance (Shigeta et al., 2001; Trzepacz and van der Mast, 2002; Cole, 2004).

## The role of the hypothalamo-pituitary axis (HPA) in delirium

In physical illness, one of the body's responses is to produce glucocorticoids. This is a protective mechanism designed to promote return to health. In certain conditions the way in which the body responds becomes maladaptive. Cortisol excess is a well described cause of neuropsychiatric abnormalities. In Cushing's syndrome, where glucocorticoid hormones are produced in excess without the usual negative-feedback control, marked changes are observed in mood and cognition. The hippocampus seems to be the area of the brain most affected by excess cortisol, owing to its high numbers of glucocorticoid receptors. Reduction in hippocampal volume has been observed in both Cushing's syndrome patients and those with major depression (Olsson 1999). Hypercortisolism has been demonstrated in delirium associated with lower respiratory infection, post-operative delirium, and in delirium following stroke (McIntosh et al., 1985; Lipowski, 1990; O'Keefe and Devlin, 1994). Abnormalities of the HPA axis similar to those described in major depression are present. This can be demonstrated using the dexamethasone suppression test. Patients with a lower respiratory tract infection will have high endogenous cortisol levels in response to the stress of the infection. In non-delirious subjects given dexamethasone, the cortisol levels dropped (normal response) in the majority of patients (6/7 patients). In the majority of delirious subjects, however, the cortisol levels were not suppressed (7/9 patients) (O'Keeffe and Devlin, 1994).

## The role of cytokines in delirium

Cytokines, when used at supraphysiological doses may lead to delirium. Interleukin-2 (IL-2), which has a central role in both cellular and humoral immunity, is the best studied of the cytokines. Delirium has been observed in patients receiving IL-2 therapy and the effect seems dose dependent (Denikoff et al., 1987; Rosenberg et al., 1989; Fenner et al., 1993). The mechanism by which IL-2 causes delirium is uncertain. EEG changes pointing to diffuse cerebral dysfunction have been observed.

Despite a considerable amount of research into the neuropathophysiology of delirium, the mechanisms remain poorly understood. The confusion was summed up by Trzepacz and van der Mast (2002): 'Certain neuroanatomical and neurotransmitter systems may represent final common pathways for the otherwise diverse aetiologies of delirium, or delirium may be the final common symptom of multiple neurotransmitter abnormalities'.

It is likely that all of the potential contributors described above have a role to play, but perhaps to different degrees in different individuals. What makes one person susceptible to delirium compared with a fellow patient with similar risk factors remains unclear.

## Other types of delirium

### Delirium tremens

This term was introduced by Sutton in 1813 and is still widely used today. It is defined as a delirious state which occurs within a week of withdrawal of alcohol. Its diagnostic criteria include marked autonomic hyperactivity and the associated features which include: vivid hallucinations which can be visual, auditory, and tactile; delusions; agitation; a coarse irregular tremor. Seizures can occur, especially if excess alcohol consumption has occurred for at least 5 years and often herald a florid delirium.

Although anecdotally common, the incidence of true delirium tremens is considered to be low. Some believe it to be less than 1% of all alcoholics undergoing withdrawal, but in specific populations such as those hospitalized for acute mental and physical disturbances associated with alcohol the incidence was as high as 40% (Lipowski, 1990). Men are affected by delirium tremens more commonly than women by four or five fold, and on average it occurs in the fifth decade of life.

Management involves the use of benzodiazepines (Trzepacz, 1999) both for symptoms and seizure treatment. Nutritional problems frequently co-exist and treatment with B vitamins, especially thiamine, is important. Although the majority of elderly patients presenting with delirium will not have an alcohol withdrawal aetiology, it is important to establish an alcohol history as the consequences of missing such a case can be devastating, due to the possible development of Wernicke's encephalopathy or Wernicke–Korsakoff syndrome. If in doubt concentrated B vitamins should be used. As the elderly population changes and alcohol problems, particularly amongst women, are destined to increase a good awareness of delirium tremens and the consequences of failing to treat should be borne in mind. Pharmacological agents used in other causes of delirium, such as haloperidol, should be used with caution.

## Benzodiazepine withdrawal

Abrupt reduction in dosage or cessation of any sedative drug may result in a withdrawal syndrome similar to that seen in alcohol withdrawal. This should be avoided with gradual reduction in dosage over months, and in some cases years. Although thought to be safe drugs a few decades ago, the benzodiazepines are highly addictive in susceptible individuals and there are still many patients on such agents decades later. Sometimes abrupt withdrawal can occur inadvertently when the patient is admitted to hospital and is unable to give a clear account of their medications (Moss, 1991; Moss and Lanctot, 1998). If the baseline medication list is in doubt one must contact the general practitioner at the earliest possibility to ensure an iatrogenic withdrawal syndrome is avoided.

## References

Anthony, J.C., LeResche, L., Niaz, V. *et al.* (1982). Limits of the 'MMSE' as a screening test for dementia and delirium among hospital patients. *Psychological Medicine*, **12**, 397–408.

American Psychiatric Association (1994). *Diagnostic and statistical manual of mental disorders*, 4th edn. APA, Washington, DC.

Baker, F.M., Wiley, C., Kokmen, E., Chandra, V., and Schoenberg, B.S. (1999). Delirium episodes during the course of clinically diagnosed Alzheimer's disease. *Journal of the National Medical Association*, **91**, 625–30.

Barberger-Gateau, P., Commenges, D., Gagnon, M. *et al.* (1992). Instrumental activities of daily living as a screening tool for cognitive impairment in elderly community dwellers. *Journal of the American Geriatrics Society*, **40**(11), 1129–34.

Beresin, E.V. (1998). Delirium in the elderly. *Journal of Geriatric Psychiatry and Neurology*, **1**, 127–43.

Bowen, J.D. and Larson, E.B. (1993). Drug induced cognitive impairment. *Drugs & Aging*, **3**, 349–57.

Breitbart, W., Marotta, R., Platt, M.M. *et al.* (1996). A double blind trial of haloperidol, chlorpromazine and lorazepam in the treatment of delirium in hospitalized AIDS patients. *American Journal of Psychiatry*, **153**, 231–237.

Breitbart, W., Narotta, R., Platt, M.M. *et al.* (1999). A double blind trial of haloperidol, chlorpromazine and lorazepam in the treatment of delirium in hospitalised AIDS patients. *American Journal Psychiatry*, **153**, 231–7.

Brenner, R.P. (1991). Utility of EEG in delirium: past views and current practice. *International Psychogeriatrics*, **3**, 211–29.

Cole, M.G. (2004). Delirium in elderly patients. *American Journal of Psychiatry*, **12**, 7–21.

Cole, M.G., McCusker, J., Bellevance, F. *et al.* (2002). Systematic detection and multidisciplinary care of delirium in older medical inpatients; a randomised trial. *Canadian Medical Association Journal*, **167**(7), 753–9.

Denikoff, K., Rubinow, D.R., Papa, M.Z. *et al.* (1987). The neuropsychiatric effects of treatment with interleukin-2 and lymphocyte-activated killer cells. *Annals of Internal Medicine*, **107**, 293–300.

Dolan, M.M., Hawkes, W.G., Zimmermen, S.I. *et al.* (2000). Delirium on hospital admission in aged hip fracture patients, prediction of mortality and 2 year functional outcomes. *Journals of Gerontology. Series A, Biological Sciences and Medical Sciences*, **55A**, M527–M534.

Dyer, C.B., Ashton, C.M., and Teasdale, T.A. (1995). Postoperative delirium. *Archives of Internal Medicine*, **155**, 461–5.

Eikelenboom, P. and Hoogendijk, W.J. (1990). Do delirium and Alzheimer's dementia share specific pathogenic mechanisms? *Dementia and Geriatric Cognitive Disorders*, **10**, 319–24.

Engel, G.L. and Romano, J. (1959). Delirium, a syndrome of cerebral insufficiency. *Journal of Chronic Diseases*, **9**, 260–77.

Evans, L.K. and Strumpf, N.E. (1989). Tying down the elderly. A review of the literature on physical restraint. *Journal of the American Geriatrics Society*, **37**, 65–74.

Fenner, M., Hanninen, E., Kirchner, H. *et al.* (1993). Neuropsychiatric symptoms during treatment with interleukin-2 and interferon-alpha [letter]. *Lancet*, **341**, 372.

Fick, D. and Foreman, M. (2000). Consequences of not recognising delirium superimposed on dementia in hospitalised elderly individuals. *Journal of Gerontological Nursing*, **26**, 30–40.

Fisher, B.W. and Flowerdew, G. (1995). A simple model for predicting postoperative delirium in older patients undergoing elective orthopaedics surgery. *Journal of the American Geriatrics Society*, **43**, 175–8.

Flacker, J.M. and Lipsitz, L.A. (1999). Serum anticholinergic activity changes with acute illness in elderly medical patients. *Journals of Gerontology. Series A, Biological Sciences and Medical Sciences*, **54**, M12–M16.

Flacker, J.M. and Marcantonio, E.R. (1998). Delirium in the elderly: optimal management. *Drugs and Ageing*, **13**, 119–30.

Folstein, M.F., Folstein, S.E., and McHugh, P.R. (1975). Mini-mental state: a preactical method for grading the cognitive state of patients for the clinician. *Journal of Psychiatric Research*, **12**, 189–98

Folstein, M.F., Bassett, S.S., Romanosski, A.L., and Nestadt, G. (1991). The epidemiology of delirium in the community: the Eastern Baltimore Mental Health Survey. *International Psychogeriatrics*, **3**, 169–76.

Foreman, M.D. (1989). Confusion in the hospitalised elderly, incidence, onset and associated features. *Research in Nursing & Health*, **12**, 21–9.

Foreman, M. and Milisen, K. (2004). Improving recognition of delirium in the elderly. *Primary Psychiatry*, **11**, 46–50.

Francis, J. and Kapoor, W.N. (1992). Prognosis after hospital discharge of older medical patients with delirium. *Journal of the American Geriatrics Society*, **40**, 601–6.

Francis, J., Martin, D., and Kappor, W.N. (1990). A prospective study of delirium in hospitalized elderly. *Journal of the American Medical Association*, **263**, 1097–101.

George, J., Bleasdale, S., and Singleton, S.J. (1997). Causes and prognosis of delirium in elderly patients admitted to district general hospital. *Age and Ageing*, **26**, 423–7.

Gillick, M.R., Serrell, N.A., and Gillick, L.S. (1982). Adverse consequences of hospitalisation in the elderly. *Social Science & Medicine*, **1982**, 1033–8.

Golinger, R.C., Peet, T., and Tune, L.E. (1987). Association of elevated plasma anticholinergic activity with delirium in surgical patients. *American Journal of Psychiatry*, **144**, 1218–20.

Gustafson, Y., Berggren, D., Brannstrom, B. *et al.* (1988). Acute confusional states in elderly patients treated for femoral neck fractures. *Journal of the American Geriatrics Society*, **36**, 525–30.

Gustafson, Y., Brannstrom, B., Berggren, D. *et al.* (1991). A geriatric anesthesiologic program to reduce acute confusional states in elderly patients treated for femoral neck fractures. *Journal of the American Geriatrics Society*, **39**, 655–62.

Han, L., McCusker, J., Cole, M., Abrahamowicz, M., Primeau, F., and Elie, M. (2001). Use of medications with anticholinergic effect predicts clinical severity of delirium symptoms in older medical in patients. *Archives of Internal Medicine*, **161**, 1099–105.

Hart, B. (1936). Delirious states. *British Medical Journal*, **2**, 745–9.

Inouye, S.K. (1994). The dilemma of delirium: clinical and research controversies regarding diagnosis & evaluation of delirium in hospitalised elderly medical patients. *American Journal of Medicine*, **97**, 278–88.

Inouye, S.K. (1997). Delirium and cognitive decline: does delirium lead to dementia? In *Cognitive decline: strategies for prevention: proceedings of a White House Conference on aging* (ed. H.M. Fillit and R.N. Butler), pp. 85–107. Greenwich Medical Media, London.

Inouye, S.K. (1998). Delirium in hospitalised older patients. *Clinical Geriatric Medicine*, **14**, 745–64.

Inouye, S.K. and Charpentier, P.A. (1996). Precipitating factors for delirium in hospitalized persona. *Journal of the American Medical Association*, **275**, 825–7.

Inouye, S.K., van Dyck, C.H., Alessi, C.A., Balkin, S., Siefal, A.P., and Horwitz, R.I. (1990). Clarifying confusion: the confusion assessment method. A new method for detection of delirium. *Annals of Internal Medicine*, **113**, 941–8.

Inouye, S.K., Viscoli, C.M., Horowitz, R.I. *et al.* (1993). A predictive model for delirium in hospitalized elderly medical patients bade on admission characteristics. *Annals of Internal Medicine*, **119**, 474–81.

Inouye, S.K., Rushing, J.T., Foreman, M.D., Palmer, R.M., and Pompei, P. (1998). Does delirium contribute to poor hospital outcomes? A three site epidemiologic study. *Journal of General Internal Medicine*, **13**, 234–42.

Inouye, S.K., Bogardus, S.T., Jr, Charpentier, P.A. *et al.* (1999). A multicomponent intervention to prevent delirium in hospitalised older patients. *New England Journal of Medicine*, **340**, 669–76.

Inouye, S.K., Foreman, M.D., Mion, L.C., Katz, K.H., and Cooney, L.M., Jr (2001). Nurses recognition of delirium and its symptoms: comparison of nurse and researcher ratings. *Archives of Internal Medicine*, **161**, 2467–73.

Jackson, J.C., Gordon, S.M., Hart, R.P., Hopkins, R.O., and Ely, E.W. (2004). The association between delirium and cognitive decline: a review of the empirical literature. *Neuropsychological Reviews*, **14**, 87–98.

Jitapunkul, S., Pillay, I., and Ebrahim, S. (1991). The Abbreviated Mental Test: its use and validity. *Age and Ageing*, **20**, 332–6.

Johnson, J.C., Kerse, N.M., Gottlieb, J.L. *et al.* (1992). Prospective versus retrospective methods of identifying patients with delirium. *Journal of the American Geriatrics Society*, **40**, 316–19.

Kellam, A.M.P. (1987). The neuroleptic malignant syndrome, so called: a survey of the world literature. *British Journal of Psychiatry*, **150**, 752–9.

Kiely, D.K., Bergmann, M.A., Jones, R.N., Murphy, K.M., Orav, E.J., and Marcantonio, E.R. (2004). Characteristics associated with delirium persistence among newly admitted post-acute facility patients. *Journals of Gerontology. Series A, Biological Sciences and Medical Sciences*, **59**, 344–9.

Koponen, H. (1991). Electroencephalographic indices for diagnosis of delirium. *International Psychogeriatrics*, **3**, 249–51.

Koponen, H., Steinback, U., Mattila, E. *et al.* (1989). Delirium among elderly persons admitted to a psychiatric hospital; clinical course during the acute stage and one-year follow up. *Acta Psychiatrica Scandinavica*, **79**, 579–85.

Levkoff, S.E., Evans, D.A., Litpzin, B. *et al.* (1992). Delirium: the occurrence and persistence of symptoms among the elderly hospitalised patients. *Archives of Internal Medicine*, **152**, 334–40.

Levkoff, S.E., Lipstin, B., Cleary, P.D. *et al.* (1996). Subsyndromal delirium. *American Journal of Geriatrics*, **4**, 320–9.

Lipowski, Z.J. (1990). *Delirium: acute confusional states*. Oxford University Press, New York.

Lofgreen, R.P., Macpherson, D.S., Granieri, R. *et al.* (1989). Mechanical restraints on the medical wards: are protective devices safe? *American Journal of Public Health*, **79**(6), 735–8.

Lundstrom, R.N., Edlind, A., and Karlsson, S. (2005). A multifactorial intervention program reduces the duration of delirium. *Journal of the American Geriatrics Society*, **53**, 622–8.

McCusker, J., Cole, M., and Dendukuri, N. *et al.* (2001). Delirium in older medical inpatients and subsequent cognitive and functional status; a prospective study. *Candian Medical Association Journal*, **165**, 575–83.

Mach, J.R., Dysken, M.W., Kuskowski, M. *et al.* (1995) Serum anticholinergic activity in hospitalised older persons with delirium: a preliminary study. *Journal of the American Geriatrics Society*, **43**, 491–5.

McIntosh, T.K., Bush, H.L., Yeston, N.S. *et al.* (1985). Beta-endorphin, cortisol and postoperative delirium: A preliminary report. *Psychoneuroendocrinology*, **10**, 303–13.

Marcantonio, E.R., Juarez, G., Gokman, L. *et al.* (1994). The relationship of post operative delirium with psychoactive medications. *Journal of the American Medical Association*, **272**, 1518–22.

Marcantonio, E.R., Flacker, J.M., Michaels, M. *et al.* (2000). Delirium is independently associated with poor functional recovery after hip fractures. *Journal of the American Geriatrics Society*, **48**, 618–24.

Marcantonio, E.R., Flacker, J.M., Wright, J., and Resnick, N.M. (2001). Reducing delirium after hip fracture: a randomised trial. *Journal of the American Geriatrics Society*, **49**, 516–22.

Marcantonio, E.R., Simon, S.E., Bergmann, M.A. *et al.* (2003). Delirium symptoms in post acute care: prevalent, persistent and associated with poor functional recovery. *Journal of the American Geriatrics Society*, **51**, 4–9.

Mattice, M. (1989). Intrahospital room transfers: a potential link to delirium in the elderly. *Perspectives*, **13**, 10–12.

Moran, J.A. and Dorevitch, M.I. (2001). Delirium in the hospitalised elderly. *Australian Journal of Hospital Pharmacy*, **31**, 35–40.

Moss, J.H. (1991). Sedative and hypnotic withdrawal states in hospitalised patients. *Lancet*, **338**, 575.

Moss, J.H. and Lanctot, K.L. (1998). Iatrogenic benzodiazepine withdrawal delirium in hospitalised older patients. *Journal of the American Geriatrics Society*, **43**, 1020–2.

Murray, A.M., Levkoff, S.E., Wetle, T.T. *et al.* (1993). Acute delirium and functional decline in the hospitalised elderly patient. *Journal of Gerontology*, **48**, M181–M186.

Murray, J.A.H. (ed.) (1897). *A new English dictionary on historical principles*, Vol. 3, p. 165. Clarendon Press, Oxford.

O'Keeffe, S.T. and Devlin, J.G. (1994). Delirium and the dexamethasone suppression test in the elderly. *Neuropsychobiology*, **30**, 153–6.

O'Keeffe, S. and Lavan, J. (1997). The prognostic significance of delirium in older hospital patients. *Journal of the American Geriatrics Society*, **45**, 174–8.

O'Keeffe, S.T., Mulkerrin, E.C., Nazeem, K. *et al.* (2005). Use of serial MMSE scores to diagnose and monitor delirium in elderly hospital patients. *Journal of the American Geriatrics Society*, **53**(5), 867–70.

Olsson, T. (1999). Activity in the hypothalamic-pituitary-adrenal axis and delirium. *Dementia and Geriatric Cognitive Disorders*, **10**, 345–9.

Pompei, P., Foreman, M., and Rudberg, M.A. (1994). Delirium in hospitalised older persons: outcomes and predictors. *Journal of the American Geriatrics Society*, **42**, 809–15.

Potter, J. and George, J. (2006). The prevention, diagnosis and management of delirium in older people: concise guidelines. *Clinical Medicine*, **6**(3), 303–8.

Rabins, P.V. and Folstein, M.F. (1982). Delirium in dementia: diagnostic criteria and fatality rates. *British Journal of Psychiatry*, **140**, 149–53.

Rahkonen, T., Elonieme-Sulkava, U., Pannila, S., Sivenius, J., and Sulkava, R. (2001). Systematic intervention for supporting community care of elderly people after a delirium episode. *International Psychogeriatrics*, **13**, 37–49.

Roche, V. (2003). Etiology and management of delirium. *American Journal of Medical Science*, **325**, 20–30.

Rockwood, K. (1989). Acute confusion in elderly medical patients. *Journal of the American Geriatrics Society*, **37**, 150–4.

Rockwood, K. (1993). The occurrence and duration of symptoms in elderly patients with delirium. *Journal Gerontology: Medical Sciences*, **48**, M162–M166.

Rockwood, K., Cosway, S., Stolee, P. *et al.* (1994). Increasing the recognition of delirium in elderly patients. *Journal of the American Geriatrics Society*, **42**, 252–6.

Rockwood, K., Cosway, S., Carver, D., Jarrett, P., Stadnyk, K., and Fisk, J. (1999). The risk of dementia and death after delirium. *Age and Ageing*, **28**, 551–6.

Rogers, M.P., Liang, M.H., Daltory, L.H. *et al.* (1989). Delirium after elective orthopaedic surgery, risk factors and natural history. *International Journal of Psychiatry in Medicine*, **19**, 109–21.

Romano, J. and Engel, G.L. (1944). Delirium.1.electroencephalographic data. *Archives of Neurology and Psychiatry*, **51**, 356–77.

Rosenberg, S., Loetz, M., and Yang, J. (1989). Experience with the use of high-dose interleukin-2 in the treatment of 652 cancer patients. *Annals of Surgery*, **210**, 474–84.

Rudberg, M.A., Pompei, P., Foreman, M.D. *et al.* (1997). The natural history of delirium in older hospitalised patients: a syndrome of heterogeneity. *Age and Ageing*, **26**, 169–74.

Saravay, S.M. and Lavin, M. (1994). Psychiatric comorbidity and length of stay in the general hospital: a critical review of outcome studies. *Psychosomatics*, **35**, 233–52.

Schor, J.D., Levkoff, S.E., Lipsitz, L.A. *et al.* (1992). Risk factors for delirium in hospitalised elderly. *Journal of the American Medical Association*, **267**, 827–31.

Shigeta, H., Yasui, A., Nimura, Y. *et al.* (2001). Postoperative delirium and melatonin levels in elderly patients. *American Journal of Surgery*, **182**, 449–54.

Simpson, C.J. and Kellett, J.M. (1987). The relationship between pre-operative anxiety and post-operative delirium. *Journal of Psychosomatic Research*, **31**, 491–7.

Sullivan-Marx, E.M. (1994). Delirium and physical restraint in the hospitalized elderly. *Image*, **26**(4), 295–300.

Treloar, A.J. and Macdonald, A.J.D. (1995). Recognition of cognitive impairment by day and night nursing staff among acute geriatric patients. *Journal of the Royal Society of Medicine*, **88**, 196–8.

Treloar, A.J. and Macdonald, A.J.D. (1997a). Outcome of delirium: Part 1 Outcome of delirium diagnosed by DSM-III-R, ICD-10 and CAMDEC and derivation of the reversible cognitive dysfunction scale among acute geriatric in patients. *International Journal of Geriatric Psychiatry*, **12**, 609–13.

Treloar, A.J. and Macdonald, A.J.D. (1997b). Outcome of delirium: Part 2: Clinical features of reversible cognitive dysfunction – are they the same as accepted definitions of delirium? *International Journal of Geriatric Psychiatry*, **12**, 614–18.

Trzepacz, P.T. (1994). The neuropathogenesis of delirium. *Psychosomatics*, **35**, 374–91.

Trzepacz, P.T. (1996). Anticholinergic model for delirium. *Seminars in Clinical Neuropsychiatry*, **1**, 294–303.

Trzepacz, P.T. (1999). Update on the neuropathogenesis of delirium. *Dementia and Geriatric Cognitive Disorders*, **10**, 330–4.

Trzepacz, P.T. and Francis, J. (1990). Low serum albumin and risk of delirium. *American Journal of Psychiatry*, **147**, 675.

Trzepacz, P. and van der Mast, R. (2002). The neuropathophysiology of delirium. In *Delirium in old age* (ed. J. Lindesay, K. Rockwood, and A. Macdonald), pp. 51–90. Oxford University Press, Oxford.

Tune, L.E., Damlouij, N., and Holland, A. (1981). Postoperative delirium is associated with elevated serum anticholinergic levels. *Lancet*, **1**, 651.

Wengel, S.P., Roccaforte, W.H., and Burke, W.J. (1998). Donepezil improves symptoms of delirium in dementia: implications for future research. *Journal of Geriatric*, **11**, 159–61.

WHO (World Health Organization) (1993). *International classification of diseases*, 10th revision (ICD-10). WHO, Geneva.

Williams, M., Campbell, E., Raynor, W.J. *et al.* (1985). Reducing acute confusional states in elderly patients with hip fractures. *Research in Nursing & Health*, **8**, 329.

# Mood disorders: the experience of a depressive illness

Anon

I shall try to convey how it felt to suffer acute depression, first describing how the illness progressed from unheeded minor symptoms to attempted suicide shortly before my seventy-seventh birthday. Then I shall describe how I fared in hospital.

## Before hospital—the onset of depression

### Minor health details

I have experienced mild insomnia since young adulthood, spending one or two hours awake between longer spells of sleep. The remedy has been not to fret. The second sleep always came along in the end.

I have also experienced something far worse: anxiety attacks consisting of extended 'butterflies in the stomach'. It is a helpless, queasy sensation like treading down or up a step which will never be there or not there while being whirled up, down, and around simultaneously in an express lift with no destination.

With anxiety attacks there were two consolations. They never lasted more than an hour or so. And they struck only occasionally over more than half a century, often before or after the beginning of a journey. Yet another consolation was that anxiety attacks and insomnia never coincided. That such a coincidence was impossible I took for granted. What I never asked myself was…

*…what would life be like if anxiety and sleeplessness should ever coexist unrelieved for a period of weeks?*

That is what was going to happen to me. That is the subject of this chapter. That is what depression means to me.

### An unpleasant episode

I am a retired author and academic, now 86 years old. My wife and I have been married for over 50 years. Before the 1990s I had no serious adult illness. But then, in December 1995, the forces of senile disintegration swooped: I had what one specialist [ENT] diagnosed as labyrinthitis, and another [neurology] as an ischaemic incident. I feel that the neurologist was right. Anyway, it began with falling over on the way to the loo one night, which seemed so comic that I laughed aloud. I was not to laugh again for a long time. For 2 days I couldn't eat, could barely drink, could not endure light, could only move about on all fours. Recovery was slow and only partial. I still have a balancing problem.

I think this attack impaired my ability to face the challenges which were to surface just over a year later.

## Stress culminates in collapse

Suicide, attempted on 11 April 1997, was preceded by about 10 weeks of exponentially escalating stress. It started in January, when prostate cancer was diagnosed.

I took the bad news as something to be coped with, not panicked about, and the focus of my angst, as things developed in the weeks after the diagnosis, was not the cancer itself but the nexus of anxieties to which it gave rise. We were already thinking of moving to a smaller, less labour-intensive house. Now we needed to move soon.

In earlier years I had coped with the stresses of house-moving, but now they terrified me. I suspect that fear of the tumour, suppressed on diagnosis, may have lurked within the fear of house-moving.

The expected relocation hassles were soon aggravated by financial, tax, family, and other worries beyond the previous norm. And yet there was nothing unfamiliar about this crisis. My strength and resourcefulness were being challenged, as often before, and so I braced myself, as often before, and even looked forward to winning a struggle which I would have preferred not to be necessary.

The difference this time was that my resistance was to prove pathetically inadequate.

## Medicine comes to the rescue

By the time when I felt the need to see a doctor an evil coincidence had occurred. This was the retirement of the GP whose patients my wife and I had been for many years, with the result that a new [to us] GP saw me and that we were strangers to each other. I reported my troubles and a prescription was issued. I did not look to see what I had been given by the pharmacy until I got home and found it was temazepam. I already knew these tablets as a mild soporific, effective in the right context. In my present plight they were like trying to quench a forest fire by spitting.

I put the tablets on a shelf unopened.

My condition grew worse. The periods of insomnia increased. Anxiety attacks became frequent. Yes, it was now that these two former inconveniences, already fully scaled ravening dragons, joined forces. By early April both were always with me, simultaneous, unrelieved, raging, nagging, seething. I had already paid a second visit to the health centre. This time a different prescription: antidepression pills. Then another evil coincidence struck. Owing to a maddening misunderstandings I couldn't get my hands on these tablets for several frantic days. Hanging on waiting for this medication was one of the most potent anxiety-provokers in the whole sequence.

I began taking the tablets. They had no evident effect.

## Desolation week [5–11 April 1997]

Nights: mostly I stood still in the dark in my loft-extension study-bedroom, trying to solve two urgent problems. First, to find a way to cancel the past and go back to when being me had been bearable. I knew that moving backwards in time wouldn't be easy. Indeed, I was certain that, outside science fiction, it had never been done before…

…Quite so. But just a moment…had the problem ever been tackled by an intellect as powerful as my own…?

…So I spent several nights frenetically striving to turn time's moving finger back. But I could not cancel one second of the past, which rushed ahead regardless. So logic decreed that I must cancel myself.

This brings us to my second nightly preoccupation. Self-destruction. But how? I would never have the courage to leap from a high place, or trudge through the moonlight to the near-by railway line and throw myself under a train—especially as my wife's keen ears would detect my footsteps on our gravelled drive in time for her to thwart my purpose. As for hanging, I am mechanically clumsy. I would get the knot wrong. There must be a better way.

At night, too, I wrote several suicide notes which I destroyed, even leaving one on the computer—a macabre, eerily flickering green in the gloom, it would have unnerved me even more had that been possible. With a palsied shudder I hit Delete.

Daytime during Desolation Week was even worse. I could tolerate neither company nor solitude. I could not sit or lie without wanting to be up and about, and vice versa. Persistence in the illusion that physical activity might relieve the anguish drove me to frenzied solitary walks, only to prove again and again the uselessness of what had once helped to cheer away the mild anxieties of the healthy brain. Though I knew that I was being treated for depression, which is what I was unbeknownst actually suffering from, I did not believe the diagnosis. Nor, indeed, was I depressed, in the layman's sense of the word. I was anxious, anxious, anxious. I did not even know that 'depression' [unlike 'madness', 'off his rocker' etc.] was a medical term, or that I was suffering from it or from any other definable illness, or that depression could be successfully treated, as my own eventually was. All I knew was that I longed, yearned, lusted, with a passion more violent than any previously experienced, in a life not without emotional turbulence, for my accursed consciousness to be terminated once and for all. I also knew that I was going to bring that about even if—so to speak—it was the last thing I did. I gave no hint of my purpose to anyone, and least of all to my wife, whose skill in diverting my many wrong-headed intentions had been honed over nearly half a century. And, harrowed though I was, I did somehow hide the full seriousness of my condition from her and from everyone I met, though she and anyone else could see with half an eye that I wasn't bubbling with high spirits.

Did I give no thought to the hurt I must cause? Of course. But decreasingly as my brain succumbed to what I have since learned to be a chemical disorder. I was also convinced that my wife and family, along with the world in general, would be well rid of whatever subspecies of Kafkaesque vermin I was metamorphosing into.

## D minus one

The small hours. I plot an experiment. This requires my wife's absence, so I wait for her to leave for her place of part-time work on the following afternoon. Glorious, sunny, oh-to-be-in-England weather. As the sound of her car dies away I sneak up the drive to the garage to examine the exhaust pipe of my own garaged car. Unlooping the hose which is part of our pool-vacuuming assemblage, I find [as hoped] that the hose fits the exhaust-pipe to perfection. I poke the other end of the hose through the car's off-side window, sit in the driver's seat, hit the ignition. Instantly a vile black fog blinds and throttles me. 'My God, I might have killed myself!' is my first, fatuous, thought as I leap out and switch off. Grotesquely, my second thought, though I'm no eco-freak, is of a billion odd pipes globe wide spewing out non-stop the mephitic gloop that I have just sampled a couple of seconds of.

I was soon reflecting that I, a person it wasn't good to have hanging around, had hit on an effective exit route from a world that wasn't that good to hang around in. So the experiment had been doubly successful. But for some reason I was still not ready for death. Needing displacement activity, I piled the car with junk to be disposed of because of our impending move, and made the umpteenth trip to the near-by municipal dump.

## D for disaster day

Another glorious spring morning. A Friday, so household routine, which all along had pulsed in dreary counterpoint to the love–death–madness farrago fermenting away up top, required me to do my laundry. No problem tossing the stuff into the washing-machine. While it was whirling I hoisted the drying apparatus on the lawn—a space-saving structure with segments of parallel plastic cord in decreasing lengths as each wedge approaches the centre. To peg my clothing, sheets etcetera through slanting sunlight on to this devilish device as it twisted erratically in the breeze—here was the perfect recipe for whipping my reeling mind into a still more frenzied tarantella.

What next? Still hoping to find relief in physical activity, I plodded out to the wood which began only a few steps from our front gate. Knowing this intimately from many years of walking, I doddered purposively out over the rough ground, there being no path from where I started. After walking desperately for a bit I halted and looked up at the canopy of branches as they twisted, waltzed, and sashayed against the sunlight up there. This would have been an abrupt reminder that I suffer from permanent slight vertigo, had I been in the habit of forgetting about that. Swaying and sick at heart, I suddenly realized that I was completely lost barely a mile from my own house. I could not orientate myself, as would have been possible formerly, by the growl of traffic on the busy road system a mile or so away because there was a growl or whine throbbing or buzzing in my ears from all of a 360-degree circle. Would I ever find the way home? Would my bones be licked clean by foxes or deer? Would I become a bogey to the children of the nearest suburb? The ravaged fibre of my psyche could still come up with such crazed speculations while I somehow dragged myself back to our house.

## Our last lunch

My wife now tells me that we had lunch together after this, and that my low spirits had clearly not lifted, but that there was no apparent serious cause for alarm. This lunch I don't remember…

…only that it was suddenly evening, that we'd had our evening meal, and that darkness had descended. Later research has shown that this was an illusion. It was in fact about 2 o'clock in the afternoon when I wished my wife good night, resisting an impish temptation to make it 'goodbye'. Why did I pretend to be going to bed just after what I thought was supper, though it was actually lunch? With maniacal guile I wanted to maximize the time between my departure and the moment when, presumably after breakfast time, an attempt might be made to resuscitate me from what I was going to do. And that was to be no 'cry for help'.

Stone dead hath no fellow.

So up the stairs to my study-bedroom I blunder in darkness which is in fact daylight, switch on the strip lighting, which does nothing to diminish the Stygian gloom clouding my eyes ['must get a new tube' crosses my mind], grope for a high shelf and bring down the saucer into which I have previously shelled out of their blister integuments…

…what else but the formerly execrated temazepam tablets, now transformed from a mockery of my condition into the means of ending it? As may have been evident above, my previous day's play-acting with the exhaust fumes had been one more displacement activity along with the earlier hanging and other fantasies and later trip to the dump. Temazepam had been the instrument of choice bobbing around up in the serotonin [a word crucial to my crisis that I didn't yet know] all along.

Sliding the tablets into an empty vodka glass, I saw them start to effervesce [there must have been a little moisture in the glass], at which point every scintilla of play-acting was quenched. I knew those tablets would become useless unless ingested instantly.

In which case I would be condemned to life!

'No way, José!' or similar idiocy flashed through my, er, mind as I gulped the pills with water, and chased them with the unexpired portion of my prescribed antidepression tablets.

# First 3 weeks in hospital. Depression comes to a climax

### Where am I?

After less than 24 hours' mercifully total unconsciousness my hopes of dying happily ever after are dashed. So what went wrong?

By about 7.30 on the evil evening of Friday 11 April my wife, as I learn later, is wondering why I have not responded to her buzzings announcing supper. She goes upstairs, finds me comatose and vomit-puddled on my futon, dials 999, rings our nearest-domiciled son. At John Radcliffe Hospital the casualty doctor tells my wife and son 'the prognosis is poor because of his age'. Wife and son watch my pulse hesitate on a video monitor until the throb perks up. I survive because [says the doctor] I have a strong constitution, but I suspect his professional skill was no less culpable.

The first thing I know is a familiar voice [my son's in fact] in the blackness asking what England's chances are of beating Australia in the pending Ashes series. An even more familiar voice replies: a voice which I do not know to be my own at the time.

'That is a ridiculous question. You know perfectly well we don't have a bat's chance in hell.' Nor did we. This was 1997.

The decisiveness, impatience with lesser intellects, and sheer intellectual rigour have my son's dear old dad written into every syllable, he explains later with his usual teasing irony. At the time of course my scathing sally was of importance as an indicator that I had escaped serious brain damage.

Some time after this exchange black nothingness lightens into grey somethingness, and I am suddenly multiply alert, while yet swimming in a sea of doziness as self-contradicting fractured notions assail me.

I'm glad to be alive. I wish I was dead. It's good to see my wife and son. I wish they weren't here, wherever here is. I wish I wasn't here either. Or anywhere else. So much for my temazepam cocktail! What went wrong? How ill am I because it feels like very? Surely this can't be that worst worst-case scenario Life after Death. It looks more like…it is…a hospital ward.

## Hospital. General observations

I was admitted on 11 April 1997 and discharged on 24 June of the same year. And if my precision in recalling dates and periods of time seems surprising, it surprises me too, because during most of my illness I could not have told you the date or the day of the week or where I was or, often, even who I was.

I spent 7 days in Edward Buzzard Ward at the John Radcliffe Hospital, followed by 67 days in Sandford Ward at another hospital.

Three points about my hospital experience.

First, nothing in this *via dolorosa* was as agonizing as the mental condition which preceded it and drove me to seek death—even though, during the run-up to the overdose, illness had so little affected me outwardly that my family thought I was just in low spirits. In fact, barely a moment in my hospital experiences, acutely distressing as they were, was as painful as *every single moment of the appalling week preceding my suicide attempt*.

Second, there was a contrast throughout my hospital stay between the hyperactivity of my brain and my external demeanour. I was sullen and uncommunicative, rarely spoke first, and did what the medical staff required, with one marked exception [see below]. This negativism was wearing off by the end of my stay and was punctured by manic interludes.

Third come hallucinations. These were lurid nightmares. But…!

…Dreams fade from memory on waking. My hallucinations still have not faded. I can recall enough to fill a large book, and this chapter contains only a tiny sampling.

## The week of the Buzzard

At Edward Buzzard I was well treated and cured of pneumonia, but remained prostrate. My mental health was rapidly deteriorating and was to do so for another 3 weeks. Coma alternated with fretful wakefulness and savage lung pain when I coughed. I could not find my way from loo back to bed or vice versa, I would wander off without knowing or remembering doing it. I even popped up in casualty once. So I was tagged with an Edward Buzzard ward wristlet and anklet.

Doctors on ward rounds saw me and individual psychiatrists saw me tête-à-tête. There were comic moments, e.g. after I had a brain scan [MRI] because this, claimed one doctor, showed me as an alcohol abuser. Would I be prepared to go on a course for treating alcohol dependency? I was speechless.

I cannot fault Edward Buzzard in terms of medical treatment, staff courtesy or kindness—only for its dinginess, its minuscule monochrome TV [dark green on light green] quacking away night and day, and perhaps for an aura emanating from the ghosts of overdosers and wrist-slashers of yesteryear.

The last day at Buzzard came 1 week after admission and was a trial since it wasn't clear until late evening whether a bed in a psychiatric ward would be available. My wife and younger daughter [then a social worker] both stayed with me all day in Buzzard where we felt threatened by visiting feral adolescents, possibly 'junkies', circling a newly admitted self-destructor in the bed on my left.

After my discharge from Buzzard late in the evening the three of us had to wait for up to an hour outside in the dark and cold of a dispensary for prescriptions to take to the new hospital. My wife had brought warm coats, but this was no setting for an incontinent [as I now was] and mentally disordered pneumonia convalescent. Then came navigation in my wife's car through the endemic severe traffic of the area. Slanting lights criss-crossed my sore eyelids and my two ladies understandably kept losing the way, especially within the new hospital's precincts—which are hard to navigate by day and at night are like a city of the dead. I think this hyper-anxious day was prejudicial to my condition.

## Sandford Ward

We might have entered paradise. Smiles from nurses, tea and sandwiches, and the Buzzard name tags snipped in no time.

Writing now in 2006 I remember Sandford as little short of ideal, not only in skilled medical treatment but also in human contact. Nurses, housekeepers, registrars, consultant-in-charge were models of consideration and friendliness. Visitors were welcome throughout the day. My wife was encouraged to seek advice on my well-being from doctors and nurses. Noticing that she was taking my dirty laundry home every day, the housekeepers relieved her of that. Nurses were patient and ingenious in proposing games, exercises, and pastimes to deploy physical and mental activity, but never forced things on anyone. The food was excellent. The bright lighting in the private rooms formed a contrast to Buzzard's baleful murk. Each room had its own wash basin and *en suite* loo shared with the occupant of the adjacent room. In short the ward was a credit to its staff and architect. True, it had two television sets. Nothing in this world is perfect.

These benefits are clear to me now, nearly 10 years later. It is also clear that they were beneficial from the moment of my admission onwards. But such was not my perception at the time. While the food was indeed excellent my appetite was poor to non-existent. The lighting in my room indeed did render it less baleful than Buzzard, but for one significant detail: the small point of light which circled non-stop round the central light fitting in the ceiling. A nurse told me that it was to show that the smoke alarm was functioning correctly…

…A likely story! That it was in fact a mini-camera designed to record my movements day and night was as plain as a barn door.

Deeply suspicious too was the conspiracy to keep me in ignorance of what the outside world was being told about me. And the public was already only too well informed, make no mistake. Take two such potent stimuli of the tabloid-reading hoi polloi as 'Suicide' and 'Oxford', and the headlines scream themselves.

DRUG-CRAZED… OXFORD THIS… SEX-RAT DON… FAILED DEATH BID… OXFORD THAT… SKULKS IN NHS HIDEOUT.

And similar, day after day. At least the staff had so far managed to keep the media away from Sandford, which showed they had retained shreds of decency. But just a moment. There's always a reason for these things. Clearly they were holding out for a bigger financial inducement.

As for their *en suite* loo, what a laugh…

…That amenity [shared with one other patient, remember] contained no fewer than four sliding catches at handle level, one inside and one outside of each of the two doors. With one of these little bolts each patient of a sharing pair could keep his oppo from coming into his own quarters. With the other little slider oppo could stop oppo intruding *in medias res*. So ingeniously were the catches dovetailed into the stainless steel of the doors that you could only tell whether a slider was engaged by trying to open the door by the handle, whether from inside or out. If, when you wanted to go, you couldn't open the door—that told you one of two things. Either your oppo was inside about his business. Or he had long ago done his business and forgotten to release the catch barring you from access…

…Forgotten!

How very unlikely! Ha ha. The idea of the inmate of a geriatric psychiatric ward forgetting something can of course be discounted out of hand!!!

Their plot was so insultingly obvious. Sandford was in cahoots with Buzzard, and had learnt—on a 'hot line' no doubt—that I had…

…begun to be plagued, as indicated above, by severe urinary urge incontinence…

…But at least I knew now why Sandford had been chosen as the ward for me. Oh, yes, it wasn't long before I saw through their little game! This was probably the only psychiatric outfit in the entire globe that boasted lavatories with the fiendish invisible sliding-catch arrangement described above. Its true purpose was to keep patients permanently worrying whether their amenity was vacant or engaged at any given moment and thus to pump up the pressures of incontinence to permanent bursting point.

Some of the best brains in the country planned this down to the last detail…

…My wife has since corrected my memory of this. She says that I was so ill during the first few weeks at Sandford that I was unaware of being incontinent, but—while remaining thus unaware—was yet capable of feeling anxiety about the potential unavailability of the loo. The fact that I began worrying about incontinence later was, she says, a sign that I cared, and that I had begun to get better. I think she is right, but add that my mental disorder was not a constant so that the process of being aware was not a constant either. Phases of lucidity punctuated the long delusional coma periods. Multiple anxieties were the keynote of both. Before the overdose anxiety had seemed a single intolerable integrated sensation. Whereas in Sandford it was *multiple anxieties* that devoured me: from outside like piranhas pouncing on a slab of blubber; from inside like wasp grubs hatching inside a live caterpillar on a TV nature programme. Even that caterpillar had better luck than I. *He* would soon die. *My* only hope now was that the cancer might move into galloping metastasis. But even the Big C let me down.

Anyway, the nurses soon moved me to a different room, one with a plastic-covered, wipeable floor, whereas my original room had a carpet…

…a carpet which soon caused me anxiety. Since I had ruined the sodden carpet in my first room I could expect a hefty bill for its replacement. Furthermore, though the hospital itself was in the National Health Service, Sandford might well be a private enclave where patients would be charged at exorbitant rates. And what of the laundering of my sheets, underpants and track-suit bottoms? I could just see some contracted up-market launderer gloating 'never give a sucker an even break' as he padded his bill.

That all this was no fantasy was proved when a nurse casually told me that she would be replaced next day by a 'bank nurse'. As that struck home my blood froze. After all, a hospital, like any other institution, is ultimately dependent on finance. If Sandford's hospital was deeply in hock to the banks, what more natural than that the banks should send round an official, posing as a nurse, to audit patients' individual liabilities? In no time these people would subpoena my accountant, ransack my desk, sell up my house and put wife and self in the street.

Thinking back to the evening of Friday 18 April, when my wife and daughter had driven me to Sandford, I couldn't remember how we had gained access. A dim recollection of being smuggled through a back door began to emerge…

…It didn't have any back door…

…How the two of them had got away with this I couldn't figure. But let's face it, they had dumped me there just to be rid of me. I was an interloper, an intruder! No thanks to my nearest and dearest!

More sinister still, my wife and son came back the very day after I was admitted. Cool as cucumbers, if you please. Which could only mean one thing.

They were both in on the act!

Such were the salient facts. You can't argue with facts.

As I mused misty details came into focus. Close to Sandford Ward is a renowned hospice, I happened to know.

What better cover for an institution less than respectable…no, let's not mince words…downright disreputable such as Sandford, the building of which had only recently been completed, than to cloak itself in an odour of sanctity by contriving—and there was contrivance written in letters of fire over the whole of this squalid business—to locate itself in close proximity to a renowned hospice?

So I began to put two and two together. And I soon noticed that, every few days, one of my fellow patients would have mysteriously disappeared, to be replaced by a stranger. Once, and once was enough, I was rash enough to ask a nurse what had happened to one of these desparecidos. 'Discharged' was the answer. Plausible enough, you say. But you didn't see the look that went with it.

And, anyway, wasn't the true explanation as plain as a pikestaff? What we had here at Sandford was an undercover unit which, for a suitable consideration, would dispose of unwanted aged relatives.

I had unmasked a clandestine euthanasia gang!

And the otherwise inexplicable construction of the shared loo fitted in here. What easier than to usher some unfortunate into one of a pair of empty rooms, shoot a jab of poisoned hypodermic, hustle the corpse through the loo into the other empty room where a large laundry trolley would 'happen' to be standing. Into the trolley with the corpse, off with it and up the ramp into a waiting van and then off to the huge boiler house which all hospitals have! Sizzle, sizzle, sizzle…and laugh all the way to the bank…

…But we must return to what is quaintly called reality.

## Visitors

Sandford's policy was of making patients' visitors welcome all day… I value that now, but didn't at the time.

Among visitors my wife was special. Though certain that she had sold out to Them, I thought she had been prudent. Why risk her life for worthless me? I got used to her visits, and became dependent on them. Often I could not or would not talk to her, but her kindness was a big factor in my recovery.

One day she said something that helped me a lot. She said that what I had done [overdosed] was a symptom of my illness, not something I was responsible for.

With other visitors it was different, especially in the early weeks. What with our numerous children, grandchildren, and friends I seemed to have more callers than the rest of the patients all told. I asked my wife to stop them coming, but she said they would take no notice. They persisted, and their affectionate loyalty mightily assisted my cure.

Why did I try to keep our children away in the early weeks?

I knew that they were in dire danger from Them. Of this I had proof one night when our youngest son was visiting. There was a nurse from the Caribbean, a colossus with bristling eyes and a voice of thunder. I was scared out of my wits by this fine nurse, as she later turned out to be. Especially as I had privately christened her 'Topsy'…

…and knew that if she found out about this she would kill me. Also, I would be 'done' for racism afterwards. Of Topsy's satanic malevolence she gave proof on the night when my son, much to my displeasure, suddenly materialized by the nurse's station.

Topsy glared. 'What is your relationship with this patient?'

He sprang to attention. 'Son'.

'Right!' snarls Topsy, picks up my six-foot-three son, inverts him, whisks him round a corner. I stand helpless as she rams him upside down into a cylindrical laundry basket, as revealed by the crunching of bone inside straining wickerwork…

…I remember it now as the most frightening moment of my life.

My children's determination to visit a creature as contemptible as myself struck me as a sign of appallingly bad judgement. I'd thought we brought them up better than that…

## Hospital under siege…

…Meanwhile a lot had been going on. All bad. Soon my pitiful suicide attempt, at first greeted with general hilarity by the public, was evoking snarls of righteous indignation.

People gathered round the hospital perimeter in cars and on foot. Some erected makeshift shelters. And soon what began with few good-humoured jeers mutated into something very different.

Oxford as a seat of learning has never been slow to fire the spleen of the unwashed, superstitiously dreading as they do the proximity of the best university in the world, and before long a chant broke out.

ELITIST SWINE… ELITIST SWINE…

Then these syllables began to be pounded out in staccato rhythm on car horns.

Before long the relatively harmless Oxford mob was joined by itinerant 'rent-a-yobbo' types from London and up north who would stop at nothing. And some of them drive BMWs!

And all I had to protect me was what time and energy the police could spare from 'politically correct' priorities for the minor matter of law and order. And a fat lot that would be once it penetrated Plod's thick skull that, PC-wise in both senses, I had committed every crime in the book, being male, white, heterosexually 'orientated', a taxpayer of unblemished pedigree, a holder of several higher degrees, and having behind me a career single-heartedly devoted to training pampered whelps from the privileged classes to conspire in keeping deserving comprehensive schoolites out of those posh, snobby, precious colleges of theirs with their antique silverware and port-sodden 'fellows'…

### …**Five days that shook the world**

We have reached Thursday 1 May 1997, the occasion of a General Election, but this blip in history is eclipsed by something more important because a nurse is asking me for a urine 'specimen'. Something I'm as well qualified to provide as any patient in history…

> …I deduce that the crunch time of my persecution is nigh. Clearly the raging mob outside the hospital can be denied no longer. They—yobbos, hysterical schoolgirls, Guardian readers, concerned senior citizens, the lot—will be allowed through the barriers to witness my public humiliation on a dais in front of Sandford. Proceedings will begin with someone pouring my own specimen over my own head.

…As I return that specimen to the nurse it occurs to me to sound her on the matter. I still remember our words *verbatim*.

'I believe I have to take part in some ceremony today?'

'I don't know about that', says nurse. 'All I know is you have a urology appointment at 3 o'clock this afternoon.'

At this point I blacked out and remained in deep coma, broken by a few short semi-lucid intervals, for 5 days. All I now remember is a few glimpses of our eldest son, who had flown over from Munich, where he works. What happened I later reconstructed from his testimony and from my wife's.

It seems that I did indeed keep my urology appointment, and without being conscious of being trundled several hundred yards there and back in a wheel-chair over roughish surfaces by a male nurse, or of seeing the specialist, or of anything else. When I am back in bed I somehow learn, still in deep coma, that the urologist has prescribed a course of tablets to be followed by a sequence of implants of the prostate-cancer inhibitor Zoladex [goserelin]. This, I knew, contains female hormones and can induce impotence. It may also promote the growth of a chap's very own rudimentary mammary protuberances. Not the ideal nostrum to feed a red-blooded, albeit septuagenarian, male!

This threat of emasculation *with knobs on* is an outrage too far. Still in deep coma I categorically refuse the urologist's tablets, also refusing my extensive other medication. I stop eating and drinking. After a day or two I am posing Sandford a problem—and this has of course to be a weekend which ends with a Bank Holiday. If I persist in my hunger and medication strike I shall have to be sectioned. And so I would have been if Sandford consultant had not come back from her holiday to rescue me. She skilfully persuaded me—without me being aware—to abandon my hunger and medication strike.

By the evening of 5 May I am through with the 5-day coma and watching Doherty beat Hendry in the final of the World Snooker Championship on TV, but unable to decode the movement of the balls as my sorely afflicted brain labours to assess precisely how afflicted it is. This process is not assisted when the channel is rezapped to the triumphalist gibberings of newly elected cabinet ministers.

## Last hospital weeks. Events outside my head

Between the 5-day crisis in early May and discharge from hospital in late June my illness lurched peristaltically towards recovery. Two aberrant episodes interrupted this sequence: one beneficial, the other malign.

### A leap forward

In the early afternoon of Saturday 17 May I'm gazing dozily at the willows outside my window and bracing myself to tidy the room behind me, cluttered with newspapers and magazines brought by my family. For several weeks, though, the process of reading has been beyond me.

I turn from the window, and…

…suddenly realise that, during the morning, I have—and without noticing it—done two *Times* crossword puzzles and read a *Spectator* from cover to cover!

It was a giant leap forward, but stopped far short of ending hallucinations and mental suffering.

### A step backwards

Awake one night I am half a-dream when a demoniac screech breaks the silence.

'TIBOR, I SHALL KILL YOU!!!'

Nurse Topsy! After that murderous midnight yelp could any doubt remain that I had been…

> …kidnapped by a medical Cosa Nostra with tentacles probing the very nerve centres of the hospital? By now, too, the Mob must be well established in Urology. Hence those female hormone tablets foisted on me, as related above…?

…I never learned how Tibor triggered Topsy's death threat. He was known to defaecate on the floor of our shared lavatory. Perhaps it was something in that line.

This episode did not help my recovery.

### Jim

As my illness receded contact with Jim, another patient, did help my recovery. He was a bit younger than I, had been a night operator at the local telephone exchange, had also plied other trades far removed from my own. His exposure to the educational process had been low compared with mine, and he had great respect—higher than my own—for intellectual prowess in general and mine in particular. This was a staple theme for mutual banter and laughter such as rarely came from anyone else in the ward.

We did crossword puzzles together. He admired my skill and I told him that my verbal dexterity is balanced by marked ineptitude in other areas of endeavour.

He was of small stature but with understated 'presence', a quiet clear voice and an air of benevolent authority. At first his easy force of personality had me typing him as the chief local representative of Them. This changed as my health improved. We became close friends.

We used to sit in the spring sunshine of Sandford's garden while I relished passively smoking his cigarettes: two old men comfortable together talking, laughing, or just sitting silent.

After we had both been discharged I wrote to thank him for the comfort and help his company had given me, and he replied that I had done the same service for him. I found this moving. Alas, I have lost touch, and can't believe he is any longer with us.

Jim is the only close friend I've ever had whose background was so different from my own. All we had in common was being about the same age and the serotonin curdle. But we were natural friends. We didn't need things in common.

### A voice from Tibor's past

My friendship with Jim was not matched among other patients. They behaved with quiet courtesy, but tended to avoid contact except for a gentle camaraderie among the ladies. From the popular misconception of a mad-house nothing could have been further removed.

Apart from the odd bizarre scene. Two still remain vivid.

Tibor, my monoglot Hungarian neighbour, was a handsome old man with bright eyes and a hooked nose—almost a senior Magyar alpha male to look at, though much stooped and, in the vernacular, completely cuckoo. I never saw him have a visitor until once when I was sitting near him in the lounge.

In struts a medium-sized beldame in a flouncy pearly-grey costume which might have been all the rage in 1850s Vienna.

Madame deposits herself opposite Tibor in one of the urine-proof armchairs. He gazes impassively, but there's an unnerving glint in his eagle's eyes. Hatred, love, fear, a wish to strangle? I couldn't read it.

Madame is addressing the old fellow in beautifully enunciated Hungarian—even-toned, confident-sounding, imperious…and sinister. She might have been reciting the terms of surrender to a beleaguered fortress. And Tibor looks as if he is ingesting this over-spiced goulash only too thoroughly. A tear appears below each eye and flows down each cheek. His face does not move, and soon the weeping is copious.

With a flick of the tongue the Visitor signals that she is through. Snapping a finger at a passing nurse she reveals an unsuspected command of English idiom.

'Bring fork!'

The voice of someone never knowingly disobeyed!

She extracts a wedge of chocolate cake from a carrier bag, rams it into Tibor's mouth and marches out like someone not planning to return. It's one way of having the last word.

Tibor champs away with relish. His tears dry up.

### Sister Dorothy

Sister Dorothy was a patient, a tiny wizened woman. I never saw her except in a wheel-chair in a brownish nun's habit. She sat splayed out as if structured like scissors fully opened.

I never heard her speak. Until one day…

…in flowed half a dozen nuns in habits like Sister Dorothy's. They cooed welcome towards the wheel-chair. Whence answer came there none.

One apple-cheeked visitor carried a small object which she held out in front of her. And spoke in tones more than dulcet. 'Sister Dorothy, this pear was picked by Sister Mary Elizabeth in our convent orchard specially for you.'

Sister Dorothy, twisting in her chair, opened her mouth as I prepared to decode bird-like tweets. What I heard, though, made me look round in panic: a deep-throated growl. Could this be, was it…yes, it was, and heard for the first time, the tiny Sister's voice!

'Grrrrrrrrrrh!'

The nuns bridled. 'Now, Sister, that's not very nice. Sister Felicity and Sister Someone Else spent a lot of time helping Sister Mary Elizabeth find the very best pear in our convent garden, just for you.'

Sister Dorothy replied in a deep, rasping, whistly bass and what sounded like broad Glaswegian. Her words related to the proffered pear. 'Tak' the bluidy thing awa'!'

Flurry of indignant twitters moderated by Christian forbearance. 'Now, Sister, that isn't very nice at all. When people take the trouble to visit people in hospital…'

'And ye can tak' yersel's wi' it!'

'Now, really, Sister…'

From the wheel-chair a string of obscenities suitable to Sauchiehall Street on a Saturday night. The visitors drift sadly away, feathers ruffled and no doubt reflecting that God moves in a mysterious way.

If my account sounds frivolous or callous please note that entertainment on this level was rare in our ward, up-staging the sit-coms, quizzes, and comics on the fool's lantern.

I don't remember the little Sister speaking again, and I hope her God has been kind to her.

## Last hospital weeks. Events inside my head

As my mind slowly recovered the hallucinations became more vivid.

There were self-aggrandizing delusions in which I was the key personality. I shall summarize two. Each has a cosmic dimension…

### …Inside the sun

I am near the core of the Sun, where it is bitterly cold, and I'm facing a wall of packed snow festooned with crimson capital letters. I blunder after them as they disappear to the right of the curved surface. The first is purely informative:

CENTRAL HELIOS

Then increasingly dire warnings tell 'personnel' not to proceed further, so I proceed further. Then comes TRESPASSERS WILL BE GASIFIED. And after that…

THE END OF THE WORLD IS NIGH.

'The sooner the better', snarl I, pressing on…only to be confronted by

RELIQUITZIAE…

…I record that monstrosity because it occurred in the hallucination, not because I can explain it or fully resolve the etymology…

…I come to a mysterious mechanical contrivance labelled

DON'T PULL ME

Below that a notice explains that hauling down a heavy metal lever at the front will detonate a nest of nuclear devices seeded round the helial core, and blow Sun and Solar System to smithereens.

A way out at last!

A lesser man might have hesitated, but not I. I jump on that lever and down it crashes with a dismal clang. I fall on the tundra surface.

Silence…

Nothingness…

But there shouldn't even be silence, dammit, and any nothingness shouldn't be the kind you wonder about. Hell's bells, yet again I haven't died happily ever after…

…Now for the second megalomaniac delusion…

### …An offer I can refuse

A buzzing in my ears resolves itself into a trio of male voices.

The Voices call themselves the Ultimate Gods and claim to inhabit an astronomical Black Hole many light years distant from the Solar System. From time immemorial they have ruled the universe as a trinity. Now they have converted to monotheism and decided to abdicate. So a single successor is urgently needed.

As they speak I begin to discern through thick mist their shadowy figures and trailing beards. They are pointing directly at me!

'We need young man.'

'But I'm seventy-seven years old.'

'So you make joke. Ha. We are seventy-seven squillion millennia old.'

They tell me about the perks. 'We make offer you can't refuse, ha ha ha. We make you sexy virtual bimbos for rumpy-pumpy.'

'Can you make me a new prostate?'

'No sweat, kiddo. Plus, you get to be immortal.' Their speech has crossed the Atlantic!

A shudder seizes me as I realize what I'm being suckered into.

'Thanks, but no thanks. Sorry, but it's get lost time, pals.'

## Ziggurat man

The following hallucination was the only one to be matched by a real-life happening.

A ziggurat, you may know, is an ancient Mesopotamian building, pyramid-shaped except that the outside is stepped…

…I found myself in an all-enveloping brownish-green robe so designed that my elevation on all sides was a narrow version of such a structure. The garment came to a peak over my head, giving it the form of a Klu Klux Klan get-up, but with stepped contours.

I was about to embark on some comedy routine to amuse my wardmates, when suddenly…

'Ziggurat Man!'

The voice of senior nurse Kate! Crisper than her wont.

I came to attention, saluted. 'Ziggurat Man present and ready for your inspection!'

'Don't give me that crap, Ziggurat Man! Just for once you have the chance to be some use. Listen to me.'

It turned out that hospital and surroundings were menaced by an immediate danger, about which she was vague. Was it meteorological, nuclear, bacterial, radiological, or even magnetic? I started to question her, but she cut me off: 'Don't waste my time.'

The nub of the threat had been identified as a spot immediately in front of the nurses' station. And there was only one way to combat that threat. Some individual with total neurological control must stand at attention on that exact spot without moving a muscle for however long it took. And it had been calculated that the heavy, symmetrical ziggurat costume was spot on to provide the 'equipoise of balance' necessary to counter any neurological tremors from inside. This meant I could remain stock still for as long as it took.

'It's an outside chance, Ziggurat Man, but there's nobody else.'

A warm my-country-needs-me glow came over me.

'I'm game, ma'am!'

'Ziggurat Man! Atten…shun!! Freeze!!!'

I snapped to attention, and at once contrived to put myself into rigor mortis. I stood unflinching, like the Roman soldier in Pompeii…

…And, by hokey, it worked! The grand old hospital remained unscathed, and there it stands to this very day—battered maybe, ramshackle undoubtedly, but gallant as ever, still dispensing elixirs of life to the weary and heavy-laden—thanks solely to yours truly. Oh yes, they go on about the boy with his finger in the dyke and the one who stood on the burning deck—more fool he, say I! But let's not forget the unsung heroes, the anonymous ones, those like me who don't go round blowing their own trumpets. And who ask for no reward but the consciousness of a job well done and the lift that comes from 'his Captain's hand on his shoulder smote'….

…I later learned that there was a particular occasion when I actually did stand motionless in front of the nurses' station for several hours, wearing an old dressing-gown, though, and not any ziggurat-like concoction. It is a feat which I, who was hardly able to stand upright for 1 minute without something to lean on, could not possibly have performed except in hypnotic coma….

That the two freezing acts, that in the hallucination and the real-life freeze reported by W, were one and the same seems to me certain. In other words, at least one of my comas was in vertical mode.

## Dance of the living dead

The following is the only hallucination which I remember as taking place *while I was still awake*, and in coma only partially. It shows my sick brain transmuting a humdrum hospital routine—the nurses' evening round with patients' medication, tea and sandwiches—into a hideous nightmare while it was occurring in reality.

Topsy [who else?] and another Caribbean nurse were on duty that night, and they duly wheeled their medication trolley into the larger patients' lounge…

…'Who's for a cuppa very HOT tea?' bellows Topsy. The sinister swerve put on the 'hot' becomes understandable when—horror of horrors—the sweet, treacly, seductive scent of rum floats into my stricken consciousness.

So our tea is laced with spirits from voodooland! So much for the Hippocratic Oath! And this is only the beginning. Electricity in the air bodes a full-blooded orgy.

Orgy? What happened was far worse.

Singing 'While Doctor's away Nursey will play', those two demon carers are tossing the contents of scores of pill boxes and phials and blister packs from their pharmaceutical store into the cauldron of mulled rum on the trolley, stirring that witches' broth with a wooden spoon. Soon they are tipsily ladling the steaming contents into tea mugs.

'Yo-ho-ho! Who's for Jamaican mulligatawny?' None dare refuse.

Still worse is to come.

Topsy and her oppo…Jumping Jehosaphat! Each hauls a decrepit geriatric upright, each whirls her skeletal partner round in a wild mazurka. Cracking of aged ribs! Poor old things, destined by their own families, remember, for imminent incineration in the hospital boilers…do they really need to be robbed in advance of every shred of dignity by those very ha ha professionals who are paid to care for them…?

Topsy starts to set up a conga. I black out….

## …Rat of the millennium

I now present a self-diminishing hallucination, the most pervasive of all my sick fancies…

…As the prospect of a new millennium loomed in the mid-1990s media barons, consortia and so on, which normally compete, decided to combine in a joint search for the 'Rat of the Millennium': someone unknown to the wider public but uniquely mean, petty, humiliation-ripe, inelegant, embarrassment-causing and the like.

The attraction lay in identifying an individual whom every other inhabitant of the globe could self-righteously denounce. And with added frisson—the Rat's name, when announced, might turn out to be your own!

It was announced that the nailing of the Rat would take place simultaneously, on worldwide television, and would be modelled on the renowned This is Your Life series. Arc-lights, camera crew, anchor persons, gaffers, first grips, and such would burst in on the lucky winner, carrying documents and grinning all over their faces. The presenter would open a large volume.

'John Smith, this is your miserable, pathetic apology for a life, you sickening little turd.'

A succession of figures from John Smith's past would then appear with a lot of 'I remember when you peed your pants at little Doris Jones's 8th birthday party, scumbag' sort of remarks, which I leave to your imaginations.

It was going to be the television scoop of all time, and it got to the point where, seemingly, nobody could think of anything else, so exciting was the prospect of the promised showdown.

And then…

…suddenly they found the perfect candidate. I shall not insult your intelligence by naming him.

So the rat hunt was over, You-know-who was cornered, and his identity inevitably leaked prematurely. Every search-light in the world accordingly homed in, on Sandford.

You remember the grid-locked lynch mob which had surrounded the hospital in early May, baying for my blood? A hard core remained, now boosted by kindred delegations from all over the world, jabbering imprecations in a hundred different tongues. When wind conditions were right fleets of air balloons drifted across, some shaped like inflated condoms, from which rowdies of every hue and ilk shrieked foul curses through loud-hailers…

…I now need to use the pseudonymous 'Professor Sidgwick Mountjoy' as if it were my own name…

…'Show yerself, Sidgwick baby', bellowed one air-borne wag.

''Ow's yer prostate, Prof?'

'Schweinhund Sietzschwieck!'

Other balloon-borne shrieks suggested in uncouth accents that I was in the habit of performing an unnatural act with a close relative.

Outside Urology a makeshift gibbet bore the legend 'Mountjoy's last neck-tie'.

At this point I must pay tribute to the sheer professionalism of Sandford's small medical staff. Throughout this appalling crisis they contrived to behave as if nothing out of the ordinary was occurring at all!!!….

…Well, of course, the visitation from the This is Your Life team, dreaded out of coma as well as in, never materialized.

The Rat delusion was in a class of its own. All the others were one-off affairs. Rat recurred uncounted times.

Though I slept better in this latter part of my hospital stay, I had long insomniac periods reviewing my life from the point of view of the Rat investigators…and dredging up hauls of autobiographical sewage with which I shall not defile these learned pages.

## Afterthought

I have tried to give a light-hearted account. So I will end by stressing what I may have underplayed: how painful were the sufferings endured in hospital, even though the depression which led to attempted suicide beforehand was even worse. But I add that the decade since that desperate act has been a happy one for me. I don't forget those who made that possible.

# Mood disorders: depressive disorders

## Robert Baldwin

## Introduction

Depression and old age are often regarded as inextricably linked. The litany of losses which older people face seems sufficient justification and supportive quotations are not difficult to find. Burton's famous 'after seventy years, all is trouble and sorrow..' comes from his *Anatomy of Melancholy* published over 300 years ago. In reality, for modern Western people at least, life as an older person is reported by the majority as having turned out be better than hoped for (Harris, 1975).

Health professionals see, in the main, older people who are most susceptible to depression, those with frailty and medical illnesses. Whilst it is true that depressive symptoms are common in healthcare practice, this can easily lead to complacency, with the danger that older people who develop depressive disorder, the topic of this chapter, may be overlooked.

## Terms and definitions

The classification of psychiatric disorders is subject to changing evidence and perhaps fashion. In this chapter 'depressive disorder' will be use to encompass all clinically significant forms of depression in later life. The terms depressive episode and major depression are used interchangeably. Box 29ii.1 outlines a classification of mood disorders from the *International Classification of Diseases* (version 10) (World Health Organization, 1993).

Both ICD-10 and the North American equivalent, the *Diagnostic and Statistical Manual of Mental Disorder*, 4th edition (DSM-IV; American Psychiatric Association, 1994) list the central symptoms of depressive episode (major depression), of which at least five should be present, including two core ones (Boxes 29ii.2 and 29ii.3). ICD-10 adds a somatic syndrome as a further subclassification (Box 29ii.4). DSM-IV adds a specifier for 'melancholia', which is almost identical to this. The somatic syndrome, or melancholia, encompasses many of the features of the older term 'endogenous' depression.

An organic depressive episode is diagnosed when a depressive episode (major depression) is present but there is evidence of a direct link between the onset of depression and either a systemic or neurological condition or an ingested substance or drug. Depression accompanying dementia may be classified here, but in DSM-IV there are separate mood specifiers for the dementias. Alcohol can precipitate or prolong major depression or depressive symptoms.

Bipolar disorder of first onset in older people is uncommon but recurrent bipolar disorder with episodes of depression is not uncommon.

Dysthymia is a chronic depression with a duration of at least 2 years and a number of symptoms from Box 29ii. 2. These range from a few to over five. It is frequently associated with chronic physical illness.

In mixed anxiety and depressive disorder symptoms of depression and anxiety are both present but below the threshold for either depressive episode or generalized anxiety disorder.

Adjustment disorder with depressive reaction is diagnosed when depressive symptoms below the threshold for a diagnosis of depressive episode begin within a month of a serious threat or loss. Symptoms usually resolve within 6 months.

The term minor depression does not appear in ICD-10 but has been proposed as a 'potential category' in DSM-IV. Either or both of the core symptoms of depressed mood and/or anhedonia are present along with one or two ancillary depressive symptoms, to a maximum of four symptoms. Individuals with minor depression

---

**Box 29ii.1** Classification of mood disorders using the International Classification of Diseases (version 10)

- Mild depressive episode (F32.0)[a]
- Moderate depressive episode (F32.1)[a]
- Severe depressive episode without psychotic symptoms (F32.2)[a]
- Severe depressive episode with psychotic symptoms (F32.3)[a]
- Recurrent depressive disorder (F33)
- Organic depressive episode (F06.32)[b]
- Bipolar affective disorder: current episode mild, moderate or severe depression with or without psychotic symptoms (F31.3–F31.5)
- Dysthymia (F34.1)
- Mixed anxiety and depressive disorder (F41.2)
- Adjustment disorder with depressive reaction (F43.20, F43.21)
- Minor depressive disorder[c]

[a] Equivalent to major depression in DSM-IV (Code 296).
[b] Equivalent to mood disorder due to a general medical condition in DSM-IV (Code 293.83).
[c] This appears as a proposal for further consideration in DSM-IV (see text).

| Box 29ii.2 DSM-IV criteria for major depressive episode |
|---|

A: Five or more of the following symptoms have been present during the same 2-week period and represent change from previous functioning; at least one of the symptoms is either (1) depressed mood or (2) loss of interest or pleasure.
*Note:* Symptoms that are clearly due to a general medical condition are not included, nor are mood-incongruent delusions or hallucinations.

1. Depressed mood most of the day, nearly every day, as indicated by either subjective report (e.g. feels sad or empty) or observation made by others (e.g. appears tearful).
2. Markedly diminished interest or pleasure in all, or almost all, activities most of the day, nearly every day (as indicated by either subjective account or observation made by others).
3. Significant weight loss when not dieting or weight gain (e.g. a change of more than 5% of body weight in a month), or decrease or increase in appetite nearly every day.
4. Insomnia or hypersomnia nearly every day.
5. Psychomotor agitation or retardation nearly every day (observable by others, not merely subjective feelings of restlessness or being slowed down).
6. Fatigue or loss of energy nearly every day.
7. Feelings of worthlessness or excessive or inappropriate guilt (which may be delusional) nearly every day (not merely self-reproach or guilt about being sick).
8. Diminished ability to think or concentrate or indecisiveness, nearly every day (either by subjective account or as observed by others).
9. Recurrent thoughts of death (not just fear of dying), recurrent suicidal ideation without a specific plan, or a suicide attempt or a specific plan for committing suicide

B: The symptoms do not meet criteria for a mixed episode.
C: The symptoms cause clinically significant distress or impairment in social, occupational, or other important areas of functioning.
D: The symptoms are not due to the direct physiological effects of a substance (e.g. a drug of abuse, a medication) or a general medical condition (e.g. hypothyroidism).
E: The symptoms are not better accounted for by bereavement, i.e. after the loss of a loved one, the symptoms persist for longer than 2 months or are characterised by marked functional impairment, morbid preoccupations with worthlessness, suicidal ideation, psychotic symptoms, or psychomotor retardation.
*Specifiers* can be coded for *severity* (mild, moderate, or severe); *psychosis* (delusions or hallucinations); and *remission* (partial or full).

| Box 29ii.3 ICD-10 depressive episode |
|---|

A: The syndrome of depression must be present for at least 2 weeks; no history of mania; and not attributable to organic disease or psychoactive substance.

**Mild depressive episode**

B: At least two of the following three symptoms must be present:
1. Depressed mood to a degree that is definitely abnormal for the individual, present for most of the day and almost every day, largely uninfluenced by circumstances, and sustained for at least 2 weeks.
2. Loss of interest or pleasure in activities that are normally pleasurable.
3. Decreased energy or increased fatigability.

C: An additional symptom or symptoms from the following (giving a total of at least four):
1. Loss of confidence or self-esteem.
2. Unreasonable feelings of self-reproach or excessive and inappropriate guilt.
3. Recurrent thoughts of death or suicide, or any suicidal behaviour.
4. Complaints or evidence of diminished ability to think or concentrate, such as indecisiveness or vacillation.
5. Change in psychomotor activity, with agitation or retardation (either subjective or objective).
6. Sleep disturbance of any type.
7. Change in appetite (decrease or increase) with corresponding weight change.

**Moderate depressive episode**

As above but giving a total of at least *six* symptoms.

**Severe depressive episode**

All *three* from Section B and *at least five* from Section C (eight symptoms in total). Severe cases may be further subdivided according to the presence or otherwise of psychosis and/or stupor.
In addition a fifth character (F32.χ1) may be added to specify the presence of a *somatic syndrome*, as in Box 29ii.4

| Box 29ii.4 Somatic syndrome of ICD-10 |
|---|

At least four of:
1. Marked loss of interest or pleasure.
2. Lack of emotional reactions to events or activities normally producing a response.
3. Wakening in the morning 2 hours or more before the usual time.
4. Depression worse in the morning.
5. Objective evidence of marked psychomotor retardation or agitation.
6. Marked loss of appetite.
7. Weight loss (5% of body weight in the past month).
8. Marked loss of libido.

will have between two and four depressive symptoms present continuously for a 2-week period. Minor depression in later life has risk factors similar to those for major depression and is associated with functional impairment approaching that of major depression (Lyness *et al.*, 2006). Minor depression is a risk factor for depressive episode (Judd *et al.*, 1998).

The term subsyndromal depression has been used in a confusing way in the literature. It may denote: all depressive disorders with symptom counts below that required for major depression, in which case it includes minor depression; or only depressions with symptom counts below that required for minor depression; or as a term interchangeable with minor depression. This is unsatisfactory. However, it is worth noting that depression is increasingly seen as a spectrum rather than a series of dichotomous disorders (Judd *et al.*, 1998). In a 3-year outcome study of depression in elderly community-dwellers, Copeland *et al.* (1992) found that 'subcase' depression was associated with a significant risk of developing a depressive syndrome.

AGECAT is a computerized diagnostic algorithm widely used in research and derived from a structured interview (the Geriatric Mental Status Schedule). Its output correlates closely with ICD and DSM categories (Copeland *et al.*, 1987).

## Epidemiology

Among older and younger community dwellers the prevalence of *depressive symptoms* exceeds that of *depressive episodes*. Early research (Kay *et al.*, 1964) found a prevalence of about 10% for depression in community residents, with only 1.3% met criteria for what would now be called a depressive episode. The latter figure is similar to that found by the influential North American Epidemiologic Catchment Area (ECA) (Blazer *et al.*, 1988). This caused controversy because a lower rate of major depression among older compared with middle-aged subjects was taken to mean that the more severe forms of depression gradually diminish with advancing age, which seemed counter-intuitive to clinical experience (Snowdon, 1990). Yet similar rates to the seminal work of Kay and colleagues were found in Australia by Henderson *et al.* (1993) who commented that this may be because they applied the diagnostic criteria of DSM and ICD strictly. For example, cases with cognitive impairment or major physical impairment could easily be excluded.

It seems likely that old age depressive disorders are not particularly well encompassed by the strict checklist approach of current operational classifications such as DSM and ICD. There is some research to support this. Prince *et al.* (1999) used the 'EURO-D' scale in 14 countries to compare symptoms of depression and identified two factors under which the majority of depressive symptoms clustered. One they called 'affective suffering', characterized by depression, tearfulness, and a wish to die, and the second was a 'motivation' factor, comprising loss of interest, poor concentration, and lack of enjoyment. It was the motivation factor which tended to increase with age rather than affective suffering, which remained constant across age groups. The term 'clinically significant depression' has been adopted by the European Collaborative (EURODEP)as a more inclusive approach: they found rates of between 8.6 and 14.1% for clinically significant depression and 1 to 4% for major depression (Copeland *et al.*, 1999). In summary, between 10 and 15% of elderly people in the community have depressive symptomatology at a given point in time and about 3% of the same community have depressive episodes meeting ICD-10 and DSM-IV criteria.

It might be thought that growing old is a major determinant of depression. However, Robert *et al.* (1997) assessed depression in an epidemiologically derived cohort of patients and found that healthy older people were not at a greater risk of depression than younger people provided the effects on mood from physical ill-health had been taken into account. In other words, the main predictor of depression was medical morbidity rather than age (although clearly the two are often associated). Rates of depression (including major depression) in long-term care facilities such as nursing homes are typically up to three times higher than among community residents (Blazer, 2003). In hospitalized elderly patients the prevalence of depressive episode ranges between 12 and 45% with an average of about 20% (Koenig *et al.*, 1988; Jackson and Baldwin, 1993). Cognitive impairment is also associated with high rates of depression. Allen and Burns (1995) calculated a prevalence of moderate to severe depressive disorder in patients with Alzheimer's disease of 20%, higher than in aged-matched community residents. Rates of depression were higher in vascular as opposed to Alzheimer-type dementia.

## Clinical presentation

Compared with younger adults, certain symptoms of depressive disorder become more frequent with advancing years. These include a preponderance of somatic complaints (Brown *et al.*, 1984; Husain *et al.*, 2005), hypochondriasis (Gurland, 1976), more psychomotor disturbance, a greater likelihood of psychotic symptoms (Meyers *et al.*, 1988; Brodaty *et al.*, 1997), more reported insomnia (Husain *et al.*, 2005), more melancholia (Brodaty *et al.*, 1991), and possibly an increased likelihood of psychotic presentations (Baldwin, 1992). Some symptoms may reduce in frequency or intensity. In a recent study of individuals between 18 and 75 years of age, older depressed adults reported less irritability and hypersomnia and were less likely to hold negative views of themselves or of their future (Husain *et al.*, 2005). Others have, however, noted few differences (Musetti *et al.*, 1989; Blazer, 2003) and it is possible that study bias (for example studying only inpatients or patients from tertiary referral centres) favouring those with more severe illness may account for some of this.

The motivational factor identified by Prince *et al.* (1999)(above) shows some similarity to the symptom profile of vascular depression, discussed later.

Another approach is to distinguish recurrent depression, usually with an onset in early adulthood, from late onset depression, often arbitrarily defined as onset after aged 60. Brodaty *et al.* (2005) examined the effect of age of onset on the phenomenology of late life depression in 810 patients referred to a specialist mood disorders service in Australia. Some clinical types, such as melancholia and psychosis, and some clinical features, such as psychomotor agitation, retardation, non-interactiveness, hypochondriasis, and severe guilt, were more common in older patients and were associated more with age than with age at onset, although this effect was more pronounced in females. In this study, subjective reports of depression were lower in older patients whereas objective measures were higher. This disparity increased markedly with age and supports the often expressed view that older patients minimize feelings of sadness.

However, where studies try to examine whether there are characteristic symptoms of old age depression by using strict diagnostic criteria, such as those outlined earlier, they risk 'defining away' any peculiarities of young versus old depression, leaving only those features which are the same at all ages. The argument thus becomes circular, unless research can demonstrate that older depressives do indeed experience symptoms not currently included in the standard classifications and descriptions of mood disorders.

Lastly, a major challenge of diagnosis in late life depression is co-morbidity, including dementia. Olin *et al.* (2002) have proposed guidelines for the diagnosis of depression in Alzheimer's disease which include symptoms not emphasized in ICD-10 or DSM-IV such as reduced positive affect, social isolation, and withdrawal.

## Diagnostic difficulties

There is then some truth in the adage that 'depression is depression at any age', at least in terms of its clinical presentation. Rather, there are factors which may modify the expression of depressive disorder in the elderly. Some of these arise from differences in how generations attribute psychological and physical health symptoms; other differences occur because of the frequent overlap of depressive symptoms and physical illness. Some of these factors may accentuate certain aspects of the clinical picture, whilst others may mask the diagnosis. The factors which lead to an altered presentation of depression in older people are summarized in Box 29ii.5.

A common difficulty arises from depression with associated physical illness (co-morbidity) leading to overlapping symptoms. DSM-IV takes an aetiological approach to mood symptoms; that is to say, the clinician must judge whether a symptom (for example reduced appetite) is due to physical illness and if so discount it in diagnosing depression. In practice this is not easy. Koenig *et al.* (1997) applied a range of strategies from the purely aetiological approach to an inclusive one and showed that they resulted in a two-fold difference in the assessed prevalence of major depression.

An individual with active rheumatoid arthritis may experience insomnia, fatigue, and poor appetite equally from his or her physical illness or an associated depression. The history is key. For example early morning wakening may emerge from a background of more generalized sleep disturbance due to pain. Questions must be appropriate. For example for those with limited mobility or exercise tolerance a question such as 'Do you feel tired even when resting?' is preferable to 'Have you no energy?'. With the patient's permission, a history from someone close to him or her may be informative, and it is important to identify prior episodes of depression, which may provide support for thinking that a current unclear presentation is a recurrence of depression.

Older people tend to *minimize feelings of sadness* when depressed (Georgotas *et al.*, 1983; Brodaty *et al.*, 2005), presumably reflecting a cohort of people brought up not to bother their doctors with emotional difficulties. Excessive worrying over health or a preoccupation with somatic symptoms is often regarded as the way in which older people make up for not complaining of depressed mood, and there is some truth in this (Brown *et al.*, 1984). Possible reasons include a heightened awareness of physiological changes due to ageing or disease, peer expectations (for example, concerning the regularity of bowel habit), or as part of a repertoire of behaviours ('abnormal illness behaviour') designed to maintain certain roles and patterns. *Hypochondriasis*, a morbid fear of bodily illness, is common in depression. Preoccupations may be delusional, occasionally achieving grotesque proportions. For example, one patient dismissed the author and instead requested an undertaker, for she believed herself dead and was convinced that her flesh had rotted. However, a patient's hypochondriacal complaints caused by depressive disorder can be quite different from bodily symptoms one might expect from a knowledge of their medical history (Kramer-Ginsberg *et al.*,1989).

There is growing awareness that depression may present predominantly with *pain*. In primary care this may occur in as many as 50% of adult presentations (Katona *et al.*, 2005). Whether it is more or less frequent in later life is not clear. The pain is often non-specific. Headache, abdominal pain, or musculoskeletal pains in the lower back, joints, and neck are common and may occur in combination so that the clinician should have a high index of suspicion in patients presenting multiple pain symptoms of unclear aetiology.

It is mistake to take at face value *neurotic symptoms of recent onset*. The sudden emergence of severe anxiety, obsessional compulsive phenomena, hysteria, or hypochondriasis in an older person not previously neurotically prone should serve as a prompt to look closely for depressive disorder, which is the usual cause. Likewise, at all levels of severity of depression, anxiety is a common accompanying symptom (Post, 1972). If it dominates the clinical picture it may mask the depressive disorder. A (literally) fatal mistake is to dismiss an act of *deliberate self-harm*, because it appears to be medically trivial. There is no consistent correlation between the medical severity of deliberate self-harm and its psychiatric seriousness. The severity of depression is not a reliable guide either. Elderly people rarely take 'manipulative' overdoses. Most have depressive disorder and *all* require psychiatric assessment. More difficult to characterize is the concept of depression presenting as 'subintentional' suicide. These individuals may be profoundly withdrawn, reject assistance, refuse food, and suffer severe weight loss. However, patients who 'turn their face to the wall' are a heterogeneous group some of whom may be severely depressed but others not clearly so. For example, some cases referred to the author turned out to have had occult carcinomas.

Lishman (1987) describes '*pseudodementia*' as 'a number of conditions (in which) a clinical picture resembling organic dementia presents for attention yet physical disease proves to be little if at all responsible'. It is, in many respects, an unsatisfactory term and one which is perhaps waning in the psychiatric lexicon. Other terms such as such as 'dementia of depression' (Pearlson *et al.*, 1989) or 'depression–executive dysfunction syndrome' (Alexopoulos *et al.*, 2002) are used. 'Pseudodementia' has been used in several different ways: when someone with depression 'fails' a routine cognitive screening test for dementia; as a particular clinical presentation [vociferous complaints of poor memory, many 'don't know' responses, and a relatively short onset (Post, 1982)]; or when cognitive impairment on neuropsychological testing has been detected in someone with major depression. Such deficits typically involve memory and attention; but specific deficits in higher cortical function, such as aphasia, agraphia, acalculia, etc., suggest an underlying dementia.

---

**Box 29ii.5** Presentation of depressive disorder in old age

- Overlap of physical and somatic psychiatric symptoms
- Minimal expression of sadness
- Somatization or disproportionate complaints associated with physical disorder
- Unexplained pain syndromes
- Neurotic symptoms of recent onset
- Deliberate self-harm (including medically 'trivial')
- 'Pseudodementia'
- Depression superimposed upon dementia
- Accentuation of abnormal personality traits
- Behaviour disorder
- Late onset alcohol dependency syndrome

Less discussed in the literature, but readily recognizable to clinicians working with older patients, is depression presenting as a *disorder of behaviour*. Pitt (1982) highlights certain patterns. These include presentations with food refusal, 'incontinence' (for example a perverse ability to eliminate in almost any place other than the toilet, unlike the incontinence of dementia), screaming and outwardly aggressive behaviour. Often the location is a residential or nursing home facility and the context one of resented dependency. A history from someone who knows the patient is crucial.

Depressive disorder may lead to an *accentuation of pre-morbid personality traits*. Such individuals may be known for their flamboyant displays. The advent of depressive disorder may lead to dramatic theatricality and ceaseless importuning, sometimes to several agencies simultaneously, for example social services, primary care, and the local accident and emergency department. An escalation in the disruptive behavioural pattern may herald the onset of depression. Other behavioural problems which may occur as 'markers' of depressive disorder in older people include *shoplifting*, and a late onset *alcohol dependence syndrome*.

Lastly a complaint of *loneliness* from an individual who has hitherto coped quite well alone, often accompanied by a request to be rehoused, should raise a suspicion of depressive disorder.

## Detecting depression

Screening instruments for depression are not a substitute for an appropriate history and examination of mental state, but where the prevalence of depression is high, as in care home settings, intermediate care, and hospital wards, a case for routine screening can be made.

The Beck Depression Inventory (Beck *et al.*, 1961) is widely used in adult populations. Both this and the Zung Depression Rating Scale, which may require adjustment of its cut-off score for 'caseness' in older people (Zung, 1967), use a multiple choice format which some elderly people find confusing. The Center for Epidemiologic Studies Depression Scale (CES-D) (Radloff, 1977) and the SelfCARE(D) (Bird *et al.*, 1987) are validated screening questionnaires in epidemiological studies which have been widely used in older subjects.

The Geriatric Depression Scale (GDS) (Yesavage *et al.*, 1983) and the Brief Assessment Schedule Depression Cards (BASDEC) (Adshead *et al.*, 1992) have been developed specifically for older patients. The BASDEC is unusual in comprising a 19-item deck of cards requiring yes/no responses. It is useful where privacy is difficult, as on an open medical ward, or where the person has expressive language problems where pointing to 'yes' or 'no' cards will suffice. The GDS is the most widely used self-rating scale both in screening individuals and in survey work. It avoids questions concerning physical depressive symptomatology, which are often poor discriminators between depression and physical ill-health, and instead focuses on the cognitive aspects of depressive disorder. It also has a simple 'yes/no' format. In the UK, the GDS has been endorsed for hospital use by the Royal College of Physicians and the British Geriatric Society (Royal College of Physicians and British Geriatric Society, 1992) and in primary care by the Royal College of General Practitioners (Williams and Wallace, 1993).

Even so, the full version has 30 questions (Box 29ii.6) and the original validation was carried out on a physically fit group of patients with depressive disorder, some of whom were as young as 55 years. A cut-off score of 11 or above indicates probable depression. The same cut-off was found to give satisfactory sensitivity and specificity in hospitalized elderly patients with concurrent medical illness (Koenig *et al.*, 1988; Jackson and Baldwin, 1993). It loses specificity in severe dementia (Burke *et al.*, 1989) but seems to perform reasonably well in dementia of mild to moderate severity (O'Riordan *et al.*, 1990). New scales, for example the Cornell Scale for Depression in Dementia (Alexopoulos *et al.*, 1988), have been introduced to address this difficult area. The latter incorporates information from a carer.

Shorter versions of the GDS have been introduced, including a 15-item version (Box 29ii.6) and a four-item one, (which utilizes questions 1, 3, 8, and 9). There is a GDS website with the various versions, bibliography and useful translated versions (http://stanford.edu/~yesavage/GDS.html). For a review of the performance

---

**Box 29ii.6**  Geriatric Depression Scale

Instructions: Choose the best answer for how you have felt over the past *week*.

 1. **Are you basically satisfied with your life?** No
 2. **Have you dropped many of your activities and interests?** Yes
 3. **Do you feel your life is empty?** Yes
 4. **Do you often get bored?** Yes
 5. Are you hopeful about the future? No
 6. Are you bothered by thoughts you can't get out of your head? Yes
 7. **Are you in good spirits most of the time?** No
 8. **Are you afraid something bad is going to happen to you?** Yes
 9. **Do you feel happy most of the time?** No
10. **Do you often feel helpless?** Yes
11. Do you often get restless and fidgety? Yes
12. **Do you prefer to stay at home, rather than going out and doing new things?** Yes
13. Do you frequently worry about the future? Yes
14. **Do you feel you have more problems with your memory than most?** Yes
15. **Do you think it is wonderful to be alive now?** No
16. Do you often feel down-hearted and blue (sad)? Yes
17. **Do you feel pretty worthless the way you are?** Yes
18. Do you worry a lot about the past? Yes
19. Do you find life very exciting? No
20. Is it hard for you to start on new projects (plans)? Yes
21. **Do you feel full of energy?** No
22. **Do you feel that your situation is hopeless?** Yes
23. **Do you think most people are better off (in their lives) than you are?** Yes
24. Do you frequently get upset over little things? Yes
25. Do you frequently feel like crying? Yes
26. Do you have trouble concentrating? Yes
27. Do you enjoy getting up in the morning? No
28. Do you prefer to avoid social gatherings (get-togethers)? Yes
29. Is it easy for you to make decisions? No
30. Is your mind as clear as it used to be? No

Notes: (1) Answers refer to responses which score '1'; (2) bracketed phrases refer to alternative ways of expressing the questions; (3) questions in bold comprise the 15-item version. Cut-off scores for possible depression: ≥11 (GDS30); ≥5 (GDS15); ≥2 (GDS4).

of several of the above instruments in primary care, see Watson and Pigmore (2003).

The use of screening questionnaires requires thinking through. A positive score should lead to a fuller assessment, but false positives, which can be both stigmatizing for the individual and misleading to the non-specialist, are bound to occur. Non-specialist staff may also be falsely reassured by a negative score in an uncomplaining, withdrawn, depressed individual. On the other hand, the managed introduction of such scales may have educational benefit. Their introduction may lead to improved detection rates, but it is yet to be demonstrated that screening programmes lead to better outcomes for depression.

### Cognitive impairment in old age depressive disorder

Memory and speed of information processing are impaired in depression (McAllister, 1981), especially on tasks involving sustained effort (Weingartner et al., 1981). Memory deficits are not confined to elderly depressed patients but they are arguably more severe than in younger subjects (Austin et al., 1992). Poor memory associated with depression usually improves with cueing, which suggests that the problem is one of unreliable retrieval of memories which have been laid down. Although the severity of deficits in depression may sometimes approach those found in Alzheimer's disease (Abas et al., 1990), in Alzheimer's disease these deficits commonly occur at the earliest (registration) stage of memory, so that the information is not merely difficult to access but non-existent, and cueing does not help. Functional imaging suggest that the areas of the brain involved in the cognitive disorder of Alzheimer's disease are different from those involved in major depression (Dolan et al., 1992).

Deficits on executive tasks (planning, initiation, and task persistence), speed of information processing, and visuospatial tasks were found to be most affected in one study of 100 patients with late life depression (Butters et al., 2004). Other studies have found greater deficits in late onset depressive disorder (Alexopoulos et al., 2000), compared with early onset, or found a different pattern of deficits. For example, Rapp et al. (2005) found attention and executive problems in late onset depressed patients but deficits in episodic memory in recurrent (early onset) depression. Possibly in recurrent depression chronic hypercortisolaemia (discussed later) may result in hippocampal damage leading to memory dysfunction, whilst in late onset depression the problem may lie in frontostriatal vascular damage leading to executive deficits. This latter pattern of cognitive disturbance—memory and attentional deficits with low effort—is similar to that found in subcortical disorders.

Two further important issues are whether neuropsychological deficits are reversible with recovery from depression and whether is there an increased risk of later dementia? Abas et al. (1990) found that disordered attention and information processing persisted in around a third of their elderly subjects after successful treatment of depression, and it is now becoming accepted that cognitive deficits often persist (Beats et al., 1996; Simpson et al., 1998; Baldwin et al., 2004), although this is not unique to older patients. Further, executive dysfunction has been linked to a poorer response to antidepressant treatment (Kalayam and Alexopoulos, 1999; Alexopoulos et al., 2000).

In an uncontrolled study, Kral and Emery (1989) reported that 39 of 44 elderly patients originally diagnosed as cases of depressive pseudodementia had developed the typical picture of Alzheimer's disease after a median period of follow-up of 8 years, even if the index affective disorder had improved with treatment. Alexopoulos et al. (1993) followed 57 depressed patients annually over an average period of 3 years. They subdivided the group according to the presence or not of 'reversible dementia', based on whether subjects met criteria for both depressive disorder and dementia with remission of dementia after improvement of the depression. Using survival analysis, there was an almost five-fold increase in the risk of developing dementia over 3 years for those presenting originally with 'reversible dementia'. In one study older patients receiving ECT had a higher risk of developing dementia, possibly underpinned by cerebrovascular disease (Brodaty et al., 2000).

Although other clinical studies have not shown higher than expected rates of dementia at follow-up, they have usually excluded patients with anything more than modest cognitive impairment at presentation (Murphy, 1983; Baldwin and Jolley, 1986; Brodaty et al., 2003). However, there is now growing evidence from epidemiological studies that depression is a risk factor for later cognitive impairment or dementia (Green et al., 2003; Sachs-Ericsson et al., 2005). Why this might be so is not clear but it is known that chronic depression is associated with hippocampal atrophy in older patients (Bell-McGinty et al., 2002) and that depressed patients may adopt unhealthy lifestyles which can aggravate the risk factors for vascular disease and hence dementia.

In summary, late life depression is frequently associated with subtle cognitive impairment which often persists, even if depression lifts. This may reflect functional or anatomical disruption to subcortical-frontal pathways or structures such as the hippocampus. In some patients this may be a harbinger of dementia, although predicting in which of these patients is as yet imprecise. Practically, those who present with cognitive impairment when depressed (for example with a Mini-Mental State Examination score below 24) might comprise an at-risk group for dementia.

## Aetiology

Aetiology can be subdivided into the three 'p's: predisposing risk factors (vulnerability to depression), precipitating factors, and perpetuating features. Many of these interact, and it is rarely the case that there is one cause for an episode of late life depression. Perpetuating factors are addressed under Management. Lastly, there are factors which protect (or 'buffer') against depression.

### Predisposing factors

#### Genetic susceptibility

The genetic contribution to depressive illness decreases with age (Brodaty et al., 2001). Hopkinson (1964) reported that the risk to first-degree relatives of probands with depressive illness was 20% when onset was early but only 8% when it was late. However, there may still be a genetic component to some of the risk factors for depression such as brain hyperintensities (Carmelli et al., 2002) or metabolic pathways, for example involving folate and homocysteine, leading to vascular disease (Hickie et al., 2001). Despite interest, no definite risk has been found with regard to the ε4 allele of the apolipoprotein E gene by contrast with its role in dementia.

## Gender and civil status

Depression across the age range is more frequent in women (Cole and Dendukuri, 2003). In Finland, Kivela *et al.* (1988) found higher rates of depression among elderly widows and divorcees.

## Past psychiatric history

A past history of depressive disorder or dysthymic disorder increases the risk of later depression (Cole and Dendukuri, 2003). Alcohol dependency and schizophrenia are associated with depression. So too, obviously, is bipolar affective disorder.

## Physical ill-health and depression

Practitioners of old age psychiatry are constantly challenged by the admixture of physical and psychiatric disorder in their patients. Indeed, for many it is a chief fascination of the specialty. More information is available in Chapter 22 on liaison psychiatry.

Ischaemic heart disease, some neurological disorders (such as Parkinson's disease and Alzheimer's disease), cerebrovascular disease (such as vascular dementia and stroke), hip fracture and chronic obstructive pulmonary disease (COPD) have all been associated with a high level of depression in older adults (Krishnan *et al.*, 2002). As discussed, pain syndromes in various conditions are also closely linked to depression. Importantly these associations are bidirectional (Lin *et al.*, 2003). Physical impairment may provoke a depressive disorder, which may in turn increase the degree of disability associated with the original physical disorder (Prince *et al.*, 1998). Likewise depression worsens the prognosis for medical morbidity, with greater mortality after myocardial infarction (Romanelli *et al.*, 2002), a poorer prognosis for heart failure in females (Williams *et al.*, 2002), increased physical decline and disability (Penninx *et al.*, 1999, 2000), increased health utilization (e.g. Unützer *et al.*, 1997), and reduced bone mineral density (Robbins *et al.*, 2001).

There are several mechanisms whereby physical disorder may lead to depression. For the neurological disorders such as the dementias, stroke, and Parkinson's disease, alteration in the brain serotonergic systems may be important. However, the wide range of disabling medical conditions along with other risk factors such as hearing and visual difficulties suggests that the meaning of the illness for the sufferer is as important as the precise body system involved. Recently, Prince *et al.* (1998) have shown that handicap—the disadvantage in society imposed by a physical impairment and the ensuing disability—is a key risk factor for depression in older people at home. The concept of handicap provides an important perspective, as handicap is as much a societal issue as a medical one. Two older people may be similarly impaired by medical illnesses but if one has limited practical support and poor transport, then she is the more handicapped. Lastly a range of disorders, some with occult presentation, can predispose to depressive disorder (see Table 29ii.1).

## Medication

Many medications (Table 29ii.1) are associated with precipitating or perpetuating depression. Dhondt *et al.* (2002) examined the Dutch LASA epidemiological database and calculated the population attributable risk percentage (PAR%) for a large number of medications. The PAR% is that part of depression in the population that is associated with the use of certain medication. For non-selective β-blockers the PAR% was 2.5%, for calcium antagonists 5%, and for benzodiazepines 15.42%. For systemic corticosteroids it was 2.95%. This does not mean that all patients on these drugs who present with depression should be switched to something else. It can be

**Table 29ii.1** Medical conditions and central-acting drugs that may cause organic depressive disorder

| Medical conditions | **Endocrine/metabolic**: hypo/hyperthyroidism; Cushing's disease; hypercalcaemia; subnutrition; pernicious anaemia<br>**Organic brain disease**: cerebrovascular disease/stroke; CNS tumours; Parkinson's disease; Alzheimer's disease and vascular dementia; multiple sclerosis; systemic lupus erythematosus<br>**Occult carcinoma**: pancreas; lung<br>**Chronic infections**: neurosyphilis; brucellosis; neurocysticercosis; myalgic encephalomyelitis; AIDS |
|---|---|
| Central-acting drugs | **Antihypertensive drugs**: β-blockers (especially non-selective); methyldopa; reserpine; clonidine; nifedipine, calcium channel agents; digoxin<br>**Steroids**<br>**Analgesic drugs**: opioids; indomethacin<br>**Anti-Parkinson**: levodopa; amantadine; tetrabenazine<br>**Psychiatric drugs**: neuroleptics; benzodiazepines<br>**Miscellaneous**: sulphonamides; alcohol; interferon |

difficult to judge whether a particular medication is the cause of depression in the way that the diagnosis of 'organic depressive episode' requires. Given the likelihood of older people receiving multiple medications, how can one be sure which one is the culprit? Ideally the clinical history will help us to understand this, but often things are less certain and it is best to review all medication and have a high index of suspicion regarding the above-mentioned groups, especially any newly prescribed medication. High alcohol intake may lead to depression or aggravate it. Late life depression is sometimes complicated by excess alcohol taken to dim the mental pain with the result that depression is made worse.

## Personality and developmental factors

Surprisingly little has been written about personality traits and the risk of developing late life depression. Roth (1955) believed that those with late onset depressive illness had more robust personalities than those with recurrent depression arising earlier in life. Post (1972) noted that severe depression was associated with less pre-morbid personality dysfunction than milder depression. He also observed that obsessional traits were over-represented in his inpatient group. However, differentiating the features of current depression from those of the pre-morbid personality can be very difficult, and even informants can provide biased accounts. More structured techniques of assessing personality, for example derived from DSM-III (Abrams *et al.*,1987), suggest that personality dysfunction, especially of the 'avoidant' and 'dependent' types, is associated with late life depression. Murphy (1982) found that a life-long lack of a capacity for intimacy, in other words a personality variable, seemed to be a risk factor for depression in later life.

Trying to correlate fixed categories of personality, such as anxious, obsessional, and so forth, with depression can be restrictive, especially as traits frequently overlap in an individual. Character and personality variables also interact with life events to alter the risk of depression (Mazure *et al.*, 2002). Positive coping styles, self-efficacy, and a high level of mastery over the environment are traits which can protect against depression (Blazer and Hybels, 2005).

In a secondary analysis of the US study 'The Maintenance Therapies in Late-life Depression Study' (Morse and Robins, 2005) investigators studied the effect of particular personality types termed 'Cluster C' (meaning avoidant, dependent, perfectionist, and/or self-defeating in nature) on the outcome of depressive disorder in patients aged 60 and above. One hundred and eighty-seven elderly patients were included, all with recurrent non-psychotic unipolar major depressions. Compared to patients with non-'Cluster C' personality, those with the trait were as likely to respond to treatment but did so more slowly and experienced greater functional impairment in instrumental activities of daily living. This is an interesting pointer, as the authors themselves mention, to identifying which patients might benefit more from a psychological approach in addition to an antidepressant. Given the limited availability of psychological interventions this could be important.

Psychotherapeutic and developmental issues are discussed elsewhere in this book. The increased awareness of childhood abuse, including sexual abuse, as a risk factor for adult depression should not be overlooked when treating elderly patients. One patient in her late 60s who presented to the author with a late onset depressive disorder with panic attacks and nightmares revealed for the first time (to a female member of the team) that she had been abused by her brothers 60 years earlier. This became an important focus of her treatment.

### Psychosocial factors

Poverty, poor social support, and social isolation predispose to depression in later life. Low socio-economic status leads to a vicious cycle, since it is linked to poorer detection of depression and poorer access to and take-up of appropriate treatments (Arean and Reynolds, 2005). Being a victim of crime, itself linked to socio-economic status, is a further risk factor (Arean and Reynolds, 2005).

Many older people have been exposed to extreme trauma, mainly as a result of war, combat, or the Holocaust. The limited evidence that there is suggests that these events may predispose to depression in later life (Averill and Beck, 2000). Although this is hard to prove, the writer experienced an upswing in older veterans presenting with affective symptoms on two major anniversaries of the Second World War. Often this appeared to be linked to physical deterioration undermining coping mechanisms.

The role of intimate social contact has been touched upon (Murphy, 1982). Research is not completely agreed over the issue of confidants. Henderson *et al.* (1986) found that although elderly depressed people living at home did not report a lack of intimate relationships, they did report lacking more general social contact. In another study (Emmerson *et al.*, 1989) it was men who more often reported poor or no confiding relationships. So strongly was this linked to depression that it almost eclipsed adverse life events in the aetiology of depressive illness, although these too were important. Further evidence for a gender effect in the perception of or availability of intimacy comes from a Finnish study which found that only females reported a link between (lack of) perceived intimacy with their spouse and depression (Pahkala, 1990).

The area is a difficult one. Firstly, there is no consensus on the meaning or measurement of intimacy. Secondly, distinctions between objective and subjective measures of support are not always made. Subjective reports of support are liable to be influenced by lowered mood. Objective measures may not be capable of differentiating which 'supports' are facilitative and healthy and which are not. Nevertheless, commentators seem agreed that it is the perception of support which is crucial (Blazer and Hybels, 2005).

### Ethnic and cultural factors

In Western societies, African-Americans, African-Caribbeans, Hispanics, Latinos, and Asians are less likely to use mental health services than are White Caucasians (Unützer *et al.*, 1999), although the degree of acculturation is also important. Acculturation is typically defined in terms of individual responses to a dominant culture. There are also differences in the rates of antidepressant prescribing, favouring Whites, but cultural factors may also influence the acceptability of such medication. These may also influence the presentation and hence likelihood of detection of depression. For example, in a study of Korean-Americans a lower level of acculturation among older adults was associated with fewer depressive symptoms, with the suggestion that the traditional cultural emphasis on self-effacement inhibited the expression of depression (Jang *et al.*, 2005).

Barriers to the uptake of mental health care among ethnic minorities include stigma, concerns about financial reimbursement (in some health systems), limited geographical access to specialist mental health services, distrust of mental health providers, and a lack of culturally appropriate services (Unützer *et al.*, 1999). Older members of minorities tend to seek help for depression not in mental health services but in primary care.

### Caregiving

This deserves special attention as a risk factor for depression, as there are opportunities for identification and treatment. In one study (Ballard *et al.*, 1996) a quarter of carers of dementia patients were depressed, and many had persistent symptoms. Factors associated with depression in carers were depression in the designated patient and problem behaviours arising from him or her. Financial strain appears to be another risk factor (Blazer and Hybels, 2005).

## Precipitating factors

### Life events

The seminal work of Brown and Harris (1978) found that only the most severely threatening life events were related to depression. Extending the methodology of Brown and Harris to the elderly Murphy (1982) found, in a population of 119 people suffering from depressive disorder, that 48% of them had experienced at least one severe life event in the preceding year compared with 23% of a control group. The events were threatening and often involved loss—such as death of a loved one, life-threatening illness to somebody close, major financial problems, and having to give up ones home suddenly. In addition major social difficulties (as distinct from abrupt life events) lasting for 2 years or more were also significantly associated with depression.

Although these findings are in line with Brown and Harris's work with younger adults, a difference was the conspicuous role of poor physical health among the elderly depressed group, either a recent grave illness or a longer-term seriously disabling one. However, a quarter of Murphy's control group had experienced a major adverse event *without* the development of depression. If adversity alone was sufficient to 'explain' depression then eventually all old people would fall victim to it. Yet most do not. Not all adverse

**Table 29ii.2** Precipitating factors in depression of later life

| Life events | Bereavement |
| --- | --- |
| | Separation |
| | Acute physical illness |
| | Medical illness or threat to life of someone close |
| | Sudden homelessness or having to move into an institution |
| | Major financial crisis |
| | Negative interactions with family member or friend |
| | Loss of 'significant other' (including a pet) |
| Chronic stress | Declining health and mobility; dependence |
| | Sensory loss, cognitive decline |
| | Housing problems |
| | Major problems affecting family member |
| | Marital difficulties |
| | Socio-economic decline |
| | Problems at work; retirement |
| | Caring for a chronically ill and dependent family member |

events are followed by depression; not all depressions are preceded by adverse life events. Therefore, a judgement, based on the psychiatric history, about past reactions to loss and so on must be made. An uncritical acceptance of an adverse life event as a trigger for depression may result in overlooking a serious underlying organic illness. Such was the near fate of a depressed recently retired school teacher. A chest radiograph resulted in an abrupt change of emphasis in treatment, from retirement counselling to a pneumonectomy!

Bereavement is one of the most frequent triggers for depressive disorder in later life (Green *et al.*, 1994) and the presentation of normal grief and depression often overlap. For a full discussion of the topic see Clayton (2004). In brief, in the first month a large number of bereaved individuals experience low mood, anorexia, insomnia, crying bouts, fatigue, loss of interest, and guilt. The latter is usually linked specifically to supposed omissions in care at the time of death rather than the ruminative guilt of depressive disorder. Suicidal thinking is rare at this stage. By 12 months somatic symptoms will have improved but low mood, often linked to important dates and poor sleep may persist. The picture can be complicated by the use of alcohol. Besides the failure of earlier symptoms to resolve, those which suggest depression rather than bereavement are: suicidal thoughts or wishing oneself dead, pervasive guilt (not merely remorse over what more might have been done to prevent death), retardation, marked feelings of worthlessness or hopelessness, 'mummification' (maintaining grief by keeping everything the same), and psychomotor retardation.

Table 29ii.2 lists the more typical antecedents and stressors associated with late life depressive disorder.

### Protective factors

Relatively little is known about factors which protect against late life depression. If lack of a confidant leads to depression, perhaps the converse is also true, a confidant may be a buffer against the social losses and isolation which engender depression. Likewise, the magnitude of handicap might be offset by appropriate support. The role of crime is as much to do with the fear of becoming a victim as being one (Arean and Reynolds, 2005), as this fear reinforces lifestyles which promote depression, such as isolation and

avoidance of outside activity. Adaptive coping styles and psychological resilience are further individual factors which may lower the chances of depression after adversity or stress (Arean and Reynolds, 2005). Resilience in this context means the ability to persevere, make sense of events, accept one's existence, and be self-reliant.

Affiliation and belonging are also important. Religious observance has been shown to protect against depression in older adults in both Western and Eastern cultures (Bosworth *et al.*, 2003; Hahn *et al.*, 2004). And just as negative life events may promote depression, positive events, such as a new grandchild, may be protective

Lastly, Blazer and Hybels (2005) have proposed that wisdom in later life may protect against depression. Wisdom is a term which has been defined in research (Blazer and Hybels, 2005) and includes characteristics such an accumulation of knowledge, understanding, and judgement as well as being able to place matters in context.

## Overview of the pathophysiology of depressive disorder in later life

The amine hypothesis of depression was proposed in the 1960s. This stated that deficiency of the amines noradrenaline and/or serotonin (5-HT) underlies depressive disorder. However, it is now clear that amine deficiency alone is not sufficient to cause depression and does not explain why antidepressant drugs fail to work in a significant minority of depressed patients. Current neurobiological approaches to aetiology recognize that other neurochemical and neurohormonal systems have roles. These include dopamine pathways, corticotropin-releasing factor (CRF), thyrotropin-releasing hormone (TRH), and growth hormone releasing factor (GHRF), along with their associated neurohormonal systems, such as the hypothalamic–pituitary–adrenal (HPA) axis. The role of immune and inflammatory responses is also recognized. Complex interactions occur between the HPA axis and the immune and inflammatory systems. Research has also explored structural and functional correlates of depressive disorder. There is insufficient space to cover all these aspects other than in broad outline, emphasizing aspects relevant to late life depression.

### Biogenic amines

Lack of noradrenaline is associated with poor attention and memory, decreased concentration, reduced socialization, and altered states of arousal. Serotonin deficiency is associated with poor impulse control, low sex drive, decreased appetite, and irritability.

The mesolimbic dopamine system is also important in mood regulation (Nestler and Carlezon, 2006) with effects on motivation, hedonia, and exploratory behaviour. Dopamine is an important substrate for reward from food, sex, and social interactions. Deficits in reward-mediated behaviour are thought to be important in depression, including perhaps the amotivational state associated with vascular depression (see below).

If advancing age were shown to be linked to decrements in biogenic amines, this might lead to an increased susceptibility to depressive disorder in later life. The evidence is mixed (Veith and Raskind, 1988; Karlsson, 1990). 3-Methoxy-4-hydroxyphenylglycol (MHPG), a metabolite of noradrenaline, may increase rather than decrease with age. 5-Hydroxy-indole acetic acid (5-HIAA), a marker for serotonin likewise may show an increase. However, these counter-intuitive findings may merely reflect increased turnover of the amine in response to reduced cell numbers. Homovanilic acid (HVA), a dopamine marker, does however decline in both ageing and depression.

A recent development in antidepressant medication has been to manipulate receptor sites rather than necessarily attempting to target levels of neuroamines directly. These sites include 5-HT receptors and $\alpha_2$ autoreceptors. Serotonin 1A (5-HT1A) receptor binding, thought to be a regulator of treatment response, may be influenced by age, and in one recent study, 5-HT1A autoreceptor function in late life depression was disturbed. It was suggested that this was linked to depression severity and predictive of resistance to treatment with SSRIs (Meltzer et al., 2004).

### Neuroendocrine disturbances

A variety of neuroendocrine changes are associated with ageing (Veith and Raskind, 1988; Schneider, 1992). At all ages depression is associated with hyperactivity and dysregulation of the HPA axis. Ageing is associated with increasing cortisol levels and cortisol non-suppression (Alexopoulos et al., 1984). Hippocampal atrophy has been linked to chronic depression and cortisol stress (O'Brien et al., 1996; Bell-McGinty et al., 2002). Repeated episodes of depression or repeated stressful life events, or both, may exacerbate neuronal damage (the 'feed-forward cascade'; Sapolsky et al., 1986). Corticotropin-releasing hormone (CRH) is secreted by the hypothalamus and in one study CRH-mRNA levels in the paraventricular nucleus of elderly depressed patients were higher than the levels in Alzheimer's disease patients (also elevated), and very much higher than the normal controls (Raadsheer et al., 1995). This has led to speculation that hyperactivation of paraventricular CRH neurons may contribute to the aetiology of late life depression.

Early life trauma may lead to long-term supersensitivity of the HPA and CRF systems, which is the basis of the 'stress-diathesis' model of depression (Heim and Nemeroff, 1999). Genetic predisposition coupled with early stress in critical phases of development may lead to an individual being more vulnerable to developing depression and anxiety with further stress exposure. How far these changes extend to older adults is not known. Murphy (1982) found no evidence that early maternal loss predisposed to late life depression. Interestingly though Thompson et al. (2001), in a study of over 800 singletons born in the 1920s and interviewed at an average age of 68, found that the odds ratio for depression among men, but not women, rose incrementally with decreasing birth weight. The authors speculate that this might be mediated by faulty programming of the HPA axis very early in life.

### Immune and inflammatory changes

Excessive or prolonged exposure to glucocorticoids can compromise the immune system and mediators of inflammation. Immune response in depressed patients, such as the number of T4 lymphocytes and mitogen responsivity, may reduce with advancing age (Schleifer et al., 1989) although there are few data regarding late life depression. Linked to the immune response is the release of cytokines such as interleukins, tumour necrosis factor, and interferons. The latter are associated with so-called 'sickness behaviour' such as fatigue, anorexia, depressed mood, hopelessness, anhedonia, and poor concentration. Pathogens, stress, and non-pathogen-induced inflammation (including brain tissue inflammation) may all cause the release of cytokines.

In one study of older people, compared with 2879 non-depressed subjects those with depression ($n = 145$) had higher median plasma levels of interleukin-6 and tumour necrosis factor. After adjustment for health and demographic variables, depressed mood was two and a half times more common in subjects with above median scores on inflammatory markers (Penninx et al., 2003). In a clinical sample Thomas et al. (2005) found elevated levels of interleukin-1[beta] but only in major depression. It is not known whether such changes are state or trait, but in the study by Thomas et al. there was an association with depression severity, suggesting a state effect.

### Structural brain changes

Using computed tomography (CT), Jacoby and Levy, (1980) identified a subgroup of patients with major depression who had ventricular enlargement (implying atrophy) and who were characterized by being older, having a later age of onset of depression, a more 'endogenous' clinical picture, and a higher death rate from extracerebral causes at 2 years (Jacoby et al., 1981). Kumar et al. (2000) studied 51 patients with late life depression and 30 control subjects. The odds of being depressed were significantly increased with: (1) smaller frontal lobe volume and (2) greater volume of brain lesions. Neither factor affected the ability of the other to predict depression, suggesting they represent independent pathways to depression. Amongst other things, these findings suggest that there may be one pathway to depression involving neurodegeneration and another via localized lesions caused by, for example, vascular disease.

The superior resolution of magnetic resonance imaging (MRI) has enabled much better visualization of small localized brain lesions, and a plethora of clinical studies demonstrating a high rate of lesions of brain deep white matter and basal ganglia in late life depression has emerged (summarized by Baldwin, 2005). This body of data is complemented by epidemiological research such as the Cardiovascular Health Study (Steffens et al., 1999, 2002) and the Rotterdam Scan Study (de Groot et al., 2000). In the Cardiovascular Health Study (after adjusting for confounders) lesions of the basal ganglia were a significant predictor of depression. In the Rotterdam Study subjects with severe white matter change had a three- to five-fold increase in the likelihood of depression.

Other structures which may atrophy in depression include the hippocampus which, as discussed, is at particular risk from hypercortisolaemia (Bell-McGinty et al., 2002); and the caudate nucleus (Beats et al., 1991).

### Functional imaging and EEG

Slowing of the alpha waves is the most common EEG change recorded after the age of 60. EEG variables measured during sleep show changes in depression similar to those of normal ageing (Veith and Raskind, 1988). These include similarities in night-time wakefulness, decreased slow wave sleep, total rapid eye movement (REM) sleep, and REM latency. Using discriminant function analysis, Reynolds et al. (1988) found that four EEG sleep variables correctly differentiated depressed from demented elderly patients in 80% of cases.

The P300 paradigm is a method which uses evoked responses to assess physiological correlates of psychomotor slowing via the EEG. It may serve as a proxy for superior limbic function, and longer latencies have been found in late life depression with executive dysfunction (Kindermann et al., 2000). This interesting technology has not yet found an application in clinical practice.

Positron emission tomography (PET) can map structure to function. Bench et al. (1992) reported focal abnormalities in regional cerebral blood flow (rCBF) using PET in middle-aged and elderly depressives. Reduced rCBF was found in the left anterior cingulate gyrus and left dorsolateral pre-frontal cortex. However, additional abnormalities were apparent in a depressed subgroup with co-existent cognitive impairment—reduced flow to the left anterior medial pre-frontal gyrus and increased flow to the cerebellar vermis. The dissociation in rCBF between depression-associated cognitive impairment and that seen in depression without such impairment is of particular interest to an understanding of depressive pseudo-dementia in elderly patients. Different functional pathways are presumably involved.

Single photon emission computed tomography (SPECT) is a more widely available than PET. It uses a radioactive tracer, such as $^{99}$Tc$^{m}$-hexamethylpropylene amine oxime. Studies of elderly depressed patients are few but support a general reduction in cerebral perfusion mainly involving the frontal cortex (Sackeim et al., 1990) but not confined to it (Philpot et al., 1993). Furthermore, the location and severity of white matter hyperintensities as visualized on MRI correlate with SPECT evidence of reduced subcortical white matter perfusion (Kobari et al., 1990). Although the direction of cause and effect is not clear, the evidence is suggestive that some of the MRI lesions visualized in late life depressions may lead to functional disturbance such as reduced cerebral perfusion. Whether these deficits normalize after the depression remits is less clear, as research findings differ (Nobler et al., 2000; Navarro et al., 2002).

How different functional circuits and neuronal networks interact is of course crucial. Detailed discussion is beyond the scope of this chapter, but Tekin and Cummings (2002) have proposed a model. Superior limbic structures may regulate attentional and cognitive aspects of depression (apathy, psychomotor disturbance, impaired attention, and dysexecutive symptoms); a ventral compartment formed of limbic, paralimbic, and subcortical structures may mediate vegetative and somatic aspects (sleep, appetite, endocrine disturbance); and the rostral cingulate area regulates interactions between these two.

## Post-mortem findings

In post-mortem studies, Thomas et al. (2000, 2001, 2002) found that deep white matter hyperintensities visualized on MRI were due to ischaemic change in all elderly depressed subjects but only a third of controls. The difference lay largely in smaller punctuate lesions which were ischaemic in depressed subjects but not so in controls (Thomas et al., 2002). Ischaemic white matter lesions tended to be found mainly in the dorsolateral pre-frontal cortex, an area known to be involved in depression. This research provides some support for the vascular depression hypothesis (below) since there was a significant increase in large vessel atheroma in the depressed group (Thomas et al., 2001). Rajkowska et al. (2005) studied the brains of 15 elderly subjects with depression and 11 control subjects. The density of pyramidal neurons in the orbitofrontal cortex of the depressed subjects was particularly low in cortical layers V and III, the origin of pre-frontostriatal, pre-frontocortical and pre-frontoamygdala projections. This suggests that the degeneration of these neurons, which was more severe than in younger depressed subjects (Rajkowska et al., 1999), may be due to lesions in the white matter which includes the projections to these neurons.

## The vascular depression hypothesis

Almost 40 years ago Post wrote: '… subtle cerebral changes may make ageing persons increasingly liable to affective disturbance' (Post, 1968). The hypothesis that vascular depression is an identifiable clinical entity was proposed by Alexopoulos et al. (1997). Using a four-point vascular risk scale, depression in 65 elderly patients was classified as either vascular or non-vascular. The minimum requirement for vascular depression was the presence of one risk factor, for example hypertension. The clinical features of the depression were analysed in three domains: symptoms, as elicited by the 17-item Hamilton depression scale (Hamilton, 1960), disability, and cognitive impairment. It was found that, compared with non-vascular cases, the vascular group had less depressive ideation, more psychomotor retardation, poorer insight, and more cognitive impairment on tests of fluency and naming. The vascular group also had greater disability and more often had a late onset (aged after 60). Krishnan et al. (2004) have proposed a refinement to the diagnosis of vascular depression. In a case–control study evaluating 139 depressed patients, 75 met MRI criteria for visually rated lesions in deep white matter or subcortical grey matter of at least 'multipunctate' or 'diffuse' grading. These patients were denoted as having 'subcortical ischaemic depression' (SID). SID patients had less family history of depression, a higher overall rating for the symptom 'lassitude', and a trend for greater functional impairment in activities of daily living. Cognitive dysfunction in vascular depression typically involves executive dysfunction, leading to slowed responses, failure of initiation and persistence in tasks, and inefficient memory (Alexopoulos et al., 2002). Such deficits do not necessarily reverse with treatment (Baldwin et al., 2004).

What is the clinical relevance of these findings? The severity of white matter lesions may predict poor response to electroconvulsive therapy (ECT) (Hickie et al., 1995; Steffens et al., 2001). Location of lesions in the frontal deep white matter and the presence of pontine lesions and numerous basal ganglia lesions are associated with a poorer response to antidepressant therapy (Simpson et al., 1998). In a 3-year follow-up study, hyperintensities in the pons and corona radiata were associated with a poorer clinical outcome; and severe periventricular hyperintensities were associated with subsequent dementia (Baldwin et al., 2000). In a 2-year follow-up study, O'Brien et al. (1998) reported that patients with the most severe hyperintensities had the worst clinical outcomes. Other research has failed to show significant differences in outcome in patients with and without vascular depression treated with selective serotonin reuptake inhibitors (SSRIs; Krishnan et al., 1998, 2001).

Interestingly, the vascular depression syndrome has no clear correlation with traditional vascular risk factors (hypertension, diabetes, etc.). These factors do not seem to reliably differentiate late onset depression from control subjects (Baldwin et al., 2004; Lloyd et al., 2004), and no consistent relationship has been found between cerebrovascular risk factors and depression severity, symptomatology, or measures of brain volume (Kumar et al., 1997; Lyness et al., 1998). One possibility is that chronic hypoperfusion may be the causal problem (Fernando et al., 2006) and this is less straightforwardly detected by 'bedside' measures of cerebrovascular health.

An intriguing notion is that if some depression is 'vascular' then treatment should not be confined to antidepressants but might include drugs aimed at the vasculature. A recent study has demonstrated that nimodipine (a drug with vasoprotective properties)

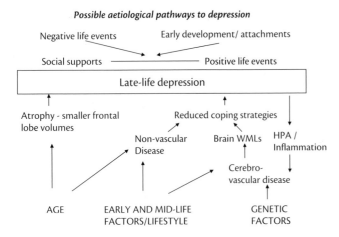

*Possible aetiological pathways to depression*

**Fig. 29ii.1** Possible aetiological pathways to depression (WML, white matter lesions (or hyperintensities); HPA, hypothalamic–pituitary–adrenal axis).

when combined with antidepressant medication led to reduced time to remission and recurrence in patients with late life depression when compared to an antidepressant/placebo combination (Tarangano *et al.*, 2005). This should be replicated.

Critics of the vascular depression hypothesis point to the heterogeneous disorders which are associated with white matter hyperintensities, the failure to identify a symptomatic subgroup corresponding to vascular depression in epidemiological surveys (Licht-Strunk *et al.*, 2004), the uncertainty regarding a vascular causal mechanism, and the abundant evidence that vascular disease and depression are linked in a bidirectional way, each increasing the risk of the other. The vascular depression hypothesis may ultimately prove too restrictive from a conceptual point of view but clinically it serves as a useful prompt that patient management should encompass both psychiatric symptoms and medical co-morbidity.

Figure 29ii.1 illustrates how multiple pathways may lead to depression and how they might interact. Some pathways are intrinsic to the brain, others arise from circumstances and life events whilst other factors may be protective. To illustrate, van den Berg *et al.* (2001) studied 132 older depressed patients and identified three distinct pathways: an early onset group associated with a family history and neuroticism, a late onset group associated with severe life stresses, and a late onset group associated with vascular risk factors.

## Management

### Assessing the patient

The clinical *history* should, with the patient's permission, include information from someone who knows him or her well in order to clarify the range and duration of symptoms, provide an estimate of pre-morbid personality and past capacity to respond to stress and loss, and describe existing supportive relationships. If there has been a past psychiatric history, sight of the relevant case notes can be very informative, for example elucidating what sort of treatment helped in past episodes. The primary care physician will often have some of this information and crucially can provide the relevant medical history.

The *mental state examination* must clarify whether suicidal ideation or delusional phenomena are present. Using a standard screening instrument such as the Mini-Mental State Examination

(Folstein *et al.* 1975), evidence of cognitive impairment should be documented to allow later comparison. Routine neuropsychological testing is not usually necessary unless dementia is suspected, and even then the findings might be equivocal in the depressed state. A *physical examination* should be carried out. This will be focused on relevant findings from the history, for example a neurological examination in patients with poor cognitive function or a system-focused examination relevant to specific symptoms brought up by the patient or linked to their medical history.

*Laboratory investigation* should include haemoglobin and red blood cell indices which may point to possible $B_{12}$ deficiency or alcohol excess. Vitamin $B_{12}$ and folate estimation should be undertaken in a first episode. Red cell folate gives more information about long-term true tissue levels of folate stores; serum folate is more affected by recent dietary fluctuations. In severe depression in older people undernutrition or even dehydration can develop quite quickly and a biochemical screen is important. The guiding principle is an awareness that elderly people have less physiological reserve. Severe depression in a 75-year-old may lead to quite serious metabolic derangement which would be unlikely in a fit 40-year-old. Elevated calcium is occasionally associated with depression, as in primary hyperparathyroidism (Peterson, 1968) or metastatic cancer. Thyroid function testing should be performed because of the well-known association of depression with hypothyroidism, which may be overlooked in the elderly, and because 'apathetic hyperthyroidism' can be mistaken for depression. Neurosyphilis can in theory present with depression. Nowadays this is exceedingly rare although the incidence of syphilis is once again on the increase in some communities. The clinician should have an adequate clinical reason for conducting neurosyphilis testing in depressive disorder, for example relevant neurological signs, and be prepared to discuss this with the patient along with relevant public health implications (for example contact tracing).

Table 29ii.3 summarizes a range of tests and their indications in a first episode of depression and a recurrence.

Regarding the *electroencephalogram* (EEG) there are no diagnostic changes specific to depression on the standard 12-lead EEG. The main benefit of an EEG clinically is to help differentiate depression from an organic brain syndrome. Other changes are discussed under Aetiology.

*Neuroimaging* in affective disorders is largely done largely to rule out a space-occupying lesion and in treatment resistant cases (see Vascular depression, above) where cerebrovascular disease may be linked to poor response.

Hypercorticolism is a well-known feature of depressive disorder. The dexamethasone suppression test (DST) measures activity of the HPA axis. In depression, non-suppression of cortisol after ingestion of dexamethasone is common and once seemed promising as a diagnostic tool for depression (Carroll *et al.*, 1981). However, non-suppression gradually increases with age itself (particularly after 75 years) and the DST does not differentiate between dementia and depression in any reliable manner (Spar and Gerner, 1982), so its use is not recommended.

### General principles of treatment

The management of depressive disorder in older people should be multimodal (involving physical and psychological modalities along with social interventions), multidisciplinary (with involvement as needed from nurses, social worker, and occupational therapists and *ad hoc* help as needed from the dietician, speech

**Table 29ii.3** Investigations for depression in later life

| Investigation | First episode | Recurrence |
| --- | --- | --- |
| Full blood count | Yes | Yes |
| Urea and electrolytes | Yes | Yes |
| Calcium | Yes | Yes |
| Thyroid function | Yes | If clinically indicated, or more than 12 months elapsed |
| B$_{12}$ | Yes | If clinically indicated, or more than 12 months elapsed |
| Folate | Yes | If clinically indicated (for example recent poor diet) |
| Liver function | Yes | If indicated (for example suspected or known alcohol misuse) |
| Syphilitic serology | If clinically indicated (for example relevant neurological symptoms) | Only if clinically indicated |
| CT (brain) | If clinically indicated | If clinically indicated |
| EEG | If clinically indicated | If clinically indicated |

**Table 29ii.4** Management goals in depression and suggested ways to achieve them

| Goal | Ways to achieve |
| --- | --- |
| Risk reduction—of suicide or harm from self-neglect | A risk assessment and monitoring of risk Prompt referral of urgent cases to a specialist |
| Remission of depressive symptoms | Providing appropriate treatment (usually an antidepressant and/or a psychological treatment) Giving the patient and his/her supporters timely education about depression and its treatment |
| To help the patient achieve optimal function | Arrange practical support Ensure access to appropriate agencies which can help |
| To treat the whole person, including somatic problems | Treat co-existing physical health problems Reduce wherever possible the effects of handicap caused by factors such as chronic disease, sensory impairment, and poor mobility Review medication and withdraw unnecessary drugs |
| To prevent relapse and recurrence | Educate the patient about staying on medication once recovered, and about signs of relapse Continuation treatment (staying on treatment after recovery) Maintenance treatment (preventive treatment) |

and language therapist, and podiatrist), and patient centred (that is starting from the patient's concerns and not merely those of the practitioner). Treatments that work are the same as for younger adults: antidepressants, psychosocial and psychological interventions—or combinations of these—and ECT (Anderson *et al.*, 2000). However, patient centredness includes giving the patient as much choice as possible regarding their treatment. In one large study (*n* = 1602) 57% of older depressed patients preferred psychological treatments to an antidepressant (Gum *et al.*, 2006) The availability of alternatives to antidepressants is limited, probably more so for older patients, so services should advocate for service developments which will facilitate true choice.

Some broad goals of treatment and ways of achieving them are shown in Table 29ii.4. The aim is to produce a remission (that is, to resolve all or almost all depressive symptoms) rather than simply improvement, as residual symptoms are strongly linked to future relapse. Since older patients consume a large number of medications, it is always worth reviewing and simplifying drug regimes, and especially so in older depressed patients who tend to have below average adherence to medication.

Given the large range of potential tasks listed in Table 29ii.4, is it realistic to expect a single practitioner, for example a primary care physician, to manage the totality of care? Probably not; and to this end a model known as collaborative care been extensively investigated in depressed patients, including older people. The components are a depression care manager (usually a nurse, psychologist, or social worker) who coordinates the care, including medication concordance. Built into the model is a requirement for regular dialogue between the primary care team and the specialist psychiatric services. The largest study to date of this model is the IMPACT trial in the USA (Unützer *et al.*, 2002). A total of 1801 depressed primary care patients (major depression, 17%; dysthymia, 30%; or both, 53%) were allocated to either usual care or active case management, including a depression care manager and planned collaboration between psychiatrist and primary care physician. There was a patient choice of problem solving treatment (PST) or an antidepressant (prescribed by the primary care physician). At 12 months, 45% of intervention patients achieved a 50% reduction in symptoms, compared to 19% of usual care subjects. This resulted in a respectable number needed to treat (NNT) of 4. (The NNT is the number of subjects to be treated in order that one more will recover than if no treatment is given.) Another large study from the USA using a similar model found an effect in reducing suicidal thinking (Bruce *et al.*, 2004). Suicide is discussed in Chapter 29iii.

Local services have their own criteria for when to refer to specialist services. Typical reasons for referral include: when the diagnosis in doubt (for example, is this dementia?); when depression is severe, as evidenced by psychotic depression, risk to health because of failure to eat or drink or suicide risk; complex therapy is indicated (for example in cases with medical co-morbidity); when first-line therapy fails (although primary care physicians may pursue a second course of an antidepressant from a different class).

# Pharmacotherapy

## Sources of treatment variability in older patients

Altered pharmacokinetics, different pharmacodynamics, a greater chance of polypharmacy and hence drug interactions, and reduced compensatory mechanisms are all important factors which bear upon treatment response in late life depression. These factors are discussed in more detail in Chapter 14 and in Lotrich and Pollock (2005). Briefly, pharmacokinetic response is affected by reduced renal clearance of both the main drug and any active metabolite, diminished microsomal metabolism (involving the P450 systems), a smaller liver mass, reduced hepatic blood flow, and age-related decrements in total albumin and plasma binding. With so many factors it is not surprising that interindividual difference in pharmacokinetics is greater than among younger adults–the same dose may have less predictable effects. There may also be genetic influences for antidepressants. For example a differential response to paroxetine and mirtazapine was reported among older depressed patients depending on whether the allele on the serotonin transporter gene was short or long (Murphy *et al.*, 2003).

Differences in pharmacodynamics may partly explain why older patients have increased sensitivity to particular groups of side-effects at relatively low concentrations of antidepressants. Examples include anticholinergic effects with tricyclic antidepressants (TCAs) and paroxetine, treatment-emergent parkinsonism with SSRIs, and possibly a higher chance of developing the syndrome of inappropriate antidiuretic hormone secretion (SIADH).

The risk of adverse events increases with the number of prescribed drugs, and older patients are likely to be on multiple medication. Oxidative metabolism via the the cytochrome P450 systems is the main mode of metabolism for most drugs. In the 2D6 enzyme system, SSRIs, especially paroxetine and fluoxetine, nefazodone (no longer available in the UK), and venlafaxine can inhibit the metabolism of drugs such as TCAs, antipsychotics, lipophilic β-blockers, some narcotic analgesics (for example codeine), some anti-arrhythmics, and triazolobenzodiazepines, such as alprazolam. Adverse interactions between SSRIs and TCAs occur because each may inhibit the metabolism of the other. In the CYP3A enzyme system, nefazodone, fluoxetine, and paroxetine can inhibit the metabolism of benzodiazepines, calcium channel blockers, cisapride, terfenadine, and theophylline and enhance that of phenytoin. Some of the diseases which underlie polypharmacy, for example inflammatory conditions, may themselves exacerbate poor drug handling.

Lastly, reduced homeostatic reserve can lead to impaired orthostatic responses, impaired thermoregulation, a greater risk of delirium, and an increased risk of falls. An unexplained finding is that SSRIs are associated with an increased risk of hip fracture and falls in the elderly (Ensrud *et al.*, 2003) and in one study more so than TCAs (odds ratio of 1.5 for TCAs and 2.2 for SSRIs) (Liu *et al.*, 1998).

### Initiating treatment in the acute phase of management

The management of depressive disorder is divided into three stages (Frank *et al.*, 1991). Acute treatment refers to the current episode, the end of which is signified by first improvement and then remission. This is usually measured in weeks. Continuation treatment is the period following remission during which treatment is designed to prevent a return of symptoms (a relapse). It is measured in months. Lastly, maintenance treatment attempts to prevent future episodes of depression and is measured in years. The following deals with the pharmacological management of an episode of depression, also called the acute treatment phase. The other stages are discussed later.

The type of depression is important. A number of studies show that psychotic depression requires either an antidepressant combined with an antipsychotic drug, or ECT (Baldwin, 1988). Second, there is some evidence that for depression severe enough to

require admission to hospital, TCAs are more effective than SSRIs (Anderson *et al.*, 2000). Third, current antidepressants are indicated for major rather than minor depression, although in one study (Williams *et al.*, 2000) minor depression when accompanied by disablement was more likely to respond to paroxetine than placebo. In the UK, the National Institute for Health and Clinical Excellence (NICE) suggests watchful waiting as the first strategy for minor depression (http://www.nice.org.uk/). Lastly, bereavement has been discussed earlier; depressive disorder complicating bereavement can be successfully treated with antidepressants (Reynolds *et al.*, 1999a).

For the older antidepressants in particular, the adage 'start low—go slow' is apt. Prolonged dose-titration is usually unnecessary with newer antidepressants, which account for the majority of prescribing in current practice.

A classification of antidepressants is shown in Table 29ii.5.

With so many antidepressants to choose from it is important to match the antidepressant to the patient, taking account of tolerability, safety, side-effects, drug interactions, and contraindications. For example the SSRIs citalopram, sertraline, and escitalopram are non-sedative and largely free from major interactions with other drugs. They are often preferred when frailty is a concern. Mirtazapine is sedative and may be helpful where insomnia is a prominent symptom. If a patient experienced a good recovery in the past with a particular antidepressant then, other things being equal, it makes clinical sense to give the same one during a recurrence.

Currently there is public concern about antidepressants. These range from fears that the risk of self-harm may be intensified during early treatment to a belief that antidepressants encourage passivity and undermine natural coping mechanisms. A further fundamental criticism is that they are simply ineffective or only marginally effective (Moncrieff and Kirsch, 2005). Media attention is likely to magnify fears. There is much polemic on both sides of the debate, but suffice it to say that involvement of the patient in

**Table 29ii.5** Classification of antidepressants

| Older TCAs | Secondary amines (nortriptyline, desipramine)<br>Tertiary amines [imipramine, amitriptyline, dosulepin (dothiepin), clomipramine] |
|---|---|
| Newer TCAs | Lofepramine |
| Atypical antidepressants | Trazodone, nefazodone[a], mianserin |
| Monoamine oxidase inhibitors (non-reversible) | Phenelzine, tranylcypromine |
| Reversible inhibitors of monoamine oxidase A ('RIMA' agents) | Moclobemide |
| Selective serotonin reuptake inhibitors (SSRIs) | Fluvoxamine, fluoxetine, paroxetine, sertraline, citalopram, escitalopram |
| Noradrenaline and specific serotonin enhancers (NASSa) | Mirtazapine |
| Noradrenaline reuptake inhibitors (NARI) | Reboxetine |
| Serotonin/noradrenaline reuptake inhibitors (SNRI) | Venlafaxine, duloxetine |

[a] Withdrawn in late 2003 following concerns regarding adverse effects on the liver.

---

**Box 29ii.7** Practical aspects of concordance in treatment

- Understanding the patient's perception of what depression is and that of his/her family and supporters.
- Explaining what depression is and what it is not (for example, 'weakness of character').
- Clarifying attribution of symptoms (for example, all due to heart, bowels, etc.).
- Explaining side-effects.
- Explaining delay in onset.
- Agreeing management plan.
- Involving family/supporters with consent.

---

decisions regarding treatment is crucial. 'Concordance' rather than 'compliance' is the vocabulary which should underpin such discussions (Box 29ii.7).

Particular difficulties arise when patients do not adhere to antidepressant medication because of persistent attribution of all symptoms to physical illness. Time should be set aside to explain carefully the nature and extent of any actual physical illness present and its likely effects, and that depression too can be considered an illness; that it is common and treatable, rather than a sign of moral weakness. Sometimes too it is necessary to examine the ways in which both the patient and his or her family understand illness and its consequences in order to shed light on what might be the rewards of invalidism. An elderly patient may 'use' physical illness and physical symptomatology to foster dependence, often in the face of social isolation. Sometimes, after the depressive component has been treated adequately, these issues linger and impede functional recovery, in which case inpatient or day patient admission may be the only way to achieve progress. Such cases require a consistent staff approach and a behavioural programme with appropriate rewards, or at the very least a carefully structured day to promote purposeful activity.

Many patients need reassurance that antidepressants are not addictive, and that depression is not 'senility' or a harbinger of dementia. They need to be warned not to expect immediate results. It may be necessary to take the treatment in stages. For example, patients can be told that antidepressants will relieve their depressive symptoms, but that further help to address a bereavement may be needed. Commonly occurring side-effects should be explained. Patients often read the package insert which can be informative but may also be rather overwhelming, so that locally produced information sheets can be helpful.

### Efficacy

In a Cochrane Systematic Review of randomized controlled trials (RCT) Wilson et al. (2001) found efficacy for antidepressants over placebo in late life major depression. However, the authors could find only 17 suitable studies (two of SSRIs). The NNT averaged 4, but was higher for SSRIs. In a further Cochrane Systematic Review of 29 studies which included patients aged over 55, using the Cochrane Depression, Anxiety and Neurosis Group (CCDAN) Controlled Trials Register (to 2003), no difference in efficacy was found between TCAs and SSRIs, but TCAs were associated with higher withdrawal rates due to side-effects. Patients receiving TCA-related antidepressants (mianserin or trazodone) had a similar withdrawal rate to SSRIs, leading the authors to conclude that

TCA-related antidepressants may offer a viable alternative to SSRIs in older depressed patients. The study also investigated 'atypical' antidepressants but were unable to make recommendations because of low statistical power. Atypicals included the important antidepressants reboxetine, venlafaxine, and mirtazapine (Mottram et al., 2006).

Several recent RCTs have produced mixed findings. Schatzberg and Cantillon (2000) failed to show any advantage over placebo of either venlafaxine or fluoxetine in patients averaging 71 years of age. Nor did Roose et al. (2004) find citalopram more effective than placebo in patients who were approximately a decade older. Kasper et al. (2005) compared escitalopram (173 patients), fluoxetine (164 patients), and placebo (180 subjects) in a study with participants aged 75. Again neither antidepressant was statistically more effective than placebo. Schneider et al. (2003) showed a modest although statistically significant advantage of sertraline over placebo in an RCT of patients of average age 70. Nelson et al. (2005) found that duloxetine was superior to placebo in an RCT of young-old (early to mid-60s). Remission rates, as opposed to response rates, were relatively low in these studies. However, the design of these trials—short duration (average 8 weeks) and inability to switch patients who were non-responsive at 4 weeks—might have contributed to these less than encouraging findings. So it is noteworthy that Rapaport et al. (2003) reported the highest response rate (68% versus 52% placebo, a significant difference) and remission rate (43% versus 26% placebo, again significant) in an RCT of controlled release paroxetine in patients of average age 70 who were treated for a longer period (12 weeks).

Some trials compare one antidepressants to another ('head-to-head' trials). Using a statistical approach which measured the efficacy of antidepressants in the elderly with an NNT analysis (using data between 1966 and 1999), Katona and Livingston (2002) found no advantage of one antidepressant over another, although wide confidence intervals were reported.

L-tryptophan may have a role as an adjunctive therapy in treatment-resistant depression but has been associated with the eosinophilic–myalgic syndrome and with a risk of the serotonin syndrome when combined with other antidepressants such as SSRIs. There are few data regarding older patients and its use has waned. Transcranial magnetic stimulation (TMS) is discussed later.

Table 29ii.6 provides an overview of the principal mode of action, side-effects, and dosaging for the main antidepressants used in old age psychiatry. The mixed findings with regard to recent antidepressant trials have caused much debate. One conclusion is that placebo treatment in RCTs comprises much more than a pill. Participants will see research personnel who may provide empathic listening and informal support. The role of 'non-specific' factors in the treatment of depressive disorder is increasingly recognized as a key component (McCusker et al., 1998). Although the individual ingredients have yet to be identified properly, factors likely to be important are: having a plausible treatment delivered by someone perceived as an expert who is enthusiastic about it and takes depression seriously; the expectation of improvement; the positive regard of the prescriber towards the patient who is listened to with empathy and encouraged to verbalize distress and, perhaps especially important in older adults, encouraging purposeful activity to counter apathy and withdrawal.

**Table 29ii.6** Mode of action, side-effect profiles, and dosages of the main antidepressants used to treat late life depression in the UK

| Drug | Main mode of action | Main side-effects | Starting dosage (mg) | Average daily dose (mg) |
|---|---|---|---|---|
| Amitriptyline | NA++, 5-HT+ | Sedation, anticholinergic, postural hypotension, tachycardia/arrhythmia | 25–50 | 75–100[a] |
| Imipramine | NA++, 5-HT+ | As for amitriptyline but less sedation | 25 | 75–100[a] |
| Nortripyline | NA++, 5-HT+ | As for amitriptyline but less sedation, anticholinergic effects and hypotension | 10 t.d.s. | 75–100[a] |
| Dothiepin | NA++, 5-HT+ | As for amitripyline | 50–75 | 75–150 |
| Mianserin | $\alpha_2$ | Sedation | 30 | 30–90 |
| Lofepramine | NA++, 5-HT+ | As for amitriptyline but less sedation, anticholinergic effects, hypotension, and cardiac problems | 70–140 | 70–210 |
| Trazodone | $5\text{-HT}_2$ | Sedation, dizziness, headache | 100 | 300 |
| Citalopram | 5-HT | Nausea, vomiting, dyspepsia, abdominal pain, diarrhoea, headache, sexual dysfunction | 20 | 20–40 |
| Sertraline | 5-HT | As for citalopram | 50 | 50–150 |
| Fluoxetine | 5-HT | As for citalopram but insomnia and agitation more common | 20 | 20 |
| Paroxetine | 5-HT | As for citalopram but sedation and anticholinergic effects may occur | 20 | 20 |
| Fluvoxamine | 5-HT | As for citalopram but nausea more common | 50–100 | 100–200 |
| Escitalopram | 5-HT | As for citalopram | 5 | 10 |
| Moclobemide | MAO | Sleep disturbance, nausea, agitation | 300 | 300–400 |
| Venlafaxine | NA, 5-HT | Nausea, insomnia, dizziness, dry mouth, somnolence, hyper- and hypotension | 75 | 150[b] |
| Duloxetine | NA, 5-HT | Nausea, insomnia, dizziness | 30 | 60 |
| Mirtazapine | $\alpha_2$ blocking selective antagonist $5\text{-HT}_2$ and $5\text{-HT}_3$ receptors | Increased appetite, weight gain, somnolence, headache | 30 | 30 |

[a] These are average doses. Some patients will require higher dosages.

[b] Titration up to higher dosages in common is specialist care.

NA, noradrenaline; 5-HT, serotonin; MAO, monoamine oxidase inhibitor.

## Efficacy of antidepressants in specific groups
### Elderly patients with dementia
A Cochrane Systematic Review of antidepressants for depression in dementia found 'weak' evidence for their effectiveness (Bains *et al.*, 2002). However, only four studies met the inclusion criteria. A more recent study (Lyketsos *et al.*, 2003) included only 44 subjects but was an RCT. It compared sertaline to placebo and showed significant improvement on the Cornell Scale for Depression in Dementia in favour of sertraline, but no change in cognition. A significant response rate was also reported by Roth *et al.* (1996) in 511 patients treated with moclobemide against placebo in patients with and

without dementia. Methodological considerations meant this study was not included in the Cochrane Review but it did demonstrate improvement in cognitive function in depressed patients with low baseline cognitive function. Similar findings have been reported for the SSRI citalopram (Nyth *et al.*, 1992). However, there is a high rate of spontaneous recovery from depression complicating dementia so that 'watchful waiting' is reasonable for mild-to-moderate cases.

### Depression in association with general systemic disease
The SSRI fluoxetine was more effective than placebo in one study of medical patients with a mixture of physical conditions; interestingly

it was as effective or possibly even more effective the more severe the underlying physical condition (Evans *et al.*, 1997). The drug was well tolerated. However, Roose *et al.* (1994), found that 22 depressed patients with heart disease with a mean age of 73 years responded less well to fluoxetine than 42 comparable patients treated with nortriptyline (mean age 70). Only 5 of the 22 fluoxetine-treated patients responded, and those with the melancholic subtype (the majority) did especially poorly. The number of dropouts in each group was similar.

In the previously-mentioned IMPACT research on collaborative care for late life depression, both physical function and pain were improved in participants who received active case management compared with usual care (Lin *et al.*, 2003; Callahan *et al.*, 2005). The Sertraline Antidepressant Heart Attack Trial (SADHART) and the Enhancing Recovery in Coronary Heart Disease (ENRICH-D), of mixed aged patients, both reported marginal benefits for sertraline over placebo, notably for patients with more severe depression, but in neither study were cardiac outcomes improved (Glassman *et al.*, 2002; Writing Committee for the ENRICHD Investigators, 2003).

Depression after stroke is common. Paranthaman and Baldwin (2006) reviewed the literature to 2005. Of 10 RCT studies (nine placebo-controlled) using antidepressants from different classes, eight showed positive results. A high rate of spontaneous recovery was evident, especially in the first 6 weeks. The effect of repetitive TMS (rTMS) (see also later) on patients with refractory post-stroke depression was studied by Jorge *et al.* (2004) in a placebo RCT. Patients were given either 10 sessions of active left pre-frontal rTMS or sham rTMS. There was a significant reduction of depressive symptoms in the treatment group and this was not influenced by the patient's age, or the type or location of stroke. Side-effects were few and mild and there were no significant changes in cognitive functioning. There is though a risk of seizures following TMS and this must be weighed carefully in stroke patients who may in any case be at increased risk. Both TCAs and SSRIs in standard dosages have been found to ameliorate post-stroke depression (Paranthaman and Baldwin, 2006).

There is evidence that some antidepressants may prevent post-stroke depression. For example, Rasmussen *et al.* (2003) studied 130 non-depressed stroke patients in an RCT with the SSRI sertraline versus placebo followed to 12 months. Sertraline was found to have significantly superior prophylactic efficacy compared with placebo and was well tolerated. Other studies have been less positive, so that it is not possible to recommend prophylactic post-stroke antidepressant medication routinely. It might be reasonable to consider this for stroke patients at high risk of depression, for example those with a prior history of depressive disorder.

Idiopathic Parkinson's disease also has a high rate of depression during its course but at the time of writing there are few controlled trials to support evidence-based recommendations for treatment. Although SSRIs are usually recommended—because they are generally well tolerated—worsening of parkinsonism may occur, although this is controversial (Dell'Agnello *et al.*, 2001).

### Depression in residential and nursing homes

The detection and management of depression in frail elderly people in residential and nursing homes is poor. In a placebo-controlled study of nortriptyline a significant benefit was seen, but a third of those entered could not tolerate the drug (Katz *et al.*, 1990). In an open-label study of SSRIs in a similar setting which included

very old subjects, the response rate for major depression was poor in those subjects who had depression complicating dementia (Trappler and Cohen, 1998). Given the high prevalence of depressive symptoms in care settings and the high rate of intolerance to older antidepressants it is advisable to use newer antidepressants but the evidence for their efficacy is not yet clear.

### Side effects of medication

Table 29ii.6 shows the main side-effects of antidepressants used to treat late life depression. Side-effects are the commonest reason for poor adherence to antidepressant medication (Mitchell, 2006).

Anticholinergic side-effects include dry mouth, blurred vision, constipation, urinary retention, and cardiotoxicity [which may be a reason for carrying out an electrocardiogram (ECG) prior to starting an older TCA]. Persistent dryness of the mouth, another anticholinergic effect, can lead to dental caries. These effects are common with TCAs and cardiac arrhythmia in overdose can be fatal. Delirium can occur and is more likely in patients who are acutely medically unwell. Postural hypotension due to adrenergic blockade is a serious problem with TCAs and histaminic effects often cause sedation and, in the longer term, weight gain. Lofepramine is a second-generation TCA less likely to cause these adverse effects.

SSRIs are safer than TCAs but they have undesirable side-effects of their own. These include nausea (around 15%), diarrhoea (around 10%), insomnia (5–15%), anxiety and/or agitation (2 to 15%), sexual dysfunction (up to 30% among younger people treated; unknown prevalence in elderly patients), headache, and, occasionally, weight loss. The main metabolite of fluoxetine is clinically active and remains so for approximately a week, possibly longer for older patients. The SSRIs have minimal impact on cognitive function in older patients with depression and there is also evidence that SSRIs and lofepramine cause less impairment than the older TCAs in cognitive skills relevant to driving. There is concern about gastrointestinal haemorrhage with SSRIs, particularly in elderly patients (van Walraven *et al.*, 2001). Caution is needed in patients treated with non-steroidal anti-inflammatory drugs (NSAIDs) or aspirin for whom SSRIs are being considered, and gastroprotective medication may be required.

Discontinuation symptoms may occur with all classes of antidepressants after several weeks of treatment and are more common and severe with antidepressants that have a short half-life. Inappropriate antidiuretic hormone secretion (IADH) is often linked to SSRIs, but may occur as a side-effect of all classes of antidepressants. There is a paucity of systematic data, but increased age, female gender, and drugs that lower sodium levels are all risk factors (Kirby and Ames, 2001). Symptoms often (but not invariably) occur when the blood sodium level falls below 130 mmol/litre. Symptoms of IADH, which include lethargy, fatigue and sleep disturbance as well as muscle cramps and headaches, overlap with those of depression and should prompt a blood test.

Moclobemide is well tolerated by older people. Although a special diet is not required, patients should be aware of the drug interactions with painkillers and other antidepressants. Co-prescriptions of moclobemide with TCAs or SSRIs should be avoided. A wash-out period of around four to five half-lives of the drug and any active metabolite is advised when transferring from a TCA or SSRI to moclobemide (but is not necessary from moclobemide to a TCA or SSRI).

Venlafaxine is generally well tolerated among older patients, particularly if the dose is increased slowly. Side-effects such as nausea and gastrointestinal disturbance tend to be transitory. Venlafaxine is known to cause hypertension, although in older patients dose-related postural hypotension can also be a significant problem. Blood pressure monitoring is recommended. Venlafaxine is not recommended in patients with heart disease likely to predispose to arrhythmia. Duloxetine, a newer dual-acting antidepressant, does not appear to be cardiotoxic although nausea can be a problem.

Mirtazapine is an interesting antidepressant which appears to enhance both noradrenergic and serotonergic function via antagonism at the pre-synaptic $\alpha_2$ receptor. Differences in pharmacodynamics and pharmacokinetics are minimal with age. The side-effect profile is similar to TCAs; weight gain and sedation can be troublesome, or useful where anorexia and insomnia are features of the patient's depression.

Of the older atypical antidepressants, mianserin has few anticholinergic or adverse cardiovascular effects, at least in normal individuals, but it is quite sedative. Concerns over blood dyscrasias necessitating regular blood counts make it inconvenient to use. Trazodone, another novel non-TCA drug, also has sedative properties and a good safety record, making it a useful alternative. There have been occasional reports of priapism associated with its use.

It is often said that older depressed patients take longer to recover than younger adults and that they therefore require longer treatment intervals with antidepressants. This may have been true of the older TCAs which required a long dose-titration period before effective dosages were achieved but it is questionable when applied to newer antidepressants. Sackeim *et al.* (2005), for example, analysed data from two comparative trials, one of sertaline versus fluoxetine and the other sertaline versus nortriptyline in patients with a mean age of 67 years. If little or no improvement (equal to or less than 30% on a recognized mood rating scale) had occurred by week 4 then recovery or remission was unlikely. This is no different from younger adults. So unless there are special factors, such as the need for a dose-titration period, non-response at 4 weeks should prompt a change in strategy (Box 29ii.8). Mottram *et al.* (2002) also found that response at 4 weeks predicted eventual recovery. A caveat though is that the above trials were of relatively younger older adults and those with more severe or unstable physical illnesses are likely to have been excluded. If, however, recovery has begun at 4 weeks then optimising the dosage and continuing with the same medication leads to substantial further recovery. In the study of Mottram *et al.* (2002), of those who eventually recovered, 61% had done so by 6 weeks and 88% by 8 weeks.

## Electroconvulsive therapy (ECT)

ECT is discussed in detail in Chapter 15. Although ECT is recognized to be effective in older patients, opinion is divided about bilateral versus unilateral delivery of ECT. High-dosage unilateral ECT leads to remission rates equal to bilateral ECT (Sackeim *et al.*, 2000) but increasing the dose causes more cognitive impairment. A compromise is to start with unilateral placement and continue with bilateral if there has been no response after four to six treatments.

A major problem with ECT is the high subsequent relapse rate, and it is unclear how best to prevent this. Sackeim *et al.* (2001) in a study of a group of patients of mixed ages reported that virtually all patients relapsed after ECT if not given ongoing medication. In their study nortripyline plus lithium offered the best protection.

## Pharmacological treatment of resistant depression

At least a third of patients do not respond to antidepressant monotherapy. Guscott and Grof (1991) have proposed a systematic approach in which key questions are posed before a move to augmentation regimes or to ECT are contemplated (Box 29ii.9). Thus, the diagnosis should be reviewed; for example an older depressed patient quietly harbouring psychotic thoughts will not recover with an antidepressant alone. Treatment adequacy, duration of treatment (at a therapeutic dose), compliance with treatment, side-effects, and psychosocial factors likely to impede recovery should all be re-evaluated.

Beyond this there exists a range of strategies (Table 29ii.7) but none are proven to be better than others. Nevertheless, clinicians often have favourite regimens with which they have developed a lot of practical expertise. The practice of increasing the dosages of drug beyond the recommended upper level is of dubious value for the SSRIs, although there may be a place for this with the dual-acting drug venlafaxine, if tolerated. Prolonging the treatment period is only realistic for patients who have already begun to respond. Measuring serum levels can be helpful for the older TCAs where a therapeutic window has been established, but is not recommended, and is not usually routinely available, for newer antidepressants.

Persistence pays. In a clinical series, Flint and Rifat (1996), using a rational stepped-care protocol, showed that sequential regimes of antidepressant therapy eventually produced improvement or recovery in over 80% of their patients.

---

**Box 29ii.8**  Strategies for the acute phase of treatment

If little or no response (<30% reduction in symptoms) by 4 weeks:
- increase the dose *or* if the dosage is optimal
- change to another antidepressant (switch class)

If partial response by 4 weeks:
- optimize dose (if not already done)
- continue and review 2–4 weekly

If little further improvement by 8 weeks:
- consider augmentation (either with medication or a psychological intervention) *or*
- consider combining antidepressants

At all stages consider ECT if indicated by severity or risks,

---

**Box 29ii.9**  A systematic approach to resistant depression

- Is the diagnosis correct?
- Was treatment adequate (duration, dose, compliance)?
- Has a stepped care pharmacological approach been used?
- Has outcome been measured appropriately?
- Has medical and/or psychiatric co-morbidity been addressed?
- Are there factors in the treatment setting (including psychosocial reinforcers) that have been overlooked?

From Guscott and Grof (1991)

**Table 29ii.7** Strategies for resistant depression

| Category | Example |
| --- | --- |
| Optimization (maximize dose/serum level/time) | Dose increase<br>Prolong course<br>Measure/adjust drug concentration |
| Substitution (substitute one antidepressant for another) | SSRI to SSRI (questionable unless to address tolerability)<br>SSRI to different class |
| Augmentation (use of a non-primary antidepressant) | Lithium or tri-iodothyronine to primary antidepressant<br>Psychological intervention |
| Combination (use two primary antidepressants together) | SSRI + TCA<br>SSRI + mirtazapine<br>Mirtazapine + venlafaxine |

## Combining antidepressants

A popular strategy at the time of writing is to combine antidepressants from different classes. Dodd *et al.* (2005) systematically reviewed the literature to January 2005, finding only eight RCTs, each with differing results. Sixteen 'open-label' trials were of varying quality and with differing antidepressant combinations. Numerous case series and chart reviews were found. Among these were several which reported adverse events from antidepressant combinations, including one case of the serotonin syndrome. It seems then that clinical practice has developed ahead of evidence. A number of treatment algorithms were also examined. Steps in these algorithms included not only combining antidepressants, but also a higher dose of a monotherapy drug, class switching of antidepressants, lithium augmentation, and ECT. The authors suggest that combination treatment works in about 50% of resistant patients treated. As there are few data specifically for the elderly on this question, we have to extrapolate from broader research like this. Popular combinations include a SSRI plus mirtazapine, a SSRI plus venlafaxine, and venlafaxine plus mirtazapine, but these should be undertaken by psychiatrists experienced with such combinations.

## Augmentation

Like ECT, lithium augmentation is an effective treatment for the management of resistant depression and, like ECT, its use in this regard has declined with the advent of newer antidepressants. Unfortunately there are no double-blind placebo-controlled trials of lithium augmentation therapy in elderly patients. In the UK in 2006, NICE released guidance (http://www.nice.org.uk/page.aspx?o=cg38niceguideline) about the management of bipolar disorder. Lithium levels of 0.6 to 0.8 mmol/litre were recommended for adults requiring maintenance lithium, and in the absence of specific recommendations for lithium augmentation in unipolar depression, this remains pragmatic guidance. Based on experience, some old age psychiatrists aim at serum levels as low as 0.35 mmol/litre, but their intention may chiefly be to minimize the risk of adverse effects. Foster (1992) reviewed the use of lithium in elderly patients and found that non-toxic side-effects are common. For example polydipsia occurred in 50–74%, polyuria in 25–58%, tremor in 33–58%, dry mouth in 53%, nausea in 33%, and memory impairment in 33%. Of concern was Foster's finding that about 11–23% of elderly patients appear to suffer acute lithium toxicity.

The NICE bipolar guidance also covers other treatments of bipolar depression. The main message is that antidepressants, if used, should be combined with a mood stabilizer or an antipsychotic because of the risk of a manic switch.

Psychological interventions are effective in both the acute and continuation stages of treatment (see below and Chapters 18) and these, too, should be considered as valid alternative strategies for augmentation treatment.

### Other strategies

Because of dietary restrictions traditional monoamine oxidase inhibitors (MAOIs) are rarely used. However, Georgotas *et al.* (1983) gave phenelzine (15–75 mg/day) to 20 elderly patients with refractory depression and achieved a 65% recovery rate, which is a reminder that under specialist care the MAOIs may still have a role. Tri-iodothyronine is usually well tolerated but the evidence seems mainly for its use in conjunction with TCAs, and thyroid function must be monitored. Tryptophan has been mentioned; usually a dose of 2–3 g is recommended.

Other reported strategies which lack definitive evidence are: lamotrigine, pindolol, the addition of an atypical antipsychotic and the addition of reboxetine to other antidepressants. (The latter is not recommended for use in older patients due to a lack of submitted evidence when the drug was licensed.)

rTMS is a reasonably effective treatment for moderate depressive episode but there have been no adequate RCTs in older patients. Frontal atrophy, as can occur in late life depression, may reduce the response to rTMS in older patients (Manes *et al.*, 2001; Fabre *et al.*, 2004). rTMS and vagal nerve stimulation are two further developments of relevance to resistant depression in later life, although there is a paucity of evidence in older patients. Some small studies have (Fabre *et al.*, 2004) and have not (Mosimann *et al.*, 2004) found benefit of rTMS in resistant depression in older patients. Intriguingly, there has been some evidence for improvement in cognitive performance, especially that linked to executive function, in mid-life and later life depressed patients treated with rTMS (Fabre *et al.*, 2004; Moser *et al.*, 2002).

Lastly, ECT is effective for resistant depression and psychosurgery is still used in a few designated centres. Success is reported, although the patients referred to these centres are usually middle aged rather than elderly.

# Psychological interventions

Cognitive behavioural therapy (CBT), interpersonal psychotherapy (IPT), problem-solving treatment (PST), and psychodynamic psychotherapy are the most widely researched forms of psychotherapy in later life practice. CBT and IPT along with family interventions are discussed elsewhere. PST deals with the here and now, focusing on current difficulties and setting future goals. It is designed to help the patient gain a sense of mastery over difficulties.

These interventions have been used successfully in older people (Gatz *et al.*, 1998; Pinquart and Sorensen, 2001), including in group format (Steuer and Hammen, 1983), but their use specifically in late life depression is less well researched although evidence is accumulating (Scogin and McElreath, 1994; Koder, *et al.*, 1996; Reynolds *et al.*, 1999a;.Karel and Hinrichsen, 2000).

A problem in the delivery of psychological interventions is consistency. Pills are the same regardless of who prescribed them, but there can be great variation in the experience, enthusiasm, and expertise of the therapist delivering a psychological intervention. Williams *et al.* (2000) encountered this in their multisite study, in which the efficacy of PST in minor depression varied markedly across sites as compared with paroxetine.

Psychological interventions also have a place in relapse prevention. Reynolds *et al.* (1999b) found that monthly IPT given in the continuation phase of treatment was more effective than routine care, and the combination of IPT with maintenance antidepressant therapy was the most effective of all. However, the same group were unable to replicate this in a later study with a group of patients on average 10 years older (Reynolds *et al.*, 2006).

Anxiety management can be a highly effective adjunctive treatment for depressed patients, especially those recovering from depression but left with residual anxiety, low confidence, or phobic avoidance, all of which can undermine functional improvement. Techniques include progressive relaxation, either alone with a commercial tape, or in groups. Graded tasks under the supervision of an occupational therapist, nurse, or psychologist can be extremely helpful.

Exercise and activity are important both to avoid depression and to counter it. Behavioural activation is a technique which can overcome the withdrawal and apathy that so often exists in late life depression. It works by helping the patient develop a schedule of activities, agreed between the patient and therapist, with or without a written diary to support implementation.

Family work is discussed in Chapter 18iv. Not only may a dysfunctional family contribute to the onset of depressive illness, but the family is often critical in ensuring a successful treatment outcome.

## Social interventions

Scogin and McElreath (1994) conducted a meta-analysis of 17 psychosocial treatments for late life depression. This included some of the interventions discussed in the previous section. They found an overall treatment effect size (comparing interventions with placebo or no treatment) of 0.78, suggesting that these treatments are effective. A caveat is that such studies often exclude mobility-impaired, frail, or otherwise unfit older adults and therefore may not be truly generalizable.

As discussed earlier, poor housing, poverty, high local rates of crime or fear of crime, and other indices of deprivation are important determinants of depression. Many factors interact: low socio-economic status is linked to poverty, poor housing, higher exposure to crime, and poorer health. Sometimes a change to better circumstances can be crucial to recovery. Generally though it is best to defer discussion of issues such as rehousing until after recovery from depression, as the patient's view may alter. The impact of these factors will also be affected by others such as the availability of social support or other resources, and individual coping styles. Interventions for each of these can be addressed as part of recovering from depression, often using a psychiatric day hospital as a focus for treatment.

Mention was made earlier of the link between handicap and depression and how the notion of handicap contains a social dimension. Social workers can help address the sources of handicap and 'sign-post' the patient with depression to resources which may help reduce this and other disadvantages. This may of course be too UK-centric a view, since in many cultures the family provides the main social framework. However, in the UK networks

of day centres, clubs, resource centres, and luncheon clubs can provide support to the depressed older person. Some have been developed specifically with minority communities in mind. They may help counter isolation which may be either a cause or effect of depression. Last but not least, effective networks exist to support care-givers, a group with a high incidence of depression.

## Prognosis

The outcome of depression can be expressed either as its 'natural history', based on aggregated data obtained from large numbers of patients, or as an outcome for a particular patient, based on various predictive variables. We know more about the former than the latter.

### Natural history

After up to 6 years' follow-up of a sample of elderly depressed patients requiring hospitalization, Post (1962, 1972) found that around 60% had either remained well or had experienced relapses with full recovery. Interestingly, the advent of TCAs during the period between these two studies made little difference to outcome. Cole and Bellavance (1997a) found similar results after reviewing the literature. Results from the community and medical wards (Cole and Bellavance, 1997b, 1999) were poorer—only a third and fifth respectively had good outcomes. Beekman *et al.* (2002) followed 277 community-dwelling subjects, aged over 55 (most over 75), from the Dutch LASA epidemiological survey. Unlike the above studies they used multiple assessments of mood (14 assessments over a 6-year period) rather than one at baseline and another at the last contact. Almost half the sample was depressed for more than 60% of the time; 23% had true remissions; 12% had remissions with recurrence; a third had a chronic–intermittent course; and a third had chronic depression. There was a gradient in outcome according to the initial diagnosis, from subthreshold depression (with the least unfavourable outcome), to major depression and dysthymia (intermediate prognosis) through to double depression (depression with dysthymia) which conferred the worst prognosis.

It is now accepted that across all age groups depressive disorder is a chronic condition, prone to recurrence. A key question is whether the poorer outcomes observed in community and hospital settings are indicative of: poor levels of detection [consistently found in community and hospital studies (Green *et al.*, 1994; Jackson and Baldwin, 1993; Koenig *et al.*, 1997)]; insufficient treatment of identified cases; or differences in risk and maintaining factors, such as medical co-morbidity. In the Liverpool Continuing Health in the Community Study (Green *et al.*, 1994) involving 1070 older participants, four vulnerability factors were associated with a poorer prognosis at 3 years: female gender, smoking, loneliness, and dissatisfaction with life.

In terms of comparative outcomes Mitchell and Subramaniam (2005) reviewed the literature between 1966 and July 2004 finding 24 publications which could be used to assess outcomes between different age groups. Although there were some contradictory findings, overall the authors concluded that episodes of depression remitted as well in later life as in other age groups, but there was a greater risk of relapse in older people. This was linked to two mechanisms: age of onset (recurrent depression from earlier life conferring a poorer prognosis) and medical co-morbidity (which worsened prognosis and was linked to a later onset). This suggests that interventions in the continuation and maintenance phases of treatment are even more important in later life.

Lastly, most prognostic studies focus on depressive symptoms and their reduction. Little is known about social outcomes, for example whether patients can resume normal social function.

## Mortality

In a systematic review of the literature from 1997 to 2001 examining the evidence linking depression to non-suicide mortality, Schulz *et al.* (2002) identified a positive link between depression and non-suicide mortality in three-quarters of studies, with a trend for the effect to be greater for elderly males than females. Following a cohort of 652 depressed and non-depressed subjects over 3.5 years, Geerlings *et al.* (2002) found that duration, chronicity, and increasing symptoms from baseline were all linked to a higher risk of death. This led them to suggest that adequate treatment may reduce this effect.

However, not all research has confirmed a link between depression and non-suicide mortality. For example for the USA, Blazer *et al.* (2001) found a high odds ratio for death following depression but this reduced to almost 1 after allowing for potential confounders such as chronic disease, health habits, cognitive impairment, functional impairment, and social support.

The arguments are probably circular. For example, physical disability is a risk factor for depression but depression itself worsens physical illness outcomes which are likely to lead to increased mortality via poor self monitoring of health and poor adherence to medical treatments.

## Prognostic factors

As a generalisation, predictive factors may be divided into *general factors* and those relevant to *characteristics of the illness* (Table 29ii.8). Adverse factors of a general kind include chronic stress associated with poor environment, crime and poverty, becoming a victim of crime, poor perceived (but not objectively lacking) social support, and supervening serious physical ill-health. Surprisingly few features of the illness itself can be directly linked with a poorer prognosis.

**Table 29ii.8** Poor outcome factors

| Illness—clinical features | Slower initial recovery |
| --- | --- |
| | More severe initial depression |
| | Duration > 2 years |
| | Three or more previous episodes (for recurrence) |
| | Previous history of dysthymia |
| | Psychotic symptoms |
| | Extensive disease of deep white matter and basal ganglia grey matter (vascular depression) |
| | Organic brain disease (for example dementia) |
| General factors | Chronic stress associated with poor environment, crime, and poverty |
| | A new physical illness |
| | Becoming a victim of crime |
| | Poor perceived (but not objectively lacking) social support |

The literature suggests that the following are important: a slow or incomplete recovery, three or more previous episodes, severity of illness, duration from onset exceeding 2 years, and the presence of organic cerebral pathology.

Another adverse outcome is of course suicide. This is covered in Chapter 29iii.

# Prevention

## Primary prevention

Avoiding depressive symptoms in later life, like so many things, is probably linked to a healthy earlier lifestyle and a certain amount of good fortune. Many but by no means all diseases of later life are associated both with depression and lifestyle factors such as diet, exercise, obesity, and good self-monitoring of health. A systematic review of the effects of exercise on depressive symptoms in later life (Sjosten and Kievla, 2006) concluded that both aerobic and non-aerobic exercise can be effective in those with clinically defined depression or even with elevated depressive symptoms falling short of disorder. Where benefits occurred this happened quite quickly but waned during follow-up. Tai Chi training seemed promising.

Whether the same logic can be applied to the prevention of major depression is less clear. Some individuals seem especially at risk. Those who lack the capacity for intimacy have already been mentioned (Murphy, 1982, 1983). Cole and Dendukuri (2003) carried out a meta-analysis of risk factors for late life depression, finding five which were robustly linked to it. These were bereavement, sleep problems, physical disability, prior depression, and female gender. They suggest that some of these are amenable to a public health preventative approach.

Specialist mental health professionals have an important role in education. Older people most vulnerable to depression will often be in touch with a home help, a warden, a district nurse, or an active case manager, and education about detection could usefully be targeted to these professionals. Another potential target group for education is the staff of nursing homes where depression is highly prevalent. Post-graduate training of general practitioners is another way of improving detection via the 'filter' of primary care.

Awareness of organizations that can help is also clearly important. These include CRUSE Bereavement Care (helpline@cruse.org.uk; http://www.crusebereavementcare.org.uk/; day by day helpline 0844 477 9400); the Bipolar Organisation [formerly the Manic Depressive Fellowship, http://www.mdf.org.uk/; telephone 08456 340 540 (UK only); 0044 207 793 2600 (rest of world)]; MIND (National Association for Mental Health; http://www.mind.org.uk/; telephone 0845 766 0163); the Depression Alliance (http://www.depressionalliance.org/; telephone 0845 123 23 20), as well as the local offices of Help The Aged and Age Concern.

## Secondary prevention

The optimum duration of continuation treatment is not known for certain. The standard 6 months recommended for younger patients is probably too short—Flint (1992) calculated the maximum risk period for relapse and recurrence to be 2 years. In another study relapses or recurrences were spread fairly evenly across this period (Old Age Depression Interest Group, 1993), although in other research the first months were especially vulnerable times, perhaps linked to treatment adherence. Expert guidelines (Alexopoulos *et al.*, 2001) recommend a minimum of 12 months of continuation treatment for a first episode, 24 months for a second, and at least 3 years for three or more episodes. Pragmatically treatment can be continued for 12 months and then the individual risk factors discussed with the patient. In psychotic depression antipsychotic medication should be continued for 6 months and gradually withdrawn if the patient is well. Ongoing medication following ECT has been discussed above.

Once a patient has recovered, there is good evidence that maintenance treatment with a TCA (Old Age Depression Interest Group, 1993), the SSRIs citalopram (Klysner *et al.*, 2002) and paroxetine (Reynolds *et al.*, 2006), or a combination of medication with a psychological treatment (Reynolds *et al.*, 1999c) are effective prevention strategies. However, in a recent trial Wilson *et al.* (2003) failed to show prophylactic benefits for sertraline. The exclusion of more severely depressed patients, who benefit most from antidepressants, may have been a factor here. Alternatively, it cannot be assumed that all antidepressants are equally effective in prophylaxis.

Another question concerns the dosage of antidepressant medication to use after remission. In patients with recurrent depression, those randomized to nortriptyline, with plasma concentrations maintained at effective treatment levels, had (significantly) fewer residual depressive symptoms and (non-significantly) fewer episodes of recurrence compared with patients on half this level of medication (Reynolds *et al.*, 1999). However, in the study of Wilson *et al.* (2003) sertraline was maintained at the therapeutic dose.

Medication prophylaxis is not the only means of prevention. For example, Ong *et al.* (1987) were able to demonstrate that a support group for discharged elderly depressives, run by a social worker and a community psychiatric nurse, resulted in a significant reduction in relapses and readmissions over a 1-year period. Mention has been made of the mixed findings for IPT in prevention of recurrence.

### Tertiary prevention

Diseases do not always get better. An arteriopath who comes to limb amputation would feel justifiably angry if health agencies abandoned him on the grounds that his illness had 'only' social implications. Yet this can happen to some depressed patients who do not get better.

The needs of such patients are poorly understood. Some benefit from a change to more supportive living accommodation such as residential care. What is clear is that the burden of care upon families is considerable. Troublesome symptoms include importuning and hypochondriacal complaints but also 'negative' features such as lack of interest, poverty of conversation, apathy, and withdrawal. The mental health of carers suffers under these circumstances, and at the very least health professionals should feel some commitment to them. Often professionals can help with basic explanations and with simple instructions about how to manage problematic behaviours. Supportive work with the carer to enable guilt to be addressed may also be needed. Although respite care is usually associated with dementia, there is occasionally a case for providing it for those with resistant depression, in order to allow the relative(s) a break.

In the UK the provision of health-funded hospital-based continuing care beds for patients with chronic mental illness was abandoned several decades ago. The emphasis may now be shifting back to a greater awareness of the needs of people with chronic disorders, of which depression may be one example, and of the services which could help them. The model of collaborative care using case managers, described earlier, could be a step in the right direction as it encourages collaboration between psychiatric services and primary care so that care does not become fragmented. There will be some ongoing need for longer-term nursing or residential care for the few patients who remain very disabled by chronic affective disorder and unable to function in the community.

## Conclusions

Depressive disorder is the most common mental health condition of later life. It can be difficult to diagnose because of physical co-morbidity which can mask depression and because of age-associated factors which modify its clinical presentation. It is important to rule out organic factors in aetiology, including alcohol and iatrogenic drugs, and to give as much attention to optimizing physical ill-health as to treating psychiatric symptoms. New research suggests that brain abnormalities, most likely vascular in nature, contribute to the onset of late onset depression. Treatment should be multimodal and multidisciplinary. Persistence pays—using a range of treatments the great majority of patients will recover. Keeping patients well is more of a challenge. After recovery, antidepressants should be continued for at least 12 months. Many patients who could benefit from long-term maintenance therapy do not receive it. Psychological treatments should be available to older depressed patients since they are as effective as antidepressants in mild to moderate depression. They should be considered as one of the options when planning augmentation therapy. With optimum management, the prognosis is at least as good as at any other time of adult life.

## References

Abas, M.A., Sahakian, B.J., and Levy, R. (1990). Neuropsychological deficits and CT scan changes in elderly depressives. *Psychological Medicine*, **20**, 507–520.

Anderson, I.M., Nutt, D.J., and Deakin, J.F.W. (2000). Evidence-based guidelines for treating depressive disorders with antidepressants, a revision of the 193 British Association for Psychopharmacology guidelines *Journal of Psychopharmacology*, **14**, 3020.

Abrams, R.C., Alexopoulos, G.S., and Young, R.C. (1987). Geriatric depression and DSMIIIR personality disorder criteria *Journal of American Geriatric Society*, **35**, 383–386.

Adshead, F., Day Cody, P., and Pitt, B. (1992). BASDEC, a novel screening instrument for depression in elderly medical inpatient. *British Medical Journal*, **305**, 397.

Alexopoulos, G.S., Young, R.C., and Kocsis, J.H. (1984). Dexamethasone suppression test in geriatric depression *Biological Psychiatry*, **19**, 1567–1571.

Alexopoulos, G.S., Abrams, R.C., Young, R.C, and Shamoian, C.A. (1988). Cornell Scale for depression in dementia *Biological Psychiatry*, **23**, 271–284.

Alexopoulos,G.S., Meyers, B.S., Young, R.C., Mattis, S., and Kakuma, T. (1993). The course of geriatric depression with reversible dementia, a controlled study *American Journal of Psychiatry*, **150**, 1693–1699.

Alexopoulos, G.S., Meyers, B.S., Young, R.C., Campbell, S., Silbersweig, D., and Charlson, M. (1997). 'Vascular depression' hypothesis. *Archives of General Psychiatry*, **54**, 915–922.

Alexopoulos, G.S., Meyer, B.S., Young, R.C. *et al.* (2000). Executive dysfunction and long-term outcomes of geriatric depression *Archives of General Psychiatry*, **57**, 285–290.

Alexopoulos, G.S., Katz, I.R., Reynolds, C.F., Carpenter, D., and Docherty, J.P. (2001). *The Expert Consensus Guidelines™: pharmacotherapy of depressive disorders in older patients.* A Postgraduate Medicine Special Report, October 2001. The McGraw-Hill Companies, Inc., New York.

Alexopoulos, G.S., Kiosses, D.N., Klimstra, S., Kalayam, B., and Bruce, M.L. (2002). Clinical presentation of the 'depression–executive dysfunction syndrome' of late life. *American Journal of Geriatric Psychiatry*, **10**, 98–106.

Allen, N.H.P. and Burns, A. (1995). The non-cognitive features of dementia. *Reviews in Clinical Gerontology*, **5**, 57–75.

American Psychiatric Association (APA). (1994). *Diagnostic and statistical manual version IV*. American Psychiatric Association, Washington, DC.

Arean, P.A. and Reynolds, C.F. (2005). The impact of psychosocial factors on late-life depression. *Biological Psychiatry*, **58**, 277–282.

Austin, M.-P., Ross, M., Murray, C., O'Carroll, R.E., Ebmeier, K.P., and Goodwin, G.M. (1992). Cognitive function in major depression. *Journal of Affective Disorders*, **25**, 21–30.

Averill, P.M. and Beck, J.G. (2000). Posttraumatic stress disorder in older adults, a conceptual review. *Journal of Anxiety Disorders*, **14**, 133–156.

Bains, J., Birks, J.S., and Dening, T.D. (2002). Antidepressants for treating depression in dementia. *Cochrane Database of Systematic Reviews* 2002, Issue 4, Art. No. CD003944. DOI: 10.1002/14651858.CD003944.

Baldwin, R. (1988). Delusional and non-delusional depression in late life, evidence for distinct subtypes. *British Journal of Psychiatry*, **152**, 39–44.

Baldwin, R.C. (1992). The nature, frequency and relevance of depressive delusions in the elderly. In *Psychopathology in the elderly* (ed. C.L.E Katona and R. Levy). Royal College of Psychiatrists, Gaskell Publications, London.

Baldwin, R.C. (2005). Is vascular depression a distinct sub-type of depressive disorder? A review of causal evidence. *International Journal of Geriatric Psychiatry*, **20**, 1–11.

Baldwin, R.C. and Jolley, D.J. (1986). The prognosis of depression in old age. *British Journal of Psychiatry*, **149**, 574–583.

Baldwin, R.C., Walker, S., Simpson, S.W., Jackson, A., and Burns, A. (2000). The prognostic significance of abnormalities seen on magnetic resonance imaging in late life depression, clinical outcome, mortality and progression to dementia at three years. *International Journal of Geriatric Psychiatry*, **15**, 1097–1104.

Baldwin, R., Jeffries, S., Jackson, A. *et al.* (2004). Treatment response in late-onset depression, relationship to neuropsychological, neuroradiological and vascular risk factors. *Psychological Medicine*, **34**, 125–136.

Ballard, C.G., Eastwood, C., Gahir, M., and Wilcock, G. (1996). A follow-up study of depression in the carers of dementia sufferers. *British Medical Journal*, **312**, 947.

Beats, B., Levy, R., and Forstl, H. (1991). Ventricular enlargement and caudate hyperdensity in elderly depressives. *Biological Psychiatry*, **30**(5), 452–8.

Beats, B.C., Sahakian, B.J., and Levy, R. (1996). Cognitive performance in tests sensitive to frontal lobe dysfunction in the elderly depressed. *Psychological Medicine*, **26**(3), 591–603.

Beck, A.T., Ward, C.H., Mendelson, M., Mock, J.E., and Erbaugh, J.(1961). An inventory for measuring depression *Archives of General Psychiatry*, **4**, 561–571.

Beekman, A.T., Geerlings, S.W., Deeg, D.J. *et al.* (2002). The natural history of late-life depression. A 6-year prospective study in the community. *Archives of General Psychiatry*, **59**, 605–611.

Bell-McGinty, S., Butters, M.A., Meltzer, C.C., Greer, P.J., Reynolds, C.F., and Becker, J.T. (2002). Brain morphometric abnormalities in geriatric depression, long term neurobiological effects of illness duration. *American Journal of Psychiatry*, **159**, 1424–1427.

Bench, C.J., Friston, K.J., Brown, R.G., Scott, L.C., Frackowiak, R.S.J., and Dolan, R.J. (1992). The anatomy of depression – focal abnormalities of cerebral blood flow in major depression. *Psychological Medicine*, **22**, 607–615.

van den Berg, M.D., Oldehinkel, A.J., Bouhuys, A.L., Brilman, E.I., Beekman, A.T.F., and Ormel, J. (2001). Depression in later life, three etiologically different subgroups. *Journal of Affective Disorders*, **65**, 19–26.

Bird, A.S., Macdonald, A.J.D., Mann, A.H., and Philpot, M.P. (1987). Preliminary experiences with the SelfCARE(D). *International Journal of Geriatric Psychiatry*, **2**, 31–38.

Blazer, D., Swartz, M., Woodbury, M., Manton, K., Hughes, D., and Gregory, L. (1988). Depressive symptoms and depressive diagnoses in a community population. Use of a new procedure for analysis of psychiatric classification. *Archives of General Psychiatry*, **45**, 1078–1084.

Blazer, D.G. (2003). Depression in late life, review and commentary. *Journals of Gerontology Series A: Biological Sciences and Medical Sciences*, **56A**, 249–265.

Blazer, D.G., II and Hybels, C.F. (2005). Origin of depression in later life. *Psychological Medicine*, **35**, 1241–1252.

Blazer, D., Hybels, C., and Pieper, C. (2001). The association of depression and mortality in elderly persons, a case for multiple independent pathways. *Journals of Gerontology Series A: Biological Sciences and Medical Sciences*, **56A**, M505–M509.

Bosworth, H.B., Park, K.S., McQuoid, D.R., Hays, J.C., and Steffens, D.C. (2003). The impact of religious practice and religious coping on geriatric depression. *International Journal of Geriatric Psychiatry*, **18**(10), 905–914.

Brodaty, H., Peters, K., Boyce, P. *et al.* (1991). Age and depression. *Journal of Affective Disorders*, **23**, 137–149.

Brodaty, H., Luscombe, G., Parker, G. *et al.* (1997). Increased rate of psychosis and psychomotor change in depression with age. *Psychological Medicine*, **27**, 1205–1213.

Brodaty, H., Hickie, I., Mason, C., and Prenter, L. (2000). A prospective follow-up study of ECT outcome in older depressed patients. *Journal of Affective Disorders*, **62**, 101–111.

Brodaty, H., Luscombe, G., Parker, G. *et al.* (2001). Early and late onset depression in old age, different aetiologies, same phenomenology. *Journal of Affective Disorders*, **66**(2–3), 225–236.

Brodaty, H., Luscombe, G., Anstey, K.J., Cramsie, J., Andrews, G., and Peisah, C. (2003). Neuropsychological performance and dementia in depressed patients after 25-year follow-up, a controlled study. *Psychological Medicine*, **33**(7), 1263–1275.

Brodaty, H., Cullen, B., Thompson, C. *et al.* (2005). Age and gender in the phenomenology of depression. *American Journal of Geriatric Psychiatry*, **13**, 589–596.

Brown, G.W. and Harris, T.O. (1978). *The social origins of depression*. Tavistock, London.

Brown, R., Sweeney, J., Loutsch, E., Kocsis, J., and Frances, A. (1984). Involutional melancholia revisited. *American Journal of Psychiatry*, **141**, 24–28.

Bruce, M.L., Have, T.R.T., Reynolds, C.F. *et al.* (2004). Reducing suicidal ideation and depressive symptoms in depressed older primary care patients, a randomized controlled trial. *Journal of the American Medical Association*, **291**, 1081–1091.

Burke, W.J., Houston, M.J., Boust, S.J., and Roccaforte, W.H. (1989). Use of the Geriatric Depression Scale in dementia of Alzheimer type. *Journal of American Geriatrics Society*, **37**, 856–860.

Butters, M.A., Whyte, E.M., Nebes, R.D. *et al.* (2004). The nature and determinants of neuropsychological functioning in late-life depression. *Archives of General Psychiatry*, **61**, 587–595.

Callahan, C.M., Kroenke, K., Counsell, S.R. *et al.* for the IMPACT Investigators (2005). Treatment of depression improves physical functioning in older adults. *Journal of the American Geriatrics Society*, **53**, 367–373.

Carmelli, D., Reed, T., and deCarli, C. (2002). A bivariate genetic analysis of cerebral white matter hyperintensities and cognitive performance in elderly male twins. *Neurobiology of Aging*, **23**, 413–420.

Carroll, B.J., Feinberg, M., Greden, J.F. *et al.* (1981). A specific laboratory test for the diagnosis of melancholia. *Archives of General Psychiatry*, **38**, 15–22.

Clayton, P.J. (2004). Bereavement and depression. In *Late-life depression* (ed. S.P. Roose and H.A. Sackeim), pp. 107–114. Oxford University Press, New York.

Cole, M.G. and Bellavance, F. (1997a). The prognosis of depression in old age. *American Journal of Geriatric Psychiatry*, **5**(1), 4–14.

Cole, M.G. and Bellavance, F. (1997b). Depression in elderly medical inpatients, a meta-analysis of outcomes. *Canadian Medical Association Journal*, **157**(8), 1055–1060.

Cole, M.G. and Dendukuri, N. (2003). Risk factors for elderly community subjects, a systematic review and meta-analysis. *American Journal of Psychiatry*, **160**, 1147–1156.

Cole, M.G., Bellavance, F., and Mansour, A. (1999). Prognosis of depression in elderly community and primary care populations, a systematic review and meta-analysis. *American Journal of Psychiatry*, **156**(8), 1182–1189.

Copeland, J.R.M., Dewey, M.E., Wood, N., Searle, R., Davidson, I.A., and McWilliam, C. (1987). Range of mental illness among the elderly in the community, prevalence in Liverpool using the GMS-AGECAT package. *British Journal of Psychiatry*, **150**, 815–823.

Copeland, J.R.M., Davidson, I.A., Dewey, M.E. *et al.* (1992). Alzheimer's disease, other dementias, depression and pseudodementia, prevalence, incidence and three-year outcome in Liverpool. *British Journal of Psychiatry*, **161**, 230–239.

Copeland, J.R.M., Beekman, A.T.F., Dewey, M.E. *et al.* (1999). Depression in Europe, geographical distribution among older people. *British Journal of Psychiatry*, **174**, 312–321.

Cuijpers, P.I.M. (1998). Psychological outreach programmes for the depressed elderly, a meta-analysis of effects and dropouts. *International Journal Geriatric Psychiatry*, **13**, 41–48.

Dell'Agnello, G., Cearvollo, R., Nuti, A. *et al.* (2001). SSRIs do not worsen Parkinson's disease. Evidence from an open-label prospective study. *Clinical Neuropharmacology*, **24**, 221–227.

Dhondt, T.D.F., Beekman, A.T.F., Deeg, D.J.H., and van Tilburg, W. (2002). Iatrogenic depression in the elderly Results from a community-based study in the Netherlands. *Social Psychiatry and Psychiatric Epidemiology*, **37**, 393–398.

Dodd, S., Horgan, D., Malhi, G.S., and Berk, M. (2005). To combine or not to combine? A literature review of antidepressant combination therapy. *Journal of Affective Disorders*, **89**(1–3), 1–11.

Dolan, R.J., Bench, C.J., Brown, R.G., Scott, L.C., Friston, K.J., and Frackowiak, R.S.J. (1992). Regional cerebral blood flow abnormalities in depressed patients with cognitive impairment. *Journal of Neurology, Neurosurgery and Psychiatry*, **55**, 768–773.

Emmerson, J.P., Burvill, P.W., Finlay-Jones, R., and Hall, W. (1989). Life events, life difficulties and confiding relationships in the depressed elderly. *British Journal of Psychiatry*, **155**, 787–792.

Ensrud, K.E., Blackwell, T., Mangione, C.M. *et al.* (2003) Central nervous system active medications and risk for fractures in older women; for the Study of Osteoporotic Fractures Research Group. *Archives of Internal Medicine*, **163**, 949–957.

Evans, M.E., Hammond, M., Wilson, K., Lye, M., and Copeland, J. (1997). Placebo-controlled treatment trial of depression in elderly physically ill patients. *International Journal of Geriatric Psychiatry*, **12**, 817–824.

Fabre, I., Galinowski, A., Oppenheim, C. *et al.* (2004). Antidepressant efficacy and cognitive effects of repetitive transcranial magnetic stimulation in vascular depression, an open trial. *International Journal of Geriatric Psychiatry*, **19**(9), 833–842.

Fernando, M.S., Simpson, J.E., Matthews, F. *et al.* (2006). MRC Cognitive Function and Ageing Neuropathology Study Group. White matter lesions in an unselected cohort of the elderly: molecular pathology suggests origin from chronic hypoperfusion injury. *Stroke*, **37**(6), 1391–1398.

Flint, A.J. (1992). The optimum duration of antidepressant treatment in the elderly. *International Journal of Geriatric Psychiatry*, **7**, 617–619.

Flint, A.J. and Rifat, S.L. (1996). The effect of sequential antidepressant treatment on geriatric depression. *Journal of Affective Disorders*, **36**, 95–105.

Folstein, M.F., Folstein, S.E., and McHugh, P.R. (1975). 'Mini-Mental State', a practical method for grading the cognitive state of patients for the clinician. *Journal of Psychiatric Research*, **12**, 185–198.

Foster, J.R. (1992). Use of lithium in elderly psychiatric patients, a review of the literature. *Lithium*, **3**, 77–93.

Frank, E., Prien, R.F., Jarrett, R.B. *et al.* (1991). Conceptualization and rationale for consensus definitions of terms in major depressive disorder. Remission, recovery, relapse, and recurrence. *Archives of General Psychiatry*, **48**(9), 851–855.

Gatz, M., Fiske, A., Fox, L.S. *et al.* (1998). Empirically validated psychological treatments for older adults. *Journal of Mental Health and Aging*, **4**, 9–46.

Geerlings, S.W., Beekman, A.T.F., Deeg, D.J.H., Twisk, J.W.R., and Van Tilburg, W. (2002). Duration and severity of depression predict mortality in older adults in the community. *Psychological Medicine*, **32**, 609–618.

Georgotas, A., Friedman, E., McCarthy, M. *et al.* (1983). Resistant geriatric depressions and therapeutic response to monoamine oxidase inhibitors. *Biological Psychiatry*, **18**, 195–205.

Geriatric Depression Scale. http://stanford.edu/~yesavage/GDS.html

Glassman, A.H., O'Connor, C.M., Califf, R.M. *et al.* (2002). Sertraline treatment of major depression in patients with acute MI or unstable angina. *Journal of the American Medical Association*, **288**, 701–709.

Green, B.H., Copeland, J.R.M., Dewey, M.E., Sharma, V., and Davidson, I.A. (1994). Factors associated with recovery and recurrence of depression in older people, a prospective study. *International Journal of Geriatric Psychiatry*, **9**, 789–795.

Green, R.C., Cupples, L.A., Kurz, A. *et al.* (2003). Depression as a Risk Factor for Alzheimer Disease, The MIRAGE Study. *Archives of Neurology*, **60**, 753–759.

de Groot, J.C., de Leeuw, F.-E., Oudkerk, M., Hofman, A., Jolles, J., and Breteler, M.M.B. (2000). Cerebral white matter lesions and depressive symptoms in elderly adults. *Archives of General Psychiatry*, **57**, 1071–1076.

Gurland, B.J. (1976). The comparative frequency of depression in various adult age groups. *Journal of Gerontology*, **31**(3), 283–92.

Gum, A.M., Arean, P.A., Hunkeler, E. *et al.* (2006). Depression treatment preferences in older primary care patients *Gerontologist*, **46**(1), 14–22.

Guscott, R. and Grof, P. (1991). The clinical meaning of refractory depression, a review for the clinician. *American Journal of Psychiatry*, **148**, 695–704.

Hahn, C.Y., Yang, M.S., Yang, M.J., Shih, C.H., and Lo, H.Y. (2004). Religious attendance and depressive symptoms among community dwelling elderly in Taiwan. *International Journal of Geriatric Psychiatry*, **19**(12), 1148–1154.

Hamilton, M. (1960). A rating scale for depression. *Journal of Neurology, Neurosurgery and Psychiatry*, **23**, 56–62.

Harris, D. (1975). *The myth and reality of aging in America*. The National Council on Aging Inc, Washington, DC.

Heim, C. and Nemeroff, C.B. (1999). The impact of early adverse experiences on brain systems involved in the pathophysiology of anxiety and affective disorders. *Biological Psychiatry*, **46**(11), 1509–1522.

Henderson, A.S., Grayson, D.A., Scott, R., Wilson, J., Rickwood, D., and Kay, D.W.K. (1986). Social support, dementia and depression among the elderly living in the Hobart community. *Psychological Medicine*, **16**, 379–390.

Henderson, A.S., Jorm, A.F., MacKinnon, A. *et al.* (1993). The prevalence of depressive disorders and the distribution of depressive symptoms in later-life, a survey using Draft ICD-10 and DSM-III-R. *Psychological Medicine*, **23**, 719–729.

Hickie, I., Scott, E., Wilhelm, K., Austin, M.-P., and Bennett, B. (1995). Subcortical hyperintensities on magnetic resonance imaging, clinical correlates and prognostic significance in patients with severe depression. *Biological Psychiatry*, **37**, 151–160.

Hickie, I., Scott, E., Naismith, S. *et al.* (2001). Late-onset depression, genetic, vascular and clinical contributions. *Psychological Medicine*, **31**(8), 1403–1412.

Hopkinson, G. (1964). A genetic study of affective illness in patients over 50. *British Journal of Psychiatry*, **110**, 244–254.

Husain, M.M., Rush, A.J., Sackeim, H.A. *et al.* (2005). Age-related characteristics of depression, a preliminary STAR*D report. *American Journal of Geriatric Psychiatry*, **13**, 852–860.

Jackson, R. and Baldwin, B. (1993). Detecting depression in elderly medically ill patients, the use of the Geriatric Depression Scale compared with medical and nursing observations. *Age and Ageing*, **22**, 349–353.

Jacoby, R.J. and Levy, R. (1980). Computed tomography in the elderly 3, affective disorder. *British Journal of Psychiatry*, **136**, 270–275.

Jacoby, R.J., Levy, R., and Bird, J.M. (1981). Computed tomography and the outcome of affective disorder, a follow-up study of elderly patients. *British Journal of Psychiatry*, **139**, 288–292.

Jang, Y., Kim, G., and Chiriboga, D. (2005). Acculturation and manifestation of depressive symptoms among Korean-American older adults. *Aging and Mental Health*, **9**(6), 500–507.

Jorge, R.E., Robinson, R.G., Tateno, A. *et al.* (2004). Repetitive transcranial magnetic stimulation as treatment of poststroke depression, a preliminary study. *Biological Psychiatry*, **55**, 398–405.

Judd, L.L., Akiskal, H.S., Maser, J.D. *et al.* (1998). A prospective 12-year study of subsyndromal and syndromal depressive symptoms in unipolar major depressive disorders. *Archives of General Psychiatry*, **55**, 694–700.

Kalayam, B. and Alexopoulos, G.S. (1999). Prefrontal dysfunction and treatment response in geriatric depression. *Archives of General Psychiatry*, **56**, 713–718.

Karel, M.J. and Hinrichsen, G. (2000). Treatment of depression in late life, psychotherapeutic interventions. *Clinical Psychology Review*, **20**(6), 707–729.

Karlsson, I. (1990). 5-HT reuptake inhibition in the elderly. In *Proceedings of the 17th CINP Congress* (ed. I. Yamashita, M. Toru, and A.J. Coppen), pp. 99–100. Raven Press, New York.

Kasper, S., de Swart, H., and Andersen, H.F. (2005). Escitalopram in the treatment of depressed elderly patients. *American Journal of Geriatric Psychiatry*, **13**, 884–891.

Katona, C. and Livingston, G. (2002). How well do antidepressants work in older people? A systematic review of number needed to treat. *Journal of Affective Disorders*, **69**(1–3), 47–52.

Katona, C., Peveler, R., Dowrick, C. *et al.* (2005). Pain symptoms in depression, definition and clinical significance. *Clinical Medicine*, **5**(4), 390–395.

Katz, I.R., Simpson, G.M., Curlik, S.M., Parmelee, P.A., and Muhly, C. (1990). Pharmacologic treatment of major depression for elderly patients in residential care settings. *Journal of Clinical Psychiatry*, **51**(Suppl. 4), 41–47.

Kay, D.W., Beamish, P., and Roth, M. (1964). Old age mental disorders in Newcastle-Upon-Tyne, Part I, a study of prevalence. *British Journal of Psychiatry*, **110**, 146–158.

Kindermann, S.S., Kalayam, B., Brown, G.G., Burdick, K.E., and Alexopoulos, G.S. (2000). Executive functions and P300 latency in elderly depressed patients and control subjects. *American Journal of Geriatric Psychiatry*, **8**(1), 57–65.

Kirby, D. and Ames, D. (2001). Hyponatraemia and selective serotonin re-uptake inhibitors in elderly patients. *International Journal of Geriatric Psychiatry*, **16**, 484–493.

Kivela, S.-L., Pahkala, K., and Laippala, P. (1988). Prevalence of depression in an elderly Finnish population. *Acta Psychiatrica Scandinavica*, **78**, 401–413.

Klysner, R., Bent-Hansen, J., Hansen, H.L. *et al.* (2002). Efficacy of citalopram in the prevention of recurrent depression in elderly patients, placebo-controlled study of maintenance therapy. *British Journal of Psychiatry*, **181**, 29–35.

Kobari, M., Meyer, J.S., and Ichijo, M. (1990). Leukoaraiosis, cerebral atrophy and cerebral perfusion in normal aging. *Archives of Neurology*, **47**, 161–165.

Koder, D.-A., Brodaty, H., Anstey, KJ. (1996). Cognitive therapy for depression in the elderly *International Journal of Geriatric Psychiatry* 11, 97–107.

Koenig, H.G., Meador, K.G., Cohen, H.J., and Blazer, D. (1988). Depression in elderly hospitalised patients with medical illness. *Archives of Internal Medicine*, **148**, 1929–1936.

Koenig, H.G., George, L.K., Peterson, B.L., Pieper, C.F. (1997). Depression in medically ill hospitalized older adults, prevalence, characteristics, and course of symptoms according to six diagnostic schemes. *American Journal of Psychiatry*, **154**(10), 1376–1383.

Kral, V.A. and Emery, O.B. (1989). Long-term follow-up of depressive pseudodementia of the aged. *Canadian Journal of Psychiatry*, **34**, 445–446.

Kramer-Ginsberg, E., Greenwald, B.S., Aisen, P.S., and Brod-Miller, C. (1989). Hypochondriasis in the elderly depressed. *Journal of the American Geriatric Society*, **37**, 507–510.

Krishnan, K.R., Hays, J.C., George, L.K., and Blazer, D.G. (1998). Six-month outcomes for MRI-related vascular depression. *Depression & Anxiety*, **8**(4), 142–146.

Krishnan, K.R.R., Doraiswamy, P.M., and Clary, C.M. (2001). Clinical and treatment response characteristics of late-life depression associated with vascular disease, a pooled analysis of two multicenter trials with sertraline. *Progress in Neuro-Psychopharmacology and Biological Psychiatry*, **25**, 347–361.

Krishnan, K.R.R., Delong, M., Kraemer, H. *et al.* (2002). Comorbidity of depression with other medical diseases in the elderly. *Biological Psychiatry*, **52**(6), 559–588.

Krishnan, K.R.R., Taylor, W.D., McQuiod, D.R. *et al.* (2004). Clinical characteristics of Magnetic Resonance Imaging-defined subcortical ischemic depression. *Biological Psychiatry*, **55**, 390–397.

Kumar, A., Miller, D., Ewbank, D. *et al.* (1997). Quantitative Anatomical measures and comorbid medical illness in late-life depression. *American Journal of Geriatric Psychiatry*, **5**(1), 15–25.

Kumar, A., Bilker, W., Jin, Z., and Udupa, J. (2000). Atrophy and high intensity lesions: complementary neurobiological mechanisms in late-life major depression. *Neuropsychopharmacology*, **22**, 264–274.

Licht-Strunk, E., Bremmer, M.A., van Marwijk, H.W.G. *et al.* (2004). Depression in older persons with versus without vascular disease in the open population, similar depressive symptom patterns, more disability. *Journal of Affective Disorders*, **83**(2–3), 155–160.

Lin, E.H., Katon, W., Von Korff, M. *et al.* and the IMPACT Investigators (2003). Effect of improving depression care on pain and functional outcomes among older adults with arthritis, a randomized controlled trial. *Journal of the American Medical Association*, **290**(18), 2428–2429.

Lishman, W.A. (1987). *Organic psychiatry*, 2nd edn. Blackwell, Oxford.

Liu, B., Anderson, G., Mittmann, N., To, T., Axcell, T., and Shear, N. (1998). Use of selective serotonin-reuptake inhibitors or tricyclic antidepressants and risk of hip fractures in elderly people. *Lancet*, **351**(9112), 1303–1307.

Lloyd, A.J., Ferrier, I.N., Barber, R., Gholkar, A., Young, A.H., and O'Brien, J.T. (2004). Hippocampal volume change in depression, late- and early-onset illness compared. *British Journal of Psychiatry*, **184**, 488–495.

Lotrich, F.E. and Pollock, B.G. (2005). Aging and clinical pharmacology, implications for antidepressants. *Journal of Clinical Pharmacology*, **45**, 1106–1122.

Lyketsos, C.G., DelCampo, L., Steinberg, M. *et al.* (2003). Treating depression in Alzheimer's disease, efficacy and safety of sertraline therapy, and the benefits of depression reduction, the DIADS. *Archives of General Psychiatry*, **60**(7), 737–746.

Lyness, J.M., Caine, E.D., Cox, C., King, D.A., Conwell, Y., and Olivares, T. (1998). Cerebrovascular risk factors and late-life major depression. *American Journal of Geriatric Psychiatry*, **6**, 5–13.

Lyness, J.M., Heo, M., Datto, C.J. *et al.* (2006). Outcomes of minor and subsyndromal depression among elderly patients in primary care settings. *Annals of Internal Medicine*, **144**(7), 496–504.

Manes, F., Jorge, R., Morcuende, M., Yamada, T., Paradiso, S., and Robinson, R. (2001). A controlled study of repetitive transcranial magnetic stimulation as a treatment of depression in the elderly. *International Psychogeriatrics*, **13**, 225–231.

McAllister, T.W. (1981). Cognitive functioning in the affective disorders. *Comprehensive Psychiatry*, **22**, 572–586.

McCusker, J., Cole, M., Keller, E. *et al.* (1998). Effectiveness of treatments of depression in older ambulatory patients. *Archives of Internal Medicine*, **158**, 705–712.

Mazure, C.M., Maciejewski, P.K., Jacobs, S.C., and Bruce, M.L. (2002). Stressful life events interacting with cognitive/personality styles to predict late-onset major depression. *American Journal of Geriatric Psychiatry*, **10**(3), 297–304.

Meltzer, C.C., Price, J.C., Mathis, C.A. *et al.* (2004). Serotonin 1A receptor binding and treatment response in late-life depression. *Neuropsychopharmacology*, **29**(12), 2258–2265.

Meyers, B.S., Greenberg, R., and Alexopoulos, G. (1988). Age of onset and studies of late-life depression. *International Journal of Geriatric Psychiatry*, **3**, 219–228.

Mitchell, A.J. (2006). Depressed patients and treatment adherence. *Lancet*, **367**, 2041–2043.

Mitchell, A.J. and Subramaniam, H. (2005). Prognosis of depression in old age compared to middle age, a systematic review of comparative studies. *American Journal of Psychiatry*, **162**, 1588–1601.

Moncrieff, J. and Kirsch, I. (2005). Efficacy of antidepressants in adults. *British Medical Journal*, **331**, 155–157.

Morse, J.Q. and Robins, C.J. (2005). Personality-life event congruence effects in late-life depression. *Journal of Affective Disorders*, **84**(1), 25–31.

Moser, D.J., Jorge, R.E., Manes, F., Paradiso, S., Benjamin, M.L., and Robinson, R.G. (2002). Improved executive functioning following repetitive transcranial magnetic stimulation. *Neurology*, **58**(8), 1288–1290.

Mosimann, U.P., Schmitt, W., Greenberg, B.D. *et al.* (2004). Repetitive transcranial magnetic stimulation, a putative add-on treatment for major depression in elderly patients. *Psychiatry Research*, **126**(2), 123–133.

Mottram, P.G., Wilson, K.C., Ashworth, L., and Abou-Saleh, M. (2002). The clinical profile of older patients' response to antidepressants–an open trial of sertraline. *International Journal of Geriatric Psychiatry*, **17**(6), 574–578.

Mottram, P., Wilson, K., and Strobl, J. (2006). Antidepressants for depressed elderly. *Cochrane Database of Systematic Reviews* 2006, Issue 1, Art. No. CD003491. DOI: 10.1002/14651858.CD003491.pub2.

Murphy, E. (1982). Social origins of depression in old age. *British Journal of Psychiatry*, **141**, 135–142.

Murphy, E. (1983). The prognosis of depression in old age. *British Journal of Psychiatry*, **142**, 111–119.

Murphy, G.M., Kremer, C., Rodrigues, H., Schatzberg, A.F. and the Mirtazepine Versus Paroxetine Study Group (2003). The apolipoprotein E epsilon4 allele and antidepressant efficacy in cognitively intact elderly depressed patients. *Biological Psychiatry*, **54**, 665–673.

Musetti, L., Perugi, G., Soriani, A., Rossi, V.M., Cassano, G.B., and Akiskal, H.P. (1989). Depression before and after age 65, a re-examination. *British Journal of Psychiatry*, **155**, 330–336.

Navarro, V., Gasto, C., Lomena, F., Mateos, J.J., Marcos, T., and Portella, M.J. (2002). Normalisation of frontal cerebral perfusion in remitted elderly major depression, a 12 month follow-up SPECT study. *NeuroImage*, **16**, 781–787.

Nestler, E.J. and Carlezon, W.A. (2006). The mesolimbic dopamine reward circuit in depression. *Biological Psychiatry*, **59**, 1151–1159.

National Institute for Health and Clinical Excellence (2006). *NICE clinical guideline 38: Bipolar disorder, the management of bipolar disorder in adults, children and adolescents, in primary and secondary care*. National Institute for Health and Clinical Excellence, London.

Nelson, J.C., Wohlreich, M.M., Mallinckrodt, C.H., Detke, M.J., Watkin, J.G., and Kennedy, J.S. (2005). Duloxetine for the treatment of major depressive disorder in older patients. *American Journal of Geriatric Psychiatry*, **13**(3), 227–235.

Nobler, M.S., Roose, S.P., and Probovnik, I. (2000). Regional cerebral blood flow in mood disorders, V. effects of antidepressant medication in late-life depression. *American Journal of Geriatric Psychiatry*, **8**, 289–296.

Nyth, A.L., Gottries, C.G., Lyby, K. *et al.* (1992). A multicenter clinical study of citalopram and placebo in elderly depressed patients with and without concomitant dementia. *Acta Psychiatrica Scandinavica*, **86**, 138–145.

O'Brien, J.T., Ames, D., and Schwietzer, I. (1996). White matter changes in depression and Alzheimer's disease, a review of magnetic resonance imaging findings. *International Journal of Geriatric Psychiatry*, **11**, 681–694.

O'Brien, J., Ames, D., Chiu, E., Schweitzer, I., Desmond, P., and Tress, B. (1998). Severe deep white matter lesions and outcome in elderly patients with major depressive disorder, follow up study. *British Medical Journal*, **317**, 982–984.

Olin, J.T., Schneider, L.S., Katz, I.R. *et al.* (2002). Provisional diagnostic criteria for depression of Alzheimer disease. *American Journal of Geriatric Psychiatry*, **10**(2), 125–128.

Ong, Y.-L., Martineau, F., Lloyd, C., and Robbins, I. (1987). Support group for the depressed elderly. *International Journal of Geriatric Psychiatry*, **2**, 119–123.

O'Riordan, T.G., Hayes, J.P., O'Neill, D., Shelley, R., Walsh, J.B., and Coakley, D. (1990). The effect of mild to moderate dementia on the Geriatric Depression Scale and on the General Health Questionnaire. *Age and Ageing*, **19**, 57–61.

Old Age Depression Interest Group (1993). How long should the elderly take antidepressants? A double blind placebo-controlled study of continuation/prophylaxis therapy with dothiepin. *British Journal of Psychiatry*, **162**, 175–182.

Pahkala, K. (1990). Social and environmental factors and depression in old age. *International Journal of Geriatric Psychiatry*, **5**, 99–113.

Paranthaman, R. and Baldwin, R.C. (2006). Treatments of psychiatric syndromes due to cerebrovascular disease. *International Review of Psychiatry*, **18**(5), 453–470.

Pearlson, G.D., Rabins, P.V., Kim, W.S. *et al.* (1989). Structural brain CT changes and cognitive deficits with and without reversible dementia ('pseudodementia'). *Psychological Medicine*, **19**, 573–584.

Penninx, B.E.H., Leveille, S., Ferrucci, L., van Eijk, J.T., and Guralnik, J.M. (1999). Exploring the effect of depression on physical disability. Longitudinal evidence from the established populations for epidemiologic studies of the elderly. *American Journal of Public Health*, **89**(9), 1346–1352.

Penninx, B.W., Deeg, D.J., van Eijk, J.T., Beekman, A.T., and Guralnik, J.M. (2000). Changes in depression and physical decline in older persons, a longitudinal perspective. *Journal of Affective Disorders*, **61**, 1–12.

Penninx, B.W.J.H., Kritchevsky, S.B., and Yaffe, K. (2003). Inflammatory Markers and Depressed Mood in Older Persons, results from the Health, Aging and Body Composition Study. *Biological Psychiatry*, **54**, 566–572.

Pinquart, M. and Sorensen, S. (2001). How effective are psychotherapeutic and other psychosocial interventions with older adults? A meta-analysis. *Journal of Mental Health and Aging*, **7**, 207–243.

Peterson, P. (1968). Psychiatric disorders in primary hyperparathyroidism. *Journal of Clinical Endocrinology and Metabolism*, **28**, 1491–1495.

Philpot, M.P., Banerjee, S., Needham-Bennett, H., Campos Costa, D., and Ell, P.J. (1993). $^{99m}$Tc-HMPAO single photon emission tomography in late life depression, a pilot study of regional cerebral blood flow at rest and during a verbal fluency task. *Journal of Affective Disorders*, **28**, 233–240.

Pitt, B. (1982). *Psychogeriatrics*, 2nd edn. Churchill Livingstone, Edinburgh.

Post, F. (1962). *The significance of affective symptoms in old age*, Maudsley Monographs 10. Oxford University Press, London.

Post, F. (1968). The factor of ageing in affective disorder. In *Recent developments in affective disorders*, Royal Medico-Psychological Association Publication No. 2 (ed. A. Coppen and A. Walk). Headley Bros., Ashford.

Post, F. (1972). The management and nature of depressive illnesses in late life, a follow-through study. *British Journal of Psychiatry*, **121**, 393–404.

Post, F. (1982). Functional disorders. In *The psychiatry of late life* (ed. R. Levy and F. Post), pp. 176–221. Blackwell, Oxford.

Prince, M.J., Harwood, R.H., Thomas, A., and Mann, A.H. (1998). A prospective population-based cohort study of the effects of disablement and social milieu on the onset and maintenance of late-life depression. The Gospel Oak Project VII. *Psychological Medicine*, **28**, 337–350.

Prince, M.J., Beekman, A.T.F., Deeg, D.J.H. *et al.* (1999). Depression symptoms in late life assessed using the EURO-D scale. Effect of age, gender and marital status in 14 European centers. *British Journal of Psychiatry*, **174**(4), 339–345.

Raadsheer, F.C., Joop, J., Van Heerikhuize, J.J., and Lucassen, P.J. (1995). Corticotropin-releasing hormone mRNA levels in the paraventricular nucleus of patients with Alzheimer's disease and depression. *Archives of General Psychiatry*, **152**, 1372–1376.

Radloff, L.S. (1977). The CES-D scale, a self-report depression scale for research in the general population. *Applied Psychological Measurement*, **1**, 385–401.

Rajkowska, G., Miguel-Hialgo, J.J., and Wei, J. (1999). Morphometric evidence for neuronal and glial prefrontal cell pathology in major depression. *Biological Psychiatry*, **45**, 1083–1084.

Rajkowska, G., Miguel-Hidalgo, J.J., Dubey, P., Stockmeier, C.A., and Krishnan, K.R. (2005). Prominent reduction in pyramidal neurons density in the orbitofrontal cortex of elderly depressed patients. *Biological Psychiatry*, **58**(4), 297–306.

Rasmussen, A., Lunde, M., Poulsen, D.L., Sorensen, K., Qvitzau, S., and Bech, P. (2003). A double-blind, placebo-controlled study of sertraline in the prevention of depression in stroke patients. *Psychosomatics*, **44**(3), 216–221.

Rapaport, M.H., Schneider, L.S., Dunner, D.L. *et al.* (2003). Efficacy of controlled release paroxetine in the treatment of late-life depression. *Journal of Clinical Psychiatry*, **64**, 1065–1074.

Rapp, M.A., Dahlman, K., Sano, M., Grossman, H.T., Haroutunian, V., and Gorman, J.M. (2005). Neuropsychological differences between late-onset and recurrent geriatric major depression. *American Journal of Psychiatry*, **162**, 691–698.

Reynolds, C.F., Kupfer, D.J., Houck, P.R. *et al.* (1988). Reliable discrimination of elderly depressed and demented patients by electroencephalographic sleep data. *Archives of General Psychiatry*, **45**, 258–264.

Reynolds, C.F., III, Miller, M.D., Pasternak, R.E. *et al.* (1999a). Treatment of bereavement-related major depressive episodes in later life: a controlled study of acute and continuation treatment with nortriptyline and interpersonal psychotherapy. *American Journal of Psychiatry*, **156**, 202–208.

Reynolds, C.F., III, Frank, E., Perel, J.M. *et al.* (1999b). Nortriptyline and Interpersonal Psychotherapy as maintenance therapies for recurrent major depression, a randomized controlled trial in patients older than 59 year. *Journal of the American Medical Association*, **281**, 39–45.

Reynolds, C.F., Perel, J.M., Frank, E. *et al.* (1999c). Three-year outcomes of maintenance nortriptyline treatment in late-life depression, a study of two fixed plasma levels. *American Journal of Psychiatry*, **156**, 1177–1181.

Reynolds, C.F., III, Dew, M.A., Pollock, B.G. *et al.* (2006). Maintenance Treatment of Major Depression in Old Age J. *New England Journal of Medicine*, **354**, 1130–1138.

Robbins, J., Hirsch, C., Whitmer, R., Cauley, J., and Harris, T. (2001). The association of bone mineral density and depression in an older population. *Journal of the American Geriatrics Society*, **49**(6), 732–736.

Robert, R.E., Kaplan, G.A., Shema, S.J., and Strawbridge, W.J. (1997). Does growing old increase the risk for depression? *American Journal of Psychiatry*, **154**, 1384–1390.

Romanelli, J., Fauerbach, J.A., Bush, D.E., and Ziegelstein, R.C. (2002). The significance of depression in older patients after myocardial infarction. *Journal of the American Geriatrics Society*, **50**(5), 817–822.

Roose, S.P., Glassman, A.H., Attia, E., and Woodring, S. (1994). Comparative efficacy of selective serotonin reuptake inhibitors and tricyclics in the treatment of melancholia. *American Journal of Psychiatry*, **151**, 1735–1739.

Roose, S.P., Sackeim, H.A., Krishnan, K.R. *et al.* (2004). Antidepressant pharmacotherapy in the treatment of depression in the very old, a randomized, placebo-controlled trial. *American Journal Psychiatry*, **161**, 2050–2059.

Roth, M. (1955). The natural history of mental disorder in old age. *Journal of Mental Science*, **101**, 281–301.

Roth, M., Mountjoy, C.Q., and Amrein, R. (1996). Moclobemide in elderly patients with cognitive decline and depression, an international double-blind placebo-controlled study. *British Journal of Psychiatry*, **168**, 149–157.

Royal College of Physicians and British Geriatric Society (1992). *Standardised assessment scales for elderly people*. Report of the Joint Workshops of the Research Unit of the Royal College of Physicians and the British Geriatric Society. Royal College of Physicians, London.

Sachs-Ericsson, N., Joiner, T., Plant, E.A., and Blazer, D.G. (2005). The influence of depression on cognitive decline in community-dwelling elderly persons. American Journal of Geriatric Psychiatry, 13, 402–408.

Sackeim, H.A., Prohovnik, I., Moeller, J.R. *et al.* (1990). Regional cerebral blood flow in mood disorders 1. Comparison of major depressives and normal controls at rest. *Archives of General Psychiatry*, **47**, 60–70.

Sackeim, H.A., Prudic, J., Devanand, D.P. *et al.* (2000). A prospective, randomized, double-blind comparison of bilateral and right unilateral electroconvulsive therapy at different stimulus intensities. *Archives of General Psychiatry*, **57**(5), 425–434.

Sackeim, H.A., Haskett, R.F., Mulsant, B.H. *et al.* (2001). Continuation pharmacotherapy in the prevention of relapse following electroconvulsive therapy, a randomized controlled trial. *Journal of the American Medical Association*, **285**(10), 1299–1307.

Sackeim, H.A., Roose, S.P., and Burt, T. (2005). Optimal length of antidepressant trials in late-life depression. *Journal of Clinical Psychopharmacology*, **25**(Suppl. 1), S34–S37.

Sapolsky, R., Krey, L., and McEwen, B. (1986). The neuroendocrinology of stress and aging, the glucocorticoid cascade hypothesis. *Endocrine Reviews*, **7**, 284–301.

Schatzberg, A.F. and Cantillon, M. (2000). Antidepressant early response and remission of venlafaxine and fluoxetine in geriatric outpatients. *European Neuropsychopharmacology*, **10**(Suppl.), S225–S226.

Schleifer, S.J., Keller, S.E., Bond, R.N., Cohen, J., and Stein, M. (1989). Major depressive disorder and immunity. Role of age, sex, severity, and hospitalization. *Archives of General Psychiatry*, **46**(1), 81–7.

Schneider, L.S. (1992). Psychobiologic features of geriatric affective disorders. *Clinics in Geriatric Medicine*, **8**, 253–265.

Schneider, L., Nelson, J.C., Clary, C.M. *et al.* (2003). An 8-week multicenter, parallel-group, double-blind, placebo-controlled study of sertraline in elderly outpatients with major depression. *American Journal Psychiatry*, **160**, 1277–1285.

Schulz, R., Drayer, R.A., and Rollman, B.L. (2002). Depression as a risk factor for non-suicide mortality in the elderly. *Biological Psychiatry*, **52**, 205–225.

Scogin, F. and McElreath, L. (1994). Efficacy of psychosocial treatments for geriatric depression, a quantitative review. *Journal of Consulting and Clinical Psychology*, **62**, 69–74.

Simpson, S., Baldwin, R.C., Jackson, A., and Burns, A. (1998). Is subcortical disease associated with a poor response to antidepressants? Neurological, neuropsychological and neuroradiological findings in late life depression. *Psychological Medicine*, **28**, 1015–1026.

Sjösten, N. and Kivelä, S.-L. (2006). The effects of physical exercise on depressive symptoms among the aged, a systematic review. *International Journal of Geriatric Psychiatry*, **21**, 410–418.

Snowdon, J. (1990). The prevalence of depression in old age. *International Journal of Geriatric Psychiatry*, **5**, 141–144.

Spar, J.E. and Gerner, R. (1982). Does the dexamethasone suppression test distinguish dementia from depression? *American Journal of Psychiatry*, **139**, 238–240.

Steffens, D.C., Helms, M.J., Krishnan, K.R.R., and Burke, G.L. (1999). Cerebrovascular disease and depression symptoms in the cardiovascular health study. *Stroke*, **30**, 2159–2166.

Steffens, D.C., Conway, C.R., Dombeck, C.B., Wagner, H.R., Tupler, L.A., and Weiner, R.D. (2001). Severity of subcortical gray matter hyperintensity predicts ECT response in geriatric depression. *Journal of ECT*, **17**, 45–49.

Steffens, D.C., Krishnan, K.R.R., Crump, C., and Burke, G.L. (2002). Cerebrovascular disease and evolution of depressive symptoms in the Cardiovascular Health Study. *Stroke*, **33**, 1636–1644.

Steuer, J.L. and Hammen, C.L. (1983). Cognitive-behavioral group therapy for the depressed elderly: issues and adaptations. *Cognitive Therapy and Research*, **7**, 285–296.

Tarangano, F.E., Bagnatti, P., Allegri, R.F. (2005). A double-blind, randomized clinical trial to assess the augmentation with nimodipine of antidepressant therapy in the treatment of vascular depression. *International Psychogeriatrics*, **17**, 487–498.

Tekin, S. and Cummings, J.L. (2002). Frontal-subcortical neuronal circuits and clinical neuropsychiatry, an update. *Journal of Psychosomatic Research*, **53**, 647–654.

Thomas, A.J., Ferrier, I.N., and Kalaria, R.N. (2000). Elevation in late-life depression of intercellular adhesion molecule-1 expression in the dorsolateral prefrontal cortex. *American Journal of Psychiatry*, **157**, 1682–1684.

Thomas, A.J., Ferrier, I.N., Kalaria, R.N., Perry, R.H., Brown, A., and O'Brien, J.T. (2001). A neuropathological study of vascular factors in late life depression. *Journal of Neurology, Neurosurgery and Psychiatry*, **70**, 83–87.

Thomas, A.J., O'Brien, J.T., Davis, S. *et al.* (2002). Ischemic basis for deep white matter hyperintensities in major depression, a neuropathological study. *Archives of General Psychiatry*, **59**, 785–792.

Thomas, A.J., Davis, S., Morris, C., Jackson, E., Harrison, R., and O'Brien, J.T. (2005). Increase in interleukin-1beta in late-life depression. *American Journal of Psychiatry*, **162**(1), 175–177.

Thompson, C., Syddall, H., Rodin, I., Osmond, C., and Barker, D.J.P. (2001). Birth weight and the risk of depressive disorder in late life. *British Journal of Psychiatry*, **179**, 450–455.

Trappler, B. and Cohen, C.I. (1998). Use of SSRIs in 'very old' depressed nursing home residents. *American Journal of Geriatric Psychiatry*, **6**, 83–89.

Unützer, J., Patrick, D.L., Simon, G. *et al.* (1997). Depressive symptoms and the cost of health services in HMO patients aged 65 years and older. A 4-year prospective study. *Journal of the American Medical Association*, **277**(20), 1618–1623.

Unützer, J., Katon, W., Sullivan, M., and Miranda, J. (1999). Treating depressed older adults in primary care, narrowing the gap between efficacy and effectiveness. *The Milbank Quarterly*, 77, 225–256.

Unützer, J., Katon, W., Callahan, C. *et al.* (2002). Collaborative care management of late-life depression in the primary care setting. *Journal of the American Medical Association*, **288**, 2836–2845.

Veith, R.C. and Raskind, M.A. (1988). The neurobiology of aging, does it predispose to depression? *Neurobiology of Aging*, **9**, 101–117.

van Walraven, C., Mamdani, M., and Wells, P. (2001). Inhibition of serotonin reuptake by antidepressants and upper gastrointestinal bleeding in elderly patients, retrospective cohort study. *British Medical Journal*, **323**, 655–658.

Watson, L.C. and Pigmore, M.P. (2003). Screening accuracy for late-life depression in primary care, a systematic review. *Journal of Family Practice*, **52**, 956–964.

Weingartner, H., Cohen, R.M., Murphy, D.L., Martello, J., and Gerdt, C. (1981). Cognitive processes in depression. *Archives of General Psychiatry*, **38**, 42–47.

Williams, E.I. and Wallace, P. (1993). Health checks for people aged 75 and over. *Occasional Paper (Royal College of General Practitioners)*, 59.

Williams, J.W., Barrett, J., Oxman, T. *et al.* (2000). Treatment of dysthymia and minor depression in primary care, a randomised controlled trial in older adults. *Journal of the American Medical Association*, **284**, 1519–1526.

Williams, S.A., Kasl, S.V., Heiat, A., Abramson, J.L., Krumholz, H.M., and Vaccarino, V. (2002). Depression and risk of heart failure among the elderly, a prospective community-based study. *Psychosomatic Medicine*, **64**, 6–12.

Wilson, K., Mottram, P., Sivanranthan, A., and Nightingale, A. (2001). Antidepressant versus placebo for depressed elderly. *Cochrane Database of Systematic Reviews* 2001, Issue 1, Art. No. CD000561. DOI: 10.1002/14651858.CD000561.

Wilson, K.C.M., Mottram, P.G., Ashworth, L., and Abou-Saleh, M.T. (2003). Older community residents with depression, long-term treatment with sertraline, randomised, double-blind, placebo-controlled study. *British Journal of Psychiatry*, **182**, 492–497.

World Health Organization (1993). *The ICD-10 classification of mental and behavioural disorders, research criteria*. WHO, Geneva.

Writing Committee for the ENRICHD Investigators (2003). Effects of treating depression and low perceived social support on clinical events after myocardial infarction, The Enhancing Recovery in Coronary Heart Disease Patients (ENRICHD). Randomized Trial. *Journal of the American Medical Association*, **289**, 3106–3116.

Yesavage, J.A, Brink, T.L, Rose, TL, and Lum, O. (1983). Development and validation of a geriatric depression screening scale, a preliminary report. *Journal of Psychiatric Research*, **17**, 37–49.

Yohannes, A.M., Roomi, J., Baldwin, R.C., and Connoly, M.J. (1998). Depression in elderly outpatients with disabling chronic obstructive pulmonary disease. *Age and Ageing*, **27**, 155–160.

Zung, W.W.K. (1967). Depression in the normal aged. *Psychosomatics*, **8**, 287–292.

# Mood disorders: suicide in older persons

## Daniel Harwood

A common lay view is that suicide in older people is an understandable and rational phenomenon driven by unbearable or terminal physical illness or other intractable problems. Psychiatrists, on the other hand, are sometimes prone to another form of oversimplification, over-emphasizing the role of mental disorder as the primary cause of suicide. Any clinician who has been involved in the care of a patient dying through suicide will know that most suicides are the end result of a complex interplay of biological, psychological, and interpersonal factors. And, on a population level, factors such as the stability and cohesion of society have a far greater effect on suicide rates than do medical or psychiatric disorder. Clinicians need a broad understanding of the determinants of suicidal behaviour in order to understand how these might impact on the patients they work with, and to inform the management of the suicidal patients under their care.

In older people, suicidality exists as a spectrum ranging from thoughts of hopelessness through deliberate self-harm, to completed suicide. There is a strong overlap in the characteristics of older people who have suicidal thoughts, those who harm themselves, and those who end their lives. As will become evident, the nature of the act itself is much less important in predicting suicide risk than the intent behind it.

## Suicidal thoughts

Older people probably do not think about ending their lives more than the younger population; a recent Australian survey of adults living in the community showed that suicidal thoughts were most frequent in the 25–44-year-old age band, and decreased with advancing age (De Leo *et al.*, 2005). Feelings of hopelessness are, however, common in older people; of a sample aged 65 and over in an Irish population, 15.5% said they had felt life was not worth living in the month prior to interview, although only 3.3% of this sample had felt an actual wish to die (Kirby *et al.*, 1997). The desire for death in older people is, as would be expected, strongly associated with depression (Forsell *et al.*, 1997), but also with physical disability, pain, sensory impairments, institutionalization, and single marital status (Jorm *et al.*, 1995; Forsell *et al.*, 1997). Readers will note the similarity of this group of risk factors to a list of the established risk factors for completed suicide, which will be discussed later in this chapter.

## Indirect self-destructive behaviour

Clinicians will be familiar with the occasional situation where a patient decides to refuse treatment, food, and fluids, withdraws from human contact, and 'turns and faces the wall' as a prelude to death. This is a form of so-called 'indirect self-destructive behaviour'. Indirect forms of self-harm are more common in nursing and residential care homes, particularly large, low-cost homes with high staff turnover (Osgood *et al.*, 1991). They are particularly frequent amongst women and the very old (Osgood *et al.*, 1991). Other risk factors for indirect self-harm include cognitive impairment, low religiosity, dissatisfaction with treatment, and loss events (Nelson and Farberow 1980; Draper *et al.*, 2002). The behaviours appear to be a substitute for overt suicidal acts in physically ill, dependent, or cognitively impaired people who are either not able to express their distress verbally or do not have easy access to methods of more direct self-harm.

## Deliberate self-harm

Most acts of deliberate self-harm in older people, however apparently trivial, are carried out with high suicidal intent. In a large survey from Oxford nearly three-quarters of older people's deliberate self-harm episodes were associated with high suicidal intent scores, a greater proportion than found in younger samples (Hawton and Harriss, 2006). It has been argued that every act of self-harm in an older person should be regarded as a 'failed suicide' and treated as such (Salib *et al.*, 2001). Doctors in England appear to follow this advice; a recent survey showed that older deliberate self-harm patients attending casualty departments were more likely to be admitted and to be referred for a psychiatric assessment than younger people (Marriott *et al.*, 2003).

Self-poisoning is the commonest method of self-harm in older people. In the recent Oxford survey, deliberate self-harm involved self-poisoning in 89% of cases. The three most frequent classes of drug used were minor tranquillizers, paracetamol and combination analgesics, and antidepressants (Hawton and Harriss, 2006). Minor tranquillizer and sedative overdose was particularly prevalent in women.

The absolute number of attempted suicides in the elderly is slightly higher in women, but the *rates* in the two genders are similar because there are fewer men than women in the older population. Other demographic risk factors associated with deliberate self-harm in older people include single or divorced marital status, and, possibly, low socio-economic group (Draper, 1996).

Older people attempting suicide are more likely to have a psychiatric illness than younger patients (Merrill and Owens, 1990). Over half will have a depressive disorder, with alcohol abuse in 5–32% and other psychiatric disorders in around 10%. A minority, probably less than 14%, will have no psychiatric illness (Draper, 1996). Personality factors associated with attempted suicide in the elderly have been under-researched, although it seems likely that personality disorder is much rarer than in the younger self-harm population.

In the Oxford study, the most frequent problems facing older deliberate self-harm patients at the time of the act were physical illness (46%), social isolation (36%), problems with family members (29%), and problems in the relationship with a partner (26%) (Hawton and Harriss, 2006). In this study problems related to bereavement were only reported by 17% of the sample, but in a review of earlier studies, grief, especially after spousal bereavement, was noted to be consistently associated with self-harm in the elderly (Draper, 1996). It must be noted that much of the research in this area has not used standardized assessments of life problems, so these findings must be interpreted with caution. However, the life problems so far found to be associated with deliberate self-harm in older people resemble those linked to completed suicide and suicidal thinking, consistent with the idea of a continuum of suicidality in older people.

An act of self-harm in an older person is a predictor of further self-harm and completed suicide. A British study found the rate of repetition of self-harm in a cohort of older deliberate self-harm patients to be 5.4% annually, lower than for younger age groups. However, the rate of completed suicide (around 6% during the 2–5-year follow-up period) was higher than for younger deliberate self-harm patients (Hepple and Quinton, 1997). In a longer-term follow-up study, the risk of suicide was found to be greatest in the first 5 years after the index attempt (Hawton and Harriss, 2006). Factors predicting suicide following deliberate self-harm in older people were male gender, a psychiatric history prior to the index attempt, persistent depression being treated by a psychiatric team, and, probably, high suicidal intent at the time of the initial episode (Hepple and Quinton, 1997; Hawton and Harriss, 2006). A history of previous deliberate self-harm at the time of the index attempt was a key independent risk factor for eventual suicide in the more recent study. Clinicians need to make a concerted effort to obtain a history of previous suicide attempts when assessing risk in older deliberate self-harm patients.

## Epidemiology of suicide

According to World Health Organization (WHO) data, suicide rates remain highest in older people in most countries submitting data to the organization (World Health Organization, 2002). However, in England and Wales, as in many other industrialized countries, the suicide rate in older people has steadily fallen between 1979 and 1999, in tandem with a rise in suicide rates in younger people, especially men, over the same time period (Gunnell et al., 2003; Pritchard and Hansen, 2005). The suicide rate in very old men (those over 85), however, has either remained static or increased over this period (Pritchard, 1996; Kelly and Bunting, 1998).

A British study has found that the decline in suicide rates in older people was temporally associated with an increase in the gross domestic product, the size of the female workforce, and the increased prescription of antidepressants (Gunnell et al. 2003).

Suicide rates show dramatic international variations. Rates in older people are very high in China, Lithuania, and other central and eastern European countries, high in the USA, Canada, and Australia, intermediate in western Europe, with low rates in Greece, Italy, Portugal, and Spain (Cantor, 2000; World Health Organization, 2002). These variations are due to a variety of factors. Countries undergoing social upheaval (such as China and central and eastern Europe) tend to experience high suicide rates, and countries where there is easy access to lethal methods of self-harm (guns in the USA and agricultural chemicals in rural China and India) may have an elevated suicide rate.

Suicide rates are prone to period effects. The Second World War, the changeover from toxic coal gas to safer North Sea gas (Murphy et al., 1986), and restrictions on barbiturate prescribing (Nowers and Irish, 1988) caused reductions in the suicide rate in older people in the UK. Cohort effects are more difficult to identify. Lindesay (1991), noted that suicide rates tend to be higher in age groups constituting larger proportions of the population, and predicted a rise in suicide rate as the 'baby boom generation' ages.

In most countries male suicides outnumber female in older age groups. In the USA, older male suicides outnumber female by 4:1 (Bharucha and Satlin 1997), in the UK the ratio is nearer 3:1 (Harwood et al., 2000; Hoxey and Shah, 2000). Rural China is an exception, with a notably high rate of suicide in older women (Pritchard and Baldwin, 2002; World Health Organization, 2002). Marriage is a protective factor against suicide, with rates higher in divorced and single older people (Smith et al., 1988; Harwood et al., 2000;). Widowers are at much greater risk of suicide than widows (Li, 1995). Suicide rates in older immigrants to the UK are influenced by their country of origin (Raleigh and Balarajan, 1992), and in the USA rates are higher in older Whites than non-Whites (Moscicki, 1995).

## Method of suicide

In general, elderly men adopt more violent methods than women, which may partly account for the sex difference in rates. Shooting is the commonest method in the USA (Kaplan et al., 1996, 1997). In a UK sample of older suicides, the two commonest modes of death were drug overdose (more common in women) accounting for 36% of deaths, and hanging (more common in men) causing 26% of deaths (Harwood et al., 2000). Paracetamol, combination analgesics, and antidepressants were the three most frequent drug classes implicated in overdose.

As already noted, pre-meditation and a high degree of suicidal intent are key features of suicidal acts in older people. In a recent study of older people dying through suicide in the UK, extensive planning prior to the act had taken place in 22%, with evidence of some degree of planning in a further 59%. Forty-two per cent of the sample had written a suicide note (Harwood et al., 2000). More than a third of this sample had a history of a suicide attempt preceding the final act (Harwood et al., 2000).

Suicide pacts are rare, accounting for only 0.6% of suicides in England and Wales, but half these pacts involve people over 65, usually married couples of higher social class (Brown and Barraclough, 1997).

# Clinical contact preceding suicide

About 50% of older suicide victims contact their general practitioner (GP) in the month before death (Harwood *et al.*, 2000), a higher rate than for younger people (Pirkis and Burgess, 1998). However, in one study, over half of these final consultations were for physical symptoms (Harwood *et al.*, 2000), so GPs might have difficulty identifying those older people at high imminent risk of suicide unless they perform an assessment of mental state and suicidal ideation.

Only around one-quarter of older people dying through suicide had had contact with a psychiatric team in the year before death in the study noted above (Harwood *et al.*, 2000). Again, this rate was much lower than for younger people dying through suicide (Pirkis and Burgess, 1998).

# Risk factors for suicide

## Neurobiology

The study of the neurobiology of suicide in older people is fraught with methodological problems (Conwell *et al.*, 1995). The most consistent research findings in the biology of suicidal behaviour in general are the associations with underactivity of the serotonin system and low serum cholesterol (Träskman-Bendz and Mann, 2000). One study on a specifically older sample showed lower concentrations of cerebrospinal fluid 5-hydroxyindoleacetic acid (5-HIAA) and homovanillic acid (HVA) in suicidal depressed patients than in depressed patients without suicidal ideation and a non-depressed control group (Jones *et al.*, 1990).

## Psychiatric disorder

A series of psychological autopsy studies from the USA, Scandinavia, and the UK has found that over 70% of older people who die through suicide are suffering from a psychiatric illness at the time of death (Conwell *et al.*, 1996; Harwood *et al.*, 2001; Waern *et al.*, 2002a). Depression is the commonest disorder, occurring in over half the suicides in older people in nearly all the published studies. Case–control studies using both deceased and living control groups have confirmed depressive disorder as a major risk factor for suicide in older people (Beautrais, 2002; Conwell *et al.*, 2000; Harwood *et al.*, 2001; Waern *et al.*, 2002a). Depression is more frequently associated with suicide in older people than in younger age groups (Conwell *et al.*, 1996). Clinicians would like to know the specific characteristics of depression predicting particularly high suicide risk, but unfortunately research findings are not conclusive. Persistent feelings of hopelessness (Dennis *et al.*, 2005), a long duration of depressive symptoms (Modestin, 1989), and poor self-reported sleep quality (Turvey *et al.*, 2002) are probably risk factors for suicide in depressed older people.

Rates of alcohol misuse in older suicide victims are higher in the USA than Britain where studies show rates of 10% or lower (Barraclough, 1971; Harwood *et al.*, 2001). Schizophrenia is an important risk factor for suicide in younger people but is found in less than 10% of older suicides (Harwood *et al.*, 2001). The role of neurotic and stress-related disorders in suicide in older people remains unclear. Most studies have reported rates of less than 10% (Conwell *et al.* 1996, 2000; Harwood *et al.* 2001) but a recent Scandinavian study found that 15% of the sample had an 'anxiety disorder' (Waern *et al.*, 2002a). The rates of dementia found in psychological autopsy studies of older suicide victims are similar to the general population rates of these disorders (Harwood *et al.*, 2001). However, this finding may mask a possible increased risk of suicide in *early* dementia, particularly if depressive symptoms are also present (Rohde *et al.*, 1995; Draper *et al.*, 1998). An interesting preliminary post-mortem study showed Alzheimer's disease pathology to be over-represented in older patients who had died through suicide compared with an age-matched control group dying through natural causes (Rubio *et al.*, 2001).

## Personality

Whilst it is clear that personality plays a key role in determining a person's suicide risk in the context of life stresses (Williams and Pollock, 2000) few studies have looked at this area in older samples. Around 15% of suicides in people aged 60 years and over are associated with a diagnosis of personality disorder (Henriksson *et al.*, 1995; Harwood *et al.*, 2001), lower rates than those found in samples of younger suicide victims. However, an additional 28% may have significant accentuation of personality traits, most notably anankastic and anxious traits. These two personality traits were found to be predictors of suicide in a case–control analysis (Harwood *et al.*, 2001); a finding consistent with US research showing a link between suicide in old age and low 'openness to experience' (methodical, rigid, and emotionally restricted traits) (Duberstein *et al.*, 1994).

## Physical illness

Physical health problems are the commonest type of life problem associated with suicide in older people. In a recent UK psychological autopsy study (Harwood *et al.*, 2006a), problems related to physical illness were felt to have contributed to the person's decision to die in 62% of the sample. In a Scandinavian case–control study serious illness affecting any organ category was found to be a predictor of suicide, with a stronger association in men (Waern *et al.*, 2002b). Visual impairment (Waern *et al.*, 2002b) and pain (Harwood *et al.*, 2006a) are two specific symptoms closely linked to suicide risk. In the latter study, pain was a factor influencing the decision to die in 24% of the sample. Physical dependence resulting from illness was found to be predictor of suicide in older people in a controlled study from the USA (Conwell *et al.*, 2000).

Studies on the suicide risk for specific disorders are often difficult to interpret due to methodological problems. There is reasonable evidence for a modest increased risk of suicide in patients with cancer (Harris and Barraclough, 1994; Waern *et al.*, 2002b). The high risk of suicide in neurological disorders, especially multiple sclerosis and epilepsy, is well established (Harris and Barraclough, 1994; Waern *et al.*, 2002b), and a Danish study showed a higher risk in patients, especially younger people, who had suffered a stroke (Stenager *et al.*, 1998). The suicide risk associated with the other common disorders of old age is less clear, although older people on medication for cardiac failure, chronic pulmonary disease, and urinary problems may have an increased risk of suicide, particularly those on multiple treatments (Juurlink *et al.*, 2004).

Depression is of course closely linked to physical illness and accounts for some, but not all, the risk of suicide associated with physical disorders (Waern *et al.*, 2002b).

## Social factors and life problems

A limited social network may increase the risk of an older person dying through suicide (Beautrais 2002), and, more specifically, the lack of a confidant may confer a particular risk (Turvey *et al.*, 2002). In a UK case–control study problems related to accommodation, often linked to worries regarding a move to more supported residential setting, was found to predict membership of the suicide group (Harwood *et al.*, 2006a). A case–control study from the USA has confirmed the importance of poor social integration as a contributory factor to suicide in people over 50 years old. The link between indicators of poor social integration (such as limited contact with family or low level of social interaction) and suicide was found to be robust and largely independent of the presence of psychiatric disorder (Duberstein *et al.*, 2004).

Interpersonal problems are a common trigger to suicide in all age groups, and were present in around half of a sample of older people dying through suicide in the UK (Harwood *et al.*, 2006a). Bereavement, although frequent in an older population, appears to be no more common as a precipitant to suicide in older compared with younger adults (Heikkinen and Lönnqvist, 1995). However, unresolved problems relating to bereavement more than a year before death emerged as a risk factor for suicide in a recent UK case–control study (Harwood *et al.*, 2006a). This study also showed that problems adjusting to retirement, and financial difficulties, were associated with suicide, particularly in the 'younger' age groups.

## Rational suicide, physician-assisted suicide, and euthanasia

Around 20% of suicides in older people are not associated with psychiatric disorder, and undoubtedly some of these are rational acts in response to insoluble life problems. A recent UK study described a sample of older people who had died through suicide and did not have a psychiatric disorder (Harwood *et al.*, 2006b). Most did not have significant physical illness, but around half the sample had abnormal personality traits. It is possible, therefore, that cognitive distortions may have contributed to their decision to die, rather than the decision being a entirely 'rational' response to life problems.

The lenient attitudes to suicide and towards euthanasia and physician-assisted suicide in The Netherlands, and, more recently, Belgium, have stimulated a debate on end-of-life issues. Pritchard (1995) argues that older people may feel a pressure to opt for death as a preferable alternative to being a burden on relatives or society. The majority of people dying as a result of euthanasia or physician-assisted suicide in The Netherlands have significant physical illness, and a recent study showed that most physicians in that country would refuse a request for euthanasia in the absence of severe disease (Rurup *et al.*, 2005). However, in Belgium, the current law allows mental suffering from a somatic *or mental* disorder to be a valid basis for euthanasia. Naudts *et al.* (2006) discuss the ethical issues for psychiatrists working in this climate.

All older patients expressing a wish to die, whether or not their wish appears 'rational', should receive an assessment for the presence of depression, and effective treatment if depression is present. The next step is the identification and assertive management of other problems which may be contributing to suicidal thinking, many of which, such as pain, social isolation, and interpersonal problems, are potentially remediable. Suicidal thinking should be seen as a symptom of distress due to problems which a patient may need help with.

## Suicide prevention

The recent National Suicide Prevention Strategy for England (Department of Health, 2002) lists specific actions in six areas of suicide prevention: availability and lethality of suicide methods, targeting of high-risk groups, promotion of well-being in the population, improvement in the media reporting of suicidal behaviour, promotion of research, and monitoring of progress in reducing suicide rates. These general measures are applicable to patients of all ages, but there are some interventions which may have more specific relevance to the older population. These will now be discussed.

The greatest potential for reducing suicide rates lies in limiting the availability of methods of suicide (Lewis *et al.*, 1997). In the USA, where most suicides in older people are inflicted by gunshot (Kaplan *et al.*, 1996, 1997), the obvious measure to reduce rates would be gun control. In most European countries where drug overdose is the commonest method of suicide in older people, limiting the use of drugs frequently implicated in acts of self-harm is more appropriate. Combination analgesics should be avoided in the elderly because of their limited effectiveness (Po and Zhang, 1997) and high lethality in overdose. The use of minor tranquillizers should be avoided other than for short-term use. Pain, anxiety, and insomnia are common symptoms of depression in older people. Doctors should be encouraged to identify and treat depression with an antidepressant or appropriate psychological treatment rather than pursuing the ineffective and potentially dangerous strategy of trying to treat symptoms of depression with tranquillizers or painkillers. Deaths through antidepressant overdose could be reduced by exercising caution in the prescription of cardiotoxic antidepressants with a high 'fatal toxicity index' (notably amitriptyline and dosulepin) (Henry *et al.*, 1995), particularly if the patient does not have a relative or carer who can ensure safe adherence to the medication.

Another approach to suicide prevention is the targeting of high-risk groups. One such group of older people are the socially isolated. An Italian study demonstrated that a service involving an alarm system to access help and regular telephone support seemed to reduce the suicide rate in a population of socially isolated elderly people (De Leo *et al.*, 1995). This intriguing study merits replication in other countries.

Older patients with depression are another group at higher risk of suicide. In order to treat depression it must first be identified. In a group of older suicide victims who had visited their family physician in the month before death, the doctor had identified psychiatric symptoms in most cases, but less than half of those with a psychiatric disorder were offered treatment (Caine *et al.*, 1996). A British primary care study showed that GPs diagnosed depression in only half of depressed older patients, and only 38% of those who were diagnosed as depressed received any treatment (Crawford *et al.*, 1998). Clearly, there remains scope for the education of GPs, and clinicians from other specialities, in the detection and treatment of depression in the elderly, especially in those with co-morbid medical conditions. The current changes in UK undergraduate and post-graduate medical training and education might allow psychiatric teachers to ensure that these areas receive priority on the new curricula.

The third group of high-risk patients who could be targeted in suicide prevention are those under the care of psychiatric services, especially older deliberate self-harm patients. All older deliberate self-harm patients should receive a thorough psychiatric assessment in view of the high suicidal intent often associated with this behaviour (see above). Multidisciplinary audit of cases of suicide under the care of a psychiatric team can usefully highlight deficits in local services. In the UK the National Confidential Inquiry, an ambitious national audit of suicides occurring among people under psychiatric care, has published a series of reports on suicide prevention in this patient group. The latest report contains a comprehensive list of recommendations, which include an overhaul of the Care Programme Approach, better training in risk assessment for all mental health workers, changes to the structure of some inpatient units, and more effective information exchange (Appleby *et al.*, 2001).

## Risk assessment

Using established risk factors in a standardized risk assessment schedule to assess suicide risk in an individual tends to produce many false-positive predictions due to the high prevalence of many of the risk factors but the relatively low rate of suicide. Risk assessment in clinical practice should adopt a more individualized approach with an interview covering the two most important risk factors for suicide in any age group—current suicidal intent and details of past suicide attempts. Protective factors must also be established; it is vital to ascertain what has prevented a suicidal patient from ending their life so far. The loss of a previously identified protective factor may signify a sudden escalation of risk. The established risk factors for suicide as discussed in this chapter also need to be covered, but more important than constructing a list of risk factors is establishing the meaning of the patient's current life experiences to that person at that point in time.

There is no substitute for a thorough psychiatric history and mental state examination as the basis for assessing suicide risk, despite the current vogue for poorly validated risk assessment schedules. As one experienced clinician and academic puts it 'perhaps our most appropriate approach should be to refine and evaluate our basic clinical skills. Suicide rates might well then look after themselves' (Morgan, 1997).

## References

Appleby, L., Shaw, J., Sherratt, J. *et al.* (2001). *Safety first: report of the National Confidential Inquiry into suicide and homicide by people with a mental illness*. Stationery Office, London.

Barraclough, B.M. (1971). Suicide in the elderly. *British Journal of Psychiatry* (special supplement 6), 87–97.

Beautrais, A.L. (2002). A case-control study of suicide and attempted suicide in older people. *Suicide and Life-threatening Behavior*, **32**, 1–9.

Bharucha, A.J. and Satlin, A. (1997). Late-life suicide: a review. *Harvard Review of Psychiatry*, **5**, 55–65.

Brown, M. and Barraclough, B. (1997). Epidemiology of suicide pacts in England and Wales, 1988–1992. *British Medical Journal*, **315**, 286–287.

Caine, E.D., Lyness, J.M., and Conwell, Y. (1996). Diagnosis of late-life depression: preliminary studies in primary care settings. *American Journal of Geriatric Psychiatry*, **4** (Suppl. 1), 545–550.

Cantor, C.H. (2000). Suicide in the Western world. In *International handbook of suicide and attempted suicide* (ed. K. Hawton and K. van Heeringen), pp. 9–28. John Wiley and Sons, Chichester.

Conwell, Y., Raby, W.N., and Caine, E.D. (1995). Suicide and aging II: the psychobiological interface. *International Psychogeriatrics*, **7**, 165–181.

Conwell, Y., Duberstein, P.R., Cox, C., Herrmann, J.H., Forbes, N.T., and Caine, E.D. (1996). Relationships of age and axis I diagnoses in victims of completed suicide: a psychological autopsy study. *American Journal of Psychiatry*, **153**, 1001–1008.

Conwell, Y., Lyness, J.M., Duberstein, P. *et al.* (2000). Completed suicide among older patients in primary care practices: a controlled study. *Journal of the American Geriatrics Society*, **48**, 23–29.

Crawford, M.J., Prince, M., Menezes, P., and Mann, A.H. (1998). The recognition and treatment of depression in older people in primary care. *International Journal of Geriatric Psychiatry*, **13**, 172–176.

De Leo, D., Carollo, G., and Dello Buono, M. (1995). Lower suicide rates associated with a Tele-Help/Tele-Check service for the elderly at home. *American Journal of Psychiatry*, **152**, 632–634.

De Leo, D., Cerin, E., Spathonis, K. *et al.* (2005). Lifetime risk of suicide ideation and attempts in an Australian community: prevalence, suicidal process, and help-seeking behaviour. *Journal of Affective Disorders*, **86**, 215–224.

Dennis, M., Wakefield, P., Molloy, C., Andrews, H., and Friedman, T. (2005). Self-harm in older people with depression: comparison of social factors, life events, and symptoms. *British Journal of Psychiatry*, **186**, 538–539.

Department of Health (2002). *National suicide prevention strategy for England*. Department of Health, London.

Draper, B. (1996). Attempted suicide in old age. *International Journal of Geriatric Psychiatry*, **11**, 577–587.

Draper, B., MacCuspie-Moore, C., and Brodaty, H. (1998). Suicidal ideation and the 'wish to die' in dementia patients: the role of depression. *Age and Ageing*, **27**, 503–507.

Draper, B., Brodaty, H., Low, L.F., Richards, V., Paton, H., and Lie, D. (2002). Self-destructive behaviors in nursing home residents. *Journal of the American Geriatrics Society*, **50**, 354–358.

Duberstein, P.R., Conwell, Y., and Caine, E.D. (1994). Age differences in the personality characteristics of suicide completers: preliminary findings from a psychological autopsy study. *Psychiatry*, **57**, 213–224.

Duberstein, P.R., Conwell, Y., Conner, K.R., Eberly, S., Evinger, J.S., and Caine, E.D. (2004). Poor social integration and suicide: fact or artifact? A case-control study. *Psychological Medicine*, **34**, 1331–1337.

Forsell, Y., Jorm, A.F., and Winblad, B. (1997). Suicidal thoughts and associated factors in an elderly population. *Acta Psychiatrica Scandinavica*, **95**, 108–111.

Gunnell, D., Middleton, N., Whitley, E., Dorling, D., and Frankel, S. (2003). Why are suicide rates rising in young men but falling in the elderly? – a time-series analysis of trends in England and Wales 1950–1998. *Social Science and Medicine*, **57**, 595–611.

Harris, E.C. and Barraclough, B.M. (1994). Suicide as an outcome for medical disorders. *Medicine*, **73**, 281–296.

Harwood, D.M.J., Hawton, K., Hope, T., and Jacoby, R. (2000). Suicide in older people: mode of death, demographic factors, and medical contact before death. *International Journal of Geriatric Psychiatry*, **15**, 736–743.

Harwood, D.M.J., Hawton, K., Hope, T., and Jacoby, R. (2001). Psychiatric disorder and personality factors associated with suicide in older people: a descriptive and case-control study. *International Journal of Geriatric Psychiatry*, **16**, 155–165.

Harwood, D.M.J., Hawton, K., Hope, T., Harriss, L., and Jacoby, R. (2006a). Life problems and physical illness as risk factors for suicide in older people: a descriptive and case-control study. *Psychological Medicine*, **36**, 1265–1274.

Harwood, D.M.J., Hawton, K., Hope, T., and Jacoby, R. (2006b). Suicide in older people without psychiatric disorder. *International Journal of Geriatric Psychiatry*, **21**, 363–367.

Hawton, K. and Harriss, L. (2006). Deliberate self-harm in people aged 60 years and over: characteristics and outcome of a 20-year cohort. *International Journal of Geriatric Psychiatry*, **21**, 572–581.

Heikkinen, M.E. and Lönnqvist, J.K. (1995). Recent life events in elderly suicide: a nationwide study in Finland. *International Psychogeriatrics*, **7**, 287–300.

Henriksson, M.M., Marttunen, M.J., Isometsä, E.T. *et al.* (1995). Mental disorders in elderly suicide. *International Psychogeriatrics*, **7**, 275–286.

Henry, J.A., Alexander, C.A., and Sener, E.K. (1995). Relative mortality from overdoses of antidepressants. *British Medical Journal*, **310**, 221–224.

Hepple, J. and Quinton, C. (1997). One hundred cases of attempted suicide in the elderly. *British Journal of Psychiatry*, **171**, 42–46.

Hoxey, K. and Shah, A. (2000). Recent trends in elderly suicide rates in England and Wales. *International Journal of Geriatric Psychiatry*, **15**, 274–279.

Jones, J.S., Stanley, B., Mann, J.J. *et al.* (1990). CSF 5-HIAA and HVA concentrations in elderly depressed patients who attempted suicide. *American Journal of Psychiatry*, **147**, 1225–1227.

Jorm, A.F., Henderson, A.S., Scott, R., Korten, A.E., Christensen, H., and Mackinnon, A.J. (1995). Factors associated with the wish to die in elderly people. *Age and Ageing*, **24**, 389–392.

Juurlink, D.N., Herrmann, N., Szalai, J.P., Kopp, A., and Redelmeier, D.A. (2004). Medical illness and the risk of suicide in the elderly. *Archives of Internal Medicine*, **164**, 1179–1184.

Kaplan, M.S., Adamek, M.E., and Geling, O. (1996). Sociodemographic predictors of firearm suicide among older white males. *Gerontologist*, **36**, 530–533.

Kaplan, M.S., Adamek, M.E., Geling, O., and Calderon, A. (1997). Firearm suicide among older women in the US. *Social Science and Medicine*, **44**, 1427–1430.

Kelly, S. and Bunting, J. (1998). Trends in suicide in England and Wales, 1982–1996. *Population Trends*, **92**, 29–41.

Kirby, M., Bruce, I., Radic, A., Coakley, D., and Lawlor, B.A. (1997). Hopelessness and suicidal feelings among the community dwelling elderly in Dublin. *Irish Journal of Psychological Medicine*, **14**, 124–127.

Lewis, G., Hawton, K., and Jones, P. (1997). Strategies for preventing suicide. *British Journal of Psychiatry*, **171**, 351–354.

Li, G. (1995). The interaction effect of bereavement and sex on the risk of suicide in the elderly: an historical cohort study. *Social Science and Medicine*, **40**, 825–828.

Lindesay, J. (1991). Suicide in the elderly. *International Journal of Geriatric Psychiatry*, **6**, 355–361.

Marriott, R., Horrocks, J., House, A., and Owens, D. (2003). Assessment and management of self-harm in older adults attending accident and emergency: a comparative cross-sectional study. *International Journal of Geriatric Psychiatry*, **18**, 645–652.

Merrill, J. and Owens, J. (1990). Age and attempted suicide. *Acta Psychiatrica Scandinavica*, **82**, 385–388.

Modestin, J. (1989). Completed suicide in psychogeriatric inpatients. *International Journal of Geriatric Psychiatry*, **4**, 209–214.

Morgan, H.G. (1997). Management of suicide risk. *Psychiatric Bulletin*, **21**, 214–216.

Mościcki, E.K. (1995). Epidemiology of suicide. *International Psychogeriatrics*, **7**, 137–148.

Murphy, E., Lindesay, J., and Grundy, E. (1986). 60 years of suicide in England and Wales: a cohort study. *Archives of General Psychiatry*, **43**, 969–976.

Naudts, K., Ducatelle, C., Kovacs, J., Laurens, K., van den Eynde, F., and van Heeringen, C. (2006). Euthanasia: the role of the psychiatrist. *British Journal of Psychiatry*, **188**, 405–409.

Nelson, F.L. and Farberow, N.L. (1980). Indirect self-destructive behavior in the elderly nursing home patient. *Journal of Gerontology*, **35**, 949–957.

Nowers, M. and Irish, M. (1988). Trends in the reported rates of suicide by self-poisoning in the elderly. *Journal of the Royal College of General Practitioners*, **38**, 67–69.

Osgood, N.J., Brant, B.A., and Lipman, A. (1991). *Suicide among the elderly in long-term care facilities.* Greenwood Press, New York.

Pirkis, J. and Burgess, B. (1998). Suicide and recency of health care contacts: a systematic review. *British Journal of Psychiatry*, **173**, 462–474.

Po, A.L.W. and Zhang, W.Y. (1997). Systematic overview of co-proxamol to assess analgesic effects of addition of dextropropoxyphene to paracetamol. *British Medical Journal*, **315**, 1565–1571.

Pritchard, C. (1995). *Suicide – the ultimate rejection.* Open University Press, Buckingham.

Pritchard, C. (1996). New patterns of suicide by age and gender in the United Kingdom and the Western World 1974–1992; an indicator of social change? *Social Psychiatry and Psychiatric Epidemiology*, **31**, 227–234.

Pritchard, C. and Baldwin, D.S. (2002). Elderly suicide rates in Asian and English-speaking countries. *Acta Psychiatrica Scandinavica*, **105**, 271–275.

Pritchard, C. and Hansen, L. (2005). Comparison of suicide in people aged 65–74 and 75+ by gender in England and Wales and the major Western countries 1979–1999. *International Journal of Geriatric Psychiatry*, **20**, 17–25.

Raleigh, V.S. and Balarajan, R. (1992). Suicide levels and trends among immigrants in England and Wales. *Health Trends*, **24**, 91–94.

Rohde, K., Peskind, E.R., and Raskind, M.A. (1995). Suicide in two patients with Alzheimer's disease. *Journal of the American Geriatrics Society*, **43**, 187–189.

Rubio, A., Vestner, A.L., Stewart, J.M., Forbes, N.T., Conwell, Y., and Cox, C. (2001). Suicide and Alzheimer's pathology in the elderly: a case-control study. *Biological Psychiatry*, **49**, 137–145.

Rurup, M.L., Muller, M.T., Onwuteaka-Philipsen, B.D., van der Heide, A., van der Wal, G., and van der Maas, P.J. (2005). Requests for euthanasia or physician-assisted suicide from older persons who do not have a severe disease: an interview study. *Psychological Medicine*, **35**, 665–671.

Salib, E., Tadros, G., and Cawley, S. (2001). Elderly suicide and attempted suicide: one syndrome. *Medical Science and Law*, **41**, 250–255.

Smith, J.C., Mercy, J.A., and Conn, J.M. (1988). Marital status and the risk of suicide. *American Journal of Public Health*, **78**, 78–80.

Stenager, E.N., Madsen, C., Stenager, E., and Boldsen, J. (1998). Suicide in stroke patients: epidemiological study. *British Medical Journal*, **316**, 1206.

Träskman-Bendz, L. and Mann, J.J. (2000). Biological aspects of suicidal behaviour. In *The international handbook of suicide and attempted suicide* (ed. K. Hawton and K. van Heeringen), pp. 65–77. John Wiley, Chichester.

Turvey, C.L., Conwell, Y., Jones, M.P. *et al.* (2002). Risk factors for late-life suicide: a prospective, community-based study. *American Journal of Geriatric Psychiatry*, **10**, 398–406.

Waern, M., Runeson, B.S., Allebeck, P. *et al.* (2002a). Mental disorder in elderly suicides: a case-control study. *American Journal of Psychiatry*, **159**, 450–455.

Waern, M., Rubenowitz, E., Runeson, B., Skoog, I., Wilhelmson, K., and Allebeck, P. (2002b). Burden of illness and suicide in elderly people: a case-control study. *British Medical Journal*, **324**, 1355–1357.

Williams, J.M.G. and Pollock, L.R. (2000). The psychology of suicidal behaviour. In *The international handbook of suicide and attempted suicide* (ed. K. Hawton and K. van Heeringen), pp. 79–93. John Wiley, Chichester.

World Health Organization (2002). *Suicide prevention (SUPRE)* (http://www.who.int/mental_health/prevention/suicide/suicideprevent/en/).

# Mood disorders: manic syndromes in old age

Kenneth I. Shulman and Nathan Herrmann

## Classification issues

The title of this chapter deliberately uses the broader and generic notion of 'syndrome' to label the heterogeneous clinical conditions under review. Mania or hypomania is fundamental to the diagnosis of bipolar disorder as conceived in DSM-IV (American Psychiatric Association, 1994). Within this context, 'bipolarity' is considered a primary mood disorder, and further refinement into bipolar I, II, or even III are shadings dependent upon the severity of manic symptomatology or the ease of their precipitation, i.e. whether spontaneous or drug induced. The available evidence suggests that the primary form of bipolarity is heavily influenced by genetic (familial) factors (Goodwin and Jamison, 1990).

Within the elderly population, however, the very high levels of co-morbidity cloud the diagnostic horizon (Shulman, 1997a). DSM-IV has established a category of 'mood disorder due to a general medical condition' (293.83) with the prescription that 'the disturbance is the direct physiologic consequence of a general medical condition'. Given the high prevalence of neurological and medical co-morbidity in old age (described below), the issue of 'direct physiologic consequence' becomes difficult indeed. The extent to which the clinician can presume a pathogenic link between mania and associated medical conditions is questionable. *A fortiori*, the assumption of an aetiological relationship is even more precarious.

Outside the formal DSM and ICD classification system lies the widely held concept of secondary mania (Krauthammer and Klerman, 1978; Brooks and Hoblyn, 2005). This concept implies that cerebral organic factors are responsible for the syndrome, an implication that is supported by the existence of a close temporal relationship between the medical or neurological condition and the manic syndrome, absence of a personal or a family history of mania, and a distinction from delirium. Interestingly, the neurological literature uses the term 'disinhibition syndrome' in a way that is virtually identical to the psychiatric notion of secondary mania and has similar implied conditions that underlie the clinical syndrome. Finally, the concept of a 'bipolar spectrum' (Akiskal, 1986) has considerable merit when applied to the elderly. Affective vulnerability (inherited or acquired) maybe expressed through temperament in adult life and in late life may interact with a variety of cerebral organic factors to produce a manic syndrome.

The high prevalence of cerebrovascular disease associated with mania led Steffens and Krishnan (1998) to propose a vascular subtype of mania similar to the subtype of vascular depression proposed by Alexopoulos *et al.* (1997). The concept of a vascular subtype of mania fits the data found in studies of elderly bipolar patients (these are discussed below). This subtype is characterized by the occurrence of a manic syndrome in the context of clinical or neuroimaging evidence for cerebrovascular disease with further evidence of neuropsychological impairment. Such clinical evidence can include stroke, transient ischaemic attack (TIA), or focal signs, while evidence from neuroimaging includes hyperintensities or silent cerebral infarctions. Impairment of cognition is most common in the area of memory or executive function. Further support for a diagnosis of the vascular subtype of mania includes late onset, a switch to mania shortly after the onset of vascular disease, negative family history, and impairment of independent activities of daily living (IADL).

Nosology remains at the heart of our understanding of disorders that have 'manic expression'. Diagnostic terms are inextricably linked to the understanding of the nature, pathogenesis, and aetiology of these syndromes. The uncertainty and fuzziness that pervades our current classification should be a stimulus for further clarification based on the best available data. Indeed, the practical question of management and prognosis will follow from our use of diagnostic terminology.

This chapter will critically review the literature on mania in late life by describing its epidemiology, pathogenesis, co-morbidity, and management. Based on the available evidence, a summary of the essential determinants of manic syndromes in old age will be presented. Following from this synthesis, a classification of subtypes is proposed as a basis for further research into the cause of these syndromes as well as their effective management. Hopefully, this approach will help to clarify the current confusion around classification and will enhance our capacity to understand these conditions.

## Epidemiology

Methodological concerns confound the data on the prevalence and incidence of mania in old age. Some of the concerns are inherent in identifying individuals with mania in the community who, similar to paranoid patients, are not readily amenable to interview or cooperation with community surveys. Compounding these problems is the diagnostic uncertainty described above.

Interestingly, there are no clinical features that are unique to old age except for the higher prevalence of cognitive dysfunction (Broadhead and Jacoby, 1990). While clinical symptoms in an elderly cohort are qualitatively similar to a mixed-age population they tend to be less severe and intense in older people.

The effect of age on hospital admission rates is opposite to the effect on community prevalence of bipolar illness. For *inpatient* psychogeriatric units relatively high 'treated prevalence' (4–8%) has been reported (Yassa *et al.*, 1988) while in a national survey, first admission rates for mania showed a modest increase in the extremes of old age (Eagles and Whalley, 1985; Spicer *et al.*, 1973). Specialized psychogeriatric units report significant numbers of elderly people with bipolar disorder, approximately 7–10 per year (Shulman and Post, 1980; Shulman *et al.*, 1992; Yassa *et al.*, 1988). In contrast, the Epidemiologic Catchment Area (ECA) study shows a negligible prevalence of mania in over 65s in *the community* (<0.1%) down from a high of 1.4% in young adults (Weissman *et al.*, 1991). Other studies of elderly cohorts also support the conclusion that there is a significant decrease in the community prevalence of mania at the extreme end of the lifespan (Tsuang, 1978; Weeke and Vaeth, 1986; Snowdon, 1991).

So, where have all the young bipolars gone? Some suggest the influence of a relatively high mortality rate from natural causes and from suicide, as well as evidence for 'burn out' of the disorder over a long-term course (Winokur, 1975; Snowdon, 1991). Given the very early age of onset of the majority of bipolar disorders (early 20s), prospective follow-up studies are not easily conducted, and the dependence on retrospective data makes this question an on-going challenge.

## Age of onset

Age of onset has been viewed as an important variable that could distinguish the subtypes of mania, and hence lead to an improved understanding of pathogenesis and aetiology (Young and Klerman, 1992; LeBoyer *et al.*, 2005). However, the cut-off used for 'late onset' has been variable (Yassa *et al.*, 1988). Wylie *et al.* (1999) have suggested that in a sample of mixed-age patients, the median age at onset could reasonably be used to set the cut-off point between 'early' and 'late' onset. In their sample of 'elderly' bipolar patients (over 60 years of age) the median age of onset was 49 years. This finding of course was influenced by the cut-off for the age considered 'elderly'. Most studies have used age 65 as the benchmark for old age, and in such samples the 'late onset' cut-off would then be likely to fall in the early to mid 50s. This was indeed the case for a study in which the mean age of elderly bipolars was 70, and the mean age of their first psychiatric hospitalization was 55 (the median age was not reported) (Shulman *et al.*, 1992). While no clear convention for 'late onset' in the elderly has been established, an age of at least 50 years would seem a reasonable marker for future use. Using a cut-off point of 49 years, Wylie *et al.* (1999) found the late onset group of elderly bipolar patients to have more psychotic features and more cerebrovascular risk factors. At the time of discharge, outcome [as measured by Brief Psychiatric Rating Scale (BPRS), Mini-Mental State Examination (MMSE), and Global Assessment] did not differ significantly between the early and late onset cases. Using a cut-off of 50 years for age at onset, Hays *et al.* (1998) also found an increase in vascular co-morbidity in their sample of elderly bipolar patients (mean age 74 years).

Late onset subjects were reported to have more psychosocial supports and also less family history of psychiatric problems; but their sample had an unusually high proportion of patients with a positive family history—83% for late onset and 88% for early onset—a difference that in fact is not significant. Previous attempts to link the age of onset with a family history of mood disorder have produced inconsistent results. Results have ranged from 24% to 88% for the presence of a positive family history (Glasser and Rabins, 1984; Stone, 1989; Broadhead and Jacoby, 1990; Snowdon, 1991; Shulman *et al.*, 1992; Hays *et al.*, 1998). The usual methodological issues arise with respect to the rigor of investigation and the criteria for a positive family history of psychiatric disorder (for example, whether only first-degree relatives are considered). Within the elderly bipolar group, there is a trend towards a higher rate of positive family history in those with an earlier age of onset (Stone, 1989; Hays *et al.*, 1998) while the converse is true for the presence of a neurological disorder: such disorder is generally associated with a very late onset of bipolar disorder (Snowdon, 1991; Shulman *et al.*, 1992; Tohen *et al.*, 1994). Even in the neurological subgroup of patients, the prevalence of a positive family history in first-degree relatives is high at 30%. Further confirmation of age 50 as the best cut-off for 'late onset' comes from a retrospective study of bipolar patients in a district inpatient service in Newcastle, UK (Moorehead and Young, 2003). The patients without a family history of psychiatric disorder were more likely to have their first admission at over 50 years of age. The authors suggest that this group may belong to a distinct aetiological subgroup.

Using a population-based data set from Denmark's nationwide registry, Kessing (2006) described a cohort of inpatients with bipolar disorder with late onset (over 50 years of age). Compared with a cohort of early onset bipolar patients, the older sample had a lower prevalence of psychotic symptoms associated with their mania, but they presented with more psychosis associated with their depression. No other significant differences between the two groups were found. This is consistent with an earlier report (Broadhead and Jacoby, 1990) showing that older bipolar (manic) patients experience less severe symptoms than younger manic patients. However, the reverse may be true for older bipolar patients who have serious depression requiring hospitalization.

A study in Finland of hospital admissions for bipolar illness reveals that almost 20% of first admissions occurred after the age of 60, with the peak admission rates being in middle age (Rasanan *et al.*, 1998). However, when the age of onset is determined by episode rather than by hospitalization, community surveys found a much earlier age of onset, at about 20 years. This is consistent with the earlier paradox reported above, in which community prevalence rates decreased while hospital prevalence rates increased with age. Community-based samples such as the ECA Study (Weissman *et al.*, 1991) and the US National Comorbidity Study (Kessler *et al.*, 1997) report the mean age of onset of bipolar disorder as 21 years. In studies of mixed-age samples of manic inpatients, the mean age of onset is higher at 30 years (Goodwin and Jamison, 1990; Tohen *et al.*, 1990). Accepting the fact of an early onset of bipolarity in the general population, it is noteworthy that very few elderly bipolar inpatients have experienced their first mania before the age of 40 (Snowdon, 1991; Shulman *et al.*, 1992). One could conclude that the early onset community-based bipolar patients burn out, or are effectively treated or die by old age; and that the late peak in first admissions for mania represent a different group—a subgroup of neurologically based manic syndromes which often require hospitalization because of their severity (psychosis) or because of the associated vascular risk factors. Further studies must carefully separate out the age of patients during the episode under study, and the age at onset of their disorder, as separate variables for analysis.

Sajatovic *et al.* (2005) studied an older bipolar group derived from a large Veterans Affairs (VA) database, the National Psychosis Registry (NPR) that includes the inpatient admissions and outpatient visits of all veterans with a diagnosis of 'psychosis' which included bipolar disorder. They defined 'earlier onset' illnesses as those occurring before the years of the initiation of the registry (1988 for inpatients and 1997 for outpatients). 'Earlier' therefore does not necessarily mean 'early onset', as exact dates of onset were not possible to determine with this database. Those whose first illness occurred during the years of the registry were considered 'new onset illness'. The authors found that overall health service use was high, including substantial general hospital (non-psychiatric) inpatient care. Patients with 'earlier onset' bipolar illness appear to use more resources than those with 'new onset' illness, suggesting a more serious disorder. However, the mean age difference between these two groups was minimal (70.0 years for 'earlier onset' versus 71.2 years for 'new onset'). Therefore, one cannot compare those groups with the early and late onset categories (defined by cut-off at age 50) used in other studies.

## Neurological co-morbidity and pathogenesis

While the neurological and psychiatric literatures have developed independently, they have resulted in a convergence of findings (Shulman, 1997b). Whether one uses the term 'disinhibition syndrome' which the neurologists prefer (Starkstein and Robinson, 1997) or 'secondary mania' (Krauthammer and Klerman, 1978), their clinical features and neurological findings are similar. Moreover, individual case reports and small case series (using either label) tend to agree in finding a predominance of heterogeneous right-hemisphere lesions (Starkstein *et al.*, 1990; Strakowski *et al.*, 1994; Verdoux and Bourgeois, 1995; Carroll *et al.*, 1996; Steffens and Krishnan, 1998). Similarly, Sackeim *et al.* (1982) noted that pathological laughing was associated with right-sided lesions while left-sided lesions tended to produce pathological crying.

Still in this vein, Pearlson (1999) has observed that 'normal mood is dependent on the integrity of the frontal, limbic, and basal ganglia circuit'. Indeed, it has been argued that this is a functional system (known as the orbitofrontal circuit) which integrates sensory input with motivational states (Zald and Kim, 1996). Evidence supporting the hypothesis that the right-sided orbitofrontal circuit mediates manic syndromes comes from a variety of sources, to be discussed below.

Disinhibition of sexuality and oral behaviour (Kluver–Bucy syndrome) have been associated with bitemporal lesions (Kling and Steklis, 1976). It is interesting therefore that a preponderance of basal temporal lesions was found in patients who developed a manic episode in the first year following head injury (Jorge *et al.*, 1993). This is consistent with the hypothesis that the inferior surface of the skull is more likely to be damaged in injuries (Starkstein and Robinson, 1997). Furthermore, patients with frontotemporal dementias distinct from Alzheimer's disease are more likely to manifest disinhibition (Neary *et al.*, 1988). Indeed in those cases of

dementia with disinhibition, the decrease in metabolic activity was greater in the orbitofrontal circuit than in parietal areas (Kumar *et al.*, 1990; Starkstein *et al.*, 1994). Thus, in an elegant synthesis of the available data, Starkstein and Robinson (1997) have suggested that disinhibition syndromes in secondary mania are produced by lesions disrupting connections within the orbitofrontal circuit. The frontal lobes modulate motivational and psychomotor behaviour; limbic connections modulate emotions; while the biogenic amine nuclei in the hypothalamus, amygdala, and brainstem modulate instinctive behaviours.

In a recent comprehensive review of published case reports involving focal unilateral cortical lesions, the trend towards right-sided lesions for mania and pseudomania was confirmed (Braun *et al.*, 1999).

In studies of mania specifically in old age, the association with a variety of neurological disorders was high (36%) compared with age- and sex-matched depressives (8%) (Shulman *et al.*, 1992). Within the manic group, patients whose first affective episode was mania were even more likely to present with coarse neurological abnormalities (71%) than were patients with a history of multiple episodes of bipolar illness (28%). Very late onset mania is strongly associated with neurological co-morbidity as well as high mortality due to cerebrovascular disease (Tohen *et al.*, 1994). Ten out of fourteen of these elderly manic patients were found to have co-morbid neurological disorders, largely due to cerebral infarctions (Tohen *et al.*, 1994).

Lesions and disorders associated with secondary mania include head injuries (Jorge *et al.*, 1993); endocrine conditions (Sweet, 1990; Lee *et al.*, 1991; Ur *et al.*, 1992); HIV (Lyketsos *et al.*, 1993); and epilepsy (Carroll *et al.*, 1996). However, reports of right-sided cerebrovascular lesions dominate the literature (Jampala and Abrams, 1983; Robinson *et al.*, 1988; Fawcett, 1991; Isles and Orrell, 1991; Cummings, 1993; Carroll *et al.*, 1996). Furthermore, Wylie *et al*, (1999) and Cassidy and Carroll (2002) both confirmed an increase in vascular risk factors among late onset manic patients. The former study included outpatients only, while the latter included hospitalized patients.

Significant cognitive dysfunction has consistently been found in association with mania in late life (Stone, 1989; Broadhead and Jacoby, 1990; Berrios and Bakshi, 1991; Dhingra and Rabins, 1991). This reflects the neurological co-morbidity described above, especially when associated with cerebrovascular disease (Steffens and Krishnan, 1998). Spicer *et al.* (1973) had hypothesized that the increase in first admission rates for mania late in life was a reflection of an increased prevalence of dementia in this subpopulation. However, none of the studies that have followed the course of mania in old age have found dementia to be more common than in age-matched controls. None the less, in the light of recent findings by Alexopoulos *et al.* (1993) with respect to pseudodementia and major depression, longer follow-up may be necessary to confirm or refute this concern.

In a study of older bipolar bipolar patients when they were euthymic, Gildengers *et al.* (2004) found that more than half scored one or more standard deviations below the mean of age- and education-matched comparison subjects. These findings were based on the use of relatively coarse cognitive screening instruments such as the MMSE and Mattis Dementia Rating Scale. Nevertheless, they strongly suggest lasting changes rather than temporary cognitive impairment due primarily to the abnormal mood state.

## Other co-morbid conditions

Two recent studies have shed some light on co-morbidity associated with late life bipolar disorders (Goldstein *et al.*, 2006; Sajatovic and Kales, 2006). Using the VA database, Sajatovic and Kales show a lower prevalence (13–30%) of substance use in older people with bipolar disorder than in mixed-age samples of bipolar patients in whom over 60% had co-morbid substance abuse. Among mixed-age bipolar patients there is an extremely high rate (92%) of lifetime co-morbid anxiety disorder, as determined by the National Comorbidity Survey. In the Epidemiologic Catchment Area (ECA) survey, patients with bipolar illness have a lifetime prevalence of 21% for panic disorder compared with 10% for people with depressive disorder. Obsessive–compulsive disorder is found in 21% of patients with bipolar disorder, compared with 12% of patients with major depression and only 2% of the general population. In the VA sample, 23% of patients had co-morbid anxiety. Further data are provided by Goldstein *et al.* (2006) derived from the National Epidemiology Survey on Alcohol-Related Conditions (NESARC). They identified 84 older bipolar patients, in whom the lifetime and 20-month co-morbid prevalence of alcohol use disorders was 38%. For generalized anxiety disorder, the elderly bipolar patients showed a 20.5% lifetime prevalence and a 9.5% 12-month prevalence. For panic disorder, 19% had lifetime prevalence while 12-month prevalence was 11.9%.

## Neuroimaging research

Recent neuroimaging research has helped to clarify the nature, more than the localization, of brain lesions (Shulman, 1997a). Neuroimaging studies have shown a preponderance of subcortical hyperintensities, decreased cerebral blood flow, and evidence of silent cerebral infarctions. Young *et al.* (1999) conducted an analysis of computed tomography in 30 older manic patients and compared them with same-age controls. The manic patients had greater cortical sulcal widening, and the authors suggested a need for further investigation of brain structure in mania in older people. The increase in subcortical (basal ganglia) hyperintensities found in the elderly bipolar population is largely localized to the inferior half of the frontal lobe (McDonald *et al.*, 1991; Woods *et al.*, 1995). More recently, McDonald *et al.* (1999) further investigated the significance of white matter hyperintensities in elderly bipolar patients. They confirmed the finding of an increase in subcortical white matter hyperintensities, but this did not correlate with evidence of cerebrovascular disease. Indeed, controlling for age, the late onset older bipolar patients had the same number of hyperintensities in deep white matter and subcortical grey nuclei as did young bipolar patients and older bipolar patients with early onset of their disorder. The authors conclude that the evidence supports the hypothesis that neuroanatomical changes in mania are present early in life. In further work using magnetic resonance imaging de Asis *et al.* (2006) found that elderly manic patients had more severe frontal deep white matter hyperintensities when compared with a same aged community group. They were unable to replicate the findings of McDonald *et al.* (1999) who found an increase in hyperintensities in the subcortical grey matter The authors hold out hope that greater clarity on the questions of number and localization of brain lesions in older bipolar patients will be possible with newer imaging techniques such as diffusion tensor imaging, functional MRI and near-infrared spectroscopy techniques.

Beyer *et al.* (2004a) found a decreased right caudate volume in older bipolar patients compared with controls which was unaffected by duration of illness. This was most pronounced in late onset older bipolar patients. This finding is significant in relation to the role of the caudate in an emotional regulation loop including the pre-frontal cortex, amygdala, thalamus, as well as other basal ganglia structures. The same group found an increase in left hippocampal volume in older bipolar patients (Beyer *et al.* 2004b). This was not associated with age of onset, mood, or cognitive status. Rather, the authors suggest that this may be associated with exposure to treatment with lithium carbonate. This could provide support for the hypothesis that lithium enhances neuroplasticity and cellular resilience in this region of the brain (Manji and Duman, 2001).

The association of hyperintensities with risk factors such as hypertension, atherosclerotic heart disease, and diabetes mellitus strengthens the relationship of mania to cerebrovascular pathology. Late onset mania has been associated with a high prevalence of silent cerebral infarctions on neuroimaging (Kobayashi *et al.*, 1991; Fujikawa *et al.*, 1995). Silent cerebral infarctions were more common in late onset mania than in age-matched patients with depression. Indeed, the proportion of manic patients over the age of 60 who had silent cerebral infarctions was greater than 20%. These patients also had a relatively low incidence of family history in first-degree relatives, consistent with the notion of secondary mania. These neuroimaging findings provide additional support to the proposal for a vascular subtype of mania (Steffens and Krishnan, 1998).

## Clinical course and outcome

Studies specifically of elderly bipolar patients reveal that by and large they experience a relatively late age of onset, at approximately 50 years. Half of the index patients were first hospitalized for the treatment of depression (Stone, 1989; Broadhead and Jacoby, 1990; Snowdon, 1991; Shulman *et al.*, 1992). A striking finding is the fact that for the elderly bipolar patients whose first episode is depression, a very long latency (mean 15 years) precedes the onset of first mania (Shulman and Post, 1980; Shulman *et al.*, 1992). Within this subgroup, almost one-quarter of the patients experienced a latency of at least 25 years between the first episode of depression and the subsequent episode of mania. In contrast to the conclusion of Perris (1966), that three consecutive depressive episodes could define unipolar depression, about half of elderly bipolars whose first episode is depression also go on to experience at least three distinct depressions before mania becomes manifest (Shulman and Post, 1980; Stone, 1989; Snowdon, 1991). It is this apparent 'conversion' to a bipolar diagnosis after many years of a unipolar course that highlights the importance of cerebral-organic changes and co-morbid neurological disorders described above.

Although the diagnosis of bipolar disorder is dependent upon a single episode of mania, most of the elderly bipolar patients experienced a clinical course that was characterized by both depressive and manic episodes. However, a small subgroup (12%) met strict criteria for a course of unipolar mania (Shulman and Tohen, 1994). This group experienced at least three distinct manic episodes without major depression, with a minimum period of 10 years' follow-up from the time of their first hospitalization for a manic episode. Interestingly, the age of onset for this subgroup was significantly lower (41 years) compared to a mean of 65 years for elderly manics.

These 'unipolar' manic patients were among the very few elderly patients whose illness began early in life. This suggests that this unique clinical course is worthy of further investigation with regard to differences in genetic vulnerability as well as pathogenesis.

Long-term clinical outcomes in elderly bipolar patients have been reported by Berrios and Bakshi (1991), Dhingra and Rabins (1991), and Shulman et al. (1992). In two of these studies, a mean of 6 years' follow-up data is available and a comparison group of elderly depressives was utilized (Dhingra and Rabins, 1991; Shulman et al., 1992). Prognosis nowadays seems to be better than in the original findings by Roth (1955), as 72% of patients still alive were considered symptom-free and living independently (Dhingra and Rabins, 1991). In this latter study, however, about a third of the original cohort had died at follow-up and a significant decline in cognition was reported in a similar proportion of patients. Shulman et al. (1992) found a significant difference in mortality in the elderly manic group. Half of the elderly manic patients had died at a mean 6-year follow-up, compared with only one-fifth of age- and sex-matched elderly patients with depression. Using a comparison group of patients with depression, Berrios and Bakshi (1991) also found that the manic patients were less likely to respond to treatment and to suffer from a higher prevalence of cerebrovascular disease together with cognitive dysfunction, leading to persistent disturbances in behaviour and psychosocial functioning. In summary, elderly manic patients experience high rates of mortality and morbidity, reflecting the underlying CNS pathology found in association with these syndromes.

# Determinants of manic illness in old age

There are four broad factors that are implicated in the manifestation of manic syndromes in old age.

1 Affective vulnerability. Despite the general pattern of less genetic loading in later onset manic illness and in manic syndromes associated with neurological disorders, this subgroup still has a very significant familial prevalence of mood disorder (50–85%) in first-degree relatives (Shulman et al., 1992; Hays et al., 1998). Clinical experience also suggests that affective vulnerability may not be based solely on genetic factors but also on the psychological sequelae of early loss and early trauma in childhood and adolescence. This merits further evaluation in future studies of bipolar disorder late in life. Paradoxically, one suspects that it is the losses of early life that are more relevant to affective disorder in old age, rather than the ubiquitous losses associated with old age.

2 Degenerative changes associated with normal ageing may be a significant factor in the apparent conversion of 'latent' bipolarity into manifest bipolar disorder. These are the middle-aged depressives who become manic after many years and multiple episodes of unipolar depression. Other determinants, however, must also be present to elicit a manic syndrome.

3 A heterogeneous group of brain lesions is associated with mania late in life, with a predominance of cerebrovascular disease including silent cerebral infarctions as well as more obvious strokes. Chronic alcoholism, brain tumours, and a variety of other metabolic conditions have also been implicated.

4 The localization of lesions to the right hemisphere and specifically to the orbitofrontal circuit seems to be critical for the manifestation of mania in old age. While not rare, manic syndromes are certainly uncommon in comparison to depression in old age. Thus, localization of CNS pathology to the right-sided orbitofrontal circuit in association with a vulnerability to mood disorder may constitute the necessary pathogenetic mechanism(s) for the development of mania in the elderly.

# Management

This section will focus only on those features of the management of bipolar disorder that are unique to the elderly. Most fundamental is the high prevalence of neurological morbidity in manic syndromes in old age and hence the need to search assiduously for localizing neurological signs and symptoms. A careful history, alert to evidence of head injury, cerebrovascular disease, and related risk factors, is essential in light of our current understanding of bipolar disorder in old age. Indeed, neuroimaging has been considered an essential component of the investigation of elderly manic patients (Van Gerpen et al., 1999). Another important consideration in old age is the need for caution in using pharmacological therapies (mood stabilizers and antimanic agents), because of their narrow therapeutic range in this age group (Shulman and Herrmann 1999).

## Mood stabilizers

### Lithium

Lithium continues to be a commonly used mood stabilizer in old age (Head and Dening, 1998; Shulman et al., 2003). This maybe a cohort effect, the elderly bipolar population having started on lithium before the introduction of newer mood stabilizing agents (particularly divalproex). Unfortunately, there are no randomised controlled trials of the use of lithium in late life—either in acute mania or maintenance therapy; though there are several open label trials and retrospective reports which suggest that even older, frail patients can be treated safely and effectively (Himmelhoch et al., 1980; Shulman and Post, 1980; Janicak, 1993; Chen et al., 1999; Fahy and Lawlor, 2001; Gildengers et al., 2005). Lithium must be used with considerable caution in the geriatric population as it is eliminated exclusively by the kidneys (Hardy et al., 1997). Normal decline in renal function (including creatinine clearance and glomerular filtration rate) will clearly affect the pharmacokinetics of lithium. Other factors include a decrease in volume of distribution and marked intra-individual variability (Hardy et al., 1987). In their study of the pharmacokinetics of lithium, lithium was excreted in older people at a rate approximately half that of younger patients. Because of these substantial changes in old age, only half the adult dose should be prescribed. For many older patients this would translate into doses of 300–600 mg per day depending on targeted serum levels (see below).

From a pharmacodynamic perspective, sensitivity to lithium is also increased in old age (Shulman and Herrmann, 1999). Adverse reactions and toxicity at 'normal' adult serum levels have been reported (Roose et al., 1979; Smith and Helms, 1982; Murray et al., 1983). However, under well-controlled conditions in a specialized geriatric clinic, lithium is reported to be safe and well tolerated (Parker et al., 1994). Nonetheless, concerns continue, depending on the patient population. Stoudemire et al. (1998) studied a medically ill elderly population who received lithium as an augmenting agent and found that it was relatively poorly tolerated in these circumstances.

Some controversy continues to revolve around the appropriate maintenance dose of lithium in old age. Recommendations have varied: Shulman et al. (1987) suggested a maintenance serum level of 0.5 mmol/litre, but in other studies higher levels were associated with better outcome (Young, 1996; Chen et al., 1999). Clinical experience of the high co-morbidity found in elderly manic patients does suggest caution and the need for better data to support recommendations on serum levels.

The adverse effects of lithium include a wide range of systemic reactions especially affecting the central nervous system (Shulman and Herrmann, 1999). These include lithium-induced tremor, aggravation of parkinsonian tremor, and spontaneous extrapyramidal symptoms. One community study found that almost a third of elderly patients on lithium were on thyroid replacement or else had elevated levels of thyroid stimulating hormone (Head and Dening, 1998), and another study of 1705 new lithium users over 65 years of age found treated hypothyroidism in almost 6% of the sample, twice the prevalence expected among a mixed-age population (Shulman et al., 2005a).

Drug interactions continue to be an on-going concern with lithium, particularly thiazide diuretics which can significantly lower lithium clearance and thereby put the patient at risk of toxicity by increasing the serum lithium levels. Other medications of concern include angiotensin-converting enzyme (ACE) inhibitors and non-steroidal anti-inflammatory drugs (NSAIDs) such as indomethacin (Shulman and Herrmann, 1999). In an observational study of 10,615 elderly lithium users, 3.9% were admitted to hospital for lithium toxicity (Juurlink et al., 2004). In this study, initiation of a loop diuretic like furosemide or an ACE inhibitor significantly increased the risk of lithium toxicity, while neither thiazide diuretics nor NSAIDs were independent risk factors.

### Anticonvulsants

Valproic acid or divalproex has emerged as a significant and viable alternative to lithium carbonate for mood stabilization. In fact, there is evidence that valproate therapy for elderly bipolar patients now occurs more frequently than even lithium (Shulman et al., 2003). Within the elderly population, only case reports (McFarland et al., 1990; Risinger et al., 1994) and case series (Kando et al. 1996; Noaghiul et al., 1998; Jeste et al., 1999; Mordecai et al., 1999; Gildengers et al., 2005) are available. Early indications are that valproate is indeed an effective and well-tolerated mood stabilizer in an elderly population. Noaghiul et al. (1998) studied 21 elderly manic patients and rated the vast majority as much improved. In this study, the average mean dose of divalproex was 1400 mg per day with an average serum level of 72 mg/litre. In another retrospective study, Chen et al. (1999) found lithium to be more effective for classic mania, while response rates in mixed mania were similar for lithium and valproate. This is the opposite of what was found by Bowden (1995) in a mixed-age population. Single case reports reflect valproate's usefulness in rapid cycling illness in old age (Gnam and Flint, 1993) and as a combination agent with lithium carbonate (Schneider and Wilcox, 1998; Goldberg et al., 2000).

While valproic acid appears reasonably well tolerated in older people, there are significant dose-dependent changes in valproate pharmacokinetics which might predispose the elderly to toxicity (Felix et al., 2003). Principal side-effects have included sedation and gastrointestinal disturbance, which can be modulated by dosage reduction (Shulman and Herrmann, 1999). Interestingly, even though valproate has been considered a safer alternative to lithium in the elderly, a recent study of 2422 elderly lithium users and 2918 valproate users found no differences in the rate of hospitalization for delirium (Shulman et al., 2005b). An under-recognized adverse event associated with valproate therapy is thrombocytopenia, which may be more common in the elderly than younger patients (Trannel et al., 2001). Potential adverse reactions can occur because of drug interactions. Valproate is highly protein bound and a weak inhibitor of cytochrome P450 2D6. Accordingly, it could inhibit the metabolism of tricyclic antidepressants and displace diazepam from protein-binding sites, thus increasing their plasma concentrations (Janicak, 1993).

The authors' clinical experience suggests that valproic acid in the form of divalproex is a very reasonable alternative mood stabilizer and is well tolerated with mean dosages ranging between 1000 and 1500 mg daily. The value of monitoring serum levels is unclear, though one retrospective series suggested that greater effectiveness was associated with increased serum levels (Niedermier and Nasrallah, 1998). Further systematic studies will be necessary to confirm these positive initial clinical impressions.

Carbamazepine, another widely used mood stabilizer, has had less exposure in an elderly population, with only a few case reports (Kellner and Neher, 1991; Schneier and Kahn, 1990). As with other mood stabilizing agents, there has been no controlled trial of its use in elderly populations. Because it is a potent inducer of cytochrome P450 2D6 and is highly protein bound, it has the potential for drug interactions (Janicak, 1993). Clinical experience also suggests that it can be highly neurotoxic in an elderly population, so for maintenance relatively low serum levels—below 9 μg/ml (Young, 1996)—have been suggested. Tariot et al. (1998) have recommended the use of carbamazepine for treatment of agitation in dementia patients, so presumably it is well tolerated in this group of patients. Interactions with other drugs used in the elderly include those that increase plasma levels of carbamazepine: fluoxetine, cimetidine, erythromycin, calcium channel blockers. Conversely, carbamazepine may decrease the plasma concentration and half-lives of alprazolam, haloperidol, theophylline, and warfarin.

A small number of reports involve the newer anticonvulsant agents. Gabapentin was used successfully to treat an elderly bipolar patient who was not tolerant of either lithium or valproate (Sheldon et al., 1998). Two case series that used gabapentin included a subsample of elderly patients (Ghaemi et al., 1998; Cabras et al., 1999). A case series of five elderly females suggested that lamotrigine improved symptoms significantly in these patients (Robillard and Conn, 2002). Lamotrigine was added to divalproex in the treatment of a rapid cycling disorder in an elderly patient (Kusumakar and Yatham, 1997); and in an open label trial of treatment-refractory bipolar disorder, a number of elderly patients appeared to tolerate lamotrigine (Calabrese et al., 1999). Finally, in a subanalysis of older subjects enrolled in a placebo-controlled trial of maintenance therapy for bipolar 1 disorder, 33 patients were treated with lamotrigine (Sajatovic et al., 2005). While lamotrigine was significantly better than placebo at delaying time to intervention for any mood disorder, the average age of these 'older' subjects was only 62. Clearly, more clinical experience and trials are required to establish the safety and efficacy of these newer agents among older bipolar patients.

## Other treatments

The typical antipsychotics which are commonly used as adjunctive treatments for bipolar disorder can cause significant side-effects, including anticholinergic effects, orthostatic hypotension, and extrapyramidal symptoms (Sajatovic et al., 2005). In contrast, atypical antipsychotics (including risperidone, olanzapine, and quetiapine) appear to be better tolerated and produce fewer extrapyramidal symptoms including tardive dyskinesia, and they are increasingly being used for elderly manic patients (Jeste et al., 1999). Atypical antipsychotics are likely to have mood stabilizing properties and can be used as monotherapy or adjunctive therapy (Young et al., 2004). Whether the well-known metabolic effects (e.g. weight gain, diabetes mellitus, hyperlipidaemia) which are associated with atypical antipsychotic treatment of younger patients occur in the elderly is unknown. Similarly, it unclear whether the risks of increased cerebrovascular adverse events and mortality, noted in elderly dementia patients treated with antipsychotics, is a concern for elderly bipolar patients (Herrmann and Lanctot, 2006).

While there are no published reports of the use of antidepressants for bipolar depression, the use of selective serotonin reuptake inhibitors and bupropion has been suggested (Sajatovic, 2002; Young et al., 2004). In a recent study comparing 1000 elderly bipolar patients treated with antidepressants with 3000 similar patients who did not receive antidepressants, the antidepressant-treated group surprisingly had significantly fewer admissions for manic or mixed episodes on follow-up (Schaffer et al., 2006).

Finally, while there are few studies of non-pharmacological approaches for the management of elderly bipolar patients, ECT, transcranial magnetic stimulation, and a variety of psychotherapeutic approaches including interpersonal psychotherapy, cognitive-behavioural therapy, family therapy, and group psychotherapy have all been recommended (Sajatovic et al., 2002).

## Summary

As a means of organizing the available evidence on manic syndromes in old age, we propose four distinct subtypes that may have heuristic value for further investigation.

1. *Primary bipolar disorder.* This includes early onset bipolar patients who remain symptomatic into old age and need ongoing management. While relatively few of these individuals appear in studies of hospitalized elderly manic patients, a community or outpatient sample may reveal a different pattern.

2. *Latent bipolar disorder.* This group consists largely of patients who have an onset of depression in middle age, suffer multiple depressive episodes, and then 'convert', after this long latency, to mania later in life. It is postulated that this conversion may be due to cerebral organic factors, including normal degenerative changes and the effects of medication.

3. *Secondary mania (disinhibition syndromes).* This group consists mainly of very late onset manic syndromes without prior history and with a lower familial pre-disposition, occurring in association with neurological or other systemic medical disorders.

4. *Unipolar mania.* This relatively small subgroup appears to have an earlier age of onset compared with other elderly bipolar patients, with persistence of only manic episodes into old age.

The element of chronic frontal disinhibition may also be relevant, but this requires further study.

## Future research

Retrospective studies have now provided enough data to support hypotheses such as those we have outlined, to improve our understanding of manic syndromes in late life. Future research on the pathogenesis of these syndromes will need to use prospective controlled studies that incorporate neuroimaging and neuropsychological testing. Specific attention to frontal lobe function and the role of disinhibition in manic syndromes will be particularly relevant. Inevitably, an integrative model will be best suited to furthering our understanding of mania, not only in old age but also for younger people with bipolar illness.

Finally, it will be useful to determine whether there is a differential response to mood stabilizers or antipsychotics according to the subtype of mania. Specifically, do manic syndromes associated with neurological co-morbidity require long-term stabilization, or can we treat these conditions with short-term antipsychotics? Are the new 'mood stabilizers' as effective as lithium in old age? Prospective systematic multicentre trials will be needed to obtain meaningful information that can inform clinical practice.

## References

Akiskal, H. (1986). The clinical significance of the 'soft' bipolar spectrum. *Psychiatric Annals*, **16**, 667–71.

Alexopoulos, G.S., Meyers, B.S., Young, R.C., Mattis, S., and Kakuma, T. (1993). The course of geriatric depression with 'reversible dementia': a controlled study. *American Journal of Psychiatry*, **150**, 1693–9.

Alexopoulos, G.S., Meyers, B.S., Young, R.C., Kakuma, T., Silbersweig, D., and Charlson, M. (1997). Clinically defined vascular depression. *American Journal of Psychiatry*, **154**, 562–5.

American Psychiatric Association (APA) (1994). *Diagnostic and statistical manual version IV*. American Psychiatric Association, Washington, DC.

Berrios, G.E. and Bakshi, N. (1991). Manic and depressive symptoms in the elderly: their relationships to treatment outcome, cognition and motor symptoms. *Psychopathology*, **24**, 31–8.

Beyer, J.L., Kuchibhatla, M., Payne M. *et al.* (2004a). Caudate volume measurement in older adults with bipolar disorder. *International Journal of Geriatric Psychiatry*, **19**, 109–14.

Beyer, J.L., Kuchibbatla, M., Payne, M. *et al.* (2004b). Hippocampal volume measurement in older adults with bipolar disorder. *American Journal Geriatric Psychiatry*, **12**(6), 613–20.

Bowden, C.L. (1995). Predictors of response to divalproex and lithium. *Journal of Clinical Psychiatry*, **56**(Suppl. 3), 25–30.

Braun, C.M.J., Larocque, C., Daigneault, S., and Montour-Proulx, I. (1999). Mania, pseudomania, depression, and pseudodepression resulting from focal unilateral cortical lesions. *Neuropsychiatry, Neuropsychology, and Behavioural Neurology*, **12**, 35–51.

Broadhead, J. and Jacoby, R. (1990). Mania in old age: a first prospective study. *International Journal of Geriatric Psychiatry*, **5**, 215.

Brooks, J.O. and Hoblyn, J.C., (2005). Secondary mania in older adults. *American Journal of Psychiatry*, **162**, 2033–8.

Cabras, P.L., Hardoy, J., Hardoy, M.C., and Carta, M.G. (1999). Clinical experience with gabapentin in patients with bipolar or schizoaffective disorder: results of an open-label study. *Journal of Clinical Psychiatry*, **60**, 245–8.

Calabrese, J.R., Bowden, C.L., McElroy, S.L. *et al.* (1999). Spectrum of activity of lamotrigine in treatment-refractory bipolar disorder. *American Journal of Psychiatry*, **156**, 1019–23.

Carroll, B.Y., Goforth, H.W., Kennedy, J.C., and Dueño, O.R. (1996). Mania due to general medical conditions: frequency, treatment, and cost. *International Journal of Psychiatry in Medicine*, **26**, 5–13.

Cassidy, F. and Carroll B.Y. (2002). Vascular risk factors in late onset mania. *Psychological Medicine*, **32**, 359–62.

Chen, S.T., Altshuler, L.L., Melnyk, K.A., Erhart, S.M., Miller, E., and Mintz, J. (1999). Efficacy of lithium vs valproate in the treatment of mania in the elderly: a retrospective study. *Journal of Clinical Psychiatry*, **60**, 181–6.

Cummings, J.L. (1993). Frontal-subcortical circuits and human behavior. *Archives of Neurology*, **50**, 873–80.

de Asis, J.M., Greenwald, B.S., Alexopoulos, G.S. *et al.* (2006). Frontal signal hyperintensities in mania in old age. *American Journal of Geriatric Psychiatry*, **14**(7), 598–604.

Dhingra, U. and Rabins, P.V. (1991). Mania in the elderly: A five-to-seven year follow-up. *Journal of the American Geriatrics Society*, **39**, 582–3.

Eagles, J.M. and Whalley, L.J. (1985). Ageing and affective disorders: the age at first onset of affective disorders in Scotland, 1996–1978. *British Journal of Psychiatry*, **147**, 180.

Fahy, S. and Lawlor, B.A. (2001). Discontinuation of lithium augmentation in an elderly cohort. *International Journal of Geriatric Psychiatry*, **16**, 1004–9.

Fawcett, R.G. (1991). Cerebral infarct presenting as mania. *Journal of Clinical Psychiatry*, **52**, 352–3.

Felix, S., Sproule, B.A., Hardy, B.G., and Naranjo, C.A. (2003). Dose-related pharmacokinetics and pharmacodynamics of valproate in the elderly. *Journal of Clinical Psychopharmacology*, **23**, 471–8.

Fujikawa, T, Yamawaki, S., and Touhouda, Y. (1995). Silent cerebral infarctions in patients with late-onset mania. *Stroke*, **26**, 946–9.

Ghaemi, S.N., Katzow, J.J., Desai, S.P., and Goodwin, F.K. (1998). Gabapentin treatment of mood disorders: a preliminary study. *Journal of Clinical Psychiatry*, **59**, 426–9.

Gildengers, A.G., Butters, M.A., Seligman, K. *et al.* (2004). Cognitive functioning in late-life bipolar disorder. *American Journal of Psychiatry*, **161**, 736–8.

Gildengers, A.G., Mulsant, B.H., Begley, A.E. *et al.* (2005). A pilot study of standardized treatment in geriatric bipolar disorder. *American Journal of Geriatric Psychiatry*, **13**, 319–23.

Glasser, M. and Rabins, P. (1984). Mania in the elderly. *Ageing*, **13**, 210–13.

Gnam, W. and Flint, A.J. (1993). New onset rapid cycling bipolar disorder in an 87 year old woman. *Canadian Journal of Psychiatry*, **38**, 324–6.

Goldberg, J.F., Sacks, M.H., and Kocsis, J.H. (2000). Lithium augmentation of divalproex in geriatric mania. *Journal of Clinical Psychiatry*, **61**, 304.

Goldstein, B.I., Herrmann, N., and Shulman, K.I. (2006). Comorbidity in bipolar disorder among the elderly; results from an epidemiological community sample. *American Journal of Psychiatry*, **163**(2), 319–21.

Goodwin, F.K. and Jamison, K.R. (1990). *Manic-depressive illness*. Oxford University Press, New York.

Hardy, B.G., Shulman, K.I., MacKenzie, S.E., Kutcher, S.P., and Silverberg, J.D. (1987). Pharmacokinetics of lithium in the elderly. *Psychopharmacology*, **7**, 153–8.

Hardy, B.G., Shulman, K.I., and Zucchero, C. (1997). Gradual discontinuation of lithium augmentation in elderly patients with unipolar depression. *Journal of Clinical Psychopharmacology*, **17**, 22–6.

Hays, J.C., Krishnan, K.R.R., George, L.K., and Blazer, D.G. (1998). Age of first onset of bipolar disorder: demographic, family history, and psychosocial correlates. *Depression and Anxiety*, **7**, 76–82.

Head, L. and Dening, T. (1998). Lithium in the over-65s: who is taking it and who is monitoring it? *International Journal of Geriatric Psychiatry*, **13**, 164–71.

Herrmann, N. and Lanctot, K.L. (2006). Atypical antipsychotics for neuropsychiatric symptoms of dementia: malignant or maligned? *Drug Safety*, **29**, 833–43.

Himmelhoch, J.M., Neil, J.F., May, S.J., Fuchs, C.Z., and Licata, S.M. (1980). Age, dementia, dyskinesis, and lithium response. *American Journal of Psychiatry*, **137**, 941–5.

Isles, L.J. and Orrell, M.W. (1991). Secondary mania after open-heart surgery. *British Journal of Psychiatry*, **159**, 280–2.

Jampala, V.S. and Abrams, R. (1983). Mania secondary to left and right hemisphere damage. *American Journal of Psychiatry*, **140**, 1197–9.

Janicak, P.G. (1993). The relevance of clinical pharmacokinetics and therapeutic drug monitoring: anticonvulsants, mood stabilizers and antipsychotics. *Journal of Clinical Psychiatry*, **54**(Suppl. 9), 35–41.

Jeste, D.V., Lacro, J.P., Bailey, A., Rockwell, E., Harris, M.J., and Caligiuri, M.P. (1999). Lower incidence of tardive dyskinesia in risperidone compared with haloperidol in older patients. *Journal of the American Geriatrics Society*, **47**, 716–19.

Jorge, R.E., Robinson, R.G., Starkstein, S.E., Arfndt, S.V., Forrester, A.W., and Geisler, F.H. (1993). Secondary mania following traumatic brain injury. *American Journal of Psychiatry*, **150**, 916–21.

Juurlink, D.N., Mamdani, M.M., Kopp, A., Rochon, P.A., and Shulman, K.I. (2004). Drug-induced lithium toxicity in the elderly: a population-based study. *Journal of the American Geriatric Society*, **52**, 794–8.

Kando, J.C., Tohen, M., Castillo, J., and Zarate, C.A. (1996). The use of valproate in an elderly population with affective symptoms. *Journal of Clinical Psychiatry*, **57**, 238–40.

Kellner, M.B. and Neher, F. (1991). A first episode of mania after age 80. *Canadian Journal of Psychiatry*, **36**, 607–8.

Kessing, L.V. (2006). Diagnostic subtypes of bipolar disorder in older versus younger adults. *Bipolar Disorders*, **8**, 56–64.

Kessler, R.C., Rubinow, D.R., Holmes, C., Abelson, J.M., and Zhao, S. (1997). The epidemiology of DSM-III-R bipolar I disorder in a general population survey. *Psychological Medicine*, **27**, 1079–89.

Kling, A. and Steklis, H.D. (1976). A neural substrate for affiliative behavior in nonhuman primates. *Brain Behaviour and Evolution*, **13**, 216–38.

Kobayashi, S., Okada, K., and Yamashita, K. (1991). Incidence of silent lacunar lesions in normal adults and its relation to cerebral blood flow and risk factors. *Stroke*, **22**, 1379–83.

Krauthammer, C. and Klerman, G.L. (1978). Secondary mania: manic syndromes associated with antecedent physical illness or drugs. *Archives of General Psychiatry*, **35**, 1333–9.

Kumar, A., Schapiro, M.D., Haxby, J.V., Grady, C.L., and Friedland, R.P. (1990). Cerebral metabolic and cognitive studies in dementia with frontal lobe behavioral features. *Journal of Psychiatric Research*, **24**, 97–109.

Kusumakar, V. and Yatham, L.N. (1997). Lamotrigine treatment of rapid cycling bipolar disorder. *American Journal of Psychiatry*, **154**, 1171–2.

Leboyer, M., Henry, C., Paillere-Martinot, M-L., and Bellivier, F. (2005). Age at onset in bipolar affective disorders: a review. *Bipolar Disorders*, **7**, 111–18.

Lee, S., Chow, C.C., Wing, Y.K., Leung, C.M., Chiu, H., and Chen, C. (1991). Mania secondary to thyrotoxicosis. *British Journal of Psychiatry*, **159**, 712–13.

Lyketsos, C.G., Hanson, A.L., Fishman, M., Rosenblatt, A., McHugh, P.R., and Treisman, G.J. (1993). Manic syndrome early and late in the course of HIV. *American Journal of Psychiatry*, **150**, 326–7.

Manji, H.K. and Duman, R.S. (2001) Impairments of neuroplasticity and cellular resilience in severe mood disorders: implications for the development of novel therapeutics. *Psychopharmacology Bulletin*, **35**, 5–49.

McDonald, W.M., Krishnan, K.R.R., Doraiswamy, P.M., and Blazer, D.G. (1991). Occurrence of subcortical hyperintensities in elderly subjects with mania. *Psychiatry Research*, **40**, 211–20.

McDonald, W.M., Tupler, L.A., Marsteller, F.A. *et al.* (1999). Hyperintense lesions on magnetic resonance images in bipolar disorder. *Biological Psychiatry*, **45**, 965–71.

McFarland, B.H., Miller, M.R., and Straumfjord, A.A. (1990). Valproate use in the older manic patient. *Journal of Clinical Psychiatry*, **51**, 479–81.

Moorehead, S.R.J. and Young, A.H., (2003). Evidence for a late onset bipolar-I disorder sub-group after 50 years. *Journal of Affective Disorders*, **73**, 271–7.

Mordecai, D.J., Sheikh, J.I., and Glick, I.D. (1999). Divalproex for the treatment of geriatric bipolar disorder. *International Journal of Geriatric Psychiatry*, **14**, 494–6.

Murray, N., Hopwood, S., Balfour, D.J.K., Ogston, S., and Hewick, D.S. (1983). The influence of age on lithium efficacy and side effects in out-patients. *Psychological Medicine*, **13**, 53–60.

Neary, D., Snowden, J.S., Northern, B. *et al.* (1988). Dementia of frontal lobe type. *Journal of Neurology, Neurosurgery and Psychiatry*, **51**, 353–61.

Niedermier, J.A. and Nasrallah, H.A. (1998). Clinical correlates of response to valproate in geriatric inpatients. *Annals of Clinical Psychiatry*, **10**, 165–8.

Noaghiul, S., Narayan, M., and Nelson, J.C. (1998). Divalproex treatment of mania in elderly patients. *American Journal of Geriatric Psychiatry*, **6**, 257–62.

Parker, K.L., Mittmann, N. Shear, N.H. *et al.* (1994). Lithium augmentation in geriatric depressed outpatients: a clinical report. *International Journal of Geriatric Psychiatry*, **9**, 995–1002.

Pearlson, G.D. (1999). Structural and functional brain changes in bipolar disorder: a selective review. *Schizophrenia Research*, **39**, 133–40.

Perris, C. (1966). A study of bipolar (manic depressive) and unipolar recurrent psychoses (IX). *Acta Psychiatrica Scandinavica*, **194**(Suppl.), 1–189.

Rasanan, P, Tiihonen, J., and Hakko, H. (1998). The incidence and onset-age of hospitalised bipolar affective disorder in Finland. *Journal of Affective Disorders*, **48**, 63–8.

Risinger, R.C., Risby, E.D., and Risch, S.C. (1994). Safety and efficacy of divalproex sodium in elderly bipolar patients. *Journal of Clinical Psychiatry*, **55**, 215.

Robillard, M. and Conn, D.K. (2002). Lamotrigine use in geriatric patients with bipolar depression. *Canadian Journal of Psychiatry*, **47**, 767–70.

Robinson, R.G., Boston, J.D., Starkstein, S.E., and Price, T.R. (1988). Comparison of mania with depression following brain injury: causal factors. *American Journal of Psychiatry*, **145**, 172–8.

Roose, S.P., Bone, S., Haidorfer, C., Dunner, D.L., and Fieve, R.R. (1979). Lithium treatment in older patients. *American Journal of Psychiatry*, **136**, 843–4.

Roth, M. (1955). The natural history of mental disorder in old age. *Journal of Mental Science*, **101**, 281–301.

Sackeim, H.A., Greenberg, M.S., Weiman, A.L., Gur, R.C., Hungerbuhler, J.P., and Geschwind, N. (1982). Hemispheric asymmetry in the expression of positive and negative emotions. *Archives of Neurology*, **39**, 210–18.

Sajatovic, M. and Kales, H.C. (2006). Diagnosis and management of bipolar disorder with comorbid anxiety in the elderly. *Journal of Clinical Psychiatry*, **67** (Suppl. 1), 21–7.

Sajatovic, M., Sultana, D., Bingham, C.R., Buckley, P., and Donenwirth, K. (2002). Gender related differences in clinical characteristics and hospital based resource utilization among older adults with schizophrenia. *International Journal of Geriatric Psychiatry*, **17**, 542–8.

Sajatovic, M., Gyulai, L, Calabrese, J.R., Thompson, T.R., Wilson, B.G., and White, R. (2005a). Maintenance treatment outcomes in older patients with bipolar 1 disorder. *American Journal of Geriatric Psychiatry*, **13**, 305–11.

Sajatovic, M., Madhusoodanan, S., and Coconcea, N. (2005b). Managing bipolar disorder in the elderly: defining the role of the newer agents. *Drugs and Aging*, **22**, 39–54.

Schaffer, A., Mamdani, M., Levitt, A., and Herrmann, N. (2006). Effect of antidepressant use on admissions to hospital among elderly bipolar patients. *International Journal of Geriatric Psychiatry*, **21**, 275–80.

Schneider, A.L. and Wilcox, C.S. (1998). Divalproex augmentation in lithium-resistant rapid cycling mania in four geriatric patients. *Journal of Affective Disorders*, **47**, 201–5.

Schneier, H.A. and Kahn, D. (1990). Selective response to carbamazepine in a case of organic mood disorder. *Journal of Clinical Psychiatry*, **51**, 485.

Sheldon, L.F., Ancill, R.J., and Holliday, S.G. (1998). Gabapentin in geriatric psychiatry patients. *Canadian Journal of Psychiatry*, **43**, 422–3.

Shulman, K.I. (1997a). Neurologic co-morbidity and mania in old age. *Clinical Neuroscience*, **4**(1), 37–40.

Shulman, K.I. (1997b). Disinhibition syndromes, secondary mania and bipolar disorder in old age. *Journal of Affective Disorders*, **46**, 175–82.

Shulman, K.I. and Herrmann, N. (1999). The nature and management of mania in old age. *Psychiatric Clinics of North America*, **22**(3), 649–65.

Shulman, K. and Post, F. (1980). Bipolar affective disorder in old age. *British Journal of Psychiatry*, **136**, 26–32.

Shulman, K.I. and Tohen, M. (1994). Unipolar mania reconsidered: evidence from an elderly cohort. *British Journal of Psychiatry*, **164**, 547–9.

Shulman, K.I., MacKenzie, S., and Hardy, B. (1987). The clinical use of lithium carbonate in old age. *Progress in Neuro-Psychopharmacology and Biological Psychiatry*, **11**, 159–64.

Shulman, K.I., Tohen, M., Satlin, A., Mallya, G., and Kalunian, D. (1992). Mania compared with unipolar depression in old age. *American Journal of Psychiatry*, **142**, 341–5.

Shulman, K. I., Rochon, P., Sykora, K. *et al.* (2003). Changing prescription patterns for lithium and divalproex in old age: shifting practice without evidence. *British Medical Journal*, **326**, 960–1.

Shulman, K.I., Sykora, K., Gill, S.S. *et al.* (2005a). New thyroxine treatment in older adults beginning lithium therapy: implications for clinical practice. *American Journal of Geriatric Psychiatry* **13**, 1–6.

Shulman, K.I., Sykora, K., Gill, S. *et al.* (2005b). Incidence of delirium in older adults newly prescribed lithium or valproate: a population based cohort study. *Journal of Clinical Psychiatry*, **66**, 424–7.

Smith, R.E. and Helms, P.M. (1982). Adverse effects of lithium therapy in the acutely ill elderly patient. *Journal of Clinical Psychiatry*, **43**, 94–9.

Snowdon, J. (1991). A retrospective case-note study of bipolar disorder in old age. *British Journal of Psychiatry*, **158**, 484–90.

Spicer, C.C., Hare, E.H., and Slater, E. (1973). Neurotic and psychotic forms of Depressive illness: evidence from age-incidence in a national sample. *British Journal of Psychiatry*, **123**, 535–41.

Starkstein, S.E. and Robinson, R.G. (1997). Mechanism of disinhibition after brain lesions. *Journal of Nervous Mental Disorder*, **185**, 108–14.

Starkstein, S.E., Mayberg, H.S., Berthier, M.L., Fedoroff, P., Price, T.R., and Robinson, R.G. (1990). Mania after brain injury: Neuroradiological and metabolic findings. *Annals of Neurology*, **27**, 652–9.

Starkstein, S.E., Migliorelli, R., Teeson, A. *et al.* (1994). The specificity of cerebral blood flow changes in patients with frontal lobe dementia. *Journal of Neurology, Neurosurgery and Psychiatry*, **57**, 790–6.

Steffens, D.C. and Krishnan, K.R.R. (1998). Structural neuroimaging and mood disorders. Recent findings, implications for classification, and future directions. *Biological Psychiatry*, **43**, 705–12.

Stone, K. (1989). Mania in the elderly. *British Journal of Psychiatry*, **155**, 220–4.

Stoudemire, A., Hill, C.D., Lewison, B.J., Marquardt, M., and Dalton, S. (1998). Lithium intolerance in a medical-psychiatric population. *General Hospital Psychiatry*, **20**, 85–90.

Strakowski, S.M., McElroy, S., Keck, P., and West, S. (1994). The co-occurrence of mania with medical and other psychiatric disorders. *International Journal of Psychiatry in Medicine*, **24**, 305–28.

Sweet, R. (1990). Case of craniopharyngioma in late life. *Journal of Neuropsychiatry*, **2**, 464–5.

Tariot, P.N., Eerb, R., Podgorski, C.A. *et al.* (1998). Efficacy and tolerability of carbamazepine for agitation and aggression in dementia. *American Journal of Psychiatry*, **155**, 54–61.

Tohen, M., Waternaux, C.M., and Tsuang, M.T. (1990). Outcome in mania: a four year prospective follow-up study utilising survival analysis. *Archives of General Psychiatry*, **47**, 1106–11.

Tohen, M., Shulman, K.I., and Satlin, A. (1994). First-episode mania in late life. *American Journal of Psychiatry*, **151**, 130–2.

Trannel, T.J., Ahmed, I., and Goebert, D. (2001). Occurrence of thrombocytopenia in psychiatric patients taking valproate. *American Journal of Psychiatry*, **158**, 128–30.

Tsuang, M.T. (1978). Suicide in schizophrenics, manics, depressives, and surgical controls. *Archives of General Psychiatry*, **35**, 153–5.

Ur, E., Turner, T.H., Godwin, T.J. *et al.* (1992). Mania in association with hydrocortisone replacement for Addison's disease. *Postgraduate Medicine*, **68**, 41–3.

Van Gerpen, M.W., Johnson, J.E., and Winstead, D.K. (1999). Mania in the geriatric patient population: a review of the literature. *American Journal of Geriatric Psychiatry*, **7**, 188–202.

Verdoux, H. and Bourgeois, M. (1995). Manies secondaires a des pathologies organiques cerebrales. *Annals of Medical Psychology*, **153**, 161–8.

Weeke, A. and Vaeth, M. (1986). Excess mortality of bipolar and unipolar manic-depressive patients. *Journal of Affective Disorders*, **11**, 227–34.

Weissman, M.M., Bruce, M.L., Leak, P.J. *et al.* (1991). Affective disorders. In *Psychiatric disorders in America: the Epidemiologic Catchment Area Study* (ed. L.N. Robins and D.A. Regier), p. 53. Free Press, New York.

Winokur, G. (1975). The Iowa 500: Heterogeneity and course in manic depressive illness (bipolar). *Comprehensive Psychiatry*, **16**, 125–31.

Woods, B.T., Yurgelun-Todd, D., Mikulis, D., and Pillay, S.S. (1995) Age-related MRI abnormalities in bipolar illness: a clinical study. *Biological Psychiatry*, **38**, 846–7.

Wylie, M.E., Mulsant, B.H., Pollock, B.G. *et al.* (1999). Age at onset in geriatric bipolar disorder. *American Journal of Geriatric Psychiatry*, **7**, 77–83.

Yassa, R., Nair, V., Nastase, C. *et al.* (1988). Prevalence of bipolar disorder in a psychogeriatric population. *Journal of Affective Disorders*, **14**, 197–201.

Young, R.C. (1996). Treatment of geriatric mania. In *Mood disorders across the life span* (ed. K.I. Shulman, M. Tohen, and S.P. Kutcher), pp. 411–25. Wiley-Liss, New York.

Young, R.C. and Klerman, G.L. (1992). Mania in late life: focus on age at onset. *American Journal of Psychiatry*, **149**, 867–76.

Young, R.C., Nambudiri, D.E., Jain, H., de Asis, J.M., and Alexopoulos, G.S. (1999). Brain computed tomography in geriatric manic disorder. *Biological Psychiatry*, **45**, 1063–5.

Young, R.C., Gyulai, L, Mulsand, B.H., Flint, A., Beyer, J.L., and Shulman, K.I. (2004). Pharmacotherapy of bipolar disorder in old age: review and recommendations. *American Journal of Geriatric Psychiatry*, **12**, 342–57.

Zald, D. and Kim, S.W. (1996). Anatomy and function of the orbital frontal cortex: I anatomy, neurocircuitry, and obsessive-compulsive disorder. *Journal of Neuropsychiatry and Clinical Neuroscience*, **8**, 125–38.

# Neurotic disorders

## James Lindesay

## Introduction

Although neurotic disorders in elderly people are common, distressing, treatable, and costly to health and social services, they have traditionally been neglected relative to other psychiatric disorders in old age, and to neuroses in younger adults. However, as psychogeriatric services develop, as the primary care sector becomes increasingly involved in the commissioning and delivery of mental health services, and as elderly people themselves become more demanding of equitable treatment, the needs of this group are becoming apparent. The growing literature reflects this: there has in recent years been a steady increase in the number of research papers, reviews, and textbooks addressing anxiety and neurotic disorders in old age. However, as this chapter makes clear, there is still much that we do not know about these interesting and important conditions.

## The concept of neurosis

The term 'neurosis' was originally coined in the 18th century to describe a group of conditions such as hysteria, melancholia, and epilepsy that were thought at that time to be due to pathology of the peripheral nerves (Cullen, 1784). By the mid-19th century this model had largely been abandoned, and attention moved to factors such as constitution and environment, with neurosis regarded as the consequence of adverse external agents acting on 'degenerate' and 'nervous' temperaments. In general terms this model still underlies our current thinking, but the unitary, dimensional concept of neurosis yielded in the second half of the 20th century to a system of specific diagnostic categories based upon patterns of symptoms. This process has been driven by the growth of biological psychiatry, clinical dissatisfaction with psychoanalysis, and the natural human need for clinicians, researchers, and service planners to deal with 'cases' (Lindesay, 1995a). Current nosological thinking is embodied in the 10th edition of the *International Classification of Diseases* (ICD-10) (World Health Organization, 1992) and the fourth edition of the *Diagnostic and Statistical Manual of Mental Disorders* (DSM-IV) (American Psychiatric Association, 1994) (Table 30.1). ICD-10 still contains a vestigial remnant of the earlier approach in its reference to 'neurotic, stress-related and somatoform disorders'; in DSM-IV, however, all mention of neurosis and the neurotic has been expunged.

Although unfashionable, and difficult to accommodate in descriptive classifications, the broad dimensional concept of neurosis is not obsolete (Andrews, 1996). Tyrer (1989, 1990) has reviewed the evidence in favour of a general neurotic syndrome, pointing out that there is considerable co-morbidity between the specific neurotic categories, and between them and other disorders such as depression. These categories are also unstable over time, and the effectiveness of treatments appears to be relatively independent of diagnosis. The dimensionality of these disorders is particularly apparent in community and primary care populations; latent trait analysis of psychological symptoms in both younger and older adults identifies independent but related dimensions of depression and anxiety underlying the manifest symptomatology (Goldberg *et al.*, 1987; Mackinnon *et al.*, 1994). An individual's symptoms during any particular episode are determined by pre-existing vulnerability, the particular factors precipitating that episode (destabilization factors), and the steps taken by the patient or the doctor to manage it (restitution factors). Most of the current diagnostic categories such as phobic disorder, dissociative disorder, or somatoform disorder result from various maladaptive attempts by patients to reduce their symptoms (Goldberg and Huxley, 1992). The population-based Amsterdam Study of the Elderly (AMSTEL) has shown that there are no differences in the vulnerability factors for anxiety, depression, and mixed anxiety/depression (Schoevers *et al.*, 2003). The value of the dimensional approach to these disorders is that it formulates them as longitudinal processes rather than just as cross-sectional episodes; this perspective is particularly important in elderly patients who often present with many years of illness experience. It also integrates the depressive component of many neurotic disorders, something that categorical classifications have never been able to do satisfactorily.

Modern nosologies are probably most appropriate in their categorization of obsessive–compulsive disorder (OCD) as a distinct disorder, although its current classification with the anxiety disorders may be inappropriate. Although a proportion of OCD patients also develop significant symptoms of depression and anxiety, it is a relatively persistent and stable diagnosis; it shows an early and specific response to treatment with serotonergic drugs, and the placebo response rate is much lower than that which occurs in depression and anxiety. OCD appears to have more in common with neurodevelopmental disorders such as Gilles de la Tourette's

**Table 30.1** Modern classifications of neurotic disorders (ICD-10 and DSM-IV)

| ICD-10 | DSM-IV |
|---|---|
| MOOD DISORDERS | MOOD DISORDERS |
| F34: *Persistent mood disorders* | *Depressive disorders* |
| Dysthymia | 300.4: Dysthymic disorder |
| NEUROTIC, STRESS-RELATED AND SOMATOFORM DISORDERS | |
| F40: *Phobic anxiety disorders* | ANXIETY DISORDERS |
| .0: Agoraphobia | 300.01: Panic disorder without agoraphobia |
| .1: Social phobia | 300.21: Panic disorder with agoraphobia |
| .2: Specific phobia | 300.22: Agoraphobia without history of panic disorder |
| F41: *Other anxiety disorders* | 300.23: Social phobia |
| | 300.29: Specific phobia |
| .0: Panic disorder | 300.3: Obsessive-compulsive disorder |
| .1: Generalized anxiety disorder | 309.81: Post-traumatic stress disorder |
| .2: Mixed anxiety and depressive disorder | 300.02: Generalized anxiety disorder |
| | 293.89: Anxiety disorder due to a general medical condition |
| F42: *Obsessive–compulsive disorder* | 292.89: Substance-induced anxiety disorder |
| F43: *Reaction to severe stress, and adjustment disorders* | |
| .0: Acute stress reaction | |
| .1: Post-traumatic stress disorder | |
| .2: Adjustment disorders | |
| F44: *Dissociative disorders* | DISSOCIATIVE DISORDERS |
| .0: Dissociative amnesia | 300.12: Dissociative amnesia |
| .1: Dissociative fugue | 300.13: Dissociative fugue |
| .2: Dissociative stupor | 300.14: Dissociative identity disorder |
| .3: Trance and possession states | 300.6: Depersonalization disorder |
| .4: Dissociative motor disorders | |
| .5: Dissociative convulsions | |
| .6: Dissociative anaesthesia and sensory loss | |
| F45: *Somatoform disorders* | SOMATOFORM DISORDERS |
| .0: Somatization disorder | 300.81: Somatization disorder |
| .1: Undifferentiated somatoform disorder | 300.11: Conversion disorder |
| .2: Hypochondriacal disorder | 300.7: Hypochondriasis |
| .3: Somatoform autonomic dysfunction | 300.7: Body dysmorphic disorder |
| .4: Persistent somatoform pain disorder | 307.80: Pain disorder associated with psychological factors |
| F46: *Other neurotic disorders* | 307.89: Pain disorder associated with both psychological factors and a general medical condition |
| .0: Neurasthenia | 300.81: Undifferentiated somatoform disorder |
| .1: Depersonalization–derealization syndrome | |

syndrome, and is due to impairment of a specific striatal–orbitofrontal neuronal circuit (Insel, 1982). This is in contrast to other anxiety disorders, which are thought to be due to disturbances in the frontal cortex–amygdala–septum–hippocampus system which mediates fear (Gray, 1982).

# Epidemiology

Neurotic disorders are uncommon primary diagnoses in hospital inpatient, outpatient, and casualty populations (Thyer *et al.*, 1985; Schwartz *et al.*, 1987), but as co-morbid disorders their prevalence in clinical populations is significant (Hocking and Koenig, 1995). The picture is rather different in primary care settings, where there is a steady accumulation of chronic psychiatric cases of all types in older age groups (Shepherd *et al.*, 1981). However, there is a marked decline in the rate of new consultations with increasing age, with new cases after the age of 65 years being only about 10% of all cases in that age group (Shepherd *et al.*, 1981; Cooper, 1986). These falls in the prevalence and incidence of neurotic disorders with age in clinical populations are not due simply to falls in the general population (see below), but to non-presentation by patients and non-recognition by clinicians; one recent study of anxiety in elderly attendees at an inner-city general practice found very high rates of generalized anxiety disorder (GAD) and agoraphobia (Krasucki *et al.*, 1999). Neurotic disorders do not pass easily through the various 'filters' on the pathway to psychiatric care (the subject's decision to consult, detection of disorder, psychiatric referral, admission to a hospital bed) (Goldberg and Huxley, 1980); factors such as the age and sex of the subject, the severity of the disorder, and the doctor's attitudes are all important impediments. However, these patients may instead be referred inappropriately to non-psychiatric specialist services for investigation and treatment (Blazer *et al.*, 1991; Beitman *et al.*, 1991). Over the last two decades there have been a number of epidemiological studies of elderly community populations that have provided information about the rates of neurotic disorder in this age group using standardized methods and operationalized diagnostic criteria. These methodological developments have greatly improved the reliability and comparability of the results, but the different rates found using different criteria indicate that their validity is still questionable. For example, in the United States Epidemiologic Catchment Area (ECA) Study, the overall 1-month prevalence of DSM-III phobic disorder was 4.8% (Regier *et al.*, 1988), but in studies using the Geriatric Mental State (GMS)/AGECAT system, diagnostic syndrome cases of phobic neurosis were very rare (Copeland *et al.*, 1987). Most of these discrepancies are probably due to differences in the diagnostic criteria used, particularly the rules governing severity thresholds and hierarchies of disorders (Lindesay and Banerjee, 1993). A more general question, still unanswered, is the extent to which the current diagnostic criteria for anxiety disorders are appropriate for the older population, who may present with more somatic symptoms (Flint, 2005a).

Table 30.2 summarizes the findings of the ECA study so far as DSM-III categories related to neurotic disorder in the elderly population are concerned. Overall, lifetime prevalence rates decreased with age, although this decline was least apparent in phobic disorder and somatization disorder; phobic disorder was the commonest psychiatric disorder identified in women over 65 years, and the second commonest after cognitive impairment in men. Females had higher period prevalence rates than males for phobic disorder, panic disorder, generalized anxiety disorder (GAD), and somatization disorder, and higher lifetime prevalence rates of OCD and somatization disorder. Most elderly subjects with neurotic disorders had developed them before their 50s, but elderly cases of phobic disorder, panic disorder, and OCD tended to be of later onset.

**Table 30.2** Prevalence and incidence rates of specific DSM-III mental disorders (ECA study)

**(a) One-month prevalence (%) (Regier et al., 1988; Blazer et al., 1991)**

|  |  | Males | Females | Total |
|---|---|---|---|---|
| Dysthymia | 65+ | 1.0 | 2.3 | 1.8 |
|  | All ages | 2.2 | 4.2 | 3.3 |
| Phobic disorder | 65+ | 2.9 | 6.1 | 4.8 |
|  | All ages | 3.8 | 8.4 | 6.2 |
| Panic disorder | 65+ | 0.0 | 0.2 | 0.1 |
|  | All ages | 0.3 | 0.7 | 0.5 |
| Obsessive–compulsive disorder | 65+ | 0.7 | 0.9 | 0.8 |
|  | All ages | 1.1 | 1.5 | 1.3 |
| Somatization | 65+ | 0.0 | 0.2 | 0.1 |
|  | All ages | 0.0 | 0.2 | 0.1 |
| Generalized anxiety disorder | 65+ | – | – | 1.9[a] |
|  | 45–64 | – | – | 3.1[a] |

**(b) Annual incidence per 100 person-years of risk (Eaton et al., 1989)**

|  |  | Males | Females | Total |
|---|---|---|---|---|
| Phobic disorder | 65+ | 2.66 | 5.52 | 4.29 |
|  | All ages | 2.33 | 5.38 | 3.98 |
| Panic disorder | 65+ | 0.00 | 0.07 | 0.04 |
|  | All ages | 0.30 | 0.76 | 0.56 |
| Obsessive–compulsive disorder | 65+ | 0.12 | 1.00 | 0.64 |
|  | All ages | 0.39 | 0.92 | 0.69 |

[a] Six-month prevalence.

Incidence rates of most neurotic disorders fell with age in both sexes, but this was least apparent for phobic disorder and OCD (Robins and Regier, 1991). The Longitudinal Aging Study Amsterdam also used DIS/DSM-III, and has reported similar prevalence rates to the ECA study for phobic disorder, panic disorder, and OCD (Beekman *et al.*, 1998). However, at 7.3%, the rate of GAD was rather higher. Within their sample (aged 55–85 years), there was little evidence of change of rates of these disorders with age.

Not surprisingly, given the more stringent case definitions employed, the prevalence rates of neurotic disorders in studies using the GMS/AGECAT system are lower than those found by DIS/DSM-III (Table 30.3). However, a significant proportion had subcase levels of anxiety, phobic, and obsessional neurosis. Age and sex differences for the case and subcase AGECAT categories were less consistent than those found by the ECA study using DSM-III criteria. A 3-year follow-up of the Liverpool sample found an incidence rate for neurotic disorders of 4.4/1000 per year (Larkin

**Table 30.3** One-month prevalence rates (%) of GMS/AGECAT neurotic disorders (Copeland *et al.*, 1987)

|  | Male | | Female | |
|---|---|---|---|---|
|  | Case | Subcase | Case | Subcase |
| Anxiety neurosis | 0.2 | 18.5 | 1.7 | 16.9 |
| Phobic neurosis | 0.0 | 3.7 | 1.2 | 5.6 |
| Obsessional neurosis | 0.0 | 2.4 | 0.2 | 1.4 |
| Hypochondriacal neurosis | 0.5 | 0.2 | 0.5 | 0.2 |

*et al.*, 1992). In their view, the findings supported the idea of a general neurotic syndrome, with the majority of affected subjects having a prolonged course and variation in the predominance of different symptoms over time.

Another study of neurotic disorders in elderly community populations is the Guy's/Age Concern survey, which looked at anxiety disorders using the Anxiety Disorder Scale which employed non-hierarchical, non-judgemental diagnostic criteria, validated against clinical diagnosis (Lindesay *et al.*, 1989). The overall 1-month prevalence was 10% for phobic disorders, and 3.7% for GAD; rates were higher in women than in men, although this was only statistically significant for phobic disorders. No subject met DSM-III criteria for panic disorder. Another community survey using the same instrument found very similar prevalence rates of anxiety disorders (Manela *et al.*, 1996). Phobic disorders in the Guy's/Age Concern sample were examined further in a case–control study (Lindesay, 1991); cases had more neurotic symptoms than controls and higher rates of previous psychiatric disorders. One-third of the cases had their onset after the age of 65 years. Phobic subjects reported higher rates of contact with their general practitioners, but only a minority were receiving any form of treatment for their anxiety.

One interesting finding of the ECA study was that elderly subjects also had lower lifetime prevalence rates of depression and neurotic disorders than did younger groups; it is unclear whether this is a genuine cohort phenomenon or merely the result of a survivor effect or non-recall of past illness episodes by older adults (Klerman, 1988). In a review of epidemiological studies over the lifespan, Jorm (2000) concludes that there is evidence that old age may reduce the risk of anxiety and depression. However, other risk factors modify this effect, and it is difficult to separate ageing from cohort effects in cross-sectional studies. If there is an age effect, it may be the result of decreased emotional responsiveness, increased emotional control, or psychological immunization to stress. The relationship between anxiety disorders and age has also been reviewed by Krasucki *et al.* (1998).

Little is known about the longer-term course and outcome of neurotic disorders in old age. In the 3-year follow up study of Larkin *et al.* (1992), only 20% of the re-interviewed elderly cases had improved. In their review of studies of general adult populations, Marks and Lader (1973) concluded that 41–59% of cases of 'anxiety neurosis' (GAD and panic) were recovered or much improved at 1- to 20-year follow-up. Noyes and Clancy (1976) found that 33% of their patient sample was unchanged or worse at 5-year follow-up, and that later age of onset of anxiety was a predictor of poor outcome, particularly in men. In a 35-year follow-up of former panic patients Coryell (1984) found that they had an excess mortality. In particular, male patients had a higher rate of deaths from cardiovascular disease. Follow-up studies of general adult phobic populations have produced similar results, with about half of the subjects showing at least some improvement (Roberts, 1964; Agras *et al.*, 1972). A Scandinavian follow-up study of inpatients with 'pure' anxiety neurosis found an increased risk of suicide and unnatural deaths in subjects who died before the age of 70 years (Allgulander and Lavori, 1991). Suicide rates were also higher than expected in those patients with anxiety and/or depressive neurosis who survived until 71 years of age. Among this group, both men and women with 'pure' anxiety neurosis had a higher than expected mortality due to cardiac causes.

The chronic nature of these disorders at all ages means that over the long term, patients with neurotic disorders are high consumers of all types of health services (Leon *et al.*, 1995; Kennedy and Schwab, 1997). In a study of elderly patients in the UK, it was estimated that mean cost per month of community care for an individual without mental health problems was £32.52, compared with £86.96 for anxiety, £85.93 for depression, and £194.70 for dementia. The total estimated UK healthcare cost due to anxiety in old age was £750 million (Livingston *et al.*, 1997).

## Transcultural epidemiology

Evidence regarding the epidemiology of anxiety disorders in late life across different cultures and ethnic groups is still very limited, with most of it coming from studies of immigrant groups in Western populations. In the ECA study, phobic disorders were more prevalent in the Black and Hispanic groups aged 65 years and older, and the prevalence of panic disorder increased with age in Hispanic females, in contrast to the other groups. Rates of GAD did not appear to differ (Robins and Regier, 1991). In the UK, a study of elderly immigrant Gujarati Asians found that they had lower rates of simple phobia than the indigenous elderly population (Lindesay *et al.*, 1997). Research in this area is fraught with methodological difficulties, however, and more work is needed.

# Associated factors

## Biological

There has to date been little research into the biological aspects of neurotic disorders in the elderly population, and we are reliant on studies of younger subjects, and studies of elderly depressed patients where there is information about 'neurotic' subgroups. There are important limitations to much of this research: the subject samples are usually highly selected and unrepresentative; the study designs are rarely longitudinal; and 'old age' is always defined chronologically rather than biologically. In the absence of markers of biological age, however, it is not possible to determine to what extent ageing is in and of itself a biological risk factor for neurotic disorders in late life (Philpot, 1995).

## Genetics

Studies of the inheritance of neurotic disorders suggest that while there is a significant genetic component to vulnerability to these disorders as a group, it is not disorder-specific, and it is environmental factors that determine the particular form of illness that patients develop (Andrews *et al.*, 1990; Hettema *et al.*, 2001).

However, there is some evidence that the genetic heritability of OCD and panic disorder may be more specific (Marks, 1986; Torgersen, 1990). Genetic factors also contribute to the personality traits associated with vulnerability to neurotic disorders, such as fearfulness and neuroticism (Bouchard *et al.*, 1990; Middeldorp *et al.*, 2005), and to measures of arousal such as the galvanic skin response (Marks, 1986). No specific genetic loci have yet been identified or replicated in independent samples, but it is proposed that genetic variation within the neuronal serotonin system, particularly the serotonin transporter molecule, 5-HTT, may underlie differences in emotional regulation and in vulnerability to affective and anxiety disorders (Hariri and Holmes, 2006). The contribution of genetic factors to affective disorders diminishes with age, but it is not known if this is also true of neurotic disorders.

## Brain structure and function

There have been many structural and functional neuroimaging studies of elderly patients with affective disorders (see Chapter 13), but they provide only limited information about neuroses. The implication of CT studies is that patients with milder forms of depression and higher anxiety scores are more likely to have normal scans (Jacoby and Levy, 1980; Alexopoulos *et al.*, 1992). Magnetic resonance imaging (MRI) studies have shown that elderly depressed patients have more subcortical grey and white matter lesions (Coffey *et al.*, 1990), but it is not known if this also true for patients with neurotic disorders. Studies of post-stroke anxiety disorders show that the distribution of lesions differs from that in patients with post-stroke affective disorders, but they are not consistent as to location; for example, Sharpe *et al.* (1990) found anxiety to be related to the size of left-hemisphere lesions, whereas Castillo *et al.* (1993) found pure anxiety states to be associated with right-hemisphere lesions. Astrom (1996) has reported that in the acute phase following a stroke, GAD with depression was associated with left-hemispheric lesions on computed tomography (CT), whereas GAD alone was associated with right-hemispheric lesions. GAD was not related to frontality of lesion, lesion volume, subcortical versus cortical lesion, or cerebral atrophy. At 3-year follow-up, cerebral atrophy on a repeat CT scan was associated with both anxiety and depression.

Recent years have seen interesting developments in the use of both structural and functional neuroimaging studies in the study of some anxiety disorders. Post-traumatic stress disorder (PTSD) has been extensively studied, and there is now good evidence from structural imaging (Kitayama *et al.*, 2005) for a reduction in hippocampal volume associated with this disorder in adults. Using magnetic resonance spectroscopy, reduced *N*-acetyl aspartate (NAA), a marker of neuronal viability, has also been found in this region in PTSD (Schuff *et al.*, 2001). Other brain regions are also involved in the functional neuroanatomy of this disorder, with evidence of decreased function in the medial and dorsolateral pre-frontal cortex, and increased function in the posterior cingulate and parahippocampal gyrus.

While structural changes in the hippocampus or elsewhere in the brain have not been found in other anxiety disorders, there is evidence of altered function in this area in panic disorder (both increased and decreased) (Bremner, 2004). In simple phobias, presentation of the feared stimulus results in altered function in the visual association cortex, hippocampus, and the anterior paralimbic cortex; these alterations appear to return to normal following cognitive behaviour therapy (Mountz *et al.*, 1989; Paquette *et al.*, 2003). There is some suggestion that there may be a more specific activation of the amygdala in social phobia (Stein *et al.*, 2002). Functional imaging studies in OCD have shown that induction of obsessional thoughts is associated with increased orbitofrontal, caudate, and anterior cingulate blood flow (Rauch *et al.*, 1994; Breiter *et al.*, 1996). To date, there have been relatively few functional imaging studies of GAD, but one positron emission tomography (PET) study (Wu *et al.*, 1991) found that provocation of anxiety was associated with a relative increase in basal ganglia metabolism, and that benzodiazepines reduced metabolism in this area, as well as in cortical and limbic areas. Metabolic changes in these areas were also correlated with changes in anxiety scores following administration of placebo. A more recent magnetic spectroscopy study has found an increased NAA/creatinine ratio in the right dorsolateral pre-frontal cortex in patients with GAD (Matthew *et al.*, 2004). In a single photon emission computed tomography (SPECT) study of older men, state anxiety was associated with lower levels of blood flow in the dorsolateral pre-frontal cortex (Tankard *et al.*, 2003).

## Psychosocial

There is considerable evidence that psychosocial factors such as prolonged adversity, life events, early experiences, and social relationships have an important influence on the onset and course of neurotic disorders at all ages. Protective factors and those determining recovery have been less extensively studied, but these also need to be identified and understood if these disorders are to be effectively treated and prevented (Lindesay, 1995b).

## Adversity

At all ages, there is a clear relationship between psychological ill-health and indicators of social adversity such as low occupational class, unemployment, poor housing, overcrowding, and limited access to amenities such as transport (Harris, 1988; Champion, 1990; Singleton *et al.*, 2001). In the elderly population, the evidence for this association is strongest in studies that use dimensional scales for measuring anxiety and depression (Himmelfarb and Murrell, 1984; Kennedy *et al.*, 1989, 1990). The relationship between adversity and categorical definitions of cases is less clear; in the ECA study there was no association between DSM-III affective disorders and socio-economic variables, and among neurotic disorders, only GAD was associated with low household income. Phobic disorders in the elderly population are associated with urban domicile in some studies (Walton *et al.*, 1990; Blazer *et al.*, 1991) but not others (Beekman *et al.*, 1998); this may not be an indicator of adversity so much as of poor social networks. Beekman *et al.* (1998) found an association between DSM-III anxiety disorders and lower levels of education. It would appear that adversity increases levels of distress, but may be less important as an aetiological factor in the development of more severe disorders.

There are several ways in which social adversity causes psychological ill-health in elderly people; for example, through increased levels of physical illness, and higher rates of adverse life events. Brown and Harris (1978) identified poor self-esteem as an important mediator between adverse social circumstances and psychiatric disorder in their study of young women. It is not clear whether this is applicable to elderly people, since self-esteem appears to be very resilient in late life (Baltes and Baltes, 1990). It may be that those who have endured a lifetime of hardship will be better equipped to cope with adversity in old age than those for whom it is a new experience (Fillenbaum *et al.*, 1985).

## Life events

Adverse life events are a significant class of provoking agent which determine the onset of some psychiatric disorders in vulnerable individuals. The best evidence comes from studies using investigator-rated events (Brown and Harris, 1978, 1989); most studies have been carried out in young adults, although Murphy (1982) has shown the importance of life events in relation to depression in elderly people. It is the meaning of the event to the individual, rather than its severity, that appears to be important (Brown *et al.*, 1987),

and different types of event in terms of their particular meaning may provoke the onset of different disorders. For example, in the Longitudinal Aging Study Amsterdam, loss events (death of partner) predicted the onset of depression, and threat events (conflict with/illness of partner) predicted anxiety (de Beurs *et al.*, 2001). Positive 'fresh start' and 'anchoring' events have also been shown to contribute to recovery in younger patients with depression and anxiety respectively (Brown *et al.*, 1992; Brown, 1993). Only some life events are followed by disorder, and only some disorders are preceded by life events, so in the individual case the occurrence of a preceding life event does not mean that there are no other aetiologically important factors, and these should always be looked for (Murphy, 1986).

Some classes of life event, such as bereavement, retirement, and institutionalization, are commoner in old age than at other times of life, but their psychological impact is still under-researched. Bereavement appears to take the same form and follow the same course in old age as it does earlier in life, with a short-term increase in the rates of depressive and anxiety disorders in the year following widowhood (Onrust and Cuijpers, 2006). The 'timeliness' of some losses in old age may reduce their impact (Davis, 1994); in one study, the only significant predictor of persistent grief in elderly men was the unexpectedness of their spouses' death (Byrne and Raphael, 1994). It is not known if psychiatric morbidity following bereavement is more or less common in elderly people compared with other age groups. Significant anxiety following bereavement in old age may be associated with the subsequent persistence of depression (Prigerson *et al.*, 1996a). Retirement is the event that defines the beginning of 'old age' for many people, and the association with mental health problems varies with age. Statutory retirement age is associated with marked reductions in depression and anxiety, whereas rates are increased in early retirees (Villamil *et al.*, 2006), perhaps due to associated physical ill-health. Institutionalization is a profound loss event, and one that is experienced by a particularly physically and mentally vulnerable part of the elderly population. Most studies have been of established residents, and while many have shown poor quality of life and high levels of depression, it is not possible to distinguish between the impact of the transitional process and the effect of the institutional environment. Longitudinal studies suggest that factors such as pre-admission vulnerability, the degree of difference between home and institution, and the amount of choice and control the individual has in the admission process are important determinants of subsequent well-being (Tobin and Liebermann, 1976).

Exposure to extreme catastrophe can cause significant psychological disturbance, and because of the close relationship of these stress reactions to acute or continuing trauma they are now classified as specific diagnoses in DSM-IV and ICD-10, notably post-traumatic stress disorder (PTSD). Little is known about the long-term effect of severely traumatic experiences, although PTSD can persist for many years. Its onset may also be delayed, sometimes manifesting itself for the first time in old age following retirement or an adverse life event (Scaturo and Hyman, 1992; Kaup *et al.*, 1994). Many people who are now elderly were exposed to severe trauma during the Second World War, and it appears that what we now call PTSD was common then and has been persistent. In one study of US ex-prisoners of war, 67% had suffered from PTSD at the time, and only 27% had fully recovered (Kluznik *et al.*, 1986). Another recent study of 800 Second World War prisoners of war found that 80% had persistent nightmares, and that those who had been imprisoned for longer periods and who had been subjected to more severe stress were more likely to meet the diagnostic criteria for PTSD (Guerrero and Crocq, 1994). Traumatic wartime experiences have an enduring effect on a significant minority of older people, particularly more vulnerable groups such as psychiatric patients or those in long-term care (Rosen *et al.*, 1989; Hermann and Eryavec, 1994), and health professionals need to be aware of this when making assessments. Now that PTSD sufferers are eligible for financial compensation, increasing numbers of veterans are coming forward for diagnosis and treatment, and psychiatric services will need to develop more effective assessment and management strategies for dealing with this problem.

### Early experience

Experiences such as early parental loss and physical and sexual abuse in childhood are significant vulnerability factors for depression and other psychiatric disorders in adult life, although their significance in old age has not been extensively studied. Depression is associated with early maternal loss in young women (Brown and Harris, 1978), but Murphy (1982) did not find any relationship between depression and parental loss in her elderly sample. So far as anxiety disorders are concerned, studies have shown a link, in both young adulthood and old age, between phobic disorders, particularly agoraphobia, and early parental loss (Faravelli *et al.*, 1985; Tweed *et al.*, 1989; Lindesay, 1991). GAD has also been linked with early parental loss in men (Zahner and Murphy, 1989). Most interest has focused on maternal loss, but there is some evidence that anxiety disorders may be related more to loss or departure of the father (Finlay-Jones, 1989; Lindesay, 1991). It appears that it is not the parental loss that is important so much as the associated experiences such as prior marital conflict or subsequent inadequate care (Tennant *et al.*, 1982). Presumably these experiences affect the developing personality and result in particular cognitive habits and 'defence styles' (Pollock and Andrews, 1989) that determine the responses to adverse events and experiences in later life. In a study of 50 elderly spousal carers of terminally ill patients, childhood adversity, together with paranoid, histrionic, or self-defeating personality styles, directly increased the odds of having a DSM-III anxiety disorder (Prigerson *et al.*, 1996b). Beekman *et al.* (1998) found that external locus of control was a significant vulnerability factor for anxiety disorders in their community sample (see Case study 1).

### Case study 1

A 77-year-old widow developed generalized agoraphobia following a mugging in the street. In addition, she had a severe but untroublesome mouse phobia which had persisted since childhood. There was no other formal psychiatric history, but she described herself as 'a lifelong worrier' who always responded to threats and challenges by avoiding them. She attributed this tendency to her disrupted childhood; her father died when she was a baby and her mother was hospitalized for long periods, with the result that the patient had spent most of her early years in children's homes.

The role of abuse in childhood in determining vulnerability to psychiatric disorder in old age is still unexplored in any detail, but general population and primary care surveys of adults of all ages indicate that childhood physical and sexual abuse have adverse

effects on both physical and mental health across the lifespan (Briere and Elliott, 2003; Spertus *et al.*, 2003). One small clinical study has suggested an association between childhood sexual abuse and panic disorder in old age (Sheikh *et al.*, 1994).

### Relationships

Cross-sectional studies usually show an association between psychological ill-health and reduced levels of social support. However, it is not clear from these whether psychiatric disorder leads to social withdrawal, or whether lack of social relationships increases vulnerability to disorder. On this point, follow-up studies are inconsistent in their findings; Blazer (1983) found that depression was associated with increased levels of social support 13 months later, whereas Oxman *et al.* (1992) found that reduced social support was associated with increased depression at 3-year follow-up. The quality of social relationships is as important as the quantity, and it appears to be the lack of an intimate confidant that particularly increases vulnerability to depression in old age (Murphy, 1982; Blazer, 1983; Kennedy *et al.*, 1989). Of course, the lack of a confidant in old age may reflect a long-standing difficulty in forming and sustaining close relationships, and Murphy (1986) has argued that it is this that increases vulnerability to life events. Regarding the association between anxiety and either the presence or absence of intimate relationships, the evidence is mixed. Some studies have not found any relationship (Finlay-Jones, 1989; Lindesay, 1991), but in the Longitudinal Aging Study Amsterdam anxiety disorders were associated with smaller contact networks and with loneliness (Beekman *et al.*, 1998).

### Physical illness

Neurotic disorders in old age are associated with increased mortality and physical morbidity in community populations (Kay and Bergmann, 1966; Lindesay, 1990; Beekman *et al.*, 1998; Ostir and Goodwin, 2006), and in both psychiatric and medical patients (Bergmann, 1971; Burn *et al.*, 1993). There are several reasons why neurotic and physical disorders are linked in old age.

#### Physical illness causing neurotic disorders

The onset of physical illness is an important life event that most elderly people have to negotiate at some time, and in most it will evoke some degree of anxiety and sadness, particularly if the illness is painful, life-threatening, or disabling. In some, this response may be sufficiently severe to qualify as an adjustment disorder (Pitt, 1995), and in a few vulnerable individuals it may trigger the onset of an anxiety or depressive disorder. For example, mild, chronic anxiety symptoms are relatively common following myocardial infarction in old age (Peach and Pathy, 1979), and in a few cases this can develop into a severe and disabling 'cardiac neurosis', often focused on somatic anxiety symptoms such as palpitations. Such anxiety about physical illness can have important behavioural consequences: the onset of agoraphobia after the age of 65 years is attributed in most cases to the experience of a physical health event such as a myocardial infarct, a fracture, or elective surgery (Lindesay, 1990). These and other traumatic experiences, such as falls or muggings, probably play a similar aetiological role to that of panic attacks in younger adults in precipitating loss of confidence, fear, and avoidance in vulnerable individuals. The fear of falling associated with balance disorders and mobility problems appears to be a common cause of disabling secondary avoidance in older adults

(Marks, 1981; Isaacs, 1992). Since the experience of physical health events is an important precipitant of agoraphobia in old age, the identification and rehabilitation of elderly medical and surgical patients at risk may be an effective preventive strategy (see Case study 2).

---

### Case study 2

An active 81-year-old widow with no previous history of psychiatric disorder sustained a minor injury after falling off a bus as it pulled away. She made a full physical recovery, but in the year following this accident she gradually lost confidence in going out by herself, and eventually became totally housebound unless accompanied by her daughter. She also developed severe episodes of free-floating anxiety associated with thoughts of the accident, and mild depression secondary to her isolation and restricted mobility. Her anxiety disorder only came to the attention of the health services because a psychiatric report was required to support her claim against the bus company.

---

A number of studies have examined the prevalence and course of anxiety following specific physical illnesses. Anxiety disorders are common following stroke, both in the acute phase and at medium- to long-term (1–5 years) follow-up (Sharpe et al., 1990; Burvill et al., 1995; Astrom, 1996; Schultz et al., 1997), with prevalence figures ranging from 5–28%. Agoraphobia is the most common disorder in this population (9–20%), followed by GAD. One- to 3-year outcome studies of post-stroke anxiety disorders show that only around a quarter to a half have resolved at 12 months. Non-resolution of symptoms at 12 months is associated with chronic course and poor functional outcome over 3 years. The presence of co-morbid depression not only adversely affects the responsiveness to treatment but also increases mortality. Follow-up studies of patients with acute myocardial infarction have also reported that depression and anxiety independently predict a higher rate of subsequent cardiac events (Frasure-Smith et al., 1995). In their review, Lenze et al. (2001) comment on the extent to which depression, anxiety, and physical disability are mutually reinforcing.

It is not only acute episodes of physical ill-health that provoke anxiety and fear in elderly people. Chronic disability due to conditions such as arthritis and sensory impairment is also associated with high rates of subjective anxiety and avoidance (Kay et al., 1987; Lindesay, 1990; Beekman et al., 1998), perhaps because they heighten the individual's sense of vulnerability and awareness of the grave consequences of possible future adverse events.

### Physical illness mimicking neurotic disorders

A number of physical disorders may present with apparently neurotic symptoms in old age, and these are considered in the discussion of the differential diagnosis of neurotic disorders below.

### Neurotic disorders mimicking physical illness

Neurotic disorders at all ages are associated with a variety of somatic symptoms such as palpitations, dysphagia, nausea, altered bowel habit, paraesthesia, and pain. It is a common clinical impression that the somatization of psychological distress is commoner in elderly patients, but to some extent this may be due to a selection bias, since it is the individuals who complain of physical symptoms of anxiety and depression who will be most likely to make it through the 'filters' and present to medical services. Anxious and depressed elderly people are also more likely to be concerned about trivial physical problems which will lead them to consult their doctors. The somatization of anxiety in elderly patients is discussed further below.

### Neurotic disorders causing physical illness

Neurotic disorders may cause physical illness by direct or indirect effects on bodily function. Most important in this respect are the higher rates of damaging behaviours such as smoking and alcohol abuse. Among younger adults, phobic anxiety is commoner in smokers than non-smokers (Haines et al., 1980); if anxious, avoidant individuals are more likely to be (or have been) smokers, it may be that the increased rates of cardiovascular and respiratory illness observed in association with anxiety disorders in elderly people are a result of this. In the Northwick Park heart study, phobic anxiety was strongly related to subsequent ischaemic heart disease in men aged 40–64 years (Haines et al., 1987). However, smoking did not explain the association in this sample, and it was suggested that anxiety-related hyperventilation might cause coronary artery spasm, or that subjects with phobic anxiety might have exaggerated hormonal responses to myocardial infarction. Kubzansky et al., (1998) have proposed on the basis of data from the Normative Aging Study that anxiety is associated with abnormal autonomic cardiac control and increased risk of arrhythmias.

## Clinical assessment and diagnosis

It is evident from the epidemiology and associations of neurotic disorder in old age that health professionals need to be more alert to the possibility of these conditions in their patients, and aware of the ways in which they may present. These disorders have psychological and somatic symptoms, and are often associated with particular disturbances of behaviour. For the most part, these are similar to those seen in younger adults, but there are some important differences in how they manifest themselves.

### Psychological symptoms

The depressive symptomatology that may accompany neurotic disorders is described in Chapter 29ii. So far as anxiety is concerned, patients' preoccupations are usually focused on topics that are of concern to most elderly people, such as physical illness, finances, crime, and the family. The fears and phobias described by elderly people are similar to those found in younger adults: animals, heights, enclosed spaces, public transport, going out of doors (Lindesay et al., 1989). Severe anxiety about death appears to be less common than might be supposed in this age group, perhaps because elderly people are more familiar with it (Kay, 1988). Clinically important worries and fears in elderly people are often dismissed as reasonable simply because of the patient's age. In fact, an elderly person's perception of their vulnerability is determined more by factors such as physical disability and the availability of social support, and it is these rather than age that should be taken into account when judging the reasonableness of fears.

The clinical features of OCD in elderly patients are broadly similar to those seen in younger adults (Kohn et al., 1997). It is rare for obsessional symptoms to appear for the first time in old age, although instances have been reported (Bajulaiye and Addonizio, 1992). More often, cases that present in old age are long-standing disorders that have never been adequately assessed or treated (Jenike, 1989). Some late onset cases may be due to external factors, such as adverse life events, that weaken an elderly individual's resistance to long-standing subclinical obsessionality (Colvin and Boddington, 1997). It is important therefore that all elderly patients receive thorough evaluation and the benefit of modern treatments as and when they present to psychogeriatric services (Austin *et al.*, 1991). In old age, the late appearance of apparently obsessional orderliness and preoccupation with routines may presage the onset of dementia, particularly if the frontal lobe is involved (Neary, 1990). Obsessional symptoms may also appear at any age following head injury or cerebral tumour; in such cases, apparently obsessional and stereotypic behaviour is not preceded by mounting anxiety or followed by a release of tension.

## Somatic symptoms

The somatic symptoms of anxiety in elderly people are also similar to those occurring at other ages. These include the full range of autonomic symptoms, muscular tension pains, motor restlessness, globus hystericus, dyspnoea, and the effects of hyperventilation. In elderly patients, however, they may be wrongly attributed by both the patient and the doctor to physical illness, with the result that their significance is missed and the patient is subjected instead to unnecessary investigations and treatments. Careful enquiry into the circumstances surrounding the onset of the symptoms, and the accompanying mood, is usually sufficient to determine their origin. Most elderly patients who misattribute the symptoms of psychological distress to physical illness will readily accept the real cause when it is explained to them, but a minority are extremely resistant and will meet the criteria for a somatization disorder. In these individuals, the somatization of psychological disturbance will usually have started early in life, but they may have been skilled at avoiding psychiatrists in youth and adulthood, only presenting to psychiatric services for the first time in old age. They are usually accompanied by a voluminous medical history of negative investigations, unhelpful treatments, and complicating iatrogenic problems. Studies of clinical populations suggest that somatization disorder does not ameliorate substantially with age (Pribor *et al.*, 1994), although as they get older these patients may transfer their concern to genuine organic symptoms.

In contrast to patients with somatization, who have multiple physical complaints and who demand relief from their distress, the focus of hypochondriacal patients is usually restricted to one or two body organs or systems. Typically, they are preoccupied with the possibility of serious illness, and their demand is for investigation rather than treatment. In elderly patients, primary hypochondriasis is usually of long standing; if it presents for the first time in old age it is more likely to be a secondary manifestation of depression or anxiety.

Hysterical symptoms in elderly patients are an important exception to the general rule that neurotic symptoms in old age have the same diagnostic significance as in younger adults. As Bergmann (1978) has said, 'it is best to assert dogmatically that primary hysterical illness does not begin in old age'. Apparently dissociative symptoms are usually due either to underlying undiagnosed physical illness or to the release of old hysterical tendencies in vulnerable personalities by organic cerebral pathology or functional psychiatric disorder (Case study 3).

---

## Case study 3

A 65-year-old man whose wife was dying of dementia was admitted to hospital following the appearance of dysphasic symptoms similar to his wife's when he was particularly distressed. Physical examination was normal, and this was initially diagnosed as a dissociative disorder, but further investigation revealed that he was suffering from neurosyphilis, and his condition greatly improved following treatment.

---

Panic in old age may also be a significant cause of misdiagnosed somatic symptoms. Despite the considerable amount of research that has been carried out into panic in recent years, little is known about this condition in the elderly population. Cross-sectional epidemiological studies suggest that it is rare, and a number of explanations have been put forward to account for this (Flint *et al.*, 1996). However, its prevalence may be underestimated by survey methodology, given the chronic episodic nature of the disorder. The limited evidence from case reports and series (Luchins and Rose, 1989; Frances and Flaherty, 1989; Sheikh *et al.*, 2004), volunteer samples (Sheikh *et al.*, 1991), and non-psychiatric patient populations (Katon, 1984; Beitman *et al.*, 1991) suggest that panic in old age is less common than in early adulthood, is commoner in women and widows, and late onset cases are less severe in terms of symptoms, levels of distress, and secondary avoidance than those whose disorder started earlier in life. Elderly panic patients tend not present to psychiatric services (Thyer *et al.*, 1985; Kenardy *et al.*, 1990), but because of the prominent physical symptoms they may be referred instead for investigation and treatment to cardiologists, neurologists, and gastroenterologists. In a study of cardiology patients with chest pain and no evidence of coronary artery disease, one-third of those aged 65 years and over met diagnostic criteria for panic disorder (Beitman *et al.*, 1991). At all ages, there is extensive co-morbidity between panic disorder and somatization disorder (Boyd *et al.*, 1984), and patients with panic are often misdiagnosed by their GPs as chronic somatizers (Katon, 1984). In late onset cases, the possibility of depression or an iatrogenic cause such as dopamine agonist treatment for Parkinson's disease should be considered.

A common somatic symptom of anxiety in elderly patients is delayed or interrupted sleep due to worry and nightmares, and this is often the presenting complaint in those who seek medical help. Daytime tiredness is common in those with GAD, and specific fears or rituals associated with bedtime may interfere with the sleep routines of phobic and obsessional patients. As a group, patients with sleep disturbance due to a neurotic disorder often have problems with chronic hypnotic, sedative, and alcohol abuse. The effective management of disturbed sleep is an important aspect of the care of these patients (see below).

## Behaviour disturbance

The psychological and somatic symptoms of anxiety and depression can have important adverse behavioural consequences. Many of the neurotic responses to somatic symptoms discussed above can be understood as forms of abnormal illness behaviour. Another important behavioural consequence of anxiety and panic is the phobic avoidance of feared objects and situations. Lifelong avoidance is unlikely to present as a problem in old age unless a change in circumstances makes this avoidance impossible, such as the death of a spouse who used to do the shopping. Late onset agoraphobic avoidance is more likely to be restricting, but if it is rewarded with the provision of domiciliary services and well-meaning family support, it will not present as a problem either. Sometimes cases present as a family problem if they become over-dependent on others for support.

Chronic psychological distress may also lead to the use and abuse of sedative drugs and alcohol. As a group, elderly people are among the heaviest consumers of psychotropic drugs, particularly repeat prescriptions of benzodiazepine tranquillizers and hypnotics (Catalan *et al.*, 1988). Less is known about the extent of alcohol abuse as a result of anxiety and depression in old age, but about one-third of elderly alcohol abusers appear to have started late in life as the result of 'stress' (Rosin and Glatt, 1971; Gurnack and Thomas, 1989). An eating disorder may re-emerge in late life as a maladaptive coping strategy in an individual who is having difficulty in adjusting to their old age (Bowler, 1995).

## Assessment scales

Over the years, a wide range of instruments have been used to identify and measure anxiety in elderly patients. Few of the available scales have been specifically developed for use with the elderly population, but some, such as the Fear Questionnaire and the State-Trait Anxiety Inventory (STAI), have been shown to have acceptable internal reliability in older people (Fuentes and Cox, 2000). More recently, some elderly-specific instruments have been developed, such as the 10-item Short Anxiety Screening Test (SAST) in medical inpatients and outpatients (Sinoff *et al.*, 1999), the four-item FEAR in elderly primary care attenders (Krasucki *et al.*, 1999), and RAID in elderly patients with dementia (Shankar *et al.*, 1999). Another recent development with promising psychometric properties is the self-report Geriatric Anxiety Inventory (GAI; Pachana *et al.*, 2006).

## Differential diagnosis

### Depression

In view of the extensive co-morbidity between neurotic disorders and depression, and the fact that depressive symptoms are often an integral component of the neurotic disorder, it is not useful to consider them as strict diagnostic alternatives. In their review of the evidence, Lenze *et al.* (2001) estimate that 85% of older adults with depression also have significant symptoms of anxiety. In studies of elderly subjects using GMS/AGECAT, anxiety disorders were 20 times more likely to occur in depressed than non-depressed subjects (Kay, 1988). Elderly subjects with phobic disorders report an increased history of depression compared with controls (Lindesay, 1990). Clinical experience suggests that late onset anxiety in elderly patients is nearly always associated with some degree of depression, but it should be borne in mind that it is the currently or previously depressed cases who will be more likely to present or be known to services.

The possibility that anxious, hypochondriacal, and obsessional individuals are also depressed (and vice versa) should always be considered, since treating one part of the problem may not alleviate the other (Blazer *et al.*, 1989). For example, if an elderly person is depressed because of the restrictions imposed by agoraphobia, it is not sufficient to prescribe antidepressants without attending to the underlying cause. Certain clinical features such as pronounced hypochondriasis, anhedonia, guilt, agitation, or panic attacks are highly indicative of associated depression requiring treatment in its own right. Co-morbid anxiety may have an adverse effect on treatment outcome, reducing responsiveness to antidepressants, and increasing discontinuation rates. Persistence of anxiety following remission of the depression is associated with quicker relapse (Flint and Rifat, 1997a,b) (Case study 4).

### Case study 4

A 79-year-old man was referred to the local psychiatric service by his general practitioner for the assessment of an anxiety state, which had developed following a minor head injury the previous year. His principal complaints were severe anxiety with both subjective and somatic symptoms, panic attacks at night, and generalized agoraphobic avoidance associated with a fear of falling. On examination, however, it was apparent that he was also severely depressed, with early morning wakening, hypochondriacal delusions, and auditory hallucinations urging him to commit suicide. He was admitted to hospital and, following treatment with an antidepressant, the depression, subjective anxiety, and panic all resolved. He was discharged home, but at follow-up he remained agoraphobic. This required further outpatient treatment with a programme of graded desensitization.

### Dementia

Krasucki *et al.* (1998) have suggested that anxiety disorders may predispose to cognitive impairment in later life, resulting in a 'diagnostic shift' towards the latter that might explain the observed decline in the prevalence of anxiety disorders with age. This idea remains speculative, although there is some epidemiological evidence to support an association, at least in the case of GAD (Manela *et al.*, 1996). It is certainly true that in the early stages dementia may reveal itself through symptoms such as anxiety or obsessionality (Wands *et al.*, 1990; Ballard *et al.*, 1994); however, it should be borne in mind that anxiety alone can impair performance on tests of cognitive function. In the later stages of dementia, anxiety is associated with agitation and is probably one of its causes (Twelftree and Qazi, 2006). Anxiety in demented patients may be associated with depressive or psychotic symptoms, or with their concerns about implications of the disorder and its impact on social functioning (Ballard *et al.*, 1996). Studies have yet to examine the possibility that the neurodegenerative process in Alzheimer's disease is itself a cause of anxiety.

The reported prevalence of anxiety symptoms and anxiety disorders in subjects with dementia ranges from 3% to 38% (Wands *et al.*, 1990; Forsell and Winblad, 1997). Whether the prevalence of anxiety in demented individuals is higher than in age-matched controls is unclear, but the evidence suggests that it is rates of symptoms rather than disorders that are elevated. There does not appear to be any correlation between anxiety and severity of cognitive impairment, but the expression of anxiety may change as the dementia progresses; in more severely demented patients anxiety may manifest itself as agitation. Patients with vascular dementia may be more prone to develop anxiety symptoms than those with Alzheimer's disease (Sultzer *et al.*, 1993).

Dementia also puts a considerable strain on carers, and their rates of anxiety symptoms and disorders have been consistently found to be significantly higher than controls (Dura *et al.*, 1991; Russo *et al.*, 1995). One study has found that carers' subjective competence is related to their neuroticism and the behaviour problems in the patient, but not to the formal support and help that they receive (Vernooij-Dassen *et al.*, 1996).

### Delirium

Although delirium in the elderly is usually relatively 'quiet', affected individuals are sometimes terrified by their hallucinations and imagined persecutions, and may present as panic rather than delirium. Panic attacks are uncommon in old age, and the abrupt onset of terror should be regarded as a sign of delirium until proved otherwise, particularly if there is evidence of cognitive impairment and the individual is physically ill. Careful examination of the mental state and a history from an informant will usually determine the presence or absence of other features of delirium, such as attentional deficits, fluctuating level of consciousness, and perceptual disturbances. Very occasionally, anxiety itself may induce delirium in vulnerable individuals.

### Paranoid states and schizophrenia

Occasionally, the fear and anxiety accompanying a functional psychosis may be mistaken for a simple anxiety state. However, a careful history and examination will usually reveal the underlying psychotic experiences and beliefs. Peculiar hypochondriacal preoccupations can sometimes be difficult to distinguish from monosymptomatic delusional disorders.

### Physical illness

In view of the important association between neurotic disorders and physical illness in old age, assessment should always include a thorough physical examination to exclude any primary physical cause of the neurotic symptoms. Some of the physical causes of neurotic symptoms in elderly patients are listed in Table 30.4. In particular, a number of important cardiovascular, respiratory, and endocrine disorders may present atypically with anxiety or depression and little else in this age group. A physical cause for neurotic symptoms should be considered if there is no psychiatric history, and no sufficient current stress in the patient's life to account for the mental disturbance. Anxiety symptoms can also be caused by prescribed drugs such as oral hypoglycaemics and corticosteroids, or by substances such as caffeine and over-the-counter preparations containing sympathomimetics (Lader, 1982). Drug withdrawal is also likely to lead to anxiety if the patient is physically dependent. Similarly, the erratic use of very short-acting hypnotics, such as triazolam, may cause rebound withdrawal during the day. In patients with a physical cause for their neurotic symptoms, these usually remit with treatment of the underlying disorder.

### Sleep disorders

At all ages, depression and anxiety are the commonest causes of sleep disturbance, and should be considered in any patient presenting with this problem (Bramble, 1995). Other causes of disturbed sleep in elderly patients include insomnia due to physical disability and pain, sleep apnoea, restless legs syndrome, and periodic leg movements syndrome. (see also Chapter 36).

## Management

Despite the greater clinical awareness of neurotic disorders in elderly patients nowadays, many still go unrecognized and untreated. In the minority who do receive treatment, this usually takes the form of medication with anxiolytic and hypnotic drugs, and few patients receive any form of psychological intervention (Lindesay *et al.*, 1991). This over-reliance on drugs and the neglect of alternatives is unfortunate, since the latter are much safer and may well be more effective in the long-term management of neurotic symptoms in this age group.

Since most cases of neurotic disorder in elderly patients are seen in primary care and general medical settings, this is where the focus

**Table 30.4** Physical causes of neurotic symptoms in the elderly (Pitt, 1995)

| | |
|---|---|
| Cardiovascular | Myocardial infarction |
| | Cardiac arrhythmias |
| | Orthostatic hypotension |
| | Mitral valve prolapse |
| Respiratory | Pneumonia |
| | Pulmonary embolism |
| | Emphysema |
| | Asthma |
| | Left-ventricular failure |
| | Hypoxia |
| | Chronic obstructive airways disease |
| | Bronchial carcinoma |
| Endocrine and metabolic | Hypo- and hyperthyroidism |
| | Hypo- and hypercalcaemia |
| | Cushing's disease |
| | Carcinoid syndrome |
| | Hypoglycaemia |
| | Insulinoma |
| | Phaeochromocytoma |
| | Hyperkalaemia |
| | Hypokalaemia |
| | Hypothermia |
| Neurological | Head injury |
| | Cerebral tumour |
| | Dementia |
| | Delirium |
| | Epilepsy |
| | Migraine |
| | Cerebral lupus erythematosus |
| | Demyelinating disease |
| | Vestibular disturbance |
| | Subarachnoid haemorrhage |
| | CNS infections |
| Dietary and drug related | Caffeine |
| | Vitamin deficiencies |
| | Anaemia |
| | Sympathomimetics |
| | Dopamine agonists |
| | Corticosteroids |
| | Withdrawal syndromes |
| | Akathisia |
| | Digoxin toxicity |
| | Fluoxetine |

of identification and treatment should be. Specialist psychogeriatric services have only a limited role in the management of these patients, particularly in the long term, but they are a valuable source of expertise and should aim to offer advice and education in appropriate management strategies to primary care and general hospital staff. For example, one group of patients who are mismanaged by most health professionals are the 'heartsink' group with long-standing mood disturbance and hypochondriacal preoccupations, persistent insomnia, and dependence on anxiolytic and hypnotic medication. While it is probably optimistic to hope for complete cure in such cases, there is much that can be done provided that there is a firm and consistent strategy. In the first place, there should be a single individual (ideally the general practitioner) responsible for coordinating the various aspects of care, and this should be made clear to all concerned, particularly the patient and their family. Two important functions of the coordinating practitioner are to rationalize existing medication and to ensure that the patient does not receive unnecessary investigations or treatments. If somatic complaints are a particular problem, the patient should be offered regular check-ups rather than consultation on demand. There is little point in engaging in battles over the cause of complaints; the best approach is simply to express understanding of the patient's distress, agree that they need help, and reassure them that they are being cared for. Once a reasonably positive relationship is established, it may eventually be possible to engage the patient in an examination of cognitions and dynamics (Case study 5).

---

### Case study 5

A 72-year-old woman was referred to the local psychogeriatric service by her exasperated GP. She and her husband had been patients of the practice for many years, both attending regularly with an ever-changing repertoire of non-specific somatic complaints. The routine of joint attendance at the surgery to complain and collect their repeat prescriptions for night sedation was broken by the sudden death of her husband from a heart attack. Subsequently, her demands on the practice escalated to the point where she was calling the GP at home at night to demand home visits. When these were refused, she started to importune the neighbours and on one occasion was taken to casualty following a collapse in the street. The psychogeriatrician's opinion was that this severe exacerbation of her long-standing anxiety state was a bereavement reaction, complicated by anger against the GP over the death of her husband. Following a joint meeting of the patient, the GP, and the psychogeriatrician, it was agreed that the GP would undertake to physically examine the patient and listen to all complaints once a week, provided that no other demands were made. The GP was also instructed in appropriate strategies for addressing the patient's anxious and angry thoughts. After 2 months, the frequency of these contacts was reduced to once a month, and the patient agreed to attempt a gradual withdrawal of her night sedation.

---

## Psychological treatments

### Cognitive behavioural

Cognitive behaviour therapy (CBT) for neurotic disorders is of proven benefit in younger adults, but its effectiveness has only recently begun to be evaluated in elderly patients. However, individual case reports and case series of successful treatments in elderly patients with GAD, phobic disorders, and OCD (Thyer, 1981; Woods and Britton, 1985; Downs et al., 1988; Colvin and Boddington, 1997; Mohlman, 2004) show that this approach can be successfully applied to this age group. CBT has also been evaluated in elderly patients with depression, prolonged grief, and panic with encouraging results (e.g. Thompson et al., 1987; King and Barrowclough, 1991). While systematic reviews have shown CBT in elderly patients with GAD to be superior to no treatment, the effect size is relatively modest at about 0.5 (Nordhus and Pallesen, 2003). It is not yet clear if CBT outperforms other interventions for late-life anxiety such as supportive therapy (Mohlman, 2004). To date, most studies have involved small numbers of young-old, well-educated females, and it is not clear to what extent the results are generalizable to other groups. CBT in elderly patients also appears to be associated with high rates of attrition (Mohlman, 2004), so retention strategies may be important to maximize the treatment effect.

CBT involves both the cognitive and behavioural approaches to conceptualizing and modifying the disturbances in thinking and behaviour that characterize neurotic disorders. Although theoretically distinct they are in practice rarely carried out in isolation, and procedures such as anxiety management training draw heavily on both models (Woods, 1995). Cognitive therapy involves identifying, evaluating, controlling, and changing the negative thoughts, cognitive distortions, and false attributions that occur in anxiety and depression. For example, in an elderly anxious patient this might involve challenging the misattribution of autonomic anxiety symptoms to physical disease, or the automatic thoughts about vulnerability that maintain agoraphobic avoidance. In behaviour therapy, on the other hand, it is the concepts of conditioning, reinforcement, and avoidance that underlie clinical strategies such as desensitization for phobic disorders and habituation for obsessional rumination. CBT may be carried out both individually and in groups. The advantages of groups are that there is better evidence for efficacy, they are more cost-effective, and they also harness useful peer support which often persists after the formal treatment has finished (Zerhusen et al., 1991). However, it can be difficult and time-consuming to assemble groups in which the members are sufficiently similar to ensure they work well together and do not exclude or scapegoat particular individuals. While the principles of applying CBT to elderly patients are the same as for younger adults, the goals and techniques may need to be adapted in some cases, for example if there is significant physical disability or cognitive impairment (Woods, 1995; Koder, 1998). It has been suggested that elderly patients are less psychologically minded and so less likely to be able to use CBT, but there is no good evidence to support this; factors such as education and socio-cultural background are probably more important in this respect. CBT may also be effective in lowering the risk of relapse by reducing underlying vulnerability factors such as neuroticism and locus of control (Andrews, 1996) (see also Chapter 18ii).

### Psychodynamics

As Martindale (1995) has pointed out, some knowledge of psychodynamics is of great value when assessing elderly patients, particularly if their disorders involve difficulties in negotiating the developmental issues of late life, or the inappropriate and maladaptive use of defence mechanisms. Formal psychodynamic treatments and techniques, particularly in group settings, are also useful in the treatment of neurotic disorders in elderly patients. These are discussed in depth in Chapter 18v.

## Physical treatments

Medication has an important role in the treatment of neurotic disorders in elderly patients, but much current practice is still insufficiently careful, rational, or discriminating. Before starting an elderly patient on any psychotropic medication there are a number of important factors to consider. First, thorough assessment and accurate diagnosis are the necessary foundations of effective management. Second, consider available non-pharmacological alternatives (see above). Medication is only one part of a comprehensive plan that also includes psychological and social interventions, patient education, lifestyle advice, bibliotherapy, and supportive counselling. In the absence of compelling evidence for a particular form of treatment, patient preference and choice are important considerations. Third, 'start low and go slow'. Many of the drugs used in the management of anxiety are less efficiently metabolized and eliminated in elderly patients. Fourth, set clear goals for the treatment at the outset. These might include: symptom relief without sedation; improvement in sleep; freedom from adverse physical and cognitive side-effects; and avoidance of physical dependence and drug interactions. Fifth, give an adequate trial of treatment. Some drugs, e.g. antidepressants, can take some weeks to have their full effect. Sixth, at the outset, decide how long the course of anxiolytic drug treatment will be. Many patients end up with repeat prescriptions merely because no thought has been given as to whether the drug is still needed. Finally, be aware of the possible adverse consequences of treatment: unpleasant or risky side-effects, drug interactions, potential for dependency and abuse, and toxicity in overdose (Suribhatla and Lindesay, 2005).

### Antidepressants

If there is any evidence of depression associated with the patient's neurotic disorder, then a trial 6–8 week course of antidepressant medication is clearly indicated. However, anxiety disorders also respond to antidepressant drugs in the absence of co-morbid depression. A selective serotonin reuptake inhibitor (SSRI) drug is the nowadays the treatment of first choice for GAD, with escitalopram having been shown to be efficacious in studies including elderly patients (Goodman et al., 2005). There is also evidence that venlafaxine is effective against GAD in this age group (Katz et al., 2002), and mixed-age studies also support the use of paroxetine and trazodone (Flint, 2005b). By extrapolation from studies in younger adults, a SSRI would also be the drug of choice for the treatment of panic disorder in an elderly patient (Flint and Gagnon, 2003). SSRIs also have a specific effect in OCD, and appear to be effective in elderly patients, although systematic studies are still lacking (Jenike, 1985; Austin et al., 1991). Although tricyclic drugs are effective against symptoms of anxiety, their use is limited by the risks they pose to physically ill patients, and their toxicity in overdose; an important exception in this respect is lofepramine (Dorman, 1988), although this drug is not licensed for use in anxiety disorders alone. The use of antidepressant medication in older adults is discussed in more detail in Chapter 29ii.

### Benzodiazepines

Although clinical opinion has turned against the use of benzodiazepines in recent years, they are still prescribed in considerable quantities to elderly patients as tranquillizers and hypnotics. Certain groups, such as those in long-term care, are particularly likely to receive these drugs (Gilbert et al., 1988). Important problems associated with the prolonged use of benzodiazepines include dependence, memory impairment, poor motor coordination, depression of respiratory drive, and paradoxical excitement (Tyrer, 1980; Curran, 1986; Fancourt and Castleden, 1986). Elderly people are particularly sensitive to these adverse effects, and the accumulation of drugs with long elimination half-lives also leads to drowsiness, delirium, depression, incontinence, falls, and fractures. In one study of elderly hospitalized patients, benzodiazepines were found to account for 29% of new episodes of acute confusion (Foy et al., 1995). Surprisingly little controlled research has been conducted

into the therapeutic effect of benzodiazepines in elderly patients, and most practice is guided by studies in younger adults and by anecdotal clinical experience (Salzman, 1991). Despite these problems, there is still a place for benzodiazepines in the management of transient, short-term anxiety symptoms in elderly patients. Drugs with short half-lives and no active metabolites, such as oxazepam, may be preferable to the long-acting agents, although there is increasing evidence that these are also problematic. For example, short-acting benzodiazepines have been shown to be associated with hip fracture and with increased incident disability in mobility and activities of daily living (Wagner et al., 2004; Gray et al., 2006). Why this should be so is not clear; it may be that they are more likely to be prescribed to high-risk patients. This reinforces the message that long-term use of these drugs is to be avoided if at all possible (Higgitt, 1988), and that they should be prescribed at the lowest effective dose.

The commonest and least justifiable reason why elderly patients are given benzodiazepines is because they complain of insomnia. Quite often this complaint is merely concern over normal changes in the quantity and pattern of sleep that occur with increasing age (Reynolds et al., 1985), and explanation and reassurance are usually all that is required. Where there is an underlying cause for the sleep disturbance, such as worry, depression, pain, or breathlessness, it is that rather than the sleeplessness that should be addressed. Psychophysiological insomnia due to tension and worry at bedtime is best managed in the first instance with a programme of advice on sleep hygiene to help the patient establish a regular sleep routine (Bramble, 1995). CBT has also been shown to be superior to zopiclone in the short-term and long-term management of insomnia in older adults (Sivertsen et al., 2006). A hypnotic should only be prescribed if other strategies are ineffective, or if the insomnia is transient.

### Azapirones

Buspirone is an azapirone anxiolytic, a $5\text{-HT}_{1A}$ partial agonist which acts differently from the benzodiazepines and has no cross-tolerance with them. Its pharmacokinetics, safety, and efficacy in elderly patients are similar to those in younger adults (Robinson et al., 1988), and its short-term use is not associated with rebound, dependence, or abuse (Lader, 1991). It appears to be well tolerated by elderly patients receiving treatment for chronic medical conditions (Bohm et al., 1990). Unlike other anxiolytics, it takes about 2 weeks to become effective, so it has a limited role in the management of acute anxiety states. It is indicated for severe, chronic GAD (Feighner, 1987), and in patients where there is a risk of dependence and abuse. Withdrawal from long-term benzodiazepine use may be facilitated by co-prescription of buspirone during the dose-reduction phase (Rickels et al., 2002). One recent study of GAD in elderly medical inpatients suggests that non-pharmacological factors may be important in determining the response to buspirone; those with high levels of both physical co-morbidity and social contacts responded better to treatment than did those who scored low on these factors (Majercsik and Haller, 2004).

### Neuroleptics

A short course of a conventional neuroleptic drug, such as haloperidol or zuclopenthixol, may be used to control severe anxiety in elderly patients, most effectively when it is due to psychotic experiences, as in delirium. However, the risk of disabling extra-pyramidal side-effects such as parkinsonism and tardive dyskinesia associated with these drugs, even in low doses, means that they are not indicated for the long-term management of anxiety in old age. The 'atypical' neuroleptics, such as sulpiride, risperidone, quetiapine, and olanzapine have a reduced incidence of side-effects, and are to be preferred if long-term management with this group of drugs is unavoidable. Aripiprazole has been proposed as an augmentation treatment for patients taking a SSRI who have significant residual anxiety symptoms (Adson et al., 2005).

### β-Blockers

These drugs are sometimes used to control the sympathetic somatic symptoms of anxiety where these are particularly troublesome (Kathol et al., 1980). However, they are contraindicated in patients with asthma, chronic obstructive airways disease, sinus bradycardia, and heart failure. These restrictions, together with side-effects such as nightmares and insomnia, limit their usefulness in this age group.

### Antihistamines

Antihistamine drugs such as hydroxyzine have long been used as anxiolytics in elderly patients. Their effect is probably due primarily to their sedative action. They are relatively safe, although hypotension can be a problem. They have a role in patients where respiratory depressant drugs are contraindicated.

### Barbiturates

The use of barbiturates and related drugs such as meprobamate and glutethimide in the treatment of mental disorder is now obsolete, but one occasionally comes across an elderly patient who is being maintained on one of these preparations. Their use is associated with many serious problems, notably physical dependency, dangerous withdrawal states, delirium, and paradoxical excitement. They are a very effective means of suicide. No patient should ever be started on a sedative or hypnotic barbiturate, and established users should be carefully weaned off these drugs. Barbiturate withdrawal should be covered with a reducing regime of phenobarbitone to prevent seizures.

## Conclusion

Our knowledge of neurotic disorders in the elderly population has improved considerably in recent years, but there is still much to be learned: about their origins, course and outcome; about their impact on other disorders and upon health services generally; and about the effectiveness of different treatment strategies. Elderly people are a very diverse group exposed to a wide range of physical, environmental, and psychosocial factors that determine vulnerability to, onset of, and recovery from neurotic disorders, and further study of this age group will almost certainly enhance our understanding of these conditions at all ages.

## References

Adson, D.E., Kushner, M.G., and Fahnhorst, T.A. (2005). Treatment of residual anxiety symptoms with adjunctive aripiprazole in depressed patients taking selective serotonin reuptake inhibitors. *Journal of Affective Disorders*, **86**, 99–104.

Agras, W.S., Chapin, N., and Oliveau, D.C. (1972). The natural history of phobia: course and prognosis. *Archives of General Psychiatry*, **26**, 315–17.

Alexopoulos, G.S., Young, R.C., and Shindeldecker, R.D. (1992). Brain computed tomography findings in geriatric depression and primary degenerative dementia. *Biological Psychiatry*, **31**, 591–9.

Allgulander, C. and Lavori, P.W. (1991). Excess mortality among 3302 patients with 'pure' anxiety neurosis. *Archives of General Psychiatry*, **48**, 599–602.

American Psychiatric Association (1994). *Diagnostic and statistical manual of mental disorders*, 4th edn. American Psychiatric Association, Washington, DC.

Andrews, G., Stewart, G., Allen, R., and Henderson, A.S. (1990). The genetics of six neurotic disorders: a twin study. *Journal of Affective Disorders*, **19**, 23–9.

Andrews, G. (1996). Comorbidity in neurotic disorders: the similarities are more important than the differences. In *Current controversies in the anxiety disorders* (ed. R.M. Rapee), pp. 3–20. Guilford Press, New York.

Astrom, M. (1996). Generalized anxiety disorder in stroke patients. A 3-year longitudinal study. *Stroke*, **27**, 270–5.

Austin, L.S., Zealberg, J.J., and Lydiard, R.B. (1991). Three cases of pharmacotherapy of obsessive-compulsive disorder in the elderly. *Journal of Nervous and Mental Disease*, **179**, 634–5.

Bajulaiye, R. and Addonizio, C. (1992). Obsessive-compulsive disorder arising in a 75-year-old woman. *International Journal of Geriatric Psychiatry*, **7**, 139–42.

Ballard, C.G., Mohan, R.N.C., Patel, A., and Graham, C. (1994). Anxiety disorder in dementia. *Irish Journal of Psychological Medicine*, **11**, 108–9.

Ballard, C.G., Boyle, A., Bowler, C., and Lindesay, J. (1996). Anxiety disorders in dementia sufferers. *International Journal of Geriatric Psychiatry*, **11**, 987–90.

Baltes, P.B. and Baltes, M.M. (1990). Psychological perspectives on successful aging: the model of selective optimization with compensation. In *Successful aging* (ed. P.B. Baltes and M.M. Baltes), pp. 1–34. Cambridge University Press, Cambridge.

Beekman, A.T.F., Bremmer, M.A., Deeg, D.J.H. et al. (1998). Anxiety disorders in later life: a report from the Longitudinal Aging Study Amsterdam. *International Journal of Geriatric Psychiatry*, **13**, 717–26.

Beitman, B.D., Kushner, M., and Grossberg, G.T. (1991). Late onset panic disorder: evidence from a study of patients with chest pain and normal cardiac evaluations. *International Journal of Psychiatry in Medicine*, **21**, 29–35.

Bergmann, K. (1971). The neuroses of old age. In *Recent developments in psychogeriatrics* (ed. D.W.K. Kay and A. Walk), pp. 39–50. Headley Bros, Ashford.

Bergmann, K. (1978). Neurosis and personality disorder in old age. In *Studies in geriatric psychiatry* (ed. A.D. Isaacs and F. Post), pp. 41–75. John Wiley and Sons, Chichester.

de Beurs, E., Beekman, A., and Geerlings, S. (2001). On becoming depressed or anxious in late life: similar vulnerability factors but different effects of life events. *British Journal of Psychiatry*, **179**, 426–31.

Blazer, D.G. (1983). The impact of late-life depression on the social network. *American Journal of Psychiatry*, **140**, 162–6.

Blazer, D.G., Hughes, D.C., and Fowler, N. (1989). Anxiety as an outcome symptom of depression in elderly and middle-aged adults. *International Journal of Geriatric Psychiatry*, **4**, 273–8.

Blazer, D.G., George, L.K., and Hughes, D. (1991). The epidemiology of anxiety disorders: an age comparison. In *Anxiety in the elderly* (ed. C. Salzman and B.D. Lebowitz), pp. 17–30. Springer, New York.

Bohm, C., Robinson, D.S., Gammans, R.E. et al. (1990). Buspirone therapy in anxious elderly patients: a controlled clinical trial. *Journal of Clinical Psychopharmacology*, **10**, 47S–51S.

Bouchard, T.J., Lykken, D.T., McGue, M., Segal, N.L., and Tellegen, A. (1990). The Minnesota study of twins reared apart. *Science*, **250**, 223–8.

Bowler, C. (1995). Eating disorders. In *Neurotic disorders in the elderly* (ed. J. Lindesay), pp. 193–204. Oxford University Press, Oxford.

Boyd, J.H., Burke, J.D., Gruenberg, E. *et al.* (1984). Exclusion criteria of DSM-III. A study of co-occurrence of hierarchy-free syndromes. *Archives of General Psychiatry*, **41**, 983–9.

Braithwaite, R. (1982). Pharmacokinetics and age. In *Psychopharmacology of old age* (ed. D. Wheatley), pp. 46–54. Oxford University Press, Oxford.

Bramble, D. (1995). Sleep and its disorders. In *Neurotic disorders in the elderly* (ed. J. Lindesay), pp. 227–43. Oxford University Press, Oxford.

Breiter, H.C., Rauch, S.L., and Kwong, K.K. (1996). Functional magnetic resonance imaging of symptom provocation in obsessive-compulsive disorder. *Archives of General Psychiatry*, **53**, 595–606.

Bremner, J.D. (2004) Brain imaging in anxiety disorders. *Expert Reviews in Neurotherapeutics*, **4**, 275–84.

Briere, J, and Elliot, D.M. (2003). Prevalence and psychological sequelae of self-reported childhood physical and sexual abuse in a general population sample of men and women. *Child Abuse and Neglect*, **27**, 1205–22.

Brown, G.W. (1993). Life events and psychiatric disorder: replications and limitations. *Psychosomatic Medicine*, **55**, 248–59.

Brown, G.W. and Harris, T.O. (1978). *Social origins of depression*. Tavistock, London.

Brown, G.W. and Harris, T.O. (ed.) (1989). *Life events and illness*. Unwin Hyman, London.

Brown, G.W., Bifulco, A., and Harris, T.O. (1987). Life events, vulnerability and onset of depression: some refinements. *British Journal of Psychiatry*, **150**, 30–42.

Brown, G.W., Lemyre, L., and Bifulco, A. (1992). Social factors and recovery from anxiety and depressive disorders: a test of the specificity hypothesis. *British Journal of Psychiatry*, **161**, 44–54.

Burn, W.K., Davies, K.N., McKenzie, F.R., Brothwell, J.A., and Wattis, J.P. (1993). The prevalence of psychiatric illness in acute geriatric admissions. *International Journal of Geriatric Psychiatry*, **8**, 175–80.

Burvill, P.W., Johnson, G.A., Jamrozik, K.D., Anderson, C.S., Stewart-Wynne, E.G., and Chakera, T.M.H. (1995) Anxiety disorders after stroke: results from the Perth Community Stroke Study. *British Journal of Psychiatry*, **166**, 328–37.

Byrne, G. and Raphael, B. (1994). A longitudinal study of bereavement phenomena in recently widowed elderly men. *Psychological Medicine*, **24**, 411–21.

Castillo, C.S., Starkstein, S.E., Federoff, J.P., Price, T.R., and Robinson, R.G. (1993). Generalised anxiety disorder after stroke. *Journal of Nervous and Mental Disease*, **181**, 102–8.

Catalan, J., Gath, D.H., Bond, A., Edmonds, G., Martin, P., and Ennis, J. (1988). General practice patients on long-term psychotropic drugs: a controlled investigation. *British Journal of Psychiatry*, **152**, 399–405.

Champion, L. (1990). The relationship between social vulnerability and the occurrence of severely threatening life events. *Psychological Medicine*, **20**, 157–61.

Coffey, C.E., Figiel, G.S., Djang, W.T., and Weiner, R.D. (1990). Subcortical hyperintensity on magnetic resonance imaging: a comparison of normal and depressed elderly subjects. *American Journal of Psychiatry*, **147**, 187–9.

Colvin, C. and Boddington, S.J.A. (1997) Behaviour therapy for obsessive-compulsive disorder in a 78-year old woman. *International Journal of Geriatric Psychiatry*, **12**, 488–91.

Cooper, B. (1986). Mental illness, disability and social conditions among old people in Mannheim. In *Mental health and the elderly* (ed. H.G. Häfner, N. Moschel, and N. Sartorius), pp.35–45. Springer, Berlin.

Copeland, J.R.M., Dewey, M.E., Wood, N., Searle, R., Davidson, I.A., and McWilliam, C. (1987). Range of mental illness among the elderly in the community: prevalence in Liverpool using the GMS-AGECAT package. *British Journal of Psychiatry*, **150**, 815–23.

Coryell, W. (1984). Mortality after thirty to forty years. Panic disorder compared with other psychiatric illnesses. In *Psychiatry update* (ed. L. Grinspoon). American Psychiatric Association, Washington, DC.

Cullen, W. (1784). *First lines of the practice of physic*. Reid and Bathgate, Edinburgh.

Curran, H.V. (1986). Tranquillising memories: a review of the effects of benzodiazepines on human memory. *Biological Psychiatry*, **23**, 179–213.

Davis, A. (1994). Life events in the normal elderly. In *Principles and practice of geriatric psychiatry* (ed. J.R.M. Copeland, M.T. Abou-Saleh, and D.G. Blazer), pp. 106–14. John Wiley and Sons, Chichester.

Dorman, T. (1988). The management of depression and the use of lofepramine in the elderly. *British Journal of Clinical Practice*, **42**, 459–64.

Downs, A.F.D., Rosenthal, T.L., and Lichstein, K.L. (1988). Modelling therapies reduce avoidance of bath-time by the institutionalised elderly. *Behaviour Therapy*, **19**, 359–68.

Dura, J.R., Stukenberg, K.W., and Kiecolt-Glaser, J.K. (1991). Anxiety and depressive disorders in adult children caring for demented parents. *Psychology and Aging*, **6**, 467–73.

Eaton, W.W., Kramer, M., Anthony, J.C., Dryman, A., Shapiro, S., and Locke, B.Z. (1989). The incidence of specific DIS/DSM-III mental disorders: data from the NIMH Epidemiologic Catchment Area program. *Acta Psychiatrica Scandinavica*, **79**, 163–78.

Faravelli, C., Webb, T., Ambonetti, A., Fonessu, F., and Sessarego, A. (1985). Prevalence of traumatic early life events in 31 agoraphobic patients with panic attacks. *American Journal of Psychiatry*, **142**, 1493–4.

Fancourt, G. and Castleden, M. (1986). The use of benzodiazepines with particular reference to the elderly. *British Journal of Hospital Medicine*, **v**, 321–5.

Feighner, J.P. (1987). Buspirone in the long-term treatment of generalized anxiety disorder. *Journal of Clinical Psychiatry*, **48**(Suppl.), 3–6.

Fillenbaum, G.G., George, L.K., and Palmore, E.B. (1985). Determinants and consequences of retirement among men of different races and economic levels. *Journal of Gerontology*, **40**, 85–94.

Finlay-Jones, R. (1989). Anxiety. In *Life events and illness* (ed. G.W. Brown and T.O. Harris), pp. 95–112. Unwin Hyman, London.

Flint, A.J. (2005a). Anxiety and its disorders in late life: moving the field forward. *American Journal of Geriatric Psychiatry*, **13**, 3–6.

Flint, A.J. (2005b). Generalised anxiety disorder in elderly patients: epidemiology, diagnosis and treatment options. *Drugs and Aging*, **22**, 101–14.

Flint, A.J., Cook, J.M., and Rabins, P.V. (1996). Why is panic disorder less frequent in late life? *American Journal of Geriatric Psychiatry*, **4**, 96–109.

Flint, A.J. and Gagnon, N. (2003). Diagnosis and management of panic disorder in older patients. *Drugs and Aging*, **20**, 881–91.

Flint, A.J. and Rifat, S.L. (1997a). Two-year outcome of elderly patients with anxious depression. *Psychiatry Research*, **66**, 23–31.

Flint, A.J. and Rifat, S.L. (1997b). Anxious depression in elderly patients. Response to antidepressant treatment. *American Journal of Geriatric Psychiatry*, **5**, 107–15.

Forsell, Y. and Winblad, B. (1997). Anxiety disorders in non-demented and demented elderly patients: prevalence and correlates. *Journal of Neurology, Neurosurgery and Psychiatry*, **62**, 294–5.

Foy, A., O'Connell, D., Henry, D. *et al.* (1995). Benzodiazepine use as a cause of cognitive impairment in elderly hospital inpatients. *Journal of Gerontology*, **50**, M99–M106.

Frances, A., and Flaherty, J.A. (1989). Elderly widow develops panic attacks, followed by depression. *Hospital and Community Psychiatry*, **40**, 19–23.

Frasure-Smith, N., Lesperance, F., and Talajic, M. (1995). The impact of negative emotions on prognosis following myocardial infarction: is it more than depression? *Health Psychology*, **14**, 388–98.

Fuentes, K. and Cox, B. (2000). Assessment of anxiety in older adults: a community-based survey and comparison with younger adults. *Behaviour Research and Therapy*, **38**, 297–309.

Gilbert, A., Quintrell, L.N., and Owen, N. (1988). Use of benzodiazepines among residents of aged-care accommodation. *Community Health Studies*, **12**, 394–9.

Goldberg, D. and Huxley, P. (1980). *Mental illness in the community*. Tavistock, London.

Goldberg, D.P., Bridges, K., Duncan-Jones, P., and Grayson, D. (1987). Dimensions of neurosis seen in primary care settings. *Psychological Medicine*, **17**, 461–70.

Goldberg, D. and Huxley, P. (1992). *Common mental disorders: a bio-social model.* Tavistock/Routledge, London.

Goodman, W.K., Bose, A., and Wang, Q. (2005). Treatment of generalized anxiety disorder with escitalopram: pooled results from double-blind, placebo-controlled trials. *Journal of Affective Disorders*, **87**, 161–7.

Gray, J. (1982). *The neuropsychology of anxiety.* Oxford University Press, Oxford.

Gray, S.L., LaCroix, A.Z., Hanlon, J.T. *et al.* (2006). Benzodiazepine use and physical disability in community-dwelling older adults. *Journal of the American Geriatrics Society*, **54**, 224–30.

Guerrero, J. and Crocq, M. (1994). Sleep disorder in the elderly: depression and PTSD. *Journal of Psychosomatic Research*, **38**(Suppl. 1), 141–50.

Gurnack, A.M. and Thomas, J.L. (1989). Behavioural factors related to elderly alcohol abuse: research and policy issues. *International Journal of Addictions*, **24**, 641–54.

Haines, A.P., Imeson, J.D., and Meade, T.W. (1980). Psychoneurotic profiles of smokers and non-smokers. *British Medical Journal*, **280**, 1422.

Haines, A.P., Imeson, J.D., and Meade, T.W. (1987). Phobic anxiety and ischaemic heart disease. *British Medical Journal*, **295**, 297–9.

Hariri, A.R. and Holmes, A. (2006). Genetics of emotional regulation: the role of the serotonin transporter in neural function. *Trends in Cognitive Science*, **10**, 182–91.

Harris, T.O. (1988). Psychosocial vulnerability to depression. In *Handbook of social psychiatry* (ed. S. Henderson and G. Burrows). Elsevier, Amsterdam.

Hermann, N. and Eryavec, G. (1994). Posttraumatic stress disorder in institutionalized World War II veterans. *American Journal of Psychiatry*, **151**, 324–31.

Hettema, J.M., Neale, M.C., and Kendler, K.S. (2001). A review and meta-analysis of the genetic epidemiology of anxiety disorders. *American Journal of Psychiatry*, **158**, 1568–78.

Higgitt, A. (1988). Indications for benzodiazepine prescriptions in the elderly. *International Journal of Geriatric Psychiatry*, **3**, 239–49.

Himmelfarb, S. and Murrell, S.A. (1984). The prevalence and correlates of anxiety symptoms in older adults. *Journal of Psychology*, **116**, 159–67.

Hocking, L.B. and Koenig, H.G. (1995). Anxiety in medically ill older patients: a review and update. *International Journal of Psychiatry in Medicine*, **25**, 221–38.

Insel, T.R. (1992). Neurobiology of obsessive-compulsive disorder: a review. *International Clinical Psychopharmacology*, **7**(Suppl. 1), 31–3.

Isaacs, B. (1992). *The challenge of geriatric medicine*, pp. 84–5. Oxford University Press, Oxford.

Jacoby, R., and Levy, R. (1980). Computed tomography in the elderly. 3. Affective disorder. *British Journal of Psychiatry*, **136**, 270–5.

Jenike, M.A. (1985). Handbook of geriatric psychopharmacology. PSG Publishing, Littleton, MA.

Jenike, M.A. (1989). Geriatric psychiatry and psychopharmacology: a clinical approach. Mosby Year Book, St Louis.

Jorm, A.F. (2000). Does old age reduce the risk of anxiety and depression? A review of epidemiological studies across the adult life span. *Psychological Medicine*, **30**, 11–22.

Kathol, R.G., Noyes, R., Slyman, D.J., Crowe, R.R., Clancy, J., and Kerbor, R. (1980). Propanolol in chronic anxiety disorders. A controlled study. *Archives of General Psychiatry*, **37**, 1361–5.

Katon, W.J. (1984). Chest pain, cardiac disease and panic disorder. *Journal of Clinical Psychiatry*, **51**, 27–30.

Katz, I.R., Reynolds, C.F., Alexopoulos, G.S., and Hackett, D. (2002). Venlafaxine ER as a treatment for generalized anxiety disorder in older adults: pooled analysis of five randomized placebo-controlled clinical trials. *Journal of the American Geriatrics Society*, **50**, 18–25.

Kaup, B.A., Ruskin, P.E., and Nyman, G. (1994). Significant life events and PTSD in elderly World War II veterans. *American Journal of Psychiatry*, **2**, 239–43.

Kay, D.W.K. (1988). Anxiety in the elderly. In *Handbook of anxiety, Vol.2: classification, etiological factors, and associated disturbances* (ed. R. Noyes, M. Roth, and G.D. Burrows), pp. 289–310. Elsevier, Amsterdam.

Kay, D.W.K., and Bergmann, K. (1966). Physical disability and mental health in old age. *Journal of Psychosomatic Research*, **10**, 3–12.

Kay, D.W.K., Holding, T.A., Jones, B., and Littler, S. (1987). Psychiatric morbidity in Hobart's dependent aged. *Australian and New Zealand Journal of Psychiatry*, **21**, 463–8.

Kenardy, J., Oei, T.P.S., and Evans, L. (1990). Neuroticism and age of onset for agoraphobia with panic attacks. *Journal of Behaviour Therapy and Experimental Psychiatry*, **21**, 193–7.

Kendler, K.S., Kessler, R.C., Heath, A.C., and Eaves, L.J. (1992). Major depression and generalized anxiety disorder. Same genes, (partly) different environments? *Archives of General Psychiatry*, **49**, 716–22.

Kennedy, B.L. and Schwab, J.J. (1997). Utilization of medical specialists by anxiety disorder patients. *Psychosomatics*, **38**, 109–12.

Kennedy, G.J., Kelman, H.R., and Thomas, C. (1989). Hierarchy of characteristics associated with depressive symptoms in an urban elderly sample. *American Journal of Psychiatry*, **146**, 220–2.

Kennedy, G.J., Kelman, H.R., and Thomas, C. (1990). The emergence of depressive symptoms in late life. The importance of declining health and increasing disability. *Journal of Community Health*, **15**, 93–104.

King, P. and Barrowclough, C. (1991). A clinical pilot study of cognitive-behavioural therapy for anxiety disorders in the elderly. *Behavioural Psychotherapy*, **19**, 337–45.

Kitayama, N., Vaccarino, V., Kutner, M., Weiss, P., and Bremner, J.D. (2005). Magnetic resonance imaging (MRI) measurement of hippocampal volume in posttraumatic stress disorder: a meta-analysis. *Journal of Affective Disorders*, **88**, 79–86.

Klerman, G. (1988). The current age of youthful melancholia: evidence for increase in depression among adolescents and young adults. *British Journal of Psychiatry*, **152**, 4–14.

Kluznik, J.C., Speed, N., Van Valkenberger, C., and McGraw, R. (1986). Forty-year follow-up of United States prisoners of war. *American Journal of Psychiatry*, **143**, 1443–5.

Koder, D. (1998). Treatment of anxiety in the cognitively impaired elderly: can cognitive-behaviour therapy help? *International Psychogeriatrics*, **10**, 173–82.

Kohn, R., Westlake, R.J., Rasmussen, S.A., Marsland, R.T., and Norman, W.H. (1997). Clinical features of obsessive-compulsive disorder in elderly patients. *American Journal of Geriatric Psychiatry*, **5**, 211–15.

Krasucki, C., Howard, R., and Mann, A. (1998). The relationship between anxiety disorders and age. *International Journal of Geriatric Psychiatry*, **13**, 79–99.

Krasucki, C., Ryan, P., Ertan, T., Howard, R., Lindesay, J., and Mann, A. (1999). The FEAR: a rapid screening instrument for generalized anxiety in elderly primary care attenders. *International Journal of Geriatric Psychiatry*, **14**, 60–8.

Kubzansky, L.D., Kawachi, I., Weiss, S.T., and Sparrow, D. (1998). Anxiety and coronary heart disease: a synthesis of epidemiological, psychological, and experimental evidence. *Annals of Behavioral Medicine*, **20**, 47–58.

Lader, M. (1982). Differential diagnosis of anxiety in the elderly. *Journal of Clinical Psychiatry*, **43**, 4–9.

Lader, M. (1991). Can buspirone induce rebound, dependence or abuse? *British Journal of Psychiatry*, **159**(Suppl. 12), 45–51.

Larkin, A.B., Copeland, J.R.M., Dewey, M.E. *et al.* (1992). The natural history of neurotic disorder in an elderly urban population. Findings from the Liverpool Longitudinal Study of Continuing Health in the Community. *British Journal of Psychiatry*, **160**, 681–6.

Lenze, E., Rodgers, J., Martire, L. *et al.* (2001). The association of late-life depression and anxiety with physical disability. A review of the literature and a prospectus for future research. *American Journal of Geriatric Psychiatry*, **9**, 113–35.

Leon, A.C., Portera, L., and Weissmann, M.M. (1995). The social costs of anxiety disorders. *British Journal of Psychiatry*, **27**(Suppl.), 19–22.

Lindesay, J. (1990). The Guy's/Age Concern Survey: physical health and psychiatric disorder in an urban elderly community. *International Journal of Geriatric Psychiatry*, **5**, 171–8.

Lindesay, J. (1991). Phobic disorders in the elderly. *British Journal of Psychiatry*, **159**, 531–41.

Lindesay, J. (1995a). Introduction: the concept of neurosis. In *Neurotic disorders in the elderly* (ed. J. Lindesay), pp. 1–11. Oxford University Press, Oxford.

Lindesay, J. (1995b). Psychosocial factors. In *Neurotic disorders in the elderly* (ed. J. Lindesay), pp. 56–71. Oxford University Press, Oxford.

Lindesay, J. and Banerjee, S. (1993). Phobic disorders in the elderly: a comparison of three diagnostic systems. *International Journal of Geriatric Psychiatry*, **8**, 387–93.

Lindesay, J., Briggs, K., and Murphy, E. (1989). The Guy's/Age Concern Survey: prevalence rates of cognitive impairment, depression and anxiety in an urban elderly community. *British Journal of Psychiatry*, **155**, 317–29.

Lindesay, J., Jagger, C., Hibbett, M., Peet, S., and Moledina, F. (1997). Knowledge, uptake and availability of health and social services among Asian Gujarati and White elderly persons. *Ethnicity and Health*, **2**, 59–69.

Livingston, G., Manela, M., and Katona, C. (1997). Cost of care for older people. *British Journal of Psychiatry*, **171**, 56–9.

Luchins, D.J. and Rose, R.P. (1989). Late-life onset of panic disorder with agoraphobia in three patients. *American Journal of Psychiatry*, **146**, 920–1.

McGuire, P.K., Bench, C.J., Frith, C.D., Marks, I.M., Frakowiak, R.S.J., and Dolan, R.J. (1994). Functional anatomy of obsessive-compulsive phenomena. *British Journal of Psychiatry*, **164**, 459–68.

Machlin, S.R., Harris, G.J., Pearlson, G.D., Hoehn-Saric, R., Jeffrey, P., and Camargo, E.E. (1991). Elevated, medial-frontal cerebral blood flow in obsessive-compulsive patients: a SPECT study. *American Journal of Psychiatry*, **148**, 1240–2.

Mackinnon, A., Christiansen, H., Jorm, A.F., Henderson, A.S., Scott, R., and Korten, A.E. (1994). A latent trait analysis of an inventory designed to detect symptoms of anxiety and depression using an elderly community sample. *Psychological Medicine*, **24**, 977–86.

Majercsik, E. and Haller, J. (2004). Interactions between anxiety, social support, health status and buspirone efficacy in elderly patients. *Progress in Neuropsychopharmacology and Biological Psychiatry*, **28**, 1161–9.

Manela, M., Katona, C., and Livingston, G. (1996). How common are the anxiety disorders in old age? *International Journal of Geriatric Psychiatry*, **11**, 65–70.

Marks, I.M. (1981). Space phobia: a pseudo-agoraphobic syndrome. *Journal of Neurology, Neurosurgery and Psychiatry*, **44**, 387–91.

Marks, I.M. (1986). Genetics of fear and anxiety disorders. *British Journal of Psychiatry*, **149**, 406–18.

Marks, I. and Lader, M. (1973). Anxiety states (anxiety neurosis): a review. *Journal of Nervous and Mental Disease*, **156**, 3–18.

Martindale, B. (1995). Psychological treatments II: psychodynamic approaches. In *Neurotic disorders in the elderly* (ed. J. Lindesay), pp. 114–137. Oxford University Press, Oxford.

Matthew, S.J., Mao, X., Coplan, J.D. *et al.* (2004). Dorsolateral prefrontal cortical pathology in generalized anxiety disorder: a proton magnetic resonance spectroscopic imaging study. *American Journal of Psychiatry*, **161**, 1119–21.

Middeldorp, C.M., Cath, D.C., Van Dyck, R., and Boomsma, D.I. (2005). The co-morbidity of anxiety and depression in the perspective of genetic epidemiology. A review of twin and family studies. *Psychological Medicine*, **35**, 611–24.

Mohlman, J. (2004). Psychosocial treatment of late-life generalized anxiety disorder: current status and future directions. *Clinical Psychology Review*, **24**, 149–69.

Mountz, J.M., Modell, J.G., Wilson, M.W. *et al.* (1989). Positron emission tomographic evaluation of cerebral blood flow during state anxiety in simple phobia. *Archives of General Psychiatry*, **46**, 501–4.

Murphy, E. (1982). Social origins of depression in old age. *British Journal of Psychiatry*, **141**, 135–42.

Murphy, E. (1986). Social factors in late life depression. In *Affective disorders in the elderly* (ed. E. Murphy), pp. 79–96. Churchill Livingstone, London.

Neary, D. (1990). Dementia of frontal lobe type. *Journal of the American Geriatrics Society*, **38**, 71–2.

Noyes, R. and Clancy, J. (1976). Anxiety neurosis: a 5-year follow up. *Journal of Nervous and Mental Disease*, **162**, 200–5.

Nordhus, I.H. and Pallesen, S. (2003). Psychological treatment of late life anxiety: an empirical review. *Journal of Consulting and Clinical Psychology*, **71**, 643–51.

Onrust, S.A. and Cuijpers, P. (2006). Mood and anxiety disorders in widowhood: a systematic review. *Aging and Mental Health*, **10**, 327–34.

Ostir, G.V. and Goodwin, J.S. (2006). High anxiety is associated with an increased risk of death in an older tri-ethnic population. *Journal of Clinical Epidemiology*, **59**, 534–40.

Oxman, T.E., Berkman, L.F., Kasl, S., Freeman, D.H., and Barratt, J. (1992). Social support and depressive symptoms in the elderly. *American Journal of Epidemiology*, **135**, 356–68.

Pachana, N.A., Byrne, G.J., Siddle, H., Koloski, N., Harley, E., and Arnold, E. (2006). Development and validation of the Geriatric Anxiety Inventory. *International Psychogeriatrics*, **18**, 1–12.

Paquette, V., Levesque, J., and Mensour, B. (2003). 'Change the mind and you change the brain': effects of cognitive-behavioral therapy on the neural correlates of spider phobia. *Neuroimage*, **18**, 401–9.

Peach, H. and Pathy, J. (1979). Disability of the elderly after myocardial infarction. *Journal of the Royal College of Physicians*, **13**, 154–7.

Philpot, M. (1995). Biological factors. In *Neurotic disorders in the elderly* (ed. J. Lindesay), pp. 72–96. Oxford University Press, Oxford.

Pitt, B. (1995). Neurotic disorders and physical illness. In *Neurotic disorders in the elderly* (ed. J. Lindesay), pp. 46–55. Oxford University Press, Oxford.

Pollock, C. and Andrews, G. (1989). The defense style associated with specific anxiety disorders. *American Journal of Psychiatry*, **146**, 455–60.

Pribor, E.F., Smith, D.S., and Yutzy, S.H. (1994). Somatization disorder in elderly patients. *American Journal of Geriatric Psychiatry*, **2**, 109–17.

Prigerson, H.G., Shear, M.K., Newsom, J.T. *et al.* (1996a). Anxiety among widowed elders: is it distinct from depression and grief? *Anxiety*, **2**, 1–12.

Prigerson, H.G., Shear, M.K., Bierhals, A.J. *et al.* (1996b). Childhood adversity, attachment and personality styles as predictors of anxiety among elderly caregivers. *Anxiety*, **2**, 234–41.

Rauch, S.L., Jenike, M.A., Alpert, N.M. *et al.* (1994). Regional cerebral blood flow measured during symptom provocation in obsessive-compulsive disorder using oxygen 15-labelled carbon dioxide and positron emission tomography. *Archives of General Psychiatry*, **51**, 62–70.

Regier, D.A., Boyd, J.H., Burke, J.D. *et al.* (1988). One-month prevalence of mental disorders in the United States. *Archives of General Psychiatry*, **45**, 977–86.

Reynolds, C.F., Kupfer, D.J., Taska, L.S. *et al.* (1985). EEG sleep in elderly depressed, demented and healthy subjects. *Biological Psychiatry*, **20**, 431–42.

Rickels, K., DeMartinis, N., Garcia-Espana, F., Greenblatt, D.J., Mandon, L.A., and Rynn, M. (2002). Imipramine and buspirone in treatment of patients with generalized anxiety disorder who are discontinuing long-term benzodiazepine therapy. *American Journal of Psychiatry*, **157**, 1973–9.

Roberts, A.H. (1964). Housebound housewives- a follow-up study of a phobic anxiety state. *British Journal of Psychiatry*, **110**, 191–7.

Robins, L. and Regier, D. (ed.) (1991). *Psychiatric disorders in America*. The Free Press, New York.

Robinson, D., Napoliello, M.J., and Shenck, L. (1988). The safety and usefulness of buspirone as an anxiolytic drug in elderly versus young patients. *Clinical Therapeutics*, **10**, 740–6.

Rosen, J., Fields, R.B., Hand, A.M., Falsettie, G., and Van Kammen, D.P. (1989). Concurrent posttraumatic stress disorder in psychogeriatric patients. *Journal of Geriatric Psychiatry and Neurology*, **2**, 65–9.

Rosin, A.J. and Glatt, M.M. (1971). Alcohol excess in the elderly. *Quarterly Journal of Studies on Alcohol*, **32**, 53–9.

Russo, J., Vitaliano, P.P., Brewer, D.D. *et al.* (1995). Psychiatric disorders in spouse caregivers of care recipients with Alzheimer's disease and matched controls: a diathesis-stress model of psychopathology. *Journal of Abnormal Psychology*, **104**, 197–204.

Salzman, C. (1991). Pharmacologic treatment of the anxious elderly patient. In *Anxiety in the elderly* (ed. C. Salzman and B.D. Lebowitz), pp. 149–73. Springer, New York.

Scaturo, D.J. and Hayman, P.M. (1992). The impact of combat trauma across the family life cycle: clinical considerations. *Journal of Trauma and Stress*, **5**, 273–88.

Schoevers, R., Beekman, A., Deeg, D., Jonker, C., and van Tilburg, W. (2003). Co-morbidity and risk patterns of depression, generalised anxiety disorder and mixed anxiety-depression in later life: results from the AMSTEL study. *International Journal of Geriatric Psychiatry*, **18**, 994–1001.

Schuff, N., Neylan, T.C., Lenoci, M.A. *et al.* (2001). Decreased hippocampal N-acetylaspartate in the absence of atrophy in posttraumatic stress disorder. *Biological Psychiatry*, **50**, 952–9.

Schultz, S.K., Castillo, C.S., Kosier, J.T., and Robinson, R.G. (1997). Generalized anxiety and depression: Assessment over 2 years after stroke. *American Journal of Geriatric Psychiatry*, **5**, 229–37.

Schwartz, G.M., Braverman, B.G., and Roth, B. (1987). Anxiety disorders and psychiatric referral in the general medical emergency room. *General Hospital Psychiatry*, **9**, 87–93.

Shankar, K.K., Walker, M., Frost, D., and Orrell, M.W. (1999). The development of a valid and reliable scale for rating anxiety in dementia. *Aging and Mental Health*, **3**, 39–49.

Sharpe, M., Hawton, K., House, A. *et al.* (1990). Mood disorders in long-term survivors of stroke: associations with brain lesion location and volume. *Psychological Medicine*, **20**, 815–28.

Sheikh, J.I., King, R.J., and Barr Taylor, C. (1991). Comparative phenomenology of early-onset versus late-onset panic attacks: a pilot survey. *American Journal of Psychiatry*, **148**, 1231–3.

Sheikh, J.I., Swales, P.J., Kravitz, J., Bail, G., and Barr Taylor, C. (1994). Childhood abuse history in older women with panic disorder. *American Journal of Geriatric Psychiatry*, **2**, 75–7.

Sheikh, J.I., Swales, P.J., Carlson, E.B., and Lindley, S.E. (2004). Aging and panic disorder: phenomenology, comorbidity, and risk factors. *American Journal of Geriatric Psychiatry*, **12**, 102–9.

Shepherd, M., Cooper, B., Brown, A.C., and Kalton, G. (1981). *Psychiatric illness in general practice*. Oxford University Press, London.

Singleton, N., Bumpstead, R., O'Brien, M., Lee, A., and Meltzer, H. (2001). *Psychiatric morbidity among adults living in private households*. The Stationery Office, London.

Sinoff, G., Ore, L., Zlotogorsky, D., and Tamir, A. (1999). Short Anxiety Screening Test: a brief instrument for detecting anxiety in the elderly. *International Journal of Geriatric Psychiatry*, **14**, 1062–71.

Sivertsen, B., Omvik, S., Pallesen, S. *et al.* (2006). Cognitive behavioural therapy vs. zopiclone for treatment of chronic primary insomnia in older adults: a randomized controlled trial. *Journal of the American Medical Association*, **28**, 2851–8.

Spertus, I.L., Yehuda, R., Wong, C.M., Halligan, S., and Seremetis, S.V. (2003). Childhood emotional abuse and neglect as predictors of psychological and physical symptoms in women presenting to a primary care practice. *Child Abuse and Neglect*, **27**, 1247–58.

Stein, M.B., Goldin, P.R., Sareen, J., Zorilla, L.T.E., and Brown, G.G. (2002). Increased amygdala activation to angry and contemptuous faces in generalized social phobia. *Archives of General Psychiatry*, **59**, 1027–34.

Sultzer, D.L., Levin, H.S., Mahler, M.E. *et al.* (1993). A comparison of psychiatric symptoms in vascular dementia and Alzheimer's disease. *American Journal of Psychiatry*, **150**, 1806–12.

Suribhatla, S. and Lindesay, J. (2005). Treatment of anxiety disorders. In *Practical old age psychopharmacology – a multi-professional approach* (ed. S. Curran and R. Bullock), pp. 165–76. Radcliffe Medical Press, Oxford.

Tankard, C.F., Waldstein, S.R., Siegel, E.L. *et al.* (2003). Cerebral blood flow and anxiety in older men: an analysis of resting anterior asymmetry and prefrontal regions. *Brain and Cognition*, **52**, 70–8.

Tennant, C., Bebbington, P., and Hurry, J. (1982). Social experiences in childhood and adult psychiatric morbidity: a multiple regression analysis. *Psychological Medicine*, **12**, 321–7.

Thompson, L.W., Gallagher, D.E., and Breckenridge, J.S. (1987). Comparative effectiveness of psychotherapies for depressed elderly. *Journal of Consulting and Clinical Psychology*, **55**, 385–90.

Thyer, B.A. (1981). Prolonged in-vivo exposure therapy with a 70 year old woman. *Journal of Behaviour Therapy and Experimental Psychiatry*, **12**, 69–71.

Thyer, B.A., Parrish, R.T., Curtis, G.C., Nesse, R.M., and Cameron, O.G. (1985). Ages of onset of DSM-III anxiety disorders. *Comprehensive Psychiatry*, **26**, 113–22.

Tiihonen, J., Kuikka, J., Bergstrom, K. *et al.* (1997). Dopamine reuptake site densities in patients with social phobia. *American Journal of Psychiatry*, **154**, 239–42.

Tobin, S.S. and Liebermann, M.A. (1976). *Last home for the aged*. Jossey-Bass, San Francisco.

Torgersen, S. (1990). Comorbidity of major depression and anxiety disorders in twin pairs. *American Journal of Psychiatry*, **147**, 1199–202.

Tweed, J.L., Schoenbach, V.J., George, L.K., and Blazer, D.G. (1989). The effects of childhood parental death and divorce on six-month history of anxiety disorders. *British Journal of Psychiatry*, **154**, 823–8.

Twelftree, H. and Qazi, A. (2006). Relationship between anxiety and agitation in dementia. *Aging and Mental Health*, **10**, 362–7.

Tyrer, P. (1980). Dependence on benzodiazepines. *British Journal of Psychiatry*, **137**, 576–7.

Tyrer, P. (1989). *Classification of neurosis*. John Wiley, Chichester.

Tyrer, P. (1990). The division of neurosis: a failed classification. *Journal of the Royal Society of Medicine*, **83**, 614–16.

Vernooij-Dassen, M.J., Persoon, J.M., and Felling, A.J. (1996). Predictors of sense of competence in caregivers of demented persons. *Social Science and Medicine*, **43**, 41–9.

Villamil, E., Huppert, F.A., and Melzer, D. (2006). Low prevalence of depression and anxiety is linked to statutory retirement ages rather than personal work exit: a national survey. *Psychological Medicine*, **36**, 999–1009.

Wagner, A.K., Zhang, F., Soumerai, S.B. *et. al.* (2004). Benzodiazepine use and hip fracture in the elderly: Who is at greatest risk? *Archives of Internal Medicine*, **164**, 1567–72.

Walton, V.A., Romans-Clarkson, S.E., Mullen, P.E., and Herbison, G.P. (1990). The mental health of elderly women in the community. *International Journal of Geriatric Psychiatry*, **5**, 257–63.

Wands, K., Merskey, H., Hachinski, V.C., Fisman, M., Fox, H., and Boniferro, M. (1990). A questionnaire investigation of anxiety and depression in early dementia. *Journal of the American Geriatrics Society*, **36**, 535–8.

Woods, R.T. (1995). Psychological treatments I: behavioural and cognitive approaches. In *Neurotic disorders in the elderly* (ed. J Lindesay), pp. 97–113. Oxford University Press, Oxford.

Woods, R.T. and Britton, P.G. (1985). *Clinical psychology with the elderly*. Croom Helm/Chapman Hall, London.

World Health Organization (1992). *International classification of diseases*, 10th revision. World Health Organization, Geneva.

Wu, J.C., Buchsbaum, M.S., Hershey, T.G., Hazlett, E., Sicotte, N., and Johnson, J.C. (1991). PET in generalised anxiety disorder. *Biological Psychiatry*, **29**, 1181–99.

Zahner, G.E.P. and Murphy, J.M. (1989). Loss in childhood: anxiety in adulthood. *Comprehensive Psychiatry*, **30**, 553–63.

Zerhusen, J.D., Boyle, K., and Wilson, W. (1991). Out of the darkness: group cognitive therapy for the elderly. *Journal of Psychosocial Nursing*, **29**, 16–20.

# Personality in later life: the effects of ageing on personality

Bob Woods and Gill Windle

## Introduction

Thirty years ago, it was not uncommon for assessment of personality to form part of a comprehensive psychogeriatric assessment. Dissatisfaction with the projective tests available and the lack of questionnaire measures of personality designed with older people in mind led to this area falling from favour (Woods and Britton, 1985). This reflected a broader trend at that time to emphasize the situation- and context-specific nature of behaviour over the influence of enduring personality traits (Digman, 1990). In this chapter, the re-emergence of personality variables as a focus for theory and research is evident, although there are few signs of a resurgence of personality assessment in the clinical domain as yet.

The major debate arising from investigations of personality and ageing has been whether personality changes as people age, or whether personality is stable across the lifespan. Early theories, developed from the perspective of psychoanalysis, provided detailed accounts of the development of personality during childhood and adolescence, but did not appear to conceive that personality could continue to develop during adulthood and accordingly had nothing to say about the development of personality in older age. More recent approaches suggest that personality can show elements of both change and consistency across the life-course. This chapter presents some of the theory and research relating to personality and ageing. It considers personality as a range of traits and resources: the characteristics or qualities within the individual which predispose the person to behave in characteristic ways across a range of situations. Knowledge of a person's personality profile helps to predict how that person will behave in any given situation, but there will, of course, be many other factors which influence the interaction between person and environment.

Although the title of the chapter may suggest a one-way direction of influence of ageing on personality, perhaps of greater interest is how personality might affect the person's experience of later life. It is now recognized that personality characteristics may provide a valuable resource, with a demonstrable impact on outcomes in health and well-being. Research regularly demonstrates that there is a positive relationship between increasing age and subjective well-being, despite the influence of apparent 'risk factors' in older age such as bereavement, ill-health, etc. which would be expected to have a cumulative negative effect on well-being. This has been termed the 'well-being paradox' (Staudinger, 2000) or the 'satisfaction paradox' (Diener et al., 1999) and the consistent identification of this across many studies, populations, and measures suggests that it is probably not simply a methodological artefact.

Whilst a substantial evidence base exists regarding these potential 'risk' factors and negative outcomes in older age, the psychological resources and capacities that underlie adaptation to changing situations, and that ultimately may serve to prevent negative outcomes, are reported to be inadequately understood (Diener et al., 1999; Staudinger et al., 1999). In response, this chapter explores the role of personality and the self as a source of psychological resilience in relation to ageing and well-being. It describes how the self is able to maintain continuity and stability and to change adaptively. Diener et al. (1999) suggest that the maintenance of well-being across the lifespan demonstrates the ability of the person to adapt positively to a wide range of conditions, highlighting the role of the individual in achieving a sense of well-being in older age. We are thus discussing a dynamic interaction between personality and ageing, which must also take into account that 'ageing' itself is not a unitary process, but covers a range of influences which change, often variably, over time.

As cognitive impairment and dementia are seen as a particular challenge to adaptation in older people, this chapter will conclude with reference to the impact of dementia on personality and, likewise, the impact of personality on the presentation of the person with dementia.

## Personality across the lifespan

The 'Big Five' five-factor model has emerged as the predominant trait model of personality (Digman, 1990), and has been described as offering a meta-theoretical framework of personality (McCrae and Costa, 1996). The five factors included in this model are:

◆ Neuroticism, including anxiety and vulnerability versus emotional stability.

- Extraversion, including warmth, gregariousness and activity versus introversion.

- Openness to experience, including broad-minded values and aesthetics.

- Agreeableness, including altruism, modesty and trust versus ruthless and hostile.

- Conscientiousness, including competence and self-discipline.

These factors form a crucial part of the self concept. With its origins in psychometrics and the study of individual differences, the five-factor model represents a scientific approach to the study of personality. It is derived from factor analyses of descriptions of personality that were obtained through self-report methods and observer ratings which have been extensively validated. Each trait represents a tendency to behave in a particular way, with individuals varying in the extent to which they show each trait. It is the consensus on this model that has underpinned the revival of research on the development of personality over the lifespan.

Based on evidence from longitudinal and cross-sectional research, using a personality measure that evaluates these five traits [the Neuroticism–Extraversion–Openness Personality Inventory (NEO-PI)], it had been previously argued that there is little or no mean level change in personality after the age of 30, despite the varied experiences that occur over the life-course (Costa and McCrae, 1992, 1994, 1997): 'Individual differences in personality traits are extremely stable in adults, even over periods of as long as three decades' (McCrae, 2002, p. 309). Such findings have been related to the proposition that personality traits are biologically determined, with environmental influences seen as less important. However, it is important to note that there are at least three forms of stability that are being discussed: changes in the absolute *level* of scores; changes in the *rank order* of individuals (consistency); and changes in the *structure* of personality (Staudinger, 2005).

The *structure* of the five-factor model does appear to be replicable across age-groups, and with similar age-trends identified across diverse cultures. McCrae *et al.* (2005) used observer ratings of personality across 50 different cultures. The raters were college students and those being rated were of college age (18–21) or adult (40–98; the mean age of the adult group was relatively young at 49.9). They found that the five-factor model of personality was consistent cross-culturally, providing further support for the argument that personality development is independent of life experiences. Similarly, the evidence for stability of *rank order* of individuals is relatively strong, with extraversion and agreeableness having slightly higher consistencies (Staudinger, 2005).

However, there is evidence that indicates that changes in mean *levels* of personality traits may occur beyond the age of 30. A meta-analysis examined aggregate change in traits within discrete age categories over the lifespan ranging from the age of 10 to 101 (Roberts *et al.*, 2006). However, the findings tell us less about personality in the oldest old: only 6 out of the 92 studies reviewed contained data on people aged 80 or over. A facet of extraversion, described as *social vitality*, decreased between the ages of 22 and 30 and again between the ages of 60 and 70, but there was no change in the years between these two age groups. A second facet of extraversion—*social dominance*—increased up to the age of 40. Beyond this age there were no significant increases or decreases. For *agreeableness* there was a trend for an increase with age up to the age of 50.

Agreeableness significantly increased further in the 50–60 cohort, and remained at this higher level. There was little or no change in *conscientiousness* in adolescence and the college period but there were significant increases within each 10 year age group from the ages of 20 through to 70. *Emotional stability* demonstrated small but positive increases earlier in life, from the ages of 10–18 through to the third decade. There was another small but significant increase in the 50–60 year period. *Openness* increased between the ages of 18 and 22 and from there it did not change until the ages of 60–70, where the mean level declined. Thus there are distinct normative changes in personality beyond the original age of 30 previously suggested by Costa and McCrae, demonstrating that there is no specific age at which personality traits stop changing—development continues. Helson *et al.* (2002) similarly emphasize increases in conscientiousness and agreeableness and reduced social vitality with age, whereas, in a 6-year longitudinal study of 223 people aged 55–85, Small *et al.* (2003) found greater increases in neuroticism with age.

In contrast to the notion that personality is biologically determined, Roberts *et al.* (2006) argue that some of the changes between and within cohorts found in their meta-analysis could be affected by aspects of the environment. For example the younger cohorts had more change in levels of social dominance, conscientiousness, and emotional stability, which could be due to the general increase in self-assertion over the past 50 years or so. In addition, societal influences such as getting married, having children, etc. could also be factors in the increased conscientiousness in the younger cohorts. They argue that such findings demonstrate that personality does not develop independently of environmental influences. If this is the case, and personality change occurs through the 'press of contingencies found in age-graded social roles' (Roberts *et al.*, 2006, p.18) then it raises questions as to how personality traits and resources might operate in the context of old age.

Roberts *et al.* use life-course patterns as an example of how personality could be expected to develop. They refer to older age as a period dominated by 'disengagement with the roles of middle adulthood and the transition out of the labour force to become a retired person, grandparent, and possibly a widower' (2006, p.19). They argue that research with younger age groups supports the theory that there are universal, societal tasks that influence age-associated role experiences, and that these are partially responsible for the changes found in their meta-analysis. The process of adaptation is likely to be affected by a number of factors, and it has been proposed that aspects of the personality may mediate (Keyes and Waterman, 2004) or moderate (Smith *et al.*, 1999) the effects of such causal factors on subjective well-being. However, personality may itself also be subject to change and development in the face of the changed circumstances of later life.

In summary, the debate continues regarding the stability of personality, particularly in relation to mean levels of specific attributes, although there is increasing acceptance that both change and stability occur (Berry and Jobe, 2002; Hooker, 2002). As with many debates regarding the role of genetic versus environmental influences, there is clearly a need to recognize the interaction of these aspects. Measures of personality traits are, of course, designed to show stability. So it is important to look also at other aspects of the self, so as to understand more fully the subtle ways in which people change—in order, perhaps, to maintain their stability.

# Lifespan development

The lifespan development perspective offers a theoretical framework which acknowledges that personality may develop from an interaction with both biology and the environment. This approach enables the 'normal' changes that occur due to the passage of time to be understood as part of 'the ageing process', by recognizing that ageing is influenced by earlier aspects of the life-course (Baltes *et al.*,1980). Seen from this point of view, human development continues throughout the entire lifespan, with old age being just another developmental phase. This psychological perspective on lifespan development has been summarized into seven propositions about the nature of human ageing (Baltes and Baltes, 1990). These are:

1 There are major differences between normal, pathological, and optimal ageing.

2 The course of ageing demonstrates much interindividual variability (heterogeneity).

3 There is much latent reserve capacity in older age.

4 There is an age-associated limitation to the range of reserve capacity.

5 Age-related decline in some aspects of cognitive functioning (speed etc.) can be compensated by pragmatic knowledge (intelligence, reasoning).

6 The balance between gains and losses becomes less positive with increasing age.

7 In old age the self remains resilient.

Underpinning these propositions are three sets of influences. The first set—normative age-graded influences—are those which have a relatively strong relationship with chronological age in terms of their onset and duration. These include biological maturation and age-related socialization such as the family life cycle, education, and occupation. They are normative, in that the timing and duration are similar across individuals.

The second set of influences—normative history graded—are biological or environmental influences that occur in similar ways to most members of a specific population cohort (e.g. wars or epidemics).

The final set of influences—non-normative life events—occur independent of age or history, and their occurrence tends to be specific to the individual. These include factors such as unemployment, illness, winning a lottery, divorce, bereavement, institutionalization, or relocation. The 'joint impact of influences of the three types, mediated through the developing individual, accounts for the nature of lifespan development, for its regularity, and also for its differential properties in terms of inter-individual differences, multi-directionality and multi dimensionality'. (Baltes *et al.*, 1980, p.76).

The lifespan developmental perspective of ageing and its seven propositions offer a comprehensive picture of ageing, encompassing decline, change, stability, and growth, reflecting the three sets of influences on ageing described previously. They also emphasize the considerable variability and flexibility of older age, described as 'differential ageing' (e.g. Baltes *et al.*, 1999).

## Erikson's life-cycle model of personality development

Typically, developmental models with their roots in psychoanalysis focused on infancy, childhood, and adolescence, with scarcely a nod towards adulthood. Erikson's eight-stage model of the life cycle stood out because it viewed personality development as continuing throughout the whole life cycle from childhood to old age (Erikson, 1963; see Table 31i.1). This model describes how individuals may accomplish each life phase, emphasizing how the self/personality/identity develops in stages and results in fulfilment, and proposes that there is a biological pre-disposition to adapt at each of these distinct stages of the life cycle. In some respects it could be described as an interactional model of personality and environment, with the developing individual being affected by societal demands and requirements.

These eight periods of the life cycle originate in childhood. At each stage there is a conflict between two forces, and if development is to be successful, the conflict needs to be resolved in order to obtain an emerging human strength. The final stage is characterized by an evaluation of life, involving looking back and assessing whether it was a meaningful experience. Acceptance of life is crucial for achieving a sense of integrity or wholeness, with wisdom being the successful outcome. Alternatively this review of life could lead to a conclusion that life was unproductive and meaningless, thereby resulting in despair.

This theory fits well with the proposition of the 'resilient self' of Baltes and Baltes (1990). It demonstrates from a lifespan developmental perspective that older age can be accompanied by the acquisition of new behaviours important for ageing (Baltes *et al.*, 1980). In terms of Erikson's eight stages, the continuing development of the self across the lifespan and the ultimate achievement of wisdom provide some explanation for the maintenance and growth of well-being in older age.

There is some empirical support for this claim. Ardelt (2000) examined the benefits of wisdom in older age, with wisdom operationalized as cognitive, affective, and reflective personality qualities. Using latent variable modelling techniques she found that when wisdom was included in the model, the influence of objective conditions on life satisfaction were not statistically significant, even though bivariate correlations between life satisfaction and objective conditions were. A previous study by Ardelt (1997) found that wisdom had a higher impact on life satisfaction in old age than physical health, income, socio-economic status, physical environment, or the extent of social relationships. Thus the developing personality exerted a strong influence on well-being in later life.

The eight-stage model introduces some important aspects of ageing. It reflects the continuous development of the self. It highlights

**Table 31i.1** Erikson's eight stages of the life cycle (Erikson 1963)

| Conflicting issues | Emerging value | Life period |
|---|---|---|
| 1. Basic trust versus mistrust | Hope | Infancy |
| 2. Autonomy versus shame and doubt | Will | Early childhood |
| 3. Initiative versus guilt | Purpose | Play age |
| 4. Industry versus inferiority | Competence | School age |
| 5. Identity versus identity (role) confusion | Fidelity | Adolescence |
| 6. Intimacy versus isolation | Love | Young adulthood |
| 7. Generativity versus stagnation | Care | Maturity |
| 8. Integrity versus despair (and disgust) | Wisdom | Old age |

the process of adaptation, which is achieved through tackling and resolving the conflicting issues at each life stage. Implicit in the model is the potential for earlier developmental tasks that are not completely resolved to resurface at later points of the life cycle. For example, the person whose sense of inferiority is managed by additional investment in industriousness, in keeping busy and active, becomes vulnerable when retirement leads to a loss of purpose, or physical health problems enforce inactivity. Or the person who learnt in infancy that others cannot be trusted finds dependency on others difficult to countenance, even though the support of others may clearly be required. Adaptation is crucial, and is dependent upon how the factors that might either constrain or enhance the ability to reach full potential are negotiated. The emphasis on the development of the self in this life cycle theory also introduces the notion of the important role that inner psychological resources central to the self might play in successfully negotiating conflicting issues and achieving well-being. Jung also emphasizes how inner exploration in older age enables individuals to find meaning and acceptance and subsequent satisfaction (Storr, 1983). This perspective also implies that there is something about the development of the self that might be optimized and maintained in older age, providing the basis from which the best interpretation of 'the good life' might be achieved.

## The ageing self—identity in later life: self-resources

If the pathway to well-being is an interplay between internal and external factors then successful adaptation at different life stages is a necessary requirement. Diener *et al.* (1999) argue that a fundamental element of modern theories of subjective well-being should be the notion of adaptation or habituation to ongoing situations. While there is broad evidence for adaptive psychological processes, especially for cognitive and affective processes, with respect to well-being in later life (Baltes and Baltes, 1990; Brandstädter and Greve, 1994; Carstensen, 1995; Heckhausen and Schulz, 1995; Moody, 2003), the basis for the presumed underlying psychological resources contributing to well-being in older people is still not well established.

Consideration of these personality resources provides the opportunity to understand how an individual copes with some of the challenges of ageing. Psychological resources that promote a sense of control, coping, and/or adaptation may change little in older age (Baltes and Baltes, 1986; Lachman, 1986; Ryff and Singer, 1996). These personal qualities are said to have a developmental trajectory, being acquired over the lifespan (Ryff and Singer, 1996).

The next subsections explore these ideas in more depth, outlining four psychological resources important to ageing (self-esteem, perceived control, self-efficacy/competence, and self acceptance). Evidence for the relationship of each with age is discussed, and their importance across a range of outcomes is presented.

### Self-esteem

Self-esteem refers to judgements of self-worth, derived from values, goals, and aspirations (Rosenberg, 1979). Self-esteem features in research as an outcome measure, an intervening variable, and as a resource to draw on when confronted with certain situations. The wide use of the concept of self-esteem is reflected in the richness of its meanings. It encompasses underlying processes of evaluation

and affection, it can be expressed as an attitude, a psychological response (in terms of 'what something feels like'), or a personality function which regulates the self when under stress (Wells and Marwell, 1976).

There is some debate within the literature regarding the maintenance of self-esteem across the lifespan. Much of the work examining the development and trajectory of self-esteem has tended to focus on childhood and adolescence, which has often produced inconsistent findings. From this younger age range, studies suggest that self-esteem may rise during adolescence (Marsh, 1989; McCarthy and Hodge, 1982), whilst others find this is not the case (Chubb *et al.*, 1997). Inconsistencies are also present in findings that have examined self-esteem across the age span. An extensive review of the literature concluded that there were no systematic age differences in self-esteem (Wylie, 1979). In contrast, others have found self-esteem to increase with age (from childhood into old age; Gove *et al.*, 1989) or not to change at all between the ages of 18 and 75 (Erdwins *et al.*, 1981). More recent research suggests it may decline in the older decades (from 70 to 103; Ranzijn *et al.*, 1998). Robbins *et al.* (2002) found that self-esteem declined sharply from childhood to adolescence, and dropped further until about the age of 22. From there it rose, increasing gradually into the sixth decade where a decline began, which was particularly marked in the 70s and 80s. Just over a quarter (26%) of the oldest cohorts reported low self-esteem (either a 1 or a 2 on a five-point scale) (Robbins *et al.*, 2002). Stronger evidence for the stability of self-esteem in older age comes from longitudinal research in the UK. This study followed a cohort of 339 people aged 65 and over, initially interviewed in 1977/78, who were finally re-interviewed during 1990/91. It was demonstrated that self-esteem remained stable at 10 and 13 years' follow-up (Coleman *et al.*, 1993).

There are a number of reasons that could explain the inconsistencies between the studies. One is the methodologies used in the studies. Robbins *et al.* (2002) undertook a large cross-sectional study ($n = 326,641$) of people age between 9 and 90 years old. This required individuals to complete an on-line questionnaire that assessed self-esteem by a single-item question (SISE). However, this method would require individuals either to own or to have access to a computer, and to be computer literate. Consequently this method could exclude a specific group of people, particularly in the oldest cohorts who are not as familiar with using computers. Ranzijn *et al.*'s (1998) analysis was undertaken on a large sample ($n = 1087$), where a very small difference can be statistically significant. Adopting more stringent criteria for significance suggested by Weber *et al.* (2003), the oldest cohort did not then have significantly lower self-esteem.

The scales chosen to measure self-esteem may also have had an effect on the findings. Ranzijn *et al.* (1998) used a revised version—the Bachman revision—of the Rosenberg self-esteem scale which comprised 10 items. Although some of the original Rosenberg items were retained, four new items were added which emphasized feelings of usefulness or competence, whereas the old (replaced) items focused on positive self-regard. In contrast, Robbins *et al.* (2002) used a single item 'I see myself as someone who has high self-esteem' rated on a five-point scale. This latter measure explicitly refers to self-esteem, whereas the former uses self-esteem as a construct that is tapped by 10 different items.

Gender differences may also have affected the findings. The study by Erdwins *et al.* (1981) focused on females only. More recently meta-analysis finds that men tend to have higher self-esteem than women, particularly in adolescence and early adulthood, although there were no differences in those aged 60 and over (Kling *et al.*, 1999). However, another meta-analysis found that there was a small but significant gender difference, with older women reporting slightly lower self-esteem compared with older men (Pinquart and Sörensen, 2001). Consequently the female focus may underestimate the average score. The upper age limit of 75 in the study of Erdwins *et al.* (1981) may also have missed the decline experienced in the oldest cohorts of Ranzijn *et al.* (1998) and Robbins *et al.* (2002). From these findings is could be concluded that self-esteem may be fairly robust, but the oldest old may experience some decline.

## Perceived control

A major determinant of positive cognitive, physical, and psychological outcomes in older adults is the perception of being in control over the immediate environment (Brandstädter and Baltes-Götz, 1990; Rowe and Kahn, 1997). Older adults seek to maintain control when facing losses associated with older age (Baltes, 1996; Fung *et al.*, 1999), consequently control could be regarded as an important psychological resource in older age. Theoretical perspectives start from the assumption that people generally feel that they have control over their lives, in that they can make decisions and take the right type of action to produce a desirable outcome and avoid undesirable ones. Possessing a sense of control enables individuals to regulate and direct events, to participate actively in life, and to be independent and have self-responsibility (Wallhagen, 1998). This is the sense in which the word 'control' will be used in the following paragraphs.

One of the earliest theories of control was proposed by Rotter (1966), derived from his theory of social learning (Rotter, 1954). Individuals with an 'internal locus of control' believe they have control over their successes and failures, whilst those who believe that their lives are controlled by other, external forces such as luck, fate, or the behaviour of another person are said to have an 'external locus of control'. Research findings support the beneficial effect of the possession of a sense of control in older people. It has been positively related to exercising and participation in leisure activities (Menec and Chipperfield, 1997) and associated with less physical disability in women recovering from surgery for fracture of the neck of the femur (Shaw *et al.*, 2003); it has also been found to predict better life satisfaction in frail older people (Abu-Bader *et al.*, 2002). Locus of control was found to mediate the relationship between age, gender, low income, and holocaust survival on the one hand, and subjective well-being (life satisfaction and mental health) on the other, in Israelis aged 75 and over (Landau and Litwin, 2001).

It is often expected that older adults will report less perceived control than younger age groups (Wolinsky and Stump, 1996). Age and gender differences in personal control have been reported, with older women having lower perceived control than men. This gender gap was greater amongst older people than in younger comparisons (Ross and Mirowsky, 2002). Mirowsky (1995) examined perceived control across an age range of 18 to 85. In the 18–50 age range it remained high, but declined with increasing age, with the oldest age groups having the lowest score. However, in a review of the literature, Schulz *et al.* (1991) reported that there was little evidence for changes in control with increasing age, and suggested

that studies which have found negative relationships between age and control reflect cohort effects as opposed to ageing effects. Another study found that older adults reported a greater sense of general control than younger and middle-aged adults, despite reporting that they faced more constraints in areas such as health and finances (Lachman and Weaver, 1998). Clearly there are some inconsistencies which do not provide unequivocal support for a decline in perceived control with increasing age.

Lachman (1986) stated that approximately one-third of studies report a negative relationship between increasing age and control, one-third a positive relationship, and one-third no association between age and control. Wolinsky *et al.* (2003) suggest that differing results could be influenced by factors such as the type of study (cross-sectional or longitudinal) and the different types of measures used to assess the construct. These authors found a significant negative relationship between age and control both cross-sectionally and longitudinally. However, the study sample was composed of chronically ill older adults, and so was not at all representative of the normally ageing population.

More recently Schulz and Heckhausen (1996, 1998) describe a lifespan theory of control. This theory posits two types of control, primary and secondary. Primary control refers to the immediate environment, where changes are made by influencing the external world. Secondary control is based within the individual, with the self being the source of change. Both types of control assist in favourable development across the lifespan, but have different paths. Primary control is thought to be most prominent in infancy and adolescence, with a peak around the age of 40–50 years, then a gradual decline into later life. Secondary control starts later in life, with a steady increase into older age (Magai, 2001). The change from primary to secondary control across the lifespan may enable greater regulatory control of emotion and well-being, providing a valuable resource in older age. The two types of control need to be assessed differently, which may explain why results differ across studies of control. Some measures may reflect secondary control more than others.

## Self-efficacy/competence

The concept of competence can be thought of as covering three broad domains: the range and level of skills, personal belief about abilities (efficacy and mastery), and the adaptive fit between skills and environmental demands (Baltes *et al.*, 1993). Personal efficacy/self-efficacy (Bandura, 1977) encompasses the belief that success can be achieved in what we want to do. It is also regarded as an evaluation based on a sense of competence (Dietz, 1996). A strong sense of efficacy increases the likelihood of a successful outcome, by affecting performance and intentions (Bandura, 1997). Estimates of predicted success or failure are derived from memories of the effects of previous activities. This theory distinguishes between outcome expectancy and behavioural expectancy: a person may believe that an action *could* lead to a specific outcome, but their previous experiences of success or failure will determine whether they believe that they are *personally* capable—or not—of achieving a desirable outcome. Crucially, beliefs concerning personal efficacy affect thought patterns and subsequent performance.

A substantial amount of research has examined the benefits of personal efficacy, although less attention has been given to its trajectory with age. In the general population, individuals with a strong sense of self-efficacy often demonstrate less psychological and physiological strain in response to stressors than do those with a poor sense of self-efficacy (Bandura et al., 1985). Other research has found that frequent daily hassles were related to a lower sense of self-efficacy and higher levels of depression (Holahan et al., 1984). A meta-analysis examining differences in psychological and physical health between caregivers and non-caregivers found that caregivers experienced more stress and depression and had lower levels of general subjective well-being and self-efficacy than non-caregivers (Pinquart and Sörensen, 2003).

Personal competence underlies the adaptive behaviour that is central to the person–environment transaction model (Lawton, 1989). This theory proposes that the person and the environment are joint determinants of behaviour and subsequent well-being. For example, older people with decreased physical functioning may need to draw on their resources and adapt their behavioural competence to the level of 'press' they experience in the environment, in order to maintain positive subjective well-being (Lawton, 1989). Demands can come from a diverse range of environmental areas, such as (1) the interpersonal, which consists of close social relationships, (2) the suprapersonal, which refers to the characteristics (age, gender, or race) of those who participate in social relationships, (3) the social, which refers to norms, values, and institutions of subgroups, society, or culture and (4) the physical environment. In this context, competence is an evaluative, cognitive process where the demands of the situation influence an individual's sense of efficacy (Wallhagen, 1998).

Welch and West (1995) describe how according to self-efficacy theory, older age is generally considered to be a time where the potential for positive effective behaviour is reduced. In a context of negative stereotypes of ageing, cognitive changes may then be interpreted as failures. Likewise, people who have experienced changes in physical functioning can find the physical environment difficult to negotiate.

The evidence for these propositions is mixed. Lachman (1991) found that older adults reported less perceived efficacy than younger adults. However, there is considerable variability in older age and there is no consistent decline in self-efficacy (Bandura, 1994). Some research has found that *higher* levels of self-efficacy are associated with increasing age (Dietz, 1996). It has been suggested that age-related changes in efficacy beliefs are more likely to be revealed using domain-linked measures (Bandura, 1997). In terms of the domain of memory, levels of perceived memory efficacy were found to predict the extent of improvement in memory performance in both young and older adults after training in mnemonic aids (Rebok and Balcerak, 1989). A study of the Italian population between the ages of 20 and 80 found that males had greater self-efficacy in the regulation of negative affect and social self-efficacy, whilst females had greater efficacy for expressing positive affect and more empathic self-efficacy. Regardless of gender, self-efficacy for positive affect, empathic, and social self-efficacy declined as age increased, although self-efficacy for negative affect increased across the age cohorts for females (Capara et al., 2003).

### Self-acceptance

Self-acceptance is described as a key dimension of positive psychological functioning (Ryff and Singer, 1996). It is viewed as an aspect of self-actualization, maturity, and optimal functioning which emphasizes the acceptance of current and past life (Ryff and Singer, 1996). It makes possible the maintenance of self-esteem

when dealing with some of the less desirable aspects of personal life (Keyes and Waterman, 2004). Self-acceptance is crucial for achieving a sense of integrity, the final stage of Erikson's model of the life cycle.

Self-acceptance has been found to remain consistent across young, mid-life, and older aged cohorts (Ryff and Singer, 1996). Another study found no age differences across average self-acceptance scores, although males reported significantly higher self-acceptance than females (Capara et al., 2003). The positive relationship between self-acceptance and subjective well-being in older adults is seen as enabling an acceptance of age-related changes (Ranzijn and Luszcz, 1999).

To summarize, the literature highlights the importance of personality resources in older age. However, less research has directly examined their trajectory into advanced older age, which raises questions as to whether there is an optimal time for their benefit. To go some way to answer this, the next section examines some of the evidence for the relationship between psychological resources and well-being in older adults.

## The importance of psychological resources to well-being

Research that has examined the influence that psychological resources have on well-being finds that they can have an intervening effect. They can increase the possibility of positive changes in health behaviours and well-being (Wells and Kendig, 1999), or can limit the potential negative influences on well-being of risk factors associated with ageing (Windle and Woods, 2004). In the latter study, a representative sample of 420 people aged 70 and above (mean age 78) were interviewed in north Wales. The impact of a number of factors on the person's life satisfaction were examined, and it emerged that physical health limitations, loneliness, housing difficulties, and being widowed or divorced were related to lower levels of life satisfaction. However, when the person's sense of environmental mastery (measured on a nine-item scale developed by Ryff, 1989) was included in the predictive model, this mitigated the effects of both physical health limitations and housing difficulties, and, to a lesser extent, of loneliness. In other words, having a strong sense of environmental mastery reduced the impact of the difficult circumstances the older person was experiencing.

The beneficial effect of self-efficacy is demonstrated in research which shows self-efficacy to diminish the negative impact of impaired functional capacity on depressive symptoms (Knipscheer et al., 2000). Self-efficacy has also been found to buffer the impact of cancer on depressive symptoms in people aged between 55 and 85 (Bisschop et al., 2004). Self-efficacy probably works through its influence on the coping processes that people require when faced with problematic situations, and on their subsequent choice of adaptive strategies (Slangen-de Kort et al., 2001).

The impact of other psychological resources on well-being has also been evaluated. Mastery has been found to improve mental health and functioning (Badger, 1993, 2001). Increases in mental health and life satisfaction scores were found to be associated with respondents who had a higher internal locus of control (Landau and Litwin, 2001). Other research has found that older adults demonstrate no reduction in psychological resources central to the self such as self-esteem or sense of personal control despite losses in functioning and the perception of such losses (Baltes and Baltes,

1986; Lachman, 1986). Self-esteem has been reported to be a strong predictor of life satisfaction in Western societies (Campbell, 1981; Lucas *et al.*, 1996). Control beliefs have been associated with well-being between the ages of 25 and 75 (Lachman and Weaver, 1998). The beneficial effects of such resources in older age may then be a key factor for well-being. Other research that has examined resources such as mastery, self-esteem, and optimism has conceptualized them as part of the core of the reserve capacity that provides a basis of resilience in older age (Gallo *et al.*, 2005). According to Bandura (1992, p.4) such 'self generated activities lie at the very heart of causal processes'. These mechanisms of personal agency can help to give meaning to many external pressures, so that they can be dealt with successfully. Atchley (1999) reports that a large proportion of respondents in a longitudinal study maintained consistent self concepts over 20 years of study, despite threats from changing life events. Consequently the self is clearly a resilient structure, once it has developed (Atchley, 1989). Taking up this theme, the following section examines the concept of resilience.

## Resilience

Resilience has been described as being 'able to recover from or adjust to misfortune or change' (Penguin English Dictionary, 2002). It can be seen as the opposite to vulnerability and encompasses personal competences across cognitive, emotional, and social domains (Tizard and Clarke, 1992). It was derived from the observation that people can still function positively although exposed to substantial stressors and risks, and recover quickly from set-backs (Rutter, 1995). Consequently resilient individuals flourish when challenged (Ryff and Singer, 2003). Psychological resilience is thought to be important in late life as a component of successful psychosocial adjustment (Wagnild and Young, 1993).

Although the definition of resilience may be generally agreed, it is harder to measure than to describe. It tends to have been measured indirectly, and functions more as a hypothetical construct in research which finds successful outcomes despite setbacks. Much of the initial research into resilience was undertaken on children. Many children in negative family environments, (e.g. with mentally ill parents (Garmezey, 1974; Rutter, 1985) or in poor socio-economic circumstances (Garmezey, 1991)) do not display maladaptive behaviours or become mentally ill themselves. They are able to function positively despite their circumstances.

More recently it has been proposed that in older people a positive response to a stressful life event is indicative of a resilient process (Hardy *et al.*, 2004). These authors found that independence in instrumental activities of daily living, positive self-ratings of health, and few depressive symptoms were independently associated with high resilience. However, they acknowledge that the conceptualization of resilience as the response to a stressful event has limitations as it cannot be measured in the absence of a significant stressful event.

On the other hand, the examination of resilience as an internal personality resource provides the opportunity to address this limitation and examine the psychological basis of why people are resilient—the central issue in understanding resilience (Ryff and Singer, 2003). This psychological perspective might allow a deeper understanding of why some individuals can remain resilient in difficult circumstances, such as some of the challenges of ageing.

Rutter (1987) described resilient individuals as possessing self-efficacy, self-esteem, and a range of problem-solving skills.

Others describe resilient individuals as possessing self-confidence, curiosity, self-discipline, self-esteem and control over the environment, and good intellectual functioning. Self-perceptions such as self-efficacy (Beardslee, 1989; Masten, 1999), and personal competence and acceptance of self and life (Wagnild and Young, 1993) are also important. These personality resources are thought to protect individuals in the face of adversity and lead to positive adaptive behaviour by acting as a protective 'buffer' (Rutter, 1987) or as compensatory factors which directly influence outcomes (Masten, 1999). In this context, resilience could be viewed as an 'umbrella' term for such psychological resources which are central to the self.

One of the earliest psychological references to the self is by William James (1890) who described the self as being two reflexive facets, one being the cause of experience ('I' the subject) and one being the contents of experience ('me' the object). Bengston *et al.* (1985) propose that it is the contents of experience that result in the self concept. These contents represent what an individual has come to regard as essential about themselves 'the sum total of the attributes, abilities, attitudes and values that an individual believes defines who he or she is' (Osborne, 1996, p.2). In this context the self is derived from an interaction of experiences, thoughts, feelings, and actions (Wells and Marwell, 1976) acquiring a diverse range of processes and resources. The emphasis on experience in the development of the self concept suggests that there may be parts of the self concept that are highly salient in older age, providing a valuable resource for the act of self-preservation originally described by James.

The way in which individuals deal with life events and experiences crucially depends upon the 'content, organisation and functioning of the self concept' (Markus and Herzog, 1991, p. 110). Seen from the developmental perspective, a person's life-time experiences are integrated into their self concept, where meaning is attached and continuity is maintained. Crucially the self concept is involved in a wide range of mental functioning such as coping, control, efficacy, competence, motivation, goal setting, and feelings. It is the 'interpretive link' (Markus and Herzog, 1991, p. 128) between circumstances and adaptation. This fits with the view that resilience facilitates adaptation via a range of psychological resources central to the self.

In line with this, continuity theory (Atchley, 1989) assumes that learning how best to adapt to change continues across the lifespan, and that well-being is achieved through adaptive choices that maintain the continuity of internal structures whilst dealing with age-associated changes. It represents a view of stability in older age as the result of the active and ongoing interplay that an individual has with their environment. Continuity theory is not a theory of successful ageing, but rather one that 'concerns itself with how people attempt to adapt and the mental frameworks they can be expected to use in doing so' (Atchley, 1999, p. 7). The implication of mental frameworks in adaptation places a focus on internal, psychological aspects of continuity, and highlights the potential for a sense of psychological resilience which may provide a basis for adaptation.

## The theory of selective optimization with compensation

The potential regulatory effect on well-being of the resilient self can be partially explained through the theory of selective

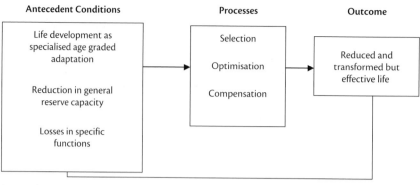

**Fig. 31i.1** Selective optimization with compensation (from Baltes and Baltes, 1990 p. 22).

Source: Baltes and Baltes (1990)

optimization with compensation (SOC; see Fig. 31i.1). The theory describes three processes which may be used in adaptation to changes occurring in later life.

*Selection* implies an adjustment of expectations to permit personal control and satisfaction (Baltes and Baltes, 1990). It involves choosing goals, life domains, or life tasks. Selection may require a restriction to fewer domains of functioning due to new responsibilities and stresses—described as elective selection—or it may occur as a consequence of or in anticipation of losses in certain areas of life, such as personal or environmental resources (loss-based selection). It may also refer to the avoidance of one domain, or a restriction of tasks or goals in one or more domains. Selection can also involve new goals, such as environmental changes (e.g. moving house due to difficulties with the current home) or a more passive type of adjustment (such as not climbing the stairs) (Baltes and Carstensen, 1999). Compensation and optimization provide the ability to maintain or even enhance chosen goals (Baltes and Carstensen, 1999). *Optimization* of behaviour occurs when losses are minimized and gains maximized, and is the desired *outcome* of the SOC process. The methods a person has for achieving their goals are refined and perfected (Baltes and Carstensen, 1999). *Compensation* is required when skills and capacity are reduced below the level required for adequate functioning. In order to maintain or even optimize that prior functioning, a present skill may be adapted into a new behaviour, or new means sought to retain that functioning (Baltes and Carstensen, 1999).

As an example of the SOC process, Baltes and Baltes (1990) describe the answer of the concert pianist Rubenstein when asked how he managed to remain a successful performer in old age. He replied that he performed fewer pieces (*selection*), he practiced more frequently (*optimization*), and he slowed his playing down before playing faster sections, in order to give the impression that they sounded faster than they really were (*compensation*). According to Herzog and Markus (1999) the theoretical perspective of the self system can assist in understanding such processes. They state that:

> The domains and dimensions that define the self provide the basis of selectivity, determining where time and energy will be invested, where efficacy and control (or the lack of it) will be experienced, what will be planned for, what will be compensated for, what will be discounted or ignored, and ultimately how individual lives accrue meaning and structure.

Herzog and Markus (1999, p.228)

In other words, the self can provide context and meaning which in turn is developed from a view of the self from the past, present, and future perspectives. This process of self-reference can maintain a positive self concept. In relation to ageing, how individuals react to changing roles and life events is dependent upon mediation by the self concept (Markus and Herzog, 1991). The concept of resilience may then represent positive functioning across the diverse range of resources which characterize the self. Given the potential for positive outcomes associated with these psychological resources, resilience, both as a process and an outcome, requires further investigation.

## Personality and dementia

If personality can indeed be thought of as showing continuity over the lifespan, with individuals showing remarkable capacity to adapt and cope with difficult life circumstances, what are the effects of a dementia on personality, and does the person's personality influence the way in which dementia presents? McCrae (2002) suggests that 'the most dramatic and best-documented changes in personality are those associated with changes in the brain, attributable to Alzheimer's disease or to traumatic brain injury'.

### Does dementia change personality?

In evaluating personality change in people with dementia, researchers must usually rely on a relative completing two personality inventories, one for how the person is now and one for a period well before the onset of the condition. This involves two assumptions; firstly that proxy reports of personality can be reliable and valid; and secondly that retrospective accounts can be accurate, and not influenced by the dementia-related changes, or by the relative's experience of caregiving. The reliability and validity of the proxy version of the NEO-PI scale has been well documented (McCrae and Costa, 2003). Evidence for the second assumption is provided by Strauss *et al.*, (1993), who report ratings of 22 people with Alzheimer's disease by two informants (the main caregiver and another relative or friend), showing substantial agreement between the raters, both in comparative rankings and in absolute level on the NEO-PI scale.

Some studies have used scales designed to be sensitive to dementia-related personality changes; for example, Aitken *et al.* (1999) used a scale that had been developed for use with people with head injuries, with 99 relatives of people with dementia rating previous and current levels on 18 dimensions. They concluded that there were changes, largely negative, across all domains, with greater changes in those having a diagnosis of vascular dementia.

A number of studies have used the NEO scale, which places the results more clearly in the context of contemporary personality research. Siegler *et al.* (1991) reported significant changes in four of the five NEO factors: higher neuroticism, lower extraversion, lower conscientiousness, and less openness; the trend towards lower agreeableness did not reach significance in this sample of 35 people with mild to moderate memory impairment. These findings were replicated in a sample of 26 people with Alzheimer's disease (Siegler *et al.*, 1994). Chatterjee *et al.* (1992) similarly reported that relatives rated people with Alzheimer's disease on the NEO scale as more neurotic, less extraverted, and less conscientious than they had been before the onset of the illness, with smaller reductions in agreeableness and openness. With the exception of conscientiousness, the changes appeared to reflect consistent systematic shifts across all patients. Similarly, Strauss *et al.* (1993) reported significant differences between pre-morbid and current NEO personality ratings for four of the five dimensions. In a UK study of 36 people with dementia, again using the NEO-PI, Williams *et al.* (1995) reported findings that are broadly consistent, with increased neuroticism and reduced extraversion and conscientiousness emerging clearly. Dawson *et al.* (2000), in a study of 50 people with Alzheimer's disease, concluded that the changes in these three areas were related only to the pre-morbid rating and not to other variables such as duration of dementia, education, age, and gender. This probably accounts for the robust finding of change in these areas across samples. The reduction in extraversion may reflect the withdrawal from social contact and social roles typically seen in dementia; the reduced conscientiousness may arise from difficulty in maintaining previous standards in view of the cognitive impairment; and the increased neuroticism may reflect the presence of increased uncertainty and vulnerability for the person with dementia.

### Does personality influence dementia presentation?

An association between pre-morbid personality, assessed using the NEO-PI, and current symptoms was reported by Chatterjee *et al.* (1992). They found that current depression was related to high levels of reported pre-morbid neuroticism, and that pre-morbid hostility was related to paranoid delusions. However, Strauss *et al.* (1997) cautioned that having the same informant rating both personality and current behavioural problems may lead to overstating their degree of association. In their sample, where personality was rated by two informants, only neuroticism and current anxiety symptoms were associated, when different informants were used for past and current ratings. Using the Munich Personality Test, with a sample of 56 people with Alzheimer's disease, Meins *et al.* (1998) found that higher levels of pre-morbid neuroticism were related to disturbed behaviour whereas low tolerance of frustration was related to depression.

There has been some considerable interest in the effect of the attachment style of the person with dementia on their behaviour and adjustment (e.g. Miesen, 1993). Attachment style in adulthood is thought to reflect early experiences of parenting, with typically three main styles identified: secure; insecure–ambivalent; and insecure–avoidant. These styles provide a basis for personality traits such as neuroticism, extraversion, and agreeableness.

Magai *et al.* (1997) report results from a group of 27 people with mid to late dementia. Relatives rated lifelong attachment style, and ratings of the person's current emotional state were made by family, care staff, and independent observers. People with dementia rated as having a secure attachment style appeared to show greater positive affect, whereas ratings of pre-morbid hostility were related to ratings of current anger, disgust, and contempt. In a much larger sample of 168 people with mid to late dementia, Magai and Cohen (1998) found that people who were rated by relatives as insecure–ambivalent had increased levels of depression and anxiety. Those rated as insecure–avoidant had higher levels of activity disturbance and paranoid symptoms. Caregivers of people rated as having secure attachment styles reported less overall burden than caregivers of people with dementia who had life-long insecure attachment styles. Browne and Shlosberg (2005), in a sample of 53 people with dementia living in care homes, found that those rated as having a life-long insecure–avoidant attachment styles showed more overt attachment behaviours (e.g. following staff, clinging onto visitors) than those rated as securely attached.

In summary, it appears that there is some evidence that aspects of pre-morbid personality are related to the current emotional state and behaviour of the person with dementia, but the precise nature of the relationship needs further exploration. Given that ratings of pre-morbid personality rely on family members as informants, using other informants for current function is essential to avoid spurious associations that reflect the impact of caregiving rather than an accurate appraisal.

## Conclusions

This chapter first presented the debate regarding stability and change in personality across the lifespan, especially in relation to the 'Big Five' five-factor model. There is much evidence, in general, for continuity and consistency, but some changes are widely accepted, such as reduced neuroticism, less extraversion, and greater conscientiousness. Lifespan developmental models emphasize that change may well be required to maintain stability in the face of changing external and internal circumstances and events, and Erikson's model provides a broad-brush approach, identifying a developmental task specific to later life, reflecting the potential for continued growth.

The model of selective optimization with compensation indicates how individuals can deal with ageing and the age-related tendencies for increased losses and fewer gains, making use of regulatory processes (Baltes, 1993). It has been proposed that the regulation of subjective well-being can occur through psychological resources that promote adaptation to adverse situations (Smith *et al.*, 1999; Staudinger *et al.*, 1999). Continuity theory would imply that a lifetime's accumulation of experience would aid the development of a resilient self over the years, and this could explain how the self might be the link between various domains of life and well-being. Resilience is presented as a concept that captures the reality of development into later life, where the self faces many difficulties, losses, and threats, and yet seeks to maintain well-being. Research that has examined the role of resources such as mastery, self-esteem, optimism, perceptions of social support, and social conflict has conceptualized these resources as the core of reserve capacity that provides a resilient basis in older age (Gallo *et al.*, 2005). Although the literature points to the importance of these psychological resources in older age, it is less clear about the maintenance of these resources in the oldest cohorts. The psychological resources that underpin resilience may provide the basis for the maintenance of well-being in older age, but it may be that there is an optimal time for their benefit.

In the context of dementia, evidence is emerging of consistent personality changes, especially relating to increased neuroticism, reduced extraversion, and conscientiousness. But the picture is less clear with respect to the association of pre-morbid personality and current behaviour, except perhaps in relation to neuroticism and depression/anxiety. There is great scope for further work exploring the self in dementia, and the influence of factors such as resilience in this most demanding of challenges.

Finally, Hooker (2002) describes a three-level model of personality, of which the first two levels have been the main focus of this chapter. Level I relates to traits, as in the five-factor model; Level II includes self-regulatory processes, such as self-efficacy and control processes. The third level reflects the person's life story, and is seen in activities with a social component such as remembering, reminiscence, and story-telling. It is also at the heart of Erikson's eighth stage, where the person's life review can enable meaning and coherence to be found in the varied experiences of a life lived. Hooker suggests that 'personality is most clearly revealed in later life', and it is ultimately in the person's life story narrative that the richness and meaning of the individual's personality can be discerned.

## References

Abu-Bader, S.H., Barusch, A.S., and Rogers, A. (2002). Predictors of life satisfaction in frail elderly. *Journal of Gerontological Social Work*, **38**(3), 3–17.

Aitken, L., Simpson, S., and Burns, A. (1999). Personality change in dementia. *International Psychogeriatrics*, **11**, 263–271.

Ardelt, M. (1997). Wisdom and life satisfaction in old age. *Journal of Gerontology: Psychological Sciences*, **52B**, 15–27.

Ardelt, M. (2000). Antecedents and effects of wisdom in old age. A longitudinal perspective on aging well. *Research on Aging*, **22**(4), 360–394.

Atchley, R.C. (1989). A continuity theory of normal aging. *The Gerontologist*, **29**(2), 183–190.

Atchley, R.C. (1999). *Continuity and adaptation in aging*. Johns Hopkins University Press, Baltimore.

Badger, T.A. (2001). Depression, psychological resources and health-related quality of life in older adults 75 and above, *Journal of Clinical Geropsychology*, **7**(3), 189–200.

Badger, T.A. (1993). Physical health impairment and depression among older adults, *Journal of Nursing Scholarship*, **25**, 325–330.

Baltes, M.M. (1996). *The many faces of dependency in old age*. Cambridge University Press, New York.

Baltes, M.M. and Baltes, P.B. (1986). *The psychology of control and aging*. Erlbaum, Hillsdale, NJ.

Baltes, M.M. and Carstensen, L.L. (1999). Social-psychological theories and their applications to aging: from individual to collective. In *Handbook of theories of aging*, Vol. 1 (ed. V.L. Bengtson and K.W. Schaie), pp. 209–226. Springer, New York.

Baltes, M.M., Mayer, U., Borchelt, M., Maas, I., and Wilms, H.U. (1993). Everyday competence in old and very old age: An inter-disciplinary perspective. *Ageing and Society*, **13**(4), 657–680.

Baltes, M.M., Mayer, U., Borchelt, M., Maas, I., and Wilms, H.U. (1999). Everyday competence in old and very old age: theoretical considerations and empirical findings. In *The Berlin Aging Study. Aging from 70 to 100* (ed. P.B. Baltes and K.U. Mayer). Cambridge University Press, Cambridge.

Baltes, P.B. (1993). The aging mind: potential and limits. *Gerontologist*, **33**, 580–594.

Baltes, P.B., Reese, R.H., and Lipsitt, L.P. (1980). Life span developmental psychology. *Annual Review of Psychology*, **31**, 65–110.

Baltes, P.B. and Baltes, M.M. (1990). Psychological perspectives on successful aging: The model of selective optimisation with compensation. In *Successful aging: perspectives from the behavioural sciences* (ed. P.B. Baltes and M.M. Baltes), pp. 1–34. Cambridge University Press, Cambridge.

Bandura, A. (1977). Self-efficacy: toward a unifying theory of behavioural change. *Psychological Review*, **84**, 191–215.

Bandura, A. (1992). Exercise of personal agency. In *Self efficacy. Thought control of action* (ed. R. Schwarzer). Hemisphere, New York.

Bandura, A. (1994). Self-efficacy. In *Encyclopedia of human behaviour*, Vol. 4 (ed. V.S. Ramachaudran), pp. 71–81. Academic Press, New York.

Bandura, A. (1997). *Self efficacy: the exercise of control*. Freeman and Company, New York.

Bandura, A., Taylor, C.B., Williams, S.L., Mefford, I.N., and Barchas, J.D. (1985). Catecholamine secretion as a function of perceived coping and self-efficacy. *Journal of Consulting and Clinical Psychology*, **53**, 406–414.

Beardslee, W.R. (1989). The role of self-understanding in resilient individuals: the development of a perspective. *American Journal of Orthopsychiatry*, **59**(2), 266–278.

Bengston, V.L., Reedy, M.N., and Gordon, C. (1985). Aging and self-conceptions: personality processes and social contexts. In *Handbook of the psychology of aging*, Vol. 2 (ed. J.E. Birren and K.W. Schaie), pp. 544–593. Van Nostrand Reinhold, New York.

Berry, J. and Jobe, J.B. (2002). At the intersection of personality and adult development. *Journal of Research in Personality*, **36**, 283–286.

Bisschop, M.I., Kriegsman, D.M.W., Beekman, A.T.F., and Deeg, D.J.H. (2004). Chronic diseases and depression: the modifying role of psychosocial resources. *Social Science and Medicine*, **59**, 721–733.

Brandstädter, J. and Baltes-Götz, B. (1990). Personal control over development and quality of life perspectives in adulthood. In *Successful aging. Perspectives from the behavioural sciences* (ed. P.B. Baltes and M.M. Baltes), pp. 197–224. Cambridge University Press, Cambridge.

Brandstädter, J. and Greve, W. (1994). The ageing self: stabilizing and protective processes. *Developmental Review*, **14**, 52–80.

Browne, C. J. and Shlosberg, E. (2005). Attachment behaviours and parent fixation in people with dementia: the role of cognitive functioning and pre-morbid attachment style. *Aging and Mental Health*, **9**(2), 153–161.

Campbell, A. (1981). *The sense of well-being in America: recent patterns and trends*. McGraw-Hill, New York.

Capara, G.V., Capara, M., and Steca, P. (2003). Personality's correlates of adult development and aging. *European Psychologist*, **8**(3), 131–147.

Carstensen, L.L. (1995). Evidence for life-span theory of socioemotional selectivity. *Current Directions in Psychological Sciences*, **4**, 151–156.

Chatterjee, A., Strauss, M.E., Smyth, K.A., and Whitehouse, P. (1992). Personality changes in Alzheimer's disease. *Archives of Neurology*, **49**, 486–491.

Chubb, N.H., Fertman, C.L., and Ross, J.L. (1997). Adolescent self-esteem and locus of control: a longitudinal study of gender and age differences. *Adolescence*, **32**, 113–129.

Coleman, P.G., Ivani-Chalian, C., and Robinson, M. (1993). Self esteem and its sources: stability and change in later life. *Ageing and Society*, **13**, 171–192.

Costa, P.T. and McCrae, R.R. (1992). Multiple uses for longitudinal personality data. *European Journal of Personality*, **6**, 85–102.

Costa, P.T., Jr and McCrae, R.R. (1994). *Revised NEO Personality Inventory (NEO-PI-R) and NEO-Five-Factor Inventory (NEO-FFI) professional manual*. Psychological Assessment Resources, Odessa, FL.

Costa, P.T. and McCrae, R.R. (1997). Longitudinal stability of adult personality. In *Handbook of personality psychology* (ed. R. Hogan, J. Johnson, and S. Briggs), pp. 269–292. Academic Press, San Diego.

Dawson, D.V., Welsh-Bohmer, K.A., and Siegler, I.C. (2000). Premorbid personality predicts level of rated personality change in patients with Alzheimer's disease. *Alzheimer Disease and Associated Disorders*, **14**, 11–19.

Diener, E., Suh, E.M., Lucas, R.E., and Smith, H.L. (1999). Subjective well-being; three decades of progress. *Psychological Bulletin*, **2**, 276–302.

Dietz, B.E. (1996). The relationship of aging to self esteem: the relative effects of maturation and role accumulation. *International Journal of Aging and Human Development*, **43**(3), 249–266.

Digman, J. (1990). Personality structure: emergence of the 5 factor model. *Annual Review of Psychology*, **41**, 417–440.

Erdwins, C.J., Mellinger, J.C., and Typer, Z.E. (1981). A comparison of different aspects of self-concept for young, middle aged and older women. *Journal of Clinical Psychology*, **37**, 484–490.

Erikson. E. (1963). *Childhood and society*. Penguin, Harmondsworth.

Fung, H.H., Carstensen, L.L., and Lutz, A.M (1999). Influence of time on social preferences: Implications for life-span development. *Psychology and Aging*, **14**(4), 595–604.

Gallo, L.C., Bogart, L.M., Vranceanu, A., and Mathews, K.A. (2005). Socioeconomic status, resources, psychological experiences and emotional responses: A test of the reserve capacity model. *Journal of Personality and Social Psychology*, **88**(2), 386–399.

Garmezey, N. (1974). The study of competence in children at risk for severe psychopathology. In *The child in his family*, Vol. 3 (ed. E.J. Anthony and C. Koupernick). Wiley, New York.

Garmezey, N. (1991). Resiliency and vulnerability of adverse developmental outcomes associated with poverty. *American Behavioural Scientist*, **34**, 416–430.

Gove, W.R., Ortega, S.T., and Style, C.B. (1989). The maturational and role perspectives on aging and self through the adult years: An empirical evaluation. *American Journal of Sociology*, **94**, 1117–1145.

Hardy, S.E., Concato, J., and Gill, T.M. (2004). Resilience of community dwelling older persons. *Journal of the American Geriatrics Society*, **52**, 257–262.

Heckhausen, J. and Schulz, R. (1995). A life-span theory of control. *Psychological Review*, **102**, 284–304.

Helson, R., Kwan, V.S.Y., John, O.P., and Jones, C. (2002). The growing evidence for personality change in adulthood: findings from research with personality inventories. *Journal of Research in Personality*, **36**, 287–306.

Herzog, A.R. and Markus, H.R. (1999). The self-concept in life-span and aging research. In *Handbook of theories of aging*, Vol. 1 (ed. V.L. Bengtson and K.W. Schaie), pp. 227–252. Springer, New York.

Holahan, C.K., Holahan, C.H, and Belk, S.S. (1984). Adjustment in aging: the roles of life stress, hassles, and self efficacy. *Health Psychology*, **3**, 315–328.

Hooker, K. (2002). New directions for research in personality and aging: a comprehensive model for linking levels, structures and processes. *Journal of Research in Personality*, **36**, 318–334.

James, W. (1890). *Principles of psychology*, Vol. 1. Henry Holt, New York.

Keyes, C.L.M. and Waterman, M.B. (2004). Dimensions of well-being and mental health in adulthood. In *Well being. Positive development across the lifecourse* (ed. M.H. Bornstein, L. Davidson, C.L.M. Keyes, and K.A. Moore). Lawrence Erlbaum Associates, Hillsdale, NJ.

Kling, K.C., Hyde, J.S., Showers, C.J., and Buswell, B. N. (1999). Gender differences in self esteem: a meta-analysis. *Psychological Bulletin*, **125**, 470–500.

Knipscheer, C.P.M., Broese van Groenou, M.I., Leene, G.J.F., Beekman, A. T.F., and Deeg, D.J.H. (2000). The effects of environmental context and personal resources on depressive symptomatology in older age: a test of the Lawton model. *Ageing and Society*, **20**, 183–202.

Lachman, M.E. (1986). Personal control in later life: stability, change and cognitive correlates. In *The psychology of control and aging* (ed. M.M. Baltes and P.B. Baltes), pp. 207–236. Erlbaum, Hillsdale, NJ.

Lachman, M.E. (1991). Perceived control over memory aging: developmental and intervention perspectives. *Journal of Social Issues*, **47**, 159–175.

Lachman, M.E. and Weaver, S.L. (1998). The sense of control as a moderator of social class differences in health and well-being. *Journal of Personality and Social Psychology*, **74**(3), 763–773.

Landau, R. and Litwin, H. (2001). Subjective well-being among the old-old: the role of health, personality and social support. *International Journal of Ageing and Human Development*, **54**(4), 265–289.

Lawton, M.P. (1989). Behaviour relevant ecological factors. In *Social structure and ageing* (ed. K.W. Schaie and C. Schooler), pp. 57–78. Lawrence Erlbaum Associates, Hillsdale, NJ.

Lucas, R.E., Diener, E., and Suh, E. (1996). Discriminant validity of well-being measures. *Journal of Personality and Social Psychology*, **71**, 616–628.

McCarthy, J.D. and Hodge, D.R. (1982). Analysis of age effects in longitudinal studies of adolescent self-esteem. *Developmental Psychology*, **18**, 372–379.

McCrae, R.R. (2002). The maturation of personality psychology: adult personality development and psychological well-being. *Journal of Research in Personality*, **36**, 307–317.

McCrae, R.R. and Costa, P.T. (1996). Towards a new generation of personality theories: theoretical contexts for the five-factor model. In *The five factor model of personality. Theoretical perspectives* (ed. J.S. Wiggins), pp. 51–87. Guildford, New York.

McCrae, R.R. and Costa, P.T. (2003). *Personality in adulthood: a five factor theory perspective*, 2nd edn. Guilford, New York.

McCrae, R.R., Costa, P.T., Jr, Lima, M.P. *et al.* (1999). Age differences in personality across the adult life span: parallels in five cultures. *Developmental Psychology*, **35**, 466–477.

McCrae, R.R., Terracciano, A., and 78 Members of the Personality Profiles of Cultures Project (2005). Universal features of personality traits from the observer's perspective: data from 50 cultures. *Journal of Personality and Social Psychology*, **88**, 547–561.

Magai, C. (2001). Emotions over the life span. In *Handbook of the psychology of aging* (ed. J.E. Birren and K.W. Schaie). Academic Press, New York.

Magai, C. and Cohen, C.I. (1998). Attachment style and emotion regulation in dementia patients and their relation to caregiver burden. *Journal of Gerontology*, **53B**(3), P147–P154.

Magai, C., Cohen, C.I., Culver, C., Gomberg, D., and Malatesta, C. (1997). Relation between premorbid personality and patterns of emotion expression in mid- to late-stage dementia. *International Journal of Geriatric Psychiatry*, **12**, 1092–1099.

Markus, H.R. and Herzog, A.R. (1991). The role of the self concept in aging. *Annual Review of Gerontology and Geriatrics*, **11**, 110–143.

Marsh, H.W. (1989). Age and sex effects in multiple dimensions of self-concept: preadolescence to adulthood. *Journal of Educational Psychology*, **81**, 417–430.

Masten, A.S. (1999). Resilience comes of age: Reflections on the past and outlook for the next generation of research. In *Resilience and development: positive life adaptations. Longitudinal research in the social and behavioral sciences* (ed. M.D. Glantz and J.L. Johnson), pp. 281–296. Kluwer, New York.

Meins, W., Frey, A., and Thiesemann, R. (1998). Premorbid personality traits in Alzheimer's disease: do they predispose to non-cognitive behavioral symptoms? *International Psychogeriatrics*, **10**, 369–378.

Menec, V.H. and Chipperfield, J.G. (1997). Remaining active in later life: the role of locus of control in senior's leisure activity participation, health and life satisfaction. *Journal of Ageing and Health*, **9**(1), 105–125.

Miesen, B.M.L. (1993). Alzheimer's disease, the phenomenon of parent fixation and Bowlby's attachment theory. *International Journal of Geriatric Psychiatry*, **8**, 147–153.

Mirowsky, J. (1995). Age and the sense of control. *Social Psychology Quarterly*, **58**(1), 31–43.

Moody, H.R. (2003). Conscious aging: a strategy for positive development in later life. In *Mental wellness in aging: strength-based approaches* (ed. J.L. Ronch and J.R.J. Goldfield). Health Professions Press, Baltimore, MD.

Osborne, R.E. (1996). *Self. An eclectic approach.* Allyn and Bacon, Needham Heights, MA.

Pinquart, M. and Sörensen, S. (2001). Gender differences in self-concept and psychological well-being in old age: a meta-analysis. *Journal of Gerontology: Psychological Sciences*, **56B**(4), 195–213.

Pinquart, M. and Sörensen, S. (2003). Differences between caregivers and non-caregivers in psychological health and physical health: a meta-analysis. *Psychology and Aging*, **18**(2), 250–267.

Ranzijn, R. and Luszcz, M. (1999). Acceptance: a key to well-being in older adults? *Australian Psychologist*, **34**(2), 94–98.

Ranzijn, R., Keeves, J., Luszcz, M., and Feather, N.T. (1998). The role of self-perceived usefulness and competence in the self-esteem of elderly adults: confirmatory factor analyses of the Bachman revision of Rosenberg's Self-Esteem Scale. *Journal of Gerontology: Psychological Sciences*, **33B**, 96–104.

Rebok, G.W. and Balcerak, L.J. (1989). Memory self efficacy and performance differences in young and old adults: the effect of mnemonic training. *Educational Gerontology*, **12**, 359–374.

Robbins, R.W., Trzesniewski, K.H., Tracy, J.L., Gosling, S.D., and Potter, J. (2002). Global self-esteem across the life span. *Psychology and Ageing*, **17**(3), 423–434.

Roberts, B. W., Walton, K.E., and Viechtbauer, W. (2006). Patterns of mean-level change in personality traits across the life course: A meta-analysis of longitudinal studies. *Psychological Bulletin*, **132**, 3–27.

Rosenberg, M. (1979). *Conceiving the self.* Basic Books, New York.

Ross, C.E. and Mirowsky, J. (2002). Age and the gender gap in the sense of personal control. *Social Psychological Quarterly*, **65**(2), 125–145.

Rotter, J.B. (1954). *Social learning theory and clinical psychology.* Prentice Hall, New York.

Rotter, J.B. (1966). Generalised expectancies for internal versus external control of reinforcement. *Psychological Monographs*, **90**, 1–28.

Rowe, J.W. and Kahn, R.L. (1997). Successful aging. *Gerontologist*, **37**(4), 433–440.

Rutter, M. (1985). Resilience in the face of adversity: protective factors and resistance to psychiatric disorder. *British Journal of Psychiatry*, **147**, 598–611.

Rutter, M. (1987). Psychosocial resilience and protective mechanisms. *American Journal of Orthopsychiatry*, **57**(3), 316–331.

Rutter, M. (1995). Psychosocial adversity: risk, resilience and recovery. *Southern African Journal of Child and Adolescent Psychiatry*, **7**, 75–88.

Ryff, C.D. (1989). In the eye of the beholder: views of psychological well-being among middle aged and older adults. *Psychology and Aging*, **4**, 195–210.

Ryff, C.D. and Singer, B. (1996). Psychological well-being: meaning, measurement and implications for psychotherapy research. *Psychotherapy and Psychosomatics*, **65**, 14–23.

Ryff, C. D. and Singer, B. (2003). Flourishing under fire: resilience as a prototype of challenged thriving. In *Flourishing: positive psychology and the life well lived* (ed. C.L.M. Keyes and J. Haidt), pp. 15–36. American Psychological Association, Washington, DC.

Schulz, R. and Heckhausen, J. (1996). A life-span model of successful aging. *American Psychologist*, **15**, 702–714.

Schulz, R. and Heckhausen, J. (1998). Emotion and control: a life-span perspective. In *Annual Review of Gerontology and Geriatrics*, **17**, 185–205.

Schulz, R., Heckhausen, J., and Locher, J. (1991). Adult development, control and adaptive functioning. *Journal of Social Issues*, **47**, 177–196.

Shaw, C., McColl, E., and Bond, S. (2003). The relationship of perceived control to outcomes in older women undergoing surgery for fractured neck of femur. *Journal of Clinical Nursing*, **12**(1), 117–123.

Siegler, I.C., Welsh, K.A., Dawson, D.V. *et al.* (1991). Ratings of personality change in patients being evaluated for memory disorders. *Alzheimer Disease and Associated Disorders*, **5**, 240–250.

Siegler, I.C., Dawson, D.V., and Welsh, K.A. (1994). Caregiver ratings of personality change in Alzheimer's disease patients: a replication. *Psychology and Aging*, **9**, 464–466.

Slangen-de Kort, Y.A.W., Midden, C.J.H., Aarts, H., and van Wagenberg, F. (2001). Determinants of adaptive behaviour among older persons: self-efficacy, importance of personal dispositions as directive mechanisms. *International Journal of Aging and Human Development*, **53**(4), 253–274.

Small, B.J., Hertzog, C., Hultsch, D.F., and Dixon, R.A. (2003). Stability and change in adult personality over 6 years: findings from the Victoria Longitudinal Study. *Journal of Gerontology*, **58B**, P166–P176.

Smith, J., Fleeson, W., Geiselmann, B., Settersten, R.A., and Kunzmann, U. (1999). Sources of well-being in very old age. In *The Berlin Ageing Study. Ageing from 70–100* (ed. P.B. Baltes and K.U. Mayer). Cambridge University Press, Cambridge.

Staudinger, U.M. (2000). Many reasons speak against it, yet many people feel good: the paradox of subjective well-being. *Psychologische Rundschau*, **51**(4), 185–197.

Staudinger, U.M. (2005). Personality and ageing. In *The Cambridge handbook of age and ageing* (ed. M.L. Johnson), pp. 237–244. Cambridge University Press, Cambridge.

Staudinger, U.M., Freund, A., Linden, M., and Maas, I. (1999). Self, personality, and life regulation: facets of resilience in old age. In *The Berlin Ageing Study. Ageing from 70–100* (ed. P.B. Baltes and K.U. Mayer), pp. 302–328. Cambridge University Press, Cambridge.

Storr, A. (1983). *Jung. Selected writings.* Fontana, London.

Strauss, M.E., Lee, M.M., and DiFilippo, J.M. (1997). Premorbid personality and behavioral symptoms in Alzheimer disease: some cautions. *Archives of Neurology*, **54**, 257–259.

Strauss, M.E., Pasupathi, M., and Chatterjee, A. (1993). Concordance between observers in descriptions of personality change in Alzheimer's disease. *Psychology and Aging*, **8**, 475–480.

Tizard, B. and Clarke. A. (1992). *Vulnerability and resilience in human development.* Kingsley Publishers, London.

Wagnild, G.M. and Young, H.M. (1993). Development and psychometric evaluation of the Resilience Scale. *Journal of Nursing Measurements*, **1**, 165–178.

Wallhagen, M.I. (1998). Perceived control theory: a re-contextualised perspective. *Journal of Clinical Geropsychology*, **4**(2), 119–140.

Weber, G., Glück, J., Sassenrath, S. *et al.* (2003). *Comparative report on self resources in advanced and old age* (http://www.bangor.ac.uk/esaw/self%20resources%20final%20report.pdf).

Welch, D.C. and West, R.L. (1995). Self efficacy and mastery – its application to issues of environmental control, cognition and aging. *Developmental Review*, **15**(2), 150–171.

Wells, E.L. and Marwell, G. (1976). *Self esteem. Its conceptualisation and measurement.* Sage Publications, London.

Wells, Y.D. and Kendig, H.L. (1999). Psychological resources and successful retirement. *Australian Psychologist*, **34**(2), 111–115.

Williams, R., Briggs, R., and Coleman, P. (1995). Carer-rated personality changes associated with senile dementia. *International Journal of Geriatric Psychiatry*, **10**, 231–236.

Windle, G. and Woods, R.T. (2004). Variations in subjective well-being: the mediating role of a psychological resource. *Ageing and Society*, **24**, 583–602.

Wolinsky, F.D. and Stump, T.E. (1996). Age and the sense of control among older adults. *Journals of Gerontology Series B: Psychological Sciences and Social Sciences*, **51**(4), 217–220.

Wolinsky, F.D., Wyrwich, K.W., Babu, A.N., Kroenke, K., and Tierney, W.M. (2003). Age, Aging, and the sense of control among older adults: A longitudinal reconsideration. *Journal of Gerontology, Series B: Psychological and Social Sciences*, **58**, 212–220.

Woods, R.T. and Britton, P.G. (1985). *Clinical psychology with the elderly*. Croom Helm/Chapman Hall, London.

Wylie, R.C. (1979). *The self-concept*. University of Nebraska Press, Lincoln, NE.

# Personality in later life: personality disorder and the effects of illness on personality

Catherine Oppenheimer

## Introduction

Clinical aspects of personality in old age fall into an area that has so far been relatively little studied, and where conceptual issues are still being hammered out.

One of these conceptual issues concerns the *framework* in which personality and its disorders should be described: is it more useful to sort people into types (the categorical approach) or to describe traits which, in various mixtures, combine to make up a person's personality (the dimensional approach)? The categorical approach may be better suited to making binary decisions: for example, whether or not this person has a mental disorder. Dimensions on the other hand are graded and quantifiable concepts, and so lend themselves much better to statistical studies, as will be seen.

Where personality disorder in old age is concerned, the literature generally follows a categorical approach, mostly using the classifications of personality set out in the current internationally accepted diagnostic schedules—DSM-IV and ICD-10—while at the same time expressing reservations about the usefulness of these categories to the study of older people (see van Alphen *et al.*, 2006a). This will be discussed later in the chapter.

By contrast, studies of the illnesses of old age that may affect the sufferer's personality have generally used the dimensional concepts that emerged from work on normal personality: in particular, the five-factor model (see Digman, 1990).

Another set of issues concerns *the meaning of words*. Personality, temperament, and character are closely related ideas; sometimes they are used almost as alternatives, but other authors are careful to make a distinction between them. For example in the Cloninger temperament and character inventory (quoted by Grucza *et al.*, 2003), temperament 'describes biases in automatic responses to emotional stimuli' while character 'relates to individual difference in the ability to control and adapt behaviour to be consistent with chosen goals and values'.

A complex model (the six-foci model) of personality has been described, in which traits operate at the most basic level, and are incorporated into 'personal action constructs' (including personal goals and imagined 'possible selves') at the next level, which in turn is incorporated into the person's own story of their unique life (Hooker and McAdams, 2003). Such a model of personality can embrace the idea of 'self-concept' (as for example in a study of changes in identity and self-concept after stroke; Ellis-Hill and

Horn, 2000). Otherwise self-concept only partially overlaps with the commoner usage of 'personality', which is based more on outward behaviours than on internal states.

The concept of 'personhood' takes us into yet more philosophical realms (see Chapter 38). There is little overlap with the concept of personality as used in the literature surveyed here, but it should be mentioned because of the question of personality change in dementia. There was a time when many clinicians in old age psychiatry were made uncomfortable by the proposition that dementia changes a person's personality. For them, that came too close to making a moral evaluation of the patient, rather than speaking with understanding about their illness and their efforts to cope with it. At worst, it seemed to imply a dismissal of the patient as no longer fully a person—dementia therefore leading to a loss of 'personhood'.

Personality has been defined in a number of ways, for example (quoted in Mychack *et al.*, 2001), for Alport in 1937 personality was 'the dynamic organisation within the individual of those psychosocial systems that determine his unique adjustments to his environment'; for Pervin in 1970 it was 'those structural and dynamic properties of an individual … as they reflect themselves in characteristic responses to situations'. McCrae and Costa (1988) define personality traits as 'a set of characteristic dispositions that determine emotional, interpersonal experiential, attitudinal and motivational styles'. The common elements to these definitions of personality appear to be the notions of pattern and structure, of individuality, and of interaction with the external world.

It might be thought that the semantic issues discussed above will become less important as different personality traits become operationalized through the use of generally accepted questionnaires and statistical methods of analysing them. To an extent this is true; a group of researchers who report their findings in terms of the 'NEO-PI, based on the Five-Factor model' will be understood by another group familiar with the same methodology. (The NEO-PI, referred to frequently below, stands for the Neuroticism–Extraversion–Openness Personality Inventory). But because of the need to communicate the findings to a wider audience, researchers give a verbal identity to the factors which emerge (validly and reliably) from the analysis of answers to questionnaires about everyday behaviours. How well that garment of words actually captures for the reader the meaning of the statistical factors, and itself translates back comprehensibly to the behaviours on which the factors are based, is an interesting question (see Digman, 1990). In the Minnesota Multiphasic Personality Inventory (MMPI), for example (as used by Golden and Golden 2003), the names of the dimensions are not particularly helpful in understanding the meaning of the personality profiles.

Nevertheless, words are important: as McCrae and Costa (1997) argue: 'The lexical approach to personality structure … adopts the hypothesis that because personality traits are so central to human interactions, all important traits will have been encoded in natural language. Thus, an analysis of trait language should yield the structure of personality itself'.

A different issue that needs also to be considered is the question of *time-scale*. How long does a pattern of responses have to last before it can be regarded as characteristic of an individual? This is a real question, and particularly so in old age. It is pertinent to the recognition of a personality disorder—does the difficulty really have to have arisen in youth in order to qualify as a personality disorder in an old person, whose early history may be impossible to confirm? And it is pertinent to the study of chronic illness, which may have profound effects on the person's pattern of response to the environment. Are those effects to be regarded as a change in personality, or as a persisting manifestation of illness (see Thompson *et al.*, 1988; Bergmann, 2002)?

The final set of issues concerns the *perspective* from which personality is described. Should the person's own view of their characteristic style be relied on, are family and friends a more reliable source of information, should the questions focus only on present patterns of behaviour, or can valid evidence be gathered about patterns in the past? There is no 'right answer' to this; studies cited later in this chapter will illustrate the value of each of these approaches, and—more interestingly—show where comparisons between the results of different approaches have yielded additional valuable information.

## Methodologies

### Dimensional measures of personality and personality change: the NEO-PI

Digman (1990) gives an excellent and very readable review of the historical background to the five-factor model of personality and of the NEO-PI based on that model, developed by McCrae and Costa at the National Institute on Aging (see also McCrae and Costa, 1987, 1997 for an illuminating discussion of the theoretical issues).

The five factors are called: neuroticism, extraversion, openness to experience, agreeableness, and conscientiousness. Each factor is further divided into six 'facets': for example, the factor of 'agreeableness' is made up of the following facets: trust, straightforwardness, altruism, compliance, modesty, and tender-mindedness.

The five factors are described (for example by Low *et al.*, 2002) as follows:

♦ Neuroticism is the general tendency to experience negative affect (e.g. fear, sadness, anger).

♦ Extraversion is the tendency to like people and to be assertive, active, and talkative.

♦ Openness to experience involves a curiosity about inner and outer worlds.

♦ Agreeableness is a tendency to be sympathetic to others and eager to help.

♦ Conscientiousness is the ability to plan, organize, and carry out tasks.

The questionnaire has gone through various revisions, but as the NEO-PI-R (Costa and McCrae, 1992) it consists of 240 items with responses made on a five-point scale ranging from 'strongly agree' to 'strongly disagree'; it is suitable both for self-rating and informant-rating, and has been translated and validated in many languages (McCrae and Costa, 1997).

The NEO-PI has been used in the majority of studies of personality change in old age (see below) and appears to be capable of detecting the changes of interest to us.

### Dimensional measures of personality and personality change: Wiggins' Interpersonal Adjectives Scale; Beck's Sociotropy Autonomy Scale; Brooks and McKinlay's personality inventory; and others

The Interpersonal Adjectives Scale (IAS) has been used in a series of studies of personality change in dementia (Mychack *et al.*, 2001; Rankin *et al.*, 2003, 2005). As described by Rankin *et al.* (2005), the scale identifies eight facets of social interaction, distributed around two orthogonal axes representing power (or dominance) and love (or affiliation). The facets are the following: assured/dominant, arrogant/calculating, cold hearted, aloof/introverted, unassured/submissive, unassuming/ingenuous, warm/agreeable, and gregarious/extraverted. The scale is accompanied by a computerized scoring program which compares the subject with a normative group. It is suitable for both subjects and informants, both retrospectively and in present time; and the comparison of these perspectives was used to good effect in these studies.

The Sociotropy Autonomy Scale (SAS) has been used in a study of dementia (Hilton and Moniz-Cook, 2004) and in a study of late onset major depression (Mazure *et al.*, 2002). The scale (Beck *et al.*, 1983) identifies what is thought to be a stable mode of personality or temperament, which at the two extreme ends of the dimension may predict vulnerability to illness or behaviour problems:

'Sociotropic' individuals … would derive their sense of worth and efficacy primarily from meaningful contacts with others, thus seeking reassurance or social contact and presenting with anxious behaviour in the absence of this. In contrast, 'autonomous' individuals have greater need for mastery and control, thus placing a strong emphasis on their own achievements. When these are placed under threat, they present with social avoidance and hostility.

Hilton and Moniz-Cook (2004)

The SAS is a 60-item self-report questionnaire, with 30 items each for the sociotropy and autonomy subscales.

Brooks and McKinlay (1983) developed an inventory to measure behavioural change after severe blunt head injury, and this inventory has been used in a number of studies of personality change in dementia (Petry *et al.*, 1988, 1989; Dian *et al.*, 1990; Aitken *et al.*, 1999; Heinik *et al.*, 1999). It consists of a list of 18 pairs of adjectives, each pair chosen to represent opposite ends of a dimension of personality (or behaviour); the informant rates the subject on a

**Table 31ii.1** Dimensions of Personality (after Brooks and McKinlay 1983)

| | |
|---|---|
| Talkative | Quiet |
| Even-tempered | Quick-tempered |
| Does things by himself | Relies on others |
| Affectionate | Cold |
| Fond of company | Dislikes company |
| Easygoing | Irritable |
| Happy | Unhappy |
| Calm | Excitable |
| Down-to-earth | Out of touch |
| Cautious | Rash |
| Enthusiastic | Listless |
| Mature | Childish |
| Sensitive | Insensitive |
| Kind | Cruel |
| Generous | Mean |
| Reasonable | Unreasonable |
| Stable | Changeable |
| Energetic | Lifeless |

five-point scale (−2 to +2) for each of the pairs. The pairs of adjectives are listed in Table 31ii.1. The statistical handling of the inventory results is discussed in Petry *et al.* (1988).

A number of other scales have been used, often in only one or two studies. Rubin *et al.* (1987) used a variety of measures, including the (informant-rated) Blessed Dementia scale, from which they selected eleven items (scored 0 or 1) relevant to personality; Bozzola *et al.* (1992) used the same items and summed the scores to produce an overall 'personality score'; Balsis *et al.* (2005) selected eight of these items. Hagberg *et al.* (2002) chose the Gordon Personality Inventory (GP:A) in preference to the NEO-PI because they found it more relevant to questions about the quality of life of older people, which was the focus of their study. Golden and Golden (2003), in comparing the effects of Alzheimer's disease, stroke, and head injury on personality, used the MMPI. Gould and Hyer (2004), studying the influence of pre-morbid personality on behavioural changes in dementia, used caregivers' ratings on Strack's Personality Adjective Check List, which yields eight dimensions of personality: introverted, inhibited, cooperative, sociable, confident, forceful, respectful, sensitive. Other authors (e.g. Stone *et al.*, 2004) have used questionnaires of their own design.

It will be apparent that there is a variety of instruments available for research in this field, and no consensus yet on their respective merits—either as analytical tools, or as a medium for dialogue with the wider world of interested professionals.

### Methods for establishing categorical distinctions: the problem of personality disorder

If the field of dimensional studies of personality change in old age is poorly developed and somewhat confusing, the situation of personality disorder research is even worse (Zimmerman, 1994; Abrams and Horowitz, 1996; Segal *et al.*, 1996; van Alphen *et al.*, 2006a).

Studies of personality disorder in old age have so far been based on the diagnostic categories of DSM-III, DSM-IV, and ICD-10, and have used the structured or semi-structured interviews, diagnostic checklists, and clinicians' consensus judgements which reflect the architecture of these diagnostic systems. As shown in the reviews noted above, there are numerous difficulties with this approach, not least the fact that the criteria and descriptions for the different personality disorders fail to reflect the realities of life in old age.

In recognition of this problem, van Alphen and colleagues are in the process of developing an age-appropriate screening instrument, the Gerontological Personality Disorders Scale (GPS). The initial version of the scale consists of two parallel sets (subject-rated and informant-rated) of 52 items, between them covering relevant aspects of the patient's habitual behaviour and biographical information, and observations of their behaviour. Interestingly, the patient's version of the scale is presented on cards, one card for each statement: for example 'I'm often taken advantage of by others' (habitual) or 'At the most I've only had one acquaintance or friend in my life' (biographical); and the patient is asked to respond (yes, no, don't know, not applicable) to each card. Preliminary results are given for the reliability and validity of this scale—tested for its ability to predict a clinical diagnosis of personality disorder—and the authors make the point that the scale is not suitable for diagnosing *specific* personality disorders (van Alphen *et al.*, 2006b).

## The effects of illness on personality in old age

It is reasonable now to make the working assumption that personality does not alter substantially as a result of age alone. There is evidence to support this view (see Chapter 31i; Costa and McCrae, 1986; Weiss *et al.*, 2005). Also, a few studies examining the effects of illness on personality have taken the additional step of using a control group of normal older people (e.g. Rubin *et al.*, 1987; Petry *et al.*, 1988, 1989; Balsis *et al.*, 2005).

In 1987, Rubin, Morris, and Berg published an analysis of personality change in a research group of 44 patients with senile dementia of the Alzheimer's type (SDAT)—which would now be called Alzheimer's disease—whom they had studied over a 50-month follow-up period. Patients, control subjects, and collateral sources (mainly spouses and children) were interviewed every 15–18 months, and information on personality changes over this time (using open-ended questions and items from the Blessed Dementia Scale) was factor-analysed and grouped into four types of change: passive, agitated, self-centred, and suspicious.

'Passive' changes tended to be present early in the dementia, whereas the frequency of 'self-centred' and 'agitated' behaviours in the patient group increased as their dementia progressed. Significantly, the authors showed that the occurrence of personality change early in the dementia did not predict a more rapid progression to severe dementia; by contrast, the presence of aphasia early in the disease did act as a marker for rapid progression.

This early study raised many of the questions that have been examined in the literature over the following 20 years; some of these will be discussed here. [Helpful general discussions may be found within the papers by (among others) Strauss *et al.* (1993, 1997), Siegler *et al.* (1991), Chatterjee *et al.* (1992), and Rankin *et al.* (2003).]

## Is there a consistent finding of personality change in dementia?

Longitudinal studies of this question, using informant ratings, include Petry *et al.* (1989) and Balsis *et al.* (2005). Petry *et al.* (1989) undertook a follow-up analysis, after approximately 3 years, of the sample of patients they described in 1988 (Petry *et al.* 1988). They showed that the progression of personality change over time was not uniform. Some personality characteristics changed markedly at the onset of the disease but relatively little thereafter (thus, patients were described as more out of touch, childish, lifeless, and reliant on others, compared with their pre-morbid selves). Other characteristics (listlessness, insensitivity, and coldness) tended to progress throughout the follow-up period; while other characteristics showed no change, or even resolved as the disease progressed.

Balsis *et al.* (2005) studied 108 volunteer participants in a longitudinal study of healthy ageing who were examined annually, with collateral information also being collected annually. During the course of this study, 68 of the participants received a clinical diagnosis of Alzheimer's disease (AD), and 14 of the participants who were not clinically demented during their life received a post-mortem diagnosis of AD. Approximately half the clinically demented group and half the 'pre-clinical' (autopsy-diagnosed) group showed some personality change, in the direction of increased rigidity, apathy, egocentricity, and impaired emotional control (on the Blessed Scale). By contrast, only a quarter of the non-demented subjects showed any personality change, most of this being limited to increased rigidity. An important point made by these authors was that '*observable personality changes may occur in the very earliest stages of the disease and precede measurable cognitive loss*' [emphasis added].

Other studies have used a cross-sectional approach, asking informants to rate the patient's personality 'in the present', and retrospectively 'before the illness' (defining this point of pre-morbid comparison differently in different studies); or to rate their perception of 'change' in personality. Studies of this kind include Bozzola *et al.* (1992), Chatterjee *et al.* (1992), Siegler *et al.* (1991, 1994), and Aitken *et al.* (1999). The studies of Siegler *et al.*, using the NEO-PI, may be taken as an example. In their 1991 study, 35 patients with memory impairment from a variety of causes (13 with AD) were assessed. The 1994 study was a replication using a new sample of 26 patients with AD. The findings on personality change were broadly consistent across these two studies, and consistent with others in the literature using similar methodology. Patients showed *increases* in neuroticism (except for the facet of 'impulsiveness'); *decreases* in extraversion (except for 'gregariousness'), in openness, and in conscientiousness; and *stability* in agreeableness. Moreover the authors commented on personality variables that did *not* appear to be affected by the dementia: impulsiveness, gregariousness, openness to fantasy, aesthetics, feelings, actions, and values. They suggested that such differential effects of the illness on the personality of patients (as reported by their caregivers) argued for the objectivity of these reports, and made it unlikely that caregiver stress was the explanation for their observations.

## Does the presence or severity of personality change correlate with the severity or the time-course of the illness?

Evidence from the different studies that have addressed this question is not consistent, but overall it would seem that the prevalence of personality change (in a group of patients) increases over time (e.g. Rubin *et al.*, 1987); and that with some aspects of personality change there is a progression over time within some individuals but not within others (Petry *et al.*, 1989). In some studies the severity of personality change correlates with the severity of the dementia (e.g. Aitken *et al.*, 1999), but a substantial number of other studies have emphasized the occurrence of personality change early in the illness, which is *not* correlated with measures of cognitive decline as the illness progresses (Petry *et al.*, 1988, 1989; Dian *et al.*, 1990; Bozzola *et al.*, 1992; Chatterjee *et al.*, 1992; Heinik *et al.*, 1999).

## Do different types of illness produce different patterns of personality change?

Most studies of personality change with disease in old age have focused on AD. However some (e.g. Siegler *et al.*, 1991) have reported on diagnostically mixed samples of attendees at a memory clinic, and others have explicitly compared patients across diagnostic groups. Glosser *et al.* (1995) compared patients with Parkinson's disease, AD, and with medical illnesses (as controls); Aitken *et al.* (1999) compared AD with multi-infarct dementia (MID); Golden and Golden (2003) compared AD, head injury, and strokes. Ellis-Hill and Horn (2000) studied self-reported self-image after stroke; Dian *et al.* (1990) compared patients with MID with controls, using the Brooks and McKinlay Scale; Stone *et al.* (2004) gathered carer perceptions of personality change after stroke, using a composite questionnaire.

There is no strong evidence from these studies for a characteristic pattern of personality change that distinguishes between AD, vascular dementia or stroke, or Parkinson's disease; although there are differences in detail between one diagnostic category and another in some of the studies (e.g. Aitken *et al.* found that their MID patients had more severe personality changes overall; and Golden and Golden found different patterns of change on the MMPI). On the other hand, Glosser *et al.* (1995) comment specifically on the similarity of personality changes in Parkinson's disease and AD (by contrast with medically ill controls), and suggest that this may represent a common pattern of behavioural adaptation across a variety of neurological disorders.

However, the evidence for a specific pattern of personality change in frontotemporal dementia (FTD) is much stronger. Barber *et al.* (1995), in an interesting post-mortem study of AD compared with FTD, interviewed the relatives of patients with autopsy-confirmed diagnoses of these two diseases (20 cases of AD, 18 cases of FTD), some 2 or 3 years after the patients' deaths. Using a specially designed questionnaire, they obtained descriptions of the patients' symptoms and behaviours, using two informants wherever possible. So different were the patterns of these informant descriptions in the two diseases, that a blind rater was able to use them to classify patients into the correct diagnostic group with 100% accuracy. Frontotemporal patients were distinguished by early personality change, loss of empathy, inappropriate affect, unconcern, and socially inappropriate behaviour; while disturbed memory and topographical orientation typified the AD patients; aggressive behaviour was commoner in AD than in FTD; and anxiety, distress and loss of confidence were described by the informants in AD but not in FTD.

Rankin *et al.* (2003) showed that a further diagnostic distinction based on personality change (measured by the IAS) can validly be made between the frontal and temporal variants of FTD and AD (as a control group). Patients with the temporal variant showed severe 'interpersonal coldness', with some loss of 'social dominance'; patients with the frontal variant had extreme loss of 'social dominance' and milder 'interpersonal coldness' (loss of nurturance and affiliation). Both subgroups of FTD showed much more marked personality change than the patients with AD. These findings were further developed by Mychack et al. (2001), where four individual patients (one with the frontal variant, one with the temporal variant, and two with AD) were described in detail, showing their differential scores on the NEO-PI, IAS, and the Interpersonal Measure of Psychopathy.

## Can reliable assessments of personality change in dementia, and of patients' pre-morbid personalities, be obtained from collateral sources?

Most of the studies of personality change in dementia use informant ratings alone, and there are few direct comparisons between self-reports and informant reports (with one illuminating exception, to be discussed later). However, the validity of informant ratings in dementia has been assessed in other ways:

First, more than one informant per patient has been sought, and their ratings compared [Strauss et al. (1993) using the NEO-PI; Barber et al. (1995) and Heinik et al. (1999), using the Brooks and McKinlay questionnaire]. These studies found good agreement between informants, both as to change in personality, and in description of the patient's personality before the onset of the disease.

Second, informants' ratings obtained at different points in time have been compared for stability over time. Thus, Strauss et al. (1997) reported on 21 informants who had rated their relative's personality when they entered other studies; a year later, they asked these same informants to rate the patient's personality again—as it was in the present, and as it had been a year earlier, when they described it before. The results showed a tendency for the retrospective ratings to be less pathological, or closer to normality, than the rating at the time had been. This tendency was found across most of the informants, and across four out of five of the NEO-PI dimensions.

Petry et al. (1989), making a similar comparison of informant ratings over time, came to a similar conclusion. They gave the name 'historical revisionism' to this tendency by relatives to perceive the past as more normal (or more positive) than it appeared at the time, and they linked it to another of their findings: the spouses of patients tended to rate their pre-morbid personality more favourably than did the spouses of control subjects. Strauss et al. (1997) discuss a variety of possible explanations for this 'normalizing tendency' in informants' retrospective evaluation of a patient's past personality, and draw important implications for the design of future studies in this field.

Nevertheless, Dawson et al. (2000), discussing the consistency in findings (using the NEO-PI) from a number of different studies on personality change in dementia, conclude that this body of evidence has 'substantially allayed concerns regarding the reliability of informant ratings of personality' in dementia.

## Can patients themselves give reliable information about their own personality?

As mentioned above, most studies of patients with AD do not attempt to obtain self-rated data on personality, assuming that the cognitive changes in the disease will make the data unreliable.

Rankin et al. (2005) tested this assumption in a study of 10 patients with AD, 12 with FTD, and 11 controls. Using the IAS, the informants were asked to rate the patients' personality both in the present and pre-morbidly; while the patients themselves were asked to rate their personality in the present. By comparison with their informants' ratings, the patients with FTD had a very inaccurate perception of their current selves, while the patients with AD had the same difficulty, only much less severely. Control subjects' ratings of themselves matched well with their informants.

To regard this finding as simply illustrating the 'loss of insight' of dementia would be to miss a clue to understanding part of what 'insight' means. The self-ratings of both the FTD patients and the patients with AD, though inaccurate about their current selves, were much closer to the informant descriptions of their pre-morbid selves. The authors describe this as a failure in a normal process of 'updating' of perception of one's self; and they regard this failure of updating as a clinical feature of these two forms of dementia.

## Does pre-morbid personality predict changes with the onset of disease?

There is a variety of studies which examine this question, either directly or incidentally, and the findings from these are mixed. To begin with, is there a characteristic personality that predicts liability to a particular disease? In a study mentioned earlier, Glosser et al. (1995) assessed current and pre-morbid personality in three groups of patients: with AD, with Parkinson's disease, and (as controls) with rheumatoid arthritis and osteoarthritis. They showed that the pre-morbid characteristics of Parkinson's and AD patients resembled each other, and that there was no characteristic 'pre-parkinsonian personality' as has sometimes been supposed. Meins and Dammast (2000), however, showed that AD patients in a memory clinic had higher pre-morbid neuroticism scores than patients in the same clinic with Parkinson's disease.

Does pre-morbid personality influence the personality changes that come with the onset of a dementia? Dawson et al. (2000) showed that pre-morbid scores on the different dimensions of the NEO-PI predicted informant-rated change in personality, such that people low in neuroticism before the onset of the dementia were perceived to have greater than average increases in neuroticism as the disease progressed; and conversely those high in conscientiousness were rated as having the greatest loss of conscientiousness when they became ill. Statistically, this was a powerful factor in determining the magnitude and direction of changes in NEO-PI scores, but it is not clear whether this tells us more about rater characteristics, about features of the disease, or about the nature of the NEO-PI itself.

Bergua et al. (2006) examined preference for routines (using a specifically designed questionnaire) in a community sample of older people followed longitudinally (the PAQUID Study). They showed that preference for routines was associated with symptoms of anxiety and depression (as cause or effect?), but also with cognitive complaints not amounting to dementia, and they showed that as time progressed, increasing cognitive impairment was associated with greater preference for routine. They suggested that the preference for routine might represent an adaptation strategy in vulnerable individuals threatened by an awareness of cognitive changes in themselves.

Several studies have also examined the relationship between pre-morbid personality and the subsequent development of psychiatric symptoms in AD. Chatterjee et al. (1992), using the NEO-PI with a research sample of AD patients, showed that pre-morbid personality does not predict change in *personality* during the illness, but does predict some of the *symptoms*. For example, patients with depressive symptoms were rated by their informants as higher in neuroticism pre-morbidly, and those with paranoid delusions were rated as having been more hostile pre-morbidly. Interestingly, those with hallucinations were rated higher pre-morbidly on 'openness to fantasy' and on 'aesthetics'.

Meins *et al.* (1998), using the Munich Personality Test for caregiver ratings of pre-morbid personality and current personality, behaviour, and mood, showed that lower levels of pre-morbid frustration tolerance were associated with depressive symptoms after the onset of AD, and high levels of pre-morbid emotional instability were associated with troublesome behaviour and personality change. Hamel *et al.* (1990), studying aggressive behaviour (broadly defined) in patients with dementia who were living with a family caregiver in the community, showed that pre-morbid aggressive behaviour was one factor (among 11 other factors) which predicted current aggressive behaviour.

Approaching this question in a different population, Low *et al.* (2002) studied residents of nursing homes who had been identified as suffering from depression or psychosis, and gathered informant ratings (on the NEO-PI) of their pre-morbid personality. Although they were able to show correlations between pre-morbid personality and current symptoms (for example, higher pre-morbid neuroticism predicted the presence of delusions), the authors questioned the reliability of their findings and raised the possibility of various methodological sources of bias. Similarly, Holst *et al.* (1997), studying patients on old age psychiatry wards who had vocally disruptive behaviour, found some limited evidence that previous neuroticism was associated with the disruptive behaviours. By contrast, Brandt *et al.* (1998) showed that pre-morbid personality had no relationship to the ability of patients with AD to adjust to placement in long-term residential care.

Lastly, Gould and Hyer (2004) studied 68 community-living patients with dementia, comparing informants' ratings (on the Personality Adjectives Checklist) of their pre-morbid personality with current behavioural and mood changes (assessed by a semi-structured interview with the primary carer). They showed that 'a premorbid personality style characterised by independence is associated with increased withdrawal once dementia occurs, and to a lesser extent, an inhibited premorbid personality style is associated with increased withdrawal and irritable behaviour'. Whether these new patterns of behaviour should be regarded as 'behavioural and psychological *symptoms* of dementia (BPSD)' or as changes in the *personality* of the patient, returns us to the semantic questions discussed at the beginning of this chapter.

Taken as a whole, studies of personality change associated with dementia (and especially, studies that are able to take a longitudinal perspective) tell us that:

1 Personality changes are consistently (though not invariably) described by the carers of people with dementia.

2 The nature of these changes does not generally reflect 'an exaggeration of the patient's previous personality', does not correlate with any demographic features of the patient, nor with the degree of cognitive impairment or the stage that the dementia has reached.

3 The changes reported by informants are not an artefact of the carer's feelings, or of the burden of care. But carers' feelings probably do influence their perception of the past personality of the person they care for, in ways that deserve further study.

4 The pattern of reported personality change in dementia is consistent enough across individuals to suggest that it is a feature of the illness itself.

5 The specificity of the changes in personality that accompany forms of dementia with a specific anatomical distribution (FTD); and the more unpredictable (but sometimes very early) occurrence of personality change in other forms of dementia (which have a less predictable location of their pathological changes, such as AD and vascular dementia), are very suggestive of a neuropathological basis to personality change (Petry *et al.*, 1988; Aitken *et al.*, 1999). Might—as Rankin *et al.* (2003) suggest—the study of AD and the other dementias lead us in the end to 'a neuroanatomy of personality'?

# Personality disorder in old age

Research on personality disorder in old age is generally acknowledged to be in its earliest stages, and the literature reflects this. There are few reliable findings as yet, but there is general agreement on the different conceptual and methodological questions that need to be resolved. These are well summarized in van Alphen *et al.* (2006a), but other helpful reviews include Kroessler (1990), Abrams and Horowitz (1996), Segal *et al.* (1996), Holroyd (2000), Bergmann (2002), and Engels *et al.* (2003).

The themes commonly raised in these reviews include:

The change in concepts and definitions of personality disorder over time; the usefulness of categorical or dimensional descriptions of disorder; the applicability (in old age) of diagnostic criteria based on younger patients; the appropriateness of different diagnostic instruments; whether ageing alters the behavioural manifestation of a stable personality trait ('heterotypical continuity'); the temporal framework for making a diagnosis of personality disorder; and the overlap between personality traits (Axis II disorders) and the symptoms of psychiatric illness (Axis I disorders).

The fundamental difficulty with 'personality disorder' as a psychiatric concept lies in the problem of drawing general lessons (important for research and clinical management) out of the uniqueness of individuals and their personal circumstances. The balance between generalization and particularity must be set differently for different purposes. Epidemiologists need clear categories to sort people into (preferably with 'points of rarity' to define their boundaries), unambiguous operational criteria, and reliable simple screening instruments; while psychotherapeutic insights concern universal psychological mechanisms that we all share—more or less—and they are best communicated through narrative and illustration.

Somewhere between those two anchor points comes the working old age psychiatrist, who needs to engage with disorders of personality because (1) they modify the expression of psychiatric illness, (2) they present as clinical problems in their own right, and (3) understanding them will help to illuminate the treatment of individuals, families, and wider groups.

## Prevalence of personality disorder in old age

The specific personality disorders are, as defined in DSM-IV: *Cluster A*, paranoid, schizoid, schizotypal; *Cluster B*, antisocial, borderline, histrionic, narcissistic; *Cluster C*, avoidant, dependent, obsessive–compulsive. (ICD-10 has a very similar list). The general definition of personality disorders (regardless of age), for example in ICD-10, includes the following elements:

> deeply ingrained and *enduring* behaviour patterns, manifesting themselves as *inflexible* responses to a broad range of personal and social situations … *significant deviations* from the way the average individual thinks, feels and particularly, relates to others … encompass *multiple domains* of behaviour and psychological functioning … frequently associated with *subjective distress* and problems in *social functioning and performance*. [emphases added]

Findings from the different studies on the prevalence of personality disorder in old age vary so much that little confidence can yet be put on the methods and criteria used, and the meta-analyses and reviews mentioned above quote a range of figures (e.g. Abrams and Horowitz, 1996; Holroyd, 2000; Bergmann, 2002; van Alphen *et al.*, 2006a). Very approximately, the prevalence of personality disorder may be up to 10% of community-living older people, and 30% or more in samples of psychiatrically ill older people.

Engels *et al.* (2003), using a cross-sectional design and a dimensional measure of personality based on the DSM and ICD categories, set out to compare the prevalence of personality disorder across age groups and between patients and healthy controls. They showed that there is no decrease with age in the overall prevalence of personality disorder, but that there is a change in the distribution of the different specific personality traits. Older community residents showed more schizoid and obsessive–compulsive traits than their younger counterparts, and among older patients there were more schizoid characteristics and fewer paranoid, impulsive, borderline, and histrionic traits, than in younger patients. Other authors describe a similar shift with age towards a preponderance of Cluster C and Cluster A disorders, and a decrease in prevalence of Cluster B (the so-called 'high energy') disorders. Engels and colleagues suggest, from their findings, that a different clustering of disorders (schizoid, schizotypal, and avoidant), with the common element of 'social discomfort' and unwillingness to seek social support, is important in older life.

## The relevance of current definitions of personality disorder in the context of old age

Many authors make the point [most strongly made by van Alphen *et al.* (2006a)] that the concepts and diagnostic criteria for personality disorder were framed with younger people in mind, and that a different set of definitions is needed for older people. The applicability of the standard criteria to older people is in question, because the social and biological changes of old age will have so much influence on the behaviours specified in the diagnostic criteria that the criteria may become unreliable. For example, a criterion related to work would be irrelevant in a retired population; while in a physically ill person, dependence on others might represent a lifesaving necessity rather than a preferred style of relationship.

Rosowsky and Gurian (1991), in a preliminary study of borderline personality disorder (BPD) in late life, showed that out of eight psychiatric outpatients identified by clinicians as having BPD, none fully met the DSM-IIIR criteria or the DIB (Diagnostic Interview for Borderlines) for the disorder. They identified some of the diagnostic features of BPD that are preserved in old age, namely: difficulty in maintaining an active social life involving groups of people; therapeutic relationships characterized by splitting, specialness, and negative countertransference; a pattern of unstable and intense interpersonal relationships; affective instability; and difficulties in the control of anger, which tends to be inappropriate, intense, and poorly managed. However, other diagnostic features of BPD generally decline in later life, namely: impulsivity, acting-out, self-mutilation, risk-taking behaviour and substance abuse; and identity disturbances (or 'lability of self'). The authors discuss the implications of this preliminary study, both for an understanding of the long-term course of BPD, and for the usefulness of current diagnostic instruments.

A point made by this study, and by other authors, is that a maladaptive trait may be expressed in one form of behaviour in youth (a behaviour that contributes to making a diagnosis of personality disorder), and the same trait may be expressed in a different way (which does not meet any criterion for the disorder) in old age. This phenomenon has been named 'heterotypical continuity' (see van Alphen *et al.*, 2006a). An example might be the misuse of prescribed medications in old age in place of self-mutilation (as part of a BPD) in youth (Rosowsky and Gurian, 1991).

A related point is made by Holroyd (2000) and Bergmann (2002) and also by other authors: traits that are maladaptive at a young age may eventually prove adaptive in the changed circumstances of old age. Most clinicians will have known patients whose dependence on others had been burdensome to their relatives, and who in the end accepted with relief the enforced dependence of physical frailty and institutional care.

## What timeframe is appropriate to the diagnosis of personality disorder in old age?

This is a question that is both methodological and real. Does the definition of personality disorder as having its onset in adolescence or young adult life still hold for personality disorder in old age? This information may be difficult to collect [and indeed Abrams and Horowitz (1996) doubted whether it had in fact been collected in many of the studies they reviewed]. The information may be irrelevant: can we be sure that there is no such thing as later onset personality disorder? Zimmerman (1994), in a thorough survey of methodological questions, has a helpful discussion of this issue. Some diagnostic instruments specify a time period over which the traits of interest should have been present, but it may be hard to distinguish between psychiatric symptoms and the manifestations of personality, if a chronic illness such as depression has extended over the whole of that time. Perhaps, in these circumstances there *is* no real distinction between illness and personality (Bergmann, 2002).

## Personality traits, disorders, and psychiatric illness

There is good evidence [for example summarized in Morse and Lynch (2004)] that adverse personality traits—not necessarily amounting to categorical personality disorder—confer vulnerability to psychiatric illness, complicate its course, delay recovery, impair cooperation with clinicians, and increase the risk of relapse. This evidence is discussed elsewhere in this book under the relevant illness (see Chapters 29ii, 30, 32), but a few studies may be cited here.

Thompson *et al.* (1988), studying patients with major depressive disorder, showed that those who scored higher (on self-rating) for personality disorder were less likely to benefit from psychotherapy. (No informant data were collected.) Prigerson *et al.* (1996) showed that a variety of personality traits, in conjunction with a history of childhood adversity, predicted the risk that an elderly carer (of a terminally ill spouse) would develop an anxiety disorder. Mazure *et al.* (2002), comparing a group of patients (with major depressive disorder) with a control group, showed that adverse life events interacted with personality style (measured by self-report on the Sociotropy Autonomy Scale) to predict the occurrence of major depression. Patients scoring higher on 'autonomy' were significantly less likely to be depressed. Rao (2003) studied consecutive referrals to a community mental health team, and showed a significant association between personality disorder and subsequent admission to hospital with depression. Monopoli and Vaccaro (2003) linked high scores for anxiety and neuroticism, with the development of hypochondriasis. Morse and Lynch (2004), using the (self-rated) Personality Disorder Inventory, found a preponderance of Cluster A and C personality disorders in a sample of patients with depression, and showed that the patients with personality disorder were four times more likely to have persistent or relapsing symptoms of their depression. They discuss the reasons why these specific disorders might be expressed in behaviours that would tend over time to intensify the disorder.

A study of personality disorder and suicide (Duberstein, 1995) merits more detailed discussion here, because it links back to the studies reviewed earlier in which informant ratings of personality were used. This report forms part of a comprehensive psychological autopsy study of 52 people (29 below the age of 50, 23 aged 50 and over) who had succeeded in committing suicide, and 52 matched controls. On informant ratings using the NEO-PI, both older and younger people who committed suicide scored higher on neuroticism than did the controls, but the older group of suicides also stood out as having lower scores on the Openness to Experience (OTE) Scale than either the young suicides or the controls at all ages. The meaning of this finding, and the clinical picture of a person low in OTE (characterized by constriction of thinking, affect, and behaviour, and rigidity of self-concept) are discussed in detail, and directions for future research are suggested. This study is valuable not only because it used informant ratings of personality (which is not common in the studies of personality disorder in old age), but also because it represents an attempt in this field to bridge the gap between quantitative findings in groups and therapeutic understanding of individuals. A more recent case–controlled study (Harwood *et al.*, 2001), likewise using retrospective informant ratings of personality, showed that anankastic and anxious personality traits were predictors of suicide, and the authors drew attention to the similarity between these personality traits and the low OTE described by Duberstein (see also Chapter 29iii).

### Understanding rather than measuring personality disorder in old age

Less quantitative than these studies but no less important clinically is the paper by Sadavoy (1987) on character pathology in the elderly. The patients discussed here correspond approximately to the category of borderline personality disorder. The impact of these personality traits and their interaction with the common life stresses of old age are clearly and simply described, from a psychodynamic perspective. Particularly helpful are the discussion of the loss of outlets for the expression of pathological traits, and of

the situation of carer and patient when the patient's conflicts over closeness and dependence play themselves out in the 'inescapable relationship'.

A similarly understanding account of the personality of older people as they respond to the stress of illness and adversity is given by Wesby (2004) and by many of the other chapters in the same handbook (Evans and Garner, 2004). Personality traits and styles of relating to others, as much as illness, are an important focus for psychotherapy in old age (see Chapter 18v).

## Self-neglect in old age, and the so-called 'Diogenes syndrome'

In 1975, Clark, Mankikar, and Gray coined the name 'Diogenes syndrome' to describe 30 patients who had been admitted to hospital with acute illness and extreme self-neglect. Although these authors were the first to use this name, the kind of patients they described—people living in circumstances of extreme self-neglect and lack of hygiene, who refuse help—were certainly not unknown before. Macmillan (1957) and Shaw (1957) had described 'social breakdown in the elderly', and subsequently (Macmillan and Shaw 1966) reported on a series of 72 people exhibiting 'senile breakdown in standards of personal and environmental cleanliness'.

Over subsequent years the literature on this pattern of self-neglect has grown, often in the form of case reports of patients coming to clinical notice, and some larger series or reviews of this literature (e.g. Johnson and Adams, 1996; Pavlou and Lachs, 2006). The review by Pavlou and Lachs is a comprehensive summary of 'a complex and sprawling literature of varying quality' on self-neglect in older adults; 54 articles are reviewed and this offers a valuable starting point for the reader who wishes to explore the subject further. Only a small sample of that literature will be referred to here.

'Diogenes syndrome' is a striking name for a memorable clinical picture, but it has been well argued that neither is this a true syndrome, nor has it any legitimate connection with the real Diogenes, the Greek cynic philosopher of the 4th century BC (e.g. Johnson and Adams, 1996; Haddad and Lefebvre, 2002). Over the years a number of alternative names have been proposed, (such as 'senile squalor syndrome', 'social breakdown of the elderly syndrome', and 'Augean Stables syndrome'), but none has captured the imagination of clinicians in the way that Diogenes does, or yet come into general usage.

Leaving aside the nomenclature, do the cases described have enough in common to constitute a diagnostic entity? To describe a syndrome implies that a cluster of symptoms and signs, time course, and outcome occur together with such regularity that a common cause for them seems likely—even if the cause is as yet unknown. Asperger's syndrome would be a good example of a 'syndrome', understood in this way. Or, in the cases of Diogenes syndrome described in the literature, are we seeing an immediately recognizable 'final common pathway' of a multitude of different causes—the combined effect of the many and various mishaps of old age?

This understanding of 'syndrome' is argued by Pavlou and Lachs (2006), who compare the syndrome of self-neglect with other common syndromes of old age such as falls or incontinence, which likewise are the visible result of a combination of the ordinary pathologies of old age—a 'category' outcome, as it were, springing from 'dimensional' causes.

Or perhaps we are taking too narrow and medical a view of the problem when we consider the patient alone: the syndrome merely reflecting a *societal* response to an unusual but autonomous choice of lifestyle. Are the patients who appear in the literature simply the most dramatic instances, at the 'medical' peak of an iceberg hidden in the community ocean, of ordinary people more or less neglecting themselves, more or less deliberately (Johnson and Adams, 1996)?

The case reports which dominate the literature cannot go far to answer these questions, and many authors in the field conclude that properly planned epidemiological, longitudinal studies will be needed to clarify the picture of self-neglect in old age (and indeed at any age). One of the obvious questions concerns the source from which the patients are drawn. In the series of Clark *et al.* (1975), the patients came to professional notice because of an episode of acute illness; other series (Macmillan and Shaw, 1966; Pavlou and Lachs, 2006) are drawn from referrals to agencies for help with hygiene and self-care.

## Clinical features of the syndrome

What are the typical features of the syndrome of 'extreme self-neglect'; which of these features reflect only ascertainment and publication bias, and which are intrinsic to the condition (if it is a 'condition')?

It has not yet earned a place in the international diagnostic schedules, but there is a reasonable 'implicit consensus' emerging in the literature, judging by the review sections of case reports (e.g. Rosenthal *et al.* 1999; Haddad and Lefebvre, 2002; Greve *et al.*, 2004; Campbell *et al.*, 2005) and more comprehensive reviews (Johnson and Adams, 1996; Pavlou and Lachs, 2006). Greve *et al.* (2004) provide a succinct and up-to-date summary of the available information.

*Necessary features* of the syndrome (in other words, implicit criteria for the diagnosis) seem to be:

1 Living in circumstances of neglected personal and environmental hygiene: dirt and squalor, sometimes to an extreme degree (human or animal faeces, putrefying food, infestations).

2 Refusal of help to remedy the situation (often coupled with apparent unawareness or denial of any problem).

3 Often—but not always—hoarding of possessions, often valueless and perceived by others as rubbish ('syllogomania'), encroaching severely on the living space of the home.

Features which are *not necessary to the diagnosis*, but have been linked with it, include the following:

1 Physical illness. Although cases ascertained in general hospitals (e.g. Clark *et al.*, 1975) have had a variety of acute medical problems, including anaemia, poor nutrition, and dehydration, other cases have been described with good physical health.

2 Social isolation. Most of the people described have lived alone, but not all; some cases are described in which there has been another member of the household, but who has not been able— for various reasons—to influence the situation. Bereavement may be a precipitating cause of self-neglect, or it may—as with dementia—serve to uncover a longstanding problem.

3 Poverty, or being unknown to helping agencies. Some of the published cases have indeed been known to agencies—brought to their attention by concerned relatives, for example; but the subjects themselves have not sought this, nor wanted help when

it was offered. Descriptions of cases often emphasize that the self-neglect was not due to lack of material resources.

4 Psychiatric illness. According to Bergmann (2002), 'What characterises Diogenes syndrome is the presence of self-neglect unaccompanied by any psychiatric disorder sufficient to account for the squalor in which patients exist'. In the literature, many patients who neglect themselves have been mentally ill, mostly with a chronic psychotic illness, or with obsessive–compulsive disorder, alcohol abuse, or dementia. But many instances where the self-neglect has no such explanation are also (understandably) described and published.

5 Personality disorder. Although there is no evidence that the syndrome of self-neglect is associated with any *specific* personality disorder, those authors who have been able to interview informants for their cases describe a variety of pre-morbid personality traits that may have contributed to the self-neglect—unfriendliness, stubbornness, aggressiveness, independence, eccentricity, paranoia, aloofness, detachedness, compulsivity, narcissism, and lack of insight (Greve *et al.*, 2004). No systematic studies of personality, using informant reports and standard measures (such as the NEO-PI) have yet been carried out for patients with the Diogenes syndrome. This is understandable, given that these patients may be unwilling to cooperate with researchers, the available standard measures may not be suitable (van Alphen and Engelen, 2005), and there may be no informants to be found. Likewise there are few longitudinal studies (even more understandably) to illuminate the path by which these patients arrive at the impossible situations in which they are found.

6 Frontal lobe dysfunction. In everyday practice, the most baffling aspect of patients with the Diogenes syndrome is their indifference to degrees of squalor and to sights and smells that are daunting even to experienced workers in the community. No exaggeration of personality traits seems sufficient to explain such denial of need, and the possibility that this is a manifestation of frontal lobe dysfunction has been explored in a number of cases (e.g. Orrell *et al.*, 1989; Campbell *et al.*, 2005); and conversely, Diogenes syndrome has been described as a possible feature of frontal lobe dementia (Gregory and Hodges, 1993).

7 Prognosis. This also is not a distinguishing feature of the condition. The hospital series show a high mortality, but the mortality is probably lower for community-living patients. Some patients decline contact and are lost to follow-up; others revert to their previous patterns of hoarding and reclusiveness when they return home from a hospital admission; some go into institutional care where the social forces exerted by the staff prevent a reversion to old patterns, but their desire for privacy and their indifference to hygiene are still detectable; some will accept just enough help when they are at home to enable them to continue living in the community for a few years.

In the end, the Diogenes syndrome remains a somewhat enigmatic and teasing concept. It seems quite clear that self-neglect, broadly considered [as in Pavlou and Lachs' (2006) review], has multiple causes, often including medical and psychiatric illness and sensory impairment. But the suspicion that there is a 'core syndrome', characterized by severe social impairment (of a very specific kind) without any obvious psychiatric or medical cause, has not yet convincingly been refuted. If there is such a core diagnostic entity, it seems likely to bear a close relationship to the lifetime personality traits of its sufferers.

# References

Abrams, R.C. and Horowitz, S.V. (1996). Personality disorders after age 50: a meta-analysis. *Journal of Personality Disorders*, **10**(3), 278–81.

Aitken, L., Simpson, S., and Burns, A. (1999). Personality change in dementia. *International Psychogeriatrics*, **11**(3), 263–71.

van Alphen, S.P.J. and Engelen, G.J.J.A. (2005). Reaction to 'Personality disorder masquerading as dementia: a case of apparent Diogenes syndrome'. *International Journal of Geriatric Psychiatry*, **20**, 189–90.

van Alphen, S.P.J., Engelen, G.J.J.A., Kuin, Y., and Derksen, J.J.L. (2006a). The relevance of a geriatric sub-classification of personality disorders in the DSM-V. *International Journal of Geriatric Psychiatry*, **21**, 205–9.

van Alphen, S.P.J., Engelen, G.J.J.A., Kuin, Y., Hoijtink, H.J.A., and Derksen, J.J.L. (2006b). A preliminary study of the diagnostic accuracy of the Gerontological Personality disorders Scale (GPS). *International Journal of Geriatric Psychiatry*, **21**, 862–8.

Balsis, S., Carpenter, B.D., and Storandt, M. (2005). Personality change precedes clinical diagnosis of dementia of the Alzheimer type. *Journal of Gerontology*, **60B**(2), 98–101.

Barber, R., Snowden, J.S., and Craufurd, D. (1995). Frontotemporal dementia and Alzheimer's disease: retrospective differentiation using information from informants. *Journal of Neurology, Neurosurgery, and Psychiatry*, **59**, 61–70.

Beck, A.T., Epstein, N., Harrison, R.P., and Emery, G.(1983). *Development of the Sociotropy-Autonomy Scale: A measure of personality factors in psychopathology*. Center for Cognitive Therapy, University of Pennsylvania, Philadelphia.

Bergmann, K.(2002). Psychiatric aspects of personality in later life. In *Psychiatry in the elderly* (ed. R. Jacoby and C. Oppenheimer), pp. 722–43. Oxford University Press, New York.

Bergua, V., Fabrigoule, C., Barberger-Gateau, P., Dartigues, J.-F., Swendsen, J., and Bouisson, J. (2006). Preference for routines in older people: associations with cognitive and psychological vulnerability. *International Journal of Geriatric Psychiatry*, **21**, 990–8.

Bozzola, F.G., Gorelick, P.B., and Freels, S. (1992). Personality changes in Alzheimer's disease. *Archives of Neurology*, **49**, 297–300.

Brandt, J., Campodonico, J.R., Rich, J.B. *et al.* (1998). Adjustment to residential placement in Alzheimer disease patients: does premorbid personality matter? *International Journal of Geriatric Psychiatry*, **13**, 509–15.

Brooks, D.N. and McKinlay, W. (1983). Personality and behavioral change after severe blunt head injury: a relative's view. *Journal of Neurology, Neurosurgery and Psychiatry*, **46**, 336–44.

Campbell, H., Tadros, G., Hanna, G., and Bhalerao, M. (2005). Diogenes syndrome: frontal lobe dysfunction or multi-factorial disorder? *Geriatric Medicine*, **35**(3), 77–9.

Chatterjee, A., Strauss, M.E., Smyth, K.A., and Whitehouse, P.J. (1992). Personality changes in Alzheimer's disease. *Archives of Neurology*, **49**, 486–91.

Clark, A.N.G., Mankikar, G.O., and Gray, I. (1975). Diogenes syndrome: a clinical study of gross neglect in old age. *The Lancet*, **I**, 366–8.

Costa, P.T. and McCrae, R.R. (1986). Personality stability and its implications for clinical psychology. *Clinical Psychology Review* **6**, 407–23.

Costa, P.T. and McCrae, R.R. (1992). *Revised NEO Personality Inventory (NEO-PI-R) and NEO Five Factor Inventory (NEO-FFI) professional manual*. Psychological Assessment Resources, Inc., Odessa, FL.

Dawson, D.V., Welsh-Bohmer, K.A., and Siegler, I.C. (2000). Premorbid personality predicts level of rated personality change in patients with Alzheimer disease. *Alzheimer Disease and Associated Disorders*, **14**(1), 11–19.

Dian, L., Cummings, J.L., Petry, S., and Hill, M.A. (1990). Personality alterations in multi-infarct dementia. *Psychosomatics*, **31**, 415–19.

Digman, J.M. (1990). Personality structure: emergence of the five-factor model. *Annual Review of Psychology*, **41**, 417–40.

Duberstein, P.R. (1995). Openness to experience and completed suicide across the second half of life. *International Psychogeriatrics*, **7**(2), 183–98.

Ellis-Hill, C.S. and Horn, S. (2000). Change in identity and self-concept: a new theoretical approach to recovery following a stroke. *Clinical Rehabilitation*, **14**, 279–87.

Engels, G.I., Duijsens, I.J., Haringsma, R., and van Putten, C.M. (2003). Personality disorders in the elderly compared to four younger age groups: a cross-sectional study of community residents and mental health patients. *Journal of Personality Disorders*, **17**(5), 447–59.

Evans, S. and Garner, J. (eds) (2004). *Talking over the years. A handbook of dynamic psychotherapy with older adults*. Brunner-Routledge, Hove and New York.

Glosser, G., Clark, C., Freundlich, B., Kliner-Krenzel, L., Flaherty, P., and Stern, M. (1995). A controlled investigation of current and premorbid personality: characteristics of Parkinson's disease patients. *Movement disorders*, **10**(2), 201–6.

Golden, Z. and Golden, C.J. (2003). The differential impacts of Alzheimer's dementia, head injury, and stroke on personality dysfunction. *International Journal of Neuroscience*, **113**, 869–78.

Gould, S.L. and Hyer, L.A. (2004). Dementia and behavioural disturbance: does premorbid personality really matter? *Psychological Reports*, **95**, 1072–8.

Gregory, C.A. and Hodges, J.R. (1993). Dementia of frontal type and the focal lobar atrophies. *International Review of Psychiatry*, **5**, 397–406.

Greve, K.W., Curtis, K.L., and Collins, B.T. (2004). Personality disorder masquerading as dementia: a case of apparent Diogenes syndrome. *International Journal of Geriatric Psychiatry*, **19**, 701–5.

Grucza, R.A., Przybeck, T.R., Spitznagel, E.L., and Cloninger, C.R. (2003). Personality and depressive symptoms: a multi-dimensional analysis. *Journal of Affective Disorders*, **74**, 123–30.

Haddad, V. and Lefebvre, V. (2002). Diogenes syndrome from myth to reality. About three cases. *La Revue de Geriatrie*, **27**, 107–14.

Hamel, M., Gold, D.P., Andres, D., Reis, M., Dastoor, D., Grauer, H., and Bergman, H.(1990). Predictors and consequences of aggressive behavior by community-based dementia patients. *The Gerontologist*, **30**(2), 206–11.

Harwood, D.M.J., Hawton, K, Hope, T., and Jacoby, R. (2001). Psychiatric disorder and personality factors associated with suicide in older people: a descriptive and case-control study. *International Journal of Geriatric Psychiatry*, **16**, 155–65.

Heinik, J., Keren, P., Vainer-Benaiah, Z., Lahav, D., and Bleich, A.(1999). Agreement between spouses and children in descriptions of personality change in Alzheimer's disease. *Israel Journal of Psychiatry and Related Sciences*, **36**(2), 88–94.

Hilton, C. and Moniz-Cook, E. (2004). Examining the personality dimensions of sociotropy and autonomy in older people with dementia: their relevance to person centred care. *Behavioural and Cognitive Psychotherapy*, **32**, 457–65.

Holroyd, S. (2000). Personality disorders in the elderly. In *New Oxford textbook of psychiatry* (ed. M.G. Gelder, J.J. Lopez-Ibor, and N. Andreasen), pp. 1655–8. Oxford University Press, New York.

Holst, G., Hallberg, I. R., and Gustafson, L. (1997). The relationship of vocally disruptive behavior and previous personality in severely demented institutionalized patients. *Archives of Psychiatric Nursing*, **11**, 14–54.

Hooker, K. and McAdams, D.P. (2003). Personality reconsidered: a new agenda for aging research. *Journal of Gerontology*, **58B**(6), 296–304.

Johnson, J. and Adams, J. (1996). Self-neglect in later life. *Health and Social Care in the Community*, **4**(4), 226–33.

Kroessler, D. (1990). Personality disorder in the elderly. *Hospital and Community Psychiatry*, **41**(12), 1325–9.

Low, L.-F., Brodaty, H., and Draper, B. (2002). A study of premorbid personality and behavioural and psychological symptoms of dementia in nursing home residents. *International Journal of Geriatric Psychiatry*, **17**, 779–83.

Mazure, C.M., Maciejewski, P.K., Jacobs, S.C., and Bruce, M.L. (2002). Stressful life events interacting with cognitive/personality styles to predict late-onset major depression. *American Journal of Geriatric Psychiatry*, **10**(3), 297–304.

Macmillan, D. (1957). The evidence of social breakdown in the elderly: (b) psychiatric aspects of social breakdown in the elderly. *Royal Society of Health Journal*, **77**(11), 830–6.

Macmillan, D. and Shaw, P. (1966), Senile breakdown in standards of personal and environmental cleanliness. *British Medical Journal*, **2**, 1032–7.

McCrae, R.R. and Costa, P.T. (1987). Validation of the five-factor model of personality across instruments and observers. *Journal of Personality and Social Psychology*, **52**(1), 81–90.

McCrae, R.R. and Costa, P.T. (1988). Age, personality, and the spontaneous self-concept. *Journal of Gerontology*, **43**, 5177–85.

McCrae, R.R. and Costa, P.T. (1997). Personality trait structure as a human universal. *American Psychologist*, **52**(5), 509–16.

Meins, W. and Dammast, J. (2000). Do personality traits predict the occurrence of Alzheimer's disease? *International Journal of Geriatric Psychiatry*, **15**, 120–4.

Meins, W., Frey, A., and Thiesemann, R. (1998). Premorbid personality traits in Alzheimer's disease: do they predispose to noncognitive behavioural symptoms? *International Psychogeriatrics*, **10**(4), 369–78.

Monopoli, J. and Vaccaro, F. (2003). The relationship of hypochondriasis measures to correlates of personality in the elderly. *Clinical Gerontologist*, **26**(3/4), 123–37.

Morse, J.Q. and Lynch, T.R. (2004). A preliminary investigation of self-reported personality disorders in late life: prevalence, predictors of depressive severity, and clinical correlates. *Aging and Mental Health*, **8**(4), 307–15.

Mychack, P., Rosen, H., and Miller, B.L. (2001). Novel applications of social-personality measures to the study of dementia. *Neurocase*, **7**, 131–43.

Orrell, M., Sahakian, B., and Bergmann, K. (1989), Self neglect and frontal lobe function. *British Journal of Psychiatry*, **155**, 101–5.

Pavlou, M.P. and Lachs, M.S. (2006). Could self-neglect in older adults be a geriatric syndrome? *Journal of the American Geriatrics Society*, **54**, 831–42.

Petry, S., Cummings, J.L., Hill, M.A., and Shapira, J. (1988). Personality alterations in dementia of the Alzheimer type. *Archives of Neurology*, **45**, 1187–90.

Petry, S., Cummings, J.L., Hill, M.A., and Shapira, J. (1989). Personality alterations in dementia of the Alzheimer type: a three-year follow-up study. *Journal of Geriatric Psychiatry and Neurology*, **4**, 203–7.

Prigerson, H.G., Shear, K., Bierhals, A.J., Zonarich, D.L., and Reynolds, C.F. (1996). Childhood adversity, attachment and personality styles as predictors of anxiety among elderly caregivers. *Anxiety*, **2**, 234–41.

Rankin, K.P., Kramer, J.H., Mychack, P., and Miller, B.L. (2003). Double dissociation of social functioning in frontotemporal dementia. *Neurology*, **60**, 266–71.

Rankin, K.P., Baldwin, E., Pace-Savitsky, C., Kramer, J.H., and Miller, B.L. (2005). Self awareness and personality change in dementia. *Journal of Neurology, Neurosurgery and Psychiatry*, **76**, 632–9.

Rao, R. (2003). Does personality disorder influence the likelihood of in-patient admission in late-life depression? *International Journal of Geriatric Psychiatry*, **18**, 960–1.

Rosenthal, M., Stelian, J., Wagner, J., and Berkman, P. (1999). Diogenes syndrome and hoarding in the elderly: case reports. *Israel Journal of Psychiatry and Related Sciences*, **36**(1), 29–34.

Rosowsky, E. and Gurian, B. (1991). Borderline personality disorder in late life. *International Psychogeriatrics*, **3**(1), 39–52.

Rubin, E.H., Morris, J.C. and Berg, L. (1987). The progression of personality changes in senile dementia of the Alzheimer's type. *Journal of the American Geriatrics Society*, **35**, 721–5.

Sadavoy, J. (1987). Character pathology in the elderly. *Journal of Geriatric Psychiatry*, **20**, 165–78.

Segal, D.L., Hersen, M., Van Hasselt, V.B., Silberman, C.S., and Roth, L. (1996). Diagnosis and assessment of personality disorders in older adults: a critical review. *Journal of Personality Disorders*, **10**(4), 384–99.

Shaw, P. (1957). The evidence of social breakdown in the elderly: a) social breakdown in the elderly. *Royal Society of Health Journal*, **77**(11), 823–30.

Siegler, I.C., Welsh, K.A., Dawson, D.V. *et al.* (1991). Ratings of personality change in patients being evaluated for memory disorders. *Alzheimer Disease and Associated Disorders*, **5**(4), 240–50.

Siegler, I.C., Dawson, D.V., and Welsh, K.A. (1994). Caregiver ratings of personality change in Alzheimer's disease patients: a replication. *Psychology and Aging*, **9**(3), 404–66.

Smith-Gamble, V., Baiyewu, O., Perkins, A.J. *et al.* (2002). Informant reports of changes in personality predict dementia in a population-based study of elderly African Americans and Yoruba. *American Journal of Geriatric Psychiatry*, **10**, 724–32.

Stone, J., Townend, E., Kwan, K., Dennis, M.S., and Sharpe, M. (2004). Personality change after stroke: some preliminary observations. *Journal of Neurology, Neurosurgery and Psychiatry*, **75**, 1708–13.

Strauss, M.E., Pasupathi, M., and Chatterjee, A. (1993). Concordance between observers in descriptions of personality change in Alzheimer's disease. *Personality and Aging*, **8**(4), 475–80.

Strauss, M.E., Stuckey, J.C., Pasupathi M., and Moore, A. (1997). Accuracy of retrospective descriptions of personality during the course of Alzheimer's disease. *Journal of Clinical Geropsychology*, **3**(2), 93–9.

Thompson, L.W., Gallagher, D., and Czirr, R. (1988). Personality disorder and outcome in the treatment of late-life depression. *Journal of Geriatric Psychiatry*, **21**, 133–46.

Weiss, A., Costa, P.T., Karuza, J., Duberstein, P.R., Friedman, B., and McCrae, R.R. (2005). Cross-sectional age differences in personality among Medicare patients aged 65 to 100. *Psychology and Aging*, **20**(1), 182–5.

Wesby, R. (2004). Inpatient dynamics: thinking, feeling and understanding. In *Talking over the years. A handbook of dynamic psychotherapy with older adults*. (ed. S. Evans and J. Garner), pp. 101–16. Brunner-Routledge, Hove and New York.

Zimmerman, M. (1994). Diagnosing personality disorders: a review of issues and research methods. *Archives of General Psychiatry*, **51**, 225–45.

# 32

# Late onset schizophrenia and very late onset schizophrenia-like psychosis

Robert Howard

## Historical development of diagnostic concepts

### Paraphrenia to late paraphrenia

The classification of schizophrenia-like and paranoid disorders in the elderly has a long and confusing history. To Kraepelin (1894) *dementia praecox* was fundamentally a disorder of emotion and volition; *paraphrenia* was characterized by hallucinations and delusions without deterioration or disturbance of affective response, and *paranoia* involved the insidious development of a permanent delusional system which resulted from internal causes and was accompanied by perfect preservation of orderly thinking, acting, and will. However, by the eighth edition of his textbook in 1913, Kraepelin was expressing serious doubts about the assumptions on which his conception of dementia praecox had been based. In some cases a complete and lasting recovery was seen and the relationship between onset and early adult life was not absolute. Indeed, Bleuler (1911) had introduced the term 'schizophrenia' in order to get away from the concept of the disorder as an adolescent mental deterioration. The notion of paraphrenia as a distinct entity was further discredited following Mayer's (1921) follow-up of Kraepelin's 78 original cases. At least 40% of the patients had developed clear signs of dementia praecox within a few years and only 36% could still be classified as paraphrenic. Many of the paraphrenics had positive family histories of schizophrenia and the presenting clinical picture of those patients who remained 'true' paraphrenics did not differ from those who were later to develop signs of schizophrenia. Thirty-one years later, Roth and Morrisey (1952) resurrected both terminology and controversy with their choice of the term *late paraphrenia* to describe patients who they believed had schizophrenia, but with an onset delayed until after the age of 55 or 60 years. The term was intended to be descriptive; to distinguish the illness from the chronic early onset schizophrenic patients seen in psychiatric institutions at the time and to emphasize the clinical similarities with the illness described by Kraepelin. Late paraphrenia was never intended to mean the same

thing as paraphrenia and Kraepelin certainly did not emphasize late age of onset as a feature of the illness.

### Late schizophrenia

Both Kraepelin (1913) and Bleuler (1911) observed that there was a relatively rare group of schizophrenics who had an onset of illness in late middle or old age and who, on clinical grounds, closely resembled those who had an onset in early adult life. Utilizing a very narrow conception of dementia praecox and specifically excluding cases of paraphrenia, Kraepelin (1913) reported that only 5.6% of 1054 patients had an onset after the age of 40 years. If the age of onset was set at 60 years or greater, only 0.2% of patients could be included.

Manfred Bleuler (1943) carried out the first specific and systematic examination of late onset patients and defined late schizophrenia as follows:

1 Onset after the age of 40.

2 Symptomatology that does not differ from that of schizophrenia occurring early in life (or if it does differ it should not do so in a clear or radical way).

3 It should not be possible to attribute the illness to a neuropathological disorder because of the presence of an amnestic syndrome or associated signs of organic brain disease.

Bleuler found that between 15% and 17% of two large series of schizophrenic patients had an onset after the age of 40. Of such late onset cases, only 4% had become ill for the first time after the age of 60. Later authors confirmed that while onset of schizophrenia after the age of 40 was unusual, onset after 60 should be considered even rarer. From 264 elderly schizophrenic patients admitted in Edinburgh in 1957, only 7 had an illness that had begun after the age of 60 (Fish, 1958). Using very broad criteria for the diagnosis of schizophrenia (including schizoaffective, paraphrenic, and other non-organic non-affective psychoses) and studying 470 first contacts with the Camberwell Register, Howard *et al.* (1993) found 29% of cases to have been aged over 44 at onset.

Kraepelin and E. Bleuler both considered late onset cases to have much in common with more typically early onset schizophrenia, and this view was supported by M. Bleuler's report (1943) of only very mild phenomenological variance from early onset cases. His 126 late onset cases were, however, symptomatically milder, had less affective flattening, and were less likely to have formal thought disorder than patients with a younger onset. Fish (1960) reported that the clinical picture presented by 23 patients with onset after the age of 40 did not differ importantly from patients who were young at onset, but believed that with increasing age at onset schizophrenia took on a more 'paraphrenic' form.

## Late paraphrenia

Kay and Roth (1961) studied a group of 39 female and 3 male patients given a diagnosis of late paraphrenia in Graylingwell Hospital between 1951 and 1955. All but six of these cases were followed-up for 5 years. The cases notes of 48 female and 9 male late paraphrenics admitted to a hospital in Stockholm between 1931 and 1940 were also collected and these cases followed up until death or until 1956. Over 40% of the Graylingwell late paraphrenics were living alone, compared with 12% of affective patients and 16% of those with organic psychoses who were of comparable ages. Late paraphrenics were also socially isolated. Although the frequency of visual impairment at presentation (15%) was no higher than in comparison groups with other diagnoses, some impairment of hearing was present in 40% of late paraphrenics and this was considered severe in 15%. Deafness was only present in 7% of affective patients. Focal cerebral disease was identified in only 8% of late paraphrenic patients at presentation. Primary delusions, feelings of mental or physical influence, and hallucinations were all prominent and the prognosis for recovery was poor. Kay and Roth concluded that, at least descriptively, late paraphrenia was a form of schizophrenia, but that its aetiology might be multifactorial.

From a detailed analysis of 1250 first admissions to a hospital in Gothenburg, Sjoegren (1964) identified 202 elderly individuals who conformed to the French concept of paraphrenia (Magnan, 1893): having well-organized and persistent paranoid delusions with hallucinations occurring in clear consciousness. Sjoegren argued cogently that, together with constitutional factors, ageing itself produces effects (feelings of isolation and loneliness, social and economic insecurity, and heightened vulnerability) which contribute to the development of paranoid reactions.

Felix Post (1966) collected a sample of 93 patients to whom he gave the non-controversial and self-explanatory label 'persistent persecutory states' and made a point of including cases regardless of coexisting organic brain change. Within this broad category he recognized three clinical sub-types: a schizophrenic syndrome (34 patients), a schizophreniform syndrome (37 patients), and a paranoid hallucinosis group (22 patients). Post regarded those patients with the schizophrenic syndrome as having a delayed form of schizophrenia with only partial expression. All of Post's patients were treated with phenothiazines and he was able to demonstrate that the condition was responsive to antipsychotic medication.

From a series of 45 female and 2 male late paraphrenics [identified using the same criteria as Kay and Roth (1961)] admitted to St Francis' Hospital in Hayward's Heath between 1958 and 1964, Herbert and Jacobson (1967) confirmed many of Kay and Roth's

(1961) observations. In addition, they found an unexpectedly high prevalence of schizophrenia among the mothers (4.4%) and siblings (13.3%) of patients.

## ICD-10 and DSM-IV: the end for late paraphrenia

Diagnostic guidelines published by authoritative organizations such as the World Health Organization (WHO) or the American Psychiatric Association (APA) reflect the views of many contemporary clinicians who were consulted at the draft and field trial stages. Inclusion or exclusion of a particular diagnosis in published diagnostic schemes thus reflects the current credence given to the nosological validity of that diagnosis plus an indication of its general usefulness in clinical practice.

Late paraphrenia, included within ICD-9, did not survive as a separate codeable diagnosis into ICD-10. Most cases are coded under schizophrenia (F20.0) (Quintal *et al.*, 1991; Howard *et al.*, 1994a), although in the diagnostic guidelines the category of delusional disorder (F22.0) is suggested as a replacement for 'paraphrenia (late)'. The distinction between cases of schizophrenia and delusional disorder within ICD-10 is very much dependent on the quality of auditory hallucinations experienced by patients and is subject to some unhelpful ageism. The guidelines for delusional disorder (F22.0) in ICD-10 state that 'Clear and persistent auditory hallucinations (voices)…are incompatible with this diagnosis'. Rather confusingly for old age psychiatrists, these same guidelines for a diagnosis of delusional disorder further suggest however, that: '…occasional or transitory auditory hallucinations, particularly in elderly patients, do not rule out this diagnosis, provided that they are not typically schizophrenic and form only a small part of the overall clinical picture'.

The inclusion within DSM-IIIR (APA, 1987) of a separate category of late onset schizophrenia for cases with an onset of illness after the age of 44 years was a reaction to the unsatisfactory and arbitrary upper age limit for onset that had hitherto prevailed for a diagnosis of schizophrenia. DSM-IV (APA, 1993) contains no separate category for late onset schizophrenia and this presumably reflects the general North American view that there is a direct continuity between cases of schizophrenia whatever their age at onset.

The author's view is that late paraphrenia has proved (at least in European psychiatry) to be a clinically useful diagnosis, the adoption of which helped to advance the recognition and study of late onset psychoses. Because of the lack of clarity regarding its relationship with schizophrenia and its failure to achieve international recognition, the survival of late paraphrenia has always been threatened and we should not mourn its demise.

## Terminology and classification for the future

The important questions now are as follows; have ICD-10 and DSM-IV been fair to abandon any facility for coding late onset within schizophrenia and the delusional disorders, and do we need diagnostic categories that distinguish the functional psychoses with onset in later life from schizophrenia? When the late onset schizophrenia international consensus group met in 1998 (Howard *et al.*, 2000), they agreed that the available evidence from the areas of epidemiology, phenomenology, and pathophysiology supported homogeneity within schizophrenia with increasing age at onset up to the age of 60 years. By contrast, schizophrenia-like psychosis with onset after the age of 60 years (i.e. what we used to call late paraphrenia) was considered to be distinct from schizophrenia. The consensus group recommended that cases with onset between 40 and 59 years be termed late onset schizophrenia and that the group with onset after 60 years should be called very late onset schizophrenia-like psychosis (VLOSLP). The latter term is long-winded and unmemorable but is at least unambiguous, and it received the unprecedented support of both European and North American old age psychiatrists.

## Clinical features

### Schizophrenic symptoms

Although Bleuler (1943) believed that it was not possible to separate early and late onset patients on clinical grounds, he acknowledged that a later onset was accompanied by less affective flattening and a more benign course. Formal thought disorder is seen in only about 5% of cases of DSM-IIIR late onset schizophrenia (Pearlson *et al.*, 1989) and could not be elicited from any of 101 late paraphrenics (Howard *et al.*, 1994a). First-rank symptoms of Schneider are seen, but are less prevalent in later onset cases. Thought insertion, thought block, and thought withdrawal seem to be particularly uncommon (Grahame, 1984; Pearlson *et al.*, 1989; Howard *et al.*, 1994a) and negative symptoms are unusual (Almeida *et al.*, 1995a).

### Delusions

Persecutory delusions usually dominate the presentation although in a series of 101 late paraphrenics, delusions of reference (76%), of control (25%), of grandiose ability (12%), and of a hypochondriacal nature (11%) were also present (Howard *et al.*, 1994a). Partition delusions are found in about two-thirds of cases. They are the belief that people, animals, materials, or radiation can pass through a structure that would normally constitute a barrier to such passage. This barrier is generally the door, ceiling, walls, or floor of a patient's home and the source of intrusion is frequently a neighbouring residence (Herbert and Jacobson, 1967; Pearlson *et al.*, 1989; Howard *et al.*, 1992).

### Affective symptoms

The coexistence of affective features in late onset schizophrenia is well recognized clinically but there have been no controlled studies comparing such features in early and late onset cases. Atypical, schizoaffective and cycloid psychoses are all characterized by affective features, tend to arise later in life, and affect women more than men (Cutting *et al.*, 1978; Kendell, 1988; Levitt and Tsuang, 1988). Among late paraphrenic patients, Post (1966) reported depressive admixtures in 60% of cases, while Holden (1987) considered that 10 of his 24 'functional' late paraphrenic patients had affective or schizoaffective illnesses. These patients also had a better outcome in terms both of institutionalization and 10-year survival compared with paranoid patients. Such observations have led to the suggestion that some later onset schizophrenics or late paraphrenics may have variants of primary affective disorder (Murray *et al.*, 1992).

### Cognitive deficits

Kay and Roth (1961) recognized that a degree of overlap between functional and organic psychoses in senescence existed and pointed out that, particularly in the elderly, it was misleading to consider psychiatric illness in isolation from other pathologies: '…we are most prone to encounter depressive psychosis after an attack of

pneumonia, manic episodes after surgical operations, paranoid disorders with and without physical illness in old people with a mild memory defect'.

Post (1966) did not exclude patients with associated organic impairment from his study and found proven organic cerebral change in 16 of his 93 cases of persistent persecutory states. He concluded that simple paranoid and schizophrenia-like syndromes could commonly complicate early dementia but that in such cases disorders of memory and concentration could clearly be seen to have preceded the emergence of persecutory symptoms.

Attempts to identify and characterize the patterns of cognitive impairment associated with these conditions began with Hopkins and Roth (1953) who administered the vocabulary subtest from the Wechsler-Bellevue Scale, a shortened form of the Raven's Progressive Matrices, and a general test of orientation and information, to patients with a variety of diagnoses. Twelve late paraphrenic patients performed as well as a group of elderly depressives and better than patients with dementia on all three tests.

Miller *et al.* (1991) have published comprehensive neuropsychological assessments of patients suffering from what they term 'late life psychosis'. These patients performed less well than age-matched controls on the Mini-Mental State Examination (MMSE), the Wechsler Adult Intelligence Scale-Revised, the Wisconsin Card Sorting Test, Logical Memory, and Visual Reproduction subtests from the Wechsler Memory Scale, a test of verbal fluency and the Warrington Recognition Memory Test. Patients were, however, not well matched with controls for educational attainment and premorbid intelligence and some of the patients clearly had affective psychoses and dementia syndromes (Miller *et al.*, 1992), so that it is probably not fair to equate them with late paraphrenics or late onset schizophrenics.

Almeida *et al.* (1995b) carried out a very detailed neuropsychological examination of 40 patients with late paraphrenia in south London. Using cluster analysis of the results he identified two groups of patients. The first was a 'functional' group characterized by impairment restricted to executive functions, in particular a computerized test assessing extra- and intra-dimensional attention set shift ability and a test of planning. Such patients had a high prevalence and severity of positive psychotic symptoms and lower scores on a scale of neurological abnormalities. A second 'organic' group of late paraphrenics showed widespread impairment of cognitive functions together with a lower frequency of positive psychotic symptoms and a high prevalence of abnormalities on neurological examination (Almeida *et al.*, 1995b).

### Stability of cognitive deficit

In his 10-year case-note follow-up study Holden (1987) considered a group of late paraphrenics who progressed to a frank dementia in the first 3 years to have 'organic' late paraphrenia. Such patients had lower scores on cognitive testing on entry to the follow-up period, a reduced female-to-male ratio, and were less likely to have first-rank symptoms than 'functional' late paraphrenics. None of the organic patients showed a full symptomatic recovery and, perhaps not surprisingly, the functional patients had a superior 10-year survival. Holden's organic group almost certainly represented patients with dementia whose non-cognitive symptoms had led their physicians to make a diagnosis of paranoid psychosis. Strikingly, only 8% of his 'functional' group of late paraphrenics developed dementia during the follow-up period so that the risk of cognitive decline in these patients would appear to have been no higher than in the elderly general population.

Brodaty et al. (2003) carried out a prospective 5-year follow-up of 19 patients with onset of DSM-IIIR schizophrenia at age 50 years or over and found that nine had developed dementia. These authors concluded from their results that late onset schizophrenia may be a prodrome of Alzheimer's disease, but it is clear that they recruited a heterogeneous population with initial MMSE scores as low as 19/30. The authors did find, however, that if they only included patients with a MMSE of 28/30 or greater, there was still a higher rate of conversion to dementia among patients (2/7) than controls (0/23).

## Aetiology

### Family studies

Reviewing the literature on family history in schizophrenia, Gottesman and Shields (1982) reported that the overall risk of schizophrenia in the relatives of an affected proband is about 10% compared with a risk of around 1% for the general population.

Kendler et al. (1987) concluded that there was no consistent relationship between age at onset and familial risk for schizophrenia, but data from patients with an onset in old age were not included in this analysis. The literature on familiality in late onset schizophrenia and related psychoses of late life is sparse and inconclusive, partly due to variations in illness definition and age at onset, but principally because of the difficulties inherent in conducting family studies in patients who often have very few surviving first-degree relatives. The results of those few studies specifically of late onset psychoses, reviewed by Castle and Howard (1992), suggest a trend for increasing age at onset of psychosis to be associated with reduced risk of schizophrenia in first-degree relatives. Thus studies involving subjects with illness onset after the age of 40 or 45 years have reported rates of schizophrenia in relatives of between 4.4% and 19.4% (Bleuler, 1943; Huber et al., 1975; Pearlson et al., 1989), while those with onsets delayed to 50 or 60 years have yielded rates of between 1.0% and 7.3% (Funding, 1961; Post, 1966; Herbert and Jacobson, 1967). More recently, two studies of patients with late onset psychosis—one study with onset after the age of 50 (Brodaty et al., 1999) and the other study with onset after 60 years (Howard et al., 1997)—have reported no increase in the prevalence of schizophrenia among relatives of patients compared with those of healthy comparison subjects. In a controlled family study involving data from 269 first-degree relatives of patients with onset after 60 and 272 relatives of healthy elderly subjects, the estimated lifetime risk for schizophrenia with an onset range of 15 to 90 years was 2.3% for the relatives of cases and 2.2% for the relatives of controls (Howard et al., 1997).

### Brain imaging

The first computed tomography (CT) study specifically to examine patients with schizophrenic symptoms with an onset in late life was by Miller et al. (1986). Five female patients, whose age at onset of symptoms ranged from 58 to 81 years, were scanned. Three of the patients had extensive cortical and subcortical infarcts and one had normal pressure hydrocephalus. The scan appearances were so decidedly abnormal that the authors entitled their paper 'Late life paraphrenia: an organic delusional syndrome'. It has to be said that selection of patients with exclusion of those with a history or clinical signs of neurological disease or dementia has not confirmed this conclusion for the majority of cases.

Rabins et al. (1987) determined ventricle-to-brain ratios (VBRs) with CT in 29 patients whose onset of illness had been over the age of 44 years. Mean VBR was 13.3% in patients and 8.6% in a group of 23 age-matched controls. Naguib and Levy (1987) prospectively identified and CT scanned 45 cases of late paraphrenia and reported an increase in VBR measurements that was strikingly similar to that of Rabins et al.'s late onset schizophrenics. Mean VBR in patients was 13.09% compared with 9.75% in controls.

Exclusion from CT studies of patients with obvious neurological signs or a history of stroke, alcohol abuse, or dementia has shown that structural abnormalities other than large ventricles in patients with late paraphrenia are probably no more common than in healthy aged controls. Despite adhering to such exclusions, however, Flint et al. (1991) found unsuspected cerebral infarction on the scans of 5 out of 16 of their late paraphrenic patients. Most of these infarcts were subcortical or frontal and they were more likely to occur in patients who had delusions but no hallucinations. The results of this study need to be interpreted with some caution, since only 16 of a collected sample of patients had actually undergone CT scanning and it is of course possible that these represented the more 'organic' cases, or at least those that were thought most likely to have some underlying structural abnormality.

Where changes in periventricular and deep white matter are concerned, however, the results of MRI studies must again be viewed with some caution. Few studies have assessed abnormalities in the white matter in any kind of standardized manner, and few have used appropriate control populations, matched for cerebrovascular risk factors. Miller et al. (1989, 1991, 1992) reported the results of structural MRI investigations in patients with what they have termed 'late life psychosis'. They found that 42% of non-demented patients with an onset of psychosis after the age of 45 (mean age at scanning 60.1 years) had white matter abnormalities on MRI, compared with only 8% of a healthy age-matched control group. The appearance of large patchy white matter lesions (WMLs) was six times more likely in the temporal lobe, and four times more common in the frontal lobes, of patients than controls (Miller et al., 1991). These authors hypothesized that, although insufficient to give rise to focal neurological signs, WMLs might produce dysfunction in the overlying frontal and temporal cortex and that this could contribute to psychotic symptomatology. They acknowledged that since WMLs in the occipital lobes could also be implicated, it might not be possible to pinpoint an isolated anatomical white matter lesion that predisposed to psychosis. When comparisons were made between those patients who had structural brain abnormalities on MRI (10) with those who did not (7), there were no significant differences on age, educational level, IQ, or performance on a wide battery of neuropsychological tests. Our own studies of white matter signal hyperintensities among patients with late paraphrenia (from whom we have tried to exclude organic cases) have suggested that they may be no more common in such patients than in healthy community-living elderly controls (Howard et al., 1995a). This finding is replicated in a sample of late onset schizophrenia patients in the USA (Symonds et al., 1997).

We reported the results of volumetric MRI studies, based on the scans of 47 patients with late paraphrenia, 31 of whom satisfied ICD-10 criteria for a diagnosis of schizophrenia and 16 for delusional disorder. While total brain volume was not reduced in the patients compared with 35 elderly community-living controls, lateral and third ventricle volumes were increased (Howard *et al.*, 1994b). Measurements of the volumes of the frontal lobes, hippocampus, parahippocampus, thalamus, and basal ganglia structures failed to demonstrate further differences between patient and control subjects. These negative results are in accord with a North American volumetric study examining the thalamus in late onset schizophrenia. Corey-Bloom *et al.* (1995) compared MRI scans of the brains of 16 late onset and 14 early onset schizophrenic patients and of 28 normal elderly controls. All subjects were over the age of 45 years. Patients with late onset schizophrenia had significantly larger lateral ventricles than normal comparison subjects, but they had significantly larger thalamic volumes than the patients with early onset schizophrenia.

Studies of cerebral blood flow in patients with a late onset schizophrenia-like illness or in patients with early dementia and paranoid symptomatology have been few. Miller *et al.* (1992) studied 18 DSM-IIIR (APA 1987) late onset schizophrenics with single photon emission tomography (SPET) using $^{99}$Tc-hexamethyl propyleneamine oxime (HMPAO) which gives a high-resolution (approximately 7 mm) qualitative image of relative cerebral perfusion. Regional cerebral blood flow was described in right and left frontal, parietal, temporal, occipital, thalamic, and basal ganglia regions. Hypoperfusion was defined as blood flow less than 66% of maximal cerebral uptake. Of the 18 schizophrenic patients in the study, 11 (61%) had MRI evidence of either WMLs or multiple strokes. Nine of these 11 had focal or multifocal deficits on SPET suggesting vascular injury. Five patients had normal SPET perfusion scans, one had an Alzheimer's disease type pattern and 12 had a pattern suggesting multi-infarct dementia. Only 4 out of 30 normal controls had abnormal SPET scans. In the light of previous suggestions that temporal and frontal dysfunction may be important in the pathogenesis of psychosis (e.g. Cummings, 1985), Miller *et al.* (1992) further evaluated regional temporal, parietal, and frontal perfusion in these patients and their controls. Thirteen of 18 late life psychosis patients, compared with 7 of 30 control subjects, had unilateral or bilateral temporal hypoperfusion ($P < 0.003$). Seven of 18 patients and 4 of 30 controls had frontal hypoperfusion ($P < 0.002$). Fifteen of 18 (83%) late life psychosis patients, compared with 27% of controls, had either frontal or temporal hypoperfusion. These results support the view of this group of workers who emphasize the contribution of vascular-based structural brain abnormalities in the aetiology of late onset schizophrenia-like psychoses.

## Sex ratio

The female preponderance of individuals who have an onset of schizophrenia or a schizophrenia-like psychosis in middle or old age is a consistent finding. Among late onset schizophrenics (onset after 40–50 years) females have been reported to constitute 66% (Bleuler, 1943), 72% (Klages, 1961), 82% (Gabriel, 1978), 85% (Marneros and Deister, 1984), or 87% (Pearlson *et al.*, 1989) of patients. In studies of patients with an illness onset at 60 years or greater, the female preponderance is even greater: 75% (Sternberg, 1972), 86% (Howard *et al.*, 1994a), 88% (Kay and Roth, 1961), or 91% (Herbert and Jacobson, 1967).

Two reports have indicated the presence of a subgroup of female schizophrenia patients with later illness onset who typically do not have a positive family history of schizophrenia (Gorwood *et al.*, 1995; Shimizu and Kurachi, 1989). Typically later illness onset, particularly in females, is associated with a milder symptom profile and better outcome, better pre-morbid social adjustment, and a lower prevalence of structural brain abnormalities than in (mostly male) patients with early illness onset. This has led to the suggestion that sex differences in schizophrenia may reflect different psychiatric disorders. Hence, Castle and Murray (1991) have suggested that early onset, typically male schizophrenia is essentially a heritable neurodevelopmental disorder, while late onset schizophrenia in females may have aetiologically more in common with affective psychosis than with the illness seen in males.

## Sensory deficits

Deafness has been experimentally (Zimbardo *et al.*, 1981) and clinically associated with the development of paranoid symptoms. Deficits of moderate to severe degree affect 40% of patients with late paraphrenia (Herbert and Jacobson, 1967; Kay and Roth, 1961) and are more prevalent than in elderly depressed patients or normal controls (Naguib and Levy, 1987; Post, 1966). Deafness associated with late life psychosis is more usually conductive than degenerative (Cooper *et al.*, 1974) and generally of early onset, long duration, bilateral, and profound (Cooper, 1976; Cooper and Curry, 1976). Corbin and Eastwood (1986) suggested that deafness may reinforce a pre-existing tendency to social isolation, withdrawal, and suspiciousness. Further, auditory hallucinations are the psychopathological phenomenon most consistently associated with deafness (Keshavan *et al.*, 1992). There are several reports of improvement in psychotic symptoms after the fitting of a hearing aid (Almeida *et al.*, 1993; Eastwood *et al.*, 1981; Khan *et al.*, 1988), although it has to be said that clinical practice suggests that this is not usually the case.

Visual impairment, most commonly a consequence of cataract or macular degeneration, is also commoner in elderly paranoid psychosis patients than those with affective disorder and there is a higher coincidence of visual and hearing impairment in paranoid than affective patients. An association between visual impairment and the presence of visual hallucinations (Howard *et al.*, 1994a) echoes Keshavan's findings with deafness.

## Pre-morbid personality and cognitive style

A consistent theme in descriptions of patients who develop paranoid psychoses late in life is the presence of abnormal personality traits; most often schizoid or paranoid personality types (Kay and Roth, 1961; Post, 1966; Kay *et al.*, 1976). Although these patients are known to experience relationship difficulties, reflected by their low rates of marriage and the apparently reduced numbers of children born to those who do marry (Kay and Roth, 1961; Herbert and Jacobson, 1967), this contrasts with their pre-morbid educational and occupational adjustment, which is often good (Pearlson and Rabins, 1988). Hence, abnormalities in personality function in these patients have a characteristic specificity. Kay and Roth (1961) reported paranoid and schizoid personality traits (characterized by jealousy, suspiciousness, emotional coldness, arrogance, egocentricity, and extreme solitariness) in 45% of patients. A further 30% were described as explosive, sensitive, or belonging to religious minority groups. Late paraphrenics were also more likely to be living alone (40%) than patients of the same age with affective disorders (12%) or organic psychoses (16%). Acknowledging that pre-morbid personality abnormality seemed almost universal in late paraphrenia, Kay and Roth (1961) identified a subgroup comprising 20% of their sample who were characterized by severely abnormal pre-morbid personalities who developed paranoid delusions but did not hallucinate. Such patients had long-standing abnormalities of personality of a kind that interfered with relationships, a high age of first admission (generally over 75 years), and delusions that were almost always confined to ideas of theft, ill-treatment, or poisoning by people in everyday contact with the patient. The onset of psychosis was often hard to date in such individuals, since relatives tended to regard symptoms as an extension and caricature of the usual personality.

Felix Post (1966) believed that the personalities of patients with persistent persecutory states could frequently be recognized as having been paranoid in early life. From 87 patients for whom he had information about pre-morbid personality function, 35 had what he termed 'paranoid traits', in that they had been quarrelsome, sensitive, suspicious, or generally hostile. He described other patients as having been odd, eccentric, histrionic, or pretentious, and in only 26 cases was he able to conclude that the pre-morbid personality had been free of significant abnormality.

Pre-morbid personality in late and mid-life paranoid psychoses and the quality of pre-morbid relationships within families and with friends were assessed retrospectively by Kay et al. (1976). This study is an important one because, through use of structured patient and informant interviews, it represented a first effort to overcome some of the problems inherent in any retrospective attempt at defining pre-morbid personality. From a consecutive series of first admissions to a psychiatric hospital the authors selected 54 cases of paranoid and 57 of affective psychosis over the age of 50. Patients and close relatives or friends were independently given a semi-structured clinical interview, designed to cover a wide range of paranoid traits. The paranoid patients were rated more highly, both by themselves and informants, on items that suggested that they had greater difficulty in establishing and maintaining satisfactory relationships pre-morbidly. They had also been significantly more shy, reserved, touchy, and suspicious and less able to display sympathy or emotion. Through principal components analysis of the results, the authors derived a 'prepsychotic schizoid personality factor', consisting of unsociability, reticence, suspiciousness, and hostility.

Retterstol (1966) has argued that since personality deviations in paranoid patients are recognizable at a very early age, factors in the childhood and adolescence of patients are important in determining a predisposition to paranoid psychosis later in life. Key experiences in the later development of paranoid psychoses are proposed to be those which provoke feelings of insecurity or which damage the self-image of an individual whose personality is already overtly sensitive. Gurian et al. (1992) have also provided evidence for the importance of childhood experiences in the development of paranoid psychosis in late life. Among nine Israeli patients with delusional disorder, these authors found a high prevalence of 'war refugees'. These were individuals who had survived the Armenian or Nazi holocausts or had been forced to leave their native country. The authors proposed an association between the presence of extremely life-threatening experiences in childhood, a failure to produce progeny, and the development of paranoid delusional symptoms in late life in response to a stressful situation such as widowhood. Just how early the threatening experience needs to be is not clear. Cervantes et al. (1989) found the risk of developing a paranoid psychosis to be doubled in immigrants from Mexico and Central America who were escaping war or political unrest

compared with those who had moved for economic reasons. Thus, the period during which a personality may be rendered sensitive to the later development of paranoid psychosis by exposure to trauma is presumably not limited to early childhood.

African- and Caribbean-born elders in the UK are at higher risk of developing psychosis after the age of 60 years (Reeves et al., 2001), and patients who are members of such migrant groups have a less marked female preponderance and are younger at psychosis onset than indigenous elders (Mitter et al., 2005).

Studies investigating the cognitive aetiology of persecutory delusions in young adults with schizophrenia have implicated abnormalities in three specific areas of social belief formation. Such patients make explicit mentalizing errors when determining the intentions of others (Corcoran et al., 1995), jump to conclusions on the basis of insufficient evidence when reasoning under conditions of uncertainty (Garety et al., 1991), and are more likely than normal subjects to attribute the cause of negative events to other people (Kaney and Bentall, 1989). When we have studied very late onset schizophrenia-like psychosis patients to see if they share these key abnormalities with schizophrenia subjects, we found that while performance on deception mentalizing tasks was impaired, patients performed as well as healthy controls on tasks involving probabilistic reasoning and attributional style (Moore et al., 2006). It is possible that mentalizing errors may contribute to the development and maintenance of persecutory delusions in very late onset schizophrenia-like psychosis, but these patients do not seem to show the wider range of cognitive biases described in younger deluded patients.

# Management/treatment

## Establishing a therapeutic relationship

Although these patients are often described as hostile and relationships with neighbours, GP, and the local police have frequently been affected by their psychotic symptoms by the time psychiatric referral is considered, the author's experience is that they are often also extremely lonely. Without entering into any kind of collusion it is always possible at least to take the time to listen to the patient's account of her persecution and it is not difficult to express sympathy for the distress she is experiencing. Sometimes a brief admission to hospital or the establishment of regular visits from the community psychiatric nurse (CPN) can be rendered acceptable as an attempt to 'get to the bottom' of whatever is going on. Once a relationship of trust and support has been established, patients will often accept medication and visits from members of the psychiatric team without really ever developing insight into their condition. Telling the patient directly that he or she has a mental illness is probably the quickest way to join a list of perceived persecutors, and hence use of the Mental Health Act should be reserved until all else has failed. Even though this may mean that the patient does not receive antipsychotic medication, the provision and maintenance of a relationship of trust with a member of staff who can absorb complaints about, for example, a patient's neighbours will do more to reduce distress than will an enforced prescription. Relatives and friends should be advised to encourage the patient to reserve discussion of such complaints to the time that the CPN visits, if this is possible. Of course, there is no single strategy which is best for all patients. For most patients, interventions delivered to their own homes (CPN or volunteer visits, home helps, and meals on wheels) seem to be most acceptable and although some will respond well to the activities and company provided by a day hospital or centre, many will decline to attend. The potential role of psychological treatments in the management of psychotic symptoms in younger patients is becoming clearer, but elderly psychotic patients are not routinely considered for these, which is unfortunate and unfair (Aguera-Ortiz and Reneses-Prieto, 1999).

## Rehousing

Since these patients are often persistent and able complainers and may have highly restricted and encapsulated delusional systems, their complaints about neighbours or the home environment are sometimes taken at face value by social services staff. It is therefore not uncommon to discover that, by the time of first psychiatric referral, a patient has been rehoused at least once in the preceding months. As a general rule, even if it results in a brief reduction of complaints from the sufferer, provision of new accommodation is followed within a few weeks by a re-emergence of symptoms. The obvious distress this causes is sufficient reason always to advise patients and social workers against such moves unless they are being considered for non-delusional reasons or following successful treatment of psychosis.

## Antipsychotic medication

Sadly, there are no reported randomized controlled trials of the use of antipsychotic medication in these patients. There are good reasons to suspect that a smaller number of late than early onset patients with schizophrenia or schizophrenia-like psychoses show a complete response to antipsychotic medication. For example, Rabins *et al.* (1984) found no, or only a partial, response to neuroleptics in 43% of schizophrenic patients with an onset after 44 years, while Pearlson *et al.* (1989) reported that 54% of their patients fell into this category. In reports of patients with late paraphrenia, the comparable rates of non-response range from 49% (Post, 1966) to 75% (Kay and Roth, 1961). The general conclusion from such studies is that while drugs relieve some target symptoms, the overall treatment response to medication is modest (Raskind and Risse, 1986).

It would be useful to know which illness parameters are associated with poor response to medication. Pearlson *et al.* (1989) found poor response to neuroleptics to be associated with the (rare) presence of thought disorder and with schizoid pre-morbid personality traits. The presence of first-rank symptoms, family history of schizophrenia, and gender had no effect on treatment response. In a late paraphrenic patient group, Holden (1987) found auditory hallucinations and affective features to predict a favourable response. This may of course simply reflect a better natural history in such patients.

Among a group of 64 late paraphrenic patients prescribed neuroleptic medication for at least 3 months, 42.2% showed no response, 31.3% a partial response, and 26.6% a full response to treatment (Howard and Levy, 1992). Compliance with medication, receiving depot rather than oral medication, and support by a CPN if the patient was an outpatient all had a positive effect on treatment response. Patients prescribed depot medication received on average a lower daily dose in chlorpromazine equivalents than those prescribed oral medication. Hence use of depot, rather than the oral route, is associated with a better response rate (a significantly higher proportion of patients treated with depot had

improved symptoms) despite the administration of smaller amounts of medication.

Clozapine has anticholinergic, hypotensive, and sedating effects and has been shown to impair memory function even in young patients; despite a couple of early positive case reports it has not found favour with those of us who regularly prescribe for older patients.

Risperidone is a benzisoxazole derivative with extremely strong binding affinity for serotonin 5-HT2 receptors, strong affinity for dopamine D2 receptors and a high affinity for alpha-1 and alpha-2 adrenergic and histamine H1 receptors. Of all the atypicals, clinical experience with risperidone in this patient group is most extensive. Activity at 5-HT2 receptors appears to be important in the treatment of complex visual hallucinations which have been traditionally regarded as treatment resistant. Risperidone has efficacy in the treatment of hallucinations and delusions in elderly patients at low doses (typically 0.5–2 mg per day). When compared with treatment with traditional neuroleptics in open-label studies, risperidone has been shown to improve cognitive function (Jeste *et al.*, 1999) and to result in a significantly lower cumulative incidence of tardive dyskinesia (Jeste *et al.*, 1998, 2000). Since the risk of developing extrapyramidal symptoms, hypotension, and somnolence increases with higher doses, prescription of more than 2 mg per day should be avoided if possible. Indeed, experience suggests that 0.5 mg b.d. is generally as much as most patients will accept and generally has good antipsychotic effect.

Olanzapine has a similar receptor binding profile to clozapine but doesn't appear to cause the anticholinergic and sedating problems seen with the latter agent, probably because it has antipsychotic activity at much lower doses. A starting dose of 2.5 mg per day is generally well tolerated and can be increased to 10 mg per day if no adverse events appear. Anecdotal evidence suggests that olanzapine is less likely to cause extrapyramidal symptoms than risperidone, but more likely to produce sedation and weight gain. This has not, however, been subjected to testing by controlled trial and the choice as to which of these two atypicals is prescribed will depend very much on individual experience.

## Guidelines for prescribing

There is no real evidence that any particular drug is more effective than others in this group of patients. The choice of drug for each individual patient should thus be based on considerations of concomitant physical illness and other treatments received, together with the specific side-effect profile of the drug (Tran-Johnson *et al.*, 1994). While there is an argument that all patients should be commenced on depot (Raskind and Risse, 1986), treatment will usually be commenced at a low dose of an oral preparation and it is easy to argue that this should be one of the atypicals because of the reduced risk of early and delayed emergent side-effects. Patients who do not respond to oral treatment (whether due to poor compliance or genuine treatment resistance) can be treated with depot. Successful treatment of patients with depot can often be at very modest doses. For example, the mean dose of prescribed depot in Howard and Levy's (1992) study was 14.4 mg of flupenthixol decanoate or 9 mg of fluphenazine decanoate every fortnight. In those patients who continue to experience psychotic symptoms after receiving depot for several weeks, the dose can be increased by 10% every 2 to 3 weeks until a response is seen or side-effects emerge. There is no reason why patients in the community should not be maintained on depot for several years so long as (and this is very important) they are monitored through examination by the prescriber for the presence of extrapyramidal side-effects at least once every 3 months, in addition to regular reports from the nurse who gives the injection. The advent of risperidone depot injections in recent years has had a disappointingly small impact on the treatment of this patient group, largely because of the high milligram daily equivalent of the lowest available dose.

## Conclusions

The history of schizophrenia and schizophrenia-like psychoses that have onset in later life is a long one, but it is only in the last three decades that any real attempts have been made to study patients with these conditions and to understand how they might relate to psychoses which arise earlier in the life cycle. The aetiological roles of pre-morbid personality functioning, degenerative, and genetic factors are still not elucidated fully, although most recent brain imaging studies indicate that gross degenerative changes are not present. If compliance with neuroleptic medication can be established and maintained, the prognosis for symptomatic improvement is good.

## References

Aguera-Ortiz, L. and Reneses-Prieto, B. (1999). The place of non-biological treatments. In *Late onset schizophrenia* (ed. R. Howard, P.V. Rabins, and D.J. Castle). Wrightson Biomedical. Petersfield.

Almeida, O., Förstl, H., Howard, R., and David, A.S. (1993). Unilateral auditory hallucinations. *British Journal of Psychiatry*, **162**, 262–264.

Almeida, O., Howard, R., Levy, R., and David, A. (1995a). Psychotic states arising in late life (late paraphrenia). Psychopathology and nosology. *British Journal of Psychiatry*, **166**, 205–214.

Almeida, O., Howard, R., Levy, R., David, A., and Morris, R. (1995b). Clinical and cognitive diversity of psychotic states arising in late life (late paraphrenia). *Psychological Medicine*, **25**, 699–714.

APA (American Psychiatric Association) (1987). *Diagnostic and statistical manual of mental disorders*, 3rd edn revised. American Psychiatric Association, Washington, DC.

APA (American Psychiatric Association) (1993). *Diagnostic and statistical manual of mental disorders*, 4th edn. American Psychiatric Association, Washington, DC.

Bleuler, E.P. (1911). *Dementia praecox or the group of schizophrenias*. Deuticke, Leipzig.

Bleuler, M. (1943). Die spatschizophrenen krankheitsbilder. *Fortschritte der Neurologie Psychiatrie*, **15**, 259–290.

Brodaty, H., Sachdev, P., Rose, N., Rylands, K., and Prenter, L. (1999). Schizophrenia with onset after age 50 years. 1. Phenomenology and risk factors. *British Journal of Psychiatry*, **175**, 410–415.

Brodaty, H., Sachdev, P., Koschere, A., Monk, D., and Cullen, B. (2003). Long-term outcome of late onset schizophrenia: 5-year follow-up study. *British Journal of Psychiatry*, **183**, 213–219.

Castle, D.J. and Howard, R. (1992) What do we know about the aetiology of late onset schizophrenia? *European Psychiatry*, **7**, 99–108.

Castle, D.J. and Murray, R.M. (1991). The neurodevelopmental basis of sex differences in schizophrenia. *Psychological Medicine*, **21**, 565–575.

Cervantes, R.C., Salgado-Snyder, V.N., and Padilla, A.M. (1989). Post-traumatic stress in immigrants from Central America and Mexico. *Hospital and Community Psychiatry*, **40**, 615–619.

Cooper, A.F. (1976). Deafness and psychiatric illness. *British Journal of Psychiatry*, **129**, 216–226.

Cooper, A.F. and Curry, A.R. (1976). The pathology of deafness in the paranoid and affective psychoses of later life. *Journal of Psychosomatic Research*, **20**, 107–114.

Cooper, A.F., Curry, A.R., Kay, D.W.K., Garside, R.F., and Roth, M. (1974). Hearing loss in paranoid and affective psychoses of the elderly. *Lancet*, **ii**, 851–854.

Corbin, S. and Eastwood, M.R. (1986) Sensory deficits and mental disorders of old age: causal or coincidental associations? *Psychological Medicine*, **16**, 251–256.

Corcoran, R., Frith, C.D., and Mercer, G. (1995). Schizophrenia, symptomatology and social inference: investigating theory of mind in people with schizophrenia. *Schizophrenia Research*, **17**, 5–13.

Corey-Bloom, J., Jernigan, T., Archibald, S., Harris, M.J., and Jeste, D.V. (1995). Quantitative magnetic resonance imaging of the brain in late-life schizophrenia. *American Journal of Psychiatry*, **152**, 447–449.

Cummings, J. (1985) Organic delusions: phenomenology, anatomical correlations and review. *British Journal of Psychiatry*, **146**, 184–197.

Cutting, J.C., Clare, A.W., and Mann, A.H. (1978). Cycloid psychosis: investigation of the diagnostic concept. *Psychological Medicine*, **8**, 637–648.

Eastwood, M.R., Corbin, S., and Reed, M. (1981). Hearing impairment and paraphrenia. *Journal of Otolaryngology*, **10**, 306–308.

Fish, F. (1958). A clinical investigation of chronic schizophrenia. *British Journal of Psychiatry*, **104**, 34–54.

Fish, F. (1960). Senile schizophrenia. *Journal of Mental Science*, **106**, 938–946.

Flint, A., Rifat, S., and Eastwood, M. (1991). Late onset paranoia: distinct from paraphrenia? *International Journal of Geriatric Psychiatry*, **6**, 103–109.

Funding, T. (1961). Genetics of paranoid psychoses in late life. *Acta Psychiatrica Scandinavica*, **37**, 267–282.

Gabriel, E. (1978). *Die Langfristige Entwicklung der Spatschizophrenien*. Karger. Basel.

Garety, P.A., Hemsley, D.R., and Wessely, S. (1991). Reasoning in deluded schizophrenic and paranoid patients. *Journal of Nervous and Mental Disorders*, **179**, 194–201.

Gorwood, P., Leboyer, M., Jay, M., Payan, C., and Feingold, J. (1995). Gender and age at onset in schizophrenia: Impact of family history. *American Journal of Psychiatry*, **152**, 208–212.

Gottesman, I.I. and Shields, J. (1982). *Schizophrenia, the epigenetic puzzle*. Cambridge University Press, Cambridge.

Grahame, P.S. (1984). Schizophrenia in old age (late paraphrenia). *British Journal of Psychiatry*, **145**, 493–495.

Gurian, B.S., Wexler, D., and Baker, E.H. (1992). Late-life paranoia: Possible associations with early trauma and infertility. *International Journal of Geriatric Psychiatry*, **7**, 277–284.

Herbert, M.E. and Jacobson, S. (1967). Late paraphrenia. *British Journal of Psychiatry* **113**, 461–467.

Holden, N. (1987). Late paraphrenia or the paraphrenias: a descriptive study with a 10-year follow-up. *British Journal of Psychiatry*, **150**, 635–639.

Hopkins, B. and Roth, M. (1953). Psychological test performance in patients over 60. Paraphrenia, arteriosclerotic psychosis and acute confusion. *Journal of Mental Science*, **99**, 451–463.

Howard, R. and Levy, R. (1992). Which factors affect treatment response in late paraphrenia? *International Journal of Geriatric Psychiatry*, **7**, 667–672.

Howard, R. and Levy, R. (1993) Personality structure in the paranoid psychoses of later life. *European Psychiatry*, **8**, 59–66.

Howard, R. and Levy, R. (1994). Charles Bonnet syndrome plus: complex visual hallucinations of Charles Bonnet type in late paraphrenia. *International Journal of Geriatric Psychiatry*, **9**, 399–404.

Howard, R., Castle, D., O'Brien, J., Almeida, O., and Levy, R. (1992a). Permeable walls, floors, ceilings and doors. Partition delusions in late paraphrenia. *International Journal of Geriatric Psychiatry*, **7**, 719–724.

Howard, R., Forstl, H., Naguib, M., Burns, A., and Levy, R. (1992b). First rank symptoms in late paraphrenia: cortical structural correlates. *British Journal of Psychiatry*, **160**, 108–109.

Howard, R., Castle, D., Wessely, S., and Murray, R. (1993). A comparative study of 470 cases of early and late onset schizophrenia. *British Journal of Psychiatry*, **163**, 353–357.

Howard, R., Almeida, O., and Levy, R. (1994a). Phenomenology, demography and diagnosis in late paraphrenia. *Psychological Medicine*, **24**, 397–410.

Howard, R., Almeida, O., Levy, R., Graves, M., and Graves, P. (1994b). Quantitative magnetic resonance imaging in delusional disorder and late onset schizophrenia. *British Journal of Psychiatry*, **165**, 474–480.

Howard, R., Cox, T., Mullen, R., Almeida, O., and Levy, R. (1995a). White matter signal hyperintensities in the brains of patients with late paraphrenia and the normal community-living elderly. *Biological Psychiatry*, **38**, 86–91.

Howard, R., Dennehey, J., Lovestone, S. *et al.* (1995b). Apolipoprotein E genotype and late paraphrenia. *International Journal of Geriatric Psychiatry*, **10**, 157–150.

Howard, R., Mellers, J., Petty, R. *et al.* (1995c). Magnetic resonance imaging of the temporal and frontal lobes, hippocampus, parahippocampal and superior temporal gyri in late paraphrenia. *Psychological Medicine*, **25**, 495–503.

Howard, R., Graham, C., Sham, P. *et al.* (1997) A controlled family study of late onset non-affective psychosis (late paraphrenia). *British Journal of Psychiatry*, **170**, 511–514.

Howard, R., Rabins, P.V., Seeman, M.V., Jeste D.V., and the International Late onset Schizophrenia Group (2000). Late onset schizophrenia and very-late onset schizophrenia-like psychosis: an international consensus. *American Journal of Psychiatry*, **157**, 172–178.

Huber, G., Gross, G., and Schuttler, R. (1975) Spät schizophrenie. *Archiv für Psychiatrie und Nervenkrankheiten*, **22**, 53–66.

Jeste, D.V., Lohr, J.B., Eastham, J.H., Rockwell, E., and Caligiuri, M.P. (1998). Adverse effects of long-term use of neuroleptics: human and animal studies. *Journal of Psychiatric Research*, **32**, 201–214.

Jeste, D.V., Lacro, J.P., Palmer, B., Rockwell, E., Harris, M.J., and Caligiuri, M.P. (1999). Incidence of tardive dyskinesia in early stages of neuroleptic treatment for older patients. *American Journal of Psychiatry*, **156**, 309–311.

Jeste, D.V., Okamoto, A., Napolitano, J, Kane, J.M., and Matinez, R.A. (2000). Low incidence of persistent tardive dyskinesia in elderly patients with dementia treated with risperidone. *American Journal of Psychiatry*, **157**, 1150–1155.

Kaney, S. and Bentall, R.P. (1989). Persecutory delusions and attributional style. *British Journal of Medical Psychology*, **62**, 191–198.

Kay, D.W.K. and Roth, M. (1961). Environmental and hereditary factors in the schizophrenias of old age ('late paraphrenia') and their bearing on the general problem of causation in schizophrenia. *Journal of Mental Science*, **107**, 649–686.

Kay, D.W.K., Cooper, A.F., Garside, R.F., and Roth, M. (1976). The differentiation of paranoid from affective psychoses by patients' premorbid characteristics. *British Journal of Psychiatry*, **129**, 207–215.

Kendell, R.E. (1988). Other functional psychoses. In *Companion to psychiatric studies* (ed. R.E. Kendell and A.K. Zealley). Churchill Livingstone, Edinburgh.

Kendler, K.S., Tsuang, M.T., and Hays, P. (1987). Age at onset in schizophrenia: a familial perspective. *Archives of General Psychiatry*, **44**, 881–890.

Keshavan, M.S., David, A.S., Steingard, S., and Lishman, W.A. (1992). Musical hallucinations: a review and synthesis. *Neuropsychiatry, Neuropsychology and Behavioural Neurology*, **5**, 211–223.

Khan, A.M., Clark, T., and Oyebode, F. (1988). Unilateral auditory hallucinations. *British Journal of Psychiatry*, **152**, 297–298.

Klages, W. (1961) *Die Spätschizophrenie*. Enke, Stuttgart.

Kraepelin, E. (1894). Die abgrenzung der paranoia. *Allgemeine Zeitschrift fuer Psychiatrie*, **50**, 1080–1081.

Kraepelin, E. (1913). *Psychiatrie, ein Lehrbuch fur Studierende und Artze*. Barth, Leipzig.

Levitt, J.J. and Tsuang, M.T. (1988). The heterogeneity of schizoaffective disorder: implications for treatment. *American Journal of Psychiatry*, **145**, 926–936.

Magnan, V. (1893). *Lecons cliniques sur les maladies mentales*. Bureaux de Progres Medical, Paris.

Marneros, A. and Deister, A. (1984). The psychopathology of 'late schizophrenia'. *Psychopathology*, **17**, 264–274.

Mayer, W. (1921). Uber paraphrene psychosen. *Zeitschrift für die Gesamte Neurologie und Psychiatrie*, **71**, 187–206.

Miller, B., Benson, F., Cummings, J.L., and Neshkes, R. (1986). Late paraphrenia: an organic delusional syndrome. *Journal of Clinical Psychiatry*, **47**, 204–207.

Miller, B.L., Lesser, I.M., Boone, K. *et al.* (1989) Brain white-matter lesions and psychosis. *British Journal of Psychiatry*, **155**, 73–78.

Miller, B.L., Lesser, I.M., Boone, K., Hill, E., Mehringer, C., and Wong, K. (1991). Brain lesions and cognitive function in late-life psychosis. *British Journal of Psychiatry*, **158**, 76–82.

Miller, B.L., Lesser, I.M., Mena, I. *et al.* (1992). Regional cerebral blood flow in late-life-onset psychosis. *Neuropsychiatry, Neuropsychology and Behavioural Neurology*, **5**, 132–137.

Mitter, P., Reeves, S., Romero-Rubiales, F., Bell, P., Stewart, R., and Howard, R. (2005). Migrant status, age, gender and social isolation in very late onset schizophrenia-like psychosis. *International Journal of Geriatric Psychiatry*, **20**, 1046–1051.

Moore, R., Blackwood, N., Corcoran, R. *et al.* (2006). Misunderstanding the intentions of others: an exploratory study of the cognitive aetiology of persecutory delusions in very late onset schizophrenia-like psychosis. *American Journal of Geriatric Psychiatry*, **14**, 410–418.

Murray, R.M., O'Callaghan, E., Castle, D.J., and Lewis, S.W. (1992). A neurodevelopmental approach to the classification of schizophrenia. *Schizophrenia Bulletin*, **18**, 319–332.

Naguib, M. and Levy, R. (1987). Late paraphrenia: neuropsychological impairment and structural brain abnormalities on computed tomography. *International Journal of Geriatric Psychiatry*, **2**, 83–90.

Pearlson, G.D. and Rabins, P.V. (1988). The late onset psychoses: possible risk factors. *Psychiatric Clinics of North America*, **11**, 15–32.

Pearlson, G.D., Kreger, L., Rabins, P. *et al.* (1989). A chart review study of late onset and early-onset schizophrenia. *American Journal of Psychiatry*, **146**, 1568–1574.

Post, F. (1966). *Persistent persecutory states of the elderly*. Pergamon, Oxford.

Quintal, M., Day-Cody, D., and Levy, R. (1991). Late paraphrenia and ICD-10. *International Journal of Geriatric Psychiatry*, **6**, 111–116.

Rabins, P.V., Pauker, S., and Thomas, J. (1984). Can schizophrenia begin after age 44? *Comprehensive Psychiatry*, **25**, 290–293.

Rabins, P.V., Pearlson, G., Jayaram, G., Steele, C., and Tune, L. (1987). Ventricle-to-brain ratio in late onset schizophrenia. *American Journal of Psychiatry*, **144**, 1216–1218.

Raskind, M.A. and Risse, S.C. (1986). Antipsychotic drugs and the elderly. *Journal of Clinical Psychiatry*, **47**, 5(Suppl.), 17–22.

Reeves, S., Sauer, J., Stewart, R., Granger, A., and Howard, R. (2001). Increased first contact rates for very late onset schizophrenia-like psychosis in African- and Caribbean-born elders. *British Journal of Psychiatry*, **179**, 172–174.

Retterstol, N. (1966). *Paranoid and paranoiac psychoses. A personal follow-up investigation with special reference to aetiological, clinical and prognostic aspects*. Oslo Universitetsforlaget/Thomas, Springfield, IL.

Roth, M. and Morrisey, J. (1952). Problems in the diagnosis and classification of mental disorders in old age. *Journal of Mental Science*, **98**, 66–80.

Shimizu, A. and Kurachi, M. (1989). Do women without a family history of schizophrenia have a later onset of schizophrenia? *Japanese Journal of Psychiatry and Neurology*, **43**, 133–136.

Sjoegren, H. (1964). Paraphrenic, melancholic and psychoneurotic states in the pre-senile and senile periods of life. *Acta Psychiatrica Scandinavica*, Suppl. 176.

Sternberg, E. (1972) Neuere forschungsergebnisse bei spatschizophrenen psychosen. *Fortschritte der Neurologie Psychiatrie*, **40**, 631–646.

Symonds, L.L., Olichney, J.M., Jernigan, T.L., Corey-Bloom, J., Healy, J.F., and Jeste, D.V. (1997). Lack of clinically significant gross structural abnormalities in MRIs of older patients with schizophrenia and related psychoses. *Journal of Neuropsychiatry and Clinical Neuroscience*, **9**, 251–258.

Tran-Johnson, T.K., Harris, M.J., and Jeste, D.V. (1994). Pharmacological treatment of schizophrenia and delusional disorder of late life. In *Principles and practice of geriatric psychiatry* (ed J.R.M. Copeland, M.T. Abou-Saleh, and D.G. Blazer), pp. 685–692. Wiley, New York.

Zimbardo, P.G., Anderson, S.M., and Kabat, L.G. (1981). Induced hearing deficit generates experimental paranoia. *Science*, **212**, 1529–1531.

# 33

# Severe and enduring mental illness in old age

*Jenny McCleery*

## Definition

Previous editions of this book have included a chapter entitled 'Graduates'—a term initially coined by Arie and Jolley (1982) for patients 'who entered hospitals for the mentally ill before modern methods of treatment were available and have grown old there' (DHSS, 1972). The majority of these patients had schizophrenia. However, as the policy of mental hospital closure has progressed in many Western countries, the term in its original sense has ceased to be useful. The large asylums have disappeared. Of those patients still living who spent long periods in such institutions, most are now living out their final years outside hospitals, and most younger patients with illnesses of a severity which could previously have led to lengthy hospital stays are now living—and ageing—'in the community'.

Although the neat administrative category of 'graduates' has disappeared, the patients have not. There remains a group of people who are entering old age having suffered from long-standing, severe mental illnesses. Their dispersal to a variety of settings and services has made them harder to identify for research or service purposes. One clinically useful way to think of this group might be as those whose illnesses have prevented them from fulfilling many of the roles of adult life—for example, forming families, maintaining work, and accumulating material resources for old age. However, what research there is that is relevant to these patients identifies them either by setting (for example, the elderly long-stay hospital patients of the hospital closure studies) or by diagnosis (predominantly schizophrenia). This chapter is very largely concerned with schizophrenia, but many of the service considerations could apply equally to patients with other long-standing, severe mental illnesses. However, the clinical aspects of other illnesses in old age are covered elsewhere in the book.

## Changing settings: from the asylum to the 'community'

Interest in the characteristics of elderly patients with chronic, severe mental illness was kindled by the policy of deinstitutionalization which gathered pace throughout the 1970s and 1980s. It became apparent that if this policy was to be pursued successfully, alternative provision would be needed for high numbers of elderly patients who had been admitted to the asylums with functional diagnoses and had remained in hospital for many years. For example, in 1975 there were 21,439 people over 65 who had been resident in English mental hospitals for more than 5 years. Between 1976 and 1986, this number fell by 15.7%. Over the same period, there was a fall of 40% in the number of younger patients in mental illness beds in England, reflecting the greater difficulty found in discharging the older patients (DHSS, 1988). Thus, as the era of the large mental hospitals drew to a close, the average age and length of stay of their occupants increased. Clifford *et al.* (1991) surveyed the population of five hospitals scheduled for closure, excluding patients with dementia. The patients who had been in hospital for at least a year had a mean duration of admission of 24.5 years and a mean age of 64.5 years, with 40% aged over 70. Seventy per cent had schizophrenia. A similar pattern of increasing age of the residents of state hospitals in the early 1990s was seen in the USA (Moak and Fisher, 1991). In both England and the USA, the elderly patients who were retained longest in closing hospitals—presumably those identified as most difficult to discharge—were characterized by increasingly severe social disability and behavioural disturbance (Jones, 1993; White *et al.*, 1997).

Although hospital closures proceeded on a massive scale, there was little systematic study of the effects of the policy on patients. An exception was the large TAPS study of the reprovision made for the patients of the Friern and Claybury hospitals in London. All patients resident in either hospital for more than a year and discharged to the community during the closure programme ($n = 670$, mean age 54, age range 19–97) were followed up for 5 years (Leff and Trieman, 2000). The overall conclusion of the study was that patients' clinical state and problems of social behaviour did not change significantly, but patients acquired new skills and friends, and were living in freer conditions, which they preferred to hospital. However, there were differences for the older patients. They tended to be housed in larger community homes with more restrictions than the younger patients. Their clinical state improved more, but they showed smaller increases than younger patients in their number of friends and confidants and acquired fewer domestic and community-living skills. A smaller study within the TAPS Project (Trieman *et al.*, 1996) examined the differences developing over 2 years between 36 patients aged over 70 who moved from Claybury Hospital to newly developed care facilities in the community and

35 similar patients who remained in the hospital. Patients moved or stayed largely for administrative rather than clinical reasons. In this case, the behaviour of the discharged patients improved slightly over time and their cognitive function deteriorated slightly; those remaining in hospital deteriorated markedly in both behaviour and cognition, perhaps because social conditions in the hospital were deteriorating as the closure programme progressed. These and other studies (e.g. Honkonen *et al.*, 1999) suggest that elderly functionally ill patients who have spent many years in mental hospitals can be successfully resettled in community facilities with the potential for gains in clinical state, behaviour, and satisfaction. However, it has been pointed out that 'the results of a particularly well planned resettlement programme may not be representative of the outcome from general policies of discharge from all psychiatric hospitals' (Double and Wong, 1991).

As asylums have closed, the focus of concern for elderly patients with severe, enduring mental illness has changed. In the middle to late 20th century, attention was directed largely to the adverse effects of institutionalization (e.g. Martin, 1955; Barton, 1959; Wing and Brown, 1970). More recently, concerned commentators have been drawing attention to the extent to which this group of patients is overlooked in research and policy (e.g. Green *et al.*, 1997; Cohen *et al.*, 2000; Royal College of Psychiatrists, 2002). The services provided for these patients are subject to wide local variations; responsibility for them is often not clearly allocated or is disputed between younger adult and old age services, or between health and social services; and there is a high risk of inappropriate placement on acute wards or in continuing care settings designed primarily for demented patients, where all the earlier problems of institutionalization may be repeated or worsened. In the worst case, elderly mentally ill patients may miss out on services altogether. The proportion of homeless people who are elderly is increasing and a significant proportion of these have psychotic illnesses (Barak and Cohen, 2003; Stergiopoulos and Herrmann, 2003).

Although patients with schizophrenia constituted the majority of long-stay patients growing old in hospital, there were significant numbers with other psychiatric diagnoses. Furthermore, only a minority of patients with a lifetime diagnosis of schizophrenia became long-term residents in mental hospitals. Many more lived outside hospitals, where they were much less visible to researchers and policy-makers. The extent of their disabilities and needs has been unclear. However, now that hospital residence can no longer be used to define the most disabled patients, a diagnosis of schizophrenia has become the only convenient label under which to attempt to investigate the population growing old with the most severe functional illnesses.

## Prevalence of schizophrenia in old age

The prevalence of schizophrenia can be estimated either from case registers of patients known to psychiatric services or from community prevalence surveys. Psychiatric case registers available for different areas of the UK until the mid-1980s found 11–60 cases of chronic psychosis in people over 65 per 100,000 total population.

There have been few prevalence studies of schizophrenia in community-dwelling elderly populations. Their findings are difficult to generalize across different sites and periods of changing care policies. Early and late onset schizophrenic illnesses are not usually distinguished in these studies. The Epidemiologic Catchment Area (ECA) studies in the USA found a lifetime prevalence of schizophrenia in people of 65 and older of 0.3%, and a 1-year prevalence of 0.2% (Keith *et al.*, 1991), but this has been criticized as an underestimate for several reasons, such as undersampling from areas of public housing where there are known to be higher rates of elderly mentally ill people (Palmer *et al.*, 1999). Community studies in Liverpool and a deprived area of Scotland have found prevalence rates of 0.12% and 0.44%, respectively (Copeland *et al.*, 1998; McNulty *et al.*, 2003). Kua (1992) found a prevalence of 0.5% for schizophrenia/paranoid diagnoses among 612 community-dwelling Chinese aged over 65 in Singapore. Looked at from a different angle, Campbell *et al.* (1990) found that elderly people (over 65) made up 12% of the prevalent cases of schizophrenia in south Camden, an inner-city area in London on one day. Older patients made up a higher proportion of prevalent cases in a study by McCreadie *et al.* (1997) in rural Scotland and inner-city London: among White patients 18–19% of men and 24–26% of women were over 60.

What conclusions can be drawn from these results? Reports of the prevalence of schizophrenia among elderly people in the community, even in studies post-dating mental hospital closures, are considerably lower than the approximately 1% lifetime prevalence usually given for schizophrenia overall. Patients with schizophrenia have an excess mortality, but this probably does not account for the whole difference. Methodological considerations mean that the reported estimates are likely to represent minimum figures. Elderly people with schizophrenia may not be in contact with psychiatric services or general practitioners, they may be more likely to refuse participation in surveys or they may be practised at concealing symptoms. Alternatively, they may have recovered, at least sufficiently to make symptoms difficult to detect.

Despite the lack of authoritative prevalence data, what all authorities agree on is that the overall ageing of the population will inevitably be paralleled by sharp increases in both the proportion of patients with schizophrenia who are elderly and the absolute numbers of elderly patients with schizophrenia.

## Outcome of schizophrenia in late life

Despite more than 100 years of intense interest in the subject, there are few certainties about the long-term outcome of schizophrenia. The difficulties of conducting the very long follow-up studies needed to understand the course of an illness like schizophrenia across the adult lifespan, and the factors which influence it, are formidable.

1 The boundaries of the diagnostic category itself are not certain and diagnostic criteria have changed with time. From Kraepelin onwards, pessimistic prognostic considerations have been incorporated into diagnostic criteria for schizophrenia, begging the question of outcome.

2 Patients available for long-term observation are unlikely to be representative of the whole population of people with schizophrenia. Maintaining contact with patients over long periods of time is hugely difficult and loss to follow-up is very unlikely to be independent of outcome.

3 Long-term studies cover eras of changing treatments, social policies, and environmental factors, all of which may affect outcome.

4 Outcome in schizophrenia is a complex construct made up of a number of different dimensions, which are not related to each other in simple ways. For example, from their influential work in the early 1970s, Strauss and Carpenter (1972) identified occupational functioning, social relations, symptoms, and hospitalization as semi-independent processes with their own predictors.

Two widely held views of the course of schizophrenia relevant to the elderly patient are (1) the pessimistic, Kraepelinian view of chronic, irreversible deterioration making late improvement or recovery exceedingly rare, and (2) the idea of 'burn out' of schizophrenic symptoms with time, defined by Bridge et al. (1978) as an amelioration of symptoms above the age of 55. To what extent do the available data support or refute these two propositions?

## Late recovery in schizophrenia

By the early 1990s, five very long-term outcome studies in schizophrenia had been reported from Europe and the USA with average lengths of follow-up ranging from 22–37 years (Bleuler, 1972; Huber et al., 1975; Tsuang et al., 1979; Ciompi, 1980; Harding et al., 1987). Patients in these studies were mainly recruited in the 1940s and 1950s and so their follow-up spanned the period of introduction of the neuroleptics. Despite methodological limitations and major differences in the patient groups and their treatment, these five studies were remarkably consistent in their findings. In all cases, outcome was highly heterogeneous, but approximately half to two-thirds of all the patients in the studies (>1300) achieved significant improvement or recovery. One of these studies, the Vermont study (Harding et al., 1987), included only patients who were already chronically ill, albeit carefully selected for an intensive rehabilitation programme, at the time of their index assessment. Studies published more recently have been broadly similar. In Cologne, 41% of patients followed up after 25 years were able to care for themselves and dependants (Marneros et al., 1992). The International Study of Schizophrenia, a 15- and 25-year follow-up study coordinated by the World Health Organization, included a much more culturally diverse sample of 1633 subjects; around 50% of surviving subjects had broadly favourable outcomes (Harrison et al., 2001). Although the effect was less striking than in the Vermont study, these investigators also found that a chronic course in the early stages of the illness did not exclude a good long-term outcome.

A criticism of many of these studies is the use of imprecise or lax criteria for improvement and recovery. In the International Study of Schizophrenia, if a relatively strict criterion for recovery was adopted (which nevertheless still allowed for 'some difficulties' in social and occupational functioning), 38% of the incident cases of schizophrenia qualified and this fell to only 16% if those who had received treatment in the past 2 years were excluded (Harrison et al., 2001). Marneros et al. (1992) found only 7% of their cohort had achieved full remission. Among 384 middle-aged and elderly outpatients with schizophrenia who were followed up over a decade, Auslander and Jeste (2004) identified only 12 (8%) who met strict criteria for sustained remission. The remitted patients had levels of positive, negative, and depressive symptoms similar to control subjects matched for age, gender, and educational level. They were, however, significantly poorer than the controls on measures of cognition, quality of well-being, and daily functioning, albeit better than matched patients who were still symptomatic.

The authors comment that their figure for the prevalence of sustained remission is likely to be an underestimate as some remitted patients declined to remain in the study, but that true recovery in older patients must be viewed as 'the exception rather than the rule'. They suggest that the continuing cognitive and functional impairments in their patients even in sustained remission from psychotic symptoms may reflect a return to pre-morbid functioning, consistent with the neurodevelopmental hypothesis of schizophrenia.

## Psychotic symptoms—is 'burn-out' a real phenomenon?

To study the course of schizophrenic symptoms or symptom dimensions over the lifespan, the ideal study design would again be longitudinal, using repeated assessments with detailed, standardized symptom-rating scales. Unfortunately, such data are lacking: what evidence there is spanning significant age ranges derives mainly from cross-sectional studies. The major limitation of these is the likelihood of cohort effects, given the very different illness durations, treatments, and social policies, including experience of institutional care, experienced by the different age groups.

The long-term follow-up studies described above did not use detailed ratings of psychotic symptoms and relied on (unstable) diagnostic categories, but their results have been interpreted as suggestive of an age-related amelioration. Ciompi (1980), for example, wrote of his results that 'the latter half of life exerts a levelling, smoothing and calming influence on schizophrenia'.

A number of cross-sectional surveys of resident populations in large mental hospitals found that their elderly and long-stay patients still exhibited a high prevalence of psychotic symptoms (e.g. Cunningham et al., 1980; Leff, 1991). However, this type of study does provide some evidence of variation in symptom profile with increasing length of stay. For example, the Friern Hospital Medical Committee (1983) survey found that as length of stay increased from 1–5 to 5–10 to >10 years, there was a decrease in the frequency of delusions and in liability to marked exacerbations, while the frequency of hallucinations stayed unchanged and negative symptoms became more common.

Among studies which have attempted detailed ratings of individual symptoms, Pfohl and Winokur's (1982) study did have a longitudinal design but relied on retrospective analysis of the medical records of 52 severely ill, chronically hospitalized patients from the 'Iowa 500' study over a 40-year period. Their results suggested a diminution of hallucinations and delusions, but persistence of negative symptoms over time.

Davidson et al. (1995) studied a large cross-sectional group of hospitalized patients divided into 10-year age bands with the oldest group aged 85 or older. They described modestly reduced positive symptoms and worse negative symptoms in older compared with younger patients. However, they noted that in their sample the severity of positive symptoms was high even among their older patients. Thus, they did not regard 'burn-out' as a useful model for their findings. Other researchers have based their descriptions on the three-factor model of schizophrenic symptoms (positive, negative, and disorganized). Among patients aged between 14 and 73, Schultz et al. (1997) found older age to be associated with lower levels of hallucinations, delusions, and some aspects of the disorganization factor (bizarre behaviour and inappropriate affect, but not formal thought disorder). They found no age effect on negative symptoms. Gur *et al.* (1996) found similar results for positive and disorganized symptoms, but again reported worse negative symptoms in the older than the younger patients.

First, then, it is clear that high levels of all schizophrenic symptoms can, and frequently do, persist into old age. Second, there is imperfect evidence, largely from cross-sectional studies, for modest changes in the symptom profile of schizophrenia with ageing. In particular, there probably is a diminution of positive symptoms. Wing and Brown (1970) had suggested that a lowered prevalence of positive symptoms in very long-stay institutionalized patients was more likely to be due to protection from the strains of everyday life than the natural course of the illness. However, Schultz *et al.* (1997) found that the institutionalized patients in their sample exhibited higher levels of hallucinations and disorganized symptoms than community-resident patients. Further, a similar age-related reduction in positive symptoms was evident among patients both inside and outside the protective environment of an institution.

## Depression

The occurrence of significant depressive symptoms among elderly patients with schizophrenia is well recognized clinically, but has received little systematic study. Writing about the results of the long-term studies of schizophrenia in Europe, Angst (1988) remarked that, with time, 'the productive schizophrenic symptoms diminish in favour of affective symptoms, mainly depression'. Assessment of depression is complicated by symptom overlap with the negative syndrome.

In New York City, of 117 community-dwelling patients aged 55 and over who had been ill for at least 10 years, 44% were reported to have depressive symptoms at a level previously associated with a need for clinical intervention—a frequency one and a half to three times higher than the level in the general older population (Cohen *et al.*, 1996). Positive psychotic symptoms were predictive of depression in these patients, but so were several non-clinical variables such as physical limitations on activity and low income that are associated with depression in the general older population. Age was negatively associated with depression. Another US study of an older population (age range 40–85) found that depressive symptoms decreased with age among outpatients with schizophrenia while increasing among normal controls (Jeste *et al.*, 2003b).

## Daily living skills

A number of studies have sought to assess the level of daily functioning of elderly patients with schizophrenia and its determinants. These studies concur with those in younger patients in showing that function is more strongly predicted by cognitive performance than by positive and negative symptoms.

Harvey *et al.* (1998) compared chronically hospitalized patients, chronically ill nursing home residents, and patients admitted to hospital from the community with an acute exacerbation of symptoms. The acutely admitted community patients had similar levels of positive symptoms to the chronically hospitalized patients, but fewer negative symptoms, better cognitive functioning, and much better adaptive functioning than the institutional residents. Regardless of the severity of symptoms, or of living situation, cognitive impairment was a stronger predictor of adaptive deficits than were symptom measures. In a study of only chronically hospitalized,

elderly patients with schizophrenia, Kurtz *et al.* (2001) showed that more severe global cognitive impairment was associated with deficits in orientation and physical self-care.

A number of studies have examined the functioning of middle-aged and elderly community-dwelling patients with schizophrenia. The patients are generally found to be unimpaired relative to healthy controls in basic daily living skills (e.g. time orientation, eating, and grooming), but to show deficits in 'higher level' skills, such as communication, transportation, shopping, finance, and medication management, during simulated tasks (e.g. Klapow *et al.*, 1997; Twamley *et al.*, 2002; Evans *et al.*, 2003; Jeste *et al.*, 2003c) and in aspects of real life functioning, such as living situation or driving (e.g. Palmer *et al.*, 2002; Twamley *et al.*, 2002). In all studies, among a variety of demographic and clinical variables, cognitive performance was the strongest predictor of adaptive functioning, with negative symptoms having a smaller predictive effect in most studies. Positive symptoms appear to be unrelated to functional status. There are some inconsistencies in results concerning the effects of depressive symptoms on functioning in older outpatients with schizophrenia. In studies such as those above, using objective measures of functioning, no relationship with depressive symptoms has been found, while an association has been reported when self-rated functional measures have been used (Jin *et al.*, 2001). In the studies that included broad neuropsychological test batteries, there was no evidence of specific relationships between cognitive and functional domains, perhaps reflecting the complex, multifaceted nature of the functional tasks being assessed.

## Cognitive functioning

If daily living skills among elderly patients with schizophrenia are most closely related to their cognitive function, what is known about the nature and development of the cognitive impairments in this group of patients? Intellectual or cognitive impairment is detectable from the earliest stages of schizophrenia and is now widely regarded as a core feature of the illness. There is a generalized intellectual impairment, but the cognitive domains most affected are language, semantic memory, and executive functioning (Harrison, 2004). It has been debated whether the cognitive impairment of schizophrenia is essentially static or whether progressive deterioration occurs after the onset of illness, and if so at what stage of the illness. Cross-sectional studies comparing cognitive function in younger and older patients with different durations of illness are again flawed by the possibility of cohort effects. In recent years, results of longitudinal studies have begun to accumulate which are able to shed more light on the trajectory of cognitive impairment over time.

Studies of mainly younger outpatients with schizophrenia, including patients assessed initially at their first episode have shown a high degree of stability in scores on neuropsychological test batteries over periods of 1 to 10 years (Censits *et al.*, 1997; Lieh-Mak and Lee, 1997; Heaton *et al.*, 2001; Hoff *et al.*, 2005), although the power of most of the studies to detect even moderate effect sizes has been poor (Kurtz, 2005). The only one of these studies to include any patients over the age of 65 was Heaton *et al.*'s and then they formed only a small proportion of the total (22/142 patients). In this study, patients were compared with healthy controls and there was no evidence of any cognitive decline in patients beyond that associated with normal ageing, although the power to detect such changes occurring specifically in older patients was low.

In contrast to these results are those in several longitudinal studies of older, chronically hospitalized patients with schizophrenia. These studies differ in using briefer, global measures of cognition rather than neuropsychological test batteries. Because of floor effects in the cognitive measures used, the poorest-functioning patients tend to be excluded. Results consistently show that significant cognitive decline can be demonstrated among older patients with poor outcomes over follow-up periods as short as 2.5 years (Harvey et al., 1999a,b; Waddington and Youssef, 1996; Friedman et al., 2001, 2002). Friedman et al. (2001), studying 107 chronically hospitalized patients aged 20–80, found that the risk of decline on the Clinical Dementia Rating Scale over 6 years of follow-up was minimal below the age of 65, but increased to 37.5% above 65 years and was 100% from 75 to 80 years. It must be emphasized that the elderly patients in these studies are not representative of the full population of elderly schizophrenics, since both higher-functioning community residents and the poorest-functioning of the institutionalized patients were excluded.

Harvey et al. (2003a) set out to study elderly schizophrenic patients with a wider range of baseline scores on cognitive and functional measures, including the most impaired, and to try to elucidate the predictors of late decline. They followed up 424 hospital and nursing home residents over 6 years, assessing cognitive function and basic daily living skills with the Alzheimer's Disease Assessment Scale–Late Version (ADAS-L), an instrument which has been validated for use in elderly schizophrenic patients and can be used in those with a Mini-Mental State Examination (MMSE) score of 0. Cognitive function declined with time in all patients, with the greatest decline in female patients, those with an early age of onset, and those with more severe negative symptoms at baseline assessment. In contrast, basic activities of daily living (ADL) skills declined only in those patients who had poorer global function at baseline. The strongest predictor of a decline in basic ADLs was a decline in cognitive function. Baseline severity and deterioration in negative symptoms were also significant predictors. The authors suggested that their results might indicate a threshold effect, with basic ADLs only affected below a certain threshold of cognitive function. They point out that such a relationship could mean a significant benefit for function from treatment leading to even a partial remediation of cognitive impairment.

We still lack data on the course of cognitive impairment in better-functioning, community-dwelling elderly patients with schizophrenia. This remains an important research question because of the evidence, discussed in the previous section, that neurocognitive deficit is also associated with impairment in 'higher level' ADLs. Thus even at the higher end of the functional range, declining cognitive abilities in elderly patients might have important functional effects.

Neuropathological studies of the brains of elderly patients with schizophrenia have failed to find any evidence for neurodegenerative processes over and above the lesions typically observed in the ageing brains of psychiatrically healthy individuals (Harrison, 2004). In particular, and contrary to early reports, there is good evidence that there is no increase in pathologically defined Alzheimer's disease among patients with schizophrenia. This holds true even among patients whose cognitive function is so impaired that they are unequivocally demented (Arnold et al., 1998; Dwork et al., 1998; Purohit et al., 1998). In the light of current neurodevelopmental theories of aetiology, it has been proposed that the brain

in schizophrenia has a 'decreased cerebral reserve' so that even the accumulating neuropathological insults of normal ageing might lead to cognitive decline (Arnold, 2001).

## Social functioning

For most people, social contact is an important part of daily life. Graham et al. (2002) compared community-dwelling groups of older adults with depression and schizophrenia and normal controls on a measure of social functioning. They found that the normal controls had better social functioning than either psychiatric group. The patients with schizophrenia had fewer contacts in their local community and fewer leisure activities than the depressed patients. In a multivariate study relating symptoms of psychosis to psychosocial factors, Patterson et al. (1997) also found that older patients with schizophrenia were less well adjusted socially than healthy controls. There was an effect of psychotic symptoms on social maladjustment, but it was mediated entirely by depression.

One factor that may be related to poorer social functioning in schizophrenic patients is their level of social skills. Patterson et al. (2001) used a brief performance-based measure involving two role plays to study social competence in middle-aged and elderly patients with schizophrenia and schizoaffective disorder. Compared with normal controls, the patients showed deficits in all aspects of social performance. Their objective social skills correlated with negative symptoms and cognitive deficits, but not with positive psychotic or depressive symptoms. They also did not correlate significantly with patients' self-reported social functioning, although they were related to self-assessed quality of well-being.

## Quality of life

There are many studies of quality of life in schizophrenia, but few focus on older patients, although there is evidence that the predictors of quality of life may change with ageing (Clipp, 2001). General models of quality of life divide predictors into three broad categories: personal characteristics (which could include measures of psychopathology), objective indicators (such as physical illness, acute stressors, or income), and subjective variables (such as assessments of one's condition relative to others or the reliability of one's social supports) (Campbell et al., 1976). Health-related quality of life is a somewhat more restricted concept than global quality of life. There are many instruments designed to measure it in different patient populations. In general terms, they aim to assess the impact of illness on subjective well-being.

Several authors have concentrated on psychiatric symptoms in older schizophrenic patients and how they predict health-related quality of life. A comparison of long-term inpatients with schizophrenia with demographically matched outpatients (Kasckow et al., 2001) found that health-related quality of life was significantly lower for the inpatients. In both groups it was predicted by the severity of psychopathology and cognitive impairment. Health-related quality of life in 199 patients with schizophrenia and schizoaffective disorder aged 45–85 was predicted by the severity of depressive symptoms and cognitive impairment (Mittal et al., 2006). Another study among similar patients found anxiety symptoms to have an even greater negative impact on health-related quality of life than did depressive symptoms (Wetherell et al., 2003).

Cohen et al. (1997) found that older people with chronic schizophrenia living in the community (n = 117) were significantly worse off than their peers in the general population with respect to a number of the usual objective indicators of well-being (income, depression, social network size, physical limitations). However, none of these were predictors of subjective well-being. Lower levels of subjective well-being were found among younger, female patients who felt lonely, lacked social contacts they could rely on, and perceived themselves as having more life difficulties, supporting the view that well-being is dependent on judgements made by the patients about themselves and others (subjective factors).

Using a broad-based, global quality of life instrument and a large number of predictor variables, Cohen *et al.* (2003) found support for the idea that psychiatric, objective, and subjective variables all contribute to the quality of life of older people with schizophrenia, to approximately the same extent that they do for the healthy elderly. The patients' quality of life was lower than that of the comparison group because of poorer scores in all three areas. The single most predictive factor was depressive symptoms, which accounted for 23% of the variance in quality of life. The authors interpret this to mean that quality of life is partly a 'state' variable, but partly a longer-term appraisal of one's life. Studies of this nature are extremely valuable when trying to identify interventions that could improve the lives of older patients.

### Movement disorders

Tardive dyskinesia (TD) is a syndrome of involuntary, choreoathetoid movements, most commonly orofacial, but also involving the musculature of the limbs and trunk. 'Tardive' refers to its well-established association with prolonged use of antipsychotics. However, identical abnormal movements also occur in a proportion of patients with schizophrenia who have never been exposed to antipsychotic drugs. Studies in untreated and treated populations most commonly identify increasing age, duration of illness, cognitive/intellectual impairment, negative symptoms, and poor outcome as risk factors for involuntary movements (Waddington, 1995; Fenton, 2000). It is therefore not surprising that the highest prevalence is found in studies of hospitalized elderly patients with chronic schizophrenia.

The prevalence of spontaneous dyskinesia in patients with schizophrenia never exposed to antipsychotic drugs is difficult to determine accurately, but it has been estimated to be approximately 40% in patients with chronic schizophrenia over 60 years of age (Fenton, 2000).

The majority of studies of the prevalence of TD in antipsychotic-exposed populations have been of age-heterogeneous, predominantly younger, patient samples. Some, however, have concentrated on the chronically ill elderly. Byne *et al.* (1998) found a prevalence of 60% in 121 inpatients over 65 (mean age 75, mean duration of illness 49 years). Quinn *et al.* (2001) studied 128 inpatients (mean age 70, age range 41–90, mean duration of illness 44 years). The prevalence of involuntary movements was 63% in patients under 65 years of age, rising to 93% in patients over 75 years, leading these authors to conclude that, if followed up for long enough, essentially 'all' schizophrenic patients will develop TD.

Cognitive impairment appears to be a stronger clinical correlate of TD than any index of the extent of antipsychotic drug exposure (Waddington, 1995; Quinn *et al.*, 2001). The relationship is strongest for orofacial movements, and may be particularly with frontal executive cognitive deficits. One possibility is that the neuropathology underlying cognitive impairment predisposes to TD following

exposure to antipsychotic drugs. The occurrence of an association between dyskinesia and cognitive functioning in antipsychotic-naïve samples argues against this as the whole explanation. Furthermore, in a longitudinal study of elderly patients with chronic schizophrenia, baseline cognitive function did not predict the emergence of TD; rather those patients who developed new orofacial dyskinesia during follow-up also demonstrated a significant decline in cognitive function, suggesting a common underlying pathology (Waddington and Youssef, 1996).

The apparently high prevalence of spontaneous dyskinesias in elderly patients, and the association of dyskinesia with aspects of the illness which respond poorly to treatment, suggest that modifying drug regimes may have only a limited impact on the problem of movement disorders in elderly patients. On the other hand, there is evidence that atypical antipsychotics have a lower propensity to cause (or precipitate) TD than typical antipsychotics, with incidence rates in studies lasting 1–2 years reduced by approximately 80% (Correll *et al.*, 2004). However, data on elderly patients with long duration of illness are extremely limited. Long-term follow-up of patients exposed to these drugs for decades will be needed to see whether they can contribute to a significant reduction in the incidence of disabling dyskinesias.

## Physical health of elderly patients with schizophrenia

Schizophrenia is associated with an increased risk of early death. Suicide is the largest single cause of premature death and is most common early in the course of the illness; this large effect leads to a very high standardized mortality rate (SMR) for young adults with schizophrenia, but the SMR falls rapidly with age over early and mid-life. Although the excess of unnatural deaths is largely in younger patients, deaths from unnatural causes (suicide, homicide, and accidents) are still more common in elderly patients with schizophrenia than in the general population. Natural-cause SMR is also increased in schizophrenia, but this too falls with age, albeit more gradually (Brown, 1997). For example, Räsänen *et al.* (2003) studied 253 psychiatric patients hospitalized for more than 6 months in northern Finland. The cohort were aged from 31 to 88 and 80% had schizophrenia. As expected, SMR was very high in the youngest patients, but it approached the level of the general population in the oldest patients.

The largest contribution to excess mortality due to natural causes in schizophrenia comes from cardiovascular disease, but SMRs from diseases of the respiratory, gastrointestinal, nervous, and endocrine systems are also elevated (Brown *et al.*, 2000; Osby *et al.*, 2000; Räsänen *et al.*, 2003; Goff *et al.*, 2005a). Morbidity is also increased (Jeste *et al.*, 1996; Enger *et al.*, 2004). In the USA, high rates of HIV and hepatitis B and C have been reported in outpatients with severe mental illness (Rosenberg *et al.*, 2001), which is likely to be of increasing importance for ageing patients in the years ahead.

There is good evidence that a large part of the excess morbidity and mortality in schizophrenia is related to potentially modifiable risk factors stemming, at least in part, from unhealthy lifestyles. Compared to the general population, people with schizophrenia are more likely to smoke, eat diets high in fat and low in fibre, and take little exercise (Brown *et al.*, 1999); they have higher rates of obesity, diabetes mellitus, hypertension, and adverse lipid profiles (Goff *et al.*, 2005a,b). Some of the newer antipsychotic drugs contribute to the high rates of obesity, diabetes, and hypertriglyceridaemia (Goff *et al.*, 2005a). Alcohol consumption has been reported to be relatively low among people with schizophrenia (Brown *et al.*, 1999), but the impact of illicit drug abuse—already significant among the younger population with severe mental illness—is likely to become increasingly significant for the health of older patients.

Thus, those patients with severe, enduring mental illness who survive to old age reach it with a high burden of ill-health. When questioned about their own perceived need for services middle-aged and elderly outpatients with psychotic illnesses assigned the highest priority to receiving help with improving their physical health and memory (Auslander and Jeste, 2002). Against this background, there is evidence of poor medical care for this population. Among Medicare patients in the USA aged 65 or more, Druss *et al.* (2001a) found schizophrenia to be associated with an increased risk of dying in the year following acute myocardial infarction, the increased risk being accounted for by the lower quality of the medical care they received. For example, patients with schizophrenia were less frequently advised to stop smoking, despite evidence that smoking cessation strategies can be safe and effective in schizophrenia (Evins *et al.*, 2001; George *et al.*, 2002). The difficulty extends to less acute services. Older patients with schizophrenia of both early and late onset have also been found to have difficulty obtaining optimal correction aids for visual and hearing deficits (Prager and Jeste, 1993).

The problem of poor medical care for elderly patients with severe mental illness is likely to be greatest where medical services are fragmented and complex to access. A system with a strong primary care service freely available to all citizens, such as the NHS in the UK, should be in a strong position to coordinate care for a variety of medical needs. Recent UK guidelines (NICE, 2002) for the care of patients with schizophrenia emphasize the importance of using primary care case registers to monitor the physical health of patients. They highlight that for many stable, elderly patients, maintaining their physical health is the most important aspect of their medical care. In other systems, psychiatrists may have to retain more responsibility for the physical health of patients with severe mental illness, following appropriate guidelines (e.g. Goff *et al.*, 2005a), or innovative ways of working with other medical care providers may be needed. Druss *et al.* (2001b) describe one such model in the USA which improved medical outcomes without increasing costs.

## Incontinence

Problems of incontinence deserve specific mention because they are very common, but poorly explained, among elderly patients with severe mental illness and are often a source of difficulty to carers. Incontinence was known to be very prevalent among elderly long-stay patients with functional illnesses in mental hospitals—typical figures in the literature were of the order of 25–50% being regularly incontinent of urine or faeces (e.g. Holloway *et al.*, 1994; Friern Hospital Medical Committee, 1983). Bonney *et al.* (1997) have proposed that detrusor hyperreflexia with associated incontinence is an intrinsic neurobiological feature of schizophrenia. Leff and Trieman (2000) noted that continence improved in some elderly patients discharged from hospital to community settings and suggested that this implied some functional component to the problem.

## Patient care

Campbell and Ananth (2002) have given an eloquent account of the deficiencies in care—particularly the indifference to patients' individual experience and therapeutic pessimism—which often surround elderly patients with severe, enduring mental illness. Their account is of care in hospital wards, but there is no reason to think that the same problems are not being replicated in many of the 'community' institutions where patients can now be found and where they may not even have medical attendants with any interest in psychiatry. It is no doubt the same pessimism that accounts for the almost complete exclusion of elderly patients from the huge international research effort into the treatment of schizophrenia.

All of the principles of good care of younger patients with schizophrenia should apply equally to managing elderly patients. In the UK, government guidelines for best practice were set out by the National Institute for Clinical Excellence in its guideline on schizophrenia (NICE, 2002). It is unclear why much of this document should not apply to older patients, although the summary states that 'the guideline concentrates on services for adults of working age with schizophrenia'. It specifically excludes those with onset after the age of 60, but the older patient with chronic schizophrenia passes unmentioned.

In broad terms, caring well for the elderly patient with severe, enduring mental illness requires—as well as a general interest in this patient group and a positive approach—an understanding of:

- how best to assess individual needs in this group of patients,
- the best medical and social interventions to address those needs, and
- the best system of care to deliver those interventions.

### Assessment of needs

A need for care was usefully defined by Wing (1992), who wrote that 'a need for care exists when an individual has an illness or impairment for which there is an effective and acceptable method of intervention'. Elderly patients with schizophrenia and other severe, enduring mental illnesses have many needs in common with younger patients, but can be expected also to differ in a number of respects related to the evolution of their illness as well as to the general physical and social consequences of ageing. Very little research has been done on the specific care needs of older patients and there is a corresponding lack of instruments for research and clinical purposes. One specifically designed instrument is the Camberwell Assessment of Need in the Elderly (Reynolds *et al.*, 2000). McNulty *et al.* (2003) assessed elderly patients with schizophrenia in a highly deprived district of Scotland using the Cardinal Needs Schedule (Marshall *et al.*, 1995), but commented that it may not be sensitive to some specific needs of elderly people with major mental illness. They found considerably higher levels of unmet need than in younger patients in the same district. Using their own instrument for patients to rate the importance of receiving care for different problems, Auslander and Jeste (2002) found that the priorities of older outpatients with psychotic illness differed from those reported for younger patients in earlier studies. Both groups assigned high priority to social relations, learning about their illness and improving sleep and mood. However the older patients gave the highest priority to improving their physical health and memory and relatively low priority to treatment for psychotic symptoms, medication management, supportive psychotherapy, and reducing rehospitalizations, perhaps because all were relatively stable outpatients. This study has significant limitations, but is an interesting attempt to extend the 'consumer perspective' to elderly patients whose views are too often given little weight.

## Medication

Antipsychotic drug treatment remains a key element in the management of psychotic illnesses as patients age, but there is an extraordinary lack of high-quality research to inform the use of these drugs in older patients. Important questions to ask are:

◆ Does the risk-to-benefit ratio of various antipsychotics differ in older patients, bearing in mind such things as the changing symptom profile, the higher incidence of drug-related movement disorders, and the increasing absolute cardiovascular risk with age?

◆ Do optimum doses differ in elderly patients and, if so, when and by how much should doses be reduced?

◆ Can any antipsychotic drugs improve the cognitive deficits in elderly patients which are so significant for functioning?

Unfortunately, the research base at present does not provide definitive answers to any of these questions.

It has been widely assumed that atypical antipsychotics should be of particular benefit to older people because of the lower risk of movement disorders with these drugs compared with typical antipsychotics. As well as reduced rates of acute extrapyramidal side-effects, there is evidence that, like younger patients, elderly patients are less likely to develop TD on atypical antipsychotics, although the rates vary quite widely between studies (0% to 13.4% incidence over 1 year). The relative risk for TD in older compared with younger adult patients taking atypical antipsychotics has been estimated to be approximately the same as on typical drugs, i.e. around a five-fold higher risk over 1 year of treatment (Correll et al., 2004). It is also important to consider other side-effects. The adverse metabolic effects associated with some atypical antipsychotics need to be considered carefully in a group already high in risk factors for cardiovascular disease.

There is evidence from open-label studies that switching elderly patients from typical antipsychotics to risperidone or olanzapine can be tolerated, with reports of improvement in clinical symptoms and extrapyramidal side-effects (Davidson et al., 2000; Barak et al., 2002a,b; Ritchie et al., 2003). A Cochrane Review aimed at estimating the effects of antipsychotic medication for people over 65 with chronic schizophrenia was able to include data from only three randomized controlled trials (RCTs), one of these being a very small trial comparing two drugs that are no longer available. Fifty-nine patients over the age of 65 were included in a large RCT comparing haloperidol and olanzapine over 6 weeks (Tollefson et al., 1997). Among these older patients, the two drugs did not differ in clinical efficacy or in the incidence of side-effects, although this subgroup analysis was clearly underpowered. In a larger 8-week RCT comparing olanzapine and risperidone in 175 elderly patients with chronic schizophrenia, there were no significant differences detected between the two drugs (Jeste et al,. 2003a).

From the descriptions of the extensive psychotic symptoms and disabilities among elderly patients prior to discharge from the asylums, often despite many years of antipsychotic treatment, it is clear that treatment resistance remains a significant problem even late

in the course of schizophrenia. Clozapine is now a well-established therapeutic option for younger treatment-resistant patients. Once again, the evidence base largely excludes the elderly. The only RCT for clozapine in this group compared it with chlorpromazine over 12 weeks in 42 patients over the age of 55 (mean age approximately 67). The patients were not selected for treatment resistance. Both drugs appeared effective with no differences between them (Howanitz et al., 1999). The elderly appear to be more at risk of clozapine-induced blood problems than younger patients (Wahlbeck et al., 1999).

Manufacturers recommend lower doses of antipsychotics in the elderly for a number of drugs. One study found that it was possible to reduce doses by about 40% in middle-aged and elderly (over 45 years) psychotic patients without significant changes in psychopathology and with an improvement in extrapyramidal side-effects (Harris et al., 1997). Old age psychiatrists are often faced with decisions about prescribing antipsychotics for elderly patients, who may have residual symptoms, and of whom the psychiatrist has little long-term knowledge. In these circumstances, there can be no alternative to careful assessment, discussion—where possible—with the patient and carers, and regular reassessment if dose reductions are made.

Among younger adults, atypical antipsychotics have been shown to have a mild remedial effect on the cognitive deficits of schizophrenia (Woodward et al., 2005). Again, the data among elderly patients are very limited, but a study of elderly patients with schizophrenia or schizoaffective disorder treated with low doses of either risperidone or olanzapine did find some improvements in cognitive test scores with both drugs (Harvey et al., 2003b). Better baseline function predicted more improvement. A study of donepezil in 20 patients with chronic schizophrenia and severe cognitive impairment failed to find any benefit for cognitive function or negative symptoms (Mazeh et al., 2006).Cognitive impairment attributable to the side-effects of anticholinergic drugs is increasingly recognized as a problem in the general elderly population. Elderly patients with chronic schizophrenia have often been taking relatively high doses of anticholinergic drugs for many years. Drimer et al. (2004) found they were able to withdraw long-term anticholinergic medication from elderly patients with schizophrenia with no increase in extrapyramidal symptoms and with an improvement in cognitive test scores.

## Psychological treatments

Psychological treatments are now a well-established treatment modality for younger patients with schizophrenia. In particular, cognitive behavioural therapy (CBT) is widely recommended, although the strength of the evidence in its favour is disputed. In its guideline, the National Institute for Clinical Excellence states that 'Psychological treatments should be an indispensable part of the treatment options available for service users and their families in the effort to promote recovery' (NICE, 2002). It recommends that CBT be available to patients with persisting psychotic symptoms, and that its use be considered for problems of poor insight and low medication adherence, all of which are prevalent among the elderly population. Other individual psychotherapeutic interventions which might be of interest for older patients, in view of their particular difficulties with social functioning and cognition, are social skills training and cognitive remediation therapy, both of which rest on a growing research literature in younger patients (Bellack, 2004).

The difficulty with making any recommendations for older patients lies, again, with the lack of treatment trials in which they are included.

It is likely that CBT interventions developed for younger adults cannot simply be transferred to older patients without modification. A number of general adaptations to CBT have been suggested for older adults, especially where compensation is needed for neuro-cognitive deficits. These include such things as multiple learning modalities, increased repetition, and graded tasks to improve retention (Arean, 1993). McQuaid et al. (2000) suggested that 'the repetitive, concrete, practice-learning model of social skills training' may be well suited to older patients with more marked cognitive impairment, but that particular beliefs about their inability to change or physical impairments might make it difficult to implement. Consequently, they developed a specific treatment combining elements of CBT and social skills training for groups. In a randomized, controlled trial of this intervention versus usual treatment in 76 outpatients with chronic schizophrenia or schizoaffective disorder aged 42–74, the intervention group performed social functioning activities more frequently, showed greater mastery of the skills included in the training, and gained in cognitive insight (Granholm et al., 2005). Another group behavioural intervention aimed at improving the living skills of middle-aged and older patients with chronic psychosis has also been piloted with promising results (Patterson et al., 2003). These studies demonstrate that psychological interventions are feasible for older patients with very long histories of illness.

## Accommodation

The relationship of the social milieu within psychiatric institutions to the disabilities of their residents was well known prior to the programme of hospital closures. The Three Hospitals Study by Wing and Brown (1970) was highly influential in demonstrating that although many patients had a core deficit 'impervious to social influence', this was amplified by an unstimulating environment and the amplification could be reversed by 'sustained effort at social enrichment'. Wing (1989) has since emphasized that 'the principles of social treatment would be likely to hold wherever the patients were treated. It could not be assumed that the environment would change for the better simply because a patient had been discharged 'to the community''. We now have very few systematic data about the environments in which elderly schizophrenic patients are living. In a sample in California, 42% of older patients with schizophrenia were living in board-and-care settings (Jeste et al., 2003b). A law passed in the USA in 1987 prohibited patients with primary psychiatric diagnoses from being admitted to nursing homes (Omnibus Budget Reconciliation Act 1987. Public Law no. 100–203). Those discharged from psychiatric hospitals in the UK largely remained in fairly institutional settings, including residential and nursing homes (Double and Wong, 1991; Holloway et al., 1994). Patterns may change as succeeding cohorts age. Older patients from ethnic minority communities may be more likely than those in majority communities to live with family members (Patterson et al., 2005).

The wide range of disabilities among the functionally ill elderly means that a wide range of different accommodation options is likely to be needed, ranging from support for those in their own homes to specialized, full-time nursing. Facilities are often most lacking for those patients in the middle range of disabilities.

Holloway et al. (1994) found that staff in hostels for the mentally ill were struggling to cope with the physical disabilities of their residents as they aged. Age may also render some patients vulnerable to exploitation and abuse by younger residents in mixed-age settings. In such circumstances, the only alternative available may be nursing home care, which is unnecessarily restrictive and expensive.

There is particular concern about the placement of ageing patients with enduring functional illnesses in settings designed primarily for patients with severe dementia where functional deterioration, dwindling communication, and incontinence may be the norm and may pass without question. Ideally each patient should have an environment where protection from excessive demands is balanced with opportunities and encouragement to achieve as high a level of daily and social functioning as possible. Wing and Brown's point that effort at creating such an environment needs to be sustained is important. The patients followed up by the TAPS Project for 5 years after discharge showed maximum gains in domestic skills in the first year, but these decreased again over the next 4 years, although not to baseline level (Leff and Trieman, 2000). The authors give two possible explanations: the placement of some of the older patients in nursing homes where opportunities for domestic skills were lost; and the taking over of tasks by staff who gradually lost patience with the patients' slowness and inefficiency. The greatest areas of unmet need among elderly patients discharged from Cane Hill Hospital were in the areas of structured activity, leisure, and companionship (Holloway et al., 1994).

## Psychiatric services

Data on the use of mental health services by older people with severe mental illness are scarce. In a study from the late 1980s, older people were shown to be low users of mental health services compared with younger people with similar mental illnesses (Goldstrom et al., 1987). Ten years later, Cuffel et al. (1996) found this relationship not to hold for patients with schizophrenia. In a study of community mental health service use in San Diego County, service use and treatment costs were highest for the youngest (18–29) and oldest (over 65) patients. However, it was possible that this result was influenced by the US system of financing health care which led to mental health care being substantially cheaper for the elderly to access.

Much discussion of psychiatric services for elderly patients with long-standing, severe functional illnesses focuses on whether their care should continue to be provided by teams for working age adults or by specialist services for older adults. These patients are probably the least well served by this demarcation of responsibilities. The only sensible conclusion is that their care should be dictated by individual needs. Many such patients have built up relationships with their care teams over many years which may be of particular importance in the absence of much other social contact. As things stand in the UK, if transferred to old age services, patients suffer not only a loss of continuity but are also at risk of missing out on a number of services which have been developed for younger adults, such as crisis management and intensive home treatment. However, the expertise of old age services in managing patients with co-morbid physical illness or cognitive deficits, and their access to service settings suited to the frail, immobile, or incontinent may be indispensable. The Royal College of Psychiatrists recommends that a lead service be identified in each area, with funding arrangements reflecting this choice, but emphasizes the vital importance of services and resource allocation being flexible enough to accommodate variations depending on individual need (Royal College of Psychiatrists, 2002). Recent government guidance also speaks out strongly in favour of needs-led services (DoH, 2005).

The teams looking after these patients need to be able to draw on a range of skills from several disciplines: general medical practice, psychiatry, social work, nursing, occupational therapy, and psychology. Access to suitable physiotherapy and occasionally speech therapy or dietetics becomes increasingly important with age. Attention needs to be given to sympathetic services in areas such as optometry, audiology, podiatry, and dentistry. Given the complexities of need, it is essential that each patient has a detailed care plan and a single professional responsible for its implementation. In the UK, it has been made clear that the care programme approach (CPA), developed for younger adults with severe mental health problems, should also be applied to older adults with severe mental illness due to schizophrenia or other psychoses (DoH, 2002). Under the CPA each patient has a care coordinator, who must be a mental health professional; and regular, multidisciplinary reviews of the patient's needs and care must be held.

## Decision-making capacity

A recurrent theme throughout this chapter has been the relative dearth of high-quality research involving elderly patients with severe, enduring mental illness. It is clear that there is a need for a substantial investment in research on treatment and service organization. Concern has been expressed about the capacity of older patients with severe mental illness to give proper consent to interventional research; this subject, however, has been fairly actively investigated in recent years. Older patients with schizophrenia are found in this, as in most other things, to be a very heterogeneous group. Although some are fully capable of consenting to participation in research studies, overall they do show deficits in relevant decision-making capacity, with cognitive impairment being the best predictor of impaired capacity (Kovnick et al., 2003; Palmer et al., 2005; Palmer and Jeste, 2006; Dunn et al., 2006a,b). A number of interventions have been shown to be useful in enhancing decision-making capacity (Dunn et al., 2002, 2006a). Further, these patients perform better than patients with mild to moderate Alzheimer's disease on tests of capacity to consent (Palmer et al., 2005). Appropriate though concern about capacity is, it should not be so great as to prevent much-needed research.

## Conclusions

The old and the severely mentally ill are both vulnerable to discrimination and social exclusion, and those with both attributes certainly risk being doubly disadvantaged. The United Nations, for its International Year of the Older Person in 1995, set out as part of the conceptual framework behind the theme 'a society for all ages' that 'generations invest in one another…guided by the twin principles of reciprocity and equity'. Older people who have been severely mentally ill for much of their adult lives have often been unable to make the economic and social contributions which are seen as the basis of reciprocity. Their care needs strongly challenge a society's commitment to equity.

Discrimination against the elderly with severe, enduring mental illnesses is evident in their relative neglect in the research literature and their exclusion from, or belated inclusion in, a number of policy initiatives and service developments for younger adults. Demographic change could work for or against these patients. As the population ages, elderly patients will increase in number and become a significantly larger proportion of the severely mentally ill. Hence, finding ways to enhance their functioning and independence may become politically more pressing. On the other hand, if their claim to investment continues to be overlooked in the face of more powerful and articulate lobbies, increasing numbers may simply be associated with deteriorating services. This is perhaps a particular risk now that they are scattered in generic community facilities for the elderly where the appropriate specialist services will be hard to develop.

In the face of widespread negative attitudes about older patients with severe mental illness, what literature there is does give some grounds for guarded optimism. A substantial number of patients with schizophrenia have a broadly favourable outcome in the long-term; and older patients are likely to be able to benefit from innovations in pharmacological and psychological treatments, if these can be effectively delivered.

## References

Angst, J. (1988). European long-term studies of schizophrenia. *Schizophrenia Bulletin*, **14**, 501–13.

Arean, P.A. (1993). Cognitive behavioral therapy with older adults. *The Behavioral Therapist*, **17**, 236–9.

Arie, T. and Jolley, D.J. (1982). Making services work: organisation and style of psychogeriatric services. In *The psychiatry of late life* (ed. R. Levy and F. Post), pp. 222–51. Blackwell, Oxford.

Arnold, S.E. (2001). Contributions of neuropathology to understanding schizophrenia in late life. *Harvard Review of Psychiatry*, **9**, 69–76.

Arnold, S.E., Trojanowski, J.Q., Gur, R.E., Blackwell, P., Han, L.Y., and Choi, C. (1998). Absence of neurodegeneration and neural injury in the cerebral cortex in a sample of elderly patients with schizophrenia. *Archives of General Psychiatry*, **55**, 225–32.

Auslander, L.A. and Jeste, D.V. (2002). Perceptions of problems and needs for service among middle-aged and elderly outpatients with schizophrenia and related psychotic disorders. *Community Mental Health Journal*, **38**, 391–402.

Auslander, L.A. and Jeste, D.V. (2004). Sustained remission of schizophrenia among community-dwelling older outpatients. *American Journal of Psychiatry*, **161**, 1490–3.

Barak, Y. and Cohen, A. (2003). Characterizing the elderly homeless: a 10-year study in Israel. *Archives of Gerontology and Geriatrics*, **37**, 147–55.

Barak, Y., Shamir, E., and Weizman, R. (2002a). Would a switch from typical antipsychotics to risperidone be beneficial for elderly schizophrenic patients? A naturalistic, long-term, retrospective, comparative study. *Journal of Clinical Psychopharmacology*, **22**, 115–20.

Barak, Y., Shamir, E., Zemishlani, H., Mirecki, I., Toren, P., and Weizman, R. (2002b). Olanzapine vs. haloperidol ini the treatment of elderly chronic schizophrenia patients. *Progress in Neuropsychopharmacology & Biological Psychiatry*, **26**, 1199–202.

Barton, R. (1959). *Institutional neurosis*. John Wright, Bristol.

Bellack, A.S. (2004). Skills training for people with severe mental illness. *Psychiatric Rehabilitation Journal*, **27**, 375–91.

Bleuler, M. (1972). *Die schizophrenen Geistesstörungen im Lichte langjähriger Kranken- und Familiengeschichten*. Georg Thieme, Stuttgart. [Translated by Clemens, S.M. (1978) as *The schizophrenic disorders: long-term patient and family studies*. Yale University Press, New Haven, CT.]

Bonney, W.W., Gupta, S., Hunter, D.R., and Arndt, S. (1997). Bladder dysfunction in schizophrenia. *Schizophrenia Research*, **25**, 243–9.

Bridge, T.P., Cannon, H.E., and Wyatt, J.R. (1978). Burned-out schizophrenia: evidence for age effects on schizophrenic symptomatology. *Journal of Gerontology*, **33**, 835–9.

Brown, S. (1997). Excess mortality of schizophrenia: a meta-analysis. *British Journal of Psychiatry*, **171**, 502–8.

Brown, S., Birtwhistle, J., Roe, L., and Thompson, C. (1999). The unhealthy lifestyle of people with schizophrenia. *Psychological Medicine*, **29**, 697–701.

Brown, S., Inskip, H., and Barraclough, B. (2000). Causes of the excess mortality of schizophrenia. *British Journal of Psychiatry*, **177**, 212–17.

Byne, W., White, L., Parrella, M., Adams, R., Harvey, P.D., and Davis, K.L. (1998). Tardive dyskinesia in a chronically institutionalized population of elderly schizophrenic patients: prevalence and association with cognitive impairment. *International Journal of Geriatric Psychiatry*, **13**, 473–9.

Campbell, A., Converse, P.E., and Rodgers, W.L. (1976). *The quality of American life*. Russell Sage Foundation, New York.

Campbell, P. and Ananth, H. (2002). Graduates. In *Psychiatry in the elderly* (ed. R. Jacoby and C. Oppenheimer), pp. 782–4. Oxford University Press, Oxford.

Campbell, P.G., Taylor, J., Pantelis, C., and Harvey, C. (1990). Studies of schizophrenia in a large mental hospital proposed for closure, and in two halves of an inner London borough served by the hospital. In *International perspectives in schizophrenia research* (ed. M. Weller), pp. 185–202. John Libbey and Sons, London.

Censits, D.M., Ragland, J.D., Gur, R.C., and Gur, R.E. (1997). Neuropsychological evidence supporting a neurodevelopmental model of schizophrenia: a longitudinal study. *Schizophrenia Research*, **24**, 289–98.

Ciompi, L. (1980). Catamnestic long-term study on the course of life and aging of schizophrenics. *Schizophrenia Bulletin*, **6**, 606–18.

Clifford, P., Charman, A., Webb, Y., and Best, S. (1991). Planning for community care: long-stay populations of hospitals scheduled for rundown or closure. *British Journal of Psychiatry*, **158**, 190–6.

Clipp, E.C. (2001). Quality of life. In *Encyclopedia of aging* (ed. G.L. Maddox), pp. 851–4. Springer, New York.

Cohen, C.I., Talavera, N., and Hartung, R. (1996). Depression among aging persons with schizophrenia who live in the community. *Psychiatric Services*, **47**, 601–7.

Cohen, C.I., Talavera, N., and Harting, R. (1997). Predictors of subjective well-being among older, community-dwelling persons with schizophrenia. *American Journal of Geriatric Psychiatry*, **5**, 145–55.

Cohen, C.I., Cohen, G.D., Blank, K. *et al.* (2000). Schizophrenia and older adults – an overview: directions for research and policy. *American Journal of Geriatric Psychiatry*, **8**, 19–28.

Cohen, C.I., Ramirez, P.M., Kehn, M., Magai, C., Eimecke, J., and Brenner, R. (2003). Assessing quality of life in older persons with schizophrenia. *American Journal of Geriatric Psychiatry*, **11**, 658–66.

Copeland, J.R.M., Dewey, M.E., Scott, A. *et al.* (1998). Schizophrenia and delusional disorder in older age: community prevalence, incidence, comorbidity and outcome. *Schizophrenia Bulletin*, **24**, 153–61.

Correll, C.U., Leucht, S., and Kane, J.M. (2004). Lower risk for tardive dyskinesia associated with second-generation antipsychotics: a systematic review of 1-year studies. *American Journal of Psychiatry*, **161**, 414–25.

Cuffell, B.J., Jeste, D.V., Halpain, M., Pratt, C., Tarke, H., and Patterson, T.L. (1996). Treatment costs and use of community mental health services for schizophrenia by age cohorts. *American Journal of Psychiatry*, **153**, 870–6.

Cunningham Owens, D.G. and Johnstone, E. (1980). The disabilities of chronic schizophrenia. *British Journal of Psychiatry*, **136**, 384–95.

DHSS (1972). *Services for mental illness related to old age*. Department of Health and Social Security Circular HM (72)71. HMSO, London.

DHSS (1988). *Mental health statistics for England*. Government Statistical Service, London.

Davidson, M., Harvey, P.D., Powchik, P. *et al.* (1995). Severity of symptoms in chronically institutionalized geriatric schizophrenic patients. *American Journal of Psychiatry*, **152**, 197–207.

Davidson, M., Harvey, P.D., Vervarcke, J. *et al.* (2000). A long-term, multicenter, open-label study of risperidone in elderly patients with psychosis. On behalf of the Risperidone Working Group. *International Journal of Geriatric Psychiatry*, **15**, 506–14.

DoH (2002). *Care management for older people with serious mental health problems*. Department of Health, London.

DoH (2005). *Securing better mental health for older adults*. Department of Health, London.

Double, D.B. and Wong, T.I. (1991). What has happened to patients from long-stay psychiatric wards? *Psychiatric Bulletin*, **15**, 735–6.

Drimer, T., Shahal, B., and Barak, Y. (2004). Effects of discontinuation of long-term anticholinergic treatment in elderly schizophrenia patients. *International Clinical Psychopharmacology*, **19**, 27–9.

Druss, B.G., Bradford, W.D., Rosenheck, R.A., Radford, M.J., and Krumholz, H.M. (2001a). Quality of medical care and excess mortality in older patients with mental disorders. *Archives of General Psychiatry*, **58**, 565–72.

Druss, B.G., Rohrbaugh, R.M., Levinson, C.M. *et al.* (2001b). Integrated medical care for patients with serious psychiatric illness: a randomized trial. *Archives of General Psychiatry*, **58**, 861–8.

Dunn, L.B., Lindamer, L.A., Palmer, B.W., Golshan, S., Schneiderman, L.J., and Jeste, D.V. (2002). Improving understanding of research consent in middle-aged and elderly patients with psychotic disorders. *American Journal of Geriatric Psychiatry*, **10**, 142–50.

Dunn, L.B., Palmer, B.W., and Keehan, M. (2006a). Understanding of placebo controls among older people with schizophrenia. *Schizophrenia Bulletin*, **32**, 137–46.

Dunn, L.B., Palmer, B.W., Keehan, M., Jeste, D.V., and Appelbaum, P.S. (2006b). Assessment of therapeutic misconception in older schizophrenia patients with a brief instrument. *American Journal of Psychiatry*, **163**, 500–6.

Dwork, A.J., Susser, E.S., Keilp, J. *et al.* (1998). Senile degeneration and cognitive impairment in chronic schizophrenia. *American Journal of Psychiatry*, **155**, 1536–43.

Enger, C., Weatherby, L., Reynolds, R.F., Glasser, D.B., and Walker, A.M. (2004). Serious cardiovascular events and mortality among patients with schizophrenia. *Journal of Nervous and Mental Disease*, **192**, 19–27.

Evans, J.D., Heaton, R.K., Paulsen, J.S., Palmer, B.W., Patterson, T., and Jeste, D.V. (2003). The relationship of neuropsychological abilities to specific domains of functional capacity in older schizophrenia patients. *Biological Psychiatry*, **53**, 422–30.

Evins, A.E., Mays, V., Cather, C. *et al.* (2001). A pilot trial of bupropion added to cognitive behavioural therapy for smoking cessation in schizophrenia. *Nicotine and Tobacco Research*, **3**, 397–403.

Fenton, W.S. (2000). Prevalence of spontaneous dyskinesia in schizophrenia. *Journal of Clinical Psychiatry*, **61**(Suppl. 4), 10–14.

Friedman, J.I., Harvey, P.D., Coleman, T. *et al.* (2001). Six-year follow-up study of cognitive and functional status across the lifespan in schizophrenia: a comparison with Alzheimer's disease and normal aging. *American Journal of Psychiatry*, **158**, 1441–8.

Friedman, J.I., Harvey, P.D., McGurk, S.R. *et al.* (2002). Correlates of change in functional status of institutionalized geriatric schizophrenic patients: focus on medical comorbidity. *American Journal of Psychiatry*, **159**, 1388–94.

Friern Hospital Medical Committee (1983). *Inpatient survey 1983*. Friern Hospital, Friern Barnet.

George, T.P., Vessicchio, J.C., Termine, A. *et al.* (2002). A placebo controlled trial of bupropion for smoking cessation in schizophrenia. *Biological Psychiatry*, **52**, 53–61.

Goff, D.C., Cather, C., Evins, A.E. *et al.* (2005a). Medical morbidity and mortality in schizophrenia: guidelines for psychiatrists. *Journal of Clinical Psychiatry*, **66**, 183–94.

Goff, D.C., Sullivan, L.M., McEvoy, J.P. *et al.* (2005b). A comparison of ten-year cardiac risk estimates in schizophrenia patients from the CATIE study and matched controls. *Schizophrenia Research*, **80**, 45–53.

Goldstrom, I., Burns, B., Kessler, L.G. *et al.* (1987). Mental health service use by elderly adults in a primary care setting. *Journal of Gerontology*, **43**, 147–53.

Graham, C., Arthur, A., and Howard, R. (2002). The social functioning of older adults with schizophrenia. *Aging & Mental Health*, **6**, 149–52.

Granholm, E., McQuaid, J.R., McClure, F.S. *et al.* (2005). A randomized, controlled trial of cognitive behavioural social skills training for middle-aged and older outpatients with chronic schizophrenia. *American Journal of Psychiatry*, **162**, 520–9.

Green, S., Girling, D.M., Lough, S., Ng, A.M.N., and Whitcher, S.K. (1997). Service provision for elderly people with long-term functional illness. *Psychiatric Bulletin*, **21**, 353–7.

Gur, R., Petty, R.G., Turetsky, B.I., and Gur, R.C. (1996). Schizophrenia throughout life: sex differences in severity and profile of symptoms. *Schizophrenia Research*, **21**, 1–12.

Harding, C.M., Brooks, G.W., Ashikaga, T. *et al.* (1987). The Vermont longitudinal study of persons with severe mental illness. II: Long-term outcome of subjects who retrospectively met DSM-III criteria for schizophrenia. *American Journal of Psychiatry*, **144**, 727–35.

Harris, M.J., Heaton, R.K., Schalz, A., Bailey, A., and Patterson, T.L. (1997). Neuroleptic dose reduction in older psychotic patients. *Schizophrenia Research*, **27**, 241–8.

Harrison, G., Hopper, K., Craig, T. *et al.* (2001). Recovery from psychotic illness: a 15- and 25-year international follow-up study. *British Journal of Psychiatry*, **178**, 506–17.

Harrison, P.J. (2004). Schizophrenia and its dementia. In *The neuropathology of dementia* (ed. M.M. Esiri, V.M.-Y. Lee, and J.Q. Trojanowski), pp. 497–508. Cambridge University Press, Cambridge.

Harvey, P.D., Howanitz, E., Parrella, M. *et al.* (1998). Symptoms, cognitive functioning and adaptive skills in geriatric patients with lifelong schizophrenia: a comparison across treatment sites. *American Journal of Psychiatry*, **155**, 1080–6.

Harvey, P.D., Parrella, M., White, L., Mohs, R.C., Davidson, M., and Davis, K.L. (1999a). Convergence of cognitive and adaptive decline in late-life schizophrenia. *Schizophrenia Research*, **35**, 77–84.

Harvey, P.D., Silverman, J.M., Mohs, R.C. *et al.* (1999b). Cognitive decline in late-life schizophrenia: a longitudinal study of geriatric chronically hospitalized patients. *Biological Psychiatry*, **45**, 32–40.

Harvey, P.D., Bertisch, H., Friedman, J.I. *et al.* (2003a). The course of functional decline in geriatric patients with schizophrenia: cognitive-functional and clinical symptoms as determinants of change. *American Journal of Geriatric Psychiatry*, **11**, 610–19.

Harvey, P.D., Napolitano, J.A., Mao, L., and Gharabawi, G. (2003b). Comparative effects of risperidone and olanzapine on cognition in elderly patients with schizophrenia or schizoaffective disorder. *International Journal of Geriatric Psychiatry*, **18**, 820–9.

Heaton, R.K., Gladsjo, J.A., Palmer, B.W., Kuck, J., Marcotte, T.D., and Jeste, D.V. (2001). Stability and course of neuropsychological deficits in schizophrenia. *Archives of General Psychiatry*, **58**, 24–32.

Hoff, A.L., Svetina, C., Shields, G., Stewart, J., and DeLisi, L.E. (2005). Ten year longitudinal study of neuropsychological functioning subsequent to a first episode of schizophrenia. *Schizophrenia Research*, **78**, 27–34.

Holloway, F., Rutherford, J., Carson, J., and Dunn, L. (1994). 'Elderly graduates' and a hospital closure programme. *Psychiatric Bulletin*, **18**, 534–7.

Honkonen, T., Saarinen, S., and Salokangas, R.K. (1999). Deinstitutionalization in Finland II: discharged patients and their psychosocial functioning. *Schizophrenia Bulletin*, **25**, 543–51.

Howanitz, E., Pardo, M., Smelson, D.A. *et al.* (1999). The efficacy and safety of clozapine versus chlorpromazine in geriatric schizophrenia. *Journal of Clinical Psychiatry*, **60**, 41–4.

Huber, G., Gross, G., and Schüttler, R. (1975). A long-term follow-up study of schizophrenia: psychiatric course of illness and prognosis. *Acta Psychiatrica Scandinavica*, **52**, 49–57.

Jeste, D.V., Gladsjo, J.A., Lindamer, L.A., and Lacro, J.P. (1996). Medical comorbidity in schizophrenia. *Schizophrenia Bulletin*, **22**, 413–30.

Jeste, D.V., Barak, Y., Madhusoodanan, S., Grossman, F., and Gharabawi, G. (2003a). International multisite double-blind trial of the atypical antipsychotics risperidone and olanzapine in 175 elderly patients with chronic schizophrenia. *American Journal of Geriatric Psychiatry*, **11**, 638–47.

Jeste, D.V., Twamley, E.W., Eyler Zorilla, L.T., Golshan, S., Patterson, T.L., and Palmer, B.W. (2003b). Aging and outcome in schizophrenia. *Acta Psychiatrica Scandinavica*, **107**, 336–43.

Jeste, S.D., Patterson, T.L., Palmer, B.W., Dolder, C.R., Goldman, S., and Jeste, D.V. (2003c). Cognitive predictors of medication adherence among middle-aged and older outpatients with schizophrenia. *Schizophrenia Research*, **63**, 49–58.

Jin, H., Zisook, S., Palmer, B.W. *et al.* (2001). Association of depressive symptoms with worse functioning in schizophrenia: a study in older outpatients. *Journal of Clinical Psychiatry*, **62**, 797–803.

Jones, D. (1993). The TAPS Project. 11: the selection of patients for reprovision. *British Journal of Psychiatry*, **162**(Suppl. 19), 36–9.

Kasckow, J.W., Twamley, E., Mulcahey, J.J. *et al.* (2001). Health-related quality of well-being in chronically hospitalized patients with schizophrenia: comparison with matched outpatients. *Psychiatry Research*, **103**, 69–78.

Keith, S.J., Regier, D.A., and Rae, D.S. (1991). Schizophrenic disorders. In *Psychiatric disorders in America* (ed. L.N. Robins and D.A. Regier), pp. 33–52. The Free Press, New York.

Klapow, J.C., Evans, J., Patterson, T.L., Heaton, R.K., Koch, W.L., and Jeste, D.V. (1997). Direct assessment of functional status in older patients with schizophrenia. *American Journal of Psychiatry*, **154**, 1022–4.

Kovnick, J.A., Appelbaum, P.S., Hoge, S.K., and Leadbetter, R.A. (2003). Competence to consent to research among long-stay inpatients with chronic schizophrenia. *Psychiatric Services*, **54**, 1247–52.

Kua, E.H.A. (1992). A community study of mental disorders in elderly Singaporean Chinese using the GMS-AGECAT package. *Australia and New Zealand Journal of Psychiatry*, **26**, 502–6.

Kurtz, M.M. (2005). Neurocognitive impairment across the lifespan in schizophrenia: an update. *Schizophrenia Research*, **74**, 15–26.

Kurtz, M.M., Moberg, P.J., Mozley, L.H. *et al.* (2001). Cognitive impairment and functional status in elderly institutionalized patients with schizophrenia. *International Journal of Geriatric Psychiatry*, **16**, 631–8.

Leff, J. (1991). Evaluation of the closure of mental hospitals. In *The closure of mental hospitals* (ed. P. Hall and I.F. Brockington), pp. 25–32. Gaskell, London.

Leff, J. and Trieman, N. (2000). Long-stay patients discharged from psychiatric hospitals. *British Journal of Psychiatry*, **174**, 217–23.

Lieh-Mak, F. and Lee, P.W. (1997). Cognitive deficit measures in schizophrenia: factor structure and clinical correlates. *American Journal of Psychiatry*, **154**(6 Suppl.), 39–46.

McCreadie, R.G., Leese, M., Tilak-Singh, D., Loftus, L., MacEwan, T., and Thornicroft, G. (1997). Nithsdale, Nunhead and Norwood: similarities and differences in prevalence of schizophrenia and utilisation of services in rural and urban areas. *British Journal of Psychiatry*, **170**, 31–6.

McNulty, S.V., Laing, D., Semple, M., Jackson, G.A., and Pelosi, A.J. (2003). Care needs of elderly people with schizophrenia. *British Journal of Psychiatry*, **182**, 241–7.

McQuaid, J.R., Granholm, E., McClure, F.S. *et al.* (2000). Development of an integrated cognitive-behavioral and social skills training intervention for older patients with schizophrenia. *Journal of Psychotherapy Practice and Research*, **9**, 149–57.

Marneros, A., Deister, A., and Rohde, A. (1992). Comparison of long-term outcome of schizophrenic, affective and schizoaffective disorders. *British Journal of Psychiatry*, **161**(Suppl. 18), 44–51.

Marriott, R.G., Neil, W., and Waddingham, S. (2006). Antipsychotic medication for elderly people with schizophrenia. Cochrane Database of Systematic Reviews 2006, Issue 1, Art. No. CD005580.DOI: 10.1002/14651858.

Marshall, M., Hogg, L., Lockwood, A. *et al.* (1995). The Cardinal Needs Schedule: a modified version of the MREC Needs for Care Schedule. *Psychological Medicine*, **25**, 605–17.

Martin, D. (1955). Institutionalisation. *Lancet*, **ii**, 1188–90.

Mazeh, D., Zemishlani, H., Barak, Y., Mirecki, I., and Paleacu, D. (2006). Donepezil for negative signs in elderly patients with schizophrenia: an add-on, double-blind, crossover, placebo-controlled study. *International Psychogeriatrics*, **18**, 429–36.

Mittal, D., Davis, C.E., Depp, C. *et al.* (2006). Correlates of health-related quality of well-being in older patients with schizophrenia. *Journal of Nervous and Mental Disease*, **194**, 335–40.

Moak, G.S. and Fisher, W.H. (1991). Geriatric patients and services in state hospitals: data from a national survey. *Hospital and Community Psychiatry*, **42**, 273–6.

NICE (2002). *Schizophrenia: core interventions in the treatment and management of schizophrenia in primary and secondary care*. National Institute for Clinical Excellence, London.

Osby, U., Correia, N., Brandt, L., Ekborn, A., and Sparen, P. (2000). Mortality and causes of death in schizophrenia in Stockholm county, Sweden. *Schizophrenia Research*, **45**, 21–8.

Palmer, B.W. and Jeste, D.V. (2006). Relationship of individual cognitive abilities to specific components of decisional capacity among middle-aged and older patients with schizophrenia. *Schizophrenia Bulletin*, **32**, 98–106.

Palmer, B.W., Heaton, S.C., and Jeste, D.V. (1999). Older patients with schizophrenia: challenges in the coming decades. *Psychiatric Services*, **50**, 1178–83.

Palmer, B.W., Heaton, R.K., Gladsjo, J.A. *et al.* (2002). Heterogeneity in functional status among older outpatients with schizophrenia: employment history, living situation, and driving. *Schizophrenia Research*, **55**, 205–15.

Palmer, B.W., Dunn, L.B., Appelbaum, P.S. *et al.* (2005). Assessment of capacity to consent to research among older patients with schizophrenia, Alzheimer disease, or diabetes mellitus: comparison of a 3-item questionnaire with a comprehensive, standardized capacity instrument. *Archives of General Psychiatry*, **62**, 726–33.

Patterson, T.L., Bucardo, J., McKibbin, C.L. *et al.* (2005). Development and pilot testing of a new psychosocial intervention for older Latinos with chronic psychosis. *Schizophrenia Bulletin*, **31**, 922–30.

Patterson, T.L., McKibbin, C., Taylor, M. *et al.* (2003). Functional Adaptation Skills Training (FAST): a pilot psychosocial intervention study in middle-aged and older patients with chronic psychotic disorders. *American Journal of Geriatric Psychiatry*, **11**, 17–23.

Patterson, T.L., Moscona, S., McKibbin, C.L., Davidson, K., and Jeste, D.V. (2001). Social skills performance assessment among older patients with schizophrenia. *Schizophrenia Research*, **48**, 351–60.

Patterson, T., Shaw, W., Semple, S. *et al.* (1997). Health-related quality of life in older patients with schizophrenia and other psychoses: relationships among psychosocial and psychiatric factors. *International Journal of Geriatric Psychiatry*, **12**, 451–61.

Pfohl, B. and Winokur, G. (1982). The evolution of symptoms in institutionalized hebephrenic/catatonic schizophrenics. *British Journal of Psychiatry*, **141**, 567–72.

Prager, S. and Jeste, D.V. (1993). Sensory impairment in late-life schizophrenia. *Schizophrenia Bulletin*, **19**, 755–72.

Purohit, D.P., Perl, D.P., Haroutunian, V., Powchik, P., Davidson, M., and Davis, K.L. (1998). Alzheimer disease and related neurodegenerative diseases in elderly patients with schizophrenia – a post-mortem neuropathologic study of 100 cases. *Archives of General Psychiatry*, **55**, 205–11.

Quinn, J., Meagher, D., Murphy, P., Kinsella, A., Mullaney, J., and Waddington, J.L. (2001). Vulnerability to involuntary movements over a lifetime trajectory of schizophrenia approaches 100%, in association with executive (frontal) dysfunction. *Schizophrenia Research*, **49**, 79–87.

Räsänen, S., Hakko, H., Viilo, K., Meyer-Rochow, V.B., and Mohring, J. (2003). Excess mortality among long-stay psychiatric patients in Northern Finland. *Social Psychiatry and Psychiatric Epidemiology*, **38**, 297–304.

Reynolds, T., Thornicroft, G., Abas, M. *et al.* (2000). Camberwell Assessment of Need for the Elderly (CANE): development, validity and reliability. *British Journal of Psychiatry*, **176**, 444–52.

Ritchie, C.W., Chiu, E., Harrigan, S. *et al.* (2003). The impact upon extra-pyramidal side effects, clinical symptoms and quality of life of a switch from conventional to atypical antipsychotics (risperidone or olanzapine) in elderly patients with schizophrenia. *International Journal of Geriatric Psychiatry*, **18**, 432–40.

Rosenberg, S.D., Goodman, L.A., Osher, F.C. *et al.* (2001). Prevalence of HIV, hepatitis B and hepatitis C in people with severe mental illness. *American Journal of Public Health*, **91**, 31–7.

Royal College of Psychiatrists (2002). *Catering for people who enter old age with enduring or relapsing mental illness ('graduates')*. Council Report CR110. Royal College of Psychiatrists, London.

Schultz, S.K., Miller, D.D., Oliver, S.E., Arndt, S., Flaum, M., and Andreasen, N.C. (1997). The life course of schizophrenia: age and symptom dimensions. *Schizophrenia Research*, **23**, 15–23.

Stergiopoulos, V. and Herrmann, N. (2003). Old and homeless: a review and survey of older adults who use shelters in an urban setting. *Canadian Journal of Psychiatry*, **48**, 374–80.

Strauss, J.S. and Carpenter, W.T., Jr (1972). The prediction of outcome in schizophrenia. I. Characteristics of outcome. *Archives of General Psychiatry*, **27**, 739–46.

Tollefson, G.D., Beasley, C.M., Tran, P.V. *et al.* (1997). Olanzapine versus haloperidol in the treatment of schizophrenia and schizoaffective disorder: results of an international collaborative trial. *American Journal of Psychiatry*, **154**, 457–65.

Trieman, N., Wills, W., and Leff, J. (1996). TAPS Project 28: does reprovision benefit elderly long-stay mental patients? *Schizophrenia Research*, **21**, 199–208.

Tsuang, M., Woolson, R., and Fleming, J. (1979). Long-term outcome of major psychoses: I. Schizophrenia and affective disorders compared with psychiatrically symptom-free surgical conditions. *Archives of General Psychiatry*, **36**, 1295–301.

Twamley, E.W., Doshi, R.R., Nayak, G.V. *et al.* (2002). Generalized cognitive impairments, ability to perform everyday tasks, and independence in community living situations of older patients with psychosis. *American Journal of Psychiatry*, **159**, 2013–20.

Waddington, J.L. (1995). Psychopathological and cognitive correlates of tardive dyskinesia in schizophrenia and other disorders treated with neuroleptics drugs. In *Behavioral neurology of movement disorders* (ed. W.J. Weiner and A.E. Lang), pp. 211–29. Raven Press, New York.

Waddington, J.L. and Youssef, H.A. (1996). Cognitive dysfunction in chronic schizophrenia followed prospectively over 10 years and its longitudinal relationship to the emergence of tardive dyskinesia. *Psychological Medicine*, **26**, 681–8.

Wahlbeck, K., Cheine, M.V., and Essali, A. (1999) Clozapine versus typical neuroleptic medication for schizophrenia. Cochrane Database of Systematic Reviews 1999, Issue 4, Art. No. CD000059. DOI: 10.1002/14651858.

Wetherell, J.L., Palmer, B.W., Thorp, S.R., Patterson, T.L., Golshan, S., and Jeste, D.V. (2003). Anxiety symptoms and quality of life in middle-aged and older outpatients with schizophrenia and schizoaffective disorder. *Journal of Clinical Psychiatry*, **64**, 1476–82.

White, L., Parrella, M., McCrystal-Simon, J., Harvey, P.D., Masiar, S.J., and Davidson, M. (1997). Characteristics of elderly psychiatric patients retained in a state hospital during downsizing: a prospective study with replication. *International Journal of Geriatric Psychiatry*, **12**, 474–80.

Wing, J.K. (1989). The concept of negative symptoms. *British Journal of Psychiatry*, **155**(Suppl. 7), 10–14.

Wing, J.K. (1992). *Epidemiologically-based mental health needs assessment. Review of research on psychiatric disorders (ICD10, F2-F6)*. Royal College of Psychiatrists, College Research Unit, London.

Wing, J.K. and Brown, G.W. (1970). *Institutionalism and schizophrenia*. Cambridge University Press, London.

Woodward, N.D., Purdon, S.E., Meltzer, H.Y., and Zald, D.H. (2005). A meta-analysis of cognitive change to clozapine, olanzapine, quetiapine and risperidone in schizophrenia. *International Journal of Neuropsychopharmacology*, **8**, 457–72.

# 34

# Alcohol and substance abuse in older people

Henry O'Connell and Brian Lawlor

## Introduction

### Alcohol use disorders

Alcohol use disorders (AUDs) are common in older people and are associated with considerable morbidity and mortality. However, clinical practice, medical research, public-health initiatives, and media attention focus primarily on how such problems affect younger people, partly because of the more clinically 'silent' nature of AUDs in older people. As a result, AUDs are less likely to be detected in older people because of a general lack of awareness and knowledge of elderly specific aspects of clinical presentation and the use of inappropriate screening instruments and diagnostic criteria that are geared towards younger people. Furthermore, even when such problems are detected in older people, they are less likely than younger people to be treated adequately or referred on to specialist treatment facilities (Khan *et al.*, 2002; O'Connell *et al.*, 2003a).

The ageing of populations worldwide means that the absolute number of older people with AUDs is on the increase and, due to worldwide cultural changes in the past three to four decades, cohorts of people reaching old age in the coming years are likely to have higher prevalence rates of AUDs than the current generations of older people.

Morbidity associated with AUDs in older people affects practically all aspects of the individual's physical, psychiatric, cognitive, and social health and well-being, and makes a substantial contribution to premature mortality. Such morbidity and mortality also has significant knock-on effects for the individual's family and carers, for healthcare professionals and service planners, and for society in general.

Therefore, it is imperative that increased attention at all levels be focused on this important area, with the aims of increasing detection rates and providing accessible, specialized, and effective treatment services, thereby preventing the development of a 'silent epidemic' of alcohol and substance use disorders in older people (Reid and Anderson, 1997; O'Connell *et al.*, 2003a).

### Medication use disorders in older people

Older people use more medications and are at a higher risk of medication use disorders (MUDs) than any other age group (Chutka *et al.*, 2004). High levels of prescribing of both psychotropic and non-psychotropic medications for older people, which may at times be inappropriate, along with variable compliance, altered pharmacokinetics, reduced functional ability, and increased levels of physical, psychiatric, and cognitive morbidity means that older people are at higher risk of developing MUDs than any other age group. As with AUDs, clinical features of MUDs may be atypical and masked by other conditions and thus go undetected and untreated (Beers *et al.*, 2000).

### Illicit drug use in older people

Illicit drug use in older people is far less of a problem in comparison to AUDs and MUDs and so will receive less attention in this chapter. However, there is emerging evidence that, as with AUDs, generations of people reaching old age in the coming decades may carry with them higher levels of illicit drug use than current and past generations of older people (Patterson and Jeste, 1999). Principles similar to those seen with AUDs and MUDs apply, in that lower levels of drug intake are required to cause harm and presentation may be atypical and thus go undetected.

### Chapter outline

This chapter covers the many elderly specific aspects of alcohol and substance use disorders and is divided in two ways. Firstly, apart from the introduction and conclusions, there are seven main sections: 'Definitions and diagnosis', 'Epidemiology', 'Aetiology, risk factors, and associations', 'Clinical features and co-morbidity', 'Clinical assessment, investigations, and screening', 'Management and prevention', and finally 'Prognosis'. Secondly, each of these seven sections is further divided into three subsections, relating to alcohol use disorders (AUDs), medication use disorders (MUDs) and the abuse of illicit substances. We have also discussed smoking in older people at the end of the chapter.

## Definitions and diagnosis

### Alcohol use disorders in older people

Alcohol use disorders (AUDs) is a general term used to include the wide spectrum of problems associated with alcohol use, from excessive consumption of alcohol above recommended 'safe' or 'healthy' levels of intake to harmful use and alcohol dependence.

Most research and clinical descriptions of alcohol status describe individuals as belonging to one of five main alcohol categories: abstinent (for a specified period of time or for their entire lifetime);

---

**Box 34.1** ICD-10 mental and behavioural disorders due to psychoactive substance use

F10.　Mental and behavioural disorders due to use of alcohol
F11.　Mental and behavioural disorders due to use of opioids
F12.　Mental and behavioural disorders due to use of cannabinoids
F13.　Mental and behavioural disorders due to use of sedatives or hypnotics
F14.　Mental and behavioural disorders due to use of cocaine
F15.　Mental and behavioural disorders due to use of other stimulants, including caffeine
F16.　Mental and behavioural disorders due to use of hallucinogens
F17.　Mental and behavioural disorders due to use of tobacco
F18.　Mental and behavioural disorders due to use of volatile solvents
F19.　Mental and behavioural disorders due to multiple drug use and use of other psychoactive substances

---

moderate drinkers, i.e. individuals who drink within recommended 'safe' or 'healthy levels' and who do not have criteria for heavy use or other AUD; individuals with 'heavy use' of alcohol (i.e. those who drink above recommended levels but without obvious negative social, behavioural or health consequences); individuals with alcohol dependence syndrome (see Boxes 34.4 and 34.5), and a fifth group whose alcohol use is problematic but milder in severity than dependence. These latter individuals may be described as being problem drinkers or having harmful use (ICD-10) or abuse (DSM-IV) of alcohol (see Box 34.3). 'Binge drinkers', i.e. individuals who do not fulfil criteria for alcohol dependence syndrome but who have a pattern of regular heavy drinking sessions associated with adverse health consequences may also be included in the latter group.

The ICD-10 (World Health Organization, 1992) and DSM-IV (American Psychiatric Association, 1994) use largely similar diagnostic criteria (see Boxes 34.4 and 34.5) and we will refer mainly to ICD-10 criteria in this chapter. AUDs and problems associated with use of other substances form section F1 of the ICD-10, 'Mental and behavioural disorders due to psychoactive substance use' (see Box 34.1).

---

**Box 34.2** ICD-10 criteria for acute intoxication

G1.　There must be clear evidence of recent use of a psychoactive substance (or substances) at sufficiently high dose levels to be consistent with intoxication.
G2.　There must be symptoms or signs of intoxication compatible with the known actions of the particular substance (or substances), as specified below, and of sufficient severity to produce disturbances in the level of consciousness, cognition, perception, affect, or behaviour that are of clinical importance.
G3.　Symptoms or signs present cannot be accounted for by a medical disorder unrelated to substance use and not better accounted for by another mental or behavioural disorder.

Acute intoxication frequently occurs in persons who have more persistent alcohol or drug-related problems in addition. Where there are such problems, e.g. harmful use, dependence syndrome, or psychotic disorder, they should also be recorded.

---

**Box 34.3** ICD-10 criteria for harmful use

A. There must be clear evidence that the substance use was responsible for (or substantially contributed to) physical or psychological harm, including impaired judgement or dysfunctional behaviour.
B. The nature of the harm should be clearly identifiable (and specified).
C. The pattern of use has persisted for at least 1 month or has occurred repeatedly within a 12-month period.
D. The disorder does not meet the criteria for any other mental or behavioural disorder related to the same drug in the same time period (except for acute intoxication).

---

The general criteria for harmful use and dependence syndrome for all substances, including alcohol, are given in Boxes 34.3–34.5. ICD-10 states that identification of the psychoactive substance (alcohol or otherwise) should be based on as many sources as possible. These include self-report data, analysis of blood and other body fluids, characteristic physical and psychological symptoms, clinical signs and behaviour, and other evidence such as a drug being in the patient's possession or reports from informed third parties.

An individual's drinking status is not static and may vary throughout life, because of changes in life circumstances and health characteristics. For example, individuals with alcohol dependence syndrome in their younger years may quit alcohol use completely

---

**Box 34.4** ICD-10 criteria for dependence syndrome

Three or more of the following manifestations should have occurred together for at least 1 month or, if persisting for periods of less than 1 month, should have occurred together repeatedly within a 12-month period:
1. A strong desire or sense of compulsion to take the substance.
2. Impaired capacity to control substance-taking behaviour in terms of its onset, termination, or levels of use, as evidenced by the substance being often taken in larger amounts or over a longer period than intended, or by a persistent desire or unsuccessful efforts to reduce or control substance use.
3. A physiological withdrawal state when substance use is reduced or ceased, as evidenced by the characteristic withdrawal syndrome for the substance, or by use of the same (or closely related) substance with the intention of relieving or avoiding withdrawal symptoms.
4. Evidence of tolerance to the effects of the substance, such that there is a need for significantly increased amounts of the substance to achieve intoxication or the desired effect, or a markedly diminished effect with continued use of the same amount of the substance.
5. Preoccupation with substance use, as manifested by important alternative pleasures or interests being given up or reduced because of substance use; or a great deal of time being spent in activities necessary to obtain, take, or recover from the effects of the substance.
6. Persistent substance use despite clear evidence of harmful consequences, as evidenced by continued use when the individual is actually aware, or may be expected to be aware, of the nature and extent of harm.

---

**Box 34.5** DSM-IV criteria for dependence syndrome

As with ICD-10, three or more of the criteria listed below must have been met in the previous 12 months to constitute a diagnosis of substance dependence.

1. Tolerance, as defined by either of the following:
   (a) need for markedly increased amounts of substance to achieve intoxication or desired effect; or
   (b) markedly diminished effect with continued use of the same amount of the substance.
2. Withdrawal, as manifested by either of the following:
   (a) characteristic withdrawal syndrome for the substance; or
   (b) the same (or a closely related) substance is taken to relieve avoiding withdrawal symptoms.
3. The substance is often taken in larger amounts or over a longer period than was intended.
4. There is a persistent desire or unsuccessful efforts to cut down or control substance use.
5. A great deal of time is spent in activities necessary to obtain the substance (e.g. visiting multiple doctors or driving long distances), using the substance (e.g. chain smoking), or recovering from its effects.
6. Important social, occupational, or recreational activities are given up or reduced because of substance use.
7. Substance use is continued despite knowledge of having a persistent physical or psychological problem that is likely to have been caused or exacerbated by the substance (e.g. current cocaine use despite recognition of cocaine-induced depression, or continued drinking despite a peptic ulcer made worse by alcohol consumption).

---

and be described as alcohol abstainers in their later years, but continue to have some of the adverse health characteristics of individuals with active alcohol dependence syndrome, such as residual physical or psychological health problems, social and occupational impairments acquired when their AUD was active, or inherent personality traits such as impulsivity, hyperactivity, or antisocial personality traits that put them at risk for other physical and mental health problems. The presence of these so-called 'sick-quitters' among non-drinkers in observational studies may in part explain the less favourable health characteristics of alcohol abstainers in comparison to moderate drinkers (see the section 'Alcohol use and health'). Furthermore, such individuals may be at risk of developing a relapse of their AUD in the context of health problems or changes in social circumstances in later life.

---

**Box 34.6** ICD-10 criteria for withdrawal state

G1. There must be clear evidence of recent cessation or reduction of substance use after repeated, and usually prolonged and/or high-dose, use of that substance.
G2. Symptoms and signs are compatible with the known feature of a withdrawal state from the particular substance or substances.
G3. Symptoms and signs are not accounted for by a medical disorder unrelated to substance use, and not better accounted for by another mental or behavioural disorder.

---

**Box 34.7** Definitions of a standard drink

A standard drink of beverage alcohol is equivalent to 12 fl oz (US 355 ml) domestic beer (alcohol content about 4%), a 5 fl oz (US 148 ml) glass of table wine (about 12% alcohol) or a mixed drink containing 1 to 1.5 fl oz (US 29–40 ml) hard liquor (about 40% alcohol).

---

Definitions of a unit of alcohol are given in Box 34.7. The recommended upper limits of alcohol intake are 14 units per week for women and 21 units per week for men, according to the Royal Colleges Report (1995). These units should not all be consumed at the one sitting. However, these recommendations relate to the general population of all ages, and 'safe' or 'healthy' levels of intake are likely to be lower for older people. Within the broadly defined group of older people, spanning as it does four decades in age, even more detailed recommendations should apply. For example, a 90-year-old woman who has multiple medical problems is unlikely to tolerate the same amount of alcohol as a fit and healthy 65-year-old man. The National Institute of Alcohol Abuse and Alcoholism recommends no more than one drink per day for older people (NIAAA, 1998) but there are no such elderly specific criteria in Europe.

There are no elderly specific criteria for AUDs described by the ICD-10 or DSM-IV. Therefore, in applying existing diagnostic criteria, AUDs in older people may be missed, as elderly people may not display classical symptoms or signs of AUDs seen in younger people such as a craving or compulsion, and signs of intoxication, changes in tolerance, withdrawal states, and other diagnostic criteria for AUDs may be atypical or masked by other health problems. Furthermore, older people may not experience the same degree of legal, family, and occupational problems associated with AUDs as seen in adults of working age, and biophysical screening measures for AUDs such as mean corpuscular volume and abnormal liver function tests may not be as sensitive in older people. Elderly people with covert AUDs may present with a wide range of seemingly unrelated problems such as unexplained falls and fractures, confusion, treatment-resistant depression, and adverse drug reactions, and the underlying AUD is likely to go undetected unless a high degree of clinical suspicion is maintained (see Table 34.2).

A stereotypical idea of the 'down and out' alcoholic with a high consumption of alcohol is also likely to lead to missed diagnoses, as older people may experience significant health problems even at relatively low levels of intake, or experience new problems in later life due to age-related reductions in tolerance, even while continuing a lifelong pattern of moderate consumption.

## Medication use disorders in older people

As with AUDs, older people are affected by a wide range of types and severity of medication use disorders (MUDs). Broadly speaking, medications may be divided into prescription-only (generally more potentially toxic) and 'over the counter' (OTC) medications. However, such a distinction may be arbitrary, as people of all ages, including older people, may experience significant problems with abuse of common OTC medications such as paracetamol or cough mixtures containing codeine.

A more useful distinction may be to divide medications into psychotropic (abuse associated more with neuropsychiatric effects) and non-psychotropic. The ICD-10 uses the same general principles of intoxication, harmful use, dependence, and withdrawal state that apply to alcohol for use of sedative and hypnotic medications (see Boxes 34.2–34.6). As with AUDs, elderly specific criteria are not cited, but the same general principles apply: older people are likely to experience harm at lower levels of use and clinical features guiding diagnosis are more likely to be atypical and masked by other health problems.

Furthermore, MUDs may be conceptualized as arising from over-use, under-use, or inappropriate use of medications (Beers *et al.*, 2000). Over-use occurs when a drug is used when no drug should be used at all. Drug misuse occurs when the wrong drug is used or a drug is used at the wrong dose, at the wrong schedule, or for the wrong duration. Under-use occurs when a drug is not used, although it is indicated.

MUDs may be further complicated due to interactions with alcohol (taken only at moderate levels or in the context of an AUD) or with illegal drugs. For example, an older person on anticoagulant treatment may be unknowingly doing themselves harm, even if their alcohol intake is moderate.

### Abuse of illicit substances in older people

ICD-10 defines specific diagnostic criteria for intoxication, harmful use, dependence, and withdrawal state for a wide range of illegal substances, including opioids, cannabinoids, cocaine, other stimulants including caffeine, hallucinogens, tobacco, and volatile solvents (see Box 34.1). As with AUDs, these diagnostic criteria may not be applicable for older people, as older people may experience harm at lower levels of use, they may not display classical features of craving or compulsion, and intoxication and withdrawal states may be masked by other medical or neuropsychiatric conditions. As with AUDs, low levels of clinical suspicion are likely to apply to older people.

## Epidemiology

### Epidemiology of alcohol use disorders in older people

Alcohol use disorders are common in older people and are associated with significant morbidity and mortality. However, the real prevalence of AUDs in older people is often underestimated for a variety of reasons, as outlined in Box 34.8.

---

**Box 34.8** Reasons for underdetection and misdiagnosis of AUDs in older people

- Older people and their families and carers are reluctant to disclose alcohol use and AUDs.
- Inaccurate recall of alcohol intake due to cognitive impairment.
- Lack of clinical suspicion on part of healthcare workers.
- Atypical and masked clinical presentation.
- Use of inappropriate screening and diagnostic instruments.
- Recommended levels of alcohol intake are inappropriately high for older people.
- Reduced likelihood of referral of older people for specialist AUD treatment.
- Therapeutic pessimism/nihilism.
- Alcohol use and AUDs in later life perceived as 'a comfort' and 'understandable'.

---

High proportions of community-dwelling older people have been reported to drink alcohol. For example, in one study of community-dwelling older people in the USA, 62% were found to drink alcohol (Mirand and Welte, 1996). However, levels of alcohol use vary widely between different populations of older people and are likely to be influenced by numerous psychosocial and socio-demographic factors such as age, clinical characteristics, social class, ethnicity, and religion.

Rates of recent alcohol use have been noted to decline after the age of 55, to 25% of people age 85 and older (Ruchlin, 1997) and, in general, levels of alcohol use and the prevalence of AUDs decline with age (Temple and Leino, 1989; Adams *et al.*, 1990; Adams and Cox, 1995). However, there have also been reports of stable (Ekerdt *et al.*, 1989) or increased (Gordon and Kannel, 1983) levels of alcohol consumption in later life.

The general decline in prevalence of AUDs with age may be due to a number of factors, including the premature deaths of those with early onset AUDs. Furthermore, age-related changes in pharmacokinetics leading to reduced physiological reserve, along with an increased prevalence of medical conditions and disabilities, may also lead to lower levels of alcohol intake in older people. Psychosocial factors such as diminished social networks, social isolation, and financial problems may also lead to reduced alcohol intake, although these factors may also lead to increased alcohol intake. An age cohort effect may exist, with the prevalence of AUDs differing between different generations, depending on the socio-cultural norms of the time. In the USA, for example, individuals reared in the Prohibition era of the 1920s, when alcohol use was outlawed and stigmatized, are likely to drink less than the so-called 'baby-boomer' generation who grew up in the more liberal climate of the 1960s and who will start to reach the age of 65 in 2011. AUDs at all levels of severity are far commoner in men than women, generally by a factor of four to six times. Other socio-demographic factors may include socio-economic group and geographical setting (i.e. urban or rural), although these relationships are not clear in older people.

Culture and ethnicity are important associations of AUDs in general adult populations and these factors are also likely to be important in older people. Therefore levels of AUDs are likely to be lower in religious or ethnic groups where alcohol use is strictly sanctioned or not allowed, such as among Muslims and Orthodox Jews. In the UK, alcohol related mortality may be marginally elevated in people of Caribbean origin, and is substantially higher in people of Irish and Indian origin (Harrison *et al.*, 1997).

The prevalence of AUDs in older people also varies depending on the restrictiveness of diagnostic criteria used and the clinical and socio-demographic characteristics of the population being studied. For example, the prevalence rate for 'excessive alcohol consumption' in a particular population will be higher than that for alcohol dependence syndrome. Community-based studies estimate the prevalence of alcohol misuse or dependence among older people as 2–4% (Adams and Cox, 1995) with much higher rates of 16% (men) and 2% (women) when looser criteria such as excessive alcohol consumption are used (UK National Digital Archive of Datasets, 1994; Greene *et al.*, 2003). Likewise, the prevalence of AUDs is higher in clinical populations such as medical or psychiatric inpatients than among primary care attendees or normal community-dwelling populations. For example, the prevalence of AUDs is higher among elderly inpatients, with estimates of 14%

for emergency department patients (Adams *et al.*, 1992), 18% for nursing home residents (Joseph *et al.*, 1995), and 23% for psychiatric inpatients (Speer and Bates, 1992).

It has been estimated that two-thirds of older people with AUDs started drinking at a younger age, with the remaining one-third having 'late onset' AUDs (Council on Scientific Affairs, 1996). Apart from the timing of onset of AUD, other key differences, with implications for clinical outcome, have also been noted to exist between these two groups: individuals with early onset AUDs are more likely to have a positive family history of AUDs, they are more likely to have antisocial personality traits, and they are more likely to have more severe AUDs with greater associated damage to their physical and psychological health and social networks. As a result, individuals with early onset AUDs may be more difficult to engage in treatment (Liberto and Oslin, 1995). In contrast, those with late onset AUDs may have higher levels of income and education and more circumscribed AUDs triggered by discrete stressful life events such as bereavement or retirement (LaGreca *et al.*, 1988). There is evidence to suggest that those with late onset AUDs have better clinical outcomes (Schutte *et al.*, 1994).

### Epidemiology of medication use disorders in older people

Older people receive more prescriptions than any other age group, and are also more likely to be dispensed multiple drug regimens (Patterson and Jeste, 1999; McGrath *et al.*, 2005). For example, although older people comprise 13% of the US population, they have been estimated to use more than 30% of prescription (Williams and Lowenthal, 1992; Avorn, 1995) and 35% of OTC drugs (Williams and Lowenthal, 1992). It has been estimated that older people use prescription and OTC medications approximately three times as much as the general population and that the estimated annual expenditure on prescription drugs by older people is four times that of younger people (Anderson *et al.*, 1993; Jeste and Palmer, 1998). While polypharmacy may be appropriate and clinically indicated in older people, the risk of adverse drug reactions has been reported to double when utilization increases from one to four medications, and the risk increases 14-fold when seven drugs are used (Cadieux, 1989; Chrischilles *et al.*, 1992). It has been estimated that older people in the USA use 5.8 prescription drugs concurrently along with 3.2 OTC drugs (Williams and Lowenthal, 1992; Sintonen, 1994; Avorn, 1995).

These high levels of medication use, along with age-related impairments in pharmacokinetics, the high levels of polypharmacy (either appropriate or not), and the fact that older people are more likely to be on long-term medications (e.g. antidiabetic or cardiovascular medication) as opposed to short-term medications (e.g. a single course of antibiotics) than is the case in younger people, mean that older people are far more likely to experience MUDs than younger people, even when medications are taken as directed. Added to this, as outlined in the previous section, medications may be over-used, under-used, used inappropriately, or used in combination with substances such as alcohol or illegal drugs that may lead to harmful drug interactions.

Benzodiazepines are the most commonly prescribed psychotropic drugs in older people, with one study of community-dwelling older people in Ireland demonstrating that 17% of participants were prescribed benzodiazepines, with use in females being twice that in males, and 18% of benzodiazepine users taking at least one other psychotropic drug. Furthermore, 52% of benzodiazepine users were prescribed a long-acting benzodiazepine (Kirby *et al.*, 1999a). It has also been reported that depression in older community-dwelling people is more likely to be detected if accompanied by anxiety symptoms, and such individuals are at risk of inappropriate treatment with benzodiazepines (Kirby *et al.*, 1999b).

Abuse of prescription drugs (most often sedative-hypnotics, anxiolytics, and analgesics) has been reported to account for 5% of visits to mental health clinic by community-dwelling elders (Jinks and Raschko, 1990) and 30% of residents of intermediate care facilities were reported as being prescribed long-acting drugs not recommended for older people (Beers *et al.*, 1988).

Misuse of drugs in older people due to poor prescribing practices is also a significant public-health problem, with 20% of community-dwelling older people receiving a drug considered inappropriate by experts and 40% of nursing home residents receiving inappropriate medication (Avorn and Gurwitz, 1995).

Use of opiate analgesia is common in older people and is liable to give rise to MUDs. Therefore, use of these medications should be carefully monitored, with due consideration of dose and careful tapering (Schneider, 2005).

### Epidemiology of illicit drug use

Lifetime prevalence rates for illicit drug dependence have been estimated as 17% for 18–29-year-olds, 4% for 30–59-year olds and less than 1% for those over the age of 60 (Hinkin *et al.*, 2002). Lifetime experience of cannabis in the 65–69-year-old age group in the UK has been reported to be 7 per 1000 (Lawlor *et al.*, 2003). The Epidemiological Catchment Area (ECA) Study found that fewer than 0.1% of older people (over the age of 65) met DSM-III criteria for illegal drug abuse or dependence in the previous month (Regier *et al.*, 1988), with corresponding rates for the same period of 3.5% for 18–24-year-olds. The ECA data suggest a lifetime prevalence rate for illegal drug use of only 1.6% for older people (Anthony and Helzer, 1991).

Several other sources of data suggest similarly low rates of illegal drug use among older people. However, the ageing of the 'baby-boomer' generation is likely to result in a cohort of older people who are healthier and have higher life expectancies than previous generations of older people, but who also carry with them higher rates of illegal drug use (Patterson and Jeste, 1999).

## Aetiology, risk factors, and associations

The aetiology, risk factors, and associations of AUDs, MUDs, and illegal substance use disorders all involve complex interactions between several factors. These factors may be described as being distal (e.g. positive family history of AUD) as opposed to proximal (e.g. recent bereavement leading to excessive drinking), they may be thought of as being fixed (e.g. female gender and risk of MUDs) as opposed to modifiable (e.g. rationalizing prescribed medication may reduce the risk of MUD), or they may be thought of as being biological/medical (e.g. age-related pharmacokinetic changes leading to relatively higher alcohol toxicity and increased risk of AUD), social (e.g. unemployed or divorced status and risk of AUDs), and psychological (e.g. antisocial personality traits or depression and risk of AUDs) in nature. Finally, risk factors can also be described in another three broad groupings: predisposing factors; factors that may increase substance exposure and consumption level; and

**Table 34.1** Risk factors for substance abuse in the elderly (from Atkinson, 2001)

| | |
|---|---|
| Predisposing factors | Family history (alcohol) |
| | Previous substance abuse |
| | Previous pattern of substance consumption (individual and cohort effects) |
| | Personality traits (sedative-hypnotics, anxiolytics) |
| Factors that may increase substance exposure and consumption level | Gender (men—alcohol, illicit drugs; women—sedative-hypnotics, anxiolytics) |
| | Chronic illness associated with pain (opioid analgesics), insomnia (hypnotic drugs), or anxiety (anxiolytics) |
| | Long-term prescribing (sedative-hypnotics, anxiolytics) |
| | Caregiver over-use of 'as needed' medication (institutionalized elderly) |
| | Life stress, loss, social isolation |
| | Negative affects (depression, grief, demoralization, anger) (alcohol) |
| | Family collusion and drinking partners (alcohol) |
| | Discretionary time, money (alcohol) |
| Factors that may increase the effects and abuse potential of substances | Age-associated drug sensitivity (pharmacokinetic, pharmacodynamic factors) |
| | Chronic medical illnesses |
| | Other medications (alcohol–drug, drug–drug interactions) |

factors that may increase the effects and abuse potential of substances (see Table 34.1).

## Aetiology, risk factors, and associations of AUDs in older people

### Biological/medical factors

While the genetics of AUDs is complex, involving the interaction of several genes (Buckland, 2001), we know that positive family history is a risk factor for AUDs in the general population and is also likely to be important in older people, in relation to both early onset (Dahmen et al., 2005) and late onset AUDs (Tiihonen et al., 1999). The genetic risk for AUDs may also overlap with risk for other mental disorders such as antisocial personality disorder, other drug use problems, anxiety disorders, and mood disorders (Nurnberger et al., 2004).

The higher prevalence of AUDs seen in clinical populations such as medical and psychiatric inpatients (see section on Epidemiology) implies that AUDs may arise as a consequence of medical conditions or indeed may play a part in the aetiology and perpetuation of medical conditions.

Age-related changes in pharmacokinetics and reductions in physiological reserve also mean that older people are more likely to encounter problems associated with alcohol intake even when consumed at moderate levels, along with having an increased risk of developing alcohol–drug interactions (NIAAA, 1998).

### Social factors

Social factors are involved in the aetiology of AUDs in older people as in all age groups, and these factors may have a two-way relationship with the development of AUDs (i.e. they may play a causative

role in the development of the AUD or arise as a consequence of the AUD).

Male gender is invariably found to be a risk factor for AUDs in all age groups and cultures, and this may simply reflect prevailing societal norms of heavier drinking among men that leads to an increased risk of developing AUDs. However, social characteristics may also reflect underlying biological/medical and psychological risk factors and associations (e.g. increased risk of AUDs in men may reflect their higher levels of antisocial personality disorder, a risk factor for AUDs in itself).

An age cohort effect may also exist, with the prevalence of AUDs differing between generations, depending on the socio-cultural norms of the time. Other important social factors include culture, ethnicity, social isolation, and marital status (see section on Epidemiology and Ekerdt et al., 1989; Bristow and Clare, 1992; Ganry et al., 2000).

### Psychological factors

Personality types and traits associated with AUDs may differ between 'early onset' and 'late onset' types. The 'early onset' type may have a stronger association with antisocial personality traits, hyperactivity, and impulsivity. 'Late onset' AUDs may have a stronger association with 'neuroticism' and depression (Mulder, 2002). Furthermore, there is emerging evidence that the personalities of lifelong non-drinkers may differ from those of moderate drinkers, being more introverted and more neurotic, thus explaining their poorer physical and psychological health characteristics as they appear on the J-shaped curve (O'Connell and Lawlor, 2005a).

AUDs in older people, as in all populations, may also have a two-way relationship with psychiatric disorders such as depression and anxiety disorders. For example, an older person may begin drinking in an effort to self-medicate depressive symptoms, or they may become depressed because of their drinking (Davidson and Ritson, 1993). Previous history of alcohol use or AUD is also important, as an individual with a resolved AUD from the past may relapse in later life in the context of changes in health characteristics or life circumstances.

AUDs are involved in the aetiology of cognitive impairment and dementia (see below), although the precise mechanisms are complex and not fully clear. However, clinical experience suggests that symptoms of AUDs may also be the first presenting problems of cognitive impairment or dementia in older people.

## Aetiology, risk factors and associations of MUDs in older people

The general principles for aetiology, risk factors, and associations for substance misuse outlined above (see Table 34.1) apply to MUDs. The much higher exposure of older people to prescribed medications (see Epidemiology above) along with age-related pharmacokinetic changes and co-morbid medical and neuropsychiatric conditions all interact to heighten the risk of MUDs in older people.

Biological and medical factors in the development of MUDs may include genetic predisposition (Nurnberger et al., 2004), chronic medical conditions requiring long-term prescribing of medication, such as pain (Helme and Katz, 1993), and age-related pharmacokinetic changes leading to an increased likelihood of developing adverse reactions to the use of medication (Beers et al., 2000). Interactions between prescribed medications and alcohol may also lead to MUDs.

The type of medication prescribed is also an important consideration. For example, benzodiazepines are among the medications most commonly implicated in MUDs in older people, and the risk of MUDs with benzodiazepines increases with higher drug potency, shorter elimination half-life, and longer duration of prescription (Kirby *et al.*, 1999a). The high prevalence of pain (estimated at 20–50% in the community-dwelling elderly; Barkin *et al.*, 2005) means that analgesics such as non-steroidal agents and opiates are likely to be misused in older people and lead to the development of MUDs.

Psychosocial factors identified to be associated with MUDs include older age, female gender, White race, lower educational level, and separated or divorced status (Swartz *et al.*, 1991). Other mental disorders associated with benzodiazepine dependence in the general population, and also likely to be relevant to older people, include depression, panic disorder, AUDs and abuse of other substances, generalized anxiety disorder, and personality disorders (Swartz *et al.*, 1991; Busto *et al.*, 1996).

## Aetiology, risk factors, and associations of illicit drug use in older people

Predictably, older opioid maintenance patients have been reported to have significantly more medical problems and worse general health, along with a later onset of use of illicit substances, than younger opioid patients (Lofwall *et al.*, 2005), and these findings are also likely to apply to older people who use other illegal drugs. Certain illegal drugs may be associated with particular conditions, such as the association seen between pain and abuse of opioids (Trafton *et al.*, 2004). As with AUDs and MUDs, genetic factors may play a role in the aetiology of illegal drug use in the general population and in older people (Kuhar *et al.*, 2001).

Important social factors may include gender (male gender being associated with a higher risk of illegal drug use), socio-economic status, and level of social supports and networks. Age cohort is also likely to be important, with 'baby-boomers' identified as carrying with them into later life a higher prevalence of illegal drug use than previous generations of older people (Patterson and Jeste, 1999).

Use of illegal drugs in the general population is associated with an increased prevalence of psychiatric illnesses and personality disorders, and this is also likely to be the case in older populations.

## Clinical features and co-morbidity

### Clinical features and co-morbidity in AUDs in older people

AUDs in older people are associated with significant morbidity and mortality, affecting practically all aspects of physical, neuropsychiatric, and social health and well-being, as summarized in Table 34.2 (Reid and Anderson, 1997; O'Connell *et al.*, 2003a).

### Physical aspects of AUDs in older people

Practically every organ system may be adversely affected by AUDs in older people, as outlined in Table 34.2. Pharmacokinetic changes in older people, with reduced physiological reserve, reduced metabolic efficiency, and an increased volume of distribution due to a higher fat to lean muscle ratio, means that alcohol intake in older people leads to relatively higher blood alcohol concentrations (Dufour and Fuller, 1995; Kalant, 1998). This increase in blood

**Table 34.2** Physical, neuropsychiatric, and socio-demographic aspects of AUDs in older people

| | |
|---|---|
| Gastrointestinal | Hepatic problems: elevated liver enzymes; fatty liver; alcoholic hepatitis; cirrhosis; malignancy<br>Gastritis, peptic ulcer disease, and bleeding<br>Oesophageal varices<br>Acute and chronic pancreatitis<br>Malignancies: mouth, pharynx, larynx, oesophagus, hepatic, colorectal, pancreatic |
| Cardiovascular | Ischaemic heart disease<br>Hypertension<br>Alcohol-induced arrhythmias<br>Congestive heart failure<br>Alcoholic cardiomyopathy |
| Haematological | Macrocytosis (acute effect of alcohol intake and due to vitamin $B_{12}$ and folate deficiency in chronic AUD)<br>Anaemia (due to gastrointestinal problems) |
| Musculoskeletal | Falls and fractures<br>Reduced bone density<br>Myopathy |
| Metabolic | Hypoglycaemia<br>Hyperuricaemia<br>Elevated lipids<br>Diabetes more difficult to control |
| Neuropsychiatric | Cognitive impairment and dementia<br>Frontal lobe impairment<br>Wernicke–Korsakoff syndrome<br>Cerebellar cortical degeneration<br>Central pontine myelinosis<br>Marchiafava–Bignami disease<br>Depression<br>Psychosis<br>Intoxication<br>Withdrawal syndrome (may be more difficult to treat in older people)<br>Suicide |
| Other: | Alcohol–drug interactions<br>Aspiration pneumonia<br>Road traffic and other accidents |
| Socio-demographic: | Male gender<br>Divorced, widowed, and single status<br>Social isolation<br>Upper and lower ends of socio-economic spectrum |

alcohol concentration is associated with a higher risk of intoxication and harmful effects. Furthermore, even when blood alcohol concentration is controlled for, alcohol-induced impairment in task performance has been demonstrated to increase with advancing age (Vogel-Sprott and Barrett, 1984).

These pharmacokinetic changes, along with the general effects of physical and cognitive ageing, increasing frailty, reduced functional ability, and higher levels of concomitant prescription drug use means that alcohol is relatively more toxic to older people than younger people. Furthermore, as outlined earlier, such toxic effects may be subtle and may be missed or mistaken for other conditions.

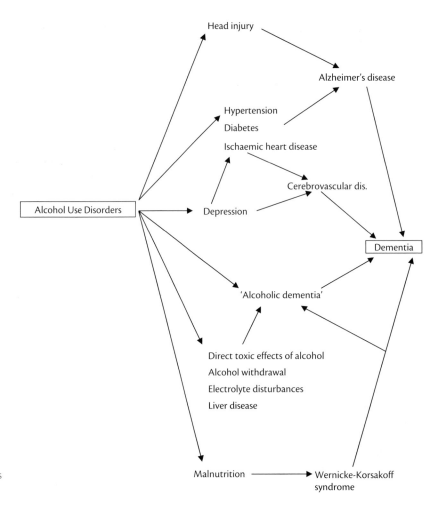

**Fig. 34.1** Relationship between AUDs and dementia.

## Neuropsychiatric aspects of AUDs in older people

AUDs in older people are associated with a wide range of mental disorders, such as depression, psychosis, withdrawal syndromes, cognitive impairment, and dementia (see Table 34.2). The relationship between alcohol use and brain damage and dementia is complex (Neiman, 1998; and see Fig. 34.1), in that AUDs may increase the risk for many types of dementia (Letenneur, 2004) and there also exist diagnostic entities known as 'alcohol-induced persisting dementia' (Box 34.9) and an amnesic syndrome associated with alcohol use (Box 34.10), while light to moderate alcohol use may protect against dementia (Ruitenberg *et al.*, 2002; see section on Alcohol use and health). Sulcal widening and ventricular enlargement have been cited as the strongest neuropathological findings in patients with 'alcohol-induced dementia', with additional evidence for peripheral neuropathy, ataxia, sparing of language, and improved prognosis when compared with other types of dementia (Smith and Atkinson, 1995).

There are several ways in which AUDs may cause cognitive impairment and dementia (see Fig. 34.1). AUDs may increase the risk for vascular dementia and Alzheimer's dementia, and these conditions probably account for most of the cognitive impairment and dementia seen in older people with AUDs. AUDs are also associated with the Wernicke–Korsakoff syndrome, an amnestic syndrome arising from thiamine deficiency due to AUDs or other causes.

AUDs in older people are frequently associated with other psychiatric disorders, most commonly depression. There may be a two-way interaction between mental disorders and alcohol use. For example, an individual with depression may begin to drink excessively, or excessive drinking may lead to depression (Davidson and Ritson, 1993). Thus, co-morbidity may arise as a result of cause or effect, i.e. older individuals who develop psychological problems in later life may drink alcohol as a form of 'self-medication' (i.e. 'late onset' AUD, see above), and put themselves at risk of developing an AUD, or individuals with AUDs may develop psychiatric disorders because of the physical, cognitive, or social consequences of their drinking. In general terms, the nature and severity of psychiatric co-morbidity is likely to differ between those with early and late onset AUDs, with the early onset group having higher levels of antisocial personality traits, a stronger family history, and more severe and complicated AUDs.

The Liverpool longitudinal community study (Saunders *et al.*, 1991) demonstrated that older men with a history of heavy drinking for 5 years or more at some time in their lives had a greater than five-fold increased risk of suffering from a psychiatric disorder. Furthermore, it was concluded that those with a current psychiatric diagnosis had significantly higher alcohol consumption and the association between heavy alcohol consumption in earlier years and psychiatric morbidity in later life was not simply explained by current drinking habits.

---

**Box 34.9** DSM-IV diagnostic criteria for alcohol-induced persisting dementia (APA, 1994)

**A.** The development of multiple deficits manifested by both:
1. Memory impairment (impaired ability to learn new information or to recall previously learned information); and
2. One or more of the following cognitive disturbances:
   (a) aphasia (language disturbance);
   (b) apraxia (impaired ability to carry out motor activities despite intact motor function);
   (c) agnosia (failure to recognize or identify objects despite intact sensory function); and/or
   (d) disturbance in executive functioning (i.e. planning, organization, sequencing, abstracting).

**B.** The cognitive deficits in criteria A1 and A2 each cause significant impairment in social or occupational functioning and represent a significant decline from a previous level of functioning.

**C.** The deficits do not occur exclusively during the course of a delirium and persist beyond the usual duration of alcohol intoxication or withdrawal.

**D.** There is evidence from the history, physical examination, or laboratory findings that the deficits are aetiologically related to the persisting effects of alcohol use.

---

In the USA, data from the National Longitudinal Alcohol Epidemiologic Survey demonstrated that major depression is three times commoner in the over 65s who have an AUD compared with those who do not (Grant and Harford, 1995) and in another survey 30% of an elderly population with AUDs were found to have concurrent psychiatric disorders (Moos *et al.*, 1998). These high levels of co-morbidity are also reflected in the observation that up to 50% of older psychiatric inpatients have been noted to be heavy users of alcohol (Atkinson and Schuckit, 1983; McGrath *et al.*, 2005).

Depression in older people with AUDs has a more complicated clinical course and has been demonstrated to be more severe and

---

**Box 34.10** Amnesic syndrome (due to alcohol or other substances) (WHO, 1992)

**A.** Memory impairment is manifest in both:
(1) a defect of recent memory (impaired learning of new material) to a degree sufficient to interfere with daily living; and
(2) a reduced ability to recall past experiences.

**B.** All of the following are absent (or relatively absent):
(1) defect in immediate recall (as tested, for example, by the digit span);
(2) clouding of consciousness and disturbance of attention, as defined in F05, criterion A of ICD-10;
(3) global intellectual decline (dementia).

**C.** There is no objective evidence from physical and neurological examination, laboratory tests, or history of a disorder or disease of the brain (especially involving bilaterally the diencephalic and medial temporal structures), other than that related to substance use, which can reasonably be presumed to be responsible for the clinical manifestations described under criterion A.

---

chronic in nature than depression without AUDs (Cook *et al.*, 1991). Such individuals may be less likely to present to or engage with mental health services and may be less compliant with any treatment strategies introduced.

Other psychiatric disorders, such as anxiety disorders, MUDs, and psychotic disorders are also important but less common co-morbidities of AUDs in older people.

In view of the high degree of psychiatric co-morbidity associated with AUDs in older people, it is not surprising that AUDs in older people are also strongly associated with suicide, due to interaction between the effects of drinking and other health factors such as depressive symptoms, medical illness, negatively perceived health status, and low social support (Blow *et al.*, 2004). In a Swedish retrospective case–control study, alcohol dependence or misuse as defined by DSM-IV was present in 35% of male and 18% of female suicides, in comparison to only 2% of male and 1% of female controls (Waern, 2003).

It must also be borne in mind that, even in the absence of a clinically diagnosable AUD, the neuropsychiatric effects of alcohol intoxication, (emotional changes, disinhibition, impulse dyscontrol, impaired judgement, and increased propensity for violent self-harm), may increase suicide risk: alcohol intoxication may be part of the individual's suicide plan, or intoxication may lead on to suicidal behaviour, particularly if the individual is currently experiencing psychological distress (O'Connell and Lawlor, 2005b).

## Clinical features and co-morbidity in MUDs in older people

Clinical features and co-morbidities associated with MUDs in older people will vary widely depending on the drug being used and patient characteristics such as age, gender, and presence of other physical and neuropsychiatric problems. An outline of clinical features and co-morbidities is given in Table 34.3.

## Clinical features and co-morbidity of illegal drug use in older people

As outlined in the section on Epidemiology, illegal drug use is uncommon in older people and there is thus a dearth of information on clinical features and co-morbidity. Such features will also vary widely depending on the drug in question and the mode of administration. For example, an elderly smoker of marijuana is likely to have different clinical features and co-morbidities from an elderly intravenous heroin user. As with AUDs and MUDs, clinical

**Table 34.3** Clinical features and co-morbidity associated with MUDs in older people

| Neuropsychiatric (all psychotropic drugs; benzodiazepines particularly prevalent) | Delirium<br>Day-time drowsiness<br>Sleep disturbance<br>Depression<br>Anxiety |
|---|---|
| Physical | Falls<br>Fractures<br>Drug–drug and drug–alcohol interactions<br>Problems related to drug metabolism (e.g. renal and hepatic impairment) |

features of illegal drug use in older people may be atypical and masked by other conditions, and problems are likely to arise at lower levels of drug use due to reduced physiological reserve, pharmacokinetic changes, and other physical and neuropsychiatric conditions.

# Clinical assessment, investigations, and screening

## Clinical assessment, investigations, and screening in AUDs

### Clinical assessment in AUDs

The assessment of AUDs in older people should be based on the standard clinical interview, mental state examination, physical examination, and collateral history if available and with the patient's consent. The standard interview and examination should be supplemented by specific questions relating to alcohol use, keeping in mind the potentially subtle and atypical nature of AUDs in older people. Questions should be framed in a sensitive and non-judgemental way, as patients may disengage and be lost to treatment and follow-up if they feel threatened by the assessment procedure.

The history should involve questions about current and past levels of alcohol use, frequency and quantity of intake, the types of alcoholic beverage consumed, and the context in which drinking takes place. Changes in levels of intake may be significant, and should be interpreted in the context of the overall history. For example, while an elderly individual may have reduced their level of alcohol intake in recent years, suggesting that they have no current AUD, this reduction may have occurred due to decreased tolerance to the effects of alcohol on a background history of a chronic AUD, and the person may continue to experience alcohol-related problems even at this lower level of intake.

Specific questions relating to the features of alcohol intoxication (Box 34.2), harmful use (Box 34.3), alcohol dependence (Boxes 34.4 and 34.5), and a previous history of alcohol withdrawals (Box 34.6) should be asked if indicated by the initial history and examination, along with specific questions relating to AUDs in older people (see Table 34.2). Concomitant medication and illegal drug use should be recorded. A family history of psychiatric illness should be elicited, focusing especially on AUDs and mood disorders. Relevant aspects of the personal and social history include early life experiences and exposure to AUDs in others, age of onset of drinking, occupational record, relationship history, and legal or forensic problems.

The mental state examination should take into account the level of alertness and a preliminary cognitive assessment or cognitive screening measure (e.g. Mini-Mental State Examination; Folstein et al., 1975); current mood state; any evidence of psychosis; ideas of hopelessness, suicide, or deliberate self-harm; and psychiatric manifestations of alcohol withdrawal (Box 34.6). The physical examination should include recording of vital signs such as blood pressure, pulse, temperature, and respiratory rate. Objective evidence of acute alcohol withdrawals should be recorded. A more detailed physical examination should be performed if indicated, focusing on the different organ systems involved in AUDs (see Table 34.2).

A collateral history is also very valuable for the overall assessment, as the person may underestimate their level of alcohol intake and associated AUD either deliberately because of embarrassment and reluctance to engage in treatment or because of faulty recall related to cognitive impairment.

### Investigations in AUDs

Following a detailed history and examination, other investigations may be indicated and should be directed by the patient's clinical status. For example, an individual admitted for treatment of alcohol withdrawals will require blood tests to check at least the following: urea and electrolytes; full blood count; liver function tests; vitamin $B_{12}$ and folate levels. Further investigations may also be indicated, depending on the clinical findings and the organ system involved (see Table 34.2). These may include the following: neuroimaging (CT or MRI brain); gastrointestinal investigations such as ultrasound, CT, or MRI examinations of the abdomen, upper gastrointestinal endoscopy, and liver biopsy; basic cardiovascular investigations such as electrocardiogram and other more detailed investigations if indicated, e.g. echocardiogram and 24-hour blood pressure monitoring.

Further psychological investigations include detailed neuropsychological assessment of cognition if impairment is detected in the initial assessment, as outlined above. Psychological assessment may also be required to assess the patient's suitability and level of motivation for addiction counselling or other psychotherapeutic interventions.

Social investigations include more detailed collateral histories if available, along with an assessment of financial status, social support, and accommodation arrangements.

### Screening for AUDs in older people

As already alluded to throughout this chapter, screening for AUDs in older people should focus on the broad spectrum of such problems and not merely clear-cut cases such as the 'down and out' alcoholic. Screening should also aim to detect the subtler but also damaging effects of AUDs in older people, such as drinking moderately while taking medications that interact with alcohol.

The main methods of screening used in older people involve self-report screening measures such as CAGE (Ewing, 1984) and AUDIT (Saunders, 1993) and elderly specific versions of self-report instruments (e.g. MAST-G; Blow, 1991), along with biophysical measures such as blood tests checking mean corpuscular volume and liver function tests. In practice, different screening measures are often used in the assessment of an individual. It is important to point out that screening instruments are designed to detect at-risk individuals but they are not diagnostic tools in themselves, their use may yield false positives and false negatives, and they should not serve as a substitute for a thorough clinical interview and examination.

A systematic review of self-report alcohol screening instruments in older people (O'Connell et al., 2004) found that CAGE (Ewing, 1984) was the most widely studied instrument, followed by MAST (Selzer, 1968) and variations of MAST, AUDIT (Saunders, 1993) and variations of AUDIT, and others. The sensitivity and specificity of self-report alcohol screening instruments was found to vary widely, depending on the prevalence of AUDs in the population under study, the clinical characteristics of the population, and the type of AUD being detected. The Cyr–Wartman (Cyr and Wartman, 1988) and CAGE questionnaires are the briefest tests and can be administered in less than 30 seconds, making these screening instruments the easiest to use. Far more research has focused on CAGE, and its sensitivity and specificity in older people are superior to those of the Cyr–Wartman questionnaire. Despite the advantage of ease of use of CAGE, deficiencies were highlighted in number of studies of elderly populations and AUDIT-5 (Philpot *et al.*, 2003), another brief test, may prove to be more useful in older people with psychiatric illness. ARPS and shARPS (Fink *et al.*, 2002) may prove to be more useful in older people with medical co-morbidity, but their use is limited by the fact that they take, respectively, 10 and 9 minutes to apply.

In order to use AUD screening in routine clinical practice, the demographic characteristics of the target population are an important consideration. For example, routinely screening all elderly women attending an active retirement centre may yield few cases of AUDs, and may prove to be a costly and intrusive exercise. However, screening of high-risk populations, such as elderly medical and psychiatric inpatients (see 'Epidemiology') is advised, as this practice may yield high levels of AUDs that direct the development of appropriate and much needed treatment services. Furthermore, ease of use, patient acceptability, and sensitivity and specificity of the screening instrument must all be taken into consideration.

As with self-report screening instruments, the utility of biophysical screening measures such as carbohydrate-deficient transferrin, liver function tests, or the mean corpuscular volume may be less reliable in older people (Luttrell *et al.*, 1997), because of higher levels of co-morbid physical illnesses leading in themselves to abnormal results.

### Clinical assessment, investigations, and screening for MUDs in older people

#### Clinical assessment in MUDs

As with AUDs, a standard clinical assessment involving a history, mental state and physical examination, and collateral history should be performed. A list of all prescribed and OTC medications being used, along with their indications for use, should be recorded. Ideally, the patient should be asked to bring with them all medications in their containers, as this will also give an indication as to levels of adherence or compliance. Any reported adverse effects should be recorded, along with symptoms and signs indicating under-use, over-use, or intermittent use of medication. Clinical features will vary depending on the medications being used.

#### Investigations in MUDs

Blood levels of some prescribed medications may be checked in order to assess levels of compliance and to establish whether the blood level is within the therapeutic window for the drug in question (e.g. lithium, carbamazepine). Other biophysical measures may also be indicated that provide proxy measures of medication compliance, such as random or fasting glucose levels and levels of glycosylated haemoglobin to assess for level of diabetes control and compliance with hypoglycaemic agents or insulin.

#### Screening in MUDs

There are no routinely used screening measures for MUDs in older people. However, use of a measure such as Beers' criteria (Beers, 1997) may be a useful addition to the overall assessment of an older person if a MUD is suspected. In a study updating Beers' criteria (Fick *et al.*, 2003), a modified Delphi method was used, which is a set of procedures and methods for formulating a group judgement for subject matter for which precise information is lacking.

Forty-eight individual medications or classes of medications that should be avoided were identified in older adults (Table 34.4) and medication to be avoided in older adults with 20 various diseases/conditions (Table 34.5). Sixty-six of the inappropriate medications identified were considered by the panel to have adverse outcomes of high severity.

### Clinical assessment, investigations, and screening for illicit drug use in older people

As with AUDs and MUDs, a thorough history of any current or past use of illicit drugs should be recorded, along with mental state and physical examinations and collateral history, if available. Further investigations will be directed by the type of drug or drugs used, the route of administration, and the clinical findings.

The low levels of illicit drug use in older people mean that screening is unwarranted in most populations except for those with particularly high risk, such as the homeless and prison inmates, or people already known to have AUDs and MUDs.

## Management and prevention

Management and prevention can be broadly divided into primary prevention, secondary prevention, and finally tertiary prevention or treatment. Primary prevention refers to the prevention of problems arising for the first time (e.g. late onset AUDs); secondary prevention aims to prevent the onset or worsening of problems in at-risk individuals (e.g. individuals with 'heavy use' of alcohol), and tertiary prevention refers to treatment for established problems (e.g. individuals with established alcohol dependence syndrome).

In considering the prevention of problems due to alcohol misuse it is important to be aware of the complex relationship between moderate alcohol consumption and health. Up to 100 epidemiological studies conducted since the 1970s have demonstrated that, in relation to physical, social, psychiatric, and cognitive health and well-being, light to moderate drinkers seem to be generally healthier than both non-drinkers and heavy drinkers or those with AUDs, a phenomenon that has been referred to as the J- or U-shaped curve (Doll *et al.*, 1994; O'Connell and Lawlor, 2005a). As a result, it has been argued that light to moderate consumption of alcohol, particularly red wine (the so-called 'French paradox'), has beneficial effects on health. Furthermore, there is some empirical evidence linking light to moderate alcohol intake and an improved profile of cardiovascular biomarkers (Rimm *et al.*, 1999).

However, there are a number of potential problems with the epidemiological evidence. Non-drinkers are a heterogeneous group, comprising both lifelong non-drinkers and individuals with a past history of AUD (so-called 'sick quitters'), and the latter group may be less healthy than moderate drinkers for reasons other than their current drinking habits (Shaper, 1995). The 'French paradox', whereby moderate intake of red wine has been proposed as the factor responsible for the lower levels of cardiovascular disease in the French compared with British and American populations, has also been questioned (Law and Wald, 1999). Moderate drinkers may also have other favourable physical (Shaper, 1995) and psychological health characteristics, such as differing personality type, in comparison with non-drinkers.

Furthermore, no controlled trials of light to moderate alcohol intake and effects on cardiovascular or other health characteristics

Table 34.4  Criteria for potentially inappropriate medication use in older adults: independent of diagnoses or conditions (from Fick et al., 2003, reproduced with permission)

| Drug | Concern | Severity rating (high or low) |
|---|---|---|
| Propoxyphene and combination products | Offers few analgesic advantages over acetaminophen, yet has the adverse effects of other narcotic drugs | Low |
| Indomethacin | Of all available nonsteroidal anti-inflammatory drugs, this drug produces the most CNS adverse effects | High |
| Pentazocine | Narcotic analgesic that causes more CNS adverse effects including confusion and hallucinations, more commonly than other narcotic drugs. Additionally it is a mixed agonist and antagonist | High |
| Trimethobenzamide | One of the least effective antiemetic drugs, yet it can cause extrapyramidal adverse effects | High |
| Muscle relaxants and antispasmodics: methocarbamol, carisoprodol, chlorzoxazone, metaxalone, cyclobenzaprine, and oxybutynin | Most muscle relaxants and antispasmodic drugs are poorly tolerated by elderly patients, since these cause anticholinergic adverse effects sedation, and weakness. Additionally, their effectiveness at doses tolerated by elderly patients is questionable | High |
| Flurazepam | This benzodiazepine hypnotic has an extremely long half-life in elderly patients (often days), producing prolonged sedation and increasing the incidence of falls and fracture. Medium-or short-acting benzodiazepines are preferable | High |
| Amitriptyline, chlordiazepoxide–amitriptyline, and perphenazine–amitriptylina | Because of its strong anticholinergic and sedation properties, amitriptyline is rarely the antidepressant of choice for elderly patients | High |
| Doxepin | Because of its strong anticholinergic and sedating properties, doxepin is rarely the antidepressant of choice for elderly patients | High |
| Meprobamate | This is a highly addictive and sedating anxiolytic. Those using meprobamate for prolonged periods may become addicted and may need to be withdrawn slowly | High |
| Doses of short-acting benzodiazepines: doses greater than lorazepam, 3 mg; oxazepam, 60 mg; alprazolam, 2 mg; temazepam, 15 mg; and triazolam, 0.25 mg | Because of increased sensitivity to benzoadiazepines in elderly patients smaller doses may be effective as well as safer. Total daily doses should rarely exceed the suggested maxima | High |
| Long-acting benzodiazepines: chlordiazepoxide, diazepam, etc | These drugs have a long half-life in elderly patients (often several days), producing prolonged sedation and increasing the risk of falls and fractures. Short- and intermediate-acting benzodiazepines are preferred if a benzodiazepine is required | High |
| Disopyramide | Of all antiarrhythmic drugs, this is the most potent negative inotrope and therefore may induce heart failure in elderly patients. It is also strongly anticholinergic. Other antiarrhythmic drugs should be used | High |
| Digoxin (should not exceed >0.125 mg/day except when treating atrial arrhythmias) | Decreased renal clearance may lead to increased risk of toxic effects | Low |
| Short-acting dipyridamole. Do not consider the long-acting dipyridamole (which has better properties than the short-acting in older adults) except with patients with artificial heart valves | May cause orthostatic hypotension | Low |
| Methyldopa and methyldopa-hydrochlorothiazide | May cause bradycardia and exacerbate depression in elderly patients | High |
| Reserpine at doses >0.25 mg | May induce depression impotence sedation and orthostatic hypotension | Low |
| Chlorpropamide | It has a prolonged half-life in elderly patients and could cause prolonged hypoglycemia. Additionally, it is the only oral hypoglycemic agent that causes SIADH | High |
| Gastrointestinal antispasmodic drugs: dicyclomic hyoscyamine (Levsin and Levsinex), propantheline, belladonna alkaloids, and clidinium– chloridiazepoxide | GI antispasmodicd drugs are highly anticholinergic and have uncertain effectiveness. These drugs should be avoided (especially for long-term use) | High |

Table 34.4 (cont.)

| Drug | Concern | Severity rating (high or low) |
|---|---|---|
| Anticholinergics and antihistamines: chlorpheniramine, diphenhydramine, hydroxyzine, cyproheptadine, promethazine, tripelennamine dexchlorphoniramine | All non-prescription and many prescription antihistamines may have potent anticholinergic properties. Non-anticholinergic antihistamines are preferred in elderly patients when treating allergic reactions | High |
| Diphenhydramine | May cause confusion and sedation. Should not be used as a hypnotic and when used to treat emergency allergic reactions, it should be used in the smallest possible dose | High |
| Ergot mesyloids and cyclandelate | Have not been shown to be effective in the doses studied | Low |
| Ferrous sulphate >325 mg/day | Doses >325 mg/day do not dramatically increase the amount absorbed but greatly increase the incidence of constipation | Low |
| All barbiturates (except phenobarbital) except when used to control seizures | Are highly addictive and cause more adverse effects than most sedative or hypnotic drugs in elderly patients | High |
| Meperidine | Not an effective oral analgesic in doses commonly used. Many cause confusion and has many disadvantages compared to other narcotic drugs | High |
| Ticlopidine | Has been shown to be no better than aspirin in preventing clotting and may be considerably more toxic. Safer more effective alternatives exist | High |
| Ketorolac | Immediate and long-term use should be avoided in older persons, since a significant number have asymptomatic GI pathological conditions | High |
| Amphetamines and anorexic agents | These drugs have potential for causing dependence, hypertension, angina, and myocardial infarction | High |
| Long-term use of full-dosage, longer half-life, non-COX-selective NSAIDs: naproxan, oxaprozin, and proxicam | Have the potential to produce GL bleeding renal failure, high blood pressure, and heart failure | High |
| Fluoxetine | Long half-life of drug and risk of producing excessive CNS stimulation sleep disturbances and increasing agitation. Safer alternatives exist | High |
| Long-term use of stimulant laxatives: bisacodyl cascara sagrada and Neoloid except in the presence of opiate analgestic use | May exacerbate bowel dysfunction | High |
| Amiodarone | Associated with QT interval problems and risk of provoking torsades de pointes. Lack of efficacy in older adults | High |
| Orphenadrine | Causes more sedation and anticholinergic adverse effects than safer alternatives | High |
| Guanethidine | May cause orthostatic hypotension. Safer alternatives exist | High |
| Guanadrel | May cause orthostatic hypotension | High |
| Cyclandelate | Lack of efficacy | Low |
| Isoxsurpine | Lack of efficacy | Low |
| Nitrofurantoin | Potential for renal impairment. Safer alternatives available | High |
| Doxazosin | Potential for hypotension, dry mouth, and urinary problems | High |
| Methyltestosterone | Potential for prostatic hypertrophy and cardiac problems | High |
| Thioridazine | Greater potential for CNS and extrapyramidal adverse effects | High |
| Mesoridazine | CNS and extrapyramidal adverse effects | High |
| Short acting nifedipine | Potential for hypotension and constipation | High |
| Clonidine | Potential for orthostatic hypotension and CNS adverse effects | Low |
| Mineral oil | Potential for aspiration and adverse effects. Safer alternatives available | High |
| Cimetidine | CNS adverse effects including confusion | Low |
| Ethacrynic acid | Potential for hypertension and fluid imbalances. Safer alternatives available | Low |

Table 34.4 (cont.)

| Drug | Concern | Severity rating (high or low) |
|---|---|---|
| Dessicated thyroid | Concerns about cardiac effects. Safer alternatives available | High |
| Amphetamines (excluding methylphenidate hydrochloride and anorexics) | CNS stimulant adverse effects | High |
| Estrogens only (oral) | Evidence of the carcinogenic (breast and endometrial cancer) potential of these agents and lack of caridoprotective effect in older women | Low |

Abbreviations: CNS, central nervous system; COX, cyclo-oxygenase; GI, gastrointestinal; NSAIDs, non-steroidal anti-inflammatory drugs; SIADH, syndrome of inappropriate antidiuretic hormone secretion.

**Table 34.5** Criteria for potentially inappropriate medication use in older adults: considering diagnoses or conditions (from Fick *et al.*, 2003, reproduced with permission)

| Disease or condition | Drug | Concern | Severity rating (high or low) |
|---|---|---|---|
| Heart failure | Disopyramide and high sodium content drugs [sodium and sodium salts (alginate bicarbonate, biphosphate, citrate phosphate, salicylate, and sulfate)] | Negative inotropic effect. Potential to promote fluid retention and exacerbation of heart failure | High |
| Hypertension | Phenylpropanclamine hydrochloride (removed from the market in 2001), pseudoephedrine diet pills, and amphetamines | May produce elevation of blood pressure secondary to sympathomimetic activity | High |
| Gastric or duodenal ulcers | NSAIDs and aspirin (>325 mg) (coxibs excluded) | May exacerbate existing ulcers or produce new/additional ulcers | High |
| Seizures or epilepsy | Clozapine, chlorpromazine, thioridazine, and thiothixene | May lower seizure thresholds | High |
| Blood clotting disorders or receiving anticoagulant therapy | Aspirin, NSAIDs, dipyridamole, ticlopidine, and clopidogrel | May prolong clotting time and elevate INR values or inhibit platelet aggregation, resulting in an increased potential for bleeding | High |
| Bladder outflow obstruction | Anticholinergics and antihistamines, gastrointestinal antispasmodics, muscle relaxants, oxybutynin, flavoxate, anticholinergics, antidepressants, decongestants, and tolterodine | May decrease urinary flow, leading to urinary retention | High |
| Stress incontinence | α-Blockers, anticholinergics, tricyclic antidepressants (imipramine hydrochloride, doxepin hydrochloride, and amitriptyline hydrochloride), and long-acting benzodiazepines | May produce polyuria and worsening of incontinence | High |
| Arrhythmias | Tricyclic antidepressants (imipramine hydrochloride, doxepin hydrochloride, and amitriptyline hydrochloride) | Concern due to pro-arrhythmic effects and ability to produce QT interval changes | High |
| Insomnia | Decongestants, theophylline, methylphenidate, MAOIs and amphetamines | Concern due to CNS stimulant effects | High |
| Parkinson's disease | Metoclopramide, conventional antipsychotics and tacrine | Concern due to their antidopaminergic cholinergic effects | High |
| Cognitive impairment | Barbiturates, anticholinergics, antispasmodics, and muscle relaxants. CNS stimulants: dextroAmphetamine, methylphenidate, methamphetamine and pemolin | Concern due to CNS-altering effects | High |
| Depression | Long-term benzodiazepine use. Sympatholytic agents: methyldopa, reserpine, and guanethidine | May produce or exacerbate depression | High |
| Anorexia and malnutrition | CNS stimulants: DextroAmphetamine, methylphenidate, methamphetamine, pemolin, and fluoxetine | Concern due to appetite-suppressing effects | High |
| Syncope or falls | Short- to intermediate-acting benzodiazepine and tricyclic antidepressants (imipramine hydrochloride, doxepin hydrochloride, and amitriptyline hydrochloride) | May produce ataxia, impaired psychomotor function, syncope, and additional falls | High |

**Table 34.5** (*cont.*)

| Disease or condition | Drug | Concern | Severity rating (high or low) |
|---|---|---|---|
| SIADH/hyponatraemia | SSRIs: fluoxetine, citalopram, fluvoxamine, paroxetine, and sertraline | May exacerbate or cause SIADH | Low |
| Seizure disorder | Bupropion | May lower seizure threshold | High |
| Obesity | Olanzapine | May stimulate appetite and increase weight gain | Low |
| COPD | Long-acting benzodiazepines: chlordiazepoxide, diazepam, etc. β-Blockers: propranolol | CNS adverse effects. May induce respiratory depression. May exacerbate or cause respiratory depression | High |
| Chronic constipation | Calcium channel blockers, anticholinergics, and tricyclic antidepressant (Imipramine hydrochloride, doxepin hydrochloride, and amitriptyline hydrochloride) | May exacerbate constipation | Low |

Abreviations: CNS, central nervous systems; COPD, chronic obstructive pulmonary disease; INR, international normalized ratio; MAOIs, monoamine oxidase inhibitors; NSAIDs, non-steroidal anti-inflammatory drugs; SIADH, syndrome of inappropriate antidiuretic hormone secretion;` SSRIs, selective serotonin reuptake inhibitors.

have been performed and such trials are likely to encounter ethical barriers due to the neuropsychiatric effects of alcohol and the existence of proven treatments in the form of conventional medication.

Therefore, despite the epidemiological and biochemical evidence for potential health benefits of light to moderate alcohol intake, there is insufficient evidence at present to support advising moderate alcohol intake for the entire population, particularly when the many potential harmful effects of excessive alcohol intake are considered.

## Management and prevention of AUDs

### Primary prevention

Primary prevention aims to prevent the development of *de novo* AUDs in older people. Primary prevention of AUDs in older people is important, considering that up to one in three older people with AUDs may have developed such problems for the first time in later life (Adams and Waskel, 1991). Clinicians should watch for the development of AUDs when an older person encounters stressful life circumstances and major changes or losses, particularly if that individual has a personal or family history of AUDs.

Primary prevention can also be seen as a strategy directed at the entire population, targeting factors such as ease of access to alcohol, restrictions on alcohol advertising, and education about the adverse effects of drinking. Such primary prevention and public health initiatives tend to be directed towards younger individuals, but they should also take into account the more clinically 'silent' AUDs that may develop in older people (O'Connell *et al.*, 2003b).

### Secondary prevention

Secondary prevention strategies should focus on older people who already have 'at-risk' drinking behaviour, either currently or in the past, and who are at risk of developing worsening problems in the context of diverse factors such as bereavement, social isolation, adjustment to retirement, and physical or psychiatric health problems. As with primary prevention, there should be a high index of clinical suspicion when assessing such people. There is emerging evidence that formalized brief psychological interventions in primary care may have a positive impact on AUDs in older people

(Blow and Barry, 2000; Fleming *et al.*, 1999). However, older people should also be referred on to specialist mental health and addiction services if problems persist.

### Tertiary prevention

Tertiary prevention involves treatment of existing AUDs. Treatment modalities can be divided into biological/medical, social, and psychological. Biological/medical treatments are most important in the acute setting, where detoxification may be required. In view of their increased physical frailty and evidence for more severe alcohol withdrawals in older people (Brower *et al.*, 1994), it is advisable to admit older people requiring detoxification, preferably to a medical ward, particularly if there is a history of alcohol withdrawal seizures or delirium tremens. Fluid and electrolyte imbalances should be corrected and cognitive state should be monitored regularly in view of the risk of developing delirium.

Care should be taken with benzodiazepine-assisted withdrawal in older people, in view of the elevated risk of over-sedation, confusion, and falls. There are no specific guidelines on benzodiazepine-assisted alcohol withdrawal in older people. However, it has been established that older people have more severe alcohol withdrawals and receive higher doses of chlordiazepoxide as a result (Liskow *et al.*, 1989). Lorazepam has been identified as the safest choice of benzodiazepine for treatment of alcohol withdrawal in older people, in view of the fact that advancing age and liver disease have little impact on its metabolism, and absorption by the intra-muscular route is predictable (Peppers, 1996). In practice, however, it is likely that there is more clinical experience with use of long-acting benzodiazepines, such as chlordiazepoxide. Use of an objective measure of alcohol withdrawal such as the Clinical Institute Withdrawal Assessment for Alcohol–Revised Version (CIWA-Ar; Taylor *et al.*, 2005) is advisable in defining the severity of alcohol withdrawal and monitoring the clinical course, although this scale is not elderly specific and areas such as 'orientation and clouding of sensorium' may be disproportionately affected in older people, especially if cognitive impairment is present (Naranjo and Sellers, 1986; see Box 34.11).

Parenteral or oral thiamine should be given to prevent development of the Wernicke–Korsakoff syndrome. A recent review has concluded

**Box 34.11** The Clinical Institute Withdrawal Assessment for Alcohol-Revised Version (CIWA-Ar (Taylor *et al.,* 2005)

Items 1–9 are scored from 0–7 and item 10 from 0–4. The maximum possible score is 67.
1. Nausea and vomiting
2. Tremor
3. Paroxysmal sweats
4. Anxiety
5. Agitation
6. Tactile disturbances
7. Auditory disturbances
8. Visual disturbances
9. Headaches and fullness in head
10. Orientation and clouding of sensorium

**Severity of alcohol withdrawal**

Mild: <10
Moderate: 10–20
Severe: 20+

that, in the emergency department setting, oral administration of thiamine is as effective as parenteral administration (Jackson and Teece, 2004). However, there are no elderly specific guidelines and individual patient characteristics must be taken into account, such as general health, ability to take oral medication, and compliance.

The three medications that are approved by the US Food and Drug Administration to promote abstinence and reduce relapse are disulfiram, acamprosate and naltrexone (Williams, 2005). However, the limited efficacy of disulfiram, combined with the potential for a more toxic side-effect profile, means that it is best avoided in older people. In contrast, naltrexone and acamprosate have been suggested as suitable agents for use in this age group (Barrick and Connors, 2002).

Social aspects of treatment include identifying and addressing problems in such diverse areas as personal finances, housing, employment, and levels of social contacts, because continuing problems in these areas may serve to perpetuate the AUD. Psychological treatments include specific psychotherapies focusing on AUDs (e.g. motivational interviewing, addiction counselling) and psychotherapies aimed at co-morbid mood or other psychiatric disorders. While there is little evidence on the effectiveness of psychotherapeutic approaches to addiction in older people, one review has concluded that only those studies involving behavioural and cognitive behavioural interventions have provided empirical support for treatment effectiveness (Schonfeld and Dupree, 1995). There is also some evidence that older people may respond better to psychotherapy in same-age settings, i.e. among other older people (Kofoed *et al.,* 1987; Schonfeld and Dupree, 1995), presumably because of a shared experience of the elderly specific aspects of AUDs.

The wide variety of elderly specific aspects of AUDs, along with a projected increase in the numbers of older people with AUDs in future years and evidence for improved treatment response in same-age settings, means that the development of screening programmes and treatment facilities geared towards older people, that may be based on population-defined sectors, is now needed. Such screening and treatment programmes should involve collaboration between old age psychiatry and geriatric medicine

and a multidisciplinary team should deliver treatment, targeting the many medical, social, and psychological aspects of AUDs in older people.

## Management and prevention of MUDs

### Primary prevention

Along with patients themselves, healthcare workers, family members, and carers all have important roles in the primary and secondary prevention of MUDs in older people. Prescriptions should be reviewed regularly with a view to simplification and rationalization if possible, and the practice of giving 'repeat prescriptions' without clinical assessment should be discouraged.

Community pharmacists should have an active role in advising on the appropriate use of prescription and OTC medications, in cautioning patients on inappropriate use and on interactions with alcohol and other medications, and in alerting the prescribing physician when over-use, under-use, or inappropriate use of medication (either iatrogenically or due to patient behaviour) is suspected.

Patients should be educated about all aspects of their medication: physical descriptions of the medication, the clinical indications, dose and frequency, and common side-effects. If the patient is unable to manage administration of their own medication due to cognitive or other impairments, then provision should be made for a family member or caregiver to arrange this.

Several physical and cognitive impairments affect the ability of an older person to open medicine containers. One study of older people age 81 years and older, living in the community and in institutions in Sweden (Beckman *et al.,* 20005), found that 14% were unable to open a screw cap bottle, 32% a bottle with a snap lid, and 10% a blister pack. Less than half of those who were unable to open one or more of the containers received help with their medication, and only 27% of those living in their own homes received help.

Dosette boxes may be useful, but it has been pointed out that those patients most in need of them are the least likely to be able to manage them, and problems may occur both with filling the devices and with the taking of medications from them (Levings *et al.,* 1999). One study found that the use of a combination pack for medication used to treat osteoporosis was associated with improved understanding of medication directions and improved patient satisfaction (Ringe *et al.,* 2006).

Active management of physical and psychiatric conditions also helps in primary prevention of MUDs. For example, adequate treatment of depression and anxiety should lead to a reduced risk of benzodiazepine over-use and adequate management of pain should lead to a reduced risk of over-use of opiates and other analgesics. Criteria such as those of Beers (Beers, 1997; Fick *et al.,* 2003; Tables 34.4 and 34.5) should be taken into account when considering the most appropriate medication to prescribe, and the ones best avoided, for a particular condition in an older person.

### Secondary prevention

Secondary prevention of MUDs in older people should focus on those with a past history of MUD, and the medical conditions and medications listed among Beers' criteria in Tables 34.4 and 34.5.

### Tertiary prevention

Tertiary prevention of MUDs in older people will depend on the medication in question and the clinical and socio-demographic profile of the patient. Admission to a medical or psychiatric ward may be required to facilitate the reduction or stopping of certain medications, e.g. benzodiazepine detoxification, as outpatient detoxification in older people may be hazardous.

## Management and prevention of illegal drug use

The relative rarity of illegal drug use in older people means that there is a dearth of information and guidelines on primary and secondary prevention. However, the ageing 'baby-boom' generation in the USA has been cited as a potential source of older illegal drug users (Patterson and Jeste, 1999) and so clinical experience in this area and the need for primary prevention strategies focused both on the individual and older people in general may increase in the future.

Secondary prevention strategies are likely to focus on those with a past history of illegal drug use, medical (e.g. pain), and psychiatric (e.g. AUDs) disorders that may increase the risk for illegal drug use, and social and environmental factors.

Tertiary prevention or treatment will depend on the drug in question and the clinical and socio-demographic characteristics of the patient.

## Prognosis

### Prognosis in AUDs

The available literature on the topic suggests that older people are at least as likely, if not more likely, to benefit from treatment of AUDs as younger people (Curtis et al., 1989; Oslin et al., 2002). However, prognosis in older people is likely to vary widely depending on a number of factors relating to the individual themselves and the nature of their AUD, the presence of family and other support systems, and the availability of treatment services, particularly services that are tailored to older people.

Individuals with late onset AUDs are generally felt to have a better prognosis than those with early onset or life-long AUDs (Babor et al., 1992). Better prognosis may be related to the shorter history and milder severity of AUDs in this group, more intact social supports, higher income levels, and the presence of potentially modifiable precipitants such as depression, bereavement reactions, or social isolation. In contrast, the elderly individual with an early onset or lifelong AUD may have accumulated significant physical, psychiatric, cognitive, and social deficits that are more difficult to address. The higher prevalence of antisocial personality disorder and the higher risk of co-morbid substance use in this group may also lead to increased difficulties in engagement with therapy.

Of particular relevance to the prognosis of AUDs in older people is the role of cognitive impairment, which is likely to act as a barrier to engaging with treatment. However, one study comparing cognitively impaired and cognitively intact outpatients enrolled in an intensive treatment programme found no significant intergroup differences in outcome; a wide range of treatment gains were seen in both groups, albeit with a higher level of treatment drop-out in the impaired group (Teichner et al., 2002).

The level of cognitive impairment is likely to be higher in the early onset AUD group, but clinical experience suggest that there may be a subgroup of individuals with late onset AUDs whose AUD arises as a *result* of cognitive impairment, with an increase in alcohol intake a behavioural manifestation of an early dementing process.

Co-morbid psychiatric illness, gender (with possibly a poorer prognosis in men), levels of social support, and the availability of alternative and healthier social outlets (which may in turn be related to factors such as culture and ethnicity) may influence motivation for the individual to change their drinking habits.

In view of the wide range of elderly specific aspects of AUDs, it makes intuitive sense that older people would be best treated by specialists in same-age settings, among other older people who may share similar problems, and there is evidence to suggest that such an approach is associated with a better outcome (Kofoed et al., 1987). However, despite the mounting evidence for the extent of AUDs in older people, elderly-specific treatment settings are few in number. Furthermore, engaging with such services may be dependent on an intuitive and motivated physician with sufficient training and expertise to identify the AUD and treat or refer appropriately.

### Prognosis in MUDs

Similar prognostic indicators that apply to AUDs are likely to be relevant to MUDs, and centre on the individual's clinical and socio-demographic characteristics, level of support, and available services. The duration of abuse and the medication or medications being abused is also of relevance. For example, an older person who has been over-using benzodiazepines for decades is more likely to encounter adverse effects and difficulties with cessation than someone who has been over-using mild analgesics because of a recent worsening of arthritic pain. As with AUDs, the relationship with the individual's physician, and the ability of the physician to identify and treat or refer appropriately, is vital. Likewise, motivation to address the MUD may be related to the individual's mental health, level of cognition, and social circumstances.

### Prognosis in illegal substance use

There is a dearth of literature in this area, but similar general principles of good and poor prognostic indicators that relate to AUDs and MUDs are likely to apply to use of illegal substances.

## Smoking in older people

Although use of tobacco (primarily through cigarette smoking) may be classified as a mental and behavioural disorder due to psychoactive substance use and may fulfil criteria for harmful use, dependence, and withdrawal states (see Boxes 34.2–34.6 above), and despite the fact that nicotine use is arguably associated with more morbidity and mortality in older people than alcohol and all other substance use disorders (Atkinson, 2001), this particular problem receives relatively little attention in the psychiatric literature. This is perhaps due to the fact that the neuropsychiatric effects of smoking are subtle and are not generally clinically significant, and there may be a perception that smoking palliates psychological distress. Indeed, a complex and circular relationship between depression, smoking, and medical illness has been described (Wilhelm et al., 2004).

We know that significant proportions of older people (approximately 10%) smoke (Bratzler et al., 2002), and this figure is likely to be higher again for older people with psychiatric disorders such as depression (Covey et al., 1998). The health impact of smoking is well documented elsewhere and includes malignancies (lung, oesophageal, bladder, etc.), cardiovascular disease (ischaemic heart disease, cerebrovascular disease, peripheral vascular disease, etc.), respiratory disease (chronic obstructive airways disease), and countless other problems. Furthermore, the effects of smoking are cumulative and age-related and it has been estimated that 70% of the excess mortality attributed to smoking in the USA occurs in those over the age of 60 (Burns, 2000).

The key message from recent research on smoking in older people is that smoking cessation is possible in this age group and is worthy of active consideration in the individual clinical setting and in a wider public-health context, in view of the considerable health benefits that are likely to accrue. LaCroix and Omenn (1992) found that older smokers who quit have a reduced risk of death compared with current smokers within 1–2 years of quitting and overall risk of death approaches that of those who never smoked after 15–20 years of abstinence. Although the benefits of smoking cessation for longevity are most pronounced in younger people, a large study of smoking cessation has demonstrated that men over the age of 65 gained 1.4–2.0 years of life and women gained 2.7–3.7 years (Taylor *et al.*, 2002).

Systematic reviews on the Cochrane database have demonstrated that nicotine replacement therapy through any mode (e.g. gum, spray, or transdermal patch) increases rates of quitting by 1.5- to 2-fold regardless of setting (Silagy *et al.*, 2004). Another such systematic review has demonstrated that the antidepressants bupropion and nortriptyline aid long-term smoking cessation but the serotonin selective reuptake inhibitors do not (Hughes *et al.*, 2007). There is a dearth of research on such pharmacological approaches to smoking cessation specifically in older populations, and it must be borne in mind that any such therapies may be associated with higher levels of adverse effects in older people. In any comprehensive approach to improving the health of older people, however, consideration should be given to pharmacological therapies, along with advice and education on the many health benefits of smoking cessation.

## Summary and conclusions

This chapter has highlighted the importance of AUDs and MUDs in older people, in terms of their prevalence and their important contribution to morbidity and mortality. AUDs are under-detected, misdiagnosed, and often completely missed in older populations. However, despite ageist and therapeutically pessimistic assumptions, AUDs in older people are as amenable to treatment as in younger people, and treating an AUD in an individual of any age can lead to significant benefits in their quality of life. Likewise, the wide variety of MUDs in older people may be associated with addiction to medication and the under-treatment and inappropriate treatment of medical and psychiatric conditions. Considering that older people are the highest consumers of prescription medications, screening and treatment programmes for MUDs should also lead to considerable improvements in quality of life, along with financial and other savings. Misuse of illicit drugs by older people is not generally a major problem at present, but it is virtually certain that consumption of illegal substances by people aged over 65 will increase in the future.

Greater awareness amongst physicians and other healthcare providers of the possibility of AUDs and MUDs in their older patients should lead to the development of more comprehensive and age-appropriate prevention and treatment strategies. At the levels of everyday clinical practice and public-health policy, greater emphasis should be placed on AUDs and MUDs in older people and further evaluation of dedicated 'same-age' treatment services and settings should be performed.

## References

Adams, S.L. and Waskel, S.A. (1991). Late onset of alcoholism among older Midwestern men in treatment. *Psychological Reports*, **68**, 432.

Adams, W.L. and Cox, N.S. (1995). Epidemiology of problem drinking among elderly people. *International Journal of Addiction*, **30**, 1693–716.

Adams, W.L., Garry, P.J., Rhyne, R. *et al.* (1990). Alcohol intake in the healthy elderly. *Journal of the American Geriatrics Society*, **38**, 211–16.

Adams, W.L., Magruder-Habib, K., Trued, S., and Broome, H.L. (1992). Alcohol abuse in elderly emergency department patients. *Journal of the American Geriatrics Society*, **40**, 1236–40.

American Psychiatric Association (1994). *Diagnostic and statistical manual of mental disorders*, 4th edn. American Psychiatric Press, Washington, DC.

Anderson, G.M., Kerluke, K.J., Pulcins, I.R. *et al.* (1993). Trends and determinants of prescription drug expenditures in the elderly: data from the British Columbia Pharmacare program. *Inquiry*, **30**(2), 199–207.

Anthony, J.C. and Helzer, J.E. (1991). Syndromes of drug abuse and dependence. In *Psychiatric disorders in America: the Epidemiologic Catchment Area Study* (ed. L.N. Robins and D.A. Regier). Free Press, New York.

Atkinson, J.H. and Schuckit, M.A. (1983). Geriatric alcohol and drug misuse and abuse. *Advances in Substance Abuse*, **3**, 195–237.

Atkinson, R.M. (2001). Alcohol and drug abuse in the elderly. In *Psychiatry in the elderly* (ed. R. Jacoby and C. Oppenheimer). Oxford University Press, Oxford.

Avorn, J. (1995). Medication use and the elderly: current status and opportunities. *Health Affairs*, **14**(1), 276–86.

Avorn, J. and Gurwitz, J.H. (1995). Drug use in the nursing home. *Annals of Internal Medicine*, **123**, 195–204.

Babor, T.F., Hofmann, M., DelBoca, F.K. *et al.* (1992). Types of alcoholics, 1. Evidence for an empirically derived typology based on indicators of vulnerability and severity. *Archives of General Psychiatry*, **49**(8), 599–608.

Barkin, R.L., Barkin, S.J., and Barkin, D.S. (2005). Perception, assessment, treatment and management of pain in the elderly. *Clinics in Geriatric Medicine*, **21**(3), 465–90.

Barrick, C. and Connors, G.J. (2002). Relapse prevention and maintaining abstinence in older adults with alcohol use disorders. *Drugs and Aging*, **19**, 583–594.

Beckman, A., Bernsten, C., Parker, M.G., Thorslund, M., and Fastbom, J. (2005). The difficulty of opening medicine containers in old age: a population-based study. *Pharmacy World and Science*, **27**(5), 393–8.

Beers, M.H. (1997). Explicit criteria for determining potentially inappropriate medication use by the elderly. An update. *Archives of Internal Medicine*, **157**(14), 1531–6.

Beers, M., Avorn, J., Soumerai, S.B. *et al.* (1988). Psychoactive medication use in intermediate-care facility residents. *Journal of the American Medical Association*, **260**, 3016–20.

Beers, M.H., Baran, R.W., and Frenia, K. (2000). Drugs and the elderly, Part 1: the problems facing managed care. *American Journal of Managed Care*, **6**, 1313–20.

Blow, F. (1991). *Michigan alcoholism screening test–geriatric version (MAST-G)*. University of Michigan Alcohol Research Center, Ann Arbor.

Blow, F.C. and Barry, K.L. (2000). Older patients with at-risk and problem drinking patterns: new developments in brief interventions. *Journal of Geriatric Psychiatry and Neurology*, **13**(3), 115–23.

Blow, F.C., Brockmann, L.M., and Barry, K.L. (2004). Role of alcohol in late-life suicide. *Alcoholism, Clinical and Experimental Research*, **28**(5, Suppl.), 48S–56S.

Bratzler, D.W., Oehlert, W.H., and Austelle, A. (2002). Smoking in the elderly—it's never too late to quit. *Journal of the Oklahoma State Medical Association*, **95**(3), 185–91.

Bristow, M.F. and Clare, A.W. (1992). Prevalence and characteristics of at risk drinkers among elderly acute medical inpatients. *British Journal of Addiction*, **87**, 291–4.

Brower, K.J., Mudd, S., Blow, F.C., Young, J.P., and Hill, E.M. (1994). Severity and treatment of alcohol withdrawal in elderly versus younger patients. *Alcoholism, Clinical and Experimental Research*, **18**(1), 196–201.

Buckland, P.R. (2001). Genetic association studies of alcoholism—problems with the candidate gene approach. *Alcohol and Alcoholism*, **36**(2), 99–103.

Burns, D.M. (2000). Cigarette smoking among the elderly: disease consequences and the benefits of cessation. *American Journal of Health Promotion*, **14**(6), 357–61.

Busto, U.E., Romach, M.K., and Sellers, E.M. (1996). Multiple drug use and psychiatric comorbidity in patients admitted to the hospital with severe benzodiazepine dependence. *Journal of Clinical Psychopharmacology*, **16**(1), 51–7.

Cadieux, R.J. (1989). Drug interactions in the elderly: How multiple drug use increases risk exponentially. *Postgraduate Medicine*, **86**, 179–86.

Chrischilles, E.A., Segar, E.T., and Wallace, R.B. (1992). Self-reported adverse drug reactions and related resource use. A study of community-dwelling persons 65 years of age and older. *Annals of Internal Medicine*, **117**, 634–40.

Chutka, D.S., Takahashi, P.Y., and Hoel, R.W. (2004). Inappropriate medications for elderly patients. *Mayo Clinic Proceedings*, **79**(1), 122–39.

Council on Scientific Affairs, American Medical Association (1996). Alcoholism in the elderly. *Journal of the American Medical Association*, **275**, 797–801.

Cook, B.L., Winokur, G., Garvey, M.J. *et al.* (1991). Depression and previous alcoholism in the elderly. *British Journal of Psychiatry*, **158**, 72–5.

Covey, L.S., Glassman, A.H., and Stetner, F. (1998). Cigarette smoking and major depression. *Journal of Addictive Diseases: the Official Journal of the ASAM, American Society of Addiction Medicine*, **17**(1), 35–46.

Curtis, J.R., Geller, G., Stokes, E.J., Levine, D.M., and Moore, R.D. (1989). Characteristics, diagnosis and treatment of alcoholism in elderly patients. *Journal of the American Geriatrics Society*, **37**(4), 310–16.

Cyr, M.G. and Wartman, S.A. (1988). The effectiveness of routine screening questions in the detection of alcoholism. *Journal of the American Medical Association*, **259**, 51–4.

Dahmen, N., Volp, M., Singer, P., Hiemke, C., and Szegedi, A. (2005). Tyrosine hydroxylase Val-81-Met polymorphism associated with early-onset alcoholism. *Psychiatric Genetics*, **15**(1), 13–16.

Davidson, K.M. and Ritson, E.B. (1993). The relationship between alcohol dependence and depression. *Alcohol and Alcoholism*, **28**, 147–55.

Doll, R., Peto, R., Hall, E., Wheatley, K., and Gray, R. (1994). Mortality in relation to consumption of alcohol: 13 years' observations on male British doctors. *British Medical Journal*, **309**(6959), 911–18.

Dufour, M. and Fuller, R.K. (1995). Alcohol in the elderly. *Annual Review of Medicine*, **46**, 123–32.

Ekerdt, D.J., DeLabry, L.O., Glynn, R.J. *et al.* (1989). Change in drinking behaviours with retirement: findings from the normative ageing study. *Journal of Studies on Alcohol*, **50**, 347–53.

Ewing, J.A. (1984). Detecting alcoholism: the CAGE questionnaire. *Journal of the American Medical Association*, **252**, 1905–7.

Fick, D.M., Cooper, J.W., Wade, W.E., Waller, J.L., Maclean, J.R., and Beers, M.H. (2003). Updating the Beers criteria for potentially inappropriate medication sue in older adults: results of a US consensus panel of experts. *Archives of Internal Medicine*, **163**(22), 2716–24.

Fink, A., Morton, S.C., Beck, J.C. *et al.* (2002). The alcohol-related problems survey: identifying hazardous and harmful drinking in older primary care patients. *Journal of the American Geriatrics Society*, **50**(10), 1717–22.

Finlayson, R.E. (1995). Misuse of prescription drugs. *International Journal of the Addictions*, **30**, 1871–901.

Fleming, M.F., Manwell, L.B., Barry, K.L., Adams, W., and Stauffacher, E.A. (1999). Brief physician advice for alcohol problems in older adults: a randomized community-based trial. *Journal of Family Practice*, **48**(5), 378–84.

Folstein, M.F., Folstein, S.E., and McHugh, P.R. (1975). 'Mini-mental state'. A practical method for grading the cognitive state of patients for the clinician. *Journal of Psychiatric Research*, **12**(3), 189–98.

Ganry, O., Joly, J., Queval, M.P., and Dubreuil, A. (2000). Prevalence of alcohol problems among elderly patients in a university hospital. *Addiction*, **95**, 107–13.

Goldstein, M.Z., Pataki, A., and Webb, M.T. (1996). Alcoholism among elderly persons. *Psychiatric Services*, **47**, 941–3.

Gordon, T. and Kannel, W.B. (1983). Drinking and its relation to smoking, BP, blood lipids and uric acid. *Archives of Internal Medicine*, **143**, 1366–74.

Grant, B.F. and Harford, T.C. (1995). Comorbidity between DSM-IV alcohol use disorders and major depression: results of a national survey. *Drug and Alcohol Dependence*, **39**, 197–206.

Greene, E., Bruce, I., Cunningham, C., Coakley, D., and Lawlor, B.A. (2003). Self-reported alcohol consumption in the Irish community dwelling elderly. *Irish Journal of Psychological Medicine*, **20**(3), 77–9.

Harrison, L., Sutton, M., and Gardiner, E. (1997). Ethnic differences in substance use and alcohol use related mortality in first generation migrants to England and Wales. *Journal of Substance Use and Misuse*, **32**, 849–76.

Helme, R.D. and Katz, B. (1993). Management of chronic pain. *Medical Journal of Australia*, **158**(7), 478–81.

Hinkin, C., Castellin, S., Dickinson-Fuhrman, E. *et al.* (2002). Screening for drug and alcohol abuse among older adults using modified version of CAGE. *American Journal of Addiction*, **10**, 319–26.

Hughes, J.R., Stead, L.F., Lancaster, T. Antidepressants for smoking cessation. *Cochrane Database of Systematic Reviews* 2007, Issue 1. Art. No.: CD000031. DOI: 10.1002/14651858.CD000031.pub3.

Jackson, R. and Teece, S. (2004). Oral or intravenous thiamine in the emergency department. *Emergency Medicine Journal*, **21**, 501–2.

Jeste, D.V. and Palmer, B. (1998). Secondary psychoses: an overview. *Seminars in Clinical Neuropsychiatry*, **3**, 2–3.

Jinks, M.J. and Raschko, R.R. (1990). A profile of alcohol and prescription drug abuse in a high risk community-based elderly population. *Annals of Pharmacotherapy*, **24**, 971–5.

Joseph, C.L., Ganzini, L., and Atkinson, R.M. (1995). Screening for alcohol use disorders in the nursing home. *Journal of the American Geriatrics Society*, **43**, 368–73.

Kalant, H. (1998). Pharmacological interactions of aging and alcohol. In *Alcohol problems and aging*, NIAAA Research Monograph no. 33 (ed. E.S.L. Gomberg, A.M. Hegedus, and R.A. Zucker), NIH publication no. 98–4163. NIAAA, Bethesda, MD.

Khan, N., Davis, P., Wilkinson, T.J., Sellman, J.D., and Graham, P. (2002). Drinking patterns among older people I the community: hidden from medical attention? *New Zealand Medical Journal*, **115**(1148), 72–5.

King, C., Van Hasselt, V., Segal, D. *et al.* (1994). Diagnosis and assessment of substance abuse in older adults. Current strategies and issues. *Addictive Behaviors*, **19**, 41–5.

Kirby, M., Denihan, A., Bruce, I., Radic, A., Coakley, D., and Lawlor, B.A. (1999a). Benzodiazepine use among the elderly in the community. *International Journal of Geriatric Psychiatry*, **14**(4), 280–4.

Kirby, M., Denihan, A., Bruce, I., Radic, A., Coakley, D., and Lawlor, B.A. (1999b). Influence of anxiety on treatment of depression in later life in primary care: questionnaire survey. *British Medical Journal*, **318**, 579–80.

Kofoed, L.L., Tolson, R.L., Atkinson, R.M., Toth, R.L., and Turner, J.A. (1987). Treatment compliance of older alcoholics: an elder-specific approach is superior to 'mainstreaming'. *Journal of Studies on Alcohol*, **48**, 47.

Kuhar, M.J., Joyce, A., and Dominguez, G. (2001). Genes in drug abuse. *Drug and Alcohol Dependence*, **62**(3), 157–62.

LaCroix, A.Z. and Omenn, G.S. (1992). Older adults and smoking. *Clinics in Geriatric Medicine*, **8**, 69–87.

LaGreca, A.J., Akers, R.L., and Dwyer, J.W. (1988). Life events and alcohol behaviors among older adults. *Gerontologist*, **28**, 552–8.

Law, M. and Wald, N. (1999). Why heart disease mortality is low in France: the time-lag explanation. *British Medical Journal*, **318**, 1471–1476.

Lawlor, D.A., Patel, R., and Ebrahim, S. (2003). Association between falls in elderly women and chronic disease and drug use. *British Medical Journal*, **327**, 712–17.

Letenneur, L. (2004). Risk of dementia and alcohol and wine consumption: a review of recent results. *Biological Research*, **37**, 189–93.

Levings, B., Szep, S., Helps, S.C. (1999). Towards the safer use of dosettes. *Journal of Quality in Clinical Practice*, **19**, 69–72.

Liberto, J.G. and Oslin, D.W. (1995). Early onset versus late onset alcoholism in the elderly. *International Journal of Addiction*, **30**, 1799–818.

Liskow, B.I., Rinck, C., Campbell, J., and DeSouza, C. (1989). Alcohol withdrawal in the elderly. *Journal of Studies on Alcohol*, **50**(5), 414–21.

Lofwall, M.R., Brooner, R.K., Bigelow, G.E., Kindbom, K., and Strain, E.C. (2005). Characteristics of older opioid maintenance patients. *Journal of Substance Abuse Treatment*, **28**(3), 265–72.

Luttrell, S., Watkin, V., Livingston, G. *et al.* (1997). Screening for alcohol misuse in older people. *International Journal of Geriatric Psychiatry*, **12**, 1151–1154.

McGrath, A., Crome, P., and Crome, I.B. (2005). Substance misuse in the older population. *Postgraduate Medical Journal*, **81**, 228–31.

Mirand, A.L. and Welte, J.W. (1996). Alcohol consumption among the elderly in a general population, Erie County, New York. *American Journal of Public Health*, **86**, 978–84.

Moos, R., Brennan, P., and Schutte, K. (1998). Life context factors, treatment, and late-life drinking behaviour. In *Alcohol problems and aging*, NIAAA Research Monograph no. 33 (ed. E.S.L. Gomberg, A.M. Hegedus, and R.A. Zucker), NIH publication no. 98–4163. NIAAA, Bethesda, MD.

Mulder, R.T. (2002). Alcoholism and personality. *Australian and New Zealand Journal of Psychiatry*, **36**, 44–52.

Naranjo, C.A. and Sellers, E.M. (1986). Clinical assessment and pharmacotherapy of the alcohol withdrawal syndrome. *Recent Developments in Alcoholism*, **4**, 265–81.

NIAAA (National Institute on Alcohol Abuse and Alcoholism). *Alcohol alert no. 40*. NIAAA, Bethesda, MD (http://pubs.niaaa.nih.gov/publications/aa40.htm).

Neiman, J. (1998). Alcohol as a risk factor for brain damage: neurologic aspects. *Alcoholism, Clinical and Experimental Research*, **22**(7, Suppl.), 346S–351S.

Nurnberger, J.I., Wiegand, R., Bucholz, K. *et al.* (2004). A family study of alcohol dependence: coaggregation of multiple disorders in relatives of alcohol-dependent probands. *Archives of General Psychiatry*, **61**(12), 1246–56.

O'Connell, H. and Lawlor, B. (2005a). Alcohol and heart disease—what do you prescribe? *Irish Medical Journal*, **98**, 230–1.

O'Connell, H. and Lawlor, B.A. (2005b). Recent alcohol intake and suicide: a neuropsychological perspective. *Irish Journal of Medical Science*, **174**, 51–4.

O'Connell, H., Chin, A.V., Cunningham, C., and Lawlor, B. (2003a). Alcohol use disorders in elderly people—redefining an age old problem in old age. *British Medical Journal*, **327**, 664–7.

O'Connell, H., Chin, A.V., and Lawlor, B.A. (2003b). Alcohol use in Ireland—can we hold our drink?'. *Irish Journal of Psychological Medicine*, **20**, 109–10.

O'Connell, H., Chin, A.V., Hamilton, F. *et al.* (2004). A systematic review of the utility of self-report alcohol screening instruments in the elderly. *International Journal of Geriatric Psychiatry*, **19**, 1074–86.

Oslin, D.W., Pettinati, H., and Volpicelli, J.R. (2002). Alcoholism treatment adherence: older age predicts better adherence and drinking outcomes. *American Journal of Geriatric Psychiatry*, **10**(6), 740–7.

Patterson, T.L. and Jeste, D.V. (1999). The potential impact of the baby-boom generation on substance abuse among elderly persons. *Psychiatric Services*, **50**(9), 1184–8.

Peppers, M.P. (1996). Benzodiazepines for alcohol withdrawal in the elderly and in patients with liver disease. *Pharmacotherapy*, **16**(1), 49–57.

Philpot, M., Pearson, N., Petratou, V., Dayanandan, R., Silverman, M., and Marshall, J. (2003). Screening for problem drinking in older people referred to a mental health service: a comparison of CAGE and AUDIT. *Aging & Mental Health*, **7**(3), 171–5.

Regier, D.A., Boyd, J.H., Burke, J.D. *et al.* (1988). One-month prevalence of mental disorders in the United States based on five Epidemiologic Catchment Area sites. *Archives of General Psychiatry*, **45**, 977–986.

Reid, M.C. and Anderson, P.A. (1997). Geriatric substance use disorders. *Medical Clinics of North America*, **81**, 999–1016.

Rimm, E.B., Williams, P., Fosher, K., Criqui, M., and Stampfer, M.J. (1999). Moderate alcohol intake and lower risk of coronary heart disease: meta-analysis of effects on lipids and haemostatic factors. *British Medical Journal*, **319**(7224), 1523–8.

Ringe, J.D., van der Geest, S.A., and Moller, G. (2006). Importance of calcium co-medication in bisphosphonate therapy of osteoporosis: an approach to improving correct intake and drug adherence. *Drugs & Aging*, **23**(7), 569–78.

Ruchlin, H.S. (1997). Prevalence and correlates of alcohol use among older adults. *Preventive Medicine*, **26**, 651–7.

Ruitenberg, A., van Sweiten, J.C., Witteman, J.C.M. *et al.* (2002). Alcohol consumption and risk of dementia: the Rotterdam study. *Lancet* **359**, 281–6.

Satre, D., Mertens, J., Arean, P. *et al.* (2003). Contrasting outcomes of older versus middle aged and younger adult chemically dependent patients in a managed care programme. *Journal of Studies on Alcohol*, **64**, 520–30.

Saunders, J.B. (1993). Development of the alcohol use disorders identification test (AUDIT) *Addiction*, **88**, 791–804.

Saunders, P.A., Copeland, J.R., Dewey, M.E. *et al.* (1991). Heavy drinking as a risk factor for depression and dementia in elderly men. Findings from the Liverpool longitudinal community study. *British Journal of Psychiatry*, **159**, 213–16.

Schneider, J.P. (2005). Chronic pain management in older adults: with coxibs under fire, what now? *Geriatrics*, **60**(5), 26–8, 30–1.

Schonfeld, L. and Dupree, L.W. (1995). Treatment approaches for older problem drinkers. *International Journal of Addiction*, **30**(13–14), 1819–42.

Schutte, K.K., Brennan, P.L., and Moos, R.H. (1994). Remission of late-life drinking problems: a 4-year follow-up. *Alcoholism, Clinical and Experimental Research*, **18**, 835–44.

Selzer, M.L. (1968). Michigan Alcoholism Screening Test (MAST): preliminary report. *University of Michigan Medical Center Journal*, **34**(3), 143–5.

Shaper, A.G. (1995). Mortality and alcohol consumption. Non-drinkers shouldn't be used as a baseline. *British Medical Journal*, **310**(6975), 325.

Silagy, C., Lancaster, T., Stead, L., Mant, D., and Fowler, G. (2004). *Cochrane Database of Systematic Reviews* 2004, Issue 3. Art. No.: CD000146. DOI: 10.1002/14651858.CD000146.pub2.

Sintonen, H. (1994). Outcomes measurement in acid-related diseases. *PharmacoEconomics*, **5**(Suppl. 3), 17–26.

Smith, D.M. and Atkinson, R.M. (1995). Alcoholism and dementia. *International Journal of Addiction*, **30**(13–14), 1843–69.

Speer, D.C. and Bates, K. (1992). Comorbid mental and substance disorders among older psychiatric patients. *Journal of the American Geriatrics Society*, **40**, 886–90.

Swartz, M., Landerman, R., George, L.K. *et al.* (1991). Benzodiazepine anti-anxiety agents: prevalence and correlates of use in a southern community. *American Journal of Public Health*, **81**, 592–6.

Taylor, D., Paton, C., and Kerwin, R. (2005). *The Maudsley 2005–2006 Prescribing Guidelines*. 8th edn. Taylor and Francis, London.

Taylor, D.H., Hasselblad, V., Henley, S.J., Thun, M.J., and Sloan, F.A. (2002). Benefits of smoking cessation for longevity. *American Journal of Public Health*, **92**, 990–6.

Teichner, G., Horner, M.D., Roitzsch, J.C., Herron, J., and Thevos, A. (2002). Substance abuse treatment outcomes for cognitively impaired and intact outpatients. *Addictive Behaviors*, **27**(5), 751–63.

Temple, M.T. and Leino, E.V. (1989). Long-term outcomes of drinking: a twenty year longitudinal study of man. *British Journal of Addiction*, **84**, 889–93.

The Royal Colleges Report (1995). Alcohol and the heart in perspective: sensible limits reaffirmed. A working group of the Royal Colleges of Physicians, Psychiatrists and General Practitioners. *Journal of the Royal College of Physicians of London*, **29**, 266–71.

Tiihonen, J., Hammikainen, T., Lachman, H. *et al.* (1999). Association between the functional variant of the catechol-O-methyltransferase (COMT) gene and type 1 alcoholism. *Molecular Psychiatry*, **4**(3), 286–9.

Trafton, J.E., Olivia, E., Horst, D. *et al.* (2004). Treatment needs associated with pain in substance use disorder patients; implications of concurrent treatment. *Drug and Alcohol Dependence*, **73**, 23–31.

UK National Digital Archive of Datasets (1994). *General household survey, UK, 1994* (http://www.ndad.nationalarchives.gov.uk/CRDA/28/DS/1/detail.html).

Vogel-Sprott, V. and Barrett, P. (1984). Age, drinking habits and the effects of alcohol. *Journal of Studies on Alcohol*, **45**, 517–21.

Waern, M. (2003). Alcohol dependence and misuse in elderly suicides. *Alcohol and Alcoholism*, **38**, 249–54.

Wilhelm, K., Arnold, K., Niven, H., and Richmond, R. (2004). Grey lungs and blue moods: smoking cessation in the context of lifetime depression history. *Australian and New Zealand Journal of Psychiatry*, **38**(11–12), 896–905.

Williams, L. and Lowenthal, D.T. (1992). Drug therapy in the elderly. *Southern Medical Journal*, **85**(2), 127–31.

Williams, S.H. (2005). Medications for treating alcohol dependence. *American Family Physician*, **72**, 1775–1780.

World Health Organization (1992). *The ICD-10 classification of mental and behavioural disorders*. World Health Organization, Geneva.

# 35

# Working with older people with intellectual difficulties

Tony Holland

## Introduction

This chapter primarily addresses three aspects of ageing as it affects people with intellectual disabilities (ID). First, the epidemiological evidence on mental and other health-related problems associated with ageing in people with ID. Second, the special circumstances of ageing in people with Down's syndrome (DS) and in those with some other syndromes associated with ID. Finally, it considers the social context of ageing and the consequent implications for services, particularly the issue of generic versus specialist provision for people with ID in later life. The fact that 'ageing' in this group of people is now being considered at all is a reflection of the positive and fundamental changes both in health status and also in societal attitudes that have occurred. Central to this chapter on ID are the issues of how 'ageing' and 'later life' are defined, the fact that there are differences in life expectancy across levels of disabilities and between different causes of ID, and the question as to whether, with respect to people with ID, access to services for older people is determined by chronological age, by the presence of illnesses generally associated with later life (such as dementia), or whether it should be defined in relationship to life expectancy and the age of the oldest portion of the particular population in question (e.g. people with DS). These issues are important in terms of understanding how the ageing process affects those in this highly heterogeneous group and to what extent it is similar to or different from ageing in the non-intellectually disabled population, and also in order to ensure that people with ID are not discriminated against when it comes to access to specialist services for older people or, for example, services for people with dementia.

Elderly people with ID who are alive now were born at a time when attitudes and the services available were very different. Medical care in the neonatal period for those with particular genetic syndromes associated with ID would have been limited and education during childhood would have been denied to many, as it only became mandatory in England for education authorities to provide education to all children (and therefore to those with ID) in the 1970s. Anecdotal reports from families of older people with ID often mention the authorities telling them to place their children in institutions and advising parents that there was little hope of a meaningful life for their son or daughter. This generation of older people with ID and their families are likely to have experienced considerable prejudice and social isolation, yet the individuals with

ID were robust enough to survive the complications of early childhood (see Atkinson *et al.*, 1997). The attitudes and the principles that now guide the support of people with ID have changed remarkably in the 30 years between the two major White Papers devoted to people with ID: 'Better services for the mentally handicapped' (Department of Health and Social Security, 1971) and 'Valuing people' (Department of Health, 2001). The first of these White Papers set the scene for the closure of long-stay institutions after major scandals and the second, in promoting social inclusion, set out four key principles that should govern the way services are provided. These are rights, independence, choice, and inclusion. It is in this context of marked social change, together with improvements in life expectancy, that ageing has now appropriately become the focus of new research and of service and policy developments.

## Background

'Intellectual disability' is becoming the more universally used term applied to a group of people who have in common evidence of developmental delay in early childhood together with evidence of intellectual, educational, and functional disabilities. Such impairments and associated disabilities extend into adult life. This term is synonymous with that of 'learning disability' used by the Department of Health in England and with other terms used in different countries and statutes, including those of 'mental handicap' and 'mental retardation' (World Health Organization, 1992; American Psychiatric Association, 1994). As a group, people with developmental ID are very heterogeneous. Those with severe and profound ID are likely to have a history of significant developmental delay and functional disabilities, such that they require care throughout their lives. Those with milder ID may be able to live independent or relatively independent lives and only require additional support through their school years or at times of particular difficulties. No single term fully encapsulates the complexity of need. The World Health Organization's classification system of impairments, disabilities, and handicaps helps to address this issue (World Health Organization, 1980). In the case of intellectual disabilities the 'impairment' reflects dysfunction of the brain, 'disability' the extent to which the individual has limited functional and social skills, as would be expected for his/her age, and the 'handicap' the disadvantage that follows. The extent of 'handicap' or disadvantage is determined by the extent to which society invests in strategies that might help to compensate for the disability, such as the level of the support offered. Thus, the term 'intellectual disability' is referring to the functional and social outcomes of a complex dynamic between a person's limitations, often predominately of biological origin, and past and present opportunities and experiences (Shakespeare, 2006).

Given the distribution and properties of formal IQ assessments approximately 2% of the population can be said to have a significant intellectual impairment (IQ < 70), and 3 to 5 per 1000 of the population have been reported to have severe or profound ID (Birch *et al.*, 1970). However, when age-specific prevalence rates for ID are considered, other factors, such as difficulties ascertaining people with ID at different stages in their lifespan and differential effects across the spectrum of disability on age-related mortality rates, influence the age-specific prevalence rates and the profiles of disability observed. Those with more severe disabilities generally have a reduced life expectancy compared with those with milder disabilities or those without such disabilities (Jacobson *et al.*, 1985; Strauss and Eyman, 1996; for review see Fryers, 2000) (Table 35.1). However, in contrast, the life expectancy of those with mild LD now approaches that of the general population (Bittles *et al.*, 2002). For this reason, at a population level, the extent of need of the group as a whole, in contrast to the general population, decreases with chronological age because of the increased mortality rates of those with the more severe disabilities. A further factor is the particular effects of ageing for people with DS who, despite significant improvements in life expectancy, continue to have a reduced mean life expectancy of approximately 50 years (see Table 35.2).

Although life expectancy for some groups of people with ID is significantly less than for those without such disabilities, overall life expectancy is improving for people with ID, as it is for the general population. In the USA it has been estimated that life expectancy for persons with ID has increased from an average of 18.5 years in 1930 to 59.1 years in 1970 and to an estimated 66.2 years in 1993 (Braddock, 1999). Again in the USA, it has been estimated that by 2020 the proportion of people with ID aged over 65 will have doubled (Janicki and Dalton, 2000). A study in Ireland estimated that

**Table 35.1** Estimates of age-specific prevalence of severe intellectual impairment in an average English district of stable population *c.* 1990 (from Fryers, 2000)

| Age (years) | Ratio/1000 population |
|---|---|
| 0–4 | ?2.5 |
| 5–9 | 3.0 |
| 10–14 | 4.0 |
| 15–19 | 4.5 |
| 20–24 | 5.0 |
| 25–34 | 4.0 |
| 35–44 | 3.0 |
| 45–54 | 2.5 |
| 55–64 | 2.0 |
| 65–74 | 1.0 |
| 75+ | Very few |

**Table 35.2** Summary of (1) estimated mean life expectancy in years for people with DS compared with men and women in the general population and (2) estimated relative mortality rates divided according to the level of disability for people with ID in general (for references see text)

**(1) Life expectancy**

|  | 1901 | | 2002 | |
|---|---|---|---|---|
|  | **Male** | **Female** | **Male** | **Female** |
| General population | 45 | 49 | 81 | 84 |
| People with DS | 9 | | 50 | |

**(2) Mortality rates**

**Mortality rates (1990s)**

| People with mild ID 1.7 that of general population |
|---|
| People with profound ID 4.1 that of general population |

by the year 2021 the total population of people with ID would have increased by 20%, of whom over a third would then be 50 years or older (McConkey *et al.*, 2006). These figures are only estimates, but if they turn out to be approximately correct they vividly illustrate how ageing must now be the focus of the policy agenda in ID.

During the lifetime of this present group of older people with ID there have also been major advances in several fields that have a direct bearing on our understanding of early development and of the causes of developmental delay. The structure of DNA was proposed as recently as 1953 (Watson and Crick, 1953) and the human chromosome complement of 23 pairs was first reported in 1956 (Levan, 1956). By the present day, many possible causes of significant developmental delay and subsequent ID have been described, including the presence of chromosome abnormalities or single gene disorders and the role of environmental factors, such as perinatal trauma or intra-uterine infections, and maternal and early childhood nutritional deficiencies, maternal alcohol abuse, or severe childhood neglect and deprivation (Kaski, 2000). DS is recognised in developed countries as the single most prevalent chromosomal syndrome associated with ID and fragile-X syndrome as the most common X-linked single gene disorder.

Although the later 20th century saw a move away from an emphasis on genetics in the field of ID, largely because of the historical context, it is now recognized that knowing the cause of a person's ID may be important in terms of informing support, as there may be particular associated health risks that may only appear in later life. Any observed specific relationship between the genotype associated with a syndrome and its particular cognitive and behavioural developmental profile and/or any specific risk for psychiatric co-morbidity has become known as the 'behavioural phenotype' of the syndrome (O'Brien and Yule 1995). In context of this chapter on ageing, this concept of a 'behavioural phenotype' is best illustrated by the relationship between DS and the high risk of Alzheimer's disease, which is unique to this particular syndrome and not to others associated with ID (see later). However, for many people with ID born some years ago the diagnosis of the cause of their ID was not possible in their childhood as knowledge was limited or investigations were not undertaken. People with mild ID, in contrast to those with more severe or profound ID, rarely have a single identifiable cause but both polygenic and social/environmental influences are important, and factors such as social deprivation are likely to be relevant. For this group of people with mild ID who numerically outnumber those with more severe or profound ID by ten to one, ageing and associated health and other problems are more likely to relate to long-term effects of social factors, such as poverty (Emerson, 2005).

The extent to which a particular cause of a person's ID predominates in any given country will vary depending upon the social, political, and economic status of that country and the resultant health and nutritional status of the general population, particularly that of mothers and newborn children. Many other factors that are socially determined and/or dependent on the extent of resources provided contribute to the actual extent of a person's disability and 'handicap' (disadvantage). These include educational, social, and health resources that might maximize abilities and determine the extent of available opportunities. Whilst biological factors might affect early development and place constraints on the ultimate level of attainment in later life, a strong message of the last 50 years has been the responsibility that society has as a whole to people with ID to ensure that meaningful opportunities, initially in education, and later in the form of supported employment or occupation and the opportunities for social inclusion, are provided. These same issues are now also important in later life when considering how people with ID should be supported and how the balance between specialist ID provision and the social inclusion of people with ID into the mainstream of services for the elderly is managed.

The heterogeneity of the group of people with ID is therefore characterized in various ways. Some will have genetically determined disorders that had a marked effect on brain development and therefore on intellectual, social, and functional abilities. Others may develop adequate living skills, are able to make their needs and wishes known through spoken language, and lead relatively independent lives, but may have poor psychological resources and are also often disadvantaged in society. Some sensory, physical, or developmental disabilities, such as cerebral palsy and autistic spectrum disorders, are also considered to be related to ID in that many individuals with these other conditions also have evidence of significant intellectual and functional impairments. All aspects from the biological functioning of the brain, to the manifestations of disability, to societal responses can play a part in the emergence of patterns of function and dysfunction during the course of development and over the lifespan. Added to this is the fact that the process of ageing should also be seen as part of the developmental trajectory and those people born with particular genetic or environmental determined disorders that affect early development may have an atypical course to their later lives and to what is, for them, 'old age'. The needs of older people with ID cannot therefore be fully appreciated without an understanding of an individual's earlier developmental trajectory and previous life experiences and opportunities.

## Physical and psychiatric co-morbidity in later life

The assessment of co-morbidity among the population of people with ID is not without its difficulties, for two main reasons. First, the definition of what is referred to as 'an intellectual disability' does not have a neat dividing line. This term refers to a continuum rather than an easily defined category and therefore, for example,

quite which side of this artificial divide (intellectual disability or no intellectual disability) a person on the borderline falls will be a matter of dispute. This issue of definition is also of great relevance when it comes to service provision (see later). Secondly, both physical and mental health problems may go unnoticed as the person affected may not be readily able to complain or, when an illness is present, it may present in atypical ways, such as a change in behaviour. These changes may not be recognized for what they really represent, i.e. psychological or physical discomfort and distress consequent upon some new pathology. This is particularly so for those with more severe ID who may have no or very limited speech. For psychiatric disorders in particular there is a debate as to whether existing diagnostic criteria, derived from typically developing populations, are appropriate and modified diagnostic systems have been developed (the DC-LD; Cooper et al., 2003). This problem of definition is confounded further by divisions between what are seen as psychiatric disorders and what are referred to as 'challenging behaviours'. These two broad problems of, first, defining and ascertaining a population sample of people with ID and, second, identifying and characterizing co-morbidity, are factors that have to be considered when comparing studies and drawing conclusions from them. These problems remain when the sample in question is older people with ID. An older population defined by their chronological age (e.g. over 64 years of age), will be very different in terms of their profile of ID from a younger group because of differential effects on mortality.

Despite the above caveats there are several studies that have reported high rates of physical illness (Cooper, 1998; Janicki et al., 2002) and of psychiatric and behavioural problems (challenging behaviour) (Jacobson, 1982; Borthwick-Duffy and Eyman, 1990; Einfeld and Tonge, 1996; Taylor et al., 2004) among adults with ID. Other studies have reported that it is among those with more severe ID that causes of death and the nature of physical co-morbidity in later life differ from those observed in the general population. For example, the leading cause of death in this group is respiratory disorders, because of the risks of aspiration and of gastro-oesophageal reflex (Janicki et al., 1999; Patja et al., 2001). In general, throughout adult life and also in later life, sensory impairments and thyroid disorders are common (Evenhuis 1995a,b; Janicki and Dalton, 1998; Kapell et al., 1998). However, it is of note that in the study of Davidson et al. (2003) the 1371 people with ID aged 40 years or older living in the group homes surveyed were generally reported to be in good health and much like others in the general population in terms of health status, with the exception of some additional disability-related problems. In comparison with general population data, they had a lower risk for cardiovascular disease-related factors. However, like the general population, over 50% were obese and diets were poor and the amount of exercise taken was limited.

With respect to psychiatric disorder and challenging behaviours those with more severe ID are reported to have prevalence rates of around 50% of which at least 20% will be seen as 'challenging behaviour' in that psychological models of causation based on learning theory are of particular relevance (Jacobson, 1982). Lifetime rates of schizophrenia are increased at 3% and anxiety disorders are particularly common (Cooper, 1997; Deb et al., 2001). There are few studies of the prevalence rates of psychiatric disorder specifically in older people with ID. For example, Day (1985), in a case note study of those aged 40 years and older in an institutional population, found that 30% had a documented psychiatric history. The rates were reported as 20% in the 99 of the 357 residents aged 65 or over. As part of the development of a psychiatric assessment tool for use with people who have an ID, Moss and Patel (1993) undertook a study of 101 older people with moderate to profound ID aged 50 years or older known to services in one catchment area. Prevalence rates of psychiatric disorder (excluding dementia) were nearly 12%, with psychotic illness and affective and anxiety disorders being the main diagnoses. The best systematic study in the UK of population of people with ID aged 65 years or older was that of Cooper (1997). Using a structured psychiatric rating scale, she undertook a study of an administrative sample of people with ID and applied established but slightly modified diagnostic criteria. The overall prevalence rate of psychiatric disorder (including lifetime affective disorder and dementia) was 68%. As with other studies of the adult ID population, rates of schizophrenia were increased at 3%, and 15% had a history of affective disorder. Again anxiety disorders were prominent, with generalized anxiety disorders at 9%, agoraphobia at 3.7%, and other phobias 3.0%. Prevalence rates of behaviour disorders were nearly 15%. At the same time she investigated prevalence rates in a younger adult population for comparison. Essentially, there is an age-related increase in affective and anxiety disorders but similar rates of schizophrenia and behaviour disorder. As would be expected, autistic spectrum disorder (being a developmental disorder and therefore present from childhood) was also similar across the age span at 6.0%.

Age-specific prevalence rates for dementia among people with ID have also been investigated. As with other psychiatric disorders the recognition that dementia may be present and its subsequent diagnosis may be more problematic, for several reasons. First, people with ID may not be able themselves to articulate that they have a new problem, such as difficulty remembering things. It therefore may be incumbent upon those supporting the person to notice that a problem exists. However, given the varied abilities of this population, unless a support worker has known someone over time, and therefore has been able to observe deterioration, any absence of skills may be misinterpreted as being due to the fact that the person has an ID. The availability of longitudinal information, ideally from a family member or else some objective record of previous abilities, is essential. The problems of diagnosis will be discussed in more detail later. A second problem is that older people with ID may never have had the opportunity to acquire more advanced living skills or the opportunity to use such skills now, so that they do not have the skills to lose or the opportunity to show that they have lost them. Therefore the process of dementia may have to be quite advanced before it is apparent. Moss and Patel (1995) found that nearly 12% of older people with ID aged 50 years and over met criteria for dementia. Excluding people with DS, just over 20% of people with ID aged 65 years and older have been found to have dementia, with the expected age-related increases in prevalence (Cooper, 1997). These and other studies suggest that the age-related rates of dementia in people with ID are similar in pattern to those found in the general population but brought forward by a few years. How this is best explained is uncertain, but it may be due to less 'reserve brain capacity' given the person's pre-existing ID or to a general non-specific effect that impaired brain development might have, much in the same way as head injury increases the risk of dementia.

## Links between the cause of the ID and atypical patterns of ageing

The social movements of the 20th century associated with ID rightfully moved away from what was seen as a biological and medically dominated view of mental deficiency or mental handicap. These perspectives had not only been tainted by the interpretations and adverse consequences predicted by the eugenics movement but they failed remotely to do justice to the individual and his/her needs and rights. The framework that guides the support of people with ID has now become more firmly rooted in the individual, and government policy is committed to the principle of full citizenship. With such positive social and attitudinal changes it has been possible to once more to consider the biological and genetic aspects and to acknowledge that different causes of ID may have very distinct effects. With advances in genetics and the identification of chromosomal and single gene disorders associated with ID, research has returned to the study of the commonalities and differences within and between people with different syndromes associated with ID.

However, other than DS, relatively little research has considered old age in people with other genetically determined syndromes, such as Angelman, fragile-X, cri-du-chat, Cornelia de Lange, Smith–Magenis, Prader–Willi, and Williams syndromes, and tuberous sclerosis and many others. All of these have their unique genotypes and are recognized as having patterns of development and/or associated profiles of skills and maladaptive behaviours that are broadly characteristic of the syndrome. Anecdotally there appear to be considerable differences in life expectancy. For example, people with fragile-X syndrome have been reported to have lived into their 70s, but those with other syndromes, such as Prader–Willi syndrome (PWS) (Whittington *et al.*, 2001), often of similar levels of intellectual disability, do not live to such ages. Whether these observations are correct requires a more systematic investigation. However, any such study will be problematic as many of the older people will not have received a formal diagnosis for the cause of their ID as, when they were children (when medical diagnoses are usually made), the tests may not have been available or the syndrome may not have been described. Thus, at present we do not know to any great degree whether specific patterns of early development associated with a specific genotype have implications for the ageing process in later life, and whether, like people with DS, there are very particular health risks in later life.

The potential problems of later life and their contrasting causes are considered below with respect to three specific conditions with very different genetic aetiologies: DS, tuberous sclerosis, and PWS. These should be considered to be illustrative of the general point that there may be as yet unexplored effects on life expectancy and health risks in later life that are particular to specific causes of a person's developmental ID. It is important that these associations are recognized as it may be possible to prevent their development, but also because when a person has limited communication ability, recognizing there is a problem and arriving at an explanation for any observed deterioration or change in behaviour can be difficult. Knowing about potential risks may at least alert carers to that possibility. In the three examples below people born with these particular syndromes have, in addition to the normal health risks associated with age, other health risks that are specific to their syndrome. These problems may develop for the first time in adult life and affect life expectancy.

## Down's syndrome and ageing

The association between DS and the risk of Alzheimer's disease (AD) was initially mainly based on neuropathological studies that found evidence of extensive plaques and neurofibrillary tangles in the brains of people with DS who died aged 30 years or older. Mann (1988) reviewed the published neuropathological studies and reported that they all described evidence of such neuropathological change in people with DS aged over 40 years. Cross-sectional clinical studies also reported evidence of decline prior to death that was indicative of dementia (e.g. Wisniewski et al., 1978; Thase et al., 1984; Zigman et al., 1987). However, it was also clear that whilst most, if not all, people with DS might have neuropathological change characteristic of AD, not all people with DS in later life developed clinical features of AD (see review by Oliver and Holland, 1986). Subsequent systematic studies looking at the age-specific prevalence of clinically diagnosed AD in people with DS have found increasing prevalence rates from age 30 years. In a study in one health district in the UK, Holland et al. (1998) identified 80 people with DS aged 30 years and over. Seventy-five agreed to take part in the study. Using an adapted version of the CAMDEX informant interview (part of the CAMDEX-DS; Ball et al., 2006), they reported rates of dementia ranging from 2.0% in the 30s to 10% between age 40–49 and 40% from 50 years onwards. Other studies have found a similar age-related increase, with prevalence rates increasing to as much as 75% in the oldest group (Lai and Williams, 1989) but never to 100%. It is of note that in all these studies it is very rare to find people with DS living into their 70s.

The CAMDEX-DS, developed for the Cambridge population-based studies of DS and AD, was modified from the original CAMDEX (Roth et al., 1986) to place greater emphasis on the importance of informant-rated loss of function in those domains known to deteriorate with the onset of AD. This was necessary, as with people who have an ID a particular level of pre-morbid function could not be assumed and people with DS may also have difficulty reporting changes in functioning themselves. This informant-based diagnostic assessment, which also includes a neuropsychological assessment (the CAMCOG-DS), diagnostic criteria, and guidance for post-diagnosis management, has been shown to be both valid and reliable (Ball et al., 2004). A longitudinal study using the CAMDEX-DS for diagnosis and the CAMCOG-DS for serial neuropsychological assessments has indicated that behavioural and personality changes precede the onset of clinically diagnosable AD, possibly by some years (Ball et al., 2006). It has been proposed that this may be a consequence of a developmentally determined reduced reserve capacity of the frontal lobes of the brain in people with DS and for this reason relatively early neuropathological change affects frontal lobe function sooner than it would in the general population.

The fact that people with DS have a reduced life expectancy of about two-thirds of that of the general population suggests that they may have an abnormal and premature ageing process. Some support for this comes from the observations that age-related sensory impairments and thyroid dysfunction are common and they, like AD, occur at a relatively early age. The differential diagnosis of apparent decline in later life in people with DS therefore includes not only AD but also the impact of sensory impairments, hypothyroidism, and also depression (see Prasher and Hall, 1996). Thus, a thorough assessment is essential when decline has been observed or is suspected.

The main hypothesis to account for the relationship between these two disorders is the presence of the β-amyloid precursor protein (APP) gene on chromosome 21 (Tanzi et al., 1987). People with DS, having trisomy 21, have three copies of this gene and therefore increased expression of this protein (Rumble et al., 1989). The assumption is that this excess deposition over time sets off a train of neuropathological events leading to plaque and tangle formation and neuronal cell death. As with the general population variants of the APOE gene have a modifying effect in a similar manner (Rubinzstein et al., 1999).

The systematic evaluation of management and treatment of AD in people with DS has not received great attention. The use of donepezil has been shown to have a modest effect for some people (Prasher et al., 2002, 2003). At present the main strategies recommended are those that are used in the general population, such as modifications of the environment, consistent and predicable approaches, and support strategies aimed at compensating for a failing memory (see section by Dodd in the CAMDEX-DS; Dodd et al., 2003).

## Tuberous sclerosis (TS)

Several of the health risks associated with TS may present in later life. This genetically determined syndrome is a multisystem condition characterized mainly by a particular skin appearance and most strikingly by nodule formation in the brain and elsewhere and the risk of renal pathology, the latter due to the development of a number of possible renal pathologies. TS is caused by mutations affecting one of two genes located on chromosomes 9 and 16 (for review see Yates, 2006) and it has a prevalence of approximately 10 per 100,000 of the population (O'Callaghan et al., 1998). TS is associated with a wide range of ID and also with epilepsy (Joinson et al., 2003). Some people have no obvious disability and are only recognized as having the condition when they have a child with the disorder and the family are investigated. Others have severe levels of intellectual disabilities and may have, for example, very poor language skills, an autistic pattern of development, and severe epilepsy. In later life, the brain 'tubers' may exert clinically significant effects, either on the circulation of the cerebrospinal fluid leading to hydrocephalus or else through transformation into malignant tumours. In addition, renal failure may develop. For people with TS and limited communication ability the effects of raised intra-cranial pressure or insidiously developing renal failure may go unnoticed. In a population-based study of adults with TS, prevalence rates of psychiatric disorder were found to be very high. Of the 60 adults identified 40% had a lifetime prevalence of mental illness with major depression, alcohol-related problems and anxiety disorders being particularly present (Raznaham et al., 2006).

Ageing for people with TS is therefore associated with risks of insidiously developing disorders, such as renal failure. Thus, regular screening is indicated and special vigilance may be required for those with tuberous sclerosis and severe ID who may have very limited speech. Epilepsy is another problem that persists into later life in TS. It may be particularly severe, multifocal and difficult to treat. Severe epilepsy has its own associated mortality, and in such cases the practical management of these risks must be carefully considered.

## Prader–Willi syndrome

PWS is a genetically determined neurodevelopmental disorder with a distinct clinical and behavioural phenotype. The syndrome results from the absence of the paternally inherited contribution of maternally imprinted genes at the chromosomal locus 15q11q13 (for review see Goldstone, 2004). Most people with the syndrome (70–75%) have a deletion of approximately 4 Mb in the paternally inherited homologue of chromosome 15. In the remainder, both copies of chromosome 15 are maternal in origin (rather than one paternal and one maternal), referred to as a maternal uniparental disomy of chromosome 15 (mUPD).

The main early clinical features of PWS include neonatal hypotonia, developmental delay, short stature, small hands and feet, hypogonadism, and dysmorphic facial features (Cassidy et al., 1997). Characteristic of the syndrome is the onset of severe hyperphagia in childhood which, if not controlled, leads to life-threatening obesity (Holland, 1998). Other behavioural characteristics include a marked propensity to temper tantrums, obsessive–compulsive behaviour, possessiveness, stubbornness, and severe skin picking (Holm et al., 1993; Holland et al., 2003). In a large population study of PWS undertaken in the UK (Thomson et al., 2006), the birth incidence and population prevalence of PWS were estimated to be 1:28,000 and 1:52,000, respectively. From these data a mortality rate of 3% per year or 7% after the age of 32 was calculated, depending on various assumptions. Nobody with confirmed PWS older than 55 years of age was found. Since then there has been increasing concern about unexpected deaths across the lifespan.

What then are the particular concerns with respect to ageing? First, whilst in childhood the potential for life-threatening obesity as a result of the marked propensity to overeat can be managed by controlling the food environment, this is much more difficult in adult life. As a result, severe obesity often develops if there is no effective supervision of the food environment. The risks of obesity-related physical disorders such as diabetes mellitus, leg ulcers, respiratory disorders, and sleep disorders increase significantly with age (Butler et al., 2002). Second, for those people with PWS due to mUPD (but much less so for those with PWS due to a deletion) the risk of psychosis increases markedly with age (Boer et al., 2002). In this study all five people aged 28 years or older with PWS due to mUPD had had periods of psychosis, in contrast to just one out of nine with PWS due to a deletion This finding of excess psychotic illness in PWS due to mUPD was subsequently also reported by Vogels et al. (2003). Third, the hypogonadal and low growth hormone status of people with PWS results in an increased risk of problems related to hormone deficiency, such as osteoporosis, Finally, people with PWS have high pain thresholds, rarely vomit, and have atypical temperature regulation (Holm et al., 1993). For these reasons the development of serious physical illness can go unnoticed until it is so advanced that it is too late to treat (e.g. appendicitis). For people with PWS ageing and later life are therefore associated with the development of very significant physical and psychiatric morbidity and an increased mortality that relates directly to the underlying pathophysiology of the syndrome. 'Old age' for this group of people at present appears to be as low as 50 years of age.

## The social context of ageing and services for people with ID in later life

As described at the beginning of this chapter, people with ID are an extremely heterogeneous group. Individuals vary greatly in the nature and extent of their disability, in the biological cause of

their ID, and in the presence or not of physical and psychiatric co-morbidity or challenging behaviour. As illustrated by the examples above, it is apparent that the trajectories of later life may be very different between syndromes. Also the age bands that might be considered to reflect 'later life' for a person with, for example, DS or with PWS, are much younger than for people with mild ID or those without such disabilities. The same is true for those with severe or profound disabilities and probably also for those with other genetically determined syndromes.

As well as this, the overall structure of the lives of people with ID is likely to have been very different. Although schooling until 19 years of age is now provided for people with special needs, the absence of proper employment opportunities in adult life, and therefore an opportunity to earn a salary, means that the social structures over the lifespan leading to retirement and receiving a pension are not present. For both biological reasons (and its impact on life expectancy) and for societal reasons, 'later life' or 'old age' for people with ID is not readily definable. For some groups of people with ID the chance of reaching 'retirement age', as defined in our society (over 65 years), is small.

Families continue to be the main care providers to their adult children with ID (Hubert and Hollins, 2000). Whilst mothers are usually the primary care providers and take the lead in day to day matters of care (such as personal care) (Toseland and McCallion, 1997) other family members, including those from the extended family, are also important (Seltzer et al., 1991). Over years of providing support, family members develop their own ways of coping with the demands upon them, such as acceptance, positive reinterpretation and growth, turning to religion, and planning for the future (Hayden and Heller, 1997). Respite care has been advocated as an important means of helping carers, although the extent to which it helps to reduce carer stress is debatable (see review by McCallion and Kolomer, 2003). Whereas in the past it was generally expected that a child with severe ID would not outlive his or her parents, with improvements in the life expectancy of people with ID it is increasingly likely that the parents (as the main carers) will themselves be reaching an advanced age and experiencing health problems and possibly financial hardships and that the adult child with ID will outlive them (Fujura, 1998). Advancing age for a person with ID is therefore increasingly associated with a greater likelihood of the death of a loved one and the subsequent grief that follows. Whilst there was in the past the view that many people with ID did not have the intellectual capacity to experience grief, it is now clearly established that people with ID do experience grief and that this may be at least as severe as that experienced by people without ID. Some individuals with ID experience increased anxiety, depression, and other symptoms of stress in the context of loss (Hollins and Esterhuyzen, 1997).

A further issue that has received increasing attention is that of the vulnerability of people with ID to neglect, exploitation, and/or abuse (Turk and Brown, 1993). In the general population the vulnerability of elderly people to such problems is now well recognized. Therefore those who are both elderly and have an ID may be at particular risk. Studies investigating the consequences of abuse are difficult but changes in behaviour and affect are recognized (Sequeira et al., 2003). Protection of vulnerable adult (POVA) procedures are now required in each district of the UK that ensure that, when such problems are alleged, appropriate action is taken with respect to the safety of the person's living environment and that treatment is available, as well as support from police officers with suitable training to work with this group. Special measures are now available if people with ID are required to give evidence in court.

## The support of older people with ID and treatment of co-morbidity

In the UK, the social care for people with ID living away from the family home is provided by a range of private and voluntary social care agencies. Community-based multidisciplinary teams are established to provide support to people in various settings ranging from living independently, through supported living, to residential care, and also to their families. The government White Paper 'Valuing people' (Department of Health, 2001) also emphasized the importance of primary care and the need to facilitate access to health services, particularly for those with more severe ID. For older people with DS, for example, the onset of dementia, possibly as early as 30 years of age, will result in new and greater needs delivered to the home setting in much the same way as would be the case for anyone developing dementia whether they had an ID or not. This is likely to be initiated through primary care services in partnership with community teams. Given the evidence of high rates of co-morbidity among people with ID, ready access to primary care and to specialist interdisciplinary teams is crucially important to provide expert assessments and advice on support and intervention strategies. In adult life, in general, and with the older population of people with ID in particular, health promotion and the detection and treatment of ill-health and the use of appropriate support strategies is crucial to the maintenance of quality of life and the prevention of placement breakdown.

## Health promotion

As mentioned above, people with milder ID have a life expectancy that is closer to that of the general population. For this group, life expectancy and age-related problems are likely to be similar to those factors that influence ageing and associated co-morbidities in the general population, such as socio-economic status, diet, smoking, and extent of physical exercise. This group of people with mild ID may benefit from the same approaches that aim to reduce health inequalities in the general population. However, for people with more severe ID, Cooper et al. (2004) have argued that strategies aimed at reducing health inequalities in the general population will bring no benefit to this group and may even have the effect of widening such inequalities. For these reasons it is necessary to have a flexible and individualized approach to health promotion and the detection and treatment of ill-health with increasing age. It is necessary to be aware of the specific risks that may be associated with ageing in those with a specific syndrome. However, at the same time, attention to appropriate levels of exercise and a healthy diet and the detection of common age-related health problems (such as sensory impairments, osteoporosis, or dementia) are also important. Conditions such as osteoporosis may be prevented through dietary supplementation, for example, and the risk of bone fractures reduced (Vanlint and Nugent, 2006) or, in the case of people with PWS, obesity-related illnesses can be prevented by an appreciation of the responsibility of carers to manage the food environment and to prevent obesity (Holland and Wong, 1999).

## Detection, treatment, and management of co-morbid illnesses and problem behaviours

For staff and carers supporting people with ID who have limited language and who cannot readily make their thoughts and feelings known, there is a responsibility for ensuring the detection and treatment of both physical and psychiatric co-morbidity when it occurs. Those supporting a person with ID should be aware that illnesses may present in atypical ways. For example, mental illnesses (such as depression) may present in people with ID as changes in behaviour (Meins 1995; Tsiouris, 2001). For those with mild intellectual disabilities, affective disorder is common. It may remain unrecognized and/or untreated over many years and it often follows a chronic course (Richardson et al., 2001). However, not all maladaptive behaviour should be seen as due to problems within the individual and therefore as 'mental health' problems. Some maladaptive behaviour has been shaped and is a form of communication that has a function to it, such as 'demand avoidance', or the behaviour is 'attention maintained' (Emerson, 2003).

For these above reasons, sound and theoretically valid assessment is the bedrock of successful intervention and treatment for behavioural and psychiatric disorder affecting older people with ID. The presentation of apparently similar behaviours (e.g. aggression) in different people may have very different aetiologies. In each case assessment aims to identify those biological, psychological, environmental, and developmentally determined factors that predispose to, precipitate, and maintain such behaviours. For people with limited language, illnesses that are fundamentally physical in nature may present in ways that incorrectly suggest a psychological origin (e.g. the presentation of self-injurious behaviour that is in fact due to pain from gastro-oesophageal reflux or toothache). Alternatively, aggression may be incorrectly treated with neuroleptic medication when a more extensive psychological assessment indicates that such outbursts occur at times of uncertainty and following changes in routine. So instead of requiring drug treatment, they could be reduced in frequency and severity by the use of appropriate communication strategies, such as signs or symbols. Figure 35.1 summarizes the stages to be followed in assessing and managing such problems and shows how, through the process of formulation, appropriate interventions can be developed. Where treatment involves the use of medication whose action is on the brain (e.g. psychiatric medications, anticonvulsants) doses will often need to be lower and should be increased carefully as responses to such medication may be atypical. Treatment of these problems is rarely just of one type and the formulation needs to identify what is required to address specific issues. These might be as diverse as environmental changes, the use of specific psychological strategies, development of skills, improvement in communication, and/or the treatment of co-morbid medical or psychiatric disorders.

## Generic or specialist services?

Although there have been substantial advances in enabling people with ID to lead more independent and inclusive lives, the reality for many is still one of dependence on others. Of course, the support of other people can also be used to help achieve greater social inclusion. The heterogeneity of the ID population and the marked differences in the extent and nature of their disabilities, and therefore of their needs across the lifespan, mean that no one model of

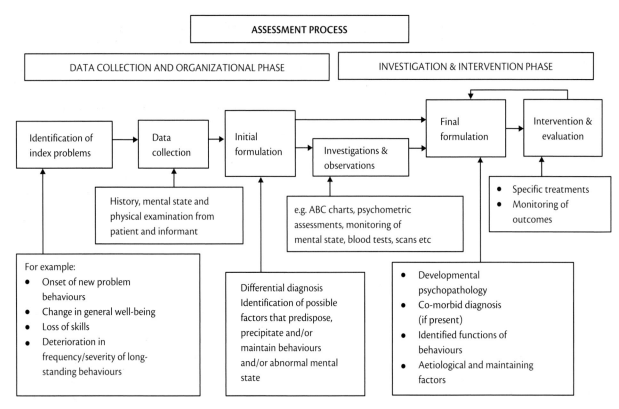

**Fig. 35.1** Schematic pathway of assessment and formulation of health and behaviour problems.

service provision will be able to meet the needs of all older people with ID. In some cases access to generic services for the elderly has been both possible and successful (Janicki *et al.*, 2002). Those with more severe ID will have lived their lives in supported settings and for them the issues is one of ageing in what is and may have been their home over many years. Services therefore must be community orientated and additional financial resources need to be available to provide additional support when it is required.

Some older people with ID may not have the capacity (ability) to make some or all the decisions in their lives that are required to be made, for example choices relating to their financial affairs or to their health and welfare (Wong *et al.*, 1999). Their lack of capacity may be lifelong or it may arise from the development of dementia in later life. The question of a person's capacity to make such decisions is important as it is crucial in the balance between the need to respect a person's autonomy, on the one hand, and the need to take decisions and/or act on their behalf, on the other. For example, those who lack capacity to understand money and to manage a budget may be at particular risk of financial exploitation. Different countries have different frameworks for managing this. In England and Wales, the provisions of the Mental Capacity Act 2005 came into force in 2007. This legislation provides the legal means for substitute decision-making when a person lacks the capacity to make the decision in question. The assessment of capacity is specific to the decision in question and to the time when the decision is to be made. An act subsequently done when someone has been found to lack capacity must be in their 'best interests'. The process for determining 'best interest' is defined in the Mental Capacity Act and in its Code of Practice (Department for Constitutional Affairs, 2005).

## Conclusion

This chapter has emphasized the complexity and heterogeneity of the group of people described as having an intellectual disability. Life expectancy remains reduced for many and there are clear health inequalities. However, there have also been fundamental changes in the principles that determine service development and in the attitudes that have determined policy and practice. In the UK these have their origins in enlightened legislation and in education policy. There is much to be discovered about how ageing specifically affects people with particular syndromes associated with ID. The experience with older people with some syndromes, such as DS, would suggest that ageing may have special risks in specific conditions and that these require informed and focused interventions. More specialist services for older people with ID may well be needed but the right of access of people with ID to generic services must also be recognized. Not to uphold fair access, in circumstances when such services are appropriate for them, is to discriminate against older people with ID.

### References

American Psychiatric Association (1994). *Diagnostic and statistical classification of disease and related health problems*, 4th edn. American Psychiatric Association, Washington, DC.

Atkinson, D., Johnston, M. *et al.* (1997). *Forgotten lives; exploring the history of learning disability*. BILD Publications, Kidderminster.

Ball, S., Holland, A. *et al.* (2004). Modified CAMDEX informant interview is a valid and reliable tool for use in the diagnosis of dementia in adults with Down's syndrome. *Journal of Intellectual Disability Research*, **48**, 611–620.

Ball, S., Holland, A.J. *et al.* (2006). Personality and behaviour changes mark the early stages of Alzheimer's disease in adults with Down's syndrome: findings from a prospective population-based study. *International Journal of Geriatric Psychiatry*, **21**, 661–673.

Birch, H., Richardson, S. *et al.* (1970). *Mental subnormality in the community: a clinical and epidemiological study.* Williams and Wilkins, Baltimore, MD.

Bittles, A., Petterson, B. *et al.* (2002). The influence of intellectual disability on life expectancy. *Journal of Gerontology Series A: Biological Sciences and Medical Sciences*, **57**, M470–M472.

Boer, H., Holland, A.J. *et al.* (2002). Psychotic illness in people with Prader–Willi syndrome due to chromosome 15 maternal uniparental disomy. *The Lancet*, **359**, 135–136.

Borthwick-Duffy, S. and Eyman, R. (1990). Who are the dually diagnosed?. *American Journal of Mental Retardation*, **94**, 586–595.

Braddock, D. (1999). Aging and developmental disabilities: demographic and policy issues affecting American families. *Mental Retardation*, **37**, 155–161.

Butler, J., Whittington, J. *et al.* (2002). Medical conditions in Prader Willi syndrome. *Developmental Medicine and Child Neurology*, **44**, 248–255.

Cassidy, S., Forsythe, M. *et al.* (1997). Comparison of phenotype between patients with Prader-Willi syndrome due to deletion 15q and uniparental disomy 15. *American Journal of Medical Genetics*, **68**, 433–440.

Cooper, S.-A. (1997). Epidemiology of psychiatric disorders in elderly compared with younger people with learning disabilities. *British Journal of Psychiatry*, **170**, 375–380.

Cooper, S.-A. (1998). A population-based cross-sectional study of social networks and demography in older compared with younger adults with learning disabilities. *Journal of Learning Disabilities for Nursing, Health and Social Care*, **2**, 212–220.

Cooper, S.-A., Melville, C. *et al.* (2003). Psychiatric diagnosis, intellectual disabilities and diagnostic criteria for psychiatric disorders for use with adults with learning disabilities/mental retardation (DC-LD). *Journal of Intellectual Disability Research*, **47**, 3–15.

Cooper, S.-A., Melville, C. *et al.* (2004). People with intellectual disabilities. Their health needs differ and need to be recognised and met. *British Medical Journal*, **329**, 414–415.

Davidson, P., Prasher, V. *et al.* (eds) (2003). *Mental health, intellectual disabilities and the aging process.* Blackwell Publishing, Oxford.

Day, K. (1985). Psychiatric disorder in the middle-aged and elderly mentally handicapped. *British Journal of Psychiatry*, **147**, 660–667.

Deb, S., Thomas, M. *et al.* (2001). Mental disorder in adults with intellectual disability. I: Prevalence of functional psychiatric illness among a community based population aged between 16 and 64 years. *Journal of Intellectual Disability Research*, **45**, 495–505.

Department for Constitutional Affairs (2005). *The Mental Capacity Act 2005 (England and Wales).* HMSO, London.

Department of Health (2001). *Valuing people: a new strategy for the 21st century.* Department of Health, London.

Department of Health and Social Security (1971). *Better services for the mentally handicapped.* DHSS, London.

Dodd, B., Holm, A. *et al.* (2003). Phonological development: a normative study of British English-speaking children. *Clinical Linguistics and Phonetics*, **8**, 617–643.

Einfeld, S. and Tonge, B. (1996). Population prevalence of psychopathology in children and adolescents with intellectual disability II: epidemiological findings. *Journal of Intellectual Disability Research*, **40**, 99–109.

Emerson, E. (2003). Prevalence of psychiatric disorders in children and adolescents with and without intellectual disability. *Journal of Intellectual Disability Research*, **47**, 51–58.

Emerson, E. (2005). Emotional and behavioural needs of children and adolescents with intellectual disabilities in an urban conurbation. *Journal of Intellectual Disability Research*, **49**, 16–24.

Evenhuis, H. (1995a). Medical aspects of ageing in a population with intellectual disability: I. Visual impairment. *Journal of Intellectual Disability Research*, **39**, 19–25.

Evenhuis, H. (1995b). Medical aspects of ageing in a population with intellectual disability: II. Hearing impairment. *Journal of Intellectual Disability Research*, **39**, 27–33.

Fryers, T. (2000). Epidemiology of mental retardation. In *New Oxford textbook of psychiatry*, Vol. 2, pp. 1941–1945. Oxford University Press, Oxford.

Fujura, G. (1998). Demography of family households. *American Journal of Mental Retardation*, **103**, 225–235.

Goldstone, A. (2004). Prader–Willi syndrome: advances in genetics, pathophysiology and treatment. *Trends in Endocrinology and Metabolism*, **15**, 12–20.

Hayden, M. and Heller, T. (1997). Support, problem-solving/coping ability, and personal burden of younger and older caregivers of adults with mental retardation. *Mental Retardation*, **35**, 364–372.

Holland, A.J. (1998). Understanding the eating disorder affecting people with Prader–Willi Syndrome. *Journal of Applied Research in Intellectual Disability*, **11**(3), 192–206.

Holland, A.J. and Wong, J. (1999). Genetically determined obesity in Prader–Willi syndrome: the ethics and legality of treatment. *Journal of Medical Ethics*, **25**, 230–236.

Holland, A.J., Hon, J. *et al.* (1998). A population-based study of the prevalence and presentation of dementia in adults with Down Syndrome. *British Journal of Psychiatry*, **172**, 493–498.

Holland, A., Whittington, J. *et al.* (2003). The paradox of Prader–Willi syndrome: a genetic model of starvation. *The Lancet*, **362**, 989–991.

Hollins, S. and Esterhuyzen, A. (1997). Bereavement and grief in adults with intellectual disabilities. *British Journal of Psychiatry*, **170**, 497–501.

Holm, V., Cassidy, S. *et al.* (1993). Prader–Willi syndrome: consensus diagnostic criteria. *Pediatrics*, **91**, 398–402.

Hubert, J. and Hollins, S. (2000). Working with elderly carers of people with intellectual disabilities and planning for the future. *Advances in Psychiatric Treatment*, **6**, 41–48.

Jacobson, J. (1982). Problem behaviour and psychiatric impairment within a developmentally disabled population. 1:Behaviour frequency. *Journal of Applied Research in Mental Retardation*, **3**, 121–139.

Jacobson, J., Sutton, M. *et al.* (1985). Demography and characteristics of aging and aged mentally retarded persons. In *Aging and developmental disabilities: issues and approaches* (ed. M. Janicki and H. Wisniewski). Brookes, Baltimore.

Janicki, M. and Dalton, A. (1998). Down's syndrome. *Dementia, Aging and Intellectual Disabilities*, **10**, 183–197.

Janicki, M. and Dalton, A. (2000). Prevalence of dementia and impact on intellectual disability services. *Mental Retardation*, **38**(3), 276–288.

Janicki, M., Dalton, A., Henderson, C., and Davidson, P. (1999). Mortality and morbidity among older adults with intellectual disability: health services considerations. *Disability and Rehabilitation*, **21**, 284–294.

Janicki, M., Anderson, D. *et al.* (2002). An overview of three critical wellness issues affecting adults with intellectual disabilities: the mind, nutrition and exercise. *Health disparities and a paradigm for health promotion: report of the Invitational Symposium on Health, Aging, and Developmental Disabilities.* University of Illinois at Chicago, Department of Human Development and Disability, Chicago.

Joinson, C., O'Callaghan, F. *et al.* (2003). Learning disability and epilepsy in an epidemiological sample of individuals with tuberous sclerosis complex. *Psychological Medicine*, **33**, 335–344.

Kapell, D., Nightingale, B. *et al.* (1998). Prevalence of chronic medical conditions in adults with mental retardation: Comparison with the general population. *Mental Retardation*, **36**(4), 269–279.

Kaski, M. (2000). Aetiology of mental retardation: general issues and prevention. In *New Oxford textbook of psychiatry*, Vol. 2, pp. 1947–1952. Oxford University Press, Oxford.

Lai, F. and Williams, R. (1989). A prospective study of Alzheimer disease in Down syndrome. *Archives of Neurology*, **46**, 849–853.

Levan, A. (1956). Chromosome studies in some human tumours and tissues of normal origin, grown *in vivo* and *in vitro* at the Sloan-Kettering Institute. *Cancer*, **9**, 648–663.

McCallion, P. and Kolomer, S.R. (2003).Understanding and addressing psychosocial concerns among aging family caregivers of persons with intellectual disabilities. In *Mental health, intellectual disabilities and the aging process* (ed. P. Davidson, V. Prasher, and M.P. Janicki), pp. 179–195. Blackwell, Oxford.

McConkey, R., Mulvany, F. *et al.* (2006). Adult persons with intellectual disabilities on the island of Ireland. *Journal of Intellectual Disability Research*, **50**(3), 227–236.

Mann, D. (1988). Alzheimer's disease and Down's syndrome. *Histopathology*, **13**, 125–137.

Meins, W. (1995). Symptoms of major depression in mentally retarded adults. *Journal of Intellectual Disability Research*, **39**, 41–46.

Moss, S. and Patel, P. (1993). Prevalence of mental illness in people with learning disability over 50 years of age, and the diagnostic importance of information from carers. *Irish Journal of Psychiatry*, **14**, 110–129.

Moss, S. and Patel, P. (1995). Psychiatric symptoms associated with dementia in older people with learning disability. *British Journal of Psychiatry*, **167**, 663–667.

O'Brien, G. and Yule, W. (eds) (1995). *Behavioural phenotypes*. Mac Keith Press, London.

O'Callaghan, F., Shiell, A. *et al.* (1998). Prevalence of tuberous sclerosis estimated by capture-recapture analysis. *The Lancet*, **351**, 1490.

Oliver, C. and Holland, A.J. (1986). Down's syndrome and Alzheimer's diseases: a review. *Psychological Medicine*, **16**, 307–322.

Patja, K., Molsa, P. *et al.* (2001). Cause-specific mortality of people with intellectual disability in a population-based. 35-year follow up study. *Journal of Intellectual Disability Research*, **45**(1), 30–40.

Prasher, V. and Hall, W. (1996). Short-term prognosis of depression in adults with Down's syndrome: association with thyroid status and effects on adaptive behaviour. *Journal of Intellectual Disability Research*, **40**(1), 32–38.

Prasher, V., Huxley, A. *et al.* (2002). A 24-week, double-blind, placebo-controlled trial of donepezil in patients with Down's syndrome and Alzheimer's disease – pilot study. *International Journal of Geriatric Psychiatry*, **17**, 270–278.

Prasher, V., Adams, C. *et al.* (2003). Long term safety and efficacy of donepezil in the treatment of dementia in Alzheimer's disease in adults with Down's syndrome: open label study. *International Journal of Geriatric Psychiatry*, **18**, 549–551.

Raznaham, A., Joinson, C. *et al.* (2006). Psychopathology in tuberous sclerosis: an overview and finding in a population-based sample of adults with tuberous sclerosis. *Journal of Intellectual Disability Research*, **50**(8), 561–569.

Richardson, S., Maughan, B. *et al.* (2001). Long-term affective disorder in people with mild learning disability. *British Journal of Psychiatry*, **179**, 523–527.

Roth, M., Tym, E. *et al.* (1986). CAMDEX-A standardised instrument for the diagnosis of mental disorder in the elderly with special reference to the early detection of dementia. *British Journal of Psychiatry*, **149**, 698–709.

Rubinzstein, D., Hon, J. *et al.* (1999). ApoE genetoype and risk of dementia in Down's syndrome. *Neuropsychiatric Genetics*, **88b**(4), 344–347.

Rumble, B., Retallack, R. *et al.* (1989). Amyloid A4 protein and its precursor in Down's syndrome and Alzheimer's disease. *New England Journal of Medicine*, **320**, 1446–1452.

Seltzer, G., Begun, A. *et al.* (1991). The impact of siblings on adults with mental retardation and their aging mothers. *Family Relations*, **40**, 310–317.

Sequeira, H., Howlin, P. *et al.* (2003). Psychological disturbance associated with sexual abuse in people with learning disabilities. *British Journal of Psychiatry*, **183**, 451–456.

Shakespeare, T. (2006). *Disability rights and wrongs*. Routledge, London.

Strauss, D. and Eyman, R. (1996). Mortality of people with mental retardation in California with and without Down syndrome 1986–1991. *American Journal of Mental Retardation*, **100**(6), 643–653.

Tanzi, R., St George-Hyslop, P. *et al.* (1987). The genetic defect in familial Alzheimer's disease is not tightly linked to the amyloid B-protein gene. *Nature*, **329**, 156–157.

Taylor, J., Hatton, C. *et al.* (2004). Screening for psychiatric symptoms: PAS-ADD Checklist norms for adults with intellectual disabilities. *Journal of Intellectual Disability Research*, **48**(1), 37–41.

Thase, M., Tigner, R. *et al.* (1984). Age-related neuropsychological deficits in Down's syndrome. *Biological Psychiatry*, **4**, 571–585.

Thomson, A., Glasson, E. *et al.* (2006). A long-term population-based clinical and morbidity review of Prader–Willi syndrome in Western Australia. *Journal of Intellectual Disability Research*, **50**(1), 69–78.

Toseland, R. and McCallion, P. (1997). Trends in caregiving intervention research. *Social Work Research*, **21**, 154–164.

Tsiouris, J. (2001). The diagnosis of depression in people with severe/ profound intellectual disability. *Journal of Intellectual Disability Research*, **45**, 115–120.

Turk, V. and Brown, H. (1993). The sexual abuse of adults with learning disabilities: results of a two-year incidence survey. *Mental Handicap Research*, **6**, 193–216.

Vanlint, S. and Nugent, M. (2006). Vitamin D and fractures in people with intellectual disability. *Journal of Intellectual Disability Research*, **50**(10), 761–767.

Vogels, A., Matthijs, G. *et al.* (2003). Chromosome 15 maternal uniparental disomy and psychosis in Prader–Willi syndrome. *Journal of Medical Genetics*, **40**(1), 72–73.

Watson, J. and Crick, F. (1953). Genetical implications of the structure of deoxyribonucleic acid. *Nature*, **171**, 964–967.

Whittington, J., Holland, A.J. *et al.* (2001). Population prevalence and estimated birth incidence and mortality rate for people with Prader Willi syndrome in one health district. *Journal of Medical Genetics*, **38**, 792–798.

Wisniewski, K., Howe, J. *et al.* (1978). Precocious aging and dementia in patients with Down's syndrome. *Biological Psychiatry*, **13**, 619–627.

Wong, J., Clare, I. *et al.* (1999). Capacity to make health care decisions: its importance in clinical practice. *Psychological Medicine*, **29**, 437–446.

World Health Organization (1980). *International classification of impairments, disabilities and handicaps*, 10th revision. WHO, Geneva.

World Health Organization (1992). *International statistical classification of disease and related health problems*, 10th revision. WHO, Geneva.

Yates, J. (2006). Tuberous sclerosis. *European Journal of Human Genetics*, **14**, 1065–1073.

Zigman, W., Schupf, N. *et al.* (1987). Premature regression of adults with Down's syndrome. *American Journal of Mental Deficiency*, **92**, 161–168.

# 36

# Sleep disorders in older people

Urs Peter Mosimann and Bradley F. Boeve

Sleep is most consistently defined as a periodic temporary loss of consciousness. Although the purpose of sleep remains unknown it clearly has a restorative effect. Sleep deprivation has been associated with impaired executive function, impaired attention, memory loss, an overall poorer quality of life, and increased health service utilization (Cricco *et al.*, 2001). Population-based studies have revealed that both sleep deprivation and sleep excess can have detrimental effects (Kripke *et al.*, 2002).

Sleep problems are common in older people. Ageing is associated with changes in sleep architecture and altered sleep habits, such as daytime napping (Phillips and Ancoli-Israel, 2001). However, these changes do not explain the extent of sleep disturbance encountered in elderly subjects. Sleep problems in the elderly are commonly indicators of poor physical or mental health (Manabe *et al.*, 2000). Foley *et al.* (2004) assessed 1506 elderly Americans (aged 55 to 84) in an epidemiological study. The majority of participants (83%) were suffering of one or more medical conditions. Depression, heart disease, pain, and memory problems were associated with insomnia, whereas obesity, lung disease, arthritis, stroke, and osteoporosis were related to sleep breathing problems, snoring, daytime somnolence, and insufficient sleep. About two-thirds of the participants with major co-morbidity complained of sleep problems and poor sleep quality. The vast majority (90%) of participants without co-morbidity reported good sleep. Sleep problems therefore should not be regarded as part of healthy ageing.

Physical frailty often goes together with poorer mobility, inactivity, and reduced daylight exposure, which are all factors that contribute to impaired sleep (Yoon *et al.*, 2003). Higher co-morbidity is a common reason for polypharmacy and many types of medication can contribute to sleep problems (Ancoli-Israel, 2005). Elderly people are also at higher risk of suffering from neurodegenerative disorders, which are commonly associated with sleep disturbance or excessive daytime sleepiness (Ohayon, 2005). Furthermore, sleep disorders can antedate neurodegenerative disorders. Recent studies (Boeve *et al.*, 2001; Postuma *et al.*, 2006) revealed, for example, that rapid eye movement (REM) sleep behaviour disorder (RBD), can precede the onset of synucleinopathies including multiple system atrophy, dementia with Lewy bodies (DLB), and Parkinson's disease (PD) by several years. RBD may therefore be an early clinical marker for these neurodegenerative disorders. Finally sleep

problems are more common in the elderly, because the prevalence of primary sleep disorders such as sleep-related breathing disorders, restless legs syndrome (RLS), periodic limb movements disorders (PLMD), and RBD increase with age (Ancoli-Israel, 2005). Sleep disorders are also common in residents of nursing homes. Up to two-thirds of residents of nursing homes complain about fragmented sleep, daytime sleepiness, or have a disturbed sleep cycle (Conn and Madan, 2006). Ambient light in multipurpose rooms, the lack of daytime activities, noise, and disruptive nursing at night are some of the reasons contributing to sleep disturbance in patients living in institutions (Alessi and Schnelle, 2000). Sleep problems are also rarely documented (Martin *et al.*, 2006), but may contribute to behavioural disturbances, such as agitation during the day (Gehrman *et al.*, 2003).

It is crucial for old age psychiatrists to be familiar with age-related changes in sleep in order to distinguish between normal sleep changes and sleep disorders. Coexisting physical and mental disorders need careful assessment and management when sleep problems are addressed. Sleep disturbance and mental disorder commonly coexist, and sleep disorders such as obstructive sleep apnoea (OSA) have overlapping symptoms with depression. Lack of libido, lethargy, and hopelessness are common in depression and OSA. The treatment of sleep disorders in elderly patients warrants careful consideration of risk and benefit because alterations in pharmacodynamics/kinetics and medication interactions mean they are susceptible to adverse events, such as an increased risk of falls and confusion (Glass *et al.*, 2005) (see Chapter 14).

This chapter is aimed at the non-sleep specialist and will review the most common sleep disorders found in elderly patients. It begins with a brief review of sleep physiology, and then gives an outline of how to take a comprehensive sleep history. Following this it provides details about the most common sleep problems in elderly patients, such as insomnia, parasomnias, daytime sleepiness, and sleep-related breathing disorders. Throughout the chapter we focus on the assessment and treatment of the sleep disorders that are most likely to be encountered in elderly patients with mental or neurodegenerative disorders. The reader with a special interest in sleep will find more detailed information in general textbooks on sleep medicine (e.g. Buysse, 2005; Carney and Berry, 2005; Kryger *et al.*, 2005; Ambrogetti *et al.*, 2006).

# The control of sleep and wakefulness

## Sleep architecture

The 'three states of being' are wakefulness, non-rapid eye movement (NREM) sleep, and REM sleep. Sleep architecture refers to the organization of sleep and the distribution of the different sleep stages during a night's sleep. It changes during a person's lifespan, with the most prominent alterations taking place before the age of 60 (Ohayon *et al.*, 2004). The sleep stages are defined by sets of electroencephalographic (EEG), electromyographic (EMG), and electro-oculographic (EOG) features (Rechtschaffen and Kales, 1968). Polysomnography (PSG) includes all these measures plus measurement of blood oxygenation and inductive plethysmography. The latter measures the circumference of the thorax and abdomen which is important for assessing inspiration and expiration. PSG is required to relate symptoms of sleep disorders to sleep stages.

## Wakefulness

Wakefulness has, compared with sleep, the greatest variability in EEG, EOG, and EMG signals. This is because these measures depend on the interaction of the subject with the environment. The characteristic EEG signal whilst awake is a low-voltage (15 to 45 µV), high-frequency (alpha 8–13 Hz and beta > 13 Hz) signal. The alpha rhythm is most prominent over the occipital pole, when the eyes are closed.

## NREM sleep

During NREM sleep, the EEG voltage increases and the frequency slows down resulting in more theta and delta activity. NREM sleep can be divided into four progressive stages: Stages 1 and 2 are the light NREM sleep stages whereas stages 3 and 4 are the deep NREM sleep stages, also called slow wave sleep (SWS) due to the characteristic high-amplitude (75 µV), slow wave delta activity. Stage 1 is the transitory stage between wakefulness and stage 2. This stage is clinically characterized by drowsiness and slow rolling eye movements (< 0.5 Hz). The EMG and EOG usually diminish in activity when stage 2 is reached. The typical EEG features of stage 2 are sleep spindles and K complexes. The latter are relatively high-amplitude biphasic waves with an initial negative component. Sleep spindles are signal complexes of gradually increasing and decreasing amplitude in the 12–14 Hz range. The number of sleep spindles and K complexes decrease in old age (Crowley *et al.*, 2002). Stage 3 and 4 sleep are characterized by delta activity (< 4 Hz) on the EEG, with stage 4 having delta wave activity for more than 50% of the time. EOG and EMG activity is usually low during SWS. In individuals above the age of 80, particularly in men, SWS declines. Most of the NREM sleep in this age group is therefore spent in stage 2 (Landolt *et al.*, 1996).

## REM sleep

High-frequency eye movements (> 1 Hz) and absence of EMG activity are the most prominent hallmarks of REM sleep. The absence of EMG activity is due to active inhibition of all muscles except the extraocular eye-muscles, diaphragm, and small muscles in the ear apparatus. The EEG characteristics of REM sleep are quite similar to wakefulness. Alpha activity is common but usually 1–2 Hz slower than during wakefulness. REM latency refers to the time elapsing between sleep onset and the first REM episode which usually ranges from 60 to 90 min. The basic characteristics of the sleep stages are summarized in Table 36.1.

**Table 36.1** Characteristic features of wakefulness, NREM and REM sleep

|  | EEG | EOG | EMG |
| --- | --- | --- | --- |
| Wakefulness | Low voltage, fast activity (occipital alpha activity) | Variable | Variable |
| NREM sleep |  |  |  |
| Stage 1 | Mixed activity | Slow eye movements < 1 Hz | Little activity towards the end of stage 1 |
| Stage 2 | K-complexes and spindles | Low activity | Low activity |
| Slow wave sleep (Stages 3 and 4) | High voltage, slow wave activity | Low activity | Low activity |
| REM sleep | Low voltage, fast activity, alpha activity | Rapid eye movements | Absence of muscle tone |

## Sleep periods

The amount of night-time sleep required decreases steadily with age, from about 16 hours in a newborn to 7 hours in a 75-year-old subject (Roffwarg *et al.*, 1966). The elderly tend to sleep less at night, their sleep becomes more fragmented and sleep latency is prolonged. Sleep latency refers to the time required from going to bed until falling asleep. Napping during daytime may help to catch up with sleep needs. The duration of sleep is more consistent in the elderly than in younger people and there is less difference in sleep duration between weekdays and weekends. Throughout a typical sleep period, the sleep stages cycle repeats approximately four to six times. Each cycle lasts 60 to 120 minutes with the sleep stages progressing from stage 1 to stage 4, followed by a period of REM sleep. The percentage of REM sleep remains stable during early and mid-life, but there is a decrease in older age, and the REM latency in older adults is often shorter. The majority of REM sleep occurs in the last few hours of the night and this may be a reason why REM sleep behaviour disorder (RBD) is more common in the early morning hours. The progression between the different sleep stages can be disrupted by periods of arousal. These periods are usually short and not remembered in young and middle-aged adults. In elderly adults, however, the arousal periods become longer and more frequent, leading to more being recalled (Klerman *et al.*, 2004). An overview of the characteristic changes in sleep architecture that occur with ageing is given in Box 36.1.

---

**Box 36.1** Sleep changes in elderly subjects (> 65 years)

♦ Reduced total sleep time
♦ More daytime napping
♦ Overall decrease in sleep efficiency (bedtime > sleep time)
♦ Changes of sleep architecture with:
    less slow wave sleep (SWS) and REM sleep
    more stage 1 and 2 sleep
    more night-time arousals and recalled awakenings
    shorter REM latency
    longer sleep latency

Transitory behavioural and perceptual phenomena on the borders of sleep are common and do not necessarily indicate disease. Jerks, involuntary head or limb movements, and hallucinations are not rare in this transition phase. Thirty seven per cent of individuals in a community-based sample of nearly 5000 people (age 15–100) experienced hallucinations whilst falling asleep (hypnagogic hallucinations) and 12.5% reported hallucinations while waking up (hypnopompic hallucinations) (Ohayon *et al.*, 1996). Transient confusion when waking up is called confusional arousal, which occurs when suddenly waking up from a deep sleep stage (Naitoh *et al.*, 1993).

## The anatomy and neurochemistry of sleep and wakefulness

Numerous brain areas and neurotransmitters are involved in the control of sleep and wakefulness (Saper *et al.*, 2005). Areas important in the generation of these states are linked with each other and are interconnected with areas vital for other functions such as breathing, cardiovascular circulation, temperature regulation, hormone production, sensory information processing, and appetite. This section will provide an overview of the most important structures and neurotransmitters involved in the generation of sleep and wakefulness.

### Systems promoting wakefulness

The ascending reticular activating system is the major *arousing system*. It consists of two major branches (Saper *et al.*, 2005), the thalamo-cortical and hypothalalmic–aminergic arousal branches.

The *thalamo-cortical arousal branch* is essential for the generation of wakefulness and REM sleep. This pathway contains cholinergic neurons, which project from the laterodorsal tegmental and the peduculopontine tegmental nuclei (LDT-PPT) via the thalamus to the cortex. The LDT-PPT system is crucial for wakefulness and arousal. The LDT-PPT nuclei are involved to some extent in the induction of REM sleep and may contribute to the loss of skeletal muscle tone during REM sleep. Cholinesterase inhibitors (ChE-I) increase REM sleep in patients with Alzheimer's disease (Moraes Wdos *et al.*, 2006), whereas treatment with drugs with anticholinergic or antimuscarinergic properties (atropine, scopolamine, and tricyclic antidepressants) can reduce REM sleep (Wilson and Argyropoulos, 2005).

The *hypothalamic-aminergic arousal branch* projects through the lateral hypothalamic nucleus to the basal forebrain. This branch of the ascending arousal system involves the serotonergic dorsal raphe nuclei (DRN), the noradrenergic locus coeruleus (LC), and the histaminergic tuberomammillary nuclei (TMN). The aminergic arousal system fires constantly during wakefulness but is suppressed during NREM sleep and is inactive in REM sleep. Aminergic transmitters, including dopamine, noradrenaline, serotonin, and histamine, are commonly modulated by psychotropic drugs. In addition to causing parkinsonism, dopamine deficiency or antagonism can lead to sleep-related movement disorders such as restless legs syndrome (RLS) and PLMD. These conditions improve upon treatment with dopamine replacement therapy (Clemens *et al.*, 2006). Substances which raise the action of noradrenaline, such as amphetamines, promote wakefulness and reduce REM sleep, whereas medications antagonizing the effects of *noradrenaline* reduce wakefulness (Nicholson *et al.*, 1989). Histamines promote wakefulness, and antihistamines which pass the blood–brain

barrier, are commonly used as over-the-counter sedatives. *Serotonin* increases SWS but reduces REM sleep. The treatment of affective disorders with selective serotonin reuptake inhibitors (SSRIs) can cause insomnia and rapid discontinuation of SSRIs can cause nightmares and parasomnias (Wilson and Argyropoulos, 2005).

### Sleep-promoting systems

The ventrolateral pre-optic area (VLPO) of the anterior hypothalamic region is the key *sleep-promoting area*. This area has reciprocal inhibitory links with both the thalamo-cortical arousal branch and the hypothalamic–aminergic arousal branch of the ascending reticular activating system. The main neurotransmitters of the VLPO are gamma-aminobutyric acid (GABA) and galanin. The extended part of the VLPO contains REM-active neurons which may be part of the circuitry switching between REM and NREM sleep (Lu *et al.*, 2006). Benzodiazepine and non-benzodiazepine hypnotics enhance GABA activity. They reduce sleep latency and night-time awakening (Bateson, 2006).

### Switching between wakefulness and sleep

In 1998 two research groups identified independently two peptides synthesized in the lateral hypothalamus. One group called the peptides orexin A and B (Sakurai *et al.*, 1998) and the other hypocretin 1 and 2 (de Lecea *et al.*, 1998). Later it became clear that orexin/hypocretin is crucial for the maintenance of wakefulness and sleep. These peptides play a key role in stabilizing the 'switch' for the maintenance of either wakefulness or sleep (Saper *et al.*, 2001, 2005). Low levels or absence of hypocretin in the cerebrospinal fluid are associated with narcolepsy (Nishino *et al.*, 2000). Other structures contributing to the transition between wakefulness and sleep are the VLPO for sleep promotion, the TMN for the promotion of wakefulness, and the suprachiasmatic nucleus (SCN), which is the site of the internal clock. Recent analyses in rodents have revealed a putative flip–flop switch for REM sleep (Lu *et al.*, 2006).

### Circadian rhythm generator

The SCN is the most powerful circadian clock in humans, and is important for wakefulness and sleep. It is linked to the VLPO and the pineal gland and synchronized by light. In addition, light suppresses the release of melatonin from the pineal gland, whereas darkness promotes its release. Circadian rhythm disorders are common in the elderly, especially in nursing homes, where dim light and immobility are major causes for inadequate light exposure (Shochat *et al.*, 2000). Degeneration of the SCN probably contributes to circadian dysrhythmias.

An overview of major transmitter systems involved in the generation of wakefulness and sleep is given in Table 36.2. This table includes only transmitters which can be influenced by psychotropic medication.

## Assessment of sleep disturbance

A comprehensive sleep history includes the views of both patient and bedpartners. The most common complaints of patients are difficulties falling asleep, remaining asleep, early morning wakening, and the lack of restorative sleep with associated excessive daytime sleepiness. Bedpartner complaints, however, refer to snoring, breath pauses, odd behaviour, and fidgety and other abnormal movements whilst being asleep. These latter symptoms are usually

**Table 36.2** Major neurotransmitters involved in the maintenance of wakefulness and sleep

| | Histamine | Serotonin | NA | Dopamine | Ach | Glutamate | GABA | Melatonin |
|---|---|---|---|---|---|---|---|---|
| Major nuclei | TMN | Raphe nucleus | Locus coeruleus | Mesencephalon, substantia nigra pars compacta | PPT-LDT, nucleus Meynert | Reticular formation | VLPO | Pineal gland |
| Major function | Arousal system (via hypothalamus forebrain) | | | | Thalamo-cortical arousal system | | Sleep induction | Circadian rhythms |
| Wakefulness | +++ | +++ | +++ | +++ | +++ | +++ | 0 | 0 |
| SWS | + | + | + | | + | + | +++ | +++ |
| REM sleep | 0 | 0 | 0 | | +++ | 0 | +++ | +++ |
| Agonizing/ enhancing effects | | SSRI | Amphetamine | Levodopa, Methyl-phenidate | ChE-I | | Benzodiazepines, Zaleplon, Zolpidem, Zopiclone, Ethanol | Melatonin, Ramelteon |
| Antagonizing/ attenuating effects | Antihistaminics | | Prazosin | Neuroleptics | Scopolamine, Atropine, TCA | Ketamine, Memantine | Flumazenil | |

Ach, acetylcholine; 5-HT, 5-hydroxytryptamine; GABA, gamma-aminobutyric acid; NA, noradrenaline; TMN, tuberomammillary nuclei; PPT-LDT, cholinergic pedunculopontine and laterodorsal tegmental nuclei; VLPO, ventrolateral pre-optic nucleus; SSRI, selective serotonin reuptake inhibitor; ChE-I, cholinesterase inhibitors; REM, rapid eye movement sleep; SWS, slow wave sleep; TCA, tricyclic antidepressants.

+++, high activity; ++, intermediate activity; +, low activity; 0, no activity.

not evident to the patient. Box 36.2 gives an overview of key areas to be covered in a comprehensive sleep history.

A sleep history assesses the *extent of the main complaints*. This includes questions about the onset, duration, and progression of the sleep complaint. It is helpful to establish why the problem is being articulated right now and whether the patient or the informant is initiating the assessment. It is essential to verify any risks involved, such the tendency to fall asleep whilst driving. Any *mental or physical disorders* co-existing with the sleep problem need attention. The relationship between the onset of the sleep disturbance and the mental or physical conditions remains to be established. It is important to clarify current medication. This review includes prescribed and over-the-counter medication such as valerian, hop, and antihistamines. Medication is commonly associated with sleep disturbance or sleepiness during daytime. It is therefore important

to establish whether the start or the discontinuation of medication is followed by disturbed sleep or daytime sleepiness. Some medication can contribute to sleep disturbance when taken before bedtime and will not affect sleep when taken in the morning, e.g. SSRIs. Common conditions and medication contributing to sleep problems are reviewed in the section on insomnia later in this chapter.

Knowledge about *current and past sleep habits* is important, since they vary from individual to individual. Some sleep complaints expressed by elderly patients may refer to altered sleep needs and habits or unrealistic expectations rather than a sleeping disorder. The assessment must include questions about pre-bed activities; the time at which the patient goes to bed; the amount of sleep; the time spent in bed awake. Clarity is needed as to whether sleep disruptions are related to toilet habits.

The *sleep environment* needs careful exploration. Noise, uncomfortable beds, a sleep disorder of the bedpartner, new neighbours, heat, and light can contribute to impaired sleep. Finally a sleep history is not complete without addressing the *daytime habits*. This part of the history establishes the timing and amount of physical exercise during the day, and the exposure to daylight. Numerous naps taken during a day can decrease the amount and quality of sleep. Clarity is also needed about nicotine, caffeine, and alcohol consumption.

## Classification of disorders of sleep and wakefulness

Three major classification systems are currently used to categorize sleep disorders. They include the *International Classification of Sleep Disorders Diagnostic and Coding Manual* (ICSD-2), the *Diagnostic and Statistical Manual of Mental Disorders*, 4th edition, text revision (DSM-IV-TR) (APA, 2005) and the *International Statistical Classification of Diseases and Related Health Problems*, 9th revision, clinical modification (ICD-9-CM) (WHO, 2003). ICSD-2 is the consensus classification of the American Academy of Sleep

---

**Box 36. 2** Key areas in a sleep history

A comprehensive sleep history includes the patient's and the bedpartner's views and establishes the
- *Main complaints*
- *Extent of the problem*: onset, chronology, duration, frequency, progression, reasons to address the problem now, impact on daily living, response to previous treatment
- *Psychiatric and medical co-morbidity*
- *Current prescribed and over the counter medication*
- *Current and past sleep habits*: pre-bed activities, bedtime, sleep duration, waking up time, getting up time, number of sleep disruption, and toilet habits during the night
- *Sleep environment*: noise, temperature, personal stressors, sleep problems of the bedpartner
- *Daytime habits*: amount of physical exercise, number and duration of daytime naps, exposure to light, smoking, alcohol, caffeine

Medicine (American Academy of Sleep Medicine, 2005). It codes sleep disorder into six main categories, including insomnia, sleep-related breathing disorders, hypersomnia, circadian rhythms sleep disorder, parasomnia, and sleep-related movement disorder. Unlike DSM-IV-TR and ICD-9-CM, it does not use an axial system for the classification and focuses on the sleep disorders only. DSM-IV-TR separates sleep disorders into primary sleep disorders including dyssomnias and parasomnias and secondary sleep disorders related to a mental disorder. ICD-9-CM distinguishes between sleep disorders of organic origin and those of mental origin. The systematic discussion of all sleep disorders is outside of the scope of this chapter and we will focus on the sleep disorders most commonly encountered in older people.

# Common sleep disorders in old age

## Insomnia

Insomnia is the most common sleep complaint in elderly individuals. It is often undiagnosed and can significantly impact upon an individual's quality of life. It contributes to illness, institutionalization, and falls (Brassington et al., 2000; McCurry and Ancoli-Israel, 2003; Avidan et al., 2005). Insomnia is an umbrella term that includes difficulties in initiating and maintaining sleep and the subjective complaint of non-restorative sleep. To fulfil restrictive clinical definitions of insomnia, symptoms need to persist over 2 weeks and contribute to impaired daytime functioning (Ohayon, 2002; APA, 2005). The prevalence varies depending on the population assessed or the diagnostic criteria applied. The prevalence of insomnia is about 30–35% in the adult population (Sateia and Nowell, 2004). In the older adult population, transient symptoms of insomnia are common (30–60% of older adults) in particular in elderly females (Foley et al., 1995). Insomnia is classified by the clinical presentation (onset, maintenance, or early morning wakening insomnia) and the association with physical or mental illnesses. Transient insomnia is defined as lasting up to 2 weeks. Intermediate insomnia ranges from 2 to 4 weeks, and chronic insomnia is defined as lasting more than 4 weeks (Nowell et al., 1997; Sateia et al., 2000). Primary (idiopathic) insomnia, unrelated to any illness exists, but is rare in elderly patients.

The pathogenesis of insomnia is multifaceted and cognitive models suggest that individual factors contribute to the *predisposition*, *precipitation*, and *perpetuation* of insomnia (Spielman et al., 1987). Predisposing factors are age, gender, weak sleep drive, and hyperarousal. Precipitating factors include pain, medical conditions, physical illness, stress, and a noisy environment. Perpetuating factors which contribute to the maintenance of insomnia include dysfunctional thoughts, such as excessive worrying about the consequences of poor sleep. Careful analysis of contributing factors and assessment of the type of insomnia are essential when developing an adequate management strategy.

Common psychiatric disorders associated with insomnia are depression, mania (Wilson and Argyropoulos, 2005) and anxiety disorders, such as obsessive–compulsive disorder (OCD), post-traumatic stress disorder (PTSD), and panic disorder (Maher et al., 2006). Insomnia can precede depression and may contribute to the onset of a depressive episode (Riemann and Voderholzer, 2003). Patients suffering from chronic insomnia are at risk of using alcohol as a sleep aid. Alcohol shortens the sleep latency but contributes to sleep fragmentation, REM sleep suppression, and early morning awakening (Stein and Friedmann, 2006). Chronic pain (Ohayon, 2005),

chronic pulmonary disease, congestive heart failure, chronic renal failure, diabetes mellitus, and hyperthyroidism are common medical causes for insomnia (Culpepper, 2006). Most medications can contribute to insomnia, particularly CNS stimulants such as dexamfetamine, methylphenidate; alpha- and beta-adrenoceptor blocking drugs, reserpine, bronchodilators, theophylline, calcium-channel blockers, corticosteroids, decongestants, bupropion, SSRIs, venlafaxine, monoamine oxidase inhibitors, and thyroid hormone. Other sleep disorders such as sleep-related breathing disorder, PLMD, RLS, or circadian rhythms disturbance are common reasons for insomnia. Insomnia and sleep fragmentation are particularly common in neurodegenerative disorders, such as PD, Alzheimer's disease, and DLB. Dysfunctional behaviour such as daytime napping, irregular sleep and wake schedules, eating in the middle of the night, nicotine, and caffeine consumption can contribute to insomnia.

### Assessment

Subjective complaints of the degree of insomnia are often greater than objective measures of insomnia in PSG sleep studies or questionnaires. A comprehensive sleep evaluation takes both subjective views and objective measures into account. The details for taking a sleep history were outlined above. Sleep diaries help to record patients' sleep pattern and disturbances prospectively. Such diaries should document the usual bed and sleep time, the timing and quantity of meals, the use of alcohol and exercise, daytime napping, and the duration and quantity of sleep each day.

Actigraphy is an alternative objective measure to a sleep log. Actigraphy uses a piezoelectric movement detector in a watch-like format, which allows the storage of movements for up to 4 weeks. It is well tolerated by elderly patients with and without cognitive impairment and helps to separate sleep from wakefulness (Ancoli-Israel et al., 2003). Actigraphy can be used by specialists to establish the pattern of sleep disturbance (sleep onset, maintenance, or early morning wakening) and to separate insomnia from circadian rhythm disturbances (advanced and delayed sleep phase syndromes). Early morning awakening is characteristic for depressed patients and needs to be distinguished from an advanced sleep phase which will be discussed later in the section on circadian sleep disorder.

Insomnia assessment involves a thorough physical examination to rule out medical conditions and a mental state examination. Routine blood tests should include thyroid function testing, since thyroid dysfunction is a common medical cause for insomnia. If insomnia persists after common causes such as depression, physical illness, and medication are excluded, patients may benefit from a referral to a specialist centre.

### Treatment

The identification and management of the underlying causes is crucial, since insomnia often improves when associated disorders are treated. Without recognizing the underlying condition, the long-term treatment is likely to fail and inappropriate treatments may be used which may worsen symptoms. For example, insomnia may worsen when the depression is treated with a stimulating antidepressant such as an SSRI. OSA needs to be excluded, before a treatment with sedative hypnotics is started. This is important because OSA and associated sleep fragmentation can worsen when treated with hypnotics. Good sleep habits and sleep hygiene and realistic goals and expectations should be enforced regardless of the cause of the insomnia.

Regardless of which treatment is used, an important facet of therapy requires the patient to hide clocks in the bedroom. When struggling to fall or stay asleep, seeing the time will almost always engender frustration and heighten the level of arousal. Therefore, patients should be instructed to either place clocks out of site or at least turn them so that the faces of clocks are not within view. An alarm should be set, and the patient should be instructed that if the alarm has not gone off yet, the patient should be sleeping. Many patients find it initially uncomfortable not knowing the time when struggling to sleep, but within days or weeks, they are better able to sleep.

### Non-pharmacological treatment of insomnia

Cognitive behavioural therapy is the most widely used psychological intervention for the treatment of insomnia. It includes cognitive therapy, education about sleep hygiene, relaxation techniques, stimulus control, and sleep restriction. *Cognitive therapy* seeks to alter dysfunctional beliefs and attitudes about sleep, such as the fear of going to bed and catastrophic thoughts around the consequences of poor sleep. Information about physiological age-related changes of sleep (see Box 36.1) may help to improve unrealistic expectations. Sleep hygiene includes: avoiding heavy meals, physical exercise, and limiting the volume of liquids prior to sleep; the restriction of caffeine, nicotine, and alcohol in the period 4 to 6 hours before bedtime; and a regular sleep schedule with reduced sleep during daytime. The National Sleep Foundation website contains helpful information about sleep hygiene for patients (http://www.sleepfoundation.org/).

*Stimulus control therapy* is based on the premise that sleep disturbances can be behaviourally conditioned. Patients with insomnia may associate the bedroom with wakefulness, frustration, and arousal. Reconditioning is needed by pairing sleep with the bedroom. Patients are advised (1) to go to bed only when sleepy and (2) to leave the bedroom when unable to fall asleep and to return to the bedroom again only when sleepy. Additional instructions include (3) to repeat this procedure throughout the night; (4) to arise in the morning at a set time, independent of the amount of sleep obtained, and (5) reduce daytime napping. Using this approach the bed becomes the place for sleep only (Bootzin and Nicassio, 1978).

*Sleep restriction therapy* curtails the amount of time spent in bed to the actual sleep time. The rationale behind this is that the bedtime in elderly adults is often much longer than the sleep time. Frustration and worrying in bed is counterproductive and raises arousal which perpetuates insomnia (Glovinsky and Spielman, 1991). In sleep restriction therapy the bedtime gets adjusted to the sleep duration. If a patient reports to sleep 6 hours then bedtime starts 6 hours before the time for getting up. A brief midday nap may be permissible, especially in the early phase of therapy.

*Relaxation techniques* are particularly helpful for individuals with tension, hyperarousal, and anxiety. Techniques such as a warm bath, progressive muscle relaxation and autogenic training help reduce muscle tension (somatic arousal), and meditation focus on reducing intrusive thoughts (cognitive arousal). The learning of relaxation techniques may require time and practice to become effective in older adults.

Three large meta-analyses have reported that cognitive behavioural therapy (CBT) is effective in treating insomnia (Morin *et al.*, 1994; Murtagh and Greenwood, 1995; Irwin *et al.*, 2006). In a meta-analysis

involving more than 2000 patients with insomnia, Morin *et al.* (1994) found that stimulus control and sleep restriction are the most effective single therapies, whereas sleep hygiene education was not effective on its own. Murtagh and Greenwood (1995) found no differences between different treatment methods. However, they reported that the therapeutic gain of non-pharmacological treatment was greater in patients regularly using sedative hypnotics. A recent meta-analysis found no difference between the different behavioural interventions in middle-aged subjects and those older than 55 years (Irwin *et al.*, 2006). A Cochrane Review found a mild beneficial effect of CBT for sleep problems for older adults (60+), especially for sleep maintenance insomnia (Montgomery and Dennis, 2003). CBT has also proved to be effective for sleep onset and sleep maintenance therapy in elderly patients (Pallesen *et al.*, 2003; Petit *et al.*, 2003). Taking the findings of these meta-analyses into account, CBT is likely to be an effective treatment for insomnia. The use of CBT may, however, be restricted in some elderly patients by medical conditions which prevent patients leaving their bed or by cognitive impairment.

### Pharmacological treatment of insomnia

The efficacy of sedative hypnotics in older adults was recently reviewed in a large meta-analysis including 24 studies involving more than 2400 participants (Glass *et al.*, 2005). Major short-term benefits of hypnotics are increased sleep time and less night-time awakening. Associated risks are adverse cognitive effects, psychomotor impairment, falls, and daytime fatigue (Conn and Madan, 2006). These risks may outweigh the benefits, particularly in patients with chronic insomnia, cognitive impairment, ataxia, or in patients with a high falls risk (Kallin *et al.*, 2004). The exposure to benzodiazepines with a long half-life in the elderly is associated with an increased risk of road traffic accidents (Hemmelgarn *et al.*, 1997). Caution with pharmacological therapies in older adults is needed because of polypharmacy and co-morbidity. Hypnotics may exacerbate coexisting medical conditions, including hepatic, respiratory, renal, and cardiac disorders. Further risks are the development of rebound insomnia, the development of tolerance, or withdrawal symptoms. Rebound insomnia is the worsening of insomnia after the stopping of hypnotic treatment. Symptoms of hypnotic withdrawal, particularly of short-acting benzodiazepines include insomnia, anxiety, loss of appetite, tremor, tinnitus, and perceptual disturbances. They may occur within a few hours after stopping a short-acting benzodiazepine or within a few days after stopping a long-acting agent such as diazepam. Gradual discontinuation is therefore recommended.

It is therefore important to restrict the use of hypnotics to patients who meet diagnostic criteria for insomnia and to keep the treatment duration short (2–4 weeks). The lowest effective dose is recommended. Short-acting hypnotics are preferred to minimize the risk of accumulating active metabolites. A patient's medical history and medication needs to be carefully reviewed before the treatments starts. Relative contraindications are a history of sleep-related breathing disorder, severe hepatic impairment, and myasthenia gravis.

Pharmacological treatment options include benzodiazepines, non-benzodiazepine hypnotics, sedating antidepressants, and melatonin agonists (Bain, 2006). The use of over-the-counter sedative drugs is often not disclosed to the treating physician unless patients are specifically asked to do so (Busto *et al.*, 2001). They include sedative antihistaminics, dietary supplements, and melatonin. The use of sedative antihistaminics such as alimemazine, diphenhydramine, and doxylamine is not recommended for elderly patients because of their anticholinergic properties which may contribute to cognitive impairment, orthostatic hypotension, falls, and urinary retention. Valerian, chamomile, hops, kava-kava, and other dietary supplements may have large variation in purity and formulation because their production is not regulated. This makes it difficult to assess their efficacy. The same is true of melatonin in countries like the USA, since the purity is not regulated by federal organizations. Other psychotropic drugs with sedative effects such as clomethiazole, chloral hydrate, and barbiturates are now rarely prescribed as hypnotics due to their side-effects, the high mortality in overdose for barbiturates, and the availability of safer treatment alternatives (Pathy *et al.*, 1986; Overstall and Oldman, 1987). These drugs will therefore not be discussed any further.

Both benzodiazepines and non-benzodiazepine hypnotics focus on GABA, the major inhibitory neurotransmitter of the CNS. They work by enhancing the activity of the GABA receptor. The products used differ with regard to half-life (nitrazepam ($t_{1/2}$ 15–30 hours), flurazepam ($t_{1/2}$ 40–100 hours), lorazepam ($t_{1/2}$ 10–20 hours), lormetazepam ($t_{1/2}$ 12–20 hours), and temazepam ($t_{1/2}$ 6–10 hours)) and zaleplon ($t_{1/2}$ 1 hour), zolpidem ($t_{1/2}$ 2.5–4 hours) and zopiclone ($t_{1/2}$ 3.5–6.5 hours). Eszopiclone is the S-isomer and zopiclone. Two benzodiazepines are used for the short-term treatment of both insomnia and anxiety (diazepam, lorazepam) (BNF, 2007). Nitrazepam, flurazepam, and diazepam are of limited use in elderly patients, due to their long elimination half-life (Klimm *et al.*, 1987). Sedative hypnotics reduce REM sleep and SWS. They decrease sleep latency, and increase total sleep duration and stage 2 sleep. Side-effects of benzodiazepines include excessive sedation, cognitive impairment, amnesia, and difficulties with motor coordination. Non-benzodiazepine sedative hypnotics were developed to overcome the adverse events of benzodiazepines and, compared with short-acting benzodiazepines, are equally effective and possibly have fewer side-effects. Whether these drugs are cost-effective remains unclear. Different controlled trials have assessed the risks and the benefits of non-benzodiazepine hypnotics in older adults (Roger *et al.*, 1993; Ancoli-Israel *et al.*, 1999; Melton *et al.*, 2005; Scharf *et al.*, 2005) and they are considered to be safe in the short term. The safety and efficacy of sedative hypnotics in the management of chronic insomnia in elderly patients remains unclear.

Melatonin agonists are newer agents used to treat insomnia. Ramelteon is a highly selective melatonin agonist and is beneficial for the treatment of chronic insomnia. A 5-week randomized, double-blind placebo-controlled trial involving 829 patients aged 65 or more showed that ramelteon reduced sleep latency without significant rebound insomnia or withdrawal effects after stopping the drug (Roth *et al.*, 2006).

Sedative antidepressants are often used to treat insomnia in depressed patients (Silber, 2005). Small case series suggest that mirtazapine and trazodone improve sleep efficiency without suppressing REM sleep (Winokur *et al.*, 2000; Saletu-Zyhlarz *et al.*, 2002). However, sedative antidepressants are not recommended for the treatment of chronic insomnia in patients without depression (Mendelson, 2005). The same is true for tricyclic antidepressants which have anticholinergic properties in addition.

Several studies have compared CBT with pharmacological therapy (McClusky *et al.*, 1991; Morin *et al.*, 1999; Jacobs *et al.*, 2004; Sivertsen *et al.*, 2006). Two studies assessed the effects of both approaches specifically in older adults. Sivertsen *et al.* (2006) examined the short- (6 weeks) and long-term effects (6 months) of cognitive behaviour therapy and zopiclone and showed that CBT is superior to zopiclone treatment in the short- and long-term management of chronic insomnia. The other study assessed the short- and long-term effects of either CBT or temazepam or the combination of both therapies. The combination therapy was the most powerful treatment for the short-term management of insomnia. All patients who received CBT had longer-lasting effects compared with temazepam treatment (Morin *et al.*, 1999). These results indicate both CBT and pharmacological treatment are effective in the short-term management of insomnia (up to a month) but that the effect of CBT may be more beneficial in the long term. However, it may take slightly longer until sleep improves when elderly patients are treated with CBT (McClusky *et al.*, 1991). Taken together, current evident suggest that CBT may be the first-line treatment, especially for chronic insomnia in patients without severe motor disability and cognitive impairment. However, the access of patients to non-pharmacological treatments is usually limited by a lack of local service provision.

## Sleep-related breathing disorders

Sleep hypopnoea and sleep apnoea refer to clinical conditions with partial or complete respiratory impairment during sleep. In middle-aged and elderly patients this is mainly caused by the obstruction of the upper airway/oropharynx. The prevalence of OSA is increasing in the Western world and this goes together with the increased prevalence of obesity. OSA affects about 20% of adults older than 60 years and is more common in men than in women (Bixler *et al.*, 2001). The prevalence plateaus after the age of 65 (Young *et al.*, 2002). Other causes are central respiration problems caused by a lack of respiration drive due to primary cardiac or neurological dysfunction and a mix of obstructive and central causes. Mixed causes for sleep apnoea or hypopnoea are frequent in elderly patients with neurodegenerative disorders such as PD and DLB. A correct and early diagnosis of sleep apnoea is important because it is a treatable condition.

Untreated OSA is associated with high mortality and morbidity (Aloia *et al.*, 2003), such as cardiovascular, cognitive, and metabolic complications and motor vehicle accidents (Philip, 2005; Barbe *et al.*, 2007). Metabolic consequences of sleep apnoeas include glucose intolerance and insulin resistance (Punjabi *et al.*, 2002) and common neuropsychological deficits are impaired vigilance and executive function (Beebe *et al.*, 2003). Sleep apnoea is associated with systemic and pulmonary hypertension (Nieto *et al.*, 2000), complex cardiac arrhythmias, and myocardial infarction (Mehra *et al.*, 2006). Severe OSA is also a risk factor for an ischaemic stroke in elderly patients (aged 70 to 100), independent of other associated cardiovascular risk factors (Munoz *et al.*, 2006). The pathophysiology contributing to these metabolic, cardiovascular, and cognitive changes is not entirely clear. It is, however, likely that intermittent hypoxia, the stress associated with apnoeas, and sleep deprivation contribute to these common complications (Bedard *et al.*, 1991). Sleepiness and impaired cognitive function undoubtedly affect the quality of life (Alchanatis *et al.*, 2005). Patients with undiagnosed OSA are at risk of using alcohol or benzodiazepines to overcome fragmented sleep, which can be the start of a vicious cycle. Both can lead to more sleep apnoea and subsequently to more sleep fragmentation.

## Assessment

Bedpartners play a crucial role in the evaluation of a patient with possible sleep apnoea and it is often the bedpartner's concerns that trigger the initial assessment. The most typical clinical symptoms associated with OSA are loud snoring, evident breathing pauses, and daytime sleepiness. Snoring itself is common in elderly patients and as a single feature it is not specific for OSA. The snoring of patients with OSA is usually loud and disturbs the bedpartner and other people living in the same household. Snorting and choking are commonly associated with snoring. Other associated symptoms are recent weight gain and complaints of a dry mouth and headaches when waking up (American Academy of Sleep Medicine, 1999). OSA is easily misinterpreted as depression, since tiredness, hopelessness, and lack of libido are common symptoms of both disorders (Ancoli-Israel et al., 1991). If the clinical history suggests sleep hypopnoea or apnoea then PSG is required to confirm the diagnosis and titrate nasal continuous positive airway pressure (CPAP) treatment.

PSG confirms the link between sleep pauses and the desaturation of oxygenated haemoglobin. Apnoeas are commonly associated with increased levels of arousal in the EEG. The apnoea/hypopnoea index (AHI) is commonly used to quantify the severity of the disorder. The AHI reflects the number of apnoeas/hypopnoeas recorded per hour's sleep. An AHI of 5–15 indicates mild, 15–30 moderate, and >30 severe OSA (American Academy of Sleep Medicine, 1999). PSG is restricted to specialist sleep centres and is relatively expensive. A portable PSG is now becoming available to diagnose OSA in the patient's home. Portable systems are cheaper, allow assessment in the natural sleep environment, and provide a small range of measures to quantify respiration during sleep such as oxygenation and ECG. A downside of portable systems is that they cannot refer apnoeas/hypopnoeas to sleep stages. This runs the risk of producing false negative results since the apnoea periods are most prominent during REM sleep. Also, technical difficulties often arise that cannot be identified and corrected as easily as PSG in a sleep disorders centre.

The multiple sleep latency test (MSLT) measures the average latency until falling asleep during four to five 20-minute naps every 2 hours during a day. Sleep onset is determined by EEG, EMG, and EOG recordings. An average sleep latency of >10 minutes is normal. A latency of <5 minutes is pathological. Latencies between 5 and 10 minutes are in the 'grey zone' of interpretation and require clinical correlation. MSLT is sometimes used either in conjunction with PSG or to determine the severity of daytime hypersomnolence. The maintenance of wakefulness test (MWT) measures the ability to remain awake at 2-hour intervals, and this test is often used to measure the effect of therapy. This is particularly important for elderly professional drivers.

## Treatment

The treatment of OSA includes dietetic advice for weight reduction and the restriction of alcohol at bedtime. Abstinence from sedatives is also important, since they may make symptoms worse. The symptomatic treatment of first choice is CPAP therapy. This treatment can improve the quality of life, daytime function, and reduce the vascular, cognitive, and metabolic complications of sleep apnoea (Aloia et al., 2003; Marshall et al., 2006). Positive airflow therapy can also reduce daytime sleepiness in patients with Alzheimer's disease (Chong et al., 2006). Oral appliances are sometimes used as a treatment strategy. They modify the position of the mandible and tongue, but are less effective in reducing the symptoms (Ferguson et al., 2006). Another form of therapy is uvulopalatopharyngoplasty (UPPP), which is more often effective than oral appliances but not as effective as CPAP. However, in those who cannot tolerate CPAP, and particularly in those who are young (and in whom decades of nightly CPAP therapy may not seem practical), UPPP may be a good choice. Other forms of treatment include surgical reconstruction of the upper airway and mandible, and tracheostomy; these are very rarely used in elderly patients. Patients with persistent daytime sleepiness despite the treatment with CPAP may benefit from treatment with modafinil (Black and Hirshkowitz, 2005; Hirshkowitz et al., 2007).

## Circadian rhythms sleep disorders

The primary intrinsic pacemaker of the circadian rhythms is the suprachiasmatic nucleus. It controls wakefulness, facilitates sleep, and synchronizes circadian rhythms with external cues such as light, physical, and social interactions. The misalignment of the circadian clock with the environmental cycle commonly results in chronic sleep disorders such as insomnia and excessive daytime sleepiness. There are four main types of circadian rhythms sleep disorder, namely the advanced sleep phase syndrome, the delayed sleep phase syndrome, the non 24-hours sleep–wake syndrome, and the irregular sleep–wake pattern. The pathogenesis of these disorders is not entirely understood, but genetic factors play an important role (Hamet and Tremblay, 2006). The prevalence rate of circadian rhythms sleep disorder in the elderly is unknown. It is likely that prevalence is underestimated in retired adults, since they are less likely to be forced to stick to working hours. This section will focus on the advanced and delayed phase syndromes. The reader interested in other circadian rhythms disorders can find further information in textbooks of sleep medicine (Carney and Berry, 2005; Kryger et al., 2005).

The circadian rhythm tends to advance with ageing (Duffy et al., 1998) and advanced sleep phase syndrome is probably the most common rhythms disorder in older adults. The *advanced sleep phase syndrome* is characterized by falling asleep several hours before conventional norms. Patients with an advanced sleep phase fall asleep between 6 and 9 p.m. and wake up after a normal sleep duration of 6 to 8 hours in the early morning (2 to 5 a.m.). This can give the false impression of early morning wakening (thereby suggesting depression) or excessive daytime sleepiness in the afternoon. Symptoms are often chronic and persist for weeks and months. The *delayed sleep phase syndrome* is less common in older adults and is characterized by a delayed sleep cycle, which usually starts after midnight. Individuals fall asleep after 2 a.m. and struggle to wake up before 10 a.m. This is a common sleep pattern of young adults. It becomes a problem when the pattern persists throughout the week. If a delayed sleep phase syndrome is found in elderly patients it is often secondary to chronic insomnia (Weitzman et al., 1981).

## Assessment

The diagnosis of circadian rhythms sleep disorder relies largely on the clinical history. It is important to establish the times when patients go to bed and when they actually fall asleep and wake up. Patients with advanced sleep phase complain of early morning wakening and excessive daytime sleepiness in the later afternoon. Those with delayed sleep phase will mention difficulties with falling asleep and excessive daytime sleepiness in the morning. The sleep phase shift and the complaints are usually chronic. Actigraphy and sleep diaries are helpful in confirming the diagnosis. The recording period should involve a period of at least 2 weeks to enable a conclusive diagnosis. Concurrent depression or chronic insomnia need to be excluded.

### Treatment

Treatment options include the exposure to bright light, pharmaco-therapy, and chronotherapy. Bright light therapy is a safe and commonly used approach to treat circadian rhythms disorders (Benloucif et al., 2006). The Standards of Practice Committee, American Academy of Sleep Medicine has developed evidenced-based recommendations for bright light therapy in the treatment of delayed and advanced sleep cycles (Chesson et al., 1999). They recommend applying bright light (2000–2500 lux, but often most effective at 10,000 lux) from 6 to 9 a.m. in delayed sleep phase syndrome and between 9 to 11 p.m. for advanced sleep phases to improve sleep cycles. Pharmacotherapy involves the early evening administration of melatonin to advance the sleep phase in delayed sleep phase syndrome (Kayumov et al., 2001). The combination of melatonin in the evening and bright light in the morning may be an even more powerful treatment (Revell et al., 2006). Chrono-therapy is behavioural therapy for highly motivated patients. The treatment strategy for advanced sleep phases is to further advance the sleep times, e.g. every 2 days for 3 hours, until a more desired sleep schedule is found. For delayed sleep phases the sleep times are delayed by 3 hours every 2 days until the desired bedtime is sched-uled (Weitzman et al., 1981). Whether this chronotherapy is suita-ble for elderly patients remains unclear. More research is also needed to clarify optimal melatonin doses and timing for elderly patients.

### Excessive daytime sleepiness

Excessive daytime sleepiness is common in elderly patients. It includes the difficulty of remaining awake during the day. Primary causes of excessive daytime sleepiness, such as narcolepsy, idio-pathic hypersomnia, and recurrent hypersomnia, are rare and these conditions are usually diagnosed before patients reach old age. Excessive daytime sleepiness in older adults develops mainly in association with disturbed sleep, neurodegenerative disorders (e.g. Alzheimer's disease and PD), and depression (Barthlen, 2002). Other common causes are medications, such as longer-acting benzodiazepines (e.g. diazepam), alcohol and sedating antidepres-sants (e.g. trazodone, mirtazapine) (Pack et al., 2006), or neuro-leptics. The overall prevalence of excessive daytime sleepiness in older adults is 15–20% (Whitney et al., 1998; Ohayon et al., 2002).

### Assessment

The diagnosis is mainly based on the sleep history. Sleep diaries and the Epworth Sleepiness Scale (John, 1991) are helpful for monitor-ing the severity of excessive daytime sleepiness. The MSLT is critical in the evaluation of excessive daytime somnolence, preferably after PSG is performed the night before to ensure at least 7 hours of total sleep time. Other specialist assessments include the maintenance of wakefulness test (MWT) (Mitler et al., 1982)—again, the MWT is used to measure the effect of therapy, and the MSLT is used for diagnostic purposes.

### Treatment

The primary focus for the treatment of excessive daytime sleepi-ness should be on its cause. Effective treatment also requires a structured and regular nocturnal sleep pattern. Different alerting agents such as modafinil, dexamfetamines, and methylphenidate are available. However, further evidence is needed to provide clear indications that these drugs are of benefit for elderly patients with secondary causes of excessive daytime sleepiness. The use of stimu-lants is often restricted by the development of tolerance risks of abuse, medication interactions, and the increased risks of cardiovascular adverse events (http://www.fda.gov/medwatch/). Inconclusive evidence has been provided for the treatment of excessive daytime sleepiness with modafinil in patients with PD (Hogl et al., 2002; Adler et al., 2003; Ondo et al., 2005). In appropriate patients, however, careful titration of modafinil or one of the standard psychostimulants can result in improved alertness and quality of life in elderly patients with and without coexisting neurological disease.

## Parasomnias

Parasomnias comprise behavioural disturbances during sleep, which manifest at the sleep–wake transition, during REM sleep or non-REM-sleep. The sleep–wake transition and non-REM sleep parasomnias include, for example, confusional arousal, night ter-rors, and sleep-walking. They manifest most frequently in child-hood or young adulthood. The REM sleep-related parasomnias include nightmare disorders (van Liempt et al., 2006) and RBD. The nightmare disorders are commonly associated with mental disorders, such as post-traumatic stress disorder or dissociative disorders. The interested reader will find more comprehensive information in textbooks of general psychiatry and sleep medicine. The focus in this section will be on RBD, since it usually manifests above the age of 50 and is important for the differential diagnosis of dementia (Plazzi et al., 1998; McKeith et al., 2005). RBD is also a supportive feature for the diagnosis of DLB (McKeith et al., 2005).

### REM sleep behaviour disorder

RBD is characterized by the lack of muscle atonia during REM sleep associated with dream-enactment behaviour (Schenck and Mahowald, 2002). Enactment involves yelling, laughing, talking, shouting, swearing, gesturing, kicking, punching, jumping, and grabbing (Gagnon et al., 2006a). Such behaviour obviously con-tributes to a significant risk of injuries to the sleeper and their bed-partner. Injuries are often the initial manifestation when RBD comes to medical attention. Questionnaire studies in the commu-nity suggest prevalence rates of 0.5–0.8% with a male prepond-erance (Ohayon et al., 1997; Chiu et al., 2000). The prevalence of RBD is, however, much higher in patients with PD (15–34%) (Comella et al., 1998; Scaglione et al., 2005), multisystem atrophy (90%) (Plazzi et al., 1997), and DLB (Boeve et al., 2004). RBD can antedate the onset of dementia by several years or decades and may therefore be an early diagnostic marker for alpha-synucleinopathies (neurodegenerative disorders with prominent alpha-synuclein depositions either with or without Lewy body formation, e.g. PD,

DLB, multisystem atrophy, and pure autonomic failure) (Boeve et al., 2001; Postuma et al., 2006).

RBD is typically a chronic sleep disorder and once it is presents it tends to persist. It usually manifests in the early hours, since there is more REM sleep in the second half of the night. The pathophysiology of RBD is complex and includes abnormalities in the brainstem such as Lewy body pathology, neuron loss, and gliosis (Uchiyama et al., 1995; Schenck et al., 1997). Different sites and transmitter systems (dopaminergic, serotonergic, noradrenergic, and cholinergic, and probably others as yet unidentified) are involved. In some patients it appears that RBD has been precipitated or aggravated by antidepressants. But this issue is controversial—some studies have reported an association, whereas others have not (Nash et al., 2003; Onofrj et al., 2003; Winkelman and James, 2004; Wilson and Argyropoulos, 2005).

### Assessment

A bedpartner's history of acting out dreams, and a history of injuries during the night are highly suggestive for RBD. The main differential diagnosis involves obstructive sleep apnoea and sleep walking, or night terrors. Obstructive sleep apnoea is usually associated with loud snoring and excessive daytime sleepiness. Sleep walkers do not enact their dreams and are typically a lot younger. Frontal epilepsy at night can sometimes be manifested by motor activity suggesting enactment behaviour; however, this is rare and not related to REM sleep. Whenever the diagnosis is in doubt, polysomnography is needed to confirm the diagnosis of RBD and to demonstrate the lack of muscle atonia in REM sleep along with either subtle or overt motor behaviour. A confirmation is particularly important whenever there is no treatment response.

### Treatment

A safe sleeping environment for patient and bedpartner is essential to minimize RBD-related injuries. It may be necessary to remove the bedside tables, since they can contribute to head injuries. The risks and benefits of antidepressants need to be reviewed, especially if there is a temporal relationship between the onset of RBD and the start of antidepressant medication. The first-line treatment for RBD is clonazepam at bedtime. There are no randomized placebo-controlled studies to assess the treatment of RBD but several open studies have reported that clonazepam is effective, usually at 0.25–0.5 mg/night (Chiu et al., 1997; Paparrigopoulos, 2005). Treatment response is usually present after the first few doses. If there is no immediate treatment response, the diagnosis will need to be reconsidered. Careful risk and benefit consideration is needed since the long-term use of clonazepam is associated with the potential development of tolerance and an increased risk of falls in patients with alpha-synucleinopathies. Risks and benefits are best discussed with the patient, and this discussion should be recorded in the patient file. Alternative treatment strategies include treatment with melatonin (3–12 mg half an hour before sleeping) (Boeve et al., 2003) and pramipexole (Paparrigopoulos, 2005). Further studies are needed to clarify whether cholinesterase inhibitors have a role in the treatment of RBD (Gagnon et al., 2006b).

## Sleep-related movement disorders

RLS is underdiagnosed in elderly patients. It is characterized by (1) the urge to move the legs, usually accompanied or caused by uncomfortable or unpleasant sensations in the legs, (2) the urge to move or unpleasant sensations begin or worsen during periods of rest or inactivity such as lying or sitting, (3) the urge to move or unpleasant sensations are partially or totally relieved by movement, and (4) the urge to move or unpleasant sensations are worse in the evening or night. The diagnosis of RLS is based purely on the clinical history and does not require PSG. A positive family history is common and symptoms usually respond well when treated with dopaminergic drugs (Allen et al., 2003). Community-based surveys suggested an overall prevalence for RLS of approximately 7–11% (Allen et al., 2005). In 80% of patients RLS is associated with periodic limb movements when asleep. The prevalence increases with age and is higher in female patients. The severity of RLS varies, but in many patients this is a pervasive and nightly occurrence. Pain related to peripheral neuropathy can get worse at night but symptoms rarely improve when the legs are moved. Another difficult differential diagnosis is the separation of RLS and akathisia. Akathisia is usually associated with long-standing treatment with dopamine antagonists such as neuroleptics (Jeste et al., 1986). The clinical presentation of akathisia and RLS is similar, and the differential diagnosis depends on the history of neuroleptic use. It is possible that some antidepressants worsen RLS, especially when co-administered with dopaminergic treatment (Yang et al., 2005; Chang et al., 2006). RLS is common in end-stage renal disease and in iron deficiency, suggesting that iron homeostasis may play a role in the development of the condition. Some patients have lower ferritin and transferrin levels in the cerebrospinal fluid, despite normal serum levels, which may suggest an iron transport deficit into the CNS (Winkelman, 2006). Iron substitution can markedly improve symptoms of RLS in patients with iron deficiency (O'Keeffe et al., 1993). A genetic component is prominent, especially when the conditions first manifests before the age of 45 years (Winkelmann and Ferini-Strambi, 2006). Further information on RLS can be found at the website of the Restless Legs Syndrome Foundation (http://www.rls.org/).

### Assessment

Complaints of patients can be discreet. They may report uncomfortable sensations such as 'creepy-crawlies', 'itchy', 'tingly', or 'nervous legs' which improve temporarily when their legs are moved. Symptoms show usually a diurnal pattern and get worse in the evening whilst sitting in the armchair watching TV or at night when trying to fall asleep. Bedpartners complain about fidgeting in bed or repetitive jerks of the legs whilst asleep. The latter reflects the common association of RLS with periodic limb movements. Iron deficiency should be assessed in many patients, particularly those who do not respond to therapy. Measurement of *ferritin* is critical—values below 50 µg/ml are most often associated with medically refractory RLS. Caution is needed if a temporal association between the start of RLS and the start of an antidepressant is found. If pharmacological treatment is required dopaminergic agents are considered to be the first-line treatments. Longer-acting dopamine agonists (e.g. pramipexole, ropinirole) are preferred to avoid rebound effects in the second half of the night. Several double-blind studies found beneficial short-term and long-term effects for the treatment of RLS with dopamine agonists (Montplaisir et al., 1999; Trenkwalder, 2006). Gabapentin (Garcia-Borreguero et al., 2002) and carbamazepine (Telstad et al., 1984) were effective for the treatment of RLS in placebo-controlled trials. One important aspect of treatment is known as augmentation—the tendency of RLS symptoms to begin earlier and earlier in the evening and afternoon; this can be seen with many agents, particularly levodopa therapy. If this occurs, a change to another agent is often necessary.

## Summary and conclusions

Sleep disturbances are common in elderly people and should not be regarded as part of normal ageing because they are commonly associated with co-existing medical disorders, pain, mental disorders (especially depression), and neurodegenerative disorders. Sleep disorders are commonly under-recognized and non-pharmacological treatment strategies are under-used. Several studies have reported beneficial effects of daily bright light exposure, which was associated with fewer night time awakenings (Shochat et al., 2000) and reduced daytime sleep (Fetveit and Bjorvatn, 2005). Other successful interventions include increased physical activity and less bedtime rest during the day. Current evidence suggests that cognitive behavioural therapy and sedative hypnotics are equally effective for the short-term treatment of insomnia, but cognitive behavioural therapy is more effective in the long term.

Additional helpful information can be found in comprehensive textbooks of sleep medicine (Buysse, 2005; Carney and Berry, 2005; Kryger et al., 2005; Ambrogetti et al., 2006) or on the websites of the World Federation of Sleep Research and Sleep Medicine Societies (http://www.wfsrs.org) or the American Academy of Sleep Medicine (http://www.aasmnet.org). Both websites have associated links to other national sleep centres. Another informative website is the of the National Sleep Foundation (http://www.sleepfoundation.org/) and the pocket version of the ICSD-2 manual can be purchased at http://www.aasmnet.org/.

## References

Adler, C.H., Caviness, J.N., Hentz, J.G., Lind, M., and Tiede, J. (2003). Randomized trial of modafinil for treating subjective daytime sleepiness in patients with Parkinson's disease. *Movement Disorders*, **18**, 287–93.

Alchanatis, M., Zias, N., Deligiorgis, N., Amfilochiou, A., Dionellis, G., and Orphanidou, D. (2005). Sleep apnea-related cognitive deficits and intelligence: an implication of cognitive reserve theory. *Journal of Sleep Research*, **14**, 69–75.

Alessi, C.A. and Schnelle, J.F. (2000). Approach to sleep disorders in the nursing home setting. [review] *Sleep Medicine Reviews*, **4**, 45–56.

Allen, R.P., Picchietti, D., Hening, W.A., Trenkwalder, C., Walters, A.S., and Montplaisi, J. (2003). Restless legs syndrome: diagnostic criteria, special considerations, and epidemiology. A report from the restless legs syndrome diagnosis and epidemiology workshop at the National Institutes of Health. *Sleep Medicine*, **4**, 101–19.

Allen, R.P., Walters, A.S., Montplaisir, J. et al. (2005). Restless legs syndrome prevalence and impact: REST general population study. *Archives of Internal Medicine*, **165**, 1286–92.

Aloia, M.S., Ilniczky, N., Di Dio, P., Perlis, M.L., Greenblatt, D.W., and Giles, D.E. (2003). Neuropsychological changes and treatment compliance in older adults with sleep apnea. *Journal of Psychosomatic Research*, **54**, 71–6.

Ambrogetti, A., Hensley, M., and Olson, L. (2006). *Sleep disorders: a clinical textbook*. MA Healthcare Ltd, London.

American Academy of Sleep Medicine (1999). Sleep-related breathing disorders in adults: recommendations for syndrome definition and measurement techniques in clinical research. The Report of an American Academy of Sleep Medicine Task Force. *Sleep*, **22**, 667–89.

American Academy of Sleep Medicine (2005). *ICSD-2 international classification of sleep disorders diagnostic and coding manual*. American Academy of Sleep Medicine, Rochester, MN.

Ancoli-Israel, S. (2005). Sleep and aging: prevalence of disturbed sleep and treatment considerations in older adults. *Journal of Clinical Psychiatry*, **66**(Suppl. 9), 24–30 (quiz 42–3).

Ancoli-Israel, S., Kripke, D.F., Klauber, M.R., Mason, W.J., Fell, R., and Kaplan, O. (1991). Sleep-disordered breathing in community-dwelling elderly. *Sleep*, **14**, 486–95.

Ancoli-Israel, S., Walsh, J. K., Mangano, R. M., and Fujimori, M. (1999). Zaleplon, a novel nonbenzodiazepine hypnotic, effectively treats insomnia in elderly patients without causing rebound effects. *Primary Care Companion to the Journal of Clinical Psychiatry*, **1**, 114–20.

Ancoli-Israel, S., Cole, R., Alessi, C., Chambers, M., Moorcroft, W., and Pollak, C. P. (2003). The role of actigraphy in the study of sleep and circadian rhythms. *Sleep*, **26**, 342–92.

APA (2005). *Diagnostic and statistical manual of mental disorders*. American Psychiatric Association, Washington, DC.

Avidan, A.Y., Fries, B.E., James, M.L., Szafara, K.L., Wright, G.T., and Chervin, R.D. (2005). Insomnia and hypnotic use, recorded in the minimum data set, as predictors of falls and hip fractures in Michigan nursing homes. *Journal of the American Geriatrics Society*, **53**, 955–62.

Bain, K.T. (2006). Management of chronic insomnia in elderly persons. *American Journal of Geriatric Pharmacotherapy*, **4**, 168–92.

Barbe, F., Sunyer, J., de la Pena, A. et al.(2007). Effect of continuous positive airway pressure on the risk of road accidents in sleep apnea patients. *Respiration*, **74**, 44–9.

Barthlen, G.M. (2002). Sleep disorders. Obstructive sleep apnea syndrome, restless legs syndrome, and insomnia in geriatric patients. *Geriatrics*, **57**, 34–9 (quiz 40).

Bateson, A.N. (2006). Further potential of the GABA receptor in the treatment of insomnia. *Sleep Medicine*, **7**(Suppl. 1), S3–S9.

Bedard, M.A., Montplaisir, J., Richer, F., Rouleau, I., and Malo, J. (1991). Obstructive sleep apnea syndrome: pathogenesis of neuropsychological deficits. *Journal of Clinical and Experimental Neuropsychology*, **13**, 950–64.

Beebe, D.W., Groesz, L., Wells, C., Nichols, A., and McGee, K. (2003). The neuropsychological effects of obstructive sleep apnea: a meta-analysis of norm-referenced and case-controlled data. *Sleep*, **26**, 298–307.

Benloucif, S., Green, K., L'Hermite-Baleriaux, M., Weintraub, S., Wolfe, L.F., and Zee, P.C. (2006). Responsiveness of the aging circadian clock to light. *Neurobiology of Aging*, **27**, 1870–9.

Bixler, E.O., Vgontzas, A.N., Lin, H.M. et al. (2001). Prevalence of sleep-disordered breathing in women: effects of gender. *American Journal of Respiratory and Critical Care Medicine*, **163**, 608–13.

Black, J.E. and Hirshkowitz, M. (2005). Modafinil for treatment of residual excessive sleepiness in nasal continuous positive airway pressure-treated obstructive sleep apnea/hypopnea syndrome. *Sleep*, **28**, 464–71.

BNF (2007). *British National Formulary*. BMJ Publishing Group and Royal Pharmacological Society, London.

Boeve, B.F., Silber, M.H., Ferman, T.J., Lucas, J.A., and Parisi, J.E. (2001). Association of REM sleep behavior disorder and neurodegenerative disease may reflect an underlying synucleinopathy. *Movement Disorders*, **16**, 622–30.

Boeve, B.F., Silber, M.H., and Ferman, T.J. (2003). Melatonin for treatment of REM sleep behavior disorder in neurologic disorders: results in 14 patients. *Sleep Medicine*, **4**, 281–4.

Boeve, B.F., Silber, M.H. and Ferman, T.J. (2004). REM sleep behavior disorder in Parkinson's disease and dementia with Lewy bodies. *Journal of Geriatric Psychiatry and Neurology*, **17**, 146–57.

Bootzin, R.R. and Nicassio, P.M. (1978). In *Progress in behavior modification*, Vol. 6 (ed. M. Hersen, R.M. Eisler, and P.M. Miller). pp. 1–45. Academic Press, New York.

Brassington, G.S., King, A.C., and Bliwise, D.L. (2000). Sleep problems as a risk factor for falls in a sample of community-dwelling adults aged 64-99 years. *Journal of the American Geriatrics Society*, **48**, 1234–40.

Busto, U.E., Sproule, B.A., Knight, K., and Herrmann, N. (2001). Use of prescription and nonprescription hypnotics in a Canadian elderly population. *Canadian Journal of Clinical Pharmacology*, **8**, 213–21.

Buysse, D.J. (2005). *Sleep disorders and psychiatry*, American Psychiatric Publishing, Washington, DC.

Carney, P.R. and Berry, R.B. (2005). *Clinical sleep disorders*, Lippincott Williams & Wilkins, Philadelphia.

Chang, C.C., Shiah, I.S., Chang, H.A., and Mao, W.C. (2006). Does domperidone potentiate mirtazapine-associated restless legs syndrome? *Progress in Neuro-Psychopharmacology and Biological Psychiatry*, **30**, 316–18.

Chesson, A.L., Jr, Littner, M., Davila, D. *et al.* (1999). Practice parameters for the use of light therapy in the treatment of sleep disorders. Standards of Practice Committee, American Academy of Sleep Medicine. *Sleep*, **22**, 641–60.

Chiu, H.F., Wing, Y.K., Chung, D.W., and Ho, C.K. (1997). REM sleep behaviour disorder in the elderly. *International Journal of Geriatric Psychiatry*, **12**, 888–91.

Chiu, H.F., Wing, Y.K., Lam, L.C. *et al.* (2000). Sleep-related injury in the elderly--an epidemiological study in Hong Kong. *Sleep*, **23**, 513–17.

Chong, M.S., Ayalon, L., Marler, M. *et al.* (2006). Continuous positive airway pressure reduces subjective daytime sleepiness in patients with mild to moderate Alzheimer's disease with sleep disordered breathing. *Journal of the American Geriatrics Society*, **54**, 777–81.

Clemens, S., Rye, D., and Hochman, S. (2006). Restless legs syndrome: revisiting the dopamine hypothesis from the spinal cord perspective. *Neurology*, **67**, 125–30.

Comella, C.L., Nardine, T.M., Diederich, N.J., and Stebbins, G.T. (1998). Sleep-related violence, injury, and REM sleep behavior disorder in Parkinson's disease. *Neurology*, **51**, 526–9.

Conn, D.K. and Madan, R. (2006). Use of sleep-promoting medications in nursing home residents: risks versus benefits. *Drugs & Aging*, **23**, 271–87.

Cricco, M., Simonsick, E.M., and Foley, D.J. (2001). The impact of insomnia on cognitive functioning in older adults. *Journal of the American Geriatrics Society*, **49**, 1185–9.

Crowley, K., Trinder, J., Kim, Y., Carrington, M., and Colrain, I.M. (2002). The effects of normal aging on sleep spindle and K-complex production. *Clinical Neurophysiology: Official Journal of the International Federation of Clinical Neurophysiology*, **113**, 1615–22.

Culpepper, L. (2006). Secondary insomnia in the primary care setting: review of diagnosis, treatment, and management. *Current Medical Research and Opinion*, **22**, 1257–68.

Duffy, J.F., Dijk, D.J., Klerman, E.B., and Czeisler, C.A. (1998). Later endogenous circadian temperature nadir relative to an earlier wake time in older people. *American Journal of Physiology*, **275**, R1478–R1487.

Ferguson, K.A., Cartwright, R., Rogers, R., and Schmidt-Nowara, W. (2006). Oral appliances for snoring and obstructive sleep apnea: a review. *Sleep*, **29**, 244–62.

Fetveit, A. and Bjorvatn, B. (2005). Bright-light treatment reduces actigraphic-measured daytime sleep in nursing home patients with dementia: a pilot study. *American Journal of Geriatric Psychiatry*, **13**, 420–3.

Foley, D.J., Monjan, A.A., Brown, S.L., Simonsick, E.M., Wallace, R.B., and Blazer, D.G. (1995). Sleep complaints among elderly persons: an epidemiologic study of three communities. *Sleep*, **18**, 425–32.

Foley, D., Ancoli-Israel, S., Britz, P., and Walsh, J. (2004). Sleep disturbances and chronic disease in older adults: results of the 2003 National Sleep Foundation Sleep in America Survey. *Journal of Psychosomatic Research*, **56**, 497–502.

Gagnon, J.F., Postuma, R.B., Mazza, S., Doyon, J., and Montplaisir, J. (2006a). Rapid-eye-movement sleep behaviour disorder and neurodegenerative diseases. *Lancet Neurology*, **5**, 424–32.

Gagnon, J.F., Postuma, R.B., and Montplaisir, J. (2006b). Update on the pharmacology of REM sleep behavior disorder. *Neurology*, **67**, 742–7.

Garcia-Borreguero, D., Larrosa, O., de la Llave, Y., Verger, K., Masramon, X., and Hernandez, G. (2002). Treatment of restless legs syndrome with gabapentin: a double-blind, cross-over study. *Neurology*, **59**, 1573–9.

Gehrman, P.R., Martin, J.L., Shochat, T., Nolan, S., Corey-Bloom, J., and Ancoli-Israel, S. (2003). Sleep-disordered breathing and agitation in institutionalized adults with Alzheimer disease. *American Journal of Geriatric Psychiatry*, **11**, 426–33.

Glass, J., Lanctot, K.L., Herrmann, N., Sproule, B.A., and Busto, U.E. (2005). Sedative hypnotics in older people with insomnia: meta-analysis of risks and benefits. *British Medical Journal*, **331**, 1169.

Glovinsky, P.B. and Spielman, A. J. (1991). In *Case studies in insomnia* (ed. P.J. Hauri), pp. 49–63. Plenum, New York.

Hamet, P. and Tremblay, J. (2006). Genetics of the sleep-wake cycle and its disorders. *Metabolism*, **55**, S7–S12.

Hemmelgarn, B., Suissa, S., Huang, A., Boivin, J.F., and Pinard, G. (1997). Benzodiazepine use and the risk of motor vehicle crash in the elderly. *Journal of the American Medical Association*, **278**, 27–31.

Hirshkowitz, M., Black, J.E., Wesnes, K., Niebler, G., Arora, S., and Roth, T. (2007). Adjunct armodafinil improves wakefulness and memory in obstructive sleep apnea/hypopnea syndrome. *Respiratory Medicine*, **101**, 616–27.

Hogl, B., Saletu, M., Brandauer, E. *et al.* (2002). Modafinil for the treatment of daytime sleepiness in Parkinson's disease: a double-blind, randomized, crossover, placebo-controlled polygraphic trial. *Sleep*, **25**, 905–9.

Irwin, M.R., Cole, J.C., and Nicassio, P.M. (2006). Comparative meta-analysis of behavioral interventions for insomnia and their efficacy in middle-aged adults and in older adults 55+ years of age. *Health Psychology*, **25**, 3–14.

Jacobs, G.D., Pace-Schott, E.F., Stickgold, R., and Otto, M.W. (2004). Cognitive behavior therapy and pharmacotherapy for insomnia: a randomized controlled trial and direct comparison. *Archives of Internal Medicine*, **164**, 1888–96.

Jeste, D.V., Wisniewski, A.A., and Wyatt, R.J. (1986). Neuroleptic-associated tardive syndromes. *Psychiatric Clinics of North America*, **9**, 183–92.

John, M. (1991). A new method for measuring daytime sleepiness: the Epworth sleepiness scale. *Sleep*, **14**, 540–5.

Kallin, K., Jensen, J., Olsson, L.L., Nyberg, L., and Gustafson, Y. (2004). Why the elderly fall in residential care facilities, and suggested remedies. *Journal of Family Practice*, **53**, 41–52.

Kayumov, L., Brown, G., Jindal, R., Buttoo, K., and Shapiro, C.M. (2001). A randomized, double-blind, placebo-controlled crossover study of the effect of exogenous melatonin on delayed sleep phase syndrome. *Psychosomatic Medicine*, **63**, 40–8.

Klerman, E.B., Davis, J.B., Duffy, J.F., Dijk, D.J., and Kronauer, R.E. (2004). Older people awaken more frequently but fall back asleep at the same rate as younger people. *Sleep*, **27**, 793–8.

Klimm, H.D., Dreyfus, J.F., and Delmotte, M. (1987). Zopiclone versus nitrazepam: a double-blind comparative study of efficacy and tolerance in elderly patients with chronic insomnia. *Sleep*, **10**(Suppl. 1), 73–8.

Kripke, D.F., Garfinkel, L., Wingard, D.L., Klauber, M.R., and Marler, M.R. (2002). Mortality associated with sleep duration and insomnia. *Archives of General Psychiatry*, **59**, 131–6.

Kryger, M.H., Roth, T., and Dement, W.C. (2005). *Principles and practice of sleep medicine*. Elsevier–W.B. Saunders, Philadelphia.

Landolt, H.P., Dijk, D.J., Achermann, P., and Borbely, A.A. (1996). Effect of age on the sleep EEG: slow-wave activity and spindle frequency activity in young and middle-aged men. *Brain Research*, **738**, 205–12.

de Lecea, L., Kilduff, T.S., Peyron, C. (1998). The hypocretins: hypothalamus-specific peptides with neuroexcitatory activity. *Proceedings of the National Academy of Sciences USA*, **95**, 322–7.

van Liempt, S., Vermetten, E., Geuze, E., and Westenberg, H. (2006). Pharmacotherapeutic treatment of nightmares and insomnia in posttraumatic stress disorder: an overview of the literature. *Annals of the New York Academy of Sciences*, **1071**, 502–7.

Lu, J., Sherman, D., Devor, M., and Saper, C. B. (2006). A putative flip-flop switch for control of REM sleep. *Nature*, **441**, 589–94.

McClusky, H.Y., Milby, J.B., Switzer, P.K., Williams, V., and Wooten, V. (1991). Efficacy of behavioral versus triazolam treatment in persistent sleep-onset insomnia. *American Journal of Psychiatry*, **148**, 121–6.

McCurry, S.M. and Ancoli-Israel, S. (2003). Sleep dysfunction in Alzheimer's disease and other dementias. *Current Treatment Options in Neurology*, **5**, 261–272.

Maher, M.J., Rego, S.A., and Asnis, G. M. (2006). Sleep disturbances in patients with post-traumatic stress disorder: epidemiology, impact and approaches to management. *CNS Drugs*, **20**, 567–90.

McKeith, I.G., Dickson, D.W., Lowe, J. et al. (2005). Diagnosis and management of dementia with Lewy bodies: third report of the DLB Consortium. *Neurology*, **65**, 1863–72.

Manabe, K., Matsui, T., Yamaya, M. et al.(2000). Sleep patterns and mortality among elderly patients in a geriatric hospital. *Gerontology*, **46**, 318–22.

Marshall, N.S., Barnes, M., Travier, N. et al. (2006). Continuous positive airway pressure reduces daytime sleepiness in mild to moderate obstructive sleep apnoea: a meta-analysis. *Thorax*, **61**, 430–4.

Martin, J.L., Webber, A.P., Alam, T., Harker, J.O., Josephson, K.R., and Alessi, C.A. (2006). Daytime sleeping, sleep disturbance, and circadian rhythms in the nursing home. *American Journal of Geriatric Psychiatry*, **14**, 121–9.

Mehra, R., Benjamin, E. J., Shahar, E. et al. (2006). Association of nocturnal arrhythmias with sleep-disordered breathing: The Sleep Heart Health Study. *American Journal of Respiratory and Critical Care Medicine*, **173**, 910–6.

Melton, S.T., Wood, J.M., and Kirkwood, C.K. (2005). Eszopiclone for insomnia. *Annals of Pharmacotherapy*, **39**, 1659–66.

Mendelson, W.B. (2005). A review of the evidence for the efficacy and safety of trazodone in insomnia. *Journal of Clinical Psychiatry*, **66**, 469–76.

Mitler, M.M., Gujavarty, K.S., and Browman, C.P. (1982). Maintenance of wakefulness test: a polysomnographic technique for evaluation treatment efficacy in patients with excessive somnolence. *Electroencephalography and Clinical Neurophysiology*, **53**, 658–61.

Montgomery, P. and Dennis, J. (2003). Cognitive behavioural interventions for sleep problems in adults aged 60+. *Cochrane Database of Systematic Reviews* 2003, Issue 1, Art. No. CD003161. DOI: 10.1002/14651858. CD003161.

Montplaisir, J., Nicolas, A., Denesle, R., and Gomez-Mancilla, B. (1999). Restless legs syndrome improved by pramipexole: a double-blind randomized trial. *Neurology*, **52**, 938–43.

Moraes Wdos, S., Poyares, D.R., Guilleminault, C., Ramos, L.R., Bertolucci, P.H., and Tufik, S. (2006). The effect of donepezil on sleep and REM sleep EEG in patients with Alzheimer disease: a double-blind placebo-controlled study. *Sleep*, **29**, 199–205.

Morin, C.M., Culbert, J.P., and Schwartz, S.M. (1994). Nonpharmacological interventions for insomnia: a meta-analysis of treatment efficacy. *American Journal of Psychiatry*, **151**, 1172–80.

Morin, C.M., Colecchi, C., Stone, J., Sood, R., and Brink, D. (1999). Behavioral and pharmacological therapies for late-life insomnia: a randomized controlled trial. *Journal of the American Medical Association*, **281**, 991–9.

Munoz, R., Duran-Cantolla, J., Martinez-Vila, E. et al. (2006). Severe sleep apnea and risk of ischemic stroke in the elderly. *Stroke*, **37**, 2317–21.

Murtagh, D.R. and Greenwood, K.M. (1995). Identifying effective psychological treatments for insomnia: a meta-analysis. *Journal of Consulting and Clinical Psychology*, **63**, 79–89.

Naitoh, P., Kelly, T., and Babkoff, H. (1993). Sleep inertia: best time not to wake up? *Chronobiology International*, **10**, 109–18.

Nash, J.R., Wilson, S.J., Potokar, J.P., and Nutt, D.J. (2003). Mirtazapine induces REM sleep behavior disorder (RBD) in parkinsonism. *Neurology*, **61**, 1161.

Nicholson, A.N., Belyavin, A.J., and Pascoe, P.A. (1989). Modulation of rapid eye movement sleep in humans by drugs that modify monoaminergic and purinergic transmission. *Neuropsychopharmacology*, **2**, 131–43.

Nieto, F.J., Young, T.B., Lind, B.K. et al. (2000). Association of sleep-disordered breathing, sleep apnea, and hypertension in a large community-based study. Sleep Heart Health Study. *Journal of the American Medical Association*, **283**, 1829–36.

Nishino, S., Ripley, B., Overeem, S., Lammers, G.J., and Mignot, E. (2000). Hypocretin (orexin) deficiency in human narcolepsy. *Lancet*, **355**, 39–40.

Nowell, P.D., Buysse, D.J., Reynolds, C.F., 3rd et al. (1997). Clinical factors contributing to the differential diagnosis of primary insomnia and insomnia related to mental disorders. *American Journal of Psychiatry*, **154**, 1412–16.

Ohayon, M.M. (2002). Epidemiology of insomnia: what we know and what we still need to learn. *Sleep Medicine Reviews*, **6**, 97–111.

Ohayon, M.M. (2005). Relationship between chronic painful physical condition and insomnia. *Journal of Psychiatric Research*, **39**, 151–9.

Ohayon, M.M., Priest, R.G., Caulet, M., and Guilleminault, C. (1996). Hypnagogic and hypnopompic hallucinations: pathological phenomena? *British Journal of Psychiatry*, **169**, 459–67.

Ohayon, M.M., Caulet, M., and Priest, R.G. (1997). Violent behavior during sleep. *Journal of Clinical Psychiatry*, **58**, 369–76 (quiz 377).

Ohayon, M.M., Priest, R.G., Zulley, J., Smirne, S., and Paiva, T. (2002). Prevalence of narcolepsy symptomatology and diagnosis in the European general population. *Neurology*, **58**, 1826–33.

Ohayon, M.M., Carskadon, M.A., Guilleminault, C., and Vitiello, M.V. (2004). Meta-analysis of quantitative sleep parameters from childhood to old age in healthy individuals: developing normative sleep values across the human lifespan. *Sleep*, **27**, 1255–73.

O'Keeffe, S.T., Noel, J., and Lavan, J.N. (1993). Restless legs syndrome in the elderly. *Postgraduate Medical Journal*, **69**, 701–3.

Ondo, W.G., Fayle, R., Atassi, F., and Jankovic, J. (2005). Modafinil for daytime somnolence in Parkinson's disease: double blind, placebo controlled parallel trial. *Journal of Neurology, Neurosurgery and Psychiatry*, **76**, 1636–9.

Onofrj, M., Luciano, A.L., Thomas, A., Iacono, D., and D'Andreamatteo, G. (2003). Mirtazapine induces REM sleep behavior disorder (RBD) in parkinsonism. *Neurology*, **60**, 113–15.

Overstall, P.W. and Oldman, P.N. (1987). A comparative study of lormetazepam and chlormethiazole in elderly in-patients. *Age and Ageing*, **16**, 45–51.

Pack, A.I., Dinges, D.F., Gehrman, P.R., Staley, B., Pack, F.M., and Maislin, G. (2006). Risk factors for excessive sleepiness in older adults. *Annals of Neurology*, **59**, 893–904.

Pallesen, S., Nordhus, I.H., Kvale, G. et al. (2003). Behavioral treatment of insomnia in older adults: an open clinical trial comparing two interventions. *Behaviour Research and Therapy*, **41**, 31–48.

Paparrigopoulos, T.J. (2005). REM sleep behaviour disorder: clinical profiles and pathophysiology. *International Review of Psychiatry*, **17**, 293–300.

Pathy, M.S., Bayer, A.J., and Stoker, M.J. (1986). A double-blind comparison of chlormethiazole and temazepam in elderly patients with sleep disturbances. *Acta Psychiatrica Scandinavica Supplement*, **329**, 99–103.

Petit, L., Azad, N., Byszewski, A., Sarazan, F.F., and Power, B. (2003). Non-pharmacological management of primary and secondary insomnia among older people: review of assessment tools and treatments. *Age and Ageing*, **32**, 19–25.

Philip, P. (2005). Sleepiness of occupational drivers. *Industrial Health*, **43**, 30–3.

Phillips, B. and Ancoli-Israel, S. (2001). Sleep disorders in the elderly. *Sleep Medicine*, **2**, 99–114.

Plazzi, G., Corsini, R., Provini, F. *et al.* (1997). REM sleep behavior disorders in multiple system atrophy. *Neurology*, **48**, 1094–7.

Plazzi, G., Cortelli, P., Montagna, P. *et al.* (1998). REM sleep behaviour disorder differentiates pure autonomic failure from multiple system atrophy with autonomic failure. *Journal of Neurology, Neurosurgery and Psychiatry*, **64**, 683–5.

Postuma, R.B., Lang, A.E., Massicotte-Marquez, J., and Montplaisir, J. (2006). Potential early markers of Parkinson disease in idiopathic REM sleep behavior disorder. *Neurology*, **66**, 845–51.

Punjabi, N.M., Sorkin, J.D., Katzel, L.I., Goldberg, A.P., Schwartz, A.R., and Smith, P.L. (2002). Sleep-disordered breathing and insulin resistance in middle-aged and overweight men. *American Journal of Respiratory and Critical Care Medicine*, **165**, 677–82.

Rechtschaffen, A. and Kales, A. (1968). *A manual of standardized terminology, techniques and scoring system for sleep stages of human subjects.* US Government Printing Office, US Public Health Service, Washington, DC.

Revell, V.L., Burgess, H.J., Gazda, C.J., Smith, M.R., Fogg, L.F., and Eastman, C.I. (2006). Advancing human circadian rhythms with afternoon melatonin and morning intermittent bright light. *Journal of Clinical Endocrinology and Metabolism*, **91**, 54–9.

Riemann, D. and Voderholzer, U. (2003). Primary insomnia: a risk factor to develop depression? *Journal of Affective Disorders*, **76**, 255–9.

Roffwarg, H.P., Muzio, J.N., and Dement, W.C. (1966). Ontogenetic development of the human sleep–dream cycle. *Science*, **152**, 604–19.

Roger, M., Attali, P., and Coquelin, J.P. (1993). Multicenter, double-blind, controlled comparison of zolpidem and triazolam in elderly patients with insomnia. *Clinical Therapeutics*, **15**, 127–36.

Roth, T., Seiden, D., Sainati, S., Wang-Weigand, S., Zhang, J., and Zee, P. (2006). Effects of ramelteon on patient-reported sleep latency in older adults with chronic insomnia. *Sleep Medicine*, **7**, 312–18.

Sakurai, T., Amemiya, A., Ishii, M. *et al.* (1998). Orexins and orexin receptors: a family of hypothalamic neuropeptides and G protein-coupled receptors that regulate feeding behavior. *Cell*, **92**, 573–85.

Saletu-Zyhlarz, G.M., Abu-Bakr, M.H., Anderer, P. *et al.* (2002). Insomnia in depression: differences in objective and subjective sleep and awakening quality to normal controls and acute effects of trazodone. *Progress in Neuro-Psychopharmacology and Biological Psychiatry*, **26**, 249–60.

Saper, C.B., Chou, T.C., and Scammell, T.E. (2001). The sleep switch: hypothalamic control of sleep and wakefulness. *Trends in Neuroscience*, **24**, 726–31.

Saper, C. B., Scammell, T. E., and Lu, J. (2005). Hypothalamic regulation of sleep and circadian rhythms. *Nature*, **437**, 1257–63.

Sateia, M.J. and Nowell, P.D. (2004). Insomnia. *Lancet*, **364**, 1959–73.

Sateia, M.J., Doghramji, K., Hauri, P.J., and Morin, C. M. (2000). Evaluation of chronic insomnia. An American Academy of Sleep Medicine review. *Sleep*, **23**, 243–308.

Scaglione, C., Vignatelli, L., Plazzi, G. *et al.* (2005). REM sleep behaviour disorder in Parkinson's disease: a questionnaire-based study. *Neurological Sciences*, **25**, 316–21.

Scharf, M., Erman, M., Rosenberg, R. *et al.*(2005). A 2-week efficacy and safety study of eszopiclone in elderly patients with primary insomnia. *Sleep*, **28**, 720–7.

Schenck, C.H. and Mahowald, M.W. (2002). REM sleep behavior disorder: clinical, developmental, and neuroscience perspectives 16 years after its formal identification in SLEEP. *Sleep*, **25**, 120–38.

Schenck, C.H., Mahowald, M.W., Anderson, M.L., Silber, M.H., Boeve, B.F., and Parisi, J.E. (1997). Lewy body variant of Alzheimer's disease (AD) identified by postmortem ubiquitin staining in a previously reported case of AD associated with REM sleep behavior disorder. *Biological Psychiatry*, **42**, 527–8.

Shochat, T., Martin, J., Marler, M., and Ancoli-Israel, S. (2000). Illumination levels in nursing home patients: effects on sleep and activity rhythms. *Journal of Sleep Research*, **9**, 373–9.

Silber, M.H. (2005). Clinical practice. Chronic insomnia. *New England Journal of Medicine*, **353**, 803–10.

Sivertsen, B., Omvik, S., Pallesen, S. *et al.* (2006). Cognitive behavioral therapy vs zopiclone for treatment of chronic primary insomnia in older adults: a randomized controlled trial. *Journal of the American Medical Association*, **295**, 2851–8.

Spielman, A.J., Caruso, L.S., and Glovinsky, P.B. (1987). A behavioral perspective on insomnia treatment. *Psychiatric Clinics of North America*, **10**, 541–53.

Stein, M.D. and Friedmann, P.D. (2006). Disturbed sleep and its relationship to alcohol use. *Substance Abuse*, **26**, 1–13.

Telstad, W., Sorensen, O., Larsen, S., Lillevold, P.E., Stensrud, P., and Nyberg-Hansen, R. (1984). Treatment of the restless legs syndrome with carbamazepine: a double blind study. *British Medical Journal (Clinical Research Ed.)*, **288**, 444–6.

Trenkwalder, C. (2006). The weight of evidence for ropinirole in restless legs syndrome. *European Journal of Neurology*, **13**(Suppl. 3), 21–30.

Uchiyama, M., Isse, K., Tanaka, K. *et al.* (1995). Incidental Lewy body disease in a patient with REM sleep behavior disorder. *Neurology*, **45**, 709–12.

Weitzman, E.D., Czeisler, C.A., Coleman, R.M. *et al.* (1981). Delayed sleep phase syndrome. A chronobiological disorder with sleep-onset insomnia. *Archives of General Psychiatry*, **38**, 737–46.

Whitney, C.W., Enright, P.L., Newman, A.B., Bonekat, W., Foley, D., and Quan, S.F. (1998). Correlates of daytime sleepiness in 4578 elderly persons: the Cardiovascular Health *Sleep*, **21**, 27–36.

WHO (2003). *International classification of diseases*, ICD 9 CM. Churchill and Livingstone, Geneva.

Wilson, S. and Argyropoulos, S. (2005). Antidepressants and sleep: a qualitative review of the literature. *Drugs*, **65**, 927–47.

Winkelman, J.W. (2006). Considering the causes of RLS. *European Journal of Neurology*, **13**(Suppl. 3), 8–14.

Winkelman, J.W. and James, L. (2004). Serotonergic antidepressants are associated with REM sleep without atonia. *Sleep*, **27**, 317–21.

Winkelmann, J. and Ferini-Strambi, L. (2006). Genetics of restless legs syndrome. *Sleep Medicine Reviews*, **10**, 179–83.

Winokur, A., Sateia, M.J., Hayes, J.B., Bayles-Dazet, W., MacDonald, M.M., and Gary, K.A. (2000). Acute effects of mirtazapine on sleep continuity and sleep architecture in depressed patients: a pilot study. *Biological Psychiatry*, **48**, 75–8.

Yang, C., White, D.P., and Winkelman, J.W. (2005). Antidepressants and periodic leg movements of sleep. *Biological Psychiatry*, **58**, 510–14.

Yoon, I.Y., Kripke, D.F., Youngstedt, S.D., and Elliott, J.A. (2003). Actigraphy suggests age-related differences in napping and nocturnal sleep. *Journal of Sleep Research*, **12**, 87–93.

Young, T., Shahar, E., Nieto, F.J. *et al.* (2002). Predictors of sleep-disordered breathing in community-dwelling adults: the Sleep Heart Health Study. *Archives of Internal Medicine*, **162**, 893–900.

# Sexuality, ethics, and medico-legal issues

# 37

# Sexuality in later life

## Walter Pierre Bouman

> When it can be done without embarrassment or evangelisation, physicians need to support and encourage the sexuality of the old. It is a mental, social, and probably a physical preservative of their status as persons, which our society already attacks in so many cruel ways.
>
> Alex Comfort

Sexuality is an essential part of any person, and expressing it is a basic human need and right of every individual regardless of age, gender, ethnicity, religion, disability, or sexual orientation. The ongoing liberalization within society of the Western developed world in particular has undoubtedly led to more positive and less restrictive attitudes and views in the population regarding many aspects of sexuality, including later life sexuality. The latter is largely reflected by the significant growth of the literature in the area of sexuality and ageing, especially in the last few decades, as well as by the growing interest shown in this topic by the media. Clinicians, researchers, educators, journalists, programme makers, and other interested parties continue to highlight the importance of sexuality and sexual health in the older population. However, there remains a clear absence of older people as a distinct and important group within national policies and directives and government-funded research agendas in the UK with regard to sexuality and sexual health. It appears to indicate that they do not matter much in this respect, resulting in this age group being effectively marginalized and clearly discriminated against.

This chapter gives a broad and general overview concerning all aspects of sexuality and ageing. It starts with discussing myths and attitudes to later life sexuality, followed by research studies in this area, sexual physiology and the effects of physical illness and medication on sexuality, taking a sexual history, the description of the main sexual problems in older people, and addressing specific issues of the lesbian, gay, bisexual, and transgender (LGBT) population. It further describes the issue of sexual abuse in older people and the topic of sexuality and dementia. The chapter concludes with a discussion of the management of a variety of sexual problems encountered in clinical practice.

Other routes into the literature are provided by textbooks (Bancroft, 1989; Schiavi, 1999; Leiblum and Rosen, 2000; Balon and Taylor Segraves, 2005) and many of the articles cited elsewhere in this chapter.

## Myths and attitudes to sexuality

Although the literature shows that there is no age limit to sexual responsiveness—sexual activity in action, reflection, and aspiration can be enjoyable into the 90s and beyond—there are many myths about sexuality and older people which affect how society views sexuality in this age group. Some myths described in both medical and fictional literature pertinent to sexuality in older people include the following. 'A woman's sex life ends with the menopause'; 'Having sex means having intercourse'; 'A diagnosis of dementia automatically invalidates the ability to consent to be sexual'; 'Sex is for the young and not for the old'; 'Older women are not sexually desirable, nor sexually capable'; 'Older people are asexual'. The media's portrayal of ageist stereotypes over long periods of time has also further perpetuated beliefs that older people are asexual.

Myths regarding sexuality may stem from transgenerational internalized social, political, religious, cultural, and moral values and the media's portrayal of later life sexuality. These myths potentially affect the attitude that society has developed towards sexuality and older people. Research shows predominantly negative attitudes to sexuality in older people, particularly among younger individuals. More recent work, however, suggests that some positive changes have occurred, and generally more positive attitudes towards ageing sexuality are being reported in the literature. This is likely to reflect our society's increasingly liberal attitude towards sexuality, together with the development of a consumer culture, with new opportunities and roles for older people (Bouman, 2005). These attitudes will be examined in more depth in the following paragraphs. It is important to bear in mind that many research studies are cross-sectional studies, which attribute variations in attitudes exclusively to the factor of age, whilst ignoring other influences such as cohort effects, sampling biases, generational differences, and the specific historical–social milieu.

## Attitudes according to age

### Young people's attitudes towards sexuality and older people

One of the first systematic studies in this area took place almost half a century ago, when Golde and Kogan (1959) used sentence completions to assess college students' attitudes toward the elderly. The one item concerning the elderly and sex almost unanimously elicited completions to the effect that for older people sex was 'negligible, unimportant'.

LaTorre and Kear (1977) used a sample of 80 Canadian undergraduates (and 40 nursing home staff), whom they asked to read accounts in which the age of the stimulus person varied. They found that sexual activity by the older person was rated as significantly less credible and less moral than sexual activity by the younger person.

Five years later, Damrosch examined attitudes toward sexually active older persons in several types of students (Damrosch, 1982; Damrosch and Fischman, 1985). Her studies involved the use of case vignettes using medical and nursing students as samples. By random assignment, half the students read that the person was sexually active; there was no mention of sexuality for the remaining students. Both studies clearly showed that students viewed the sexually active older person as significantly more mentally alert, cheerful, and better adjusted, with warmer family relations, and as someone whom they would like better as a patient. Other studies have by and large also generated a more positive stance towards later life sexuality (Quinn-Krach and Van Hoozer, 1988; Hillman and Stricker 1996).

### Middle-aged people's attitudes towards sexuality and older people

White and Catania (1982) found that middle-aged children of older people present generally positive attitudes toward later life sexuality. However, the specific sample studied (participants in a sexuality and ageing course) may explain the positiveness of the attitude found. More than 10 years later, Poulin and Mishara (1994) compared the attitudes of adult children toward the sexuality of their older parents with their parent's own attitudes toward sexuality. They found that in general, attitudes toward sexuality were positive among parents and their adult children. However, adult children had significantly more positive attitudes than their parents, which may reflect a cohort effect.

### Older people's attitudes towards later life sexuality

Sadly, ageism has infiltrated so deeply into the belief system of our society that many older patients see themselves as too old for sex. They tend to have a relative lack of formal knowledge about sexual functioning and physiology, because they were raised during a time when scientific sexual information was not readily available or widely discussed. Their beliefs and sexual language are frequently different from those of the current culture (Cheadle, 1991). A common finding in most studies from the 1950s onwards was the poor self-image of older people: they saw themselves as less attractive than younger people, and less entitled to the enjoyment of sexual pleasure. Their attitudes were conservative, they were poorly informed, and they felt uncomfortable in discussing sex with an interviewer. More recent studies show more positive attitudes. Portnova et al. (1984) questioned 60- to 90-year-old women to determine their attitudes toward other sexually active older people. The women were asked to respond to one of eight variations of a vignette depicting a sexually active older couple. The vignette variations depicted the sexual couple alternatively as married, single, or widowed; as being the respondent's friend, family member, or church member; and as living either independently or in a nursing home. Results indicated that the women's attitudes were generally positive in all of the eight social relationships identified. Attitudes were somewhat more positive toward sexual activity by older people who were married than by those who were single. Likewise, attitudes were slightly more positive concerning sexual activity by older people living independently than by nursing home residents. One of the largest samples ever assembled for a later life sexuality study to date was produced by Brecher et al. (1984), who found that the majority of their respondents had a positive attitude towards later life sexuality. Almost two decades later Gott and Hinchliff's study (2003) yielded similar results.

## Attitudes among health professional towards later life sexuality

Negative attitudes towards sexuality and old age are not uncommon among health professionals. Ageist stereotypes commonly affect the development of health policies. This is notably exemplified by two recent Department of Health directives, the National Service Framework (NSF) for Older People (Department of Health, 2001a) and the National Sexual Health Strategy (Department of Health, 2001b). Both documents set out the policy and service development agenda for the coming years in their respective areas. However, it is striking that neither make any reference to sex or sexual health in later life. The NSF for older people does not discuss sexual health, and the sexual health strategy does not mention older people and is very youth-focused. The assumption appears to be that there is no need to develop policy in this area because it is probably irrelevant, or certainly unimportant, to the lives of older people, despite clear evidence to the contrary (Gott and Hinchliff, 2003); for example, individuals aged 50 years or more continue to account for at least 10% of AIDS cases reported annually in the UK (Knodel et al., 2002). Studies of the sexual behaviour of older adults have suggested that they are less aware of sexually transmitted infections (including HIV) and of prevention strategies, and are more likely to practise unprotected sex (Stall and Catania, 1994; Mahar and Sherrard, 2005).

Another example of how health researchers have failed to challenge age-related stereotyping, with many researchers imposing upper age limits around studies of sexually related issues, is the development of the latest national survey of sexual attitudes and lifestyles (Johnson et al. 2001). Despite being considered by the Department of Health to provide a sound evidence base for policy-making in key areas of public-health, this study only recruited participants up to 44 years of age. Similarly, a large-scale study of adult sexual behaviour in the USA imposed an upper age limit of 59 years on participation (Laumann et al. 1999). Placing older people (indeed, those from 45 upwards) outside the remit of national, population-based surveys of sexuality and sexual health issues serves not only to reinforce the notion that sex is not relevant to older people, but is also a blatant denial of an important public health issue (Gott, 2005). The issue of sexuality and sexual health in older people appears to be another domain deeply infiltrated by ageism among health professionals, despite the fact that 'rooting out age discrimination' is an explicit policy imperative of the NSF for older people (Department of Health, 2001a).

## Attitudes among doctors and nurses

There is a dearth of research when it comes to studying the attitudes of doctors to later life sexuality. A topic which has recently received relatively more attention in the literature, however, is the attitudes of doctors towards taking a sexual history in (older) patients as part of their overall clinical assessment (Temple-Smith *et al.*, 1999; Bouman and Arcelus, 2001; Gott *et al.*, 2004) (see 'Taking a sexual history' below).

Very little is known about nurses' attitudes towards discussing sexual issues with older patients. Most of the early (but sparse) literature describes rather negative attitudes among nurses towards later life sexuality (Burnside, 1976; Webb, 1988; Parke, 1991): enrolled nurses have been found to have significantly more negative attitudes than registered nurses (Smook, 1992). Over the last 15 years in particular there has been a growing recognition within the nursing profession of the need to change these negative attitudes towards sexuality and sexual health. The setting of educational standards within nurse training and the work of academic nurses are important sources for such changes.

Since the early 1990s, a large number of articles and books, reports, policies, and guidelines addressing sexuality and nursing have been published in the UK with the overall aim of developing a greater knowledge and positive attitudes towards sexuality and sexual health within the nursing profession (Luketich, 1991; Waterhouse and Metcalfe, 1991; UKCC, 1992; Matocha and Waterhouse, 1993; Van Ooijen and Charnock, 1994; Waterhouse, 1996; Peate, 1999; Bailey and Bunter, 2000; Cort *et al.*, 2001). The Royal College of Nursing made a clear statement and commitment in this respect more than a decade ago: 'The development of sexual health policy and practice guidelines is essential if nurses are to feel confident and supported in promoting sexual health and if service users are to have confidence that their sexual health rights are not denied' (RCN, 1996).

The development of nursing theory toward a more holistic approach has led to the sexuality (amongst other issues) of the patient playing an integral part in the interactions of care (Koh, 1999; Peate, 1999).

## Attitudes in residential and nursing homes towards later life sexuality

### Attitudes of residents

There is also a limited amount of scientific data on attitudes toward sexuality of residents living in residential and nursing homes. Residents in residential and nursing home facilities do show a higher incidence and level of severity of physical and psychiatric disorders compared with their counterparts living in the community (Morley and Kaiser, 1989; Burns *et al.*, 1990), which is one of the many barriers to expressing their sexuality.

There are only two studies which specifically investigate attitudes toward later life sexuality among people living in residential homes. Story (1989) compared the knowledge and attitude scores of 133 people in residential care with 133 university students. She found that general attitudes of both residents and students toward the sexuality of older people were very positive, but their attitude toward specific sexual behaviours, such as masturbation and sex outside of marriage, were less positive.

The other existing study to date concerns residents in residential and nursing care and focuses upon their views and attitudes towards 'social and sexual intimacy' (Bullard-Poe *et al.*, 1994). Forty-five

male residents aged 44–99 years rated social intimacy as the most important form of intimacy and sexual intimacy as the least important (although this was still rated as midway between somewhat and moderately important). In addition, strong associations were found between quality of life and non-sexual physical intimacy which they conclude shows that 'intimacy contributes to quality of life'.

In 1979, Wasow and Loeb reported that most of the 63 nursing home residents they studied admitted to having sexual thoughts and fantasies. Eighty-one per cent of males and 75% of females said that older people should be allowed to have sex, but most were not actively engaged in sexual activity at the time of the interview because of lack of opportunity. The persistence of desire despite infirmity and institutionalization is in agreement with the work of White (1982), who found more nursing home residents desired sex than were sexually active.

Both studies are consistent with other reports on nursing home residents demonstrating that sexual interest is usually present and positive attitudes are held toward later life sexuality in this population, despite severe functional disability (Szasz, 1983; McCartney *et al.*, 1987; Paunonen and Haggman-Laitila, 1990; Mulligan and Palguta, 1991; Johnson, 1996; Aizenberg *et al.* 2002).

The lack of privacy in nursing homes is a major obstacle to sexual expression. Not surprisingly, many residents report that because of a lack of privacy and inhibiting staff attitudes, they have little opportunity to experience intimacy (Deacon *et al.* 1995).

### Attitudes among staff

Attitudes and actions of care staff in residential and nursing homes impact directly on the expression of sexuality by the residents in these homes (Eddy, 1986). Care staff often come from varied social, moral, cultural, educational, and religious backgrounds, which may influence their perception of and attitudes toward residents' needs, and lead to inconsistent care. In dealing with issues of sexuality and sexual health in care facilities, staff should be guided by their duty to create an environment that will help residents fulfil their needs and desires, while maintaining dignity and protecting the rights of both competent and incompetent residents (Lichtenberg and Strzepek, 1990; Hajjar and Kamel, 2003a,b). Although the earlier description of societal attitudes toward later life sexuality appears to show them to be predominantly negative, some positive changes have occurred more recently. Research with care staff has revealed attitudes which are both negative or restrictive (LaTorre and Kear, 1977; Wasow and Loeb, 1979; Glass *et al.*, 1986; Commons *et al.*, 1992; Nay, 1992; Fairchild *et al.*, 1996; Bauer, 1999) and positive or permissive (Kaas, 1978; White and Catania, 1982; Luketich, 1991; Damrosch and Cogliano, 1994; Livini, 1994; Holmes *et al.*, 1997; Walker *et al.*, 1998; Bouman *et al.*, 2007). The mixed results of the research published in the last three decades should be seen in the context of the heterogeneity of the groups and the care facilities sampled, as well as the different measurements being used. There are many specific factors predictive of individuals' attitudes regarding later life sexuality. Several researchers have indicated that a young age (Bouman *et al.*, 2007), strong religious beliefs (Story, 1989; Gibson *et al.*, 1999), and experience of negative interactions with older people (Glass *et al.*, 1986) may be related to more negative attitudes of care staff; whilst, having received more vocational training (White and Catania, 1982; Aja and Self, 1986; Sullivan-Miller, 1987), a higher level of education and socio-economic background (Glass *et al.*, 1986;

Walker and Harrington, 2002), and having more work experience (Sullivan-Miller,1987; Walker and Harrington, 2002; Bouman *et al.*, 2007) generally predict more positive attitudes of care staff. Various researchers have also acknowledged that self-selection and response bias potentially limit the generalizability of these findings, and that liberal attitudes do not necessarily translate into permissive behaviour (Hillman and Stricker, 1994; Holmes *et al.*, 1997; Gibson *et al.*, 1999; Bouman *et al.*, 2006).

## Studies in sexuality and older people

The collection of objective data on sexual behaviour began with Kinsey and his colleagues (Kinsey *et al.* 1948, 1953) and continued with Masters and Johnson (1966, 1970), by the direct observation of volunteers in the laboratory, obtaining information on the sexual physiology of aged men and women which has never yet, in its detail or objectivity, been surpassed. Since then, a growing number of studies have focused specifically on older people, of which those revealing the most significant impact upon understandings of sexuality and ageing will be addressed. However, important methodological difficulties inherent in sexological research should be considered before the findings of the studies can be discussed.

### Methodological considerations for sexual research and ageing

Several methodological problems need to be considered in the evaluation of sexuality and ageing. They include issues of sampling, research strategies, and the scope of sexual measures and assessment procedures. A pervasive question is the contribution of disease to the sexual changes noted in studies of ageing individuals. The relationship between ageing and disease, and the extent to which they are considered as separable rather than inseparable constructs, have important implications for research strategy. The view that illness is an *intrinsic* component of ageing leads to design studies where subjects are included without regard to health status or to the assessment of age-related changes on a healthy–unhealthy continuum. In contrast, the view that ageing and disease are *distinct* constructs leads to studies where individuals are screened for all identifiable medical illnesses, with the expectation that age-related differences or changes then identified represent 'normal' or non-pathological ageing. The study of such a specific group of older people provides valuable information but is not generally applicable to the population at large. Most recent studies of ageing and sexual behaviour gather health status data, but many fail to take full account of this information in the analysis and interpretation of results.

Studies of ageing and sexual behaviour are largely cross-sectional in design, sampling different age cohorts and interpreting any differences across age groups as a longitudinal trend. This approach confounds the effects of the widely divergent cultural and developmental experiences of younger and older cohorts with the effects of ageing. Similarly, individuals older than 65 years are frequently considered as a single older cohort, ignoring the cultural heterogeneity within this group. Longitudinal studies, in which serial assessments are carried out on a given group of subjects at specified intervals, have their own limitations, however, since they confound the effect of ageing and the temporal changes in societal attitudes concerning sexuality.

Two major problems in sexological research, including studies of ageing, are the inadequate characterization of the populations investigated and the drawing of conclusions from small, non-representative and non-random samples. There is controversy as to the magnitude and direction of participation bias in studies which explore sensitive issues such as sexual behaviour. In general, people who volunteer for sexual studies have higher levels of education and less conservative sexual attitudes than non-volunteers. The extent to which the results of studies of ageing sexual behaviour are influenced by a differential, age-dependent participation bias is not known.

Furthermore, most studies of sexual behaviour and ageing focus predominantly on coital activity and erectile capacity. They tend to be unidimensional and orientated towards sexual performance, neglecting the importance of motivational, cognitive, and affective factors. Phenomenologically relevant aspects of the sexuality of older people such as sexual interest, sexual expectations and beliefs, satisfaction, and enjoyment are frequently ignored. There is a need for operational definition and measurement of these constructs, as they evolve and influence the sexual experiences of those who are growing old. Several sexual measures have been applied to the study of ageing and sexuality, but the validity of some of these tests, developed in studies of younger subjects, needs to be re-established in samples of older members of the population (Schiavi, 1999).

### Kinsey *et al.*: Sexual behaviour in the human male and female (1948, 1953)

Kinsey used the taxonomic method, which had served him so well as a zoologist in his studies of insects, as the scientific approach needed to name, describe, and classify human sexual behaviours in such a way as to establish norms of behaviour for entire populations. Lengthy interviews were conducted with 5300 men aged 10–80 years and 5940 women aged up to 90 years. The two resulting books describe the research findings according to types, frequencies, sources, and socio-demographic correlates of 'sexual outlet', which was defined as orgasm resulting from masturbation, nocturnal emissions, petting to climax, pre-marital intercourse, marital intercourse, and homosexual outlet. With regard to later life sexuality in males, Kinsey *et al.* (1948) reported that there was no abrupt cut-off of sexual capacity, but rather a gradual decline in all measures of 'sexual outlet'. They concluded that they did not have enough evidence to isolate factors associated with this decline, but postulated that it could be related to physiological factors, psychological factors, reduced availability of partners, or preoccupation with 'social or business functions'. Five years later, in their second book they reported that 'the female sexual capacity rises gradually to their maximum point and then stays more or less on a level until after fifty-five or sixty years of age'. The potential to investigate what happens to women after this point was clearly limited by the small sample size of participants over 60, although the authors were confident to conclude that 'individuals who have reached old age are no longer as capable of responding [sexually] as they were at an earlier age' (Kinsey *et al.* 1953).

Criticisms of Kinsey's work in relation to later life sexuality have focused mainly upon the small numbers of older people over the age of 60 included in both the male study (approximately 3% of the sample) and the female study (approximately 1% of the sample). Later authors have also argued that drawing conclusions regarding interactions between ageing and sexuality from cross-sectional data is problematic, because it does not allow for the confounding nature of the cohort effects to be explored (George and Weiler, 1981).

In the specific context of later life sexuality, Gott (2005) challenges the authors' beliefs that: (1) sexuality is a biological 'essence'; (2) sex consists mainly of those acts related to intercourse; (3) orgasm, particularly for men, is the 'most precise and scientific indicator of a sexual experience'; (4) gender differences in sexual behaviours are 'natural'; (5) the notion that sex is healthy; and (6) the idea that the best way to understand sexuality is to classify particular sexual behaviours. Nevertheless Kinsey's methodological framework and beliefs regarding sexuality have set a precedent which underpins most subsequent research in sexuality to this day.

### Masters and Johnson: *Human Sexual Response* (1966) and *Human Sexual Inadequacy* (1970)

Their landmark research project had a significant impact upon beliefs about sexuality and ageing, although their sample size was small. The authors aimed to explore the nature and causes of possible sexual dysfunction at all ages by addressing the following research question: 'What physical reactions develop as the human male and female respond to effective sexual stimulation?'. A sample of 382 female and 312 male participants aged 18–89 years was recruited and subjected to a series of laboratory tests, including 'artificial coition' where female participants were penetrated by electronically powered plastic penises. Data from this research was used to develop Master and Johnson's most far-reaching legacy—the concept of the 'human sexual response cycle'.

In relation to later life sexuality, the authors investigated 34 women and 39 men over the age of 50 over a period of 4 years. In view of the small sample size they said that they were only able to 'suggest clinical impression rather than to establish biological fact' (Masters and Johnson, 1966). Like Kinsey, they clearly considered the essence of sexuality to lie in biology. Perhaps the most important clinical impression they offer is that physiological ageing processes do not preclude sexual activity in later life, and that ageing may even bring potential benefits to sexual response—an idea as radical today as it was at the time.

### The Duke University Center for the Study of Aging and Human Development (Newman and Nichols, 1960; Verwoerdt *et al.*, 1969a,b; Pfeiffer and Davis, 1972; Pfeiffer *et al.*, 1972; George and Weiler, 1981)

The first longitudinal study at Duke University Medical Center consisted of a sample of 260 male and female community volunteers, who were aged 60 years and older at the first test date in 1955. The same studies were repeated between 1959 and 1961 and again in 1964. The sample included both those who had never married or were widowed and those who had intact marriages. The authors focused on the frequency of sexual activity (defined as sexual intercourse), degree of sexual interest, gender differences in sexual activity and interest, and patterns of sexual activity over time. They concluded: (1) that sexual activity declines gradually over time for both women and men. Approximately 60% of married subjects aged 60–69, nearly the same proportion of those aged 70–74, and 25% of those aged 75 and over were sexually active. Even in extreme old age sexual activity did not disappear: one-fifth of the men in their 80s and 90s reported intercourse once a month or less; (2) that sexual interest declines over time, albeit more slowly than sexual activity. In all age groups interest was more common than activity; (3) that men are more sexually active than women, although the gap narrows at advanced ages; and (4) that sexual activity among women is heavily dependent on the availability of a functionally capable, socially sanctioned male partner. In addition, discontinuation of sexual activity among both men and women is most commonly attributed to the man.

The second longitudinal study consisted of 502 men and women, who were aged 46 to 71 years at the first test date. The research design included four test dates at 2-year intervals. The results were similar to those reported in the earlier studies, but added that (1) older persons reported lower levels of sexual interest and activity than younger persons; and (2) at all ages, men reported higher levels of sexual activity and interest than women. In a re-analysis of the data, George and Weiler (1981) studied both aggregate and intra-individual levels of sexual activity within their sample and showed that levels of sexual intercourse among older people do not decline to the extent that was previously believed. Rather, the identification of *cohort differences* in sexual interest and activity led the authors to conclude that these may be more pronounced than ageing effects *per se*. In other words, the modal pattern is to maintain a relatively stable level of sexual activity throughout a lifetime up to the age of around 70 or older; for some individuals, however, activity will decrease, and for others it will increase for a while. The investigators also asked their subjects in whom the level of sexual activity had *declined* to suggest why this occurred. Men tended to give as reasons the onset of illness and the loss of a partner, whilst women reported loss of the partner, illness of the partner, and illness in themselves. Loss of a partner is both commoner and more of a handicap for women, in that women survive longer than men, and tend to be younger than their husbands.

### Persson (1980)

Persson's study of older people living in Gothenburg, Sweden, was the first to be based on a representative community sample. It involved 166 men and 266 women aged 70 of whom 46% and 16%, respectively, reported current sexual intercourse. Interestingly, questions regarding masturbation were not included as this was thought to be too provocative. For men, associations were identified between current sexual intercourse and better sleep, better mental health, and a more positive attitude towards sex in later life. For women, associations were identified between current sexual intercourse and having a comparatively young husband, low levels of anxiety, better mental health, satisfaction with marriage, positive experience of sexual intercourse, and a positive attitude towards sex in later life.

### Starr and Weiner: *The Starr–Weiner Report on Sex and Sexuality in the Mature Years* (1981)

The authors surveyed 800 women and men between the ages of 60 and 91 years who were recruited from civic agencies and senior centres across the USA, where sessions on sexuality and ageing were presented by the authors. Attendees were given a 50-item open-ended questionnaire to complete at home and return to the researchers. Although the overall response rate was low (14%) and the sample is likely to be highly self-selected, Starr and Weiner's report is worthwhile mentioning as they wanted to go beyond the Kinsey model adopted up to that time of quantifying the frequency of sexual interest and activity. They recognized that frequency of orgasm or ejaculation is not the ultimate measure of good sex. Results showed that age was not related to sexual satisfaction. In their sample, 97% reported that they liked sex, 75% felt that sex was the same or better than when they were younger, and 80% were 'currently sexually active', although this term was not clearly defined. Less than half (44% of men and 47% of women) reported that they masturbated. More than 80% of the respondents believed that sex is important for both physical and mental well-being.

### Brecher and The Editors of Consumer Reports
#### Books: *Love, Sex, and Aging* (1984)

The authors conducted their research again in the USA, obtaining the largest sample ever assembled to this date for a study of later life sexuality. Their sample involved 4226 women and men aged 50–93, resulting in a total response rate of 41.6%, who were recruited via the Consumer Union to which they were subscribers. The participants completed self-administered questionnaires, which explored a more diverse range of behaviours, attitudes, and beliefs within the context of sexual relationships than previous studies, including marital, non-marital, extra-marital, and post-marital relationships, both homosexual as well as heterosexual. Although the authors acknowledge that their sample is self-selected and unlikely to be representative for the population as a whole, their results render some interesting findings, which had not been explicitly addressed previously. The following findings were among those reported: (1) sex was rated as more important by men than by women within marriage; (2) unmarried men and women who were sexually active after the age of 50 reported greater life satisfaction than those who were not sexually active; (3) more men than women had been involved in a homosexual relationship after age 50; (4) while fewer men and women were sexually active (including engaging in sexual intercourse) in their 80s than younger group participants, a significant proportion were sexually active (60% of men and 40% of women in this sample); (5) more men than women after age 60 masturbated (47% of men and 36% of women in this sample); (6) approximately 50% of men and women engaged in fellatio and/or cunnilingus after age 50, with the vast majority reporting to enjoy this type of sexual activity; (7) 13% of women and 15% of men reported having used a vibrator after age 50; (8) 16% of heterosexual men and women reported that since the age of 50, they have had their anus stimulated during sexual activity. The authors note that they failed to find a single discussion of this last topic on their comment pages, suggesting that anal sex, unlike masturbation, cunnilingus, fellatio, and the use of vibrators is still taboo as a topic of discussion, even among those who engage in it and enjoy it.

Overall Brecher *et al.* state: 'The panorama of love, sex and aging here presented is far richer and more diverse than the stereotype of life after 50, or than the view presented by earlier studies of aging.... Hence the question arises: if life after 50 is in fact so sexually rich and diverse for so many, why has this been kept a secret? Why haven't older people said so before? One reason is that few have ever been asked'.

### Bretschneider and McCoy (1988)

This research represented a cross-sectional, volunteer study, involving 100 men and 102 women aged 80 and over living in a residential home in the USA. The overall response rate was a third of the people approached. Within this group for both men and women the most common sexual activity was touching and caressing (82% of men and 64% of women at least sometimes), followed by masturbation (72% of men and 40% of women at least sometimes), followed by sexual intercourse (63% of men and 30% of women at least sometimes). In addition, 88% of men and 71% of women still fantasized or daydreamed about being close, affectionate, and intimate with the opposite sex. Of these activities, only the frequency and enjoyment of touching and caressing showed a significant decline from the 80s to the 90s, with further analyses revealing a significant decline in this activity for men but not for women.

### Bullard-Poe, Powell, and Mulligan (1994)

This study explored intimacy and its contribution to life satisfaction in older men living in a Veterans Affairs nursing home in the USA. Forty-five participants with a mean age of 70 and a mean Mini-Mental State Examination score of 22 (Folstein *et al.*, 1975) rated social intimacy as the most important form of intimacy and sexual–physical intimacy as the least important, although this was still ranked as midway between 'somewhat' and 'moderately' important. Furthermore, despite being more cognitively and functionally impaired, married participants consistently rated all forms of intimacy higher in importance than did the unmarried group. In addition, the authors found strong associations between quality of life and non-sexual physical intimacy, intellectual intimacy, and current experiences of intimacy, and they conclude that intimacy makes an important contribution to the quality of life. Although this study represents a highly selected population with a small sample size, the authors highlight the importance of social and sexual intimacy to a particular group of older people often forgotten and disenfranchised by society.

### Massachusetts Male Aging Study (Feldman *et al.*, 1994)

This was a survey of erectile function among 1709 randomly sampled men aged between 40 and 70 in Massachusetts, using a self-administered questionnaire. Questions included the subjects' satisfaction with their relationship and sex life, their partners' satisfaction with them, and frequency of sexual activity. Results showed the prevalence of erectile dysfunction to be strongly related to age. In men aged 40, 5% suffered from complete erectile dysfunction, while 15% did so at the age of 70. Moderate erectile dysfunction occurred in 17% of 40-year-olds and 34% of 70-year-olds. The most important medical and psychosocial risk factors for erectile dysfunction were heart disease, hypertension, diabetes mellitus, medication associated with these diseases, a low level of high-density lipoprotein, and psychological measures of anger, depression, and low dominance. Smoking intensified the effects of cardiovascular risk, whilst alcohol intake exerted a minor effect and obesity no effect.

### Skoog (1996)

This study describes another representative community sample of 321 85-year-olds without dementia living in Gothenburg, Sweden. The subjects were 223 women, of whom 21 were married and 98 men, of whom 55 were married. Overall, 13% of men and 1% of women reported currently engaging in sexual intercourse, although in those who were married, this figure rose to 22% of male and 10% of female participants. By contrast with the rates for intercourse, however, a much higher rate of sexual interest was expressed, reported by 37% of unmarried men and 46% of married men, whilst 15% of unmarried women and 24% of married women reported having sexual feelings.

### Gott: *Sexuality, Sexual Health and Ageing* (2005)

Gott's work represents a departure from previous studies, as it focuses in great depth on older people's own attitudes towards the role and value of sex in later life through a collection of quality of life measures, followed by semi-structured interviews. She described a randomly chosen sample comprising 44 men and women aged 50 to 92 years recruited from a general practice in the UK. Her results particularly highlighted how older people adapt and reprioritize sex when faced with barriers to remaining sexually active, such as not having a sexual partner and having poor health status. All her participants with a current sexual partner attributed at least some importance to sex, with many rating sex as very or extremely important. Her study refuted the widely held belief that if older people are not sexually active, sex is not important to them.

### Other studies

Many surveys have complemented the findings discussed here. Some are based on samples from the general (aged) population, for example: Diokno et al. (1990)—clinical interviews of 1956 participants aged 60 years and older, who were identified by a probability sample of 13,912 households in the USA; Marsiglio and Donnelly (1991)—a randomly selected cross-sectional survey with face-to-face interviews and a self-administered questionnaire with 807 married people over 60 years as part of the National Survey of Families and Households in the United States; Panser et al. (1995)—a self-administered questionnaire of 1993 men aged 40–79 years randomly selected as part of the Olmsted County Study of urinary symptoms and health status among men in the USA; Helgason et al. (1996)—an age-stratified community sample with a questionnaire survey of 319 men in Sweden; Minichiello et al. (1996)—844 older people drawn randomly from the electoral role in Australia as part of a general health survey; Davey Smith et al. (1997)—a 20-year follow-up study of 2512 men in Wales as an 'add-on' to a study of cardiovascular mortality; Dello Buono et al. (1998a)—335 people aged 65–106 recruited through their GPs in Padua, Italy, as part of an international study conducted by the World Health Organization.

Other studies have targeted specific groups: Ehrenfeld et al. (1997)—a study of nursing observations of 160 patients with dementia in long-term care in Israel; Matthias et al. (1997)—1216 community recipients of Medicare in the USA; Archibald (1998)—a survey of sexuality and dementia in 23 social service residential care homes in the UK, using managers' reports; Dello Buono et al. (1998b)—38 centenarians, as a subgroup of the study mentioned above; Bortz and Wallace (1999)—1002 members of the 50+ Fitness Association, a selected group of physically active and highly motivated Americans.

Many of the findings from these studies echo those of earlier ones. Many older people continue to engage in and enjoy a wide range of sexual activities, whilst others do not for a variety of reasons. Age, gender, the availability of a partner, living conditions, social context, and physical as well as mental health are important factors in influencing sexual interest and activity.

Finally, it is worthwhile mentioning a number of books which offer a wealth of both information and education. They describe later life sexuality issues including single-case accounts of older men and women, whose individual and intimate stories reflect the broad spectrum and diversity of the findings discussed before (Hite 1976, 1981; Greengross and Greengross, 1989; Blank, 2000; Gross, 2000).

## Sexual physiology and ageing

### The human sexual response cycle

The human sexual response cycle is mediated by the complex interplay of psychological, environmental, and physiological (hormonal, vascular, muscular, and neurological) factors. The initial phase of the human sexual response cycle is interest and desire, followed by the four successive phases described by Masters and Johnson (1966): arousal, plateau, orgasm, and resolution characterized by genital and extra-genital changes. Basson (2000) redefined the linear progression of sexual response described by Masters and Johnson. Her model postulates that the sexual cycle in women is cyclical rather than linear and that arousal and desire are interchangeable. In this model, the starting point for sexuality is the desire for intimacy and closeness rather then a need for physical sexual release. Many women are satisfied with an intimate encounter which does not necessarily include intercourse or orgasm.

The *desire phase* of the sexual response cycle is characterized by sexual fantasies and the desire to have sexual activity. It is a subjective state, which may be triggered by both internal and external sexual cues and is dependent on adequate neuroendocrine functioning.

The *arousal or excitement phase* is mediated by the parasympathetic nervous system and is characterized by a subjective sense of pleasure and the appearance of vaginal lubrication in women and penile tumescence leading to erection in men. Testosterone plays a major role in desire and arousal in both men and women.

The *orgasm phase* is a myotonic response mediated by the sympathetic nervous system. It consists of a peaking of sexual pleasure, with the release of sexual tension and the rhythmic contraction of the perineal muscles and the pelvic reproductive organs. In women, orgasm is characterized by 3 to 15 involuntary contractions of the lower third of the vagina and by strong sustained contractions of the uterus, flowing from the fundus downward to the cervix. In men, a subjective sense of ejaculatory inevitability triggers orgasm with emission of semen. It is also associated with four to five rhythmic spasms of the prostate, seminal vesicles, vas, and urethra. Both women and men have involuntary contractions of the internal and external sphincters.

The *resolution phase* consists of the disgorgement of blood from the genitalia (detumescence) and the body returns to a resting state. It is further characterized by a subjective sense of well-being and a feeling of relaxation. After orgasm, men have a refractory period, which may last from several minutes to many hours; in this period they cannot be stimulated to further orgasm. Many women do not have a refractory period and are thus capable of multiple and successive orgasms. There is wide variability in the way people respond sexually, and each phase can be affected by ageing, illness, medication, alcohol, illicit drugs, as well as psychological and relationship factors. The diagnostic classification of sexual disorders both in the ICD-10 (World Health Organization, 1992) and DSM-IV (American Psychiatric Association, 1994) are based on the sexual response cycle.

### Hormonal changes and ageing

In women, the most salient biochemical markers of sexual maturation and senescence are the age-related changes in the level of oestrogen and testosterone. The structural integrity of the female genitalia is predominantly maintained by oestrogen. Vaginal dryness and atrophy, dyspareunia, and urinary tract symptoms in older women suggest a lack of oestrogen.

In healthy men, testosterone production remains relatively stable until the fifth decade, when a gradual decline in testosterone production begins in many men. It is probably mainly a result of testicular ageing, although a rise in sex hormone-binding globulin

(SHBG) and testosterone-binding and a relative failure of the hypothalamo-pituitary axis to drive the testis also contribute (Bancroft, 1989). The decline in circulating testosterone occurring in ageing men is responsible for the decrease in desire, but not erectile function, although clinically it may be difficult to distinguish reliably between the two complaints.

More detailed reviews on this topic are available elsewhere (Mooradian and Greiff, 1990; Schiavi, 1999; Leiblum and Rosen, 2000; Brincat *et al.*, 2002).

### Sexual response and ageing

In both sexes, as one ages, the speed and intensity of the various vasocongestive responses to sexual stimulation tend to be reduced (Masters and Johnson, 1966). Table 37.1 reflects the main changes in sexual response with age in women and Table 37.2 describes these changes in ageing men.

Whilst the overall decline of the sexual responses may seem stark and dreary, it is important to remember that this process tends to develop extremely gradually, allowing a couple or an individual to adjust to a less intense, but not necessarily less enjoyable, form of sexual activity. In fact, several cross-sectional studies have shown that sexual satisfaction does not decline with age, despite decrements in sexual function and behaviour (McKinlay and Feldman, 1994; Schiavi *et al.*, 1994).

## Effects of physical illness and medication on sexuality

One of the commonest reasons given by older people for ending sexual activity is the onset of physical illness, which may operate through a number of different mechanisms. Physical illness may generate unfounded anxieties about the *risks* of sexual activity (as in heart disease or stroke); it may make intercourse *difficult*, exhausting, or painful [as in respiratory disease, arthritis, and (sexually transmitted) infection]; or it may impair *responsiveness* of the sexual organs (as in diabetes mellitus or peripheral vascular disease). Physical illness may further undermine *self-confidence* and the feeling of attractiveness (as in mutilating operations such as mastectomy or colostomy), and it may have a direct effect in reducing sexual *desire* (as in depression, chronic renal or hepatic failure, and Parkinson's disease).

Older people in general are more likely to suffer from a variety of chronic diseases which may impact on their sexual function.

They also commonly undergo surgery, which may influence sexual function, either because of psychological sequelae or as a result of organic damage (Table 37.3). In addition, a significant proportion of older people take medication, and often there is considerable polypharmacy. The list of drugs that can interfere with sexual function is very long: among them should be noted antidepressants and antipsychotics, benzodiazepines, antihypertensive medication, thiazide diuretics, statins, and anticonvulsants (Zeiss, 1997; Thomas, 2003; Taylor *et al.*, 2005).

Where drug-induced sexual dysfunction is suspected, discontinuing the suspected medication or substituting with a different agent can usually resolve the question. Much less commonly, medication can enhance (or over-stimulate) sexual function, which has been described with levodopa (Uitti *et al.*, 1989) and trazodone (Garbell, 1986; Sullivan, 1988).

## Taking a sexual history

The effects of mental illness on sexual functioning, the psychological impact of sexual dysfunction on mental health, and the effects of psychotropic medication on sexuality all suggest that high rates of sexual dysfunction will be found among psychiatric patients (Bancroft, 1989; Wylie *et al.*, 2002; Macdonald *et al.*, 2003; Taylor *et al.*, 2005). Given the effects of ageing and physical illness on sexual response as well as the increased sensitivity of older people to the side-effects of medication, it is likely that sexual dysfunction will find its highest prevalence in the older age group. Hence it is vital that a sexual history forms part of any comprehensive psychiatric assessment. But are members of the medical profession knowledgeable and comfortable enough about sexual health to be able to take a sexual history? If undergraduate medical training is anything to go by, the omens are poor. The National Sexual Health Strategy commented that 'there are a number of important gaps in sexual health training and education, including inadequate, patchy or absent sexual health training in undergraduate medical curricula' (Department of Health, 2001b). Surveys of medical schools in the UK and USA have shown that time devoted to sexual health is limited and decreasing (FitzGerald *et al.*, 2003; Solursh, 2003; Wylie *et al.*, 2003). Furthermore, many post-graduate psychiatric training programmes fail to teach a broad range of human sexuality issues,

**Table 37.1** Sexual response and the effects of ageing in women

| |
| --- |
| Decreased sexual desire |
| Increased time required to become sexually aroused |
| Vaginal lubrication response is slower and less marked |
| Less intense orgasms |
| Increased need for stimulation to become orgasmic |
| No change in the ability to have orgasms |
| Less likely to be multi-orgasmic |
| Resolution following orgasm is more rapid |

Based on Bancroft, J. (1989) Human sexuality and its problems, 2nd edn, pp. 282–98. Churchill Livingstone, Edinburgh with permission.

**Table 37.2** Sexual response and the effects of ageing in men

| |
| --- |
| Decreased sexual desire |
| Erection takes longer to develop and may require more direct tactile stimulation |
| Period of sustaining an erection gets shorter |
| Nocturnal erections and emissions are less frequent |
| Less marked scrotal and testicular changes associated with arousal |
| Production of less pre-ejaculatory mucus |
| Ejaculation becomes less powerful with fewer contractions and seminal fluid volume is reduced |
| The point of ejaculatory inevitability becomes more difficult to recognise |
| Resolution is more rapid |
| The refractory period is markedly longer |

Based on Bancroft, J. (1989) Human sexuality and its problems, 2nd edn, pp. 282–98. Churchill Livingstone, Edinburgh, with permission.

**Table 37.3** Physical illnesses and surgery associated with sexual dysfunction

| Cardiovascular | Angina pectoris |
|---|---|
| | Myocardial infarction |
| | Hypertension |
| | Peripheral vascular insufficiency (atherosclerosis) |
| | Vascular surgery (aorto-iliac/aorto-femoral bypass) |
| Endocrine | Primary hypogonadism |
| | Hypogonadotrophic hypogonadism |
| | Hyperprolactinaemia |
| | Thyroid disorders |
| | Addison's disease |
| | Cushing's syndrome |
| | Post-surgical: gonadectomy |
| Metabolic | Diabetes mellitus |
| | Chronic renal insufficiency |
| | Chronic hepatic insufficiency |
| Neurological Central | Temporal lobe pathology |
| | Multiple sclerosis |
| | Parkinson's disease |
| | Amyotrophic lateral sclerosis |
| | Cerebrovascular lesions (stroke) |
| | Sleep disorders (apnoea) |
| | Alzheimer's disease |
| | Tumours and traumatic lesions (brain and spinal cord) |
| Neurological peripheral | |
| Degenerative | Diabetic neuropathy |
| | Alcoholic neuropathy |
| Post-surgical | Transurethral surgeries |
| | Radical prostatectomy |
| | Abdomino-perineal resection |
| | Bilateral lumbar sympathectomy |
| Anatomical | Peyronie's disease |
| | Post-surgical (mastectomy, hysterectomy, genital tumours) |
| Other systemic conditions | Chronic obstructive pulmonary disease |
| | Arthritis |
| | Obesity |

Based on Schiavi, R.C. (1999). Aging and male sexuality. Cambridge University Press, Cambridge, with permission.

and expert supervision and clinical training opportunities are lacking (Sansone and Wiederman, 2000). Consequently it is perhaps unsurprising that, according to the sparse existing literature on this topic, psychiatrists generally fail to take a sexual history from their patients.

Singh and Beck (1997) reported that no sexual history was taken in 73% of adult psychiatric inpatients and only one patient had a detailed sexual history taken. Similarly, a review of current practice of consultant psychiatrists revealed that a sexual history is often omitted in the psychiatric assessment of elderly men, and that these patients do not receive appropriate referral and treatment (Bouman and Arcelus 2001).

Many clinicians lack confidence about their ability to take an appropriate sexual history. In part, the discomfort lies in the clinician's feelings of embarrassment together with the patient's embarrassment and ambivalence about bringing up the topic. Too often the result is a complete avoidance of the topic. However,

Ende *et al.* (1989) noted that more than 91% of patients thought it was appropriate for their doctor to take a sexual history. It is also not uncommon for patients to present with some other problem or condition, whilst the underlying precipitant is a sexual problem.

The principles of taking a sexual history are not altered by the age of the patient. Risen (1995) and Tomlinson (1998) give an excellent account of these, which are summarized below:

1 Understanding the barriers to taking a sexual history, which include:

- Lack of knowledge other than one's own experience. Sole reliance on one's own sexual background and experience is problematic as a clinical point of reference and may encourage a judgemental point of view regarding the patient's sexual problems. Gaining clinical experience offers the privilege of hearing about many sexual lives and broadens the clinician's frame of reference.

- Fear of the affects generated by taking a sexual history. Taking a sexual history invites and encourages an intimacy that can feel simultaneously embarrassing, exciting, anxiety provoking, and disturbing to both patient and clinician. However, with experience one develops a professional distance, which inhibits and deflects more personal internal responses. If the doctor's attitude is matter of fact, then the patient will relax and become matter of fact too.

- Choice of sexual vocabulary. Should we use vernacular terms or only medical terms? The former method risks sounding too crude or offensive, whilst the latter may cause misunderstanding by the patient. Both can cause problems in getting an accurate history, but clinicians must use very careful judgement in deciding which terminology to use. 'Let me know if you're not sure what I am asking?' or 'Use your own words and I'll tell you if I don't understand' are helpful interventions.

- Ageism has infiltrated so deeply into the belief system of our society that many older patients as well as clinicians view older people as too old for sex, despite research indicating that a significant proportion of older people remain sexually active well into advanced old age (Bretschneider and McCoy, 1988; Bergstrom-Walan and Nielsen, 1990).

2 Ensuring that the patient is seated comfortably in a private clinic room, which is free from interruption.

3 Assuring the patient of complete confidentiality. This must take place very early in the assessment, and especially if personal secrets are disclosed, such as extra-marital relationships.

4 Interviewing both partners in a relationship is always more valuable, but patients often prefer to discuss things alone at first. A warm invitation for the partner, coupled with the observation that a sexual problem tends not to be the patient's problem alone, can put the patient's worries into perspective.

5 The ideal time for taking a sexual history is when the clinician collects psychosocial and developmental information. The advantage of taking a sexual history at an early stage, regardless of whether or not a sexual problem exists, is that it gives the patient permission to speak of sexual issues in the future.

6 Using open and non-threatening questions first, which allow the patient to describe and reflect on their sexual functioning.

'What is the role of sexuality in your life right now?' and 'Are you experiencing any sexual problems or concerns?' are useful openings. Open questions, which encourage patients to tell their sexual story using their own language, are the most useful. They can be followed by closed, more specific questions to establish exact details. Judgemental questions, such as 'Don't you think you're past that sort of thing now?' should be avoided.

7   Taking a thorough psychosocial history, which includes the history from childhood, quality of relationships in the family, role of religion, family attitudes regarding sexuality and gender, the sources of sexual information, close friendships and relationships, and especially a history of the current relationship, which should establish the good periods of the couple's relationship, and what they valued in each other then.

8   Taking a medical and psychiatric history. A large proportion of sexual problems have an organic aetiology, although the interaction with psychological, social, and relationship factors should be borne in mind. Psychiatric illness, neurological conditions, diabetes mellitus, heart disease, other hormone deficiencies, operations and trauma, pain, and many other conditions may significantly affect sexual function.

9   Asking about medical and recreational drugs. Many medications, especially psychotropics and hypotensives, as well as the quantity and frequency of alcohol and nicotine intake, can have a profound effect on sexual function. Illicit drugs tend to have a deleterious long-term effect.

10  Formulating the problem in terms of predisposing, precipitating, and maintaining factors as well as a management plan, which should then be discussed and agreed with the patient or couple.

Like any other member of the public, clinicians will at times grapple with their own sexual issues and have varying views and value systems about sexual matters and morality. It does not absolve us from the responsibility to be well informed about sexual health in order to educate and help our patients, at the same time as adopting a neutral and non-censorious position

The clinical competency of the clinician in talking about sexual issues, and the level of training received in dealing with sexuality in its broadest sense, is a major factor in determining how sexual problems present or whether they are presented at all! One can only speculate on the number of patients who set out to seek advice for their sexual difficulty, but fail because of the discouraging response from the clinician involved. Although clinicians may feel awkward and unskilled, the very willingness to discuss sexual issues offers the patient an opportunity that society rarely provides. Giving patients permission to talk about their sexual lives may be therapeutic in itself. In this context, it is also entirely appropriate for the clinician to tell the patient that he needs to consider the problem further, or to ask for advice from another colleague, and to arrange a follow-up appointment for the patient. Beyond this, suitable training in psychosexual therapy or medicine is available, either as a diploma or higher degree in various institutions in the UK, or possibly as a special interest at local genito-urinary medicine, sexual health or gynaecology services (Mathers et al., 1994).

### Further assessment of sexual problems

When a sexual problem is diagnosed following a comprehensive sexual history, further assessment should include a thorough physical examination as well as blood investigations, which generally comprise full blood count, liver function, thyroid function, fasting blood glucose, cholesterol, prolactin, testosterone, and sex hormone-binding globulin (SHBG). Other specific tests may be appropriate (e.g. follicle-stimulating hormone, luteinizing hormone, free testosterone). The use of validated self-report questionnaires, such as the Golombok Rust Inventory of Sexual Satisfaction (GRISS) (Rust and Golombok, 1986), the Brief Index of Sexual Functioning for Women (BISF-W) (Taylor et al., 1994), and the International Inventory of Erectile Function (IIEF) (Rosen et al., 1997), are sometimes of relevance, and are a useful tool in facilitating the diagnostic process. The IIEF also measures improvement in response to treatment.

Interviewing the partner is vital, and its importance should be explained to the patient. Some clinicians prefer to see each partner individually at first, followed by time with the couple together, although there are no hard and fast rules regarding this issue. When the assessment is completed, a careful and unhurried explanation is given to the couple concerning the nature of the problem, the likely reasons why it arose, the factors that may be perpetuating it, and the various treatment options available. This explanation needs to be thought through beforehand, so that it can be presented in a way that does not lay blame on either partner, leaving room for positive steps to be taken. Even where nothing else is possible, there is usually scope for helping communication and understanding between the partners. The formulation of the problem is followed by time and encouragement for the couple to ask questions, through which the doctor is satisfied that they have both understood what has been said.

## Sexual problems and ageing

Having considered the various research findings in the area of sexuality and ageing and the clinical assessment, what are the main sexual problems complained of by older people?

In many respects, the complaints differ little from those of younger people who seek help for their sexual or relationship problems, and may have emotional or physical origins, or both. Fear of poor performance, lack of, or diminished, sexual desire, difficulty becoming sexually aroused either physically or psychologically, difficulty maintaining an erection, difficulty achieving orgasm, and pain or discomfort with sexual exchange, especially during intercourse, as well as a lack of opportunities for sexual encounters are among the most common of the complaints that older people present with (Bretschneider and McCoy, 1988; Feldman et al., 1994; Leiblum and Taylor Seagraves, 2000). Sexual dysfunction may also arise simply from a lack of information about the normal age-related changes in sexual physiology. A slower onset of erectile function, or a reduced need to ejaculate, may be interpreted by the man as the onset of impotence, or by the woman as a sign of declining interest in her; and their fearful or offended reactions can then aggravate the difficulty. Similarly, a reduced vaginal lubrication response may cause pain and discomfort during intercourse leading the woman to avoid further sexual intimacy, which may be interpreted by the man as a rejection of the love he wants to express. In addition to these problems, older people may mourn or regret changes in their body—its size, shape, and firmness may differ significantly from the past. They may complain, as well, about the changing body of their partner, the reduction in, or loss of, passion and attention given to emotional and sexual intimacy, sexual boredom, jealousy of younger potential rivals, and changes in sexual urgency or intensity. Menopause, surgery, and various losses, both psychological and physical can exacerbate these complaints.

Frequently, physical and psychological factors will interact in bringing about sexual dysfunction. In a man who already feels insecure and pessimistic about his sexual function, one experience of difficulty attaining or maintaining an erection may be sufficient to precipitate psychogenic impotence, with performance anxiety creating a self-fulfilling prophecy. Convinced that he will fail in intercourse, he may avoid occasions for making love, and for showing physical affection in any other way, for fear of being expected to go further. The less he is able to talk to his partner about his fear and his reasons for avoiding intercourse, the greater the risk of chronic impotence and potential relationship problems.

Similarly, if illness has reduced the capacity to respond to sexual stimulation, and this is something the couple cannot understand or discuss, then they cannot resolve this difficulty. In a relationship where the assumption was that the man always takes the active role in lovemaking, his partner may be quite unused to stroking his penis as part of their preparation for intercourse, and so cannot help him if this is what he requires.

Another, often more dramatic, scenario occurs when there is a transition from an equal partnership to one of caregiver and patient due to severe illness. The ill partner may lose the self-esteem which reassures him that he is still contributing to the relationship; or the caring partner may think it unkind and selfish to make demands on the sexual responsiveness of the one who is ill. Particularly if there is a lack of communication around sexual issues, sexual relationship changes may never be adequately worked out. But even simple actions can have far-reaching effects, such as when a couple decide they should sleep apart so as to give the ill partner a better night's rest, resulting in a potential reduction of closeness and intimacy.

Despite prevailing preconceptions, many older people are willing and open to address their sexual difficulties. In fact, many indicate they would enjoy greater sexual experimentation in their relationship (Brecher et al., 1984). Research suggests that if sex was a source of pleasure and gratification during early and middle adulthood, it will probably continue to be an important source of life satisfaction as one grows older. On the other hand, it must be acknowledged that there remain many older people who grew up in fundamental and traditional households in which sexually proscriptive values and beliefs persist. For these individuals, sex is sanctioned primarily for procreation; sexual behaviours other than intercourse, such as oral–genital sex, are considered unnatural; sexual relations outside marriage are forbidden; and masturbation is sinful. For such individuals, the opportunity to 'retire' from an active sexual life may be ardently anticipated and easily accepted.

## Lesbian, gay, bisexual, and transgender issues and ageing

Research on older lesbian, gay, bisexual, and transgender (LGBT) individuals has been slow to accumulate in the literature, which has undoubtedly been compounded by methodological difficulties in this largely invisible group. While research in the area of ageing and LGBT is limited, studies in the area of ageing transgender individuals are virtually non-existent. The characteristics of the current older LGBT generation are typically defined by the historical and societal events which occurred during their developmental periods—a time when LGBT people were socially defined as mentally ill within a medical framework, and faced considerable discrimination in both health and social service systems, and in society as a whole. This has resulted in feelings of great stigma and shame, which continue to shape their lives, often requiring them, as a vital coping mechanism, to keep their sexual or gender orientation hidden for fear of discrimination.

Most research on older LGBT individuals is based on convenience samples of urban, well-educated, relatively affluent, physically and mentally healthy adults, who are affiliated with social and recreational groups for LGBT people and who are willing to self-identify as LGBT. Meyer and Colten (1999) have shown that gay men recruited into research from LGBT community sources are significantly different from those obtained by random sampling procedures, especially in terms of the former having greater social contact with LGBT people and lower internalized homophobia. Nonetheless, interest in and desire for some form of physical intimacy is characteristic of most older homosexual men and women (Wahler and Gabbay, 1997), whilst for the most part, sexual partners of this group tend to be within a decade of their own age (Pope and Schultz, 1990). Sexual practices among older gay and bisexual men are generally similar to their younger counterparts, although they are less likely to have anal intercourse with casual partners (Van de Ven et al., 1997).

Social support is found to be particularly important for older LGBT people, not only because of its positive influence on changes in physical and mental health related to ageing in general, but also because social support can serve a unique function in mitigating the impact of the stigmatization which older LGBT people experience due to their sexual or gender orientation. Dorfman et al. (1995) reported on a sample of 108 older individuals between 60 and 93 years old, of whom 56 were lesbian or gay men and 52 were heterosexuals. No significant differences were found between the two groups with regard to depression and social support; for both groups, larger social networks were associated with less depression. The sources of social support varied: the gay sample received significantly more support from friends, whereas the heterosexual group derived more support from family. In a similar study, Grossman et al. (2000) confirmed these findings and also reported that lesbian, gay, and bisexual older people living with a partner were less lonely and rated their physical and mental health more positively then those who lived alone. Furthermore, participants were more satisfied with support from those who knew of their sexual orientation. Wojciechowski (1998), in a review on the literature on older lesbians, also highlighted the vulnerability of couples who have not been publicly recognized to interference by others in decisions about their care, in bereavement, and in their property rights.

Although in Canada and in some European countries, including the UK, partnership or marriage between same-sex couples is legally recognized, similar couples from other countries do not have access to these rights, which include next of kinship, pension and tenancy rights, and inheritance tax advantages. They may, understandably, worry about legal and financial consequences when one partner becomes ill, requires institutional care or dies.

## Sexual abuse

There is a dearth of published studies regarding sexual abuse in older people, although the general consensus in the literature appears to be that this type of abuse may occur more frequently than is generally recognized. Teaster and Roberto (2004) developed a profile of sexual abuse cases among individuals aged 60 and over receiving attention from adult protective services in Virginia, USA over a 5-year period. They identified 82 individuals experiencing sexual abuse. Most victims were women between the ages of 70 and 89 residing in a nursing home. Typically, sexual abuse involved instances of sexualized kissing and inappropriate fondling and touching. The majority of perpetrators were nursing home residents and in most situations, witnesses to the sexual abuse were other residents. Clearly it highlights the need for clear policies and procedures for monitoring and protecting vulnerable older people in care facilities. Generally, sexual abuse may happen to any older person and occur in any setting, be it at home, on a medical ward, or in residential or nursing homes, perpetrated by a spouse, formal or informal carers or staff, other residents, or complete strangers. Haddad and Benbow (1993) discuss the risk of sexual abuse of individuals with dementia. They define sexual abuse as occurring when an individual initiates a sexual relationship with a person with dementia without that person's informed consent. People with dementia may be physically frail and unable to resist sexual advances, and may not be able to report abuse when it occurs. Without a high index of suspicion and without addressing the issue explicitly, sexual abuse will easily be missed (Warner, 2000).

## Sexuality and dementia

There is limited empirical information about the impact of dementia on sexual function, despite the high prevalence of dementia, and despite the concerns often expressed by spouses, partners, and carers. Zeiss *et al.* (1990), in an uncontrolled survey of 55 men with Alzheimer's disease (AD), found that in 53% of these men the reported onset of erectile dysfunction occurred at the same time as the cognitive impairment started. This was not related to age, degree of cognitive impairment, physical illness, or medication. There are no published studies regarding the prevalence of female sexual dysfunction in dementia.

### Dementia and sexuality in established relationships

The onset of dementia does not erase sexuality, but rather alters sexual behaviour and expression in many patients, which can be extremely distressing to both the patient and their partner. Despite these difficulties, many couples want to maintain a sexual relationship, experiencing sexual intimacy as a source of comfort, reassurance, and mutual support. The more the partner can retain the ability to view the patient as a person with whom to enjoy sexuality, the more likely that the relationship can endure with some quality. Some partners, however, may lose sexual attraction and interest as the disease progresses and as they adapt themselves to the role of carer, whilst others may seek sexual satisfaction elsewhere, through private masturbation, prostitutes, or a relationship outside the dyad. This may lead to guilt, especially if the patient is still living at home. This is a particularly difficult area to manage, as partners are understandably reluctant to talk about it. If they do, a non-judgemental supportive approach is vital (Warner, 2000).

Duffy (1995) interviewed 38 spouses of patients with AD over a 1-year period to assess the impact of the disease and its progression on the couples' pattern of sexual behaviour. The patients were categorized by their partners as moderately impaired, requiring assistance with common activities of daily living. Most of the healthy spouses acknowledged that their sexual relationship had changed since the onset of the disease, but there were few reports of behaviours characterized as bizarre or inappropriately expressed outside the marital relationship. Common sources of distress were: awkward sequencing of sexual activity, requests for activities outside the couple's sexual repertoire, and lack of regard for the sexual satisfaction of the healthy partner. Additional problems in established relationships include loss of sexual interest, increased sexual demands, or inadequate sexual advances by the patient with dementia, and marital strain or loss of intimacy resulting from the patient's cognitive and behavioural decline (Haddad and Benbow, 1993). Some carers will express concerns that their partner with dementia may not have the capacity to consent to sexual relations.

Litz *et al.* (1990) found a high rate of erectile dysfunction in partners of patients with dementia and postulated that this may be due to the additional stress placed on the relationship by the illness.

Derouesne *et al.* (1996) reported the findings of two surveys of community-dwelling married couples, where one individual had a diagnosis of AD. The first, a survey of 135 couples, found that 80% of spouses reported a change in the patient's sexual activity. This was not linked to degree of cognitive impairment or gender of the patient. The second study reported the results of a questionnaire about sexual relations before and after the onset of AD. Indifference to sexual activity was common among patients (63% of respondents). Most respondents who reported a change in sexual activity noted a decrease in sexual activity.

Although increased sexual demands were rare in this study (only 8% of respondents), this problem may be more common in other types of dementia, especially frontal lobe dementia and Pick's disease. Furthermore, increased sexual demands may be particularly upsetting for carers, and very difficult to discuss with others (Warner, 2000). Another survey of 40 spouses of patients with dementia found that nine (23%) couples were sexually active (Ballard *et al.*, 1997). Of those no longer sexually active, almost 40% were dissatisfied by the absence of a sexual relationship.

Wright (1998) conducted a 5-year follow-up study of two groups of couples, one in which one partner had dementia and a control group where neither partner was ill. At baseline the partners in the two groups reported the same levels of affection and sexual activity, but over the 5 years, while reported affection remained steady for the control spouses, it declined in the spouses in the dementia group, except, interestingly, when the individual with dementia had been admitted to institutional care, after which affection in the spouse recovered significantly. Fewer couples with a partner with dementia maintained sexual activity (27% at 5 years after onset of dementia) compared with control spouses (of whom 82% were sexually active at the same period). However, in those partnerships with dementia where sexual activity was maintained, the mean frequency of sexual contact was higher than in controls, and demands for frequent contact were reported by 50% of their carers. Sexual activity in these couples was also related to the spouses' physical health and absence of depression, but not to the cognitive state of the partner with dementia. Counselling about the reasons for the patient's altered sexual behaviour, and an explanation that this is related to the dementia, may help to reassure partners and alleviate their distress. It is important to emphasize that a lack of sexual activity should not preclude physical intimacy, and that physical intimacy, such as kissing and cuddling, is unlikely to result in sexually inappropriate behaviour by the patient (Davies *et al.*, 1992).

## Dementia and sexuality in new relationships

A person with dementia may attempt to start a sexual relationship with a new partner, which inevitably raises issues of competency. This is not an uncommon occurrence, particularly within institutional settings like a residential or nursing home. Although this behaviour may be difficult to cope with for health and social care staff and family alike, it requires careful thought about individuals' rights and serious attention to the complex task of determining the capacity of the patient (and the other party) to make informed judgements regarding new relationships. As Collopy (1988) has pointed out, competency is always context specific and no diagnosis, not even dementia, precludes a patient's capacity to reach competent decisions in specific areas. In order to facilitate decisions regarding a patient's ability to consent to sexual relationships, Lichtenberg and Strzepek (1990) developed a structured assessment process, which provides a helpful framework for clinicians. This includes ascertaining the patient's awareness of the nature of the relationship, the ability to avoid exploitation, and the awareness of potential risks. They also describe the specific steps involved in their assessment process, and acknowledge the difficulties which can result from complaints by family, visitors, or even other staff as a result of the implementation of a caring and respectful policy such as their own.

If a patient is deemed competent to understand, consent to, and form a relationship with another competent adult, then the choice is primarily for the patient to make, and preventing a patient from doing so would be a violation of their basic human rights. Staff may have a role in supporting this decision (for example by ensuring access to private space). If a patient in institutional care is not competent to decide, staff have a duty of care towards the patient to ensure that no harm results. Whether a non-competent patient should be allowed to engage in a sexual relationship is a difficult decision to make and will need to be carefully considered in the light of the person's background and previous choices, and the nature of the contact. A discussion with the patient's family may be helpful.

## Sexual expression in institutional care

Sexual expression is not limited to intercourse and should be interpreted broadly to reflect a wide range of physical acts, which include intercourse, masturbation, oral sex, fondling, kissing, and hugging as well as a person's need for closeness, tenderness, and warmth. Although health and social care staff are generally reported to show a positive attitude towards sexual expression of residents in residential and nursing homes (Holmes *et al.*, 1997; Bouman *et al.*, 2006), it remains debatable whether these positive attitudes are consistent with the implemented policies in institutional care in general and with the actual behaviour of staff in particular. Cultural values, personal beliefs, and, especially, inadequate training provide obstacles for staff (as well as carers) in confidently and sensitively responding to residents' sexual expression. In this context, Warner (2000) rightly points out that few care homes provide their residents with double beds, and many such facilities have quite draconian rules disallowing sex, in keeping with acute hospitals of all disciplines. He further advocates that in cases where competency to engage in sexual activity is established in both individuals, appropriate facilities (a double bed, time in private, condoms, water-based lubrication,

and, if desired, sex toys) should be provided by care facilities for their residents.

## Inappropriate sexual behaviour in dementia

Inappropriate sexual behaviours can be defined as sexual behaviours which are not suited to their context and which impair the care of the patient in a given environment (Black *et al.*, 2005). There is sometimes a fine line between appropriate and inappropriate sexual behaviour, which often depends on the values of the staff and relatives of the patient concerned. Underlying the assessment of 'appropriateness' are the often pervasive bias of ageism, the stereotypical view of older adults as asexual, and, particularly in the medical literature, the notion that sexuality in dementia tends to be a problem rather than a normal human form of expression in the context of a specific condition.

Inappropriate sexual behaviour is not particularly common in dementia. Burns *et al.* (1990) found that 7% of 178 people with AD living at home, in residential care, or in hospital showed sexually inappropriate behaviour with about equal frequency in men (8%) and women (7%). There was a significant positive association with severity of dementia. In a review of the literature, Cummings and Victoroff (1990) found few references to inappropriate sexual behaviour in patients diagnosed with AD, noting that between 2% and 7% displayed this difficulty, but reported that as many as 14% may show an increase in libido. Zeiss *et al.* (1996) conducted an observational study of 40 men with dementia living in long-term care facilities. Inappropriate sexual behaviours (defined as sexually explicit comments, touching someone other than a partner on the breast or genitals, and exposing breasts or genitals in public) were only briefly noted in 18% of patients. Ambiguous sexual behaviours, such as appearing not fully dressed in public, occurred in less than 4% of the 1800 time segments coded. There was no evidence of sexually aggressive behaviours toward staff or other residents.

Various authors (Haddad and Benbow, 1993; Black *et al.*, 2005) have classified inappropriate sexual behaviours into common types, which include:

1 Inappropriate sexual talk. This is the most common form of inappropriate behaviour and involves using sexually explicit language in a manner that is out of keeping with the patient's premorbid personality.

2 Sexual acting out. These include clear sexual acts that occur inappropriately, either solitary, or involving staff or other residents, in private or in public areas. Examples are acts of grabbing, exposing, publicly masturbating and fondling, making sexual advances toward staff, and getting uninvitedly into bed with other residents.

3 Implied sexual acts. These include openly reading pornographic material or requesting unnecessary genital care.

4 False sexual allegations. Deliberate dishonesty excluded, these may occur as part of a variety of psychopathological symptoms occurring in dementia such as hallucinations and delusions. The possibility that a patient's allegations are true must always be considered.

Clear assessment of the type of behaviours displayed is paramount for a balanced management plan to be developed. This includes the frequencies of the behaviours, what they are, when and where they occur, and with whom. A simple and convenient general method of recording behaviours is the ABC system, where staff record the antecedents (A), behaviours (B), and consequences (C) (Wells, 1997). Alternatively, a more complex standardized system such as dementia care mapping could be utilized (Kitwood and Bredin, 1992). The effects of interventions to alter sexual inappropriate behaviours cannot be properly evaluated without clear baseline records.

### Lesbian, gay, bisexual, and transgender issues

There are no studies examining the health and social care needs of LGBT individuals with dementia. Some authors discuss the specific needs of this group in relation to their sexual or gender orientation, particularly when they require institutional care, whilst others have highlighted the difficulties this group encounters, which includes less understanding and tolerance as well as discrimination by other family members, health and social care staff as well as other residents (Brotman et al., 2003; Pachankis and Goldfried, 2004; Johnson et al., 2005). If the dementia is HIV related, patient and carer have to come to terms with being HIV positive, as well as with the diagnosis of dementia. Many older LGBT people express a variety of concerns about discrimination in health and social care services, including residential and nursing homes, whilst a significant proportion would prefer to live in an exclusively LGBT facility, which is seen as more sensitive to their needs (Quam and Whitford, 1992).

In the UK, the Alzheimer's Society Lesbian and Gay Network supports the needs of people with dementia and carers who identify themselves as LGBT, through a telephone help-line service and a website (http://www.alzheimers.org.uk/Gay_Carers), which offers a wealth of information pertinent to this specific group.

## Management of sexual problems

### Education

Most authors on sexuality and ageing, from Masters and Johnson (1966) onwards, have emphasized the necessity of disseminating accurate information about normal sexual physiology and about the acceptability of sexual feelings and behaviour in later life so as to dispel harmful attitudes and preconceptions. The publication of books (Hite 1976, 1981; Greengross and Greengross, 1989; Blank, 2000; Gross, 2000) and magazines easily accessible to the general public, and programmes on radio and television are important vehicles for this process. The education of health and social care professionals is also vital. There are a number of papers in the literature discussing the value of educational programmes regarding sexuality and ageing. White and Catania (1982) were the first to describe the effects of a formal educational programme for residents, their families, and the care staff of a residential home; a four-fold increase in sexual activity was reported by the study group of residents following the programme. Mayers and McBride (1998) describe a 3-hour workshop for care staff in geriatric long-term care homes, followed up by questionnaires to assess the usefulness of the workshop. Participants found it valuable and enjoyable. Sadly, however, the untrained care staff found it hard to get away from their work, and so it was mainly senior staff who attended. This is a problem often encountered in the UK by health and social care staff who try to set up teaching programmes in residential and nursing homes; and it re-emphasizes the crucial importance of a real and practical commitment to education by the managers of

care homes. Walker and Harrington (2002) evaluated staff training materials designed to improve staff knowledge and attitudes about sexuality. Results indicated significant improvement in knowledge and attitudes of staff regarding the topics of three training modules: the need for sexuality and intimacy, sexuality and dementia, and sexuality and ageing. A large proportion of participants (>90%) reported finding the education useful and interesting.

The Dementia Services Development Centre (http://www.dementia.stir.ac.uk/) has produced a book and a video on sexuality and dementia for staff education. Counsel and Care (advice@counselandcare.org.uk) have issued a thoughtful guide for care homes regarding sex and relationships.

### Prevention

The sexual difficulties which can occur following illness or surgery, or as a consequence of medication, might be alleviated or prevented if better-informed health professionals discussed with their patients beforehand any sexual implications of their condition or treatment. Lawton and Hacker (1989) reported that, among the women referred to their clinic for gynaecological cancers, at least a third of the women over the age of 70 who had radical surgery were still sexually active; and they emphasized the importance of pre-operative counselling that encompasses the sexuality of older patients. Thorpe et al. (1994) found that in only 30% of their sample of men undergoing prostatectomy was there a record of pre-operative counselling about the possibility of retrograde ejaculation following surgery. Moreover, men over 70 were significantly less likely to have been advised on the sexual consequences of their operation than younger men in the study. Rees et al. (2002) discuss the importance of counselling after stroke. Finally, it is crucial to educate and inform older people about safe sex practices. Many older adults who resume dating in later life have been hitherto sexually monogamous and may be unaware or naïve about sexually transmitted infections, including HIV/AIDS.

### Common sexual problems

Many sexual difficulties, especially those arising in untroubled relationships and related to physical illness, can be helped by relatively simple advice. It is important to have an open and frank discussion about how certain medical conditions can affect sexual functioning and what precautions the couple may need to take. Topics may include: (1) when to resume intercourse after a myocardial infarction or stroke; (2) identifying different positions and different timing for analgesic medication for intercourse when arthritis or pain is a problem; and (3) how long to wait before resuming sexual activity and how much activity to attempt after surgery. It should be pointed out that weakness may hinder usual sexual activity and 'going slow' may be the optimum approach. Concrete examples, such as 'if you can walk a flight of stairs without shortness of breath, you can resume intercourse' may be helpful. With patients or partners who have undergone mutilative surgery, mastectomy, or ostomies, it is important to address fears of causing pain and the need to respond to fears of rejection because of drastic changes in body image. The healthy partner may be reluctant to discuss feelings of revulsion or contagion (Szwabo, 2003).

Following the loss of a partner, older people may find themselves facing sexual activity with a new partner, which can be a very stressful prospect. Concerns about personal desirability, attractiveness and sex appeal, about sexual performance, and about the risks of acquiring sexually transmitted infections, are often real and significant. Advice on open communication and sexual education, particularly about practising safe sex, is paramount. The older adult may need encouragement to tell a new partner how nervous they are: such open and positive communication will not only make them feel safer, but will also set the stage for enhanced sexual communication in general.

If intercourse is no longer a possibility, masturbation should be discussed as another source of self-pleasuring and as an appropriate activity to enhance individual or couple-pleasuring activities. Depending upon the individual's religious and cultural background, masturbation may not be perceived as an appropriate or comfortable option. For those without partners, masturbation may be the only option. Addressing the subject, and giving implicit permission, may be all that is needed to enable the patient to start engaging in sexual activity again.

If medication is implicated in causing sexual dysfunction, a discussion should take place about the feasibility of a change in dosage, or of changing to a different type of medication, or simply explaining that sexual response may take longer to develop, which will require more time and foreplay to achieve an adequate sexual response.

Dyspareunia due to vaginal dryness and atrophy may need advice on lubricants and prescription of low-dose vaginal oestrogens.

Erectile dysfunction is the most common sexual complaint in older men. The oral phosphodiesterase type 5 (PDE5) inhibitors, which include sildenafil (Viagra), tadalafil (Cialis) and vardenafil (Levitra) have revolutionized the treatment of erectile dysfunction as a convenient and safe alternative to more invasive treatment options. In addition, modification of risk factors, which include diabetes mellitus, hypertension, cardiovascular disease, depression, prostatic hypertrophy, smoking, medication, a sedentary lifestyle, drug and alcohol misuse, is an essential part of first-line treatment for erectile dysfunction, to improve erectile function and the patient's response to treatment. Despite the efficacy and tolerability of PDE5 inhibitors 30–35% of patients fail to respond (McMahon *et al.*, 2006). Educating patients on the correct use of these drugs can increase efficacy (Atiemo *et al.*, 2003). Other treatment options are generally provided by specialist services following rigorous assessment procedures. They include self-administration (by intra-cavernosal injection) of vasodilator medication, intra-urethral alprostadil by application of a microsuppository into the distal urethra, androgen replacement, psychosexual counselling, vacuum constrictor devices, and penile prosthesis implantation. Despite the growing clinical evidence that combination treatment may be successful in men for whom monotherapy fails, research is lacking to establish the benefits, optimal dosage, possible adverse effects, and acceptability to patients of these treatments (Bouman, 2006).

## Specialist services

Where the psychological and relationship issues contributing to a sexual problem are too time-consuming or complex for the primary care or psychiatry services to deal with, help may be sought from Relate (http://www.relate.org.uk/), or (in some areas) from psychosexual clinics provided through the local genito-urinary medicine or psychiatric service. The British Association of Sexual and Relationship (BASRT; http://www.basrt.org.uk/) holds a list of all accredited psychosexual therapists; they also approve training programmes for psychosexual therapy in various institutions in the UK.

Where the physical issues contributing to a sexual problem are beyond the expertise of primary care or psychiatric services, specialist advice may be obtained from a variety of specialities, which include genito-urinary medicine, urology, gynaecology, andrology, and sexual medicine.

## Inappropriate sexual behaviour in dementia

Harris and Wier (1998) and Black *et al.* (2005) offer a comprehensive overview of various treatment strategies to reduce unacceptable sexual behaviours. They distinguish two primary approaches in this area: psychological intervention and pharmacotherapy. In general, pharmacotherapy should only be considered when all other interventions have failed. The choice of treatment also depends upon the urgency of the situation, the type of behaviour, and the underlying medical conditions of the patient.

The main psychological intervention consists of behavioural modification which includes a range of approaches, such as removing reinforcement during the undesired behaviour and increasing reinforcement of appropriate alternative behaviours. Other approaches include distraction as a useful technique for some patients, whilst others may benefit from avoidance of external cues such as over-stimulating radio or television programmes. In patients with a tendency to expose themselves or masturbate in public, the use of modified clothing that makes it difficult to undress may change this type of behaviour. For sexual misinterpretations or other inappropriate behaviours, giving simple and repeated explanations of why such behaviour is unacceptable may be helpful. In institutional care, the provision of private rooms or home visits may help to reduce the frequency of inappropriate sexual behaviours by satisfying the patient's normal sex drive. Although all these interventions are often time-consuming, they lack the often significant side-effects associated with pharmacotherapy.

Currently no medication is licensed in the UK for the treatment of inappropriate sexual behaviour in patients with dementia and no systematic studies in this area have been reported. Most of the literature stems from case reports or case series. The classes of medications that have been found to be useful in the treatment of these behaviours include serotonin reuptake inhibitors, antipsychotics, mood stabilizers, and hormonal agents, such as anti-androgens, oestrogens, and luteinizing hormone releasing hormone (LHRH) agonists (Series and Dégano, 2005).

## References

Aizenberg, D., Weizman, A., and Barak, Y. (2002). Attitudes toward sexuality among nursing home residents. *Sexuality and Disability*, **20**(3), 185–9.

Aja, A. and Self, D. (1986). Alternate methods of changing nursing home staff attitudes towards sexual behavior of the aged. *Journal of Sex Education and Therapy*, **12**, 37–41.

American Psychiatric Association (1994). *Diagnostic and statistical manual of mental disorders*, 4th edn. American Psychiatric Association, Washington, DC.

Archibald, C. (1998). Sexuality, dementia and residential care: managers report and response. *Health and Social Care in the Community*, **6**, 95–101.

Atiemo, H.O., Szostak, M.J., and Sklar, G.N. (2003). Salvage of sildenafil failures referred from primary care physicians. *Journal of Urology*, **170**, 2356–8.

Bailey, S. and Bunter, H. (2000). Sexual activity policies. *Mental Health Nursing*, **20**, 12–15.

Ballard, C.G., Solis, M., Gahir, M. *et al.* (1997). Sexual relationships in married dementia sufferers. *International Journal of Geriatric Psychiatry*, **12**, 447–51.

Balon, R. and Taylor Segraves, R. (2005). *Handbook of sexual dysfunction*. Taylor and Francis, Boca Raton.

Bancroft, J. (1989). *Human sexuality and its problems*, 2nd edn, pp.282–98, 614–17. Churchill Livingstone, Edinburgh.

Basson, R. (2000). The female sexual response: a different model. *Journal of Sex & Marital Therapy*, **26**, 51–65.

Bauer, M. (1999). Global aging: their only privacy is between their sheets: privacy and the sexuality of elderly nursing home residents. *Journal of Gerontological Nursing*, **28**, 37–41.

Bergstrom-Walan, M-B. and Nielsen, H.H. (1990). Sexual expression among 60–80-year-old men and women: a sample from Stockholm, Sweden. *Journal of Sex Research*, **27**(2), 289–95.

Black, B., Muralee, S., and Tampi, R.R. (2005). Inappropriate sexual behaviours in dementia. *Journal of Geriatric Psychiatry and Neurology*, **18**, 155–62.

Blank, J. (2000). *Still doing it. Women & men over 60 write about their sexuality*. Down There Press, San Francisco, CA.

Bortz, W.M. and Wallace, D.H. (1999). Physical fitness, aging, and sexuality. *Western Journal of Medicine*, **170**, 167–9.

Bouman, W.P. (2005). Keeping sex alive in later years. In *Sexual health and the menopause* (ed. J.M. Tomlinson, M. Rees, and T. Mander), pp. 1–7. RSM Press, London.

Bouman, W.P. (2006). Sex and the sexagenarian-plus. *Geriatric Medicine*, **36**(12), 42–6.

Bouman, W.P. and Arcelus, J. (2001). Are psychiatrists guilty of ageism when it comes to taking a sexual history? *International Journal of Geriatric Psychiatry*, **16**, 27–31.

Bouman, W.P., Arcelus, J., and Benbow, S.M. (2006). Nottingham Study of Sexuality & Ageing (NoSSA I). Attitudes regarding sexuality and older people: a review of the literature. *Sexual and Relationship Therapy*, **21**, 149–61.

Bouman, W.P., Arcelus J., and Benbow S.M. (2007). Nottingham Study of Sexuality & Ageing (NoSSA II). Attitudes of care staff regarding sexuality and residents: a study in residential and nursing homes. *Sexual and Relationship Therapy*, **22**, 45–61.

Brecher, E.M. and the Editors of Consumer Reports Books. (1984). *Love, sex and aging: a Consumers Union report*. Little, Brown, Boston, MA.

Bretschneider, J.G. and McCoy, N.L. (1988). Sexual interest and behavior in healthy 80- to 102-year-olds. *Archives of Sexual Behavior*, **17**, 109–29.

Brincat, M., Muscat Baron, Y., and Galea, R. (2002). The menopause. In *Gynecology*, 2nd edn (ed. R.W. Shaw, W.P. Soutter, and S.L. Stanton), pp.373–392. Churchill Livingstone, London.

Brotman, S., Ryan, B., and Cormier, R. (2003). The health and social service needs of gay and lesbian elders and their families in Canada. *The Gerontologist*, **43**, 192–202.

Bullard-Poe, L., Powell, C., and Mulligan, T. (1994). The importance of intimacy to men living in a nursing home. *Archives of Sexual Behavior*, **23**, 231–6.

Burns, A., Jacoby, R., and Levy, R. (1990). Psychiatric phenomena in Alzheimer's disease. IV: disorders of behaviour. *British Journal of Psychiatry*, **157**, 86–94.

Burnside, I.M. (1976). *Nursing and the aged*. McGraw Hill, New York.

Cheadle, M.J. (1991). The screening sexual history. *Clinics in Geriatric Medicine*, **7**(1), 9–13.

Collopy, B. (1988). Autonomy in long term care: some crucial distinctions. *Gerontologist*, **28**, 10–18.

Commons, M., Bohn, J., Godon, L., Hauser, M., and Guthel, T. (1992). Professionals' attitudes towards sex between institutionalised patients. *American Journal of Psychotherapy*, **46**, 571–8.

Cort, E.M., Attenborough, J., and Watson, J.P. (2001). An initial exploration of community mental health nurses' attitudes to and experience of sexuality-related issues in their work with people experiencing mental health problems. *Journal of Psychiatric and Mental Health Nursing*, **8**, 489–500.

Cummings, J.L. and Victoroff, J.I. (1990). Noncognitive neuropsychiatric syndromes in Alzheimer's disease. *Neuropsychiatry, Neuropsychology, & Behavioral Neurology*, **3**, 140–58.

Damrosch, S.P. (1982). Nursing students' attitudes toward sexually active older persons. *Nursing Research*, **31**, 252–5.

Damrosch, S.P. and Fischman, S.H. (1985). Medical students' attitudes toward sexually active older patients. *Journal of the American Geriatrics Society*, **33**, 852–5.

Damrosch, S.P. and Cogliano, J. (1994). Attitudes of nursing home licensed practical nurses toward sexually active, older residents. *Journal of Women and Aging*, **6**, 123–33.

Davey Smith, G., Frankel, S., and Yarnell, J. (1997). Sex and death: are they related? Findings from the Caerphilly Cohort Study. *British Medical Journal*, **315**, 1641–4.

Davies, H.D., Zeiss, A., and Tinklenberg, J.R. (1992). 'Till death do us part': intimacy and sexuality in the marriages of Alzheimer's patients. [see comments] *Journal of Psychosocial Nursing and Mental Health Services*, **30**, 5–10.

Deacon, S., Minichiello, V., and Plummer, D. (1995). Sexuality and older people: revisiting the assumptions. *Educational Gerontology*, **21**, 497–513.

Dello Buono, M., Zachi, P.C., Padoani, W. *et al.* (1998a). Sexual feelings and sexual life in an Italian sample of 335 elderly 65 to 106-year-olds. *Archives of Gerontology and Geriatrics*, Suppl. **6**, 155–62.

Dello Buono, M., Urciuoli, O., and De Leo, D. (1998b). Quality of life and longevity: a study of centenarians. *Age and Ageing*, **27**, 207–16.

Department of Health (2001a). *National service framework for older people*. HSMO, London.

Department of Health (2001b). *National sexual health strategy*. HSMO, London.

Derouesne, C., Guigot, J., Chermat, V., Winchester, N., and Lacomblez, L. (1996). Sexual behavioural changes in Alzheimer's disease. *Alzheimer Disease and Associated Disorders*, **10**, 86–92.

Diokno, A.C., Brown, M.B., and Herzog, A.R. (1990). Sexual function in the elderly. *Archives of Internal Medicine*, **150**, 197–200.

Dorfman, R., Walters, K., Burke, P. *et al.* (1995). Old, sad and alone: the myth of the aging homosexual. *Journal of Gerontological Social Work*, **24**, 29–44.

Duffy, L.M. (1995). Sexual behavior and marital intimacy in Alzheimer's couples: a family theory perspective. *Sexuality and Disability*, **13**, 239–54.

Eddy, D.M. (1986). Before and after attitudes toward aging in a BSN program. *Journal of Gerontological Nursing*, **12**, 117–22.

Ehrenfeld, M., Tabak, N., Bronner, G., and Bergman, R. (1997). Ethical dilemmas concerning sexuality of elderly patients suffering from dementia. *International Journal of Nursing Practice*, **3**, 255–9.

Ende, J., Kazis, L., Ash, A., and Moskowitz, M.A. (1989). Measuring patients' desire for autonomy: decision-making and information-seeking preferences among medical patients. *Journal of General Internal Medicine*, **4**, 23–30.

Fairchild, S.K., Carrino, G.E., and Ramirez, M. (1996). Social workers' perceptions of staff attitudes toward resident sexuality in a random sample of New York State nursing homes: a pilot study. *Journal of Gerontological Social Work*, **26**, 153–70.

Feldman, H.A., Goldstein, I., Hatzichristou, D.G., Krane, R.J., and McKinlay, J.B. (1994). Impotence and its medical and psychosocial correlates: results of the Massachusetts male aging study. *Journal of Urology*, **151**, 54–61.

FitzGerald, M., Crowley, T., Greenhouse, P., Probert, C., and Horner, P. (2003). Teaching sexual history taking to medical students and examining it: experience in one medical school and a national survey. *Medical Education*, **37**, 94–8.

Folstein, M.F., Folstein, S.E., and McHugh, P.R. (1975). Mini-mental state: a practical method of grading the cognitive state of patients for the clinician. *Journal of Psychiatric Research*, **12**, 189–98.

Garbell, N. (1986). Increased libido in women receiving trazodone. *American Journal of Psychiatry*, **143**, 781–2.

George, L.K. and Weiler, S.J. (1981). Sexuality in middle and later life; the effects of age, cohort and gender. *Archives of General Psychiatry*, **38**, 919–23.

Gibson, M.C., Bol, N., Woodbury, M.G., Beaton, C., and Janke, C. (1999). Comparison of caregivers', residents', and community-dwelling spouses' opinions about expressing sexuality in an institutional setting. *Journal of Gerontological Nursing*, **25**(4), 30–9.

Glass, J.C., Mustian, R.D., and Carter, L.R. (1986). Knowledge and attitudes of health-care providers toward sexuality in the institutionalised elderly. *Educational Gerontology*, **12**(5), 465–75.

Golde, P. and Kogan, N. (1959). A sentence completion procedure for assessing attitudes toward old people. *Journal of Gerontology*, **14**, 355–60.

Gott, M. and Hinchliff, S. (2003). How important is sex in later life? The views of older people. *Social Science & Medicine*, **56**,1617–28.

Gott, M., Galena, E., Hinchliff, S., and Elford, H. (2004). 'Opening a can of worms': GP and practice nurse barriers to talking about sexual health in primary care. *Family Practice*, **21**, 528–36.

Gott, M. (2005). *Sexuality, sexual health and ageing*. Open University Press, Maidenhead.

Greengross, W. and Greengross, S. (1989). *Living loving & ageing. Sexual and personal relationships in later life*. Age Concern England, Mitcham.

Gross, Z.H. (2000). *Seasons of the heart. Men and women talk about love, sex, and romance after 60*. New World Library, Novato, CA.

Grossman, A.H., D'Augelli, A.R., and Hershberger, S.L. (2000). Social support networks of lesbian, gay, and bisexual adults 60 years of age and older. *Journal of Gerontology*, **55**, 171–9.

Guthrie, C. (1999). Nurses' perceptions of sexuality relating to patient care. *Journal of Clinical Nursing*, **8**, 313–21.

Haddad, P.M. and Benbow, S.M. (1993). Sexual problems associated with dementia: Part 1. Problems and their consequences. *International Journal of Geriatric Psychiatry*, **8**, 547–51.

Hajjar, R.R. and Kamel, H.K. (2003a). Sexuality in the nursing home, part 1: attitudes and barriers to sexual expression. *Journal of the American Medical Directors Association*, **4**,152–6.

Hajjar, R.R. and Kamel, H.K. (2003b). Sex and the nursing home. *Clinics in Geriatric Medicine*, **19**, 575–86.

Harris, L. and Wier, M. (1998). Inappropriate sexual behavior in dementia: a review of the treatment literature. *Sexuality and Disability*, **16**, 205–17.

Hayter, M. (1996). Is non-judgemental care possible in the context of nurses' attitudes to patients' sexuality? *Journal of Advanced Nursing*, **24**, 662–6.

Helgason, A.R., Adolfsson, J., Dickman, P. *et al.* (1996). Sexual desire, erection, orgasm and ejaculatory functions and their importance to elderly Swedish men: a population-based study. *Age and Ageing*, **25**, 285–91.

Hillman, J.L. and Stricker, G. (1994). A linkage of knowledge and attitudes toward elderly sexuality: not necessarily a uniform relationship. *Gerontologist*, **34**, 256–260.

Hillman, J.L. and Stricker, G. (1996). College students' attitudes toward elderly sexuality: a two factor solution. *Canadian Journal on Aging*, **15**, 543–558.

Hite, S. (1976). *The Hite report: a nationwide study of female sexuality*. Macmillan Publishing Company, New York.

Hite, S. (1981). *The Hite report: a nationwide study of male sexuality*. Alfred A. Knopf, New York.

Holmes, D., Reingold, J., and Teresi, J. (1997). Sexual expression and dementia. Views of caregivers: a pilot study. *International Journal of Geriatric Psychiatry*, **12**, 695–701.

Johnson, A.A., Mercer, C.H., Erens, B. *et al.* (2001). Sexual behaviour in Britain: partnerships, practices, and HIV behaviours. *The Lancet*, **358**, 1835–42.

Johnson, B. (1996). Older adults and sexuality: a multidimensional perspective. *Journal of Gerontological Nursing*, **22**, 6–15.

Johnson, M.J., Jackson, N.C., Kenneth Arnette, J., and Koffman, S.D. (2005). Gay and lesbian perceptions of discrimination in retirement care facilities. *Journal of Homosexuality*, **49**, 83–102.

Kaas, M.J. (1978). Sexual expression of the elderly in nursing homes. *Gerontologist*, **18**, 372–8.

Kinsey, A.C., Pomeroy, W.B., and Martin, C.E. (1948). *Sexual behaviour in the human male*. W.B. Saunders, Philadelphia.

Kinsey, A.C., Pomeroy, W.B., Martin, C.E., and Gebhard, P.H. (1953). *Sexual behaviour in the human female*. W.B. Saunders, Philadelphia.

Kitwood, T. and Bredin, K. (1992). A new approach to the evaluation of dementia care. *Journal of Advances in Health and Nursing Care*, **1**, 41–60.

Knodel, J., Watkins, S., and VanLandingham, M. (2002). *AIDS and older persons: an international perspective*. PSC Research Report No. 02–495. Population Studies Center, University of Michigan, Ann Arbor, MI.

Koh, A. (1999). Non-judgemental care as a professional obligation. *Nursing Standard*, **13**, 38–41.

LaTorre, R.A. and Kear, K. (1977). Attitudes toward sex in the aged. *Archives of Sexual Behavior*, **6**, 203–13.

Laumann, E.O., Paik, A.M.A., and Rosen, R.C. (1999). Sexual dysfunction in the United States: prevalence and predictors. *Journal of the American Medical Association*, **281**, 537–44.

Lawton, F.G. and Hacker, N.F. (1989). Sex and the elderly. [letter] *British Medical Journal*, **299**, 1279.

Leiblum, S.R. and Rosen, R.C. (2000). *Principles and practice of sex therapy*, 3rd edn. Guildford Press, New York.

Leiblum, S.R. and Taylor Seagraves, R. (2000). Sex therapy with aging adults. In *Principles and practice of sex therapy*, 3rd edn (ed. S.R. Leiblum and R.C. Rosen), pp. 423–48. Guildford Press, New York.

Lichtenberg, P.A. and Strzepek, D.M. (1990). Assessment of institutionalized dementia patients' competencies to participate in intimate relationships. *Gerontologist*, **30**, 117–20.

Litz, B.T., Zeiss, A.M., and Davies, H.D. (1990). Sexual concerns of male spouses of female Alzheimer's disease patients. *Gerontologist*, **30**, 113–16.

Livini, M.D. (1994). Nurses' attitudes toward sexuality and dementia. *American Journal of Geriatric Psychiatry*, **2**, 338–45.

Luketich, G.F. (1991). Sex and the elderly: what do nurses know? *Educational Gerontology*, **17**, 573–80.

McCartney, J.R., Izeman, H., Rogers, D., and Cohen, N. (1987). Sexuality and the institutionalised elderly. *Journal of the American Geriatrics Society*, **35**, 331–3.

Macdonald, S., Halliday, J., MacEwan, T. *et al.* (2003). Nithsdale Schizophrenia Surveys 24: sexual dysfunction. case-control study. *British Journal of Psychiatry*, **182**, 50–6.

McKinlay, J.B. and Feldman, H.A. (1994). Age-related variations in sexual activity and interest in normal men: results from the Massachusetts Male Aging Study. In *Sexuality across the life course* (ed. A.S. Rossi), pp.261–85. University of Chicago Press, Chicago.

McMahon, C.N., Smith, C.J., and Shabsigh, R. (2006). Treating erectile dysfunction when PDE5 inhibitors fail. *British Medical Journal*, **332**, 589–92.

Mahar, F. and Sherrard, J. (2005). Sexually transmitted infections. In *Sexual health and the menopause* (ed. J.M. Tomlinson, M. Rees, and T. Mander), pp. 55–62. RSM Press, London.

Marsiglio, W. and Donnelly, D. (1991). Sexual relations in later life: a national study of married persons. *Journal of Gerontology*, **46**, S338–S344.

Masters, W.H. and Johnson, V.E. (1966). *Human sexual response*. Little, Brown, Boston.

Masters, W.H. and Johnson, V.E. (1970). *Human sexual inadequacy*. Little Brown, Boston.

Mathers, N., Bramley, M., Draper, K., Snead, S., and Tobert, A. (1994). Assessment of training in psychosexual medicine. *British Medical Journal*, **308**, 969–72.

Matocha, L.K. and Waterhouse, J. (1993). Current nursing practice related to sexuality. *Research in Nursing and Health*, **16**, 371–8.

Matthias, R.E., Lubben, J.E., Atchison, K.A., and Schweitzer, S.O. (1997). Sexual activity and satisfaction among very old adults: results from a community-dwelling Medicare population survey. *The Gerontologist*, **37**, 6–14.

Mayers, K.S. and McBride, D. (1998). Sexuality training for caretakers of geriatric residents in long term care facilities. *Sexuality and Disability*, **16**, 227–36.

Meyer, I.H. and Colten, M.E. (1999). Sampling gay men: random digit dialling versus sources in the gay community. *Journal of Homosexuality*, **37**, 99–110.

Minichiello, V., Plummer, D., and Seal, A. (1996). The 'asexual' older person? Australian evidence. *Venereology*, **9**, 180–8.

Mooradian, A.D. and Greiff, V. (1990). Sexuality in older women. *Archives of Internal Medicine*, **150**, 1033–8.

Morley, J.E. and Kaiser, F.E. (1989). Sexual function with advancing age. *Medical Clinics of North America*, **73**, 1483–95.

Mulligan, T. and Palguta, R.F. (1991). Sexual interest, activity, and satisfaction among male nursing home residents. *Archives of Sexual Behavior*, **20**, 199–204.

Nay R. (1992). Sexuality and aged women in nursing homes. *Geriatric Nursing*, **13**, 312–14.

Newman, G. and Nichols, C.R. (1960). Sexual activities and attitudes in older persons. *Journal of the American Medical Association*, **173**, 33–5.

Pachankis, J.E. and Goldfried, M.R. (2004). Clinical issues in working with lesbian, gay, and bisexual clients. *Psychotherapy: Theory, Research, Practice, Training*, **41**, 227–46.

Panser, L.A., Rhodes, T., Girman, C.J. *et al.* (1995). Sexual function of men ages 40 to 79 years: the Olmsted County Study of urinary symptoms and health status among men. *Journal of the American Geriatrics Society*, **43**, 1107–11.

Parke, F. (1991). Sexuality in later life. *Nursing Times*, **87**, 40–2.

Paunonen, M. and Haggman-Laitila, A. (1990). Sexuality and the satisfaction of sexual needs. a study on the attitudes of aged home-nursing clients. *Scandinavian Journal of Caring Sciences*, **4**, 163–8.

Peate, I. (1999). The need to address sexuality in older people. *British Journal of Community Nursing*, **4**, 174–80.

Persson, G. (1980). Sexuality in a 70-year-old urban population. *Journal of Psychosomatic Research*, **24**, 335–42.

Pfeiffer, E. and Davis, G.C. (1972). Determinants of sexual behavior in middle and old age. *Journal of the American Geriatrics Society*, **20**, 151–8.

Pfeiffer, E., Verwoerdt, A., and Davis, G.C. (1972). Sexual behavior in middle life. *American Journal of Psychiatry*, **128**, 82–7.

Pope, M. and Schultz, R. (1990). Sexual attitudes and behavior in midlife and aging homosexual males. *Journal of Homosexuality*, **20**, 169–77.

Portnova, M., Young, E., and Newman, M. (1984). Elderly women's attitudes toward sexual activity among their peers. *Health Care International*, **5**, 289–98.

Poulin, N. and Mishara, B.L. (1994). A comparison of adult attitudes toward their parents' sexuality and their parents' attitudes. *Canadian Journal on Aging*, **13**, 96–103.

Quam, J.K. and Whitford, G.S. (1992). Adaptation and age-related expectations of older gay and lesbian adults. *Gerontologist*, **32**, 367–74.

Quinn-Krach, P. and Van Hoozer, H. (1988). Sexuality of the aged and the attitudes and knowledge of nursing students. *Journal of Nursing Education*, **27**, 359–63.

RCN (1996). *Sexual health: key issues within mental health services*. Royal College of Nursing, London.

Rees, J., Wilcox, J.R., and Cuddihy, R.A. (2002). Psychology in rehabilitation of older adults. *Reviews in Clinical Gerontology*, **12**, 343–56.

Risen, C.B. (1995). A guide to taking a sexual history. *Psychiatric Clinics of North America*, **18**, 39–53.

Rosen, R.C., Riley, A., Wagner, G., Osterloh, I.H., Kirkpatrick, J., and Mishra, A. (1997). The international index of erectile function (IIEF): a multidimensional scale for assessment of erectile dysfunction. *Urology*, **49**, 822–30.

Rust, J. and Golombok, S. (1986). *The Golombok–Rust inventory of sexual satisfaction*. NFER-Nelson Publishing Company, Windsor.

Sansone, R.A. and Wiederman, M.W. (2000). Sexuality training for psychiatry residents: a national survey of training directors. *Journal of Sex & Marital Therapy*, **26**, 249–56.

Schiavi, R.C. (1999). *Aging and male sexuality*. Cambridge University Press, Cambridge.

Schiavi, R.C., Mandeli, J., and Schreiner-Engel, P. (1994). Sexual satisfaction in healthy aging men. *Journal of Sex and Marital Therapy*, **20**, 3–13.

Series, H. and Dégano, P. (2005). Hypersexuality in dementia. *Advances in Psychiatric Treatment*, **11**, 424–31.

Singh, S.P. and Beck, A. (1997). No sex please, we're British. *Psychiatric Bulletin*, **21**, 99–101.

Skoog, J. (1996). Sex and Swedish 85-year olds. *New England Journal of Medicine*, **334**, 1140–1.

Smook, K. (1992). Nurses' attitudes towards the sexuality of older people: an investigative study. *Nursing Practice*, **6**, 15–17.

Solursh, D.S., Ernst, J.L., Lewis, R.W. *et al.* (2003). The human sexuality education of physicians in North American medical schools. *International Journal of Impotence Research*, **15**(Suppl. 5), 41–5.

Stall, R. and Catania, J. (1994). AIDS risk behaviours among late middle-aged and elderly Americans. National AIDS behavioural surveys. *Archives of Internal Medicine*, **154**, 57–63.

Starr, B.D. and Weiner, M.B. (1981). *The Starr–Weiner report on sex & sexuality in the mature years*. Stein and Day, New York.

Story, M.D. (1989). Knowledge and attitudes about the sexuality of older adults among retirement home residents. *Educational Gerontology*, **15**, 515–26.

Sullivan, G. (1988). Increased libido in three men treated with trazodone. *Journal of Clinical Psychiatry*, **49**, 202–3.

Sullivan-Miller, B. (1987). Dealing with attitudes and preconceived notions. *Provider*, **13**, 24–6.

Szasz, G. (1983). Sexual incidents in an extended care unit for aged men. *Journal of the American Geriatrics Society*, **31**, 407–11.

Szwabo, P.A. (2003). Counseling about sexuality in the older person. *Clinics in Geriatric Medicine*, **19**, 595–604.

Taylor, D., Paton, C., and Kerwin, R. (2005). *The South London and Maudsley NHS Trust & Oxleas NHS Trust 2005–2006 prescribing guidelines*, 8th edn, pp. 99–103, 169–70. Taylor & Francis, London.

Taylor, J.F., Rosen, R.C., and Leiblum, S.R. (1994). Self-report of female sexual function: psychometric evaluation of the Brief Index of Sexual Functioning for Women. *Archives of Sexual Behavior*, **23**, 627–43.

Teaster, P.B. and Roberto, K.A. (2004). Sexual abuse of older adults: APS cases and outcomes. *Gerontologist*, **44**, 788–96.

Temple-Smith, M.J., Mulvey, G., and Keogh, L. (1999). Attitudes to taking a sexual history in general practice in Victoria, Australia. *Sexual Transmitted Infections*, **75**, 41–4.

Thomas, D.R. (2003). Medication and sexual function. *Clinics in Geriatric Medicine*, **19**, 553–62.

Thorpe, A.C., Cleary, R., Coles, J., Reynolds, J., Vernon, S., and Neal, D.E. (1994). Written consent about sexual function in men undergoing transurethral prostatectomy. *British Journal of Urology*, **74**, 479–84.

Tomlinson, J. (1998). ABC of sexual health: taking a sexual history. *British Medical Journal*, **317**, 1573–6.

Uitti, R.J., Tanner, C.M., Rajput, A.H., Goetz, C.G., Klawans, H.L., and Thiessen, B. (1989). Hypersexuality with antiparkinsonian therapy. *Clinical Neuropharmacology*, **12**, 375–83.

UKCC (1992). *The code of professional conduct for the nurse, midwife and health visitor*. UKCC, London.

Van de Ven, P., Rodden, P., Crawford, J., and Kippax, S. (1997). A comparative demographic and sexual profile of older homosexually active men. *Journal of Sex Research*, **34**, 349–60.

Van Ooijen, E. and Charnock, A. (1994). *Sexuality and patient care: a guide for nurses and teachers*. Chapman Hall, London.

Verwoerdt, A., Pfeiffer, E., and Wang, H-S. (1969a). Sexual behavior in senescence. changes in sexual activity and interest of aging men and women. *Journal of Geriatric Psychiatry*, **2**, 163–80.

Verwoerdt, A., Pfeiffer, E., and Wang, H-S. (1969b). Sexual behavior in senescence. II. Patterns of sexual activity and interest. *Geriatrics*, **24**, 137–54.

Wahler, J. and Gabbay, S. (1997). Gay male aging: a review of the literature. *Journal of Gay and Lesbian Social Services*, **6**, 1–20.

Walker, B.L. and Harrington, D. (2002). Effects of staff training on staff knowledge and attitudes about sexuality. *Educational Gerontology*, **28**, 639–54.

Walker, B.L., Osgood, N.J., Richardson, J.P., and Ephross, P.H. (1998). Staff and elderly knowledge and attitudes toward elderly sexuality. *Educational Gerontology*, **24**, 471–90.

Warner, J. (2000). Sexuality and dementia. In *Dementia*, 2nd edn (ed. J. O'Brien, D. Ames, and A. Burns), pp. 267–71. Arnold, London.

Wasow, M. and Loeb, M. (1979). Sexuality in nursing homes. *Journal of the American Geriatrics Society*, **27**, 73–9.

Waterhouse, J. (1996). Nurse practice related to sexuality: a review and recommendations. *Nursing Times Research*, **1**, 412–19.

Waterhouse, J. and Metcalfe, M. (1991). Attitudes toward nurses discussing sexual concerns with patients. *Journal of Advanced Nursing*, **16**, 1048–54.

Webb, C. (1985). *Sexuality, nursing and health*. John Wiley and Sons, Chichester.

Webb, C. (1988). A study of nurses' knowledge & attitudes about sexuality in health care. *International Journal of Nursing Studies*, **25**, 235–44.

Wells, A. (1997). *Cognitive therapy of anxiety disorders*. John Wiley and Sons, Chichester.

White, C.B. (1982). Sexual interest, attitudes, knowledge, and sexual history in relation to sexual behavior in the institutionalised aged. *Archives of Sexual Behavior*, **11**, 11–21.

White, C.B. and Catania, J.A. (1982). Psychoeducational intervention for sexuality with the aged, family members of the aged, and people who work with the aged. *Journal of Aging and Human Development*, **15**, 121–38.

Wojciechowski, C. (1998). Issues in caring for older lesbians. *Journal of Gerontological Nursing*, **24**, 28–33.

World Health Organization (1992). *International classification of diseases and related health problems*, ICD-10. World Health Organization, Geneva.

Wright, L.K. (1998). Affection and sexuality in the presence of Alzheimer's disease: a longitudinal study. *Sexuality and Disability*, **16**, 167–79.

Wylie, K.R., Steward, D., Seivewright, N., Smith, D., and Walters, S. (2002). Prevalence of sexual dysfunction in three psychiatric outpatient settings: a drug misuse service, an alcohol misuse service and a general adult psychiatry clinic. *Sexual and Relationship Therapy*, **17**, 149–60.

Wylie, K., Hallam-Jones, R., and Daines, B. (2003). Review of an undergraduate medical school training programme in human sexuality. *Medical Teacher*, **25**, 291–5.

Zeiss, A.M., Davies, H.D., Wood, M., and Tinklenberg, J.R. (1990). The incidence and correlates of erectile problems in patients with Alzheimer's disease. *Archives of Sexual Behaviour*, **19**, 325–31.

Zeiss, A.M. (1997). Sexuality and aging: normal changes and clinical problems. *Topics in Geriatric Rehabilitation*, **12**, 11–27.

Zeiss, A.M., Davies, H.D., and Tinklenberg, J.R. (1996). An observational study of sexual behavior in demented male patients. *Journals of Gerontology Series A: Biological Sciences and Medical Sciences*, **51**, M325–M329.

# 38

# Ethics and old age psychiatry

Julian C. Hughes and Clive Baldwin

## Introduction

It would not be entirely fashionable to say that ethics is about what we become as human beings. The pressing ethical issues in the practice of old age psychiatry normally come in the form of questions such as: Will the outcome from this treatment be good? What is the right thing to do for this patient? Such questions conform to the more fashionable approaches of moral philosophy that stress consequences and duties. In other words, it is more fashionable in ethics to ask questions about what we do rather than about what we become.

Thus consequentialists, in judging whether an action is good or bad, tend to look at outcomes. For instance, utilitarians (the most common type of consequentialist) regard actions that maximize happiness as good; and, in the classic formulations of Jeremy Bentham (1748–1832) and John Stuart Mill (1806–1873), happiness is conceived as pleasure or the absence of pain. Meanwhile, deontologists, such as Immanuel Kant (1724–1804), emphasize duties and the correlative rights that go with them. In other words, if someone has a right to good-quality care, someone else has a duty to provide it. According to Kant, our duties and rights can be determined by reason in a way that provides us with 'categorical imperatives' to act in one way rather than another. So, much of modern moral philosophy has been concerned with the consequences of actions and the rules that govern them.

Hence, there are good reasons to regard consequentialism and deontology as very reasonable theories to explain and guide actions and decisions in healthcare. Sometimes it will be absolutely correct to think of consequences and duties in determining what we do for our patients. If the consequence of giving this tablet (say an antipsychotic) is that we hugely increase the chances that a man will have a stroke, it might not be the right thing to do. If we are aware that this woman with dementia is being financially and physically abused, we have a duty to act to protect her.

Clinicians are used to thinking in these ways, which are useful in that they bring together the clinical and the ethical. Both these aspects come into the decision about the antipsychotic and involve similar factors, such as the likely outcome (including the good and bad consequences) as well as the views of the man himself. Similarly, the protection of vulnerable adults is both a clinical and an ethical duty based on the rational ground that we would want to be protected ourselves if we were vulnerable. But it also involves a propensity to protect people who are less fortunate or frailer than ourselves; in other words it reflects some sort of basic human instinct. Thinking of consequences and duties, therefore, will often be very helpful and, clinically, to the point. We might wish to note that already in this initial foray into the world of clinical practice, we have brought into the discussion something about taking into account the views of the person concerned and something about basic human instincts. We shall park these ideas for a moment.

Instead, it is inevitable that we should mention the principles of autonomy, beneficence, non-maleficence, and justice (Beauchamp and Childress, 2001). Inevitable because they have become ubiquitous in discussions of medical ethics; inevitable because they are useful; and inevitable because they follow from a mixture of consequentialist and deontological considerations (Gillon, 1986). The use of the four principles has sometimes been referred to as 'principlism' and, again, this approach often squares well with clinical practice: of course we wish to avoid harming (in accordance with the principle of non-maleficence) the man who needs the antipsychotic and of course we wish to do good (in accordance with beneficence) to the vulnerable woman who is being abused.

Because the four principles are so commonly known and discussed in the literature, we shall not discuss them further, except for the special case of autonomy. But it is worth noting that it is easy enough to expand the four principles to include others such as confidentiality and truthfulness. For instance, Vallis and Boyd (2002) identified three further relevant principles in connection with end-of-life decisions: protective responsibility, responsibility for narrative integrity, and candour.

So far we have mentioned two major ethical theories and principlism, with the possibility that the latter can be added to. The fact is that theories of and approaches to clinical ethics multiply (see for instance Table 36.1 in Hughes (2002) and our discussions of the different theories and approaches in Hughes and Baldwin (2006)). This leads to a profound question for moral philosophers, which is of some significance to practitioners. It also causes a strategic concern within this chapter.

The profound question is to do with how we decide between the various moral theories. Do we have to become consequentialists and always answer our moral dilemmas by appeal to something akin to the greatest happiness for the greatest number? Or should we all be deontologists and simply insist that there is a duty to tell the truth, for instance about the diagnosis, whatever the consequences? Alternatively, if we are all to become advocates of the four principles, by what means shall we decide between autonomy and beneficence when they clash (when, for example, the person with delusions does not wish to take antipsychotic medication)? If, however, we are told that we do not need to commit to a particular theory, but that it is acceptable to pick and choose between theories depending on the exact nature of the dilemma, then it is more than justified to ask on what basis such a choice should be made.

The trouble is that this profound question is also practical. We really might be faced by the person with late onset schizophrenic symptoms who insists that no medication is required but who seems to be placing him- or herself at risk on account of the mental illness. Whether we force the issue by using compulsory powers will be decided by whether we feel at the time that autonomy or beneficence wins out (although, as we shall see, the idea that there is a true conflict between these principles may be an aberration). This, in turn, might be decided on the basis of consequences, or on the basis of the person's right to receive care and our duty to provide it. These different possibilities seem to suggest that there is no objective certainty underpinning our ethical decisions.

Our inclination is, indeed, to be eclectic and to pick and choose between different moral approaches (Hughes and Baldwin, 2006). We would also have an inclination to suggest that this sort of eclecticism can still be underpinned by something more objective than might at first appear possible. Fortunately, since it would be very difficult, this is not the place for us to defend such a view. However, the problem of the multifarious moral theories and approaches does raise a strategic concern. For how are we to deal with the plethora of theories as well as the plethora of clinical issues within a single chapter? Our strategy will be to direct the reader to broader texts in the field of medical ethics in order to find further discussion of the various approaches and theories (Beauchamp and Childress, 2001; Hope *et al.*, 2003; Campbell *et al.*, 2005; Ashcroft *et al.*, 2007), whilst we focus on virtue and narrative ethics.

This focus is not entirely random. Our hope is that whilst considering some of the ethical issues that arise in old age psychiatry we shall give a sense of how virtue theory and the narrative approach can provide both a useful practical framework and an objective basis for moral discourse. Of course, we shall merely be gesturing at the objective basis that virtue ethics implies. The focus will not be narrow because virtue theory underpins a variety of approaches. Nor could it be narrow, given the great breadth of practice in old age psychiatry, where it must be routine to keep in view the biological, psychological, social, and spiritual aspects of care.

The broad sweep of relevant considerations in this field recalls our parked items: the views of the person concerned and something about basic human instincts. We noted how these notions appeared as soon as we started talking, even in a sketchy way, about real cases. This was not coincidental, but essential, because ethical issues will not usually be solved without some consideration being given to the views of the person concerned. This is an element of 'perspectivism', but reflects the importance of the narrative history of the person. Talk of 'basic human instincts' is close to talk of the virtues. Importantly, it is a way of noting that decisions in clinical practice reflect something deep about us as human beings. And this calls to mind the extent to which we might be changed by our decisions, because they reflect what we are becoming, which was the unfashionable idea with which we began. Hence, although we shall

be interested in the consequences of actions and the rules that govern them, the focus we have adopted means that the discussion will be more about the narratives of our lives and about what we become rather than purely about what we do.

In due course we shall set out the various ethical issues that arise in old age psychiatry generally, by reviewing some of the recent literature and by considering some of the ethical issues that arise for carers of people with dementia. We need an overview of virtue and narrative ethics, but we shall first say something about the notion of autonomy.

## Autonomy

Of the four principles autonomy is generally regarded as being central: it tends to (but does not invariably) trump the others (Wolpe, 1998). There are good reasons for giving it such pre-eminence. After all, much of the impetus behind the development of biomedical ethics has been a concern to recognize the rights of patients to be involved in the decisions made about them. Partly because of the success of medical ethics in embedding its central messages in good practice, most doctors would regard it as useful and routine to involve patients in the decisions that affect them. Respect for autonomy reflects things that we value deeply, such as liberty and agency: being free to act as individuals is basic to our sense of ourselves as persons.

Thus, given its importance, and particularly because it is of the utmost relevance when we think of people whose ability to make decisions for themselves is impaired, it might seem odd not to give it more emphasis in our discussion. Well, it will undoubtedly be a notion that recurs. Our discussion in terms of virtues and narrative is decidedly not irrelevant to the notion of respect for autonomy, as Beauchamp and Childress (2001) acknowledge in their chapter on moral character. They suggest there is a rough, imperfect correspondence between the principle of respect for autonomy and the virtue of 'respectfulness'. Autonomy is likely to continue to crop up in this chapter, both because it links to various virtue terms and because, at least in part, our emphasis on narrative helps to stress the degree to which people should be allowed to live their lives as they choose.

Concerning the virtues, autonomy links not only to 'respectfulness', but also to some of the other virtues Beauchamp and Childress highlight (e.g. concern, caring, and sympathy), as well as to charity and humility. According to Pellegrino and Thomasma (1993, pp. 131–2):

> …if we look at autonomy as a derivative of the integrity of the person and not as an isolated ethical principle, the presumed conflict between autonomy and beneficence should disappear. …Paternalism involves the physician's usurpation of the patient's moral claim as a human being to decide what is in his or her own best interests. This violates the integrity of the person and under no circumstances could be a beneficent act. Rather, to be beneficent, respect for the patient's values and choices is essential.

According to these authors, there is a connection, via the virtue of benevolence, rather than a conflict between the principles of autonomy and beneficence. And, of course, within the space of our moral lives, their notion of benevolence links to Beauchamp and Childress's notion of respectfulness. So there are connections to be made between respect for autonomy and the virtues, as well as between the concept of autonomy and a person's narrative history.

We wish, however, to be slightly more critical of autonomy before we proceed further. Our moral lives are complex. Part of the function of moral theorizing is to lay open this complicated landscape through which clinicians have to navigate. We should not overlook the complexity, which was well demonstrated by Collopy (1988). This work has been taken further by Agich (2003) who presents an effective case in favour of the argument that, especially in the context of long-term care for older people, autonomy and dependency go hand in hand. If dependency helps to maintain the person's functional integrity in ways that the person values, then dependency (on medication or other forms of professional care) is not simply consistent with respecting the person's autonomy, but it becomes the way in which such respect must be played out. For, as Agich (2003, p. 174) suggests: 'The concept of autonomy properly understood requires that individuals be seen in essential interrelationship with others and the world'. He also makes the point that (Agich 2003, p. 165):

> Autonomy fundamentally importantly involves the way individuals live their lives; it is found in the nooks and crannies of everyday experience; it is found in the way that individuals interact and not exclusively in the idealized paradigm of choice or decision-making that dominates ethical analysis.

We should regard ethical claims based on autonomy, therefore, with a critical eye. Whilst freedom for people to make their own decisions is crucial—and in connection with the frail and vulnerable is an important gauge of the depth of civility—properly understood autonomy frequently entails dependency. Hence our inclination to discuss the ethical issues that arise in old age psychiatry without recourse to the four principles, but with an emphasis on a mixture of virtue ethics and narrativity.

## Virtue ethics

According to virtue ethics, we ought to do what the *virtuous person* would do. The virtuous person is someone who has the virtues, where these are regarded as dispositions to live well or flourish as a human being. Virtues are inner dispositions that lead to human flourishing. In other words, these are the dispositions that help us to excel in the ways that humans should excel. Just as a 'good' egg will conform to certain criteria, so too the virtues pick out the attributes required for a person to be a good human being. The pressing questions to be answered concern how we know who the virtuous people are, and, therefore, how we know what the virtues are.

It is worth noting that those who first raised the flag of virtue ethics in the modern period did so because of the deep malaise they saw in modern moral philosophy. In the late 1950s, Elizabeth Anscombe pointed out that the language of morality had become disconnected from the intellectual and cultural context in which it made sense (Anscombe, 1981). Discussions in moral philosophy, therefore, often appear vacuous as a result. Continuing this theme, MacIntyre (1985) highlighted the extent to which modern moral philosophy was failing to provide 'a shared, public rational justification for morality' (p. 50). MacIntyre characterizes the virtues as those dispositions that sustain us in our quest for human goods. He sees these goods as being worked out in historically embedded, shared practices and traditions (or narratives). Without such practices and traditions the arguments in moral philosophy cannot be ended, because there is no grounding beyond the arguments themselves. Alternatively, we might say that the language of morals remains vacuous unless it is embedded in a moral life that makes some sense, as it were, beyond itself; for which it requires a shared communal understanding of what a humanly good life must be like.

Hursthouse (1999) provides some straightforward answers to the question about how we know what constitutes the virtuous life: if you do not know what the virtuous person would do in a particular circumstance, you should ask a virtuous person.

> This is far from being a trivial point, for it gives a straightforward explanation of an important aspect of our moral life, namely the fact that we do not always act as 'autonomous', utterly self-determining agents, but quite often seek moral guidance from people we think are morally better than ourselves.
>
> Hursthouse (1999, p. 35)

It is worth noting a significant parallel. It will often be the case in clinical practice that a junior will consult a senior over a tricky problem. The significance of the parallel is partly that we know whom to consult. We recognize expertise, and this is no less so in the sphere of ethically problematic cases than it is in clinically problematic ones. Just as we can know that Dr Smith is the person to speak to about psychopharmacology, we can also know that we should approach Dr Khan with our knotty ethical dilemma. The parallel runs deeper, because the problematic cases, concerning which the young consultant might wish to seek help, are not usually solely problems of fact. The dose of a drug can always be looked up. But the problematic cases are typically those where there are conflicts at the level of values. [Hence the increasing emphasis on values-based practice as the counterpart to evidence based practice (Fulford, 2004).] Perhaps a family is split over whether or not a patient should be treated at all. So then, in seeking help, the young consultant is likely to look to someone who not only knows about the treatment but who is also practically wise. The virtues are acquired over time with training and by experience. All of which suggests that, in reality, we do know who the virtuous people are and, indeed, we can discriminate between the virtues. So-and-so is scrupulously honest; so-and-so is wise.

Hursthouse (1999) is keen to stress that we do have this shared sort of practical knowledge of the virtues. We know, for instance, that the good person (and the good doctor) will tend to be honest, charitable, and true to her word. We would not expect the virtuous person to lie through her teeth. In addition, Hursthouse combats the complaint that virtue ethics tells us too much about what the person is or might become and not enough about the rules that guide action:

> Not only does each virtue generate a prescription – do what is honest, charitable, generous – but each vice a prohibition – do not do what is dishonest, uncharitable, mean.
>
> Hursthouse (1999, p. 36)

But she goes on to suggest that there are some good reasons why virtue ethics concentrates on the *agent* more than the *act*. For one thing, whereas there might be a tendency in other ethical theories to speak as if it were always possible to determine the right action, this tends to ignore those cases where it is reasonable to regard every action as undesirable. Whilst concentrating on the act can be a way of ignoring this aspect of the dilemma, virtue ethics grasps the nettle. The virtuous reactions to some actions ought to include regret, guilt, sadness, and the like, even if the action were the one that had to be taken. Not to manifest these reactions would be to demonstrate the vice of callousness and a lack of compassion. On this point it is worth quoting Hursthouse (1999, p.48) at length:

> Although I am, personally, sympathetic to doctors rather than otherwise, one does hear occasional hair-raising stories about the arrogance and callousness of some. What people often complain about is not whatever decision the doctors made, but the manner in which they delivered it or acted on it. No expressions of regret, no expression of concern over whether anything could be done to make it less likely that such decisions would have to be made in the future; having made (what they take to be) the morally right decision, they seem to think that they can review their own conduct with complete satisfaction. But if someone dies, or suffers, or undergoes frightful humiliation as a result of their decision, even supposing it is unquestionably correct, surely regret is called for. A dose of virtue ethics might make them concentrate more on how they should respond, rather than resting content with the thought that they have made the right decision.

Virtue ethics does emphasize, therefore, the agent—even if this allows us to characterize virtuous and vicious acts—and in so doing stresses the importance of what we become by what we do. Virtue ethics will inform much of the rest of the discussion in this chapter.

## Narrative ethics

Narrative has become increasingly influential as an analytical and methodological tool across a range of disciplines. Its effects can be traced not only through the arts and humanities, but through the social sciences, and even into the natural and pure sciences. It should come as little surprise, then, that narrative has also found a home in ethical discourse. Narrative, however, owes its ubiquity to its rather nebulous nature. The fact that narrative can mean so many things—not all of them consistent with one another—means that it can travel easily, but not always with consensus or clarity. Different disciplines can use it, different philosophical and methodological frameworks can draw on it, and different professional groups can put it into practice in a variety of ways.

So it is with narrative in ethical discourse. For some, narrative is a means by which to gather (and inform) deep or thick data about a particular case and thus to inform decision-making from within a particular ethical framework. For instance, accessing the details of the story might provide the informational base on which to make a decision located within a principlist framework (Davis, 1991). For others, narrative may be a means of accessing the subjective worlds of stakeholders and thus enabling decision-making participants to understand each other's points of view. Enhanced communication enhances ethical decision-making. Everyone has a perspective on the situation which needs to be taken into account when making the right decision. This is more than just eliciting data, but takes account of multiple voices. These voices may then be worked into univocal practice decisions or polyphonic stories as pedagogic aids. These two approaches have in common a view of narrative as a source of raw data for either making ethical decisions or for ethical analysis; thus narrative becomes a means to an end.

There are, however, other approaches that take narrative far more seriously, viewing narrative both as a way of knowing (an epistemology) and as a way of being (an ontology). Of course, not everyone accepts the centrality of narrative to human life (Lamarque, 2004; Strawson, 2004), but that is for another day. As epistemology, narrative helps us understand the world we live in (Spence, 1982;

Polkinghorne, 1988; Bruner, 1994). As ontology, it locates us as narrative beings in a narrative world (Schwandt, 1997; Bruner, 2004). One may choose to hold to narrative epistemology but not ontology, or vice versa, or to hold to both. This last approach, the one that we take here, is what we call 'deep narrative'.

This deep narrative approach insists that we know ourselves and our world in and through narrative. In this approach there is no pre-narrativized experience, for it is through narrative that we formulate our experience (Bruner, 2004). For us, as for Barthes:

> [N]arrative is present in every age, in every place, in every society; it begins with the very history of mankind and there nowhere is nor has been a people without narrative. [N]arrative is international, transhistorical, transcultural: it is simply there, like life itself.
>
> Barthes (1977, p. 79); cited in Rankin (2002, p.3)

The implications of this approach for the practice of ethics are manifold, but we shall deal with only three. First, it suggests that ethical behaviour and decision-making is a matter of character rather than a subset of decision-making theory. As such, narrative ethics relates well to virtue theory and focuses primarily on the person making the decision rather than the decision itself. For some people, for example, should they become unable to decide for themselves, faced with having to make a decision, it is more important *who* makes the decision than what is decided. Second, there is a sense of narrative necessity: the right decision emerges from the narrative itself rather than being imposed upon the narrative. This narrative necessity is what makes most sense given the characters, the context, and trajectory of the narrative. So, for example, the decision to accept extra care may be necessitated by the unfolding narrative if the narrative and its characters are to maintain their unity, coherence, credibility, and trajectory. Third, narrative ethics are always relational, always and inevitably involving others. Ethics is thus essentially worked out *between* individuals rather than simply *by* them. Fourth, this approach locates individual narratives within wider narratives and social practices. We are not simply the stories we tell about ourselves but also the stories others tell about us (whether these wider narratives are at the level of the individual, the institution or society). And the virtues are what sustain our part in the total story (Schneewind, 1982).

The primary difficulty for the narrative approach is how to evaluate competing narratives. Given that there can be disagreement over something as relatively simple as a horse race (Goodman, 1980) it is unsurprising to find disagreement in more complex matters such as the practice of psychiatry (Baldwin, 2005a). In such cases it is not simply a matter of subsuming one narrative into another, for the two may well be incommensurable (Baldwin, 2004). Neither can the problem be resolved by recourse to 'facts', as it is perfectly possible to construct a coherent and persuasive narrative in the absence of such (Baldwin, 2005b). And it is not enough to have recourse to our place in the 'total story' as the total story itself, while providing unity to one story, may itself be undesirable.

How then do we judge better from worse narratives? Hauerwas and Burrell (1977) go some way to providing us with narrative criteria for making such evaluations. They propose four criteria for preferring some narratives over others. To be preferable, to warrant our allegiance, narratives must have:

1 the power to release us from destructive alternatives;

2 ways of seeing through current distortions;

**3** room to keep us from having to resort to violence;

**4** a sense for the tragic: how meaning transcends power.

Destructive alternatives and current distortions do not have to be physical acts but can be located in discourse. Certain meta-narratives can damage identity (Nelson, 2001). The meta- (or master) narratives of some medical conditions may fall into these categories—for example, witness the meta-narrative of dementia as cognitive decline and loss of self. Similarly, violence is not limited to physical acts, but can be found in policies and procedures that take precedence over,

> the moral task…to learn to continue to do the right, to care for this immediate patient, even when we have no assurance that it will be the successful thing to do.
>
> Hauerwas and Burrell (1977, p.188)

Thus we return to the development of the virtues. For MacIntyre (1985), the virtues are those dispositions that sustain us in our quest for human goods, goods which, we would argue, include Hauerwas and Burrell's four narrative criteria.

> Stories, then, help us, as we hold them, to relate to our world and our destiny: the origins and goals of our lives, as they embody in narrative form specific ways of acting out that relatedness. So in allowing ourselves to adopt and be adopted by a particular story, we are in fact assuming a set of practices which will shape the ways we relate to our world and destiny.
>
> Hauerwas and Burrell (1977, p.186)

Having outlined virtue and narrative ethics, we now wish to put them into practice by showing how they can add depth to discussions of various ethical issues arising in old age psychiatry. In order to structure the ethical issues, we have attempted to follow what might be a patient's pathway. Although we shall be discussing issues that arise in a number of conditions in old age, we have used as our raw data quotes from carers of people with dementia. This allows us to get closer to the real experience of people. Fuller details of the research can be found elsewhere (Baldwin *et al.*, 2004, 2005).

## Perceptions of illness

Diseases can appear insidiously or suddenly. The perception of illness may initially be only a sense that something is not quite right. Later on, when a diagnosis has been made, the early signs might seem obvious. The theme of this section is the place of values in diagnosis. We shall start by considering the concepts of denial and lack of insight and move on to think more about the specific diagnosis of mild cognitive impairment (MCI). In doing so we shall draw out the importance of evaluative judgements in the labelling of diseases. Behind the value judgements lie deep concerns about the nature of our lives and it is here that our discussion of narrative and virtues will reappear.

In *Moral theory and medical practice*, Fulford's (1989) 'ethics-based view of medicine' stressed,

> …that the conceptual structure of medicine is essentially evaluative (rather than factual) in nature, and, second, that the particular kind of value which is expressed by medical terms is derived via 'illness' (rather than 'disease') from 'failure of action' (rather than 'failure of function').
>
> Fulford (1989, p. 260)

Fulford was keen to stress that this did not mean facts were unimportant, but many problems in the practice of medicine will have to be solved by attending to values rather than facts.

Fulford's first point, therefore, is very clear in the practice of old age psychiatry. Many of the really problematic issues, both clinically and ethically, require careful negotiation because of the values involved. For instance, whether someone goes into long-term care, or whether they should be compulsorily detained under mental health legislation, or whether a drug with particular side-effects should be started, or whether confidential information should be shared, such issues are decided on the basis of some important facts, but crucially on the basis of values. Hence the importance of values-based practice (Fulford, 2004).

Fulford's second point is pertinent to our immediate discussion. What comes first is 'failure of action' or 'ordinary doing'. This is then understood in terms of illness, which takes precedence over the more biomedical understanding of disease as a 'failure of function'. Hence, depression is not just neurochemical dysfunction, but low mood, loss of pleasure, loss of energy, with lethargy, poor concentration, disturbed sleep and the like. In fact, depression involves disruptions to the person's ability to do things day to day. The judgements about these symptoms are evaluative. There is no clear, objective boundary between ordinary unhappiness and clinical depression. Fulford has also persuasively agued that there are similar conceptual difficulties over psychotic experiences such as delusions.

It is commonplace that people with early dementia often do not recognize that they have a problem. This raises several difficulties in support of Fulford's analysis that are ethical as well as clinical. It is not too difficult to suggest reasons why the person should be told there is a problem: for example, it offers the possibility of coming to terms with what is happening, of making plans for future care, of sorting out affairs, and of accepting medication and other forms of help. Nevertheless, we have to recognize that the process of being assessed and, as it were, having the disease and the status of illness thrust upon you, which is how it might seem to the person concerned, is upsetting:

> So at that stage the doctor had made a diagnosis of borderline dementia but trying to explain that to my mum was very difficult. She obviously wanted to know why this doctor was coming into her house and talking to her and asking her all these silly questions. And, at that stage the doctor did say, 'I feel there's something wrong with your memory', and she completely denied that and got very upset. [son]

However, there are two important points. First, as Hursthouse suggested, a 'dose of virtue ethics' might come in handy inasmuch as this will focus attention on *how* things are done, even if *what* is done is easily justified. Secondly, we can see how the status of illness in the case of dementia is largely a public matter. Sometimes the patient will recognize what Fulford called a failure of 'ordinary doing'—people are aware that they are forgetful—but often it is others who define the problem and seek help, sometimes without the full cooperation of the person concerned. The illness occupies a public space and is defined by shared evaluative judgements. It affects, therefore, others in an intimate way and in a problematic way, because they then find themselves at odds with the understanding of the person concerned.

> It's funny in a way but if the person denies [it] completely to themselves it does put an extra burden on the person who is looking after

them. Not in terms of dealing with the denial but taking that on board for themselves. Acceptance of the disease can be quite hard for both the patient and the relative or the carer and I think once the carer has realized that something's wrong [and] the other person still completely denies it, to some extent you assume that responsibility for them as well as the other day to day or physical responsibilities and that can be an extra strain. [son]

For those concerned the problem becomes one of negotiating between the different understandings (one might say the different narratives) of what is going on. This can be a strain for all concerned, especially when it is not just the person with dementia who denies what is happening but the carer too. It becomes more of a strain when risks start to become apparent. This reveals the extent to which the public space in which these things happen is also a realm of values and meanings. It is because of evaluative judgements that people feel they must act; but different judgements (perhaps based on different facts reflecting different values) entail that there can be clashes, which then have to be negotiated.

And I was dealing with *her* denial of it as well, which was *really* difficult and that's the only time when I really felt alienated from the family because what I said to my husband about them, or about his father, his mother would deny: 'Oh no he would never do that, my husband would never hit me, he would never push me. He is a sweet person; he would never be that unkind to me'. [daughter-in-law]

The clash of viewpoints, reflecting different judgements, is shown in the next quote where the ethical issue for the carer concerns whether anything can be done and the sense of impotence comes from the underlying wish to respect the person. The difficulties cannot simply be framed in terms of the need to respect the person's autonomy, however, nor can the problem be understood merely in terms of a clash of principles (autonomy versus beneficence). The real issues here are the nature of relationship, the way in which the person's narrative is co-created, the issue of dependency, which is intrinsic to the relationship and reflects the autonomous decisions that led to it, as well as the standing of the people concerned as agents situated in a world where free choices can (and cannot) be made.

I felt a tremendous feeling of anger towards him that I knew something was happening to him and sometimes I would say to him 'You know something's happening to you don't you?' And he didn't say yes but he didn't say no, and I tried to play it down although I had this awful gut feeling that it was tremendously serious. …Impotent fury I think would aptly describe the way I felt. Very, quite I felt quite depressed.… Here was he going along with his life as he wanted it and I was knowing something was going drastically wrong and yet unable to get him to do anything about it. [partner]

In some sense, in dementia but also in other psychiatric conditions, the judgement about illness is made by others. The social and cultural aspects of disease are much more prominent in psychiatric conditions, even at the level of diagnosis. But similar aspects are at play in relation to ageing itself. The boundary between normal and pathological ageing is not at all clear and the end result is a feeling of uncertainty.

Yes, I put a lot of it down to the fact that, at that stage I thought we were both getting older… And I just assumed, that every now and then, everybody does have a slight lapse of memory.…but I just had the feeling that things were very different in some way and I couldn't pick it up. [husband]

These sorts of uncertainty come to the fore when we turn to debates about MCI (see Chapter 26). One of the ethical issues associated with MCI is whether giving someone this diagnosis might ever be harmful (and sometimes unwarranted). As in the case of dementia itself, there is at least some evidence that this might be true. Corner and Bond (2006) quote the case of Rose, who was told that she had a dementia that was 'very mild, not really dementia'. Her husband Ron described matters thus:

When we were told that that Rose had this dementia we were just devastated, that's the only word for it. Our world came crashing down around us and…we cried for days. We couldn't bring ourselves to talk to…the kids…or anyone about it. It was too shameful for Rose. She didn't want anyone to know. …That was oh, eighteen months ago now, and really she's no different to then. But every time she's even a bit forgetful, we're thinking 'Is this it then?', even though we're not quite sure what 'it' is or will be. …We've just been turned upside down by it. …You picture these people who are vegetable…it's horrific.

At a more conceptual level, given that the biology shows no discontinuity from normal to abnormal ageing, the implications of accepting our diagnostic categories need to be thought through. As Kirkwood (2006) suggests:

Although there have been unquestionable benefits from the labelling of neurodegenerative conditions such as [Alzheimer's disease] as distinct clinical entities, not least the removal of some of the stigma previously associated with 'senile dementia', the biology of ageing suggests that too rigid an approach to classification is of doubtful validity and may even get in the way of understanding what is really going on.

The very diagnosis of Alzheimer's disease is questionable at a cultural as well as at a biological level. Whilst the diagnosis has to be accepted as useful in numerous ways, it may also be—especially if the scientific standing of subtypes of dementia as 'natural kinds' is in doubt (see Graham and Ritchie, 2006)—that it focuses the research agenda in ways that might be unhelpful (e.g. the search for a genetic explanation for a condition that might be heterogeneous). Moving one step back in biological terms, to try to find the precursor of Alzheimer's disease, simply increases the social, cultural, and ethical difficulties. These themes are developed by Whitehouse (2006), who makes a link between diagnostic categories and our quality of life and death:

At the hundredth anniversary of the first case of what we have come to call Alzheimer's disease [AD], perhaps it is time to reflect on the individual and social advantages and disadvantages of these labels on the continuum of cognitive aging. The process of social deconstruction (i.e. ending AD as a label) cannot eliminate the suffering that accompanies the loss of cognitive capacity as we age but it can allow us to think of these processes in richer and deeper ways than the medical model allows us. We need to imagine different, perhaps wiser, visions and values about aging processes in our brains that respect our limits as mortal creatures and as scientists. Perhaps by pursuing this exercise in humility we can recognize that, although some suffering may be inevitable in life, the stories we tell about brain aging can dramatically affect the quality of our lives and of our deaths.

One link between brain ageing and the quality of our lives and deaths is provided by just the evaluative judgements with which we commenced this section. How we think of brain ageing is itself value-laden. In part this will reflect social judgements to do with what is and is not accepted as normal within everyday life: 'notions of the social good *are* the conceptual background that permit the judgment of normal or pathological' (Sadler, 2005, p. 239). According to Sadler (2005) there needs to be a balance between technological practice (which involves efficiency, productivity, economy, and the like) and poietic practice (which concerns creativity, tradition, nature, and connectedness). Poietic practice brings in values; but 'value-commitments' pepper psychiatric practice. The important point here is that at stake are ultimate questions about the meaning of life.

If a particular behaviour is seen as a sign of disease and degeneration, the person's life might be discounted or downgraded. But if our mode of living sets some value on age and being older, a degree of forgetfulness might be tolerated. As Bavidge (2006, p. 49) has put it:

> The elderly have been around the block, seen it all before, and developed habitual ways of responding. Their interests and behaviour are motivated by different ambitions, concerns, and anxieties from those of the young. …But there are also distinctive and valuable qualities in the experience and the attitudes of the elderly who have been in similar situations many times before.

Bavidge offers the corrective:

> We should think of old age as offering alternative rather than impaired ways of experiencing life [ibid.].

In stressing the poietic, Sadler (2005) wishes to draw our attention back 'towards questions that matter to us the most, the ones concerning how we should live' (p. 345). In so doing, he also makes a link to that which human life aims at, what Aristotle called *eudaimonia*, or human flourishing. And in order to flourish well in a distinctively human way, we require the virtues.

So, the argument runs as follows: illnesses involve evaluative judgements, which are decided upon in the public realm. What should count here cannot be solely determined by technological considerations. For what is required is some shared sense of the human goods towards which we should be striving. We are helped in this endeavour by the virtues, which pick out just what comprises human flourishing. For instance charity is likely to make us more tolerant and less inclined to condemn odd behaviour; and courage will give us the determination to stand up for and advocate on behalf of people who are different. Virtuous perceptions of ageing will not become so narrow and mean spirited that we wish to disregard older people and the contributions they might make to society. We should take a broader narrative view of the person's overall accomplishments and evaluate failures of 'ordinary doing' in the context of his or her life as a whole. Although at some stage cognitive dysfunction and ageing, like alcohol misuse and depression, will be pathological, we should feel more inclined to preserve the person's abilities to cope for themselves in creative and nurturing ways.

## Help-seeking

At some stage of an illness help is normally sought, but—especially in the case of severe mental disorders—not always by the person concerned. The crucial ethical issue raised is then confidentiality. The details of the illness have been imparted to someone else and confidences need to be respected, but if the person with the presumed illness has not presented him- or herself, the issue of confidentiality is immediately more problematic. In discussing this issue we shall focus on the virtue of *phronesis* or practical wisdom. This is the virtue that allows people to determine the correct action by judgements of a practical nature about what is good or bad for human beings. In a distinct way it is the virtue that is crucial for clinicians. It also makes an immediate link with ideas around narrative ethics; because clinicians, if they are to be successful, will normally recognize the utility and inevitability of entering into the person's story if they are to be helpful.

### Confidentiality

In the field of dementia there are conflicting views and experiences. One husband, caring for his wife, could see no problems whatsoever:

> I can't think of any occasion where I was concerned about confidentiality and indeed I suppose I can't say I would have been concerned if confidentiality had been broken…I can think of possible advantageous aspects of breaking confidentiality.

Nevertheless, some carers describe doctors seeming to hide behind the principle of confidentiality to the detriment of the patient. They say that doctors refuse to tell them things concerning which they might be able to help. Yet, complained one daughter, when real problems arise the doctors say: 'There you are, you're the relatives, you deal with it'. The same daughter went on to say:

> I think with something like dementia and something that is going to involve long term *chronic* deterioration in somebody, if you're going to get a good effective support for the patient you *have* to get the relatives – or whoever is going to do the caring – on board as soon as possible. And to make it *feel* that they're part of some kind of plan.

Many doctors would be inclined to share information, but a distinction can be made between sharing information between professionals and sharing information with others, including family. Tracy *et al.* (2004) found discordant views amongst those involved in community care. Professionals were keen that good practice guidelines should be followed. For instance, clear notes should be kept and reasons for actions recorded. But, for the sake of the patient's best interests, these Canadian professionals stated that bending the rules was common practice. And, as far as the patients interviewed were concerned, there were no concerns about professionals sharing information between themselves. Tracy *et al.* (2004) state that their efforts to suggest a problem over the privacy of the patients' records, as far as other professionals might be concerned, met with 'bemused dismissal'. One participant in their study with dementia said:

> So what? So what? I don't think that's important. It's only important if you are doing something wrong. I mean, I don't care how many people know what specific medication I'm taking.

In the same study the professionals recognized potential problems about sharing information with families, because families might have dissenting members and they might fool the professionals. On the whole, however, it was thought that the risks were worth taking for the sake of the patients. The difficulties were seen as a natural concomitant of dealing with complicated family dynamics in the community. When it came to the views of the people with dementia, however, their desire 'to maintain control over the decision to contact and disclose information to family members was palpable' (Tracy *et al.* 2004). One of the participants with dementia stated:

> Why would the doctor have to call? [tone of irritation] If I wanted anybody in my family to know about my problem, to know that I needed help, or to ask them for help, I can do that myself. Why would anybody else do it? It's wrong that somebody else would do it other than me.

Tracy *et al.* (2004) discuss the discordance between the views of the family carers and the professionals on the one hand and the views of the people with dementia on the other in terms of a conflict between the principles of autonomy and beneficence. They solve the dilemma by plumping for 'the values and preferences of those experiencing an illness first hand'. They assert that the concept of 'the *expert patient*' should take precedence over the views of '*professional experts*'; they wish to reclaim the ground for 'the people'.

This is all very well, but it is interesting that no real arguments are offered to support these assertions beyond some politically correct hand waving in the direction of 'the people'. One obvious argument against these assertions is that it would be odd if, on the grounds of respecting the views of the person with dementia, he or she came to harm. It is also paradoxical that respect for autonomy might involve respecting the non-autonomous decisions of the person: 'non-autonomous' in that they are made—in the case of some—without insight and without the requisite capacity for the person to exercise true autonomy. A further flaw in the argument of Tracy *et al.* (2004) is that the dichotomy between professionals and non-professionals should not, perhaps, be made without critical thought. As far as confidentiality goes, for instance, what are the important ethical differences between the care worker at the day centre and the caring daughter? If people with dementia are motivated to allow professional carers to share information, what are the grounds for this? And might not the same motivating forces be applicable to family carers? In brief, it is possible to criticize the assertions made in Tracy *et al.* (2004), because the grounds are not evidently supported.

Furthermore, there is a real conflict in perspectives here. The person with dementia, when it is suggested that a relative might be contacted, is adamantly against the suggestion. The carer of the person with dementia points out with vehemence the ways in which he or she could help the person they care about if they were kept informed. It is quite difficult to say that one perspective (or narrative) is wrong; they both encapsulate important concerns. What is required of the clinician are practical wisdom and a means to bring together the different narratives in a way that makes sense. Perhaps there are ways to accommodate all concerned, for example by involving the family carer with the person with dementia from the beginning. The thought of the doctor ringing up a relative who was not present at the assessment to impart confidential information is understandably shocking. But maybe it is not so shocking to have the relative with you during the process of assessment. When it is apparent that one side of the dilemma is clearly wrong a judgement will have to be made based on practical wisdom, which will itself come from experience and practical knowledge (about prognosis, legal frameworks, guidelines, and the like) and should aim at allowing the people concerned the greatest chance of human flourishing. Other virtues may be required, such as the courage to advocate for the person with dementia. But, as this daughter makes plain, practical wisdom will be exercised more easily in the context of relationships, where it will be easier to negotiate with those concerned:

> I think that it is a very difficult area because there are people who would take advantage of the situation…but by and large I think the doctor and the relatives need to make some sort of relationship. The doctor needs to be prepared to do that, or try to do it and so does the relative. And if it's clear to the doctor that you are doing your best and acting in what you perceive to be the best interests and you're not breaking any law and you're not doing anything about which he should have severe concerns, I see no problem with why he can't discuss the situation with you. …If a person is dealing, caring for another person who is totally dependent upon them and a professional

withholds information that would make their life easier – and I don't mean just necessarily in a practical sense, but more bearable perhaps – then I think that professional should have the right and the courage to work with them and tell them. But then I think you see we should all be working together in these things.

The notion of working together itself suggests a practical working out, depending on the exact circumstances of the case, but this is being done in a spirit of mutual engagement. Practical wisdom suggests such an engagement, which is also a way of saying that entering into the narratives of those concerned is a way of influencing, co-creating, how things develop.

If we shift attention to the case of someone with late onset schizophrenia, the same considerations apply. For instance, in Tracy *et al.* (2004) one of the physicians said:

> In the community, you often have to make a judgement on the basis of very limited information. Say the scenario is a paranoid person living alone who refuses to let anybody in the door and there's increasing concern by community health professionals that they're dangerous or they're at risk. That is a very difficult area where you just have to use common sense.

'Common sense', when it is guided by experience and aimed at human good—the best interests of the patient say—approximates to practical wisdom. 'To possess phronesis', say Widdershoven and Widdershoven-Heerding (2003) 'one has to show it in one's actions, situated in time, place, circumstance, and history…this type of wisdom includes a certain attitude, a certain condition, obtained by practice' (p. 110). A social worker in Tracy *et al.* (2004) exemplified this attitude in discussing risk and the need to break confidentiality:

> Usually the greater the risk, the more liberal I am in terms of talking to people because I'm not going to risk the health and safety of a client for the rules of privacy or whatever.…So you stretch the rules of confidentiality depending on how risky the situation is.

The person with paranoid delusions may be dangerous and for that reason it may become necessary to inform others (family, neighbours, or even the police) of the potential risks. Being involved in the narrative means that these people have roles to play and need to be directed, but only to the degree that practical wisdom deems necessary. Equally, however, the clinician must recognize the crucial role of the protagonist, who will want to exercise some control over how things will go. It may not always be possible to agree, but things are likely to go better if the clinician can see things from the person's point of view.

The issue here is to do with relationships, empathy, and communication. Even the person with schizophrenia will respond better if he or she is understood to the degree that this is possible. Attention to demeanour is another way of creating the appropriate atmosphere with the person; and demeanour reflects the inner dispositions, such as love, from which the virtues, such as charity, spring. Empathy, or putting your self in the shoes of others, is another manifestation of the narrative approach: being able to understand someone's story from his or her perspective. It may also require the exercise of various virtues: a degree of courage or fortitude, being able to stick with people, along with compassion and fidelity. The gay partner of someone with dementia felt the lack of empathy fairly forcibly in a number of his encounters with professionals:

> And I think that this is the problem with medical staff and professionals as a whole.…It isn't sufficient for them simply to say that they

accepted in some equal opportunities way the nature of a gay relationship. There needs to be an empathy there that sees both partners through any decisions or any situations that are going to occur in the future. Because if you have that empathy then you can foresee any problems that might occur. But if you don't have that empathy then you simply abide by the letter of the law and that will provide unnecessary problems.

True empathy and seeing the person as located in a narrative should encourage professionals to look ahead in a way that will be helpful to carers as well as to people with dementia, so that help is given appropriately. This sort of practical help is a way of showing compassion as well as wisdom.

What is required, when the person or his or her relative seeks help, is a trusting engagement that recognizes the complexity of the narratives in which we are embedded. So confidences will need to be established between all those involved.

> Confidentiality is a token of the trust that should exist as an element of this mutual engagement, but not necessarily as an overriding principle. This trust, therefore, exists within a shared context in which others are likely to become involved as a matter of routine and for the good of the patient.
>
> Hughes and Louw (2002a)

Negotiating how confidential information is shared will be a matter of practical wisdom based on the knowledge of particular circumstances and contexts. In emphasizing real world practical judgements, and engagement with people's narratives, we are putting aside those approaches that privilege particular principles or theories. Instead there is practical working out to be done, which can often seem to upset the tidier theories and legalistic approaches of some conceptions of medical ethics.

> I think there's some huge experience out there in the real world, people learn all sorts of practical ways of managing. And some of it doesn't necessarily sit *easily* with professional ethics but you're dealing with people,… And I'm not sure that the classic ethics of the medical profession actually apply….. You have to manage patients in their world. It takes stress and conflict out of the process, not entirely, but it makes the whole process more manageable. [son]

Whether or not it amounts to telling lies, accessing the worlds of people with schizophrenia, severe depression, or dementia is the first task of the professional.

# Diagnosis

## Assessment and defectology

The first step on the road to diagnosis is assessment. We are apt to forget that this process requires some form of valid consent (see below), which may or may not be possible. Kapp (2006) outlines the legal options in America, but concludes that 'bumbling through' rather than invoking formal legal procedures might be the 'most ethically sensible' strategy,

> where there are no obvious conflicts of interest and all involved parties appear to be working to protect and promote the best interests and, to the extent feasible, the autonomy of the individual in whom dementia is suspected.

Professionals are also apt to forget that assessment is stressful. One of the ways in which it is stressful is that it raises ethical concerns, as we have seen, about being assessed in the first place. Matters become worse if the assessment is itself upsetting, especially if it is demeaning.

> So somebody going into her house and asking her a lot of questions about the mini-mental test score, for instance, which has got questions which are fairly obvious to anybody who's not very demented…that they're asking you about your memory. And when you can't answer those questions, as happened with mum, she got very uptight and quite, not aggressive, but the realisation there was something wrong and that she wasn't giving the doctor the answers that she wanted made her get quite anti about it really. A bit 'bolshie' I suppose. [son]

This sort of response is not uncommon. In a pilot study of the ethical issues that arise for carers of people with dementia, several mentioned how upsetting cognitive testing could be and one recommended that a conversation would be a better way to test someone while showing them respect (Hughes *et al.*, 2002a). Similar concerns and annoyance emerge in the discussions between Sabat (2001) and people with dementia. Indeed, when performed without thought, cognitive testing can be termed 'defectology' because of its tendency to emphasize the defects in a person's life rather than the persisting abilities. Whilst cognitive assessment is important, the question should be how it might be done virtuously. A hopeful suggestion is that it might be more acceptable if it were embedded in the context of taking a narrative history. Understanding the person as such, through narrative, might naturally involve some aspects of testing. But to test without the narrative background is not to understand the person at all, it is simply to apply a technique.

## Diagnostic disclosure

To be told that you have any serious disease is terrible. In the case of dementia there are particular concerns because of the nature of the disease. In a systematic review, Bamford *et al.* (2004), found wide variations in terms of people's beliefs and attitudes to the disclosure of the diagnosis, with reported practice also being variable. Although many of the studies had methodological shortcomings, they showed that the impact of the diagnosis could be both positive and negative. Bamford *et al.* (2004) commented that the meaning of disclosure and the perspectives of people with dementia have been relatively ignored.

The views of older people presenting with memory problems have recently been studied by Elson (2006) who found that 86% wanted to know the cause of their problems. However, only one person out of the 36 interviewed had considered the possibility of Alzheimer's disease and only 69% said they would want to know if they had Alzheimer's disease. Whilst, on the one hand, Elson (2006) suggests it can no longer be justified to tell the carers but not the person with dementia, the paper suggests that a significant proportion of people fear the diagnosis of Alzheimer's. Hence there is a great need to be cautious in judgements about whether or not and how to tell someone the diagnosis of any form of dementia.

In our study of carers of people with dementia, although most of the participants seemed to favour telling the truth, there was a range of views. Here, for instance, is a daughter who was adamantly against the diagnosis being given to her mother because of the anticipated bad consequences:

> I think it was right, absolutely right to keep the diagnosis from her. I have no hesitation; it was absolutely the right thing to do because she knew what the word was and she knew what it meant and she would

have been absolutely panic stricken if she'd thought she'd got it. It would have been awful.

But another daughter felt differently:

They have a right to know. They need to know what's happening to them. Otherwise it's awful when you don't know what is going on and you don't know what is happening to you. In my mother's case, she was so distressed because she thought everybody was stealing her things. Nobody was stealing her things; she just couldn't remember where she put them. And so they should be told because like, for example, now I can reason with her.

We should note that this daughter, like other carers, speaks in terms of rights. Similarly, there is a real concern about consequences. To this ex-wife, who also uses the language of rights, the consequences seemed to be beneficial:

Yes I do think people have a right. They have a right to make decisions about how they will live out the end of their lives. It gives them the opportunity to say goodbye. It gives them the opportunity to actually exercise some power over what happens.

It is certainly possible to discuss the ethical issues in terms of consequences or in terms of rights (to which there are correlative duties). The problem with these approaches is that they do not seem to settle the argument. For it is true that the consequences of telling the truth might be good or bad. If, alternatively, it is pointed out that there is a duty to tell the truth because the person has a right to know, it could be retorted that the duty of care—given the risk of harm—would suggest that there should not be a frank disclosure of the diagnosis.

This might be taken to suggest that all that is required is more empirical work to determine whether, in fact, there are more harmful or beneficial consequences associated with disclosure. But such empirical work still does not answer the question for the individual in front of us and does not give regard to whether the person in front of us wants to know or not.

Perhaps it is more to do with the way in which people are told things: the manner and speed of disclosure:

I don't feel you can tell everything too quickly, you have to take it gradually as well. So I was just answering the question. I let her dictate the pace really, to be honest. [daughter]

In which case, however, we are no longer talking of consequences or rights and duties. Instead we are looking at the manner in which the thing was done and, to cut to the chase, this is where Hursthouse's 'dose of virtue ethics' might again come in handy. For we might wish to say that the key thing is it should be done as the virtuous person would do it. It is certainly possible to talk in terms of the virtues in connection with diagnostic disclosure and the most obvious relevant virtue is that of honesty. But does this mean telling the truth, come what may? Well, perhaps the important point is that the virtues connect and overlap. Carers tend to take a broad view. They are naturally aware of how a particular decision fits into the person's whole life scheme:

In my mother's case I tried to ascertain whether she wanted to know. My view was that she possibly didn't, but my previous experience of dealing with her was that she dealt better when she knew what was going on than when she didn't. She didn't like thinking things were going wrong and not knowing what it was, whether that was a social thing or medical thing. [daughter]

Hence, from the perspective of the person with dementia, it might well be that the narrative can make no sense because the whole story is not being told. It might be objected that the story makes no sense to the person because of the cognitive impairment, but this is to beg the question. Even without cognitive impairment, how could anyone form a coherent narrative view without having the whole story?

If they want to know they have the right to be told and this was the case with my mother. She wanted to know and she wasn't told. She was still able to reason up to a point. How was she able to understand the situation if she wasn't told? This was part of the problem. She could not understand why she needed help, why she couldn't stay in her flat, because she had no understanding of her illness. [daughter]

Although this daughter started by talking of rights, her real concern was that her mother could not understand. The problem is the way in which the lack of truthfulness intrudes into the already complicated picture to make things worse.

If we start to think in terms of a narrative perspective, whereby the person's lifetime concerns and values are taken seriously and considered, it also becomes clearer that honesty is not the only virtue we should be considering. What often seems to be at issue for carers is the nature of the relationship they have with the person with dementia, which is based on the nature of the relationship over time. The issue becomes more one of fidelity, of being true to the person, rather than simply, in a disconnected way, either telling or not telling the truth on one particular occasion.

At the time the neurologist and most of my in-laws and almost everyone else told me that my wife should not be told what the true problem was. I disagree now emphatically with that. It removed any scope for me to combine with her to combat the problems she had. It also meant that I had to do a variety of pretty awful things by subterfuge. I had to remove her driving licence, her bank cards at different stages, cheque books, all kinds of things like this without being able to tell her the reason I was doing this. And this of course caused an incredible amount of bad feeling and really ruined our relationship in many ways. Even though I was the person that she really depended upon she didn't like me, I think for most of the remaining time because of all these things that I'd done: I was the obstacle in the way of her life in many ways.

One has a sense in this husband's words of a fractured narrative: the mutuality of their lives was destroyed by the deceit that came to exist between them. Just as the earlier carer spoke of understanding, perhaps what is required, whether or not this amounts to a disclosure of the exact diagnosis, is a shared understanding of what is happening. Thus, in the quote that follows, even though the wife concerned did not wish her husband to know the exact diagnosis (which entails that the truth is not told), there is a sense of persisting honesty and, thereby, a persisting mutuality:

So we didn't need anybody saying that he'd got dementia, he knew we kept on talking about the fact that his memory was going. But I didn't want him to know the sort of things that were going to happen and I didn't want him to hear the word Alzheimer's. But he was fully aware of the fact that his brain was not working the way it should and it was getting worse.

The persisting honesty comes from the recognition that there is a problem and the mutuality is seen in the way this understanding is shared. But there is also a sense here of the broader virtue of fidelity, which implies faithfulness and loyalty as well as conformity to the truth. In saying this we are making the point that virtues overlap. To be true in the sense of showing fidelity, especially in the face of adverse circumstances, sometimes requires courage and a sort of practical wisdom, which allows the person to make judgements on the basis of experience about how to navigate through the difficulties that inevitably emerge.

Concerning the professional, May (1994) suggests:

> The virtues with which the professional dispenses the truth may condition the very reality he or she offers the patient. …The professional relationship, though less comprehensive and intimate than marriage, is similarly promissory and fiduciary. …The moral question for the professional becomes not simply a question of telling truths, but of *being true to his promises*. Conversely, the total situation for the patient includes not only his disease but also whether others ditch him or stand by him in extremity. …The fidelity of the professional *per se* will not eliminate the disease…but it can affect mightily the context in which the trouble runs its course.

Of course, diagnostic disclosure could be debated in terms of autonomy: some arguing that, in order to respect autonomy, the person should be told; and others that we respect the person's autonomy by paying attention to his or her choices, including the choice not to be told. Once we leave this theoretical debate, however, albeit autonomy is highly relevant as a background feature, what actually counts is the carer's detailed understanding of the person cared for. Carers are required to make decisions that draw upon their practical wisdom together with their embeddedness in the narrative of the person with dementia's life; it is not a straightforward matter of simply respecting autonomous wishes, because—for one thing—these have to be discerned.

Practical wisdom, which has been referred to as the virtue of prudence, can also suggest, especially if the diagnosis is made late, that disclosure is pointless if the person is unlikely to understand what it means. Prudence should also suggest some thought be given to who might give the diagnosis, under what circumstances, and how, and this should to be combined with fidelity, which suggests the need to be faithful to the person's wishes. Moreover, it should not be overlooked that the person with dementia is also capable of exercising the virtues, including the virtue of practical wisdom:

> In my wife's case it was helpful to know the diagnosis. She was puzzled and wanted to know what was happening. So when it was explained to her she said, 'Right, what do we do?' [husband]

### Genetic testing

Connected to the issue of giving the diagnosis is the issue of genetic testing. Many carers ask about the genetic risks associated with having someone in the family with dementia. Few people are tested, other than in the context of early onset dementias with a strong family history. Neumann *et al.* (2001) have usefully reviewed the literature in a study of public attitudes to genetic testing. They found that 79% of people across all ages would take a completely predictive test, whereas only 45% would take a test where there was a one in ten chance of the test being incorrect. Participants in this American study who did not want the test were concerned at the prospect of having to live with the news (69%), the lack of preventative treatment (61%), with only 30% being concerned about confidentiality or privacy. This could be taken to suggest that prudence was more important to these participants than principles. The practical nature of their responses was also shown by their inclination to sign advance directives (84%), spend more time with their families (80%), and sort out their finances (74%) if they received a positive test. Meanwhile, Malpas (2005) has argued that,

on the grounds of autonomy, people *ought* to know their genetic status. But this merely serves to demonstrate (in line with our earlier comments), either the limited nature of autonomy as a principle, or the importance of characterizing autonomy in an entirely richer way.

### Summary

Much of the discussion in this section would be relevant to other conditions, such as late onset schizophrenia. What has emerged is the extent to which the virtues overlap. In addition, we have seen how the right decision—the decision that the virtuous person would take—cannot be divorced from context and a detailed knowledge of the person with dementia. We have glimpsed the importance of how this knowledge is embedded in relationships extending over time. This is the narrative view of the person, which remains important as we proceed to think about treatment.

## Treatment

The story of the person with a disease is usually that they will require treatment. In the normal course of events this requires consent and the ground for this requirement is autonomy. Our proposal in this section is that the ethical basis of treatment is a relationship and shared understanding [a very similar conclusion is evident in Dyer and Bloch (1987)]. Once again, a richer description of the crucial ethical issues comes from a broader view of the situation, rather than a more limited, atomistic, and legalistic view. Albeit briefly, we shall first discuss consent and capacity in general, and then consider four issues: covert medication, compulsion, resource allocation, and research.

### Consent and capacity

For consent to be fully valid it should be informed, competent, non-coerced, and continuing. Each of these elements raises difficulties. These difficulties have been discussed previously in the literature in the context of the treatment of dementia (Hughes, 2000), whilst the broader ethical and legal issues around consent can be found elsewhere (e.g. Hope *et al.*, 2003). Nevertheless it is still worth noting that the difficulties are all to do with judgements of value: How much information needs to be given? How much competence is required? Where does cajoling end and coercing begin? What constitutes continuing consent? In this field laws can help, but individual judgements on the ground are ultimately what are generally required. These difficulties are seen most strikingly in the judgements that have to be made about competence or capacity (see Chapter 42).

The concept of capacity is vitally important, partly because of its complexity. At first blush it seems straightforward: decisional capacity is defined in terms of the person's ability to understand, recall, weigh up, and communicate about a particular decision. One problem is simply that, once again, we can ask how much understanding, recall, weighing up? In addition, the problem with this understanding of capacity is that it is too cognitive. From the legal point of view this is very congenial, because a cognitive description of capacity lends itself to cognitive (objective) tests. But in a study of judgements concerning competence to consent to treatment what we find are diverse views, probably reflecting different values (Vellinga *et al.*, 2004). This study appears to show some support for using vignettes to determine capacity, possibly because this method taps into everyday experience and, to this extent, is less like a formal test.

In the UK it has been made plain that you can still have capacity and yet make irrational decisions, whereas some commentators have questioned the extent to which this is true: for example, Culver and Gert (2004) who argue that to be competent the person needs to be able to make a rational decision as without some degree of basic rationality it is difficult, if not impossible, to weigh things up appropriately. They went on to say that 'the ability to make a rational decision has intellectual, affective, and volitional components' (Culver and Gert, 2004). Whether or not their point about rationality is correct, it has certainly been recognized for a while that capacity involves an emotional element as well as intellectual discernment (Charland, 1998). In which case, the clinician ought to be bringing to bear an awareness of the emotional and volitional aspects of competency or capacity assessments. This is most naturally achieved by taking a broad view of what is required for the person to weigh things up. In other words, a person may be able to demonstrate that they are weighing things up by a mixture of what they can do and how they react as well as by what they know.

A good example of this is where an assessment of the person's capacity to make a decision about going home after a hospital inpatient admission is required. What would be the knowledge required to demonstrate this capacity? Much more pertinent is the result of the occupational therapy home assessment and the person's emotional response to home. So a broad assessment of capacity will be required, involving the multidisciplinary team, and a cognitive test will not suffice. But there is more to it than that. As Brindle and Holmes (2005) have commented, 'the presence or absence of capacity is frequently a secondary issue and its absence should not be used as a justification for disregarding individual choice'. One of the principles in assessing capacity is that the person's ability to participate in decision-making should be encouraged. In dementia, decision-making capacity is easily eroded simply by the way in which the person is regarded, because it is too easy to undermine the person's self-hood and ability to convey meaning (Sabat, 2005). What is required, on the part of the person making the assessment of capacity, is the ability to form empathic relationships and achieve a shared understanding to the extent that this is possible. This is quite different from the ability to think up legalistic cognitive tests.

People who make decisions for those who lack capacity must act in the person's best interests, but defining this is difficult. It also smacks of paternalism. This can be avoided by following the sort of procedure set out in the Mental Capacity Act 2005, which applies to England and Wales, in which attention has to be paid to the person's present and past wishes, including anything applicable set out in an advance directive, to their beliefs and values, and to the views of other people involved in the person's care or acting for the person under a lasting power of attorney or having been appointed by a court. Despite the estimation of best interests being prescribed in this fashion, at least in England and Wales, the possibility of paternalism is still present. The difficulty is to do with knowing what the person him or herself would have wanted under the circumstances.

## Covert medication

A good example of this is the issue of covert medication. Treloar *et al.* (2000) found that in 71% of the 34 residential, nursing, and inpatient units they studied medication was sometimes given covertly. They concluded that, even if the practice could be justified, the secrecy and poor recording that surrounded it was a cause of concern. They later opined that, 'in exceptional circumstances' the duty of care might require that covert medication be used (Treloar *et al.*, 2001), provided there were a transparent procedure, which should involve: an explicit determination that the person lacks capacity to make the decision about medication; discussion with relatives, advocates and other professionals; proper care planning and recording, to allow monitoring and auditing. These papers helped to shape and sharpen practice in the UK.

Many carers are in broad agreement with the policy of covert medication under certain circumstances:

> …if somebody is exhibiting certain signs and symptoms that are…really bad in a variety of ways, then…I think the ordinary ethics sometimes have to go out of the window. You know I wouldn't dream of expecting somebody who is compos mentis to have medication in a surreptitious manner, or any treatment. But I think to expect people who have dementia to be able to think rationally and reasonably about their medication, it's a bit like putting people back in the community with schizophrenia and not helping them to keep up their medication. Left to their own devices they won't do it and then they're back with the all the problems that they had before. [partner]

But not everyone agrees:

> I think you have to try to be as honest as you can, and keep talking about what the drugs are and what they're doing. …Sometimes, when she was really angry, it was tempting to slip a sedative into her tea or something, but I didn't. I'm really against anything being done surreptitiously. [husband]

We see here the possibility of a tension between the virtues of honesty and compassion. However, it is not obviously true that the husband who favours honesty lacks compassion; and it is not true that the partner who understands the need for covert medication actually lacks honesty; indeed, the husband went on to say that he had never had to resort to this sort of deceit. But it is possible that the option of honesty might become extraordinarily difficult, if the person were tormented but unwilling to comply with any medication.

If we return to the idea that the ethical basis of treatment is relationship and shared understanding, then honesty should be maintained for as long as possible. It will be possible for as long as there is a shared understanding. The tendency to position the person with dementia, however, in such a way that there is no chance of shared understanding is strong. It is all too easy to miss the person's meaning. The result is a manifestation of 'malignant positioning', which is the tendency to emphasize the person's defects and, according to Sabat (2006, pp. 291–2):

> Malignant positioning can lead to the creation of story lines that confirm the initial positioning of the person in question. …any actions of such people are quite easily construed as being pathological.

If the narrative reflects the virtue of compassion it is less likely to lead to malignant positioning and more likely to achieve a shared understanding. It may be the case, at some point, that there can be no possibility of such an understanding; yet even then we would still have the potential to fall back on the notion of relationship to underpin our treatment decisions. It may be in this context that covert medication could be ethically justified, for the relationship is likely to have, or to be able to call upon, a narrative history. And in this context compassion might involve being true (and honest in some sense) to the way the person once was, to his or her previous values and beliefs. Medication might then be given covertly both with compassion and without overt deceit (i.e. lies may not need to be told if the person is truly at a stage where shared understanding is impossible), yet also with openness and fidelity, so that elements of honesty are maintained, even if the relevance of this virtue under these 'exceptional circumstances' (to borrow from Treloar *et al.*, 2001) is lessened. But, according to our analysis, the 'exceptional circumstances' will be *extreme*: they will occur when the possibility of shared understanding no longer exists. The important ethical caveat is that we should be aware of the extent to which we are prone to presume the person's ability to share meaning and understanding is absent when it is really present (Sabat, 2001). It may be that the problem is located in neither the behaviour nor the pathology at which the medication is aimed, but in the 'malignant social psychology' that is so often ignored (Kitwood, 1997).

## Compulsion

Shared understanding and relationships become much more difficult when a person is psychotic with delusions. It is under this sort of extreme circumstance that compulsory detention and treatment might be required. However, as with covert medication, the circumstances need to be extreme. The same discussion of the possibility of shared understandings and relationships still applies. In the case of psychosis, these understandings and relationships might still be possible in other ways.

> Mrs Rodgers, a widow living alone, believes that her young neighbours are terrorists who intend to kill her because they know that she has uncovered their plot. They now watch her all the time looking for a good opportunity to do away with her. Hence, she will not go out for food because she does not wish to leave her property unguarded or expose herself to their assault. She refuses medication because she becomes suspicious that it might be poisoned.

It may or may not be possible to rid Mrs Rodgers completely of her delusions. In the short term it will certainly be difficult to establish a relationship with her if her paranoia comes, as it seems to have done, to involve clinical staff, and there is little prospect of shared understanding. Compulsory treatment seems inevitable.

Nonetheless, a relationship of sorts might slowly be established and she might come to understand that she is, at least, looked after in the hospital and that the ward staff are generally kind to her. In other words, if the staff involved treat her appropriately, she may come to accept their support. Appropriate treatment is likely to involve medication, but it will also involve the right sort of approach, and thus manifests the requisite virtues. Staff will have to show her a good deal of charity and benevolence; they should be just towards her and act with integrity in the face of her accusations and unwillingness to comply with medication. With this approach there should develop, albeit tentatively, a relationship that is likely to be therapeutic. If so, to this extent, it will be possible to talk of relationship and shared understanding.

However, there are two cautionary notes. First, although it is usually possible to form a therapeutic relationship even in such a case, it may still be that the narratives of the staff and of Mrs Rodgers remain incommensurable; even if the staff appreciate her perspective, they may not be able to share it. If no true therapeutic alliance can be established, the need for some form of compulsory treatment

will persist. The staff must still act with compassion, honesty, and integrity towards her, but some forms of compulsion may continue to have to be used. Treating her within a legal framework, with the protections that this provides, is part of what it is to act with professional integrity.

But the second cautionary note is that we cannot be complacent in the knowledge that we are acting within the law. Steinert *et al.* (2005) compared attitudes to compulsory admission and treatment in schizophrenia in four European countries. The differences between countries were highly significant. Participants in Hungary and England were much more likely to agree with compulsion, whereas people in Germany and Switzerland were less likely to do so. The authors concluded that traditions and personal attitudes, perhaps fashioned by a mixture of political and media pressure, underpinned the use of compulsory procedures. It may be, then, that from within our own professional and legal frameworks we do not notice the extent to which we are acting in ways that do not show respect and compassion.

The history of psychiatric abuse, for instance in the former Soviet Union (Bloch, 1991), should mean that we are attuned to the possibility of going too far in the exercise of our civil powers. To appeal to the political system that gives legitimacy to our practice is precisely what the Soviet doctors (and the Nazis) were able to do. In a potentially corrective manner the notion of human flourishing, which is the aim of the virtues, suggests creativity, inspiration, difference, diversity, and even dissent perhaps.

Returning to the notion of capacity, some have suggested that it should be used as the yardstick to decide whether compulsory treatment is warranted. That is, according to this viewpoint, mental health legislation should simply be mental capacity legislation. The important argument in favour of this idea is that it would help to ameliorate some of the stigma of mental illness. If a person lacks capacity, whether through a mental illness or through some physical disorder (a head injury or stroke for instance), they would—under such proposals—be dealt with in accordance with capacity legislation. Contrariwise, if someone with a mental illness were nevertheless able to demonstrate decisional capacity then, just as would be the case if they were capacitous but physically ill, he or she would be free to make the decision. There would be no distinction in the way that people were dealt with whether they had a mental or physical illness (Doyal and Sheather, 2005).

The reason for returning to our discussion of capacity is that Dickenson and Fulford (2000) have worried that the adoption of generic criteria of incapacity might be 'a recipe for the values of the majority being imposed on the minority'. Dickenson and Fulford (2000, p. 88) continue:

> …as the abuse of psychiatry in the former USSR showed …the risks here will be especially large if the value judgements concerned are not recognized for what they are – if the generic incapacity criteria are thought to be objective scientific criteria and a matter solely for expert witnesses to determine.

The concern is that capacity judgements carry with them the aura of being objective, whereas their value commitments are profound and complex. In connection with anorexia nervosa, but in keeping with our comments above about the importance of professional virtues, Tan and Hope (2006) state:

> …capacity is not the main factor in determining whether patients feel they benefit from compulsory treatment. Instead, respect from and

trust in professionals and the context are all important in determining whether compulsory treatment is experienced as helpful and appropriate.

Meanwhile, the decision to move someone with only mild to moderate dementia into long-term care can be made with alacrity on the basis of a single assessment of capacity and with no real checks (Stewart, 2006). This should help to reinforce the message that the attributes of the physician will be vital in terms of allowing the person with dementia to participate as fully as possible in the decisions that are being made.

This has been referred to as 'geriatric assent', which requires that particular virtues are cultivated. Coverdale *et al.* (2006) highlight *self-effacement*, which involves supporting the patient's values; *self-sacrifice*, which does away with self-interest and allows the psychiatrist to tolerate foreboding when risks have to be taken; and *steadiness*, a virtue suggested by the Scottish physician-ethicist, Dr John Gregory (1724–1773), which involves self-control in the face of risks. 'Steadiness' has also been called 'detached concern', which leads us to add that it needs to be complemented by the virtues of compassion and humility if it is not to be felt as coldness.

This takes us back to Mrs Rodgers with her paranoid delusions. If we are going to treat her against her wishes it is as well to do so within a legal and professional framework. But the putative objectivity of these frameworks does not establish their justice. The use of compulsion, remember, is determined by traditions and personal attitudes (Steinert *et al.*, 2005). Legal and professional frameworks can become perverted. The value judgements involved in estimations of mental incapacity and mental illness are diverse rather than shared and, to avoid the possibility of minority views and attitudes being ignored, legal and professional frameworks must allow room for diversity. This requires just those virtues that will help to make possible for Mrs Rodgers shared understandings and relationships, which will be therapeutic and which, moreover, provide the underpinning ethical basis to treatment.

## Resource allocation

In case the idea that the interests of the minority might be subsumed by those of the majority seems unduly pessimistic, consider the words of a highly influential health economist arguing in favour of rationing on the basis of age: 'So the values of the citizenry as a whole must override the values of a particular interest group within it' (Williams, 1997). Opposing this view, the similarly influential geriatrician Grimley Evans (1997) argued against, '…the exclusion from treatment on the basis of a patient's age without reference to his or her physiological condition'. Grimley Evans (1997) was keener to stress, 'the equality of citizens in their relation to the institutions of the state' and 'the uniqueness of individuals regardless of their physical or mental attributes'. The arguments about rationing and old age continue [and have been discussed briefly in Hope and Oppenheimer (1997) and in Hughes (2002); with a more sustained critique in Lesser (1999)], and the main arguments have been summarized by Clarke (2001), who plumps for the 'prudential lifespan argument', which 'defends rationing by age in certain circumstances'. She argues:

> Rationing life-sustaining treatment by age, unlike differential treatment by race or gender, does not create inequalities between persons when it is applied over a lifespan because we all age. Therefore, denying older people access to highly technical life-sustaining treatment

could enhance lifetime well-being and in certain circumstances be both prudent and just.

Clarke (2001)

Welfare economics has been dominated by the quality adjusted life years (QALY) approach, which is broadly utilitarian, and according to which resource allocation decisions should be aimed at maximizing QALYs. This is the approach used in England and Wales by the National Institute for Health and Clinical Excellence (NICE). It has led, at the time of writing, to the determination that cholinesterase inhibitors, whilst showing modest efficacy, are not cost-effective for everyone with Alzheimer's disease. The allegation has long been that QALYs are inherently ageist because, all other things being equal, they discriminate against someone precisely because they are old. A newer approach, which is gaining favour, is to look at capabilities. As described by Anand (2005), this theory has at its core '…the idea that what people can do (capabilities), as opposed to what they actually do (functionings), should be the focus of well-being evaluations and government policy'.

Although considering capabilities will bring into the discussion factors related to age, this is not necessarily discriminatory. Rather, the approach offers a framework to accommodate considerations of well-being, and allows recognition of how the capabilities that people wish to develop can vary across the population in a number of ways.

Anand (2005) describes how the capabilities approach can be applied to individual medical decisions, but an inherent difficulty at the macroeconomic level of resource allocation is that the approach finally makes suggestions that are applicable to populations. The obvious complaint is that the decisions made are likely, as in the case of the NICE guidance on the use of cholinesterase inhibitors, to be unjust towards particular individuals. Furthermore, the decisions themselves reflect political commitments that are not inevitably protective of minority interests. As Oppenheimer (1999, p. 324) has commented:

> The obvious absurdity and inhumanity of the proposition (when it is starkly put) that 'older people are nothing more than a drain on society' doesn't unfortunately prevent it creeping in, half-believed and mostly unspoken, to the political and administrative decisions which affect the allocation of resources to illness in old age – and especially to the dementing illnesses.

She goes on to say: 'Alertness to ethical issues in old age psychiatry brings a constant realization that…our patients are unwanted and unloved' (p. 325).

Although resource allocation is crucial to treatment—as people with dementia (and their carers) who will not be able to receive cholinesterase inhibitors because of NICE guidance know, and as those who ought to be receiving psychological therapies for conditions such as depression and anxiety should know – it is unconcerned by the need for relationships and shared understandings since it does not deal with individuals. There can, of course, be a degree of mutual understanding over allocation issues on the basis of public information and social consensus. But there is rarely a unanimous opinion and dissenting voices, reflecting diverse views and values, should be heard. The views of older people need to be accommodated (Bowling *et al.*, 2002; Werntoft *et al.*, 2005); and the evidence that individual older people suffer from ageism (e.g. Bond *et al.*, 2003) yet will benefit from treatment and investigation (e.g. Yoong and Heymann, 2005) should be highlighted. But the voices of dissent might only be heard at the level of the individual clinical encounter, where relationships and shared understandings certainly will count, and where older people with unmet needs who suffer from inequity will still deserve support and advocacy.

## Research

The potential for people to participate in research occurs at any stage of the illness. But it often arises in connection with treatment, when it can raise particular problems related to consent. Once again, this can seem like a thoroughly legalistic concern, but our emphasis will remain on the need for understanding and relationship.

Whilst on the one hand there are increasingly stringent safeguards covering research on people who lack capacity, on the other there are more people speaking out in favour of lessening the regulation in case beneficial research is stifled (Barron *et al.*, 2004; Hougham, 2005).

A survey of professionals and lay people serving on research ethics committees in Sweden showed fairly uniform responses (for instance in connection with the balancing of risks and benefits), but some statistically significant differences emerged (Peterson and Wallin, 2003). The lay people tended to be against legal proxies and proxies who did not have knowledge of the person's previous values; experts were more willing to allow people with moderate to severe dementia to enter placebo-controlled trials. The differences might be explained by saying that the experts were more able to assess and tolerate risk, but were less attuned to the importance of values and relationships. It might also be that experts are simply less impressed by the need for protection.

Pucci *et al.* (2001) found that 70% of patients with mild to moderate Alzheimer's disease deemed to be eligible for a randomized control trial were unable to demonstrate a minimal understanding of the research procedures. Meanwhile, 70% of the caregivers, without evidence of cognitive or thought disorders, were found unable to demonstrate an understanding of basic elements of the research. Pucci *et al.* (2001) wondered whether this implied that exhaustive accounts of research methodology might be irrelevant to potential research participants. Instead it might be more beneficial to focus on consent 'discussions' (Hougham, 2005), or the sort of 'assent' referred to by Coverdale *et al.* (2006).

Sugarman *et al.* (2001) considered the very different motivations that lay behind proxies giving consent for someone to participate in research. They state:

> Proxies indicated that understanding the research was not as important as their hopes for the benefits it might bring, and their trust in the doctors and institutions conducting the research.

The researchers were struck by the lack of clarity concerning who actually made the decisions to participate. One proxy, speaking of the research participant's understanding, said:

> She had a very general global idea of what we were talking about and it did not run counter to something she was willing to do.
>
> Sugarman *et al.* (2001)

But should we be troubled by a degree of vagueness? Surrogate decision-making, even when the risks and burdens for the participants

are significant, seems to be acceptable to people who are at risk of developing dementia (Kim *et al.* 2005). According to Kim *et al* (2005) lay people are capable of appreciating risk, tend to accept it, but would be more protective towards a loved one than towards themselves. The use of surrogates for research, when supported by 'assent discussions' involving the person with dementia, therefore, might seem like a very reasonable way forward. One surprising finding in Sugarman *et al.* (2001) was that the respondents did not seem to put much weight on the commonly used distinction (cf. Mental Capacity Act 2005) between research that directly benefits the participant and that which does not do so.

The uncertainties about proxy consent might well be diminished if research advance directives were used. Stocking *et al.* (2006) showed that this would be acceptable to patients and proxies. On the whole, in the context of joint discussions, the patients were willing to 'defer future decisions to trusted proxies'. This was true even amongst a group who had previously said they would not cede their decision-making to the proxies. If, however, the reason for not wishing to be enrolled in a study was because of discomfort they were more likely to retain decisional control. Patients also handed over control even when they disagreed with the proxy during a separate initial interview. Stocking *et al.* (2006) concluded that the tendency to defer control of decision-making should be reassuring to researchers, who have to rely on proxy advice, 'but it is important to stay mindful that a sizeable minority do wish to retain control of their decisions'.

On the one hand, therefore, it is possible to have considerable sympathy with those who feel that research is becoming over-regulated. It is entirely reasonable to point to the benefits and acceptability of more relaxed, informal procedures, which would indeed recognize the importance of the person's well-established relationships and would do justice to the extent to which there can be shared understandings even if legal tests might not be satisfied. On the other hand, however, the dissenting voices still need to be heard and protected because, although public altruism is strong, it needs nurturing and 'public trust is fragile and needs to be protected' (Cayton and Denegri, 2003)

## Summary

Cayton and Denegri's (2003) emphasis on 'communication with, respect for and partnership with patients and research participants' chimes well with our theme of relationship and shared understanding being the ethical bedrock of treatment. So, too, does their championing of 'the relationship of trust that exists between patients and their doctors, nurses and therapists'.

# Developments

Chronic deteriorating diseases have to be lived with. As dementia progresses a number of different issues can arise that all create a similar dilemma, which is mainly to do with safety and the need to balance risks against and benefits.

> We have to balance this risk versus personal safety, and sometimes I think people – myself included – we look at the risks more than allowing a person a little bit of freedom which might have a risk attached to it. [wife]

This encapsulates a good aspiration, which is to allow the person with dementia as much freedom as possible. And yet, as is shown by studies of restraint (Kirkevold *et al.*, 2004), far too often care is provided in a way that undermines freedom. By so doing it undermines personhood too. In this area, therefore, there are marked clashes involving ethical principles and theories.

## Wandering

The classic case is wandering. (We should note in passing the very important point that terms such as 'wandering' do no service to people with dementia because of the implication that the behaviour lacks purpose and meaning, whereas it might have both. Furthermore, there are good research reasons to discriminate between so-called 'challenging behaviours' rather than lump them together.) This husband made the decision to keep his wife safe, but then had to reap the consequences in terms of her frustration and alarm at discovering she was, in effect, imprisoned:

> Well I felt bad about locking the doors but on the other hand I realised that it was for her protection. I couldn't let her out. And the thing then, you see, was once she knew that I'd got the door locked then of course she'd start to thump the door and thump me and scream and call for the police and all sorts of things. And I had a terrible job to try and calm her down.

Alternatively, another husband plumped for freedom:

> Well, I used to say to the carers who came in, 'Don't stop my wife going out at all, just go with her'. It's quite simple really; stop them getting into danger, yes, by whatever means you have to but certainly not restrict their freedom. Definitely not. Let her go is my philosophy. If it's raining take an umbrella, but don't restrict what she wants to do, because she's not a prisoner, she's my wife. So, yeah, plenty of freedom but with care.

Now it certainly should not be presumed that the first husband was wrong, because it is often the case that the dangers associated with people 'wandering' are very real. Nevertheless, first, there may be other ways to deal with wandering beyond mere incarceration. Secondly, even if in many cases the means of preventing wandering, such as electronic tagging, could be ethically justified, there remain libertarian concerns (Hughes and Louw, 2002b). Once more we have to be in the business, from the ethical perspective, of recognizing diversity and vulnerability.

In a systematic review of the non-pharmacological means of preventing wandering in dementia, Robinson *et al.* (2006) also considered the ethical implications and acceptability of various methods. From the ethical point of view, where conclusions were based on both the literature review and focus groups, exercise and distraction therapies were the most acceptable interventions, raising no ethical concerns. Physical restraints were considered unacceptable. And there were considerable ethical concerns expressed over the use of electronic tagging and tracking devices and physical barriers. Interestingly, some of these concerns may represent cohort effects. For example, older people with dementia in the focus group said that electronic devices, such as mobile phones, might be more confusing for them, whereas they would not object to identity cards because they remembered having to carry them in the Second World War.

## Driving

Driving is taken for granted by many of us, but losing the ability to drive means more to people than just having to find a new way to get around. The loss of this ability involves a loss of individual independence and a constriction of the person's world:

> Losing the car was incredibly traumatic for my mother because it summed everything up for her. It was independence, freedom, being in control of herself. I think it was all put into driving. [daughter]

Some people with dementia and their carers find it easier to come to terms with the loss of driving if the person has been thoroughly assessed at a driving assessment centre rather than if they are simply told (seemingly) on a whim not to drive. This makes sense because of the evidence that people in the milder stages of dementia can still drive safely (see Chapter 44). The process of assessment, when undertaken with care, can be a way of recognizing the person's standing as an individual who requires respect, even if unsafe driving has to be stopped (Snyder, 2005).

## Inappropriate behaviour

A variety of behaviours in dementia are regarded as 'inappropriate' or 'challenging'. Family carers can be sophisticated in their responses to such behaviours (Baldwin *et al.*, 2005, pp. 29–33). But you should ask who the problem is a problem for, because it makes a difference if a third party is concerned. On the other hand, there is no reason to put up with stigmatizing responses. Sometimes it is best to 'go with the flow', if for instance the person wishes to dress in an unconventional fashion. Where there is violence, however, or inappropriate sexual behaviour, it becomes necessary to intervene. Again the ethical issue concerns the point at which the intervention should come; but also the manner of intervention and how it is delivered need to be considered.

## Going into long-term care

One of the most difficult responses to the deterioration of behaviour in dementia is when the carer has to think about long-term care. This is a cause of considerable guilt on the part of family carers and emphasizes the differences in perspective between family and professional carers (Hughes *et al.*, 2002a). Family carers carry a considerable burden, and it may be that some of this reflects the ethical issues with which they have to deal (Hughes *et al.*, 2002b). Professionals do not tend to make the sort of promises that this daughter describes and do not, therefore, experience the remorse she must then feel:

> Now we had promised Mum that we would never put her in a home, so you have to renege on your promises. [daughter]

The guilt that goes along with these decisions is not something professionals can share, because they do not share the reciprocal relationship that the carer experiences.

Carers do, of course, recognize the benefits of long-term care, sometimes in terms of the improvement in relationships:

> Because somebody else was providing the physical care, we were then better able to maintain our relationship with her, I think. [daughter]

It certainly remains true that carers can stay involved. They often feel the need to advocate on behalf of the person they love:

> So as a relative you have to be the advocate for your relative and make sure she's not harmed in any way. [daughter]

But the need to advocate is, in part, a reflection of the poor quality of care often provided in 'care' homes (Ballard *et al.*, 2001). A more radical point is simply this: if people do not wish to go into long-term care—in the absence of reasons for compulsion—they ought not to be forced:

> I don't honestly think, unless people are a danger to themselves or other people, that they should be forced to live somewhere that they don't want to live. [wife]

And yet, for many older people the reality is that they must put up with unstimulating environments and low levels of care in institutions because there is seemingly neither the will, nor are there the resources, to support them in their own homes or to improve the quality of care in institutions. So the choice facing the carers of some people with dementia is whether to risk unsafe behaviour at home (violence say) or see the person they care for being 'placed' into a safer, but restricted, environment, one in which the risks to the person's individuality are significantly increased beyond those caused by their brain pathology.

### Weighing up

The dilemmas in this section can readily be discussed in terms of the principles of medical ethics; but it is hard to see on what basis we shall be able to say that we should respect the person's autonomy here, but be beneficent there. We might apply the utilitarian felicific calculus to work out which option will maximize pleasure; or we might wish to appeal to this or that duty. These options will supposedly tell us the right action to take. And this is what is wrong with them.

Not only are the definitions of pleasure or duty arguable, but the suggestion that the outcome of the dilemma is 'right' should, if we have really engaged with the dilemma from the perspectives of those concerned, cause us to pause.

According to virtue ethics the key thing is going to be some conception of the good life for human beings. If someone is placed in a dilemma between two options where neither seems good, even if he or she makes what many would consider to be the *right* decision (e.g. to put mother into a home), it may be *difficult* to describe the action as *good*. It is important to note that virtue ethics might equally suggest the person should seek some alternative: perhaps enough complaints in the right political direction will encourage the local social services to find more money for adequate support at home. But it may be that the right decision, in a sense, leaves one's life marred. Hursthouse (1999, pp. 76–7), discussing tragic dilemmas, puts it thus:

> …to say that there are some dilemmas from which even a virtuous agent cannot emerge having acted well is just to say that there are some from which even a virtuous agent cannot emerge with her life unmarred…simply in virtue of the fact that her life presented her with *this* choice, and was thereby marred, or perhaps even ruined.

If, after a long and happy marriage, a husband finds himself having to restrain his wife physically, use medication to sedate her, and finally agree to her being admitted into an institution, his life may be ruined. At any point it could be argued that the virtuous agent might have acted differently—with more courage, charity, or practical wisdom—but this is not inevitable. The circumstances (and narrative) are tragic to the extent that it was inevitable that this virtuous man had to act as he did. He did not thereby act badly, because he did not take the decisions lightly, as the callous husband would have done, instead he felt immense regret and pain.

This view is encouraged by the narrative approach, which seeks to understand the meaning of actions from the context of the persons involved. Hence we have a more human account of these dilemmas, in which the need for fortitude and fidelity and the other virtues come into play, and where the possibility of regret is acknowledged. But so too is the possibility that the same virtues might allow someone to pick themselves up and continue to seek the good in life despite its tragedies.

## Endings

> I wish I knew more abut what the bitter end might look like, because I'm the sort of person who needs to, needs to know. I'm not frightened by it. I might not like the sound of it, but I need to know what's up ahead because I think if you're forewarned, you're forearmed. [wife]

Old age psychiatry often deals with death (Black and Jolley, 1990). In the case of dementia this is inevitable, but decisions about (for instance) suspending life-sustaining treatment crop up in other areas. For instance, in liaison psychiatry, if someone is refusing treatment questions might arise concerning whether the person has capacity or whether he or she is depressed. The decision about how energetically to treat someone with marked depressive symptoms who is also severely ill physically and likely to die is never easy.

The notion of palliative care in dementia has been gaining ground (Hughes *et al.*, 2005). The evidence base for a number of the decisions that arise in this context is building (Volicer and Hurley, 1998; Hughes, 2006a). These include decisions about how to treat fevers, the use of artificial nutrition and hydration, the place of resuscitation, and the recognition and treatment of pain. Much of the relevant literature, including ethical issues, has recently been reviewed (Robinson *et al.*, 2005). Exactly how palliative care should be provided in the context of dementia is not obvious (Sampson *et al.*, 2005). The nature of the ethical issues, however, and the philosophical motivation underlying the need for palliative care in dementia is clearer (Purtilo and ten Have, 2004), and it is to these topics that we shall turn before concluding.

The ethical question in the context of palliative care is typically: how far should we go? One way to frame this question is in terms of the doctrine of ordinary and extraordinary means, according to which it is morally obligatory to take ordinary means, but not to take extraordinary. Procedures should be regarded as extraordinary when they,

> …no longer correspond to the real situation of the patient, either because they are by now disproportionate to any expected results or because they impose an excessive burden on the patient and…family.
>
> John Paul II (1995)

To forego investigations or treatment under this sort of circumstance is to express 'acceptance of the human condition in the face of death' (John Paul II, 1995).

The notion of 'the real situation of the patient', presented here in a Catholic doctrine, is at the heart of the issue from other perspectives too. For instance, on the grounds that tube feeding is otiose in people with advanced dementia, Gillick (2001) used the Jewish distinction between being moribund (*goses*) and being in an incurable state (*treifah*) to argue that in severe dementia artificial nutrition and hydration would be neither natural, nor necessary. The judgement required here would be easily recognized from a secular viewpoint too: few people would wish to stop worthwhile treatment too soon, but 'the face of death' also has to be accepted.

What is required, therefore, is a proper appreciation of the full context and situation of any particular patient. This sounds remarkably like the recommendation that the person's narrative (medical, cultural, social, religious, and so on) must be taken into consideration and entered into. One way in which this can be done is if the person has completed an advance statement of values (see Rich, 1991). Such a statement goes further than an advance refusal of treatment in that it need not be as specific concerning the exact nature of the refusal and the circumstances of its application. The worry about advance refusals of treatment, which is how advance directives are normally conceived, is their specific nature. This entails that they can easily be ignored on the grounds that the circumstances that apply at the time are not the ones anticipated in the advance refusal; or they might be used without discrimination, even though the circumstances might have subtly altered. Nevertheless, advance directives (with or without broader statements of value) have gradually been accepted as an important way for people to plan their care (Vollman, 2001). The evidence (from a vignette study in Europe) is that a relatively large number of doctors do not act in accordance with the previously expressed wishes of patients, but that this varies within and between countries (Richter *et al.*, 2001). Similarly, in Japan, physicians report a wide variety of concerns over the use of 'living wills' (Masuda *et al.*, 2003). A possible conclusion, therefore, is that advance directives can only be regarded as one means to achieving the end of better communication with and more respect for patients and their values. Understanding the person's narrative more fully is a way of gaining some purchase on the values that permeate the person's life.

Broadly speaking, then, the question about how far we should go has to be answered by pointing to where we are in the trajectory of the person's life. Whilst this may seem unobjectionable, some people have the concern that judgements will be made about the quality of the person's life. This concern is evident again in different religious traditions, for instance both Catholic (Jeffery, 2001) and Jewish (Kunin, 2003). And it reflects a more general concern that quality of life is a multifaceted and complex notion: a concern that flies in the face of the trend to try to measure it by operationalized tests (Bond and Corner, 2004).

What we now naturally come to, therefore, are the underlying philosophical motivations for encouraging palliative care in dementia (Hughes, 2006b). The main motivation is the desire to continue to think of the individual person. In which case, these comments broaden in their relevance to include people in general and, therefore, should be relevant to all older people, *especially* if they are vulnerable through mental illness.

To be a person is to be situated in numerous fields, picked out by one's personal narrative and the narratives with which one's own story interacts. It is also to be an embodied agent (Hughes, 2001). Both notions are important: our agency links with our sense of autonomy; and the fact of our embodiment means that we are not separate from our biological narratives, which will be as crucial to our lives as our psychosocial histories. This broad conceptualization of personhood is relevant to discussions of a range of ethical issues (Hughes, 2002); it supports, for instance, the requirement that assessment of quality of life needs to be individualized and open in the way that the possibilities of personhood are uncircumscribed: there are always different ways to exercise personhood (Hughes, 2003).

The situated embodied agent view of the person builds on and is supported by those philosophies that reject a narrow account of personal identity (Lesser, 2006), and those that use broader conceptions (e.g. Merleau-Ponty's ideas about the 'body subject') of personhood (Matthews, 2006). These broader approaches, which stand over against 'hypercognitivism', also encourage the holism that is part and parcel of a hospice approach (Post, 2000) and should engender respect for older people even in the face of forgetfulness (Post, 2006). This is more than theorizing, however, because the broader approach affects our understanding of what it is to be person-centred (Brooker, 2004). In turn this alerts us to the need to maintain the person's self-hood through our approach (Sabat, 2006) and to focus on the person's abilities and strengths as a citizen (Downs *et al.*, 2006). The broad view of the person encourages a narrative approach. We understand people through the stories they tell. In dementia this might require greater efforts of interpretation, but meaning-making remains possible (Widdershoven and Berghmans, 2006).

The possibility of controlling how the person's story might end requires again a focus on 'the real situation'. Whether assisted dying should be allowed in any form will depend on views about the human goods we should be aiming at. There can be little doubt that palliative care, where the aim is to decrease suffering, increase well-being, and not to hasten death but not to prevent it, would be in keeping with a virtuous approach. The worry about voluntary assisted euthanasia is that by removing the prohibition on intentional killing of the innocent, it unpicks the fabric of civil society (Keown, 2002). In so doing it makes non-voluntary euthanasia more likely, because there could be no *principled* objection to it. But it also undermines common, current judgements about ways in which we can flourish as human beings: by courage or fortitude, by charity, compassion, humility, steadfastness, and by the avoidance of light mindedness.

## Conclusion

In this chapter we have discussed a number of ethical issues that arise in the practice of old age psychiatry, along with some of the underlying philosophy. We have commended a narrative and virtue ethics approach. One of the benefits of this approach is that it requires us to get down to the nitty-gritty of clinical practice. The voices of family carers have helped us in this regard. They help to confirm the view that most ethical difficulties are not to be found in the major dilemmas that are frequently debated, but in the narratives of our ordinary lives (Komesaroff, 1995). It is here that we can exercise the virtues—by compassionate caring and understanding—and flourish as human beings.

> But if you can do more coaxing and keep your patience then that's a good thing, that is really a good thing. Because they don't know they are irritating you, they just think they're doing whatever they want to do I suppose. ...It's having a lot of patience and doing it with a good heart. Well, you must do it with a good heart because you love them I suppose. [husband]

## Acknowledgements

This chapter makes use of quotes from carers interviewed by Clive Baldwin during research undertaken at Ethox, University of Oxford, between 2001 and 2004. The quotes are used with permission of the participants in the research. We should like to express our gratitude to the Alzheimer's Society who funded the research, and to acknowledge very warmly our collaborators: Professor Tony Hope, Professor Robin Jacoby, and Sue Ziebland. The opinions expressed in this chapter are, however, our own. Further details of the research are contained in our references as cited.

## References

Agich, G.J. (2003). *Dependence and autonomy in old age: an ethical framework for long-term care*. Cambridge University Press, Cambridge.

Anand, P. (2005). Capabilities and health. *Journal of Medical Ethics*, **31**, 299–303.

Anscombe, G.E.M. (1981). Modern moral philosophy. In *The philosophical papers of G.E.M. Anscombe, volume three: ethics, religion and politics*, pp. 26–42. Blackwell, Oxford. (First published in 1958, *Philosophy*, **33**, 1–19.)

Ashcroft, R.E., Dawson, A., Draper, H., and McMillan, J. R.(eds) (2007). *Principles of health care ethics*, 2nd edn. John Wiley & Sons, Chichester.

Baldwin, C. (2004). Competing narratives in cases of alleged Munchausen syndrome by proxy. In *Narrative research in health and illness* (ed. V. Skultans, B. Horowitz, and T. Greenhalgh), pp. 205–22. British Medical Journal, London.

Baldwin, C. (2005a). Narrative, ethics and people with severe mental illness. *Australian and New Zealand Journal of Psychiatry*, **39**, 1022–9.

Baldwin, C. (2005b). Who needs fact when you've got narrative? The case of P,C&S vs United Kingdom. *International Journal for the Semiotics of the Law*, **18**, 217–41.

Baldwin, C., Hope, T., Hughes, J., Jacoby, R., and Ziebland, S. (2004). Ethics and dementia: the experience of family carers. *Progress in Neurology and Psychiatry*, **8**, 24–8.

Baldwin, C., Hope, T., Hughes, J., Jacoby, R., and Ziebland, S. (2005). *Making difficult decisions: the experience of caring for someone with dementia*. Alzheimer's Society, London.

Ballard, C., Fossey, J., Chithramohan, R., *et al.* (2001). Quality of care in private sector and NHS facilities for people with dementia: cross sectional survey. *British Medical Journal*, **323**, 426–7.

Bamford, C., Lamont, S., Eccles, M., Robinson, L., May, C., and Bond, J. (2004). Disclosing a diagnosis of dementia: a systematic review. *International Journal of Geriatric Psychiatry*, **19**, 151–69.

Barron, J.S., Duffey, P.L., Byrd, L.J., Campbell, R., and Ferrucci, L. (2004). Informed consent for research participation in frail older persons. *Aging Clinical and Experimental Research*, **16**, 79–85.

Barthes, R. (1977). Introduction to the structural analysis of narratives. In *Image, music, text: essays* (transl. S. Heath), pp. 79–124. Fontana Press, London.

Bavidge, M. (2006). Ageing and human nature. In *Dementia: mind, meaning, and the person* (ed. J.C. Hughes, S.J. Louw, and S.R. Sabat), pp. 41–53. Oxford University Press, Oxford.

Beauchamp, T.L. and Childress, J.F. (2001). *Principles of biomedical ethics*, 5th edn. Oxford University Press, Oxford.

Black, D. and Jolley, D. (1990) Slow euthanasia? The deaths of psychogeriatric patients. *British Medical Journal*, **300**, 1321–3.

Bloch, S. (1991). The political misuse of psychiatry in the Soviet Union. In *Psychiatric ethics*, 2nd edn (ed. S. Bloch and P. Chodoff), pp. 493–515. Oxford University Press, Oxford.

Bond, J. and Corner, L. (2004). *Quality of life and older people*. Open University Press, Maidenhead.

Bond, M., Bowling, A., McKee, D. *et al.* (2003). Does ageism affect the management of ischaemic heart disease? *Journal of Health Services Research and Policy*, **8**, 40–7.

Bowling, A., Mariotto, A., and Evans, O. (2002). Are older people willing to give up their place in the queue for cardiac surgery to a younger person? *Age and Ageing*, **31**, 187–92.

Brindle, N. and Holmes, J. (2005). Capacity and coercion: dilemmas in the discharge of older people with dementia from general hospital settings. *Age and Ageing*, **34**, 16–20.

Brooker, D. (2004). 'What is person centred care?' *Reviews in Clinical Gerontology*, **13**, 215–22.

Bruner, J. (1994). *Acts of meaning*. Harvard University Press, Cambridge, MA.

Bruner, J. (2004). Life as narrative. *Social Research*, **71**, 691–710.

Campbell, A., Gillett, G., and Jones, G. (2005). *Medical ethics*, 4th edn. Oxford University Press Australia and New Zealand, Melbourne.

Cayton, H. and Denegri, S. (2003). Is what's mine my own? *Journal of Health Services Research & Policy*, **8**(Suppl. 1), S1:33–5.

Charland, L.C. (1998). Appreciation and emotion: theoretical reflections on the MacArthur Treatment Competence Study. *Kennedy Institute of Ethics Journal*, **8**, 359–76.

Clarke, C.M. (2001). Rationing scarce life-sustaining resources on the basis of age. *Journal of Advanced Nursing*, **35**, 799–804.

Collopy, B.J. (1988). Autonomy in long term care: some crucial distinctions. *Gerontologist*, **28**(Suppl.), 10–17.

Corner, L. and Bond, J. (2006). The impact of the label of mild cognitive impairment on the individual's sense of self. *Philosophy, Psychiatry, & Psychology*, **13**, 3–12.

Coverdale, J., McCullough, L.B., Molinari, V., and Workman, R. (2006). Ethically justified clinical strategies for promoting geriatric assent. *International Journal of Geriatric Psychiatry*, **21**, 151–7.

Culver, C.M. and Gert, B. (2004). Competence. In *The philosophy of psychiatry: a companion* (ed. J. Radden), pp. 258–70. Oxford University Press, Oxford.

Davis, D.S. (1991). Rich cases: the ethics of thick description. *Hastings Center Report*, **21**, 12–17.

Dickenson, D. and Fulford, Bill (K.W.M.) (2000). *In two minds: a casebook of psychiatric ethics*. Oxford, Oxford University Press.

Downs, M., Clare, L., and Mackenzie, J. (2006). Understandings of dementia: explanatory models and their implications for the person with dementia and therapeutic effort. In *Dementia: mind, meaning, and the person* (ed. J.C. Hughes, S.J. Louw, and S.R. Sabat), pp. 235–58. Oxford University Press, Oxford.

Doyal, L. and Sheather, J. (2005). Mental health legislation should respect decision making capacity. *British Medical Journal*, **331**, 1467–9.

Dyer, A.R. and Bloch, S. (1987). Informed consent and the psychiatric patient. *Journal of Medical Ethics*, **13**, 12–16.

Elson, P. (2006). Do older adults presenting with memory complaints wish to be told if later diagnosed with Alzheimer's disease? *International Journal of Geriatric Psychiatry*, **21**, 419–25.

Fulford, K.W.M. (1989). *Moral theory and medical practice*. Cambridge University Press, Cambridge.

Fulford, K.W.M. (Bill) (2004). Facts/values. Ten principles of values-based medicine. In *The philosophy of psychiatry: a companion* (ed. J. Radden), pp. 205–34. Oxford University Press, Oxford.

Gillick, M.R. (2001). Artificial nutrition and hydration in the patient with advanced dementia: is withholding treatment compatible with traditional Judaism? *Journal of Medical Ethics*, **27**, 12–15.

Gillon, R. (1986) *Philosophical medical ethics*. John Wiley and Sons, Chichester.

Goodman, N. (1980). Twisted tales, or, story, study, and symphony. In *On narrative* (ed. W.J.T. Mitchell), pp. 99–115. University of Chicago Press, Chicago.

Graham, J.E. and Ritchie, K. (2006). Mild cognitive impairment: ethical considerations for nosological flexibility in human kinds. *Philosophy, Psychiatry, & Psychology*, **13**, 31–43.

Grimley Evans, J. (1997). The rationing debate: rationing health care by age: the case against. *British Medical Journal*, **314**, 822–5.

Hauerwas, S. and Burrell, D. (1977). From system to story: an alternative pattern for rationality in ethics. In *Truthfulness and tragedy: further investigations in Christian ethics* 9ed. S. Hauerwas), pp.15–39. University of Notre Dame Press, Notre Dame, IN.

Hope, T. and Oppenheimer, C. (1997). Ethics and the psychiatry of old age. In *Psychiatry in the elderly*, 2nd edn (ed. R. Jacoby and C. Oppenheimer), pp. 709–35. Oxford University Press, Oxford.

Hope, T., Savulescu, J., and Hendrick, J. (2003) *Medical ethics and law: the core curriculum*. Churchill Livingstone, Edinburgh.

Hougham, G.W. (2005). Waste not, want not: cognitive impairment should not preclude research participation. *American Journal of Bioethics*, **5**, 36–7.

Hughes, J.C. (2000). Ethics and the anti-dementia drugs. *International Journal of Geriatric Psychiatry*, **15**, 538–43.

Hughes, J.C. (2001). Views of the person with dementia. *Journal of Medical Ethics*, **27**, 86–91.

Hughes, J.C. (2002). Ethics and the psychiatry of old age. In *Psychiatry in the elderly*, 3rd edn (ed. R. Jacoby and C. Oppenheimer), pp. 863–95. Oxford University Press, Oxford.

Hughes, J.C. (2003). Quality of life in dementia: an ethical and philosophical perspective. *Expert Review of Pharmacoeconomics and Outcomes Research*, **3**, 525–34.

Hughes, J.C. ed. (2006a). *Palliative care in severe dementia*. Quay Books, London.

Hughes, J.C. (2006b). Beyond hypercognitivism: a philosophical basis for good quality palliative care in dementia. *Les cahiers de la fondation médéric Alzheimer*, **2**, 17–23.

Hughes, J.C. and Baldwin, C. (2006) *Ethical issues in dementia care: making difficult decisions*. Jessica Kingsley, London.

Hughes, J.C. and Louw, S.J. (2002a). Confidentiality and cognitive impairment: professional and philosophical ethics. *Age and Ageing*, **31**, 147–50.

Hughes, J.C. and Louw, S. J. (2002b). Electronic tagging of people with dementia who wander. *British Medical Journal*, **325**, 847–8.

Hughes, J.C., Hope, T., Reader, S., and Rice, D. (2002a). Dementia and ethics: a pilot study of the views of informal carers. *Journal of the Royal Society of Medicine*, **95**, 242–6.

Hughes, J.C., Hope, T., Savulescu, J., and Ziebland, S. (2002b). Carers, ethics and dementia: a survey and review of the literature. *International Journal of Geriatric Psychiatry*, **17**, 35–40.

Hughes, J.C., Robinson, L., and Volicer, L. (2005). Specialist palliative care in dementia. *British Medical Journal*, **330**, 57–8.

Hursthouse, R. (1999). *On virtue ethics*. Oxford University Press, Oxford.

Jeffery, P. (2001). *Going against the stream: ethical aspects of ageing and care*. The Liturgical Press, Collegeville, MN.

John Paul II (1995). *Evangelium vitae*. Libreria Editrice Vaticana, Vatican City.

Kapp, M.B. (2006). Informed consent implications of diagnostic evaluations for dementia. *American Journal of Alzheimer's Disease and Other Dementias*, **21**, 24–7.

Keown, J. (2002). *Euthanasia, ethics and public policy: an argument against legalisation*. Cambridge University Press, Cambridge.

Kim, S.Y.H., Kim, H.M., McCallum, C., and Tariot, P.N. (2005). What do people at risk for Alzheimer disease think about surrogate consent for research? *Neurology*, **65**, 1395–401.

Kirkevold, Ø., Sandvik, L., and Engedal, K. (2004). Use of constraints and their correlates in Norwegian nursing homes. *International Journal of Geriatric Psychiatry*, **19**, 980–8.

Kitwood, T. (1997). *Dementia reconsidered: the person comes first*. Open University Press, Buckingham.

Kirkwood, T.B.L. (2006). Alzheimer's disease, MCI, and the biology of intrinsic ageing. *Philosophy, Psychiatry, & Psychology*, **13**, 79–82.

Komesaroff, P.A. (1995). From bioethics to microethics: ethical debate and clinical medicine. In *Troubled bodies: critical perspectives on postmodernism, medical ethics and the body* (ed. P.A. Komesaroff), pp. 62–86. Duke University Press, Durham, NC.

Kunin, J. (2003). Withholding artificial feeding from the severely demented: merciful or immoral? Contrasts between secular and Jewish perspectives. *Journal of Medical Ethics*, **29**, 208–12.

Lamarque, P.V. (2004). On not expecting too much from narrative. *Mind and Language*, **19**, 393–408.

Lesser, A.H. (ed.) (1999). *Ageing, autonomy and resources*. Ashgate, Aldershot.

Lesser, A.H. (2006). Dementia and personal identity. In *Dementia: mind, meaning, and the person* (ed. J.C. Hughes, S.J. Louw, and S.R. Sabat), pp. 55–61. Oxford University Press, Oxford.

Macintyre, A. (1985). *After virtue: a study in moral theory*, 2nd edn. Duckworth, London.

Malpas, P. (2005). The right to remain in ignorance about genetic information – can such a right be defended in the name of autonomy? *The New Zealand Medical Journal*, **118** (1220) (http://www.nzma.org.nz/journals/118-1220/1611/).

Masuda, Y., Fetters, M.D., Hattori, A. *et al.* (2003). Physicians' reports on the impact of living wills at the end of life in Japan. *Journal of Medical Ethics*, **29**, 248–52.

Matthews, E. (2006). Dementia and the identity of the person. In *Dementia: mind, meaning, and the person* (ed. J.C. Hughes, S.J. Louw, and S.R. Sabat), pp.163–77. Oxford University Press, Oxford.

May, W.F. (1994). The virtues in a professional setting. In *Medicine and moral reasoning* (ed. K.W.M. Fulford, G.R. Gillett, and J.M. Soskice), pp. 75–91. Cambridge University Press, Cambridge.

Nelson, H.L. (2001). *Damaged identities, narrative repair*. Cornell University Press, Ithaca, NY.

Neumann, P.J., Hammitt, J.K., Mueller, C. *et al.* (2001). Public attitudes about genetic testing for Alzheimer's disease. *Health Affairs*, **20**, 252–64.

Oppenheimer, C. (1999). Ethics in old age psychiatry. In *Psychiatric ethics*, 3rd edn (ed. S. Bloch, P. Chodoff, and S.A. Green), pp. 317–43. Oxford University Press, Oxford.

Pellegrino, E.D. and Thomasma, D.C. (1993). *The virtues in medical practice*. Oxford University Press, New York.

Peterson, G. and Wallin, A. (2003). Alzheimer disease ethics – informed consent and related issues in clinical trials: results of a survey among the members of the research ethics committees in Sweden. *International Psychogeriatrics*, **15**, 157–70.

Polkinghorne, D.E. (1988). *Narrative knowing and the human sciences*. SUNY Press, Albany, NY.

Post, S.G. (2000). *The moral challenge of Alzheimer disease: ethical issues from diagnosis to dying*, 2nd edn. Johns Hopkins University Press, Baltimore, MD.

Post, S.G. (2006). *Respectare*: moral respect for the lives of the deeply forgetful. In *Dementia: mind, meaning, and the person* (ed. J.C. Hughes, S.J. Louw, and S.R. Sabat), pp. 223–34. Oxford University Press, Oxford.

Pucci, E., Belardinelli, N., Borsetti, G., Rodriguez, D., and Signorino, M. (2001). Information and competency for consent to pharmacologic clinical trials in Alzheimer disease: an empirical analysis in patients and family caregivers. *Alzheimer Disease and Associated Disorders*, **15**, 146–54.

Purtilo, R.B. and ten Have, H.A.M.J. (2004). *Ethical foundations of palliative care for Alzheimer disease*. Johns Hopkins University Press, Baltimore, MD.

Rankin, J. (2002). What is narrative? Ricoeur, Bakhtin, and process approaches. *Concrescence: The Australasian Journal of Process Thought*, **3**, 1–12.

Rich, B.A. (1991). The values history: a new standard of care. *Emory Law Review*, **40**, 1109–81.

Richter, J., Eisemann, M., and Zgonnikova, E. (2001). Doctors' authoritarianism in end-of-life treatment decisions. A comparison between Russia, Sweden and Germany. *Journal of Medical Ethics*, **27**, 186–91.

Robinson, L., Hughes, J., Daley, S., Keady, J., Ballard, C., and Volicer, L. (2005). End-of-life care and dementia. *Reviews in Clinical Gerontology*, **15**, 135–48.

Robinson, L., Hutchings, D., Corner, L. *et al.* (2006). A systematic literature review of the effectiveness of non-pharmacological interventions to prevent wandering in dementia and evaluation of the ethical implications and acceptability of their use. *Health Technology Assessment*, **10**, 26(August).

Sabat, S.R. (2001). *The experience of Alzheimer's disease: life through a tangled veil*. Blackwell, Oxford.

Sabat, S.R. (2005). Capacity for decision-making in Alzheimer's disease: selfhood, positioning and semiotic people. *Australian and New Zealand Journal of Psychiatry*, **39**, 1030–5.

Sabat, S.R. (2006). Mind, meaning, and personhood in dementia: the effects of positioning. In *Dementia: mind, meaning, and the person* (ed. J.C. Hughes, S.J. Louw, and S.R. Sabat), pp. 287–302. Oxford University Press, Oxford.

Sadler, J.Z. (2005). *Values and psychiatric diagnosis*. Oxford University Press, Oxford.

Sampson, E., Ritchie, C., Lai, R., Raven, P., and Blanchard, M.A. (2005). A systematic review of the scientific evidence for the efficacy of a palliative-care approach in dementia. *International Psychogeriatrics*, **17**, 31–40.

Schneewind, J.B. (1982). Virtue, narrative and community: MacIntyre and morality. *The Journal of Philosophy*, **79**, 653–63.

Schwandt, T.A. (1997). *Qualitative inquiry: a dictionary of terms*. Sage, Thousand Oaks CA.

Snyder, C.H. (2005). Dementia and driving: autonomy versus safety. *Journal of the American Academy of Nurse Practitioners*, **17**, 393–402.

Spence, D.P. (1982). *Narrative truth and historical truth: meaning and interpretation in psychoanalysis*. W.W. Norton, New York.

Steinert, T., Lepping, P., Baranyai, R., Hoffmann, M., and Leherr, H. (2005). Compulsory admission and treatment in schizophrenia: a study of ethical attitudes in four European countries. *Social Psychiatry and Psychiatric Epidemiology*, **40**, 635–41.

Stewart, R. (2006). Mental health legislation and decision-making capacity (letter). *British Medical Journal*, **332**, 118–19.

Stocking, C.B., Hougham, G.W., Danner, D.D., Patterson, M.B., Whitehouse, P.J., and Sachs, G.A. (2006). Speaking of research advance directives: planning for future research participation. *Neurology*, **66**, 1361–6.

Strawson, G. (2004) Against narrativity. *Ratio*, **17**(4), 428–52.

Sugarman, J., Cain, C., Wallace, R., and Welsh-Bohmer K.A. (2001). How proxies make decisions about research for patients with Alzheimer's disease. *Journal of the American Geriatrics Society*, **49**, 1110–19.

Tan, J.O.A. and Hope, T. (2006). Mental health legislation and decision-making capacity. [letter] *British Medical Journal*, **332**, 119.

Tracy, C.S., Drummond, N., Ferris, L.E. *et al.* (2004). To tell or not to tell? Professional and lay perspectives on the disclosure of personal health information in community-based dementia care. *Canadian Journal on Aging/La Revue canadienne du vieillissement*, **23**, 203–15.

Treloar, A., Beats, B., and Philpot, M. (2000). A pill in the sandwich: covert medication in food and drink. *Journal of the Royal Society of Medicine*, **93**, 408–11.

Treloar, A., Philpot, M., and Beats, B. (2001). Concealing medication in patients' food. *Lancet*, **357**, 62–4.

Vallis, J. and Boyd, K. (2002). Ethics and end-of-life decision-making. In *Palliative care for older people in care homes* (ed. J. Hockley and D. Clark), pp. 120–37. Open University Press, Buckingham.

Vellinga, A., Smit, J.H., van Leeuwen, E., van Tilburg, W., and Jonker, C. (2004). Competence to consent to treatment of geriatric patients: judgements of physicians, family members and the vignette method. *International Journal of Geriatric Psychiatry*, **19**, 645–54.

Volicer, L. and Hurley, A. (eds) (1998). *Hospice care for patients with advanced progressive dementia*. Springer, New York.

Vollmann, J. (2001). Advance directives in patients with Alzheimer's disease: ethical and clinical considerations. *Medicine, Health Care and Philosophy*, **4**, 161–7.

Werntoft, E., Hallberg, I.R., Elmstahl, S., and Edberg, A.K. (2005). Older people's views of prioritization in health care. *Aging Clinical and Experimental Research*, **17**, 402–11.

Whitehouse, P.J. (2006). Demystifying the mystery of Alzheimer's as late, no longer MCI. *Philosophy, Psychiatry, & Psychology*, **13**, 87–8.

Widdershoven, G.A.M. and Berghmans, R.L.P. (2006). Meaning-making in dementia: a hermeneutic perspective. In *Dementia: mind, meaning, and the person* (ed. J.C. Hughes, S.J. Louw, and S.R. Sabat), pp. 179–91. Oxford University Press, Oxford.

Widdershoven, G.A.M. and Widdershoven-Heerding, I. (2003). Understanding dementia: a hermeneutic perspective. In *Nature and narrative: an introduction to the new philosophy of psychiatry* (ed. K.W.M. Fulford, K. Morris, J.Z. Sadler, and G. Stanghellini), pp. 103–11. Oxford University Press, Oxford.

Williams, A. (1997). The rationing debate: rationing health care by age: the case for. *British Medical Journal*, **314**, 820–2.

Wolpe, P.R. (1998). The triumph of autonomy in American bioethics: a sociological view. In *Bioethics and society: constructing the ethical enterprise* (ed. R. DeVries and J. Subedi), pp. 38–59. Prentice Hall, Upper Saddle River, NJ.

Yoong, K.K.Y. and Heymann, T. (2005). Colonoscopy in the very old: why bother? *Postgraduate Medical Journal*, **81**, 196–7.

# 39

# Elder maltreatment

Rolf D. Hirsch and Bodo R. Vollhardt

## Introduction

Although elder maltreatment is not a new phenomenon, it has only been given attention in the medical literature in the last three decades, after case descriptions of 'granny battering' were published by a major medical journal (Burston, 1975). Whereas child abuse and spouse abuse had been an issue of concern to society and research since the 1960s and 1970s, the topic of elder maltreatment was recognized only in the 1980s. Limited coverage in the medical literature has been accompanied by limited attention to this topic by the medical profession. Thus, whereas prevalence data suggest that elder abuse is encountered daily by a busy clinician seeing between 20 and 40 older patients a day (Lachs and Pillemer, 2004), 79% of surveyed primary care physicians denied having seen a case of elder abuse in the past 12 months (Kennedy, 2004). Thus, many cases of elder abuse may go undetected through the healthcare system, leaving a dire need for help unattended.

One of the main reasons why physicians are unfamiliar with the problem of elder maltreatment may be a lack of medical education. In a nationwide survey of American emergency physicians (Jones *et al.*, 1997a) only 25% of the respondents indicated that they had received training during the residency on the topic of elder maltreatment, whereas 63% and 87% had received training on spouse abuse and child abuse, respectively. Furthermore, they did not attend continuing medical education on this topic when they went into speciality practice. It was also found that despite requirements for mandatory reporting, applicable state laws were generally not known. That inadequate familiarity of physicians with the problem of elder abuse is not confined to the USA, has been shown by McCreadie *et al.* (2000) in a survey of British general practitioners. Only 39% of the respondents indicated some familiarity with the issue, but 72% indicated interest in additional training and education.

Any situation involving maltreatment of an elderly person is usually complex and multifactorial. Most such situations have a prior history. Usually more than one type of maltreatment is involved (for example physical and psychological abuse). Often, the situation is compounded by passivity and helplessness by all involved, and by unfamiliarity with the possibilities for remedial action. The following case gives an example:

Mr K., a 66-year-old gentleman, has been cared for at home by his wife since he suffered a stroke 2 years ago. A mild dementia has also been present since that time. In the past several weeks, Mr K. has developed a third-degree pressure ulcer. The apartment is in disarray and has became increasingly filthy. Home care has been provided in the last few months and the GP has been making weekly visits to Mr K. who has been suffering pains lately. Subsequently, he has been rather restless, frequently moaning and groaning. His wife has been desperate and has indicated that she cannot take the situation any longer.

The presence in this case of a pressure ulcer indicates the possibility of negligent care. This judgement, however, depends on assessing whether the pressure ulcer could have been prevented and whether timely and adequate treatment was given. Other questions raised by the situation concern the presence of risk factors and whether these had been recognized and adequately attended to. Have preventive routines been used appropriately, such as attention to mobility, sufficient turning, attendance to urinary incontinence? Was it at all appropriate to attempt home care in that setting? Had attention been given to the wife who was overburdened with the situation? The answers to such questions will depend on subjective perceptions and judgements and do not lend themselves easily to an objective decision. The complexity involved may prevent an acknowledgement that a situation of maltreatment is present and, consequently, the opportunity to take appropriate remedial action may be missed.

Elder persons who are dependent on care, especially those suffering from additional psychiatric problems, are usually without the means to help themselves when they are maltreated. They may react with disturbing behaviour, which may then be followed by more maltreatment, for example being placed in restraints. The role of physicians in caring for these patients calls for an awareness of the indicators of maltreatment, familiarity with assessment techniques, as well as knowledge about helpful interventions. These are geared more towards prevention, treatment, and rehabilitation for all parties involved in the maltreatment situation, and less towards a search for perpetrators and their punishment.

## Definition and types of maltreatment

The problem of elder maltreatment has been an issue for politicians, researchers, and professionals from social sciences, law, psychology, and health services alike. Each profession dealing with this problem has tended to produce its own views and definitions, with different shades of meaning, resulting in a disparate terminology and a lack of comparability for data obtained from service providers, statutory agencies, and researchers. This is true even for statute definitions in the USA, where no single term describing elder abuse is used uniformly across all states (Daly and Jogerst, 2001). Definitions have been based on legal, psychological or socio-cultural perspectives. For example, if elder maltreatment is viewed as a crime, the definition of elder maltreatment will then be based on the components *intent*, *injury*, and *causation*. A psychological understanding of this view will include motivational aspects, the role of aggression on the part of the perpetrator, and the harmful consequences for the victim. Whereas these definitions focus on individual aspects, other approaches place the problem into a societal context. Such a perspective emphasizes the role of cultural and social perceptions, and the violation of existing social norms and cultural standards. For practical use, different terms have been established:

*Abuse* is the generic term for statutory use as well as the preferred term in the medical literature. It covers both acts of commission—physical, psychological, sexual, and financial types of damage and infringements—as well as acts of omission—neglect and abandonment. Referring to acts of commission, abuse denotes a corrupt practice, improper or excessive treatment (Merriam-Webster, 2003). There are two aspects of an abuse situation that are encompassed in definitions. One is the concept of a vulnerable adult, i.e. a person in need of care, not able to live independently without help. This aspect is emphasized, for example, in the definition from the National Council on Elder Abuse (NCEA), as given on their website:

> Elder abuse is a term referring to any knowing, intentional, or negligent act by caregiver or any other person that causes harm or a serious risk of harm to a vulnerable adult.

This definition covers adults vulnerable by mental or physical handicaps who cannot help themselves and are therefore in need for protection. Another aspect inherent to a caring relationship is the expectation of trust. This feature is stressed as crucial by the definition from Action on Elder Abuse on their website which is included in the Toronto Declaration (World Health Organization, 2002a):

> …a single or repeated act or lack of appropriate action, occurring within any relationship where there is an expectation of trust, which causes harm or distress to an older person.

The definition excludes strangers as perpetrators of abuse, thereby posing a legal distinction between crime and abuse. This definition of elder abuse and neglect is the most widely accepted and is endorsed by the World Health Organization (WHO) and the International Network for the Prevention of Elder Abuse (INPEA).

*Neglect* refers to acts of omission which result in a failure to provide support for the basic essentials of physical and emotional health and for basic functions in activities of daily living (ADL). Subsumed under this term are active (intentional or reckless) as well as passive acts (lack of knowledge or skills). In the USA, only paid caregivers are liable for neglect, while informal carers such as family members or friends are usually exonerated.

*Self-neglect*, referring to a failure to attend to one's own basic needs or self-care tasks, has been included under the term of neglect

as well. Whereas self-neglect represents the most frequently reported form of elder abuse and neglect in US statistics, this inclusion may be challenged, because of distinct features and risk factors which are generally not shared by victims of abuse and neglect (Longres, 1995; O'Brian *et al.*, 1999; Abrams *et al.*, 2002;). NCEA excludes from this category persons who are mentally competent, so as to include under this term only persons considered to be vulnerable adults and therefore in need for protection under federal statues.

*Mistreatment* indicates any kind of harmful, improper, or incorrect treatment, including all types of abuse and neglect. A panel of the National Research Council has suggested that this term should be used for research, as it avoids the incongruous use of legal definitions. According to this panel, 'elder mistreatment' refers to

> …(a) intentional actions that cause harm or create a serious risk of harm (whether or not harm is intended) to a vulnerable elder by a caregiver or other person who stands in a trust relationship to the elder or (b) failure by a caregiver to satisfy the elders basic needs or to protect the elder from harm.

This term is meant to exclude cases of 'self-neglect' as well as cases of victimization by strangers (National Research Council, 2002).

*Maltreatment* denotes a cruel or rough treatment (Merriam-Webster, 2003 ) and was a term originally introduced in the literature on child abuse. This term is included in the 10th revision of the *International Statistical Classification of Diseases and Related Health Problems* (ICD-10) of the WHO (World Health Organization, 1992) to cover maltreatment cases encountered in medical practice. In this chapter we will use predominantly the term maltreatment as a generic term, and abuse as a special type of maltreatment, in accordance with the nomenclature in ICD-10. A total of six different types of maltreatment are listed in the ICD-10 (see Table 39.1); however, none are supplied with a definition. In this chapter we are therefore using working definitions for the different types of maltreatment discussed (Table 39.2).

*Violence*, denoting an exertion of physical force so as to injure or abuse (Merriam-Webster, 2003) has been mostly used in the literature on family violence. Implied in this term is usually a violation as well, and violence has been viewed within a broader context of the violation of human rights (Krug *et al.*, 2002). Galtung (1990) points out that in addition to violation of human rights, violence may also be viewed as an infringement of basic human needs, including the need for well-being, for personal identity, and personal freedom. Such an infringement is brought about by structural and cultural forces. This perspective sets a useful frame of reference for dealing with elder maltreatment. Rather than being only an interpersonal event, it may also be influenced by a variety of situational and environmental factors. In the nursing home such

**Table 39.1** ICD-10 codes for elder maltreatment

| T 74.- | Maltreatment syndromes |
|--------|------------------------|
| T 74.0 | Neglect or abandonment |
| T 74.1 | Physical abuse |
| T 74.2 | Sexual abuse |
| T 74.3 | Psychological abuse |
| T 74.8 | Other maltreatment syndromes |
| T 74.9 | Maltreatment syndrome, unspecified |

**Table 39.2** Types of elder maltreatment (compiled from Aravanis *et al.* 1992; Fillit and Picariello, 1998; National Council on Elder Abuse, 2000)

| Type of abuse | Definition | Examples | Medical indications |
|---|---|---|---|
| Physical abuse | Forceful acts inflicting pain, injury or impairment | Hitting, pushing, shoving, inappropriate use of drugs or restraints; force feeding, physical punishment | Unexplained bruises or lacerations, injuries bilateral or in various stages of healing, broken eyeglasses, signs of having been restrained, serum drug levels indicating over-medication |
| Sexual abuse | Any kind of forced intimate or sexual contact with a person | Sexual explicit advances such as touching, exposure, assault | Bruises around breasts or genitals, vaginal or rectal bleeding, unexplained venereal disease |
| Psychological (emotional) abuse | Verbal or non-verbal conduct resulting in anguish or distress | Threats, harassment, intimidation, insults, behaviour expressing disinterest in a person, infantilizing behaviour | A sudden change in behaviour of the elder person involving agitation, anxiety, depression, withdrawal, or other unusual behaviour |
| Financial exploitation | Unauthorized use of an elder's funds or property for the personal gain of the caregiver | Withdrawal from bank account, stealing money or possessions, pressuring elder for signature on documents | Substandard care despite availability of adequate financial resources, unfilled prescriptions for medication or for rehabilitation aids |
| Neglect | Failure to provide care for basic needs, optimal function or medical treatments | Inadequate food, fluids, hygiene, clothing, shelter, personal safety, healthcare | Dehydration, malnutrition, bed sores, poor hygiene of person and/or of living environment, inadequate medication administration, unsafe home |
| Violation of personal rights | Ignoring elder's rights or capabilities to make own decisions | Not involving an elder in decision-making, inappropriate handling of guardianship | Forced placement in nursing home, limiting the social contacts of elder |

structural factors may include, among others, inadequate staffing or failure to provide supervision for the support of the nursing staff. Cultural forces arise from beliefs that may be expressed, for example, in views that the elderly are no longer capable of handling their own affairs. In this model, maltreatment may be viewed as the result of an action by a person influenced by structural and cultural forces (Fig. 39.1).

The triangular model, by emphasizing cultural and structural forces as antecedents for maltreatment, tends to de-emphasize personal aspects such as the personality and motivation of the perpetrator, without ignoring the personal responsibility of the maltreating person. The pragmatic implications of this understanding lead to a frame of reference for remedial interventions based on four tenets:

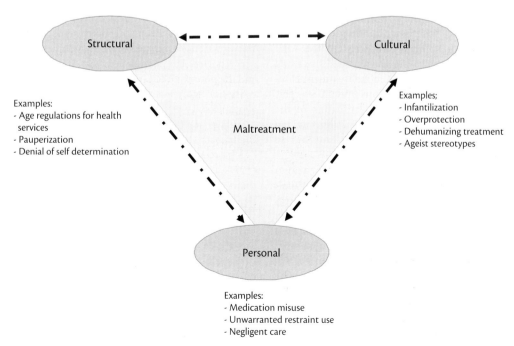

**Fig. 39.1** The triangular maltreatment model (adapted from Galtung, 1990; Hirsch, 2000).

- maltreatment is defined as an avoidable infringement of basic human needs. By virtue of its neutrality this definition permits a non-stigmatizing approach to critical situations and the uncovering and clear presentation of underlying facts in order to allow remedial action;

- maltreatment is understood as something that has developed from many sources, each of which may be corrected;

- the approach to assessment needs to be multidimensional;

- a polarized state of 'victim and perpetrator' is avoided.

## The scope of the problem

### Incidence

Mandatory reporting of elder maltreatment to Adult Protective Services (the APS) in the USA has provided yearly statistics (collected by the NCEA) on the incidence rates of elder maltreatment in US federal states. According to the APS, the number of reports of elder mistreatment has increased steadily. In 1986 117,000 cases were reported and in 2004, in the latest available survey from US states that keep separate statistics on elder abuse (32 out of 52 states in all), the number of cases was 253,426. Rather than implying that maltreatment has increased in the USA, higher reporting rates may reflect increased awareness of this problem in the general population and/or more acceptance of the option to report elder abuse. Different recording of abuse reports, different definitions of abuse, and different criteria for case definitions across US states do not allow exact figures on the incidence of maltreatment in the USA.

At present, the best available estimate of actual incidence rates of elder maltreatment in the USA has been provided by the National Elder Abuse Incidence Study (NEAIS). Based on a representative sample of persons aged 60+ not living in institutions, this study relies on data collected prospectively and on a single definition case identification (NCEA and Westat. Inc., 1998). In addition to reports received by the APS agencies, data were collected from specially trained reporters (the sentinels) working in community agencies serving seniors. These sentinels were in a position to collect four times as many cases as those officially reported to the APS. Excluding cases of self-neglect, which were also recorded, this study shows an incidence of approximately 1.2% of maltreatment cases in the elder population not living in institutions in the USA. This study has done pioneer work in allowing an estimation of the extent of unreported cases (the so-called iceberg effect) by showing that for each case of elder maltreatment reported, at least four go unreported.

The reports of elder maltreatment to the APS had a confirmation rate of 49%, indicating perhaps not so much the absence of maltreatment, but rather the difficulties of case identification. Whereas physicians and nursing staff from hospitals had filed 8% of all reports, their confirmation rate was highest, reaching 86%. In 90% of confirmed cases, the maltreatment was committed by a member of the family; in order of frequency by adult children (47%), spouses (19%), and other members of the family (24%). The majority of victims were women (67%) in need of care and cognitively impaired. Those over 80 years of age were over-represented. Types of maltreatment included different forms of neglect (49%), emotional abuse (35%), financial exploitation (30%), and physical abuse (26%) (all figures rounded).

In another study from Iowa, where the duty to report is mandatory only for cases involving professional carers, reports made to the APS over a period of 10 years (Jogerst *et al.*, 2000) were analysed. Cases of self-neglect were not included. The confirmation rate of 26.5% was comparatively low. The average yearly incidence rate was 1.27% and was correlated with the population census and with rates of reported child abuse, among others.

The data from these two studies provide the most reliable basis at present to estimate maltreatment incidence rates in the USA. However, methodological constraints limit their generalizability. This problem has not been overcome, as can be inferred from the last available survey (Teaster *et al.*, 2006). From data on abuse reports in 52 US states, only 32 have recorded data on elder abuse separately and only 24 states provide information whether abuse as reported was in fact substantiated. When substantiation rates are given, it is apparent that these differ by a factor of 10, apparently related to state-specific differences in statutory criteria for case identification.

### Prevalence

Methodological problems with non-representative data collection, selection bias, and focus on different aspects on maltreatment are even more prominent in prevalence studies on estimates of elder maltreatment. We shall consider studies of the prevalence of maltreatment in the community and in both domestic and institutional care of patients with dementia.

### Community

Prevalence estimates of elder maltreatment in the community range between 1.2% (Kurrle *et al.*, 1997) and 10.8% (Hirsch and Brendebach, 1999), depending on the method chosen. Most of these estimates are based on self-reports and have been collected retrospectively over different periods of time. Maltreatment after the age of 65 years was reported by 3.2% of those interviewed by telephone in a study by Pillemer and Finkelhor (1988). Whereas this estimate has been frequently used as an indicator for the prevalence of elder maltreatment in the population at large, this figure, due to a narrow definition and exclusion of some types of maltreatment, has been considered as too conservative, with the true prevalence estimated to be many times greater than the numbers reported. The authors highlight the role of maltreating spouses and the poor state of health of those maltreated.

Studies with a similar design have been done in Canada (Podnieks, 1990), England (Ogg and Bennett, 1992), Finland (Kivelä *et al.*, 1992), Germany (Wetzels *et al.* 1995; Hirsch and Brendebach, 1999), and The Netherlands (Comijs *et al.*, 1998).

A more standardized procedure has been utilized by Kurrle *et al.* (1997) in Australia. These authors employed a geriatric assessment that included psychological and social evaluations. Their sample was recruited from an outpatient geriatric programme, where patients presented for medical evaluation. Data on maltreatment were collected retrospectively as well as prospectively. A 1-year prevalence of 1.2% was found. The majority of the victims were care-recipients with physical (67%) or cognitive impairment (37%). In 87% of the cases, maltreatment had been committed at home by family members (spouses in 38% of cases, adult children in 43%). Recorded in the order of frequency, psychological and physical abuse, financial exploitation, and neglect were noted. The majority of subjects (65% of all cases) had suffered more than one type of maltreatment.

Estimates of prevalence have also been based on data from the APS agencies. In an epidemiological longitudinal study, Lachs *et al.* (1996) sampled reports for suspected maltreatment from subjects in the cohort. During an 11-year period, 6.4% of the subjects were reported to the APS agencies. Maltreatment was confirmed in 75% of the cases, resulting in a 11-year prevalence of 4.6%. In 73% of the cases, self-neglect was the cause of maltreatment leaving a prevalence of 1.3% for all other forms of maltreatment. Other than self-neglect, the types of maltreatment included, in the order of frequency, neglect, abuse, and financial exploitation.

### Domestic care of dementia patients

Table 39.3 gives an overview of empirical studies of maltreatment in the domestic care of dementia patients. This population has been shown to carry a special risk for maltreatment. Because of severe impairments in memory and communication in the persons afflicted, most of the studies have chosen to obtain information from the caregivers. Since one might question the reliability of this kind of information, alternative methods of assessment have been employed such as anonymous questionnaires or covert ratings pre-formed by visiting home services. With appropriate techniques, however, data obtained by personal interview do not contradict the data from studies that have used different methods. Contrary to expectations, caregivers were open to a suggestion for a personal interview and were willing to talk about this problem in a way that appeared to the investigator to be non-defensive (Pillemer and Moore, 1989; Homer and Gilleard, 1990; Pillemer and Suitor, 1992). All studies reviewed have worked with quantitative methods, have used similar definitions of maltreatment, and collected data with the help of valid measurements. The findings of these studies agree on a number of important points:

- different types of maltreatment are associated with different risk factors;
- reciprocity of maltreatment may be encountered following an established pattern of past spousal relationship;
- psychological abuse is the most frequent form of maltreatment, followed by physical abuse;
- abuse of the caregiver is encountered two to four times as frequently as abuse of the care recipient.

Many caregivers are found to be depressed and burdened as a consequence of the caregiving context and the symptoms of dementia in the person they care for. However, not all studies have found a clear-cut relationship between abuse and care burden or cognitive impairment. Another important finding of these studies has been a pattern of reactivity for abuse (Hamel *et al.*, 1990). An abusive pattern established in the pre-morbid relationship frequently underlies mutual abuse in cases of dementia at home (Keene *et al.*, 1999; Lyketsos *et al.*, 2000) and may be expected to increase the risk for abuse in these situations.

### Institutional care of the dependent elder

Despite public awareness of elder maltreatment in hospitals and nursing homes, little is actually known about the true prevalence of institutional maltreatment. For different reasons research in this area has been difficult. Impairments in memory and communication render interviews with care recipients unreliable, while reporting bias and the need to cover up what might be an offence under penal law make it difficult to evaluate information obtained during interviews of staff. The diversity of organizations and structures in institutions may not be comparable, thereby making representative sampling difficult to achieve. Perhaps the only common

**Table 39.3** Maltreatment in domestic dementia care

| Authors | Methods | Prevalence | Significant findings |
|---|---|---|---|
| Homer and Gilleard (1990) | Structured interview and rating scales obtained from 51 Cgs and their 43 Crs, referred for respite care | Overall 6-month prevalence for abuse 45%, including emotional abuse 42%; physical abuse 47%, neglect 12% | Alcoholism and depression scores (Cg); problem behaviour (Cr), abusive pre-morbid relationship (Cg and Cr). Mental impairment (Cr) non-significant for maltreatment |
| Paveza *et al.* (1992) | Questionnaire and telephone interview obtained from 184 Cgs referred from a multisite dementia registry | Overall prevalence for violence since dementia diagnosis 17%; 16% directed at Cg; 5% at Cr; 5% in Cd | Depression scores (Cg), living with immediate family but without the spouse (Cr). Cognitive or functional impairment non-significant for maltreatment |
| Pillemer and Suitor (1992) | Structured interview and rating scales obtained from 236 Cgs referred from different dementia screening sites | For unspecified time period, 6% of the Cgs had used violence; 25% had been subjected to it; 19% had violent feelings | Actual violence: mutual violence (Cd), spouse status and age (Cg). Violent feelings: care demands, ADL impairment, behavioural problems (Cr), mutual violence, living together (Cd) |
| Coyne *et al.* (1993) | Postal questionnaires obtained from 342 Cgs picked up from a phone helpline | Throughout Cd, 12% of Cgs had perpetrated abuse; 33% had been subjected to it | Longer care, more daily care hours (Cd); functional impairment (Cr), depression scores (Cg) |
| Cooney and Mortimer (1995) | Postal questionnaires obtained from 67 Cgs members of a volunteer organization | Overall 1-year prevalence 55%, including 52% emotional abuse; 12% physical abuse; 12% neglect | Physical abuse: psychological symptoms (Cg), longer caring relationship and mutual abuse, not related: Cr variables. Verbal abuse: abusive pre-morbid relationship, mutual abuse (Cd), social isolation (Cg) |
| Mendonica *et al.* (1996) | Ratings by visiting nurses on 82 observed family Cds | Emotional abuse 11%, physical abuse 5%, financial exploitation 5%, various forms of neglect 5% | Physical neglect predicts physical abuse, and psychosocial neglect emotional abuse. Financial exploitation predicts emotional abuse |

Cg, caregiver; Cr, care receiver; Cd, care dyad; ADL, activities of daily living. All numbers are rounded.

characteristics of institutions are those of a total institution (Goffman, 1961) in being governed by administrative regulations, standards, and routines that impinge on the autonomy and privacy of clients. In this setting the boundaries between institutional routines and acts of maltreatment may be difficult to distinguish in a given case. Glendenning (1999) has therefore distinguished institutional or institutionalized maltreatment from individual acts of maltreatment in institutions.

Given these difficulties, indirect indicators may be used for an estimate of the prevalence of maltreatment in institutions. Suitable indicators for this purpose are prescribing practices for psychoactive drugs and the use of mechanical restraints. Another approach may be to determine the prevalence of putative indicators for negligent care, such as pressure ulcers.

### Nursing homes

Table 39.4 combines findings from two studies that have looked at the prevalence of maltreatment in a sample from different nursing homes in a given area. Different methods of data collection notwithstanding, some conclusions reached by the studies were in agreement. Maltreatment can be related to characteristics of the residents, problems in the interaction between staff and residents, and work satisfaction of the staff. These studies have also found that aggression by a resident frequently precedes staff maltreatment and that there may be mutually aggressive interactions between residents and staff. Other studies have added further details to this point. With a questionnaire completed anonymously by 126 nursing assistants, Goodridge *et al.* (1996) found a 1-month reported prevalence of 84% for psychological abuse suffered by nursing assistants and a corresponding figure of 58% for physical abuse. Commenting on these findings, Goodridge *et al.* note dryly:

> On average, a nursing assistant in this health care facility may expect to be physically assaulted by residents 9.3 times per month and verbally assaulted 11.3 times per month.

Similar results were obtained by Hagen and Sayers (1995). In a 200-bed facility, these authors found an 8-day-prevalence of 182 reported acts of physical aggression by residents against nursing assistants, 6% of which resulted in physical injuries. Most of these incidents occurred during routine nursing care such as dressing and changing (48%), turning and transfer (22%), assisting in meals (8%), and bathing (7%) (all figures rounded).

As Goodridge *et al.* (1996) have shown in their analysis, a situation involving maltreatment of an elder dependent needs to be viewed in the situational context brought about by extreme working conditions and responsibilities unmatched by the level of training. Although nursing assistants or untrained carers take a central role in the care of residents, they receive little appreciation, are underpaid, and are frequently viewed as dispensable at will. While frequently encountering conflict situations with residents, they have usually not received training on interpersonal aspects of nursing care nor on techniques of conflict resolution. Therefore resident abuse in institutions needs to be viewed in the context of the institutional structures in the setting. Healthcare Canada (1994, as quoted by Goodridge *et al.*, 1996) define systemic abuse as:

> Harmful situations created, permitted, or facilitated by procedures and processes within institutions including situations where institutions do not provide or structure resources in a manner that allows recognized standards of care to be met.

## Medical interventions as infringements of basic human needs

### Mechanical restraints

The successful implementation of nationwide restraint reduction programmes in nursing homes in the USA under the regulations of the Omnibus Budget Reconciliation Act 987 (OBRA-87) has clearly shown that the restraint practice in use until then had been excessive. From an average of 40% the rate of restraints has been

**Table 39.4** Maltreatment in nursing homes

| Author | Methods | Prevalence | Significant findings |
|---|---|---|---|
| Pillemer and Moore (1989) | Structured telephone-interview of 677 nurses and nursing-aides from different nursing homes | One-year prevalence rates for: Maltreatment observed by staff: 36% physical abuse, 81% psychological abuse. Maltreatment committed: 10% physical and 40% psychological abuse | Abuse associated with less work satisfaction, burn-out symptoms, aggressive behaviour of patients, younger age of care professional, negative attitudes towards patient, staff–patient conflict. Psychological abuse also related to personal life stress of caregiver. No association between abuse and size of facility, staff quality |
| Schneider (1990) | Questionnaires from 205 administrators and nursing staff selected by administrators from different nursing homes | No time period specified. Resident to resident: psychological aggression often 2–7%, sometimes 6–37%; physical aggression often 1%, sometimes 2–3% Resident to staff: psychological aggression often 2–3%, sometimes 8–31%; physical aggression often 1%, sometimes Staff to resident: psychological aggression often 1–2%, sometimes 2–11%; physical aggression often 0%, sometimes 6% | Aggression related to: Residents variables: cognitive impairment and social competence Staff variables: work and life satisfaction, stressors Structural variables: staffing level, size of facility, census of local town Milieu variables: general level of aggression increased in care milieu with number of aggressive acts (violence escalation) |
| Allen *et al.* (2003) | 3443 Nursing home complaints to the state long-term ombudsman programme | 2-year prevalence rate: 23% care complaints, 8% abuse complaints: physical abuse 41%, psychological abuse 19%, gross abuse 19% | 87% of abuse complaints substantiated. 53% of state facilities without abuse complaints, 12% had 3 or more complaints. Facility size positively correlated with documented abuse and care concerns |

reduced in US nursing homes to an average of 11% in 2001 (Department of Health and Human Services, 2003). Even this figure may be viewed as excessive when considering restraint rates of 4% and below in nursing homes in another American study (Neufeld *et al.*, 1999). The practice of using restraints has been shown to depend on institutional characteristics such as the geographical location, staffing levels, and staff knowledge and attitudes. Educational efforts to improve knowledge about alternatives to restraint, such as case conferences and supervised management of difficult cases or providing special care units to residents suffering from dementia, has enabled the use of restraints to be limited. Whereas considerable reduction in the use of restraints has taken place, no higher incidence of serious falls has been observed, and the changes accomplished have not led to higher use of psychotropic drugs nor to the need for higher staffing levels (Evans *et al.*, 1997; Neufeld *et al.*, 1999).

Despite these successful changes, traditional beliefs continue to influence decision-making about the use of restraints. It is still argued by some that mechanical restraints prevent falls, but in fact use of restraints is poorly correlated with standardized fall assessment (Karlson *et al.*, 1997), and the risk of falls is increased by the use of mechanical restraints, especially at the point when they are discontinued (Tinetti *et al.*, 1992; Arbesman and Wright, 1999; Kron *et al.*, 2003).

Another frequent reason given for the use of restraint has been to control disturbed behaviour and agitation, particularly in residents suffering from dementia. Experience has shown however, that restraint use will not control consistently disturbed behaviour but may in fact worsen agitation, and cause anxiety and anguish. It has also been documented that restraints are associated with objective indices for subsequent intellectual decline, immobility, and loss of physical function as well as increased morbidity (Evans and Strumpf, 1989). There has also been documentation of lethal complications of restraint use (Parker and Miles, 1997). Moreover, it has been shown that the decision to place an elder dependent in restraints may not so much reflect the special risk of that person but features of the institution itself—such as staff-to-resident ratio, reimbursement rates, particular institutional philosophies, and prevailing myths (Strumpf and Evans, 1991; Phillips *et al.*, 1996; Castle *et al.*, 1997). This body of research may be taken as empirical evidence for the relevance of the triangular model proposed by Galtung, considering that mechanical restraints are infringements of basic human needs and that their use:

◆ may frequently be avoided;

◆ may depend more on the structure of the care setting rather than on the individual risk profile of the resident;

◆ may be influenced by cultural attitudes and perceptions.

The current restraint practice in different settings is reflected in point prevalence rates. As reported in the literature, the corresponding figures for geropsychiatric institutions range from 24% to 45% (De Santis *et al.*, 1997; Kranzhoff and Hirsch, 1997; Karlson *et al.*, 1998) from 4% to 22% in nursing homes (Karlson *et al.*, 1997; Neufeld *et al.*, 1999) and between 17% and 18% in acute geriatric care (Robins *et al.*, 1987; Karlson *et al.*, 1998). The spread of these figures highlights the role of extraneous factors in the practice of over-using and misusing mechanical restraints in institutional elder care.

## Use of psychoactive drugs in nursing homes

The use of psychoactive drugs in nursing homes is common practice: between 17% and 78% of residents will receive at least one prescription of a psychoactive drug (Llorente *et al.*, 1998; Schmidt *et al.*, 1998). The use of psychoactive drugs has been criticized because of inappropriate choices, hazardous combinations, and failure to discontinue prescriptions at an appropriate time (Board of Directors of the American Association for Geriatric Psychiatry, 1992). Such misuse is more prevalent in institutions with less adequate treatment resources (Svarstad and Mount, 1991; Riedel-Heller *et al.*, 1999). Whereas neuroleptics, hypnotics, and especially benzodiazepines are over-used, antidepressants are under-used, despite the well-known high prevalence of depression in nursing homes. This prescription practice points to a use of psychoactive drugs that is geared more to the control of unspecific symptoms than to the specific treatment of a diagnosed psychiatric illness. This disturbing finding may be indicative of inadequate geropsychiatric care in nursing home. In response to this problem, guidelines have been established by OBRA-87 for the use of psychoactive drugs in US nursing homes, including the requirements for specific indications for drug use, schedules for the reduction and discontinuation of drugs, the employment of non-drug treatment alternatives such as behavioural interventions, and prohibition of as-needed schedules. These regulations have been quite successful in restricting the use of psychoactive drugs, especially when combined with educational programmes. Efforts to reduce the use of psychoactive drugs by offering a visiting consulting service and medical education programmes have been successful in other countries as well, but to a lesser extent than achieved under the OBRA-87 regulations in the USA (Schmidt *et al.*, 1998; Snowdon, 1999).

## Putative indicators of neglect: pressure ulcers

Pressure ulcers are generally considered to be preventable, and their presence a putative indicator of negligent care. Long ago, Florence Nightingale (1849) considered them 'generally the fault not of the disease but of the nursing'. This traditional view may be upheld by studies that have established a relationship between pressure ulcer and institutional parameters such as staffing level, number of beds, geographical location, inadequacies in nursing care, in wound treatment, and in medical documentation, as well as a general lack of quality care (Rudman *et al.*, 1993; Bergstrom *et al.*, 1996; Spector and Fortinsky, 1998; Berlowitz *et al.*, 1999; Heinemann *et al.*, 2000). Despite the availability of standards for risk assessment and preventive measures, these are frequently not used and considerable shortcomings in the prevention and treatment of pressure ulcers may be found in nursing home care (Bergstrom *et al.*, 1996; Heinemann *et al.*, 2000). Pressure ulcers have been found more frequently in institutions which have other adverse outcomes such as medication errors, a more rapid decline of physical function, and higher levels of disturbing behaviours of residents, typically associated with lower staffing levels and higher staff turnover (Rudman *et al.*, 1993; Blegen *et al.*, 1998; Ooi *et al.*, 1999).

These studies underline the significance of pressure ulcers as a possible sign of neglect in the institutional care of dependent older persons. Even though the prevalence and incidence rates reported in the literature may not be fully comparable because different risk profiles in the samples are not adjusted for comparison, the available raw data indicate an incidence for pressure ulcer stage 2 or above of between 0% and 15%, and up to more than 38% (Bergstrom *et al.*, 1992; Rudman *et al.*, 1993). The reported prevalence rates for all stages of pressure ulcers vary between 12% and more than 83% (Spector and Fortinsky, 1998; Bours *et al.*, 1999). Whereas some of the variation in these figures may be accounted for by different risk profiles, these figures nevertheless point to inconsistencies in standards of care, and specifically the lack of quality care in some long-term care institutions. To expect a prevalence of 0%, however, may be unrealistic. This was demonstrated by Hagisawa and Barbenel (1999), who studied the development of pressure ulcers in a setting with adequate staffing levels, established schedules for routine risk assessment, and regular preventive measures. In this setting, annual rates for pressure ulcer development were over 4% (incidence) and over 5% (prevalence).

# Causes and consequences

## Causal models and risk factors

Prevalence studies have identified a number of associations between a maltreatment event and factors in the surrounding situation. These factors are often considered to be risk markers, implying that the likelihood of a maltreatment event is increased in their presence, without the implication of a causal relationship. The diversity and multiplicity of reported risk markers suggest that quite different attendant circumstances may be involved in maltreatment. In an overview of the literature Jones *et al.* (1997b) list 19 risk markers for the parties in a maltreatment situation—victims, perpetrators and their mutual relationship—as well as 14 factors pertaining to the situational context of the maltreatment event. Reis and Nahmiash (1998) were able to isolate, by discriminant function analysis, 'indicators for abuse' related to the person maltreated (including a past history of being abused and social isolation) and the person maltreating. The latter include mental health problems and inexperience with caregiving, underdeveloped empathic skills, troubled personal and social relationships, and financial dependence on the care recipient. From the complex tangle of diverse factors, an overview by the NCEA on their website lists four risk categories: caregiver stress; impairment of the dependent elder; cycle of violence; and personal problems of the abuser. The relevance of most of these markers in predicting maltreatment has not been well established. In the only published study with a longitudinal prospective design, Lachs *et al.* (1997) found the variables of age, race, poverty, impairments of ADL and cognitive function, as well as the trajectory of cognitive decline, to discriminate the abused from the other subjects in the cohort. Most of the cases were referred for self-neglect to the APS, however, and the authors caution that the sample may not have been representative.

## Personal factors

### Cycle of violence

Many studies trying to identify risk markers have been based on existing explanatory models. The first such model was developed in child abuse research. It postulates that violent behaviour is learned in the family and is then passed on to the next generation. This hypothesis was adapted to elder maltreatment and led to a number of earlier studies. More recently a large-scale population study has been able to demonstrate an association between elder maltreatment and child abuse in the community at large, but has not analysed this pattern for individual families (Jogerst *et al.*, 2000). A family dynamic has been identified in spousal relationships, in a pattern of mutual abuse which turns worse when one spouse becomes dependent as a consequence of dementia (Homer and Gilleard, 1990; Coyne *et al.*, 1993). Another lead has been the consistent finding of adult children as the perpetrators of elder maltreatment. There is no study, however, that has looked for a transgenerational transmission of violent behaviour as the cause of maltreatment in these cases. Rather, the dynamics of interpersonal aggression in elder maltreatment have more often been shown to be reactive, either to aggressive behaviour in the context of dementia, or else in response to caregiver burden. This kind of aggression dynamic is not confined to families but is also prevalent in institutional care, where there may be mutual abuse between residents and staff (Pillemer and Moore, 1989; Schneider, 1990).

### Impairment of a dependent elder

Another model has been developed from the observation that elder maltreatment is most prevalent in care dyads. For this paradigm, prospective studies have identified risk markers of functional impairment of physical and cognitive abilities, psychiatric symptoms such as confusion and depression, as well as recent deterioration in cognitive function (Lachs *et al.*, 1997; National Council On Elder Abuse and Westat Inc.1998). Care dependence has also been shown to be a risk marker in large-scale community studies (Pillemer and Finkelhor, 1988; Podnieks, 1990). However, findings have been less consistent in this regard in the domestic care of dementia patients. Presumably other factors may increase the risk for maltreatment in this setting including, for example, disruptive behaviour of the care recipient or stress symptoms of the caregiver (Paveza *et al.*, 1992; Cooney and Mortimer, 1995).

### Caregiver stress

Care requirements of the dependent elder will place high emotional, physical, and financial demands on the caregiver. The burden resulting is a continual challenge to the personal limits of stress tolerance of the carer. The constant pressure of care demands and the necessity to defer one's own needs as well as obligations to family, work, and friends may lead to exhaustion and social isolation as well as to emotional stress symptoms (Coyne *et al.*, 1993). Burden notwithstanding, it is frequently not the caregiving context in and of itself, but the added presence of other factors that raise an existing risk situation to a critical level and precipitate maltreatment. Such factors may include specific living arrangements, lack of support for the task of caring, and financial or emotional dependency. Situational trigger events, external stresses, or illness of the caregiver may also acutely raise risk (Jones *et al.*, 1997b; Kleinschmid, 1997). In institutional care, the caregiver's burden is also frequently found to be an antecedent for maltreatment. Of special importance in this regard is the burn-out syndrome of the nursing staff (Pillemer and Moore, 1989). In addition, stresses in the personal life of the staff, and institutional factors as well as the situational context have also been described (Schneider, 1990; Goodridge *et al.*, 1996; Glendenning, 1999).

### Personal problems of the person maltreating

In addition to stress symptoms arising from the caregiver burden, many studies have uncovered personal problems of the maltreating person, including alcoholism and psychiatric illness. Social isolation, and emotional and material dependence on the care recipient have also been described, as summarized by Jones *et al.* (1997b) and Kleinschmidt (1997). These factors are interdependent, but, given a cross-sectional study design, it has not been possible to establish whether the factors are antecedents or consequences. Undoubtedly, however, such factors identify persons in trouble who lack the emotional stability to endure the stress of caregiving. Many of the perpetrators are weak and helpless themselves and it may be justified, considering the specifics of a given case, to view a perpetrator as a victim of attendant circumstances, being unable to take charge of a difficult and overwhelming situation.

## Structural factors

Studies from a social psychology perspective have illuminated the role of factors that may increase the potential for violence and maltreatment in institutions. Pertinent in this context are the observations by Goffman (1961). Given the situation of institutionalized persons who have to live in a secluded environment cut off from society and whose regulated life, administered and enforced by the rules of the institution, is devoid of privacy and self-determination, this constellation tends to create a schism between superordinates in a role of power and subordinates, dependent and powerless, stripped of personal identity and self-esteem. The inherent asymmetry of power tends to develop a dynamic conducive to violence on both sides, by oppositional self-assertion and protest on the part of the subordinates, and by feelings of superiority demonstrated in forceful and coercive action on the part of the superordinates. Asymmetry of power, and distance in a relationship shaped by authoritarian structure, favours violence, as also shown by Milgram (1974). His experiment has been seen as an indication that people tend to follow obedience to duties towards an authority more than their conscience, especially, when the responsibility for a duty has been delegated to them by the authority. This applies to educated and psychologically stable persons as well, as shown in the Stanford experiment by Zimbardo (Haney *et al.*, 1973). There, mock prisoners were stripped of their personal identity and their personal belongings and subjected to treatment designed to signal to them their loss of power and control. This design elicited sadistic and humiliating behaviour on the part of the mock guardians. Taken together, these findings indicate that the potential for abusive, and even sadistic, behaviour may be stimulated in almost anyone, given a facilitative, or even permissive, situation.

## Cultural factors

Negative stereotypical assumptions about old age are the basis for ageist attitudes, frequently expressed in demeaning language that portrays negative images of the physical and mental characteristics of old age, and the economic drain and burden to society imposed by the aged as a group. Such views represent a form of 'symbolic violence' (Bourdieu and Passeron, 1977) and purport to provide justification for the social and economic disadvantages in society, and abusive treatment in daily suffered by older people (World Health Organization, 2002a). Such attitudes may result from a deficit model of aging or a biased perception of elder's lives, or may be an expression of unacknowledged aversion or even aggression against old age. Even professional discourse is not free from ageist

bias, and by focusing on old age, neglect of the professional care of the older person is frequently committed.

## A working model for maltreatment

In sum, the literature on risk factors suggests that a one-dimensional approach is not adequate to account for maltreatment. Every maltreatment has its own history and carries along its own risk factors. Drawing on available evidence, Jones *et al.* (1997b) have formulated a multidimensional explanatory model, offering a useful tool for educational purposes as well as for professional work with a maltreated elder. However, this model does not account for the structural factors of a maltreatment situation. In our own work (Hirsch *et al.*, 2002) we favour a model in which we assume that every caregiver has the individual potential for a maltreatment behaviour in a given situation. The threshold of such behaviour is influenced by personal values and structural factors connected with the caring situation, as well as by the personal characteristics of all people involved in the situation and the kind of relationships among them. The trigger point may be extraneous, such as disturbing behaviour of the dependent, e.g. incontinence or communication problems, or acute stress on the caretaker from any source.

## Consequences of maltreatment

Field studies from nursing homes have described emotional reactions to maltreatment, especially maltreatment by neglect (Schneider, 1994). These have included depressive symptoms with feelings of helplessness and social withdrawal, suicidal thoughts, and regressive symptoms; but no psychiatric assessment or standardized evaluation has been reported. Single case studies, as reviewed by Wolf (1997), have indicated the presence of depression, and post-traumatic stress disorder has also been mentioned. A more systematic approach has been taken by Comijs *et al.* (1998), who reported follow-up data on 43 maltreated subjects. Most of these indicated reactions of anger, disappointment, or grief, and one in four reported having reacted with aggressive behaviour in turn. In the study by Hirsch and Brendebach (1999), only 5 of the 44 subjects who reported having suffered maltreatment indicated the absence of any emotional sequelae, whereas all others reported significant emotional distress, including anxiety, feelings of humiliation, and being unable to forget. Only one subject reported an aggressive response to the event. Long-term consequences included avoiding or completely breaking contact with the maltreating person.

In addition to emotional distress reactions, physical effects bearing on mortality have been reported by Lachs *et al.* (1998). During longitudinal follow-up for 9 years, maltreatment as confirmed by the APS was shown to be an independent predictor of early death, all other known mortality risk factors being controlled for.

# Taking steps against maltreatment
## Prevention

Considering the multiplicity of causes for elder maltreatment and realizing that an act of maltreatment has many harbingers, it is apparent that with appropriate measures there are possibilities for their reduction, if not prevention altogether. Suitable approaches may be levelled at the people and the environment in a maltreatment situation, at the professionals serving clients at risk, and at the policy-makers in institutions dealing with elderly. Whereas all these approaches are geared at the personal level, the structural and cultural aspects of the maltreatment situation need to be addressed as well. Fundamental to prevention is the societal condemnation of maltreatment as well as effective protective services for its vulnerable members.

Since maltreatment is usually not a single event but an ongoing pattern, prevention is the conceptual basis for casework in maltreatment cases, and the orientation mark for interventions. The objective for prevention is to reduce the potential for maltreatment at different points of time:

+ *Primary prevention* of maltreatment is geared towards prevention of future occurrences of maltreatment. This can be achieved by educational programmes to improve the recognition of maltreatment, the awareness of factors that have an influence on the potential for abuse as well as remedial measures. Examples include education for families and caregivers on care issues; media coverage questioning patronizing attitudes towards the old, challenging beliefs that violence is unavoidable, emphasizing alternatives to violent behaviour; implementation of screening protocols and reporting procedures for maltreatment for professional services.
+ *Secondary prevention* of maltreatment is geared towards limiting the harmful consequences of a maltreatment event, once it has occurred. Then treatment of physical and psychological symptoms is needed, as well as provision of immediate protection for the victim. Effective protection in the long run can only be achieved if the causes of the actual occurrence have been made transparent and remedial actions have been implemented. Accordingly, secondary prevention consists of attention to the medical, psychological, and legal needs of the victim, crisis intervention, as well as an assessment for required changes as the basis to prevent future recurrence.
+ Long-term care plans for the victim, considered as *tertiary prevention*, are intended to prevent lasting after-effects of an abuse event and to reduce the potential for recurrence. This includes systemic therapy to neutralize conflicted relationships in families, counselling and case management for difficult care situations, and provision of de-escalation techniques and assertiveness training.

At the first suspicion of a maltreatment, any witness needs to take the situation seriously and be prepared to take appropriate action, such as involving third parties. General practitioners in particular have an important role in this regard, since they will be among the first to make pertinent observations, to hear about 'family news', to notice stress symptoms or changes in physical and psychological functioning indicative of maltreatment.

In institutions, prevention is geared towards the staff, their collaboration with one another, and their support from supervisors and administrators. The existence of structures fostering a supportive work environment, the interpersonal climate, and good role models from among their supervisors will contribute to this goal, as much as warmth and support for the clients and the institutional philosophy and human values reflected by it.

Of special importance is continuing professional development for all professionals working with the elderly. Such programmes may help in the self-awareness of one's own violent impulses, to develop a sense for situations where maltreatment may occur, and to understand how to deal with such situations in a helpful and professional way. Many approaches to the prevention of elder maltreatment have come into existence, encompassing a broad range from penal law and mandatory reporting to regional services, run by statutory agencies as well as by voluntary organizations, providing information and help at various levels (Kemshall and Pritchard, 1996; Pritchard, 1996; California Department of Justice, 2002; National Council On Elder Abuse, 2002; The Home Care Companion, 2006). The International Network for the Prevention of Elder Abuse (INPEA), founded in 1997, documents prevention programmes internationally. Unfortunately, there has been little research to evaluate the effects of such approaches. However, from the experience in practical work with prevention programmes, empirical support exists for the efficacy of such approaches (Görgen *et al.*, 2002).

## Assessment

A multistep procedure is required to understand how a maltreatment situation came about, and to determine what kinds of interventions may be helpful. In any case of suspected maltreatment it is necessary to gather in a systematic way the facts about the situation and about the people involved (Table 39.5). In addition, an evaluation has to be made of whether the maltreated person wants changes made in the situation or is afraid of them, especially when dreaded consequences of such changes include retaliation or abandonment. In some relationships in which dysfunctional patterns have been entrenched over a long period, there is great reluctance to accept help from outside.

If it is possible to overcome such barriers, then an evaluation of the people involved and the contextual (structural and cultural) givens of the situation is needed. All these aspects are brought into focus by an assessment (Table 39.6). It serves the purpose of uncovering existing maltreatment patterns, finding the points amenable to intervention, and exploring available sources of help. In the majority of cases, antecedents have gone unrecognized for some time. This aspect requires exploration as much as those factors that have precipitated or aggravated the event.

**Table 39.5** Points to clarify when maltreatment is suspected

| |
|---|
| Why is the report being made now (trigger)? |
| When and where did the situation take place? |
| Who is involved/who else was present in the situation? |
| What are the objective facts? |
| Is there more than one perpetrator present? |
| What types of maltreatment are present? |
| Has this event occurred before? |
| Is the current situation likely to continue? |
| Are future occurrences likely? |
| What personal consequences did the event have? |
| How does the person reporting feel about the event? |
| What would the person reporting like to see happening? |
| Is the report credible? |

**Table 39.6** Assessment of elder maltreatment

| Person afflicted | Maltreatment aspects | Others involved | Contextual factors |
|---|---|---|---|
| *Personal characteristics:* | *Specific details:* | *Perpetrator:* | *Structural factors:* |
| Identifying data | Objective signs of abuse or neglect | Identifying data | Adequacy of accommodation |
| Physical examination | Type, frequency, and intensity of maltreatment | Physical and emotional state | Adequacy of care, acceptance for outside services |
| Mental state examination | Antecedents of current maltreatment situation | Living arrangement, relationship to person maltreated | Financial resources |
| ADL—function and physical condition | History of previous maltreatment | Financial or emotional dependence on person maltreated | |
| Socio-economic situation | Likelihood of recurrence | Perceived need for changes | |
| Care and treatment needs, adequacy of services provided | | | |
| Living arrangement, relationship to perpetrator | | | |
| *Motivation for change:* | *Interpersonal aspects:* | *Third persons in the situation:* | *Cultural factors:* |
| Personal view of situation and of need for help and protection | Previous relationship patterns | Behaviour in situation (permissive or interventional) | 'Punitive' moral values |
| Fears of retaliation, of changes in the relationship, of consequences for the perpetrator | Mutual dependence | Fear of perpetrator and of retaliation | Concepts about care needs |
| Motivation for change and for interventions involved | | View of maltreatment situation | Concepts of ageing and of elder needs |
| Interest in seeing perpetrator punished | | Future involvement | |

## Interventions

Maltreatment may be contagious, and a situation not worked through and resolved will usually be repeated. Professional help is usually needed to resolve a maltreatment situation and to stabilize the results. Rarely will one intervention suffice to correct a problem; more typically, several interventions in collaborative work by several professional groups are required. Physicians, by virtue of the respect and public trust they enjoy, have a special role in this task.

Unfortunately many maltreatment situations, by the time they come to light, have been in existence for a long time and have developed into a chronic problem. It may therefore be quite difficult to achieve more than partial success. Some victimized clients tend to complain but may be reluctant to consider any changes. Others may be unwilling to accept help because of the fear that maltreatment may increase when a third party becomes involved. In such situations, too, mitigation rather than changes may be achieved.

## Families

Maltreatment in families may be a visible manifestation of a destructive pattern in the relationship between family members that has been present for some time. In such families, spouses frequently share a similar background with difficult relationships, including violence, in their families of origin. They are tied together by similar conflicts in their relationship, as well as by weak communication skills. In such a relationship it is often not possible to differentiate between 'victim' and 'perpetrator' and it may not be appropriate to look for the one guilty party. Violence has become part of the ordinary and has shown up regularly in many different ways.

Stress levels have increased and an acute crisis has arisen. Often, one member has escaped or left already, by illness, admission to a hospital or to a nursing home, or by death.

A troubled person seeking help should be encouraged on the initial contact to talk about all their concerns. Prior to any kind of intervention planning it is important to satisfy concerns for safety. The plan must ensure that maltreatment can be, in effect, stopped immediately. This can mean separation of the parties involved, either by admission to a hospital or referral to a shelter. Further steps are:

- An attempt needs to be made to arrange for an interview with all involved, alone and together. Such an interview needs to be conducted in a neutral atmosphere. Blame and prejudice need to be avoided, but it may be appropriate for all parties to share their own observations. The focus should be on patterns of maltreatment, and how they relate to patterns of interactions in the family. Strategies for communication skills and conflict-solving techniques, typically absent or underdeveloped in such families, need to be emphasized and potentials for change in the family system pointed out.

- Available local resources that need to be utilized may include counselling services, self-help groups, family support groups, psychosocial services, psychiatric community services, as well as pastoral counselling. The guideline for all such interventions is the basic principle of help before punishment.

- If it becomes apparent that social support will not be enough or will be unlikely to succeed in stopping the maltreatment, referral for legal services may be required.

◆ Having an opportunity to talk about their problems and their fears in a private and protected atmosphere may be a significant relief for many families, and may create grounds for the building of trust which allows a working alliance to be established, aimed at making and stabilizing necessary changes. Specific interventions following an initial interview depend on the type and intensity of maltreatment, the options agreeable to the parties involved, and their expectations, their value systems and availability of social support systems.

## Domestic care for dependent elders

Care dependence of an older person usually means a critical life event for the family. Typically, it has the most severe consequences for daughters and daughters-in-law, since male family members rarely feel under an obligation to involve themselves directly with the ongoing care. Females in the family usually have to change their lives altogether, and they bear extremes of emotional and physical burden. A critical point is reached when they can no longer maintain their own autonomy because of guilt feelings, unresolved conflicts from their past relationship with the dependent elder, or other conflicts resulting from consequences imposed on their personal lives by caregiving. Such troubled caregivers will tend to drift into social isolation, while at the same time becoming increasingly overburdened. Care burden alone is rarely the cause of maltreatment, but often, the carer has become enmeshed with the person dependent on care in what may be considered a symbiotic life situation. Social withdrawal and rejection of outside help may have followed, and a climate fostering violent feelings and maltreatment may have been in existence for some time. In this situation it is mandatory to disentangle the care dyad, to involve other family members in the ongoing care, and to organize additional community service, as needed. Referral to a support group may be helpful and contact with the general practitioner in charge is required, to make him or her aware of the critical situation and to discuss possible helpful resources. In addition, local arrangements for reprieve (e.g. day care, respite care) may be helpful.

## Institutional care

Every institution has its own rules and regulations, its own philosophy reflecting the values and goals of services. Structural forces in an institution influence the work life of the staff just as much as the life of the clients (residents or patients) being served in that institution. Such structural influences include availability of a single room versus shared accommodation, convenience of times for meals and basic care, protection of privacy. Coercive measures (restraints, drugs, compulsory admissions) may turn into maltreatment if not used in the interest of the client's health and in support of their general level of function. Incidents involving pressure ulcers, dehydration, or malnutrition need to be routinely reviewed to rule out maltreatment. Problems between clients and staff involving allegations of maltreatment need to be referred for mandatory review by a neutral committee, composed of different professional groups and administrative staff as well as lay persons from the community.

Interventions against maltreatment in institutions may include, on a *personal level*:

◆ Education on types of maltreatment, their manifestations in the institutional setting, as well as corrective interventions, exposing prevailing myths on restraint, staff liability for client falls, etc.

◆ Discussion in team meetings to address the potential for maltreatment in daily routines, exemplifying maltreatment situations in institutions analysing sources, and reflecting how to reduce the likelihood of such occurrences.

◆ Helping staff to examine their own feelings about difficult clients (e.g. recognizing helplessness, resentment, anger, anxiety, and insecurity) and finding ways of ensuring that such feelings do not get in the way of caring for such clients.

On a *structural level* interventions may include:

◆ Review care plans and treatment routines and staff working schedules for their suitability to the needs of clients.

◆ Implement stress-reduction programmes, increase work satisfaction for staff.

◆ Implement continuous team supervision, in which the potential of work routines for maltreatment or the liability of work routines to bring about maltreatment can be analysed, appropriate changes planned, and the effects of such changes reviewed.

◆ Improve the environment, with attention to safety, orientation aids, and quality of life for the clients.

On a *cultural level* interventions may include:

◆ Emphasize equal status and dignity of both physical and psychiatric illness, of patients both young and old, and of care as well as treatment for old people.

◆ Achieve a shift in models of care: from a task-oriented model to a model based on human needs and relationship; and from a biomedical to a psychosocial model for the treatment and care of old people.

## Society

Maltreatment is a violation of basic human rights. To prevent such violations, democratic constitutions have been brought into existence. For the international community, conventions have been formulated to assert the obligation placed on each state to protect its citizens. Looking at such international conventions it is striking how little consideration has been given to concerns for the elderly until recent times. The convention for the political rights of women was formulated in 1952, the declaration of rights for children in 1959, and of mentally retarded persons in 1975. In 1982 an international congress in Vienna convened to deal with the rights of the elderly and formulated recommendations (United Nations, 1983). Only since then has international awareness and concern for the issue of elder maltreatment increased, promoted by international institutions and prominently by the World Health Organization (2002b). Against the background of demographic development, with a rapidly growing ageing population worldwide, this issue will become more prominent, since the proportion of those in need of care is increasing exponentially with time.

# Concluding remarks

Maltreatment is not inherently unavoidable but it can be prevented. The multifaceted presentation of maltreatment in its physical, emotional, social, structural, and cultural dimensions requires a discriminating view for an understanding of the causal web as well as for the recognition of points for intervention. In the family context, it may often be difficult to distinguish between victim and perpetrator. Maltreatment usually indicates the existence of a destructive relationship pattern, adverse personality characteristics, external stressors, and internal conflicts, as well as social isolation and inadequate support. Therefore, help before punishment is the basic principle for interventions. In the institutional context, it is important to consider not only staff maltreatment, but resident aggression as well as institutional abuse.

Maltreatment, when encountered, needs to be confronted, and alternative ways of handling a situation pursued. Attitudes of denial or of trying to explain it away will encourage more maltreatment. Unfortunately, the needs for counselling, for support, and for services for those afflicted are still not being met. The physician, in the dual role of the patient's advocate and the patient's therapist, has a special responsibility to be aware of maltreatment, to be able to recognize risk factors and the signs of its presence, and to be familiar with the process of assessing for maltreatment and arranging helpful interventions.

## References

Abrams, R.C., Lachs, M., McAvay G. et al. (2002). Predictors of self-neglect in community dwelling elders. American Journal of Psychiatry, 159, 1724–1730.

Allen, P.D., Kellett, K., and Gruman, C. (2003). Elder abuse in Connecticut's nursing homes. Journal of Elder Abuse and Neglect, 15, 19–42.

Action on Elder Abuse (2006). What is abuse (http://www.elderabuse.org.uk/; accessed 16 May 2007).

Arbesman, R.C. and Wright, C. (1999). Mechanical restraints, rehabilitation therapies, and staffing adequacy as risk factors for falls in an elderly hospitalized population. Rehabilitation Nursing, 24, 122–128.

Bergstrom, N., Braden, B., Kemp, N., Champagne, M., and Ruby E. (1996). Multi-site study of incidence of pressure ulcers and the relationship between risk level, demographic characteristics, diagnoses, and prescription of preventive interventions. Journal of the American Geriatrics Society, 44, 22–30.

Berlowitz, D.R., Anderson, J.J. Brandeis, G.H., Lehner, L.A., Brand, H.K., Ash, A.S., and Moskowitz, M.A. (1999). Pressure ulcer development in the VA: characteristics of nursing homes providing best care. American Journal of Medical Quality, 14, 39–44.

Blegen, M.A., Goode, C.J., and Reed, L. (1998). Nurse staffing and patient outcomes. Nursing Research, 47, 43–50.

Board of Directors of the American Association for Geriatric Psychiatry (1992). Position statement. Psychotherapeutic medications in the nursing home. Journal of the American Geriatrics Society, 40, 946–949.

Bourdieu, P. and Passeron, J.(1977). Reproduction in education, society and culture. Sage, London.

Bours, G. J., Halfens, R. J., Lubbers, M., and Haalboom, J. R. (1999). The development of a national registration form to measure the prevalence of pressure ulcers in the Netherlands. Ostomy Wound Management, 45(11), 28–33, 36–38, 40.

Burston, G.R. (1975). Granny-battering. [Letter to the Editor] British Medical Journal, 3(5983), 592.

California Attorney General's Office. Elder and dependent adult abuse (http://safestate.org/index.cfm?navID=11; accessed 16 May 2007).

Castle, N.G., Fogel B., and Mor, V. (1997). Risk factors for physical restraint use in nursing homes: pre- and post-implementation of the Nursing Home Reform Act. Gerontologist, 37, 737–747.

Comijs, H., Pot, A.M., Smit, H.H., Bouter, L.M., and Jonker, C. (1998). Elder abuse in the community: prevalence and consequences. Journal of the American Geriatrics Society, 46, 885–888.

Cooney, C. and Mortimer, A. (1995). Elder abuse and dementia-a pilot study. International Journal of Social Psychiatry, 41, 276–283.

Coyne, A.C., Reichman, W.E., and Berbig, L.J. (1993). The relationship between dementia and elder abuse. American Journal of Psychiatry, 150, 643–646.

Daly, J.M. and Jogerst, G. (2001). Statute definitions of elder abuse. Journal of Elder Abuse and Neglect, 13, 39–57.

Department of Health and Human Services (2003). Nursing homes deficiency trends and survey and certification process consistency (http://oig.hhs.gov/oei/reports/oei-02-01-00600.pdf; accessed 16 May 2007).

Deutsches Institut für Menschenrechte (2006). Soziale Menschenrechte älterer Personen in der Pflege. Deutsches Institut für Menschenrechte (2 Aufl.), Bad Honnef, Berlin (available at http://www.institut-fuer-menschenrechte.de).

DeSantis, J., Engberg, S., and Rogers, J. (1997). Geropsychiatric restraint use. Journal of the American Geriatrics Society, 45, 1515–1518.

Evans, L.K. and Strumpf, N.E. (1989). Tying down the elderly. Journal of the American Geriatrics Society, 37, 65–74.

Evans, L.K., Strump, N.E., Allen-Taylor, S.L., Capezuti, E., Maislin, G., and Jacobsen, B.(1997). A clinical trial to reduce restraints in nursing homes. Journal of the American Geriatrics Society, 45, 67–68.

Galtung, J. (1990). Cultural violence. Journal of Peace Research, 27, 291–305.

Glendenning, F. (1999). Elder abuse and neglect in residential settings: the need for inclusiveness in elder abuse research. Journal of Elder Abuse and Neglect, 10, 1–11.

Görgen, Th., Kreuzer, A., Nägele, B., and Krause, S. (2002). Gewalt gegen Ältere im persönlichen Nahraum. Schriftenreihe des Bundesministeriums für Familie, Senioren, Frauen und Jugend, Band 217. Stuttgart.

Goffman, E. (1961). Asylums: essays on the social situations of mental patients and other inmates. Anchor, Garden City, NY.

Goodridge, D.M., Johnston, P., and Thompson, M. (1996). Conflict and aggression as stressors in the work environment of nursing assistants: implications for institutional elder abuse. Journal of Elder Abuse and Neglect, 8, 49–67.

Hagen, B.F. and Sayers, D. (1995). When caring leaves bruises. Journal of Gerontological Nursing, 21(11), 7–16.

Hagisawa, S. and Barbenel, J. (1999). The limits of pressure sore prevention. Journal of the Royal Society of Medicine, 92, 576–578.

Hamel, M., Gold, P.D., Andres, D. et al. (1990): Predictors and consequences of aggressive behavior by community-based dementia patients. The Gerontologist, 30, 206–211.

Haney, C., Banks, C., and Zimbardo, P.(1973). Interpersonal dynamics in a simulated prison. International Journal of Criminology and Penology, 1, 69–97.

Heinemann A., Lockemann U., Matschke, J., Tsokos M., and Pueschel K. (2000). Dekubitus im Umfeld der Sterbephase: Epidemiologische, medizinrechtliche und ethische Aspekte. Deutsche Medizinische Wochenschrift, 125(3), 45–51.

Hirsch, R.D.(2000). Definition und Abgrenzung von Gewalt und Aggression. In Aggression im Alter (ed. R.D. Hirsch, J. Bruder, and H. Radebold), pp. 15–43. Chudek–Druck, Bornheim-Sechtem.

Hirsch, R.D. and Brendebach, C. (1999). Gewalt gegen alte Menschen in der Familie: Untersuchungsergebnisse der "Bonner HsM–Studie". Zeitschrift für Gerontologie und Geriatrie, 32, 449–455.

Hirsch, R.D., Erkens, F., Flötgen, P., Frießner, K., Halfen, M., and Vollhardt, B. (2002). Handeln statt Misshandeln: Rückblick–Entwicklung–Aktivitäten 1997–2002. Bonner Schriftenreihe "Gewalt im Alter", Band 10. Mabuse, Frankfurt.

Homer, A.C. and Gilleard, C. (1990). Abuse of elderly people by their carers. British Medical Journal, 301, 1359–1362.

Jogerst,G.J., Dawson, J.D., Hartz, A.J., Ely, J.W., and Schweitzer, L.A. (2000). Community characteristics associated with elder abuse. Journal of the American Geriatrics Society, 48, 513–518.

Jones, J.S., Veenstra, T.R., Seamon, J.P., and Krohmer, J. (1997a). Elder mistreatment: national survey of emergency physicians. Annals of Emergency Medicine, 30, 473–479.

Jones, J.S., Holstege, C., and Holstege, H. (1997b). Elder abuse and neglect: understanding the causes and potential risk factors. *American Journal of Emergency Medicine*, **15**, 579–583.

Karlson, S., Nyberg, L., and Sandman, P.O. (1997). The use of physical restraints in elder care in relation to fall risk. *Scandinavian Journal of Caring Science*, **11**, 238–242.

Karlson, S., Bucht, G., and Sandman, P.O. (1998). Physical restraints in geriatric care. *Scandinavian Journal of Caring Science*, **12**, 48–56.

Keene, J., Hope, T., Fairburn. C.G., Jacoby, R., Oedling, K., and Ware, C.J.G. (1999). National history of aggressive behaviour in dementia. *International Journal of Geriatric Psychiatry*, **14**, 541–548.

Kemshall, H. and Pritchard, J. (1996). *Good practice in risk assessment and risk management*. Kingsley Publishers, London.

Kennedy, R.D. (2004). Elder abuse and neglect: the experience, knowledge, and attitudes of primary care physicians. *Family Medicine*, **37**, 481–485.

Kivelä, S.L., Köngäs-Savaro, P., Kesti, E., Pahkala, K., and Ijäs, M.-L. (1992). Abuse in old age-epidemiological data from Finland. *Journal of Elder Abuse and Neglect*, 4(3), 1–8.

Kleinschmidt, K.C. (1997). Elder abuse: a review. *Annals of Emergency Medicine*, **30**, 463–472.

Kranzhoff, E.U. and Hirsch, R.D. (1997). Problemfeld "Fixierung" in der Gerontopsychiatrie. *Zeitschrift für Gerontologie und Geriatrie*, **30**, 321–326.

Kron, M., Loy, S., Sturm, E., Nikolaus, Th., and Becker, C. (2003). Risk indicators for falls in institutionalized frail elderly. *American Journal of Epidemiology*, **158**, 645–653.

Krug, E.G., Dahlberg, L.L., Mercy, J.A., Zwi, A.B., and Lozano, R. (2002). *World report on violence and health*. World Health Organization, Geneva.

Kurrle, S.E., Sadler, P.M., Lockwood, K., and Cameron, I.D. (1997). Elder abuse: prevalence, intervention and outcomes in patients referred to for aged care assessment teams. *Medical Journal of Australia*, **166**, 119–122.

Lachs, M.S. and Pillemer, K. (2004). Elder abuse. *Lancet*, **364**, 1263–1272.

Lachs, M.S., Williams, C., O'Brien, S., Hurst, L., and Horwitz, R. (1996). Older adults. An 11-year longitudinal study of adult protective service use. *Archives of Internal Medicine*, **156**, 449–453.

Lachs, M.S., Williams, C., O'Brien, M.S., Hurst, L., and Horwitz, R. (1997). Risk factors for reported elder abuse and neglect: a nine-year observational cohort study. *The Gerontologist*, **37**, 469–474.

Lachs, M.S., Williams, C., O'Brien, S., Pillemer, K.A., and Charlson, M.E. (1998). The mortality of elder mistreatment. *Journal of the American Medical Association*, **280**, 428–432.

Llorente, M.D., Olsen, E.J., Leyva, O., Silverman, M.A., Lewis J.E., and Rivreo, J. (1998). Use of antipsychotic drugs in nursing homes: current compliance with OBRA regulations. *Journal of the American Geriatrics Society*, **46**, 198–201.

Longres, J.F. (1995). Self-neglect among the elderly. *Journal of Elder Abuse and Neglect*, **7**, 69–86.

Lyketsos, C.G., Steinberg, M., Tschanz, J.T., Norton, M.C., Steffens, D.C., and Breitner, J.C. (2000). Mental and behavioral disturbances in dementia: findings from the Cache County Study on Memory in Aging. *American Journal of Psychiatry*, **157**, 708–714.

McCreadie, C., Bennett, G., Gilthrope, M.S., Houghton, G., and Tinker, A. (2000). Elder abuse: do general practitioners know or care? *Journal of the Royal Society of Medicine*, **93**, 67–71.

Merriam-Webster (2005). *Merriam-Webster collegiate dictionary*, 11th edn. Merriam-Webster, Springfield, MA.

Milgram, S. (1974). *Obedience to authority. An experimental view*. Harper, New York.

National Center on Elder Abuse (NCEA) in collaboration with Westat Inc. (1998). *The National Elder Abuse Incidence Study; final report September 1998* (http://www.aoa.gov/eldfam/Elder_Rights/Elder_Abuse/ABuseReport_Full.pdf; accessed 16 May 2007).

National Center on Elder Abuse (2002). Development training programs on elder abuse prevention for in-home helpers www.elderabusecenter.org/pdf/familiy/training.pdf (visited September 5, 2006).

National Center on Elder Abuse (NCEA). *What is elder abuse?* (http://www.elderabusecenter.org/; accessed 16 May 2007).

National Research Council (2002). Concepts, definitions, and guidelines for measurement. Panel report, panel to review risk and prevalence of elder abuse and neglect. In *National Research Council: elder mistreatment: abuse, neglect, and exploitation in an aging America* (ed. R.J. Bonnie and R.B. Wallace), pp. 34–59. National Academy Press, Washington, DC.

Neufeld, R.R., Libow, L., Foley, W.J., Dunbar, J. M., Cohen, C., and Breuer, B. (1999). Restraint reduction reduces serious injuries among nursing home residents. *Journal of the American Geriatrics Society*, **47**, 1202–1207.

Nightingale, F. (1849). *Notes on nursing: what it is and is not*. Duckworth Press, Philadelphia (1978).

Ogg, J. and Bennett, G. (1992): Elder abuse in Britain. *British Medical Journal*, **305**, 998–999.

Ooi, W.L., Morris, J.N., Brandeis, G.H., Hossian, M., and Lipsitz, L.A. (1999). Nursing home characteristics and the development of pressure sores and disruptive behaviour. *Age and Ageing*, **28**, 45–52.

Parker, K. and Miles, S.H. (1997). Death caused by bedrails. *Journal of the American Geriatrics Society*, **45**, 797–802.

Paveza, G.J., Cohen, D., Eisdorfer, C. et al. (1992). Severe family violence and Alzheimer's disease: prevalence and risk factors. *The Gerontologist*, **32**, 493–497.

Phillips, C.D., Hawes, C., Mor, V., Fries, B.E., Morris, J.N., and Nennstiel, M.E. (1996). Facility and area variation affecting the use of physical restraints in nursing homes. *Medical Care*, **34**, 1149–1162.

Pillemer, K. and Finkelhor, D. (1988): The prevalence of elder abuse: a random sample survey. *The Gerontologist*, **28**, 51–57.

Pillemer, K. and Moore, D.W. (1989). Abuse of patients in nursing homes: findings from a survey of staff. *The Gerontologist*, **29**, 314–320.

Pillemer, K. and Suitor, J.J. (1992).Violence and violent feelings: what causes them among family caregivers? *Journal of Gerontology*, **47**, S165–S172.

Podnieks, E. (1990). *National survey on abuse of the elderly in Canada, The Ryerson Study*. Ryerson Polytechnic Institute, Toronto.

Pritchard, J. (1996). *Working with elder abuse. A training manual for home care, residential and day care staff*. Kingsley Publishers, London.

Reis, M. and Nahmiash, D. (1998). Validation of the Indicators of Abuse (IOA) screen. *The Gerontologist*, **38**, 471–480.

Riedel-Heller, S.G., Stelzner, G., Schork, A., and Angermeyer, M.C. (1999). Gerontopsychiatrische Kompetenz ist gefragt. *Psychiatrische Praxis*, **26**, 273–276.

Robins, L.J., Boyko, E., Lane, J., and Jahnigen, D.W. (1987). Binding the elderly: a prospective study of the use of mechanical restraints in an acute care hospital. *Journal of the American Geriatrics Society*, **35**, 290–296.

Rovner, B.W., Edelman, B.A., Cox, M.P., and Shmuely, Y. (1992). The impact of antipsychotic drug regulations on psychoactive prescribing practices in nursing homes. *American Journal of Psychiatry*, **149**, 1390–1392.

Rudman, D., Mattson, D. E., Alverno, L., Richardson, T.J., and Rudman, I. W. (1993). Comparison of clinical indicators in two nursing homes. *Journal of the American Geriatrics Society*, **41**, 1317–1325.

Schmidt, I., Claesson, C.B., Westerholm, B., Nilson, L.G., and Svarstad, B.L. (1998). The impact of regular multidisciplinary team interventions on psychoactive prescribing in Swedish nursing homes. *Journal of the American Geriatrics Society*, **46**, 77–82.

Schneider, H.D. (1990). Bewohner und Personal als Quellen und Ziele von Gewalttätigkeit in Altersheimen. *Zeitschrift für Gerontologie*, **23**, 186–196.

Schneider, H.J. (1994). *Kriminologie der Gewalt*. Hirzel, Stuttgart.

Snowdon, J. (1999). A follow-up survey of psychotropic drug use in Sydney nursing homes. *Medical Journal of Australia*, **170**, 299–301.

Spector, W.D. and Fortinsky, R.H. (1998). Pressure ulcer prevalence in Ohio nursing homes: clinical and facility correlates. *Journal of Aging and Health*, **10**, 62–80.

Strumpf, N.E. and Evans, L.K. (1991). The ethical problems of prolonged physical restraint. *Journal of Gerontological Nursing*, **17**, 27–30.

Svarstad, B.L. and Mount, J.K. (1991). Nursing home resources and tranquilizer use among the institutionalized elderly. *Journal of the American Geriatrics Society*, **39**, 869–875.

Teaster P.B., Dugar, T.A., Mendiondo, M.S., Abner, E.L., Cecil, K.A., and Otto. J.M. (2006). *The 2004 survey of state adult protective services: abuse of adults 60 years of age and older*. accessed September 14, 2006 at www.elderabusecenter.org/pdf/2–14–06 Final 60+Report.pdf

The Home Care Companion (2006). *Elder abuse training program* (http://www.homecarecompanion.com/eatp.html; accessed 16 May 2007).

Tinetti, M., Liu, W., and Ginter, S. (1992). Mechanical restraint use and fall related injuries among residents of skilled nursing facilities. *Annals of Internal Medicine*, **116**, 369–374.

United Nations (1983). Wiener Internationaler Aktionsplan zur Frage des Alterns. *Weltversammlung zur Frage des Alterns, 26. Juli–6. August 1992, Vienna*. United Nations, New York.

Wetzels, P. and Greve, W. (1996). Alte Menschen als Opfer innerfamiliärer Gewalt-Ergebnisse einer kriminologischen Dunkelfeldstudie. *Zeitschrift für Gerontologie und Geriatrie*, **29**, 191–200.

Wolf, R.S. (1997). Elder abuse and neglect: an update. *Reviews in Clinical Gerontology*, **7**, 177–182.

World Health Organization (1992). *International statistical classification of diseases and related health problems*, 10th revision, Vol. 1. World Health Organization, Geneva.

World Health Organization (2002a). *The Toronto Declaration on the global prevention of elder abuse*. World Health Organization, Geneva.

World Health Organization (2002b). *Missing voices. Views of elder people on elder abuse*. World Health Organization, Geneva.

# 40

# Psychiatric aspects of crime and the elderly

## Seena Fazel

Increasing interest has been directed towards older offenders over the last decade. Demographic trends of rising numbers of older people in Western countries have partly driven this, as have the large numbers of older men who have accumulated in jails and prisons. A steady stream of articles in the media has highlighted this issue, some describing an 'elderly crime wave' and others the development of 'grandpa jails' in certain countries.

## How many older offenders?

In England and Wales, there were 2174 indictable offences in those aged over 60 in 2003 (Home Office, 2000). This represents 0.7% of all indictable offences—a figure that has not changed significantly since 1993 (Fazel and Jacoby, 2002). The absolute number of offences has also remained at a similar level. However, official statistics may not represent the true picture of antisocial behaviour in older people, particularly if the police disproportionately drop charges or caution offenders. But data from the Home Office do not support this, since the caution per conviction ratio is not significantly different by age band (Home Office, 2000).

Despite the numbers or proportion of crimes committed by older persons not appearing to have increased over the last decade, the number of sentenced prisoners aged 60 and above has more than doubled from 536 in 1994 to 1528 in 2004 (Home Office, 2005). This partly reflects overall increases in the sentenced population in England and Wales, which rose from 36,000 to 61,000 over the same time period. However, the proportion of men who were aged over 59 in prison has also doubled over this period to 2.6% (see Table 40. 1).

A similar trend has been observed in America, where the number of prisoners aged 55 and over has increased from 48,800 in 1999 to 71,900 in 2004 (Beck, 2000; Harrison and Beck, 2005). In Canada, the growth in the population of older offenders in prison is more than ten times the growth in the population of younger offenders (Uzoaba, 1998).

The number of receptions (i.e. incidence) of elderly men to prisons in England and Wales has also increased, but not as fast the numbers inside prison (i.e. prevalence). In 1998, there were 661 receptions of those aged over 59 to prison, compared with 339 in 1993 (Fazel and Jacoby, 2002). This reflects what criminologists call 'punitive bifurcation' whereby those in prison are staying in for longer sentences, while the admission rates are growing less quickly.

There were only 20 sentenced women aged over 60 in prison in 2004 in England and Wales, which represents only 0.6% of the female sentenced population. Between 1997 and 2004, the sentenced population of women aged over 50 increased from 60 to 172, and these women were serving longer sentences (HM Inspectorate of Prisons, 2004).

## What sort of crime?

Table 40. 2 shows the offence categories for convictions for men of all ages in 2003. Sexual offences in older men are the largest single offence category with 22% of all indictable offences in that age group. Theft and handling make up 21% of the offences in older men. In the women, the pattern is quite different. The crimes making up the largest proportion of their offences are theft and handling (46%) and fraud and forgery (28%).

Sexual offences as a proportion of all offences committed by a respective age group increases from young to old (in contrast to theft and handling). This is also reflected in prison where over half of the elderly sentenced male prisoners in England and Wales are sexual offenders—a proportion that has been increasing over the last decade. In 1993, 43% of the sentenced male prison population in England and Wales of over 59s were sexual offenders, and this had risen in 1998 to 49%, and in 2004 to 57% (Table 40. 3). Large numbers of incarcerated elderly sexual offenders are

**Table 40.1** Rise in population of men aged 60 and over in prison establishments in England and Wales from 1994 to 1999 expressed as a percentage of males of all ages (Home Office, 2000). For 2000 onwards the proportion is for sentenced prisoners only (Prison Statistics, Home Office)

| Year | 1994 | 1995 | 1996 | 1997 | 1998 | 1999 | 2000 | 2001 | 2002 | 2003 | 2004 |
|------|------|------|------|------|------|------|------|------|------|------|------|
| % of all ages | 1.51 | 1.59 | 1.69 | 1.75 | 1.80 | 2.15 | 2.20 | 2.30 | 2.40 | 2.52 | 2.62 |

**Table 40.2** Indictable offences in England and Wales in those aged 60 and over, in 2003 (Home Office, 2005, IOS 263-05)

| Offence category | Men | | Women | |
|---|---|---|---|---|
| | n | % | n | % |
| Violence against the person | 257 | 13.6 | 29 | 10.4 |
| Sexual offences | 409 | 21.6 | 1 | 0.4 |
| Burglary | 23 | 1.2 | 0 | 0.0 |
| Robbery | 7 | 0.4 | 1 | 0.4 |
| Theft and handling stolen goods | 402 | 21.2 | 129 | 46.1 |
| Fraud and forgery | 245 | 12.9 | 78 | 27.9 |
| Criminal damage | 42 | 2.2 | 6 | 2.1 |
| Drug offences | 124 | 6.5 | 12 | 4.3 |
| Other indictable offences | 309 | 16.3 | 17 | 6.1 |
| Indictable motoring offences | 76 | 4.0 | 7 | 2.5 |
| Total | 1894 | 100.0 | 280 | 100.0 |

also found in other Western countries. In Canada, for example, half of the male sentenced prison population aged over 59s are sexual offenders (Uzoaba, 1998). In the state of Florida, 34% of new receptions aged 65 and older in 2004–2005 were for sexual offences (State of Florida Correctional Medical Authority, 2005).

One of the reasons for this is that sexual offences in older adults are probably viewed more seriously by the courts than other offences in older people. Another likely contribution to this proportion is that with longer sentences being given to sexual crimes, many men are growing old in prison.

## Psychiatric associations

To date, no population studies of crime in older persons have been conducted. Overall, the information on psychiatric associations is limited, and most surveys are from selected samples at various stages in the criminal justice system. Some of these provide information for the development and planning of forensic psychiatric and prison healthcare services. Studies examining the pattern of psychiatric morbidity in older offenders referred for assessment and treatment (Heinik et al., 1994; Barak et al., 1995), and differences between older and younger offenders, can be useful in this regard. The largest of this type of study was conducted in Sweden, and examined psychiatric diagnoses in 203 older criminals referred for inpatient assessment prior to sentencing, comparing them with younger referrals (Fazel and Grann, 2002). In offenders aged over 60, 31% had a psychotic illness and 15% had substance abuse or dependence (see Table 40. 4).

In addition, investigations of referral patterns for older offenders to secure hospitals finds them to be surprisingly low considering

**Table 40.3** Proportion of sentenced men imprisoned in England and Wales in 2004 for sexual offences as percentage of all offences for respective age group (Home Office, 2005, IOS 263-05)

| All ages | 21–24 | 25–29 | 30–39 | 40–49 | 50–59 | 60+ |
|---|---|---|---|---|---|---|
| 9.9 | 3.5 | 4.0 | 8.4 | 18.0 | 34.2 | 57.4 |

the degree of psychiatric morbidity in this group. Using data from 7 out of the 14 health regions in England and Wales from 1988–1994, it was found that only 2% of all admissions to secure hospital were of individuals above the age of 60 and there was no increase in the number of older men being admitted over the study period (Coid et al., 2002). This is similar to the proportion of referrals in the over 65s (1.4%) to a large medium-security unit in London during 1990–2002 (Tomar et al., 2005).

## Psychiatric morbidity of older prisoners

A number of studies over the last decade have investigated the mental health of prisoners. The largest of these is a study of sentenced men in England and Wales (Fazel et al., 2001a), which found that one in three prisoners over the age of 60 had a potentially treatable mental illness (see Table 40.5). Using a standardized semi-structured diagnostic instrument, the Geriatric Mental State Schedule, the main findings were that 32% (95% CI, 26–38%) had a diagnosis of mental illness, and 30% (24–36%) had a diagnosis of personality disorder. In total, 53% (46–60%) of the sample had a psychiatric diagnosis (mental illness or personality disorder). Rates of psychosis and depression combined (30%) were higher in these older men than in surveys of adult male prisoners of all ages where typically one in seven prisoners have a treatable mental illness (Fazel and Danesh, 2002).

The prevalence of depression was higher than that found in younger male prisoners, which is typically around 10%

**Table 40.4** Principal psychiatric diagnoses in older individuals referred for forensic psychiatric assessment in Sweden, 1988–2000 (from Fazel and Grann, 2002)

| Psychiatric diagnosis | All ages | Age 60 and over | Age 65 and over |
|---|---|---|---|
| Dementia | 19 (0.3%) | 15 (7.1%)** | 9 (8.7%)** |
| Schizophrenia | 849 (11.6%) | 15 (7.1%)* | 5 (4.9%)* |
| Affective psychoses | 270 (3.7%) | 14 (6.7%)* | 4 (3.9%) |
| Toxic psychoses | 160 (2.2%) | 5 (2.4%) | 3 (2.9%) |
| Other organic psychoses | 250 (3.4%) | 8 (3.8%) | 5 (4.9%) |
| Other psychoses | 767 (10.5%) | 25 (11.9%) | 15 (4.6%) |
| All psychoses | 2296 (31.4%) | 67 (31.4%) | 41 (39.8%) |
| Personality disorder | 2364 (32.4%) | 41 (19.5%)** | 23 (22.3%)* |
| Alcohol/drug abuse/dependence | 916 (12.5%) | 31 (14.8%) | 13 (12.6%) |
| Depressive and anxiety disorders | 398 (5.5%) | 16 (7.6%) | 9 (8.7%) |
| Sexual disorders | 118 (1.6%) | 6 (2.9%) | 3 (2.9%) |
| Cerebral lesions | 107 (1.5%) | 10 (4.8%)** | 2 (1.9%) |
| Mental retardation | 165 (2.3%) | 4 (1.9%) | 1 (1.0%) |
| Others | 647 (8.9%) | 13 (6.2%) | 7 (6.8%) |
| No diagnosis | 271 (3.7%) | 7 (3.3%) | 4 (3.9%) |
| Column total | 7301 (100%) | 210 (100%) | 103 (100%) |

Note: In the column 'Age 60 and over', the c2-test (d.f. = 1) compared those aged 60+ with those under 60. In the column 'Age 65 and over', the c2-test (d.f. = 1) compared those aged 65+ with those under 65.

* P < 0.05; ** P < 0.001.

**Table 40.5** Psychiatric diagnoses in male sentenced prisoners aged over 60 (*n* = 203)

| Diagnoses | % of prisoners |
|---|---|
| Psychoses: | |
| Depressive | 4 |
| Other | 1 |
| Total | 5 |
| Neuroses: | |
| Depressive | 25 |
| Hypochondriasis | 1 |
| Total | 26 |
| Organic disorders: | |
| Dementia | 1 |
| DSM-IV personality disorder: | |
| Antisocial personality disorder | 8 |
| Any personality disorder | 30 |
| Current substance abuse/dependence | 5 |
| Total psychiatric morbidity[a] | 53 |

a The total is less than the sum of individual disorders because some prisoners had more than one disorder.

(Fazel and Danesh, 2002). This prevalence was also higher than in a large community study of older men that used the same diagnostic instrument, and which found that 6% had a depressive illness (Saunders *et al.*, 1993). In the older prisoner study, the risk of being diagnosed with depression was higher in those with a past psychiatric history (relative risk 2.1), and those with poor self-reported physical health (relative risk 2.2), consistent with known risk factors in the community for depression in older adults (Copeland *et al.*, 1999). The standardized mortality ratio for suicide in male prisoners aged over 60 is five times that of men in the general population of similar age, a proportionate excess that was similar to prisoners in younger age groups (Fazel *et al.*, 2005).

Research on older women in prison has been more limited. No differences between older women and older men were found in the rates of recorded mental illness in a study using medical records (17% in the women compared with 16% in the male inmates) (Regan *et al.*, 2002). Another investigation of 120 older women inmates in the USA found that 16% reported one or more impairments in activities of daily living, and described high rates of chronic medical illnesses (Williams *et al.*, 2006).

## Alcohol and substance abuse

Alcohol abuse and dependence is a particular problem in older prisoners. In a UK study of remand prisoners, Taylor and Parrott (1988) reported a steady increase with age in the numbers of prisoners experiencing alcohol withdrawal symptoms and one-third of prisoners over 65 reported such symptoms. A large American study in Iowa State Prison found that 71% of inmates aged over 55 years reported a substance misuse problem compared with over 90% of younger age groups. It also found that in comparison with younger prisoners, older inmates were more likely to abuse alcohol solely, as distinct from multiple substances (Arndt *et al.*, 2002).

## Sex offenders

Older sex offenders have been the focus of a number of studies. These have shown that recidivism rates tend to be lower than in younger sex offenders discharged from criminal justice and secure hospital settings in the USA, Canada, and the UK (Hanson, 2002; Barbaree *et al.*, 2003; Langan *et al.*, 2003). Possible explanations for this include lower sexual arousal in older men (Barbaree *et al.*, 2003) and increased self-control with age (Hanson, 2002). Cohort effects may also be relevant. A recent report described recidivism among mainly Canadian sex offenders released from prison and leaving secure hospitals, and investigated differences in rates of recidivism (without accounting for time at risk) by comparing rapists, incest offenders, and extra-familial child molesters (Hanson, 2002). It found potentially interesting differences. This work suggested that rates of recidivism were negatively correlated with age in rapists, but this was less apparent in other types of sexual offenders. This has been replicated in a study of all prisoners released in the USA in 1994, where it was found that rates of repeat sexual offending in child molesters were similar across age bands. However, age 45 and over was taken as the oldest age group (Langan *et al.*, 2003). A study of all sex offenders released from Swedish prisons has also explored age-related factors, and found that the rate of recidivism at 9 years post-release was 6.7% in the over 55-year-olds compared with 43% in those aged under 25. This study yielded some preliminary findings on differences in the risk factors for repeat offending. Having a stranger victim was the strongest risk factor in the over 55s, whereas it appeared not to be associated with recidivism in the under 25s (Fazel *et al.*, 2006).

In older prisoners incarcerated for sexual offences, the prevalence rates of mental illness are similar to those of other older male inmates. However, elderly sex offenders had more schizoid, obsessive–compulsive, and avoidant personality traits, supporting the view that sex offending in the elderly may be associated more with personality factors than with mental illness or organic brain disease (Fazel *et al.*, 2002a).

## Service and treatment implications

As stated above, prison research has shown that around 5% of older male inmates suffer from a psychotic illness. This represents a large number of psychotic inmates, and is consistent with the 4% found in a systematic review of surveys of prisoners of all ages (Fazel and Danesh, 2002). If this is extrapolated to the total elderly prison population, then the 5% with psychosis represents around 70–80 elderly sentenced men who would be psychotic at any one time in English and Welsh prisons in 2004, almost all with a depressive psychosis. Most psychiatrists would wish to see these individuals transferred to a hospital—whether secure or not—for treatment.

Similarly, around 400 elderly inmates in English and Welsh prisons would be suffering from a major (non-psychotic) clinical depression, most of whom could probably be treated appropriately within the prison setting. However, there need to be substantial improvements in prison healthcare for this to happen. In a recent study in English and Welsh prisons, only 18% of the depressed prisoners were being treated with antidepressants (Fazel *et al.*, 2004). Three-quarters of this sample were being prescribed some medication, mostly for physical disorders, and elderly prisoners were therefore in regular contact with prison doctors for their physical health needs. These contacts should provide ample opportunity for assessment and treatment of psychiatric illness within the prison setting. Similar problems with undertreatment have been found in the USA, and in one study, 13 out of 16 older inmates with active psychiatric disorders received no treatment at all (Koenig *et al.*, 1995).

Nevertheless, this population poses particular challenges for prison health services. Older depressed men may not come to the attention of prison medical staff as they sit quietly in their cells, not causing any problems for prison officers nor posing a security risk. A number of possible improvements in the prison service may assist.

First, improvements in the identification of depression in older inmates need to be considered. This may include improved training among prison staff and better screening of older prisoner receptions. Such educational interventions, though, are not sufficient. The Hampshire Depression Project, a randomized controlled trial of an educational intervention for the detection and treatment of depression in primary care in the UK, did not find that an educational programme based on clinical practice guidelines improved the recognition or outcome of depression in a community setting (Thompson *et al.*, 2000). Regular review of prisoners' medical records, with a view to aligning medication regimes with identified illnesses, would be a simple but effective intervention (Fazel *et al.*, 2004). However, structural changes to the delivery of healthcare in prisons are required; they have been shown to improve outcomes in the US prison system. In an impressive initiative to improve the medical care of all inmates in the state of Texas, a form of managed care (a general term for the activity of organizing doctors, hospitals, and other providers into groups in order to improve the quality and cost-effectiveness of healthcare) was introduced. Part of the model was that two Texan medical schools assumed responsibility for the delivery of medical care for prisoners. This included direct university involvement in primary ambulatory care clinics in each prison, prison hospitals at a regional level, and a prison hospital on an academic medical campus. Among the psychiatric services available were group and individual psychotherapy, psychotropic medication, and crisis-intervention counselling. A key part of the success of this initiative, it was argued, was the integration of prison health services with an academic medical school and its affiliated hospitals. Other areas that were highlighted included the use of standard disease-management guidelines, a common formulary, specific training for doctors, use of chronic care clinics, and technologies such as telemedicine and electronic medical records (Raimer and Stobo, 2004).

There is increasing support for separate prison wings for older prisoners. In the USA, in 1998, there were at least 12 states that had set up separate facilities for older prisoners. In the UK there are currently three—HMPs Frankland, Kingston, and Wymott. Older prisoners differ from younger inmates in the extent of their medical problems and disabilities (Fazel *et al.*, 2001b), and in their psychosocial needs as well as the psychiatric problems described above. High rates of victimization by younger inmates is a concern noted in the wide-ranging 2004 study from the Inspectorate of Prisons in England and Wales which interviewed 442 older men and 47 women (HM Inspectorate of Prisons, 2004). The physical condition and structure of a prison—designed for young, active inmates—can create significant problems for older, frailer inmates, and particularly for those with limited mobility. A range of measures to improve the physical environment of prisons was suggested

in the Inspectorate's report. These include housing such prisoners on lower landings, separate regimes, and improved training for prison staff (HM Inspectorate of Prisons, 2004). Another study has highlighted some improvements specifically for older women prisoners (Wahidin, 2003). There are various arguments for and against age-segregated facilities. In favour is the likelihood of less victimization and a sense of greater safety, the relative ease of organizing separate regimes, and the wishes of older prisoners as reported in several US studies on age-segregated facilities. Further, the 'institutional thoughtlessness' of current prison regimes is believed to magnify existing problems (Crawley and Sparks, 2005). However, against these arguments is the view that older prisoners provide a normalizing influence for younger ones; that segregation may lead to neglect of this group of inmates; that specialist facilities are likely to be further away from home; and a possible problem with a lack of social stimulation and participation in prison activities (Howse, 2003).

Another area of consideration is sentencing policy for the elderly. Much debate has been generated over the policies of successive UK governments, and the problems of incarcerating persons who pose little risk to the public. This problem is exemplified in the case of individuals who develop dementia whilst in custody (Fazel *et al.*, 2002b). Recidivism research in a variety of criminal justice and mental health settings has shown low rates of reoffending by older criminals (Bonta *et al.*, 1998; Hanson, 2002). Whether psychiatric risk factors are important in predicting reoffending in older offenders remains uncertain, and this area is a research priority in the future. Some researchers have called for national strategies to address these inter-related issues (Crawley and Sparks, 2005).

Outside prison, the development of specialist services for older offenders could be considered. In the UK, a number of authors have considered the development of supraregional medium-security units, which may be able to focus their treatment regimes more appropriately to older offenders and provide a safer setting. In particular, the admission of older individuals with dementia to normal medium- and low-security units would be problematic as the medical and allied healthcare staff would have had little training and experience in dealing with such patients. The problem, though, may be that supraregional units are likely be quite far away from the family, carers, and friends of these patients, and also from the community settings to where they will eventually be discharged.

As demographic changes continue to suggest that increasing numbers of older men and women will come into contact with the criminal justice system in Western countries, responding to the mental health needs of older offenders is an important challenge for psychiatry, public health, and prison health. Successful interventions to meet these needs in one country are likely to have implications wider afield and attract the attention of prison health services in other jurisdictions as they gradually face up to this relatively new challenge.

## Acknowledgements

I am grateful to Robin Jacoby and Catherine Oppenheimer for helpful comments on previous drafts.

## References

Arndt, S., Turvey, C., and Flaum, M. (2002). Older offenders, substance abuse, and treatment. *American Journal of Geriatric Psychiatry*, **10**, 733–739.

Barak, Y., Perry, T., and Elizur, A. (1995). Elderly criminals: a study of first criminal offence in old age. *International Journal of Geriatric Psychiatry*, **10**, 511–516.

Barbaree, H., Blanchard, R., and Langton, C. (2003). The development of sexual aggression through the life span: the effect of age on sexual arousal and recidivism among sex offenders. *Annals of the New York Academy of Sciences*, **989**, 59–71.

Beck, A. (2000). *Prison and jail inmates at midyear 1999*. Bureau of Justice Statistics Bulletin, Washington, DC.

Bonta, J., Law, M., and Hanson, K. (1998). The prediction of criminal and violent recidivism among mentally disordered offenders: a meta-analysis. *Psychological Bulletin*, **123**, 123–142.

Coid, J., Fazel, S., and Kahtan, N. (2002). Elderly patients admitted to secure forensic psychiatry services. *Journal of Forensic Psychiatry*, **13**, 416–427.

Copeland, J., Chen, R., Dewey, M. *et al.* (1999). Community-based case-control study of depression in older people. *British Journal of Psychiatry*, **175**, 340–347.

Crawley, E. and Sparks, R. (2005). Hidden Injuries? Researching the experiences of older men in English prisons. *The Howard Journal*, **44**, 345–356.

Fazel, S. and Danesh, J. (2002). Serious mental disorder in 23 000 prisoners: a systematic review of 62 surveys. *Lancet*, **359**, 545–550.

Fazel, S. and Grann, M. (2002). Older criminals: a descriptive study of psychiatrically examined offenders in Sweden. *International Journal of Geriatric Psychiatry*, **17**, 907–913.

Fazel, S. and Jacoby, R. (2002). Psychiatric aspects of crime and the elderly. In *Psychiatry in the elderly*, 3rd edn (ed. R. Jacoby and C. Oppenheimer), pp. 919–931. Oxford University Press, Oxford.

Fazel, S., Hope, T., O'Donnell, I., and Jacoby, R. (2001a). Hidden psychiatric morbidity in elderly prisoners. *British Journal of Psychiatry*, **179**, 535–539.

Fazel, S., O'Donnell, I., Hope, T., Piper, M., and Jacoby, R. (2001b). Health of elderly male prisoners: worse than younger prisoners, worse than the general population. *Age and Ageing*, **30**, 403–407.

Fazel, S., Hope, T., O'Donnell, I., and Jacoby, R. (2002a). Psychiatric, demographic, and personality characteristics of elderly sex offenders. *Psychological Medicine*, **32**, 219–226.

Fazel, S., McMillan, J., and O'Donnell, I. (2002b). Dementia in prison: ethical and legal implications. *Journal of Medical Ethics*, **28**, 156–159.

Fazel, S., Hope, T., O'Donnell, I., and Jacoby, R. (2004). Unmet treatment needs of older prisoners: a primary care survey. *Age and Ageing*, **33**, 396–398.

Fazel, S., Benning, R., and Danesh, J. (2005). Suicides in male prisoners in England and Wales, 1978–2003. *Lancet*, **366**, 1301–1302.

Fazel, S., Langstrom, N., Sjostedt, G., and Grann, M. (2006). Risk factors for criminal recidivism in older sexual offenders. *Sexual Abuse: a Journal of Research and Treatment*, **18**, 159–167.

Hanson, K. (2002). Recidivism and age: follow-up data from 4,673 offenders. *Journal of Interpersonal Violence*, **17**, 1046–1062.

Harrison, P. and Beck, A. (2005). *Prisoners in 2004*, Bureau of Justice Statistics Bulletin NCJ 210677. Bureau of Justice, Washington, DC.

Heinik, J., Kimhi, R., and Hes, J. (1994). Dementia and crime: a forensic psychiatry unit study in Israel. *International Journal of Geriatric Psychiatry*, **9**, 491–494.

HM Inspectorate of Prisons (2004). *'No problems – old and quiet': older prisoners in England and Wales*. HMSO, London.

Home Office (2000). *Prison Statistics England and Wales 1999*, Cm 4805. Stationery Office, London.

Home Office (2005). *Prison statistics 2004: England and Wales*. HMSO, London.

Howse, K. (2003). *Growing old in prison: a scoping study on older prisoners*. Prison Reform Trust, London.

Koenig, H., Johnson, S., Bellard, J., Denker, M., and Fenlon, R. (1995). Depression and anxiety disorder among older inmates at a federal correctional facility. *Psychiatric Services*, **46**, 399–401.

Langan, P., Schmitt, E., and Durose, M. (2003). *Recidivism of sex offenders released from prison in 1994*, Bureau of Justice Statistics Bulletin NCJ 198281. US Department of Justice, Washington, DC.

Raimer, B. and Stobo, J. (2004). Health care delivery in the Texas prison system: the role of academic medicine. *Journal of the American Medical Association*, **292**, 485–489.

Regan, J., Alderson, A., and Regan, W. (2002). Psychiatric disorders in aging prisoners. *Clinical Gerontologist*, **26**, 117–124.

Saunders, P., Copeland, J., Dewey, M., Gilmore, C., Larkin, B., Phaterpekar, H., and Scott, A. (1993). The prevalence of dementia, depression and neurosis in later life: the Liverpool MRC-ALPHA study. *International Journal of Epidemiology*, **22**, 838–847.

State of Florida Correctional Medical Authority (2005). *Report on elderly and aging inmates in the Florida Department of Corrections*. Correctional Medical Authority, Tallahassee, FL.

Taylor, P. and Parrott, J. (1988). Elderly offenders: a study of age-related factors among custodially remanded prisoners. *British Journal of Psychiatry*, **152**, 340–346.

Thompson, C., Kimmoth, A., Stevens, L., Peveler, R., Stevens, A., and Osler, K. (2000). Effect of a clinical practice guideline and practice based education on detection and outcome on depression in primary care: Hampshire Depression Project randomised controlled trial. *Lancet*, **355**, 185–191.

Tomar, R., Treasaden, I., and Shah, A. (2005). Is there a case for a specialist forensic psychiatry service for the elderly? *International Journal of Geriatric Psychiatry*, **20**, 51–56.

Uzoaba, J. (1998). *Managing older offenders: where do we stand?*. Correctional Service of Canada, Ottawa.

Wahidin, A. (2003). Doing hard time. Older women in prison. *Prison Service Journal*, **145**, 25–29.

Williams, B., Lindquist, K., Sudore, R., Strupp, H., Willmott, D., and Walter, L. (2006). Being old and doing time: functional impairment and adverse experiences of geriatric female prisoners. *Journal of the American Geriatric Society*, **54**, 702–707.

# 41

# Testamentary capacity

## Harvey D. Posener and Robin Jacoby

...Sed omni
Membrorum damno major dementia, quae nec
Nomina servorum nec vultum agnoscit amici,
Cum quo praeterita coenavit nocte, nec illos
Quos genuit, quos eduxit. Nam codice saevo
Haeredes vetat esse suos: bona tota feruntur
Ad Phialen. Tantum artificis valet halitus oris,
Quod steterat multis in carcere fornicis annis.

But worse than any physical disablement is the dementia that cannot remember servants' names nor recognize the face of a friend with whom he has dined on the previous evening, nor even the children whom he fathered and raised himself. By a cruel testament he forbids his own flesh and blood to be his heirs; all his possessions go to Phiale. So potent was the breath of her mouth that stood on sale at the brothel for many years.

Juvenal, *Satire 10, c.* AD 125

Testamentary capacity, or being of sound disposing mind, is the capacity to make a legally valid Will. Thus, whether or not a person has testamentary capacity is a legal and not a medical test.

In England and Wales the execution of Wills (signing them as required in the presence of witnesses) is governed by various Acts of Parliament, such as the Wills Acts (1837, 1861, 1963, and 1968), and in some circumstances the Mental Health Act 1983. As regards testamentary capacity in particular, these statutes are augmented by a large amount of case law. For a clear and concise account of testamentary capacity from the legal standpoint, in which specific cases are referenced, the reader is referred to Volume I, Chapter 4 of the *Eighth Edition of Williams on Wills* (Sherrin *et al.*, 2002).

The importance of case law in this area is exemplified by the fact that the classic statement of the law still remains the case of *Banks* v. *Goodfellow* which was decided in 1870. The trial concerned the validity of a Will made by John Banks leaving the bulk of his estate to his niece. From the facts it appeared that John Banks had made his Will in 1863. He had been confined as a lunatic for some months in 1841 and from that time he remained subject to a delusion that he was personally molested by a man who had long been dead and that he was pursued by evil spirits whom he believed to be visibly present. These delusions were shown to have existed between 1841 and the date of his death in 1865. His estate was considerable (15 houses). The Court came to the conclusion that Mr Banks's Will was valid on the basis that partial unsoundness of mind, which did not actually influence the way in which somebody disposed of their property, did not make a person incapable of validly disposing of his property by a Will.

The then Lord Chief Justice Cockburn stated:

> It is essential...that a testator [testator for a male; testatrix for a female] shall understand the nature of the act and its effects; shall understand the extent of the property of which he is disposing; shall be able to comprehend and appreciate claims to which he ought to give effect; and with a view to the latter object no disorder of mind shall poison his affections, pervert his sense of right and prevent the exercise of his natural faculties – that no insane delusion shall influence his Will in disposing of the property and bring about a disposal of it which, if the mind had been sound, would not have been made.

This still remains the basis of the law in the UK today. Identical or very similar tests for testamentary capacity are used in North American, Australian, and New Zealand jurisdictions. Indeed in *Banks* v. *Goodfellow*, Lord Chief Justice Cockburn was essentially restating the earlier decision of a New Jersey Court.

There is nothing in these criteria to prevent a testator from acting in a capricious or frivolous way, or out of mean or even bad motives. As long as testamentary capacity can be established the Will will be valid (*Boughton and Marston* v. *Knight and Others* 1873). It may, however, be hard to distinguish between capriciousness and lack of testamentary capacity, and it would probably necessitate an examination of the evidence relating to how the testator behaved throughout his life to come to any valid conclusions. As this is a medical textbook it is not the place to go in detail into *inofficious* Wills, a term for those that make inadequate or unfair provision for dependants who might expect to benefit. However, whilst English law does permit a testator with capacity 'unfettered discretion' (see below) there are safeguards contained in statute to prevent, in certain specified circumstances, a dependant or close relative being left destitute. Peisah (2005) has argued that an inofficious Will might sometimes raise the suspicion of incapacity.

The criteria for testamentary capacity can therefore be broken down into three distinct elements:

1 The testator must understand the nature of the act and its effects.

2 The testator must be aware of the *extent* of the property being disposed of.

**3** The testator must be able to understand the nature and extent of the claims upon him both of those whom he is including in his Will and those whom he is excluding.

# The nature of the act

The act of making a Will involves understanding that the testator is entering into a document which will take effect upon his death and that the Will will operate in law after his death to determine who receives his estate. That until such time as he dies he can change his Will. There is now case law which does allow the courts to limit this right to some extent in cases where the testator has made representations to third parties where those third parties have relied upon those representations to their detriment. This doctrine is known as *proprietary estoppel* (see *Gillett* v. *Holt* 2000). An example can be found in the case of *Jennings* v. *Rice and Other* (2002). In that case Mr Jennings provided care to an elderly lady on the basis that 'this will all be yours one day' or words to that effect; her will left nothing to him and the court intervened to make an appropriate award to him, in that case £200,000 which was considerably less than her estate which was £1,225,000 net.

The testator should know:

- whom he has appointed as executors in his Will (if any);

- to whom he has made gifts;

- the extent of those gifts;

- and whether those gifts are made outright or conditional upon the occurrence of some event.

In short, and at the risk of stating the obvious, but perhaps overlooked at times, the testator should know and understand the contents of his Will. In addition, the testator should understand that the Will will operate to revoke any previous Will that he has made. He should, therefore, be aware of the differences between his old Will and his new Will and should be aware of the reasons for the changes.

It is clear from a consideration of the above points that, the more complex the Will (and the more complex the estate of the testator), the greater will be the degree of mental capacity required to constitute testamentary capacity in that particular individual (*Park* v. *Park* 1954) (Shulman *et al.* 2005). The case cited here is of particular interest because the testator was deemed to have had the capacity to marry but lack the capacity to make a Will. Both acts took place on 30 May 1949, the marriage at 11.30 and the Will at 14.30 during the wedding reception!—a nice illustration of the task-specificity of competence (see Chapter 42) and an example of the higher mental capacity required for Will-making, even though as a matter of law the act of marriage will result in the revocation of a previous Will (save in cases where that Will was entered into 'in contemplation of marriage').

## Extent of the property

It is not necessary for a testator to know the exact value of his estate. However, a testator should understand the extent of the property that is owned solely by him and whether he owns any property jointly with another person, and if so whether upon his death the property will form part of his estate or will simply pass to the surviving joint owner by operation of law. He should be aware of whether there are any assets that will pass outside of his estate as a result of his death. For instance are there any life policies held upon trust for third parties? Does he have a life interest in a Trust that will now pass to a third party as a result of his death (over which he may or may not have a right to determine who receives the capital and/or income)?

## The claims of others

It is worth while setting out again the last part of the test in *Banks* v. *Goodfellow*:

> it is essential…that a testator…shall be able to comprehend and appreciate claims to which he ought to give effect; and with a view to the latter object that no disorder of mind shall poison his affections, pervert his sense of right or prevent the exercise of his natural faculties – that no insane delusion shall influence his Will in disposing of the property and bring about a disposal of it which, if the mind had been sound, would not have been made

A testator should be capable of understanding the claims to which he ought to give effect and—if he intends to prefer one beneficiary to another—the reasons why. For example, one potential beneficiary might be financially much better off than another. A testator may have given gifts to one beneficiary during his lifetime but not another. One potential beneficiary's financial needs may be much greater than another, perhaps one potential beneficiary is suffering from either a physical or mental disability which would increase his claim upon the testator's bounty (see the example of Mrs C., below). However, as has been stated previously, a testator may act capriciously provided that this capriciousness is not caused or influenced by a mental disorder, such as dementia. For example, in the case of *Beal et al.* v. *Henri et al.* (1951) a man disinherited his wife and daughters and left his estate to his mistress. In life he had always been 'eccentric, acted absurdly and foolishly, had wrong headed notions and was extremely difficult to live with. He was also under [a] delusion…'. The court dismissed the claim of his wife and daughters that the Will was invalid, ruling that 'the testator's delusion…, his eccentricity and bad character did not show that he did not appreciate the moral claims on him and did not act in the exercise of his true will in disposing of his property'. In other words his eccentricity and bad character did not in his particular case invalidate his testamentary capacity.

It might seem that this case from 1951 was supported by a much more recent one (*Sharp & Bryson* v. *Adam and Others* 2006) which came to the appeal where Lord Justice May stated 'English Law "leaves everything to the unfettered discretion of the testator" on the assumption that "the instincts, affections and common sentiments of mankind may safely be trusted to secure, on the whole a better disposition of the property of the dead" than stereotyped and inflexible rules'. The latter phrase is clearly a side-swipe at the Napoleonic Code in France and other parts of Europe where the concept of mandatory heirs restricts testamentary freedom to a much greater degree than does English law. However, in this very case the Court of Appeal upheld a judgement against the Will that excluded completely the testator's two daughters even though the solicitor who drew up the disputed Will meticulously observed Templeman's 'golden rule' (and saw to the testator's execution of his Will 'in a quite exemplary fashion'). (For the 'Golden Rule' see below under 'Prospective assessment'). The judgement hinged on *Banks* v. *Goodfellow*, because the testator was deemed to have suffered mental impairment due to multiple sclerosis, and the court ruled that the deceased could not satisfy that element of *Banks*

v. *Goodfellow* which states (in abbreviated form) 'that no disorder of mind…shall…bring about a disposal…which, if the mind had been sound, would not have been made'.

It is obvious from a consideration of the elements of testamentary capacity that are set out above, and from an analysis of what the testator must understand, that the degree of capacity required is relatively high (see *Re Beaney* 1978). *Banks* v. *Goodfellow* is actually a test which sets out in legal detail the more general proposition that it is a general requirement of the law that for a juristic act to be valid the person performing it should have the mental capacity (with the assistance of such explanation as shall have been given to him) to understand the nature and effect of that act (see, for example, Lord Justice Peter Gibson in *Hoff and Other* v. *Atherton* 2003).

## Impact of delusions on testamentary capacity

As Lord Chief Justice Cockburn indicated in the case of *Banks* v. *Goodfellow*, 'no insane delusion shall influence his Will'. In other words, delusional disorder directly affecting the three criteria for a sound disposing mind, and in particular the third criterion (awareness of those who have a claim on the testator's bounty) can invalidate a Will. Thus, the Will of a man who disinherits his wife and children because of a delusional belief that they are electronically programmed to steal his money for Al-Qa'eda, would not be valid. However, a valid Will is not invalidated by subsequent mental disorder which impairs testamentary capacity. For instance, a Will made by a healthy person at 55 is not invalidated by very severe dementia at 75.

Nor does insanity *at the time of making a Will* in itself invalidate the Will. In the case of *O'Neil et al.* v. *Royal Trust Co. and McClure et al.* (1946) a woman was bequeathed her husband's estate by him with the request that she in turn bequeath it to his great nieces. After his death, however, she made a first Will which went against his wishes. Later, she was admitted (for many years) to a private mental hospital with a chronic delusional and hallucinatory psychosis—no diagnosis is stated in the law report but the description strongly suggests paranoid schizophrenia. She was deemed incapable of handling her own financial affairs and legal measures were implemented to manage them on her behalf. Whilst in the mental hospital she made another Will revoking the previous one and fulfilling her husband's request. The Court upheld this last Will because there was no evidence that her delusions or hallucinations had influenced her decision to make the Will or determine its contents. In short she passed the *Banks* v. *Goodfellow* test. Indeed, the case of *Banks* v. *Goodfellow*, discussed above, was directly on the point of delusions and the court held the Will to be valid.

The judiciary may take a different view of what delusions are, compared with psychiatrists who define them as 'fixed, false beliefs of morbid origin that are inconsistent with the believer's cultural or educational background'. This has relevance to testamentary capacity in cases where parents form intense feelings against their children. There are two 19th century judgements where what appear to have been overvalued ideas led the respective judges to regard them as so unnatural that they were deemed a disorder of the mind, i.e. delusional. In *Dew* v. *Clark & Clark* (1826) (before *Banks* v. *Goodfellow*) Nicholl J held that the testator, Ely Stott, had held a long and persistent dislike of his only daughter to the extent that it was a delusion. 'For the prominent feature of the deceased's insanity, in respect of the daughter, was aversion or antipathy to the daughter – so pleaded and so proved'. In *Boughton* v. *Knight* (1873) (after *Banks* v. *Goodfellow*) Hannen J stated:

> If a woman believes she is one of the persons of the Trinity, and that the gentleman to whom she leaves the bulk of her property is another person of the Trinity, what more need be said? But a very different question no doubt arises where the nature of the delusion which is said to exist is this – when it is alleged that a totally false, unfounded, unreasonable, because unreasoning, estimate of another person's character is formed. That is necessarily a more difficult question. It is unfortunately a thing not unknown that parents – and in justice I am bound to say it is more frequently the case with fathers than mothers – that they take unduly harsh views of the characters of their children, sons especially. That is not unknown. But there is a limit beyond which one feels that it ceases to be a question of harsh, unreasonable judgement of character, and that the repulsion a parent exhibits towards one or more of his children must proceed from some mental defect in himself. It is so contrary to the whole current of human nature that a man should not only form a harsh judgement of his children, but that he should put that into practice so as to do them injury or deprive them of advantages which most men desire above all things to confer upon their children. I say there is a point at which such repulsion and aversion are themselves evidence of unsoundness of mind.

In our experience this sort of case still crops up but, as far as we are aware, has not recently been tested in court. An example from our practice is of an elderly testatrix who had for many years so disliked her daughter-in-law that she had taken against her only son, accusing him, wrongly, of neglecting her. Her beliefs were easily understood within the context of her dependent and paranoid personality. Within 5 years of her death she developed a delusional parasitosis, the content of which made no reference whatsoever to her son and which responded to treatment with risperidone. She made a Will excluding her son and leaving all her money to charities. After her death the son challenged the Will on the grounds that her beliefs about him were 'insane delusions' that had poisoned her natural affections towards him. The psychiatrist argued that the testatrix's beliefs about her son were overvalued ideas that were understandable within her personality and pointed out the contrast with the genuine delusions, unrelated to the son, that were manifestations of the delusional parasitosis. In the event, the matter was settled out of court and was not, therefore, tested before a judge.

## Dementia

Dementia is the condition *par excellence* which affects testamentary capacity and taxes the expertise of the old age psychiatrist. From a consideration of the points set out above it should be quite clear that the various medical tests for dementia are not directly relevant to the question of testamentary capacity, nor indeed are the criteria for mental disorder under the Mental Health Act 1983. In other words, a diagnosis of dementia is not a criterion for testamentary incapacity, nor does having dementia automatically remove the capacity for someone to make a Will. For example, it would certainly be possible for a patient to have moderately severe dementia, scoring about 15 on the Mini-Mental State Examination (MMSE) (Folstein *et al.*, 1975) and still have testamentary capacity, although it is virtually invariable that those with very severe dementia are not capable of making a valid Will. To labour the point even more, patients with dementia may be unsure as to the exact date and location, fail the serial subtraction test, and fail to copy the interlocking pentagons accurately and yet pass the *Banks* v. *Goodfellow* test, namely be aware of the nature of the act and the effect of making a Will, be aware of the extent of their property and of the claims of others. Conversely, a patient may not fulfil the criteria for dementia and yet not have testamentary capacity. For example, a man with Korsakov's syndrome has such an impaired memory that he fails to recall or retain the information that his son has died and that he has grandchildren who might have a claim on his bounty. In conclusion, the tests for dementia are not the same as those for testamentary capacity.

To stress the point further in the case of *Hoff and Others* v. *Atherton* (2003) the judge noted that *both* experts in the case accepted that it is possible for a particular individual to have testamentary capacity despite suffering from mild to moderate dementia and this was also noted in the judgement of Lord Justice Peter Gibson in the Court of Appeal in that case (albeit without comment).

## Undue influence

A Will can be declared invalid if it can be proven that the testator was subject to undue influence in making it. Elderly people, especially those suffering from dementia, are clearly vulnerable to undue influence from a variety of sources, not least from relatives, carers, and indeed advisors. Some professional care agencies do not allow their staff to reside permanently with an elderly client, but rotate them every few weeks, for fear, among other things, that they may try to influence the client into changing a Will or giving them money in some other way. Many old age psychiatrists know of cases where a younger woman (a so-called 'gold-digger') develops a relationship with an elderly mentally frail, wealthy man (sometimes the genders are reversed) which ends in marriage or a new Will in which the man's children are disinherited. However, undue influence is extremely difficult to prove to the standard required by a court, and it rarely succeeds in a claim against a disputed Will. One reason for this is that courts require coercion to be established.

## Want of knowledge and approval

A Will may be declared invalid if a court finds that the testator did not fully understand and approve its contents. This is termed 'want of knowledge and approval'. Such an understanding needs to include the implications of a bequest. For example, in *Carapeto* v. *Good* (2002) the testatrix intended to leave her house to the couple who had looked after her for a number of years. A major issue in the case was whether her solicitors—she was a serial Will maker—had explained to her the need to leave the couple enough money, in addition to the house, in order to pay the inheritance tax. Otherwise, the carers would have had to sell the house to pay the tax, thus negating her intention that they should have a home. Although the testatrix was in this case found to have testamentary capacity, it is clear that one reason for a testator not to have knowledge and approval is that he lacks the mental capacity to have it. It can be seen, therefore, that although testamentary capacity, want of knowledge and approval, and undue influence are legal entities that ultimately require a legal solution, i.e. the decision of a court, their psychiatric aspects overlap to a considerable extent.

This is perhaps best illustrated in the classic case concerning want of knowledge and approval, *Wintle* v. *Nye* (1959). The testatrix was a rather worldly-naïve elderly lady and a relative of

Lieutenant-Colonel Alfred Wintle.[1] She was bamboozled into leaving the bulk of her estate to a crooked solicitor, called Nye. Wintle is said to have removed the latter's trousers and horse-whipped him outside a London Club, for which assault he was imprisoned. On being released he challenged the Will and lost in the court of first instance and also in the Court of Appeal. But appearing before the House of Lords as a litigant in person, he won the case principally on the grounds of want of knowledge and approval. Their Lordships, however, were not unaware of the other aspects of the case, such as the fraudulent influence of Nye on the testatrix.

## Delirium

The testamentary capacity of patients with delirious states also requires some consideration, because litigation may occur when a Will has been made or altered during the patient's terminal illness.

The psychiatrist may be asked, on such occasions, to examine case records, the statements of witnesses, and diagnostic and laboratory reports as the basis for an expert opinion. Regrettably, physicians and surgeons rarely make any record of the patient's mental state. The nursing notes are often much more informative; for example, 'confused and unable to understand what is going on all afternoon – pulled out her drip tube and was continuously restless'. Such observations should be related as far as possible to the relevant time at which instructions for the Will were given or it was signed.

Other factors need to be noted: the mental state before admission to hospital—was there evidence of cerebral vulnerability such as a history of strokes or blackouts in the presence of hypertension? What was the nature of the terminal illness and the likelihood of consequent severe metabolic disturbance; did laboratory investigations indicate electrolyte imbalance, failing renal and hepatic function, severe anaemia, or evidence of fulminating infection?

An estimate can be made of the likelihood of severe clouding of consciousness at the probable time, taking into account the clinical findings, for any pre-existing cerebral vulnerability—the greater the vulnerability the less the metabolic insult needed to provoke delirium—and for contemporaneous accounts of the mental state. The presence of moderately severe delirium is likely to impair judgement, it can account for persecutory ideas, and is likely to make the patient unaware of the facts that are necessary to be of sound disposing mind.

## Lucid intervals

As a general rule the testator must be of sound disposing mind both when giving instructions for a Will to be drawn up, and when it is executed. However, it is of course perfectly possible for the mental capacity of a testator to vary from time to time, and indeed in some cases drugs can be used temporarily to increase the mental capacity of a testator, for example naloxone to reverse the effects of opioids. Provided that (for whatever reason) the mental capacity of

---

[1] Wintle was one of those colourful eccentrics whose life story is a joy to behold. The reader is strongly advised to confirm this at http://en.wikipedia.org/wiki/Alfred_Wintle

the testator has increased, whether as a result of a natural cause or of medical treatment so that at the time the Will is executed he does have testamentary capacity, according to the *Banks* v. *Goodfellow* test, then that Will may be valid.

There is a converse position where testamentary capacity can be proved at the time that instructions are given for the preparation of a Will, but during the time that it takes for the Will to be prepared the testator's mental capacity diminishes. Normally, for a Will to be valid it is necessary to show that the testator had testamentary capacity both when the instructions to draw up the Will were given *and* when the Will was executed. Where capacity changes from full to diminished between instructions and execution it is necessary for the testator to understand that he is engaged in executing the Will for which he has given instructions. In those circumstances and at the time the Will is executed, it is not necessary for the testator even to remember the instructions that he gave to draw up the Will nor indeed to be capable of understanding them, as long as he does understand that he is executing the Will for which he has given instructions. In the case of *Flynn* v. *Flynn and Others* (1982) the testator signed a codicil to his Will when he was gravely ill following a myocardial infarction and only 1 day before he died. The validity of the codicil was contested on the grounds that he was too ill to have had testamentary capacity when he signed it. The judge dismissed the claim ruling, *inter alia*: that there was ample evidence the codicil had been drawn up on the testator's instructions well before he fell ill; that he clearly had full testamentary capacity when he gave the instructions; and that he knew what he was signing.

## Medical opinion

### Prospective assessment

Old age psychiatrists and general practitioners are most likely to be asked to give their opinions as to testamentary capacity in cases of presumed or established dementia. Opinions are sought both *prospectively* and *retrospectively*, i.e. before or after a Will has been made—in the latter case usually after the testator's death. A competent solicitor should obtain an opinion any time he acts for an aged client. A very important contribution to practice in the area of prospective assessment is the so-called 'Templeman's golden rule', enunciated by Mr Justice (later Lord Justice) Templeman in the case of Simpson 1977.

> In the case of an aged testator or a testator who has suffered a serious illness, there is one golden rule which should always be observed, however straightforward matters may appear, and however difficult or tactless it may be to suggest that precautions be taken: the making of a will by such a testator ought to be witnessed or approved by a medical practitioner who satisfied himself of the capacity and understanding of the testator, and records and preserves his examination and finding.

Clearly, this is an instruction to solicitors to obtain a medical opinion on testamentary capacity. However, since it takes two to tango, doctors should ensure that they know their own steps. All old age psychiatrists should be familiar with them, but other doctors, especially GPs, should make sure that they are at least briefed by the solicitor (Jacoby and Steer, 2007).

Medical practitioners should not certify testamentary capacity prospectively solely on the basis of medical tests, but on the relevant legal criteria. If a doctor decides to make a statement as to someone's testamentary capacity he should:

♦ examine the patient specifically in relation to the *Banks* v. *Goodfellow* criteria;

and, bearing in mind the points under the various headings previously discussed:

♦ ensure that he has been briefed, usually by an instructing solicitor, on the known facts, e.g. the extent of the state, who potential beneficiaries might be, and so on;

♦ make contemporaneous notes of the examination;

♦ and record the reasons for his conclusions.

One point needs to be stressed here. Adherence to the 'golden rule' does not usurp the function of the court which may decide against a Will, in spite of meticulous evidence from a doctor, as in the case of *Sharp & Bryson* v. *Adam and Others*. However, as a general observation, adherence to the 'golden rule' provides powerful evidence that a Will is valid. Conversely, if the 'golden rule' is not followed, it does not mean that the Will is necessarily invalid.

### Case 1

Mrs C was a woman of 90 years of age. She had three daughters, two of whom were married and comfortably off. She lived with the third daughter who was unmarried and had only part-time jobs. She had previously made a Will leaving her considerable estate in equal parts to her three daughters. She asked her solicitor to draw up a new Will leaving everything to her unmarried daughter. The solicitor asked an old age psychiatrist to examine her and give an opinion on her capacity to make a new Will. The psychiatrist found that she had marked memory impairment and scored 21 on the MMSE. However, she very clearly fulfilled the three *Banks* v. *Goodfellow* criteria, and in particular explained (in relation to the third) that her unmarried daughter was in greater need of the money than her sisters, who were not only comfortably off, but had also received financial help in the past. The psychiatrist checked with the solicitor that the woman had given an accurate account of the extent of her property, and he recorded his findings, giving his opinion that she was capable of making a valid Will. The solicitor drew up the Will and asked the psychiatrist to witness its execution. The psychiatrist examined the woman again, immediately before she signed the Will, recorded his findings, and satisfied himself that she had retained testamentary capacity before he formally witnessed her signature. This case has not been tested in Court and is unlikely to be so, which was the whole point of the solicitor's request for the psychiatrist's opinion. However, we believe that an action to contest the Will would not succeed because of the careful evaluation that took place before it was drawn up and executed, and indeed it would be necessary to show that the factual statements made by Mrs C to the psychiatrist were wrong.

It is not possible to furnish specific rules that could determine whether somebody has testamentary capacity or not. But it is absolutely essential to address the peculiar characteristics of each individual case and to judge from the whole character of the testator whether he does or did have testamentary capacity or not. However, if solicitors were more widely to observe the 'golden rule' having doctors examine their clients with specific reference to the three *Banks* v. *Goodfellow* criteria and make careful notes of their findings, the number of disputes arising after the testator's death could probably be greatly reduced.

## Retrospective assessment

Much case law in relation to testamentary capacity arises out of Wills that are contested in court after the testator's death. A doctor's opinion may be sought either as the testator's former medical attendant (witness as to fact), or as an expert witness. As the former medical attendant, his opinions are admissible in evidence only as to the facts he has observed himself. Since these opinions are based on his case notes, and because lawyers seek to pick holes in such documents, the value of carefully and legibly recorded observations cannot be over-emphasized.

## Experts' reports for contentious probate

As an expert witness who never examined the testator, a doctor may be asked to study the case records and other relevant documents. If these are put before the court and *proved in evidence*, the opinion of the expert witness is admissible as to the facts therein. He may also give his opinion as to matters of general relevance, for example the clinical features, treatment, and prognosis of conditions such as dementia and delirium.

Old age psychiatrists are now often asked by solicitors to write reports on the testamentary capacity of deceased testators whose Wills are being challenged. A medical opinion may be sought by either party, but a doctor is required to give an independent opinion whether or not it is favourable to the side that instructs him. Indeed, in England and Wales, under Part 35 of the Civil Procedure Rules (Practice Direction – Experts and Assessors) doctors must acknowledge that their primary duty is to the court. Where each side submits a report it is now common practice for courts to direct their respective authors to confer (usually done by telephone) and try and reach as much agreement as possible. They then have to issue a joint report for the court specifying where they agree and where they disagree.

Experts' reports differ in layout and content. We are glad that in this age of tick-box forms such reports are not yet standardized. We therefore offer the following points on report writing in a spirit of advice rather than prescription. Also, it is not and not meant to be a comprehensive list of instructions.

- A title page setting out: the expert's name and address; the instructing solicitors' and the expert's respective office references; the date; the testator's name, date of birth and date of death; and the name and address of instructing solicitors.

- All paragraphs of the report should be numbered to make it easy for the judge, counsel, and others to locate particular points.

- It is usual for the expert to begin the report with an account of who he is and how he claims expertise. A curriculum vitae may be appended to the report.

- It is now almost universal for an expert formally to declare his duties and obligations to the Court. Some prefer a short and some a long form, examples of both of which are given below.

  A. In accordance with part 35 of the Civil Procedure Rules (Practice Direction – Experts and Assessors) I declare that my primary duty as an expert, over and above any duties I may owe to the party or parties by whom I have been engaged, is to assist the Court. I confirm that I have complied and shall continue to comply with this duty.

  B. In accordance with part 35 of the Civil Procedure Rules (Practice Direction – Experts and Assessors) I declare that:

    I understand that my primary duty is to the Court rather than the party that engaged me.

    I have endeavoured in my report and in my opinion to be accurate and to cover all relevant issues.

    I have endeavoured to include in my report those matters of which I have knowledge or I have been made aware that might adversely affect the validity of my opinion.

    I have indicated the sources of all the information that I have used.

    I have not, without forming an independent view, included or excluded anything that has been suggested by others (in particular my instructing lawyers).

    I will notify those instructing me immediately and confirm in writing if, for any reason, my report requires correction or clarification or qualification.

    I understand that: my report subject to any corrections made before swearing as to its correctness will form evidence to be given by me under oath; I may be cross examined on my report by a cross examiner assisted by an expert; I am likely to be the subject of adverse criticism by the Judge if the Court concludes that I have not taken reasonable care in the preparation of this report and the opinions I have formed.

    I have not entered into any arrangement where the amount or payment of my fees is any way dependent upon the outcome of this case.

    I believe that the facts stated in this report are true and that the opinions I have expressed are true.

- A paragraph explicitly summarizing solicitors' instructions helps not only the court but also the expert by concentrating his attention on what precisely he is required to give his opinion. A copy of the solicitors' letter of instruction may be appended to the report.

- A complete list of the documents read should be appended to the report.

- It is helpful to provide a brief outline of the background to the case to include biographical details of the testator, who the parties are, and how the Will came to be written.

- All but invariably the deceased's medical history is highly relevant to the issue of testamentary capacity. It should be described in enough detail, including a list of medication, to support the opinions expressed later in the report.

- Most lawyers do not fully understand the medical conditions that are relevant to the case, e.g. dementia and delirium. Also, many do not understand the difference between dementia and Alzheimer's disease. They greatly appreciate a brief explanation of the relevant conditions at an appropriate place in the report.

• Experts are commonly faced with partisan witness statements. It should be remembered that none is strictly speaking valid until *proved in evidence*, i.e. accepted by the court. It is advisable, therefore, for the expert to use them to build an argument only with circumspection and adding a caveat, as the following (fictitious) example shows: 'John Smith states that for the last six months of her life the testatrix did not recognise him and did not know that he had been her neighbour for 40 years. If this statement is proved in evidence, in my opinion, it strongly supports the diagnosis of dementia'.

• The crux of any expert's report on testamentary capacity amounts essentially to whether or not the testator fulfilled the *Banks* v *Goodfellow* tests. However, an expert who writes his report bearing in mind that he may have to defend every opinion in Court is least likely to be embarrassed. Bearing in mind that his duty is to the Court it is better, not to be dogmatic and not to be shy of admitting ignorance of a particular matter.

## Case 2

Mr B was a Czech who had come to England during the Second World War and stayed on. He worked as a builder and later bought houses one at a time, renovated them, and sold them at a profit which he used to buy the next house. By the end of his life he had an estate worth somewhat over a million pounds.

Mr B had a daughter, Anna, by a Czech woman whom he never married and who left him after a few years. He subsequently married another Czech woman by whom he had a son and a daughter. His wife left him, too. Anna was brought up by her mother, although she had continued contact with her father until his death. The other two children stayed with Mr B when their mother left. Mr B acknowledged all three of his children who helped him with his business to some extent. The daughters did the clerical and administrative work, especially because their father had a relatively poor command of English. The son's help was intermittent because he aspired to be a musician and probably abused alcohol and drugs.

Mr B was a lifelong smoker and suffered from severe chronic obstructive pulmonary disease (COPD). In the 3 years prior to his death he suffered four clinically established cerebrovascular accidents (CVAs). These left him with dysarthria, dysphasia, and ataxia. There was dispute between the parties in the case (see below) about whether he suffered cognitive impairment. Anna claimed that he could no longer comprehend figures and had a poor grasp of his business. The other two children asserted that his cognitive function was unimpaired.

Three months before he died he was admitted to hospital in a confused state. In the accident and emergency department he had a cardio-respiratory arrest and was resuscitated and taken to the intensive care unit (ICU). He was unconscious for a week and then over the next few days regained consciousness via a delirious state characterized by violent aggression. He remained in hospital for 2 months before discharge, by which time he was able to dress himself, move about, and attend to his personal hygiene. The hospital notes stated that he could communicate his needs but his cognitive state was not tested because his command of English was poor and he was persistently dysarthric and dysphasic.

A few days after he went home his son and younger daughter arranged for a Will to be drawn up by a solicitor who received the instructions via them in Mr B's presence because, they stated, he could not speak English well enough and had suffered strokes. Previously Mr B had refused his children's' request that he write a Will. The solicitor did not seek a medical opinion on Mr B's testamentary capacity but said that on the one occasion when he met him, he 'appeared lucid'. Mr B's Will left £70,000 to Anna and the residue of his estate (approximately £1 million) to be divided between the other two children.

About a month after executing the Will Mr B was admitted to hospital with an exacerbation of COPD and died the following day. The elder daughter, Anna, challenged the Will on the grounds of lack of testamentary capacity, undue influence on Mr B by her siblings, and want of knowledge and approval.

The expert instructed by Anna's solicitors based his opinion mostly on the voluminous medical records, although there were statements from the children and various others stating either that Mr B's cognitive function was severely impaired or that it was not impaired at all. The expert gave his opinion that the series of CVAs had caused some permanent brain damage and that this had probably been exacerbated by the cardio-respiratory arrest followed by a week's period of unconsciousness. He stated further that, had Mr B's mental state been formally examined and his cognitive function tested at the time he made the Will, he would probably have shown evidence of vascular dementia. With regard to testamentary capacity, the expert stated that he could not give a firm opinion because there was no evidence to point either way whether Mr B could have passed the *Banks* v. *Goodfellow* tests. However, he stated his opinion that, in view of the likelihood of some degree of vascular brain damage, it was not safe to assume that Mr B did have testamentary capacity at the time he made his Will.

The two younger children of Mr B did not obtain the opinion of an expert. In the event, the parties settled out of court.

### Lessons from this case

The solicitor who drew up the Will showed poor practice by not following the 'golden rule' and would probably have been seriously criticized by the judge had the case come to trial (and indeed he might have exposed himself to a professional negligence claim).

The solicitor's opinion that Mr B 'appeared lucid' was of little or no value since he did not attempt to satisfy himself that the deceased fully understood the contents of the Will or why Mr B was excluding Anna in favour of the other two children.

That the parties settled out of court is common and probably sensible. Litigation is very expensive and one or other of the parties risks a large bill for costs if a trial takes place.

Probate cases are rarely clear-cut and are often 'messy' like this one, with conflicting evidence from the partisan witnesses, and incomplete medical information.

The expert did not say more than he was able to. Because someone was likely to have suffered from vascular dementia, one may not assume that he lacked testamentary capacity. Nevertheless, in this case it was unsafe to assume that the deceased *did* have testamentary capacity. The onus of proof is on those propounding the Will, i.e. the son and younger daughter in this case, to show that the testator has the necessary capacity. Furthermore the test for proof is not 'beyond reasonable doubt' (as in criminal cases) but 'on the balance of probability'. In a recent case with similarities to this one the court did not uphold a Will because it accepted the opinion of one of the experts that on the balance of probability it was unsafe to assume that the deceased did have testamentary capacity (*Westendorp* v. *Warwick* 2006).

## Wills under the Mental Capacity Act 2005

Sections 18(1)(i) and 18(2), and paragraphs 1 of 4 to Schedule 2 of the Mental Capacity Act 2005 provide for a nominated judge of the Court of Protection to order an 'authorised person' to execute a will on behalf of a person who lacks the capacity to make a valid will for himself. In an important common-sense ruling (Re D(J)1982), Sir Robert Megarry, then the Vice-Chancellor stated that 'the Court will regard the disposition of the estate subjectively from the patient's point of view and will, so to speak sit in his armchair and make for him a will that he or she is likely to have made'. This is clearly a useful and important provision for those with dementia whose estates are large enough and whose dependants would otherwise have difficulties with probate if the patients were to die intestate.

## References

Folstein, M.F., Folstein, S.E., and McHugh, P.R. (1975). 'Mini-mental state'. A practical method for grading the mental state of patients for the clinician. *Journal of Psychiatric Research*, **12**, 189–98.

Jacoby, R. and Steer, P. (2007). How to assess capacity to make a will. *British Medical Journal*, **335**, 155–7.

Peisah, C. (2005). Reflection on changes in defining testamentary capacity. *International Psychogeriatrics*, **17**, 709–12.

Sherrin, C.H., Barlow, R.F.D., Wallington, R.A., Meadway, S.L., and Waterworth, M. (2002). *Williams on Wills*, Vol 1, *The law of Wills*, Ch. 4, pp. 35–50. Butterworth, London.

Shulman K.I., Cohen, C.A., and Hull, I (2005). Psychiatric issues in retrospective challenges of testamentary capacity. *International Journal of Geriatric Psychiatry*, **20**, 63–9.

## Legal cases

*Banks* v. *Goodfellow* [1870]. 5. LR QB 549.

*Beal et al.* v. *Henri et al.* [1951]. *Dominion Law Reports*, **1**, 260–5.

*Boughton and Marston* v. *Knight and Others* [1873]. LR III Courts of Probate and Divorce 64–80.

*Carapeto* v. *Good*, [2002] WTLR 1305.

*Dew* v. *Clark & Clark* [1826] *English Reports* Vol. CLXII containing Addams Vol. 3, 410–456.

*Flynn* v. *Flynn and Others* [1982]. *All England Law Reports*, **1**, 882–92.

*Gillett* v. *Holt* [2000] 2 All ER 289.

*Hoff and Others* v. *Atherton* [2003] EWCA Civ 1554.

*Jennings* v. *Rice and Other* [2002] EWCA Civ 159.

*O'Neil et al.* v. *Royal Trust Co. and McClure et al.* [1946]. *Dominion Law Reports*, **4**, 545.

*Park* v. *Park* [1953]. All ER 408.

*Re Beaney* [1978] 2 All ER 595 Ch. D.

*Re D(J)* [1982] 2 All ER 37.

*Re Simpson* [1977] *Solicitors Journal*, **121**, 224.

*Sharp & Bryson* v. *Adam and Others* [2006] WTLR 1059.

*Westendorp* v. *Warwick* [2006] All ER (d) 248.

*Wintle* v. *Nye* [1959] 1 WLR 284.

# 42

# Competence

## Seena Fazel

The doctrine of informed consent—that adults have the right to make decisions about their own lives—is a basic ethical and legal principle in medicine and the law. There are three essential components to informed consent: (1) a decision must be made on the basis of adequate information; (2) it must be voluntary; and (3) the person making it must be competent to do so. The last of these, competence, is particularly important in old age psychiatry as many conditions encountered in this speciality compromise a person's competence. Competence is the clinical term for the legal concept of capacity, and the one that I shall use in the remainder of this chapter.

This chapter will examine four major areas: the relevance of competence to old age psychiatry, definitions and concepts of competence, the different competencies, and their assessment.

## The relevance of competence

Competence is particularly important in old age psychiatry for several reasons. There are increasing numbers of older people in the community, whose competence may be compromised. Further, the policies of de-institutionalization and community care mean that there are more individuals with severe mental illness in the community, for whom issues such as consent to treatment and hospitalization will occasionally arise. In addition, decision-making ability may be altered in a number of illnesses that affect patients who are cared for by old age psychiatrists. Delirium, dementia, very late onset schizophrenia, affective disorders, and age-related cognitive decline all have the potential to compromise the decision-making ability of elderly persons. Although, many other medical specialities, such as oncology, geriatrics, and neurology, will care for these and other conditions that impair competence, it is psychiatrists who are usually consulted on whether these individuals have retained their competence, and what influence, if any, mental illness might have had on their decision-making ability. Governments in some jurisdictions have been giving competence a more central role in mental health legislation which will lead to increasing requests for competence assessments by doctors. This has occurred, for example, in England and Wales, where the Mental Capacity Act was introduced in October 2007, and in Scotland, where the Mental Health (Care and Treatment) Act partly bases decisions about detention in hospital on the patient's competence to consent to treatment.

## Basic concepts

### Presumption of competence

In England and Wales, and in most other common law jurisdictions, adults are presumed to be competent to give or withhold consent unless proven otherwise. Therefore, healthcare interventions carried out on individuals who have not given their consent, even if intended for an individual's best interests, may constitute an assault. This does not detract from the doctrine of necessity, which makes it justifiable to intervene medically when competence is unknown, providing the intervention is reasonable and necessary, such as the treatment of unconscious patients in casualty departments. The presumption of competence exists even if the decisions might be detrimental to the health of a person. This was exemplified in England and Wales in the landmark case of *Re: C* [all legal cases cited in this essay are fully referenced in Kennedy and Grubb (1998)], a patient at Broadmoor Hospital suffering from schizophrenia, who refused to have his leg amputated although the consensus of medical advice was that he was endangering his life by not undergoing the operation. The courts upheld his right to refuse medical treatment on the basis that he was competent to make that decision.

### Approaches to determining competence

#### Outcome approach

This approach focuses on the decision being made as the criterion for determining competence. Here, an individual who makes a decision contrary to conventional medical wisdom or the wishes of those giving treatment is viewed as incompetent. This approach has been rejected by case law in many jurisdictions, as it contradicts the principle of self-determination and undermines autonomy. The legal position therefore implies that individuals have the right to make decisions about their health even when this is likely to lead to a worse outcome. The ruling in *Re: T* states that if a person has capacity, they may refuse any treatment, including a lifesaving one (Kennedy and Grubb, 1998).

#### Status approach

This approach determines competence decisions based purely on the 'status' of the decision-maker. Here, if someone, for example, has a particular psychiatric diagnosis or is below a certain age, they are deemed incompetent. The status approach is problematic as it assumes that all those assigned a particular diagnosis or belonging to a certain population are similar to each other. Also, it does not account for the fact that competence depends on the nature of the task. In England and Wales, the status approach has been rejected by case law and by the Mental Health Act Code of Practice. Some doctors, however, seem, erroneously, to favour a status approach in some contexts. In a US survey of doctors, 72% said that a diagnosis of dementia automatically rendered someone incompetent, and 66% reported that depression established incompetence and 71% that psychosis did so (Markson *et al.*, 1994). By contrast, empirical research has given no support to the status approach. For example, 20% of those with dementia in one community sample were capable of completing advance directives (Fazel *et al.*, 1999b), and 48% of inpatients with an acute schizophrenic episode were competent to make treatment decisions (Grisso and Appelbaum, 1995). Some have argued that those with mild depression are more competent than others in general as they bring a 'depressive realism' to their decision-making (Sullivan and Youngner, 1994). Nevertheless, mental health legislation does incorporate some elements of the status approach; for example, in deeming patients detained under Section 3 of the Mental Health Act 1983 incompetent to give consent to certain treatments, such as ECT.

### Functional approach

This is the favoured approach among US and UK legal jurisdictions, and is supported by most researchers in the field. It is based on establishing the extent to which a person has the understanding, knowledge, and skills required to make a particular decision. *Competence is therefore decision-specific and time-specific, rather than global or permanent.* When asked to perform competence assessments, clinicians should be asking, 'Is the individual competent for this task at this time?' rather than 'Is this individual competent or not?' An important consequence of the functional approach is that the clinician's focus should be towards enabling or enhancing competence by improving the relevant functional abilities, rather than simply administering a test.

### Threshold for capacity

One of the difficulties with a functional approach is that there is uncertainty about the threshold for a certain decision. Some have argued for a fixed threshold for certain capacities, similar to the ability to pass a sight test for driving, but there will be differences as doctors and cultures hold different views on where the balance exists between upholding the autonomy of individuals and protecting them from harm. The threshold for competence for some decisions will be higher than for others. There is also case law in England and Wales that indicates that the more serious the decision, the higher the competence threshold (cf. *Re: T*). Some have also argued that the threshold for capacity is also dependent on the diagnosis of the individual concerned. This view proposes that those with a psychiatric diagnosis or learning disability should have a higher threshold for competence as they are in greater need of protection (Fazel *et al.*, 1999b). It is self-evident that there are many individuals in the community who are not competent to perform certain tasks, and society feels a particular responsibility to those who are at risk of harm. Others have argued that the correct threshold for competence may vary from case to case, depending on the clinical consequences of accepting or refusing a treatment, in addition to the risks and benefits of treatment alternatives, in individual cases (Drane, 1984).

### Abilities relevant to competence

The core abilities relevant to decision-making have been clarified in the research literature, in law, and in medicine (Appelbaum & Grisso, 1988). The four main abilities are:

1 Understanding information relevant to the decision. This is more than the reception, storage, and retrieval of information. It involves comprehension in 'broad terms' of the nature and purpose of the information presented. One of the ways to test this ability is by asking the individual to paraphrase the information relevant to their decision. In addition, they should be able to identify the choices available to them.

2 Manipulating information rationally. This ability tests whether an individual is able to compare the benefits and risks of the various treatment options. This standard should focus on the process by which the decision is made, rather than the outcome of the decision. The person's decision should be internally coherent, and a 'rational product' of their underlying beliefs, regardless of whether the clinician agrees or disagrees with these beliefs. It can be tested by asking individuals the reasons for their choice.

3 Appreciating the situation and its consequences. This standard refers to a person recognizing that they have a disorder or problem about which they need to make a decision on an emotional level in addition to an intellectual one, and have to relate it to their own personal situation. In other words, it tests whether an individual can appreciate the information about the likely consequences of a decision for them and for their family, and assign a value to each benefit and risk.

4 Communicating choices. This standard tests the ability to communicate and maintain choices. It is more than the physical act of communicating choices, and individuals who frequently change their choices without reason are unlikely to be deemed competent. This can be tested by repeating the question about their decision on a number of occasions.

## Types of competence in the elderly

For any given task, the specific requisite abilities must be established, the threshold for each ability determined, and valid and reliable instruments developed to aid in the assessment of these competencies. Some of the instruments that have been validated in the elderly have used clinical vignettes as part of the assessment procedure, and this appears to be a promising approach. Various competencies are now reviewed and I have focused on those that can be used in routine clinical practice. Fitness to plead and testamentary capacity are outlined elsewhere in this volume (Chapters 40 and 41). Other capacities, such as to make a gift, litigate, enter into a contract, vote, and enter into personal relationships are discussed in a recent publication (British Medical Association and The Law Society, 2004).

### Consent to medical treatment

Consent to medical treatment is probably the most requested competence assessment for clinicians and consequently the most researched. The criteria for this competence are closely related to the general abilities outlined above. Research has shown that the three standards—understanding, appreciation, and reasoning—are the three essential components in assessing competence, and that using one standard alone will not identify those who perform badly on the others (Grisso and Appelbaum, 1995). A study by Marson *et al.* (1996) showed that the fourth standard (communicating choice) does not distinguish between those who are competent and those who are incompetent to make treatment decisions in Alzheimer's disease, and is, therefore, the least stringent standard. Another study in older adults using three different instruments found that understanding treatment information was impaired in older adults in all three, whereas appreciation and reasoning were impaired using one or two instruments (Moye *et al.*, 2004). There are various instruments that have been devised to test competence to consent to treatment, the merits of which have been reviewed recently (Dunn *et al.*, 2006). For research purposes, the MacArthur tool [the MacArthur Competence Assessment Tool–Treatment (MacCAT-T)] is validated in a variety of populations but may be too time-consuming for routine clinical practice (Grisso *et al.*, 1997). In addition, it has been criticized for requiring substantial training (Dunn *et al.*, 2006). Another instrument which has been developed for use with medical inpatients is the Aid to Capacity Evaluation (see Table 42.1) (Etchells *et al.*, 1999). Although it does not explicitly test the domain of expressing a choice, it appears simple to use in clinical work. Its named questions are suggested examples rather than rigid prompts.

Investigations that have examined the proportion of older adults who are competent to consent to treatment are limited. A recent work using three instruments concluded that most individuals with mild dementia were competent, and highlighted the need for strategies to compensate for memory problems and planning (Moye *et al.*, 2004). This investigation found that around 78–89% of those with mild dementia were within normal limits for understanding treatment information, 76–98% for appreciation of the consequences of treatment choices, 83–100% for reasoning, and 89–96% for expressing a choice. Even on the most difficult domains of appreciation and understanding, around 50% of those with moderate dementia were within normal limits.

Some studies have examined the neuropsychological correlates of competence in patients with Alzheimer's disease. In general, these investigations have demonstrated that competence to consent to treatment is associated with more intact executive and frontal lobe function. The criterion of understanding the treatment situation and treatment options is correlated with abstractive capacity and with semantic (but not verbal) memory (Marson *et al.*, 1996). The criterion of appreciating the consequences of treatment choices is correlated with verbal fluency and visuomotor tracking (Marson *et al.*, 1996). The criterion of reasoning is correlated with verbal fluency [and not Mini-Mental State Examination (MMSE) score or verbal memory (Marson *et al.*, 1995)]. The least stringent standard, of making a treatment choice, is inversely correlated with auditory comprehension and dysnomia (Marson *et al.*, 1996).

## Consent to research

There are no instruments to test consent to research specifically in the elderly, and most researchers have used the general criteria for consent to treatment and applied them to the consent to research. But there is one validated instrument, the MacArthur Competence Assessment Tool for Clinical Research, that has been used in patients with Alzheimer's disease. As regards decisions to be made without covert pressure on potential participants to take part, guidelines published by the Royal College of Psychiatrists in the

**Table 42.1** Competence to consent to treatment: The Aid to Capacity Evaluation[a]

| | |
|---|---|
| 1. Medical condition: | What problems are you having right now? What problem is bothering you most? Why are you in the hospital? Do you have [name problem here]? |
| 2. Proposed treatment: | What is the treatment for [your problem]? What else can we do to help you? Can you have [proposed treatment]? |
| 3. Alternatives: | Are there any other [treatments]? What other options do you have? Can you have [alternative treatment]? |
| 4. Option of refusing proposed treatment (including withholding or withdrawing proposed treatment): | Can you refuse [proposed treatment]? Can we stop [proposed treatment]? |
| 5. Consequences of accepting proposed treatment: | What could happen to you if you have [proposed treatment]? Can [proposed treatment] cause problems/side-effects? Can [proposed treatment] help you live longer? |
| 6. Consequences of refusing proposed treatment: | What could happen to you if you don't have [proposed treatment]? Could you get sicker/die if you don't have [proposed treatment]? What could happen if you have [alternative treatment]? (If alternatives are available) |
| 7a. The person's decision is affected by depression: | Can you help me understand why you've decided to accept/refuse treatment? Do you feel that you're being punished? Do you think you're a bad person? Do you have any hope for the future? Do you deserve to be treated? |
| 7b. The person's decision is affected by psychosis: | Can you help me understand why you've decided to accept/refuse treatment? Do you think anyone is trying to hurt/harm you? Do you trust your doctor/nurse? |

[a] The complete ACE with training materials is on the website (http://www.utoronto.ca/jcb/disclaimers/ACE.pdf).

UK recommend that payment of fees or rewards to healthy volunteers or patients, beyond expenses incurred in taking part in the research, should be avoided. The guidelines also recommend a period of reflection between explanation of the research study and the final decision, as well as an assessment of the mental state of the potential participant (Royal College of Psychiatrists, 1990). Research using the MacArthur tool has found that 62% of patients with mild to moderate Alzheimer's disease were not competent to consent to research, while an older adult comparison group were all found to be competent (Kim *et al.*, 2002). Other research supports the finding that older patients without dementia tend to make the right decisions about participating in research (Stanley *et al.*, 1984). The latter study suggested the following three areas as a basis for evaluating this competence:

◆ Reasonable outcome of decision (determined by assessing willingness to participate in higher-risk/low-benefit studies).

- Quality of reasoning of the decision (determined by showing evidence of appropriate weighing of risks and benefits).
- Comprehension of the consent information.

## Consent to hospitalization

The American Psychiatric Association appointed a taskforce to draw up some guidelines on the assessment of the competence to consent to hospitalization, which suggested that two standards should be used. First, the patient must be able to communicate the choice to be voluntarily hospitalized. Secondly, the patient must understand important information regarding his or her hospitalization, such as awareness of being admitted to a psychiatric hospital, and that release may not be automatic (Appelbaum *et al.*, 1998). A useful assessment tool for the elderly has been developed (see Table 42.2) (Levine *et al.*, 1994). The latter authors examined competence to consent to hospitalization in a sample of elderly patients admitted to a psychiatric hospital, and found it to be correlated with their MMSE score and hostility rating on the Brief Psychiatric Rating Scale (BPRS). Interestingly, anxiety and depression on the BPRS were correlated with higher scores on the competence questionnaire. In studies with younger psychiatric patients, correlates of incompetence to consent to hospitalization were older age and the chronicity of the psychiatric condition (Appelbaum *et al.*, 1998).

## Financial competence

Financial capacity comprises a range of cognitive abilities important to the independent functioning of the elderly. Loss of financial capacity has important consequences for patients with dementia and their families. There are the economic consequences of not paying bills, and mismanaging one's accounts. The loss of this capacity may also lead to financial exploitation. This can take the form of consumer fraud, and also undue influence exerted by relatives or third parties. With the long-term funding of residential and nursing care moving gradually into the private sector, the pressures on older people to protect their assets are increasing. Research examining financial competence in the elderly (Marson *et al.*, 2000) identifies six domains of financial activity that should be assessed: basic monetary skills; financial conceptual knowledge; cash transactions; chequebook management; bank statement management; and financial judgement (see Table 42.3).

**Table 42.2** An aid to assessing competence to consent to hospitalization

| |
|---|
| Some people come to hospital of their own free will and others do not; how about yourself? |
| What type of hospital ward are you on? |
| What sort of problem are you here for? |
| Why do you feel that you need to be in hospital for this problem? |
| What kind of treatment will you receive in the hospital? |
| If you felt you were ready to leave the hospital and your doctor did not agree, how would you go about leaving? |
| What if your doctor still feels you are not ready? |
| Is there someone with whom you could speak about your legal rights as a patient in the hospital? |

**Table 42.3** An aid to assessing financial competence in the elderly

| Domain 1: Basic monetary skills | Identify specific coins and currency<br>Indicate relative monetary value of coins and/or currency<br>Accurately count groups of coins and/or currency |
|---|---|
| Domain 2: Financial conceptual knowledge | Define a variety of simple financial concepts<br>Practical application/computation using financial concepts |
| Domain 3: Cash transactions | Enter into simulated one-item transaction; verify change<br>Enter into simulated three-item transaction; verify change<br>Obtain exact change for vending machine use; verify change |
| Domain 4: Chequebook management | Identify and explain parts of check and check register<br>Enter into simulated transaction and make payment by check |
| Domain 5: Bank statement management | Identify and explain parts of a bank statement<br>Identify aspects of specific transactions on bank statement |
| Domain 6: Financial judgement | Detect and explain risks in mail fraud solicitation<br>Understand investment situation/options; make investment decision |

A related investigation found that individuals with mild cognitive impairment demonstrated impairments in aspects of financial competence including: conceptual knowledge; cash transactions; bank statement management; bill payment; and overall financial capacity. However, 63% were considered to be financially competent; whereas 22% of patients with Alzheimer's disease were considered financial incompetent (Griffith *et al.*, 2003).

## Advance directives

It is anticipated that the use of advance directives or 'living wills' will increase significantly over the next few decades. A number of commentators, including the British Medical Association (1994), have argued that dementia is one clinical situation for which an advance directive could potentially be useful. An important question is whether individuals with dementia are competent to complete an advance directive. In assessing this competence, it is necessary to test whether an individual is capable of understanding actual possible future situations. An instrument which has good psychometric properties and is patient-centred has been developed to test this competence (see Box 42.1) (Fazel *et al.*, 1999a). In this approach, patients are not regarded as incompetent because of cognitive impairment (such as memory difficulties), which is not critical to competence, but can interfere with assessment procedures. It was found that 20% of those with dementia were competent to complete advance directives. In patients with mild to moderate dementia, those who were competent had significantly higher estimated pre-morbid IQs than those who were incompetent (Fazel *et al.*, 1999b).

**Box 42.1** An aid to assessing competence to complete an advance directive

### Clinical vignettes

1. You are in hospital recovering from a sudden stroke. It has left you half-paralysed from which you are unlikely to improve. You cannot speak but you can understand. You cannot swallow food safely. There is a high risk that food directly enters your windpipe and makes you choke. Your doctor explains that, in order to feed you adequately and safely, he needs to use a feeding tube which passes through your nose into stomach. This is likely to make you live longer but you need the tube all the time. The other alternative is that you are kept comfortable, but without a feeding tube.

2. You are in a nursing home. Over the past few years you have become forgetful and occasionally confused. You have Alzheimer's dementia. You are able to recognize relatives and nursing home staff. You are in good physical health. You seem happy and contented. However, your memory problems are going to get worse. One day you pass some blood from your bowel. You can leave it and not have any tests. Or your doctor can organize for you to have some tests to see where the bleeding is coming from, followed by surgery if a cancer is found.

### Questions

1. Can you give a summary of the situation?   Chronic problem (1), Acute problem (1)
2. What treatment would you want if you were in this situation?   Clear answer (not scored)
3. Can you name one other option open to you?   Another treatment option (1)
4. What are the reasons for your choice?   One valid reason (1)
5. What are the problems associated with your choice of treatment?   One problem (1)
6. What will this decision mean for you and your family?   For them (1), For their family (1)
7. What short-term effect will the treatment have?   Short-term effect (1)
8. Can you think of a long-term effect?   Long-term effect (1)
9. Can you repeat what treatment you want?   Repeats answer to question 2 (1)

## The assessment of competence

The use of the tools and instruments described above should not undermine the importance of the clinical assessment of competence, which is the gold standard, and such tools should be seen only as supplementary aids. Clinical assessment should aim to enable those who are partially competent to complete the decisions that they face, and clinical style should reflect this approach.

A systematic assessment should include the following steps. The clinician needs to be aware of the relevant legal test, if there is one, that will have to be applied. Relevant background information then needs to be gathered. All relevant medical and psychiatric records prior to the assessment should be read. The examination of the person should aim to establish a diagnosis, if one exists, and identify any disabilities that may be present. The nature of these disabilities should be clarified—how transient they are,

and what impact they may have on the person's ability to fulfil the relevant legal test. This may involve the advice of a clinical psychologist (for cognitive impairment) and an occupational therapist (for physical disabilities). An examination of the person's mental state is also required with particular attention to mood, possible delusions, and any cognitive deficits. A history from an informant is most likely to be useful in the diagnostic process and to identify the underlying values and goals of the person whose competence is in question. An understanding of the progression of the patient's disease and possible response to treatment is also relevant. After assessment, the clinician needs to make a clear distinction between any diagnosis and disability that exists and how this affects the person's competence. (British Medical Association and The Law Society, 2004).

### Ways to enable competence

A report by the British Medical Association and The Law Society (2004) identified a number of ways to enhance the competence of those who are being assessed. Any treatable medical condition that affects competence should be treated before a final assessment is made.

- If a person's condition is likely to improve, such as in delirium, the assessment of capacity should, if possible, be delayed.

- In conditions such as dementia, where competence may fluctuate, the assessment should detail the level of capacity during periods of maximal and minimal disability.

- Some physical conditions that do not directly affect the mental state can interfere with competence, such as problems with communication. There should, therefore, be an assessment of speech, language function, hearing, and sight; and any disabilities discovered corrected before a conclusion about competence is reached.

- Care should be taken to provide the best location and timing for a competence assessment. Anxiety can compromise competence, and it may be appropriate to alleviate it by assessing the person in their own home. The presence of a third party may also enhance the competence of some persons.

- Education about the nature of the proposed decision may enhance competence. It is important for the clinician to re-explain, and, if necessary, use an information sheet clarifying those aspects of the decision that have not been fully understood. Presenting consent material in small packages may help. Simplifying consent information and using illustrations may also be necessary.

## Decision-making for incompetent individuals

Two approaches exist to decision-making in those who are found to be incompetent: advance directives and proxy decision-making by others. Both are increasingly used in clinical practice but have important limitations.

### Advance directives

An advance directive for medical care or 'living will' is a statement made by a person when competent about healthcare that they would want to receive if they become incompetent. There are three types of advance directive: an instruction directive; a proxy directive; and a values directive. An instruction directive is specific and often takes the form of an advance refusal of treatment. For example, 'if I develop severe dementia, and can no longer attend to any of my personal needs, and no longer recognize my close relatives, I do not wish to have any medical treatment that might prolong my life'. In a proxy directive the writer donates power to make decisions on his or her behalf to someone else, say a spouse or offspring. In a values directive, a statement of general values is made of which people are asked to take account in the event of the writer becoming incompetent. For example, someone might write:

> The following words by Arthur Hugh Clough coincide with my values. Please adhere to them if I become incompetent to make decisions on medical treatment:
>
> Thou shalt not kill
>
> But need'st not strive
>
> Officiously
>
> To keep alive.

Instruction directives in the form of advance refusals of treatment have had validity in common law in England and Wales for some years, but now have statute validity under the new Mental Capacity Act 2005 (see below under Decision-making by proxy). In themselves, proxy directives have no validity in English law, but the new Mental Capacity Act makes some provision for proxy healthcare decision-making (again, see below). A values directive has no validity in law, but any good multidisciplinary psychiatry team would take a patient's values into account when deciding on treatment.

Advance directives have been widely advocated as a means of extending the autonomy of patients to situations when they are incompetent. The main problems with advance directives are that people, whether competent or not, are not well placed to make decisions concerning their future incompetent selves, and it is often difficult to apply broad principles established in an advance directive to rapidly changing and unanticipated clinical events (Hope, 1992). Nevertheless, the informal use of advance directives, including psychiatric ones, as an aid to autonomy is becoming more common and supported in some UK National Institute for Health and Clinical Excellence guidelines.

### Decision-making by proxy

Under the new Mental Capacity Act 2005 for England and Wales, implemented in October 2007, enduring power of attorney (EPA) will be replaced by a new lasting power of attorney (LPA) which will permit attorneys to make some proxy healthcare decisions for the donor of the LPA (see Chapter 43). At the time of writing the full extent of these powers to make proxy healthcare decisions is not clear, and the new Act will need time to 'bed down'. It is not yet clear, for example, how potentially controversial life or death decisions will be handled. Until now proxy decision-making has been based on 'best interests' or 'substituted judgement'. In England and Wales, the 'best interests' test has been favoured. As no person or court can give consent to treatment for an adult who is incompetent, the only legal framework that exists is the common law doctrine of necessity. Here the normative standard is that treatment of an incompetent adult may be carried out if, in accordance with a practice accepted at the time by a responsible body of appropriately skilled medical opinion, it is necessary and in the 'best interests' of the person (Wong *et al.*, 1999). This approach also permits other

action, such as the admission to hospital of a person who lacks competence to make this decision, but is not objecting, without use of the Mental Health Act (1983) (the Bournewood ruling; see footnote 1 in Chapter 43). Some commentators have argued for broadening the definition of best interests, for example 'to save their lives or to ensure improvement or prevent deterioration in their physical or mental health'. They also argue that the wishes of the individual before they became incompetent and the views of significant others should be taken into account, and that the 'least restrictive' treatment option should be chosen (Law Commission, 1995).

There are two main problems with the 'substituted judgement' approach. The first is that potential proxies, such as family members, have been found to poorly predict the healthcare preferences of those that later become incompetent. Secondly, conflicts of interest among family members may lead some proxies to compromise the best interests of the person who has become incompetent. There are no clear ways of resolving the differing opinions of family members that may arise in the course of deciding on a treatment for an incompetent person (Wong *et al.*, 1999).

## Conclusion

This chapter has argued for the relevance of competence to old age psychiatry. The basic concepts of competence—the presumption of competence, the centrality of the functional approach, and the four general abilities of competence—have been outlined. The specific competencies of consent to medical treatment, to participate in research, to consent to hospitalization, to manage one's finances, and to complete advance directives have been discussed and tools described that can aid in the assessment of these competences. The role of the clinician has been examined, with emphasis on the importance of a comprehensive examination of the mental state and ways that the assessing clinician can enhance competence. The tools and instruments that have been developed to aid in the assessment of the specific competences should inform rather than undermine the clinical assessment of competence, which remains the gold standard.

## Acknowledgement

I am very grateful to Robin Jacoby and Catherine Oppenheimer for their comments.

## References

Appelbaum, B., Appelbaum, P., and Grisso, T. (1998). Competence to consent to voluntary psychiatric hospitalization: a test of a standard proposed by APA. *Psychiatric Services*, **49**, 1193–1196.

Appelbaum, P. and Grisso, T. (1988). Assessing patients' capacities to consent to treatment. *New England Journal of Medicine*, **319**, 1635–1638.

British Medical Association (1994). *Statement on advance directives.* BMA, London.

British Medical Association and The Law Society (2004). *Assessment of mental capacity: guidance for doctors and lawyers*, 2nd edn. BMJ Books, London.

Drane, J. (1984). Competency to give an informed consent: a model for making clinical assessments. *Journal of the American Medical Association*, **252**, 925–927.

Dunn, L.B., Nowrangi, M.A., Palmer, B.W., Jeste, D.V., and Saks, E.R. (2006). Assessing decisional capacity for clinical research or treatment: a review of instruments. *American Journal of Psychiatry*, **163**, 1323–1334.

Etchells, E., Darzins, P., Silberfeld, M. *et al.* (1999). Assessment of patient capacity to consent to treatment. *Journal of General Internal Medicine*, **14**, 27–34.

Fazel, S., Hope, T., and Jacoby, R. (1999a). Assessment of competence to complete advance directives: validation of a patient centred approach. *British Medical Journal*, **318**, 493–497.

Fazel, S., Hope, T., and Jacoby, R. (1999b). Dementia, intelligence, and the competence to complete advance directives. *Lancet*, **354**, 48.

Griffith, H.R., Belue, K., Sicola, A. *et al.* (2003). Impaired financial abilities in mild cognitive impairment: a direct assessment approach. *Neurology*, **11**, 449–457.

Grisso, T. and Appelbaum, P. (1995). Comparison of standards for assessing patients' capacities to make treatment decisions. *American Journal of Psychiatry*, **152**, 1033–1037.

Grisso, T., Appelbaum, P., and Hill-Fotouhi, C. (1997). The MacCAT-T: A clinical tool to assess patients' capacities to make treatment decisions. *Psychiatric Services*, **48**, 1415–1419.

Hope, R. (1992). Advance directives about medical treatment. *British Medical Journal*, **304**, 398.

Kennedy, I. and Grubb, T. (1998). *Principles of medical law*. Oxford University Press, Oxford.

Kim, S.Y.H., Cox, C., and Caine, E.D. (2002). Impaired decision-making ability in subjects with Alzheimer's disease and willingness to participate in research. *American Journal of Psychiatry*, **159**, 797–802.

Law Commission (1995). *Mental incapacity*. HMSO, London.

Levine, S., Bryne, K., Wilets, I., Fraser, M., Leal, D., and Kato, K. (1994). Competency of geropsychiatric patients to consent to voluntary hospitalization. *American Journal of Geriatric Psychiatry*, **2**, 300–308.

Markson, L., Kern, D., Annas, G., and Glantz, L. (1994). Physician assessment of patient competence. *Journal of the American Geriatrics Society*, **42**, 1074–1080.

Marson, D., Cody, H.A., Ingram, K., and Harrell, L. (1995). Neuropsychologic predictors of competency in Alzheimer's disease using a rational reasons legal standard. *Archives of Neurology*, **52**, 955–959.

Marson, D., Chatterjee, A., Ingram, K., and Harrell, L. (1996). Toward a neurologic model of competency: cognitive predictors of capacity to consent in Alzheimer's disease using three different legal standards. *Neurology*, **46**, 666–672.

Marson, D., Sawrie, S., Synder, S. *et al.* (2000). Assessing financial capacity in patients with Alzheimer disease. *Archives of Neurology*, **57**, 877–884.

Moye, J., Karel, M.J., Azar, A.R., and Gurrera, R.J. (2004). Capacity to consent to treatment: empirical comparison of three instruments in older adults with and without dementia. *The Gerontologist*, **44**, 166–175.

Royal College of Psychiatrists (1990). Guidelines for research ethics committees on psychiatric research involving human subjects. *Psychiatric Bulletin*, **14**, 48–61.

Stanley, B., Guido, J., Stanley, M., and Shortell, D. (1984). The elderly patient and informed consent. *Journal of the American Medical Association*, **252**, 1302–1306.

Sullivan, M. and Youngner, S. (1994). Depression, competence, and the right to refuse lifesaving medical treatment. *American Journal of Psychiatry*, **151**, 971–978.

Wong, J., Clare, I., Gunn, M., and Holland, A. (1999). Capacity to make health care decisions: its importance in clinical practice. *Psychological Medicine*, **29**, 437–446.

# 43

# The legal framework in the British Isles for making decisions on behalf of mentally incapacitated people

Denzil Lush

This chapter provides a brief overview of the legal arrangements for appointing substitute decision-makers in the four principal jurisdictions in the British Isles. It considers first the Mental Capacity Act 2005, which applies in England and Wales; secondly, the Adults with Incapacity (Scotland) Act 2000; thirdly, Northern Ireland, and finally, the legislation in the Republic of Ireland.

## Mental Capacity Act 2005

The Mental Capacity Act 2005, which applies in England and Wales, received the Royal Assent on 7 April 2005, and came fully into force on 1 October 2007. At the time this book was going to print, none of the rules, regulations, prescribed forms, and practice notes had been published, so unfortunately it has not been possible to provide any detailed information on procedure.

The Mental Capacity Act provides a framework for deciding whether people have the capacity to make decisions for themselves, and for making decisions on their behalf where they lack capacity. The principles on which the legislation is based are set out in section 1 and are as follows:

◆ A person must be assumed to have capacity unless it is established that he lacks capacity.

◆ A person is not to be treated as unable to make a decision unless all practical steps to help him to do so have been taken without success.

◆ A person is not to be treated as unable to make a decision merely because he makes an unwise decision.

◆ An act done or decision made for or on behalf of a person who lacks capacity must be done or made in his best interests.

◆ Before the act is done, or the decision is made, regard must be had to whether the purpose for which it is needed can be as effectively achieved in a way that is less restrictive of the person's rights and freedom of action.

During what was then the Mental Capacity Bill's second reading in the House of Lords on 10 January 2005, the Rt Rev. Dr Peter Selby, Bishop of Worcester, said:

[Section] 1 contains a statement about a vision of humanity and how humanity is to be regarded. I hope children in generations to come will study that as one of the clearest and most eloquent expressions of what we think a human being is and how a human being is to be treated.

In addition to the principles listed above, sections 2(3) and 3(1) of the Act provide that, when deciding whether someone lacks capacity, and, if so, determining what is in his best interests, it should not be established merely on the basis of:

◆ the person's age or appearance, or

◆ a condition of his, or an aspect of his behaviour, which might lead others to make unjustified assumptions about his capacity, or what might be in his best interests.

### Assessing capacity

Sections 2 and 3 of the Mental Capacity Act 2005 set out the requirements for assessing whether someone lacks capacity. 'A person lacks capacity in relation to a matter if at the material time he is unable to make a decision for himself in relation to the matter because of an impairment of, or disturbance in the functioning of the mind or brain' [section 2(1)]. This 'diagnostic threshold' covers a wide range of disorders, including psychiatric illness, learning disability, dementia, acquired head injury, and toxic confusional state, which may affect the functioning of the mind or brain causing someone to be unable to make a decision.

The definition in section 2(1) also envisages that capacity is:

◆ 'time-specific', focusing on the particular time when a decision has to be made—so the loss of capacity can be temporary, partial, or fluctuating, and

♦ 'decision-specific' or 'function specific', concentrating on the particular function to which the decision relates, rather than the ability to make decisions generally. So, someone may lack capacity in relation to one particular matter, but not necessarily another.

The actual test for capacity is a 'functional test' that looks at the decision-making process as a whole. Section 3 provides that a person who satisfies the diagnostic threshold is unable to make a decision for himself if he is unable to:

♦ understand the information relevant to the decision, including information about the reasonably foreseeable consequences of (a) deciding one way or another or (b) failing to make the decision; wherever necessary, the information should be explained to him in a way that is appropriate to his circumstances, such as using simple language or visual aids;

♦ retain that information, though the fact that he is able to retain the information for only a short period does not prevent him from being regarded as able to make the decision;

♦ use or weigh that information as part of the process of making the decision; or

♦ communicate his decision, whether by talking, using sign language, or any other means.

People suffering from 'locked in syndrome', for example, may be able to understand, retain, and use information as part of the decision-making process, and therefore technically not lack the capacity to make a decision, but be completely unable to communicate their decision. The Act treats such a person as someone who is unable to make a decision for him or herself. Any residual ability to communicate—such as blinking an eye to indicate 'yes' or 'no' in answer to a question—would exclude a person from this category. A good illustration of the practical application of these principles, particularly in relation to communication problems, can be found in *Re AK (Medical Treatment: Consent)* [2001] 1 FLR 129:

AK, who was 19, suffered from motor neuron disease, and for the last 2 years had been kept alive on a ventilator. For the last 3 months his only means of communicating was through moving one eyelid, by means of which he was able to answer questions with a 'yes', by the minimal movement of his eyelid, or 'no' by the absence of any movement of his eyelid. Using this method of communication, he had asked his mother, and subsequently the doctors treating him, to remove the ventilator 2 weeks after he lost the ability to communicate. He was aware that this would result in his death, and the doctors treating him sought a declaration that it would be lawful to discontinue the treatment in accordance with AK's directive. On 10 August 2000 Mr Justice Hughes granted the declaration sought.

From a practical point of view, the interesting feature of this case is the communication difficulties, and the strenuous efforts that were taken to establish that AK understood the nature and effect of his decision to refuse medical treatment. On 3 August 2000 two specialists, a consultant anaesthetist and a consultant in palliative care, visited him. Mr Justice Hughes described their visit as follows: 'Under careful questioning of a kind which I am satisfied took considerable pains to ensure they received only definitive and certain answers, Dr M and Dr S received again the same expression of wish. Dr M was, as Dr S no doubt had been before, at pains to satisfy himself that there was no question of AK being affected by any drugs at the time he gave his expression of wishes, that there was no question of coercion or pressure exerted upon him or felt by him and, although formal tests in the circumstances of AK's condition were impossible, that there was no sign that he was suffering from the kind of depression which might vitiate his

consent. Dr M satisfied himself that AK had a clear understanding of what was involved and that what was involved was his death. He also satisfied himself that AK had had explained to him the possible future discovery of the kind of preventive treatment to which I have already referred together with its limitations.'

## Best interests

Section 1(5) of the Mental Capacity Act 2005 sets out the principle that any act done or decision made under the Act for or on behalf of a person who lacks capacity must be in their best interests. Section 4 provides a checklist of points that the person making the decision must consider when deciding what is in someone's best interests. These are:

♦ whether they are likely to have capacity in relation to the matter in question in the future; this is in case the decision can be put off until the person can make it himself. Even if the decision cannot be delayed, it is likely to be influenced by whether the person concerned will always lack capacity or is likely to regain capacity;

♦ the need to permit and encourage them to participate, or to improve their ability to participate in the decision-making process;

♦ their past and present wishes and feelings (and, in particular, any relevant written statement they made when they had capacity), the beliefs and values that would be likely to influence their decision, and any other factors they would consider if they were able to do so;

♦ if it is practicable and appropriate to consult them, the views of others, such as family members, carers, and anyone else who has an interest in their welfare; and

♦ whether the purpose for which any act or decision is needed can be as effectively achieved in a manner less restrictive of their freedom of action.

Section 4(5) applies to decisions on whether life-sustaining treatment is in the best interests of the person concerned, and provides that the decision-maker must not be motivated by a desire to bring about the person's death.

## General defence in civil and criminal law

Sections 5 to 8 were originally described by the Law Commission as a 'general authority to act', and have been described by one of the authors of a textbook on the Act as 'the least formalistic and most innovative of the legal devices in the Mental Capacity Act' (Bartlett, 2005, p. 37, para. 2.49). The essential thrust of the provision is that people who act in connection with the care or treatment of someone who lacks capacity should be protected from liability for so doing, provided that such care or treatment is in the best interests of the person concerned and is performed without negligence.

Acts in connection with care might include, for example:

♦ physical assistance such as washing, dressing, toileting, and feeding;

♦ other help, such as doing the shopping, buying essential goods, arranging services required for the person's care;

♦ clearing someone's house when they have moved into residential care, washing someone's clothes, taking their car to a garage to be repaired.

Acts in connection with treatment would include, for example:

- diagnostic tests and examinations;
- medical treatment;
- dental treatment;
- nursing care.

## Lasting powers of attorney

Sections 9 to 14 create a new statutory form of power of attorney, 'lasting powers of attorney' (LPAs), which replace 'enduring powers of attorney' (EPAs). A power of attorney is a document in which an individual (called 'the donor') appoints one or more other persons to be his or her attorney(s). Unlike an ordinary power of attorney, which is automatically revoked by the donor's subsequent incapacity, EPAs and LPAs remain in force after the donor becomes mentally incapacitated, but only if they are registered.

Enduring powers of attorney had been available in England and Wales since March 1986, when the Enduring Powers of Attorney Act 1985 came into force. The 1985 Act has been repealed by the Mental Capacity Act 2005, and it is no longer possible to create an EPA, but the legal effect of existing EPAs is preserved and integrated into the new scheme by section 66(3) and Schedule 4 of the Act.

The main differences between EPAs and LPAs are summarized in Table 43.1.

Schedule 1 governs the creation, registration, and cancellation of LPAs. A lasting power of attorney must be in the prescribed form. It must also contain a certificate in a prescribed form, signed by a person of a 'prescribed description', confirming that the donor understood the purpose of the LPA and the scope of the authority conferred under it. Who persons of a 'prescribed description' may be has yet to be decided, but they might be similar to the category of persons who are entitled to certify photographs in passport applications.

## Court-appointed deputies

Where a person who has not made a LPA lacks the capacity to make a decision about his personal welfare or property and affairs, section 16 of the Act enables the Court of Protection to appoint a 'deputy' to make that decision for him. Deputies are equivalent in many respects to 'receivers' under the old legislation.

**Table 43.1** Comparison of enduring with lasting powers of attorney (© Denzil Lush)

| Enduring power of attorney | Lasting power of attorney |
|---|---|
| **Creating an EPA**<br>An EPA:<br>- must be in the prescribed form | **Creating a LPA**<br>A LPA:<br>- must be in the prescribed form<br>- may contain the names of persons the donor wishes to be notified of any application to register it, or must contain a statement that there are no such persons<br>- must contain a certificate by a person of a prescribed description to the effect that the donor understands the purpose of the instrument and the scope of authority conferred under it. |
| **Decisions the attorney(s) can make**<br>Unless the donor puts in any restrictions, the attorney(s) can do anything with the donor's property and financial affairs that a donor can lawfully do by an attorney, but the attorney(s) cannot make decisions about the donor's personal welfare | **Decisions the attorney(s) can make**<br>Unless the donor puts in any restrictions, the attorney(s) can make decisions about the donor's:<br>- property and financial affairs<br>- personal welfare (including giving or refusing consent to treatment), but only when the donor lacks, or the attorney reasonably believes that the donor lacks, the capacity to make such decisions at the time the decision has to be made |
| **When the instrument comes into operation**<br>Unless the donor expressly states that the EPA will not come into operation until he or she has become mentally incapable, an EPA comes into operation as soon as it has been executed by the donor and attorney(s)<br>It will remain in operation after the donor has become mentally incapable, provided it is registered | **When the instrument comes into operation**<br>The attorney(s) cannot act under a LPA unless it is registered with the Public Guardian<br>It can be registered with the Public Guardian before the donor becomes mentally incapacitated, but the attorney(s) can only make personal welfare decisions that the donor is incapable of making at the time |
| **The duty of the attorney(s)**<br>The attorney(s) under an EPA have a duty to apply to the Court of Protection for the registration of the instrument if they have reason to believe that the donor is, or is becoming, mentally incapable<br>The attorney(s) under an EPA have no statutory duty, though they probably have a duty at common law, to act in the donor's best interests | **The duty of the attorney(s)**<br>The attorney(s) under a LPA have no statutory duty to apply to the Public Guardian for the registration of the instrument<br>The attorney(s) under a LPA have a statutory duty:<br>- to act in accordance with the principles set out in section 1 of the Mental Capacity Act 2005<br>- to act in the donor's best interests; and<br>- to have regard to the guidance in the Code of Practice |

**Table 43.1**   *(cont.)*

| Enduring power of attorney | Lasting power of attorney |
|---|---|
| **The donor's ability to make decisions** | **The donor's ability to make decisions** |
| Until an EPA is registered, both the donor and the attorney have concurrent authority to make decisions about the donor's property and financial affairs | The donor can carry on making decisions, provided he or she has the capacity to do so |
| If the EPA is registered, in theory, the donor can still make decisions about his or her property and financial affairs, if he or she is capable of making them at the time | The attorney(s) can only make personal welfare decisions that the donor is incapable of making, or which they reasonably believe the donor is incapable of making, at the time |
| **Registering the power** | **Registering the power** |
| The attorney(s) have a duty to apply to the Court of Protection for the registration of the instrument, when they have reason to believe that the donor is, or is becoming, mentally incapable | Either the donor or the attorney(s) can apply to the Public Guardian to register the LPA. The application can be made prior to the onset of the donor's incapacity |
| Before applying to the court, the attorney(s) must give written notice (on form EP1) of their intention to apply for the registration of the power to: | Before making the application, whoever makes it must notify the persons named by the donor as being entitled to receive notification of the application |
| ◆ the donor personally, | Whoever makes the application, the Public Guardian will give notice that the application has been received to |
| ◆ any co-attorney(s), and | ◆ the donor, and |
| ◆ at least three of the donor's relatives from a list which specifies an order of priority | ◆ the attorney(s) |
| Those who receive notice of the application to register can object to the registration on the grounds that: | The donor's relatives will not be automatically notified, unless the donor has named them as being persons who are entitled to receive notice of the application |
| ◆ the power was not valid as an EPA; | The donor, the attorney(s) and the named persons may object to the registration of the instrument on the grounds that: |
| ◆ the power no longer subsists; | ◆ fraud or undue pressure was used to induce the donor to create the power; or |
| ◆ the application is premature, because the donor is not yet becoming mentally incapable; | ◆ the attorney(s) have behaved, are behaving, or are proposing to behave in a way that would contravene their authority or would not be in the donor's best interests |
| ◆ fraud or undue pressure was used to induce the donor to create the power; | |
| ◆ having regard to all the circumstances, the attorney is unsuitable to be the donor's attorney | |
| **Revoking the power** | **Revoking the power** |
| The Court of Protection must confirm the revocation of a registered EPA if it is satisfied that the donor has done whatever is necessary in law to effect an express revocation of the power and was mentally capable of revoking a power of attorney when he did so | The donor may, at any time when he has the capacity to do so, revoke the LPA |
| | The court may determine any question relating to whether a LPA has been revoked or has otherwise come to an end |
| | The dissolution or annulment of a marriage or a civil partnership will terminate the appointment of an attorney or revoke the power, unless the instrument provides that it will not do so |

The powers relating to the person's property and affairs include all necessary powers for managing and administering their estate. Powers in respect of a person's personal welfare include:

◆ deciding where they are to live;

◆ deciding what contact, if any, they are to have with specified persons;

◆ making an order prohibiting a named person from having contact; and

◆ giving or refusing consent to the carrying out or continuation of healthcare.

Section 16(4) of the Act, however, provides

◆ a decision by the court is to be preferred to the appointment of a deputy to make a decision, and

◆ the powers conferred on a deputy should be as limited in scope and duration as is reasonably practicable in the circumstances.

## Advance decisions to refuse treatment

Sections 24 to 26 provide a statutory framework, with various safeguards, whereby people can make an advance decision (or 'living will') to refuse treatment if they lose capacity in future. An advance decision will have no application to any treatment that a healthcare provider considers necessary to sustain life unless certain formalities have been complied with. These are that the advance decision must

◆ be written, signed, and witnessed, and

◆ include an express statement that the decision is to apply 'even if life is at risk' [section 25(5)].

## Independent mental capacity advocates

Sections 35 to 41, which were a last-minute amendment to the draft legislation, deal with the appointment and functions of independent mental capacity advocates (IMCAs), who will represent the views of people who have no family or friends to support them and who lack the capacity to consent to the proposals where:

- the National Health Service is proposing to provide serious medical treatment [section 37(1)]; or

- the person is being placed in, or arrangements are being made for a change in, NHS accommodation (section 38), or accommodation provided by a local authority (section 39).

## Code of practice

Guidance on the Act is contained in the Code of Practice (sections 42 and 43). The following people have a duty to follow this guidance, and any failure to do so would be considered by the courts in any relevant legal proceedings:

- donees of a LPA

- deputies appointed by the court

- persons carrying out intrusive research as part of an approved research project

- an IMCA

- persons acting in a professional capacity

- persons who receive remuneration.

Although this legal duty does not apply to relatives and unpaid carers, they would nevertheless be expected to follow the code as a matter of good practice.

## Court of Protection

Section 45 of the Mental Capacity Act 2005 abolished the former Court of Protection, which was an office of the Supreme Court, and replaced it with a new superior court of record, also known as the Court of Protection, which is able to deal with all areas of decision-making for people who lack capacity. Thus it combines the personal welfare and healthcare jurisdiction previously exercised by the Family Division of the High Court with the property and financial decision-making jurisdiction of the former Court of Protection. The court has a centralized administration office and registry in London, but contested matters can be heard at a number of venues throughout England and Wales.

Section 46 describes the judges of the Court of Protection. The court has a President and Vice-President. The President of the Family Division and the Chancellor of the High Court have been appointed President and Vice-President, respectively. There is also a Senior Judge, who is based at the court's central registry, and the other judges have been nominated from various levels of the judiciary from High Court judges to circuit judges and district judges.

The main functions of the Court of Protection are to:

- make declarations as to whether or not someone has the capacity to make a particular decision [section 15(1)];

- make declarations as to the lawfulness or otherwise or any act done, or yet to be done, in relation to a person [section 15(1)(c)];

- make single, one-off orders [section 16(2)(a)]; for example, an order authorizing the execution of a statutory will, or an order for the sale of a house and the investment of the net proceeds of sale;

- appoint a deputy to make decisions in relation to the matter(s) in which a person lacks the capacity to make a decision [section 16(2)(b)];

- resolve various issues involving LPAs (sections 22 and 23), and EPAs (Schedule 4);

- make a declaration as to whether an advance decision to refuse treatment exists, is valid, or is applicable to a particular treatment [section 26(4)];

- grant permission to persons who are not automatically entitled to make an application to the court (section 50);

- exercise an appellate jurisdiction in *Bournewood*-type cases[1] in which an individual has been deprived of his or her liberty.

## Office of the Public Guardian

Section 57 of the Mental Capacity Act 2005 provides for the creation of a new, statutory office-holder known as the Public Guardian. Section 58 confers on the Public Guardian various functions, such as:

- establishing and maintaining registers of LPAs and deputies appointed by the court;

- supervising deputies appointed by the court;

- directing a visit by a Court of Protection Visitor;

- receiving security, reports, and accounts; and

- complaints handling.

Section 59, which was a last-minute amendment to the legislation, provides for the appointment of the Public Guardian Board, whose duty is to scrutinize and review the way in which the Public Guardian discharges his functions.

## The Hague Convention on the International Protection of Adults

On 13 January 2000 The Hague Conference on Private International Law adopted a Convention on the International Protection of Adults. There is an important distinction between the adoption of a convention by the Conference, and its signing and ratification by member states, and its entry into force. By signing a convention, a contracting state expresses in principle its intention to become a party to it. By ratifying a convention, a state places itself under a

---

[1] HL, a 48-year-old man with autism had been in long-term care at Bournewood Hospital in Surrey, before moving in with Mr & Mrs E in 1994. They cared for him and treated him as one of their family. In July 1997 he became agitated whilst attending a day centre and was readmitted informally to Bournewood Hospital. Mr and Mrs E disagreed with the admission and mounted a legal challenge in October 1997. The court ruled that HL's 'informal' admission was illegal and that the Mental Health Act (MHA) should have been used. The Court of Appeal upheld this decision on 2 December 1997. The grounds for the ruling were that although HL did not actively disagree with the admission, he lacked the capacity to do so. The House of Lords overturned the Court of Appeal's judgement, stating that it was against the spirit of the MHA automatically to enforce detention if the patient lacked capacity. HL and his carers then took the case to the European Court of Human Rights which ruled that his treatment in a hospital amounted to detention and that this constituted a deprivation of liberty under Article 5 of the European Convention on Human Rights.

legal obligation to apply it. A convention finally enters into force when three instruments of ratification have been deposited with the Dutch Ministry of Foreign Affairs. The Hague Convention on the International Protection of Adults has been signed by four states—The Netherlands, France, Germany, and the UK—but so far only the UK has ratified it. Section 63 and Schedule 3 of the Mental Capacity Act 2005 give effect to this Convention as regards England and Wales.

## Scotland

### Adults with Incapacity (Scotland) Act 2000

The Adults with Incapacity (Scotland) Act 2000 was the fourth enactment passed by the then newly devolved Scottish Parliament. Like the Mental Capacity Act 2005 in England and Wales, the Scottish legislation was the culmination of a long period of public consultation, including a report from the Scottish Law Commission.

Part 2 of the Adults with Incapacity (Scotland) Act 2000 enables people in Scotland to create a continuing power of attorney in respect of their property and finances and/or a welfare power of attorney in respect of personal welfare decisions. There is no prescribed form of continuing power or welfare power, but the document must contain a prescribed form of certificate, completed by a solicitor stating that he or she is satisfied that the granter understood the nature and effect of the power. The attorney has no authority to act under power until it has been registered with the Public Guardian. The Sheriff Court exercises various supervisory functions over attorneys acting under continuing and welfare powers, and can require them to be supervised by the Public Guardian or (in the case of welfare powers) the local authority, and can order them to produce accounts for audit by the Public Guardian. The ultimate sanction is that the Sheriff Court can revoke a continuing or welfare power of attorney.

Part 6 of the Adults with Incapacity (Scotland) Act 2000 empowers the Sheriff Court to make either a 'one-off' intervention order or appoint a guardian to manage the property and finances of an adult with incapacity. Applications for such orders must be accompanied by at least two medical reports, in a prescribed form, completed not more than 30 days before the application is lodged. At least one of the medical reports must be completed by a medical practitioner who is approved for the purposes of section 20 of the Mental Health (Scotland) Act 1984 as having special expertise in the diagnosis or treatment of mental disorder. Guardianship orders may be limited in time. It is also possible for the court to appoint interim guardians, joint guardians, and substitute guardians. Intervention orders and guardianship orders must be registered with the Public Guardian. A guardian is required to submit to the Public Guardian an inventory of the estate within 3 months of his appointment, together with a management plan; is expected to account annually; and to provide caution (insurance) against any claims of mishandling funds.

## Northern Ireland

In Northern Ireland the management of mentally incapacitated patients' affairs is controlled by the High Court through the Office of Care and Protection. The relevant legislation is Part VIII of the Mental Health (Northern Ireland) Order 1986 and the Enduring Powers of Attorney (Northern Ireland) Order 1987. A *controller* is appointed to manage a patient's financial affairs. The Office of Care and Protection issues a *Handbook for Controllers*, which can be obtained from the address below.

## Ireland

In the Republic of Ireland the management of the property and affairs of mentally incapacitated adults (known as 'wards of court') is overseen by the President of the High Court, who has delegated the day-to-day administration of wardship matters to the Registrar of Wards of Court and his staff. The wardship legislation is contained in the Lunacy Regulation (Ireland) Act 1871, and in order to be taken into wardship, a person must be declared to be 'of unsound mind and incapable of managing his person or property'. Most commonly, wardship proceedings are taken by a family member in the High Court under section 15 of the Act. This involves petitioning the court to conduct an inquiry into whether to admit a person to wardship. The petition is accompanied by supporting affidavits from two medical practitioners, attesting that the person is of unsound mind and unable to manage their affairs.

After the President of the High Court has made an order bringing a person into wardship, he generally appoints a committee (i.e. a person to whom the affairs of the ward are 'committed') to act on the ward's behalf. The committee is authorized to receive the income of the ward; must enter into security with an approved insurance company, and file annual accounts for all sums received and disbursed.

It has been possible to make an enduring power of attorney in the Republic of Ireland since 1 August 1996, when Part II of the Powers of Attorney Act, 1996 came into force. The legislation is broadly similar to the now repealed Enduring Powers of Attorney Act 1985 in England and Wales, except that the donor can authorize an attorney to make personal welfare decisions on his or her behalf. The power must be in a form prescribed by the Minister for Justice. The attorney must apply for the power to be registered with the Office of Wards of Court when he or she has reason to believe that the donor is, or is becoming, mentally incapable. Certain people are entitled to be notified of the attorney's intention to register the power, and there are five grounds on which an objection to registration might be sustained.

In June 2003 The Law Reform Commission published a consultation paper on *Law and the Elderly* (LRC CP 23–2003), followed in May 2005 by a consultation paper on *Vulnerable Adults and the Law: Capacity* (LRC CP 37–2005), both of which broadly recommend reforms that would bring Irish Law in line with the capacity legislation recently enacted in Great Britain.

### Bibliography

Ashton, G., Letts, P., Oates, L., and Terrell, M. (2006). *Mental capacity: the new law.* Jordan Publishing, Bristol.

Bartlett, P. (2005). *Blackstone's guide to the Mental Capacity Act 2005.* Oxford University Press, Oxford.

Greaney, N., Morris, F., and Taylor, B. (2005). *Mental Capacity Act 2005: a guide to the new law.* The Law Society, London.

Jones, R. (2005). *Mental Capacity Act manual.* Thomson, Sweet & Maxwell, London.

O'Neill, A.-M. (2004). *Wards of Court in Ireland.* FirstLaw, Dublin.

Ward, A. (2003). *Adult incapacity.* W Green, Edinburgh.

Ward, A. (2006). *Adults with incapacity legislation.* W Green, Edinburgh.

## Websites

Pre-Legislative Scrutiny Committee reported on the draft Mental Incapacity Bill. http://www.publications.parliament.uk/pa/jt/jtdmi.htm

Mental Capacity Act 2005. http://www.hmso.gov.uk/acts/acts2005/20050009.htm

Explanatory notes to Mental Capacity Act 2005. http://www.opsi.gov.uk/acts/en2005/2005en09.htm

## Addresses

### England and Wales

Office of the Public Guardian, Archway Tower, 2 Junction Road, London N19 5SZ; Tel: 020 7664 7430; Fax: 0870 739 5780 (UK callers) or +44 207 664 7000 (for callers outside UK)

Document Exchange: DX 141150 Archway 2; E-mail: custserv@guardianship.gsi.gov.uk; website: http://www.guardianship.gov.uk/

### Scotland

The Office of the Public Guardian, Hadrian House, Callendar Business Park, Callendar Road, Falkirk FK1 1XR; Tel: 01324 678300; Fax: 01324 678301

DX 550360 Falkirk 3; E-mail: opg@scotcourts.gov.uk; website: http://www.publicguardian-scotland.gov.uk/

### Northern Ireland

The Office of Care and Protection, 2nd Floor, Royal Courts of Justice, Chichester Street, PO Box 410, Belfast BT1 3JF; Tel: 028 9072 4733; Fax: 028 9032 2782; E-mail: officeofcareandprotection@courtsni.gov.uk; website: http://www.courtsni.gov.uk

### Ireland

The Office of Wards of Court, 3rd Floor, 15/24 Phoenix Street North, Smithfield, Dublin 7; Tel: +353 (0) 1 888 6189 or 6140; Fax: + 353 (0) 1 872 4063; website: http://www.citizensinformation.ie/categories/justice/courts-system/office_of_wards_of_court/

# 44

# Driving and psychiatric illness in later life

Desmond O'Neill

## Overview of mobility and health

Mobility and driving evoke a curious response in healthcare personnel. With most areas of function we assess and treat people so as to maximize that function. The literature on driving and disease, however, is almost totally biased in favour of the identification of those who should not drive rather than maximizing health and function so that older people can participate and integrate maximally with society. This matter assumes great importance in view of the dramatic rise in the proportion of older people in our society. It is further emphasized by the enormous increase in the proportion of older people who wish to continue driving. At the White House Conference on Ageing in 1971, transportation was rated as third in importance in older people's lives, after health and finance (Carp et al., 1980). This high ranking persisted in the 2005 White House Conference on Ageing, with access to transportation ranked ahead of Medicaid and Medicare (White House Conference on Aging, 2005).

Some of the negative attitudes to older drivers stem from a more widespread failure to appreciate the idiosyncratic approach of our society to mobility and safety. At its most marked, a landmark study in the 1960s showed that American motorists felt that they were more likely to be involved in a nuclear catastrophe than in a fatal car crash. Despite high-profile campaigns to promote safety on our roads by way of exhortations to reduce speed and avoid alcohol, at virtually every level of transport policy mobility takes priority over safety. If safety were paramount, the speed limit would be 20 miles per hour and governors would be fitted to car engines to prevent this speed limit from being breached. It is also likely that we would have a more graduated entry to driving while in the late teens or early 20s. This is because youth and inexperience breed risky driving behaviours that cause crashes Unfortunately, however, the emphasis of many European governments is to stigmatize older drivers (White and O'Neill, 2000). Older drivers are forced to undergo regular medical checks in most countries of the European Union, despite evidence that this practice is harmful (Hakamies-Blomqvist et al., 1996; Langford et al., 2004) or ineffective (Rock, 1998). This ageist legislation is not based on any factual evidence and reflects the weakness of organized advocacy for older people in Europe. This is despite the fact that older drivers have one of the best safety records of any group of drivers in society (Evans, 1988).

Sometimes a U-shaped curve is displayed showing that older drivers have a higher crash risk per mile than do younger drivers (Broughton, 1988). This is spurious for several reasons. Not only do they drive considerably fewer miles than their younger peers, but at least two studies have shown that this finding is an artefact of low mileage—if low mileage is controlled for in comparisons with younger drivers, the difference in crash rate disappears (Hakamies-Blomqvist et al., 2002; Langford et al., 2006). Also, older people tend to drive on roads which are inherently more dangerous—rural and suburban highways are more dangerous than motorways. Finally, old people are more fragile and are more likely to suffer death or serious injury for a given severity of crash than young people are (Brorsson, 1989).

## Health and driving

There is a famous illustration in the pharmacology textbook by Goodman and Gilman which illustrates the process of absorbing a new medication into medical practice. This oscillates from an initial enthusiastic acceptance to a sceptical rejection and finally results in a reasoned assessment of the positive and negative aspects of the drug (Fig. 44.1). This is a similar process to that which occurs when healthcare professionals encounter the concept of driving and illness for the first time. At the outset, working in an environment where a highly selected population are much more likely to have a high burden of disease, it is it inevitable that the potential risks should be perceived rather than the impact on mobility (O'Neill et al., 1992). As the researchers in the area gain perspective, a totally different concept comes to the fore, that of the major threat posed to the mobility of older people by age-related disease (Metz, 2000). Finally, the fusion of both points of view is achieved, whereby an enabling process is developed which encompasses the mechanisms for helping those who can no longer drive to seek alternative methods of transport, secure in the knowledge that they had due process in a thorough evaluation and remediation (O'Neill, 2000). In a welcome development for the new millennium, this approach has been adopted by the Organization for Economic Cooperation and Development (OECD, 2001), the European Conference of Ministers of Transport (CEMT, 2001), and the US Transportation Research Board (Transportation Research Board, 2004).

Driving is a health-related issue: there is a consistent pattern in many countries around the world of cessation of driving relating to illness and loss of function (Campbell et al., 1993; Forrest et al., 1997;

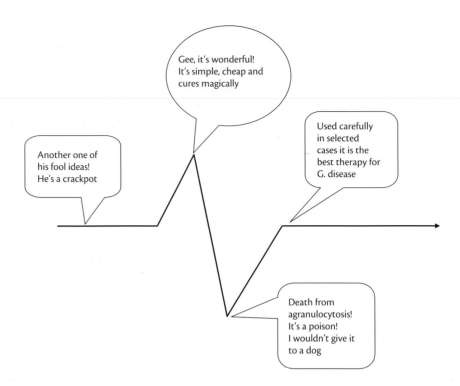

**Fig. 44.1** Oscillations in the development of a drug.

Kostyniuk *et al.*, 1998), although driving may persist after other socially useful patterns of mobility have been affected (Hjorthol, 2001). This pattern is reflected in several studies of dementia and driving (Foley *et al.*, 2000). Older people tend not to discuss concerns about driving with healthcare providers (Johnson, 1998): this is a cause of concern as it is possible that remediable medical causes of driving cessation may not be addressed. Lack of access to transportation, and in particular to driving, is associated with reduced access to healthcare (Hughes-Cromwick *et al.*, 2006) as well as earlier admission to nursing home care (Freeman *et al.*, 2006).

Although all people with progressive illnesses such as the dementias will eventually undergo decline in cognition, function, and behaviour, it is not clear that this poses a public health risk, despite a somewhat one-sided review of current studies (Dubinsky *et al.*, 2000). It is more likely that the process of reducing mileage and eventual withdrawal from driving protects the general public from the harmful effects of the illness on driving safety (Trobe *et al.*, 1996; Carr *et al.*, 2000). Indeed, focus groups of those associated with Alzheimer's disease—those with the illness, caregivers and professionals—were almost unanimous in saying that those with mild AD should continue to drive (Perkinson *et al.*, 2005).

## Skills and resources needed for automobility assessment

Many professionals working in the psychiatry of old age feel at a loss when confronted with older people who have both psychiatric illness and drive a car. They often do not realize that the many skills used in clinical decision-making also form the basis for making decisions on driving and mobility. These skills are founded in multidisciplinary assessment, an enabling philosophy, and advocacy for older people in the face of nihilism and ageism. In practice, these same skills are seen in the integration of clinical assessment and

input from the multidisciplinary team in the calculation of risk in other areas of clinical practice such as deciding on discharge to home. Elements of the decision-making process include careful multidisciplinary evaluation, discussion with carers, and perhaps a trial visit home. The elements of this process are very similar to the assessment of fitness to drive. Not only may relatives place security before independence but a psychometric model is also unlikely to be helpful. This often surprises clinicians: while psychometric support is important in backing up our diagnostic abilities, it is rarely of help when making decisions about function. For example, the decision that the patient is no longer fit to remain at home and requires placement in a nursing home is much more likely to be taken on the basis of measures of function and behaviour than on psychometric measures.

The premise that the expertise of those who practise psychiatry with older people already contains some of the elements necessary for mobility assessments is not a charter for dilettantism. Rather, it is a challenge to us to develop the extra resources required to ensure that we have adequate support when making decisions about enhancing the safe mobility of older people. This has many parallels with the task of assessing safety at home or capacity to manage financial affairs: in these cases, it is good practice to liaise with an occupational therapist or a neuropsychologist. There has also been a failure to capitalize on the rich level of knowledge of psychiatrists: many of the studies of their practice have been more concerned to highlight their lack of knowledge of the driving regulations rather than to draw on their collective wisdom (Elwood, 1998). It is likely that their estimates of the parameters of safe mobility in their patient groups would have equal if not greater validity than current driving regulations which are often arbitrary and sometimes counterintuitive and unfair.

At a minimum, the assessment of the impact of psychiatric illness on mobility in later life requires a careful medical and psychiatric assessment, a collateral history and access to occupational therapy and/or neuropsychology as well as access to a specialist driver assessment. There may be a case for developing services at a regional level, particularly for those cases where decision-making is not clear after the first assessment. A specific concern relates to the funding of such services: although the mobility/risk problem is clearly health-related in origin, Medicare in the USA will not refund specialist driving assessment and the attendant cost may deter older drivers from seeking help. The psychiatrist will also need to know the local regulations on fitness to drive, on the obligations of the patient to disclose relevant illness to the driver licensing authority and insurance company, and an awareness of the local requirements for physician disclosure, if any.

## Models of driving behaviour

Driving is an over-learned skill with a significant behavioural component (Ranney, 1994). The most significant advance in this area has been the understanding that a purely cognitive model of driving ability does not adequately reflect the complexity and hierarchical nature of the driving task. We also know that clinicians working with a range of diseases, including dementia, may not accurately predict the road testing ability of drivers (Heikkila *et al.*, 1998). Driver behaviour is complex and one of the simplest and most easily applicable models has been the hierarchy of Michon which uses strategic, tactical, and operational factors (Michon, 1985). The strategic level is the choice of whether or not to travel, the tactical decision is whether or not to overtake, and the operational level is what to do when overtaking and faced with an oncoming car. The strategic and tactical levels are probably more important in terms of driving safety than the operational level. This concept has been operationalized for brain damage (head injury and stroke) in the driving model of Galski, which adds a behavioural observational element to a battery of cognitive tests and a primitive simulator (Galski *et al.*, 1993). It has also been operationalized more closely in a driver screening battery

**Table 44.1** Framework for driver assessment

| History: | Patient, family/informant |
| | Driving history |
| Examination: | Functional status |
| | Other illnesses and drugs |
| | Vision |
| | Mental status testing |
| | Diagnostic formulation and prioritization |
| | Disease severity and fluctuations |
| Remediation | |
| Re-assess | |
| In-depth cognitive/perceptual testing + on-road assessment | |
| Overall evaluation of hazard: | Strategic |
| | Tactical |
| | Operational |
| Advice to patient/carer + driver licensing authority | |
| If driving too hazardous, consider alternative mobility strategies | |

(De Raedt and Ponjaert-Kristoffersen, 2000). The most common framework for driver assessment is shown in Table 44.1.

Not all levels of assessment will be required by all patients: a patient with a homonymous hemianopia is barred from driving throughout the European Union, and referral to the social worker to plan alternative transportation is appropriate. Equally, a mild cognitive defect may only require a review by the physician and occupational therapist. The overall interdisciplinary assessment should attempt to provide solutions to both maintaining activities and exploring transport needs. The on-road test may be helpful as it may demonstrate deficits to a patient or a carer who is ambiguous about the patient stopping driving. At a therapeutic level, members of the team may be able to help the patient come to terms with the losses associated with stopping driving. The occupational therapist may be able to maximize the patient's activities and function and help focus on preserved areas of achievement, while the social worker can advise on alternative methods of transport. This team approach to assessment should save time and valuable resources for occupational therapy, neuropsychology, and road driver assessors.

In addition to the usual work-up, the medical assessment should include a driving history from patient and carer. Although Hunt *et al.* (1993) have shown a poor correlation between carer assessment and on-road driving performance, this single small study is insufficient to allow one to discount the collateral history. The Folstein Mini-Mental State Examination (MMSE) would perhaps be the most reasonable choice from the simple screening measures of cognitive impairment: a near-consensus paper in 1994 suggested that those who score 17 or less on a MMSE require further assessment in a formal way (Hakamies-Blomqvist *et al.*, 1996). The choice of cut-off at a relatively low score reflects in part the unease among the participants that reliance on a simple test such as the MMSE would over-simplify the complex task of appropriate assessment of older people with dementia.

The next stage of testing described in the literature has been performed mainly by occupational therapists and neuropsychologists. None of the studies has been sufficiently large to have a reasonable predictive value or to determine cut-off points on neuropsychological test batteries. This situation is parallel to that in memory clinics where there is a wide variation in the test batteries used. It is likely that the important elements of successful assessment are the choice of key domains, familiarity with a test battery, and the development of an understanding and close liaison between the physician and the occupational therapist and/or neuropsychologist. A wide range of tests has been correlated with driving behaviour, but few have been sufficiently robust to calculate cut-off points for risky driving. All of these tests can be criticized for taking an over-cognitive view of the driving task.

Specific tests which show correlation with driving ability in more than one study include the MMSE (above), the Trail Making Test (Maag, 1984; Janke and Eberhard, 1998; Mazer *et al.*, 1998; Stutts, 1998), and a range of tests of visual attention (Klavora *et al.*, 1995; Duchek *et al.*, 1998; Marottoli *et al.* 1998; Owsley *et al.*, 1998; Trobe, 1998), including the Useful Field of View® [a composite measure of pre-attentive processing, incorporating speed of visual information processing, ability to ignore distracters (selective attention) and ability to divide attention (Ball *et al.*, 1991)], and the Driving Scenes Test of the Neuropsychological Assessment Battery (Brown *et al.*, 2005). A range of other tests have been assessed in single studies; an interesting one is traffic sign recognition (Carr *et al.*, 1991) and a comprehensive review is available from the US National Highway Transportation Safety Administration (Staplin *et al.*, 1999).

In conjunction with the clinical assessment and collateral history, these tests will help to decide which patients require on-road testing, as well as those who are likely to be too dangerous to test! The other interesting aspect is that there may be a disparity between scores on a test battery and the clinical assessment of the neuropsychologist. In a small paper by Fox *et al.* (1997), the neuropsychological test scores and the neuropsychological prediction were not found to be significantly associated, suggesting that the clinicians made their decisions on items not formally measured in the neuropsychological test battery.

On-road driver testing is the gold standard and should be offered to all patients who are not clearly dangerous when driving and who do not disqualify from driving for other reasons such as homonymous hemianopia or convulsions. At least three different road tests have been devised, but the numbers of drivers put through these are still relatively small with 27 patients in the Sepulveda Road Test (Fitten *et al.*, 1995), 65 in the Washington University Road Test (Hunt *et al.*, 1997), and 155 in the Alberta Road Test (Dobbs *et al.*, 1998). The assessor will require a full clinical report, and may choose to use one of the recently developed scoring systems for on-road testing of patients with dementia. A limited number of countries offer a medical advisory service, for example, the Medical Section of the Driver and Vehicle Licensing Agency (DVLA) in the UK.

## Functional illness

The role of illness other than dementia has been even less widely studied, apart from alcohol dependency. The overall impression from the literature is that the added risk from schizophrenia and affective disorders is small, although the issue is complicated by the use of psychoactive medications (Soyka *et al.*, 2005). The emphasis on risk rather than on mobility is similar to the rest of the field, and it is likely that those with psychiatric illness have less mobility than the population as a whole. Butteglieri and Guenette (1967) found that subjects with psychiatric illness had accident and violation records similar to the general population. Patients with schizophrenia and depot neuroleptics show a worse driving performance on a driving test than unmedicated normal controls (Wylie *et al.*, 1993), but concrete evidence of increased crash risk is not available. A Swiss study in 1978 of mostly young and middle-aged people with schizophrenia showed more violations and accidents in those with delusions of a religious type, but results were favourable in those with a cautious, anxious character (Sacher, 1978).

The role of psychiatric intervention has only been assessed in one study. Eelkema *et al.* (1970) found that those with alcohol dependency had higher than normal crash rates both before and after hospitalization, whereas those classified as suffering from psychotic and psychoneurotic disorders had higher rates prior to hospitalization and lower afterwards. No one in any of the groups was older than 70, which is a recurring issue in the literature in this area. In one small study of schizophrenia, one-third of older subjects were current drivers (Palmer *et al.*, 2002). The one paper dealing with depression and driving in old age is limited to two case reports and is highly conjectural. The use of car crashes as a means of suicide is considered to occur in a very small proportion

of crashes, despite a suggestion from early studies that this might be a more marked problem. Studies by Tabachnik *et al.* (1966), Schmidt *et al.* (1977), and Isherwood *et al.* (1982) have subsequently shown the risk to be small.

So where does this leave the clinician in this area? Key considerations are likely to be the severity and stability of the patient's condition, their insight, impulsiveness, and ability to react appropriately in a strategic and operational fashion. Ideally, medications will be minimized, with due caution over neuroleptics or long-acting benzodiazepines (see below).

## Medications

An area of increasing debate over the last 20 years has been the potential impact of psychoactive medications on driver safety. This interest has paralleled studies showing an impact of these medications on other injuries (Ray *et al.*, 1992), notably falls. A number of studies have suggested that physicians should be concerned about diminished driving skills and increased crash risk with these medications (Ray *et al.*, 1993; Hemmelgarn *et al.*, 1997). In terms of numbers of prescriptions, the main groups implicated are the benzodiazepines (Hemmelgarn *et al.*, 1997) and antidepressants (Ray *et al.*, 1992). If a true increased risk can be established and quantified, by medication type and dosage, restrictions either in prescribing or on driving (or both) may be an achievable component of a crash-prevention strategy.

Demonstrating cause and effect has been problematic. Separating the effects of the disease from those of the medications is not easy: depression, anxiety, and insomnia may have an impact on driving behaviour that might be ameliorated by pharmacological treatment, although current evidence suggests this is likely to be true for depression only. Studies on volunteers do not replicate clinical experience. There is a mini-industry of tests of reaction time or braking time, comparing psychoactive medications. As we have previously seen, operational or reaction factors are less important in driving safety than strategic or tactical factors, so it is very difficult to give any significant weight to these tests. There is also a danger in trying to extrapolate from these tests to a real impact on safety.

A parallel here is the theoretical differences between tricyclic antidepressants (TCAs) and selective serotoninergic reuptake inhibitors (SSRIs) in relation to the risk of falls. Although SSRIs would seem to have theoretical advantages, clinical studies have not been able to show any difference in fall rates between older people on TCAs or SSRIs (Thapa *et al.*, 1998). Similarly, epidemiological studies of car crashes have difficulty in matching controls with cases, in the exclusion of fatalities (which are more likely to involve alcohol and possibly psychoactive drugs), unreliability in medication recall at interview, lack of diagnostic categorization prior to the crash, and failure to control for the many variables which affect crash risk.

The use of large prescribing databases has helped to reduce uncertainty about prescribed medications among subjects in epidemiological studies. Hemmelgarn *et al.* (1997) showed an increased risk of crash of 1.5 in the first week of use of long-acting benzodiazepines among older drivers compared with 1.29 with chronic use and no increased risk among those on short-acting benzodiazepines. A further methodological refinement is reported in a study of a crash population where just over 1% of drivers in a first-ever crash were current users of benzodiazepines (Barbone *et al.*, 1998). The authors used a technique whereby subjects act as their own controls, eliminating the difficulty of finding matching controls and reducing some of the associated confounding effects. The finding of an almost 50% increase in crash risk in users of benzodiazepines should be interpreted cautiously where older drivers are concerned The risk was concentrated in younger drivers (under 45), and was increased greatly by the presence of alcohol. The study showed no association with increased risk in the elderly, a group who are most sensitive to the effects of benzodiazepines. This is noteworthy if confirmed by other studies, as it suggests that benzodiazepines affect crash risk by mechanisms other than those which have been traditionally measured by psychometric tests. The lack of association with TCAs found in the study is also a departure from existing data. The restriction of the study to first-time crashes limits its contribution to the understanding of those drivers who may demonstrate repeatedly risky driving behaviour.

Universal advice against driving while taking benzodiazepines is not yet supported by this study, but it should accelerate both epidemiological and policy interest in the subject, as well as clinical caution. An expansion of this style of study should be encouraged, to include all crashes and injury and death, not only in motorists, but also pedestrians and cyclists. Prospective studies are also needed, perhaps at the time of peri-marketing clinical trials (Ray, 1992). In the interim, those who prescribe benzodiazepines need to recognize that most adult patients are drivers or potential drivers. Active consideration should be given to whether the illness is likely to affect driving skills and whether the patient has a past crash history. The patient should be advised not to drive if they cannot abstain from alcohol while on treatment with benzodiazepines. Most importantly, the prescriber should query whether the patient really needs a benzodiazepine, and if they do, does it need to be long-acting.

## Practical guidelines

In advising a patient who is also a driver the psychiatrist must first ask how the the patient's illness affects their mobility. A secondary goal is to assess the potential safety risk. The procedures outlined in Table 44.1 should be carried out, and ideally any permanent decisions on driving should be made when the patient's condition is stabilized and optimized. An interim decision will have to be made until the assessment is completed, and this may involve asking the patient to desist from driving temporarily. Some countries have reasonably well-developed schemata for helping clinicians: increasingly, they have recognized the value of specialist opinion. For example, the mostly excellent 'At a glance' leaflets from the UK driver licensing authorities (http://www.dvla.gov.uk/media/pdf/medical/aagv1.pdf) have moved on from an assumption that hospitalization is the norm for significant psychiatric illness to a model based more on ambulatory care, with reference made to specialist opinion. Some of the criteria of the driver licensing authorities also seem unnecessarily strict, and as the field of driver assessment matures it will be important that professional organizations make representations to driver licensing authorities to ensure that the regulations are fair. Guidelines from the Association for the Advancement of Automotive Medicine stress the importance of leaving many of the decisions to the specialist, assuming appropriate assessment back-up (Dobbs, 2002). In the interim, physicians

who feel that the regulations hinder the health, well-being, and mobility of their patient unnecessarily may need to consult their medical defence organization about the clash of ethical responsibilities that they experience.

In some cases it may be apparent that there are no concerns about driving safety or, conversely, that the patient is too unstable or compromised to drive safely. In cases where the judgement lies in between, a full assessment including an on-road driving test may be required. Once a decision has been made, the psychiatrist needs to inform the patient of their responsibility to report to the local driver licensing authorities and/or their insurance company: this discussion should be documented in the clinical notes. I tend to phrase this by suggesting to the patient that they review their insurance policy documentation. Patients' responsibilities vary enormously from jurisdiction to jurisdiction. Failure to inform the patient of the relevant requirement may expose the doctor to criticism or even litigation. The psychiatrist also needs to be aware of any statutory requirements for physicians to report illnesses such as dementia to driver licensing authorities, as is the case in California and most Canadian provinces. Reporting a driver when one lacks confidence that there will be a fair and sensitive assessment by the driver licensing authority can pose an ethical dilemma. It is of some interest that the rate of reporting to the Californian Department of Motor Vehicles (DMV) of drivers with dementia by physicians did not increase after the institution of the relevant law. It is also notable that living in a jurisdiction with mandatory reporting did not have an impact on driving cessation in Alzheimer's disease, raising a question over the usefulness of mandatory reporting, which may have the unintended effect of deterring patients with dementia from reporting to their physician (Herrmann *et al.*, 2006).

If the assessment points to safe driving practice, the decision to allow continued driving entails several further judgements on the part of the doctor. These are:

- interval before review
- possible restriction
- driving accompanied
- licensing authority reporting relationship
- insurance reporting responsibility.

Since dementia is a progressive illness and affective disorders and alcohol dependency are recurrent or relapsing diseases, it is prudent to make any declaration of fitness to drive subject to regular review. For dementia, my own practice is to review again in 6 months, or sooner if any deterioration is reported by the carer: some support is given for this approach in one of the longitudinal studies of driving and dementia (Duchek *et al.*, 2003). Following evidence that the crash rate is reduced if the driver is accompanied (Bédard *et al.*, 1996), it could be sensible to restrict the patient to driving only when there is someone else in the car, using the co-pilot paradigm (Shua-Haim and Gross, 1996). There is also preliminary evidence from the state of Utah that those drivers with restricted driving licences have lower crash rates (Vernon *et al.*, 2002). Patients should be advised to avoid traffic congestion as well as driving at night and in bad weather. The patient and carers should be advised to acquaint themselves with the requirements of local driver licensing authorities as well as the policy of their motor insurance company. All of the above should be clearly recorded in the medical notes.

## How do older drivers with dementia deal with driving cessation when driving is no longer possible?

There is strong evidence that most drivers with dementia not only limit their own driving and cease driving voluntarily (Foley *et al.*, 2000) but also are amenable to pressure from family and physicians. In one of the largest studies 18% stopped driving of their own accord, 23% because of physicians, 42% because of family members, and the rest by a combination of interventions (Trobe *et al.*, 1996). In a recent study, factors predictive of driving cessation included global deterioration, lower level of cognition (Talbot *et al.*, 2005) and some interesting trends on neuropsychiatric behaviour. Agitation made it less likely that a patient would cease driving, whereas apathy and hallucinations made it more likely (Herrmann *et al.*, 2006). Living in rural areas is associated with later cessation of driving (Talbot *et al.*, 2005). There are no studies of how patients with dementia compensate for the transport needed to fulfil their social, occupational, and health needs, and considerable concern exists that these needs are not met adequately (Taylor and Tripodes, 2001). Psychological adaptation to cessation of driving may be helped by diagnosis and psychotherapeutic input, but this has not been tested in a randomized controlled trial. In a single case study, the patient's feelings and fears about giving up driving were explored with him (Bahro *et al.*, 1995). The intervention was designed with the patient as collaborator rather than patient, and by dealing with the events at an emotional rather than at an intellectual level. The patient was able to grieve about the disease and in particular about the loss of his car. This in turn enabled him to redirect his attention to other meaningful activities that did not involve driving. Although this approach may be hampered by the deficits of dementia, it reflects a more widespread trend towards sharing the diagnosis of dementia with the patient.

## What should doctors advise for those patients they assess as unfit to drive?

If the assessment supports driving cessation, patients and carers should be advised of this, and a social worker consulted to help maximize transportation options. Giving up driving can have a considerable effect on lifestyle. Normal elderly drivers accept that their physician's advice would be very influential in deciding to give up driving (Rabbitt *et al.*, 1996), and many patients with dementia will respond to advice from families or physicians.

The way we deal with driving reflects how we help the patient to deal with the reality of the deficits caused by dementia. If the positive and collaborative approach described above is not successful, confidentiality may have to be broken for a small minority of cases. Most professional associations for physicians accept that the principle of confidentiality is covered to a degree by a 'common good' principle of protecting third parties when direct advice to the patient is ignored (American Medical Association, 1999). Removal of the driving licence is not likely to have much effect on these patients, and the vehicle may need to be disabled (Donnelly and Karlinsky, 1990) and all local repair services warned not to respond to calls from the patient!

In the event of a decision to advise cessation of driving, advice from a medical social worker may be helpful in planning strategies for using alternative modes of travel. This may be difficult in a rural setting: one estimate of community transport exclusively for older people in the USA was $5.14 for a one-way trip in 1983 (Rosenbloom, 1993), and the political system has not woken up to the need for adequate para-transit, i.e. tailored, affordable, and reliable assisted transport which is acceptable to older adults with physical and/or mental disability (Freund, 2000). Tailored transport (para-transit) is expensive, but may have benefits in reducing institutionalization and in improving quality of life.

## Screening for dementia among older drivers

Despite the lack of convincing evidence for an older driver 'problem', ageist policies in many jurisdictions have led to screening programmes for older drivers. In the absence of reliable and sensitive assessment tools, this approach is flawed, as illustrated by data from Scandinavia (Hakamies-Blomqvist *et al.*, 1996). In Finland there is regular age-related medical certification of fitness to drive, whereas Sweden has no routine medical involvement in licence renewal. The number of older people dying in car crashes in Finland is no less than in Sweden but the number of those dying as pedestrians and cyclists is higher, possibly in part by unnecessarily removing drivers from their cars. Equally in Australia, the state with the lowest number of crashes among older drivers is that which does not undertake age-based medical screening of older drivers (Langford *et al.*, 2004). A more minimalist and less medical approach using very simple measures, such as a vision test and a written skill examination, may be more helpful (Levy *et al.*, 1995): unfortunately this approach is also associated with a reduction in the number of older drivers, a possible negative health impact (Levy, 1995). Another approach is opportunistic health screening, perhaps of those older drivers with traffic violations (Johansson *et al.*, 1996). It remains to be seen whether these and other screening policies reduce mobility among older people, a practical and civil rights issue of great importance.

## References

American Medical Association (1999). *Ethical and judicial affairs report*, pp. 182–4. American Medical Association, Chicago.

Bahro, M., Silber, E. *et al.* (1995). Giving up driving in Alzheimer's disease – an integrative therapeutic approach. *International Journal of Geriatric Psychiatry*, **10**, 871–4.

Ball, K., Owsley, C. *et al.* (1991). Visual and cognitive predictors of driving problems in older adults. *Experimental Aging Research*, **17**(2), 79–80.

Barbone, F., McMahon, A. *et al.* (1998). Association of road-traffic accidents with benzodiazepine use. *Lancet*, **352**, 1331–6.

Bédard, M., Molloy, M. *et al.* (1996). Should demented patients drive alone? *Journal of American Geriatrics Society*, **44**, S9.

Brorsson, B. (1989). Age and injury severity. *Scandinavian Journal of Social Medicine*, **17**, 287–90.

Broughton, J. (1988). *The variation of car driver's risk with age*. Transport and Road Research Laboratory, Crowthorne.

Brown, L.B., Stern, R.A. *et al.* (2005). Driving scenes test of the Neuropsychological Assessment Battery (NAB) and on-road driving performance in aging and very mild dementia. *Archives of Clinical Neuropsychology*, **20**(2), 209–15.

Buttiglieri, M.W. and Guenette, M. (1967). Driving record of neuropsychiatric patients. *Journal of Applied Psychology*, **51**(2), 96–100.

Campbell, M.K., Bush, T.L. *et al.* (1993). Medical conditions associated with driving cessation in community-dwelling, ambulatory elders. *Journal of Gerontology*, **48**(4), S230–S234.

Carp, F.M., Byerts, T. *et al.* (1980). Transportation. *The Gerontologist*, **12**, 11–16.

Carr, D., Madden, D. *et al.* (1991). The use of traffic identification signs to identify drivers with dementia. *Journal of the American Geriatrics Society*, **39**, A62.

Carr, D.B., Duchek, J. *et al.* (2000). Characteristics of motor vehicle crashes of drivers with dementia of the Alzheimer type. [see comments] *Journal of the American Geriatrics Society*, **48**(1), 18–22.

CEMT (2001). *Report on transport and ageing of the population.* CEMT, Paris.

De Raedt, R. and Ponjaert-Kristoffersen, I. (2000). Can strategic and tactical compensation reduce crash risk in older drivers? *Age and Ageing*, **29**(6), 517–21.

Dobbs, A.R., Heller, R.B. *et al.* (1998). A comparative approach to identify unsafe older drivers. *Accident Analysis and Prevention*, **30**(3), 363–70.

Dobbs, B.D. (2002). *Medical conditions and driving: current knowledge.* Association for the Advancement of Automotive Medicine, Chicago, IL.

Donnelly, R.E. and Karlinsky, H. (1990). The impact of Alzheimer's disease on driving ability: a review. *Journal of Geriatric Psychiatry and Neurology*, **3**(2), 67–72.

Dubinsky, R.M., Stein, A.C. *et al.* (2000). Practice parameter: risk of driving and Alzheimer's disease (an evidence-based review): report of the quality standards subcommittee of the American Academy of Neurology. *Neurology*, **54**(12), 2205–11.

Duchek, J.M., Hunt, L. *et al.* (1998). Attention and driving performance in Alzheimer's disease. *Journals of Gerontology B: Psychological Sciences and Social Sciences*, **53**(2), 130–41.

Duchek, J.M., Carr, D.B. *et al.* (2003). Longitudinal driving performance in early-stage dementia of the Alzheimer type. *Journal of the American Geriatrics Society*, **51**(10), 1342–7.

Eelkema, R., Brosseau, J. *et al.* (1970). A statistical study on the relationship between mental illness and traffic accidents. *American Journal of Public Health*, **60**, 459–69.

Elwood, P. (1998). Driving, mental illness and the role of the psychiatrist. *Irish Journal of Psychological Medicine*, **15**(2), 49–51.

Evans, L. (1988). Older driver involvement in fatal and severe traffic crashes. *Journal of Gerontology*, **43**(6), S186–S193.

Fitten, L.J., Perryman, K.M. *et al.* (1995). Alzheimer and vascular dementias and driving. A prospective road and laboratory study. [see comments] *Journal of the American Medical Association*, **273**(17), 1360–5.

Foley, D.J., Masaki, K.H. *et al.* (2000). Driving cessation in older men with incident dementia. *Journal of the American Geriatrics Society*, **48**(8), 928–30.

Forrest, K.Y., Bunker, C.H. *et al.* (1997). Driving patterns and medical conditions in older women. *Journal of the American Geriatrics Society*, **45**(10), 1214–18.

Fox, G.K., Bowden, S.C. *et al.* (1997). Alzheimer's disease and driving: prediction and assessment of driving performance. *Journal of the American Geriatrics Society*, **45**(8), 949–53.

Freeman, E.E., Gange, S.J. *et al.* (2006). Driving status and risk of entry into long-term care in older adults. American Journal of Public Health, **96**(7), 1254–9.

Freund, K. (2000). *Independent transportation network: alternative transportation for the elderly. Transportation News*, **206**, 3–12.

Galski, T., Bruno, R.L. *et al.* (1993). Prediction of behind-the-wheel driving performance in patients with cerebral brain damage: a discriminant function analysis. *American Journal of Occupational Therapy*, **47**(5), 391–6.

Hakamies-Blomqvist, L., Johansson, K. *et al.* (1996). Medical screening of older drivers as a traffic safety measure – a comparative Finnish-Swedish Evaluation study. *Journal of the American Geriatrics Society*, **44**, 650–3.

Hakamies-Blomqvist, L., Ukkonen, T. *et al.* (2002). Driver ageing does not cause higher accident rates per mile. *Transportation Research Part F, Traffic Psychology and Behaviour*, **5**, 271–4.

Heikkila, V.M., Turkka, J. *et al.* (1998). Decreased driving ability in people with Parkinson's disease. *Journal of Neurology, Neurosurgery and Psychiatry*, **64**(3), 325–30.

Hemmelgarn, B., Suissa, S. *et al.* (1997). Benzodiazepine use and the risk of motor vehicle crash in the elderly. [see comments] *Journal of the American Medical Association*, **278**(1), 27–31.

Herrmann, N., Rapoport, M.J. *et al.* (2006). Predictors of driving cessation in mild-to-moderate dementia. *Canadian Medical Association Journal*, **175**(6), 591–5.

Hjorthol, R. (2001). *Mobility in an ageing society.* OECD, Paris.

Hughes-Cromwick, P., Mull, H. *et al.* (2006). *Cost-effectiveness of access to nonemergency medical transportation: comparison of transportation and healthcare costs and benefits.* TRB, Washington, DC.

Hunt, L., Morris, J.C. *et al.* (1993). Driving performance in persons with mild senile dementia of the Alzheimer type. *Journal of the American Geriatrics Society*, **41**(7), 747–52.

Hunt, L.A., Murphy, C.F. *et al.* (1997). Reliability of the Washington University Road Test. A performance-based assessment for drivers with dementia of the Alzheimer type. *Archives of Neurology*, **54**(6), 707–12.

Isherwood, J., Adam, K.S. *et al.* (1982). Live event stress, psychosocial factors, suicide attempt and auto-accident proclivity. *Journal of Psychosomatic Research*, **26**, 371–83.

Janke, M.K. and Eberhard, J.W. (1998). Assessing medically impaired older drivers in a licensing agency setting. *Accident Analysis and Prevention*, **30**(3), 347–61.

Johansson, K., Bronge, L. *et al.* (1996). Can a physician recognize an older driver with increased crash risk potential? *Journal of the American Geriatrics Society*, **44**(10), 1198–204.

Johnson, J.E. (1998). Older rural adults and the decision to stop driving: the influence of family and friends. *Journal of Community Health Nursing*, **15**(4), 205–16.

Klavora, P., Gaskovski, P., *et al.* (1995). The effects of Dynavision rehabilitation on behind-the-wheel driving ability and selected psychomotor abilities of persons after stroke. *American Journal of Occupational Therapy*, **49**(6), 534–42.

Kostyniuk, L., Shope, J. *et al.* (1998). *The process of reduction and cessation of driving among older drivers: a review of the literature*, p. 50. University of Michigan Transport Research Institute, Ann Arbor, MI.

Langford, J., Fitzharris, M. *et al.* (2004). Some consequences of different older driver licensing procedures in Australia. *Accident Analysis and Prevention*, **36**(6), 993–1001.

Langford, J., Methorst, R. *et al.* (2006). Older drivers do not have a high crash risk–a replication of low mileage bias. *Accident Analysis and Prevention*, **38**(3), 574–8.

Levy, D.T. (1995). The relationship of age and state license renewal policies to driving licensure rates. *Accident Analysis and Prevention*, **27**(4), 461–7.

Levy, D.T., Vernick, J.S. *et al.* (1995). Relationship between driver's license renewal policies and fatal crashes involving drivers 70 years or older. [see comments] *Journal of the American Medical Association*, **274**(13), 1026–30.

Maag, F. (1984). [The effects of mental diseases and behavior problems on the driving of motor vehicles]. *Revue Médicale de la Suisse Romande (Lausanne)*, **104**(11), 879–91.

Marottoli, R.A., Richardson, E.D. *et al.* (1998). Development of a test battery to identify older drivers at risk for self-reported adverse driving events. [see comments] *Journal of the American Geriatrics Society*, **46**(5), 562–8.

Mazer, B.L., Korner-Bitensky, N.A. *et al.* (1998). Predicting ability to drive after stroke. *Archives of Physical Medicine and Rehabilitation*, **79**(7), 743–50.

Metz, D. (2000). Mobility of older people and their quality of life. *Transport Policy*, **7**(7), 149–52.

Michon, J.A. (1985). A critical review of driver behaviour models: what do we know, what should we do? In *Human behaviour and traffic safety* (ed. L. Evans and R.C. Schwing), pp. 487–525. Plenum, New York.

O'Neill, D. (2000). Safe mobility for older people. *Reviews in Clinical Gerontology*, **10**, 181–92.

O'Neill, D., Neubauer, K. *et al.* (1992). Dementia and driving. *Journal of the Royal Society of Medicine*, **85**(4), 199–202.

OECD (2001). *Ageing and transport: mobility needs and safety issues*. OECD, Paris.

Owsley, C., Ball, K. *et al.* (1998). Visual processing impairment and risk of motor vehicle crash among older adults. *Journal of the American Medical Association*, **279**(14), 1083–8.

Palmer, B.W., Heaton, R.K. *et al.* (2002). Heterogeneity in functional status among older outpatients with schizophrenia: employment history, living situation, and driving. *Schizophrenia Research*, **55**(3), 205–15.

Perkinson, M.A., Berg-Weger, M.L. *et al.* (2005). Driving and dementia of the Alzheimer type: beliefs and cessation strategies among stakeholders. *The Gerontologist*, **45**(5), 676–85.

Rabbitt, P., Carmichael, A. *et al.* (1996). *When and why older drivers give up driving*. A Foundation for Road Safety Research, Basingstoke.

Ranney, T.A. (1994). Models of driving behaviour: a review of their evolution. *Accident Analysis and Prevention*, **26**(6), 733–50.

Ray, W.A. (1992). Psychotropic drugs and injuries among the elderly: a review. *Journal of Clinical Psychopharmacology*, **12**(6), 386–96.

Ray, W.A., Fought, R.L. *et al.* (1992). Psychoactive drugs and the risk of injurious motor vehicle crashes in elderly drivers. *American Journal of Epidemiology*, **136**(7), 873–83.

Ray, W.A., Thapa, P.B. *et al.* (1993). Medications and the older driver. *Clinics in Geriatric Medicine*, **9**(2), 413–38.

Rock, S.M. (1998). Impact from changes in Illinois drivers license renewal requirements for older drivers. *Accident Analysis and Prevention*, **30**(1), 69–74.

Rosenbloom, S. (1993). Transportation needs of the elderly population. *Clinics in Geriatric Medicine*, **9**(2), 297–310.

Sacher, P. (1978). [Schizophrenia and the ability to drive]. *Schweizerische Medizinische Wochenschrift*, **108**(10), 373–9.

Schmidt, C.W., Shaffer, J.N. *et al.* (1977). Suicide by vehicular crash. *American Journal of Psychiatry*, **134**, 175–8.

Shua-Haim, J.R. and Gross, J.S. (1996). The 'co-pilot' driver syndrome. [see comments] *Journal of the American Geriatrics Society*, **44**(7), 815–17.

Soyka, M., Hock, B. *et al.* (2005). Less impairment on one portion of a driving-relevant psychomotor battery in buprenorphine-maintained than in methadone-maintained patients: results of a randomized clinical trial. *Journal of Clinical Psychopharmacology*, **25**(5), 490–3.

Staplin, L.S., Lococo, K.H. *et al.* (1999). *Safe mobility for older people notebook*. National Highway Traffic Safety Administration, Washington, DC.

Stutts, J.C. (1998). Do older drivers with visual and cognitive impairments drive less? *Journal of the American Geriatrics Society*, **46**(7), 854–61.

Tabachnik, N., Litman, R. *et al.* (1966). Comparative study of accidental and suicidal death. *Archives of General Psychiatry*, **14**, 60–8.

Talbot, A., Bruce, I. *et al.* (2005). Driving cessation in patients attending a memory clinic. *Age and Ageing*, **34**(4), 363–8.

Taylor, B.D. and Tripodes, S. (2001). The effects of driving cessation on the elderly with dementia and their caregivers. *Accident Analysis and Prevention*, **33**(4), 519–28.

Thapa, P., Gideon, P. *et al.* (1998). Antidepressants and the risk of falls among nursing home residents. *New England Journal of Medicine*, **24**, 875–82.

Transportation Research Board (2004). *Transportation in an aging society: a decade of experience*. Transportation Research Board, Washington, DC.

Trobe, J.D. (1998). Test of divided visual attention predicts automobile crashes among older adults. [editorial] *Archives of Ophthalmology*, **116**(5), 665.

Trobe, J.D., Waller, P.F. *et al.* (1996). Crashes and violations among drivers with Alzheimer disease. *Archives of Neurology*, **53**(5), 411–16.

Vernon, D.D., Diller, E.M. *et al.* (2002). Evaluating the crash and citation rates of Utah drivers licensed with medical conditions, 1992–1996. *Accident Analysis and Prevention*, **34**, 237–46.

White House Conference on Aging (2005). *2005 White House Conference on Aging. The booming dynamics of aging: from awareness to action*. US Department of Health and Human Services, Washington, DC (http://www.whcoa.gov/).

White, S. and O'Neill, D. (2000). Health and relicencing policies for older drivers in the European Union. *Gerontology*, **46**(3), 146–52.

Wylie, K.R., Thompson, D.J. *et al.* (1993). Effects of depot neuroleptics on driving performance in chronic schizophrenic patients. *Journal of Neurology, Neurosurgery and Psychiatry*, **56**(8), 910–13.

# Index